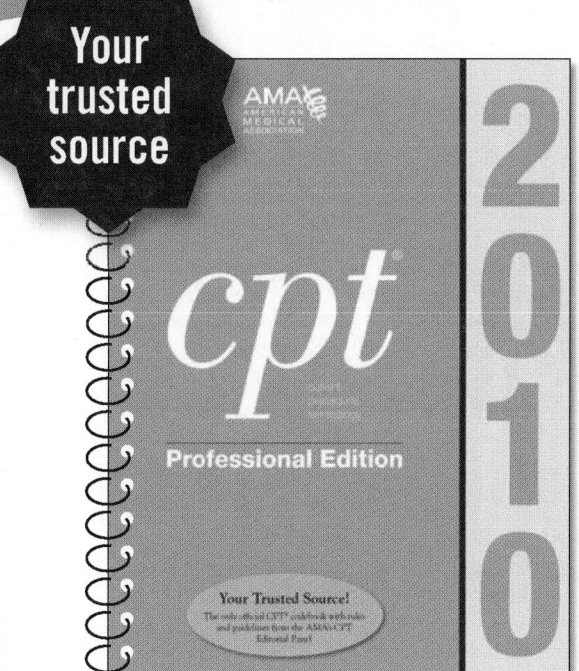
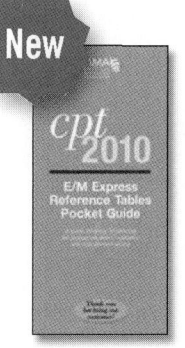

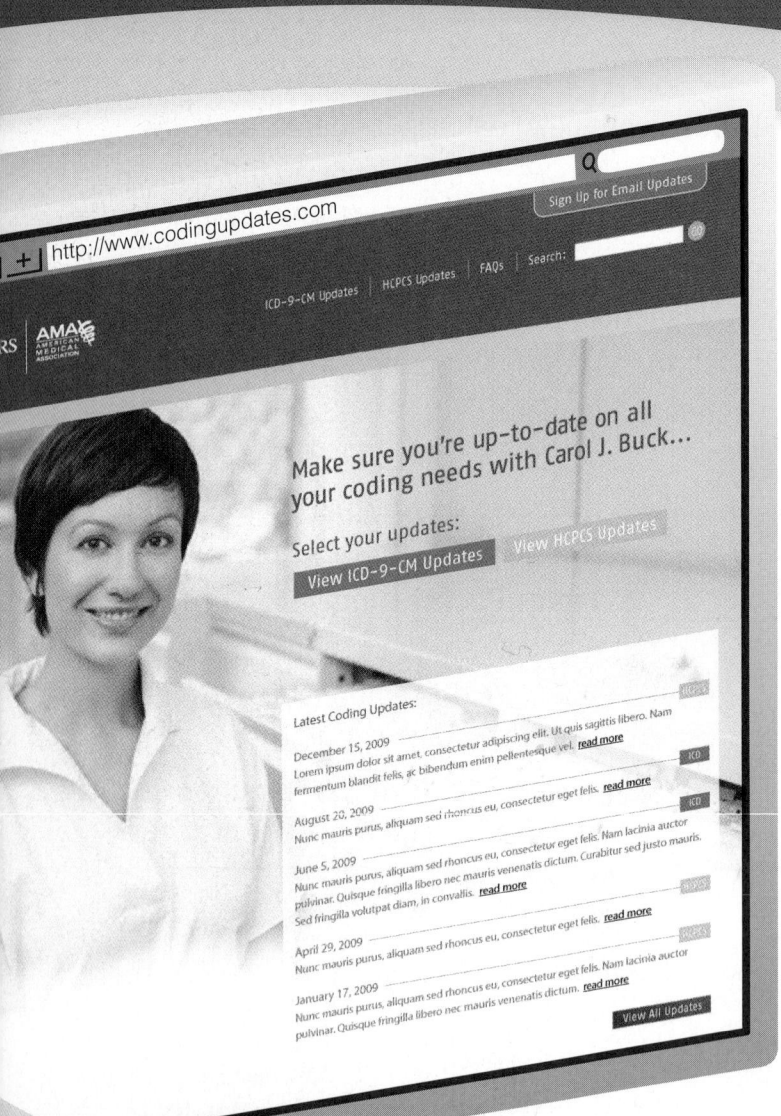
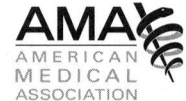

PROFESSIONAL EDITION

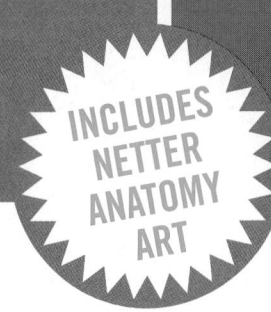
INCLUDES NETTER ANATOMY ART

2010

ICD-9-CM

VOLUMES 1 & 2

FOR PHYSICIANS

PROFESSIONAL EDITION

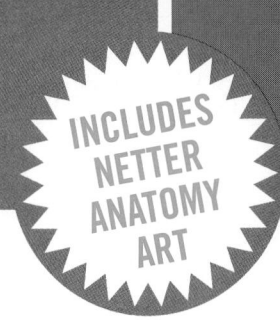
INCLUDES NETTER ANATOMY ART

2010
ICD-9-CM
VOLUMES 1 & 2

FOR PHYSICIANS

Carol J. Buck
MS, CPC-I, CPC, CPC-H, CCS-P

Program Director, Retired
Medical Secretary Programs
Northwest Technical College
East Grand Forks, Minnesota

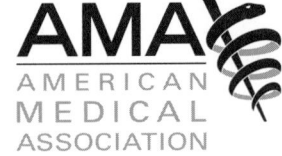
AMA
AMERICAN
MEDICAL
ASSOCIATION

SAUNDERS
ELSEVIER

SAUNDERS
ELSEVIER

3251 Riverport Lane
Maryland Heights, Missouri 63043

2010 ICD-9-CM FOR PHYSICIANS, VOLUMES 1 & 2, PROFESSIONAL EDITION   ISBN: 978-1-4377-0208-8 (spiral)
978-1-4377-1434-0 (softbound)

Notice

Knowledge and best practice in this field are constantly changing. As new research and experience broaden our knowledge, changes in practice, treatment, and drug therapy may become necessary or appropriate. Readers are advised to check the most current information provided (i) on procedures featured or (ii) by the manufacturer of each product to be administered, to verify the recommended dose or formula, the method and duration of administration, and contraindications. It is the responsibility of the practitioner, relying on his or her own experience and knowledge of the patient, to make diagnoses, to determine dosages and the best treatment for each individual patient, and to take all appropriate safety precautions. To the fullest extent of the law, neither the Publisher nor the Author assumes any liability for any injury and/or damage to persons or property arising out of or related to any use of the material contained in this book.

The Publisher

ISBN: 978-1-4377-0208-8 (spiral)
978-1-4377-1434-0 (softbound)

Publisher: Michael S. Ledbetter
Developmental Editor: Jenna Johnson
Publishing Services Manager: Pat Joiner-Myers

Printed in the United States of America

Last digit is the print number: 9 8 7 6 5 4 3 2 1

COLLABORATORS

Technical Collaborators:

Jacqueline Klitz Grass, MA, CPC
Coding Specialist
Grand Forks, North Dakota

Nancy Maguire, ACS, CRT, PCS, FCS, CPC, CPC-H, HCS-D, APC, AFC
Physician Consultant for Auditing and Education
Universal City, Texas

Technical Assistant:

Judith Neppel, RN, MS
Executive Director
Minnesota Rural Health Association
University of Minnesota, Crookston
Crookston, Minnesota

Lynn-Marie D. Wozniak, MS, RHIT
Product Manager
New York

Elsevier/MC Strategies Revenue Cycle, Coding and Compliance Staff

"Experts in providing e-learning on revenue cycle, coding and compliance."

Deborah Neville, RHIA, CCS-P
Director
Minnesota

Elizabeth Wheeler, RHIA, CCS-P
Product Manager
New York

Lynn-Marie D. Wozniak, MS, RHIT
Product Manager
New York

Therese M. Jorwic, MPH, RHIA, CCS, CCS-P, FAHIMA
Product Specialist
Illinois

Sandra L. Macica, MS, RHIA, CCS, ROCC
Product Specialist
New York

CONTENTS

GUIDE TO USING THE 2010 ICD-9-CM FOR PHYSICIANS, VOLUMES 1 & 2, PROFESSIONAL EDITION

Medical coding has long been a part of the health care profession. Through the years medical coding systems have become more complex and extensive. Today, medical coding is an intricate and immense process that is present in every health care setting. The increased use of electronic submissions for health care services only increases the need for coders who understand the coding process.

2010 ICD-9-CM for Physicians, Volumes 1 & 2, Professional Edition was developed to help meet the needs of students preparing for a career in medical coding by offering a comprehensive coding text at a reasonable price. This text combines the official coding guidelines and Volumes 1 and 2 of the ICD-9-CM in one book.

All material strictly adheres to the latest government versions available at the time of printing.

ILLUSTRATIONS AND ITEMS

The ICD-9-CM, Volume 1, Tabular List contains illustrations, pictures, and items to assist you in understanding difficult terminology, diseases/conditions, or coding in a specific category. Items are always printed in ▬▬ ink so the added material is not mistaken for official notations or instructions. ▬▬ ink is used for other annotations in the text. Your ideas on what other descriptions or illustrations should be in future editions of this text are always appreciated.

Annotated

Throughout the volumes, revisions, additions, and deleted words or codes are indicated by the following symbols:

◀▥ **Revised:** Revisions within the line or code from the previous edition are indicated by the arrow.

◀ **New:** Additions to the previous edition are indicated by the triangle.

~~deleted~~ **Deleted:** Deletions from previous edition are struck through.

ICD-9-CM, Volume 2, Index to Diseases Symbol

▬▬ **Omit code:** Identifies a term that is not reported. The words *omit code* are highlighted in ▬▬ for easier reference in Volume 1.

ICD-9-CM, Volume 1, Tabular List Symbols

❶ **First Listed:** The number 1 inside a circle appears before V codes that may be listed as the first code according to the V Code Table in the *ICD-9-CM Official Guidelines for Coding and Reporting.*

½ **First Listed or Additional:** The 1/2 inside a circle appears before V codes that may be listed as the first code and may also be listed as an additional V code according to the V Code Table in the *ICD-9-CM Official Guidelines for Coding and Reporting.*

❷ **Additional Only:** The number 2 inside a circle appears before V codes that may only be listed as an additional code. These codes may not be listed as a first code according to the V Code Table in the *ICD-9-CM Official Guidelines for Coding and Reporting.*

● **Use Additional Digit(s):** The red dot cautions that the code requires additional digit(s) to ensure the greatest specificity.

■ **Nonspecific Code:** These have a square before the code to indicate that although these codes are valid as a principal (first-listed) diagnosis, they are usually too general to be used as a first-listed diagnosis for Medicare, and you should continue to seek a code that is more specific.

● **Not a first-listed DX:** The blue dot before a code indicates that the code should not be reported as the first-listed (primary) diagnosis.

OGCR **OGCR:** The Official Guidelines for Coding and Reporting symbol indicates the placement of a portion of a guideline as that guideline pertains to the code by which it is located. The complete OGCR are located in Part I.

Coding Clinic identifies the year, quarter, and page number that presents information about an ICD-9-CM code in the American Hospital Association's *Coding Clinic.*

Excludes: Terms following the word "Excludes" are to be coded elsewhere and are highlighted in ▭ for easier reference.

Includes: This note appears immediately to further define or give examples of the content of codes and is highlighted in ▭ for easier reference.

Use additional: The words indicate an instructional note that another code may be needed, and are highlighted in ▭ for easier reference.

Code first: The words indicate an instructional note that directs the coder to sequence the underlying condition before the manifestation. "Code first" is highlighted in ▭ for easier reference.

Omit code: Identifies a term that is not reported. The words "omit code" are highlighted in ▭ for easier reference.

Age conflict: The Medicare Code Editor detects inconsistencies between a patient's age and diagnosis. For example, a 5-year-old patient with benign prostatic hypertrophy or a 78-year-old pregnant female. The diagnosis is clinically and virtually impossible in a patient of the stated age. Therefore, either the diagnosis or the age is presumed to be incorrect. There are four age categories for diagnoses in the Medicare Code Editor:

N • **Newborn.** Age of 0 years; a subset of diagnoses intended only for newborns and neonates (e.g., fetal distress, perinatal jaundice).

P • **Pediatric.** Age range is 0–17 years (e.g., Reye's syndrome, routine child health exam).

M • **Maternity.** Age range is 12–55 years (e.g., diabetes in pregnancy, antepartum pulmonary complication).

A • **Adult.** Age range is 15–124 years (e.g., senile delirium, mature cataract).

♀ ♂ **Sex conflict:** Medicare Code Editor detects inconsistencies between a patient's sex and diagnosis. For example, a male patient with cervical cancer (diagnosis) or a female patient with a prostatectomy (procedure). In both instances, the indicated diagnosis or the procedure conflicts with the stated sex of the patient. Therefore, the patient's diagnosis, procedure, or sex is presumed to be incorrect.

SYMBOLS AND CONVENTIONS

ICD-9-CM, Volumes 1 & 2
Symbols Used to Identify New, Revised, or Deleted Material

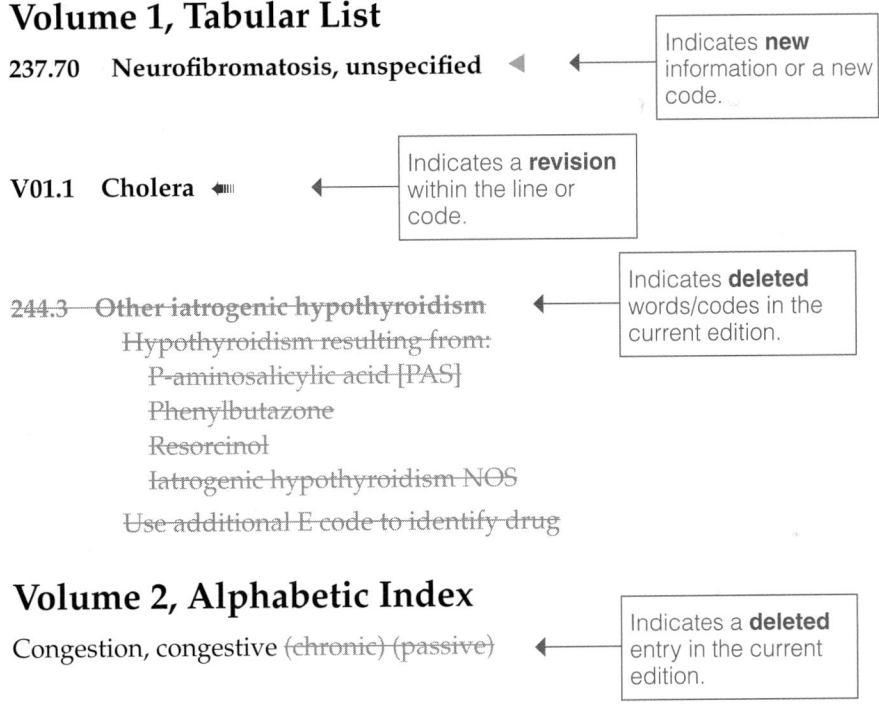

Volume 1, Tabular List

237.70   Neurofibromatosis, unspecified ◀

*Indicates **new** information or a new code.*

V01.1   Cholera ◀▥

*Indicates a **revision** within the line or code.*

~~244.3   Other iatrogenic hypothyroidism~~
~~Hypothyroidism resulting from:~~
~~P-aminosalicylic acid [PAS]~~
~~Phenylbutazone~~
~~Resorcinol~~
~~Iatrogenic hypothyroidism NOS~~
~~Use additional E code to identify drug~~

*Indicates **deleted** words/codes in the current edition.*

Volume 2, Alphabetic Index

Congestion, congestive ~~(chronic) (passive)~~

*Indicates a **deleted** entry in the current edition.*

Codes or index entries are for purposes of illustration only and may not be current.

Symbols for Volume 1, Tabular List

Use Additional Digit(s): The red dot cautions you that the code requires additional digit(s) to ensure the greatest specificity.

● **237.7   Neurofibromatosis**
von Recklinghausen's disease

■ **237.70   Neurofibromatosis,unspecified**

Nonspecific Code: These codes have a square before them to indicate that although these codes are valid as a principal (first-listed) diagnosis, they are usually too general to be used as a first-listed diagnosis for Medicare, and you should continue to seek a code that is more specific.

First Listed: This symbol appears before V codes that are acceptable as first listed codes according to the V Code Table in the *ICD-9-CM Official Guidelines for Coding and Reporting.*

❶ **V46.13   Encounter for weaning from respirator [ventilator]**

First Listed or Additional: This symbol appears before V codes that may be either first listed or additional codes according to the V Code Table in the *ICD-9-CM Official Guidelines for Coding and Reporting.*

Additional Only: This symbol appears before V codes that may be reported as additional codes, not as first listed codes according to the V Code Table in the *ICD-9-CM Official Guidelines for Coding and Reporting.*

V46.14   Mechanical complication of respirator [ventilator]

❷ **V46.11   Dependence on respirator, status**

007.4   Cryptosporidiosis
Coding Clinic: 1997, Q4, P30-31

Indicates a Volume 1 reference in the American Hospital Association *Coding Clinic for ICD-9-CM.*

Medicare Code Editor **Newborn** edit (age 0 years) indicating diagnoses intended only for newborns and neonates (e.g., fetal distress, perinatal jaundice).

747.83   Persistent fetal circulation   **N**

783.41   Failure to thrive   **P**

Medicare Code Editor **Pediatric** edit (age 0-17 years), e.g., Reye's syndrome, routine child health examination.

Medicare Code Editor **Maternity** edit (age 12-55 years) e.g., diabetes in pregnancy, antepartum pulmonary complications.

632   Missed abortion   **M**

256.31   Premature menopause   **A**

Medicare Code Editor **Adult** edit (age 15-124 years), e.g., senile delirium, mature cataract.

Codes or index entries are for purposes of illustration only and may not be current.

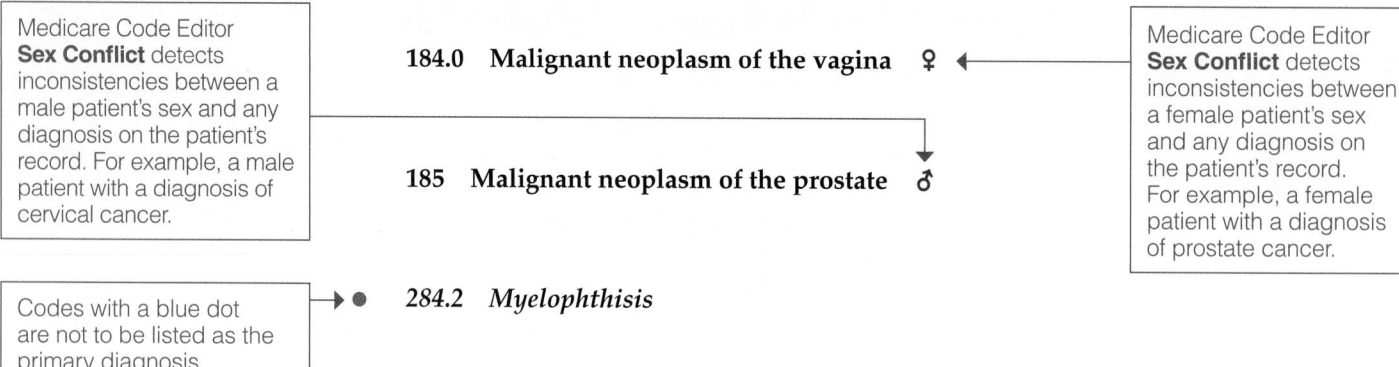

Medicare Code Editor
Sex Conflict detects inconsistencies between a male patient's sex and any diagnosis on the patient's record. For example, a male patient with a diagnosis of cervical cancer.

184.0   **Malignant neoplasm of the vagina**   ♀

185   **Malignant neoplasm of the prostate**   ♂

Medicare Code Editor
Sex Conflict detects inconsistencies between a female patient's sex and any diagnosis on the patient's record. For example, a female patient with a diagnosis of prostate cancer.

Codes with a blue dot are not to be listed as the primary diagnosis.

● 284.2   *Myelophthisis*

Codes or index entries are for purposes of illustration only and may not be current.

Conventions for Volume 1, Tabular List
2. NEOPLASMS (140–239)

Notes define terms or give coding instructions.

→ **Notes**
1. Content
   This chapter contains the following broad groups:
   140–195 Malignant neoplasms, stated or presumed to be primary, of specified sites, except of lymphatic and hematopoietic tissue

510   **Empyema**

Use additional code to identify infectious organism (041.0–041.9) ◄

"Use additional" directs you to use an additional code to give a more complete picture of the diagnosis.

Code first: The words indicate an instructional note that directs the coder to sequence the underlying condition before the manifestation.

366.4   **Cataract associated with other disorders**
 366.41   *Diabetic cataract*
→ *Code first diabetes (249.5, 250.5)*

A code with this note may be principal (first listed) if no causal condition is applicable or known.

428   **Heart failure**
→ *Code, if applicable, heart failure due to hypertension first (402.0–402.9, with fifth-digit 1 or 404.0–404.9 with fifth-digit 1 or 3)*

Terms following the word "Excludes" are to be coded elsewhere. The term "Excludes" means "Do Not Code Here."

150.2   **Abdominal esophagus**
→ **Excludes** *adenocarcinoma (151.0)*
            cardio-esophageal junction (151.0)

The "Includes" note appears to further define, or give example of, the contents of the code.

087   **Relapsing fever**
→ **Includes** recurrent fever

474   **Chronic disease of tonsils and adenoids**

"and" indicates a code that can be assigned if either of the conditions is present or if both of the conditions are present.

366.4   **Cataract associated with other disorders**

"with" indicates a code that can be used only if both conditions are present.

Codes or index entries are for purposes of illustration only and may not be current.

● **420.0** *Acute pericarditis in disease classified elsewhere*

Identifies manifestations that are not sequenced as the first diagnosis.

244.8 Other specified acquired hypothyroidism
Secondary hypothyroidism NEC ◄

NEC means Not Elsewhere Classifiable and is to be used only when the information at hand specifies a condition but there is no more specific code for that condition.

Bold type is used for all codes and titles.

159.0 Intestinal tract, part unspecified
Intestine NOS ◄

NOS means Not Otherwise Specified and is the equivalent of "unspecified."

426.89 Other
Dissociation:
atrioventricular [AV] ◄

Brackets are used to enclose synonyms, alternative wording, or explanatory phrases.

158.8 Specified parts of peritoneum
Cul-de-sac (of Douglas) ◄
Mesentery

Parentheses are used to enclose supplementary words that may be present or absent in the statement of a disease without affecting the code.

628.4 Of cervical or vaginal origin
Infertility associated with: ◄
anomaly of cervical mucus
congenital structural anomaly

A colon is used after an incomplete term that needs one or more of the modifiers that follow in order to make it assignable to a given category.

Conventions for Volume 2, Alphabetic Index

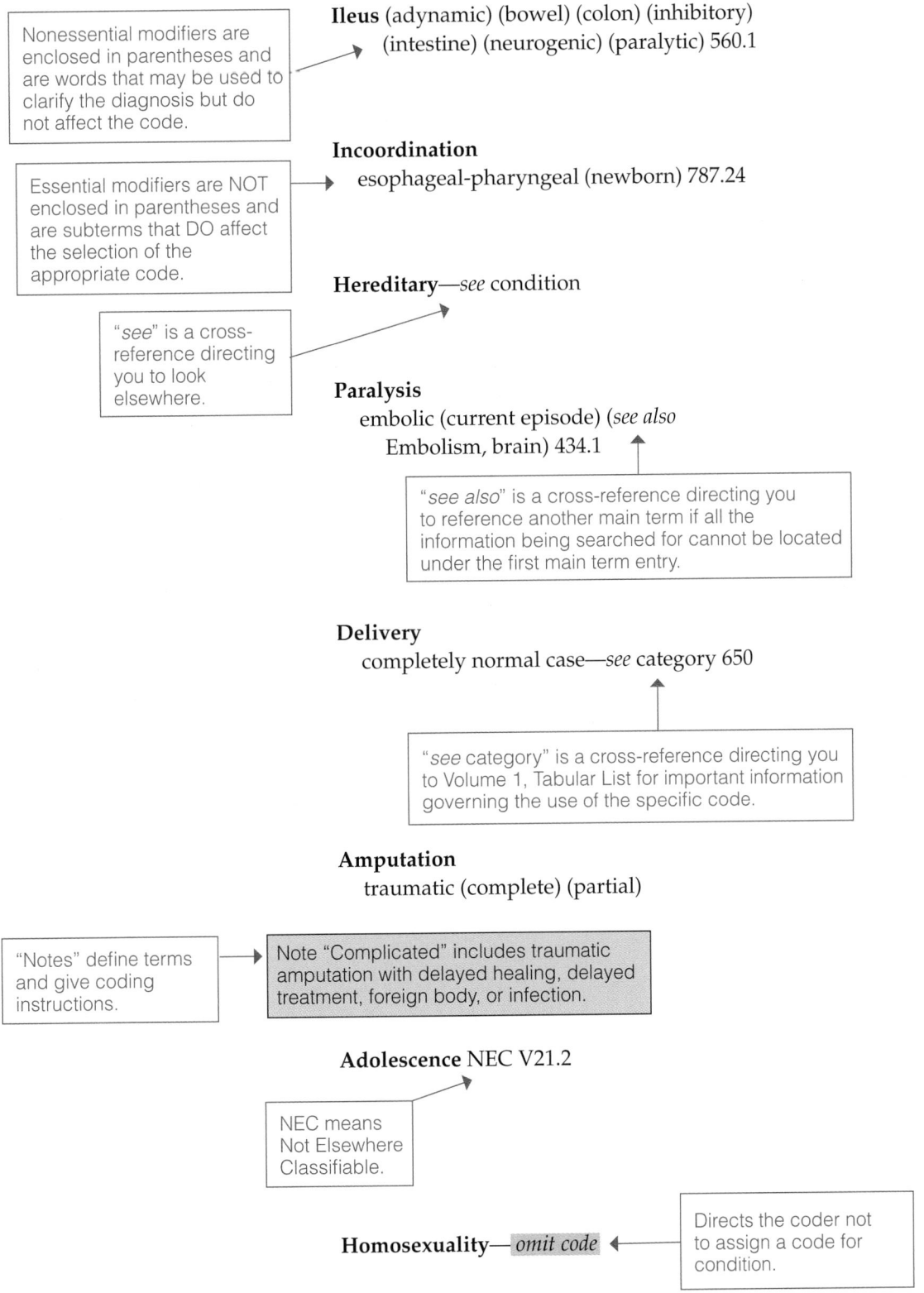

Ileus (adynamic) (bowel) (colon) (inhibitory) (intestine) (neurogenic) (paralytic) 560.1

Nonessential modifiers are enclosed in parentheses and are words that may be used to clarify the diagnosis but do not affect the code.

Incoordination
esophageal-pharyngeal (newborn) 787.24

Essential modifiers are NOT enclosed in parentheses and are subterms that DO affect the selection of the appropriate code.

Hereditary—*see* condition

"*see*" is a cross-reference directing you to look elsewhere.

Paralysis
embolic (current episode) (*see also* Embolism, brain) 434.1

"*see also*" is a cross-reference directing you to reference another main term if all the information being searched for cannot be located under the first main term entry.

Delivery
completely normal case—*see* category 650

"*see* category" is a cross-reference directing you to Volume 1, Tabular List for important information governing the use of the specific code.

Amputation
traumatic (complete) (partial)

"Notes" define terms and give coding instructions.

Note "Complicated" includes traumatic amputation with delayed healing, delayed treatment, foreign body, or infection.

Adolescence NEC V21.2

NEC means Not Elsewhere Classifiable.

Homosexuality— *omit code*

Directs the coder not to assign a code for condition.

Codes or index entries are for purposes of illustration only and may not be current.

GUIDE TO THE 2010 ICD-9-CM UPDATES

VOLUME 1 CHANGES EFFECTIVE OCTOBER 1, 2009

1. INFECTIOUS AND PARASITIC DISEASES (001-139)

Revise **Excludes** *influenza (487.0-487.8, 488.0-488.1)*

008 Intestinal infections due to other organisms

008.6 Enteritis due to specified virus

008.63 Norwalk virus
Add Norovirus

Revise **008.65 Calicivirus**

035 Erysipelas

Revise **Excludes** *postpartum or puerperal erysipelas (670.8)*

037 Tetanus

Excludes *tetanus:*
Revise *puerperal (670.8)*

041 Bacterial infection in conditions classified elsewhere and of unspecified site

Revise **041.3** ~~Friedländer's bacillus~~ Klebsiella pneumoniae
Delete ~~Infection by Klebsiella pneumoniae~~

041.8 Other specified bacterial infections

Revise **041.86 Helicobacter pylori** ~~(H. pylori)~~ [H. pylori]

046 Slow virus infections and prion diseases of central nervous system

046.1 Jakob-Creutzfeldt disease

Add Use additional code to identify dementia:
Add with behavioral disturbance (294.11)
Add without behavioral disturbance (294.10)

Revise **VIRAL DISEASES GENERALLY ACCOMPANIED BY EXANTHEM (050-059)**

078 Other diseases due to viruses and Chlamydiae

078.8 Other specified diseases due to viruses and Chlamydiae

078.89 Other specified diseases due to viruses
Delete ~~Tanapox~~

190 Malignant neoplasm of eye

Add **Excludes** *dark area on retina and choroid (239.81)*
Add *retinal freckle (239.81)*

196 Secondary and unspecified malignant neoplasm of lymph nodes

Add **Excludes** *secondary neuroendocrine tumor of (distant) lymph nodes (209.71)*

197 Secondary malignant neoplasm of respiratory and digestive systems

Add **Excludes** *secondary neuroendocrine tumor of liver (209.72)*
Add *secondary neuroendocrine tumor of respiratory organs (209.79)*

198 Secondary malignant neoplasm of other specified sites

Add **Excludes** *secondary neuroendocrine tumor of other specified sites (209.79)*

199 Malignant neoplasm without specification of site

Add **Excludes** *malignant (poorly differentiated) neuroendocrine carcinoma, any site (209.30)*
Revise *malignant (poorly differentiated) neuroendocrine tumor, any site (209.30)*
Revise *neuroendocrine carcinoma (high grade), any site (209.30)*

199.2 Malignant neoplasm associated with transplanted organ

Revise Use additional code for specific malignancy ~~site~~

MALIGNANT NEOPLASM OF LYMPHATIC AND HEMATOPOIETIC TISSUE (200-208)

Add **Excludes** *autoimmune lymphoproliferative syndrome (279.41)*

202 Other malignant neoplasms of lymphoid and histiocytic tissue

202.0 Nodular lymphoma
Lymphoma:
Revise follicular (giant) (large cell)

202.1 Mycosis fungoides
Add **Excludes** *peripheral T-cell lymphoma (202.7)*

209 Neuroendocrine tumors
Add **Excludes** *benign pancreatic islet cell tumors (211.7)*
Revise *malignant pancreatic islet cell tumors (157.4)*

209.3 Malignant poorly differentiated neuroendocrine tumors

209.30 Malignant poorly differentiated neuroendocrine carcinoma, any site
Add **Excludes** *Merkel cell carcinoma (209.31-209.36)*

New code **209.31 Merkel cell carcinoma of the face**
Merkel cell carcinoma of the ear
Merkel cell carcinoma of the eyelid, including canthus
Merkel cell carcinoma of the lip

New code   **209.32 Merkel cell carcinoma of the scalp and neck**

New code   **209.33 Merkel cell carcinoma of the upper limb**

New code   **209.34 Merkel cell carcinoma of the lower limb**

New code   **209.35 Merkel cell carcinoma of the trunk**

New code   **209.36 Merkel cell carcinoma of other sites**
                     Merkel cell carcinoma of the buttock
                     Merkel cell carcinoma of the genitals
                     Merkel cell carcinoma NOS

New sub   **209.7 Secondary neuroendocrine tumors**
                     Secondary carcinoid tumors

New code   **209.70 Secondary neuroendocrine tumor, unspecified site**

New code   **209.71 Secondary neuroendocrine tumor of distant lymph nodes**
                     Mesentery metastasis of neuroendocrine tumor

New code   **209.72 Secondary neuroendocrine tumor of liver**

New code   **209.73 Secondary neuroendocrine tumor of bone**

New code   **209.74 Secondary neuroendocrine tumor of peritoneum**

New code   **209.75 Secondary Merkel cell carcinoma**
                     Merkel cell carcinoma nodal presentation
                     Merkel cell carcinoma visceral metastatic presentation
                     Secondary Merkel cell carcinoma, any site

New code   **209.79 Secondary neuroendocrine tumor of other sites**

          238 Neoplasm of uncertain behavior of other and unspecified sites and tissues

              238.7 Other lymphatic and hematopoietic tissues

                     238.72 Low grade myelodysplastic syndrome lesions
Add   Refractory anemia with excess blasts-1 (RAEB-1)

                     238.73 High grade myelodysplastic syndrome lesions
Delete   ~~Refractory anemia with excess blasts-1 (RAEB-1)~~

          239 Neoplasms of unspecified nature

              239.8 Other specified sites
New code   **239.81 Retina and choroid**
                     Dark area on retina
                     Retinal freckle

New code   **239.89 Other specified sites**

          251 Other disorders of pancreatic internal secretion

              251.3 Postsurgical hypoinsulinemia
Add   Use additional code to identify (any associated):
Add   acquired absence of pancreas (V45.79)
Add   insulin use (V58.67)
Add   secondary diabetes mellitus (249.00-249.91)
Add   **Excludes** *transient hyperglycemia post procedure (790.29)*
                                  transient hypoglycemia post procedure (251.2)

          269 Other nutritional deficiencies

              269.8 Other nutritional deficiency
                     Excludes *feeding problems (783.3)*
Revise   *newborn (779.31-779.34)*

          270 Disorders of amino-acid transport and metabolism
Revise   **Excludes** *gout (274.00-274.9)*

          272 Disorders of lipoid metabolism
              272.2 Mixed hyperlipidemia
Add   Combined hyperlipidemia
Add   Elevated cholesterol with elevated triglycerides NEC

              272.4 Other and unspecified hyperlipidemia
Delete   ~~Combined hyperlipidemia~~

          274 Gout
              274.0 Gouty arthropathy
New code   **274.00 Gouty arthropathy, unspecified**
New code   **274.01 Acute gouty arthropathy**
                     Acute gout
                     Gout attack
                     Gout flare
                     Podagra

New code   **274.02 Chronic gouty arthropathy without mention of tophus (tophi)**
                     Chronic gout

New code   **274.03 Chronic gouty arthropathy with tophus (tophi)**
                     Chronic tophaceous gout
                     Gout with tophi NOS

              274.8 Gout with other specified manifestations
                 274.82 Gouty tophi of other sites
Add   **Excludes** *gout with tophi NOS (274.03)*
Add   *gouty arthropathy with tophi (274.03)*

          277 Other and unspecified disorders of metabolism
              277.2 Other disorders of purine and pyrimidine metabolism
Revise   **Excludes** *gout (274.00-274.9)*

              277.8 Other specified disorders of metabolism
New code   **277.88 Tumor lysis syndrome**
                     Spontaneous tumor lysis syndrome
                     Tumor lysis syndrome following antineoplastic drug therapy
                     Use additional E code to identify cause, if drug-induced

279 Disorders involving the immune mechanism

279.4 Autoimmune disease, not elsewhere classified

Delete   ~~Autoimmune disease NOS~~

New code   **279.41 Autoimmune lymphoproliferative syndrome**
ALPS

New code   **279.49 Autoimmune disease, not elsewhere classified**
Autoimmune disease NOS

279.5 Graft-versus-host disease

Code first underlying cause, such as:

Revise   complication of blood transfusion (999.89)

Revise   complication of transplanted organ ~~(bone marrow)~~ (996.80-996.89)

285 Other and unspecified anemias

285.2 Anemia of chronic disease

Revise   Anemia in (due to) (with) chronic illness

285.22 Anemia in neoplastic disease

Add   **Excludes** *anemia due to antineoplastic chemotherapy (285.3)*

New code   **285.3 Antineoplastic chemotherapy induced anemia**
Anemia due to antineoplastic chemotherapy

Excludes *anemia due to drug NEC – code to type of anemia*
anemia in neoplastic disease (285.22)
aplastic anemia due to antineoplastic chemotherapy (284.89)

290 Dementias

290.0 Senile dementia, uncomplicated

Revise   **Excludes** *mild memory disturbances, not amounting to dementia, associated with senile brain disease (310.8)*

294 Persistent mental disorders due to conditions classified elsewhere

294.1 Dementia in conditions classified elsewhere

Code first any underlying physical condition as:
dementia in:

Revise   Jakob-Creutzfeldt disease (046.11-046.19)

294.8 Other persistent mental disorders due to conditions classified elsewhere

Revise   **Excludes** *mild memory disturbances, not amounting to dementia (310.8)*

305 Nondependent abuse of drugs

305.1 Tobacco use disorder

Delete   [0-3]

307 Special symptoms or syndromes, not elsewhere classified

307.0 Stuttering

Revise   **Excludes** *dysphasia (784.59)*
Add   *stuttering (fluency disorder) due to late effect of cerebrovascular accident (438.14)*

310 Specific nonpsychotic mental disorders due to brain damage

310.1 Personality change due to conditions classified elsewhere

Delete   **Excludes** ~~*memory loss of unknown cause (780.93)*~~
Add   *mild cognitive impairment (331.83)*
Add   *postconcussion syndrome (310.2)*
Add   *signs and symptoms involving emotional state (799.21-799.29)*

310.8 Other specified nonpsychotic mental disorders following organic brain damage

Add   **Excludes** *memory loss of unknown cause (780.93)*

331 Other cerebral degenerations

331.7 Cerebral degeneration in diseases classified elsewhere

Excludes *cerebral degeneration in:*
Revise   *Jakob-Creutzfeldt disease (046.11-046.19)*

331.8 Other cerebral degeneration

331.83 Mild cognitive impairment, so stated

Add   **Excludes** *cognitive impairment due to skull fracture (800-801, 803-804)*

333 Other extrapyramidal disease and abnormal movement disorders

333.2 Myoclonus

Add   Palatal myoclonus
Delete   ~~Progressive myoclonic epilepsy~~
Delete   ~~Unverricht-Lundborg disease~~
Add   **Excludes** *progressive myoclonic epilepsy (345.1)*
Add   *Unverricht-Lundborg disease (345.1)*

345 Epilepsy and recurrent seizures

The following fifth-digit subclassification is for use with categories 345.0, .1, .4-.9:

  1   with intractable epilepsy

Add   pharmacoresistant (pharmacologically resistant)
Add   poorly controlled
Add   refractory (medically)
Add   treatment resistant

Add   **Excludes** *hippocampal sclerosis (348.81)*
Add   *mesial temporal sclerosis (348.81)*
Add   *temporal sclerosis (348.81)*

345.1 Generalized convulsive epilepsy

Add   Progressive myoclonic epilepsy
Add   Unverricht-Lundborg disease

348 **Other conditions of brain**

    348.8 Other conditions of brain

Delete   ~~Cerebral:~~

Delete   ~~calcification~~

Delete   ~~fungus~~

New code   **348.81 Temporal sclerosis**

                       Hippocampal sclerosis

                       Mesial temporal sclerosis

New code   **348.89 Other conditions of brain**

                       Cerebral:

                         calcification

                         fungus

359 **Muscular dystrophies and other myopathies**

    359.2 Myotonic disorders

           359.22 Myotonia congenita

Add   Myotonia levior

           359.29 Other specified myotonic disorder

Delete   ~~Myotonia levior~~

New sub   **359.7 Inflammatory and immune myopathies, NEC**

New code   **359.71 Inclusion body myositis**

                       IBM

New code   **359.79 Other inflammatory and immune myopathies, NEC**

                       Inflammatory myopathy NOS

372 **Disorders of conjunctiva**

    372.0 Acute conjunctivitis

New code   **372.06 Acute chemical conjunctivitis**

                       Acute toxic conjunctivitis

                       Use additional E code to identify the chemical or toxic agent

                       Excludes   *burn of eye and adnexa (940.0-940.9)*

                                   chemical corrosion injury of eye (940.2-940.3)

    372.3 Other and unspecified conjunctivitis

           372.34 Pingueculitis

Add   **Excludes**   *pinguecula (372.51)*

    372.5 Conjunctival degenerations and deposits

           372.51 Pinguecula

Add   **Excludes**   *pingueculitis (372.34)*

403 **Hypertensive chronic kidney disease**

Revise   **Excludes**   *acute ~~renal~~ kidney failure (584.5-584.9)*

413 **Angina pectoris**

    413.9 Other and unspecified angina pectoris

                       Angina:

Add   equivalent

Add   Use additional code(s) for symptoms associated with angina equivalent

415 **Acute pulmonary heart disease**

    415.1 Pulmonary embolism and infarction

Add   **Excludes**   *chronic pulmonary embolism (416.2)*

Add   *personal history of pulmonary embolism (V12.51)*

416 **Chronic pulmonary heart disease**

New code   **416.2 Chronic pulmonary embolism**

                       Use additional code, if applicable, for associated long-term (current) use of anticoagulants (V58.61)

                       Excludes   *personal history of pulmonary embolism (V12.51)*

438 **Late effects of cerebrovascular disease**

    438.1 Speech and language deficits

New code   **438.13 Dysarthria**

New code   **438.14 Fluency disorder**

                       Stuttering

445 **Atheroembolism**

    445.8 Of other sites

           445.81 Kidney

Revise   Use additional code for any associated acute ~~renal~~ kidney failure or chronic kidney disease (584, 585)

453 **Other venous embolism and thrombosis**

Delete   **Excludes**   ~~*that with inflammation, phlebitis, and thrombophlebitis (451.0-451.9)*~~

Revise   **453.2 Of inferior vena cava**

Revise   **453.4 Acute venous embolism and thrombosis of deep vessels of lower extremity**

Revise   **453.40 Acute venous embolism and thrombosis of unspecified deep vessels of lower extremity**

Revise   **453.41 Acute venous embolism and thrombosis of deep vessels of proximal lower extremity**

Revise   **453.42 Acute venous embolism and thrombosis of deep vessels of distal lower extremity**

New sub   **453.5 Chronic venous embolism and thrombosis of deep vessels of lower extremity**

                       Use additional code, if applicable, for associated long-term (current) use of anticoagulants (V58.61)

                       Excludes   *personal history of venous thrombosis and embolism (V12.51)*

New code   **453.50 Chronic venous embolism and thrombosis of unspecified deep vessels of lower extremity**

New code   **453.51 Chronic venous embolism and thrombosis of deep vessels of proximal lower extremity**

New code   **453.52 Chronic venous embolism and thrombosis of deep vessels of distal lower extremity**

New code   **453.6 Venous embolism and thrombosis of superficial vessels of lower extremity**

                       Saphenous vein (greater) (lesser)

New sub | **453.7 Chronic venous embolism and thrombosis of other specified vessels**

Use additional code, if applicable, for associated long-term (current) use of anticoagulants (V58.61)

Excludes *personal history of venous thrombosis and embolism (V12.51)*

New code | **453.71 Chronic venous embolism and thrombosis of superficial veins of upper extremity**
Antecubital vein
Basilic vein
Cephalic vein

New code | **453.72 Chronic venous embolism and thrombosis of deep veins of upper extremity**
Brachial vein
Radial vein
Ulnar vein

New code | **453.73 Chronic venous embolism and thrombosis of upper extremity, unspecified**

New code | **453.74 Chronic venous embolism and thrombosis of axillary veins**

New code | **453.75 Chronic venous embolism and thrombosis of subclavian veins**

New code | **453.76 Chronic venous embolism and thrombosis of internal jugular veins**

New code | **453.77 Chronic venous embolism and thrombosis of other thoracic veins**
Brachiocephalic (innominate)
Superior vena cava

New code | **453.79 Chronic venous embolism and thrombosis of other specified veins**

Revise | **453.8 Acute venous embolism and thrombosis of other specified veins**

New code | **453.81 Acute venous embolism and thrombosis of superficial veins of upper extremity**
Antecubital vein
Basilic vein
Cephalic vein

New code | **453.82 Acute venous embolism and thrombosis of deep veins of upper extremity**
Brachial vein
Radial vein
Ulnar vein

New code | **453.83 Acute venous embolism and thrombosis of upper extremity, unspecified**

New code | **453.84 Acute venous embolism and thrombosis of axillary veins**

New code | **453.85 Acute venous embolism and thrombosis of subclavian veins**

New code | **453.86 Acute venous embolism and thrombosis of internal jugular veins**

New code | **453.87 Acute venous embolism and thrombosis of other thoracic veins**
Brachiocephalic (innominate)
Superior vena cava

New code | **453.89 Acute venous embolism and thrombosis of other specified veins**

487 Influenza
Add | Influenza caused by unspecified influenza virus

Excludes *Hemophilus influenzae [H. influenzae]:*
Add | *influenza due to 2009 H1N1 [swine] influenza virus (488.1)*
Revise | *influenza due to identified avian influenza virus (488.0)*
Add | *influenza due to identified novel H1N1 influenza virus (488.1)*

Revise | **488 Influenza due to certain identified ~~avian~~ influenza viruses**

Delete | ~~Note: Influenza caused by influenza viruses that normally infect only birds and, less commonly, other animals~~

Revise | **Excludes** *influenza caused by ~~other~~ unspecified influenza viruses (487.0-487.8)*

New code | **488.0 Influenza due to identified avian influenza virus**
Avian influenza
Bird flu
Influenza A/H5N1

New code | **488.1 Influenza due to identified novel H1N1 influenza virus**
2009 H1N1 [swine] influenza virus
Novel 2009 influenza H1N1
Novel H1N1 influenza
Novel influenza A/H1N1
Swine flu

536 Disorders of function of stomach

536.2 Persistent vomiting
Add | **Excludes** *bilious emesis (vomiting) (787.04)*
Add | *vomiting of fecal matter (569.87)*

567 Peritonitis and retroperitoneal infections
Excludes *peritonitis:*
Revise | *puerperal (670.8)*

569 Other disorders of intestine
New sub | **569.7 Complications of intestinal pouch**
New code | **569.71 Pouchitis**
Inflammation of internal ileoanal pouch

New code | **569.79 Other complications of intestinal pouch**

569.8 Other specified disorders of intestine
New code | **569.87 Vomiting of fecal matter**

572 Liver abscess and sequelae of chronic liver disease

Revise — **572.2 Hepatic ~~coma~~ encephalopathy**
Delete — ~~Hepatic encephalopathy~~
Add — Hepatic coma

Revise — **584 Acute ~~renal~~ kidney failure**
Add — **Includes** Acute renal failure

Revise — **584.5 Acute kidney failure ~~W~~with lesion of tubular necrosis**

Revise — **584.6 Acute kidney failure ~~W~~with lesion of renal cortical necrosis**

Revise — **584.7 Acute kidney failure ~~W~~with lesion of renal medullary [papillary] necrosis**

Revise — **584.8 Acute kidney failure ~~W~~with other specified pathological lesion in kidney**

Revise — **584.9 Acute kidney failure ~~Acute renal failure~~, unspecified**

587 Renal sclerosis, unspecified
Revise — **Includes** Atrophy of kidney
Delete — ~~Atrophy of kidney~~

611 Other disorders of breast

611.8 Other specified disorders of breast

611.82 Hypoplasia of breast
Add — **Excludes** *congenital absence of breast (757.6)*

614 Inflammatory disease of ovary, fallopian tube, pelvic cellular tissue, and peritoneum
Revise — **Excludes** *major infection following delivery (670.0-670.8)*

615 Inflammatory diseases of uterus, except cervix
Revise — **Excludes** *following delivery (670.0-670.8)*
Revise — *hyperplastic endometritis (621.30-621.35)*

621 Disorders of uterus, not elsewhere classified

621.3 Endometrial hyperplasia
Delete — ~~Hyperplasia (adenomatous) (cystic) (glandular) of endometrium~~ ~~Hyperplastic endometritis~~

621.30 Endometrial hyperplasia, unspecified
Add — Hyperplasia (adenomatous) (cystic) (glandular) of endometrium
Add — Hyperplastic endometritis

621.31 Simple endometrial hyperplasia without atypia
Add — **Excludes** *benign endometrial hyperplasia (621.34)*

621.32 Complex endometrial hyperplasia without atypia
Add — **Excludes** *benign endometrial hyperplasia (621.34)*

621.33 Endometrial hyperplasia with atypia
Add — **Excludes** *endometrial intraepithelial neoplasia [EIN] (621.35)*

New code — **621.34 Benign endometrial hyperplasia**
New code — **621.35 Endometrial intraepithelial neoplasia [EIN]**
Excludes *malignant neoplasm of endometrium with endometrial intraepithelial neoplasia [EIN] (182.0)*

624 Noninflammatory disorders of vulva and perineum
Revise — **Excludes** *condyloma acuminatum (078.11)*

639 Complications following abortion and ectopic and molar pregnancies
Revise — **639.3 Kidney failure**
Revise — Renal (kidney):

646 Other complications of pregnancy, not elsewhere classified

646.6 Infections of genitourinary tract in pregnancy
Revise — **Excludes** *major puerperal infection (670.0-670.8)*

649 Other conditions or status of the mother complicating pregnancy, childbirth, or the puerperium

649.3 Coagulation defects complicating pregnancy, childbirth, or the puerperium
Revise — Conditions classifiable to 286, 287, 289
Revise — Use additional code to identify the specific coagulation defect (286.0-286.9, 287.0-287.9, 289.0-289.9)

669 Other complications of labor and delivery, not elsewhere classified
Revise — **669.3 Acute ~~renal~~ kidney failure following labor and delivery**

670 Major puerperal infection
[0,2,4]
Delete — ~~Use 0 as fourth digit for category 670~~
Delete — ~~Puerperal:~~
Delete — ~~endometritis~~
Delete — ~~fever (septic)~~
Delete — ~~pelvic:~~
Delete — ~~cellulitis~~
Delete — ~~sepsis~~
Delete — ~~peritonitis~~
Delete — ~~pyemia~~
Delete — ~~salpingitis~~
Delete — ~~septicemia~~

Revise sub — **670.0 Major puerperal infection, unspecified**
[0,2,4]

New sub — **670.1 Puerperal endometritis**
[0,2,4]

New sub — **670.2 Puerperal sepsis**
[0,2,4] Puerperal pyemia

New sub — **670.3 Puerperal septic thrombophlebitis**
[0,2,4]

New sub — **670.8 Other major puerperal infection**
[0,2,4] Puerperal:
pelvic cellulitis
peritonitis
salpingitis

671 Venous complications in pregnancy and the puerperium

Add   **Excludes** *personal history of venous complications prior to pregnancy, such as:*
Add   *thrombophlebitis (V12.52)*
Add   *thrombosis and embolism (V12.51)*

671.2 Superficial thrombophlebitis
Add   Phlebitis NOS
Add   Thrombosis NOS

671.3 Deep phlebothrombosis, antepartum
Add   Use additional code to identify the deep vein thrombosis (453.40-453.42, 453.50-453.52, 453.72-453.79, 453.82-453.89)

Add   Use additional code for long term (current) use of anticoagulants, if applicable (V58.61)

671.4 Deep phlebothrombosis, postpartum
Add   Use additional code to identify the deep vein thrombosis (453.40-453.42, 453.50-453.52, 453.72-453.79, 453.82-453.89)

Add   Use additional code for long term (current) use of anticoagulants, if applicable (V58.61)

671.9 Unspecified venous complication
Delete   ~~Phlebitis NOS~~
Delete   ~~Thrombosis NOS~~

INFECTIONS OF SKIN AND SUBCUTANEOUS TISSUE (680-686)

        Excludes *certain infections of skin classified under "Infectious and Parasitic Diseases," such as:*
Revise   *viral warts (078.10-078.19)*

707 Chronic ulcer of skin

707.0 Pressure ulcer

707.03 Lower back
Add   Coccyx

712 Crystal arthropathies
Revise   **Excludes** *gouty arthropathy (274.00-274.03)*

713 Arthropathy associated with other disorders classified elsewhere

713.0 Arthropathy associated with other endocrine and metabolic disorders
        Excludes *arthropathy associated with:*
Revise   *gouty arthropathy (274.00-274.03)*

727 Other disorders of synovium, tendon, and bursa

727.01 Synovitis and tenosynovitis in diseases classified elsewhere
Revise   **Excludes** *gouty (274.00-274.03)*

733 Other disorders of bone and cartilage

733.1 Pathologic fracture
Add   Chronic fracture

756 Other congenital musculoskeletal anomalies

756.7 Anomalies of abdominal wall
New code   **756.72 Omphalocele**
                    Exomphalos
New code   **756.73 Gastroschisis**

           756.79 Other congenital anomalies of abdominal wall
Delete   ~~Exomphalos~~
Delete   ~~Gastroschisis~~
Delete   ~~Omphalocele~~

757 Congenital anomalies of the integument
Revise   **757.6 Specified congenital anomalies of breast**
Revise   Congenital a~~A~~bsent breast or nipple
Add   **Excludes** *micromastia (611.82)*

762 Fetus or newborn affected by complications of placenta, cord, and membranes

762.3 Placental transfusion syndromes
Revise   Use additional code to indicate resultant condition in ~~fetus or~~ newborn:

768 Intrauterine hypoxia and birth asphyxia

768.5 Severe birth asphyxia
Revise   **Excludes** *hypoxic-ischemic encephalopathy (HIE) (768.70-768.73)*

768.6 Mild or moderate birth asphyxia
Revise   **Excludes** *hypoxic-ischemic encephalopathy (HIE) (768.70-768.73)*

768.7 Hypoxic-ischemic encephalopathy (HIE)
New code   **768.70 Hypoxic-ischemic encephalopathy, unspecified**
New code   **768.71 Mild hypoxic-ischemic encephalopathy**
New code   **768.72 Moderate hypoxic-ischemic encephalopathy**
New code   **768.73 Severe hypoxic-ischemic encephalopathy**

772 Fetal and neonatal hemorrhage
Add   **Excludes** *fetal hematologic conditions complicating pregnancy (678.0)*
Revise   **772.0 Fetal blood loss affecting newborn**

776 Hematological disorders of newborn
Revise   **Includes** disorders specific to the ~~fetus or~~ newborn though possibly originating in utero
Revise   **776.9 Unspecified hematological disorder specific to ~~fetus or~~ newborn**

777 Perinatal disorders of digestive system

777.5 Necrotizing enterocolitis in newborn
Delete   ~~Pseudomembranous enterocolitis in newborn~~

777.51 Stage I necrotizing enterocolitis in newborn
Add   Necrotizing enterocolitis without pneumatosis, without perforation

779 **Other and ill-defined conditions originating in the perinatal period**

Revise   779.3 <u>Disorder of stomach function and</u> feeding problems in newborn

Delete   ~~Regurgitation of food in newborn~~
Delete   ~~Slow feeding in newborn~~
Delete   ~~Vomiting in newborn~~

New code   779.31 **Feeding problems in newborn**
Slow feeding in newborn

Excludes *feeding problem in child over 28 days old (783.3)*

New code   779.32 **Bilious vomiting in newborn**

Excludes *bilious vomiting in child over 28 days old (787.04)*

New code   779.33 **Other vomiting in newborn**
Regurgitation of food in newborn

Excludes *vomiting in child over 28 days old (536.2, 787.01-787.03, 787.04)*

New code   779.34 **Failure to thrive in newborn**

Excludes *failure to thrive in child over 28 days old (783.41)*

780 **General symptoms**

780.0 **Alteration of consciousness**

Add   **Excludes** *alteration of consciousness due to:*
Add   *intracranial injuries (850.0-854.19)*
Add   *skull fractures (800.00-801.99, 803.00-804.99)*

780.9 **Other general symptoms**

780.93 **Memory loss**

Add   **Excludes** *memory loss due to:*
Add   *intracranial injuries (850.0-854.19)*
Add   *skull fractures (800.00-801.99, 803.00-804.99)*
Revise   *mild memory disturbance due to organic brain damage (310.8)*

783 **Symptoms concerning nutrition, metabolism, and development**

783.3 **Feeding difficulties and mismanagement**

Revise   **Excludes** *feeding disturbance or problems: in newborn (779.31-779.34)*

783.4 **Lack of expected normal physiological development in childhood**

783.41 **Failure to thrive**

Add   **Excludes** *failure to thrive in newborn (779.34)*

784 **Symptoms involving head and neck**

Revise   784.4 **Voice ~~disturbance~~ and resonance disorders**

Revise   784.40 **Voice ~~disturbance~~ and resonance disorder, unspecified**

New code   784.42 **Dysphonia**
Hoarseness

New code   784.43 **Hypernasality**

New code   784.44 **Hyponasality**

Revise   784.49 **Other voice and resonance disorders**

Delete   ~~Dsyphonia~~
Delete   ~~Hoarseness~~
Delete   ~~Hypernasality~~
Delete   ~~Hyponasality~~

784.5 **Other speech disturbance**

Delete   ~~Dysarthria~~
Delete   ~~Dysphasia~~
Delete   ~~Slurred speech~~

Add   **Excludes** *speech disorder due to late effect of cerebrovascular accident (438.10-438.19)*

New code   784.51 **Dysarthria**

Excludes *dysarthria due to late effect of cerebrovascular accident (438.13)*

New code   784.59 **Other speech disturbance**
Dysphasia
Slurred speech
Speech disturbance NOS

787 **Symptoms involving digestive system**

787.0 **Nausea and vomiting**

Excludes *vomiting*
Add   *fecal matter (569.87)*
Revise   *of newborn (779.32, 779.33)*
Add   *persistent (536.2)*

New code   787.04 **Bilious emesis**
Bilious vomiting

Excludes *bilious emesis (vomiting) in newborn (779.32)*

789 **Other symptoms involving abdomen and pelvis**

789.0 **Abdominal pain**
[0-7, 9]

Delete   ~~Colic:~~
~~NOS~~
~~infantile~~

Delete   ~~**Excludes** renal colic (788.0)~~

New code   789.7 **Colic**
Colic NOS
Infantile colic

Excludes *colic in adult and child over 12 months old (789.0)*
renal colic (788.0)

790 **Nonspecific findings on examination of blood**

790.01 **Precipitous drop in hematocrit**
Add   Drop in hemoglobin

Revise   793   **Nonspecific (abnormal) findings on radiological and other examination of body structure**

793.8   **Breast**

New code   793.82   **Inconclusive mammogram**
Dense breasts NOS
Inconclusive mammogram NEC
Inconclusive mammography due to dense breasts
Inconclusive mammography NEC

Revise   793.89   **Other (abnormal) findings on radiological examination of breast**

Revise   793.9   **Other**

793.99   **Other nonspecific (abnormal) findings on radiological and other examinations of body structure**

795   **Other and nonspecific abnormal cytological, histological, immunological and DNA test findings**

795.0   **Abnormal Papanicolaou smear of cervix and cervical HPV**

Revise   **Excludes**   *carcinoma in situ in situ of cervix (233.1)*

795.3   **Nonspecific positive culture findings**
795.39   **Other nonspecific positive culture findings**

Add   **Excludes**   *colonization status (V02.0-V02.9)*

796   **Other nonspecific abnormal findings**

796.7   **Abnormal cytologic smear of anus and anal HPV**

Revise   **Excludes**   *severe anal dysplasia (histologically confirmed) (230.5, 230.6)*

799   **Other ill-defined and unknown causes of morbidity and mortality**

Revise   799.2   **Nervousness Signs and symptoms involving emotional state**
Delete   "Nerves"

Add   **Excludes**   *anxiety (293.84, 300.00-300.09)*
Add   *depression (311)*

New code   799.21   **Nervousness**
Nervous

New code   799.22   **Irritability**
Irritable

New code   799.23   **Impulsiveness**
Impulsive
Excludes   *impulsive neurosis (300.3)*

New code   799.24   **Emotional lability**

New code   799.25   **Demoralization and apathy**
Apathetic

New code   799.29   **Other signs and symptoms involving emotional state**

799.8   **Other ill-defined conditions**

New code   799.82   **Apparent life threatening event in infant**
ALTE
Apparent life threatening event in newborn and infant

Use additional code(s) for associated signs and symptoms

Excludes   *signs and symptoms associated with a confirmed diagnosis-code to confirmed diagnosis*

FRACTURE OF SKULL (800-804)

Add   **Includes**   traumatic brain injury due to fracture of skull

813   **Fracture of radius and ulna**

813.4   **Lower end, closed**

Revise   813.45   **Torus fracture of radius (alone)**
Add   **Excludes**   *Torus fracture of radius and ulna (813.47)*

New code   813.46   **Torus fracture of ulna (alone)**
Excludes   *Torus fracture of radius and ulna (813.47)*

New code   813.47   **Torus fracture of radius and ulna**

832   **Dislocation of elbow**

Revise   The following fifth-digit subclassification is for use with category 832 subcategories 832.0 and 832.1:

New code   832.2   **Nursemaid's elbow**
Subluxation of radial head

INTRACRANIAL INJURY, EXCLUDING THOSE WITH SKULL FRACTURE (850-854)

Add   **Includes**   traumatic brain injury without skull fracture

854   **Intracranial injury of other and unspecified nature**

Revise   **Includes**   injury:
Revise   brain injury NOS
Revise   intracranial injury
Add   traumatic brain NOS

OPEN WOUNDS (870-897)

Delete   Use additional code to identify infection

945   **Burn of lower limb(s)**

945.0   **Unspecified degree**
Revise   [0-6, 9]

945.1   **Erythema [first degree]**
Revise   [0-6, 9]

945.2   **Blisters, epidermal loss [second degree]**
Revise   [0-6, 9]

945.3   **Full-thickness skin loss [third degree NOS]**
Revise   [0-6, 9]

945.4   **Deep necrosis of underlying tissues [deep third degree] without mention of loss of a body part**
Revise   [0-6, 9]

945.5   **Deep necrosis of underlying tissues [deep third degree] with loss of a body part**
Revise   [0-6, 9]

969 Poisoning by psychotropic agents

969.0 Antidepressants

Delete ~~Amitriptyline~~
Delete ~~Imipramine~~
Delete ~~Monoamine oxidase [MAO] inhibitors~~

New code 969.00 Antidepressant, unspecified

New code 969.01 Monoamine oxidase inhibitors
                   MAOI

New code 969.02 Selective serotonin and
                   norepinephrine reuptake inhibitors
                   SSNRI antidepressants

New code 969.03 Selective serotonin reuptake
                   inhibitors
                   SSRI antidepressants

New code 969.04 Tetracyclic antidepressants

New code 969.05 Tricyclic antidepressants

New code 969.09 Other antidepressants

969.7 Psychostimulants

Delete ~~Amphetamine~~
Delete ~~Caffeine~~

New code 969.70 Psychostimulant, unspecified

New code 969.71 Caffeine

New code 969.72 Amphetamines
                   Methamphetamines

New code 969.73 Methylphenidate

New code 969.79 Other psychostimulants

974 Poisoning by water, mineral, and uric acid
     metabolism drugs

974.1 Purine derivative diuretics

Revise **Excludes** *caffeine (969.71)*

995 Certain adverse effects not elsewhere classified

995.2 Other and unspecified adverse effect of
       drug, medicinal and biological substance
       (due) to correct medicinal substance
       properly administered

New code 995.24 Failed moderate sedation during
                   procedure
                   Failed conscious sedation during
                   procedure

995.9 Systemic inflammatory response syndrome
       (SIRS)

995.92 Severe sepsis

                   Use additional code to specify
                   acute organ dysfunction,
                   such as:
Revise   acute ~~renal~~ kidney failure
                   (584.5-584.9)

995.94 Systemic inflammatory response
        syndrome due to non-infectious
        process with acute organ
        dysfunction

                   Use additional code to specify
                   acute organ dysfunction,
                   such as:
Revise   acute ~~renal~~ kidney failure
                   (584.5-584.9)

996 Complications peculiar to certain specified
     procedures

996.4 Mechanical complication of internal
       orthopedic device, implant, and graft

Revise   996.43 ~~Prosthetic joint implant failure~~
                    Broken prosthetic joint implant

           996.47 Other mechanical complication of
                    prosthetic joint implant
Add   Prosthetic joint implant failure
                    NOS

996.7 Other complications of internal
       (biological) (synthetic) prosthetic device,
       implant, and graft

                   Use additional code to identify
                   complication, such as:
Add   venous embolism and thrombosis
                   (453.2-453.9)

997 Complications affecting specified body systems,
     not elsewhere classified

997.3 Respiratory complications

           997.31 Ventilator associated pneumonia
Add   Ventilator associated pneumonitis

997.4 Digestive system complications

           Excludes *specified gastrointestinal
                         complications classified
                         elsewhere, such as:*
Add   *complications of intestinal pouch
                         (569.71-569.79)*
Add   *pouchitis (569.71)*

997.5 Urinary complications
Revise   Renal (kidney):

999 Complications of medical care, not elsewhere
     classified

999.6 ABO incompatibility reaction

           Excludes *minor blood group antigens
                         reactions (Duffy) (E) (K(ell))
Add   (Kidd) (Lewis) (M) (N) (P)
                         (S) (999.89)*

V07 Need for isolation and other prophylactic
     measures

V07.5 Prophylactic use of agents affecting
       estrogen receptors and estrogen levels

           V07.52 Prophylactic use of aromatase
                    inhibitors
                    Prophylactic use of:
Revise   exemestane ~~exemestar~~
                    (Aromasin)

V10 Personal history of malignant neoplasm

Delete   ~~Code first any continuing functional activity, such as:~~

Delete   ~~carcinoid syndrome (259.2)~~

V10.0 Gastrointestinal tract

Add   **Excludes**   *personal history of malignant carcinoid tumor (V10.91)*

Add   *personal history of malignant neuroendocrine tumor (V10.91)*

V10.1 Trachea, bronchus, and lung

Add   **Excludes**   *personal history of malignant carcinoid tumor (V10.91)*

Add   *personal history of malignant neuroendocrine tumor (V10.91)*

V10.8 Personal history of malignant neoplasm of other sites

Add   **Excludes**   *personal history of malignant carcinoid tumor (V10.91)*

Add   *personal history of malignant neuroendocrine tumor (V10.91)*

Revise   V10.9 Other and ~~U~~unspecified personal history of malignant neoplasm

New code   V10.90 Personal history of unspecified malignant neoplasm

Add   Personal history of malignant neoplasm NOS

Excludes   *personal history of malignant carcinoid tumor (V10.91)*
personal history of malignant neuroendocrine tumor (V10.91)
personal history of Merkel cell carcinoma (V10.91)

New code   V10.91 Personal history of malignant neuroendocrine tumor
"Personal history of malignant carcinoid tumor NOS
Personal history of malignant neuroendocrine tumor NOS
Personal history of Merkel cell carcinoma NOS

Code first any continuing functional activity, such as:
carcinoid syndrome (259.2)

V12 Personal history of certain other diseases

V12.5 Diseases of circulatory system

V12.54 Transient ischemic attack (TIA), and cerebral infarction without residual deficits

Add   **Excludes**   *history of traumatic brain injury (V15.52)*

V15 Other personal history presenting hazards to health

V15.0 Allergy, other than to medicinal agents

Revise   V15.06 Allergy to insects <u>and arachnids</u>

V15.5 Injury

New code   V15.52 History of traumatic brain injury

Excludes   *personal history of cerebrovascular accident (cerebral infarction) without residual deficits (V12.54)*

V15.8 Other specified personal history presenting hazards to health

New code   V15.80 History of failed moderate sedation
History of failed conscious sedation

New code   V15.83 Underimmunization status
Delinquent immunization status
Lapsed immunization schedule status

Revise   V15.84 <u>Contact with and (suspected) exposure to</u> ~~Exposure to~~ asbestos

Revise   V15.85 <u>Contact with and (suspected) exposure to</u> ~~Exposure to~~ potentially hazardous body fluids

Revise   V15.86 <u>Contact with and (suspected) exposure to</u> ~~Exposure to~~ lead

V20 Health supervision of infant or child

    V20.2 Routine infant or child health check

Delete   ~~Initial and subsequent routine newborn check~~

Add   Health check for child over 28 days old

Add   **Excludes** *health check for child under 29 days old (V20.31-V20.32)*

Add   *newborn health supervision (V20.31-V20.32)*

New sub   **V20.3 Newborn health supervision**

        Health check for child under 29 days old

        Excludes *health check for child over 28 days old (V20.2)*

New code   **V20.31 Health supervision for newborn under 8 days old**

        Health check for newborn under 8 days old

New code   **V20.32 Health supervision for newborn 8 to 28 days old**

        Health check for newborn 8 to 28 days old

        Newborn weight check

V23 Supervision of high-risk pregnancy

    V23.8 Other high-risk pregnancy

        V23.86 Pregnancy with history of in utero procedure during previous pregnancy

Revise   **Excludes** *management of pregnancy affected by in utero procedure during current pregnancy (679.0-679.1)*

V26 Procreative management

    V26.4 General counseling and advice

New code   **V26.42 Encounter for fertility preservation counseling**

        Encounter for fertility preservation counseling prior to cancer therapy

        Encounter for fertility preservation counseling prior to surgical removal of gonads

    V26.8 Other specified procreative management

New code   **V26.82 Encounter for fertility preservation procedure**

        Encounter for fertility preservation procedure prior to cancer therapy

        Encounter for fertility preservation procedure prior to surgical removal of gonads

V45 Other postprocedural states

    V45.7 Acquired absence of organ

        V45.71 Acquired absence of breast and nipple

Add   **Excludes** *congenital absence of breast and nipple (757.6)*

V53 Fitting and adjustment of other device

Revise   **V53.5 Other <u>gastrointestinal</u> appliance and <u>device</u>**

New code   **V53.50 Fitting and adjustment of intestinal appliance and device**

New code   **V53.51 Fitting and adjustment of gastric lap band**

New code   **V53.59 Fitting and adjustment of other gastrointestinal appliance and device**

V54 Other orthopedic aftercare

    V54.1 Aftercare for healing traumatic fracture

Add   **Excludes** *aftercare following joint replacement (V54.81)*

    V54.2 Aftercare for healing pathologic fracture

Add   **Excludes** *aftercare following joint replacement (V54.81)*

V57 Care involving use of rehabilitation procedures

Revise   **V57.3 Speech-<u>language</u> therapy**

V60 Housing, household, and economic circumstances

    V60.8 Other specified housing or economic circumstances

New code   **V60.81 Foster care (status)**

New code   **V60.89 Other specified housing or economic circumstances**

V61 Other family circumstances

    V61.0 Family disruption

        V61.01 Family disruption due to family member on military deployment

Add   **Excludes** *family disruption due to family member on non-military extended absence from home (V61.08)*

New code   **V61.07 Family disruption due to death of family member**

        Excludes *bereavement (V62.82)*

New code   **V61.08 Family disruption due to other extended absence of family member**

        Excludes *family disruption due to family member on military deployment (V61.01)*

	V61.2	Parent-child problems
New code	V61.23	Counseling for parent-biological child problem
		Concern about behavior of biological child
		Parent-biological child conflict
		Parent-biological child relationship problem
New code	V61.24	Counseling for parent-adopted child problem
		Concern about behavior of adopted child
		Parent-adopted child conflict
		Parent-adopted child relationship problem
New code	V61.25	Counseling for parent (guardian)-foster child problem
		Concern about behavior of foster child
		Parent (guardian)-foster child conflict
		Parent (guardian)-foster child relationship problem
Revise	V61.29	Other <u>parent-child problems</u>
Delete		~~Problem concerning adopted or foster child~~
	V61.4	Health problems within family
New code	V61.42	Substance abuse in family

V62 Other psychosocial circumstances

	V62.8	Other psychological or physical stress, not elsewhere classified
	V62.82	Bereavement, uncomplicated
Add		**Excludes** *family disruption due to death of family member (V61.07)*

V65 Other persons seeking consultation

	V65.1	Person consulting on behalf of another person
Revise	V65.11	Pediatric pre-birth visit for expect<u>ant</u> ~~mother~~ <u>parent(s)</u>
		Pre-adoption visit for adoptive parent(s)

Add V70 General medical examination

	V70.0	Routine general medical examination at a health care facility
Revise		**Excludes** *health checkup of infant or child <u>over 28 days old</u> (V20.2)*
Add		*health supervision of newborn 8 to 28 days old (V20.32)*
Add		*health supervision of newborn under 8 days old (V20.31)*

V72 Special investigations and examinations

Add		**Excludes** *health supervision of newborn 8 to 28 days old (V20.32)*
Add		*health supervision of newborn under 8 days old (V20.31)*
Revise		*routine examination of infant or child <u>over 28 days old</u> (V20.2)*

	V72.5	Radiological examination, not elsewhere classified
Delete		**Excludes** ~~examination for suspected tuberculosis (V71.2)~~
Add		*radiologic examinations as part of pre-procedural testing (V72.81-V72.84)*

	V72.6	Laboratory examination
Add		Encounters for blood and urine testing
Delete		**Excludes** ~~that for suspected disorder (V71.0-V71.9)~~
New code	V72.60	Laboratory examination, unspecified
New code	V72.61	Antibody response examination
		Immunity status testing
		Excludes *encounter for allergy testing (V72.7)*
New code	V72.62	Laboratory examination ordered as part of a routine general medical examination
		Blood tests for routine general physical examination
New code	V72.63	Pre-procedural laboratory examination
		Blood tests prior to treatment or procedure
		Pre-operative laboratory examination
New code	V72.69	Other laboratory examination
	V72.8	Other specified examinations
Add		**Excludes** *pre-procedural laboratory examinations (V72.63)*
	V72.83	Other specified preoperative examination
Add		Examination prior to chemotherapy

V80 Special screening for neurological, eye, and ear diseases

	V80.0	Neurological conditions
New code	V80.01	Traumatic brain injury
New code	V80.09	Other neurological conditions

V87   Other specified personal exposures and history presenting hazards to health

    V87.3   Contact with and (suspected) exposure to other potentially hazardous substances

New code   V87.32   Contact with and (suspected) exposure to algae bloom

    V87.4   Personal history of drug therapy

New code   V87.43   Personal history of estrogen therapy

New code   V87.44   Personal history of inhaled steroid therapy

New code   V87.45   Personal history of systemic steroid therapy
        Personal history of steroid therapy NOS

New code   V87.46   Personal history of immunosuppression therapy

        Excludes   *personal history of steroid therapy (V87.44, V87.45)*

Revise   **SUPPLEMENTARY CLASSIFICATION OF EXTERNAL CAUSES OF INJURY AND POISONING (E000-E999)**

Revise section: Machinery accidents [other than those connected with transport] are classifiable to category E919, in which the fourth digit allows a broad classification of the type of machinery involved. ~~If a more detailed classification of type of machinery is required, it is suggested that the "Classification of Industrial Accidents according to Agency," prepared by the International Labor Office, be used in addition; it is included in this publication.~~

Categories for "late effects" of accidents and other external causes are to be found at E929, E959, E969, E977, E989, and E999.

~~Definitions and examples related to transport accidents~~

New section   **EXTERNAL CAUSE STATUS (E000)**

Add   **Note:**   A code from category E000 should be used in conjunction with the external cause code(s) assigned to a record to indicate the status of the person at the time the event occurred. A single code from category E000 should be assigned for an encounter.

New category   E000   **External cause status**

New code   E000.0   **Civilian activity done for income or pay**
        Civilian activity done for financial or other compensation

        Excludes   *military activity (E000.1)*

New code   E000.1   **Military activity**

        Excludes   *activity of off duty military personnel (E000.8)*

New code   E000.8   **Other external cause status**
        Activity NEC
        Hobby not done for income
        Leisure activity
        Off-duty activity of military personnel
        Recreation or sport not for income or while a student
        Student activity
        Volunteer activity

        Excludes   *civilian activity done for income or compensation (E000.0)*
        military activity (E000.1)

New code   E000.9   **Unspecified external cause status**

New section   **ACTIVITY (E001-E030)**

Note: Categories E001 to E030 are provided for use to indicate the activity of the person seeking healthcare for an injury or health condition, such as a heart attack while shoveling snow, which resulted from, or was contributed to, by the activity. These codes are appropriate for use for both acute injuries, such as those from chapter 17, and conditions that are due to the long-term, cumulative effects of an activity, such as those from chapter 13. They are also appropriate for use with external cause codes for cause and intent if identifying the activity provides additional information on the event.

These codes should be used in conjunction with other external cause codes for external cause status (E000) and place of occurrence (E849).

This section contains the following broad activity categories:

E001   Activities involving walking and running

E002   Activities involving water and water craft

E003   Activities involving ice and snow

E004   Activities involving climbing, rappelling, and jumping off

E005   Activities involving dancing and other rhythmic movement

E006   Activities involving other sports and athletics played individually

E007   Activities involving other sports and athletics played as a team or group

E008   Activities involving other specified sports and athletics

E009   Activity involving other cardiorespiratory exercise

E010   Activity involving other muscle strengthening exercises

E011 Activities involving computer technology and electronic devices

E012 Activities involving arts and handcrafts

E013 Activities involving personal hygiene and household maintenance

E014 Activities involving person providing caregiving

E015 Activities involving food preparation, cooking and grilling

E016 Activities involving property and land maintenance, building and construction

E017 Activities involving roller coasters and other types of external motion

E018 Activities involving playing musical instrument

E019 Activities involving animal care

E029 Other activity

E030 Unspecified activity

E001 Activities involving walking and running

New category **Excludes** *walking an animal (E019.0)*
walking or running on a treadmill (E009.0)

New code **E001.0 Walking, marching and hiking**
Walking, marching and hiking on level or elevated terrain
Excludes *mountain climbing (E004.0)*

New code **E001.1 Running**

New category **E002 Activities involving water and water craft**

Excludes *activities involving ice (E003.0-E003.9)*
boating and other watercraft transport accidents (E830-E838)

New code **E002.0 Swimming**

New code **E002.1 Springboard and platform diving**

New code **E002.2 Water polo**

New code **E002.3 Water aerobics and water exercise**

New code **E002.4 Underwater diving and snorkeling**
SCUBA diving

New code **E002.5 Rowing, canoeing, kayaking, rafting and tubing**
Canoeing, kayaking, rafting and tubing in calm and turbulent water

New code **E002.6 Water skiing and wake boarding**

New code **E002.7 Surfing, windsurfing and boogie boarding**

New code **E002.8 Water sliding**

New code **E002.9 Other activity involving water and watercraft**
Activity involving water NOS
Parasailing
Water survival training and testing

New category **E003 Activities involving ice and snow**

Excludes *shoveling ice and snow (E016.0)*

New code **E003.0 Ice skating**
Figure skating (singles) (pairs)
Ice dancing
Excludes *ice hockey (E003.1)*

New code **E003.1 Ice hockey**

New code **E003.2 Snow (alpine) (downhill) skiing, snow boarding, sledding, tobogganing and snow tubing**
Excludes *cross country skiing (E003.3)*

New code **E003.3 Cross country skiing**
Nordic skiing

New code **E003.9 Other activity involving ice and snow**
Activity involving ice and snow NOS

New category **E004 Activities involving climbing, rappelling and jumping off**
Excludes *hiking on level or elevated terrain (E001.0)*
jumping rope (E006.5)
sky diving (E840-E844)
trampoline jumping (E005.3)

New code **E004.0 Mountain climbing, rock climbing and wall climbing**

New code **E004.1 Rappelling**

New code **E004.2 BASE jumping**
Building, Antenna, Span, Earth jumping

New code **E004.3 Bungee jumping**

New code **E004.4 Hang gliding**

New code **E004.9 Other activity involving climbing, rappelling and jumping off**

New category **E005 Activities involving dancing and other rhythmic movement**
Excludes *martial arts (E008.4)*

New code **E005.0 Dancing**

New code **E005.1 Yoga**

New code **E005.2 Gymnastics**
Rhythmic gymnastics
Excludes *trampoline (E005.3)*

New code **E005.3 Trampoline**

New code **E005.4 Cheerleading**

New code **E005.9 Other activity involving dancing and other rhythmic movements**

New category	E006	Activities involving other sports and athletics played individually

Excludes *dancing (E005.0)*
gymnastic (E005.2)
trampoline (E005.3)
yoga (E005.1)

New code   E006.0   **Roller skating (inline) and skateboarding**

New code   E006.1   **Horseback riding**

New code   E006.2   **Golf**

New code   E006.3   **Bowling**

New code   E006.4   **Bike riding**

Excludes *transport accident involving bike riding (E800-E829)*

New code   E006.5   **Jumping rope**

New code   E006.6   **Non-running track and field events**

Excludes *running (any form) (E001.1)*

New code   E006.9   **Other activity involving other sports and athletics played individually**

Excludes *activities involving climbing, rappelling, and jumping (E004.0-E004.9)*
activities involving ice and snow (E003.0-E003.9)
activities involving walking and running (E001.0-E001.9)
activities involving water and watercraft (E002.0-E002.9)

New category	E007	Activities involving other sports and athletics played as a team or group

Excludes *ice hockey (E003.1)*
water polo (E002.2)

New code   E007.0   **American tackle football**
Football NOS

New code   E007.1   **American flag or touch football**

New code   E007.2   **Rugby**

New code   E007.3   **Baseball**
Softball

New code   E007.4   **Lacrosse and field hockey**

New code   E007.5   **Soccer**

New code   E007.6   **Basketball**

New code   E007.7   **Volleyball (beach) (court)**

New code   E007.8   **Physical games generally associated with school recess, summer camp and children**
Capture the flag
Dodge ball
Four square
Kickball

New code   E007.9   **Other activity involving other sports and athletics played as a team or group**
Cricket

New category	E008	Activities involving other specified sports and athletics

New code   E008.0   **Boxing**

New code   E008.1   **Wrestling**

New code   E008.2   **Racquet and hand sports**
Handball
Racquetball
Squash
Tennis

New code   E008.3   **Frisbee**
Ultimate frisbee

New code   E008.4   **Martial arts**
Combatives

New code   E008.9   **Other specified sports and athletics activity**

Excludes *sports and athletics activities specified in categories E001-E007*

New category	E009	Activity involving other cardiorespiratory exercise

Activity involving physical training

New code   E009.0   **Exercise machines primarily for cardiorespiratory conditioning**
Elliptical and stepper machines
Stationary bike
Treadmill

New code   E009.1   **Calisthenics**
Jumping jacks
Warm up and cool down

New code   E009.2   **Aerobic and step exercise**

New code   E009.3   **Circuit training**

New code   E009.4   **Obstacle course**
Challenge course
Confidence course

New code   E009.5   **Grass drills**
Guerilla drills

New code   E009.9   **Other activity involving other cardiorespiratory exercise**

Excludes *activities involving cardio-respiratory exercise specified in categories E001-E008*

New category	E010	Activity involving other muscle strengthening exercises

New code   E010.0   **Exercise machines primarily for muscle strengthening**

New code   E010.1   **Push-ups, pull-ups, sit-ups**

New code   E010.2   **Free weights**
Barbells
Dumbbells

New code   E010.3   **Pilates**

New code   E010.9   **Other activity involving other muscle strengthening exercises**

Excludes *activities involving muscle strengthening specified in categories E001-E009*

New category | **E011 Activities involving computer technology and electronic devices**

> **Excludes** *electronic musical keyboard or instruments (E018.0)*

New code | **E011.0 Computer keyboarding**
Electronic game playing using keyboard or other stationary device

New code | **E011.1 Hand held interactive electronic device**
Cellular telephone and communication device
Electronic game playing using interactive device

> **Excludes** *electronic game playing using keyboard or other stationary device (E011.0)*

New code | **E011.9 Other activity involving computer technology and electronic devices**

New category | **E012 Activities involving arts and handcrafts**

> **Excludes** *activities involving playing musical instrument (E018.0-E018.3)*

New code | **E012.0 Knitting and crocheting**

New code | **E012.1 Sewing**

New code | **E012.2 Furniture building and finishing**
Furniture repair

New code | **E012.9 Activity involving other arts and handcrafts**

New category | **E013 Activities involving personal hygiene and household maintenance**

> **Excludes** *activities involving cooking and grilling (E015.0-E015.9)*
> *activities involving property and land maintenance, building and construction (E016.0-E016.9)*
> *activity involving persons providing caregiving (E014.0-E014.9)*
> *dishwashing (E015.0)*
> *food preparation (E015.0)*
> *gardening (E016.1)*

New code | **E013.0 Personal bathing and showering**

New code | **E013.1 Laundry**

New code | **E013.2 Vacuuming**

New code | **E013.3 Ironing**

New code | **E013.4 Floor mopping and cleaning**

New code | **E013.5 Residential relocation**
Packing up and unpacking involved in moving to a new residence

New code | **E013.8 Other personal hygiene activity**

New code | **E013.9 Other household maintenance**

New category | **E014 Activities involving person providing caregiving**

New code | **E014.0 Caregiving involving bathing**

New code | **E014.1 Caregiving involving lifting**

New code | **E014.9 Other activity involving person providing caregiving**

New category | **E015 Activities involving food preparation, cooking and grilling**

New code | **E015.0 Food preparation and clean up**
Dishwashing

New code | **E015.1 Grilling and smoking food**

New code | **E015.2 Cooking and baking**
Use of stove, oven and microwave oven

New code | **E015.9 Other activity involving cooking and grilling**

New category | **E016 Activities involving property and land maintenance, building and construction**

New code | **E016.0 Digging, shoveling and raking**
Dirt digging
Raking leaves
Snow shoveling

New code | **E016.1 Gardening and landscaping**
Pruning, trimming shrubs, weeding

New code | **E016.2 Building and construction**

New code | **E016.9 Other activity involving property and land maintenance, building and construction**

New category | **E017 Activities involving roller coasters and other types of external motion**

New code | **E017.0 Rollercoaster riding**

New code | **E017.9 Other activity involving external motion**

New category | **E018 Activities involving playing musical instrument**
Activity involving playing electric musical instrument

New code | **E018.0 Piano playing**
Musical keyboard (electronic) playing

New code | **E018.1 Drum and other percussion instrument playing**

New code | **E018.2 String instrument playing**

New code | **E018.3 Wind and brass instrument playing**

New category | **E019 Activities involving animal care**

> **Excludes** *horseback riding (E006.1)*

New code | **E019.0 Walking an animal**

New code | **E019.1 Milking an animal**

New code | **E019.2 Grooming and shearing an animal**

New code | **E019.9 Other activity involving animal care**

New category | **E029 Other activity**

New code | **E029.0 Refereeing a sports activity**

New code | **E029.1 Spectator at an event**

New code | **E029.2 Rough housing and horseplay**

New code | **E029.9 Other activity**

New code | **E030 Unspecified activity**

New section | **TRANSPORT ACCIDENTS (E800-E848)**

Add | Definitions and examples related to transport accidents

(a) A transport accident (E800-E848) is any accident involving a device designed primarily for, or being used at the time primarily for, conveying persons or goods from one place to another.

WATER TRANSPORT ACCIDENTS (E830-E838)

The following fourth-digit subdivisions are for use with categories E830-E838 to identify the injured person:

New
fourth-
digit sub
.7 Occupant of military watercraft, any type

E876 Other and unspecified misadventures during medical care

Revise
E876.5 Performance of ~~inappropriate~~ wrong operation (procedure) on correct patient

Add
Wrong device implanted into correct surgical site

Add
Excludes *correct operation (procedure) performed on wrong body part (E876.7)*

New code
E876.6 Performance of operation (procedure) on patient not scheduled for surgery
Performance of operation (procedure) intended for another patient
Performance of operation (procedure) on wrong patient

New code
E876.7 Performance of correct operation (procedure) on wrong side/body part
Performance of correct operation (procedure) on wrong side
Performance of correct operation (procedure) on wrong site

E918 Caught accidentally in or between objects
Excludes *injury caused by:*
Add
mechanism or component of firearm and air gun (E928.7)

E919 Accidents caused by machinery
Excludes *injury caused by:*
Add
mechanism or component of firearm and air gun (E928.7)

E920 Accidents caused by cutting and piercing instruments or objects
Add
Excludes *injury caused by mechanism or component of firearm and air gun (E928.7)*

E922 Accident caused by firearm and air gun missile
Add
Excludes *injury caused by mechanism or component of firearm and air gun (E928.7)*

E923 Accident caused by explosive material
Add
Excludes *injury caused by mechanism or component of firearm and air gun (E928.7)*

E927 Overexertion and strenuous and repetitive movements or loads
Add
Use additional code to identify activity (E001-E030)

E928 Other and unspecified environmental and accidental causes
New code
E928.7 Mechanism or component of firearm and air gun
Injury due to:
explosion of gun parts
recoil
Pierced, cut, crushed, or pinched by slide trigger mechanism, scope or other gun part
Powder burn from firearm or air gun
Excludes *accident caused by firearm and air gun missile (E922.0-E922.9)*

DRUGS, MEDICINAL AND BIOLOGICAL SUBSTANCES CAUSING ADVERSE EFFECTS IN THERAPEUTIC USE (E930-E949)

Revise
Excludes *administration with suicidal or homicidal intent or intent to harm, or in circumstances classifiable to ~~E980-E989~~ (E950.0-E950.5, E962.0, E980.0-E980.5)*

INJURY RESULTING FROM OPERATIONS OF WAR (E990-E999)

Revise
Includes injuries to military personnel and civilians caused by war and civil
insurrections and occurring during the time of war and insurrection, and peacekeeping missions

E990 Injury due to war operations by fires and conflagrations
E990.0 From gasoline bomb
Add
Incendiary bomb
New code
E990.1 From flamethrower
New code
E990.2 From incendiary bullet
New code
E990.3 From fire caused indirectly from conventional weapon
Excludes *fire aboard military aircraft (E994.3)*

E991 Injury due to war operations by bullets and fragments
Add
Excludes *injury due to bullets and fragments due to war operations, but occurring after cessation of hostilities (E998.0)*
injury due to explosion of artillery shells and mortars (E993.2)
injury due to explosion of improvised explosive device [IED] (E993.3-E993.5)
injury due to sea-based artillery shell (E992.3)

New code
E991.4 Fragments from munitions
Fragments from:
artillery shell
bombs, except antipersonnel
detonation of unexploded ordnance [UXO]
grenade
guided missile
land mine
rockets
shell

New code
E991.5 Fragments from person-borne improvised explosive device [IED]

New code
E991.6 Fragments from vehicle-borne improvised explosive device [IED]
IED borne by land, air, or water transport vehicle

New code
E991.7 Fragments from other improvised explosive device [IED]
Roadside IED

New code
E991.8 Fragments from weapons
Fragments from:
artillery
autocannons
automatic grenade launchers
missile launchers
mortars
small arms

	E991.9	Other and unspecified fragments
Delete		~~Fragments from:~~
		~~artillery shell~~
		~~bombs, except antipersonnel~~
		~~grenade~~
		~~guided missile~~
		~~land mine~~
		~~rockets~~
		~~shell~~
Revise		Shrapnel <u>NOS</u>

E992 Injury due to war operations by explosion of marine weapons

Delete		~~Depth charge~~
		~~Marine mines~~
		~~Mine NOS, at sea or in harbor~~
		~~Sea-based artillery shell~~
		~~Torpedo~~
		~~Underwater blast~~
New code	E992.0	**Torpedo**
New code	E992.1	**Depth charge**
New code	E992.2	**Marine mines**
		Marine mines at sea or in harbor
New code	E992.3	**Sea-based artillery shell**
New code	E992.8	**Other by other marine weapons**
New code	E992.9	**Unspecified marine weapon**
		Underwater blast NOS

E993 Injury due to war operations by other explosion

Delete		~~Accidental explosion of munitions being used in war~~
		~~Accidental explosion of own weapons~~
		~~Air blast NOS~~
		~~Blast NOS~~
		~~Explosion NOS~~
		~~Explosion of:~~
		~~artillery shell~~
		~~breech block~~
		~~cannon block~~
		~~mortar bomb~~
		~~Injury by weapon burst~~
Add		Injuries due to direct or indirect pressure or air blast of an explosion occurring during war operations
Add		**Excludes** *injury due to fragments resulting from an explosion (E991.0-E991.9)*
Add		*injury due to detonation of unexploded ordnance but occurring after cessation of hostilities (E998.0-E998.9)*
Add		*injury due to nuclear weapons (E996.0-E996.9)*
New code	E993.0	**Aerial bomb**
New code	E993.1	**Guided missile**
New code	E993.2	**Mortar**
		Artillery shell
New code	E993.3	**Person-borne improvised explosive device [IED]**
New code	E993.4	**Vehicle-borne improvised explosive device [IED]**
		IED borne by land, air, or water transport vehicle
New code	E993.5	**Other improvised explosive device [IED]**
		Roadside IED
New code	E993.6	**Unintentional detonation of own munitions**
		Unintentional detonation of own ammunition (artillery) (mortars)

New code	E993.7	**Unintentional discharge of own munitions launch device**
		Unintentional explosion of own:
		Autocannons
		Automatic grenade launchers
		Missile launchers
		Small arms
New code	E993.8	**Other specified explosion**
		Bomb
		Grenade
		Land mine
New code	E993.9	**Unspecified explosion**
		Air blast NOS
		Blast NOS
		Blast wave NOS
		Blast wind NOS
		Explosion NOS

E994 Injury due to war operations by destruction of aircraft

Delete		~~Airplane:~~
		~~burned~~
		~~exploded~~
		~~shot down~~
		~~Crushed by falling airplane~~
New code	E994.0	**Destruction of aircraft due to enemy fire or explosives**
		Air to air missile
		Explosive device placed on aircraft
		Rocket propelled grenade [RPG]
		Small arms fire
		Surface to air missile
New code	E994.1	**Unintentional destruction of aircraft due to own onboard explosives**
New code	E994.2	**Destruction of aircraft due to collision with other aircraft**
New code	E994.3	**Destruction of aircraft due to onboard fire**
New code	E994.8	**Other destruction of aircraft**
New code	E994.9	**Unspecified destruction of aircraft**

E995 Injury due to war operations by other and unspecified forms of conventional warfare

Delete		~~Battle wounds~~
		~~Bayonet injury~~
		~~Drowned in war operations~~
New code	E995.0	**Unarmed hand-to-hand combat**
		Excludes *intentional restriction of airway (E995.3)*
New code	E995.1	**Struck by blunt object**
		Baton (nightstick)
		Stave
New code	E995.2	**Piercing object**
		Bayonet
		Knife
		Sword
New code	E995.3	**Intentional restriction of air and airway**
		Intentional submersion
		Strangulation
		Suffocation
New code	E995.4	**Unintentional drowning due to inability to surface or obtain air**
		Submersion
New code	E995.8	**Other forms of conventional warfare**
New code	E995.9	**Unspecified form of conventional warfare**

	E996	**Injury due to war operations by nuclear weapons**
Delete		~~Blast effects~~
		~~Exposure to ionizing radiation from nuclear weapons~~
		~~Fireball effects~~
		~~Heat~~
		~~Other direct and secondary effects of nuclear weapons~~
Add		Dirty bomb NOS
Add		**Excludes** *late effects of injury due to nuclear weapons (E999.1, E999.0)*
New code	**E996.0**	**Direct blast effect of nuclear weapon**
		Injury to bodily organs due to blast pressure
New code	**E996.1**	**Indirect blast effect of nuclear weapon**
		Injury due to being thrown by blast
		Injury due to being struck or crushed by blast debris
New code	**E996.2**	**Thermal radiation effect of nuclear weapon**
		Burns due to thermal radiation
		Fireball effects
		Flash burns
		Heat effects
New code	**E996.3**	**Nuclear radiation effects**
		Acute radiation exposure
		Beta burns
		Fallout exposure
		Radiation sickness
		Secondary effects of nuclear weapons
New code	**E996.8**	**Other effects of nuclear weapons**
New code	**E996.9**	**Unspecified effect of nuclear weapon**

	E997	**Injury due to war operations by other forms of unconventional warfare**
New code	**E997.3**	**Weapon of mass destruction [WMD], unspecified**
	E998	**Injury due to war operations but occurring after cessation of hostilities**
New code	**E998.0**	**Explosion of mines**
New code	**E998.1**	**Explosion of bombs**
New code	**E998.8**	**Injury due to other war operations but occurring after cessation of hostilities**
New code	**E998.9**	**Injury due to unspecified war operations but occurring after cessation of hostilities**

PROFESSIONAL EDITION

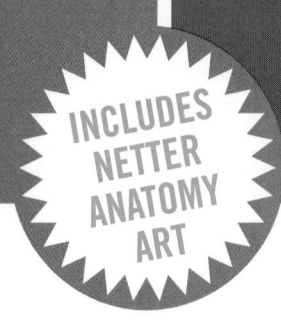

2010

ICD-9-CM

VOLUMES 1 & 2

FOR PHYSICIANS

PART I

Introduction

ICD-9-CM BACKGROUND

The International Classification of Diseases, 9th Revision, Clinical Modification (ICD-9-CM) is based on the official version of the World Health Organization's 9th Revision, International Classification of Diseases (ICD-9). ICD-9 is designed for the classification of morbidity and mortality information for statistical purposes, and for the indexing of hospital records by disease and operations, for data storage and retrieval. The historical background of the International Classification of Diseases may be found in the Introduction to ICD-9 (Manual of the International Classification of Diseases, Injuries, and Causes of Death, World Health Organization, Geneva, Switzerland, 1977).

ICD-9-CM is a clinical modification of the World Health Organization's International Classification of Diseases, 9th Revision (ICD-9). The term "clinical" is used to emphasize the modification's intent: to serve as a useful tool in the area of classification of morbidity data for indexing of medical records, medical care review, and ambulatory and other medical care programs, as well as for basic health statistics. To describe the clinical picture of the patient, the codes must be more precise than those needed only for statistical groupings and trend analysis.

COORDINATION AND MAINTENANCE COMMITTEE

Annual modifications are made to the ICD-9-CM through the ICD-9-CM Coordination and Maintenance Committee (C&M). The Committee is made up of representatives from two Federal Government agencies, the National Center for Health Statistics and the Health Care Financing Administration. The Committee holds meetings twice a year which are open to the public. Modification proposals submitted to the Committee for consideration are presented at the meetings for public discussion. Those modification proposals which are approved are incorporated into the official government version of the ICD-9-CM and become effective for use October 1 of the year following their presentation. The C&M also prepares updates for use April 1 of each year. To date, no April 1 updates have been released.

CHARACTERISTICS OF ICD-9-CM

ICD-9-CM far exceeds its predecessors in the number of codes provided. The disease classification has been expanded to include health-related conditions and to provide greater specificity at the fifth-digit level of detail. These fifth digits are not optional; they are intended for use in recording the information substantiated in the clinical record.

Volume I of ICD-9-CM contains five appendices:

Appendix A   Morphology of Neoplasms
Appendix B   Glossary of Mental Disorders (Deleted in 2004)
Appendix C   Classification of Drugs by American Hospital Formulary Service List Number and Their ICD-9-CM Equivalents
Appendix D   Classification of Industrial Accidents According to Agency
Appendix E   List of Three-Digit Categories

These appendices are included as a reference to the user in order to provide further information about the patient's clinical picture, to further define a diagnostic statement, to aid in classifying new drugs, or to reference three-digit categories.

Volume 2 of ICD-9-CM contains many diagnostic terms which do not appear in Volume 1 since the index includes most diagnostic terms currently in use.

The Disease Classification

ICD-9-CM is totally compatible with its parent system, ICD-9, thus meeting the need for comparability of morbidity and mortality statistics at the international level. A few fourth-digit codes were created in existing three-digit rubrics only when the necessary detail could not be accommodated by the use of a fifth-digit subclassification. To ensure that each rubric of ICD-9-CM collapses back to its ICD-9 counterpart, the following specifications governed the ICD-9-CM disease classification:

Specifications for the Tabular List

1. Three-digit rubrics and their contents are unchanged from ICD-9.
2. The sequence of three-digit rubrics is unchanged from ICD-9.
3. Unsubdivided three-digit rubrics are subdivided where necessary to:
   a) Add clinical detail
   b) Isolate terms for clinical accuracy
4. The modification in ICD-9-CM is accomplished by the addition of a fifth digit to existing ICD-9 rubrics.
5. The optional dual classification in ICD-9 is modified.
   a) Duplicate rubrics are deleted:
      1) Four-digit manifestation categories duplicating etiology entries.
      2) Manifestation inclusion terms duplicating etiology entries.
   b) Manifestations of diseases are identified, to the extent possible, by creating five-digit codes in the etiology rubrics.
   c) When the manifestation of a disease cannot be included in the etiology rubrics, provision for its identification is made by retaining the ICD-9 rubrics used for classifying manifestations of disease.
6. The format of ICD-9-CM is revised from that used in ICD-9.
   a) American spelling of medical terms is used.
   b) Inclusion terms are indented beneath the titles of codes.
   c) Codes not to be used for principal tabulation of disease are printed with the notation, "Code first underlying disease."

Specifications for the Alphabetic Index

1. Format of the Alphabetic Index follows the format of ICD-9.
2. When two codes are required to indicate etiology and manifestation, the manifestation code appears in brackets, e.g., diabetic cataract 250.5X [366.41]. The etiology code is always sequenced first followed by the manifestation code.

The following guidelines were the most current at the time of publication. Check the website at http://codingupdates.com for the latest updates to the Guidelines.

ICD-9-CM OFFICIAL GUIDELINES FOR CODING AND REPORTING

Effective October 1, 2008
Narrative changes appear in bold text
Items underlined have been moved within the guidelines since October 1, 2007
The guidelines include the updated V Code Table

The Centers for Medicare and Medicaid Services (CMS) and the National Center for Health Statistics (NCHS), two departments within the U.S. Federal Government's Department of Health and Human Services (DHHS) provide the following guidelines for coding and reporting using the International Classification of Diseases, 9th Revision, Clinical Modification (ICD-9-CM). These guidelines should be used as a companion document to the official version of the ICD-9-CM as published on CD-ROM by the U.S. Government Printing Office (GPO).

These guidelines have been approved by the four organizations that make up the Cooperating Parties for the ICD-9-CM: the American Hospital Association (AHA), the American Health Information Management Association (AHIMA), CMS, and NCHS. These guidelines are included on the official government version of the ICD-9-CM, and also appear in "Coding Clinic for ICD-9-CM" published by the AHA.

These guidelines are a set of rules that have been developed to accompany and complement the official conventions and instructions provided within the ICD-9-CM itself. These guidelines are based on the coding and sequencing instructions in Volumes I, II and III of ICD-9-CM, but provide additional instruction. Adherence to these guidelines when assigning ICD-9-CM diagnosis and procedure codes is required under the Health Insurance Portability and Accountability Act (HIPAA). The diagnosis codes (Volumes 1-2) have been adopted under HIPAA for all healthcare settings. Volume 3 procedure codes have been adopted for inpatient procedures reported by hospitals. A joint effort between the healthcare provider and the coder is essential to achieve complete and accurate documentation, code assignment, and reporting of diagnoses and procedures. These guidelines have been developed to assist both the healthcare provider and the coder in identifying those diagnoses and procedures that are to be reported. The importance of consistent, complete documentation in the medical record cannot be overemphasized. Without such documentation accurate coding cannot be achieved. The entire record should be reviewed to determine the specific reason for the encounter and the conditions treated.

The term encounter is used for all settings, including hospital admissions. In the context of these guidelines, the term provider is used throughout the guidelines to mean physician or any qualified health care practitioner who is legally accountable for establishing the patient's diagnosis. Only this set of guidelines, approved by the Cooperating Parties, is official.

The guidelines are organized into sections. Section I includes the structure and conventions of the classification and general guidelines that apply to the entire classification, and chapter-specific guidelines that correspond to the chapters as they are arranged in the classification. Section II includes guidelines for selection of principal diagnosis for non-outpatient settings. Section III includes guidelines for reporting additional diagnoses in non-outpatient settings. Section IV is for outpatient coding and reporting.

ICD-9-CM Official Guidelines for Coding and Reporting

Section I. Conventions, general coding guidelines and chapter specific guidelines

A. Conventions for the ICD-9-CM
- 1. Format:
- 2. Abbreviations
  - a. Index abbreviations
  - b. Tabular abbreviations
- 3. Punctuation
- 4. Includes and Excludes Notes and Inclusion terms
- 5. Other and Unspecified codes
  - a. "Other" codes
  - b. "Unspecified" codes
- 6. Etiology/manifestation convention ("code first", "use additional code" and "in diseases classified elsewhere" notes)
- 7. "And"
- 8. "With"
- 9. "See" and "See Also"

B. General Coding Guidelines
- 1. Use of Both Alphabetic Index and Tabular List
- 2. Locate each term in the Alphabetic Index
- 3. Level of Detail in Coding
- 4. Code or codes from 001.0 through V89
- 5. Selection of codes 001.0 through 999.9
- 6. Signs and symptoms
- 7. Conditions that are an integral part of a disease process
- 8. Conditions that are not an integral part of a disease process
- 9. Multiple coding for a single condition
- 10. Acute and Chronic Conditions
- 11. Combination Code
- 12. Late Effects
- 13. Impending or Threatened Condition
- **14. Reporting Same Diagnosis Code More than Once**
- **15. Admissions/Encounters for Rehabilitation**
- **16. Documentation for BMI and Pressure Ulcer Stages**

C. Chapter-Specific Coding Guidelines
- 1. Chapter 1: Infectious and Parasitic Diseases (001-139)
  - a. Human Immunodeficiency Virus (HIV) Infections
  - b. Septicemia, Systemic Inflammatory Response Syndrome (SIRS), Sepsis, Severe Sepsis, and Septic Shock
  - **c. Methicillin Resistant *Staphylococcus aureus* (MRSA) Conditions**

2. Chapter 2: Neoplasms (140-239)
   a. Treatment directed at the malignancy
   b. Treatment of secondary site
   c. Coding and sequencing of complications
   d. Primary malignancy previously excised
   e. Admissions/Encounters involving chemotherapy, immunotherapy and radiation therapy
   f. Admission/encounter to determine extent of malignancy
   g. Symptoms, signs, and ill-defined conditions listed in Chapter 16 associated with neoplasms
   h. Admission/encounter for pain control/management
   i. Malignant neoplasm associated with transplanted organ
3. Chapter 3: Endocrine, Nutritional, and Metabolic Diseases and Immunity Disorders (240-279)
   a. Diabetes mellitus
4. Chapter 4: Diseases of Blood and Blood Forming Organs (280-289)
   a. Anemia of chronic disease
5. Chapter 5: Mental Disorders (290-319)
   Reserved for future guideline expansion
6. Chapter 6: Diseases of Nervous System and Sense Organs (320-389)
   a. Pain - Category 338
7. Chapter 7: Diseases of Circulatory System (390-459)
   a. Hypertension
   b. Cerebral infarction/stroke/cerebrovascular accident (CVA)
   c. Postoperative cerebrovascular accident
   d. Late Effects of Cerebrovascular Disease
   e. Acute myocardial infarction (AMI)
8. Chapter 8: Diseases of Respiratory System (460-519)
   a. Chronic Obstructive Pulmonary Disease [COPD] and Asthma
   b. Chronic Obstructive Pulmonary Disease [COPD] and Bronchitis
   c. Acute Respiratory Failure
   d. Influenza due to identified avian influenza virus (avian influenza)
9. Chapter 9: Diseases of Digestive System (520-579)
   Reserved for future guideline expansion
10. Chapter 10: Diseases of Genitourinary System (580-629)
    a. Chronic kidney disease
11. Chapter 11: Complications of Pregnancy, Childbirth, and the Puerperium (630-679)
    a. General Rules for Obstetric Cases
    b. Selection of OB Principal or First-listed Diagnosis
    c. Fetal Conditions Affecting the Management of the Mother
    d. HIV Infection in Pregnancy, Childbirth and the Puerperium
    e. Current Conditions Complicating Pregnancy
    f. Diabetes mellitus in pregnancy
    g. Gestational diabetes
    h. Normal Delivery, Code 650
    i. The Postpartum and Peripartum Periods
    j. Code 677, Late effect of complication of pregnancy
    k. Abortions

12. Chapter 12: Diseases Skin and Subcutaneous Tissue (680-709)
    a. **Pressure ulcer stage codes**
13. Chapter 13: Diseases of Musculoskeletal and Connective Tissue (710-739)
    a. Coding of Pathologic Fractures
14. Chapter 14: Congenital Anomalies (740-759)
    a. Codes in categories 740-759, Congenital Anomalies
15. Chapter 15: Newborn (Perinatal) Guidelines (760-779)
    a. General Perinatal Rules
    b. Use of codes V30-V39
    c. Newborn transfers
    d. Use of category V29
    e. Use of other V codes on perinatal records
    f. Maternal Causes of Perinatal Morbidity
    g. Congenital Anomalies in Newborns
    h. Coding Additional Perinatal Diagnoses
    i. Prematurity and Fetal Growth Retardation
    j. Newborn sepsis
16. Chapter 16: Signs, Symptoms and Ill-Defined Conditions (780-799)
    Reserved for future guideline expansion
17. Chapter 17: Injury and Poisoning (800-999)
    a. Coding of Injuries
    b. Coding of Traumatic Fractures
    c. Coding of Burns
    d. Coding of Debridement of Wound, Infection, or Burn
    e. Adverse Effects, Poisoning and Toxic Effects
    f. Complications of care
    g. SIRS due to Non-infectious Process
18. Classification of Factors Influencing Health Status and Contact with Health Service (Supplemental V01-**V89**)
    a. Introduction
    b. V codes use in any healthcare setting
    c. V Codes indicate a reason for an encounter
    d. Categories of V Codes
    e. V Code Table
19. Supplemental Classification of External Causes of Injury and Poisoning (E-codes, E800-E999)
    a. General E Code Coding Guidelines
    b. Place of Occurrence Guideline
    c. Adverse Effects of Drugs, Medicinal and Biological Substances Guidelines
    d. Multiple Cause E Code Coding Guidelines
    e. Child and Adult Abuse Guideline
    f. Unknown or Suspected Intent Guideline
    g. Undetermined Cause
    h. Late Effects of External Cause Guidelines
    i. Misadventures and Complications of Care Guidelines
    j. Terrorism Guidelines

Section I. Conventions, general coding guidelines and chapter specific guidelines

The conventions, general guidelines and chapter-specific guidelines are applicable to all health care settings unless otherwise indicated.

A. Conventions for the ICD-9-CM

The conventions for the ICD-9-CM are the general rules for use of the classification independent of the guidelines. These conventions are incorporated within the index and tabular of the ICD-9-CM as instructional notes. The conventions are as follows:

1. **Format:**

    The ICD-9-CM uses an indented format for ease in reference

2. **Abbreviations**

    a. **Index abbreviations**

    NEC "Not elsewhere classifiable"
    This abbreviation in the index represents "other specified" when a specific code is not available for a condition the index directs the coder to the "other specified" code in the tabular.

    b. **Tabular abbreviations**

    NEC "Not elsewhere classifiable"
    This abbreviation in the tabular represents "other specified". When a specific code is not available for a condition the tabular includes an NEC entry under a code to identify the code as the "other specified" code.
    (See Section I.A.5.a. "Other" codes").

    NOS "Not otherwise specified"
    This abbreviation is the equivalent of unspecified.
    (See Section I.A.5.b., "Unspecified" codes)

3. **Punctuation**

    [ ] Brackets are used in the tabular list to enclose synonyms, alternative wording or explanatory phrases. Brackets are used in the index to identify manifestation codes.
    (See Section I.A.6. "Etiology/manifestations")

    ( ) Parentheses are used in both the index and tabular to enclose supplementary words that may be present or absent in the statement of a disease or procedure without affecting the code number to which it is assigned. The terms within the parentheses are referred to as nonessential modifiers.

    : Colons are used in the Tabular list after an incomplete term which needs one or more of the modifiers following the colon to make it assignable to a given category.

4. **Includes and Excludes Notes and Inclusion terms**

    Includes: This note appears immediately under a three-digit code title to further define, or give examples of, the content of the category.

    Excludes: An excludes note under a code indicates that the terms excluded from the code are to be coded elsewhere. In some cases the codes for the excluded terms should not be used in conjunction with the code from which it is excluded. An example of this is a congenital condition excluded from an acquired form of the same condition. The congenital and acquired codes should not be used together. In other cases, the excluded terms may be used together with an excluded code. An example of this is when fractures of different bones are coded to different codes. Both codes may be used together if both types of fractures are present.

Inclusion terms: List of terms is included under certain four and five digit codes. These terms are the conditions for which that code number is to be used. The terms may be synonyms of the code title, or, in the case of "other specified" codes, the terms are a list of the various conditions assigned to that code. The inclusion terms are not necessarily exhaustive. Additional terms found only in the index may also be assigned to a code.

5. **Other and Unspecified codes**

   a. **"Other" codes**

      Codes titled "other" or "other specified" (usually a code with a 4th digit 8 or fifth-digit 9 for diagnosis codes) are for use when the information in the medical record provides detail for which a specific code does not exist. Index entries with NEC in the line designate "other" codes in the tabular. These index entries represent specific disease entities for which no specific code exists so the term is included within an "other" code.

   b. **"Unspecified" codes**

      Codes (usually a code with a 4th digit 9 or 5th digit 0 for diagnosis codes) titled "unspecified" are for use when the information in the medical record is insufficient to assign a more specific code.

6. **Etiology/manifestation convention ("code first", "use additional code" and "in diseases classified elsewhere" notes)**

   Certain conditions have both an underlying etiology and multiple body system manifestations due to the underlying etiology. For such conditions, the ICD-9-CM has a coding convention that requires the underlying condition be sequenced first followed by the manifestation. Wherever such a combination exists, there is a "use additional code" note at the etiology code, and a "code first" note at the manifestation code. These instructional notes indicate the proper sequencing order of the codes, etiology followed by manifestation.

   In most cases the manifestation codes will have in the code title, "in diseases classified elsewhere." Codes with this title are a component of the etiology/ manifestation convention. The code title indicates that it is a manifestation code. "In diseases classified elsewhere" codes are never permitted to be used as first listed or principal diagnosis codes. They must be used in conjunction with an underlying condition code and they must be listed following the underlying condition.

   There are manifestation codes that do not have "in diseases classified elsewhere" in the title. For such codes a "use additional code" note will still be present and the rules for sequencing apply.

   In addition to the notes in the tabular, these conditions also have a specific index entry structure. In the index both conditions are listed together with the etiology code first followed by the manifestation codes in brackets. The code in brackets is always to be sequenced second.

   The most commonly used etiology/manifestation combinations are the codes for Diabetes mellitus, category 250. For each code under category 250 there is a use additional code note for the manifestation that is specific for that particular diabetic manifestation. Should a patient have more than one manifestation of diabetes, more than one code from category 250 may be used with as many manifestation codes as are needed to fully describe the patient's complete diabetic condition. The category 250 diabetes codes should be sequenced first, followed by the manifestation codes.

   "Code first" and "Use additional code" notes are also used as sequencing rules in the classification for certain codes that are not part of an etiology/ manifestation combination.

   See - Section I.B.9. "Multiple coding for a single condition".

7. **"And"**

The word "and" should be interpreted to mean either "and" or "or" when it appears in a title.

8. **"With"**

The word "with" in the alphabetic index is sequenced immediately following the main term, not in alphabetical order.

9. **"See" and "See Also"**

The "see" instruction following a main term in the index indicates that another term should be referenced. It is necessary to go to the main term referenced with the "see" note to locate the correct code.

A "see also" instruction following a main term in the index instructs that there is another main term that may also be referenced that may provide additional index entries that may be useful. It is not necessary to follow the "see also" note when the original main term provides the necessary code.

B. **General Coding Guidelines**

1. **Use of Both Alphabetic Index and Tabular List**

Use both the Alphabetic Index and the Tabular List when locating and assigning a code. Reliance on only the Alphabetic Index or the Tabular List leads to errors in code assignments and less specificity in code selection.

2. **Locate each term in the Alphabetic Index**

Locate each term in the Alphabetic Index and verify the code selected in the Tabular List. Read and be guided by instructional notations that appear in both the Alphabetic Index and the Tabular List.

3. **Level of Detail in Coding**

Diagnosis and procedure codes are to be used at their highest number of digits available.

ICD-9-CM diagnosis codes are composed of codes with 3, 4, or 5 digits. Codes with three digits are included in ICD-9-CM as the heading of a category of codes that may be further subdivided by the use of fourth and/or fifth digits, which provide greater detail.

A three-digit code is to be used only if it is not further subdivided. Where fourth-digit subcategories and/or fifth-digit subclassifications are provided, they must be assigned. A code is invalid if it has not been coded to the full number of digits required for that code. For example, Acute myocardial infarction, code 410, has fourth digits that describe the location of the infarction (e.g., 410.2, Of inferolateral wall), and fifth digits that identify the episode of care. It would be incorrect to report a code in category 410 without a fourth and fifth digit.

ICD-9-CM Volume 3 procedure codes are composed of codes with either 3 or 4 digits. Codes with two digits are included in ICD-9-CM as the heading of a category of codes that may be further subdivided by the use of third and/or fourth digits, which provide greater detail.

4. **Code or codes from 001.0 through V89.09**

The appropriate code or codes from 001.0 through V89.09 must be used to identify diagnoses, symptoms, conditions, problems, complaints or other reason(s) for the encounter/visit.

5. **Selection of codes 001.0 through 999.9**

   The selection of codes 001.0 through 999.9 will frequently be used to describe the reason for the admission/encounter. These codes are from the section of ICD-9-CM for the classification of diseases and injuries (e.g., infectious and parasitic diseases; neoplasms; symptoms, signs, and ill-defined conditions, etc.).

6. **Signs and symptoms**

   Codes that describe symptoms and signs, as opposed to diagnoses, are acceptable for reporting purposes when a related definitive diagnosis has not been established (confirmed) by the provider. Chapter 16 of ICD-9-CM, Symptoms, Signs, and Ill-defined conditions (codes 780.0 - 799.9) contain many, but not all codes for symptoms.

7. **Conditions that are an integral part of a disease process**

   Signs and symptoms that are associated routinely with a disease process should not be assigned as additional codes, unless otherwise instructed by the classification.

8. **Conditions that are not an integral part of a disease process**

   Additional signs and symptoms that may not be associated routinely with a disease process should be coded when present.

9. **Multiple coding for a single condition**

   In addition to the etiology/manifestation convention that requires two codes to fully describe a single condition that affects multiple body systems, there are other single conditions that also require more than one code. "Use additional code" notes are found in the tabular at codes that are not part of an etiology/manifestation pair where a secondary code is useful to fully describe a condition. The sequencing rule is the same as the etiology/manifestation pair - , "use additional code" indicates that a secondary code should be added.

   For example, for infections that are not included in chapter 1, a secondary code from category 041, Bacterial infection in conditions classified elsewhere and of unspecified site, may be required to identify the bacterial organism causing the infection. A "use additional code" note will normally be found at the infectious disease code, indicating a need for the organism code to be added as a secondary code.

   "Code first" notes are also under certain codes that are not specifically manifestation codes but may be due to an underlying cause. When a "code first" note is present and an underlying condition is present the underlying condition should be sequenced first.

   "Code, if applicable, any causal condition first", notes indicate that this code may be assigned as a principal diagnosis when the causal condition is unknown or not applicable. If a causal condition is known, then the code for that condition should be sequenced as the principal or first-listed diagnosis.

   Multiple codes may be needed for late effects, complication codes and obstetric codes to more fully describe a condition. See the specific guidelines for these conditions for further instruction.

10. **Acute and Chronic Conditions**

    If the same condition is described as both acute (subacute) and chronic, and separate subentries exist in the Alphabetic Index at the same indentation level, code both and sequence the acute (subacute) code first.

11. **Combination Code**

A combination code is a single code used to classify:
Two diagnoses, or
A diagnosis with an associated secondary process (manifestation)
A diagnosis with an associated complication

Combination codes are identified by referring to subterm entries in the Alphabetic Index and by reading the inclusion and exclusion notes in the Tabular List.

Assign only the combination code when that code fully identifies the diagnostic conditions involved or when the Alphabetic Index so directs. Multiple coding should not be used when the classification provides a combination code that clearly identifies all of the elements documented in the diagnosis. When the combination code lacks necessary specificity in describing the manifestation or complication, an additional code should be used as a secondary code.

12. **Late Effects**

A late effect is the residual effect (condition produced) after the acute phase of an illness or injury has terminated. There is no time limit on when a late effect code can be used. The residual may be apparent early, such as in cerebrovascular accident cases, or it may occur months or years later, such as that due to a previous injury. Coding of late effects generally requires two codes sequenced in the following order: The condition or nature of the late effect is sequenced first. The late effect code is sequenced second.

An exception to the above guidelines are those instances where the code for late effect is followed by a manifestation code identified in the Tabular List and title, or the late effect code has been expanded (at the fourth and fifth-digit levels) to include the manifestation(s). The code for the acute phase of an illness or injury that led to the late effect is never used with a code for the late effect.

13. **Impending or Threatened Condition**

Code any condition described at the time of discharge as "impending" or "threatened" as follows:

If it did occur, code as confirmed diagnosis.

If it did not occur, reference the Alphabetic Index to determine if the condition has a subentry term for "impending" or "threatened" and also reference main term entries for "Impending" and for "Threatened."

If the subterms are listed, assign the given code.

If the subterms are not listed, code the existing underlying condition(s) and not the condition described as impending or threatened.

14. **Reporting Same Diagnosis Code More than Once**

Each unique ICD-9-CM diagnosis code may be reported only once for an encounter. This applies to bilateral conditions or two different conditions classified to the same ICD-9-CM diagnosis code.

15. **Admissions/Encounters for Rehabilitation**

When the purpose for the admission/encounter is rehabilitation, sequence the appropriate V code from category V57, Care involving use of rehabilitation procedures, as the principal/first-listed diagnosis. The code for the condition for which the service is being performed should be reported as an additional diagnosis.

Only one code from category V57 is required. Code V57.89, Other specified rehabilitation procedures, should be assigned if more than one type of rehabilitation is performed during a single encounter. A procedure code should be reported to identify each type of rehabilitation therapy actually performed.

16. **Documentation for BMI and Pressure Ulcer Stages**

    For the Body Mass Index (BMI) and pressure ulcer stage codes, code assignment may be based on medical record documentation from clinicians who are not the patient's provider (i.e., physician or other qualified healthcare practitioner legally accountable for establishing the patient's diagnosis), since this information is typically documented by other clinicians involved in the care of the patient (e.g., a dietitian often documents the BMI and nurses often documents the pressure ulcer stages). However, the associated diagnosis (such as overweight, obesity, or pressure ulcer) must be documented by the patient's provider. If there is conflicting medical record documentation, either from the same clinician or different clinicians, the patient's attending provider should be queried for clarification.

    The BMI and pressure ulcer stage codes should only be reported as secondary diagnoses. As with all other secondary diagnosis codes, the BMI and pressure ulcer stage codes should only be assigned when they meet the definition of a reportable additional diagnosis (see Section III, Reporting Additional Diagnoses).

C. **Chapter-Specific Coding Guidelines**

    In addition to general coding guidelines, there are guidelines for specific diagnoses and/or conditions in the classification. Unless otherwise indicated, these guidelines apply to all health care settings. Please refer to Section II for guidelines on the selection of principal diagnosis.

    1. **Chapter 1: Infectious and Parasitic Diseases (001-139)**

        a. **Human Immunodeficiency Virus (HIV) Infections**

            1) **Code only confirmed cases**

                Code only confirmed cases of HIV infection/illness. This is an exception to the hospital inpatient guideline Section II, H.

                In this context, "confirmation" does not require documentation of positive serology or culture for HIV; the provider's diagnostic statement that the patient is HIV positive, or has an HIV-related illness is sufficient.

            2) **Selection and sequencing of HIV codes**

                (a) **Patient admitted for HIV-related condition**

                    If a patient is admitted for an HIV-related condition, the principal diagnosis should be 042, followed by additional diagnosis codes for all reported HIV-related conditions.

                (b) **Patient with HIV disease admitted for unrelated condition**

                    If a patient with HIV disease is admitted for an unrelated condition (such as a traumatic injury), the code for the unrelated condition (e.g., the nature of injury code) should be the principal diagnosis. Other diagnoses would be 042 followed by additional diagnosis codes for all reported HIV-related conditions.

                (c) **Whether the patient is newly diagnosed**

                    Whether the patient is newly diagnosed or has had previous admissions/encounters for HIV conditions is irrelevant to the sequencing decision.

                (d) **Asymptomatic human immunodeficiency virus**

                    V08 Asymptomatic human immunodeficiency virus [HIV] infection, is to be applied when the patient without any documentation of symptoms is listed as being "HIV positive," "known HIV," "HIV test positive," or similar terminology. Do not use this code if the term "AIDS" is used or if the patient is treated for any HIV-related illness or is described as having any condition(s) resulting from his/her HIV positive status; use 042 in these cases.

(e) **Patients with inconclusive HIV serology**

Patients with inconclusive HIV serology, but no definitive diagnosis or manifestations of the illness, may be assigned code 795.71, Inconclusive serologic test for Human Immunodeficiency Virus [HIV].

(f) **Previously diagnosed HIV-related illness**

Patients with any known prior diagnosis of an HIV-related illness should be coded to 042. Once a patient has developed an HIV-related illness, the patient should always be assigned code 042 on every subsequent admission/encounter. Patients previously diagnosed with any HIV illness (042) should never be assigned to 795.71 or V08.

(g) **HIV Infection in Pregnancy, Childbirth and the Puerperium**

During pregnancy, childbirth or the puerperium, a patient admitted (or presenting for a health care encounter) because of an HIV-related illness should receive a principal diagnosis code of 647.6X, Other specified infectious and parasitic diseases in the mother classifiable elsewhere, but complicating the pregnancy, childbirth or the puerperium, followed by 042 and the code(s) for the HIV-related illness(es). Codes from Chapter 15 always take sequencing priority.

Patients with asymptomatic HIV infection status admitted (or presenting for a health care encounter) during pregnancy, childbirth, or the puerperium should receive codes of 647.6X and V08.

(h) **Encounters for testing for HIV**

If a patient is being seen to determine his/her HIV status, use code V73.89, Screening for other specified viral disease. Use code V69.8, Other problems related to lifestyle, as a secondary code if an asymptomatic patient is in a known high risk group for HIV. Should a patient with signs or symptoms or illness, or a confirmed HIV related diagnosis be tested for HIV, code the signs and symptoms or the diagnosis. An additional counseling code V65.44 may be used if counseling is provided during the encounter for the test.

When a patient returns to be informed of his/her HIV test results use code V65.44, HIV counseling, if the results of the test are negative.

If the results are positive but the patient is asymptomatic use code V08, Asymptomatic HIV infection. If the results are positive and the patient is symptomatic use code 042, HIV infection, with codes for the HIV related symptoms or diagnosis. The HIV counseling code may also be used if counseling is provided for patients with positive test results.

b. **Septicemia, Systemic Inflammatory Response Syndrome (SIRS), Sepsis, Severe Sepsis, and Septic Shock**
   1) **SIRS, Septicemia, and Sepsis**
      (a) The terms *septicemia* and *sepsis* are often used interchangeably by providers, however they are not considered synonymous terms. The following descriptions are provided for reference but do not preclude querying the provider for clarification about terms used in the documentation:

      (i) Septicemia generally refers to a systemic disease associated with the presence of pathological microorganisms or toxins in the blood, which can include bacteria, viruses, fungi or other organisms.

      (ii) Systemic inflammatory response syndrome (SIRS) generally refers to the systemic response to infection, trauma/burns, or other insult (such as cancer) with symptoms including fever, tachycardia, tachypnea, and leukocytosis.

      (iii) Sepsis generally refers to SIRS due to infection.

      (iv) Severe sepsis generally refers to sepsis with associated acute organ dysfunction.

      (b) **The Coding of SIRS, sepsis and severe sepsis**

      The coding of SIRS, sepsis and severe sepsis requires a minimum of 2 codes: a code for the underlying cause (such as infection or trauma) and a code from subcategory 995.9 Systemic inflammatory response syndrome (SIRS).

      (i) The code for the underlying cause (such as infection or trauma) must be sequenced before the code from subcategory 995.9 Systemic inflammatory response syndrome (SIRS).

      (ii) Sepsis and severe sepsis require a code for the systemic infection (038.xx, 112.5, etc.) and either code 995.91, Sepsis, or 995.92, Severe sepsis. If the causal organism is not documented, assign code 038.9, Unspecified septicemia.

      (iii) Severe sepsis requires additional code(s) for the associated acute organ dysfunction(s).

      (iv) If a patient has sepsis with multiple organ dysfunctions, follow the instructions for coding severe sepsis.

      (v) Either the term sepsis or SIRS must be documented to assign a code from subcategory 995.9.

      (vi) *See Section I.C.17.g), Injury and poisoning, for information regarding systemic inflammatory response syndrome (SIRS) due to trauma/burns and other non-infectious processes.*

      (c) Due to the complex nature of sepsis and severe sepsis, some cases may require querying the provider prior to assignment of the codes.

2) **Sequencing sepsis and severe sepsis**

(a) **Sepsis and severe sepsis as principal diagnosis**

If sepsis or severe sepsis is present on admission, and meets the definition of principal diagnosis, the systemic infection code (e.g., 038.xx, 112.5, etc) should be assigned as the principal diagnosis, followed by code 995.91, Sepsis, or 995.92, Severe sepsis, as required by the sequencing rules in the Tabular List. Codes from subcategory 995.9 can never be assigned as a principal diagnosis. A code should also be assigned for any localized infection, if present.

If the sepsis or severe sepsis is due to a postprocedural infection, see Section I.C.1.b.10 for guidelines related to sepsis due to postprocedural infection.

(b) **Sepsis and severe sepsis as secondary diagnoses**

When sepsis or severe sepsis develops during the encounter (it was not present on admission), the systemic infection code and code 995.91 or 995.92 should be assigned as secondary diagnoses.

(c) **Documentation unclear as to whether sepsis or severe sepsis is present on admission**

Sepsis or severe sepsis may be present on admission but the diagnosis may not be confirmed until sometime after admission. If the documentation is not clear whether the sepsis or severe sepsis was present on admission, the provider should be queried.

3) **Sepsis/SIRS with Localized Infection**

If the reason for admission is both sepsis, severe sepsis, or SIRS and a localized infection, such as pneumonia or cellulitis, a code for the systemic infection (038.xx, 112.5, etc) should be assigned first, then code 995.91 or 995.92, followed by the code for the localized infection. If the patient is admitted with a localized infection, such as pneumonia, and sepsis/SIRS doesn't develop until after admission, see guideline I.C.1.b.2.b).

If the localized infection is postprocedural, *see Section I.C.1.b.10 for guidelines related to sepsis due to postprocedural infection.*

Note: The term urosepsis is a nonspecific term. If that is the only term documented then only code 599.0 should be assigned based on the default for the term in the ICD-9-CM index, in addition to the code for the causal organism if known.

4) **Bacterial Sepsis and Septicemia**

In most cases, it will be a code from category 038, Septicemia, that will be used in conjunction with a code from subcategory 995.9 such as the following:

(a) **Streptococcal sepsis**

If the documentation in the record states streptococcal sepsis, codes 038.0, Streptococcal septicemia, and code 995.91 should be used, in that sequence.

(b) **Streptococcal septicemia**

If the documentation states streptococcal septicemia, only code 038.0 should be assigned, however, the provider should be queried whether the patient has sepsis, an infection with SIRS.

5) **Acute organ dysfunction that is not clearly associated with the sepsis**

If a patient has sepsis and an acute organ dysfunction, but the medical record documentation indicates that the acute organ dysfunction is related to a medical condition other than the sepsis, do not assign code 995.92, Severe sepsis. An acute organ dysfunction must be associated with the sepsis in order to assign the severe sepsis code. If the documentation is not clear as to whether an acute organ dysfunction is related to the sepsis or another medical condition, query the provider.

6) **Septic shock**

(a) **Sequencing of septic shock**

Septic shock generally refers to circulatory failure associated with severe sepsis, and, therefore, it represents a type of acute organ dysfunction.

For all cases of septic shock, the code for the systemic infection should be sequenced first, followed by codes 995.92 and 785.52. Any additional codes for other acute organ dysfunctions should also be assigned. As noted in the sequencing instructions in the Tabular List, the code for septic shock cannot be assigned as a principal diagnosis.

(b) **Septic Shock without documentation of severe sepsis**

Septic shock indicates the presence of severe sepsis.

Code 995.92, Severe sepsis, must be assigned with code 785.52, Septic shock, even if the term severe sepsis is not documented in the record. The "use additional code" note and the "code first" note in the tabular support this guideline.

7) **Sepsis and septic shock complicating abortion and pregnancy**

Sepsis and septic shock complicating abortion, ectopic pregnancy, and molar pregnancy are classified to category codes in Chapter 11 (630-639).

See section I.C.11.

8) **Negative or inconclusive blood cultures**

Negative or inconclusive blood cultures do not preclude a diagnosis of septicemia or sepsis in patients with clinical evidence of the condition, however, the provider should be queried.

9) **Newborn sepsis**

See Section I.C.15.j for information on the coding of newborn sepsis.

10) **Sepsis due to a Postprocedural Infection**

(a) **Documentation of causal relationship**

As with all postprocedural complications, code assignment is based on the provider's documentation of the relationship between the infection and the procedure.

(b) **Sepsis due to postprocedural infection**

In cases of postprocedural sepsis, the complication code, such as code 998.59, Other postoperative infection, or 674.3x, Other complications of obstetrical surgical wounds should be coded first followed by the appropriate sepsis codes (systemic infection code and either code 995.91or 995.92). An additional code(s) for any acute organ dysfunction should also be assigned for cases of severe sepsis.

11) **External cause of injury codes with SIRS**

Refer to Section I.C.19.a.7 for instruction on the use of external cause of injury codes with codes for SIRS resulting from trauma.

12) Sepsis and Severe Sepsis Associated with Non-infectious Process

In some cases, a non-infectious process, such as trauma, may lead to an infection which can result in sepsis or severe sepsis. If sepsis or severe sepsis is documented as associated with a non-infectious condition, such as a burn or serious injury, and this condition meets the definition for principal diagnosis, the code for the non-infectious condition should be sequenced first, followed by the code for the systemic infection and either code 995.91, Sepsis, or 995.92, Severe sepsis. Additional codes for any associated acute organ dysfunction(s) should also be assigned for cases of severe sepsis. If the sepsis or severe sepsis meets the definition of principal diagnosis, the systemic infection and sepsis codes should be sequenced before the non-infectious condition. When both the associated non-infectious condition and the sepsis or severe sepsis meet the definition of principal diagnosis, either may be assigned as principal diagnosis.

See Section I.C.1.b.2)(a) for guidelines pertaining to sepsis or severe sepsis as the principal diagnosis.

Only one code from subcategory 995.9 should be assigned. Therefore, when a non-infectious condition leads to an infection resulting in sepsis or severe sepsis, assign either code 995.91 or 995.92. Do not additionally assign code 995.93, Systemic inflammatory response syndrome due to non-infectious process without acute organ dysfunction, or 995.94, Systemic inflammatory response syndrome with acute organ dysfunction.

See Section I.C.17.g for information on the coding of SIRS due to trauma/burns or other non-infectious disease processes.

c. **Methicillin Resistant *Staphylococcus aureus* (MRSA) Conditions**

1) **Selection and sequencing of MRSA codes**

(a) **Combination codes for MRSA infection**

When a patient is diagnosed with an infection that is due to methicillin resistant *Staphylococcus aureus* (MRSA), and that infection has a combination code that includes the causal organism (e.g., septicemia, pneumonia) assign the appropriate code for the condition (e.g., code 038.12, Methicillin resistant Staphylococcus aureus septicemia or code 482.42, Methicillin resistant pneumonia due to Staphylococcus aureus). Do not assign code 041.12, Methicillin resistant Staphylococcus aureus, as an additional code because the code includes the type of infection and the MRSA organism. Do not assign a code from subcategory V09.0, Infection with microorganisms resistant to penicillins, as an additional diagnosis.

See Section C.1.b.1 for instructions on coding and sequencing of septicemia.

(b) **Other codes for MRSA infection**

When there is documentation of a current infection (e.g., wound infection, stitch abscess, urinary tract infection) due to MRSA, and that infection does not have a combination code that includes the causal organism, select the appropriate code to identify the condition along with code 041.12, Methicillin resistant Staphylococcus aureus, for the MRSA infection. Do not assign a code from subcategory V09.0, Infection with microorganisms resistant to penicillins.

(c) **Methicillin susceptible Staphylococcus aureus (MSSA) and MRSA colonization**

The condition or state of being colonized or carrying MSSA or MRSA is called colonization or carriage, while an individual person is described as being colonized or being a carrier. Colonization means that MSSA or MSRA is present on or in the body without necessarily causing illness. A positive MRSA colonization test might be documented by the provider as "MRSA screen positive" or "MRSA nasal swab positive".

Assign code V02.54, Carrier or suspected carrier, Methicillin resistant Staphylococcus aureus, for patients documented as having MRSA colonization. Assign code V02.53, Carrier or suspected carrier, Methicillin susceptible Staphylococcus aureus, for patient documented as having MSSA colonization. Colonization is not necessarily indicative of a disease process or as the cause of a specific condition the patient may have unless documented as such by the provider.

Code V02.59, Other specified bacterial diseases, should be assigned for other types of staphylococcal colonization (e.g., S. *epidermidis*, S. *saprophyticus*). Code V02.59 should not be assigned for colonization with any type of *Staphylococcus aureus* (MRSA, MSSA).

(d) **MRSA colonization and infection**

If a patient is documented as having both MRSA colonization and infection during a hospital admission, code V02.54, Carrier or suspected carrier, Methicillin resistant *Staphylococcus aureus*, and a code for the MRSA infection may both be assigned.

2. **Chapter 2: Neoplasms (140-239)**

<u>General guidelines</u>

Chapter 2 of the ICD-9-CM contains the codes for most benign and all malignant neoplasms. Certain benign neoplasms, such as prostatic adenomas, may be found in the specific body system chapters. To properly code a neoplasm it is necessary to determine from the record if the neoplasm is benign, in-situ, malignant, or of uncertain histologic behavior. If malignant, any secondary (metastatic) sites should also be determined.

The neoplasm table in the Alphabetic Index should be referenced first. However, if the histological term is documented, that term should be referenced first, rather than going immediately to the Neoplasm Table, in order to determine which column in the Neoplasm Table is appropriate. For example, if the documentation indicates "adenoma," refer to the term in the Alphabetic Index to review the entries under this term and the instructional note to "see also neoplasm, by site, benign." The table provides the proper code based on the type of neoplasm and the site. It is important to select the proper column in the table that corresponds to the type of neoplasm. The tabular should then be referenced to verify that the correct code has been selected from the table and that a more specific site code does not exist.

See Section I. C. 18.d.4. for information regarding V codes for genetic susceptibility to cancer.

a. **Treatment directed at the malignancy**

If the treatment is directed at the malignancy, designate the malignancy as the principal diagnosis.

The only exception to this guideline is if a patient admission/encounter is solely for the administration of chemotherapy, immunotherapy or radiation therapy, assign the appropriate V58.x code as the first-listed or principal diagnosis, and the diagnosis or problem for which the service is being performed as a secondary diagnosis.

b. **Treatment of secondary site**

When a patient is admitted because of a primary neoplasm with metastasis and treatment is directed toward the secondary site only, the secondary neoplasm is designated as the principal diagnosis even though the primary malignancy is still present.

c. **Coding and sequencing of complications**

Coding and sequencing of complications associated with the malignancies or with the therapy thereof are subject to the following guidelines:

1) **Anemia associated with malignancy**

When admission/encounter is for management of an anemia associated with the malignancy, and the treatment is only for anemia, the appropriate anemia code (such as code 285.22, Anemia in neoplastic disease) is designated as the principal diagnosis and is followed by the appropriate code(s) for the malignancy.

Code 285.22 may also be used as a secondary code if the patient suffers from anemia and is being treated for the malignancy.

2) **Anemia associated with chemotherapy, immunotherapy and radiation therapy**

When the admission/encounter is for management of an anemia associated with chemotherapy, immunotherapy or radiotherapy and the only treatment is for the anemia, the anemia is sequenced first followed by code E933.1. The appropriate neoplasm code should be assigned as an additional code.

3) **Management of dehydration due to the malignancy**

When the admission/encounter is for management of dehydration due to the malignancy or the therapy, or a combination of both, and only the dehydration is being treated (intravenous rehydration), the dehydration is sequenced first, followed by the code(s) for the malignancy.

4) **Treatment of a complication resulting from a surgical procedure**

When the admission/encounter is for treatment of a complication resulting from a surgical procedure, designate the complication as the principal or first-listed diagnosis if treatment is directed at resolving the complication.

d. **Primary malignancy previously excised**

When a primary malignancy has been previously excised or eradicated from its site and there is no further treatment directed to that site and there is no evidence of any existing primary malignancy, a code from category V10, Personal history of malignant neoplasm, should be used to indicate the former site of the malignancy. Any mention of extension, invasion, or metastasis to another site is coded as a secondary malignant neoplasm to that site. The secondary site may be the principal or first-listed with the V10 code used as a secondary code.

e. **Admissions/Encounters involving chemotherapy, immunotherapy and radiation therapy**

   1) **Episode of care involves surgical removal of neoplasm**

   When an episode of care involves the surgical removal of a neoplasm, primary or secondary site, followed by adjunct chemotherapy or radiation treatment during the same episode of care, the neoplasm code should be assigned as principal or first-listed diagnosis, using codes in the 140-198 series or where appropriate in the 200-203 series.

   2) **Patient admission/encounter solely for administration of chemotherapy, immunotherapy and radiation therapy**

   If a patient admission/encounter is solely for the administration of chemotherapy, immunotherapy or radiation therapy assign code V58.0, Encounter for radiation therapy, or V58.11, Encounter for antineoplastic chemotherapy, or V58.12, Encounter for antineoplastic immunotherapy as the first-listed or principal diagnosis. If a patient receives more than one of these therapies during the same admission more than one of these codes may be assigned, in any sequence.

   The malignancy for which the therapy is being administered should be assigned as a secondary diagnosis.

   3) **Patient admitted for radiotherapy/chemotherapy and immunotherapy and develops complications**

   When a patient is admitted for the purpose of radiotherapy, immunotherapy or chemotherapy and develops complications such as uncontrolled nausea and vomiting or dehydration, the principal or first-listed diagnosis is V58.0, Encounter for radiotherapy, or V58.11, Encounter for antineoplastic chemotherapy, or V58.12, Encounter for antineoplastic immunotherapy followed by any codes for the complications.

f. **Admission/encounter to determine extent of malignancy**

   When the reason for admission/encounter is to determine the extent of the malignancy, or for a procedure such as paracentesis or thoracentesis, the primary malignancy or appropriate metastatic site is designated as the principal or first-listed diagnosis, even though chemotherapy or radiotherapy is administered.

g. **Symptoms, signs, and ill-defined conditions listed in Chapter 16 associated with neoplasms**

   Symptoms, signs, and ill-defined conditions listed in Chapter 16 characteristic of, or associated with, an existing primary or secondary site malignancy cannot be used to replace the malignancy as principal or first-listed diagnosis, regardless of the number of admissions or encounters for treatment and care of the neoplasm.

   See section I.C.18.d.14, Encounter for prophylactic organ removal.

h. **Admission/encounter for pain control/management**

   See Section I.C.6.a.5 for information on coding admission/encounter for pain control/management.

i. **Malignant neoplasm associated with transplanted organ**

   A malignant neoplasm of a transplanted organ should be coded as a transplant complication. Assign first the appropriate code from subcategory 996.8, Complications of transplanted organ, followed by code 199.2, Malignant neoplasm associated with transplanted organ. Use an additional code for the specific malignancy.

3. **Chapter 3: Endocrine, Nutritional, and Metabolic Diseases and Immunity Disorders (240-279)**

a. **Diabetes mellitus**

Codes under category 250, Diabetes mellitus, identify complications/manifestations associated with diabetes mellitus. A fifth-digit is required for all category 250 codes to identify the type of diabetes mellitus and whether the diabetes is controlled or uncontrolled.

See I.C.3.a.7 for secondary diabetes

1) **Fifth-digits for category 250:**

The following are the fifth-digits for the codes under category 250:

0   type II or unspecified type, not stated as uncontrolled

1   type I, [juvenile type], not stated as uncontrolled

2   type II or unspecified type, uncontrolled

3   type I, [juvenile type], uncontrolled

The age of a patient is not the sole determining factor, though most type I diabetics develop the condition before reaching puberty. For this reason type I diabetes mellitus is also referred to as juvenile diabetes.

2) **Type of diabetes mellitus not documented**

If the type of diabetes mellitus is not documented in the medical record the default is type II.

3) **Diabetes mellitus and the use of insulin**

All type I diabetics must use insulin to replace what their bodies do not produce. However, the use of insulin does not mean that a patient is a type I diabetic. Some patients with type II diabetes mellitus are unable to control their blood sugar through diet and oral medication alone and do require insulin. If the documentation in a medical record does not indicate the type of diabetes but does indicate that the patient uses insulin, the appropriate fifth-digit for type II must be used. For type II patients who routinely use insulin, code V58.67, Long-term (current) use of insulin, should also be assigned to indicate that the patient uses insulin. Code V58.67 should not be assigned if insulin is given temporarily to bring a type II patient's blood sugar under control during an encounter.

4) **Assigning and sequencing diabetes codes and associated conditions**

When assigning codes for diabetes and its associated conditions, the code(s) from category 250 must be sequenced before the codes for the associated conditions. The diabetes codes and the secondary codes that correspond to them are paired codes that follow the etiology/manifestation convention of the classification *(See Section I.A.6., Etiology/manifestation convention)*. Assign as many codes from category 250 as needed to identify all of the associated conditions that the patient has. The corresponding secondary codes are listed under each of the diabetes codes.

(a) **Diabetic retinopathy/diabetic macular edema**

Diabetic macular edema, code 362.07, is only present with diabetic retinopathy. Another code from subcategory 362.0, Diabetic retinopathy, must be used with code 362.07. Codes under subcategory 362.0 are diabetes manifestation codes, so they must be used following the appropriate diabetes code.

5) Diabetes mellitus in pregnancy and gestational diabetes

(a) For diabetes mellitus complicating pregnancy, see Section I.C.11.f., Diabetes mellitus in pregnancy.

(b) For gestational diabetes, see Section I.C.11, g., Gestational diabetes.

6) Insulin pump malfunction

(a) Underdose of insulin due insulin pump failure

An underdose of insulin due to an insulin pump failure should be assigned 996.57, Mechanical complication due to insulin pump, as the principal or first listed code, followed by the appropriate diabetes mellitus code based on documentation.

(b) Overdose of insulin due to insulin pump failure

The principal or first listed code for an encounter due to an insulin pump malfunction resulting in an overdose of insulin, should also be 996.57, Mechanical complication due to insulin pump, followed by code 962.3, Poisoning by insulins and antidiabetic agents, and the appropriate diabetes mellitus code based on documentation.

7) Secondary Diabetes Mellitus

Codes under category 249, Secondary diabetes mellitus, identify complications/manifestations associated with secondary diabetes mellitus. Secondary diabetes is always caused by another condition or event (e.g., cystic fibrosis, malignant neoplasm of pancreas, pancreatectomy, adverse effect of drug, or poisoning).

(a) Fifth-digits for category 249:

A fifth-digit is required for all category 249 codes to identify whether the diabetes is controlled or uncontrolled.

(b) Secondary diabetes mellitus and the use of insulin

For patients who routinely use insulin, code V58.67, Long-term (current) use of insulin, should also be assigned. Code V58.67 should not be assigned if insulin is given temporarily to bring a patient's blood sugar under control during an encounter.

(c) Assigning and sequencing secondary diabetes codes and associated conditions

When assigning codes for secondary diabetes and its associated conditions (e.g. renal manifestations), the code(s) from category 249 must be sequenced before the codes for the associated conditions. The secondary diabetes codes and the diabetic manifestation codes that correspond to them are paired codes that follow the etiology/manifestation convention of the classification. Assign as many codes from category 249 as needed to identify all of the associated conditions that the patient has. The corresponding codes for the associated conditions are listed under each of the secondary diabetes codes. For example, secondary diabetes with diabetic nephrosis is assigned to code 249.40, followed by 581.81.

(d) **Assigning and sequencing secondary diabetes codes and its causes**

The sequencing of the secondary diabetes codes in relationship to codes for the cause of the diabetes is based on the reason for the encounter, applicable ICD-9-CM sequencing conventions, and chapter-specific guidelines.

If a patient is seen for treatment of the secondary diabetes or one of its associated conditions, a code from category 249 is sequenced as the principal or first-listed diagnosis, with the cause of the secondary diabetes (e.g. cystic fibrosis) sequenced as an additional diagnosis.

If, however, the patient is seen for the treatment of the condition causing the secondary diabetes (e.g., malignant neoplasm of pancreas), the code for the cause of the secondary diabetes should be sequenced as the principal or first-listed diagnosis followed by a code from category 249.

(i) **Secondary diabetes mellitus due to pancreatectomy**

For postpancreatectomy diabetes mellitus (lack of insulin due to the surgical removal of all or part of the pancreas), assign code 251.3, Postsurgical hypoinsulinemia. A code from subcategory 249 should not be assigned for secondary diabetes mellitus due to pancreatectomy. Code also any diabetic manifestations (e.g. diabetic nephrosis 581.81).

(ii) **Secondary diabetes due to drugs**

Secondary diabetes may be caused by an adverse effect of correctly administered medications, poisoning or late effect of poisoning.

See section I.C.17.e for coding of adverse effects and poisoning, and section I.C.19 for E code reporting.

4. Chapter 4: Diseases of Blood and Blood Forming Organs (280-289)

a. **Anemia of chronic disease**

Subcategory 285.2, Anemia in chronic illness, has codes for anemia in chronic kidney disease, code 285.21; anemia in neoplastic disease, code 285.22; and anemia in other chronic illness, code 285.29. These codes can be used as the principal/first listed code if the reason for the encounter is to treat the anemia. They may also be used as secondary codes if treatment of the anemia is a component of an encounter, but not the primary reason for the encounter. When using a code from subcategory 285 it is also necessary to use the code for the chronic condition causing the anemia.

1) **Anemia in chronic kidney disease**

When assigning code 285.21, Anemia in chronic kidney disease, it is also necessary to assign a code from category 585, Chronic kidney disease, to indicate the stage of chronic kidney disease.

See I.C.10.a. Chronic kidney disease (CKD).

2) **Anemia in neoplastic disease**

When assigning code 285.22, Anemia in neoplastic disease, it is also necessary to assign the neoplasm code that is responsible for the anemia. Code 285.22 is for use for anemia that is due to the malignancy, not for anemia due to antineoplastic chemotherapy drugs, which is an adverse effect.

See I.C.2.c.1 Anemia associated with malignancy.

See I.C.2.c.2 Anemia associated with chemotherapy, immunotherapy and radiation therapy.

See I.C.17.e.1. Adverse effects.

5. **Chapter 5: Mental Disorders (290-319)**

    Reserved for future guideline expansion

6. **Chapter 6: Diseases of Nervous System and Sense Organs (320-389)**

    a. **Pain - Category 338**

    1) **General coding information**

        Codes in category 338 may be used in conjunction with codes from other categories and chapters to provide more detail about acute or chronic pain and neoplasm-related pain, unless otherwise indicated below.

        If the pain is not specified as acute or chronic, do not assign codes from category 338, except for post-thoracotomy pain, postoperative pain, neoplasm related pain, or central pain syndrome.

        A code from subcategories 338.1 and 338.2 should not be assigned if the underlying (definitive) diagnosis is known, unless the reason for the encounter is pain control/ management and not management of the underlying condition.

        (a) **Category 338 Codes as Principal or First-Listed Diagnosis**

        Category 338 codes are acceptable as principal diagnosis or the first-listed code:

        - When pain control or pain management is the reason for the admission/encounter (e.g., a patient with displaced intervertebral disc, nerve impingement and severe back pain presents for injection of steroid into the spinal canal). The underlying cause of the pain should be reported as an additional diagnosis, if known.

        - When an admission or encounter is for a procedure aimed at treating the underlying condition (e.g., spinal fusion, kyphoplasty), a code for the underlying condition (e.g., vertebral fracture, spinal stenosis) should be assigned as the principal diagnosis. No code from category 338 should be assigned.

        - When a patient is admitted for the insertion of a neurostimulator for pain control, assign the appropriate pain code as the principal or first listed diagnosis. When an admission or encounter is for a procedure aimed at treating the underlying condition and a neurostimulator is inserted for pain control during the same admission/encounter, a code for the underlying condition should be assigned as the principal diagnosis and the appropriate pain code should be assigned as a secondary diagnosis.

        (b) **Use of Category 338 Codes in Conjunction with Site Specific Pain Codes**

        (i) **Assigning Category 338 Codes and Site-Specific Pain Codes**

            Codes from category 338 may be used in conjunction with codes that identify the site of pain (including codes from chapter 16) if the category 338 code provides additional information. For example, if the code describes the site of the pain, but does not fully describe whether the pain is acute or chronic, then both codes should be assigned.

(ii) **Sequencing of Category 338 Codes with Site-Specific Pain Codes**

The sequencing of category 338 codes with site-specific pain codes (including chapter 16 codes), is dependent on the circumstances of the encounter/admission as follows:

- If the encounter is for pain control or pain management, assign the code from category 338 followed by the code identifying the specific site of pain (e.g., encounter for pain management for acute neck pain from trauma is assigned code 338.11, Acute pain due to trauma, followed by code 723.1, Cervicalgia, to identify the site of pain).

- If the encounter is for any other reason except pain control or pain management, and a related definitive diagnosis has not been established (confirmed) by the provider, assign the code for the specific site of pain first, followed by the appropriate code from category 338.

2) **Pain due to devices, implants and grafts**

Pain associated with devices, implants or grafts left in a surgical site (for example painful hip prosthesis) is assigned to the appropriate code(s) found in Chapter 17, Injury and Poisoning. Use additional code(s) from category 338 to identify acute or chronic pain due to presence of the device, implant or graft (338.18-338.19 or 338.28-338.29).

3) **Postoperative Pain**

Post-thoracotomy pain and other postoperative pain are classified to subcategories 338.1 and 338.2, depending on whether the pain is acute or chronic. The default for post-thoracotomy and other postoperative pain not specified as acute or chronic is the code for the acute form.

Routine or expected postoperative pain immediately after surgery should not be coded.

(a) **Postoperative pain not associated with specific postoperative complication**

Postoperative pain not associated with a specific postoperative complication is assigned to the appropriate postoperative pain code in category 338.

(b) **Postoperative pain associated with specific postoperative complication**

Postoperative pain associated with a specific postoperative complication (such as painful wire sutures) is assigned to the appropriate code(s) found in Chapter 17, Injury and Poisoning. If appropriate, use additional code(s) from category 338 to identify acute or chronic pain (338.18 or 338.28). If pain control/management is the reason for the encounter, a code from category 338 should be assigned as the principal or first-listed diagnosis in accordance with *Section I.C.6.a.1.a above*.

(c) **Postoperative pain as principal or first-listed diagnosis**

Postoperative pain may be reported as the principal or first-listed diagnosis when the stated reason for the admission/encounter is documented as postoperative pain control/management.

(d) Postoperative pain as secondary diagnosis

Postoperative pain may be reported as a secondary diagnosis code when a patient presents for outpatient surgery and develops an unusual or inordinate amount of postoperative pain.

The provider's documentation should be used to guide the coding of postoperative pain, as well as *Section III. Reporting Additional Diagnoses* and *Section IV. Diagnostic Coding and Reporting in the Outpatient Setting.*

See Section II.I.2 for information on sequencing of diagnoses for patients admitted to hospital inpatient care following post-operative observation.

See Section II.J for information on sequencing of diagnoses for patients admitted to hospital inpatient care from outpatient surgery.

See Section IV.A.2 for information on sequencing of diagnoses for patients admitted for observation.

4) Chronic pain

Chronic pain is classified to subcategory 338.2. There is no time frame defining when pain becomes chronic pain. The provider's documentation should be used to guide use of these codes.

5) Neoplasm Related Pain

Code 338.3 is assigned to pain documented as being related, associated or due to cancer, primary or secondary malignancy, or tumor. This code is assigned regardless of whether the pain is acute or chronic.

This code may be assigned as the principal or first-listed code when the stated reason for the admission/encounter is documented as pain control/pain management. The underlying neoplasm should be reported as an additional diagnosis.

When the reason for the admission/encounter is management of the neoplasm and the pain associated with the neoplasm is also documented, code 338.3 may be assigned as an additional diagnosis.

See Section I.C.2 for instructions on the sequencing of neoplasms for all other stated reasons for the admission/encounter (except for pain control/ pain management).

6) Chronic pain syndrome

This condition is different than the term "chronic pain," and therefore this code should only be used when the provider has specifically documented this condition.

7. Chapter 7: Diseases of Circulatory System (390-459)

a. Hypertension

Hypertension Table

The Hypertension Table, found under the main term, "Hypertension", in the Alphabetic Index, contains a complete listing of all conditions due to or associated with hypertension and classifies them according to malignant, benign, and unspecified.

1) Hypertension, Essential, or NOS

Assign hypertension (arterial) (essential) (primary) (systemic) (NOS) to category code 401 with the appropriate fourth digit to indicate malignant (.0), benign (.1), or unspecified (.9). Do not use either .0 malignant or .1 benign unless medical record documentation supports such a designation.

2) **Hypertension with Heart Disease**

Heart conditions (425.8, 429.0-429.3, 429.8, 429.9) are assigned to a code from category 402 when a causal relationship is stated (due to hypertension) or implied (hypertensive). Use an additional code from category 428 to identify the type of heart failure in those patients with heart failure. More than one code from category 428 may be assigned if the patient has systolic or diastolic failure and congestive heart failure.

The same heart conditions (425.8, 429.0-429.3, 429.8, 429.9) with hypertension, but without a stated causal relationship, are coded separately. Sequence according to the circumstances of the admission/encounter.

3) **Hypertensive Chronic Kidney Disease**

Assign codes from category 403, Hypertensive chronic kidney disease, when conditions classified to category 585 are present. Unlike hypertension with heart disease, ICD-9-CM presumes a cause-and-effect relationship and classifies chronic kidney disease (CKD) with hypertension as hypertensive chronic kidney disease.

Fifth digits for category 403 should be assigned as follows:

- 0 with CKD stage I through stage IV, or unspecified.
- 1 with CKD stage V or end stage renal disease.

The appropriate code from category 585, Chronic kidney disease, should be used as a secondary code with a code from category 403 to identify the stage of chronic kidney disease.

See Section I.C.10.a for information on the coding of chronic kidney disease.

4) **Hypertensive Heart and Chronic Kidney Disease**

Assign codes from combination category 404, Hypertensive heart and chronic kidney disease, when both hypertensive kidney disease and hypertensive heart disease are stated in the diagnosis. Assume a relationship between the hypertension and the chronic kidney disease, whether or not the condition is so designated. Assign an additional code from category 428, to identify the type of heart failure. More than one code from category 428 may be assigned if the patient has systolic or diastolic failure and congestive heart failure.

Fifth digits for category 404 should be assigned as follows:

- 0 without heart failure and with chronic kidney disease (CKD) stage I through stage IV, or unspecified
- 1 with heart failure and with CKD stage I through stage IV, or unspecified
- 2 without heart failure and with CKD stage V or end stage renal disease
- 3 with heart failure and with CKD stage V or end stage renal disease

The appropriate code from category 585, Chronic kidney disease, should be used as a secondary code with a code from category 404 to identify the stage of kidney disease.

See Section I.C.10.a for information on the coding of chronic kidney disease.

5) **Hypertensive Cerebrovascular Disease**

First assign codes from 430-438, Cerebrovascular disease, then the appropriate hypertension code from categories 401-405.

6) **Hypertensive Retinopathy**

Two codes are necessary to identify the condition. First assign the code from subcategory 362.11, Hypertensive retinopathy, then the appropriate code from categories 401-405 to indicate the type of hypertension.

7) **Hypertension, Secondary**

Two codes are required: one to identify the underlying etiology and one from category 405 to identify the hypertension. Sequencing of codes is determined by the reason for admission/ encounter.

8) **Hypertension, Transient**

Assign code 796.2, Elevated blood pressure reading without diagnosis of hypertension, unless patient has an established diagnosis of hypertension. Assign code 642.3x for transient hypertension of pregnancy.

9) **Hypertension, Controlled**

Assign appropriate code from categories 401-405. This diagnostic statement usually refers to an existing state of hypertension under control by therapy.

10) **Hypertension, Uncontrolled**

Uncontrolled hypertension may refer to untreated hypertension or hypertension not responding to current therapeutic regimen. In either case, assign the appropriate code from categories 401-405 to designate the stage and type of hypertension. Code to the type of hypertension.

11) **Elevated Blood Pressure**

For a statement of elevated blood pressure without further specificity, assign code 796.2, Elevated blood pressure reading without diagnosis of hypertension, rather than a code from category 401.

b. **Cerebral infarction/stroke/cerebrovascular accident (CVA)**

The terms stroke and CVA are often used interchangeably to refer to a cerebral infarction. The terms stroke, CVA, and cerebral infarction NOS are all indexed to the default code 434.91, Cerebral artery occlusion, unspecified, with infarction. Code 436, Acute, but ill-defined, cerebrovascular disease, should not be used when the documentation states stroke or CVA.

See Section I.C.18.d.3 for information on coding status post administration of tPA in a different facility within the last 24 hours.

c. **Postoperative cerebrovascular accident**

A cerebrovascular hemorrhage or infarction that occurs as a result of medical intervention is coded to 997.02, Iatrogenic cerebrovascular infarction or hemorrhage. Medical record documentation should clearly specify the cause- and-effect relationship between the medical intervention and the cerebrovascular accident in order to assign this code. A secondary code from the code range 430-432 or from a code from subcategories 433 or 434 with a fifth digit of "1" should also be used to identify the type of hemorrhage or infarct.

This guideline conforms to the use additional code note instruction at category 997. Code 436, Acute, but ill-defined, cerebrovascular disease, should not be used as a secondary code with code 997.02.

d. Late Effects of Cerebrovascular Disease

1) Category 438, Late Effects of Cerebrovascular disease

Category 438 is used to indicate conditions classifiable to categories 430-437 as the causes of late effects (neurologic deficits), themselves classified elsewhere. These "late effects" include neurologic deficits that persist after initial onset of conditions classifiable to 430-437. The neurologic deficits caused by cerebrovascular disease may be present from the onset or may arise at any time after the onset of the condition classifiable to 430-437.

2) Codes from category 438 with codes from 430-437

Codes from category 438 may be assigned on a health care record with codes from 430-437, if the patient has a current cerebrovascular accident (CVA) and deficits from an old CVA.

3) Code V12.54

Assign code V12.54, Transient ischemic attack (TIA), and cerebral infarction without residual deficits (and not a code from category 438) as an additional code for history of cerebrovascular disease when no neurologic deficits are present.

e. Acute myocardial infarction (AMI)

1) ST elevation myocardial infarction (STEMI) and non ST elevation myocardial infarction (NSTEMI)

The ICD-9-CM codes for acute myocardial infarction (AMI) identify the site, such as anterolateral wall or true posterior wall. Subcategories 410.0-410.6 and 410.8 are used for ST elevation myocardial infarction (STEMI). Subcategory 410.7, Subendocardial infarction, is used for non ST elevation myocardial infarction (NSTEMI) and nontransmural MIs.

2) Acute myocardial infarction, unspecified

Subcategory 410.9 is the default for the unspecified term acute myocardial infarction. If only STEMI or transmural MI without the site is documented, query the provider as to the site, or assign a code from subcategory 410.9.

3) AMI documented as nontransmural or subendocardial but site provided

If an AMI is documented as nontransmural or subendocardial, but the site is provided, it is still coded as a subendocardial AMI. If NSTEMI evolves to STEMI, assign the STEMI code. If STEMI converts to NSTEMI due to thrombolytic therapy, it is still coded as STEMI.

See Section I.C.18.d.3 for information on coding status post administration of tPA in a different facility within the last 24 hours.

8. Chapter 8: Diseases of Respiratory System (460-519)

See I.C.17.f. for ventilator-associated pneumonia.

a. Chronic Obstructive Pulmonary Disease [COPD] and Asthma

1) Conditions that comprise COPD and Asthma

The conditions that comprise COPD are obstructive chronic bronchitis, subcategory 491.2, and emphysema, category 492. All asthma codes are under category 493, Asthma. Code 496, Chronic airway obstruction, not elsewhere classified, is a nonspecific code that should only be used when the documentation in a medical record does not specify the type of COPD being treated.

2) **Acute exacerbation of chronic obstructive bronchitis and asthma**

The codes for chronic obstructive bronchitis and asthma distinguish between uncomplicated cases and those in acute exacerbation. An acute exacerbation is a worsening or a decompensation of a chronic condition. An acute exacerbation is not equivalent to an infection superimposed on a chronic condition, though an exacerbation may be triggered by an infection.

3) **Overlapping nature of the conditions that comprise COPD and asthma**

Due to the overlapping nature of the conditions that make up COPD and asthma, there are many variations in the way these conditions are documented. Code selection must be based on the terms as documented. When selecting the correct code for the documented type of COPD and asthma, it is essential to first review the index, and then verify the code in the tabular list. There are many instructional notes under the different COPD subcategories and codes. It is important that all such notes be reviewed to assure correct code assignment.

4) **Acute exacerbation of asthma and status asthmaticus**

An acute exacerbation of asthma is an increased severity of the asthma symptoms, such as wheezing and shortness of breath. Status asthmaticus refers to a patient's failure to respond to therapy administered during an asthmatic episode and is a life threatening complication that requires emergency care. If status asthmaticus is documented by the provider with any type of COPD or with acute bronchitis, the status asthmaticus should be sequenced first. It supersedes any type of COPD including that with acute exacerbation or acute bronchitis. It is inappropriate to assign an asthma code with 5th digit 2, with acute exacerbation, together with an asthma code with 5th digit 1, with status asthmatics. Only the 5th digit 1 should be assigned.

b. **Chronic Obstructive Pulmonary Disease [COPD] and Bronchitis**

1) **Acute bronchitis with COPD**

Acute bronchitis, code 466.0, is due to an infectious organism. When acute bronchitis is documented with COPD, code 491.22, Obstructive chronic bronchitis with acute bronchitis, should be assigned. It is not necessary to also assign code 466.0. If a medical record documents acute bronchitis with COPD with acute exacerbation, only code 491.22 should be assigned. The acute bronchitis included in code 491.22 supersedes the acute exacerbation. If a medical record documents COPD with acute exacerbation without mention of acute bronchitis, only code 491.21 should be assigned.

c. **Acute Respiratory Failure**

1) **Acute respiratory failure as principal diagnosis**

Code 518.81, Acute respiratory failure, may be assigned as a principal diagnosis when it is the condition established after study to be chiefly responsible for occasioning the admission to the hospital, and the selection is supported by the Alphabetic Index and Tabular List. However, chapter-specific coding guidelines (such as obstetrics, poisoning, HIV, newborn) that provide sequencing direction take precedence.

2) **Acute respiratory failure as secondary diagnosis**

Respiratory failure may be listed as a secondary diagnosis if it occurs after admission, or if it is present on admission, but does not meet the definition of principal diagnosis.

3) Sequencing of acute respiratory failure and another acute condition

When a patient is admitted with respiratory failure and another acute condition, (e.g., myocardial infarction, cerebrovascular accident, **aspiration pneumonia**), the principal diagnosis will not be the same in every situation. **This applies whether the other acute condition is a respiratory or nonrespiratory condition.** Selection of the principal diagnosis will be dependent on the circumstances of admission. If both the respiratory failure and the other acute condition are equally responsible for occasioning the admission to the hospital, and there are no chapter-specific sequencing rules, the guideline regarding two or more diagnoses that equally meet the definition for principal diagnosis *(Section II, C.)* may be applied in these situations.

If the documentation is not clear as to whether acute respiratory failure and another condition are equally responsible for occasioning the admission, query the provider for clarification.

d. Influenza due to identified avian influenza virus (avian influenza)

Code only confirmed cases of avian influenza. This is an exception to the hospital inpatient guideline Section II, H. (Uncertain Diagnosis).

In this context, "confirmation" does not require documentation of positive laboratory testing specific for avian influenza. However, coding should be based on the provider's diagnostic statement that the patient has avian influenza.

If the provider records "suspected or possible or probable avian influenza," the appropriate influenza code from category 487 should be assigned. Code 488, Influenza due to identified avian influenza virus, should not be assigned.

9. Chapter 9: Diseases of Digestive System (520-579)

Reserved for future guideline expansion

10. Chapter 10: Diseases of Genitourinary System (580-629)

a. Chronic kidney disease

1) Stages of chronic kidney disease (CKD)

The ICD-9-CM classifies CKD based on severity. The severity of CKD is designated by stages I-V. Stage II, code 585.2, equates to mild CKD; stage III, code 585.3, equates to moderate CKD; and stage IV, code 585.4, equates to severe CKD. Code 585.6, End stage renal disease (ESRD), is assigned when the provider has documented end-stage-renal disease (ESRD).

If both a stage of CKD and ESRD are documented, assign code 585.6 only.

2) Chronic kidney disease and kidney transplant status

Patients who have undergone kidney transplant may still have some form of CKD, because the kidney transplant may not fully restore kidney function. Therefore, the presence of CKD alone does not constitute a transplant complication. Assign the appropriate 585 code for the patient's stage of CKD and code V42.0. If a transplant complication such as failure or rejection is documented, see section I.C.17.f.2.b for information on coding complications of a kidney transplant. If the documentation is unclear as to whether the patient has a complication of the transplant, query the provider.

3) Chronic kidney disease with other conditions

Patients with CKD may also suffer from other serious conditions, most commonly diabetes mellitus and hypertension. The sequencing of the CKD code in relationship to codes for other contributing conditions is based on the conventions in the tabular list.

See I.C.3.a.4 for sequencing instructions for diabetes.

See I.C.4.a.1 for anemia in CKD.

See I.C.7.a.3 for hypertensive chronic kidney disease.

See I.C.17.f.2.b, Kidney transplant complications, for instructions on coding of documented rejection or failure.

11. Chapter 11: Complications of Pregnancy, Childbirth, and the Puerperium (630-679)

a. General Rules for Obstetric Cases

1) Codes from chapter 11 and sequencing priority

Obstetric cases require codes from chapter 11, codes in the range 630-679, Complications of Pregnancy, Childbirth, and the Puerperium. Chapter 11 codes have sequencing priority over codes from other chapters. Additional codes from other chapters may be used in conjunction with chapter 11 codes to further specify conditions. Should the provider document that the pregnancy is incidental to the encounter, then code V22.2 should be used in place of any chapter 11 codes. It is the provider's responsibility to state that the condition being treated is not affecting the pregnancy.

2) Chapter 11 codes used only on the maternal record

Chapter 11 codes are to be used only on the maternal record, never on the record of the newborn.

3) Chapter 11 fifth-digits

Categories 640-648, 651-676 have required fifth-digits, which indicate whether the encounter is antepartum, postpartum and whether a delivery has also occurred.

4) Fifth-digits, appropriate for each code

The fifth-digits, which are appropriate for each code number, are listed in brackets under each code. The fifth-digits on each code should all be consistent with each other. That is, should a delivery occur all of the fifth-digits should indicate the delivery.

b. Selection of OB Principal or First-listed Diagnosis

1) Routine outpatient prenatal visits

For routine outpatient prenatal visits when no complications are present codes V22.0, Supervision of normal first pregnancy, and V22.1, Supervision of other normal pregnancy, should be used as the first-listed diagnoses. These codes should not be used in conjunction with chapter 11 codes.

2) Prenatal outpatient visits for high-risk patients

For prenatal outpatient visits for patients with high-risk pregnancies, a code from category V23, Supervision of high-risk pregnancy, should be used as the first-listed diagnosis. Secondary chapter 11 codes may be used in conjunction with these codes if appropriate.

3) Episodes when no delivery occurs

In episodes when no delivery occurs, the principal diagnosis should correspond to the principal complication of the pregnancy, which necessitated the encounter. Should more than one complication exist, all of which are treated or monitored, any of the complications codes may be sequenced first.

4) When a delivery occurs

When a delivery occurs, the principal diagnosis should correspond to the main circumstances or complication of the delivery. In cases of cesarean delivery, the selection of the principal diagnosis should correspond to the reason the cesarean delivery was performed unless the reason for admission/encounter was unrelated to the condition resulting in the cesarean delivery.

5) Outcome of delivery

An outcome of delivery code, V27.0-V27.9, should be included on every maternal record when a delivery has occurred. These codes are not to be used on subsequent records or on the newborn record.

c. Fetal Conditions Affecting the Management of the Mother

1) Codes from category 655

Known or suspected fetal abnormality affecting management of the mother, and category 656, Other fetal and placental problems affecting the management of the mother, are assigned only when the fetal condition is actually responsible for modifying the management of the mother, i.e., by requiring diagnostic studies, additional observation, special care, or termination of pregnancy. The fact that the fetal condition exists does not justify assigning a code from this series to the mother's record.

See I.C.18.d. for suspected maternal and fetal conditions not found

2) In utero surgery

In cases when surgery is performed on the fetus, a diagnosis code from category 655, Known or suspected fetal abnormalities affecting management of the mother, should be assigned identifying the fetal condition. Procedure code 75.36, Correction of fetal defect, should be assigned on the hospital inpatient record.

No code from Chapter 15, the perinatal codes, should be used on the mother's record to identify fetal conditions. Surgery performed in utero on a fetus is still to be coded as an obstetric encounter.

d. HIV Infection in Pregnancy, Childbirth and the Puerperium

During pregnancy, childbirth or the puerperium, a patient admitted because of an HIV-related illness should receive a principal diagnosis of 647.6X, Other specified infectious and parasitic diseases in the mother classifiable elsewhere, but complicating the pregnancy, childbirth or the puerperium, followed by 042 and the code(s) for the HIV-related illness(es).

Patients with asymptomatic HIV infection status admitted during pregnancy, childbirth, or the puerperium should receive codes of 647.6X and V08.

e. Current Conditions Complicating Pregnancy

Assign a code from subcategory 648.x for patients that have current conditions when the condition affects the management of the pregnancy, childbirth, or the puerperium. Use additional secondary codes from other chapters to identify the conditions, as appropriate.

f. Diabetes mellitus in pregnancy

Diabetes mellitus is a significant complicating factor in pregnancy. Pregnant women who are diabetic should be assigned code 648.0x, Diabetes mellitus complicating pregnancy, and a secondary code from category 250, Diabetes mellitus, **or category 249, Secondary diabetes** to identify the type of diabetes.

Code V58.67, Long-term (current) use of insulin, should also be assigned if the diabetes mellitus is being treated with insulin.

g. Gestational diabetes

Gestational diabetes can occur during the second and third trimester of pregnancy in women who were not diabetic prior to pregnancy. Gestational diabetes can cause complications in the pregnancy similar to those of pre-existing diabetes mellitus. It also puts the woman at greater risk of developing diabetes after the pregnancy. Gestational diabetes is coded to 648.8x, Abnormal glucose tolerance. Codes 648.0x and 648.8x should never be used together on the same record.

Code V58.67, Long-term (current) use of insulin, should also be assigned if the gestational diabetes is being treated with insulin.

h. Normal Delivery, Code 650

1) Normal delivery

Code 650 is for use in cases when a woman is admitted for a full-term normal delivery and delivers a single, healthy infant without any complications antepartum, during the delivery, or postpartum during the delivery episode. Code 650 is always a principal diagnosis. It is not to be used if any other code from chapter 11 is needed to describe a current complication of the antenatal, delivery, or perinatal period. Additional codes from other chapters may be used with code 650 if they are not related to or are in any way complicating the pregnancy.

2) Normal delivery with resolved antepartum complication

Code 650 may be used if the patient had a complication at some point during her pregnancy, but the complication is not present at the time of the admission for delivery.

3) V27.0, Single liveborn, outcome of delivery

V27.0, Single liveborn, is the only outcome of delivery code appropriate for use with 650.

i. The Postpartum and Peripartum Periods

1) Postpartum and peripartum periods

The postpartum period begins immediately after delivery and continues for six weeks following delivery. The peripartum period is defined as the last month of pregnancy to five months postpartum.

2) Postpartum complication

A postpartum complication is any complication occurring within the six-week period.

3) Pregnancy-related complications after 6 week period

Chapter 11 codes may also be used to describe pregnancy-related complications after the six-week period should the provider document that a condition is pregnancy related.

4) Postpartum complications occurring during the same admission as delivery

Postpartum complications that occur during the same admission as the delivery are identified with a fifth digit of "2." Subsequent admissions/encounters for postpartum complications should be identified with a fifth digit of "4."

5) **Admission for routine postpartum care following delivery outside hospital**

When the mother delivers outside the hospital prior to admission and is admitted for routine postpartum care and no complications are noted, code V24.0, Postpartum care and examination immediately after delivery, should be assigned as the principal diagnosis.

6) **Admission following delivery outside hospital with postpartum conditions**

A delivery diagnosis code should not be used for a woman who has delivered prior to admission to the hospital. Any postpartum conditions and/or postpartum procedures should be coded.

j. **Code 677, Late effect of complication of pregnancy**

1) **Code 677**

Code 677, Late effect of complication of pregnancy, childbirth, and the puerperium is for use in those cases when an initial complication of a pregnancy develops a sequelae requiring care or treatment at a future date.

2) **After the initial postpartum period**

This code may be used at any time after the initial postpartum period.

3) **Sequencing of Code 677**

This code, like all late effect codes, is to be sequenced following the code describing the sequelae of the complication.

k. **Abortions**

1) **Fifth-digits required for abortion categories**

Fifth-digits are required for abortion categories 634-637. Fifth-digit 1, incomplete, indicates that all of the products of conception have not been expelled from the uterus. Fifth-digit 2, complete, indicates that all products of conception have been expelled from the uterus.

2) **Code from categories 640-648 and 651-659**

A code from categories 640-648 and 651-659 may be used as additional codes with an abortion code to indicate the complication leading to the abortion.

Fifth digit 3 is assigned with codes from these categories when used with an abortion code because the other fifth digits will not apply. Codes from the 660-669 series are not to be used for complications of abortion.

3) **Code 639 for complications**

Code 639 is to be used for all complications following abortion. Code 639 cannot be assigned with codes from categories 634-638.

4) **Abortion with Liveborn Fetus**

When an attempted termination of pregnancy results in a liveborn fetus assign code 644.21, Early onset of delivery, with an appropriate code from category V27, Outcome of Delivery. The procedure code for the attempted termination of pregnancy should also be assigned.

5) **Retained Products of Conception following an abortion**

Subsequent admissions for retained products of conception following a spontaneous or legally induced abortion are assigned the appropriate code from category 634, Spontaneous abortion, or 635 Legally induced abortion, with a fifth digit of "1" (incomplete). This advice is appropriate even when the patient was discharged previously with a discharge diagnosis of complete abortion.

12. **Chapter 12: Diseases Skin and Subcutaneous Tissue (680-709)**
    a. **Pressure ulcer stage codes**
       1) **Pressure ulcer stages**

          Two codes are needed to completely describe a pressure ulcer: A code from subcategory 707.0, Pressure ulcer, to identify the site of the pressure ulcer and a code from subcategory 707.2, Pressure ulcer stages.

          The codes in subcategory 707.2, Pressure ulcer stages, are to be used as an additional diagnosis with a code(s) from subcategory 707.0, Pressure Ulcer. Codes from 707.2, Pressure ulcer stages, may not be assigned as a principal or first-listed diagnosis. The pressure ulcer stage codes should only be used with pressure ulcers and not with other types of ulcers (e.g., stasis ulcer).

          The ICD-9-CM classifies pressure ulcer stages based on severity, which is designated by stages I-IV and unstageable.

       2) **Unstageable pressure ulcers**

          Assignment of code 707.25, Pressure ulcer, unstageable, should be based on the clinical documentation. Code 707.25 is used for pressure ulcers whose stage cannot be clinically determined (e.g., the ulcer is covered by eschar or has been treated with a skin or muscle graft) and pressure ulcers that are documented as deep tissue injury but not documented as due to trauma. This code should not be confused with code 707.20, Pressure ulcer, stage unspecified. Code 707.20 should be assigned when there is no documentation regarding the stage of the pressure ulcer.

       3) **Documented pressure ulcer stage**

          Assignment of the pressure ulcer stage code should be guided by clinical documentation of the stage or documentation of the terms found in the index. For clinical terms describing the stage that are not found in the index, and there is no documentation of the stage, the provider should be queried.

       4) **Bilateral pressure ulcers with same stage**

          When a patient has bilateral pressure ulcers (e.g., both buttocks) and both pressure ulcers are documented as being the same stage, only the code for the site and one code for the stage should be reported.

       5) **Bilateral pressure ulcers with different stages**

          When a patient has bilateral pressure ulcers at the same site (e.g., both buttocks) and each pressure ulcer is documented as being at a different stage, assign one code for the site and the appropriate codes for the pressure ulcer stage.

       6) **Multiple pressure ulcers of different sites and stages**

          When a patient has multiple pressure ulcers at different sites (e.g., buttock, heel, shoulder) and each pressure ulcer is documented as being at different stages (e.g., stage 3 and stage 4), assign the appropriate codes for each different site and a code for each different pressure ulcer stage.

       7) **Patients admitted with pressure ulcers documented as healed**

          No code is assigned if the documentation states that the pressure ulcer is completely healed.

8) **Patients admitted with pressure ulcers documented as healing**

Pressure ulcers described as healing should be assigned the appropriate pressure ulcer stage code based on the documentation in the medical record. If the documentation does not provide information about the stage of the healing pressure ulcer, assign code 707.20, Pressure ulcer stage, unspecified.

If the documentation is unclear as to whether the patient has a current (new) pressure ulcer or if the patient is being treated for a healing pressure ulcer, query the provider.

9) **Patient admitted with pressure ulcer evolving into another stage during the admission**

If a patient is admitted with a pressure ulcer at one stage and it progresses to a higher stage, assign the code for highest stage reported for that site.

13. **Chapter 13: Diseases of Musculoskeletal and Connective Tissue (710-739)**

   a. **Coding of Pathologic Fractures**

      1) **Acute Fractures vs. Aftercare**

         Pathologic fractures are reported using subcategory 733.1, when the fracture is newly diagnosed. Subcategory 733.1 may be used while the patient is receiving active treatment for the fracture. Examples of active treatment are: surgical treatment, emergency department encounter, evaluation and treatment by a new physician.

         Fractures are coded using the aftercare codes (subcategories V54.0, V54.2, V54.8 or V54.9) for encounters after the patient has completed active treatment of the fracture and is receiving routine care for the fracture during the healing or recovery phase. Examples of fracture aftercare are: cast change or removal, removal of external or internal fixation device, medication adjustment, and follow up visits following fracture treatment.

         Care for complications of surgical treatment for fracture repairs during the healing or recovery phase should be coded with the appropriate complication codes.

         Care of complications of fractures, such as malunion and nonunion, should be reported with the appropriate codes.

         See Section I. C. 17.b for information on the coding of traumatic fractures.

14. **Chapter 14: Congenital Anomalies (740-759)**

   a. **Codes in categories 740-759, Congenital Anomalies**

      Assign an appropriate code(s) from categories 740-759, Congenital Anomalies, when an anomaly is documented. A congenital anomaly may be the principal/first listed diagnosis on a record or a secondary diagnosis.

      When a congenital anomaly does not have a unique code assignment, assign additional code(s) for any manifestations that may be present.

      When the code assignment specifically identifies the congenital anomaly, manifestations that are an inherent component of the anomaly should not be coded separately. Additional codes should be assigned for manifestations that are not an inherent component.

      Codes from Chapter 14 may be used throughout the life of the patient. If a congenital anomaly has been corrected, a personal history code should be used to identify the history of the anomaly. Although present at birth, a congenital anomaly may not be identified until later in life. Whenever the condition is diagnosed by the physician, it is appropriate to assign a code from codes 740-759.

      For the birth admission, the appropriate code from category V30, Liveborn infants, according to type of birth should be sequenced as the principal diagnosis, followed by any congenital anomaly codes, 740-759.

15. Chapter 15: Newborn (Perinatal) Guidelines (760-779)

For coding and reporting purposes the perinatal period is defined as before birth through the 28th day following birth. The following guidelines are provided for reporting purposes. Hospitals may record other diagnoses as needed for internal data use.

a. General Perinatal Rules

1) Chapter 15 Codes

They are <u>never</u> for use on the maternal record. Codes from Chapter 11, the obstetric chapter, are never permitted on the newborn record. Chapter 15 code may be used throughout the life of the patient if the condition is still present.

2) Sequencing of perinatal codes

Generally, codes from Chapter 15 should be sequenced as the principal/first-listed diagnosis on the newborn record, with the exception of the appropriate V30 code for the birth episode, followed by codes from any other chapter that provide additional detail. The "use additional code" note at the beginning of the chapter supports this guideline. If the index does not provide a specific code for a perinatal condition, assign code 779.89, Other specified conditions originating in the perinatal period, followed by the code from another chapter that specifies the condition. Codes for signs and symptoms may be assigned when a definitive diagnosis has not been established.

3) Birth process or community acquired conditions

If a newborn has a condition that may be either due to the birth process or community acquired and the documentation does not indicate which it is, the default is due to the birth process and the code from Chapter 15 should be used. If the condition is community-acquired, a code from Chapter 15 should not be assigned.

4) Code all clinically significant conditions

All clinically significant conditions noted on routine newborn examination should be coded. A condition is clinically significant if it requires:

- clinical evaluation; or
- therapeutic treatment; or
- diagnostic procedures; or
- extended length of hospital stay; or
- increased nursing care and/or monitoring; or
- has implications for future health care needs

Note: The perinatal guidelines listed above are the same as the general coding guidelines for "additional diagnoses", except for the final point regarding implications for future health care needs. Codes should be assigned for conditions that have been specified by the provider as having implications for future health care needs. Codes from the perinatal chapter should not be assigned unless the provider has established a definitive diagnosis.

b. Use of codes V30-V39

When coding the birth of an infant, assign a code from categories V30-V39, according to the type of birth. A code from this series is assigned as a principal diagnosis, and assigned only once to a newborn at the time of birth.

c. Newborn transfers

If the newborn is transferred to another institution, the V30 series is not used at the receiving hospital.

d. **Use of category V29**

1) **Assigning a code from category V29**

Assign a code from category V29, Observation and evaluation of newborns and infants for suspected conditions not found, to identify those instances when a healthy newborn is evaluated for a suspected condition that is determined after study not to be present. Do not use a code from category V29 when the patient has identified signs or symptoms of a suspected problem; in such cases, code the sign or symptom.

A code from category V29 may also be assigned as a principal code for readmissions or encounters when the V30 code no longer applies. Codes from category V29 are for use only for healthy newborns and infants for which no condition after study is found to be present.

2) **V29 code on a birth record**

A V29 code is to be used as a secondary code after the V30, Outcome of delivery, code.

e. **Use of other V codes on perinatal records**

V codes other than V30 and V29 may be assigned on a perinatal or newborn record code. The codes may be used as a principal or first-listed diagnosis for specific types of encounters or for readmissions or encounters when the V30 code no longer applies.

See Section I.C.18 for information regarding the assignment of V codes.

f. **Maternal Causes of Perinatal Morbidity**

Codes from categories 760-763, Maternal causes of perinatal morbidity and mortality, are assigned only when the maternal condition has actually affected the fetus or newborn. The fact that the mother has an associated medical condition or experiences some complication of pregnancy, labor or delivery does not justify the routine assignment of codes from these categories to the newborn record.

g. **Congenital Anomalies in Newborns**

For the birth admission, the appropriate code from category V30, Liveborn infants according to type of birth, should be used, followed by any congenital anomaly codes, categories 740-759. Use additional secondary codes from other chapters to specify conditions associated with the anomaly, if applicable.

Also, see Section I.C.14 for information on the coding of congenital anomalies.

h. **Coding Additional Perinatal Diagnoses**

1) **Assigning codes for conditions that require treatment**

Assign codes for conditions that require treatment or further investigation, prolong the length of stay, or require resource utilization.

2) **Codes for conditions specified as having implications for future health care needs**

Assign codes for conditions that have been specified by the provider as having implications for future health care needs.

Note: This guideline should not be used for adult patients.

3) **Codes for newborn conditions originating in the perinatal period**

Assign a code for newborn conditions originating in the perinatal period (categories 760-779), as well as complications arising during the current episode of care classified in other chapters, only if the diagnoses have been documented by the responsible provider at the time of transfer or discharge as having affected the fetus or newborn.

i. **Prematurity and Fetal Growth Retardation**

Providers utilize different criteria in determining prematurity. A code for prematurity should not be assigned unless it is documented. The 5th digit assignment for codes from category 764 and subcategories 765.0 and 765.1 should be based on the recorded birth weight and estimated gestational age.

A code from subcategory 765.2, Weeks of gestation, should be assigned as an additional code with category 764 and codes from 765.0 and 765.1 to specify weeks of gestation as documented by the provider in the record.

j. **Newborn sepsis**

Code 771.81, Septicemia [sepsis] of newborn, should be assigned with a secondary code from category 041, Bacterial infections in conditions classified elsewhere and of unspecified site, to identify the organism. A code from category 038, Septicemia, should not be used on a newborn record. **Do not assign code 995.91, Sepsis, as c**ode 771.81 describes the sepsis. **If applicable, use additional codes to identify severe sepsis (995.92) and any associated acute organ dysfunction.**

16. **Chapter 16: Signs, Symptoms and Ill-Defined Conditions (780-799)**

Reserved for future guideline expansion

17. **Chapter 17: Injury and Poisoning (800-999)**

a. **Coding of Injuries**

When coding injuries, assign separate codes for each injury unless a combination code is provided, in which case the combination code is assigned. Multiple injury codes are provided in ICD-9-CM, but should not be assigned unless information for a more specific code is not available. These codes are not to be used for normal, healing surgical wounds or to identify complications of surgical wounds.

The code for the most serious injury, as determined by the provider and the focus of treatment, is sequenced first.

1) **Superficial injuries**

Superficial injuries such as abrasions or contusions are not coded when associated with more severe injuries of the same site.

2) **Primary injury with damage to nerves/blood vessels**

When a primary injury results in minor damage to peripheral nerves or blood vessels, the primary injury is sequenced first with additional code(s) from categories 950-957, Injury to nerves and spinal cord, and/or 900-904, Injury to blood vessels. When the primary injury is to the blood vessels or nerves, that injury should be sequenced first.

b. Coding of Traumatic Fractures

The principles of multiple coding of injuries should be followed in coding fractures. Fractures of specified sites are coded individually by site in accordance with both the provisions within categories 800-829 and the level of detail furnished by medical record content. Combination categories for multiple fractures are provided for use when there is insufficient detail in the medical record (such as trauma cases transferred to another hospital), when the reporting form limits the number of codes that can be used in reporting pertinent clinical data, or when there is insufficient specificity at the fourth-digit or fifth-digit level. More specific guidelines are as follows:

1) Acute Fractures vs. Aftercare

Traumatic fractures are coded using the acute fracture codes (800-829) while the patient is receiving active treatment for the fracture. Examples of active treatment are: surgical treatment, emergency department encounter, and evaluation and treatment by a new physician.

Fractures are coded using the aftercare codes (subcategories V54.0, V54.1, V54.8, or V54.9) for encounters after the patient has completed active treatment of the fracture and is receiving routine care for the fracture during the healing or recovery phase. Examples of fracture aftercare are: cast change or removal, removal of external or internal fixation device, medication adjustment, and follow up visits following fracture treatment.

Care for complications of surgical treatment for fracture repairs during the healing or recovery phase should be coded with the appropriate complication codes.

Care of complications of fractures, such as malunion and nonunion, should be reported with the appropriate codes.

Pathologic fractures are not coded in the 800-829 range, but instead are assigned to subcategory 733.1. *See Section I.C.13.a for additional information.*

2) Multiple fractures of same limb

Multiple fractures of same limb classifiable to the same three-digit or four-digit category are coded to that category.

3) Multiple unilateral or bilateral fractures of same bone

Multiple unilateral or bilateral fractures of same bone(s) but classified to different fourth-digit subdivisions (bone part) within the same three-digit category are coded individually by site.

4) Multiple fracture categories 819 and 828

Multiple fracture categories 819 and 828 classify bilateral fractures of both upper limbs (819) and both lower limbs (828), but without any detail at the fourth-digit level other than open and closed type of fractures.

5) Multiple fractures sequencing

Multiple fractures are sequenced in accordance with the severity of the fracture. The provider should be asked to list the fracture diagnoses in the order of severity.

c. Coding of Burns

Current burns (940-948) are classified by depth, extent and by agent (E code). Burns are classified by depth as first degree (erythema), second degree (blistering), and third degree (full-thickness involvement).

1) Sequencing of burn and related condition codes

Sequence first the code that reflects the highest degree of burn when more than one burn is present.

a. When the reason for the admission or encounter is for treatment of external multiple burns, sequence first the code that reflects the burn of the highest degree.

b. When a patient has both internal and external burns, the circumstances of admission govern the selection of the principal diagnosis or first-listed diagnosis.

c. When a patient is admitted for burn injuries and other related conditions such as smoke inhalation and/or respiratory failure, the circumstances of admission govern the selection of the principal or first-listed diagnosis.

2) Burns of the same local site

Classify burns of the same local site (three-digit category level, 940-947) but of different degrees to the subcategory identifying the highest degree recorded in the diagnosis.

3) Non-healing burns

Non-healing burns are coded as acute burns.

Necrosis of burned skin should be coded as a non-healed burn.

4) Code 958.3, Posttraumatic wound infection

Assign code 958.3, Posttraumatic wound infection, not elsewhere classified, as an additional code for any documented infected burn site.

5) Assign separate codes for each burn site

When coding burns, assign separate codes for each burn site. Category 946 Burns of Multiple specified sites, should only be used if the location of the burns are not documented. Category 949, Burn, unspecified, is extremely vague and should rarely be used.

6) **Assign codes from category 948, Burns**

Burns classified according to extent of body surface involved, when the site of the burn is not specified or when there is a need for additional data. It is advisable to use category 948 as additional coding when needed to provide data for evaluating burn mortality, such as that needed by burn units. It is also advisable to use category 948 as an additional code for reporting purposes when there is mention of a third-degree burn involving 20 percent or more of the body surface.

In assigning a code from category 948:

Fourth-digit codes are used to identify the percentage of total body surface involved in a burn (all degree).

Fifth-digits are assigned to identify the percentage of body surface involved in third-degree burn.

Fifth-digit zero (0) is assigned when less than 10 percent or when no body surface is involved in a third-degree burn.

Category 948 is based on the classic "rule of nines" in estimating body surface involved: head and neck are assigned nine percent, each arm nine percent, each leg 18 percent, the anterior trunk 18 percent, posterior trunk 18 percent, and genitalia one percent. Providers may change these percentage assignments where necessary to accommodate infants and children who have proportionately larger heads than adults and patients who have large buttocks, thighs, or abdomen that involve burns.

7) **Encounters for treatment of late effects of burns**

Encounters for the treatment of the late effects of burns (i.e., scars or joint contractures) should be coded to the residual condition (sequelae) followed by the appropriate late effect code (906.5-906.9). A late effect E code may also be used, if desired.

8) **Sequelae with a late effect code and current burn**

When appropriate, both a sequelae with a late effect code, and a current burn code may be assigned on the same record (when both a current burn and sequelae of an old burn exist).

d. **Coding of Debridement of Wound, Infection, or Burn**

Excisional debridement involves surgical removal or cutting away, as opposed to a mechanical (brushing, scrubbing, washing) debridement.

For coding purposes, excisional debridement is assigned to code 86.22.

Nonexcisional debridement is assigned to code 86.28.

e. **Adverse Effects, Poisoning and Toxic Effects**

The properties of certain drugs, medicinal and biological substances or combinations of such substances, may cause toxic reactions. The occurrence of drug toxicity is classified in ICD-9-CM as follows:

1) **Adverse Effect**

When the drug was correctly prescribed and properly administered, code the reaction plus the appropriate code from the E930-E949 series. Codes from the E930-E949 series must be used to identify the causative substance for an adverse effect of drug, medicinal and biological substances, correctly prescribed and properly administered. The effect, such as tachycardia, delirium, gastrointestinal hemorrhaging, vomiting, hypokalemia, hepatitis, renal failure, or respiratory failure, is coded and followed by the appropriate code from the E930-E949 series.

Adverse effects of therapeutic substances correctly prescribed and properly administered (toxicity, synergistic reaction, side effect, and idiosyncratic reaction) may be due to (1) differences among patients, such as age, sex, disease, and genetic factors, and (2) drug-related factors, such as type of drug, route of administration, duration of therapy, dosage, and bioavailability.

2) **Poisoning**

(a) **Error was made in drug prescription**

Errors made in drug prescription or in the administration of the drug by provider, nurse, patient, or other person, use the appropriate poisoning code from the 960-979 series.

(b) **Overdose of a drug intentionally taken**

If an overdose of a drug was intentionally taken or administered and resulted in drug toxicity, it would be coded as a poisoning (960-979 series).

(c) **Nonprescribed drug taken with correctly prescribed and properly administered drug**

If a nonprescribed drug or medicinal agent was taken in combination with a correctly prescribed and properly administered drug, any drug toxicity or other reaction resulting from the interaction of the two drugs would be classified as a poisoning.

(d) **Interaction of drug(s) and alcohol**

When a reaction results from the interaction of a drug(s) and alcohol, this would be classified as poisoning.

(e) **Sequencing of poisoning**

When coding a poisoning or reaction to the improper use of a medication (e.g., wrong dose, wrong substance, wrong route of administration) the poisoning code is sequenced first, followed by a code for the manifestation. If there is also a diagnosis of drug abuse or dependence to the substance, the abuse or dependence is coded as an additional code.

See Section I.C.3.a.6.b. if poisoning is the result of insulin pump malfunctions and Section I.C.19 for general use of E-codes.

3) **Toxic Effects**

(a) **Toxic effect codes**

When a harmful substance is ingested or comes in contact with a person, this is classified as a toxic effect. The toxic effect codes are in categories 980-989.

(b) **Sequencing toxic effect codes**

A toxic effect code should be sequenced first, followed by the code(s) that identify the result of the toxic effect.

(c) **External cause codes for toxic effects**

An external cause code from categories E860-E869 for accidental exposure, codes E950.6 or E950.7 for intentional self-harm, category E962 for assault, or categories E980-E982, for undetermined, should also be assigned to indicate intent.

f. **Complications of care**

1) **Complications of care**

(a) **Documentation of complications of care**

As with all procedural or postprocedural complications, code assignment is based on the provider's documentation of the relationship between the condition and the procedure.

2) <u>Transplant complications</u>

(a) <u>Transplant complications other than kidney</u>

Codes under subcategory 996.8, Complications of transplanted organ, are for use for both complications and rejection of transplanted organs. A transplant complication code is only assigned if the complication affects the function of the transplanted organ. Two codes are required to fully describe a transplant complication, the appropriate code from subcategory 996.8 and a secondary code that identifies the complication.

Pre-existing conditions or conditions that develop after the transplant are not coded as complications unless they affect the function of the transplanted organs.

See I.C.18.d.3) for transplant organ removal status

See I.C.2.i for malignant neoplasm associated with transplanted organ.

(b) **Chronic kidney disease and** kidney transplant complications

Patients who have undergone kidney transplant may still have some form of chronic kidney disease (CKD) because the kidney transplant may not fully restore kidney function. Code 996.81 should be assigned for documented complications of a kidney transplant, such as transplant failure or rejection **or other transplant complication.** Code 996.81 should not be assigned for post kidney transplant patients who have chronic kidney (CKD) unless a transplant complication such as transplant failure or rejection is documented. If the documentation is unclear as to whether the patient has a complication of the transplant, query the provider.

For patients with CKD following a kidney transplant, but who do not have a complication such as failure or rejection, *see section I.C.10.a.2, Chronic kidney disease and kidney transplant status.*

3) **Ventilator associated pneumonia**

(a) **Documentation of Ventilator associated Pneumonia**

As with all procedural or postprocedural complications, code assignment is based on the provider's documentation of the relationship between the condition and the procedure.

Code 997.31, Ventilator associated pneumonia, should be assigned only when the provider has documented ventilator associated pneumonia (VAP). An additional code to identify the organism (e.g., Pseudomonas aeruginosa, code 041.7) should also be assigned. Do not assign an additional code from categories 480-484 to identify the type of pneumonia.

Code 997.31 should not be assigned for cases where the patient has pneumonia and is on a mechanical ventilator but the provider has not specifically stated that the pneumonia is ventilator-associated pneumonia.

If the documentation is unclear as to whether the patient has a pneumonia that is a complication attributable to the mechanical ventilator, query the provider.

(b) **Patient admitted with pneumonia and develops VAP**

A patient may be admitted with one type of pneumonia (e.g., code 481, Pneumococcal pneumonia) and subsequently develop VAP. In this instance, the principal diagnosis would be the appropriate code from categories 480-484 for the pneumonia diagnosed at the time of admission. Code 997.31, Ventilator associated pneumonia, would be assigned as an additional diagnosis when the provider has also documented the presence of ventilator associated pneumonia.

g. **SIRS due to Non-infectious Process**

The systemic inflammatory response syndrome (SIRS) can develop as a result of certain non-infectious disease processes, such as trauma, malignant neoplasm, or pancreatitis. When SIRS is documented with a noninfectious condition, and no subsequent infection is documented, the code for the underlying condition, such as an injury, should be assigned, followed by code 995.93, Systemic inflammatory response syndrome due to noninfectious process without acute organ dysfunction, or 995.94, Systemic inflammatory response syndrome due to non-infectious process with acute organ dysfunction. If an acute organ dysfunction is documented, the appropriate code(s) for the associated acute organ dysfunction(s) should be assigned in addition to code 995.94. If acute organ dysfunction is documented, but it cannot be determined if the acute organ dysfunction is associated with SIRS or due to another condition (e.g., directly due to the trauma), the provider should be queried.

When the non-infectious condition has led to an infection that results in SIRS, *see Section I.C.1.b.12 for the guideline for sepsis and severe sepsis associated with a non-infectious process.*

18. **Classification of Factors Influencing Health Status and Contact with Health Service (Supplemental V01-V89)**

Note: The chapter specific guidelines provide additional information about the use of V codes for specified encounters.

a. **Introduction**

ICD-9-CM provides codes to deal with encounters for circumstances other than a disease or injury. The Supplementary Classification of Factors Influencing Health Status and Contact with Health Services (V01.0 - **V89.09**) is provided to deal with occasions when circumstances other than a disease or injury (codes 001-999) are recorded as a diagnosis or problem.

There are four primary circumstances for the use of V codes:

1) A person who is not currently sick encounters the health services for some specific reason, such as to act as an organ donor, to receive prophylactic care, such as inoculations or health screenings, or to receive counseling on health related issues.

2) A person with a resolving disease or injury, or a chronic, long-term condition requiring continuous care, encounters the health care system for specific aftercare of that disease or injury (e.g., dialysis for renal disease; chemotherapy for malignancy; cast change). A diagnosis/symptom code should be used whenever a current, acute, diagnosis is being treated or a sign or symptom is being studied.

3) Circumstances or problems influence a person's health status but are not in themselves a current illness or injury.

4) Newborns, to indicate birth status

b. **V codes use in any healthcare setting**

V codes are for use in any healthcare setting. V codes may be used as either a first listed (principal diagnosis code in the inpatient setting) or secondary code, depending on the circumstances of the encounter. Certain V codes may only be used as first listed, others only as secondary codes.

See Section I.C.18.e, V Code Table.

c. **V Codes indicate a reason for an encounter**

They are not procedure codes. A corresponding procedure code must accompany a V code to describe the procedure performed.

d. Categories of V Codes

1) Contact/Exposure

Category V01 indicates contact with or exposure to communicable diseases. These codes are for patients who do not show any sign or symptom of a disease but have been exposed to it by close personal contact with an infected individual or are in an area where a disease is epidemic. These codes may be used as a first listed code to explain an encounter for testing, or, more commonly, as a secondary code to identify a potential risk.

2) Inoculations and vaccinations

Categories V03-V06 are for encounters for inoculations and vaccinations. They indicate that a patient is being seen to receive a prophylactic inoculation against a disease. The injection itself must be represented by the appropriate procedure code. A code from V03-V06 may be used as a secondary code if the inoculation is given as a routine part of preventive health care, such as a well-baby visit.

3) Status

Status codes indicate that a patient is either a carrier of a disease or has the sequelae or residual of a past disease or condition. This includes such things as the presence of prosthetic or mechanical devices resulting from past treatment. A status code is informative, because the status may affect the course of treatment and its outcome. A status code is distinct from a history code. The history code indicates that the patient no longer has the condition.

A status code should not be used with a diagnosis code from one of the body system chapters, if the diagnosis code includes the information provided by the status code. For example, code V42.1, Heart transplant status, should not be used with code 996.83, Complications of transplanted heart. The status code does not provide additional information. The complication code indicates that the patient is a heart transplant patient.

The status V codes/categories are:

V02   Carrier or suspected carrier of infectious diseases

        Carrier status indicates that a person harbors the specific organisms of a disease without manifest symptoms and is capable of transmitting the infection.

V07.5X   Prophylactic use of agents affecting estrogen receptors and estrogen level

        This code indicates when a patient is receiving a drug that affects estrogen receptors and estrogen levels for prevention of cancer.

V08   Asymptomatic HIV infection status

        This code indicates that a patient has tested positive for HIV but has manifested no signs or symptoms of the disease.

V09   Infection with drug-resistant microorganisms

        This category indicates that a patient has an infection that is resistant to drug treatment. Sequence the infection code first.

V21	Constitutional states in development
V22.2	Pregnant state, incidental

This code is a secondary code only for use when the pregnancy is in no way complicating the reason for visit. Otherwise, a code from the obstetric chapter is required.

V26.5x	Sterilization status
V42	Organ or tissue replaced by transplant
V43	Organ or tissue replaced by other means
V44	Artificial opening status
V45	Other postsurgical states

Assign code V45.87, Transplant organ removal status, to indicate that a transplanted organ has been previously removed. This code should not be assigned for the encounter in which the transplanted organ is removed. The complication necessitating removal of the transplant organ should be assigned for that encounter.

See section I.C17.f.2. for information on the coding of organ transplant complications.

Assign code V45.88, Status post administration of tPA (rtPA) in a different facility within the last 24 hours prior to admission to the current facility, as a secondary diagnosis when a patient is received by transfer into a facility and documentation indicates they were administered tissue plasminogen activator (tPA) within the last 24 hours prior to admission to the current facility.

This guideline applies even if the patient is still receiving the tPA at the time they are received into the current facility.

The appropriate code for the condition for which the tPA was administered (such as cerebrovascular disease or myocardial infarction) should be assigned first.

Code V45.88 is only applicable to the receiving facility record and not to the transferring facility record.

V46	Other dependence on machines
V49.6	Upper limb amputation status
V49.7	Lower limb amputation status

Note: Categories V42-V46, and subcategories V49.6, V49.7 are for use only if there are no complications or malfunctions of the organ or tissue replaced, the amputation site or the equipment on which the patient is dependent.

V49.81	Postmenopausal status
V49.82	Dental sealant status
V49.83	Awaiting organ transplant status

V58.6x Long-term (current) drug use

Codes from this subcategory indicate a patient's continuous use of a prescribed drug (including such things as aspirin therapy) for the long-term treatment of a condition or for prophylactic use. It is not for use for patients who have addictions to drugs. **This subcategory is not for use of medications for detoxification or maintenance programs to prevent withdrawal symptoms in patients with drug dependence (e.g., methadone maintenance for opiate dependence). Assign the appropriate code for the drug dependence instead.**

Assign a code from subcategory V58.6, Long-term (current) drug use, if the patient is receiving a medication for an extended period as a prophylactic measure (such as for the prevention of deep vein thrombosis) or as treatment of a chronic condition (such as arthritis) or a disease requiring a lengthy course of treatment (such as cancer). Do not assign a code from subcategory V58.6 for medication being administered for a brief period of time to treat an acute illness or injury (such as a course of antibiotics to treat acute bronchitis).

V83 Genetic carrier status

Genetic carrier status indicates that a person carries a gene, associated with a particular disease, which may be passed to offspring who may develop that disease. The person does not have the disease and is not at risk of developing the disease.

V84 Genetic susceptibility status

Genetic susceptibility indicates that a person has a gene that increases the risk of that person developing the disease.

Codes from category V84, Genetic susceptibility to disease, should not be used as principal or first-listed codes. If the patient has the condition to which he/she is susceptible, and that condition is the reason for the encounter, the code for the current condition should be sequenced first. If the patient is being seen for follow-up after completed treatment for this condition, and the condition no longer exists, a follow-up code should be sequenced first, followed by the appropriate personal history and genetic susceptibility codes. If the purpose of the encounter is genetic counseling associated with procreative management, a code from subcategory V26.3, Genetic counseling and testing, should be assigned as the first-listed code, followed by a code from category V84. Additional codes should be assigned for any applicable family or personal history.

See Section I.C. 18.d.14 for information on prophylactic organ removal due to a genetic susceptibility.

V86 Estrogen receptor status

V88 Acquired absence of other organs and tissue

4) **History (of)**

There are two types of history V codes, personal and family. Personal history codes explain a patient's past medical condition that no longer exists and is not receiving any treatment, but that has the potential for recurrence, and therefore may require continued monitoring. The exceptions to this general rule are category V14, Personal history of allergy to medicinal agents, and subcategory V15.0, Allergy, other than to medicinal agents.

A person who has had an allergic episode to a substance or food in the past should always be considered allergic to the substance.

Family history codes are for use when a patient has a family member(s) who has had a particular disease that causes the patient to be at higher risk of also contracting the disease.

Personal history codes may be used in conjunction with follow-up codes and family history codes may be used in conjunction with screening codes to explain the need for a test or procedure. History codes are also acceptable on any medical record regardless of the reason for visit. A history of an illness, even if no longer present, is important information that may alter the type of treatment ordered.

The history V code categories are:

V10	Personal history of malignant neoplasm
V12	Personal history of certain other diseases
V13	Personal history of other diseases
	Except: V13.4, Personal history of arthritis, and V13.6, Personal history of congenital malformations. These conditions are life-long so are not true history codes.
V14	Personal history of allergy to medicinal agents
V15	Other personal history presenting hazards to health
	Except: V15.7, Personal history of contraception.
V16	Family history of malignant neoplasm
V17	Family history of certain chronic disabling diseases
V18	Family history of certain other specific diseases
V19	Family history of other conditions
V87	**Other specified personal exposures and history presenting hazards to health**

5) **Screening**

Screening is the testing for disease or disease precursors in seemingly well individuals so that early detection and treatment can be provided for those who test positive for the disease. Screenings that are recommended for many subgroups in a population include: routine mammograms for women over 40, a fecal occult blood test for everyone over 50, an amniocentesis to rule out a fetal anomaly for pregnant women over 35, because the incidence of breast cancer and colon cancer in these subgroups is higher than in the general population, as is the incidence of Down's syndrome in older mothers.

The testing of a person to rule out or confirm a suspected diagnosis because the patient has some sign or symptom is a diagnostic examination, not a screening. In these cases, the sign or symptom is used to explain the reason for the test.

A screening code may be a first listed code if the reason for the visit is specifically the screening exam. It may also be used as an additional code if the screening is done during an office visit for other health problems. A screening code is not necessary if the screening is inherent to a routine examination, such as a pap smear done during a routine pelvic examination.

Should a condition be discovered during the screening then the code for the condition may be assigned as an additional diagnosis.

The V code indicates that a screening exam is planned. A procedure code is required to confirm that the screening was performed.

The screening V code categories:

V28	Antenatal screening
V73-V82	Special screening examinations

6) Observation

There are three observation V code categories. They are for use in very limited circumstances when a person is being observed for a suspected condition that is ruled out. The observation codes are not for use if an injury or illness or any signs or symptoms related to the suspected condition are present. In such cases the diagnosis/symptom code is used with the corresponding E code to identify any external cause.

The observation codes are to be used as principal diagnosis only. The only exception to this is when the principal diagnosis is required to be a code from the V30, Live born infant, category. Then the V29 observation code is sequenced after the V30 code. Additional codes may be used in addition to the observation code but only if they are unrelated to the suspected condition being observed.

Codes from subcategory V89.0, Suspected maternal and fetal conditions not found, may either be used as a first listed or as an additional code assignment depending on the case. They are for use in very limited circumstances on a maternal record when an encounter is for a suspected maternal or fetal condition that is ruled out during that encounter (for example, a maternal or fetal condition may be suspected due to an abnormal test result). These codes should not be used when the condition is confirmed. In those cases, the confirmed condition should be coded. In addition, these codes are not for use if an illness or any signs or symptoms related to the suspected condition or problem are present. In such cases the diagnosis/symptom code is used.

Additional codes may be used in addition to the code from subcategory V89.0, but only if they are unrelated to the suspected condition being evaluated.

Codes from subcategory V89.0 may not be used for encounters for antenatal screening of mother. *See Section I.C.18.d., Screening).*

For encounters for suspected fetal condition that are inconclusive following testing and evaluation, assign the appropriate code from category 655, 656, 657 or 658.

The observation V code categories:

V29   Observation and evaluation of newborns for suspected condition not found

For the birth encounter, a code from category V30 should be sequenced before the V29 code.

V71   Observation and evaluation for suspected condition not found

V89   Suspected maternal and fetal conditions not found

7) Aftercare

Aftercare visit codes cover situations when the initial treatment of a disease or injury has been performed and the patient requires continued care during the healing or recovery phase, or for the long-term consequences of the disease. The aftercare V code should not be used if treatment is directed at a current, acute disease or injury. The diagnosis code is to be used in these cases. Exceptions to this rule are codes V58.0, Radiotherapy, and codes from subcategory V58.1, Encounter for chemotherapy and immunotherapy for neoplastic conditions. These codes are to be first listed, followed by the diagnosis code when a patient's encounter is solely to receive radiation therapy or chemotherapy for the treatment of a neoplasm. Should a patient receive both chemotherapy and radiation therapy during the same encounter code V58.0 and V58.1 may be used together on a record with either one being sequenced first.

The aftercare codes are generally first listed to explain the specific reason for the encounter. An aftercare code may be used as an additional code when some type of aftercare is provided in addition to the reason for admission and no diagnosis code is applicable. An example of this would be the closure of a colostomy during an encounter for treatment of another condition.

Aftercare codes should be used in conjunction with any other aftercare codes or other diagnosis codes to provide better detail on the specifics of an aftercare encounter visit, unless otherwise directed by the classification. The sequencing of multiple aftercare codes is discretionary.

Certain aftercare V code categories need a secondary diagnosis code to describe the resolving condition or sequelae, for others, the condition is inherent in the code title.

Additional V code aftercare category terms include fitting and adjustment, and attention to artificial openings.

Status V codes may be used with aftercare V codes to indicate the nature of the aftercare. For example code V45.81, Aortocoronary bypass status, may be used with code V58.73, Aftercare following surgery of the circulatory system, NEC, to indicate the surgery for which the aftercare is being performed. Also, a transplant status code may be used following code V58.44, Aftercare following organ transplant, to identify the organ transplanted. A status code should not be used when the aftercare code indicates the type of status, such as using V55.0, Attention to tracheostomy with V44.0, Tracheostomy status.

See Section I. B.16 Admissions/Encounter for Rehabilitation

The aftercare V category/codes:

V51.0 **Encounter for breast reconstruction following mastectomy**

V52 Fitting and adjustment of prosthetic device and implant

V53 Fitting and adjustment of other device

V54 Other orthopedic aftercare

V55 Attention to artificial openings

V56 Encounter for dialysis and dialysis catheter care

V57 Care involving the use of rehabilitation procedures

V58.0 Radiotherapy

V58.11 Encounter for antineoplastic chemotherapy

V58.12 Encounter for antineoplastic immunotherapy

V58.3x Attention to dressings and sutures

V58.41 Encounter for planned post-operative wound closure

V58.42 Aftercare, surgery, neoplasm

V58.43 Aftercare, surgery, trauma

V58.44 Aftercare involving organ transplant

V58.49 Other specified aftercare following surgery

V58.7x Aftercare following surgery

V58.81 Fitting and adjustment of vascular catheter

V58.82 Fitting and adjustment of non-vascular catheter

V58.83 Monitoring therapeutic drug

V58.89 Other specified aftercare

8) Follow-up

The follow-up codes are used to explain continuing surveillance following completed treatment of a disease, condition, or injury. They imply that the condition has been fully treated and no longer exists. They should not be confused with aftercare codes that explain current treatment for a healing condition or its sequelae. Follow-up codes may be used in conjunction with history codes to provide the full picture of the healed condition and its treatment. The follow-up code is sequenced first, followed by the history code.

A follow-up code may be used to explain repeated visits. Should a condition be found to have recurred on the follow-up visit, then the diagnosis code should be used in place of the follow-up code.

The follow-up V code categories:

V24	Postpartum care and evaluation
V67	Follow-up examination

9) Donor

Category V59 is the donor codes. They are used for living individuals who are donating blood or other body tissue. These codes are only for individuals donating for others, not for self donations. They are not for use to identify cadaveric donations.

10) Counseling

Counseling V codes are used when a patient or family member receives assistance in the aftermath of an illness or injury, or when support is required in coping with family or social problems. They are not necessary for use in conjunction with a diagnosis code when the counseling component of care is considered integral to standard treatment.

The counseling V categories/codes:

V25.0	General counseling and advice for contraceptive management
V26.3	Genetic counseling
V26.4	General counseling and advice for procreative management
V61.**X**	Other family circumstances
V65.1	Person consulted on behalf of another person
V65.3	Dietary surveillance and counseling
V65.4	Other counseling, not elsewhere classified

11) Obstetrics and related conditions

See Section I.C.11., the Obstetrics guidelines for further instruction on the use of these codes.

V codes for pregnancy are for use in those circumstances when none of the problems or complications included in the codes from the Obstetrics chapter exist (a routine prenatal visit or postpartum care). Codes V22.0, Supervision of normal first pregnancy, and V22.1, Supervision of other normal pregnancy, are always first listed and are not to be used with any other code from the OB chapter.

The outcome of delivery, category V27, should be included on all maternal delivery records. It is always a secondary code.

V codes for family planning (contraceptive) or procreative management and counseling should be included on an obstetric record either during the pregnancy or the postpartum stage, if applicable.

Obstetrics and related conditions V code categories:

V22	Normal pregnancy
V23	Supervision of high-risk pregnancy

Except: V23.2, Pregnancy with history of abortion. Code 646.3, Habitual aborter, from the OB chapter is required to indicate a history of abortion during a pregnancy.

V24	Postpartum care and evaluation
V25	Encounter for contraceptive management

Except V25.0x

(See Section I.C.18.d.11, Counseling)

V26	Procreative management

Except V26.5x, Sterilization status, V26.3 and V26.4

(See Section I.C.18.d.11., Counseling)

V27	Outcome of delivery
V28	Antenatal screening

(See Section I.C.18.d.6., Screening)

12) Newborn, infant and child

See Section I.C.15, the Newborn guidelines for further instruction on the use of these codes.

Newborn V code categories:

V20	Health supervision of infant or child
V29	Observation and evaluation of newborns for suspected condition not found

(See Section I.C.18.d.7, Observation)

V30-V39	Liveborn infant according to type of birth

13) Routine and administrative examinations

The V codes allow for the description of encounters for routine examinations, such as, a general check-up, or, examinations for administrative purposes, such as, a pre-employment physical. The codes are not to be used if the examination is for diagnosis of a suspected condition or for treatment purposes. In such cases the diagnosis code is used. During a routine exam, should a diagnosis or condition be discovered, it should be coded as an additional code. Pre-existing and chronic conditions and history codes may also be included as additional codes as long as the examination is for administrative purposes and not focused on any particular condition.

Pre-operative examination V codes are for use only in those situations when a patient is being cleared for surgery and no treatment is given.

The V codes categories/code for routine and administrative examinations:

V20.2	Routine infant or child health check

Any injections given should have a corresponding procedure code.

V70	General medical examination
V72	Special investigations and examinations

Codes V72.5 and V72.6 may be used if the reason for the patient encounter is for routine laboratory/radiology testing in the absence of any signs, symptoms, or associated diagnosis. If routine testing is performed during the same encounter as a test to evaluate a sign, symptom, or diagnosis, it is appropriate to assign both the V code and the code describing the reason for the non-routine test.

14) **Miscellaneous V codes**

The miscellaneous V codes capture a number of other health care encounters that do not fall into one of the other categories. Certain of these codes identify the reason for the encounter, others are for use as additional codes that provide useful information on circumstances that may affect a patient's care and treatment.

Prophylactic Organ Removal

For encounters specifically for prophylactic removal of breasts, ovaries, or another organ due to a genetic susceptibility to cancer or a family history of cancer, the principal or first listed code should be a code from subcategory V50.4, Prophylactic organ removal, followed by the appropriate genetic susceptibility code and the appropriate family history code.

If the patient has a malignancy of one site and is having prophylactic removal at another site to prevent either a new primary malignancy or metastatic disease, a code for the malignancy should also be assigned in addition to a code from subcategory V50.4. A V50.4 code should not be assigned if the patient is having organ removal for treatment of a malignancy, such as the removal of the testes for the treatment of prostate cancer.

Miscellaneous V code categories/codes:

V07	Need for isolation and other prophylactic measures
	Except V07.5, Prophylactic use of agents affecting estrogen receptors and estrogen levels
V50	Elective surgery for purposes other than remedying health states
V58.5	Orthodontics
V60	Housing, household, and economic circumstances
V62	Other psychosocial circumstances
V63	Unavailability of other medical facilities for care
V64	Persons encountering health services for specific procedures, not carried out
V66	Convalescence and Palliative Care
V68	Encounters for administrative purposes
V69	Problems related to lifestyle
V85	Body Mass Index

15) Nonspecific V codes

Certain V codes are so non-specific, or potentially redundant with other codes in the classification, that there can be little justification for their use in the inpatient setting. Their use in the outpatient setting should be limited to those instances when there is no further documentation to permit more precise coding. Otherwise, any sign or symptom or any other reason for visit that is captured in another code should be used.

Nonspecific V code categories/codes:

V11   Personal history of mental disorder

        A code from the mental disorders chapter, with an in remission fifth-digit, should be used.

V13.4   Personal history of arthritis

V13.6   Personal history of congenital malformations

V15.7   Personal history of contraception

V23.2   Pregnancy with history of abortion

V40   Mental and behavioral problems

V41   Problems with special senses and other special functions

V47   Other problems with internal organs

V48   Problems with head, neck, and trunk

V49   Problems with limbs and other problems

     Exceptions:

        V49.6   Upper limb amputation status

        V49.7   Lower limb amputation status

        V49.81   Postmenopausal status

        V49.82   Dental sealant status

        V49.83   Awaiting organ transplant status

V51.8   **Other a**ftercare involving the use of plastic surgery

V58.2   Blood transfusion, without reported diagnosis

V58.9   Unspecified aftercare

     See Section IV.K. and Section IV.L. of the Outpatient guidelines.

V CODE TABLE
October 1, 2008 (FY2009)
Items in bold indicate a new entry or change from the October 2007 table
Items underlined have been moved within the table since October 2007

The V code table below contains columns for 1st listed, 1st or additional, additional only, and non-specific. Each code or category is listed in the left hand column, and the allowable sequencing of the code or codes within the category is noted under the appropriate column.

As indicated by the footnote in the "1st Dx Only" column, the V codes designated as first-listed only are generally intended to be limited for use as a first-listed only diagnosis, but may be reported as an additional diagnosis in those situations when the patient has more than one encounter on a single day and the codes for the multiple encounters are combined, or when there is more than one V code that meets the definition of principal diagnosis (e.g., a patient is admitted to home healthcare for both aftercare and rehabilitation and they equally meet the definition of principal diagnosis). The V codes designated as first-listed only should not be reported if they do not meet the definition of principal or first-listed diagnosis.

See Section II and Section IV.A for information on selection of principal and first-listed diagnosis.

See Section II.C for information on two or more diagnoses that equally meet the definition for principal diagnosis.

Code(s)	Description	1st Dx Only[1]	1st or Add'l Dx[2]	Add'l Dx Only[3]	Non-Specific Diagnosis[4]
V01.X	Contact with or exposure to communicable diseases		X		
V02.X	Carrier or suspected carrier of infectious diseases		X		
V03.X	Need for prophylactic vaccination and inoculation against bacterial diseases		X		
V04.X	Need for prophylactic vaccination and inoculation against certain diseases		X		
V05.X	Need for prophylactic vaccination and inoculation against single diseases		X		
V06.X	Need for prophylactic vaccination and inoculation against combinations of diseases		X		
V07.0	**Isolation**		X		
V07.1	**Desensitization to allergens**		X		
V07.2	**Prophylactic immunotherapy**		X		
V07.3X	**Other prophylactic chemotherapy**		X		
V07.4	**Hormone replacement therapy (postmenopausal)**			X	
V07.5X	**Prophylactic use of agents affecting estrogen receptors and estrogen levels**			X	
V07.8	**Other specified prophylactic measure**		X		
V07.9	**Unspecified prophylactic measure**				X
V08	Asymptomatic HIV infection status		X		
V09.X	Infection with drug resistant organisms			X	
V10.X	Personal history of malignant neoplasm		X		
V11.X	Personal history of mental disorder				X
V12.X	Personal history of certain other diseases		X		
V13.0X	Personal history of other disorders of urinary system		X		
V13.1	Personal history of trophoblastic disease		X		
V13.2X	Personal history of other genital system and obstetric disorders		X		
V13.3	Personal history of diseases of skin and subcutaneous tissue		X		
V13.4	Personal history of arthritis				X
V13.5X	Personal history of other musculoskeletal disorders		X		

[1] Generally for use as first listed only but may be used as additional if patient has more than one encounter on one day or there is more than one reason for the encounter
[2] These codes may be used as first listed or additional codes
[3] These codes are only for use as additional codes
[4] These codes are primarily for use in the nonacute setting and should be limited to encounters for which no sign or symptom or reason for visit is documented in the record. Their use may be as either a first listed or additional code.

Code(s)	Description	1st Dx Only[1]	1st or Add'l Dx[2]	Add'l Dx Only[3]	Non-Specific Diagnosis[4]
V13.61	Personal history of hypospadias			X	
V13.69	Personal history of congenital malformations				X
V13.7	Personal history of perinatal problems		X		
V13.8	Personal history of other specified diseases		X		
V13.9	Personal history of unspecified disease				X
V14.X	Personal history of allergy to medicinal agents			X	
V15.0X	Personal history of allergy, other than to medicinal agents			X	
V15.1	Personal history of surgery to heart and great vessels			X	
V15.2X	**Personal history of surgery to other organs**			X	
V15.3	Personal history of irradiation			X	
V15.4X	Personal history of psychological trauma			X	
V15.5X	Personal history of injury			X	
V15.6	Personal history of poisoning			X	
V15.7	Personal history of contraception				X
V15.81	Personal history of noncompliance with medical treatment			X	
V15.82	Personal history of tobacco use			X	
V15.84	Personal history of exposure to asbestos			X	
V15.85	Personal history of exposure to potentially hazardous body fluids			X	
V15.86	Personal history of exposure to lead			X	
V15.87	Personal history of extracorporeal membrane oxygenation [ECMO]			X	
V15.88	History of fall		X		
V15.89	Other specified personal history presenting hazards to health			X	
V16.X	Family history of malignant neoplasm		X		
V17.X	Family history of certain chronic disabling diseases		X		
V18.X	Family history of certain other specific conditions		X		
V19.X	Family history of other conditions		X		
V20.X	Health supervision of infant or child	X			
V21.X	Constitutional states in development			X	
V22.0	Supervision of normal first pregnancy	X			
V22.1	Supervision of other normal pregnancy	X			
V22.2	Pregnancy state, incidental			X	
V23.X	Supervision of high-risk pregnancy		X		
V24.X	Postpartum care and examination	X			
V25.X	Encounter for contraceptive management		X		
V26.0	Tuboplasty or vasoplasty after previous sterilization		X		
V26.1	Artificial insemination		X		
V26.2X	Procreative management investigation and testing		X		
V26.3X	Procreative management, genetic counseling and testing		X		
V26.4X	Procreative management, genetic counseling and advice		X		
V26.5X	Procreative management, sterilization status			X	
V26.81	Encounter for assisted reproductive fertility procedure cycle	X			
V26.89	Other specified procreative management		X		

[1]Generally for use as first listed only but may be used as additional if patient has more than one encounter on one day or there is more than one reason for the encounter
[2]These codes may be used as first listed or additional codes
[3]These codes are only for use as additional codes
[4]These codes are primarily for use in the nonacute setting and should be limited to encounters for which no sign or symptom or reason for visit is documented in the record. Their use may be as either a first listed or additional code.

GUIDELINES - V CODE TABLE

Code(s)	Description	1st Dx Only[1]	1st or Add'l Dx[2]	Add'l Dx Only[3]	Non-Specific Diagnosis[4]
V26.9	Unspecified procreative management		X		
V27.X	Outcome of delivery			X	
V28.X	Encounter for antenatal screening of mother		X		
V29.X	Observation and evaluation of newborns for suspected condition not found		X		
V30.X	Single liveborn	X			
V31.X	Twin, mate liveborn	X			
V32.X	Twin, mate stillborn	X			
V33.X	Twin, unspecified	X			
V34.X	Other multiple, mates all liveborn	X			
V35.X	Other multiple, mates all stillborn	X			
V36.X	Other multiple, mates live- and stillborn	X			
V37.X	Other multiple, unspecified	X			
V39.X	Unspecified	X			
V40.X	Mental and behavioral problems				X
V41.X	Problems with special senses and other special functions				X
V42.X	Organ or tissue replaced by transplant			X	
V43.0	Organ or tissue replaced by other means, eye globe			X	
V43.1	Organ or tissue replaced by other means, lens			X	
V43.21	Organ or tissue replaced by other means, heart assist device			X	
V43.22	Fully implantable artificial heart status		X		
V43.3	Organ or tissue replaced by other means, heart valve			X	
V43.4	Organ or tissue replaced by other means, blood vessel			X	
V43.5	Organ or tissue replaced by other means, bladder			X	
V43.6X	Organ or tissue replaced by other means, joint			X	
V43.7	Organ or tissue replaced by other means, limb			X	
V43.8X	Other organ or tissue replaced by other means			X	
V44.X	Artificial opening status			X	
V45.0X	Cardiac device in situ			X	
V45.1X	Renal dialysis status			X	
V45.2	Presence of cerebrospinal fluid drainage device			X	
V45.3	Intestinal bypass or anastomosis status			X	
V45.4	Arthrodesis status			X	
V45.5X	Presence of contraceptive device			X	
V45.6X	States following surgery of eye and adnexa			X	
V45.7X	Acquired absence of organ		X		
V45.8X	Other postprocedural status			X	
V46.0	Other dependence on machines, aspirator			X	
V46.11	Dependence on respiratory, status			X	
V46.12	Encounter for respirator dependence during power failure	X			
V46.13	Encounter for weaning from respirator [ventilator]	X			
V46.14	Mechanical complication of respirator [ventilator]		X		
V46.2	Other dependence on machines, supplemental oxygen			X	

[1]Generally for use as first listed only but may be used as additional if patient has more than one encounter on one day or there is more than one reason for the encounter
[2]These codes may be used as first listed or additional codes
[3]These codes are only for use as additional codes
[4]These codes are primarily for use in the nonacute setting and should be limited to encounters for which no sign or symptom or reason for visit is documented in the record. Their use may be as either a first listed or additional code.

Code(s)	Description	1st Dx Only[1]	1st or Add'l Dx[2]	Add'l Dx Only[3]	Non-Specific Diagnosis[4]
V46.3	**Wheelchair dependence**			X	
V46.8	Other dependence on other enabling machines			X	
V46.9	Unspecified machine dependence				X
V47.X	Other problems with internal organs				X
V48.X	Problems with head, neck and trunk				X
V49.0	Deficiencies of limbs				X
V49.1	Mechanical problems with limbs				X
V49.2	Motor problems with limbs				X
V49.3	Sensory problems with limbs				X
V49.4	Disfigurements of limbs				X
V49.5	Other problems with limbs				X
V49.6X	Upper limb amputation status		X		
V49.7X	Lower limb amputation status		X		
V49.81	Asymptomatic postmenopausal status (age-related) (natural)		X		
V49.82	Dental sealant status			X	
V49.83	Awaiting organ transplant status			X	
V49.84	Bed confinement status		X		
V49.85	Dual sensory impairment			X	
V49.89	Other specified conditions influencing health status		X		
V49.9	Unspecified condition influencing health status				X
V50.X	Elective surgery for purposes other than remedying health states		X		
V51.0	**Encounter for breast reconstruction following mastectomy**	X			
V51.8	**Other aftercare involving the use of plastic surgery**				X
V52.X	Fitting and adjustment of prosthetic device and implant		X		
V53.X	Fitting and adjustment of other device		X		
V54.X	Other orthopedic aftercare		X		
V55.X	Attention to artificial openings		X		
V56.0	Extracorporeal dialysis	X			
V56.1	Encounter for fitting and adjustment of extracorporeal dialysis catheter		X		
V56.2	Encounter for fitting and adjustment of peritoneal dialysis catheter		X		
V56.3X	Encounter for adequacy testing for dialysis		X		
V56.8	Encounter for other dialysis and dialysis catheter care		X		
V57.X	Care involving use of rehabilitation procedures	X			
V58.0	Radiotherapy	X			
V58.11	Encounter for antineoplastic chemotherapy	X			
V58.12	Encounter for antineoplastic immunotherapy	X			
V58.2	Blood transfusion without reported diagnosis				X
V58.3X	Attention to dressings and sutures		X		
V58.4X	Other aftercare following surgery		X		
V58.5	Encounter for orthodontics				X
V58.6X	Long term (current) drug use			X	
V58.7X	Aftercare following surgery to specified body systems, not elsewhere classified		X		

[1]Generally for use as first listed only but may be used as additional if patient has more than one encounter on one day or there is more than one reason for the encounter
[2]These codes may be used as first listed or additional codes
[3]These codes are only for use as additional codes
[4]These codes are primarily for use in the nonacute setting and should be limited to encounters for which no sign or symptom or reason for visit is documented in the record. Their use may be as either a first listed or additional code.

Code(s)	Description	1st Dx Only[1]	1st or Add'l Dx[2]	Add'l Dx Only[3]	Non-Specific Diagnosis[4]
V58.8X	Other specified procedures and aftercare		X		
V58.9	Unspecified aftercare				X
V59.X	Donors	X			
V60.X	Housing, household, and economic circumstances			X	
V61.X	Other family circumstances		X		
V62.X	Other psychosocial circumstances			X	
V63.X	Unavailability of other medical facilities for care		X		
V64.X	Persons encountering health services for specified procedure, not carried out			X	
V65.X	Other persons seeking consultation without complaint or sickness		X		
V66.0	Convalescence and palliative care following surgery	X			
V66.1	Convalescence and palliative care following radiotherapy	X			
V66.2	Convalescence and palliative care following chemotherapy	X			
V66.3	Convalescence and palliative care following psychotherapy and other treatment for mental disorder	X			
V66.4	Convalescence and palliative care following treatment of fracture	X			
V66.5	Convalescence and palliative care following other treatment	X			
V66.6	Convalescence and palliative care following combined treatment	X			
V66.7	Encounter for palliative care			X	
V66.9	Unspecified convalescence	X			
V67.X	Follow-up examination		X		
V68.X	Encounters for administrative purposes	X			
V69.X	Problems related to lifestyle		X		
V70.0	Routine general medical examination at a health care facility	X			
V70.1	General psychiatric examination, requested by the authority	X			
V70.2	General psychiatric examination, other and unspecified	X			
V70.3	Other medical examination for administrative purposes	X			
V70.4	Examination for medicolegal reasons	X			
V70.5	Health examination of defined subpopulations	X			
V70.6	Health examination in population surveys	X			
V70.7	Examination of participant in clinical trial		X		
V70.8	Other specified general medical examinations	X			
V70.9	Unspecified general medical examination	X			
V71.X	Observation and evaluation for suspected conditions not found	X			
V72.0	Examination of eyes and vision		X		
V72.1X	Examination of ears and hearing		X		
V72.2	Dental examination		X		
V72.3X	Gynecological examination		X		
V72.4X	Pregnancy examination or test		X		
V72.5	Radiological examination, NEC		X		
V72.6	Laboratory examination		X		
V72.7	Diagnostic skin and sensitization tests		X		
V72.81	Preoperative cardiovascular examination		X		

[1]Generally for use as first listed only but may be used as additional if patient has more than one encounter on one day or there is more than one reason for the encounter
[2]These codes may be used as first listed or additional codes
[3]These codes are only for use as additional codes
[4]These codes are primarily for use in the nonacute setting and should be limited to encounters for which no sign or symptom or reason for visit is documented in the record. Their use may be as either a first listed or additional code.

Code(s)	Description	1ˢᵗ Dx Only[1]	1ˢᵗ or Add'l Dx[2]	Add'l Dx Only[3]	Non-Specific Diagnosis[4]
V72.82	Preoperative respiratory examination		X		
V72.83	Other specified preoperative examination		X		
V72.84	Preoperative examination, unspecified		X		
V72.85	Other specified examination		X		
V72.86	Encounter for blood typing		X		
V72.9	Unspecified examination				X
V73.X	Special screening examination for viral and chlamydial diseases		X		
V74.X	Special screening examination for bacterial and spirochetal diseases		X		
V75.X	Special screening examination for other infectious diseases		X		
V76.X	Special screening examination for malignant neoplasms		X		
V77.X	Special screening examination for endocrine, nutritional, metabolic and immunity disorders		X		
V78.X	Special screening examination for disorders of blood and blood-forming organs		X		
V79.X	Special screening examination for mental disorders and developmental handicaps		X		
V80.X	Special screening examination for neurological, eye, and ear diseases		X		
V81.X	Special screening examination for cardiovascular, respiratory, and genitourinary diseases		X		
V82.X	Special screening examination for other conditions		X		
V83.X	Genetic carrier status		X		
V84.X	Genetic susceptibility to disease			X	
V85	Body mass index			X	
V86	Estrogen receptor status			X	
V87.0X	**Contact with and (suspected) exposure to hazardous metals**		X		
V87.1X	**Contact with and (suspected) exposure to hazardous aromatic compounds**		X		
V87.2	**Contact with and (suspected) exposure to other potentially hazardous chemicals**		X		
V87.3X	**Contact with and (suspected) exposure to other potentially hazardous substances**		X		
V87.4X	**Personal history of drug therapy**			X	
V88.0X	**Acquired absence of cervix and uterus**			X	
V89.0X	**Suspected maternal and fetal anomalies not found**		X		

[1]Generally for use as first listed only but may be used as additional if patient has more than one encounter on one day or there is more than one reason for the encounter
[2]These codes may be used as first listed or additional codes
[3]These codes are only for use as additional codes
[4]These codes are primarily for use in the nonacute setting and should be limited to encounters for which no sign or symptom or reason for visit is documented in the record. Their use may be as either a first listed or additional code.

19. Supplemental Classification of External Causes of Injury and Poisoning (E-codes, E800-E999)

Introduction: These guidelines are provided for those who are currently collecting E codes in order that there will be standardization in the process. If your institution plans to begin collecting E codes, these guidelines are to be applied. The use of E codes is supplemental to the application of ICD-9-CM diagnosis codes. E codes are never to be recorded as principal diagnoses (first-listed in non-inpatient setting) and are not required for reporting to CMS.

External causes of injury and poisoning codes (E codes) are intended to provide data for injury research and evaluation of injury prevention strategies. E codes capture how the injury or poisoning happened (cause), the intent (unintentional or accidental; or intentional, such as suicide or assault), and the place where the event occurred.

Some major categories of E codes include:

> transport accidents
>
> poisoning and adverse effects of drugs, medicinal substances and biologicals
>
> accidental falls
>
> accidents caused by fire and flames
>
> accidents due to natural and environmental factors
>
> late effects of accidents, assaults or self injury
>
> assaults or purposely inflicted injury
>
> suicide or self inflicted injury

These guidelines apply for the coding and collection of E codes from records in hospitals, outpatient clinics, emergency departments, other ambulatory care settings and provider offices, and nonacute care settings, except when other specific guidelines apply.

a. General E Code Coding Guidelines

1) Used with any code in the range of 001-V89

An E code may be used with any code in the range of 001-V89, which indicates an injury, poisoning, or adverse effect due to an external cause.

2) Assign the appropriate E code for all initial treatments

Assign the appropriate E code for the initial encounter of an injury, poisoning, or adverse effect of drugs, not for subsequent treatment.

External cause of injury codes (E-codes) may be assigned while the acute fracture codes are still applicable.

See Section I.C.17.b.1 for coding of acute fractures.

3) Use the full range of E codes

Use the full range of E codes to completely describe the cause, the intent and the place of occurrence, if applicable, for all injuries, poisonings, and adverse effects of drugs.

4) Assign as many E codes as necessary

Assign as many E codes as necessary to fully explain each cause. If only one E code can be recorded, assign the E code most related to the principal diagnosis.

5) The selection of the appropriate E code

The selection of the appropriate E code is guided by the Index to External Causes, which is located after the alphabetical index to diseases and by Inclusion and Exclusion notes in the Tabular List.

6) **E code can never be a principal diagnosis**

An E code can never be a principal (first listed) diagnosis.

7) **External cause code(s) with systemic inflammatory response syndrome (SIRS)**

An external cause code is not appropriate with a code from subcategory 995.9, unless the patient also has an injury, poisoning, or adverse effect of drugs.

b. **Place of Occurrence Guideline**

Use an additional code from category E849 to indicate the Place of Occurrence for injuries and poisonings. The Place of Occurrence describes the place where the event occurred and not the patient's activity at the time of the event.

Do not use E849.9 if the place of occurrence is not stated.

c. **Adverse Effects of Drugs, Medicinal and Biological Substances Guidelines**

1) **Do not code directly from the Table of Drugs**

Do not code directly from the Table of Drugs and Chemicals. Always refer back to the Tabular List.

2) **Use as many codes as necessary to describe**

Use as many codes as necessary to describe completely all drugs, medicinal or biological substances.

3) **If the same E code would describe the causative agent**

If the same E code would describe the causative agent for more than one adverse reaction, assign the code only once.

4) **If two or more drugs, medicinal or biological substances**

If two or more drugs, medicinal or biological substances are reported, code each individually unless the combination code is listed in the Table of Drugs and Chemicals. In that case, assign the E code for the combination.

5) **When a reaction results from the interaction of a drug(s)**

When a reaction results from the interaction of a drug(s) and alcohol, use poisoning codes and E codes for both.

6) **If the reporting format limits the number of E codes**

If the reporting format limits the number of E codes that can be used in reporting clinical data, code the one most related to the principal diagnosis. Include at least one from each category (cause, intent, place) if possible.

If there are different fourth digit codes in the same three digit category, use the code for "Other specified" of that category. If there is no "Other specified" code in that category, use the appropriate "Unspecified" code in that category.

If the codes are in different three digit categories, assign the appropriate E code for other multiple drugs and medicinal substances.

7) **Codes from the E930-E949 series**

Codes from the E930-E949 series must be used to identify the causative substance for an adverse effect of drug, medicinal and biological substances, correctly prescribed and properly administered. The effect, such as tachycardia, delirium, gastrointestinal hemorrhaging, vomiting, hypokalemia, hepatitis, renal failure, or respiratory failure, is coded and followed by the appropriate code from the E930-E949 series.

d. Multiple Cause E Code Coding Guidelines

If two or more events cause separate injuries, an E code should be assigned for each cause. The first listed E code will be selected in the following order:

E codes for child and adult abuse take priority over all other E codes.

See Section I.C.19.e., Child and Adult abuse guidelines.

E codes for terrorism events take priority over all other E codes except child and adult abuse

E codes for cataclysmic events take priority over all other E codes except child and adult abuse and terrorism.

E codes for transport accidents take priority over all other E codes except cataclysmic events and child and adult abuse and terrorism.

The first-listed E code should correspond to the cause of the most serious diagnosis due to an assault, accident, or self-harm, following the order of hierarchy listed above.

e. Child and Adult Abuse Guideline

1) Intentional injury

When the cause of an injury or neglect is intentional child or adult abuse, the first listed E code should be assigned from categories E960-E968, Homicide and injury purposely inflicted by other persons, (except category E967). An E code from category E967, Child and adult battering and other maltreatment, should be added as an additional code to identify the perpetrator, if known.

2) Accidental intent

In cases of neglect when the intent is determined to be accidental E code E904.0, Abandonment or neglect of infant and helpless person, should be the first listed E code.

f. Unknown or Suspected Intent Guideline

1) If the intent (accident, self-harm, assault) of the cause of an injury or poisoning is unknown

If the intent (accident, self-harm, assault) of the cause of an injury or poisoning is unknown or unspecified, code the intent as undetermined E980-E989.

2) If the intent (accident, self-harm, assault) of the cause of an injury or poisoning is questionable

If the intent (accident, self-harm, assault) of the cause of an injury or poisoning is questionable, probable or suspected, code the intent as undetermined E980-E989.

g. Undetermined Cause

When the intent of an injury or poisoning is known, but the cause is unknown, use codes: E928.9, Unspecified accident, E958.9, Suicide and self-inflicted injury by unspecified means, and E968.9, Assault by unspecified means.

These E codes should rarely be used, as the documentation in the medical record, in both the inpatient outpatient and other settings, should normally provide sufficient detail to determine the cause of the injury.

h. Late Effects of External Cause Guidelines

1) Late effect E codes

Late effect E codes exist for injuries and poisonings but not for adverse effects of drugs, misadventures and surgical complications.

2) Late effect E codes (E929, E959, E969, E977, E989, or E999.1)

A late effect E code (E929, E959, E969, E977, E989, or E999.1) should be used with any report of a late effect or sequela resulting from a previous injury or poisoning (905-909).

3) Late effect E code with a related current injury

A late effect E code should never be used with a related current nature of injury code.

4) Use of late effect E codes for subsequent visits

Use a late effect E code for subsequent visits when a late effect of the initial injury or poisoning is being treated. There is no late effect E code for adverse effects of drugs.

Do not use a late effect E code for subsequent visits for follow-up care (e.g., to assess healing, to receive rehabilitative therapy) of the injury or poisoning when no late effect of the injury has been documented.

i. Misadventures and Complications of Care Guidelines

1) Code range E870-E876

Assign a code in the range of E870-E876 if misadventures are stated by the provider.

2) Code range E878-E879

Assign a code in the range of E878-E879 if the provider attributes an abnormal reaction or later complication to a surgical or medical procedure, but does not mention misadventure at the time of the procedure as the cause of the reaction.

j. Terrorism Guidelines

1) Cause of injury identified by the Federal Government (FBI) as terrorism

When the cause of an injury is identified by the Federal Government (FBI) as terrorism, the first-listed E-code should be a code from category E979, Terrorism. The definition of terrorism employed by the FBI is found at the inclusion note at E979. The terrorism E-code is the only E-code that should be assigned. Additional E codes from the assault categories should not be assigned.

2) Cause of an injury is suspected to be the result of terrorism

When the cause of an injury is suspected to be the result of terrorism a code from category E979 should not be assigned. Assign a code in the range of E codes based circumstances on the documentation of intent and mechanism.

3) Code E979.9, Terrorism, secondary effects

Assign code E979.9, Terrorism, secondary effects, for conditions occurring subsequent to the terrorist event. This code should not be assigned for conditions that are due to the initial terrorist act.

4) Statistical tabulation of terrorism codes

For statistical purposes these codes will be tabulated within the category for assault, expanding the current category from E960-E969 to include E979 and E999.1.

Section II. Selection of Principal Diagnosis

The circumstances of inpatient admission always govern the selection of principal diagnosis. The principal diagnosis is defined in the Uniform Hospital Discharge Data Set (UHDDS) as "that condition established after study to be chiefly responsible for occasioning the admission of the patient to the hospital for care."

The UHDDS definitions are used by hospitals to report inpatient data elements in a standardized manner. These data elements and their definitions can be found in the July 31, 1985, Federal Register (Vol. 50, No, 147), pp. 31038-40.

Since that time the application of the UHDDS definitions has been expanded to include all non-outpatient settings (acute care, short term, long term care and psychiatric hospitals; home health agencies; rehab facilities; nursing homes, etc).

In determining principal diagnosis the coding conventions in the ICD-9-CM, Volumes I and II take precedence over these official coding guidelines.

(See Section I.A., Conventions for the ICD-9-CM)

The importance of consistent, complete documentation in the medical record cannot be overemphasized. Without such documentation the application of all coding guidelines is a difficult, if not impossible, task.

A. Codes for symptoms, signs, and ill-defined conditions

Codes for symptoms, signs, and ill-defined conditions from Chapter 16 are not to be used as principal diagnosis when a related definitive diagnosis has been established.

B. Two or more interrelated conditions, each potentially meeting the definition for principal diagnosis.

When there are two or more interrelated conditions (such as diseases in the same ICD-9-CM chapter or manifestations characteristically associated with a certain disease) potentially meeting the definition of principal diagnosis, either condition may be sequenced first, unless the circumstances of the admission, the therapy provided, the Tabular List, or the Alphabetic Index indicate otherwise.

C. Two or more diagnoses that equally meet the definition for principal diagnosis

In the unusual instance when two or more diagnoses equally meet the criteria for principal diagnosis as determined by the circumstances of admission, diagnostic workup and/or therapy provided, and the Alphabetic Index, Tabular List, or another coding guidelines does not provide sequencing direction, any one of the diagnoses may be sequenced first.

D. Two or more comparative or contrasting conditions.

In those rare instances when two or more contrasting or comparative diagnoses are documented as "either/or" (or similar terminology), they are coded as if the diagnoses were confirmed and the diagnoses are sequenced according to the circumstances of the admission. If no further determination can be made as to which diagnosis should be principal, either diagnosis may be sequenced first.

E. A symptom(s) followed by contrasting/comparative diagnoses

When a symptom(s) is followed by contrasting/comparative diagnoses, the symptom code is sequenced first. All the contrasting/comparative diagnoses should be coded as additional diagnoses.

F. Original treatment plan not carried out

Sequence as the principal diagnosis the condition, which after study occasioned the admission to the hospital, even though treatment may not have been carried out due to unforeseen circumstances.

G. Complications of surgery and other medical care

When the admission is for treatment of a complication resulting from surgery or other medical care, the complication code is sequenced as the principal diagnosis. If the complication is classified to the 996-999 series and the code lacks the necessary specificity in describing the complication, an additional code for the specific complication should be assigned.

H. Uncertain Diagnosis

If the diagnosis documented at the time of discharge is qualified as "probable", "suspected", "likely", "questionable", "possible", or "still to be ruled out", or other similar terms indicating uncertainty, code the condition as if it existed or was established. The bases for these guidelines are the diagnostic workup, arrangements for further workup or observation, and initial therapeutic approach that correspond most closely with the established diagnosis.

Note: This guideline is applicable only to inpatient admissions to short-term, acute, long-term care and psychiatric hospitals.

I. Admission from Observation Unit

1. Admission Following Medical Observation

When a patient is admitted to an observation unit for a medical condition, which either worsens or does not improve, and is subsequently admitted as an inpatient of the same hospital for this same medical condition, the principal diagnosis would be the medical condition which led to the hospital admission.

2. Admission Following Post-Operative Observation

When a patient is admitted to an observation unit to monitor a condition (or complication) that develops following outpatient surgery, and then is subsequently admitted as an inpatient of the same hospital, hospitals should apply the Uniform Hospital Discharge Data Set (UHDDS) definition of principal diagnosis as "that condition established after study to be chiefly responsible for occasioning the admission of the patient to the hospital for care."

J. Admission from Outpatient Surgery

When a patient receives surgery in the hospital's outpatient surgery department and is subsequently admitted for continuing inpatient care at the same hospital, the following guidelines should be followed in selecting the principal diagnosis for the inpatient admission:

- If the reason for the inpatient admission is a complication, assign the complication as the principal diagnosis.
- If no complication, or other condition, is documented as the reason for the inpatient admission, assign the reason for the outpatient surgery as the principal diagnosis.
- If the reason for the inpatient admission is another condition unrelated to the surgery, assign the unrelated condition as the principal diagnosis.

Section III. Reporting Additional Diagnoses

GENERAL RULES FOR OTHER (ADDITIONAL) DIAGNOSES

For reporting purposes the definition for "other diagnoses" is interpreted as additional conditions that affect patient care in terms of requiring:

> clinical evaluation; or
> therapeutic treatment; or
> diagnostic procedures; or
> extended length of hospital stay; or
> increased nursing care and/or monitoring.

The UHDDS item #11-b defines Other Diagnoses as "all conditions that coexist at the time of admission, that develop subsequently, or that affect the treatment received and/or the length of stay. Diagnoses that relate to an earlier episode which have no bearing on the current hospital stay are to be excluded." UHDDS definitions apply to inpatients in acute care, short-term, long term care and psychiatric hospital setting. The UHDDS definitions are used by acute care short-term hospitals to report inpatient data elements in a standardized manner. These data elements and their definitions can be found in the July 31, 1985, Federal Register (Vol. 50, No, 147), pp. 31038-40.

Since that time the application of the UHDDS definitions has been expanded to include all non-outpatient settings (acute care, short term, long term care and psychiatric hospitals; home health agencies; rehab facilities; nursing homes, etc).

The following guidelines are to be applied in designating "other diagnoses" when neither the Alphabetic Index nor the Tabular List in ICD-9-CM provide direction. The listing of the diagnoses in the patient record is the responsibility of the attending provider.

A. Previous conditions

If the provider has included a diagnosis in the final diagnostic statement, such as the discharge summary or the face sheet, it should ordinarily be coded. Some providers include in the diagnostic statement resolved conditions or diagnoses and status-post procedures from previous admission that have no bearing on the current stay. Such conditions are not to be reported and are coded only if required by hospital policy.

However, history codes (V10-V19) may be used as secondary codes if the historical condition or family history has an impact on current care or influences treatment.

B. Abnormal findings

Abnormal findings (laboratory, x-ray, pathologic, and other diagnostic results) are not coded and reported unless the provider indicates their clinical significance. If the findings are outside the normal range and the attending provider has ordered other tests to evaluate the condition or prescribed treatment, it is appropriate to ask the provider whether the abnormal finding should be added.

Please note: This differs from the coding practices in the outpatient setting for coding encounters for diagnostic tests that have been interpreted by a provider.

C. Uncertain Diagnosis

If the diagnosis documented at the time of discharge is qualified as "probable", "suspected", "likely", "questionable", "possible", or "still to be ruled out" or other similar terms indicating uncertainty, code the condition as if it existed or was established. The bases for these guidelines are the diagnostic workup, arrangements for further workup or observation, and initial therapeutic approach that correspond most closely with the established diagnosis.

Note: This guideline is applicable only to inpatient admissions to short-term, acute, long-term care and psychiatric hospitals.

Section IV. Diagnostic Coding and Reporting Guidelines for Outpatient Services

These coding guidelines for outpatient diagnoses have been approved for use by hospitals/providers in coding and reporting hospital-based outpatient services and provider-based office visits.

Information about the use of certain abbreviations, punctuation, symbols, and other conventions used in the ICD-9-CM Tabular List (code numbers and titles), can be found in Section IA of these guidelines, under "Conventions Used in the Tabular List." Information about the correct sequence to use in finding a code is also described in Section I.

The terms encounter and visit are often used interchangeably in describing outpatient service contacts and, therefore, appear together in these guidelines without distinguishing one from the other.

Though the conventions and general guidelines apply to all settings, coding guidelines for outpatient and provider reporting of diagnoses will vary in a number of instances from those for inpatient diagnoses, recognizing that:

> The Uniform Hospital Discharge Data Set (UHDDS) definition of principal diagnosis applies only to inpatients in acute, short-term, long-term care and psychiatric hospitals.

> Coding guidelines for inconclusive diagnoses (probable, suspected, rule out, etc.) were developed for inpatient reporting and do not apply to outpatients.

A. Selection of first-listed condition

In the outpatient setting, the term first-listed diagnosis is used in lieu of principal diagnosis.

In determining the first-listed diagnosis the coding conventions of ICD-9-CM, as well as the general and disease specific guidelines take precedence over the outpatient guidelines.

Diagnoses often are not established at the time of the initial encounter/visit. It may take two or more visits before the diagnosis is confirmed.

The most critical rule involves beginning the search for the correct code assignment through the Alphabetic Index. Never begin searching initially in the Tabular List as this will lead to coding errors.

1. Outpatient Surgery

When a patient presents for outpatient surgery, code the reason for the surgery as the first-listed diagnosis (reason for the encounter), even if the surgery is not performed due to a contraindication.

2. Observation Stay

When a patient is admitted for observation for a medical condition, assign a code for the medical condition as the first-listed diagnosis.

When a patient presents for outpatient surgery and develops complications requiring admission to observation, code the reason for the surgery as the first reported diagnosis (reason for the encounter), followed by codes for the complications as secondary diagnoses.

B. Codes from 001.0 through V89

The appropriate code or codes from 001.0 through **V89** must be used to identify diagnoses, symptoms, conditions, problems, complaints, or other reason(s) for the encounter/visit.

C. Accurate reporting of ICD-9-CM diagnosis codes

For accurate reporting of ICD-9-CM diagnosis codes, the documentation should describe the patient's condition, using terminology which includes specific diagnoses as well as symptoms, problems, or reasons for the encounter. There are ICD-9-CM codes to describe all of these.

D. **Selection of codes 001.0 through 999.9**

The selection of codes 001.0 through 999.9 will frequently be used to describe the reason for the encounter. These codes are from the section of ICD-9-CM for the classification of diseases and injuries (e.g. infectious and parasitic diseases; neoplasms; symptoms, signs, and ill-defined conditions, etc.).

E. **Codes that describe symptoms and signs**

Codes that describe symptoms and signs, as opposed to diagnoses, are acceptable for reporting purposes when a diagnosis has not been established (confirmed) by the provider. Chapter 16 of ICD-9-CM, Symptoms, Signs, and Ill-defined conditions (codes 780.0 - 799.9) contain many, but not all codes for symptoms.

F. **Encounters for circumstances other than a disease or injury**

ICD-9-CM provides codes to deal with encounters for circumstances other than a disease or injury. The Supplementary Classification of factors Influencing Health Status and Contact with Health Services (V01.0- **V89**) is provided to deal with occasions when circumstances other than a disease or injury are recorded as diagnosis or problems. *See Section I.C. 18 for information on V-codes.*

G. **Level of Detail in Coding**

   1. **ICD-9-CM codes with 3, 4, or 5 digits**

   ICD-9-CM is composed of codes with either 3, 4, or 5 digits. Codes with three digits are included in ICD-9-CM as the heading of a category of codes that may be further subdivided by the use of fourth and/or fifth digits, which provide greater specificity.

   2. **Use of full number of digits required for a code**

   A three-digit code is to be used only if it is not further subdivided. Where fourth-digit subcategories and/or fifth-digit subclassifications are provided, they must be assigned. A code is invalid if it has not been coded to the full number of digits required for that code.

   See also discussion under Section I.b.3., General Coding Guidelines, Level of Detail in Coding.

H. **ICD-9-CM code for the diagnosis, condition, problem, or other reason for encounter/visit**

List first the ICD-9-CM code for the diagnosis, condition, problem, or other reason for encounter/visit shown in the medical record to be chiefly responsible for the services provided. List additional codes that describe any coexisting conditions. In some cases the first-listed diagnosis may be a symptom when a diagnosis has not been established (confirmed) by the physician.

I. **Uncertain diagnosis**

Do not code diagnoses documented as "probable", "suspected," "questionable," "rule out," or "working diagnosis" or other similar terms indicating uncertainty. Rather, code the condition(s) to the highest degree of certainty for that encounter/visit, such as symptoms, signs, abnormal test results, or other reason for the visit.

Please note: This differs from the coding practices used by short-term, acute care, long-term care and psychiatric hospitals.

J. **Chronic diseases**

Chronic diseases treated on an ongoing basis may be coded and reported as many times as the patient receives treatment and care for the condition(s)

K. Code all documented conditions that coexist

Code all documented conditions that coexist at the time of the encounter/visit, and require or affect patient care treatment or management. Do not code conditions that were previously treated and no longer exist. However, history codes (V10-V19) may be used as secondary codes if the historical condition or family history has an impact on current care or influences treatment.

L. Patients receiving diagnostic services only

For patients receiving diagnostic services only during an encounter/visit, sequence first the diagnosis, condition, problem, or other reason for encounter/visit shown in the medical record to be chiefly responsible for the outpatient services provided during the encounter/visit. Codes for other diagnoses (e.g., chronic conditions) may be sequenced as additional diagnoses.

For encounters for routine laboratory/radiology testing in the absence of any signs, symptoms, or associated diagnosis, assign V72.5 and V72.6. If routine testing is performed during the same encounter as a test to evaluate a sign, symptom, or diagnosis, it is appropriate to assign both the V code and the code describing the reason for the non-routine test.

For outpatient encounters for diagnostic tests that have been interpreted by a physician, and the final report is available at the time of coding, code any confirmed or definitive diagnosis(es) documented in the interpretation. Do not code related signs and symptoms as additional diagnoses.

Please note: This differs from the coding practice in the hospital inpatient setting regarding abnormal findings on test results.

M. Patients receiving therapeutic services only

For patients receiving therapeutic services only during an encounter/visit, sequence first the diagnosis, condition, problem, or other reason for encounter/visit shown in the medical record to be chiefly responsible for the outpatient services provided during the encounter/visit. Codes for other diagnoses (e.g., chronic conditions) may be sequenced as additional diagnoses.

The only exception to this rule is that when the primary reason for the admission/encounter is chemotherapy, radiation therapy, or rehabilitation, the appropriate V code for the service is listed first, and the diagnosis or problem for which the service is being performed listed second.

N. Patients receiving preoperative evaluations only

For patients receiving preoperative evaluations only, sequence first a code from category V72.8, Other specified examinations, to describe the pre-op consultations. Assign a code for the condition to describe the reason for the surgery as an additional diagnosis. Code also any findings related to the pre-op evaluation.

O. Ambulatory surgery

For ambulatory surgery, code the diagnosis for which the surgery was performed. If the postoperative diagnosis is known to be different from the preoperative diagnosis at the time the diagnosis is confirmed, select the postoperative diagnosis for coding, since it is the most definitive.

P. Routine outpatient prenatal visits

For routine outpatient prenatal visits when no complications are present, codes V22.0, Supervision of normal first pregnancy, or V22.1, Supervision of other normal pregnancy, should be used as the principal diagnosis. These codes should not be used in conjunction with chapter 11 codes.

GUIDELINES - SECTION IV.P

Appendix I
Present on Admission Reporting Guidelines

Introduction

These guidelines are to be used as a supplement to the *ICD-9-CM Official Guidelines for Coding and Reporting* to facilitate the assignment of the Present on Admission (POA) indicator for each diagnosis and external cause of injury code reported on claim forms (UB-04 and 837 Institutional).

These guidelines are not intended to replace any guidelines in the main body of the *ICD-9-CM Official Guidelines for Coding and Reporting*. The POA guidelines are not intended to provide guidance on when a condition should be coded, but rather, how to apply the POA indicator to the final set of diagnosis codes that have been assigned in accordance with Sections I, II, and III of the official coding guidelines. Subsequent to the assignment of the ICD-9-CM codes, the POA indicator should then be assigned to those conditions that have been coded.

As stated in the Introduction to the ICD-9-CM Official Guidelines for Coding and Reporting, a joint effort between the healthcare provider and the coder is essential to achieve complete and accurate documentation, code assignment, and reporting of diagnoses and procedures. The importance of consistent, complete documentation in the medical record cannot be overemphasized. Medical record documentation from any provider involved in the care and treatment of the patient may be used to support the determination of whether a condition was present on admission or not. In the context of the official coding guidelines, the term "provider" means a physician or any qualified healthcare practitioner who is legally accountable for establishing the patient's diagnosis.

These guidelines are not a substitute for the provider's clinical judgment as to the determination of whether a condition was/was not present on admission. The provider should be queried regarding issues related to the linking of signs/symptoms, timing of test results, and the timing of findings.

General Reporting Requirements

All claims involving inpatient admissions to general acute care hospitals or other facilities that are subject to a law or regulation mandating collection of present on admission information.

Present on admission is defined as present at the time the order for inpatient admission occurs — conditions that develop during an outpatient encounter, including emergency department, observation, or outpatient surgery, are considered as present on admission.

POA indicator is assigned to principal and secondary diagnoses (as defined in Section II of the Official Guidelines for Coding and Reporting) and the external cause of injury codes.

Issues related to inconsistent, missing, conflicting or unclear documentation must still be resolved by the provider.

If a condition would not be coded and reported based on UHDDS definitions and current official coding guidelines, then the POA indicator would not be reported.

Reporting Options

Y - Yes

N - No

U - Unknown

W – Clinically undetermined

Unreported/Not used **(or "1" for Medicare usage)** – (Exempt from POA reporting)

For more specific instructions on Medicare POA indicator reporting options, refer to http://www.cms.hhs.gov/HospitalAcqCond/02_Statute_Regulations _Program_Instructions.asp#TopOfPage

Reporting Definitions

Y = present at the time of inpatient admission

N = not present at the time of inpatient admission

U = documentation is insufficient to determine if condition is present on admission

W = provider is unable to clinically determine whether condition was present on admission or not

Timeframe for POA Identification and Documentation

There is no required timeframe as to when a provider (per the definition of "provider" used in these guidelines) must identify or document a condition to be present on admission. In some clinical situations, it may not be possible for a provider to make a definitive diagnosis (or a condition may not be recognized or reported by the patient) for a period of time after admission. In some cases it may be several days before the provider arrives at a definitive diagnosis. This does not mean that the condition was not present on admission. Determination of whether the condition was present on admission or not will be based on the applicable POA guideline as identified in this document, or on the provider's best clinical judgment.

If at the time of code assignment the documentation is unclear as to whether a condition was present on admission or not, it is appropriate to query the provider for clarification.

Assigning the POA Indicator

Condition is on the "Exempt from Reporting" list

Leave the "present on admission" field blank if the condition is on the list of ICD-9-CM codes for which this field is not applicable. This is the only circumstance in which the field may be left blank.

POA Explicitly Documented

Assign Y for any condition the provider explicitly documents as being present on admission.

Assign N for any condition the provider explicitly documents as not present at the time of admission.

Conditions diagnosed prior to inpatient admission

Assign "Y" for conditions that were diagnosed prior to admission (example: hypertension, diabetes mellitus, asthma)

Conditions diagnosed during the admission but clearly present before admission

Assign "Y" for conditions diagnosed during the admission that were clearly present but not diagnosed until after admission occurred.

Diagnoses subsequently confirmed after admission are considered present on admission if at the time of admission they are documented as suspected, possible, rule out, differential diagnosis, or constitute an underlying cause of a symptom that is present at the time of admission.

Condition develops during outpatient encounter prior to inpatient admission

Assign Y for any condition that develops during an outpatient encounter prior to a written order for inpatient admission.

Documentation does not indicate whether condition was present on admission

Assign "U" when the medical record documentation is unclear as to whether the condition was present on admission. "U" should not be routinely assigned and used only in very limited circumstances. Coders are encouraged to query the providers when the documentation is unclear.

Documentation states that it cannot be determined whether the condition was or was not present on admission

Assign "W" when the medical record documentation indicates that it cannot be clinically determined whether or not the condition was present on admission.

Chronic condition with acute exacerbation during the admission

If the code is a combination code that identifies both the chronic condition and the acute exacerbation, see POA guidelines pertaining to combination codes.

If the combination code only identifies the chronic condition and not the acute exacerbation (e.g., acute exacerbation of CHF), assign "Y."

Conditions documented as possible, probable, suspected, or rule out at the time of discharge

If the final diagnosis contains a possible, probable, suspected, or rule out diagnosis, and this diagnosis was suspected at the time of inpatient admission, assign "Y."

If the final diagnosis contains a possible, probable, suspected, or rule out diagnosis, and this diagnosis was based on symptoms or clinical findings that were not present on admission, assign "N".

Conditions documented as impending or threatened at the time of discharge

If the final diagnosis contains an impending or threatened diagnosis, and this diagnosis is based on symptoms or clinical findings that were present on admission, assign "Y".

If the final diagnosis contains an impending or threatened diagnosis, and this diagnosis is based on symptoms or clinical findings that were not present on admission, assign "N".

Acute and Chronic Conditions

Assign "Y" for acute conditions that are present at time of admission and N for acute conditions that are not present at time of admission.

Assign "Y" for chronic conditions, even though the condition may not be diagnosed until after admission.

If a single code identifies both an acute and chronic condition, see the POA guidelines for combination codes.

Combination Codes

Assign "N" if any part of the combination code was not present on admission (e.g., obstructive chronic bronchitis with acute exacerbation and the exacerbation was not present on admission; gastric ulcer that does not start bleeding until after admission; asthma patient develops status asthmaticus after admission)

Assign "Y" if all parts of the combination code were present on admission (e.g., patient with diabetic nephropathy is admitted with uncontrolled diabetes)

If the final diagnosis includes comparative or contrasting diagnoses, and both were present, or suspected, at the time of admission, assign "Y".

For infection codes that include the causal organism, assign "Y" if the infection (or signs of the infection) was present on admission, even though the culture results may not be known until after admission (e.g., patient is admitted with pneumonia and the provider documents pseudomonas as the causal organism a few days later).

Same Diagnosis Code for Two or More Conditions

When the same ICD-9-CM diagnosis code applies to two or more conditions during the same encounter (e.g. bilateral condition, or two separate conditions classified to the same ICD-9-CM diagnosis code):

Assign "Y" if all conditions represented by the single ICD-9-CM code were present on admission (e.g. bilateral fracture of the same bone, same site, and both fractures were present on admission)

Assign "N" if any of the conditions represented by the single ICD-9-CM code was not present on admission (e.g. dehydration with hyponatremia is assigned to code 276.1, but only one of these conditions was present on admission).

Obstetrical conditions

Whether or not the patient delivers during the current hospitalization does not affect assignment of the POA indicator. The determining factor for POA assignment is whether the pregnancy complication or obstetrical condition described by the code was present at the time of admission or not.

If the pregnancy complication or obstetrical condition was present on admission (e.g., patient admitted in preterm labor), assign "Y".

If the pregnancy complication or obstetrical condition was not present on admission (e.g., 2nd degree laceration during delivery, postpartum hemorrhage that occurred during current hospitalization, fetal distress develops after admission), assign "N".

If the obstetrical code includes more than one diagnosis and any of the diagnoses identified by the code were not present on admission assign "N".

(e.g., Code 642.7, Pre-eclampsia or eclampsia superimposed on pre-existing hypertension).

If the obstetrical code includes information that is not a diagnosis, do not consider that information in the POA determination.

(e.g. Code 652.1x, Breech or other malpresentation successfully converted to cephalic presentation should be reported as present on admission if the fetus was breech on admission but was converted to cephalic presentation after admission (since the conversion to cephalic presentation does not represent a diagnosis, the fact that the conversion occurred after admission has no bearing on the POA determination).

Perinatal conditions

Newborns are not considered to be admitted until after birth. Therefore, any condition present at birth or that developed in utero is considered present at admission and should be assigned "Y". This includes conditions that occur during delivery (e.g., injury during delivery, meconium aspiration, exposure to streptococcus B in the vaginal canal).

Congenital conditions and anomalies

Assign "Y" for congenital conditions and anomalies. Congenital conditions are always considered present on admission.

External cause of injury codes

Assign "Y" for any E code representing an external cause of injury or poisoning that occurred prior to inpatient admission (e.g., patient fell out of bed at home, patient fell out of bed in emergency room prior to admission)

Assign "N" for any E code representing an external cause of injury or poisoning that occurred during inpatient hospitalization (e.g., patient fell out of hospital bed during hospital stay, patient experienced an adverse reaction to a medication administered after inpatient admission)

Categories and Codes Exempt from Diagnosis Present on Admission Requirement

Effective Date: October 1, 2008

Note: "Diagnosis present on admission" for these code categories are exempt because they represent circumstances regarding the healthcare encounter or factors influencing health status that do not represent a current disease or injury or are always present on admission

137-139, Late effects of infectious and parasitic diseases

268.1, Rickets, late effect

326, Late effects of intracranial abscess or pyogenic infection

412, Old myocardial infarction

438, Late effects of cerebrovascular disease

650, Normal delivery

660.7, Failed forceps or vacuum extractor, unspecified

677, Late effect of complication of pregnancy, childbirth, and the puerperium

905-909, Late effects of injuries, poisonings, toxic effects, and other external causes

V02, Carrier or suspected carrier of infectious diseases

V03, Need for prophylactic vaccination and inoculation against bacterial diseases

V04, Need for prophylactic vaccination and inoculation against certain viral diseases

V05, Need for other prophylactic vaccination and inoculation against single diseases

V06, Need for prophylactic vaccination and inoculation against combinations of diseases

V07, Need for isolation and other prophylactic measures

V10, Personal history of malignant neoplasm

V11, Personal history of mental disorder

V12, Personal history of certain other diseases

V13, Personal history of other diseases

V14, Personal history of allergy to medicinal agents

V15.01-V15.09, Other personal history, Allergy, other than to medicinal agents

V15.1, Other personal history, Surgery to heart and great vessels

V15.2, Other personal history, Surgery to other major organs

V15.3, Other personal history, Irradiation

V15.4, Other personal history, Psychological trauma

V15.5, Other personal history, Injury

V15.6, Other personal history, Poisoning

V15.7, Other personal history, Contraception

V15.81, Other personal history, Noncompliance with medical treatment

V15.82, Other personal history, History of tobacco use

V15.88, Other personal history, History of fall

V15.89, Other personal history, Other

V15.9 Unspecified personal history presenting hazards to health

V16, Family history of malignant neoplasm

V17, Family history of certain chronic disabling diseases

V18, Family history of certain other specific conditions

V19, Family history of other conditions

V20, Health supervision of infant or child

V21, Constitutional states in development

V22, Normal pregnancy

V23, Supervision of high-risk pregnancy

V24, Postpartum care and examination

V25, Encounter for contraceptive management

V26, Procreative management

V27, Outcome of delivery

V28, Antenatal screening

V29, Observation and evaluation of newborns for suspected condition not found

V30-V39, Liveborn infants according to type of birth

V42, Organ or tissue replaced by transplant

V43, Organ or tissue replaced by other means

V44, Artificial opening status

V45, Other postprocedural states

V46, Other dependence on machines

V49.60-V49.77, Upper and lower limb amputation status

V49.81-V49.84, Other specified conditions influencing health status

V50, Elective surgery for purposes other than remedying health states

V51, Aftercare involving the use of plastic surgery

V52, Fitting and adjustment of prosthetic device and implant

V53, Fitting and adjustment of other device

V54, Other orthopedic aftercare

V55, Attention to artificial openings

V56, Encounter for dialysis and dialysis catheter care

V57, Care involving use of rehabilitation procedures

V58, Encounter for other and unspecified procedures and aftercare

V59, Donors

V60, Housing, household, and economic circumstances

V61, Other family circumstances

V62, Other psychosocial circumstances

V64, Persons encountering health services for specific procedures, not carried out

V65, Other persons seeking consultation

V66, Convalescence and palliative care

V67, Follow-up examination

V68, Encounters for administrative purposes

V69, Problems related to lifestyle

V70, General medical examination

V71, Observation and evaluation for suspected condition not found

V72, Special investigations and examinations

V73, Special screening examination for viral and chlamydial diseases

V74, Special screening examination for bacterial and spirochetal diseases

V75, Special screening examination for other infectious diseases

V76, Special screening for malignant neoplasms

V77, Special screening for endocrine, nutritional, metabolic, and immunity disorders

V78, Special screening for disorders of blood and blood-forming organs

V79, Special screening for mental disorders and developmental handicaps

V80, Special screening for neurological, eye, and ear diseases

V81, Special screening for cardiovascular, respiratory, and genitourinary diseases

GUIDELINES - APPENDIX I

V82, Special screening for other conditions

V83, Genetic carrier status

V84, Genetic susceptibility to disease

V85, Body Mass Index

V86, Estrogen receptor status

V87.4, Personal history of drug therapy

V88, Acquired absence of cervix and uterus

V89, Suspected maternal and fetal conditions not found

E800-E807, Railway accidents

E810-E819, Motor vehicle traffic accidents

E820-E825, Motor vehicle nontraffic accidents

E826-E829, Other road vehicle accidents

E830-E838, Water transport accidents

E840-E845, Air and space transport accidents

E846-E848, Vehicle accidents not elsewhere classifiable

E849.0-E849.6, Place of occurrence

E849.8-E849.9, Place of occurrence

E883.1, Accidental fall into well

E883.2, Accidental fall into storm drain or manhole

E884.0, Fall from playground equipment

E884.1, Fall from cliff

E885.0, Fall from (nonmotorized) scooter

E885.1, Fall from roller skates

E885.2, Fall from skateboard

E885.3, Fall from skis

E885.4, Fall from snowboard

E886.0, Fall on same level from collision, pushing, or shoving, by or with other person, In sports

E890.0-E890.9, Conflagration in private dwelling

E893.0, Accident caused by ignition of clothing, from controlled fire in private dwelling

E893.2, Accident caused by ignition of clothing, from controlled fire not in building or structure

E894, Ignition of highly inflammable material

E895, Accident caused by controlled fire in private dwelling

E897, Accident caused by controlled fire not in building or structure

E898.0-E898.1, Accident caused by other specified fire and flames

E917.0, Striking against or struck accidentally by objects or persons, in sports without subsequent fall

E917.1, Striking against or struck accidentally by objects or persons, caused by a crowd, by collective fear or panic without subsequent fall

E917.2, Striking against or struck accidentally by objects or persons, in running water without subsequent fall

E917.5, Striking against or struck accidentally by objects or persons, object in sports with subsequent fall

E917.6, Striking against or struck accidentally by objects or persons, caused by a crowd, by collective fear or panic with subsequent fall

E919.0-E919.1, Accidents caused by machinery

E919.3-E919.9, Accidents caused by machinery

E921.0-E921.9, Accident caused by explosion of pressure vessel

E922.0-E922.9, Accident caused by firearm and air gun missile

E924.1, Caustic and corrosive substances

E926.2, Visible and ultraviolet light sources

E928.0-E928.8, Other and unspecified environmental and accidental causes

E929.0-E929.9, Late effects of accidental injury

E959, Late effects of self-inflicted injury

E970-E978, Legal intervention

E979, Terrorism

E981.0-E981.8, Poisoning by gases in domestic use, undetermined whether accidentally or purposely inflicted

E982.0-E982.9, Poisoning by other gases, undetermined whether accidentally or purposely inflicted

E985.0-E985.7, Injury by firearms, air guns and explosives, undetermined whether accidentally or purposely inflicted

E987.0, Falling from high place, undetermined whether accidentally or purposely inflicted, residential premises

E987.2, Falling from high place, undetermined whether accidentally or purposely inflicted, natural sites

E989, Late effects of injury, undetermined whether accidentally or purposely inflicted

E990-E999, Injury resulting from operations of war

POA Examples

General Medical Surgical

1. Patient is admitted for diagnostic work-up for cachexia. The final diagnosis is malignant neoplasm of lung with metastasis.

   Assign "Y" on the POA field for the malignant neoplasm. The malignant neoplasm was clearly present on admission, although it was not diagnosed until after the admission occurred.

2. A patient undergoes outpatient surgery. During the recovery period, the patient develops atrial fibrillation and the patient is subsequently admitted to the hospital as an inpatient.

   Assign "Y" on the POA field for the atrial fibrillation since it developed prior to a written order for inpatient admission.

3. A patient is treated in observation and while in Observation, the patient falls out of bed and breaks a hip. The patient is subsequently admitted as an inpatient to treat the hip fracture.

   Assign "Y" on the POA field for the hip fracture since it developed prior to a written order for inpatient admission.

4. A patient with known congestive heart failure is admitted to the hospital after he develops decompensated congestive heart failure.

   Assign "Y" on the POA field for the congestive heart failure. The ICD-9-CM code identifies the chronic condition and does not specify the acute exacerbation.

5. A patient undergoes inpatient surgery. After surgery, the patient develops fever and is treated aggressively. The physician's final diagnosis documents "possible postoperative infection following surgery."

   Assign "N" on the POA field for the postoperative infection since final diagnoses that contain the terms "possible", "probable", "suspected" or "rule out" and that are based on symptoms or clinical findings that were not present on admission should be reported as "N".

6. A patient with severe cough and difficulty breathing was diagnosed during his hospitalization to have lung cancer.

   Assign "Y" on the POA field for the lung cancer. Even though the cancer was not diagnosed until after admission, it is a chronic condition that was clearly present before the patient's admission.

7. A patient is admitted to the hospital for a coronary artery bypass surgery. Postoperatively he developed a pulmonary embolism.

   Assign "N" on the POA field for the pulmonary embolism. This is an acute condition that was not present on admission.

8. A patient is admitted with a known history of coronary atherosclerosis, status post myocardial infarction five years ago is now admitted for treatment of impending myocardial infarction. The final diagnosis is documented as "impending myocardial infarction."

   Assign "Y" to the impending myocardial infarction because the condition is present on admission.

9. A patient with diabetes mellitus developed uncontrolled diabetes on day 3 of the hospitalization.

   Assign "N" to the diabetes code because the "uncontrolled" component of the code was not present on admission.

10. A patient is admitted with high fever and pneumonia. The patient rapidly deteriorates and becomes septic. The discharge diagnosis lists sepsis and pneumonia. The documentation is unclear as to whether the sepsis was present on admission or developed shortly after admission.

    Query the physician as to whether the sepsis was present on admission, developed shortly after admission, or it cannot be clinically determined as to whether it was present on admission or not.

11. A patient is admitted for repair of an abdominal aneurysm. However, the aneurysm ruptures after hospital admission.

    Assign "N" for the ruptured abdominal aneurysm. Although the aneurysm was present on admission, the "ruptured" component of the code description did not occur until after admission.

12. A patient with viral hepatitis B progresses to hepatic coma after admission.

    Assign "N" for the viral hepatitis B with hepatic coma because part of the code description did not develop until after admission.

13. A patient with a history of varicose veins and ulceration of the left lower extremity strikes the area against the side of his hospital bed during an inpatient hospitalization. It bleeds profusely. The final diagnosis lists varicose veins with ulcer and hemorrhage.

    Assign "Y" for the varicose veins with ulcer. Although the hemorrhage occurred after admission, the code description for varicose veins with ulcer does not mention hemorrhage.

14. The nursing initial assessment upon admission documents the presence of a decubitus ulcer. There is no mention of the decubitus ulcer in the physician documentation until several days after admission.

    Query the physician as to whether the decubitus ulcer was present on admission, or developed after admission. Both diagnosis code assignment and determination of whether a condition was present on admission must be based on provider documentation in the medical record (per the definition of "provider" found at the beginning of these POA guidelines and in the introductory section of the ICD-9-CM Official Guidelines for Coding and Reporting). If it cannot be determined from the provider documentation whether or not a condition was present on admission, the provider should be queried.

15. **A urine culture is obtained on admission. The provider documents urinary tract infection when the culture results become available a few days later.**

    Assign "Y" to the urinary tract infection since the diagnosis is based on test results from a specimen obtained on admission. It may not be possible for a provider to make a definitive diagnosis for a period of time after admission. There is no required timeframe as to when a provider must identify or document a condition to be present on admission.

16. **A patient tested positive for Methicillin resistant Staphylococcus (MRSA) on routine nasal culture on admission to the hospital. During the hospitalization, he underwent insertion of a central venous catheter and later developed an infection and was diagnosed with MRSA sepsis due to central venous catheter infection.**

    Assign "Y" to the positive MRSA colonization. Assign "N" for the MRSA sepsis due to central venous catheter infection since the patient did not have a MRSA infection at the time of admission.

Obstetrics

1. A female patient was admitted to the hospital and underwent a normal delivery.

    Leave the "present on admission" (POA) field blank. Code 650, Normal delivery, is on the "exempt from reporting" list.

2. Patient admitted in late pregnancy due to excessive vomiting and dehydration. During admission patient goes into premature labor

    Assign "Y" for the excessive vomiting and the dehydration.

    Assign "N" for the premature labor

3. Patient admitted in active labor. During the stay, a breast abscess is noted when mother attempted to breast feed. Provider is unable to determine whether the abscess was present on admission

    Assign "W" for the breast abscess.

4. Patient admitted in active labor. After 12 hours of labor it is noted that the infant is in fetal distress and a Cesarean section is performed

   Assign "N" for the fetal distress.

5. **Pregnant female was admitted in labor and fetal nuchal cord entanglement was diagnosed. Physician is queried, but is unable to determine whether the cord entanglement was present on admission or not.**

   Assign "W" for the fetal nuchal cord entanglement.

Newborn

1. A single liveborn infant was delivered in the hospital via Cesarean section. The physician documented fetal bradycardia during labor in the final diagnosis in the newborn record.

   Assign " Y" because the bradycardia developed prior to the newborn admission (birth).

2. A newborn developed diarrhea which was believed to be due to the hospital baby formula.

   Assign " N" because the diarrhea developed after admission.

3. **A newborn born in the hospital, birth complicated by nuchal cord entanglement.**

   Assign "Y" for the nuchal cord entanglement on the baby's record. Any condition that is present at birth or that developed in utero is considered present at admission, including conditions that occur during delivery.

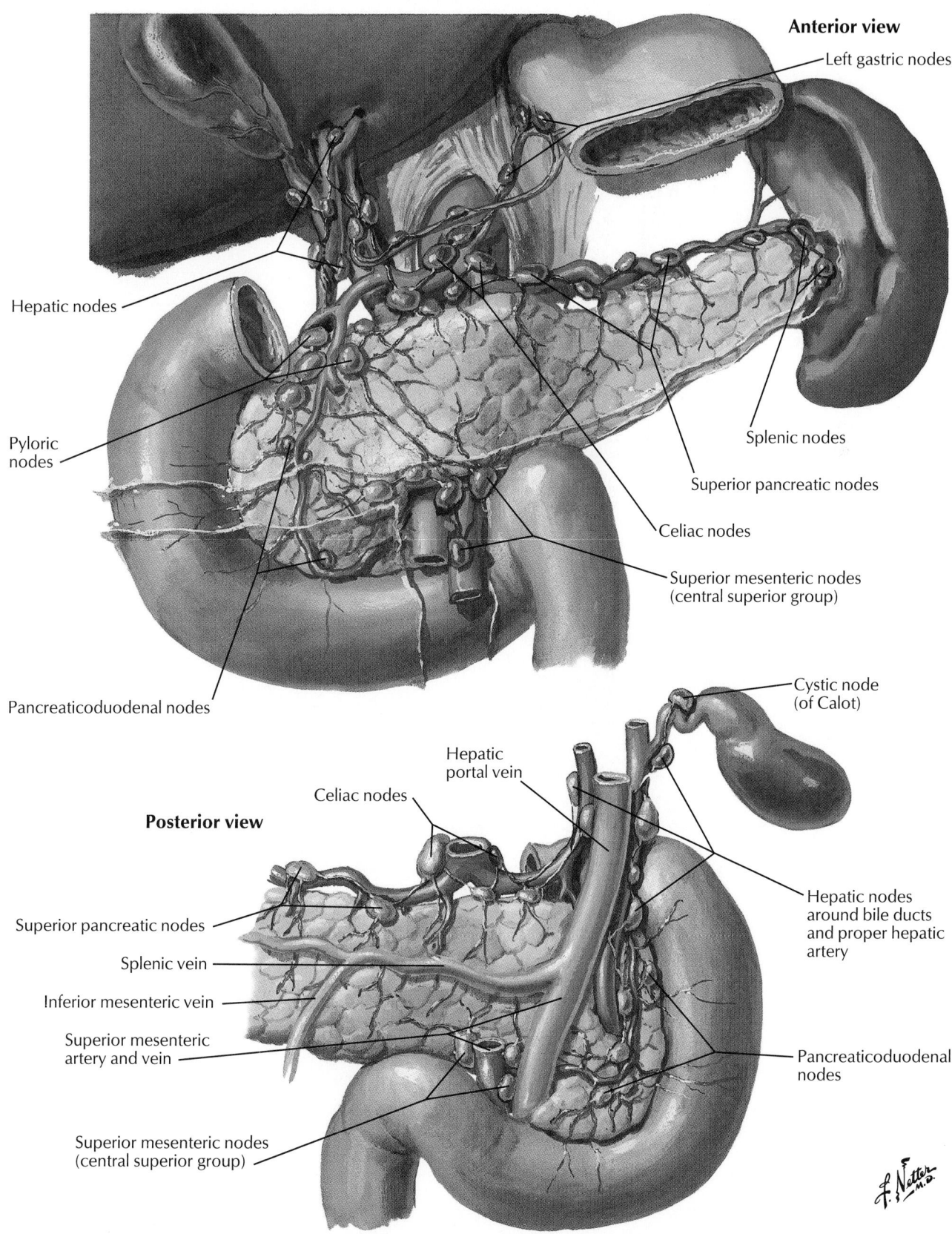

Anterior view

Left gastric nodes

Hepatic nodes

Pyloric nodes

Splenic nodes

Superior pancreatic nodes

Celiac nodes

Superior mesenteric nodes (central superior group)

Pancreaticoduodenal nodes

Cystic node (of Calot)

Hepatic portal vein

Celiac nodes

Posterior view

Superior pancreatic nodes

Splenic vein

Inferior mesenteric vein

Superior mesenteric artery and vein

Superior mesenteric nodes (central superior group)

Hepatic nodes around bile ducts and proper hepatic artery

Pancreaticoduodenal nodes

Plate 315 Lymph Vessels and Nodes of Pancreas. (Netter: Atlas of Human Anatomy, 4 ed, 2006, Saunders.)

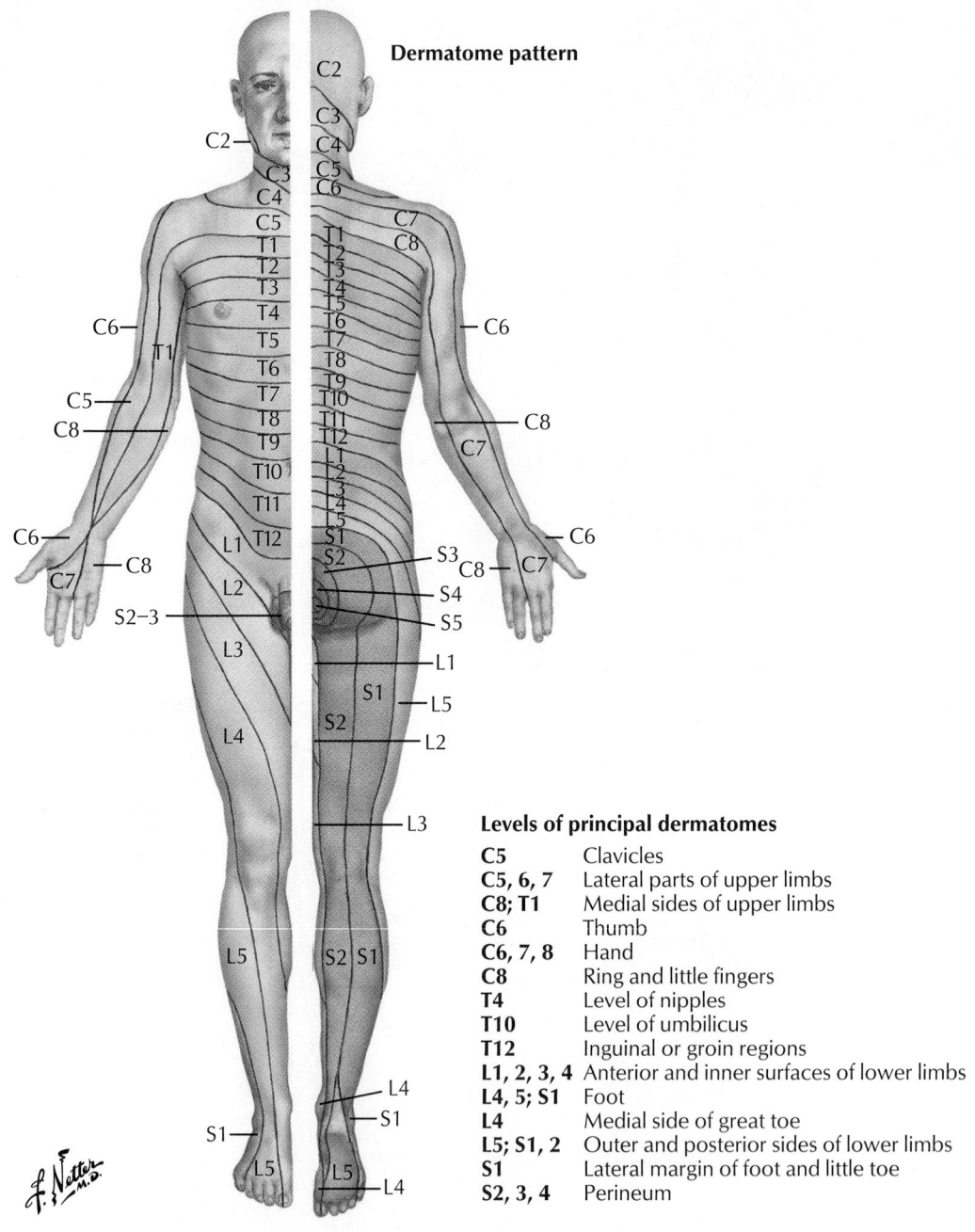

Dermatome pattern

Levels of principal dermatomes

C5	Clavicles
C5, 6, 7	Lateral parts of upper limbs
C8; T1	Medial sides of upper limbs
C6	Thumb
C6, 7, 8	Hand
C8	Ring and little fingers
T4	Level of nipples
T10	Level of umbilicus
T12	Inguinal or groin regions
L1, 2, 3, 4	Anterior and inner surfaces of lower limbs
L4, 5; S1	Foot
L4	Medial side of great toe
L5; S1, 2	Outer and posterior sides of lower limbs
S1	Lateral margin of foot and little toe
S2, 3, 4	Perineum

Plate 164   Dermatomes. (Netter: Atlas of Human Anatomy, 4 ed, 2006, Saunders.)

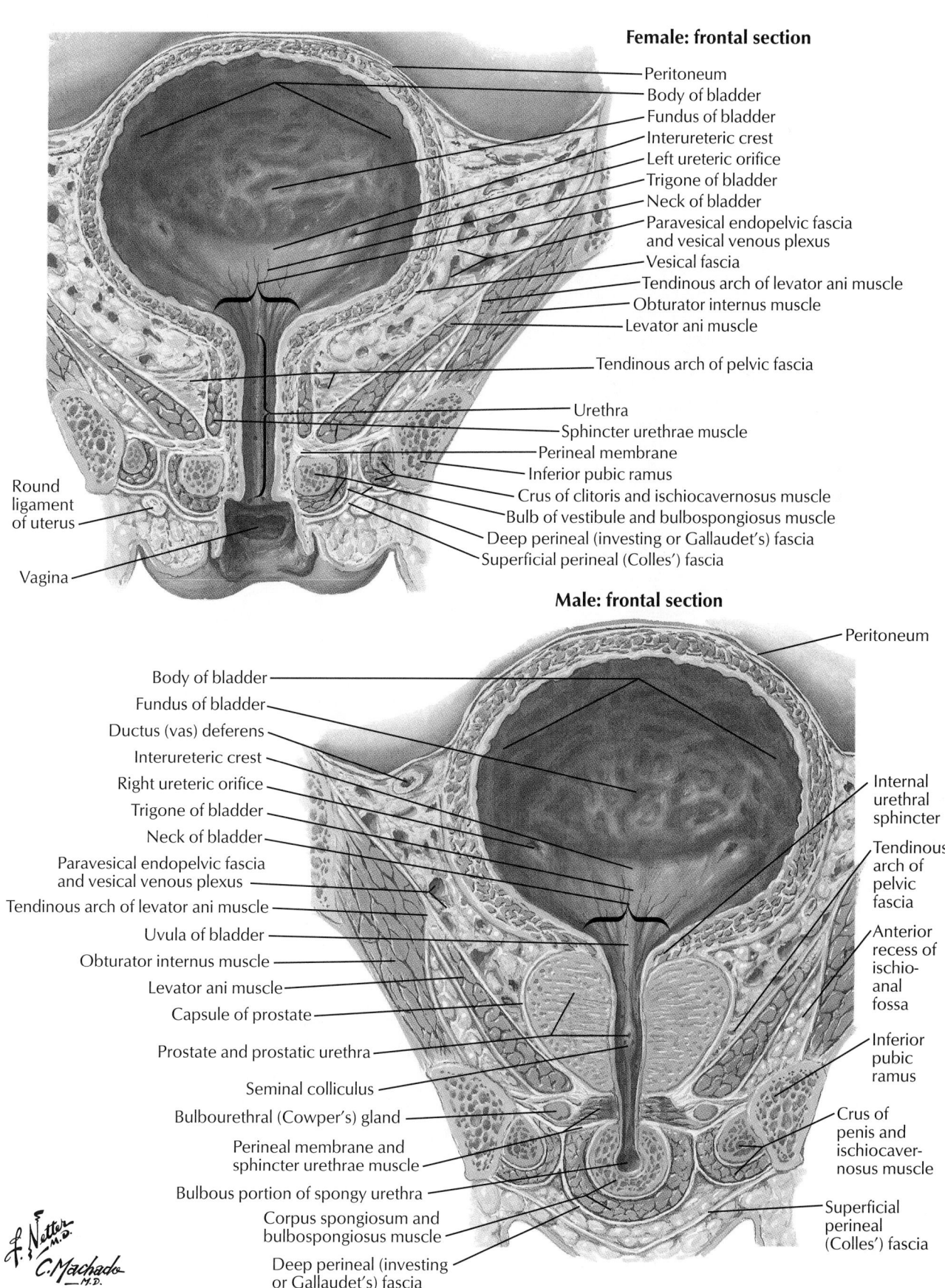

Female: frontal section

Peritoneum
Body of bladder
Fundus of bladder
Interureteric crest
Left ureteric orifice
Trigone of bladder
Neck of bladder
Paravesical endopelvic fascia and vesical venous plexus
Vesical fascia
Tendinous arch of levator ani muscle
Obturator internus muscle
Levator ani muscle

Tendinous arch of pelvic fascia

Urethra
Sphincter urethrae muscle
Perineal membrane
Inferior pubic ramus
Crus of clitoris and ischiocavernosus muscle
Bulb of vestibule and bulbospongiosus muscle
Deep perineal (investing or Gallaudet's) fascia
Superficial perineal (Colles') fascia

Round ligament of uterus

Vagina

Male: frontal section

Peritoneum

Body of bladder
Fundus of bladder
Ductus (vas) deferens
Interureteric crest
Right ureteric orifice
Trigone of bladder
Neck of bladder
Paravesical endopelvic fascia and vesical venous plexus
Tendinous arch of levator ani muscle
Uvula of bladder
Obturator internus muscle
Levator ani muscle
Capsule of prostate
Prostate and prostatic urethra
Seminal colliculus
Bulbourethral (Cowper's) gland
Perineal membrane and sphincter urethrae muscle
Bulbous portion of spongy urethra
Corpus spongiosum and bulbospongiosus muscle
Deep perineal (investing or Gallaudet's) fascia

Internal urethral sphincter
Tendinous arch of pelvic fascia
Anterior recess of ischio-anal fossa
Inferior pubic ramus
Crus of penis and ischiocavernosus muscle
Superficial perineal (Colles') fascia

Plate 366 Urinary Bladder: Female and Male. (Netter: Atlas of Human Anatomy, 4 ed, 2006, Saunders.)

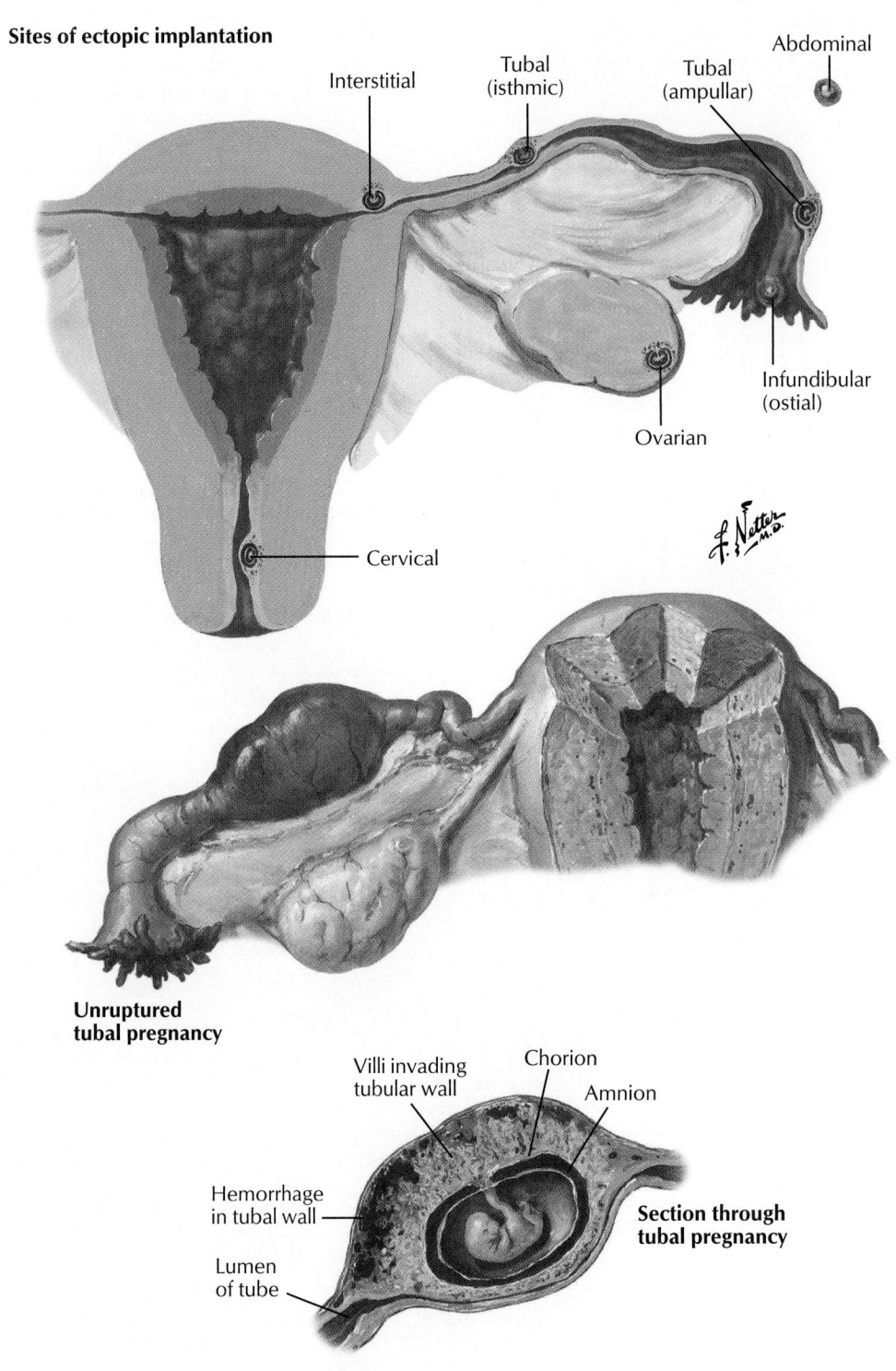

Sites of ectopic implantation

Interstitial

Tubal (isthmic)

Tubal (ampullar)

Abdominal

Infundibular (ostial)

Ovarian

Cervical

Unruptured tubal pregnancy

Villi invading tubular wall

Chorion

Amnion

Hemorrhage in tubal wall

Section through tubal pregnancy

Lumen of tube

Plate 375   Ectopic Pregnancy. (Netter: Atlas of Human Anatomy, 4 ed, 2006, Saunders.)

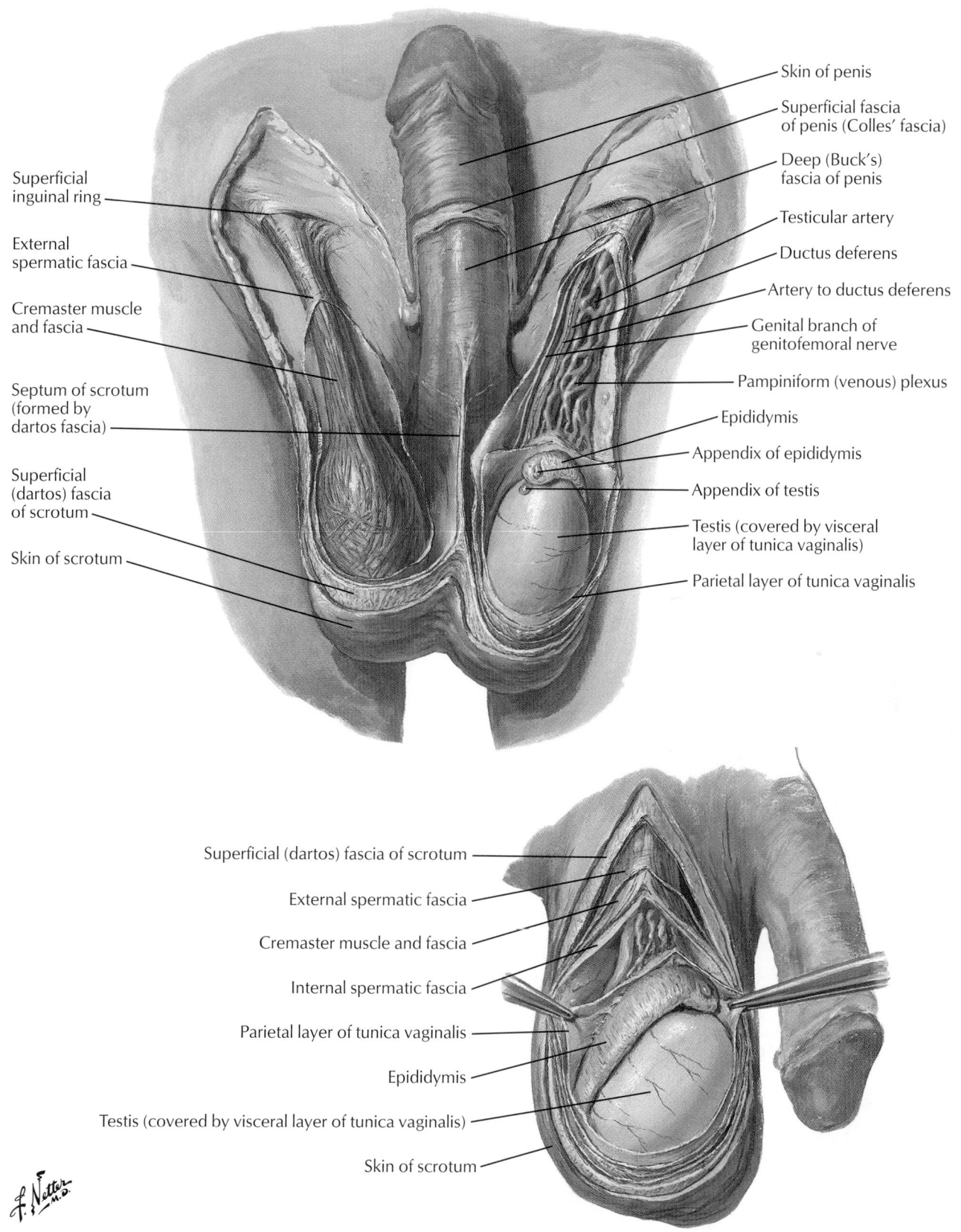

Skin of penis

Superficial fascia of penis (Colles' fascia)

Deep (Buck's) fascia of penis

Testicular artery

Ductus deferens

Artery to ductus deferens

Genital branch of genitofemoral nerve

Pampiniform (venous) plexus

Epididymis

Appendix of epididymis

Appendix of testis

Testis (covered by visceral layer of tunica vaginalis)

Parietal layer of tunica vaginalis

Superficial inguinal ring

External spermatic fascia

Cremaster muscle and fascia

Septum of scrotum (formed by dartos fascia)

Superficial (dartos) fascia of scrotum

Skin of scrotum

Superficial (dartos) fascia of scrotum

External spermatic fascia

Cremaster muscle and fascia

Internal spermatic fascia

Parietal layer of tunica vaginalis

Epididymis

Testis (covered by visceral layer of tunica vaginalis)

Skin of scrotum

Plate 387 Scrotum and Contents. (Netter: Atlas of Human Anatomy, 4 ed, 2006, Saunders.)

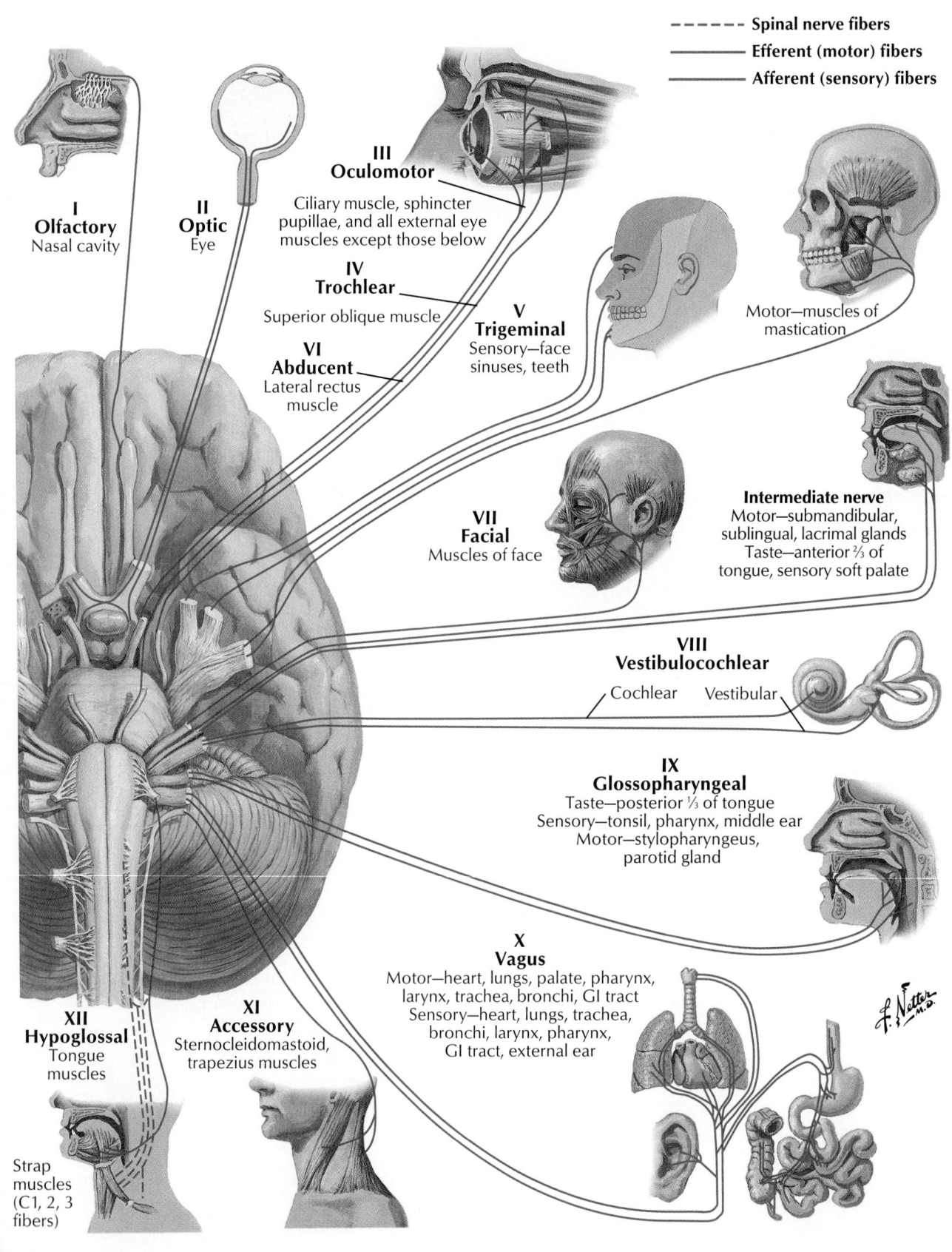

Spinal nerve fibers - - - - -
Efferent (motor) fibers ————
Afferent (sensory) fibers ————

I
Olfactory
Nasal cavity

II
Optic
Eye

III
Oculomotor
Ciliary muscle, sphincter pupillae, and all external eye muscles except those below

IV
Trochlear
Superior oblique muscle

VI
Abducent
Lateral rectus muscle

V
Trigeminal
Sensory—face sinuses, teeth

Motor—muscles of mastication

VII
Facial
Muscles of face

Intermediate nerve
Motor—submandibular, sublingual, lacrimal glands
Taste—anterior ⅔ of tongue, sensory soft palate

VIII
Vestibulocochlear
Cochlear   Vestibular

IX
Glossopharyngeal
Taste—posterior ⅓ of tongue
Sensory—tonsil, pharynx, middle ear
Motor—stylopharyngeus, parotid gland

X
Vagus
Motor—heart, lungs, palate, pharynx, larynx, trachea, bronchi, GI tract
Sensory—heart, lungs, trachea, bronchi, larynx, pharynx, GI tract, external ear

XII
Hypoglossal
Tongue muscles

Strap muscles (C1, 2, 3 fibers)

XI
Accessory
Sternocleidomastoid, trapezius muscles

Plate 118   Cranial Nerves (Motor and Sensory Distribution): Schema. (Netter: Atlas of Human Anatomy, 4 ed, 2006, Saunders.)

Superior view

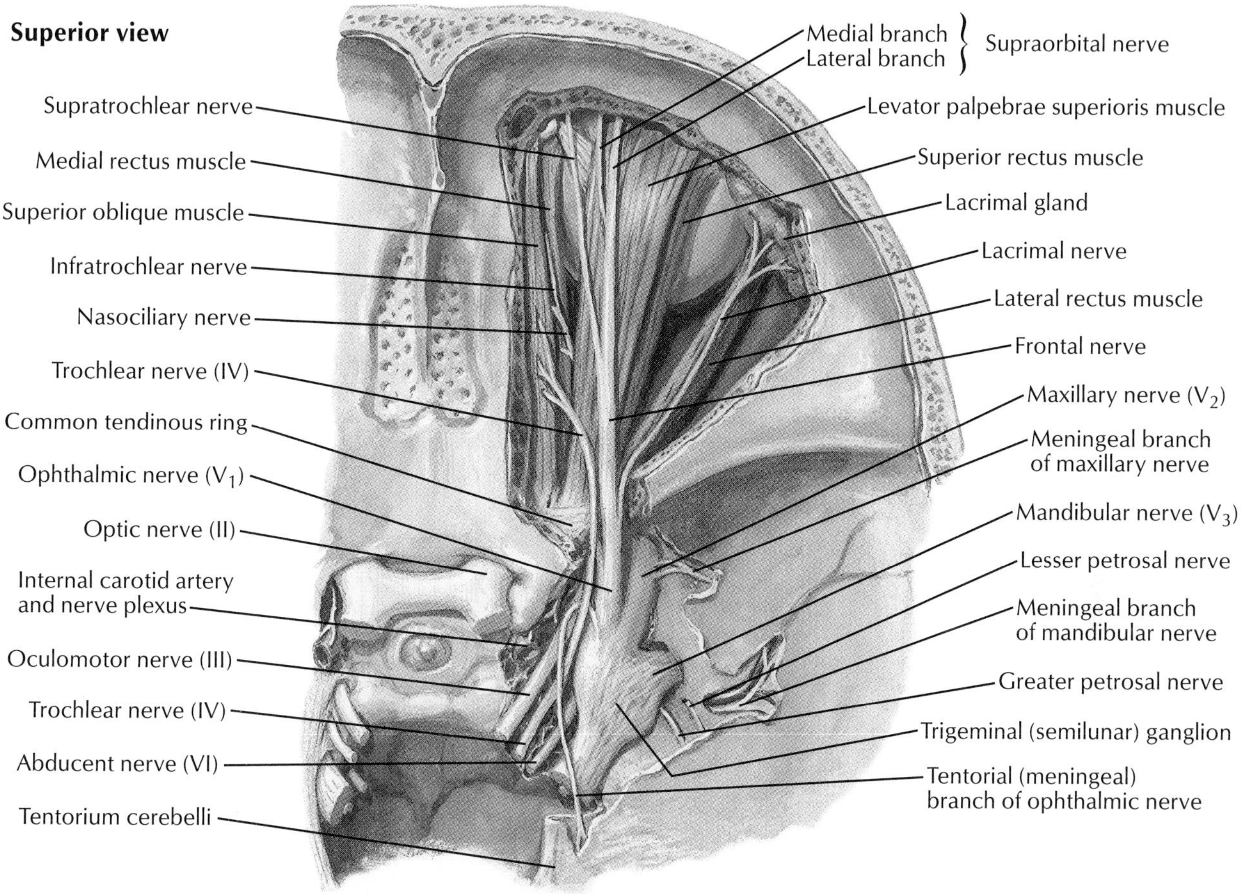

Supratrochlear nerve

Medial rectus muscle

Superior oblique muscle

Infratrochlear nerve

Nasociliary nerve

Trochlear nerve (IV)

Common tendinous ring

Ophthalmic nerve (V₁)

Optic nerve (II)

Internal carotid artery and nerve plexus

Oculomotor nerve (III)

Trochlear nerve (IV)

Abducent nerve (VI)

Tentorium cerebelli

Medial branch
Lateral branch
} Supraorbital nerve

Levator palpebrae superioris muscle

Superior rectus muscle

Lacrimal gland

Lacrimal nerve

Lateral rectus muscle

Frontal nerve

Maxillary nerve (V₂)

Meningeal branch of maxillary nerve

Mandibular nerve (V₃)

Lesser petrosal nerve

Meningeal branch of mandibular nerve

Greater petrosal nerve

Trigeminal (semilunar) ganglion

Tentorial (meningeal) branch of ophthalmic nerve

Superior view:
levator palpebrae superioris, superior rectus, and superior oblique muscles partially cut away

Supratrochlear nerve *(cut)*

Supraorbital nerve branches *(cut)*

Infratrochlear nerve

Anterior ethmoidal nerve

Optic nerve (II)

Posterior ethmoidal nerve

Superior branch of oculomotor nerve (III) *(cut)*

Nasociliary nerve

Internal carotid plexus

Trochlear nerve (IV) *(cut)*

Oculomotor nerve (III)

Abducent nerve (VI)

Long ciliary nerves

Short ciliary nerves

Lacrimal nerve

Ciliary ganglion

Parasympathetic root of ciliary ganglion (from inferior branch of oculomotor nerve)

Sympathetic root of ciliary ganglion (from internal carotid plexus)

Sensory root of ciliary ganglion (from nasociliary nerve)

Branches to inferior and medial rectus muscles

Abducent nerve (VI)

Inferior branch of oculomotor nerve (III)

Lacrimal nerve

Frontal nerve *(cut)*

Ophthalmic nerve (V₁)

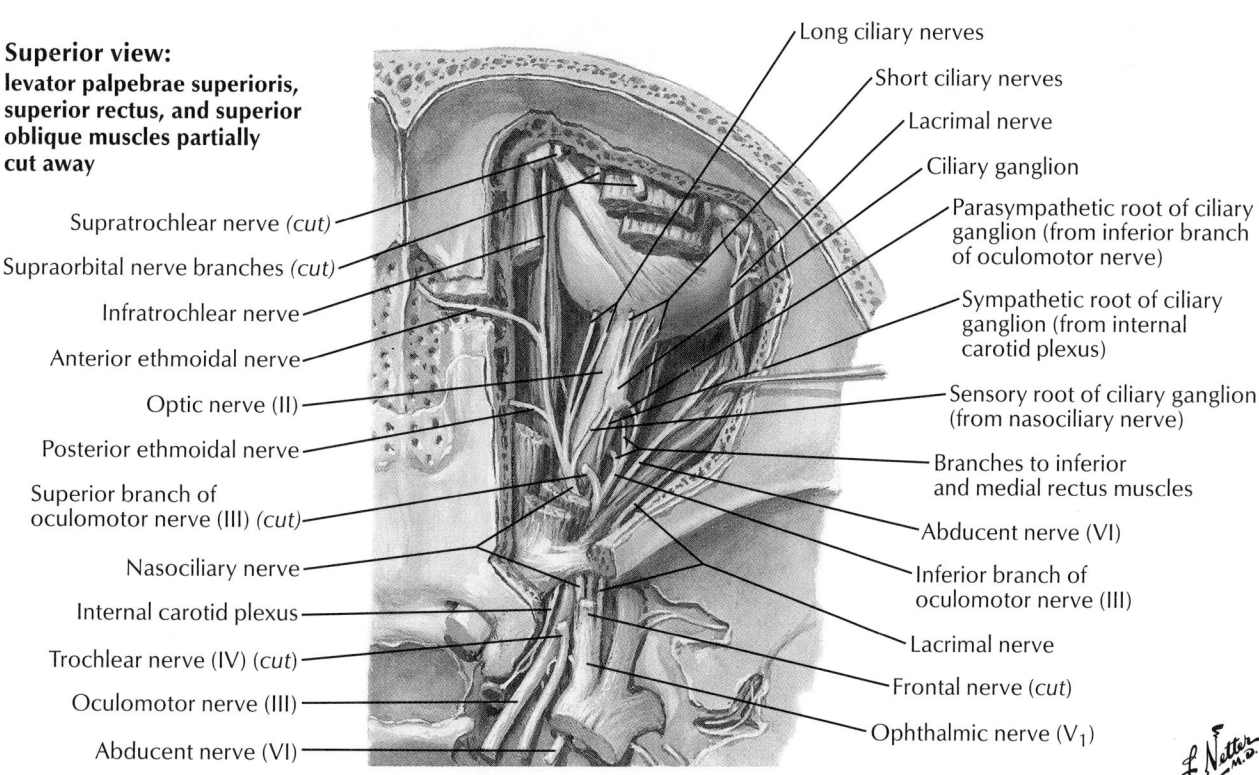

Plate 86 Nerves of Orbit. (Netter: Atlas of Human Anatomy, 4 ed, 2006, Saunders.)

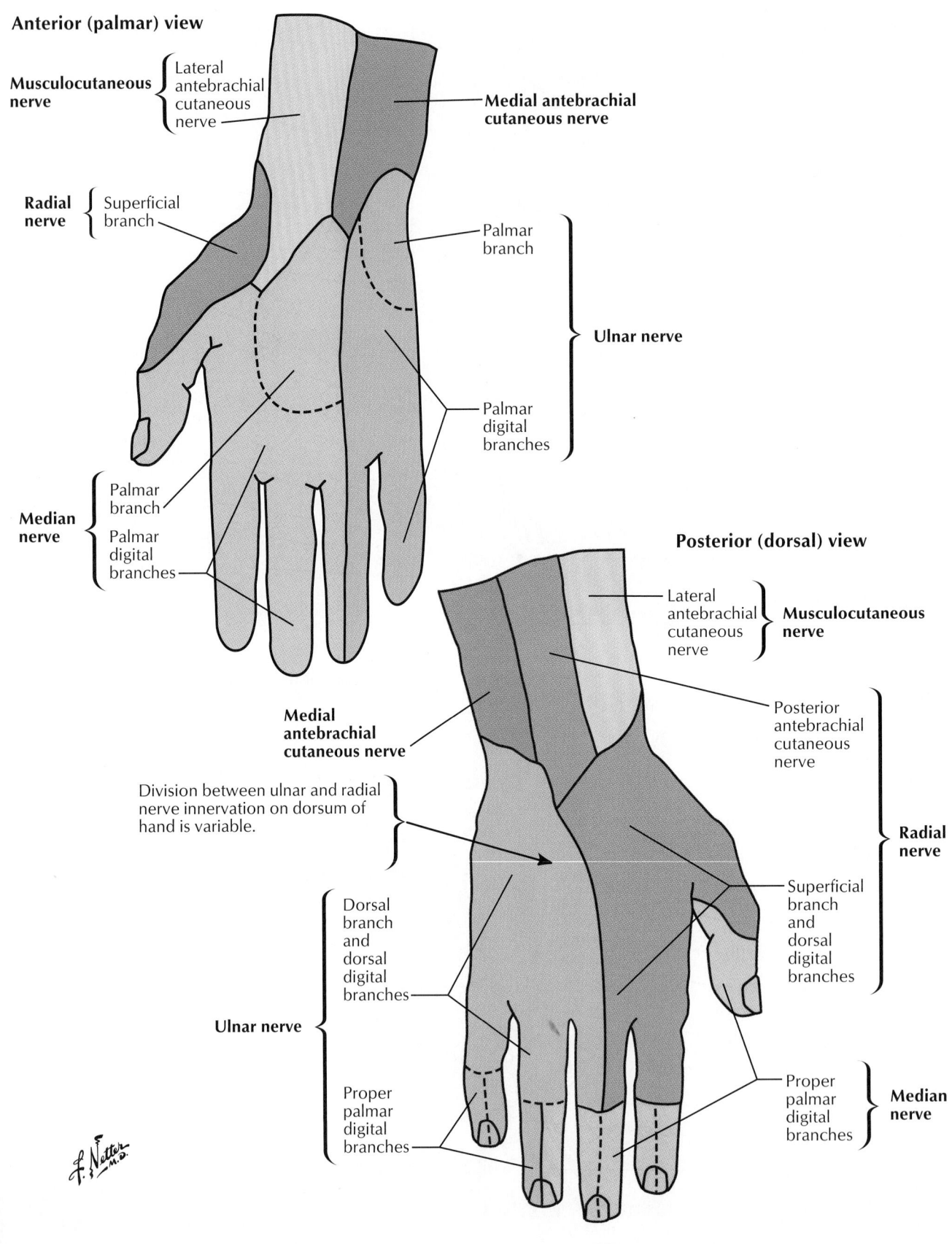

Anterior (palmar) view

Musculocutaneous nerve { Lateral antebrachial cutaneous nerve

Medial antebrachial cutaneous nerve

Radial nerve { Superficial branch

Palmar branch

Ulnar nerve

Palmar digital branches

Median nerve {
Palmar branch
Palmar digital branches

Posterior (dorsal) view

Lateral antebrachial cutaneous nerve } **Musculocutaneous nerve**

Medial antebrachial cutaneous nerve

Posterior antebrachial cutaneous nerve

Division between ulnar and radial nerve innervation on dorsum of hand is variable.

Radial nerve

Superficial branch and dorsal digital branches

Dorsal branch and dorsal digital branches

Ulnar nerve

Proper palmar digital branches

Proper palmar digital branches } **Median nerve**

f. Netter M.D.

Plate 472   Cutaneous Innervation of Wrist and Hand. (Netter: Atlas of Human Anatomy, 4 ed, 2006, Saunders.)

Anterior view

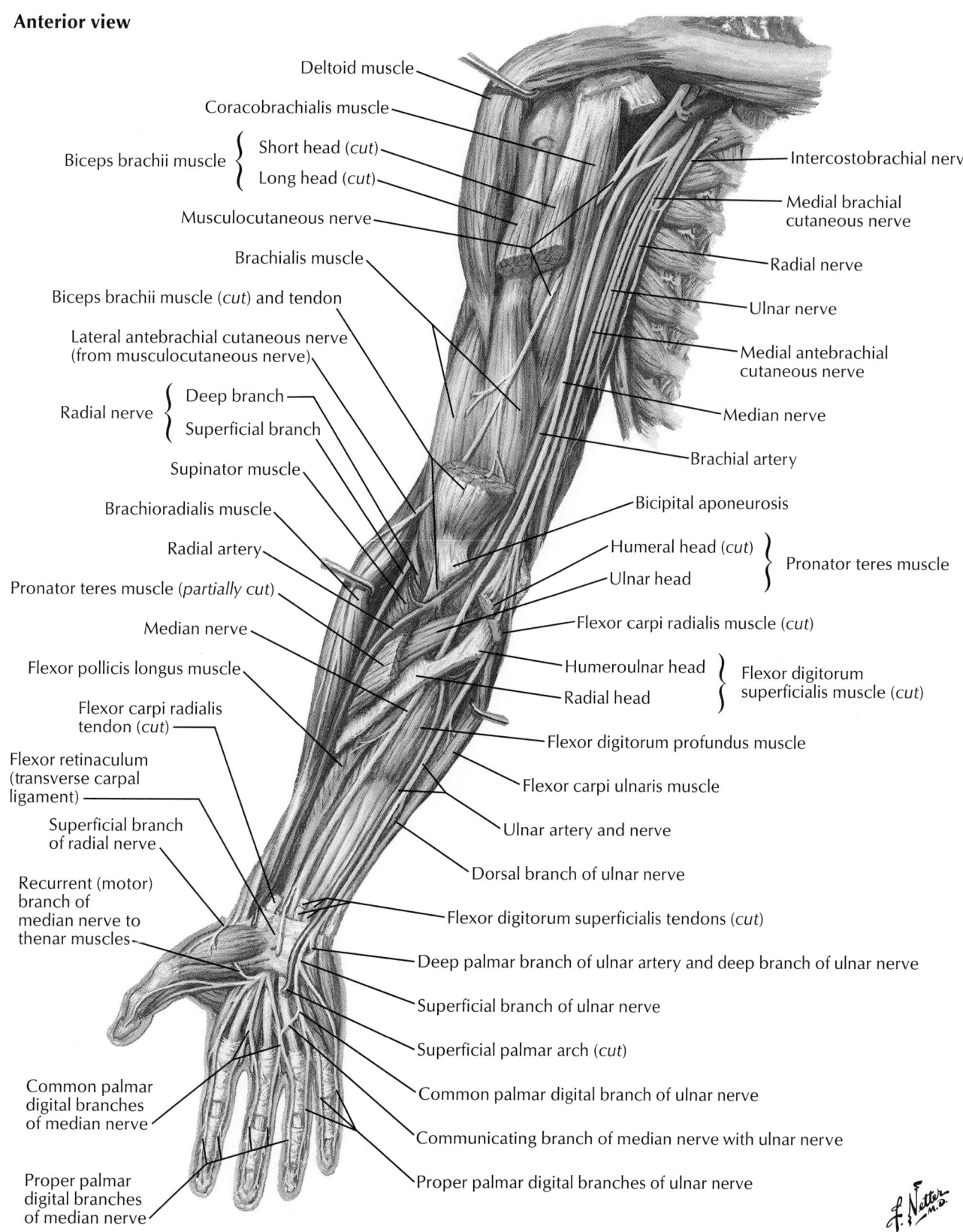

Deltoid muscle

Coracobrachialis muscle

Biceps brachii muscle
- Short head (*cut*)
- Long head (*cut*)

Musculocutaneous nerve

Brachialis muscle

Biceps brachii muscle (*cut*) and tendon

Lateral antebrachial cutaneous nerve (from musculocutaneous nerve)

Radial nerve
- Deep branch
- Superficial branch

Supinator muscle

Brachioradialis muscle

Radial artery

Pronator teres muscle (*partially cut*)

Median nerve

Flexor pollicis longus muscle

Flexor carpi radialis tendon (*cut*)

Flexor retinaculum (transverse carpal ligament)

Superficial branch of radial nerve

Recurrent (motor) branch of median nerve to thenar muscles

Common palmar digital branches of median nerve

Proper palmar digital branches of median nerve

Intercostobrachial nerve

Medial brachial cutaneous nerve

Radial nerve

Ulnar nerve

Medial antebrachial cutaneous nerve

Median nerve

Brachial artery

Bicipital aponeurosis

Humeral head (*cut*)
Ulnar head
} Pronator teres muscle

Flexor carpi radialis muscle (*cut*)

Humeroulnar head
Radial head
} Flexor digitorum superficialis muscle (*cut*)

Flexor digitorum profundus muscle

Flexor carpi ulnaris muscle

Ulnar artery and nerve

Dorsal branch of ulnar nerve

Flexor digitorum superficialis tendons (*cut*)

Deep palmar branch of ulnar artery and deep branch of ulnar nerve

Superficial branch of ulnar nerve

Superficial palmar arch (*cut*)

Common palmar digital branch of ulnar nerve

Communicating branch of median nerve with ulnar nerve

Proper palmar digital branches of ulnar nerve

Plate 473   Arteries and Nerves of Upper Limb. (Netter: Atlas of Human Anatomy, 4 ed, 2006, Saunders.)

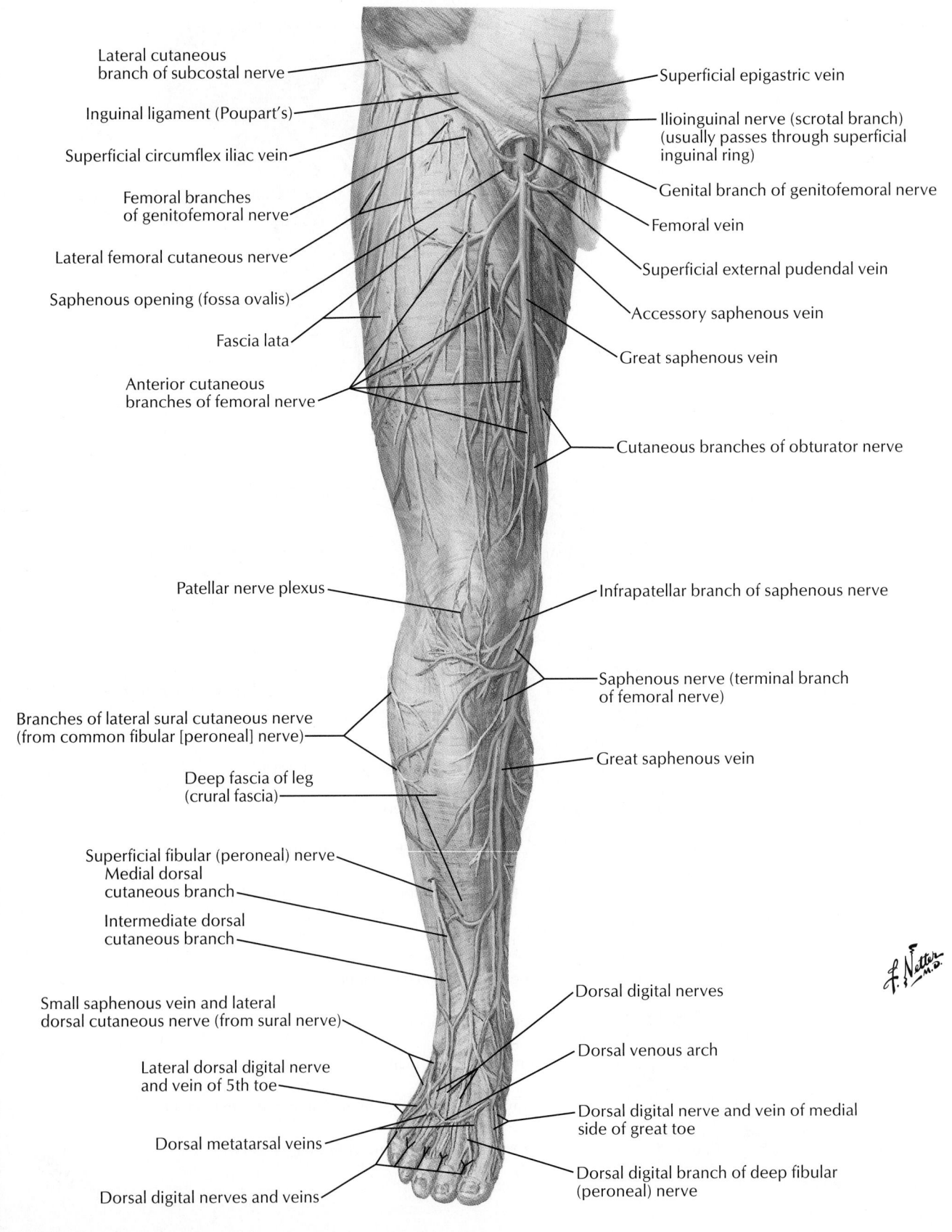

Lateral cutaneous branch of subcostal nerve

Inguinal ligament (Poupart's)

Superficial circumflex iliac vein

Femoral branches of genitofemoral nerve

Lateral femoral cutaneous nerve

Saphenous opening (fossa ovalis)

Fascia lata

Anterior cutaneous branches of femoral nerve

Patellar nerve plexus

Branches of lateral sural cutaneous nerve (from common fibular [peroneal] nerve)

Deep fascia of leg (crural fascia)

Superficial fibular (peroneal) nerve
Medial dorsal cutaneous branch

Intermediate dorsal cutaneous branch

Small saphenous vein and lateral dorsal cutaneous nerve (from sural nerve)

Lateral dorsal digital nerve and vein of 5th toe

Dorsal metatarsal veins

Dorsal digital nerves and veins

Superficial epigastric vein

Ilioinguinal nerve (scrotal branch) (usually passes through superficial inguinal ring)

Genital branch of genitofemoral nerve

Femoral vein

Superficial external pudendal vein

Accessory saphenous vein

Great saphenous vein

Cutaneous branches of obturator nerve

Infrapatellar branch of saphenous nerve

Saphenous nerve (terminal branch of femoral nerve)

Great saphenous vein

Dorsal digital nerves

Dorsal venous arch

Dorsal digital nerve and vein of medial side of great toe

Dorsal digital branch of deep fibular (peroneal) nerve

Plate 544   Superficial Nerves and Veins of Lower Limb: Anterior View. (Netter: Atlas of Human Anatomy, 4 ed, 2006, Saunders.)

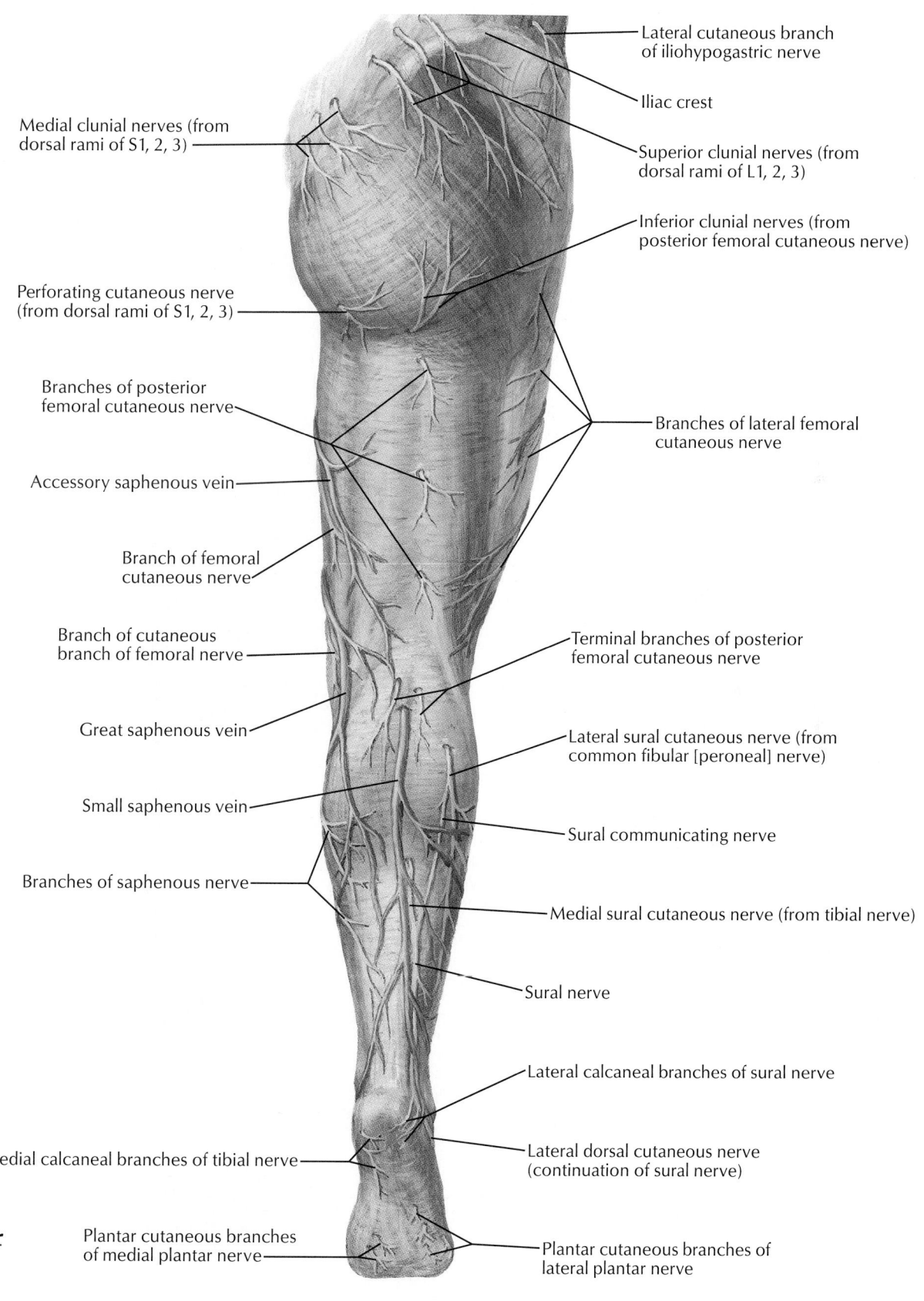

Lateral cutaneous branch of iliohypogastric nerve

Iliac crest

Medial clunial nerves (from dorsal rami of S1, 2, 3)

Superior clunial nerves (from dorsal rami of L1, 2, 3)

Inferior clunial nerves (from posterior femoral cutaneous nerve)

Perforating cutaneous nerve (from dorsal rami of S1, 2, 3)

Branches of posterior femoral cutaneous nerve

Branches of lateral femoral cutaneous nerve

Accessory saphenous vein

Branch of femoral cutaneous nerve

Branch of cutaneous branch of femoral nerve

Terminal branches of posterior femoral cutaneous nerve

Great saphenous vein

Lateral sural cutaneous nerve (from common fibular [peroneal] nerve)

Small saphenous vein

Sural communicating nerve

Branches of saphenous nerve

Medial sural cutaneous nerve (from tibial nerve)

Sural nerve

Lateral calcaneal branches of sural nerve

Medial calcaneal branches of tibial nerve

Lateral dorsal cutaneous nerve (continuation of sural nerve)

Plantar cutaneous branches of medial plantar nerve

Plantar cutaneous branches of lateral plantar nerve

Plate 545   Superficial Nerves and Veins of Lower Limb: Posterior View. (Netter: Atlas of Human Anatomy, 4 ed, 2006, Saunders.)

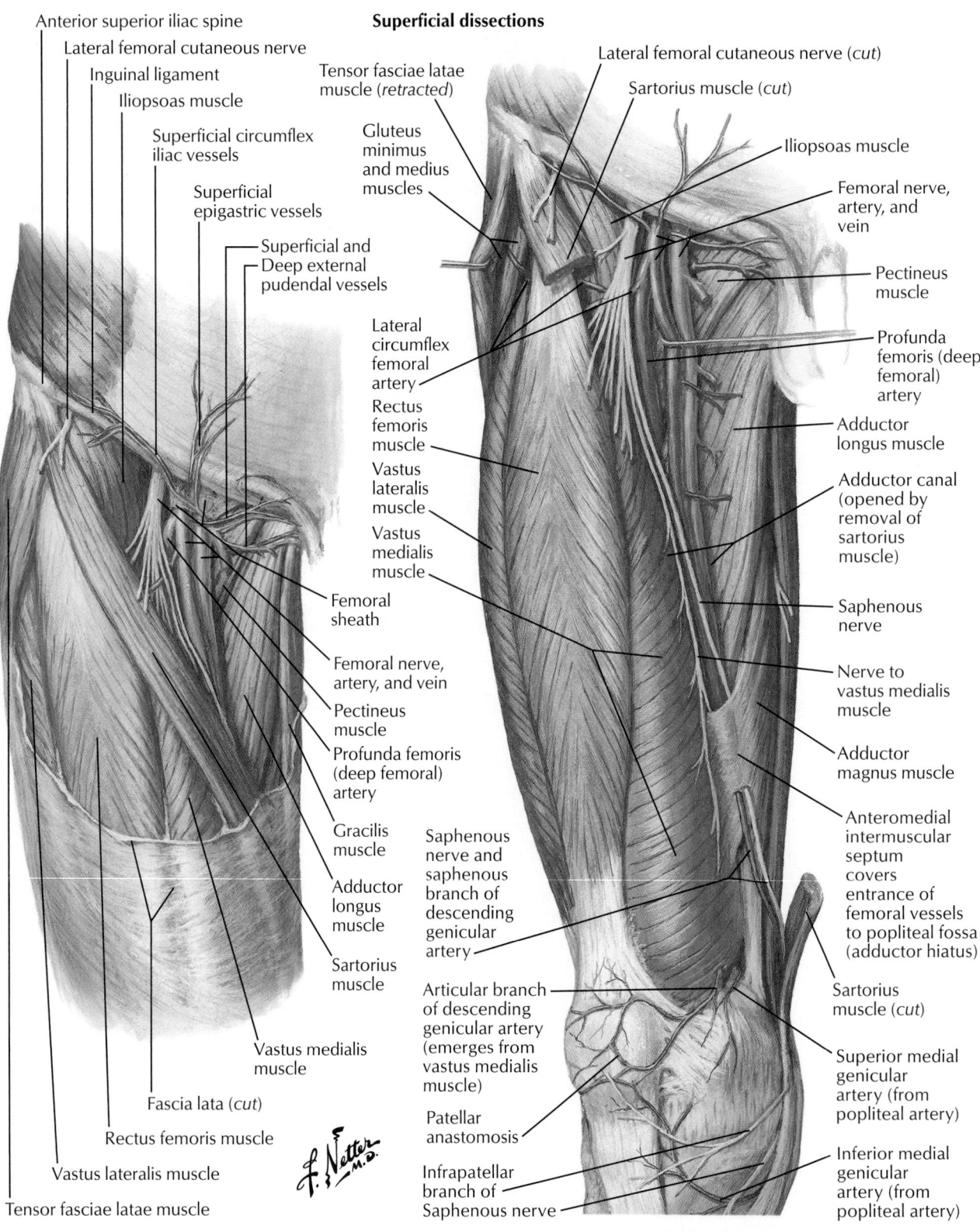

Anterior superior iliac spine
Lateral femoral cutaneous nerve
Inguinal ligament
Iliopsoas muscle
Superficial circumflex iliac vessels
Superficial epigastric vessels
Superficial and Deep external pudendal vessels

Superficial dissections

Tensor fasciae latae muscle (*retracted*)
Gluteus minimus and medius muscles
Lateral circumflex femoral artery
Rectus femoris muscle
Vastus lateralis muscle
Vastus medialis muscle
Femoral sheath
Femoral nerve, artery, and vein
Pectineus muscle
Profunda femoris (deep femoral) artery
Gracilis muscle
Adductor longus muscle
Sartorius muscle
Vastus medialis muscle
Fascia lata (*cut*)
Rectus femoris muscle
Vastus lateralis muscle
Tensor fasciae latae muscle

Lateral femoral cutaneous nerve (*cut*)
Sartorius muscle (*cut*)
Iliopsoas muscle
Femoral nerve, artery, and vein
Pectineus muscle
Profunda femoris (deep femoral) artery
Adductor longus muscle
Adductor canal (opened by removal of sartorius muscle)
Saphenous nerve
Nerve to vastus medialis muscle
Adductor magnus muscle
Anteromedial intermuscular septum covers entrance of femoral vessels to popliteal fossa (adductor hiatus)
Sartorius muscle (*cut*)
Superior medial genicular artery (from popliteal artery)
Inferior medial genicular artery (from popliteal artery)

Saphenous nerve and saphenous branch of descending genicular artery
Articular branch of descending genicular artery (emerges from vastus medialis muscle)
Patellar anastomosis
Infrapatellar branch of Saphenous nerve

Plate 500 Arteries and Nerves of Thigh: Anterior View. (Netter: Atlas of Human Anatomy, 4 ed, 2006, Saunders.)

96

Deep dissection

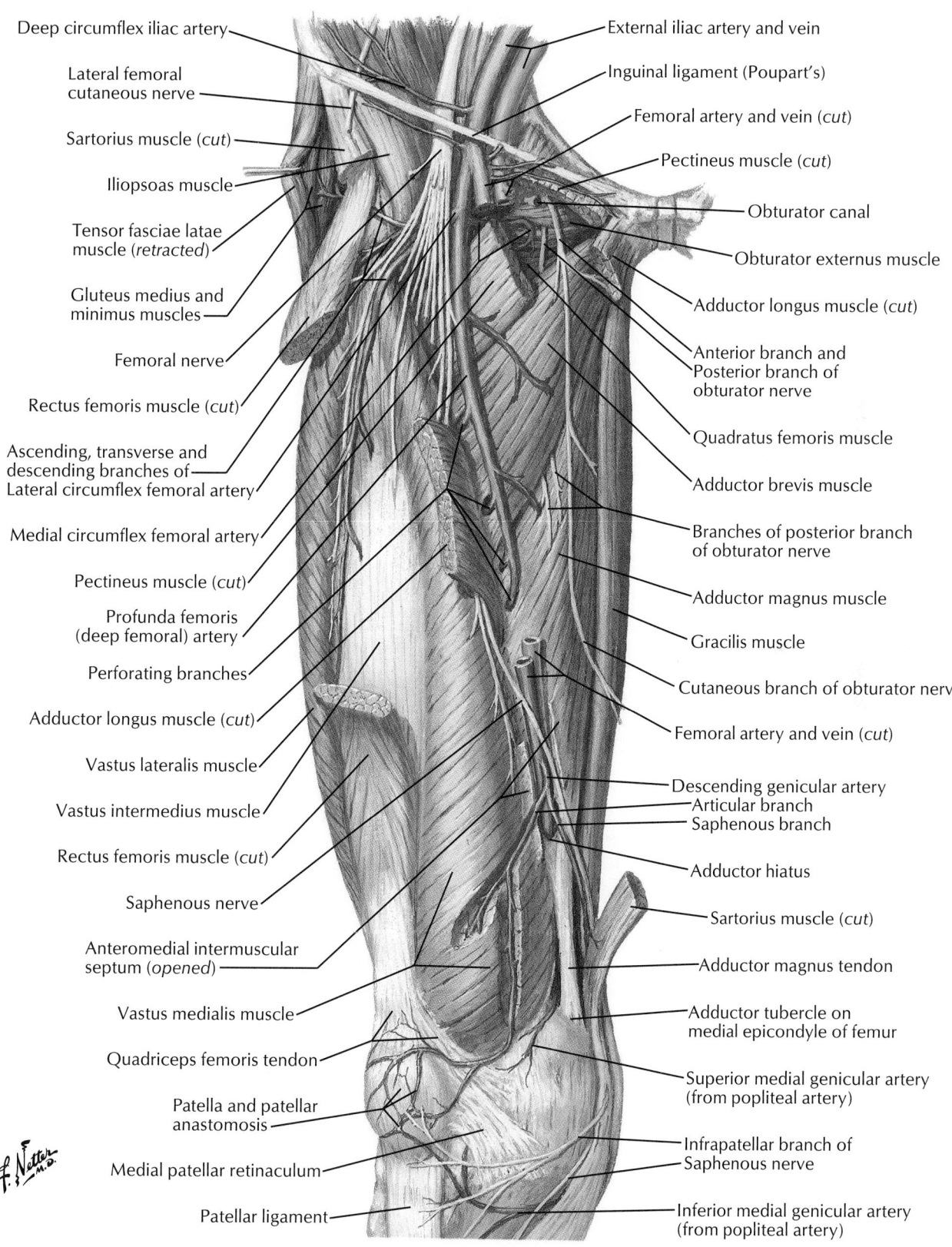

Deep circumflex iliac artery

Lateral femoral cutaneous nerve

Sartorius muscle (*cut*)

Iliopsoas muscle

Tensor fasciae latae muscle (*retracted*)

Gluteus medius and minimus muscles

Femoral nerve

Rectus femoris muscle (*cut*)

Ascending, transverse and descending branches of Lateral circumflex femoral artery

Medial circumflex femoral artery

Pectineus muscle (*cut*)

Profunda femoris (deep femoral) artery

Perforating branches

Adductor longus muscle (*cut*)

Vastus lateralis muscle

Vastus intermedius muscle

Rectus femoris muscle (*cut*)

Saphenous nerve

Anteromedial intermuscular septum (*opened*)

Vastus medialis muscle

Quadriceps femoris tendon

Patella and patellar anastomosis

Medial patellar retinaculum

Patellar ligament

External iliac artery and vein

Inguinal ligament (Poupart's)

Femoral artery and vein (*cut*)

Pectineus muscle (*cut*)

Obturator canal

Obturator externus muscle

Adductor longus muscle (*cut*)

Anterior branch and Posterior branch of obturator nerve

Quadratus femoris muscle

Adductor brevis muscle

Branches of posterior branch of obturator nerve

Adductor magnus muscle

Gracilis muscle

Cutaneous branch of obturator nerve

Femoral artery and vein (*cut*)

Descending genicular artery
Articular branch
Saphenous branch

Adductor hiatus

Sartorius muscle (*cut*)

Adductor magnus tendon

Adductor tubercle on medial epicondyle of femur

Superior medial genicular artery (from popliteal artery)

Infrapatellar branch of Saphenous nerve

Inferior medial genicular artery (from popliteal artery)

Plate 501   Arteries and Nerves of Thigh: Anterior View. (Netter: Atlas of Human Anatomy, 4 ed, 2006, Saunders.)

Deep dissection

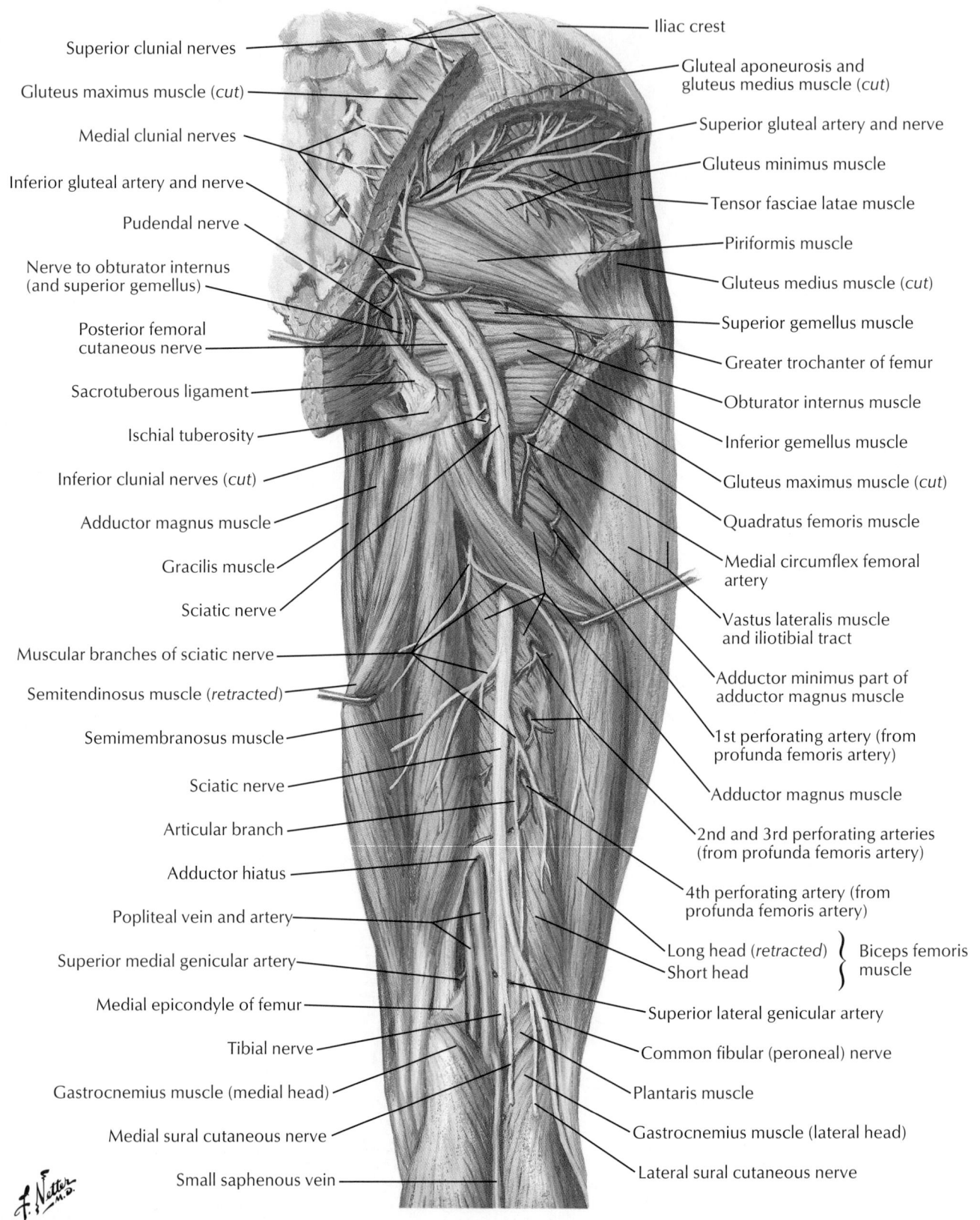

Superior clunial nerves

Gluteus maximus muscle (*cut*)

Medial clunial nerves

Inferior gluteal artery and nerve

Pudendal nerve

Nerve to obturator internus (and superior gemellus)

Posterior femoral cutaneous nerve

Sacrotuberous ligament

Ischial tuberosity

Inferior clunial nerves (*cut*)

Adductor magnus muscle

Gracilis muscle

Sciatic nerve

Muscular branches of sciatic nerve

Semitendinosus muscle (*retracted*)

Semimembranosus muscle

Sciatic nerve

Articular branch

Adductor hiatus

Popliteal vein and artery

Superior medial genicular artery

Medial epicondyle of femur

Tibial nerve

Gastrocnemius muscle (medial head)

Medial sural cutaneous nerve

Small saphenous vein

Iliac crest

Gluteal aponeurosis and gluteus medius muscle (*cut*)

Superior gluteal artery and nerve

Gluteus minimus muscle

Tensor fasciae latae muscle

Piriformis muscle

Gluteus medius muscle (*cut*)

Superior gemellus muscle

Greater trochanter of femur

Obturator internus muscle

Inferior gemellus muscle

Gluteus maximus muscle (*cut*)

Quadratus femoris muscle

Medial circumflex femoral artery

Vastus lateralis muscle and iliotibial tract

Adductor minimus part of adductor magnus muscle

1st perforating artery (from profunda femoris artery)

Adductor magnus muscle

2nd and 3rd perforating arteries (from profunda femoris artery)

4th perforating artery (from profunda femoris artery)

Long head (*retracted*) ⎱ Biceps femoris
Short head ⎰ muscle

Superior lateral genicular artery

Common fibular (peroneal) nerve

Plantaris muscle

Gastrocnemius muscle (lateral head)

Lateral sural cutaneous nerve

Plate 502   Arteries and Nerves of Thigh: Posterior View. (Netter: Atlas of Human Anatomy, 4 ed, 2006, Saunders.)

Horizontal section

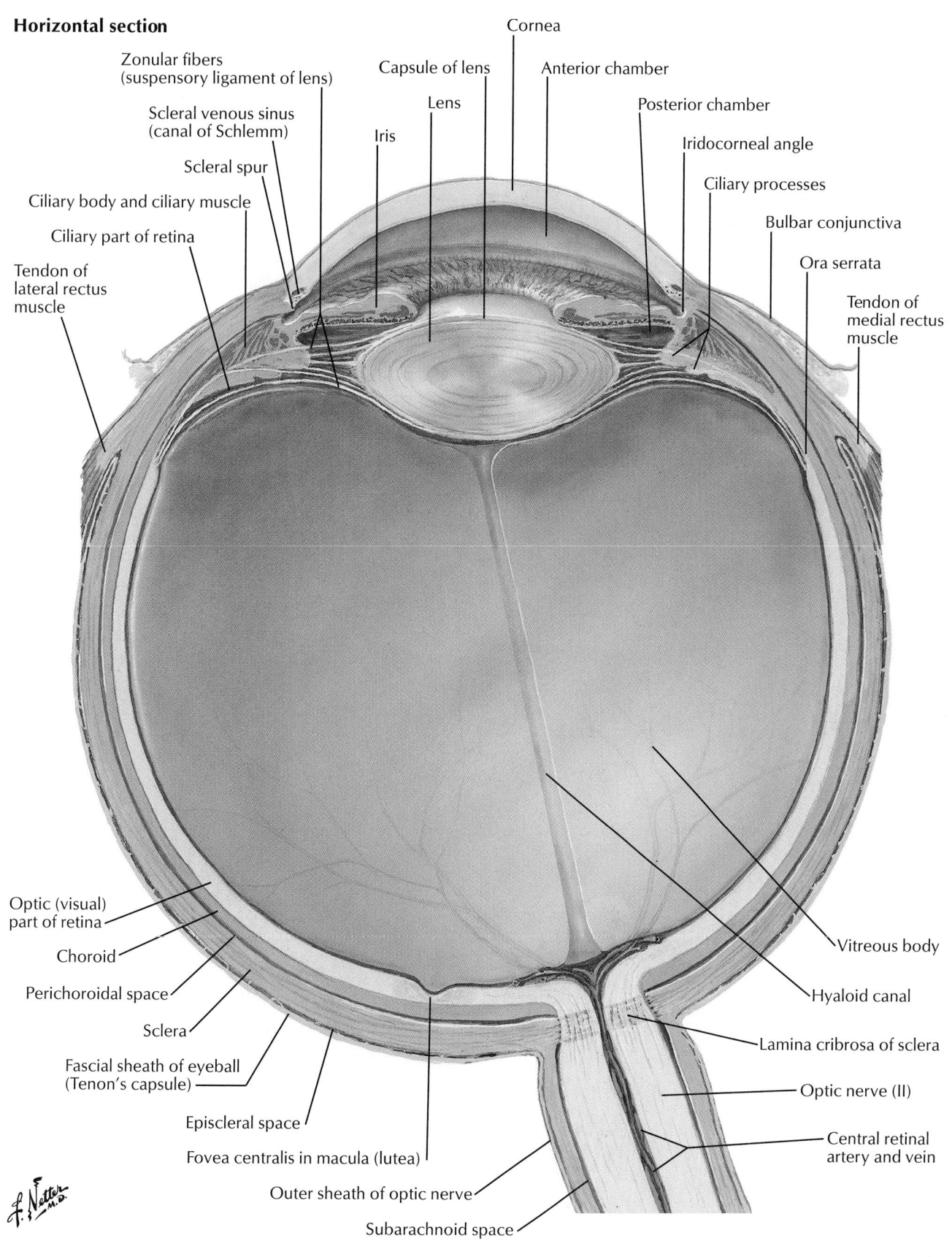

Zonular fibers (suspensory ligament of lens)

Capsule of lens

Cornea

Anterior chamber

Scleral venous sinus (canal of Schlemm)

Lens

Posterior chamber

Scleral spur

Iris

Iridocorneal angle

Ciliary body and ciliary muscle

Ciliary processes

Ciliary part of retina

Bulbar conjunctiva

Tendon of lateral rectus muscle

Ora serrata

Tendon of medial rectus muscle

Optic (visual) part of retina

Choroid

Perichoroidal space

Sclera

Fascial sheath of eyeball (Tenon's capsule)

Episcleral space

Fovea centralis in macula (lutea)

Outer sheath of optic nerve

Subarachnoid space

Vitreous body

Hyaloid canal

Lamina cribrosa of sclera

Optic nerve (II)

Central retinal artery and vein

Plate 87   Eyeball. (Netter: Atlas of Human Anatomy, 4 ed, 2006, Saunders.)

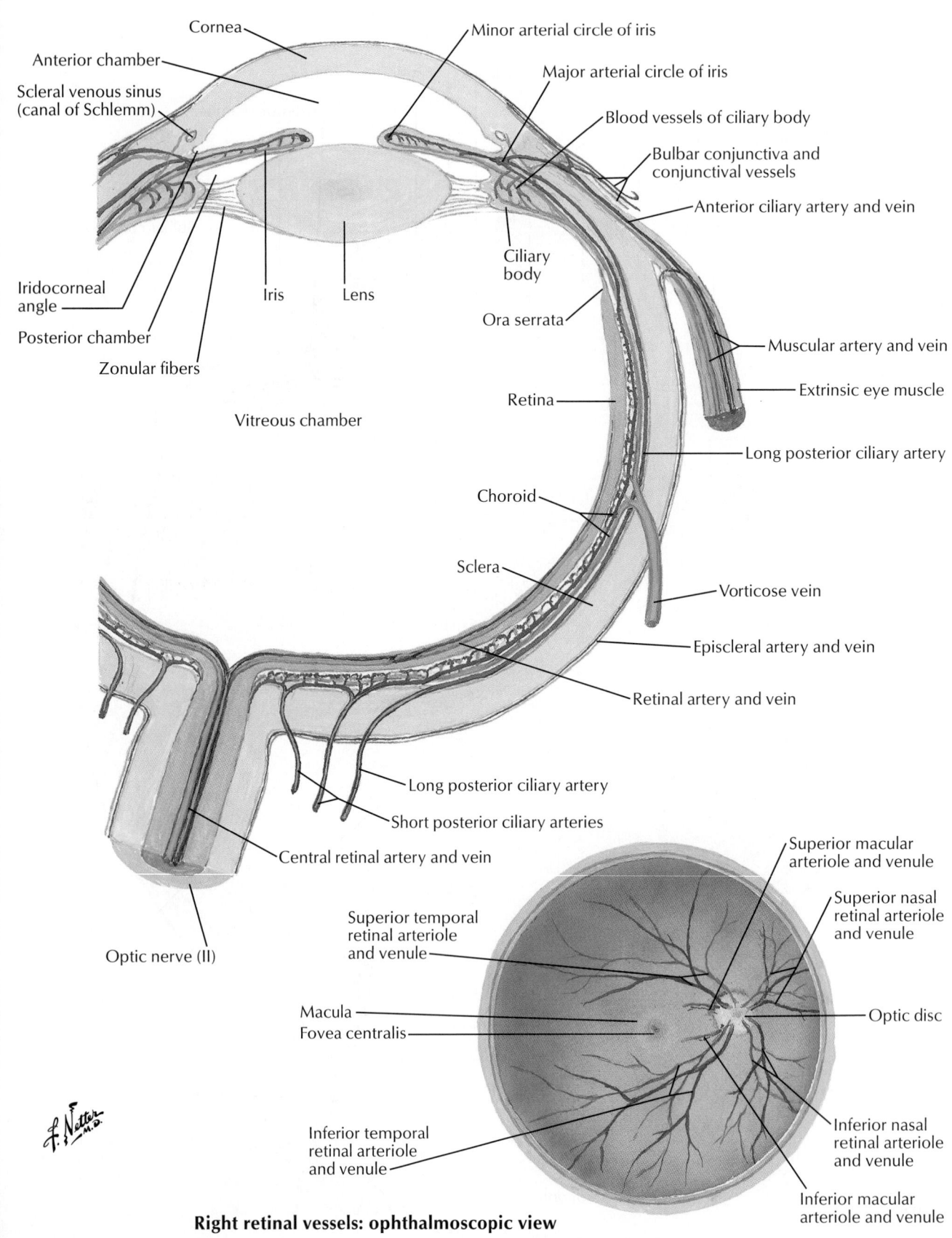

Cornea

Minor arterial circle of iris

Anterior chamber

Major arterial circle of iris

Scleral venous sinus
(canal of Schlemm)

Blood vessels of ciliary body

Bulbar conjunctiva and
conjunctival vessels

Anterior ciliary artery and vein

Ciliary
body

Iridocorneal
angle

Iris   Lens

Ora serrata

Muscular artery and vein

Posterior chamber

Extrinsic eye muscle

Zonular fibers

Retina

Long posterior ciliary artery

Vitreous chamber

Choroid

Sclera

Vorticose vein

Episcleral artery and vein

Retinal artery and vein

Long posterior ciliary artery

Short posterior ciliary arteries

Central retinal artery and vein

Optic nerve (II)

Superior macular
arteriole and venule

Superior nasal
retinal arteriole
and venule

Superior temporal
retinal arteriole
and venule

Macula

Optic disc

Fovea centralis

Inferior nasal
retinal arteriole
and venule

Inferior temporal
retinal arteriole
and venule

Inferior macular
arteriole and venule

Right retinal vessels: ophthalmoscopic view

Plate 90   Intrinsic Arteries and Veins of Eye. (Netter: Atlas of Human Anatomy, 4 ed, 2006, Saunders.)

NETTER ANATOMY PLATE

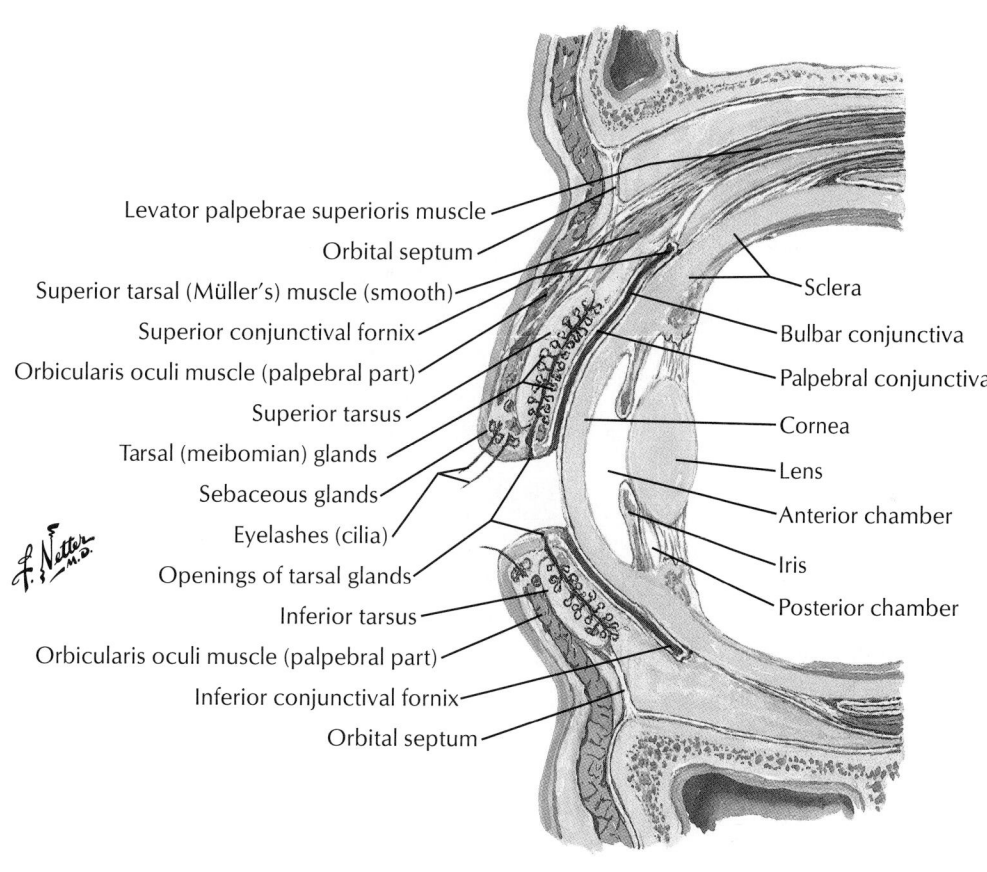

Levator palpebrae superioris muscle
Orbital septum
Superior tarsal (Müller's) muscle (smooth)
Superior conjunctival fornix
Orbicularis oculi muscle (palpebral part)
Superior tarsus
Tarsal (meibomian) glands
Sebaceous glands
Eyelashes (cilia)
Openings of tarsal glands
Inferior tarsus
Orbicularis oculi muscle (palpebral part)
Inferior conjunctival fornix
Orbital septum

Sclera
Bulbar conjunctiva
Palpebral conjunctiva
Cornea
Lens
Anterior chamber
Iris
Posterior chamber

Plate 81, Middle   Eyelid. (Netter: Atlas of Human Anatomy, 4 ed, 2006, Saunders.)

Superior palpebral conjunctiva:
tarsal (meibomian) glands
shining through

Seen through { Pupil
cornea { Iris

Corneoscleral junction
(corneal limbus)

Bulbar conjunctiva
over sclera

Inferior conjunctival fornix

Inferior palpebral conjunctiva:
tarsal glands shining through

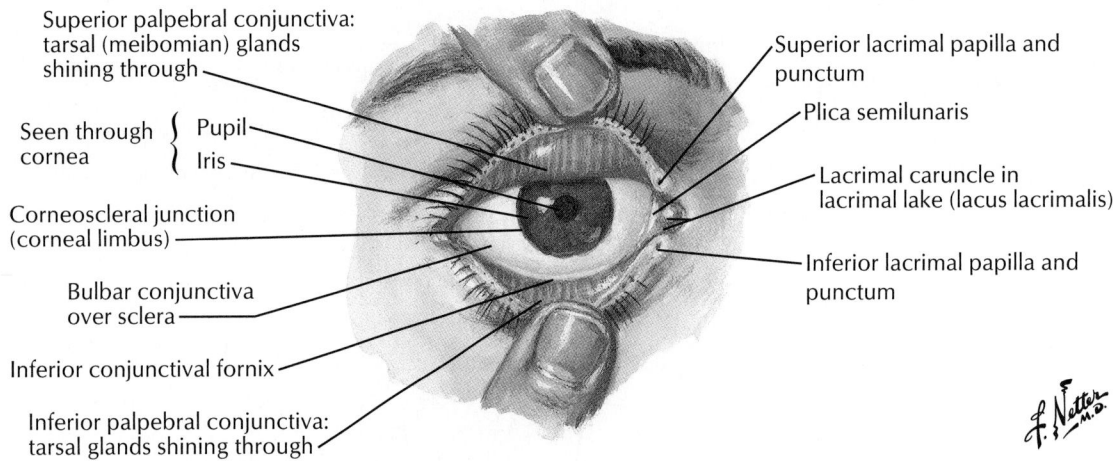

Superior lacrimal papilla and
punctum

Plica semilunaris

Lacrimal caruncle in
lacrimal lake (lacus lacrimalis)

Inferior lacrimal papilla and
punctum

Plate 81, Upper Eyelid. (Netter: Atlas of Human Anatomy, 4 ed, 2006, Saunders.)

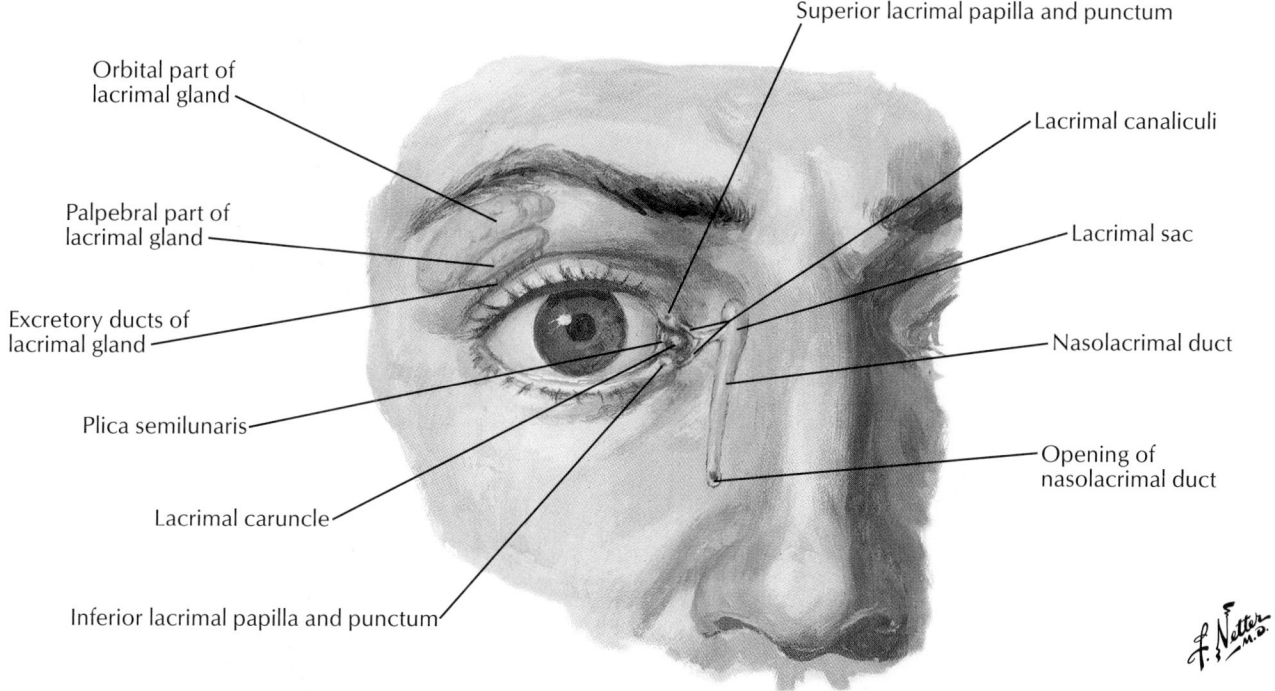

Orbital part of
lacrimal gland

Palpebral part of
lacrimal gland

Excretory ducts of
lacrimal gland

Plica semilunaris

Lacrimal caruncle

Inferior lacrimal papilla and punctum

Superior lacrimal papilla and punctum

Lacrimal canaliculi

Lacrimal sac

Nasolacrimal duct

Opening of
nasolacrimal duct

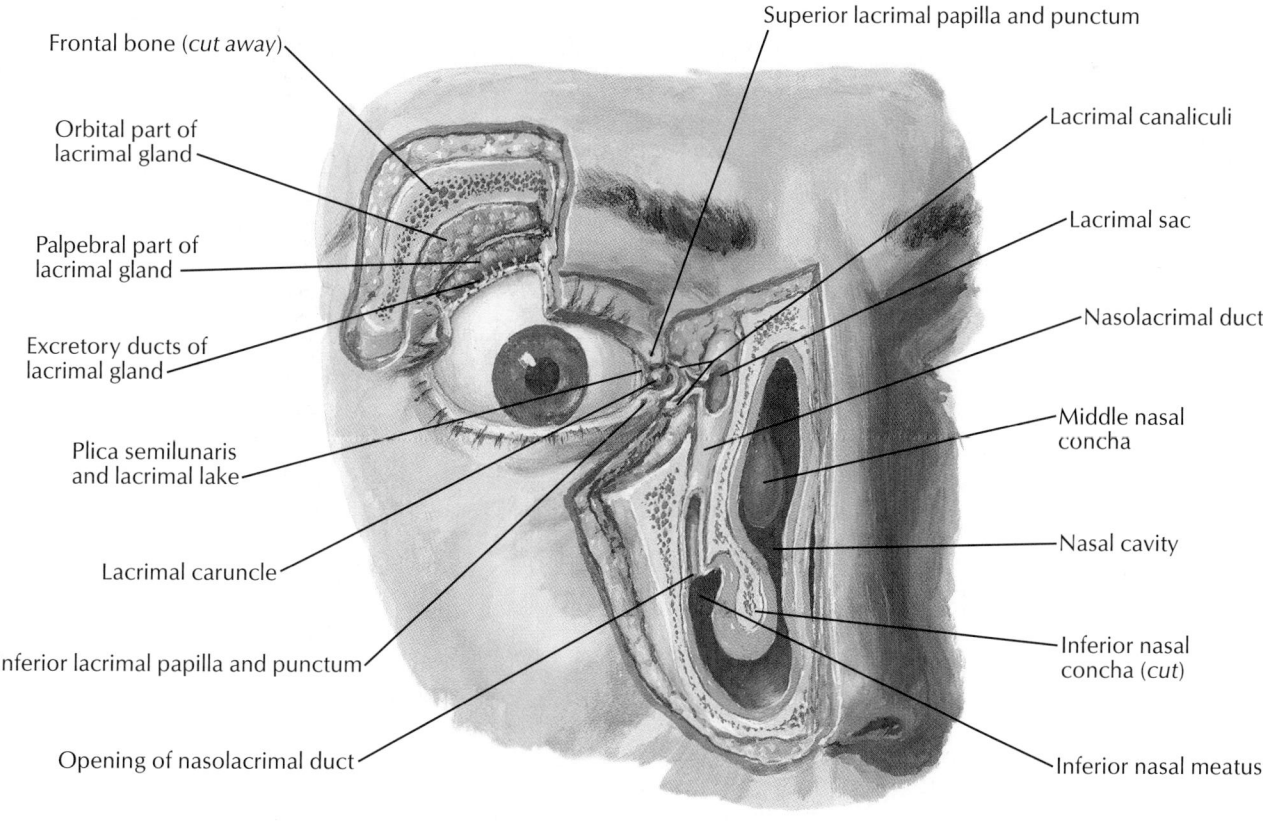

Frontal bone (*cut away*)

Orbital part of
lacrimal gland

Palpebral part of
lacrimal gland

Excretory ducts of
lacrimal gland

Plica semilunaris
and lacrimal lake

Lacrimal caruncle

Inferior lacrimal papilla and punctum

Opening of nasolacrimal duct

Superior lacrimal papilla and punctum

Lacrimal canaliculi

Lacrimal sac

Nasolacrimal duct

Middle nasal
concha

Nasal cavity

Inferior nasal
concha (*cut*)

Inferior nasal meatus

Plate 82 Lacrimal Apparatus. (Netter: Atlas of Human Anatomy, 4 ed, 2006, Saunders.)

Frontal section

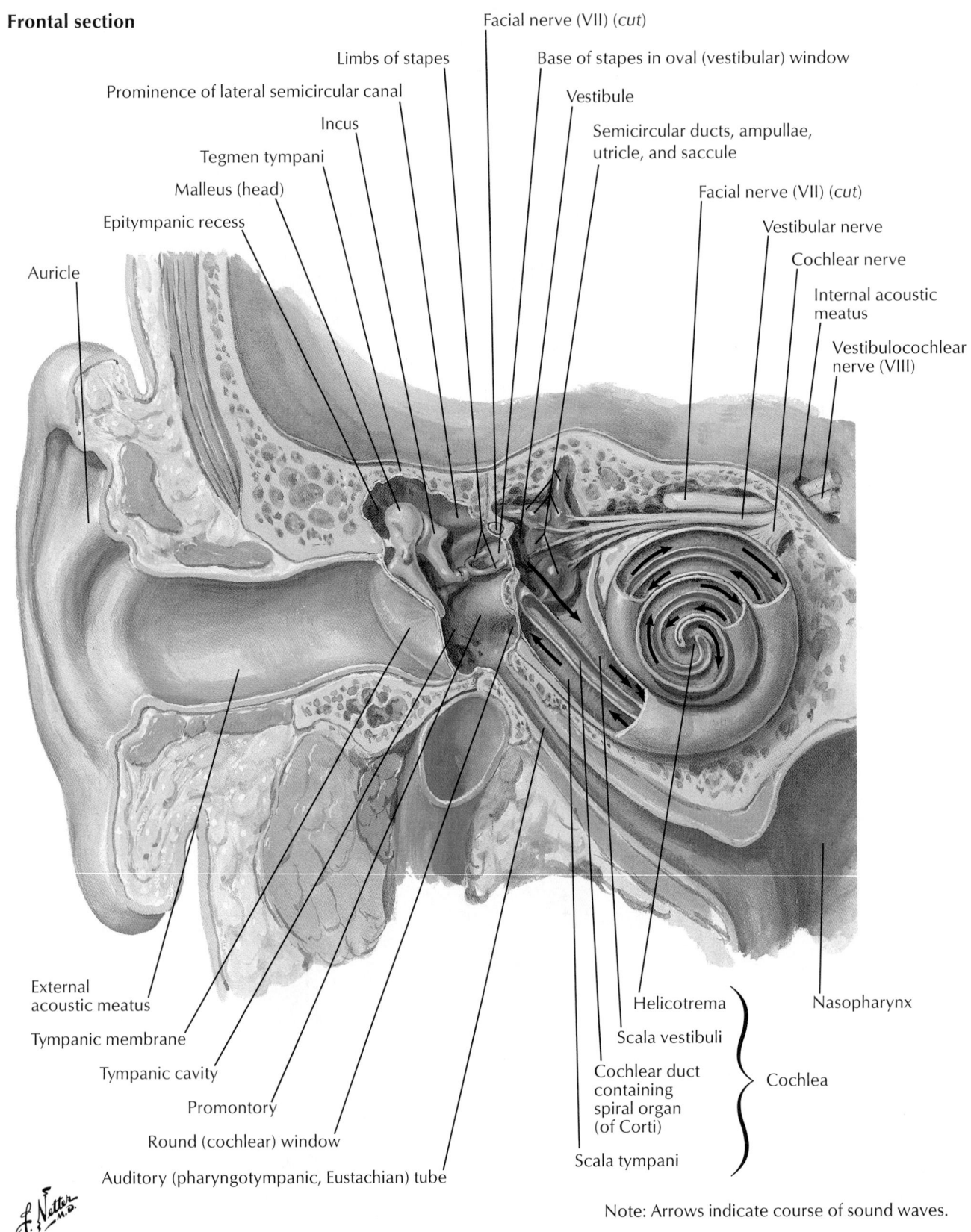

Limbs of stapes

Prominence of lateral semicircular canal

Incus

Tegmen tympani

Malleus (head)

Epitympanic recess

Auricle

Facial nerve (VII) *(cut)*

Base of stapes in oval (vestibular) window

Vestibule

Semicircular ducts, ampullae, utricle, and saccule

Facial nerve (VII) *(cut)*

Vestibular nerve

Cochlear nerve

Internal acoustic meatus

Vestibulocochlear nerve (VIII)

External acoustic meatus

Tympanic membrane

Tympanic cavity

Promontory

Round (cochlear) window

Auditory (pharyngotympanic, Eustachian) tube

Helicotrema

Scala vestibuli

Cochlear duct containing spiral organ (of Corti)

Scala tympani

Nasopharynx

Cochlea

Note: Arrows indicate course of sound waves.

Plate 92 Pathway of Sound Reception. (Netter: Atlas of Human Anatomy, 4 ed, 2006, Saunders.)

Medial wall of tympanic cavity: lateral view

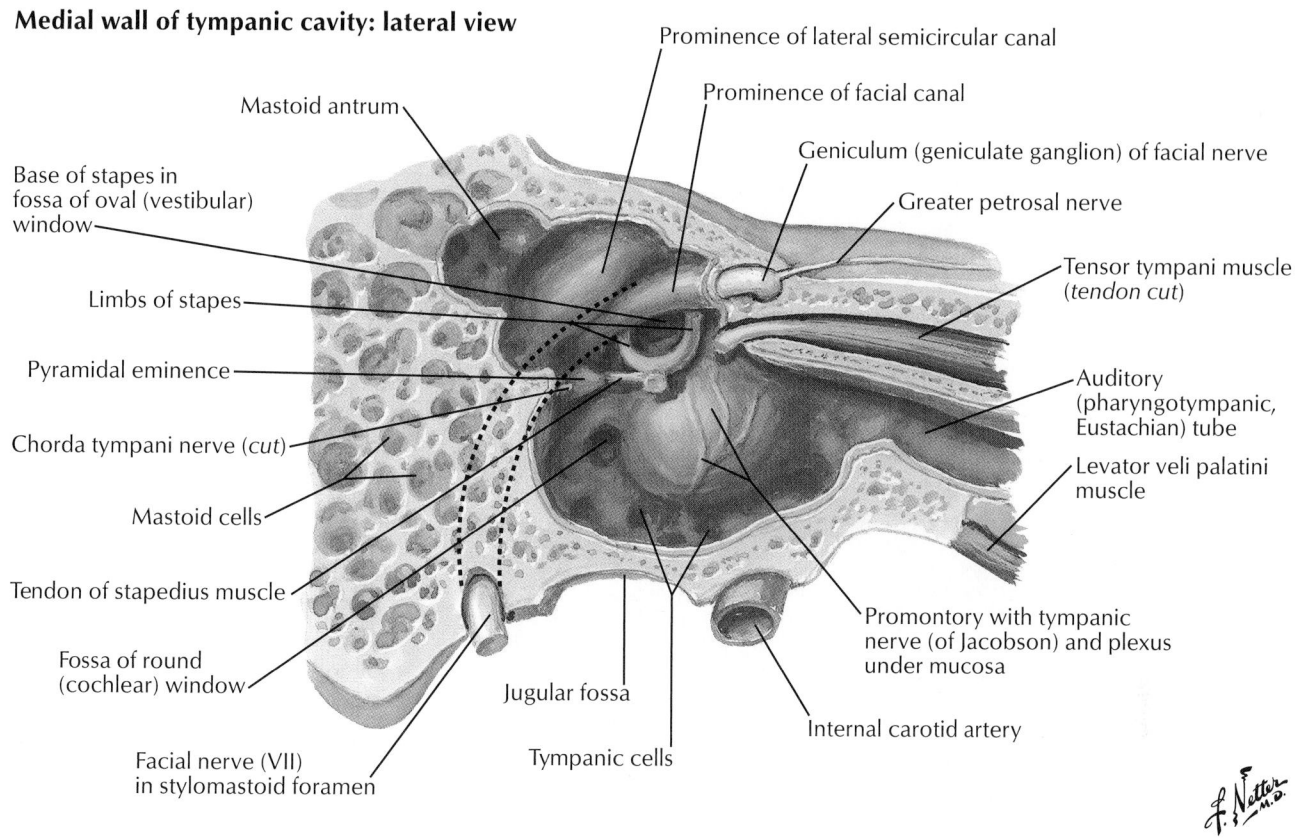

Mastoid antrum

Prominence of lateral semicircular canal

Prominence of facial canal

Geniculum (geniculate ganglion) of facial nerve

Greater petrosal nerve

Base of stapes in fossa of oval (vestibular) window

Limbs of stapes

Pyramidal eminence

Chorda tympani nerve (*cut*)

Mastoid cells

Tendon of stapedius muscle

Fossa of round (cochlear) window

Facial nerve (VII) in stylomastoid foramen

Jugular fossa

Tympanic cells

Tensor tympani muscle (*tendon cut*)

Auditory (pharyngotympanic, Eustachian) tube

Levator veli palatini muscle

Promontory with tympanic nerve (of Jacobson) and plexus under mucosa

Internal carotid artery

Plate 94 Tympanic Cavity. (Netter: Atlas of Human Anatomy, 4 ed, 2006, Saunders.)

Dissected right bony labyrinth (otic capsule): membranous labyrinth removed

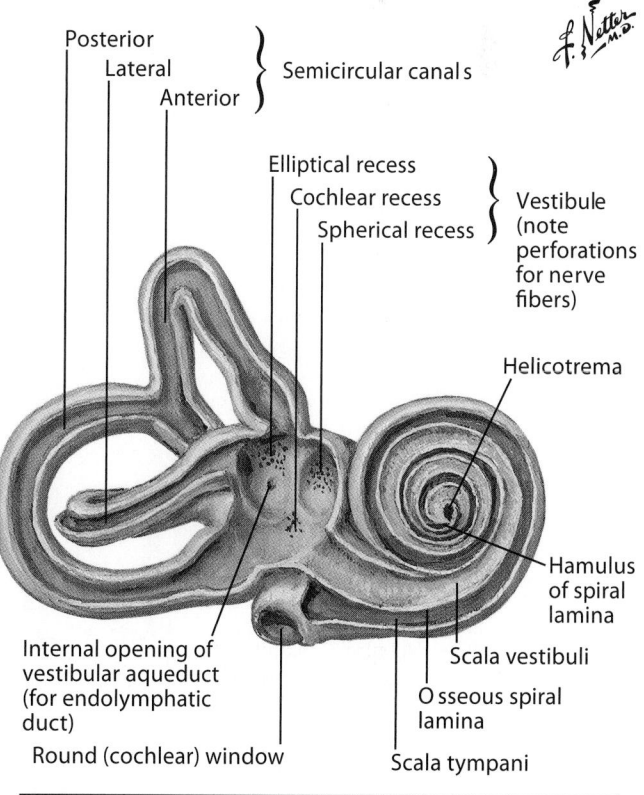

Posterior
Lateral
Anterior
Semicircular canals

Elliptical recess
Cochlear recess
Spherical recess
Vestibule (note perforations for nerve fibers)

Helicotrema

Internal opening of vestibular aqueduct (for endolymphatic duct)

Round (cochlear) window

Hamulus of spiral lamina

Scala vestibuli

Osseous spiral lamina

Scala tympani

Otoscopic view of right tympanic membrane

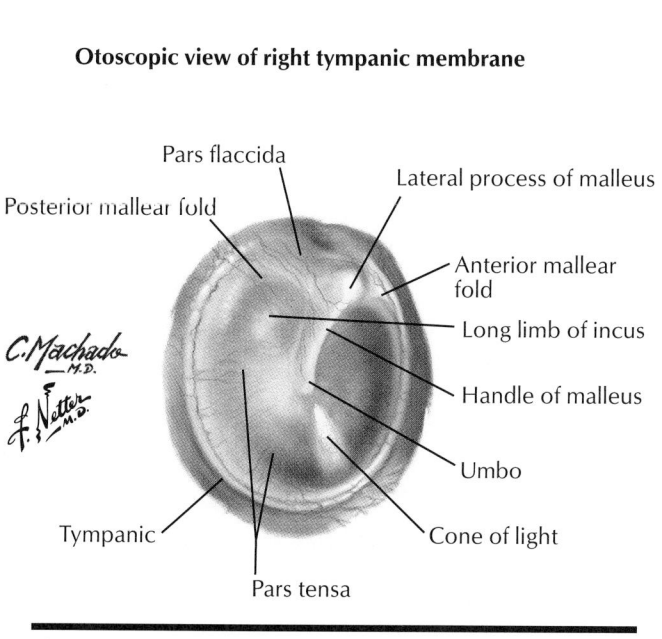

Pars flaccida

Posterior mallear fold

Lateral process of malleus

Anterior mallear fold

Long limb of incus

Handle of malleus

Umbo

Cone of light

Tympanic

Pars tensa

Plate 93 Tympanic Cavity. (Netter: Atlas of Human Anatomy, 4 ed, 2006, Saunders.)

Plate 95 Bony Membranous Labyrinth. (Netter: Atlas of Human Anatomy, 4 ed, 2006, Saunders.)

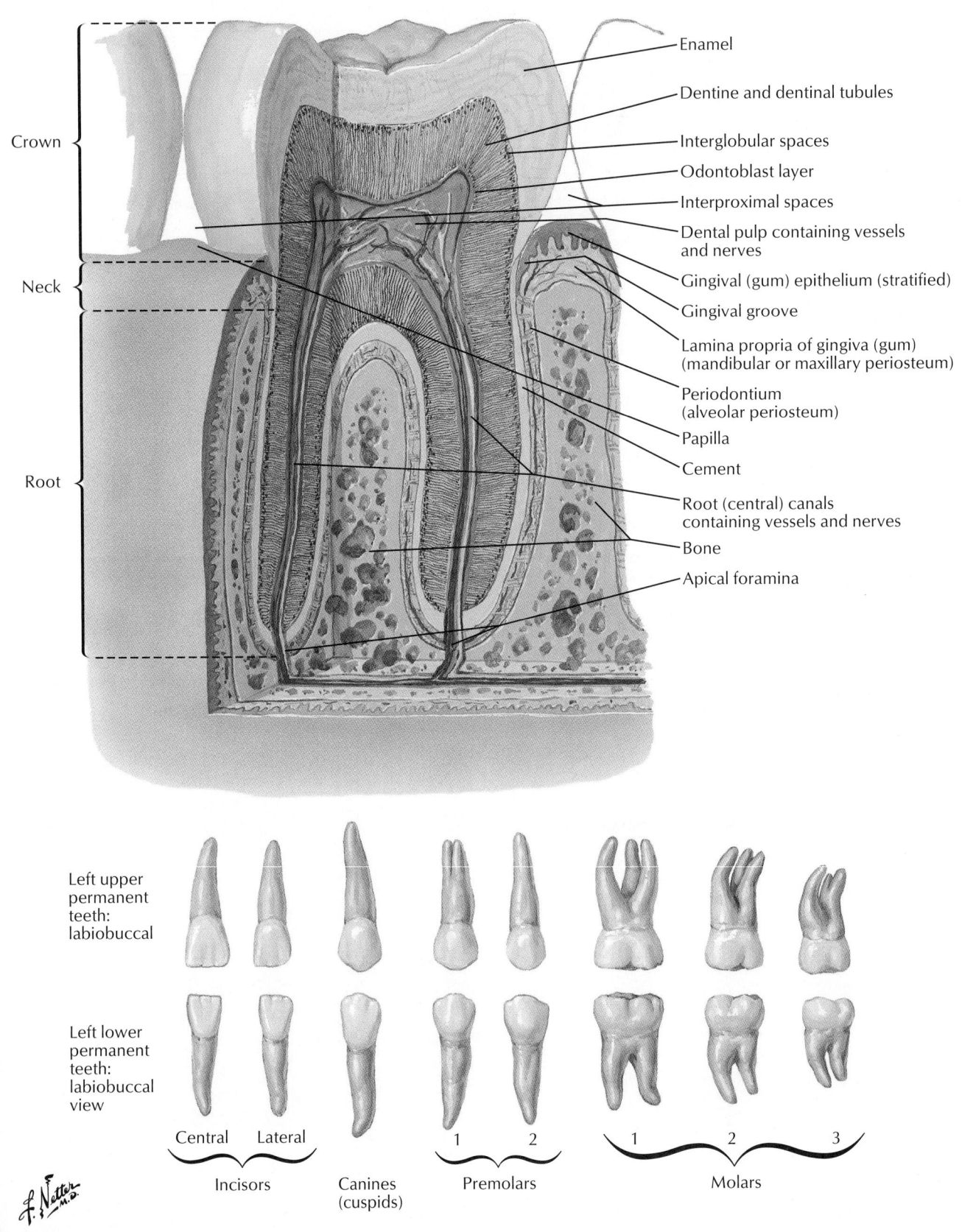

Crown

Neck

Root

Enamel

Dentine and dentinal tubules

Interglobular spaces

Odontoblast layer

Interproximal spaces

Dental pulp containing vessels and nerves

Gingival (gum) epithelium (stratified)

Gingival groove

Lamina propria of gingiva (gum) (mandibular or maxillary periosteum)

Periodontium (alveolar periosteum)

Papilla

Cement

Root (central) canals containing vessels and nerves

Bone

Apical foramina

Left upper permanent teeth: labiobuccal

Left lower permanent teeth: labiobuccal view

Central   Lateral

Incisors

Canines (cuspids)

1   2

Premolars

1   2   3

Molars

Plate 57 Teeth. (Netter: Atlas of Human Anatomy, 4 ed, 2006, Saunders.)

Tongue

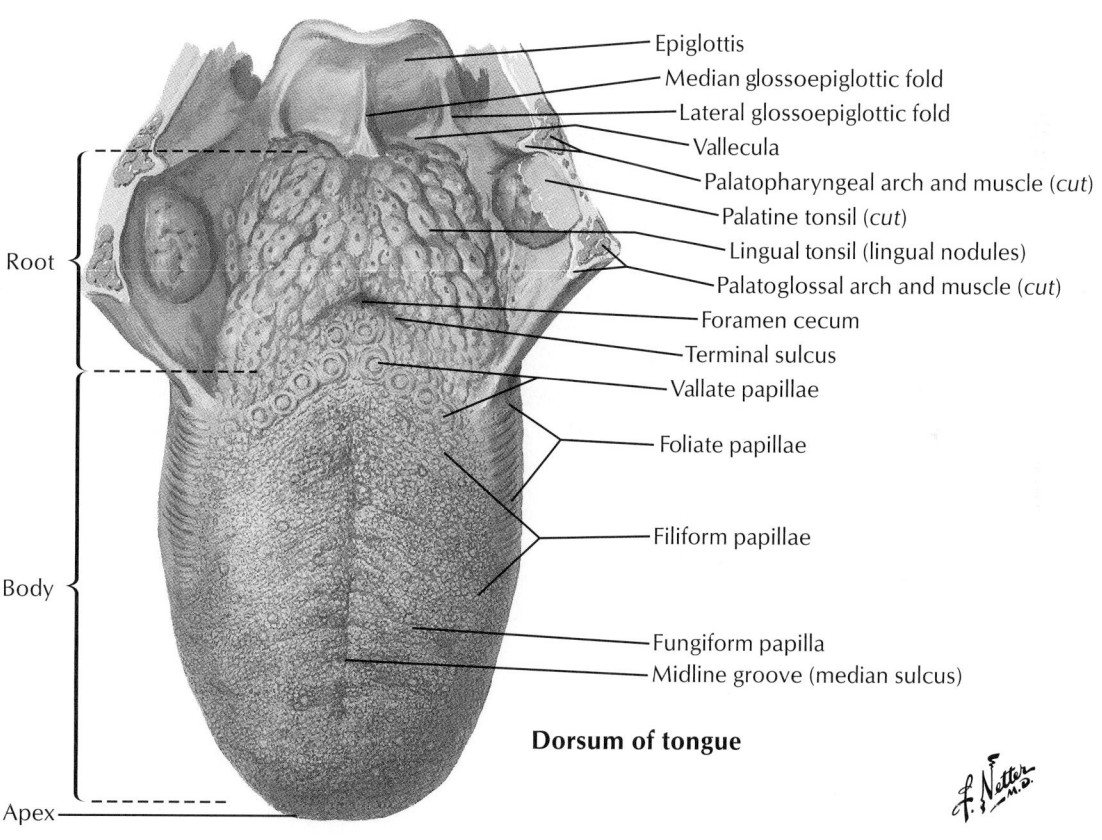

Epiglottis
Median glossoepiglottic fold
Lateral glossoepiglottic fold
Vallecula
Palatopharyngeal arch and muscle (*cut*)
Palatine tonsil (*cut*)
Lingual tonsil (lingual nodules)
Palatoglossal arch and muscle (*cut*)
Foramen cecum
Terminal sulcus
Vallate papillae
Foliate papillae
Filiform papillae
Fungiform papilla
Midline groove (median sulcus)

Root

Body

Apex

Dorsum of tongue

Plate 58   Tongue. (Netter: Atlas of Human Anatomy, 4 ed, 2006, Saunders.)

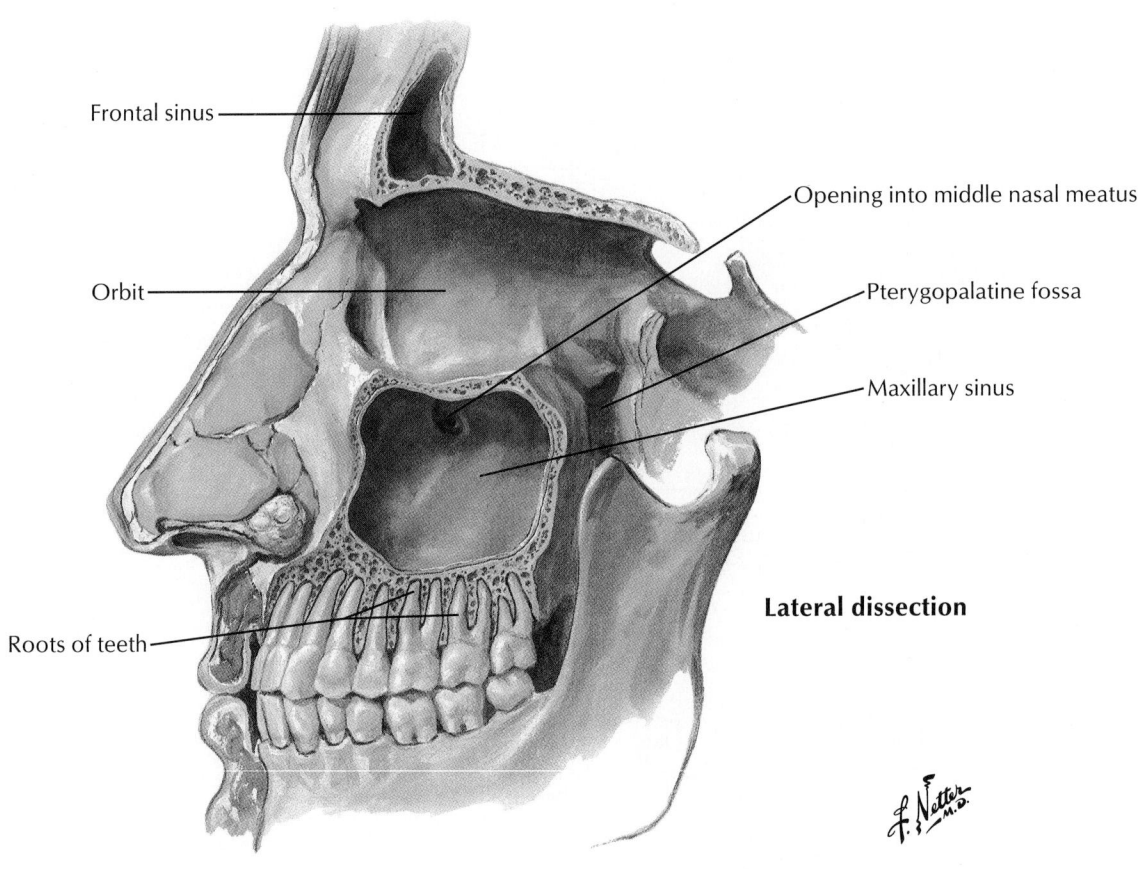

Frontal sinus

Opening into middle nasal meatus

Orbit

Pterygopalatine fossa

Maxillary sinus

Lateral dissection

Roots of teeth

Plate 49 Paranasal Sinuses. (Netter: Atlas of Human Anatomy, 4 ed, 2006, Saunders.)

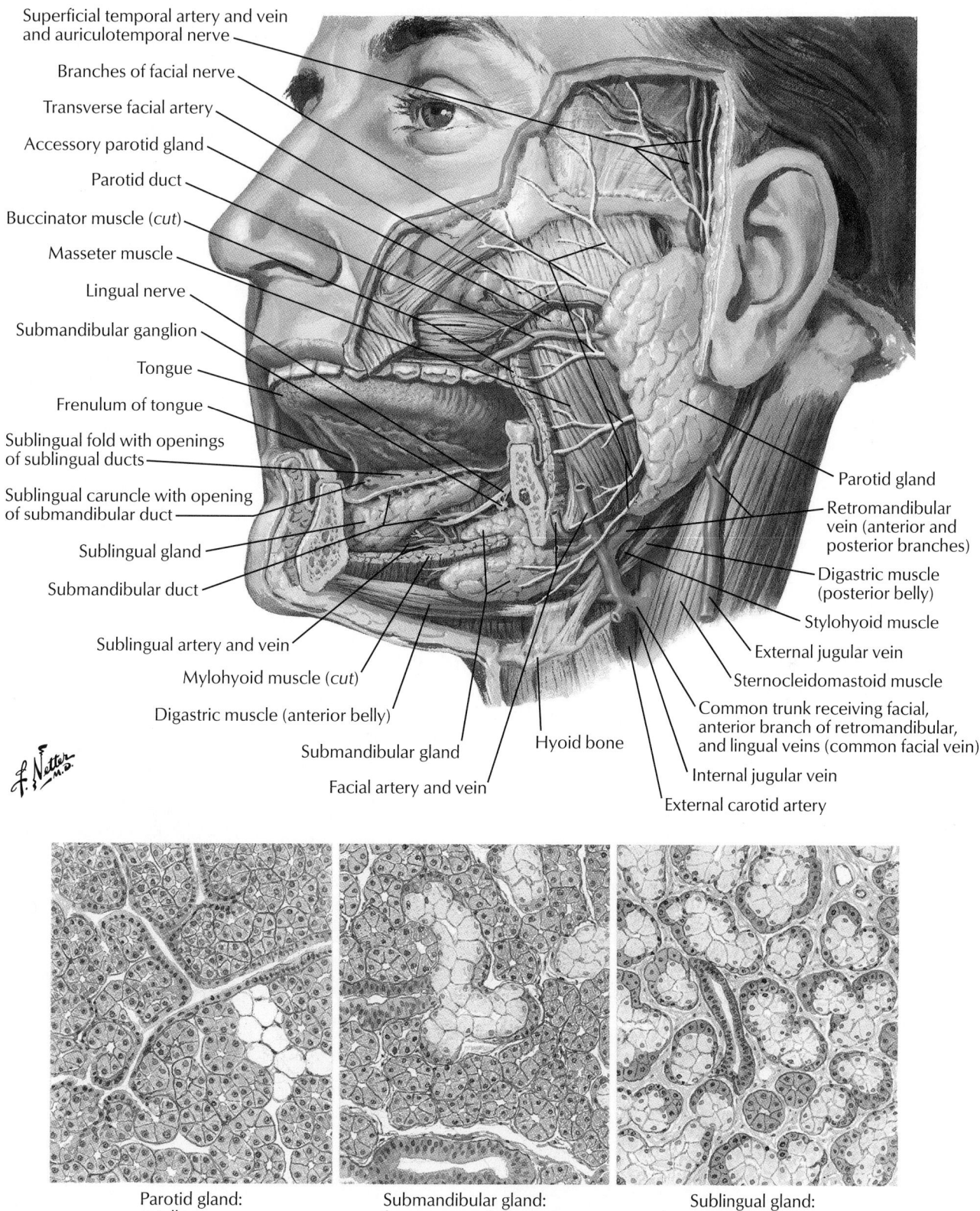

Superficial temporal artery and vein and auriculotemporal nerve

Branches of facial nerve

Transverse facial artery

Accessory parotid gland

Parotid duct

Buccinator muscle (cut)

Masseter muscle

Lingual nerve

Submandibular ganglion

Tongue

Frenulum of tongue

Sublingual fold with openings of sublingual ducts

Sublingual caruncle with opening of submandibular duct

Sublingual gland

Submandibular duct

Sublingual artery and vein

Mylohyoid muscle (cut)

Digastric muscle (anterior belly)

Submandibular gland

Facial artery and vein

Hyoid bone

Parotid gland

Retromandibular vein (anterior and posterior branches)

Digastric muscle (posterior belly)

Stylohyoid muscle

External jugular vein

Sternocleidomastoid muscle

Common trunk receiving facial, anterior branch of retromandibular, and lingual veins (common facial vein)

Internal jugular vein

External carotid artery

Parotid gland: totally serous

Submandibular gland: mostly serous, partially mucous

Sublingual gland: almost completely mucous

Plate 61 Salivary Glands. (Netter: Atlas of Human Anatomy, 4 ed, 2006, Saunders.)

Right coronary artery: left anterior oblique view

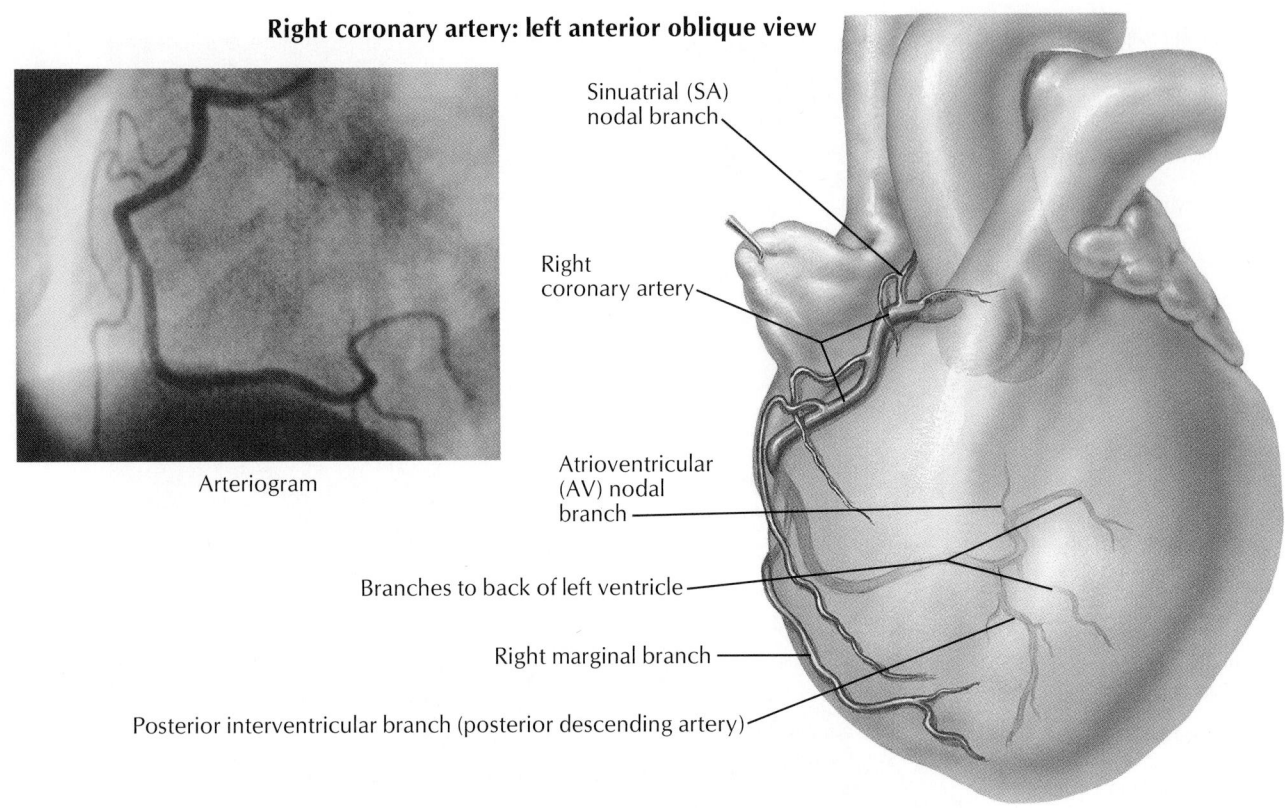

Sinuatrial (SA) nodal branch

Arteriogram

Right coronary artery

Atrioventricular (AV) nodal branch

Branches to back of left ventricle

Right marginal branch

Posterior interventricular branch (posterior descending artery)

Right coronary artery: right anterior oblique view

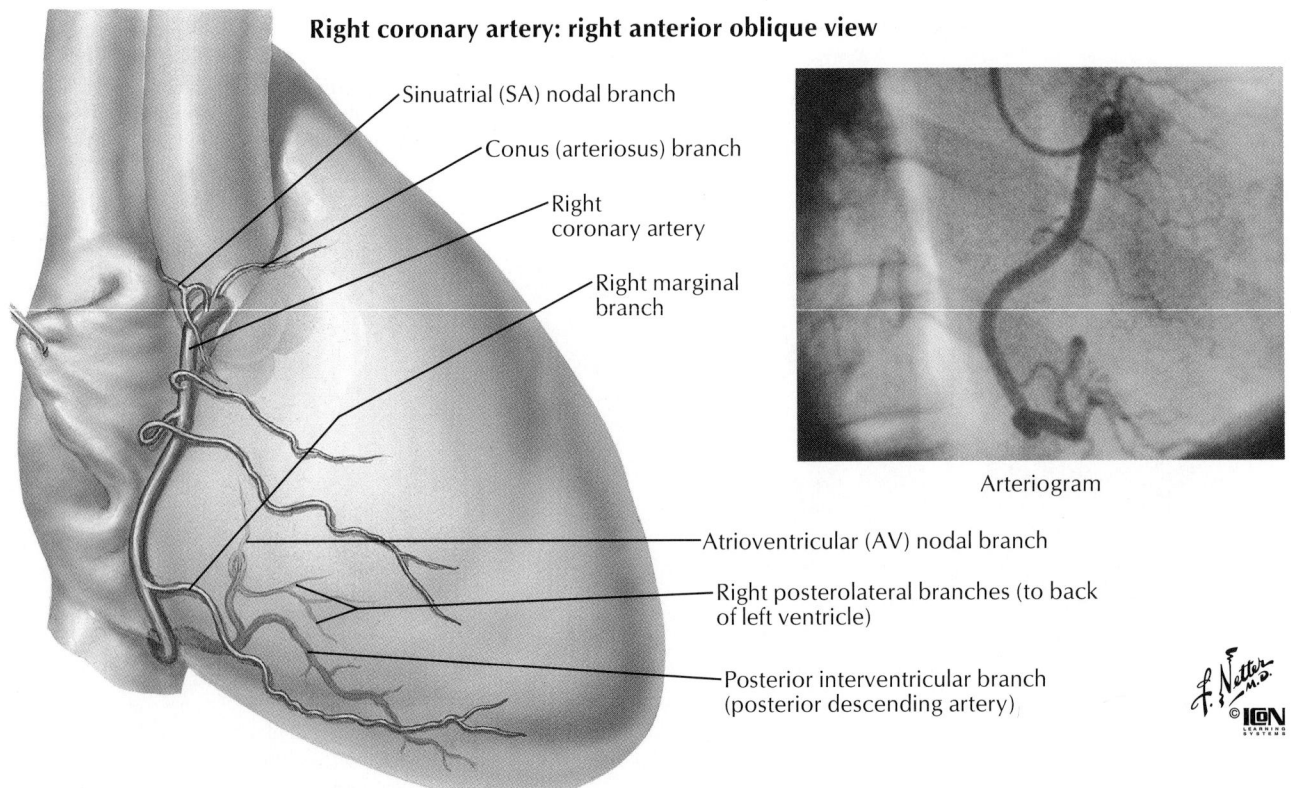

Sinuatrial (SA) nodal branch

Conus (arteriosus) branch

Right coronary artery

Right marginal branch

Arteriogram

Atrioventricular (AV) nodal branch

Right posterolateral branches (to back of left ventricle)

Posterior interventricular branch (posterior descending artery)

Plate 218   Coronary Arteries: Arteriographic Views. (Netter: Atlas of Human Anatomy, 4 ed, 2006, Saunders.)

Left coronary artery: left anterior oblique view

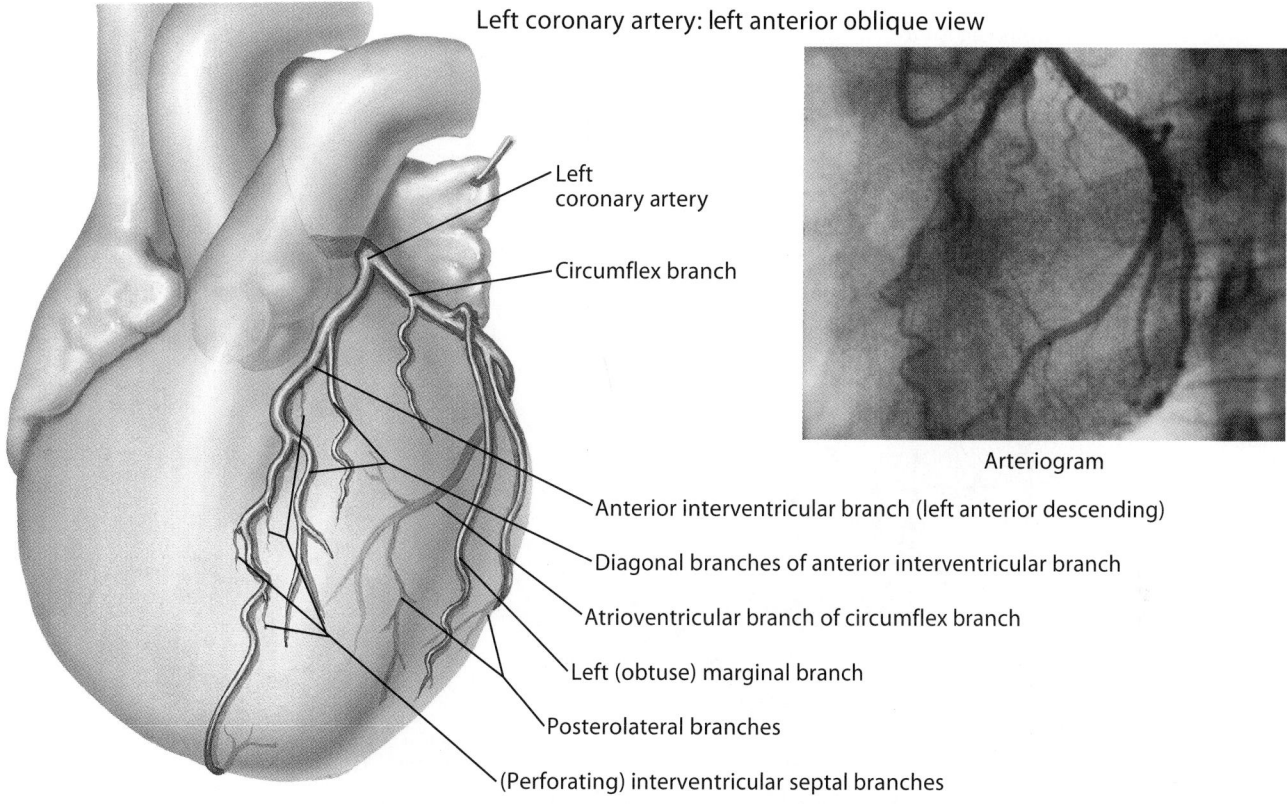

Left coronary artery

Circumflex branch

Arteriogram

Anterior interventricular branch (left anterior descending)

Diagonal branches of anterior interventricular branch

Atrioventricular branch of circumflex branch

Left (obtuse) marginal branch

Posterolateral branches

(Perforating) interventricular septal branches

Left coronary artery: right anterior oblique view

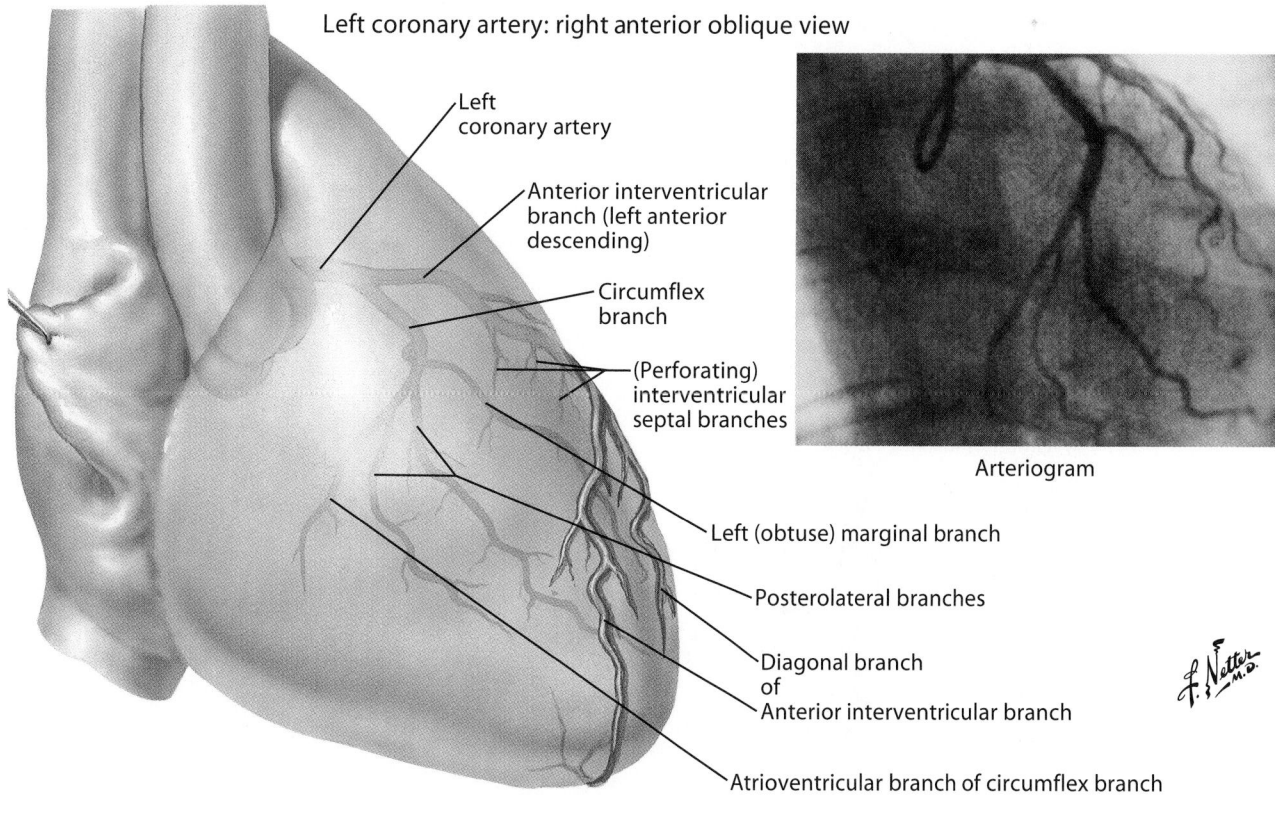

Left coronary artery

Anterior interventricular branch (left anterior descending)

Circumflex branch

(Perforating) interventricular septal branches

Arteriogram

Left (obtuse) marginal branch

Posterolateral branches

Diagonal branch of Anterior interventricular branch

Atrioventricular branch of circumflex branch

Plate 219 Coronary Arteries: Arteriographic Views. (Netter: Atlas of Human Anatomy, 4 ed, 2006, Saunders.)

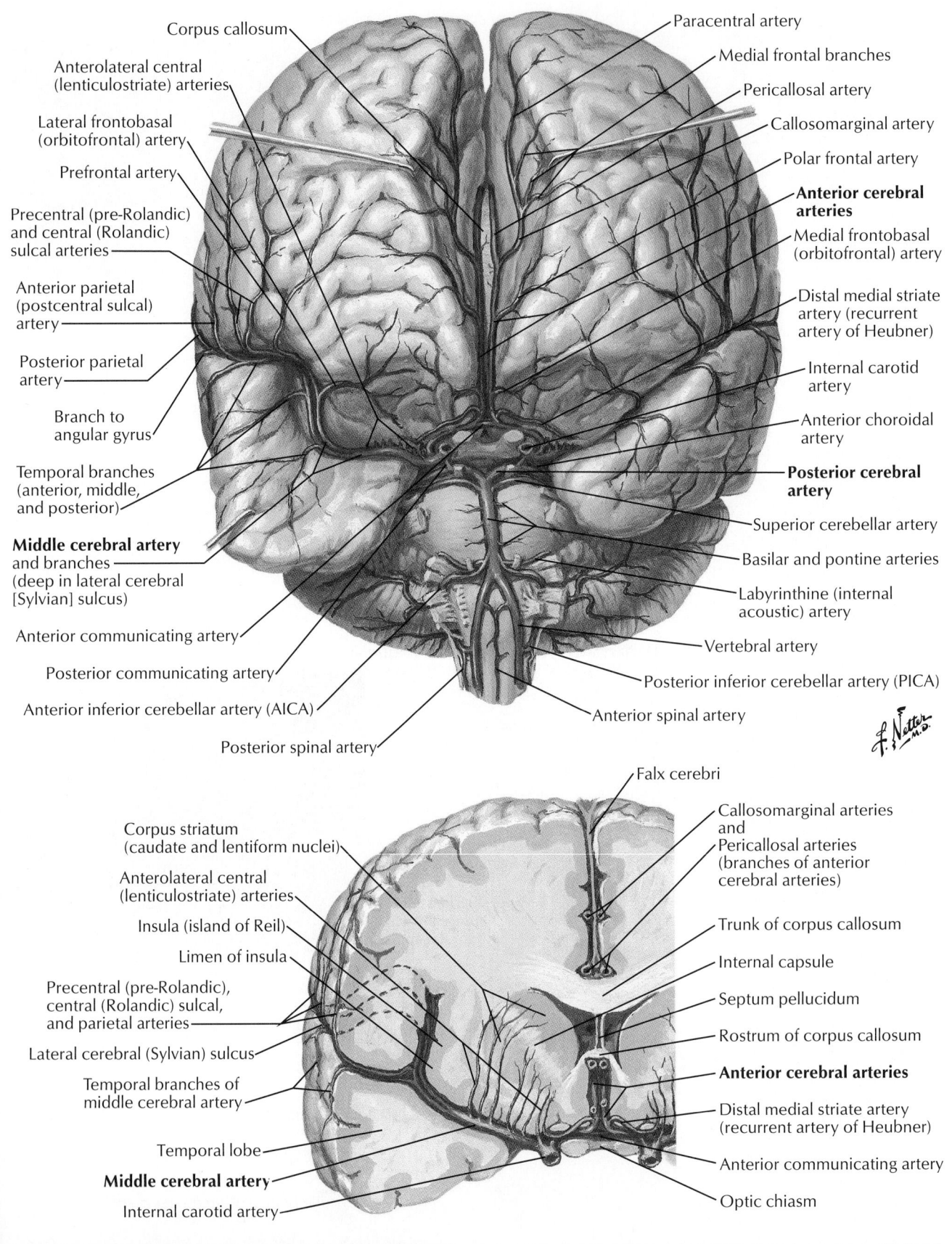

Corpus callosum

Anterolateral central
(lenticulostriate) arteries

Lateral frontobasal
(orbitofrontal) artery

Prefrontal artery

Precentral (pre-Rolandic)
and central (Rolandic)
sulcal arteries

Anterior parietal
(postcentral sulcal)
artery

Posterior parietal
artery

Branch to
angular gyrus

Temporal branches
(anterior, middle,
and posterior)

Middle cerebral artery
and branches
(deep in lateral cerebral
[Sylvian] sulcus)

Anterior communicating artery

Posterior communicating artery

Anterior inferior cerebellar artery (AICA)

Posterior spinal artery

Paracentral artery

Medial frontal branches

Pericallosal artery

Callosomarginal artery

Polar frontal artery

**Anterior cerebral
arteries**

Medial frontobasal
(orbitofrontal) artery

Distal medial striate
artery (recurrent
artery of Heubner)

Internal carotid
artery

Anterior choroidal
artery

**Posterior cerebral
artery**

Superior cerebellar artery

Basilar and pontine arteries

Labyrinthine (internal
acoustic) artery

Vertebral artery

Posterior inferior cerebellar artery (PICA)

Anterior spinal artery

Falx cerebri

Corpus striatum
(caudate and lentiform nuclei)

Anterolateral central
(lenticulostriate) arteries

Insula (island of Reil)

Limen of insula

Precentral (pre-Rolandic),
central (Rolandic) sulcal,
and parietal arteries

Lateral cerebral (Sylvian) sulcus

Temporal branches of
middle cerebral artery

Temporal lobe

Middle cerebral artery

Internal carotid artery

Callosomarginal arteries
and
Pericallosal arteries
(branches of anterior
cerebral arteries)

Trunk of corpus callosum

Internal capsule

Septum pellucidum

Rostrum of corpus callosum

Anterior cerebral arteries

Distal medial striate artery
(recurrent artery of Heubner)

Anterior communicating artery

Optic chiasm

Plate 141 Arteries of Brain: Frontal View and Section. (Netter: Atlas of Human Anatomy, 4 ed, 2006, Saunders.)

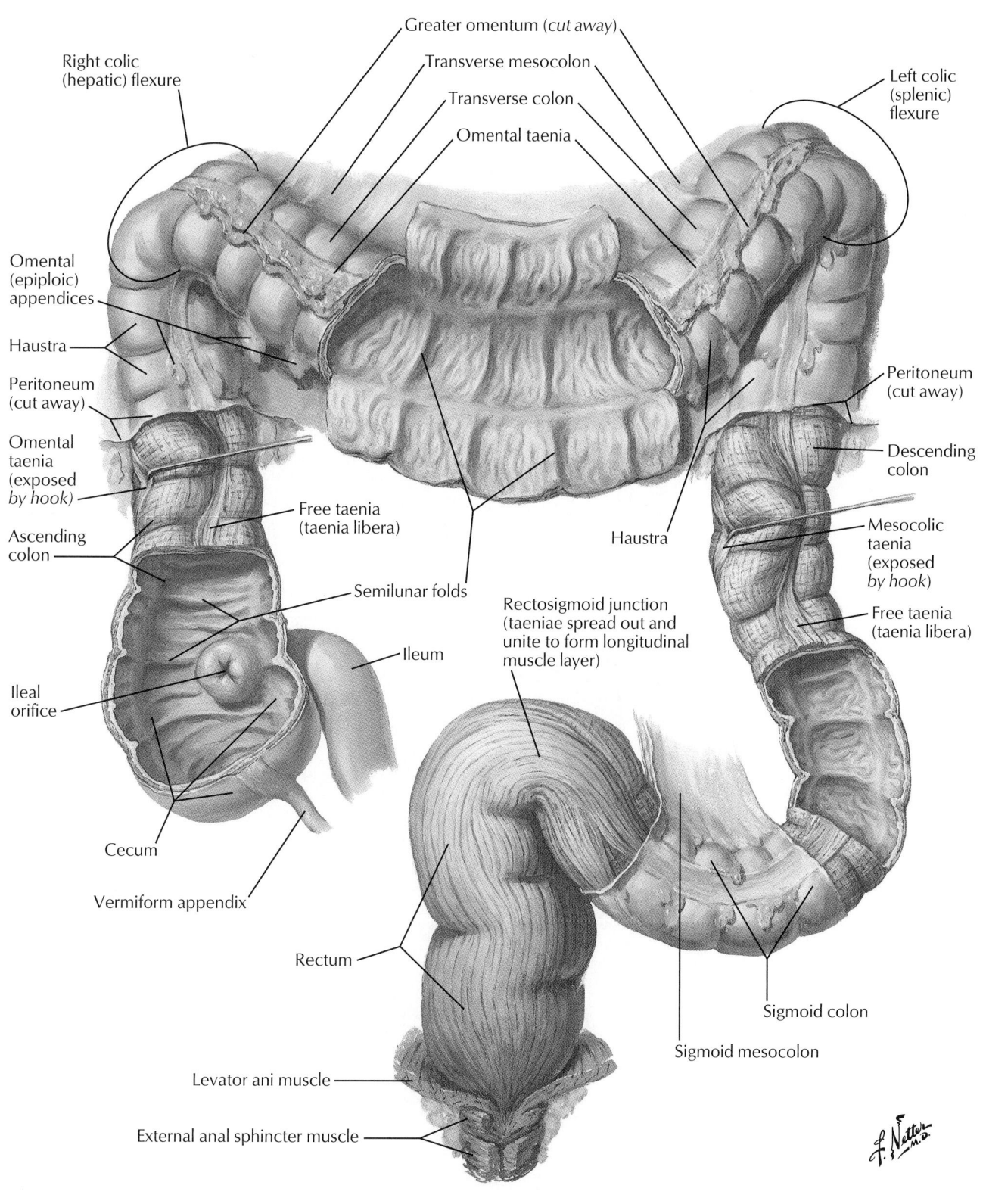

Right colic (hepatic) flexure

Greater omentum (*cut away*)

Transverse mesocolon

Transverse colon

Omental taenia

Left colic (splenic) flexure

Omental (epiploic) appendices

Haustra

Peritoneum (cut away)

Omental taenia (exposed *by hook*)

Ascending colon

Free taenia (taenia libera)

Semilunar folds

Haustra

Peritoneum (cut away)

Descending colon

Mesocolic taenia (exposed *by hook*)

Free taenia (taenia libera)

Ileum

Rectosigmoid junction (taeniae spread out and unite to form longitudinal muscle layer)

Ileal orifice

Cecum

Vermiform appendix

Rectum

Sigmoid colon

Sigmoid mesocolon

Levator ani muscle

External anal sphincter muscle

Plate 284   Mucosa and Musculature of Large Intestine. (Netter: Atlas of Human Anatomy, 4 ed, 2006, Saunders.)

Transverse Section: T3–4 Intervertebral Disc, Manubrium

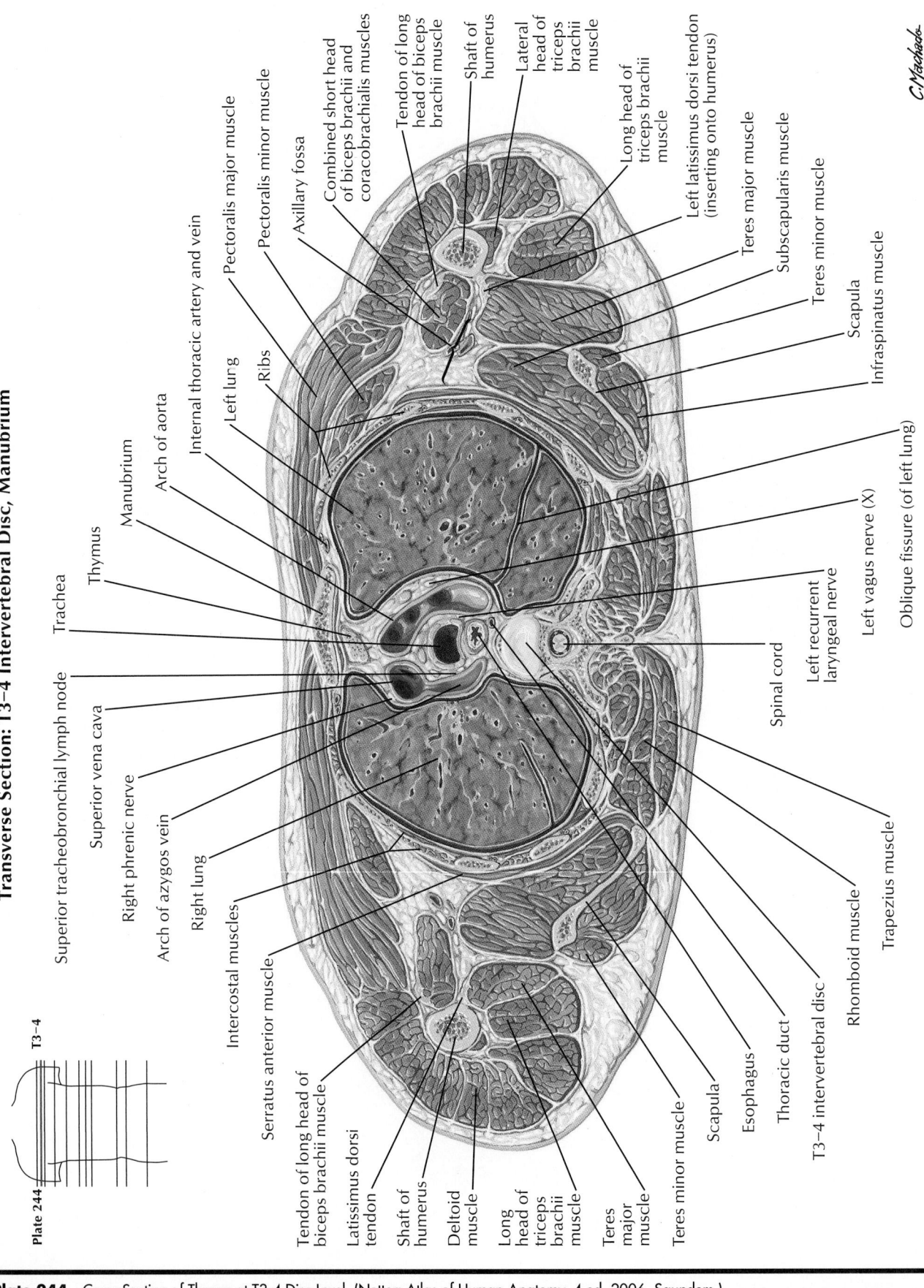

Superior tracheobronchial lymph node

Trachea

Thymus

Manubrium

Arch of aorta

Internal thoracic artery and vein

Pectoralis major muscle

Pectoralis minor muscle

Axillary fossa

Combined short head of biceps brachii and coracobrachialis muscles

Tendon of long head of biceps brachii muscle

Shaft of humerus

Lateral head of triceps brachii muscle

Long head of triceps brachii muscle

Left latissimus dorsi tendon (inserting onto humerus)

Teres major muscle

Subscapularis muscle

Teres minor muscle

Scapula

Infraspinatus muscle

Left lung

Ribs

Oblique fissure (of left lung)

Left vagus nerve (X)

Left recurrent laryngeal nerve

Spinal cord

Trapezius muscle

Rhomboid muscle

T3–4 intervertebral disc

Thoracic duct

Esophagus

Scapula

Teres minor muscle

Teres major muscle

Long head of triceps brachii muscle

Deltoid muscle

Shaft of humerus

Latissimus dorsi tendon

Tendon of long head of biceps brachii muscle

Serratus anterior muscle

Intercostal muscles

Right lung

Arch of azygos vein

Right phrenic nerve

Superior vena cava

Superior tracheobronchial lymph node

Plate 244

T3–4

Plate 244   Cross Section of Thorax at T3-4 Disc Level. (Netter: Atlas of Human Anatomy, 4 ed, 2006, Saunders.)

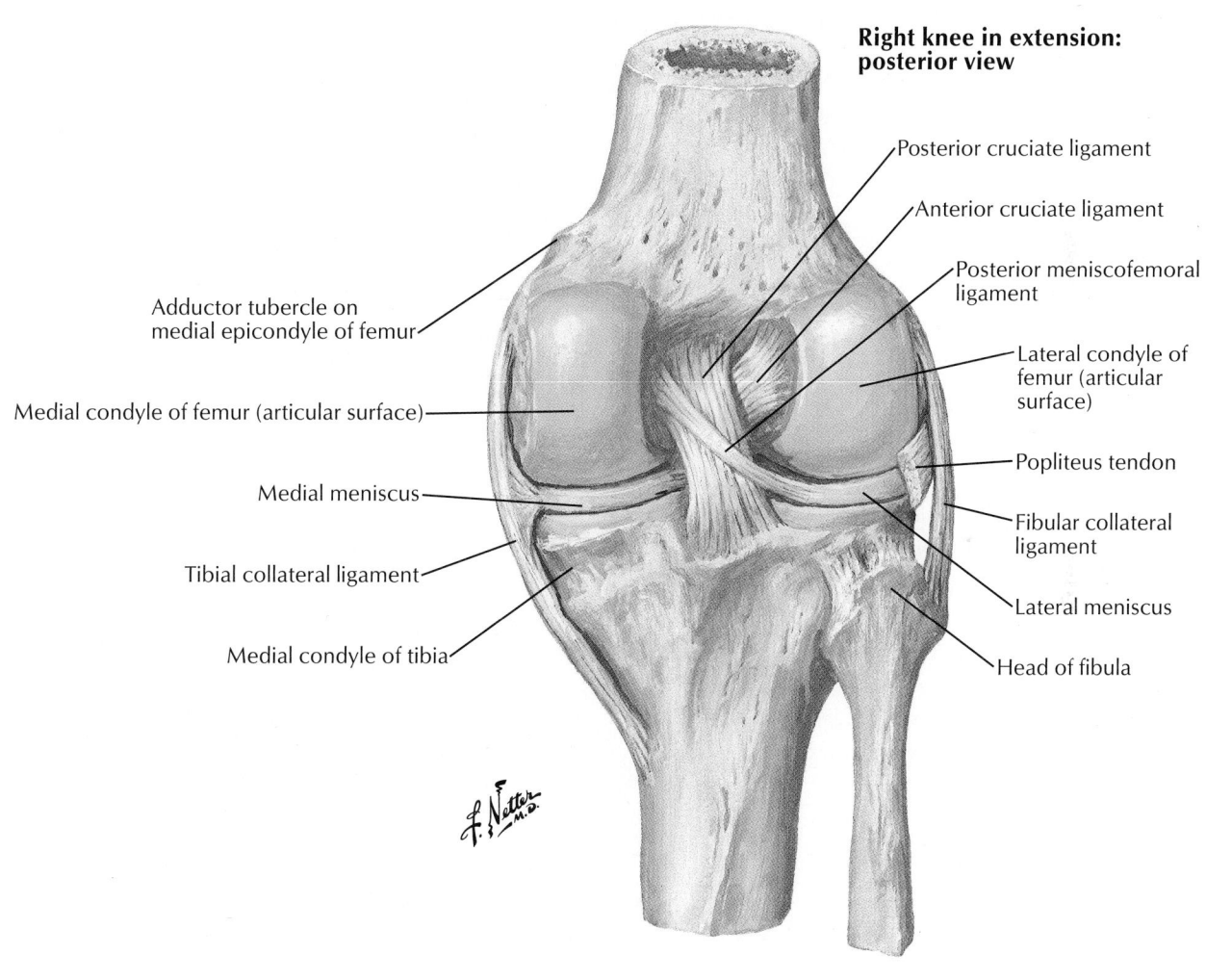

Right knee in extension: posterior view

Posterior cruciate ligament

Anterior cruciate ligament

Posterior meniscofemoral ligament

Lateral condyle of femur (articular surface)

Popliteus tendon

Fibular collateral ligament

Lateral meniscus

Head of fibula

Adductor tubercle on medial epicondyle of femur

Medial condyle of femur (articular surface)

Medial meniscus

Tibial collateral ligament

Medial condyle of tibia

Plate 509   Knee: Cruciate and Collateral Ligaments. (Netter: Atlas of Human Anatomy, 4 ed, 2006, Saunders.)

Paramedian (sagittal) dissection

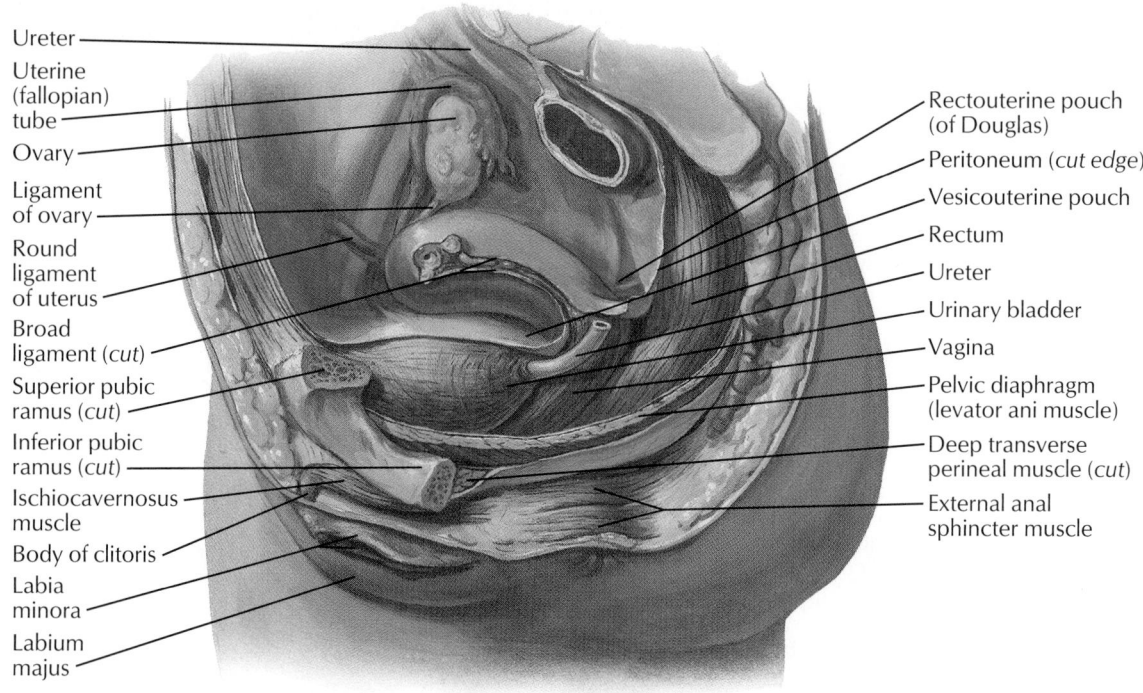

Ureter

Uterine (fallopian) tube

Ovary

Ligament of ovary

Round ligament of uterus

Broad ligament (*cut*)

Superior pubic ramus (*cut*)

Inferior pubic ramus (*cut*)

Ischiocavernosus muscle

Body of clitoris

Labia minora

Labium majus

Rectouterine pouch (of Douglas)

Peritoneum (*cut edge*)

Vesicouterine pouch

Rectum

Ureter

Urinary bladder

Vagina

Pelvic diaphragm (levator ani muscle)

Deep transverse perineal muscle (*cut*)

External anal sphincter muscle

Median (sagittal) section

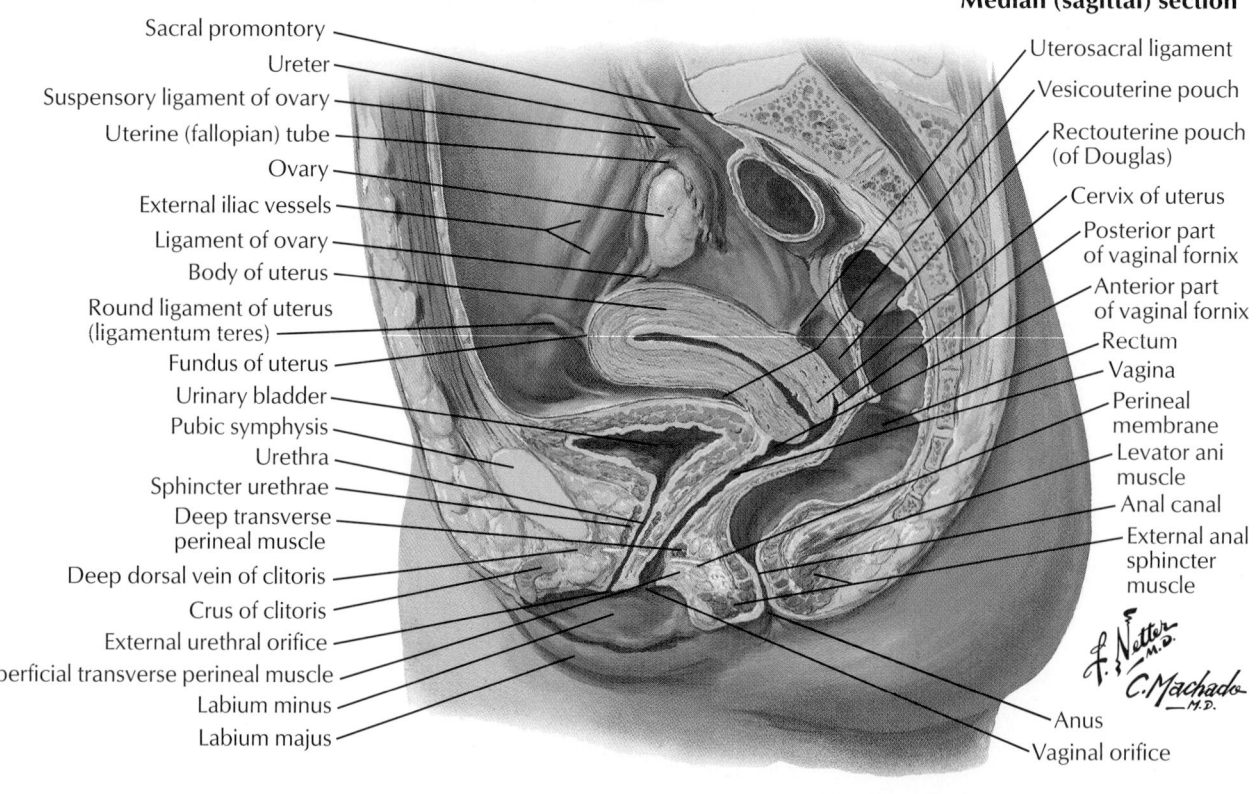

Sacral promontory

Ureter

Suspensory ligament of ovary

Uterine (fallopian) tube

Ovary

External iliac vessels

Ligament of ovary

Body of uterus

Round ligament of uterus (ligamentum teres)

Fundus of uterus

Urinary bladder

Pubic symphysis

Urethra

Sphincter urethrae

Deep transverse perineal muscle

Deep dorsal vein of clitoris

Crus of clitoris

External urethral orifice

Superficial transverse perineal muscle

Labium minus

Labium majus

Uterosacral ligament

Vesicouterine pouch

Rectouterine pouch (of Douglas)

Cervix of uterus

Posterior part of vaginal fornix

Anterior part of vaginal fornix

Rectum

Vagina

Perineal membrane

Levator ani muscle

Anal canal

External anal sphincter muscle

Anus

Vaginal orifice

Plate 360 Pelvic Viscera and Perineum: Female. (Netter: Atlas of Human Anatomy, 4 ed, 2006, Saunders.)

PART II

Alphabetic Index
Volume 2

A

A

AAT (alpha-1 antitrypsin) deficiency 273.4
AAV (disease) (illness) (infection) - *see*
    Human immunodeficiency virus
    (disease) (illness) (infection)
Abactio - *see* Abortion, induced
Abactus venter - *see* Abortion, induced
Abarognosis 781.99
Abasia (-astasia) 307.9
    atactica 781.3
    choreic 781.3
    hysterical 300.11
    paroxysmal trepidant 781.3
    spastic 781.3
    trembling 781.3
    trepidans 781.3
Abderhalden-Kaufmann-Lignac
    syndrome (cystinosis) 270.0
Abdomen, abdominal - *see also* condition
    accordion 306.4
    acute 789.0●
    angina 557.1
    burst 868.00
    convulsive equivalent (*see also*
        Epilepsy) 345.5●
    heart 746.87
    muscle deficiency syndrome 756.79
    obstipum 756.79
Abdominalgia 789.0●
    periodic 277.31
Abduction contracture, hip or other
    joint - *see* Contraction, joint
Abercrombie's syndrome (amyloid
    degeneration) 277.39
Aberrant (congenital) - *see also*
    Malposition, congenital
    adrenal gland 759.1
    blood vessel NEC 747.60
        arteriovenous NEC 747.60
        cerebrovascular 747.81
        gastrointestinal 747.61
        lower limb 747.64
        renal 747.62
        spinal 747.82
        upper limb 747.63
    breast 757.6
    endocrine gland NEC 759.2
    gastrointestinal vessel (peripheral) 747.61
    hepatic duct 751.69
    lower limb vessel (peripheral) 747.64
    pancreas 751.7
    parathyroid gland 759.2
    peripheral vascular vessel NEC 747.60
    pituitary gland (pharyngeal) 759.2
    renal blood vessel 747.62
    sebaceous glands, mucous membrane,
        mouth 750.26
    spinal vessel 747.82
    spleen 759.0
    testis (descent) 752.51
    thymus gland 759.2
    thyroid gland 759.2
    upper limb vessel (peripheral) 747.63
Aberratio
    lactis 757.6
    testis 752.51
Aberration - *see also* Anomaly
    chromosome - *see* Anomaly,
        chromosome(s)
    distantal 368.9
    mental (*see also* Disorder, mental,
        nonpsychotic) 300.9

Abetalipoproteinemia 272.5
Abionarce 780.79
Abiotrophy 799.89
Ablatio
    placentae - *see* Placenta, ablatio
    retinae (*see also* Detachment, retina)
        361.9
Ablation
    pituitary (gland) (with hypofunction)
        253.7
    placenta - *see* Placenta, ablatio
    uterus 621.8
Ablepharia, ablepharon, ablephary
    743.62
Ablepsia - *see* Blindness
Ablepsy - *see* Blindness
Ablutomania 300.3
Abnormal, abnormality, abnormalities -
    see also Anomaly
    acid-base balance 276.4
        fetus or newborn - *see* Distress, fetal
    adaptation curve, dark 368.63
    alveolar ridge 525.9
    amnion 658.9●
        affecting fetus or newborn 762.9
    anatomical relationship NEC 759.9
    apertures, congenital, diaphragm
        756.6
    auditory perception NEC 388.40
    autosomes NEC 758.5
        13 758.1
        18 758.2
        21 or 22 758.0
        D_1 758.1
        E_3 758.2
        G 758.0
    ballistocardiogram 794.39
    basal metabolic rate (BMR) 794.7
    biosynthesis, testicular androgen
        257.2
    blood level (of)
        cobalt 790.6
        copper 790.6
        iron 790.6
        lead 790.6
        lithium 790.6
        magnesium 790.6
        mineral 790.6
        zinc 790.6
    blood pressure
        elevated (without diagnosis of
            hypertension) 796.2
        low (*see also* Hypotension) 458.9
            reading (incidental) (isolated)
                (nonspecific) 796.3
    blood sugar 790.29
    bowel sounds 787.5
    breathing behavior - *see* Respiration
    caloric test 794.19
    cervix (acquired) NEC 622.9
        congenital 752.40
        in pregnancy or childbirth 654.6●
            causing obstructed labor 660.2●
                affecting fetus or newborn
                    763.1
    chemistry, blood NEC 790.6
    chest sounds 786.7
    chorion 658.9●
        affecting fetus or newborn 762.9
    chromosomal NEC 758.89
        analysis, nonspecific result 795.2
        autosomes (*see also* Abnormal,
            autosomes NEC) 758.5

Abnormal, abnormality, abnormalities
    (*Continued*)
    chromosomal NEC (*Continued*)
        fetal, (suspected) affecting
            management of pregnancy
            655.1●
        sex 758.81
    clinical findings NEC 796.4
    communication - *see* Fistula
    configuration of pupils 379.49
    coronary
        artery 746.85
        vein 746.9
    cortisol-binding globulin 255.8
    course, Eustachian tube 744.24
    creatinine clearance 794.4
    dentofacial NEC 524.9
        functional 524.50
        specified type NEC 524.89
    development, developmental NEC
        759.9
        bone 756.9
        central nervous system 742.9
    direction, teeth 524.30
    dynia (*see also* Defect, coagulation)
        286.9
    Ebstein 746.2
    echocardiogram 793.2
    echoencephalogram 794.01
    echogram NEC - *see* Findings,
        abnormal, structure
    electrocardiogram (ECG) (EKG) 794.31
    electroencephalogram (EEG) 794.02
    electromyogram (EMG) 794.17
        ocular 794.14
    electro-oculogram (EOG) 794.12
    electroretinogram (ERG) 794.11
    erythrocytes 289.9
        congenital, with perinatal jaundice
            282.9 [774.0]
    eustachian valve 746.9
    excitability under minor stress 301.9
    fat distribution 782.9
    feces 787.7
    fetal heart rate - *see* Distress, fetal
    fetus NEC
        affecting management of
            pregnancy - *see* Pregnancy,
            management affected by, fetal
        causing disproportion 653.7●
            affecting fetus or newborn 763.1
            causing obstructed labor 660.1●
                affecting fetus or newborn
                    763.1
    findings without manifest disease - *see*
        Findings, abnormal
    fluid
        amniotic 792.3
        cerebrospinal 792.0
        peritoneal 792.9
        pleural 792.9
        synovial 792.9
        vaginal 792.9
    forces of labor NEC 661.9●
        affecting fetus or newborn 763.7
    form, teeth 520.2
    function studies
        auditory 794.15
        bladder 794.9
        brain 794.00
        cardiovascular 794.30
        endocrine NEC 794.6
        kidney 794.4

Abnormal, abnormality, abnormalities
   (Continued)
   function studies (Continued)
      liver 794.8
      nervous system
         central 794.00
            peripheral 794.19
      oculomotor 794.14
      pancreas 794.9
      placenta 794.9
      pulmonary 794.2
      retina 794.11
      special senses 794.19
      spleen 794.9
      thyroid 794.5
      vestibular 794.16
   gait 781.2
      hysterical 300.11
   gastrin secretion 251.5
   globulin
      cortisol-binding 255.8
      thyroid-binding 246.8
   glucagon secretion 251.4
   glucose 790.29
      in pregnancy, childbirth, or
         puerperium 648.8●
         fetus or newborn 775.0
      non-fasting 790.29
   gravitational (G) forces or states 994.9
   hair NEC 704.2
   hard tissue formation in pulp 522.3
   head movement 781.0
   heart
      rate
         fetus, affecting liveborn infant
            before the onset of labor 763.81
            during labor 763.82
            unspecified as to time of onset
               763.83
         intrauterine
            before the onset of labor 763.81
            during labor 763.82
            unspecified as to time of onset
               763.83
         newborn
            before the onset of labor 763.81
            during labor 763.82
            unspecified as to time of onset
               763.83
      shadow 793.2
      sounds NEC 785.3
   hemoglobin (see also Disease,
      hemoglobin) 282.7
      trait - see Trait, hemoglobin,
         abnormal
   hemorrhage, uterus - see Hemorrhage,
      uterus
   histology NEC 795.4
   increase in
      appetite 783.6
      development 783.9
   involuntary movement 781.0
   jaw closure 524.51
   karyotype 795.2
   knee jerk 796.1
   labor NEC 661.9●
      affecting fetus or newborn 763.7
   laboratory findings - see Findings,
      abnormal
   length, organ or site, congenital - see
      Distortion
   liver function test 790.6
   loss of height 781.91
   loss of weight 783.21

Abnormal, abnormality, abnormalities
   (Continued)
   lung shadow 793.1
   mammogram 793.80
      calcification 793.89
      calculus 793.89
      microcalcification 793.81
   Mantoux test 795.5
   membranes (fetal)
      affecting fetus or newborn 762.9
      complicating pregnancy 658.8●
   menstruation - see Menstruation
   metabolism (see also condition) 783.9
   movement 781.0
      disorder NEC 333.90
         sleep related, unspecified 780.58
         specified NEC 333.99
      head 781.0
      involuntary 781.0
      specified type NEC 333.99
   muscle contraction, localized 728.85
   myoglobin (Aberdeen) (Annapolis)
      289.9
   narrowness, eyelid 743.62
   optokinetic response 379.57
   organs or tissues of pelvis NEC
      in pregnancy or childbirth 654.9●
         affecting fetus or newborn
            763.89
         causing obstructed labor 660.2●
            affecting fetus or newborn
               763.1
   origin - see Malposition, congenital
   palmar creases 757.2
   Papanicolaou (smear)
      anus 796.70
         with
            atypical squamous cells
               cannot exclude high grade
                  squamous
                     intraepithelial lesion
                     (ASC-H) 796.72
               of undetermined
                  significance (ASC-US)
                  796.71
            cytologic evidence of
               malignancy 796.76
            high grade squamous
               intraepithelial lesion
               (HGSIL) 796.74
            low grade squamous
               intraepithelial lesion
               (LGSIL) 796.73
         glandular 796.70
         specified finding NEC 796.79
      cervix 795.00
         with
            atypical squamous cells
               cannot exclude high grade
                  squamous
                     intraepithelial lesion
                     (ASC-H) 795.02
               of undetermined
                  significance (ASC-US)
                  795.01
            cytologic evidence of
               malignancy 795.06
            high grade squamous
               intraepithelial lesion
               (HGSIL) 795.04
            low grade squamous
               intraepithelial lesion
               (LGSIL) 795.03
         nonspecific finding NEC 795.09

Abnormal, abnormality, abnormalities
   (Continued)
   Papanicolaou (smear) (Continued)
      other site 796.9
      vagina 795.10
         with
            atypical squamous cells
               cannot exclude high grade
                  squamous
                     intraepithelial lesion
                     (ASC-H) 795.12
               of undetermined
                  significance (ASC-US)
                  795.11
            cytologic evidence of
               malignancy 795.16
            high grade squamous
               intraepithelial lesion
               (HGSIL)795.14
            low grade squamous
               intraepithelial lesion
               (LGSIL) 795.13
         glandular 795.10
         specified finding NEC 795.19
   parturition
      affecting fetus or newborn 763.9
      mother - see Delivery, complicated
   pelvis (bony) - see Deformity, pelvis
   percussion, chest 786.7
   periods (grossly) (see also
      Menstruation) 626.9
   phonocardiogram 794.39
   placenta - see Placenta, abnormal
   plantar reflex 796.1
   plasma protein - see Deficiency, plasma,
      protein
   pleural folds 748.8
   position - see also Malposition
      gravid uterus 654.4●
         causing obstructed labor 660.2●
            affecting fetus or newborn
               763.1
   posture NEC 781.92
   presentation (fetus) - see Presentation,
      fetus, abnormal
   product of conception NEC 631
   puberty - see Puberty
   pulmonary
      artery 747.3
      function, newborn 770.89
      test results 794.2
      ventilation, newborn 770.89
         hyperventilation 786.01
   pulsations in neck 785.1
   pupil reflexes 379.40
   quality of milk 676.8●
   radiological examination 793.99
      abdomen NEC 793.6
      biliary tract 793.3
      breast 793.89
         mammogram NOS 793.80
         mammographic
            calcification 793.89
            calculus 793.89
            microcalcification 793.81
      gastrointestinal tract 793.4
      genitourinary organs 793.5
      head 793.0
      image test inconclusive due to
         excess body fat 793.91
      intrathoracic organ NEC 793.2
      lung (field) 793.1
      musculoskeletal system 793.7
      retroperitoneum 793.6

Abnormal, abnormality, abnormalities
  (Continued)
  radiological examination *(Continued)*
    skin and subcutaneous tissue 793.99
    skull 793.0
  red blood cells 790.09
    morphology 790.09
    volume 790.09
  reflex NEC 796.1
  renal function test 794.4
  respiration signs - *see* Respiration
  response to nerve stimulation 794.10
  retinal correspondence 368.34
  rhythm, heart - *see also* Arrhythmia
    fetus - *see* Distress, fetal
  saliva 792.4
  scan
    brain 794.09
    kidney 794.4
    liver 794.8
    lung 794.2
    thyroid 794.5
  secretion
    gastrin 251.5
    glucagon 251.4
  semen 792.2
  serum level (of)
    acid phosphatase 790.5
    alkaline phosphatase 790.5
    amylase 790.5
    enzymes NEC 790.5
    lipase 790.5
  shape
    cornea 743.41
    gallbladder 751.69
    gravid uterus 654.4●
      affecting fetus or newborn
        763.89
      causing obstructed labor 660.2●
        affecting fetus or newborn
          763.1
    head (*see also* Anomaly, skull) 756.0
    organ or site, congenital NEC - *see*
      Distortion
  sinus venosus 747.40
  size
    fetus, complicating delivery 653.5●
      causing obstructed labor 660.1●
    gallbladder 751.69
    head (*see also* Anomaly, skull) 756.0
    organ or site, congenital NEC - *see*
      Distortion
    teeth 520.2
  skin and appendages, congenital NEC
    757.9
  soft parts of pelvis - *see* Abnormal,
    organs or tissues of pelvis
  spermatozoa 792.2
  sputum (amount) (color) (excessive)
    (odor) (purulent) 786.4
  stool NEC 787.7
    bloody 578.1
      occult 792.1
    bulky 787.7
    color (dark) (light) 792.1
    content (fat) (mucus) (pus) 792.1
    occult blood 792.1
  synchondrosis 756.9
  test results without manifest disease -
    see Findings, abnormal
  thebesian valve 746.9
  thermography - *see* Findings, abnormal,
    structure
  threshold, cones or rods (eye) 368.63

Abnormal, abnormality, abnormalities
  (Continued)
  thyroid-binding globulin 246.8
  thyroid product 246.8
  toxicology (findings) NEC 796.0
  tracheal cartilage (congenital) 748.3
  transport protein 273.8
  ultrasound results - *see* Findings,
    abnormal, structure
  umbilical cord
    affecting fetus or newborn 762.6
    complicating delivery 663.9●
    specified NEC 663.8●
  union
    cricoid cartilage and thyroid
      cartilage 748.3
    larynx and trachea 748.3
    thyroid cartilage and hyoid bone
      748.3
  urination NEC 788.69
    psychogenic 306.53
    stream
      intermittent 788.61
      slowing 788.62
      splitting 788.61
      weak 788.62
    urgency 788.63
  urine (constituents) NEC 791.9
  uterine hemorrhage (*see also*
    Hemorrhage, uterus) 626.9
    climacteric 627.0
    postmenopausal 627.1
  vagina (acquired) (congenital)
    in pregnancy or childbirth 654.7●
      affecting fetus or newborn
        763.89
      causing obstructed labor 660.2●
        affecting fetus or newborn
          763.1
  vascular sounds 785.9
  vectorcardiogram 794.39
  visually evoked potential (VEP)
    794.13
  vulva (acquired) (congenital)
    in pregnancy or childbirth 654.8●
      affecting fetus or newborn
        763.89
      causing obstructed labor 660.2●
        affecting fetus or newborn
          763.1
  weight
    gain 783.1
      of pregnancy 646.1●
        with hypertension - *see*
          Toxemia, of pregnancy
    loss 783.21
  x-ray examination - *see* Abnormal,
    radiological examination
Abnormally formed uterus - *see* Anomaly,
  uterus
Abnormity (any organ or part) - *see*
  Anomaly
ABO
  hemolytic disease 773.1
  incompatibility reaction 999.6
Abocclusion 524.20
Abolition, language 784.69
Aborter, habitual or recurrent NEC
  without current pregnancy 629.81
  current abortion (*see also* Abortion,
    spontaneous) 634.9●
    affecting fetus or newborn 761.8
  observation in current pregnancy
    646.3●

Abortion (complete) (incomplete)
  (inevitable) (with retained products
  of conception) 637.9●

Note 01   Use the following fifth-digit
subclassification with categories 634-637:

0   unspecified
1   incomplete
2   complete

---

  with
    complication(s) (any) following
      previous abortion - *see*
      category 639
    damage to pelvic organ (laceration)
      (rupture) (tear) 637.2●
    embolism (air) (amniotic fluid)
      (blood clot) (pulmonary)
      (pyemic) (septic) (soap) 637.6●
    genital tract and pelvic infection
      637.0●
    hemorrhage, delayed or excessive
      637.1●
    metabolic disorder 637.4●
    renal failure (acute) 637.3●
    sepsis (genital tract) (pelvic organ)
      637.0●
      urinary tract 637.7●
    shock (postoperative) (septic)
      637.5●
    specified complication NEC 637.7●
    toxemia 637.3●
    unspecified complication(s) 637.8●
    urinary tract infection 637.7●
  accidental - *see* Abortion, spontaneous
  artificial - *see* Abortion, induced
  attempted (failed) - *see* Abortion, failed
  criminal - *see* Abortion, illegal
  early - *see* Abortion, spontaneous
  elective - *see* Abortion, legal
  failed (legal) 638.9
    with
      damage to pelvic organ
        (laceration) (rupture) (tear)
        638.2
      embolism (air) (amniotic fluid)
        (blood clot) (pulmonary)
        (pyemic) (septic) (soap)
        638.6
      genital tract and pelvic infection
        638.0
      hemorrhage, delayed or excessive
        638.1
      metabolic disorder 638.4
      renal failure (acute) 638.3
      sepsis (genital tract) (pelvic
        organ) 638.0
        urinary tract 638.7
      shock (postoperative) (septic)
        638.5
      specified complication NEC 638.7
      toxemia 638.3
      unspecified complication(s) 638.8
      urinary tract infection 638.7
  fetal indication - *see* Abortion, legal
  fetus 779.6
  following threatened abortion - *see*
    Abortion, by type
  habitual or recurrent (care during
    pregnancy) 646.3●
    with current abortion (*see also*
      Abortion, spontaneous) 634.9●
      affecting fetus or newborn 761.8
    without current pregnancy 629.81

◀ New   ◀▥ Revised   ~~deleted~~ Deleted   ● Use Additional Digit(s)   ▭ Omit code

Abortion *(Continued)*
  homicidal - *see* Abortion, illegal
  illegal 636.9●
    with
      damage to pelvic organ
          (laceration) (rupture) (tear)
          636.2●
      embolism (air) (amniotic fluid)
          (blood clot) (pulmonary)
          (pyemic) (septic) (soap)
          636.6●
      genital tract and pelvic infection
          636.0●
      hemorrhage, delayed or excessive
          636.1●
      metabolic disorder 636.4●
      renal failure 636.3●
      sepsis (genital tract) (pelvic
          organ) 636.0●
        urinary tract 636.7●
      shock (postoperative) (septic)
          636.5●
      specified complication NEC
          636.7●
      toxemia 636.3●
      unspecified complication(s)
          636.8●
      urinary tract infection 636.7●
    fetus 779.6
  induced 637.9●
    illegal - *see* Abortion, illegal
    legal indications - *see* Abortion, legal
    medical indications - *see* Abortion,
        legal
    therapeutic - *see* Abortion, legal
  late - *see* Abortion, spontaneous
  legal (legal indication) (medical
      indication) (under medical
      supervision) 635.9●
    with
      damage to pelvic organ
          (laceration) (rupture) (tear)
          635.2●
      embolism (air) (amniotic fluid)
          (blood clot) (pulmonary)
          (pyemic) (septic) (soap)
          635.6●
      genital tract and pelvic infection
          635.0●
      hemorrhage, delayed or excessive
          635.1●
      metabolic disorder 635.4●
      renal failure (acute) 635.3●
      sepsis (genital tract) (pelvic
          organ) 635.0●
        urinary tract 635.7●
      shock (postoperative) (septic)
          635.5●
      specified complication NEC
          635.7●
      toxemia 635.3●
      unspecified complication(s)
          635.8●
      urinary tract infection 635.7●
    fetus 779.6
  medical indication - *see* Abortion,
      legal
  mental hygiene problem - *see* Abortion,
      legal
  missed 632
  operative - *see* Abortion, legal
  psychiatric indication - *see* Abortion,
      legal
  recurrent - *see* Abortion, spontaneous

Abortion *(Continued)*
  self-induced - *see* Abortion, illegal
  septic - *see* Abortion, by type, with
      sepsis
  spontaneous 634.9●
    with
      damage to pelvic organ
          (laceration) (rupture) (tear)
          634.2●
      embolism (air) (amniotic fluid)
          (blood clot) (pulmonary)
          (pyemic) (septic) (soap)
          634.6●
      genital tract and pelvic infection
          634.0●
      hemorrhage, delayed or excessive
          634.1●
      metabolic disorder 634.4●
      renal failure 634.3●
      sepsis (genital tract) (pelvic
          organ) 634.0●
        urinary tract 634.7●
      shock (postoperative) (septic)
          634.5●
      specified complication NEC
          634.7●
      toxemia 634.3●
      unspecified complication(s)
          634.8●
      urinary tract infection 634.7●
    fetus 761.8
    threatened 640.0●
      affecting fetus or newborn
          762.1
  surgical - *see* Abortion, legal
  therapeutic - *see* Abortion, legal
  threatened 640.0●
    affecting fetus or newborn 762.1
  tubal - *see* Pregnancy, tubal
  voluntary - *see* Abortion, legal
Abortus fever 023.9
Aboulomania 301.6
Abrachia 755.20
Abrachiatism 755.20
Abrachiocephalia 759.89
Abrachiocephalus 759.89
Abrami's disease (acquired hemolytic
    jaundice) 283.9
Abramov-Fiedler myocarditis (acute
    isolated myocarditis) 422.91
Abrasion - *see also* Injury, superficial, by
    site
  cornea 918.1
  dental 521.20
    extending into
      dentine 521.22
      pulp 521.23
    generalized 521.25
    limited to enamel 521.21
    localized 521.24
  teeth, tooth (dentifrice) (habitual)
      (hard tissues) (occupational)
      (ritual) (traditional) (wedge
      defect) (*see also* Abrasion, dental)
      521.20
Abrikossov's tumor (M9580/0) - *see also*
    Neoplasm, connective tissue, benign
  malignant (M9580/3) - *see* Neoplasm,
      connective tissue, malignant
Abrism 988.8
Abruption, placenta - *see* Placenta,
    abruptio
Abruptio placentae - *see* Placenta,
    abruptio

Abscess (acute) (chronic) (infectional)
    (lymphangitic) (metastatic)
    (multiple) (pyogenic) (septic) (with
    lymphangitis) (*see also* Cellulitis)
    682.9
  abdomen, abdominal
    cavity 567.22
    wall 682.2
  abdominopelvic 567.22
  accessory sinus (chronic) (*see also*
      Sinusitis) 473.9
  adrenal (capsule) (gland) 255.8
  alveolar 522.5
    with sinus 522.7
  amebic 006.3
    bladder 006.8
    brain (with liver or lung abscess)
        006.5
    liver (without mention of brain or
        lung abscess) 006.3
      with
        brain abscess (and lung
            abscess) 006.5
        lung abscess 006.4
    lung (with liver abscess) 006.4
      with brain abscess 006.5
    seminal vesicle 006.8
    specified site NEC 006.8
    spleen 006.8
  anaerobic 040.0
  ankle 682.6
  anorectal 566
  antecubital space 682.3
  antrum (chronic) (Highmore) (*see also*
      Sinusitis, maxillary) 473.0
  anus 566
  apical (tooth) 522.5
    with sinus (alveolar) 522.7
  appendix 540.1
  areola (acute) (chronic) (nonpuerperal)
      611.0
    puerperal, postpartum 675.1●
  arm (any part, above wrist) 682.3
  artery (wall) 447.2
  atheromatous 447.2
  auditory canal (external) 380.10
  auricle (ear) (staphylococcal)
      (streptococcal) 380.10
  axilla, axillary (region) 682.3
    lymph gland or node 683
  back (any part) 682.2
  Bartholin's gland 616.3
    with
      abortion - *see* Abortion, by type,
          with sepsis
      ectopic pregnancy (*see also*
          categories 633.0-633.9)
          639.0
      molar pregnancy (*see also*
          categories 630-632)
          639.0
    complicating pregnancy or
        puerperium 646.6●
    following
      abortion 639.0
      ectopic or molar pregnancy
          639.0
  bartholinian 616.3
  Bezold's 383.01
  bile, biliary, duct or tract (*see also*
      Cholecystitis) 576.8
  bilharziasis 120.1
  bladder (wall) 595.89
    amebic 006.8

◀ New   ◀▦ Revised   ~~deleted~~ Deleted   ● Use Additional Digit(s)   ▨ Omit code

Abscess *(Continued)*
   bone (subperiosteal) *(see also*
      Osteomyelitis) 730.0●
     accessory sinus (chronic) *(see also*
      Sinusitis) 473.9
     acute 730.0●
     chronic or old 730.1●
     jaw (lower) (upper) 526.4
     mastoid - *see* Mastoiditis, acute
     petrous *(see also* Petrositis)
      383.20
     spinal (tuberculous) *(see also*
      Tuberculosis) 015.0●
      [730.88]
      nontuberculous 730.08
   bowel 569.5
   brain (any part) 324.0
     amebic (with liver or lung abscess)
      006.5
     cystic 324.0
     late effect - *see* category 326
     otogenic 324.0
     tuberculous *(see also* Tuberculosis)
      013.3●
   breast (acute) (chronic) (nonpuerperal)
     611.0
     newborn 771.5
     puerperal, postpartum 675.1●
     tuberculous *(see also* Tuberculosis)
      017.9●
   broad ligament (chronic) *(see also*
     Disease, pelvis, inflammatory)
     614.4
     acute 614.3
   Brodie's (chronic) (localized) *(see also*
     Osteomyelitis) 730.1●
   bronchus 519.19
   buccal cavity 528.3
   bulbourethral gland 597.0
   bursa 727.89
     pharyngeal 478.29
   buttock 682.5
   canaliculus, breast 611.0
   canthus 372.20
   cartilage 733.99
   cecum 569.5
     with appendicitis 540.1
   cerebellum, cerebellar 324.0
     late effect - *see* category 326
   cerebral (embolic) 324.0
     late effect - *see* category 326
   cervical (neck region) 682.1
     lymph gland or node 683
     stump *(see also* Cervicitis) 616.0
   cervix (stump) (uteri) *(see also*
     Cervicitis) 616.0
   cheek, external 682.0
     inner 528.3
   chest 510.9
     with fistula 510.0
     wall 682.2
   chin 682.0
   choroid 363.00
   ciliary body 364.3
   circumtonsillar 475
   cold (tuberculous) - *see also*
     Tuberculosis, abscess
     articular - *see* Tuberculosis, joint
   colon (wall) 569.5
   colostomy or enterostomy 569.61
   conjunctiva 372.00
   connective tissue NEC 682.9
   cornea 370.55
     with ulcer 370.00

Abscess *(Continued)*
   corpus
     cavernosum 607.2
     luteum *(see also* Salpingo-oophoritis)
      614.2
   Cowper's gland 597.0
   cranium 324.0
   cul-de-sac (Douglas') (posterior) *(see*
     also Disease, pelvis,
     inflammatory) 614.4
     acute 614.3
   dental 522.5
     with sinus (alveolar) 522.7
   dentoalveolar 522.5
     with sinus (alveolar) 522.7
   diaphragm, diaphragmatic 567.22
   digit NEC 681.9
   Douglas' cul-de-sac or pouch *(see also*
     Disease, pelvis, inflammatory)
     614.4
     acute 614.3
   Dubois' 090.5
   ductless gland 259.8
   ear
     acute 382.00
     external 380.10
     inner 386.30
     middle - *see* Otitis media
   elbow 682.3
   endamebic - *see* Abscess, amebic
   entamebic - *see* Abscess, amebic
   enterostomy 569.61
   epididymis 604.0
   epidural 324.9
     brain 324.0
     late effect - *see* category 326
     spinal cord 324.1
   epiglottis 478.79
   epiploon, epiploic 567.22
   erysipelatous *(see also* Erysipelas) 035
   esophagostomy 530.86
   esophagus 530.19
   ethmoid (bone) (chronic) (sinus) *(see*
     also Sinusitis, ethmoidal) 473.2
   external auditory canal 380.10
   extradural 324.9
     brain 324.0
     late effect - *see* category 326
     spinal cord 324.1
   extraperitoneal - *see* Abscess,
     peritoneum
   eye 360.00
   eyelid 373.13
   face (any part, except eye) 682.0
   fallopian tube *(see also* Salpingo-
     oophoritis) 614.2
   fascia 728.89
   fauces 478.29
   fecal 569.5
   femoral (region) 682.6
   filaria, filarial *(see also* Infestation,
     filarial) 125.9
   finger (any) (intrathecal) (periosteal)
     (subcutaneous) (subcuticular)
     681.00
   fistulous NEC 682.9
   flank 682.2
   foot (except toe) 682.7
   forearm 682.3
   forehead 682.0
   frontal (sinus) (chronic) *(see also*
     Sinusitis, frontal) 473.1
   gallbladder *(see also* Cholecystitis,
     acute) 575.0

Abscess *(Continued)*
   gastric 535.0●
   genital organ or tract NEC
     female 616.9
      with
       abortion - *see* Abortion, by
        type, with sepsis
       ectopic pregnancy *(see also*
        categories 633.0-633.9)
        639.0
       molar pregnancy *(see also*
        categories 630-632)
        639.0
      following
       abortion 639.0
       ectopic or molar pregnancy
        639.0
      puerperal, postpartum,
       childbirth 670.8● ◀▥
     male 608.4
   genitourinary system, tuberculous *(see*
     also Tuberculosis) 016.9●
   gingival 523.30
   gland, glandular (lymph) (acute) NEC
     683
   glottis 478.79
   gluteal (region) 682.5
   gonorrheal NEC *(see also* Gonococcus)
     098.0
   groin 682.2
   gum 523.30
   hand (except finger or thumb) 682.4
   head (except face) 682.8
   heart 429.89
   heel 682.7
   helminthic *(see also* Infestation, by
     specific parasite) 128.9
   hepatic 572.0
     amebic *(see also* Abscess, liver,
      amebic) 006.3
     duct 576.8
   hip 682.6
     tuberculous (active) *(see also*
      Tuberculosis) 015.1●
   ileocecal 540.1
   ileostomy (bud) 569.61
   iliac (region) 682.2
     fossa 540.1
   iliopsoas 567.31
     tuberculous *(see also* Tuberculosis)
      015.0● *[730.88]*
   infraclavicular (fossa) 682.3
   inguinal (region) 682.2
     lymph gland or node 683
   intersphincteric (anus) 566
   intestine, intestinal 569.5
     rectal 566
   intra-abdominal *(see also* Abscess,
     peritoneum) 567.22
     postoperative 998.59
   intracranial 324.0
     late effect - *see* category 326
   intramammary - *see* Abscess, breast
   intramastoid *(see also* Mastoiditis,
     acute) 383.00
   intraorbital 376.01
   intraperitoneal 567.22
   intraspinal 324.1
     late effect - *see* category 326
   intratonsillar 475
   iris 364.3
   ischiorectal 566
   jaw (bone) (lower) (upper) 526.4
     skin 682.0

◀ New   ◀▥ Revised   ~~deleted~~ Deleted   ● Use Additional Digit(s)   ▨ Omit code

Abscess *(Continued)*
  joint *(see also* Arthritis, pyogenic)
    711.0●
    vertebral (tuberculous) *(see also*
      Tuberculosis) 015.0● *[730.88]*
    nontuberculous 724.8
  kidney 590.2
    with
      abortion - *see* Abortion, by type,
        with urinary tract infection
      calculus 592.0
      ectopic pregnancy *(see also*
        categories 633.0-633.9)
        639.8
      molar pregnancy *(see also*
        categories 630-632) 639.8
      complicating pregnancy or
        puerperium 646.6●
        affecting fetus or newborn
          760.1
    following
      abortion 639.8
      ectopic or molar pregnancy
        639.8
  knee 682.6
    joint 711.06
    tuberculous (active) *(see also*
      Tuberculosis) 015.2●
  labium (majus) (minus) 616.4
    complicating pregnancy, childbirth,
      or puerperium 646.6●
  lacrimal (passages) (sac) *(see also*
    Dacryocystitis) 375.30
    caruncle 375.30
    gland *(see also* Dacryoadenitis)
      375.00
  lacunar 597.0
  larynx 478.79
  lateral (alveolar) 522.5
    with sinus 522.7
  leg, except foot 682.6
  lens 360.00
  lid 373.13
  lingual 529.0
    tonsil 475
  lip 528.5
  Littre's gland 597.0
  liver 572.0
    amebic 006.3
      with
        brain abscess (and lung
          abscess) 006.5
        lung abscess 006.4
      due to Entamoeba histolytica 006.3
      dysenteric *(see also* Abscess, liver,
        amebic) 006.3
      pyogenic 572.0
      tropical *(see also* Abscess, liver,
        amebic) 006.3
  loin (region) 682.2
  lumbar (tuberculous) *(see also*
    Tuberculosis) 015.0● *[730.88]*
    nontuberculous 682.2
  lung (miliary) (putrid) 513.0
    amebic (with liver abscess) 006.4
      with brain abscess 006.5
  lymph, lymphatic, gland or node
    (acute) 683
    any site, except mesenteric 683
    mesentery 289.2
  lymphangitic, acute - *see* Cellulitis
  malar 526.4
  mammary gland - *see* Abscess, breast
  marginal (anus) 566

Abscess *(Continued)*
  mastoid (process) *(see also* Mastoiditis,
    acute) 383.00
    subperiosteal 383.01
  maxilla, maxillary 526.4
    molar (tooth) 522.5
      with sinus 522.7
    premolar 522.5
    sinus (chronic) *(see also* Sinusitis,
      maxillary) 473.0
  mediastinum 513.1
  meibomian gland 373.12
  meninges *(see also* Meningitis) 320.9
  mesentery, mesenteric 567.22
  mesosalpinx *(see also* Salpingo-
    oophoritis) 614.2
  milk 675.1●
  Monro's (psoriasis) 696.1
  mons pubis 682.2
  mouth (floor) 528.3
  multiple sites NEC 682.9
  mural 682.2
  muscle 728.89
    psoas 567.31
  myocardium 422.92
  nabothian (follicle) *(see also* Cervicitis)
    616.0
  nail (chronic) (with lymphangitis) 681.9
    finger 681.02
    toe 681.11
  nasal (fossa) (septum) 478.19
    sinus (chronic) *(see also* Sinusitis)
      473.9
  nasopharyngeal 478.29
  nates 682.5
  navel 682.2
    newborn NEC 771.4
  neck (region) 682.1
    lymph gland or node 683
  nephritic *(see also* Abscess, kidney)
    590.2
  nipple 611.0
    puerperal, postpartum 675.0●
  nose (septum) 478.19
    external 682.0
  omentum 567.22
  operative wound 998.59
  orbit, orbital 376.01
  ossifluent - *see* Abscess, bone
  ovary, ovarian (corpus luteum) *(see also*
    Salpingo-oophoritis) 614.2
  oviduct *(see also* Salpingo-oophoritis)
    614.2
  palate (soft) 528.3
    hard 526.4
  palmar (space) 682.4
  pancreas (duct) 577.0
  paradontal 523.30
  parafrenal 607.2
  parametric, parametrium (chronic) *(see
    also* Disease, pelvis,
    inflammatory) 614.4
    acute 614.3
  paranephric 590.2
  parapancreatic 577.0
  parapharyngeal 478.22
  pararectal 566
  parasinus *(see also* Sinusitis) 473.9
  parauterine *(see also* Disease, pelvis,
    inflammatory) 614.4
    acute 614.3
  paravaginal *(see also* Vaginitis) 616.10
  parietal region 682.8
  parodontal 523.30

Abscess *(Continued)*
  parotid (duct) (gland) 527.3
    region 528.3
  parumbilical 682.2
    newborn 771.4
  pectoral (region) 682.2
  pelvirectal 567.22
  pelvis, pelvic
    female (chronic) *(see also* Disease,
      pelvis, inflammatory) 614.4
      acute 614.3
    male, peritoneal (cellular tissue) - *see*
      Abscess, peritoneum
    tuberculous *(see also* Tuberculosis)
      016.9●
  penis 607.2
    gonococcal (acute) 098.0
      chronic or duration of 2 months
        or over 098.2
  perianal 566
  periapical 522.5
    with sinus (alveolar) 522.7
  periappendiceal 540.1
  pericardial 420.99
  pericecal 540.1
  pericemental 523.30
  pericholecystic *(see also* Cholecystitis,
    acute) 575.0
  pericoronal 523.30
  peridental 523.30
  perigastric 535.0●
  perimetric *(see also* Disease, pelvis,
    inflammatory) 614.4
    acute 614.3
  perinephric, perinephritic *(see also*
    Abscess, kidney) 590.2
  perineum, perineal (superficial) 682.2
    deep (with urethral involvement)
      597.0
    urethra 597.0
  periodontal (parietal) 523.31
    apical 522.5
  periosteum, periosteal *(see also*
    Periostitis) 730.3●
    with osteomyelitis *(see also*
      Osteomyelitis) 730.2●
      acute or subacute 730.0●
      chronic or old 730.1●
  peripleuritic 510.9
    with fistula 510.0
  periproctic 566
  periprostatic 601.2
  perirectal (staphylococcal) 566
  perirenal (tissue) *(see also* Abscess,
    kidney) 590.2
  perisinuous (nose) *(see also* Sinusitis)
    473.9
  peritoneum, peritoneal (perforated)
    (ruptured) 567.22
    with
      abortion - *see* Abortion, by type,
        with sepsis
      appendicitis 540.1
      ectopic pregnancy *(see also*
        categories 633.0-633.9)
        639.0
      molar pregnancy *(see also*
        categories 630-632) 639.0
    following
      abortion 639.0
      ectopic or molar pregnancy 639.0
    pelvic, female *(see also* Disease,
      pelvis, inflammatory) 614.4
      acute 614.3

◀ New ◀▥ Revised ~~deleted~~ Deleted ● Use Additional Digit(s) ▦ Omit code

Abscess *(Continued)*
  umbilicus NEC 682.2
    newborn 771.4
  upper arm 682.3
  upper respiratory 478.9
  urachus 682.2
  urethra (gland) 597.0
  urinary 597.0
  uterus, uterine (wall) *(see also*
      Endometritis)* 615.9
    ligament *(see also* Disease, pelvis,
        inflammatory) 614.4
      acute 614.3
    neck *(see also* Cervicitis) 616.0
  uvula 528.3
  vagina (wall) *(see also* Vaginitis) 616.10
  vaginorectal *(see also* Vaginitis) 616.10
  vas deferens 608.4
  vermiform appendix 540.1
  vertebra (column) (tuberculous) *(see
      also* Tuberculosis) 015.0● *[730.88]*
    nontuberculous 730.0●
  vesical 595.89
  vesicouterine pouch *(see also* Disease,
      pelvis, inflammatory) 614.4
  vitreous (humor) (pneumococcal)
      360.04
  vocal cord 478.5
  von Bezold's 383.01
  vulva 616.4
    complicating pregnancy, childbirth,
        or puerperium 646.6●
  vulvovaginal gland *(see also* Vaginitis)
      616.3
  web-space 682.4
  wrist 682.4
Absence (organ or part) (complete or
    partial)
  acoustic nerve 742.8
  adrenal (gland) (congenital) 759.1
    acquired V45.79
  albumin (blood) 273.8
  alimentary tract (complete) (congenital)
      (partial) 751.8
    lower 751.5
    upper 750.8
  alpha-fucosidase 271.8
  alveolar process (acquired) 525.8
    congenital 750.26
  anus, anal (canal) (congenital) 751.2
  aorta (congenital) 747.22
  aortic valve (congenital) 746.89
  appendix, congenital 751.2
  arm (acquired) V49.60
    above elbow V49.66
    below elbow V49.65
    congenital *(see also* Deformity,
        reduction, upper limb) 755.20
      lower - *see* Absence, forearm,
          congenital
      upper (complete) (partial) (with
          absence of distal elements,
          incomplete) 755.24
        with
          complete absence of distal
              elements 755.21
          forearm (incomplete)
              755.23
  artery (congenital) (peripheral) NEC
      (see also Anomaly, peripheral
      vascular system) 747.60
    brain 747.81
    cerebral 747.81
    coronary 746.85

Absence *(Continued)*
  artery NEC *(Continued)*
    pulmonary 747.3
    umbilical 747.5
  atrial septum 745.69
  auditory canal (congenital) (external)
      744.01
  auricle (ear) (with stenosis or atresia of
      auditory canal), congenital 744.01
  bile, biliary duct (common) or passage
      (congenital) 751.61
  bladder (acquired) V45.74
    congenital 753.8
  bone (congenital) NEC 756.9
    marrow 284.9
      acquired (secondary) 284.89
      congenital 284.09
      hereditary 284.09
      idiopathic 284.9
    skull 756.0
  bowel sounds 787.5
  brain 740.0
    specified part 742.2
  breast(s) (acquired) V45.71
    congenital 757.6
  broad ligament (congenital) 752.19
  bronchus (congenital) 748.3
  calvarium, calvaria (skull) 756.0
  canaliculus lacrimalis, congenital
      743.65
  carpal(s) (congenital) (complete)
      (partial) (with absence of distal
      elements, incomplete) *(see also*
      Deformity, reduction, upper limb)
      755.28
    with complete absence of distal
        elements 755.21
  cartilage 756.9
  caudal spine 756.13
  cecum (acquired) (postoperative)
      (posttraumatic) V45.72
    congenital 751.2
  cementum 520.4
  cerebellum (congenital) (vermis)
      742.2
  cervix (acquired) (uteri) V88.01
    with remaining uterus V88.03
    and uterus V88.01
    congenital 752.49
  chin, congenital 744.89
  cilia (congenital) 743.63
    acquired 374.89
  circulatory system, part NEC 747.89
  clavicle 755.51
  clitoris (congenital) 752.49
  coccyx, congenital 756.13
  cold sense *(see also* Disturbance,
      sensation) 782.0
  colon (acquired) (postoperative) V45.72
    congenital 751.2
  congenital
    lumen - *see* Atresia
    organ or site NEC - *see* Agenesis
    septum - *see* Imperfect, closure
  corpus callosum (congenital) 742.2
  cricoid cartilage 748.3
  diaphragm (congenital) (with hernia)
      756.6
    with obstruction 756.6
  digestive organ(s) or tract, congenital
      (complete) (partial) 751.8
    acquired V45.79
    lower 751.5
    upper 750.8

Absence *(Continued)*
  ductus arteriosus 747.89
  duodenum (acquired) (postoperative)
      V45.72
    congenital 751.1
  ear, congenital 744.09
    acquired V45.79
    auricle 744.01
    external 744.01
    inner 744.05
    lobe, lobule 744.21
    middle, except ossicles 744.03
      ossicles 744.04
    ossicles 744.04
  ejaculatory duct (congenital) 752.89
  endocrine gland NEC (congenital)
      759.2
  epididymis (congenital) 752.89
    acquired V45.77
  epiglottis, congenital 748.3
  epileptic (atonic) (typical) *(see also*
      Epilepsy) 345.0●
  erythrocyte 284.9
  erythropoiesis 284.9
    congenital 284.01
  esophagus (congenital) 750.3
  eustachian tube (congenital) 744.24
  extremity (acquired)
    congenital *(see also* Deformity,
        reduction) 755.4
    lower V49.70
    upper V49.60
  extrinsic muscle, eye 743.69
  eye (acquired) V45.78
    adnexa (congenital) 743.69
    congenital 743.00
    muscle (congenital) 743.69
  eyelid (fold), congenital 743.62
    acquired 374.89
  face
    bones NEC 756.0
    specified part NEC 744.89
  fallopian tube(s) (acquired)
      V45.77
    congenital 752.19
  femur, congenital (complete)
      (partial) (with absence of
      distal elements, incomplete)
      (see also Deformity, reduction,
      lower limb) 755.34
    with
      complete absence of distal
          elements 755.31
      tibia and fibula (incomplete)
          755.33
  fibrin 790.92
  fibrinogen (congenital) 286.3
    acquired 286.6
  fibula, congenital (complete)
      (partial) (with absence of
      distal elements, incomplete)
      (see also Deformity, reduction,
      lower limb) 755.37
    with
      complete absence of distal
          elements 755.31
      tibia 755.35
        with
          complete absence of distal
              elements 755.31
          femur (incomplete) 755.33
            with complete absence
                of distal elements
                755.31

Absence *(Continued)*
 finger (acquired) V49.62
  congenital (complete) (partial) *(see also* Deformity, reduction, upper limb) 755.29
   meaning all fingers (complete) (partial) 755.21
   transverse 755.21
 fissures of lungs (congenital) 748.5
 foot (acquired) V49.73
  congenital (complete) 755.31
 forearm (acquired) V49.65
  congenital (complete) (partial) (with absence of distal elements, incomplete) *(see also* Deformity, reduction, upper limb) 755.25
   with
    complete absence of distal elements (hand and fingers) 755.21
    humerus (incomplete) 755.23
 fovea centralis 743.55
 fucosidase 271.8
 gallbladder (acquired) V45.79
  congenital 751.69
 gamma globulin (blood) 279.00
 genital organs
  acquired V45.77
  congenital
   female 752.89
    external 752.49
    internal NEC 752.89
   male 752.89
    penis 752.69
 genitourinary organs, congenital NEC 752.89
 glottis 748.3
 gonadal, congenital NEC 758.6
 hair (congenital) 757.4
  acquired - *see* Alopecia
 hand (acquired) V49.63
  congenital (complete) *(see also* Deformity, reduction, upper limb) 755.21
 heart (congenital) 759.89
  acquired - *see* Status, organ replacement
 heat sense *(see also* Disturbance, sensation) 782.0
 humerus, congenital (complete) (partial) (with absence of distal elements, incomplete) *(see also* Deformity, reduction, upper limb) 755.24
  with
   complete absence of distal elements 755.21
   radius and ulna (incomplete) 755.23
 hymen (congenital) 752.49
 ileum (acquired) (postoperative) (posttraumatic) V45.72
  congenital 751.1
 immunoglobulin, isolated NEC 279.03
  IgA 279.01
  IgG 279.03
  IgM 279.02
 incus (acquired) 385.24
  congenital 744.04
 internal ear (congenital) 744.05
 intestine (acquired) (small) V45.72
  congenital 751.1
   large 751.2

Absence *(Continued)*
 intestine *(Continued)*
  large V45.72
   congenital 751.2
 iris (congenital) 743.45
 jaw - *see* Absence, mandible
 jejunum (acquired) V45.72
  congenital 751.1
 joint, congenital NEC 755.8
 kidney(s) (acquired) V45.73
  congenital 753.0
 labium (congenital) (majus) (minus) 752.49
 labyrinth, membranous 744.05
 lacrimal apparatus (congenital) 743.65
 larynx (congenital) 748.3
 leg (acquired) V49.70
  above knee V49.76
  below knee V49.75
  congenital (partial) (unilateral) *(see also* Deformity, reduction, lower limb) 755.31
   lower (complete) (partial) (with absence of distal elements, incomplete) 755.35
    with
     complete absence of distal elements (foot and toes) 755.31
     thigh (incomplete) 755.33
      with complete absence of distal elements 755.31
   upper - *see* Absence, femur
 lens (congenital) 743.35
  acquired 379.31
 ligament, broad (congenital) 752.19
 limb (acquired)
  congenital (complete) (partial) *(see also* Deformity, reduction) 755.4
   lower 755.30
    complete 755.31
    incomplete 755.32
    longitudinal - *see* Deficiency, lower limb, longitudinal
    transverse 755.31
   upper 755.20
    complete 755.21
    incomplete 755.22
    longitudinal - *see* Deficiency, upper limb, longitudinal
    transverse 755.21
  lower NEC V49.70
  upper NEC V49.60
 lip 750.26
 liver (congenital) (lobe) 751.69
 lumbar (congenital) (vertebra) 756.13
  isthmus 756.11
  pars articularis 756.11
 lumen - *see* Atresia
 lung (bilateral) (congenital) (fissure) (lobe) (unilateral) 748.5
  acquired (any part) V45.76
 mandible (congenital) 524.09
 maxilla (congenital) 524.09
 menstruation 626.0
 metacarpal(s), congenital (complete) (partial) (with absence of distal elements, incomplete) *(see also* Deformity, reduction, upper limb) 755.28
  with all fingers, complete 755.21

Absence *(Continued)*
 metatarsal(s), congenital (complete) (partial) (with absence of distal elements, incomplete) *(see also* Deformity, reduction, lower limb) 755.38
  with complete absence of distal elements 755.31
 muscle (congenital) (pectoral) 756.81
  ocular 743.69
 musculoskeletal system (congenital) NEC 756.9
 nail(s) (congenital) 757.5
 neck, part 744.89
 nerve 742.8
 nervous system, part NEC 742.8
 neutrophil 288.00
 nipple (congenital) 757.6
  acquired V45.71
 nose (congenital) 748.1
  acquired 738.0
 nuclear 742.8
 ocular muscle (congenital) 743.69
 organ
  of Corti (congenital) 744.05
  or site
   acquired V45.79
   congenital NEC 759.89
 osseous meatus (ear) 744.03
 ovary (acquired) V45.77
  congenital 752.0
 oviduct (acquired) V45.77
  congenital 752.19
 pancreas (congenital) 751.7
  acquired (postoperative) (posttraumatic) V45.79
 parathyroid gland (congenital) 759.2
 parotid gland(s) (congenital) 750.21
 patella, congenital 755.64
 pelvic girdle (congenital) 755.69
 penis (congenital) 752.69
  acquired V45.77
 pericardium (congenital) 746.89
 perineal body (congenital) 756.81
 phalange(s), congenital 755.4
  lower limb (complete) (intercalary) (partial) (terminal) *(see also* Deformity, reduction, lower limb) 755.39
   meaning all toes (complete) (partial) 755.31
   transverse 755.31
  upper limb (complete) (intercalary) (partial) (terminal) *(see also* Deformity, reduction, upper limb) 755.29
   meaning all digits (complete) (partial) 755.21
   transverse 755.21
 pituitary gland (congenital) 759.2
 postoperative - *see* Absence, by site, acquired
 prostate (congenital) 752.89
  acquired V45.77
 pulmonary
  artery 747.3
  trunk 747.3
  valve (congenital) 746.01
  vein 747.49
 punctum lacrimale (congenital) 743.65

◀ New   ◀ Revised   ~~deleted~~ Deleted   ● Use Additional Digit(s)   ▨ Omit code

Absence (Continued)
  radius, congenital (complete) (partial)
      (with absence of distal elements,
      incomplete) 755.26
    with
      complete absence of distal
          elements 755.21
      ulna 755.25
        with
          complete absence of distal
              elements 755.21
          humerus (incomplete) 755.23
  ray, congenital 755.4
    lower limb (complete) (partial) (see
        also Deformity, reduction,
        lower limb) 755.38
      meaning all rays 755.31
      transverse 755.31
    upper limb (complete) (partial) (see
        also Deformity, reduction,
        upper limb) 755.28
      meaning all rays 755.21
      transverse 755.21
  rectum (congenital) 751.2
    acquired V45.79
  red cell 284.9
    acquired (secondary) 284.81
    congenital 284.01
    hereditary 284.01
    idiopathic 284.9
  respiratory organ (congenital) NEC
      748.9
  rib (acquired) 738.3
    congenital 756.3
  roof of orbit (congenital) 742.0
  round ligament (congenital) 752.89
  sacrum, congenital 756.13
  salivary gland(s) (congenital) 750.21
  scapula 755.59
  scrotum, congenital 752.89
  seminal tract or duct (congenital)
      752.89
    acquired V45.77
  septum (congenital) - see also Imperfect,
      closure, septum
    atrial 745.69
      and ventricular 745.7
    between aorta and pulmonary
        artery 745.0
    ventricular 745.3
      and atrial 745.7
  sex chromosomes 758.81
  shoulder girdle, congenital (complete)
      (partial) 755.59
  skin (congenital) 757.39
  skull bone 756.0
    with
      anencephalus 740.0
      encephalocele 742.0
      hydrocephalus 742.3
        with spina bifida (see also
            Spina bifida) 741.0●
      microcephalus 742.1
  spermatic cord (congenital) 752.89
  spinal cord 742.59
  spine, congenital 756.13
  spleen (congenital) 759.0
    acquired V45.79
  sternum, congenital 756.3
  stomach (acquired) (partial)
      (postoperative) V45.75
    with postgastric surgery syndrome
        564.2
    congenital 750.7

Absence (Continued)
  submaxillary gland(s) (congenital)
      750.21
  superior vena cava (congenital)
      747.49
  tarsal(s), congenital (complete)
      (partial) (with absence of distal
      elements, incomplete) (see also
      Deformity, reduction, lower
      limb) 755.38
  teeth, tooth (congenital) 520.0
    with abnormal spacing 524.30
    acquired 525.10
      with malocclusion 524.30
      due to
        caries 525.13
        extraction 525.10
        periodontal disease 525.12
        trauma 525.11
  tendon (congenital) 756.81
  testis (congenital) 752.89
    acquired V45.77
  thigh (acquired) 736.89
  thumb (acquired) V49.61
    congenital 755.29
  thymus gland (congenital) 759.2
  thyroid (gland) (surgical) 246.8
    with hypothyroidism 244.0
    cartilage, congenital 748.3
    congenital 243
  tibia, congenital (complete) (partial)
      (with absence of distal elements,
      incomplete) (see also Deformity,
      reduction, lower limb) 755.36
    with
      complete absence of distal
          elements 755.31
      fibula 755.35
        with
          complete absence of distal
              elements 755.31
          femur (incomplete)
              755.33
            with complete absence
                of distal elements
                755.31
  toe (acquired) V49.72
    congenital (complete) (partial)
        755.39
      meaning all toes 755.31
      transverse 755.31
    great V49.71
  tongue (congenital) 750.11
  tooth, teeth (congenital) 520.0
    with abnormal spacing 524.30
    acquired 525.10
      with malocclusion 524.30
      due to
        caries 525.13
        extraction 525.10
        periodontal disease 525.12
        trauma 525.11
  trachea (cartilage) (congenital) (rings)
      748.3
  transverse aortic arch (congenital)
      747.21
  tricuspid valve 746.1
  ulna, congenital (complete) (partial)
      (with absence of distal elements,
      incomplete) (see also Deformity,
      reduction, upper limb) 755.27
    with
      complete absence of distal
          elements 755.21

Absence (Continued)
  ulna, congenital (Continued)
    with (Continued)
      radius 755.25
        with
          complete absence of distal
              elements 755.21
          humerus (incomplete)
              755.23
  umbilical artery (congenital) 747.5
  ureter (congenital) 753.4
    acquired V45.74
  urethra, congenital 753.8
    acquired V45.74
  urinary system, part NEC, congenital
      753.8
    acquired V45.74
  uterus (acquired) V88.01
    with remaining cervical stump
        V88.02
    and cervix V88.01
    congenital 752.3
  uvula (congenital) 750.26
  vagina, congenital 752.49
    acquired V45.77
  vas deferens (congenital) 752.89
    acquired V45.77
  vein (congenital) (peripheral) NEC (see
      also Anomaly, peripheral vascular
      system) 747.60
    brain 747.81
    great 747.49
    portal 747.49
    pulmonary 747.49
  vena cava (congenital) (inferior)
      (superior) 747.49
  ventral horn cell 742.59
  ventricular septum 745.3
  vermis of cerebellum 742.2
  vertebra, congenital 756.13
  vulva, congenital 752.49
Absentia epileptica (see also Epilepsy)
    345.0●
Absinthemia (see also Dependence)
    304.6●
Absinthism (see also Dependence)
    304.6●
Absorbent system disease 459.89
Absorption
  alcohol, through placenta or breast
      milk 760.71
  antibiotics, through placenta or breast
      milk 760.74
  anticonvulsants, through placenta or
      breast milk 760.77
  antifungals, through placenta or breast
      milk 760.74
  anti-infective, through placenta or
      breast milk 760.74
  antimetabolics, through placenta or
      breast milk 760.78
  chemical NEC 989.9
    specified chemical or substance - see
        Table of Drugs and Chemicals
    through placenta or breast milk
        (fetus or newborn) 760.70
      alcohol 760.71
      anticonvulsants 760.77
      antifungals 760.74
      anti-infective agents 760.74
      antimetabolics 760.78
      cocaine 760.75
      "crack" 760.75
      diethylstilbestrol [DES] 760.76

Absorption (Continued)
  chemical NEC (Continued)
    through placenta or breast milk
        (Continued)
      hallucinogenic agents 760.73
      medicinal agents NEC 760.79
      narcotics 760.72
      obstetric anesthetic or analgesic
          drug 763.5
      specified agent NEC 760.79
      suspected, affecting
          management of
          pregnancy 655.5●
  cocaine, through placenta or breast
      milk 760.75
  drug NEC (see also Reaction, drug)
    through placenta or breast milk
        (fetus or newborn) 760.70
      alcohol 760.71
      anticonvulsants 760.77
      antifungals 760.74
      anti-infective agents 760.74
      antimetabolics 760.78
      cocaine 760.75
      "crack" 760.75
      diethylstilbestrol (DES) 760.76
      hallucinogenic agents 760.73
      medicinal agents NEC 760.79
      narcotics 760.72
      obstetric anesthetic or analgesic
          drug 763.5
      specified agent NEC 760.79
      suspected, affecting
          management of
          pregnancy 655.5●
  fat, disturbance 579.8
  hallucinogenic agents, through
      placenta or breast milk 760.73
  immune sera, through placenta or
      breast milk 760.79
  lactose defect 271.3
  medicinal agents NEC, through
      placenta or breast milk 760.79
  narcotics, through placenta or breast
      milk 760.72
  noxious substance - see Absorption,
      chemical
  protein, disturbance 579.8
  pus or septic, general - see Septicemia
  quinine, through placenta or breast
      milk 760.74
  toxic substance - see Absorption,
      chemical
  uremic - see Uremia
Abstinence symptoms or syndrome
  alcohol 291.81
  drug 292.0
  neonatal 779.5
Abt-Letterer-Siwe syndrome (acute
    histiocytosis X) (M9722/3)
    202.5●
Abulia 799.89
Abulomania 301.6
Abuse
  adult 995.80
    emotional 995.82
    multiple forms 995.85
    neglect (nutritional) 995.84
    physical 995.81
    psychological 995.82
    sexual 995.83
  alcohol (see also Alcoholism) 305.0●
    dependent 303.9●
    nondependent 305.0●

Abuse (Continued)
  child 995.50
    counseling
      perpetrator
        non-parent V62.83
        parent V61.22
      victim V61.21
    emotional 995.51
    multiple forms 995.59
    neglect (nutritional) 995.52
    physical 995.54
      shaken infant syndrome 995.55
    psychological 995.51
    sexual 995.53
  drugs, nondependent 305.9●

Note 02   Use the following fifth-digit
subclassification with the following
codes: 305.0, 305.2-305.9:

0   unspecified
1   continuous
2   episodic
3   in remission

---

    amphetamine type 305.7●
    antidepressants 305.8●
    anxiolytic 305.4●
    barbiturates 305.4●
    caffeine 305.9●
    cannabis 305.2●
    cocaine type 305.6●
    hallucinogens 305.3●
    hashish 305.2●
    hypnotic 305.4●
    inhalant 305.9●
    LSD 305.3●
    marijuana 305.2●
    mixed 305.9●
    morphine type 305.5●
    opioid type 305.5●
    phencyclidine (PCP) 305.9●
    sedative 305.4●
    specified NEC 305.9●
    tranquilizers 305.4●
  spouse 995.80
  tobacco 305.1
Acalcerosis 275.40
Acalcicosis 275.40
Acalculia 784.69
  developmental 315.1
Acanthocheilonemiasis 125.4
Acanthocytosis 272.5
Acanthokeratodermia 701.1
Acantholysis 701.8
  bullosa 757.39
Acanthoma (benign) (M8070/0) - see also
    Neoplasm, by site, benign
  malignant (M8070/3) - see Neoplasm,
    by site, malignant
Acanthosis (acquired) (nigricans) 701.2
  adult 701.2
  benign (congenital) 757.39
  congenital 757.39
  glycogenic
    esophagus 530.89
  juvenile 701.2
  tongue 529.8
Acanthrocytosis 272.5
Acapnia 276.3
Acarbia 276.2
Acardia 759.89
Acardiacus amorphus 759.89
Acardiotrophia 429.1
Acardius 759.89

Acariasis 133.9
  sarcoptic 133.0
Acaridiasis 133.9
Acarinosis 133.9
Acariosis 133.9
Acarodermatitis 133.9
  urticarioides 133.9
Acarophobia 300.29
Acatalasemia 277.89
Acatalasia 277.89
Acatamathesia 784.69
Acataphasia 784.59   ◀▥
Acathisia 781.0
  due to drugs 333.99
Acceleration, accelerated
  atrioventricular conduction 426.7
  idioventricular rhythm 427.89
Accessory (congenital)
  adrenal gland 759.1
  anus 751.5
  appendix 751.5
  atrioventricular conduction 426.7
  auditory ossicles 744.04
  auricle (ear) 744.1
  autosome(s) NEC 758.5
    21 or 22 758.0
  biliary duct or passage 751.69
  bladder 753.8
  blood vessels (peripheral) (congenital)
      NEC (see also Anomaly,
      peripheral vascular system)
      747.60
    cerebral 747.81
    coronary 746.85
  bone NEC 756.9
    foot 755.67
  breast tissue, axilla 757.6
  carpal bones 755.56
  cecum 751.5
  cervix 752.49
  chromosome(s) NEC 758.5
    13-15 758.1
    16-18 758.2
    21 or 22 758.0
    autosome(s) NEC 758.5
    D_1 758.1
    E_3 758.2
    G 758.0
    sex 758.81
  coronary artery 746.85
  cusp(s), heart valve NEC 746.89
    pulmonary 746.09
  cystic duct 751.69
  digits 755.00
  ear (auricle) (lobe) 744.1
  endocrine gland NEC 759.2
  external os 752.49
  eyelid 743.62
  eye muscle 743.69
  face bone(s) 756.0
  fallopian tube (fimbria) (ostium)
      752.19
  fingers 755.01
  foreskin 605
  frontonasal process 756.0
  gallbladder 751.69
  genital organ(s)
    female 752.89
      external 752.49
      internal NEC 752.89
    male NEC 752.89
      penis 752.69
  genitourinary organs NEC 752.89

◀ New   ◀▥ Revised   ~~deleted~~ Deleted   ● Use Additional Digit(s)   ▨ Omit code

Accessory (Continued)
  heart 746.89
    valve NEC 746.89
      pulmonary 746.09
  hepatic ducts 751.69
  hymen 752.49
  intestine (large) (small) 751.5
  kidney 753.3
  lacrimal canal 743.65
  leaflet, heart valve NEC 746.89
    pulmonary 746.09
  ligament, broad 752.19
  liver (duct) 751.69
  lobule (ear) 744.1
  lung (lobe) 748.69
  muscle 756.82
  navicular of carpus 755.56
  nervous system, part NEC 742.8
  nipple 757.6
  nose 748.1
  organ or site NEC - see Anomaly,
    specified type NEC
  ovary 752.0
  oviduct 752.19
  pancreas 751.7
  parathyroid gland 759.2
  parotid gland (and duct) 750.22
  pituitary gland 759.2
  placental lobe - see Placenta, abnormal
  preauricular appendage 744.1
  prepuce 605
  renal arteries (multiple) 747.62
  rib 756.3
    cervical 756.2
  roots (teeth) 520.2
  salivary gland 750.22
  sesamoids 755.8
  sinus - see Condition
  skin tags 757.39
  spleen 759.0
  sternum 756.3
  submaxillary gland 750.22
  tarsal bones 755.67
  teeth, tooth 520.1
    causing crowding 524.31
  tendon 756.89
  thumb 755.01
  thymus gland 759.2
  thyroid gland 759.2
  toes 755.02
  tongue 750.13
  tragus 744.1
  ureter 753.4
  urethra 753.8
  urinary organ or tract NEC 753.8
  uterus 752.2
  vagina 752.49
  valve, heart NEC 746.89
    pulmonary 746.09
  vertebra 756.19
  vocal cords 748.3
  vulva 752.49
Accident, accidental - see also condition
  birth NEC 767.9
  cardiovascular (see also Disease,
    cardiovascular) 429.2
  cerebral (see also Disease,
    cerebrovascular, acute) 434.91
  cerebrovascular (current) (CVA) (see
    also Disease, cerebrovascular,
    acute) 434.91
    aborted 434.91
    embolic 434.11
    healed or old V12.54

Accident, accidental (Continued)
  cerebrovascular (Continued)
    hemorrhagic - see Hemorrhage,
      brain
    impending 435.9
    ischemic 434.91
    late effect - see Late effect(s) (of)
      cerebrovascular disease
    postoperative 997.02
    thrombotic 434.01
  coronary (see also Infarct, myocardium)
    410.9●
  craniovascular (see also Disease,
    cerebrovascular, acute) 436
  during pregnancy, to mother, affecting
    fetus or newborn 760.5
  heart, cardiac (see also Infarct,
    myocardium) 410.9●
  intrauterine 779.89
  vascular - see Disease, cerebrovascular,
    acute
Accommodation
  disorder of 367.51
    drug-induced 367.89
    toxic 367.89
  insufficiency of 367.4
  paralysis of 367.51
    hysterical 300.11
  spasm of 367.53
Accouchement - see Delivery
Accreta placenta (without hemorrhage)
  667.0●
  with hemorrhage 666.0●
Accretio cordis (nonrheumatic) 423.1
Accretions on teeth 523.6
Accumulation secretion, prostate 602.8
Acephalia, acephalism, acephaly 740.0
Acephalic 740.0
Acephalobrachia 759.89
Acephalocardia 759.89
Acephalocardius 759.89
Acephalochiria 759.89
Acephalochirus 759.89
Acephalogaster 759.89
Acephalostomus 759.89
Acephalothorax 759.89
Acephalus 740.0
Acetonemia 790.6
  diabetic 250.1●
    due to secondary diabetes 249.1●
Acetonglycosuria 982.8
Acetonuria 791.6
Achalasia 530.0
  cardia 530.0
  digestive organs congenital NEC 751.8
  esophagus 530.0
  pelvirectal 751.3
  psychogenic 306.4
  pylorus 750.5
  sphincteral NEC 564.89
Achard-Thiers syndrome (adrenogenital)
  255.2
Ache(s) - see Pain
Acheilia 750.26
Acheiria 755.21
Achillobursitis 726.71
Achillodynia 726.71
Achlorhydria, achlorhydric 536.0
  anemia 280.9
  diarrhea 536.0
  neurogenic 536.0
  postvagotomy 564.2
  psychogenic 306.4
  secondary to vagotomy 564.2

Achloroblepsia 368.52
Achloropsia 368.52
Acholia 575.8
Acholuric jaundice (familial)
  (splenomegalic) (see also
  Spherocytosis) 282.0
  acquired 283.9
Achondroplasia 756.4
Achrestic anemia 281.8
Achroacytosis, lacrimal gland 375.00
  tuberculous (see also Tuberculosis)
    017.3●
Achroma, cutis 709.00
Achromate (congenital) 368.54
Achromatopia 368.54
Achromatopsia (congenital) 368.54
Achromia
  congenital 270.2
  parasitica 111.0
  unguium 703.8
Achylia
  gastrica 536.8
    neurogenic 536.3
    psychogenic 306.4
  pancreatica 577.1
Achylosis 536.8
Acid
  burn - see also Burn, by site
    from swallowing acid - see Burn,
      internal organs
  deficiency
    amide nicotinic 265.2
    amino 270.9
    ascorbic 267
    folic 266.2
    nicotinic (amide) 265.2
    pantothenic 266.2
  intoxication 276.2
  peptic disease 536.8
  stomach 536.8
    psychogenic 306.4
Acidemia 276.2
  arginosuccinic 270.6
  fetal
    affecting management of pregnancy
      656.3●
    before onset of labor, in liveborn
      infant 768.2
    during labor and delivery, in
      liveborn infant 768.3
    intrauterine 656.3●
    unspecified as to time of onset, in
      liveborn infant 768.4
  newborn 775.81
  pipecolic 270.7
Acidity, gastric (high) (low) 536.8
  psychogenic 306.4
Acidocytopenia 288.59
Acidocytosis 288.3
Acidopenia 288.59
Acidosis 276.2
  diabetic 250.1●
    due to secondary diabetes
      249.1●
  fetal, affecting management of
    pregnancy 656.8●
  fetal, affecting newborn 775.81
  kidney tubular 588.89
  lactic 276.2
  metabolic NEC 276.2
    with respiratory acidosis 276.4
      of newborn 775.81
    late, of newborn 775.7
  newborn 775.81

Acidosis (Continued)
  renal
    hyperchloremic 588.89
    tubular (distal) (proximal) 588.89
  respiratory 276.2
    complicated by
      metabolic acidosis 276.4
        of newborn 775.81
      metabolic alkalosis 276.4
Aciduria 791.9
  arginosuccinic 270.6
  beta-aminoisobutyric (BAIB) 277.2
  glutaric
    type I 270.7
    type II (type IIA, IIB, IIC) 277.85
    type III 277.86
  glycolic 271.8
  methylmalonic 270.3
    with glycinemia 270.7
  organic 270.9
  orotic (congenital) (hereditary)
    (pyrimidine deficiency) 281.4
Acladiosis 111.8
  skin 111.8
Aclasis
  diaphyseal 756.4
  tarsoepiphyseal 756.59
Acleistocardia 745.5
Aclusion 524.4
Acmesthesia 782.0
Acne (pustular) (vulgaris) 706.1
  agminata (see also Tuberculosis) 017.0●
  artificialis 706.1
  atrophica 706.0
  cachecticorum (Hebra) 706.1
  conglobata 706.1
  conjunctiva 706.1
  cystic 706.1
  decalvans 704.09
  erythematosa 695.3
  eyelid 706.1
  frontalis 706.0
  indurata 706.1
  keloid 706.1
  lupoid 706.0
  necrotic, necrotica 706.0
    miliaris 704.8
  neonatal 706.1
  nodular 706.1
  occupational 706.1
  papulosa 706.1
  rodens 706.0
  rosacea 695.3
  scorbutica 267
  scrofulosorum (Bazin) (see also
    Tuberculosis) 017.0●
  summer 692.72
  tropical 706.1
  varioliformis 706.0
Acneiform drug eruptions 692.3
Acnitis (primary) (see also Tuberculosis)
  017.0●
Acomia 704.00
Acontractile bladder 344.61
Aconuresis (see also Incontinence) 788.30
Acosta's disease 993.2
Acousma 780.1
Acoustic - see condition
Acousticophobia 300.29
Acquired - see condition
Acquired immune deficiency
  syndrome - see Human
  immunodeficiency virus (disease)
  (illness) (infection)

Acquired immunodeficiency
  syndrome - see Human
  immunodeficiency virus (disease)
  (illness) (infection)
Acragnosis 781.99
Acrania 740.0
Acroagnosis 781.99
Acroasphyxia, chronic 443.89
Acrobrachycephaly 756.0
Acrobystiolith 608.89
Acrobystitis 607.2
Acrocephalopolysyndactyly 755.55
Acrocephalosyndactyly 755.55
Acrocephaly 756.0
Acrochondrohyperplasia 759.82
Acrocyanosis 443.89
  newborn 770.83
    meaning transient blue hands and
    feet - *omit code*
Acrodermatitis 686.8
  atrophicans (chronica) 701.8
  continua (Hallopeau) 696.1
  enteropathica 686.8
  Hallopeau's 696.1
  perstans 696.1
  pustulosa continua 696.1
  recalcitrant pustular 696.1
Acrodynia 985.0
Acrodysplasia 755.55
Acrohyperhidrosis (see also
  Hyperhidrosis) 780.8
Acrokeratosis verruciformis 757.39
Acromastitis 611.0
Acromegaly, acromegalia (skin) 253.0
Acromelalgia 443.82
Acromicria, acromikria 756.59
Acronyx 703.0
Acropachy, thyroid (see also
  Thyrotoxicosis) 242.9●
Acropachyderma 757.39
Acroparesthesia 443.89
  simple (Schultz's type) 443.89
  vasomotor (Nothnagel's type) 443.89
Acropathy thyroid (see also
  Thyrotoxicosis) 242.9●
Acrophobia 300.29
Acroposthitis 607.2
Acroscleriasis (see also Scleroderma) 710.1
Acroscleroderma (see also Scleroderma)
  710.1
Acrosclerosis (see also Scleroderma)
  710.1
Acrosphacelus 785.4
Acrosphenosyndactylia 755.55
Acrospiroma, eccrine (M8402/0) - see
  Neoplasm, skin, benign
Acrostealgia 732.9
Acrosyndactyly (see also Syndactylism)
  755.10
Acrotrophodynia 991.4
Actinic - see also condition
  cheilitis (due to sun) 692.72
    chronic NEC 692.74
    due to radiation, except from sun
      692.82
  conjunctivitis 370.24
  dermatitis (due to sun) (see also
    Dermatitis, actinic) 692.70
  due to
    roentgen rays or radioactive
      substance 692.82
    ultraviolet radiation, except from
      sun 692.82
    sun NEC 692.70

Actinic (Continued)
  elastosis solare 692.74
  granuloma 692.73
  keratitis 370.24
  ophthalmia 370.24
  reticuloid 692.73
Actinobacillosis, general 027.8
Actinobacillus
  lignieresii 027.8
  mallei 024
  muris 026.1
Actinocutitis NEC (see also Dermatitis,
  actinic) 692.70
Actinodermatitis NEC (see also
  Dermatitis, actinic) 692.70
Actinomyces
  israelii (infection) - see
    Actinomycosis
  muris-ratti (infection) 026.1
Actinomycosis, actinomycotic 039.9
  with
    pneumonia 039.1
  abdominal 039.2
  cervicofacial 039.3
  cutaneous 039.0
  pulmonary 039.1
  specified site NEC 039.8
  thoracic 039.1
Actinoneuritis 357.89
Action, heart
  disorder 427.9
    postoperative 997.1
  irregular 427.9
    postoperative 997.1
    psychogenic 306.2
Active - see condition
Activity decrease, functional 780.99
Acute - see also condition
  abdomen NEC 789.0●
  gallbladder (see also Cholecystitis,
    acute) 575.0
Acyanoblepsia 368.53
Acyanopsia 368.53
Acystia 753.8
Acystinervia - see Neurogenic, bladder
Acystineuria - see Neurogenic, bladder
Adactylia, adactyly (congenital) 755.4
  lower limb (complete) (intercalary)
    (partial) (terminal) (see also
    Deformity, reduction, lower limb)
    755.39
    meaning all digits (complete)
      (partial) 755.31
    transverse (complete) (partial)
      755.31
  upper limb (complete) (intercalary)
    (partial) (terminal) (see also
    Deformity, reduction, upper limb)
    755.29
    meaning all digits (complete)
      (partial) 755.21
    transverse (complete) (partial)
      755.21
Adair-Dighton syndrome (brittle bones
  and blue sclera, deafness) 756.51
Adamantinoblastoma (M9310/0) - see
  Ameloblastoma
Adamantinoma (M9310/0) - see
  Ameloblastoma
Adamantoblastoma (M9310/0) - see
  Ameloblastoma
Adams-Stokes (-Morgagni) disease or
  syndrome (syncope with heart
  block) 426.9

◀ New   ◀▥ Revised   ~~deleted~~ Deleted   ● Use Additional Digit(s)   ▨ Omit code

Adaptation reaction (*see also* Reaction, adjustment) 309.9
ADEM (acute disseminated encephalomy-elitis)(postinfectious) 136.9 *[323.61]*
  infectious 136.9 *[323.61]*
  noninfectious 323.81
Addiction - *see also* Dependence
  absinthe 304.6●
  alcoholic (ethyl) (methyl) (wood) 303.9●
    complicating pregnancy, childbirth, or puerperium 648.4●
      affecting fetus or newborn 760.71
    suspected damage to fetus affecting management of pregnancy 655.4●
  drug (*see also* Dependence) 304.9●
  ethyl alcohol 303.9●
  heroin 304.0●
  hospital 301.51
  methyl alcohol 303.9●
  methylated spirit 303.9●
  morphine (-like substances) 304.0●
  nicotine 305.1
  opium 304.0●
  tobacco 305.1
  wine 303.9●
Addison's
  anemia (pernicious) 281.0
  disease (bronze) (primary adrenal insufficiency) 255.41
    tuberculous (*see also* Tuberculosis) 017.6●
  keloid (morphea) 701.0
  melanoderma (adrenal cortical hypofunction) 255.41
Addison-Biermer anemia (pernicious) 281.0
Addison-Gull disease - *see* Xanthoma
Addisonian crisis or melanosis (acute adrenocortical insufficiency) 255.41
Additional - *see also* Accessory
  chromosome(s) 758.5
    13-15 758.1
    16-18 758.2
    21 758.0
    autosome(s) NEC 758.5
    sex 758.81
Adduction contracture, hip or other joint - *see* Contraction, joint
Adenasthenia gastrica 536.0
Aden fever 061
Adenitis (*see also* Lymphadenitis) 289.3
  acute, unspecified site 683
    epidemic infectious 075
  axillary 289.3
    acute 683
    chronic or subacute 289.1
  Bartholin's gland 616.89
  bulbourethral gland (*see also* Urethritis) 597.89
  cervical 289.3
    acute 683
    chronic or subacute 289.1
  chancroid (Ducrey's bacillus) 099.0
  chronic (any lymph node, except mesenteric) 289.1
    mesenteric 289.2
  Cowper's gland (*see also* Urethritis) 597.89
  epidemic, acute 075
  gangrenous 683
  gonorrheal NEC 098.89

Adenitis (*Continued*)
  groin 289.3
    acute 683
    chronic or subacute 289.1
  infectious 075
  inguinal (region) 289.3
    acute 683
    chronic or subacute 289.1
  lymph gland or node, except mesenteric 289.3
    acute 683
    chronic or subacute 289.1
    mesenteric (acute) (chronic) (nonspecific) (subacute) 289.2
  mesenteric (acute) (chronic) (nonspecific) (subacute) 289.2
    due to Pasteurella multocida (P. septica) 027.2
  parotid gland (suppurative) 527.2
  phlegmonous 683
  salivary duct or gland (any) (recurring) (suppurative) 527.2
  scrofulous (*see also* Tuberculosis) 017.2●
  septic 289.3
  Skene's duct or gland (*see also* Urethritis) 597.89
  strumous, tuberculous (*see also* Tuberculosis) 017.2●
  subacute, unspecified site 289.1
  sublingual gland (suppurative) 527.2
  submandibular gland (suppurative) 527.2
  submaxillary gland (suppurative) 527.2
  suppurative 683
  tuberculous - *see* Tuberculosis, lymph gland
  urethral gland (*see also* Urethritis) 597.89
  venereal NEC 099.8
  Wharton's duct (suppurative) 527.2
Adenoacanthoma (M8570/3) - *see* Neoplasm, by site, malignant
Adenoameloblastoma (M9300/0) 213.1
  upper jaw (bone) 213.0
Adenocarcinoma (M8140/3) - *see also* Neoplasm, by site, malignant

---

Note 03   The list of adjectival modifiers below is not exhaustive. A description of adenocarcinoma that does not appear in this list should be coded in the same manner as carcinoma with that description. Thus, "mixed acidophil-basophil adenocarcinoma," should be coded in the same manner as "mixed acidophil-basophil carcinoma," which appears in the list under "Carcinoma."

Except where otherwise indicated, the morphological varieties of adenocarcinoma in the list below should be coded by site as for "Neoplasm, malignant."

---

  with
    apocrine metaplasia (M8573/3)
    cartilaginous (and osseous) metaplasia (M8571/3)
    osseous (and cartilaginous) metaplasia (M8571/3)
    spindle cell metaplasia (M8572/3)
    squamous metaplasia (M8570/3)

Adenocarcinoma (*Continued*)
  acidophil (M8280/3)
    specified site - *see* Neoplasm, by site, malignant
    unspecified site 194.3
  acinar (M8550/3)
  acinic cell (M8550/3)
  adrenal cortical (M8370/3) 194.0
  alveolar (M8251/3)
    and
        epidermoid carcinoma, mixed (M8560/3)
        squamous cell carcinoma, mixed (M8560/3)
  apocrine (M8401/3)
    breast - *see* Neoplasm, breast, malignant
    specified site NEC - *see* Neoplasm, skin, malignant
    unspecified site 173.9
  basophil (M8300/3)
    specified site - *see* Neoplasm, by site, malignant
    unspecified site 194.3
  bile duct type (M8160/3)
    liver 155.1
    specified site NEC - *see* Neoplasm, by site, malignant
    unspecified site 155.1
  bronchiolar (M8250/3) - *see* Neoplasm, lung, malignant
  ceruminous (M8420/3) 173.2
  chromophobe (M8270/3)
    specified site - *see* Neoplasm, by site, malignant
    unspecified site 194.3
  clear cell (mesonephroid type) (M8310/3)
  colloid (M8480/3)
  cylindroid type (M8200/3)
  diffuse type (M8145/3)
    specified site - *see* Neoplasm, by site, malignant
    unspecified site 151.9
  duct (infiltrating) (M8500/3)
    with Paget's disease (M8541/3) - *see* Neoplasm, breast, malignant
    specified site - *see* Neoplasm, by site, malignant
    unspecified site 174.9
  embryonal (M9070/3)
  endometrioid (M8380/3) - *see* Neoplasm, by site, malignant
  eosinophil (M8280/3)
    specified site - *see* Neoplasm, by site, malignant
    unspecified site 194.3
  follicular (M8330/3)
    and papillary (M8340/3) 193
    moderately differentiated type (M8332/3) 193
    pure follicle type (M8331/3) 193
    specified site - *see* Neoplasm, by site, malignant
    trabecular type (M8332/3) 193
    unspecified type 193
    well differentiated type (M8331/3) 193
  gelatinous (M8480/3)
  granular cell (M8320/3)
  Hürthle cell (M8290/3) 193
  in
    adenomatous
        polyp (M8210/3)
        polyposis coli (M8220/3) 153.9

Adenocarcinoma *(Continued)*
  in *(Continued)*
    polypoid adenoma (M8210/3)
    tubular adenoma (M8210/3)
    villous adenoma (M8261/3)
  infiltrating duct (M8500/3)
    with Paget's disease (M8541/3) -
      see Neoplasm, breast,
      malignant
    specified site - *see* Neoplasm, by site,
      malignant
    unspecified site 174.9
  inflammatory (M8530/3)
    specified site - *see* Neoplasm, by site,
      malignant
    unspecified site 174.9
  in situ (M8140/2) - *see* Neoplasm, by
    site, in situ
  intestinal type (M8144/3)
    specified site - *see* Neoplasm, by site,
      malignant
    unspecified site 151.9
  intraductal (noninfiltrating)
    (M8500/2)
    papillary (M8503/2)
      specified site - *see* Neoplasm, by
        site, in situ
      unspecified site 233.0
    specified site - *see* Neoplasm, by site,
      in situ
    unspecified site 233.0
  islet cell (M8150/3)
    and exocrine, mixed (M8154/3)
      specified site - *see* Neoplasm, by
        site, malignant
      unspecified site 157.9
    pancreas 157.4
    specified site NEC - *see* Neoplasm,
      by site, malignant
    unspecified site 157.4
  lobular (M8520/3)
    specified site - *see* Neoplasm, by site,
      malignant
    unspecified site 174.9
  medullary (M8510/3)
  mesonephric (M9110/3)
  mixed cell (M8323/3)
  mucinous (M8480/3)
  mucin-producing (M8481/3)
  mucoid (M8480/3) - *see also* Neoplasm,
    by site, malignant
    cell (M8300/3)
      specified site - *see* Neoplasm, by
        site, malignant
      unspecified site 194.3
  nonencapsulated sclerosing (M8350/3)
    193
  oncocytic (M8290/3)
  oxyphilic (M8290/3)
  papillary (M8260/3)
    and follicular (M8340/3) 193
    intraductal (noninfiltrating)
      (M8503/2)
      specified site - *see* Neoplasm, by
        site, in situ
      unspecified site 233.0
    serous (M8460/3)
      specified site - *see* Neoplasm, by
        site, malignant
      unspecified site 183.0
  papillocystic (M8450/3)
    specified site - *see* Neoplasm, by site,
      malignant
    unspecified site 183.0

Adenocarcinoma *(Continued)*
  pseudomucinous (M8470/3)
    specified site - *see* Neoplasm, by site,
      malignant
    unspecified site 183.0
  renal cell (M8312/3) 189.0
  sebaceous (M8410/3)
  serous (M8441/3) - *see also* Neoplasm,
    by site, malignant
    papillary
      specified site - *see* Neoplasm, by
        site, malignant
      unspecified site 183.0
  signet ring cell (M8490/3)
  superficial spreading (M8143/3)
  sweat gland (M8400/3) - *see* Neoplasm,
    skin, malignant
  trabecular (M8190/3)
  tubular (M8211/3)
  villous (M8262/3)
  water-clear cell (M8322/3) 194.1
Adenofibroma (M9013/0)
  clear cell (M8313/0) - *see* Neoplasm, by
    site, benign
  endometrioid (M8381/0) 220
    borderline malignancy (M8381/1)
      236.2
    malignant (M8381/3) 183.0
  mucinous (M9015/0)
    specified site - *see* Neoplasm, by site,
      benign
    unspecified site 220
  prostate 600.20
    with
      other lower urinary tract
        symptoms (LUTS) 600.21
      urinary
        obstruction 600.21
        retention 600.21
  serous (M9014/0)
    specified site - *see* Neoplasm, by site,
      benign
    unspecified site 220
  specified site - *see* Neoplasm, by site,
    benign
  unspecified site 220
Adenofibrosis
  breast 610.2
  endometrioid 617.0
Adenoiditis 474.01
  acute 463
  chronic 474.01
    with chronic tonsillitis 474.02
Adenoids (congenital) (of nasal fossa) 474.9
  hypertrophy 474.12
  vegetations 474.2
Adenolipomatosis (symmetrical) 272.8
Adenolymphoma (M8561/0)
  specified site - *see* Neoplasm, by site,
    benign
  unspecified 210.2
Adenoma (sessile) (M8140/0) - *see also*
  Neoplasm, by site, benign

Note 04 Except where otherwise
indicated, the morphological varieties
of adenoma in the list below should
be coded by site as for "Neoplasm,
benign."

  acidophil (M8280/0)
    specified site - *see* Neoplasm, by site,
      benign
    unspecified site 227.3

Adenoma *(Continued)*
  acinar (cell) (M8550/0)
  acinic cell (M8550/0)
  adrenal (cortex) (cortical) (functioning)
    (M8370/0) 227.0
    clear cell type (M8373/0) 227.0
    compact cell type (M8371/0) 227.0
    glomerulosa cell type (M8374/0)
      227.0
    heavily pigmented variant
      (M8372/0) 227.0
    mixed cell type (M8375/0) 227.0
  alpha cell (M8152/0)
    pancreas 211.7
    specified site NEC - *see* Neoplasm,
      by site, benign
    unspecified site 211.7
  alveolar (M8251/0)
  apocrine (M8401/0)
    breast 217
    specified site NEC - *see* Neoplasm,
      skin, benign
    unspecified site 216.9
  basal cell (M8147/0)
  basophil (M8300/0)
    specified site - *see* Neoplasm, by site,
      benign
    unspecified site 227.3
  beta cell (M8151/0)
    pancreas 211.7
    specified site NEC - *see* Neoplasm,
      by site, benign
    unspecified site 211.7
  bile duct (M8160/0) 211.5
  black (M8372/0) 227.0
  bronchial (M8140/1) 235.7
    carcinoid type (M8240/3) - *see*
      Neoplasm, lung, malignant
    cylindroid type (M8200/3) - *see*
      Neoplasm, lung, malignant
  ceruminous (M8420/0) 216.2
  chief cell (M8321/0) 227.1
  chromophobe (M8270/0)
    specified site - *see* Neoplasm, by site,
      benign
    unspecified site 227.3
  clear cell (M8310/0)
  colloid (M8334/0)
    specified site - *see* Neoplasm, by site,
      benign
    unspecified site 226
  cylindroid type, bronchus (M8200/3) -
    see Neoplasm, lung, malignant
  duct (M8503/0)
  embryonal (M8191/0)
  endocrine, multiple (M8360/1)
    single specified site - *see* Neoplasm,
      by site, uncertain behavior
    two or more specified sites 237.4
    unspecified site 237.4
  endometrioid (M8380/0) - *see also*
    Neoplasm, by site, benign
    borderline malignancy (M8380/1) -
      see Neoplasm, by site,
      uncertain behavior
  eosinophil (M8280/0)
    specified site - *see* Neoplasm, by site,
      benign
    unspecified site 227.3
  fetal (M8333/0)
    specified site - *see* Neoplasm, by site,
      benign
    unspecified site 226

◄ New   ◄▥ Revised   ~~deleted~~ Deleted   ● Use Additional Digit(s)   ▨ Omit code

Adenoma *(Continued)*
　follicular (M8330/0)
　　specified site - *see* Neoplasm, by site,
　　　benign
　　unspecified site 226
　hepatocellular (M8170/0) 211.5
　Hürthle cell (M8290/0) 226
　intracystic papillary (M8504/0)
　islet cell (functioning) (M8150/0)
　　pancreas 211.7
　　specified site NEC - *see* Neoplasm,
　　　by site, benign
　　unspecified site 211.7
　liver cell (M8170/0) 211.5
　macrofollicular (M8334/0)
　　specified site NEC - *see* Neoplasm,
　　　by site, benign
　　unspecified site 226
　malignant, malignum (M8140/3) - *see*
　　　Neoplasm, by site, malignant
　mesonephric (M9110/0)
　microfollicular (M8333/0)
　　specified site - *see* Neoplasm, by site,
　　　benign
　　unspecified site 226
　mixed cell (M8323/0)
　monomorphic (M8146/0)
　mucinous (M8480/0)
　mucoid cell (M8300/0)
　　specified site - *see* Neoplasm, by site,
　　　benign
　　unspecified site 227.3
　multiple endocrine (M8360/1)
　　single specified site - *see* Neoplasm,
　　　by site, uncertain behavior
　　two or more specified sites 237.4
　　unspecified site 237.4
　nipple (M8506/0) 217
　oncocytic (M8290/0)
　oxyphilic (M8290/0)
　papillary (M8260/0) - *see also*
　　　Neoplasm, by site, benign
　　intracystic (M8504/0)
　papillotubular (M8263/0)
　Pick's tubular (M8640/0)
　　specified site - *see* Neoplasm, by site,
　　　benign
　　unspecified site
　　　female 220
　　　male 222.0
　pleomorphic (M8940/0)
　polypoid (M8210/0)
　prostate (benign) 600.20
　　with
　　　other lower urinary tract
　　　　symptoms (LUTS)
　　　　　600.21
　　　urinary
　　　　obstruction 600.21
　　　　retention 600.21
　rete cell 222.0
　sebaceous, sebaceum (gland) (senile)
　　　(M8410/0) - *see also* Neoplasm,
　　　skin, benign
　　disseminata 759.5
　Sertoli cell (M8640/0)
　　specified site - *see* Neoplasm, by site,
　　　benign
　　unspecified site
　　　female 220
　　　male 222.0
　skin appendage (M8390/0) - *see*
　　　Neoplasm, skin, benign
　sudoriferous gland (M8400/0) - *see*
　　　Neoplasm, skin, benign

Adenoma *(Continued)*
　sweat gland or duct (M8400/0) - *see*
　　　Neoplasm, skin, benign
　testicular (M8640/0)
　　specified site - *see* Neoplasm, by site,
　　　benign
　　unspecified site
　　　female 220
　　　male 222.0
　thyroid 226
　trabecular (M8190/0)
　tubular (M8211/0) - *see also* Neoplasm,
　　　by site, benign
　　papillary (M8460/3)
　　Pick's (M8640/0)
　　　specified site - *see* Neoplasm, by
　　　　site, benign
　　　unspecified site
　　　　female 220
　　　　male 222.0
　tubulovillous (M8263/0)
　villoglandular (M8263/0)
　villous (M8261/1) - *see* Neoplasm, by
　　　site, uncertain behavior
　water-clear cell (M8322/0) 227.1
　wolffian duct (M9110/0)
Adenomatosis (M8220/0)
　endocrine (multiple) (M8360/1)
　　single specified site - *see* Neoplasm,
　　　by site, uncertain behavior
　　two or more specified sites 237.4
　　unspecified site 237.4
　erosive of nipple (M8506/0) 217
　pluriendocrine - *see* Adenomatosis,
　　　endocrine
　pulmonary (M8250/1) 235.7
　　malignant (M8250/3) - *see*
　　　Neoplasm, lung, malignant
　specified site - *see* Neoplasm, by site,
　　　benign
　unspecified site 211.3
Adenomatous
　cyst, thyroid (gland) - *see* Goiter,
　　　nodular
　goiter (nontoxic) (*see also* Goiter,
　　　nodular) 241.9
　　toxic or with hyperthyroidism
　　　242.3●
Adenomyoma (M8932/0) - *see also*
　　Neoplasm, by site, benign
　prostate 600.20
　　with
　　　other lower urinary tract
　　　　symptoms (LUTS) 600.21
　　　urinary
　　　　obstruction 600.21
　　　　retention 600.21
Adenomyometritis 617.0
Adenomyosis (uterus) (internal) 617.0
Adenopathy (lymph gland) 785.6
　inguinal 785.6
　mediastinal 785.6
　mesentery 785.6
　syphilitic (secondary) 091.4
　tracheobronchial 785.6
　　tuberculous (*see also* Tuberculosis)
　　　012.1●
　　　primary, progressive 010.8●
　tuberculous (*see also* Tuberculosis,
　　　lymph gland) 017.2●
　　tracheobronchial 012.1●
　　　primary, progressive 010.8●
Adenopharyngitis 462
Adenophlegmon 683

Adenosalpingitis 614.1
Adenosarcoma (M8960/3) 189.0
Adenosclerosis 289.3
Adenosis
　breast (sclerosing) 610.2
　vagina, congenital 752.49
Adentia (complete) (partial) (*see also*
　　Absence, teeth) 520.0
Adherent
　labium (minus) 624.4
　pericardium (nonrheumatic) 423.1
　　rheumatic 393
　placenta 667.0●
　　with hemorrhage 666.0●
　prepuce 605
　scar (skin) NEC 709.2
　tendon in scar 709.2
Adhesion(s), adhesive (postinfectional)
　　(postoperative)
　abdominal (wall) (*see also* Adhesions,
　　　peritoneum) 568.0
　amnion to fetus 658.8●
　　affecting fetus or newborn 762.8
　appendix 543.9
　arachnoiditis - *see* Meningitis
　auditory tube (Eustachian) 381.89
　bands - *see also* Adhesions,
　　　peritoneum
　　cervix 622.3
　　uterus 621.5
　bile duct (any) 576.8
　bladder (sphincter) 596.8
　bowel (*see also* Adhesions, peritoneum)
　　　568.0
　cardiac 423.1
　　rheumatic 398.99
　cecum (*see also* Adhesions, peritoneum)
　　　568.0
　cervicovaginal 622.3
　　congenital 752.49
　　postpartal 674.8●
　　　old 622.3
　cervix 622.3
　clitoris 624.4
　colon (*see also* Adhesions, peritoneum)
　　　568.0
　common duct 576.8
　congenital - *see also* Anomaly, specified
　　　type NEC
　　fingers (*see also* Syndactylism,
　　　　fingers) 755.11
　　labium (majus) (minus) 752.49
　　omental, anomalous 751.4
　　ovary 752.0
　　peritoneal 751.4
　　toes (*see also* Syndactylism, toes)
　　　　755.13
　　tongue (to gum or roof of mouth)
　　　　750.12
　conjunctiva (acquired) (localized)
　　　372.62
　　congenital 743.63
　　extensive 372.63
　cornea - *see* Opacity, cornea
　cystic duct 575.8
　diaphragm (*see also* Adhesions,
　　　peritoneum) 568.0
　due to foreign body - *see* Foreign body
　duodenum (*see also* Adhesions,
　　　peritoneum) 568.0
　　with obstruction 537.3
　ear, middle - *see* Adhesions, middle ear
　epididymis 608.89
　epidural - *see* Adhesions, meninges

Adhesion(s) (Continued)
  epiglottis 478.79
  Eustachian tube 381.89
  eyelid 374.46
    postoperative 997.99
      surgically created V45.69
  gallbladder (see also Disease,
      gallbladder) 575.8
  globe 360.89
  heart 423.1
    rheumatic 398.99
  ileocecal (coil) (see also Adhesions,
      peritoneum) 568.0
  ileum (see also Adhesions, peritoneum)
      568.0
  intestine (postoperative) (see also
      Adhesions, peritoneum) 568.0
    with obstruction 560.81
      with hernia - see also Hernia, by
        site, with obstruction
        gangrenous - see Hernia, by
        site, with gangrene
  intra-abdominal (see also Adhesions,
      peritoneum) 568.0
  iris 364.70
    to corneal graft 996.79
  joint (see also Ankylosis) 718.5●
  kidney 593.89
  labium (majus) (minus), congenital
      752.49
  liver 572.8
  lung 511.0
  mediastinum 519.3
  meninges 349.2
    cerebral (any) 349.2
      congenital 742.4
    congenital 742.8
    spinal (any) 349.2
      congenital 742.59
    tuberculous (cerebral) (spinal) (see
        also Tuberculosis, meninges)
        013.0●
  mesenteric (see also Adhesions,
      peritoneum) 568.0
  middle ear (fibrous) 385.10
    drum head 385.19
      to
        incus 385.11
        promontorium 385.13
        stapes 385.12
      specified NEC 385.19
  nasal (septum) (to turbinates)
      478.19
  nerve NEC 355.9
    spinal 355.9
      root 724.9
        cervical NEC 723.4
        lumbar NEC 724.4
        lumbosacral 724.4
        thoracic 724.4
  ocular muscle 378.60
  omentum (see also Adhesions,
      peritoneum) 568.0
  organ or site, congenital NEC -
      see Anomaly, specified type
      NEC
  ovary 614.6
    congenital (to cecum, kidney, or
        omentum) 752.0
  parauterine 614.6
  parovarian 614.6
  pelvic (peritoneal)
    female (postoperative)
        (postinfection) 614.6

Adhesion(s) (Continued)
  pelvic (Continued)
    male (postoperative) (postinfection)
        (see also Adhesions,
        peritoneum) 568.0
      postpartal (old) 614.6
      tuberculous (see also Tuberculosis)
        016.9●
  penis to scrotum (congenital) 752.69
  periappendiceal (see also Adhesions,
      peritoneum) 568.0
  pericardium (nonrheumatic) 423.1
    rheumatic 393
    tuberculous (see also Tuberculosis)
        017.9● [420.0]
  pericholecystic 575.8
  perigastric (see also Adhesions,
      peritoneum) 568.0
  periovarian 614.6
  periprostatic 602.8
  perirectal (see also Adhesions,
      peritoneum) 568.0
  perirenal 593.89
  peritoneum, peritoneal (fibrous)
      (postoperative) 568.0
    with obstruction (intestinal) 560.81
      with hernia - see also Hernia, by
        site, with obstruction
        gangrenous - see Hernia, by
        site, with gangrene
    duodenum 537.3
    congenital 751.4
    female (postoperative)
        (postinfective) 614.6
    pelvic, female 614.6
    pelvic, male 568.0
    postpartal, pelvic 614.6
    to uterus 614.6
  peritubal 614.6
  periureteral 593.89
  periuterine 621.5
  perivesical 596.8
  perivesicular (seminal vesicle) 608.89
  pleura, pleuritic 511.0
    tuberculous (see also Tuberculosis,
        pleura) 012.0●
  pleuropericardial 511.0
  postoperative (gastrointestinal tract)
      (see also Adhesions, peritoneum)
    eyelid 997.99
      surgically created V45.69
    pelvic, female 614.9
    pelvic, male 568.0
    urethra 598.2
  postpartal, old 624.4
  preputial, prepuce 605
  pulmonary 511.0
  pylorus (see also Adhesions,
      peritoneum) 568.0
  Rosenmüller's fossa 478.29
  sciatic nerve 355.0
  seminal vesicle 608.89
  shoulder (joint) 726.0
  sigmoid flexure (see also Adhesions,
      peritoneum) 568.0
  spermatic cord (acquired) 608.89
    congenital 752.89
  spinal canal 349.2
    nerve 355.9
      root 724.9
        cervical NEC 723.4
        lumbar NEC 724.4
        lumbosacral 724.4
        thoracic 724.4

Adhesion(s) (Continued)
  stomach (see also Adhesions,
      peritoneum) 568.0
  subscapular 726.2
  tendonitis 726.90
    shoulder 726.0
  testicle 608.89
  tongue (congenital) (to gum or roof of
      mouth) 750.12
    acquired 529.8
  trachea 519.19
  tubo-ovarian 614.6
  tunica vaginalis 608.89
  ureter 593.89
  uterus 621.5
    to abdominal wall 614.6
      in pregnancy or childbirth 654.4●
        affecting fetus or newborn
        763.89
  vagina (chronic) (postoperative)
      (postradiation) 623.2
  vaginitis (congenital) 752.49
  vesical 596.8
  vitreous 379.29
Adie (-Holmes) syndrome (tonic pupillary
    reaction) 379.46
Adiponecrosis neonatorum 778.1
Adiposa dolorosa 272.8
Adiposalgia 272.8
Adiposis 278.0●
  cerebralis 253.8
  dolorosa 272.8
  tuberosa simplex 272.8
Adiposity 278.02
  heart (see also Degeneration,
      myocardial) 429.1
  localized 278.1
Adiposogenital dystrophy 253.8
Adjustment
  prosthesis or other device - see Fitting
      of
  reaction - see Reaction, adjustment
Administration, prophylactic
  antibiotics V07.39
  antitoxin, any V07.2
  antivenin V07.2
  chemotherapeutic agent NEC V07.39
  chemotherapy NEC V07.39
  diphtheria antitoxin V07.2
  fluoride V07.31
  gamma globulin V07.2
  immune sera (gamma globulin) V07.2
  passive immunization agent V07.2
  RhoGAM V07.2
Admission (encounter)
  as organ donor - see Donor
  by mistake V68.9
  for
    adequacy testing (for)
      hemodialysis V56.31
      peritoneal dialysis V56.32
    adjustment (of)
      artificial
        arm (complete) (partial)
            V52.0
        eye V52.2
        leg (complete) (partial) V52.1
      brain neuropacemaker V53.02
      breast
        implant V52.4
          exchange (different
              material) (different
              size) V52.4
        prosthesis V52.4

◀ New ◀▥ Revised ~~deleted~~ Deleted ● Use Additional Digit(s) ▨ Omit code

Admission (Continued)
  for (Continued)
    adjustment (of) (Continued)
      cardiac device V53.39
        defibrillator, automatic
          implantable V53.32
        pacemaker V53.31
          carotid sinus V53.39
      catheter
        non-vascular V58.82
        vascular V58.81
      cerebral ventricle
        (communicating)
        shunt V53.01
      colostomy belt V55.3
      contact lenses V53.1
      cystostomy device V53.6
      dental prosthesis V52.3
      device, unspecified type V53.90
        abdominal V53.59 ◀▥
        cardiac V53.39
          defibrillator, automatic
            implantable V53.32
          pacemaker V53.31
        carotid sinus V53.39
        cerebral ventricle
          (communicating)
          shunt V53.01
        gastrointestinal NEC V53.59 ◀
        insulin pump V53.91
        intestinal V53.50 ◀
        intrauterine contraceptive V25.1
        nervous system V53.09
        orthodontic V53.4
        other device V53.99
        prosthetic V52.9
          breast V52.4
          dental V52.3
          eye V52.2
          specified type NEC V52.8
        special senses V53.09
        substitution
          auditory V53.09
          nervous system V53.09
          visual V53.09
        urinary V53.6
      dialysis catheter
        extracorporeal V56.1
        peritoneal V56.2
      diaphragm (contraceptive) V25.02
      gastric lap band V53.51 ◀
      gastrointestinal appliance and
        device NEC V53.59 ◀
      growth rod V54.02
      hearing aid V53.2
      ileostomy device V55.2
      intestinal appliance and ~~or~~ device
        ~~NEC~~ V53.50 ◀▥
      intrauterine contraceptive device
        V25.1
      neuropacemaker (brain)
        (peripheral nerve) (spinal
        cord) V53.02
      orthodontic device V53.4
      orthopedic (device) V53.7
        brace V53.7
        cast V53.7
        shoes V53.7
      pacemaker
        brain V53.02
        cardiac V53.31
        carotid sinus V53.39
        peripheral nerve V53.02
        spinal cord V53.02

Admission (Continued)
  for (Continued)
    adjustment (of) (Continued)
      prosthesis V52.9
        arm (complete) (partial) V52.0
        breast V52.4
        dental V52.3
        eye V52.2
        leg (complete) (partial) V52.1
        specified type NEC V52.8
      spectacles V53.1
      wheelchair V53.8
    adoption referral or proceedings
      V68.89
    aftercare (see also Aftercare) V58.9
      cardiac pacemaker V53.31
      chemotherapy (oral) (intravenous)
        V58.11 ◀▥
      dialysis
        extracorporeal (renal) V56.0
        peritoneal V56.8
        renal V56.0
      fracture (see also Aftercare,
        fracture) V54.9
      medical NEC V58.89
      organ transplant V58.44
      orthopedic V54.9
        specified care NEC V54.89
      pacemaker device
        brain V53.02
        cardiac V53.31
        carotid sinus V53.39
        nervous system V53.02
        spinal cord V53.02
      postoperative NEC V58.49
        wound closure, planned V58.41
      postpartum
        immediately after delivery
          V24.0
        routine follow-up V24.2
      postradiation V58.0
      radiation therapy V58.0
      removal of
        non-vascular catheter V58.82
        vascular catheter V58.81
      specified NEC V58.89
      surgical NEC V58.49
        wound closure, planned V58.41
    antineoplastic
      chemotherapy (oral) (intravenous)
        V58.11 ◀▥
      immunotherapy V58.12
    artificial insemination V26.1
    assisted reproductive fertility
      procedure cycle V26.81
    attention to artificial opening (of)
      V55.9
      artificial vagina V55.7
      colostomy V55.3
      cystostomy V55.5
      enterostomy V55.4
      gastrostomy V55.1
      ileostomy V55.2
      jejunostomy V55.4
      nephrostomy V55.6
      specified site NEC V55.8
        intestinal tract V55.4
        urinary tract V55.6
      tracheostomy V55.0
      ureterostomy V55.6
      urethrostomy V55.6
    battery replacement
      cardiac pacemaker V53.31
    blood typing V72.86
      Rh typing V72.86

Admission (Continued)
  for (Continued)
    boarding V65.0
    breast
      augmentation or reduction V50.1
      implant exchange (different
        material) (different size)
        V52.4
      reconstruction following
        mastectomy V51.0
      removal
        prophylactic V50.41
        tissue expander without
          synchronous insertion of
          permanent implant V52.4
    change of
      cardiac pacemaker (battery) 53.31
      carotid sinus pacemaker V53.39
      catheter in artificial opening - see
        Attention to, artificial,
        opening
      drains V58.49
      dressing
        wound V58.30
          nonsurgical V58.30
          surgical V58.31
      fixation device
        external V54.89
        internal V54.01
      Kirschner wire V54.89
      neuropacemaker device (brain)
        (peripheral nerve) (spinal
        cord) V53.02
      nonsurgical wound dressing
        V58.30
      pacemaker device
        brain V53.02
        cardiac V53.31
        carotid sinus V53.39
        nervous system V53.02
      plaster cast V54.89
      splint, external V54.89
      Steinmann pin V54.89
      surgical wound dressing V58.31
      traction device V54.89
      wound packing V58.30
        nonsurgical V58.30
        surgical V58.31
    checkup only V70.0
    chemotherapy, (oral) (intravenous)
      antineoplastic V58.11 ◀▥
    circumcision, ritual or routine (in
      absence of medical indication)
      V50.2
    clinical research investigation
      (control) (normal comparison)
      (participant) V70.7
    closure of artificial opening - see
      Attention to, artificial, opening
    contraceptive
      counseling V25.09
        emergency V25.03
        postcoital V25.03
      management V25.9
        specified type NEC V25.8
    convalescence following V66.9
      chemotherapy V66.2
      psychotherapy V66.3
      radiotherapy V66.1
      surgery V66.0
      treatment (for) V66.5
        combined V66.6
        fracture V66.4
        mental disorder NEC V66.3
        specified condition NEC V66.5

Admission *(Continued)*
  for *(Continued)*
    cosmetic surgery NEC V50.1
      breast reconstruction following
        mastectomy V51.0
      following healed injury or
        operation V51.8
    counseling *(see also* Counseling)
      V65.40
      without complaint or sickness
        V65.49
      contraceptive management
        V25.09
        emergency V25.03
        postcoital V25.03
      dietary V65.3
      exercise V65.41
      fertility preservation (prior to
        cancer therapy) (prior to
        surgical removal of gonads)
        V26.42 ◀
      for
        nonattending third party
          V65.19
        pediatric pre-birth visit for
          expectant mother
          V65.11 ◀▥
          pre-adoption visit for
            adoptive parent(s)
            V65.11 ◀
          pre-birth visit for expectant
            parent(s) V65.11 ◀
        victim of abuse
          child V61.21
          partner or spouse V61.11
      genetic V26.33
      gonorrhea V65.45
      HIV V65.44
      human immunodeficiency virus
        V65.44
      injury prevention V65.43
      insulin pump training V65.46
      natural family planning
        procreative V26.41
        to avoid pregnancy V25.04
      procreative management
        V26.49
        using natural family planning
          V26.41
      sexually transmitted disease NEC
        V65.45
        HIV V65.44
      specified reason NEC V65.49
      substance use and abuse V65.42
      syphilis V65.45
      victim of abuse
        child V61.21
        partner or spouse V61.11
    desensitization to allergens V07.1
    dialysis V56.0
      catheter
        fitting and adjustment
          extracorporeal V56.1
          peritoneal V56.2
        removal or replacement
          extracorporeal V56.1
          peritoneal V56.2
      extracorporeal (renal) V56.0
      peritoneal V56.8
      renal V56.0
    dietary surveillance and counseling
      V65.3
    drug monitoring, therapeutic
      V58.83
    ear piercing V50.3

Admission *(Continued)*
  for *(Continued)*
    elective surgery
      breast
        augmentation or reduction
          V50.1
        reconstruction following
          mastectomy V51.0
        removal, prophylactic V50.41
      circumcision, ritual or routine (in
        absence of medical
        indication) V50.2
      cosmetic NEC V50.1
        breast reconstruction following
          mastectomy V51.0
        following healed injury or
          operation V51.8
      ear piercing V50.3
      face-lift V50.1
      hair transplant V50.0
      plastic
        breast reconstruction following
          mastectomy V51.0
        cosmetic NEC V50.1
        following healed injury or
          operation V51.8
      prophylactic organ removal
        V50.49
        breast V50.41
        ovary V50.42
      repair of scarred tissue (following
        healed injury or operation)
        V51.8
      specified type NEC V50.8
    end-of-life care V66.7
    examination *(see also* Examination)
      V70.9
      administrative purpose NEC V70.3
      adoption V70.3
      allergy V72.7
      antibody response V72.61 ◀
      at health care facility V70.0
      athletic team V70.3
      camp V70.3
      cardiovascular, preoperative
        V72.81
      clinical research investigation
        (control) (participant) V70.7
      dental V72.2
      developmental testing (child)
        (infant) V20.2
      donor (potential) V70.8
      driver's license V70.3
      ear V72.19
      employment V70.5
      eye V72.0
      follow-up (routine) - *see*
        Examination, follow-up
      for admission to
        old age home V70.3
        school V70.3
      general V70.9
        specified reason NEC V70.8
      gynecological V72.31
      health supervision (child) (infant)
        V20.2 ◀▥
        child (over 28 days old)
          V20.2 ◀
        infant (over 28 days old)
          V20.2 ◀
        newborn ◀
          8 to 28 days old V20.32 ◀
          under 8 days old V20.31 ◀
      hearing V72.19
        following failed hearing
          screening V72.11

Admission *(Continued)*
  for *(Continued)*
    examination*(Continued)*
      immigration V70.3
      infant routine V20.2 ◀▥
        8 to 28 days old V20.32 ◀
        over 28 days old, routine
          V20.2 ◀
        under 8 days old V20.31 ◀
      insurance certification V70.3 ◀
      laboratory V72.60 ◀▥
        ordered as part of a routine
          general medical
          examination V72.62 ◀
        pre-operative V72.63 ◀
        pre-procedural V72.63 ◀
        specified NEC V72.69 ◀
      marriage license V70.3
      medical (general) *(see also*
        Examination, medical) V70.9
      medicolegal reasons V70.4
      naturalization V70.3
      pelvic (annual) (periodic) V72.31
      postpartum checkup V24.2
      pregnancy (possible)
        (unconfirmed) V72.40
        negative result V72.41
        positive result V72.42
      preoperative V72.84
        cardiovascular V72.81
        respiratory V72.82
        specified NEC V72.83
      preprocedural V72.84
        cardiovascular V72.81
        general physical V72.83
        respiratory V72.82
        specified NEC V72.83
      prior to chemotherapy V72.83 ◀
      prison V70.3
      psychiatric (general) V70.2
        requested by authority V70.1
      radiological NEC V72.5
      respiratory, preoperative V72.82
      school V70.3
      screening - *see* Screening
      skin hypersensitivity V72.7
      specified type NEC V72.85
      sport competition V70.3
      vision V72.0
      well baby and child care V20.2
    exercise therapy V57.1
    face-lift, cosmetic reason V50.1
    fertility preservation (prior to cancer
      therapy) (prior to surgical
      removal of gonads) V26.82 ◀
    fitting (of)
      artificial
        arm (complete) (partial) V52.0
        eye V52.2
        leg (complete) (partial) V52.1
      biliary drainage tube V58.82
      brain neuropacemaker V53.02
      breast V52.4
        implant V52.4
        prosthesis V52.4
      cardiac pacemaker V53.31
      catheter
        non-vascular V58.82
        vascular V58.81
      cerebral ventricle (communicating)
        shunt V53.01
      chest tube V58.82
      colostomy belt V55.2
      contact lenses V53.1
      cystostomy device V53.6
      dental prosthesis V52.3

◀ New   ◀▥ Revised   deleted Deleted   ● Use Additional Digit(s)   ▥ Omit code

Admission *(Continued)*
  for *(Continued)*
    fitting *(Continued)*
      device, unspecified type V53.90
        abdominal V53.59 ◀
        cerebral ventricle
          (communicating) shunt
          V53.01
        gastrointestinal NEC V53.59 ◀
        insulin pump V53.91
        intestinal V53.50 ◀
        intrauterine contraceptive
          V25.1
        nervous system V53.09
        orthodontic V53.4
        other device V53.99
        prosthetic V52.9
          breast V52.4
          dental V52.3
          eye V52.2
        special senses V53.09
        substitution
          auditory V53.09
          nervous system V53.09
          visual V53.09
      diaphragm (contraceptive)
        V25.02
      fistula (sinus tract) drainage tube
        V58.82
      gastric lap band V53.51 ◀
      gastrointestinal appliance and
        device NEC V53.59 ◀
      growth rod V54.02
      hearing aid V53.2
      ileostomy device V55.2
      intestinal appliance and or device
        NEC V53.50 ◀
      intrauterine contraceptive device
        V25.1
      neuropacemaker (brain)
        (peripheral nerve) (spinal
        cord) V53.02
      orthodontic device V53.4
      orthopedic (device) V53.7
        brace V53.7
        cast V53.7
        shoes V53.7
      pacemaker
        brain V53.02
        cardiac V53.31
        carotid sinus V53.39
        spinal cord V53.02
      pleural drainage tube V58.82
      portacath V58.81
      prosthesis V52.9
        arm (complete) (partial) V52.0
        breast V52.4
        dental V52.3
        eye V52.2
        leg (complete) (partial) V52.1
        specified type NEC V52.8
      spectacles V53.1
      wheelchair V53.8
    follow-up examination (routine)
      (following) V67.9
      cancer chemotherapy V67.2
      chemotherapy V67.2
      high-risk medication NEC V67.51
      injury NEC V67.59
      psychiatric V67.3
      psychotherapy V67.3
      radiotherapy V67.1
      specified surgery NEC V67.09
      surgery V67.00
        vaginal pap smear V67.01

Admission *(Continued)*
  for *(Continued)*
    follow-up examination *(Continued)*
      treatment (for) V67.9
        combined V67.6
        fracture V67.4
        involving high-risk medication
          NEC V67.51
        mental disorder V67.3
        specified NEC V67.59
    hair transplant, for cosmetic reason
      V50.0
    health advice, education, or
      instruction V65.4
    hearing conservation and treatment
      V72.12
    hormone replacement therapy
      (postmenopausal) V07.4
    hospice care V66.7
    immunizations (childhood)
      appropriate for age V20.2 ◀
    immunotherapy, antineoplastic
      V58.12
    insertion (of)
      subdermal implantable
        contraceptive V25.5
    insulin pump titration V53.91
    insulin pump training V65.46
    intrauterine device
      insertion V25.1
      management V25.42
    investigation to determine further
      disposition V63.8
    in vitro fertilization cycle V26.81
    isolation V07.0
    issue of
      disability examination certificate
        V68.01
      medical certificate NEC V68.09
      repeat prescription NEC V68.1
        contraceptive device NEC
          V25.49
    kidney dialysis V56.0
    lengthening of growth rod V54.02
    mental health evaluation V70.2
      requested by authority V70.1
    natural family planning counseling
      and advice
      procreative V26.41
      to avoid pregnancy V25.04
    nonmedical reason NEC V68.89
    nursing care evaluation V63.8
    observation (without need for
      further medical care) *(see also*
      Observation) V71.9
      accident V71.4
      alleged rape or seduction V71.5
      criminal assault V71.6
      following accident V71.4
        at work V71.3
      foreign body ingestion V71.89
      growth and development
        variations, childhood
        V21.0
      inflicted injury NEC V71.6
      ingestion of deleterious agent or
        foreign body V71.89
      injury V71.6
      malignant neoplasm V71.1
      mental disorder V71.09
      newborn - *see* Observation,
        suspected, condition,
        newborn
      rape V71.5
      specified NEC V71.89

Admission *(Continued)*
  for *(Continued)*
    observation *(Continued)*
      suspected
        disorder V71.9
          abuse V71.81
          accident V71.4
            at work V71.3
          benign neoplasm V71.89
          cardiovascular V71.7
          exposure
            anthrax V71.82
            biological agent NEC
              V71.83
            SARS V71.83
          heart V71.7
          inflicted injury NEC V71.6
          malignant neoplasm V71.1
          mental NEC V71.09
          neglect V71.81
          specified condition NEC
            V71.89
          tuberculosis V71.2
        maternal and fetal problem not
          found
          amniotic cavity and
            membrane V89.01
          cervical shortening V89.05
          fetal anomaly V89.03
          fetal growth V89.04
          oligohydramnios V89.01
          other specified NEC V89.09
          placenta V89.02
          polyhydramnios V89.01
        tuberculosis V71.2
    occupational therapy V57.21
    organ transplant, donor - *see* Donor
    ovary, ovarian removal, prophylactic
      V50.42
    palliative care V66.7
    Papanicolaou smear
      cervix V76.2
        for suspected malignant
          neoplasm V76.2
        no disease found V71.1
        routine, as part of
          gynecological
          examination V72.31
        to confirm findings of recent
          normal smear following
          initial abnormal smear
          V72.32
      vaginal V76.47
        following hysterectomy for
          malignant condition
          V67.01
    passage of sounds or bougie in
      artificial opening - *see*
      Attention to, artificial, opening
    paternity testing V70.4
    peritoneal dialysis V56.32
    physical therapy NEC V57.1
    plastic surgery
      breast reconstruction following
        mastectomy V51.0
      cosmetic NEC V50.1
      following healed injury or
        operation V51.8
    postmenopausal hormone
      replacement therapy V07.4
    postpartum observation
      immediately after delivery
        V24.0
      routine follow-up V24.2
    poststerilization (for restoration)
      V26.0

◀ New   ◀⁞⁞ Revised   ~~deleted~~ Deleted   ● Use Additional Digit(s)   ▨ Omit code   **137**

Admission *(Continued)*
  for *(Continued)*
    procreative management V26.9
      assisted reproductive fertility
          procedure cycle V26.81
      in vitro fertilization cycle V26.81
      specified type NEC V26.89
    prophylactic
      administration of
        antibiotics V07.39
        antitoxin, any V07.2
        antivenin V07.2
        chemotherapeutic agent NEC
            V07.39
        chemotherapy NEC V07.39
        diphtheria antitoxin V07.2
        fluoride V07.31
        gamma globulin V07.2
        immune sera (gamma
            globulin) V07.2
        RhoGAM V07.2
        tetanus antitoxin V07.2
      breathing exercises V57.0
      chemotherapy NEC V07.39
        fluoride V07.31
      measure V07.9
        specified type NEC V07.8
      organ removal V50.49
        breast V50.41
        ovary V50.42
    psychiatric examination (general)
        V70.2
      requested by authority V70.1
    radiation management V58.0
    radiotherapy V58.0
    reconstruction following
        mastectomy V51.0
    reforming of artificial opening -
        see Attention to, artificial,
        opening
    rehabilitation V57.9
      multiple types V57.89
      occupational V57.21
      orthoptic V57.4
      orthotic V57.81
      physical NEC V57.1
      specified type NEC V57.89
      speech(-language) V57.3   ◀▥
      vocational V57.22
    removal of
      breast tissue expander without
          synchronous insertion of
          permanent implant V52.4
      cardiac pacemaker V53.31
      cast (plaster) V54.89
      catheter from artificial opening -
          see Attention to, artificial,
          opening
      cerebral ventricle
          (communicating) shunt
          V53.01
      cystostomy catheter V55.5
      device
        cerebral ventricle
            (communicating)
            shunt V53.01
        fixation
          external V54.89
          internal V54.01
        intrauterine contraceptive
            V25.42
        traction, external V54.89
      drains V58.49
      dressing
        wound V58.30
          nonsurgical V58.30
          surgical V58.31

Admission *(Continued)*
  for *(Continued)*
    removal of *(Continued)*
      fixation device
        external V54.89
        internal V54.01
      intrauterine contraceptive device
          V25.42
      Kirschner wire V54.89
      neuropacemaker (brain)
          (peripheral nerve) (spinal
          cord) V53.02
      nonsurgical wound dressing
          V58.30
      orthopedic fixation device
        external V54.89
        internal V54.01
      pacemaker device
        brain V53.02
        cardiac V53.31
        carotid sinus V53.39
        nervous system V53.02
      plaster cast V54.89
      plate (fracture) V54.01
      rod V54.01
      screw (fracture) V54.01
      splint, traction V54.89
      staples V58.32
      Steinmann pin V54.89
      subdermal implantable
          contraceptive V25.43
      surgical wound dressing V58.31
      sutures V58.32
      traction device, external V54.89
      ureteral stent V53.6
      wound packing V58.30
        nonsurgical V58.30
        surgical V58.31
    repair of scarred tissue (following
        healed injury or operation)
        V51.8
    reprogramming of cardiac
        pacemaker V53.31
    respirator [ventilator] dependence
        during
          mechanical failure V46.14
          power failure V46.12
        for weaning V46.13
    restoration of organ continuity
        (poststerilization) (tuboplasty)
        (vasoplasty) V26.0
    Rh typing V72.86
    routine infant and child vision and
        hearing testing V20.2   ◀
    sensitivity test - *see also* Test, skin
      allergy NEC V72.7
      bacterial disease NEC V74.9
      Dick V74.8
      Kveim V82.89
      Mantoux V74.1
      mycotic infection NEC V75.4
      parasitic disease NEC V75.8
      Schick V74.3
      Schultz-Charlton V74.8
    social service (agency) referral or
        evaluation V63.8
    speech(-language) therapy V57.3   ◀▥
    sterilization V25.2
    suspected disorder (ruled out)
        (without need for further
        care) - *see* Observation
    terminal care V66.7
    tests only - *see* Test
    therapeutic drug monitoring V58.83
    therapy
      blood transfusion, without
          reported diagnosis V58.2

Admission *(Continued)*
  for *(Continued)*
    therapy *(Continued)*
      breathing exercises V57.0
      chemotherapy, antineoplastic
          V58.11
        prophylactic NEC V07.39
          fluoride V07.31
      dialysis (intermittent) (treatment)
        extracorporeal V56.0
        peritoneal V56.8
        renal V56.0
        specified type NEC V56.8
      exercise (remedial) NEC V57.1
        breathing V57.0
      immunotherapy, antineoplastic
          V58.12
      long-term (current) drug use
          NEC V58.69
        antibiotics V58.62
        anticoagulants V58.61
        anti-inflammatories, non-
            steroidal (NSAID) V58.64
        antiplatelets V58.63
        antithrombotics V58.63
        aspirin V58.66
        high-risk medications NEC
            V58.69
        insulin V58.67
        methadone V58.69
        opiate analgesic V58.69
        steroids V58.65
      occupational V57.21
      orthoptic V57.4
      physical NEC V57.1
      radiation V58.0
      speech(-language) V57.3   ◀▥
      vocational V57.22
    toilet or cleaning
      of artificial opening - *see*
          Attention to, artificial,
          opening
      of non-vascular catheter V58.82
      of vascular catheter V58.81
    tubal ligation V25.2
    tuboplasty for previous sterilization
        V26.0
    ultrasound, routine fetal V28.3
    vaccination, prophylactic (against)
      arthropod-borne virus, viral NEC
          V05.1
        disease NEC V05.1
        encephalitis V05.0
      Bacille Calmette Guérin (BCG)
          V03.2
      BCG V03.2
      chickenpox V05.4
      cholera alone V03.0
        with typhoid-paratyphoid
            (cholera + TAB) V06.0
      common cold V04.7
      dengue V05.1
      diphtheria alone V03.5
      diphtheria-tetanus-pertussis
          (DTP) (DTaP) V06.1
        with
          poliomyelitis (DTP polio)
              V06.3
          typhoid-paratyphoid
              (DTP + TAB) V06.2
      diphtheria-tetanus [Td] [DT]
          without pertussis V06.5
      disease (single) NEC V05.9
        bacterial NEC V03.9
          specified type NEC V03.89
        combinations NEC V06.9
          specified type NEC V06.8

◀ New   ◀▥ Revised   ~~deleted~~ Deleted   ● Use Additional Digit(s)   ▨ Omit code

Admission (Continued)
for (Continued)
vaccination, prophylactic (Continued)
disease (Continued)
specified type NEC V05.8
viral NEC V04.89
encephalitis, viral, arthropod-borne V05.0
Hemophilus influenzae, type B [Hib] V03.81
hepatitis, viral V05.3
human papillomavirus (HPV) V04.89
immune sera (gamma globulin) V07.2
influenza V04.81
with
Streptococcus pneumoniae [pneumococcus] V06.6
Leishmaniasis V05.2
measles alone V04.2
measles-mumps-rubella (MMR) V06.4
mumps alone V04.6
with measles and rubella (MMR) V06.4
not done because of contraindication V64.09
pertussis alone V03.6
plague V03.3
pneumonia V03.82
poliomyelitis V04.0
with diphtheria-tetanus-pertussis (DTP polio) V06.3
rabies V04.5
respiratory syncytial virus (RSV) V04.82
rubella alone V04.3
with measles and mumps (MMR) V06.4
smallpox V04.1
specified type NEC V05.8
Streptococcus pneumoniae [pneumococcus] V03.82
with
influenza V06.6
tetanus toxoid alone V03.7
with diphtheria [Td] [DT] V06.5
and pertussis (DTP) (DTaP) V06.1
tuberculosis (BCG) V03.2
tularemia V03.4
typhoid alone V03.1
with diphtheria-tetanus-pertussis (TAB + DTP) V06.2
typhoid-paratyphoid alone (TAB) V03.1
typhus V05.8
varicella (chicken pox) V05.4
viral encephalitis, arthropod-borne V05.0
viral hepatitis V05.3
yellow fever V04.4
vasectomy V25.2
vasoplasty for previous sterilization V26.0
vision examination V72.0
vocational therapy V57.22
waiting period for admission to other facility V63.2
undergoing social agency investigation V63.8
well baby and child care V20.2
x-ray of chest
for suspected tuberculosis V71.2
routine V72.5

Adnexitis (suppurative) (see also Salpingo-oophoritis) 614.2
Adolescence NEC V21.2
Adoption
agency referral V68.89
examination V70.3
held for V68.89
Adrenal gland - see condition
Adrenalism 255.9
tuberculous (see also Tuberculosis) 017.6 ●
Adrenalitis, adrenitis 255.8
meningococcal hemorrhagic 036.3
Adrenarche, precocious 259.1
Adrenocortical syndrome 255.2
Adrenogenital syndrome (acquired) (congenital) 255.2
iatrogenic, fetus or newborn 760.79
Adrenoleukodystrophy 277.86
neonatal 277.86
x-linked 277.86
Adrenomyeloneuropathy 277.86
Adventitious bursa - see Bursitis
Adynamia (episodica) (hereditary) (periodic) 359.3
Adynamic
ileus or intestine (see also Ileus) 560.1
ureter 753.22
Aeration lung, imperfect, newborn 770.5
Aerobullosis 993.3
Aerocele - see Embolism, air
Aerodermectasia
subcutaneous (traumatic) 958.7
surgical 998.81
surgical 998.81
Aerodontalgia 993.2
Aeroembolism 993.3
Aerogenes capsulatus infection (see also Gangrene, gas) 040.0
Aero-otitis media 993.0
Aerophagy, aerophagia 306.4
psychogenic 306.4
Aerosinusitis 993.1
Aerotitis 993.0
Affection, affections - see also Disease
sacroiliac (joint), old 724.6
shoulder region NEC 726.2
Afibrinogenemia 286.3
acquired 286.6
congenital 286.3
postpartum 666.3 ●
African
sleeping sickness 086.5
tick fever 087.1
trypanosomiasis 086.5
Gambian 086.3
Rhodesian 086.4
Aftercare V58.9
amputation stump V54.89
artificial openings - see Attention to, artificial, opening
blood transfusion without reported diagnosis V58.2
breathing exercise V57.0
cardiac device V53.39
defibrillator, automatic implantable V53.32
pacemaker V53.31
carotid sinus V53.39
carotid sinus pacemaker V53.39
cerebral ventricle (communicating) shunt V53.01
chemotherapy (oral) (intravenous) session (adjunctive) (maintenance) V58.11 ◀▥
defibrillator, automatic implantable cardiac V53.32

Aftercare (Continued)
exercise (remedial) (therapeutic) V57.1
breathing V57.0
extracorporeal dialysis (intermittent) (treatment) V56.0
following surgery NEC V58.49
for
injury V58.43
neoplasm V58.42
organ transplant V58.44
trauma V58.43
joint replacement V54.81
of
circulatory system V58.73
digestive system V58.75
genital organs V58.76
genitourinary system V58.76
musculoskeletal system V58.78
nervous system V58.72
oral cavity V58.75
respiratory system V58.74
sense organs V58.71
skin V58.77
subcutaneous tissue V58.77
teeth V58.75
urinary system V58.76
spinal - see Aftercare, following surgery, of, specified body system
wound closure, planned V58.41
fracture V54.9
healing V54.89
pathologic
ankle V54.29
arm V54.20
lower V54.22
upper V54.21
finger V54.29
foot V54.29
hand V54.29
hip V54.23
leg V54.24
lower V54.26
upper V54.25
pelvis V54.29
specified site NEC V54.29
toe(s) V54.29
vertebrae V54.27
wrist V54.29
traumatic
ankle V54.19
arm V54.10
lower V54.12
upper V54.11
finger V54.19
foot V54.19
hand V54.19
hip V54.13
leg V54.14
lower V54.16
upper V54.15
pelvis V54.19
specified site NEC V54.19
toe(s) V54.19
vertebrae V54.17
wrist V54.19
removal of
external fixation device V54.89
internal fixation device V54.01
specified care NEC V54.89
gait training V57.1
for use of artificial limb(s) V57.81
internal fixation device V54.09
involving
dialysis (intermittent) (treatment)
extracorporeal V56.0
peritoneal V56.8
renal V56.0

Aftercare *(Continued)*
  involving *(Continued)*
    gait training V57.1
      for use of artificial limb(s) V57.81
    growth rod
      adjustment V54.02
      lengthening V54.02
    internal fixation device V54.09
    orthoptic training V57.4
    orthotic training V57.81
    radiotherapy session V58.0
    removal of
      drains V58.49
      dressings
        wound V58.30
          nonsurgical V58.30
          surgical V58.31
      fixation device
        external V54.89
        internal V54.01
      fracture plate V54.01
      nonsurgical wound dressing
        V58.30
      pins V54.01
      plaster cast V54.89
      rods V54.01
      screws V54.01
      staples V58.32
      surgical wound dressings V58.31
      sutures V58.32
      traction device, external V54.89
      wound packing V58.30
        nonsurgical V58.30
        surgical V58.31
  neuropacemaker (brain) (peripheral
    nerve) (spinal cord) V53.02
  occupational therapy V57.21
  orthodontic V58.5
  orthopedic V54.9
    change of external fixation or
      traction device V54.89
    following joint replacement V54.81
    internal fixation device V54.09
    removal of fixation device
      external V54.89
      internal V54.01
    specified care NEC V54.89
  orthoptic training V57.4
  orthotic training V57.81
  pacemaker
    brain V53.02
    cardiac V53.31
    carotid sinus V53.39
    peripheral nerve V53.02
    spinal cord V53.02
  peritoneal dialysis (intermittent)
    (treatment) V56.8
  physical therapy NEC V57.1
    breathing exercises V57.0
  radiotherapy session V58.0
  rehabilitation procedure V57.9
    breathing exercises V57.0
    multiple types V57.89
    occupational V57.21
    orthoptic V57.4
    orthotic V57.81
    physical therapy NEC V57.1
    remedial exercises V57.1
    specified type NEC V57.89
    speech(-language) V57.3
    therapeutic exercises V57.1
    vocational V57.22
  renal dialysis (intermittent) (treatment)
    V56.0

Aftercare *(Continued)*
  specified type NEC V58.89
    removal of non-vascular cathether
      V58.82
    removal of vascular catheter V58.81
  speech(-language) therapy V57.3 ◀▥
  stump, amputation V54.89
  vocational rehabilitation V57.22
After-cataract 366.50
  obscuring vision 366.53
  specified type, not obscuring vision
    366.52
Agalactia 676.4●
Agammaglobulinemia 279.00
  with lymphopenia 279.2
  acquired (primary) (secondary) 279.06
  Bruton's X-linked 279.04
  infantile sex-linked (Bruton's)
    (congenital) 279.04
  Swiss-type 279.2
Aganglionosis (bowel) (colon) 751.3
Age (old) *(see also* Senile) 797
Agenesis - *see also* Absence, by site,
  congenital
  acoustic nerve 742.8
  adrenal (gland) 759.1
  alimentary tract (complete) (partial)
    NEC 751.8
    lower 751.2
    upper 750.8
  anus, anal (canal) 751.2
  aorta 747.22
  appendix 751.2
  arm (complete) (partial) *(see also*
    Deformity, reduction, upper limb)
    755.20
  artery (peripheral) NEC *(see also*
    Anomaly, peripheral vascular
    system) 747.60
    brain 747.81
    coronary 746.85
    pulmonary 747.3
    umbilical 747.5
  auditory (canal) (external) 744.01
  auricle (ear) 744.01
  bile, biliary duct or passage 751.61
  bone NEC 756.9
  brain 740.0
    specified part 742.2
  breast 757.6
  bronchus 748.3
  canaliculus lacrimalis 743.65
  carpus NEC *(see also* Deformity,
    reduction, upper limb) 755.28
  cartilage 756.9
  cecum 751.2
  cerebellum 742.2
  cervix 752.49
  chin 744.89
  cilia 743.63
  circulatory system, part NEC 747.89
  clavicle 755.51
  clitoris 752.49
  coccyx 756.13
  colon 751.2
  corpus callosum 742.2
  cricoid cartilage 748.3
  diaphragm (with hernia) 756.6
  digestive organ(s) or tract (complete)
    (partial) NEC 751.8
    lower 751.2
    upper 750.8
  ductus arteriosus 747.89
  duodenum 751.1

Agenesis *(Continued)*
  ear NEC 744.09
    auricle 744.01
    lobe 744.21
  ejaculatory duct 752.89
  endocrine (gland) NEC 759.2
  epiglottis 748.3
  esophagus 750.3
  Eustachian tube 744.24
  extrinsic muscle, eye 743.69
  eye 743.00
    adnexa 743.69
  eyelid (fold) 743.62
  face
    bones NEC 756.0
    specified part NEC 744.89
  fallopian tube 752.19
  femur NEC *(see also* Absence, femur,
    congenital) 755.34
  fibula NEC *(see also* Absence, fibula,
    congenital) 755.37
  finger NEC *(see also* Absence, finger,
    congenital) 755.29
  foot (complete) *(see also* Deformity,
    reduction, lower limb) 755.31
  gallbladder 751.69
  gastric 750.8
  genitalia, genital (organ)
    female 752.89
      external 752.49
      internal NEC 752.89
    male 752.89
      penis 752.69
  glottis 748.3
  gonadal 758.6
  hair 757.4
  hand (complete) *(see also* Deformity,
    reduction, upper limb) 755.21
  heart 746.89
    valve NEC 746.89
      aortic 746.89
      mitral 746.89
      pulmonary 746.01
  hepatic 751.69
  humerus NEC *(see also* Absence,
    humerus, congenital) 755.24
  hymen 752.49
  ileum 751.1
  incus 744.04
  intestine (small) 751.1
    large 751.2
  iris (dilator fibers) 743.45
  jaw 524.09
  jejunum 751.1
  kidney(s) (partial) (unilateral) 753.0
  labium (majus) (minus) 752.49
  labyrinth, membranous 744.05
  lacrimal apparatus (congenital) 743.65
  larynx 748.3
  leg NEC *(see also* Deformity, reduction,
    lower limb) 755.30
  lens 743.35
  limb (complete) (partial) *(see also*
    Deformity, reduction) 755.4
    lower NEC 755.30
    upper 755.20
  lip 750.26
  liver 751.69
  lung (bilateral) (fissures) (lobe)
    (unilateral) 748.5
  mandible 524.09
  maxilla 524.09
  metacarpus NEC 755.28
  metatarsus NEC 755.38

Agenesis *(Continued)*
  muscle (any) 756.81
  musculoskeletal system NEC 756.9
  nail(s) 757.5
  neck, part 744.89
  nerve 742.8
  nervous system, part NEC 742.8
  nipple 757.6
  nose 748.1
  nuclear 742.8
  organ
    of Corti 744.05
    or site not listed - *see* Anomaly,
        specified type NEC
  osseous meatus (ear) 744.03
  ovary 752.0
  oviduct 752.19
  pancreas 751.7
  parathyroid (gland) 759.2
  patella 755.64
  pelvic girdle (complete) (partial) 755.69
  penis 752.69
  pericardium 746.89
  perineal body 756.81
  pituitary (gland) 759.2
  prostate 752.89
  pulmonary
    artery 747.3
    trunk 747.3
    vein 747.49
  punctum lacrimale 743.65
  radioulnar NEC *(see also* Absence,
      forearm, congenital) 755.25
  radius NEC *(see also* Absence, radius,
      congenital) 755.26
  rectum 751.2
  renal 753.0
  respiratory organ NEC 748.9
  rib 756.3
  roof of orbit 742.0
  round ligament 752.89
  sacrum 756.13
  salivary gland 750.21
  scapula 755.59
  scrotum 752.89
  seminal duct or tract 752.89
  septum
    atrial 745.69
    between aorta and pulmonary
        artery 745.0
    ventricular 745.3
  shoulder girdle (complete) (partial)
      755.59
  skull (bone) 756.0
    with
      anencephalus 740.0
      encephalocele 742.0
      hydrocephalus 742.3
        with spina bifida *(see also*
            Spina bifida) 741.0●
      microcephalus 742.1
  spermatic cord 752.89
  spinal cord 742.59
  spine 756.13
    lumbar 756.13
      isthmus 756.11
      pars articularis 756.11
  spleen 759.0
  sternum 756.3
  stomach 750.7
  tarsus NEC 755.38
  tendon 756.81
  testicular 752.89
  testis 752.89

Agenesis *(Continued)*
  thymus (gland) 759.2
  thyroid (gland) 243
    cartilage 748.3
  tibia NEC *(see also* Absence, tibia,
      congenital) 755.36
  tibiofibular NEC 755.35
  toe (complete) (partial) *(see also*
      Absence, toe, congenital) 755.39
  tongue 750.11
  trachea (cartilage) 748.3
  ulna NEC *(see also* Absence, ulna,
      congenital) 755.27
  ureter 753.4
  urethra 753.8
  urinary tract NEC 753.8
  uterus 752.3
  uvula 750.26
  vagina 752.49
  vas deferens 752.89
  vein(s) (peripheral) NEC *(see also*
      Anomaly, peripheral vascular
      system) 747.60
    brain 747.81
    great 747.49
    portal 747.49
    pulmonary 747.49
  vena cava (inferior) (superior) 747.49
  vermis of cerebellum 742.2
  vertebra 756.13
    lumbar 756.13
      isthmus 756.11
      pars articularis 756.11
  vulva 752.49
Ageusia *(see also* Disturbance, sensation)
    781.1
Aggressiveness 301.3
Aggressive outburst *(see also* Disturbance,
    conduct) 312.0●
  in children or adolescents 313.9
Aging skin 701.8
Agitated - *see* condition
Agitation 307.9
  catatonic *(see also* Schizophrenia) 295.2●
Aglossia (congenital) 750.11
Aglycogenosis 271.0
Agnail (finger) (with lymphangitis) 681.02
Agnosia (body image) (tactile) 784.69
  verbal 784.69
    auditory 784.69
      secondary to organic lesion 784.69
    developmental 315.8
    secondary to organic lesion 784.69
  visual 368.16
    object 368.16
    suspected
Agoraphobia 300.22
  with panic disorder 300.21
Agrammatism 784.69
Agranulocytopenia *(see also*
    Agranulocytosis) 288.09
Agranulocytosis (angina) *(see also*
    Neutropenia) 288.09   ◀▥
  chronic 288.09
  cyclical 288.02
  due to infection 288.04   ◀
  genetic 288.01
  infantile 288.01
  periodic 288.02
  pernicious 288.09
Agraphia (absolute) 784.69
  with alexia 784.61
  developmental 315.39
Agrypnia *(see also* Insomnia) 780.52

Ague *(see also* Malaria) 084.6
  brass-founders' 985.8
  dumb 084.6
  tertian 084.1
Agyria 742.2
Ahumada-del Castillo syndrome
    (nonpuerperal galactorrhea and
    amenorrhea) 253.1
AIDS 042
AIDS-associated retrovirus (disease)
    (illness) 042
  infection - *see* Human
      immunodeficiency virus,
      infection
AIDS-associated virus (disease) (illness)
    042
  infection - *see* Human
      immunodeficiency virus,
      infection
AIDS-like disease (illness) (syndrome)
    042
AIDS-related complex 042
AIDS-related conditions 042
AIDS-related virus (disease) (illness) 042
  infection - *see* Human
      immunodeficiency virus,
      infection
AIDS virus (disease) (illness) 042
  infection - *see* Human
      immunodeficiency virus,
      infection
Ailment, heart - *see* Disease, heart
Ailurophobia 300.29
AIN I [anal intraepithelial neoplasia I]
    (histologically confirmed) 569.44
AIN II [anal intraepithelial neoplasia II]
    (histologically confirmed) 569.44
AIN III [anal intraepithelial neoplasia III]
    230.6
  anal canal 230.5
Ainhum (disease) 136.0
Air
  anterior mediastinum 518.1
  compressed, disease 993.3
  embolism (any site) (artery) (cerebral)
      958.0
    with
      abortion - *see* Abortion, by type,
          with embolism
      ectopic pregnancy *(see also*
          categories 633.0-633.9) 639.6
      molar pregnancy *(see also*
          categories 630-632) 639.6
    due to implanted device - *see*
        Complications, due to
        (presence of) any device,
        implant, or graft classified to
        996.0-996.5 NEC
    following
      abortion 639.6
      ectopic or molar pregnancy 639.6
      infusion, perfusion, or
          transfusion 999.1
    in pregnancy, childbirth, or
        puerperium 673.0●
    traumatic 958.0
  hunger 786.09
    psychogenic 306.1
  leak (lung) (pulmonary) (thorax) 512.8
    iatrogenic 512.1
    postoperative 512.1
  rarefied, effects of - *see* Effect, adverse,
      high altitude
  sickness 994.6

Airplane sickness 994.6
Akathisia, acathisia 781.0
  due to drugs 333.99
  neuroleptic-induced acute 333.99
Akinesia algeria 352.6
Akiyami 100.89
Akureyri disease (epidemic
    neuromyasthenia) 049.8
Alacrima (congenital) 743.65
Alactasia (hereditary) 271.3
Alagille syndrome 759.89
Alalia 784.3
  developmental 315.31
    receptive-expressive 315.32
  secondary to organic lesion 784.3
Alaninemia 270.8
Alastrim 050.1
Albarrán's disease (colibacilluria) 791.9
Albers-Schönberg's disease (marble
    bones) 756.52
Albert's disease 726.71
Albinism, albino (choroid) (cutaneous)
    (eye) (generalized) (isolated)
    (ocular) (oculocutaneous) (partial)
    270.2
Albinismus 270.2
Albright (-Martin) (-Bantam) disease
    (pseudohypoparathyroidism)
    275.49
Albright (-McCune) (-Sternberg)
    syndrome (osteitis fibrosa
    disseminata) 756.59
Albuminous - see Condition
Albuminuria, albuminuric (acute)
    (chronic) (subacute) 791.0
  Bence-Jones 791.0
  cardiac 785.9
  complicating pregnancy, childbirth, or
    puerperium 646.2●
    with hypertension - see Toxemia, of
      pregnancy
    affecting fetus or newborn 760.1
  cyclic 593.6
  gestational 646.2●
  gravidarum 646.2●
    with hypertension - see Toxemia, of
      pregnancy
    affecting fetus or newborn 760.1
  heart 785.9
  idiopathic 593.6
  orthostatic 593.6
  postural 593.6
  pre-eclamptic (mild) 642.4●
    affecting fetus or newborn 760.0
    severe 642.5●
      affecting fetus or newborn 760.0
  recurrent physiologic 593.6
  scarlatinal 034.1
Albumosuria 791.0
  Bence-Jones 791.0
  myelopathic (M9730/3) 203.0●
Alcaptonuria 270.2
Alcohol, alcoholic
  abstinence 291.81
  acute intoxication 305.0●
    with dependence 303.0●
  addiction (see also Alcoholism) 303.9●
  maternal
    with suspected fetal damage
      affecting management of
      pregnancy 655.4●
    affecting fetus or newborn 760.71
  amnestic disorder, persisting 291.1
  anxiety 291.89

Alcohol, alcoholic (Continued)
  brain syndrome, chronic 291.2
  cardiopathy 425.5
  chronic (see also Alcoholism) 303.9●
  cirrhosis (liver) 571.2
  delirium 291.0
    acute 291.0
    chronic 291.1
    tremens 291.0
    withdrawal 291.0
  dementia NEC 291.2
  deterioration 291.2
  drunkenness (simple) 305.0●
  hallucinosis (acute) 291.3
  induced
    circadian rhythm sleep disorder
      291.82
    hypersomnia 291.82
    insomnia 291.82
    mental disorder 291.9
      anxiety 291.89
      mood 291.89
      sexual 291.89
      sleep 291.82
      specified type 291.89
    parasomnia 291.82
    persisting
      amnestic disorder 291.1
      dementia 291.2
    psychotic disorder
      with
        delusions 291.5
        hallucinations 291.3
    sleep disorder 291.82
  insanity 291.9
  intoxication (acute) 305.0●
    with dependence 303.0●
    pathological 291.4
  jealousy 291.5
  Korsakoff's, Korsakov's, Korsakow's
    291.1
  liver NEC 571.3
    acute 571.1
    chronic 571.2
  mania (acute) (chronic) 291.9
  mood 291.89
  paranoia 291.5
  paranoid (type) psychosis 291.5
  pellagra 265.2
  poisoning, accidental (acute) NEC 980.9
    specified type of alcohol - see Table
      of Drugs and Chemicals
  psychosis (see also Psychosis, alcoholic)
    291.9
    Korsakoff's, Korsakov's, Korsakow's
      291.1
    polyneuritic 291.1
    with
      delusions 291.5
      hallucinations 291.3
  related disorder 291.9
  withdrawal symptoms, syndrome NEC
    291.81
    delirium 291.0
    hallucinosis 291.3
Alcoholism 303.9●

Note 05   Use the following fifth-digit
subclassification with category 303:

0	unspecified
1	continuous
2	episodic
3	in remission

Alcoholism (Continued)
  with psychosis (see also Psychosis,
    alcoholic) 291.9
  acute 303.0●
  chronic 303.9●
    with psychosis 291.9
  complicating pregnancy, childbirth, or
    puerperium 648.4●
    affecting fetus or newborn 760.71
  history V11.3
  Korsakoff's, Korsakov's, Korsakow's
    291.1
  suspected damage to fetus affecting
    management of pregnancy
    655.4●
Alder's anomaly or syndrome (leukocyte
    granulation anomaly) 288.2
Alder-Reilly anomaly (leukocyte
    granulation) 288.2
Aldosteronism (primary) 255.10
  congenital 255.10
  familial type I 255.11
  glucocorticoid-remediable 255.11
  secondary 255.14
Aldosteronoma (M8370/1) 237.2
Aldrich (-Wiskott) syndrome (eczema-
    thrombocytopenia) 279.12
Aleppo boil 085.1
Aleukemic - see condition
Aleukia
  congenital 288.09
  hemorrhagica 284.9
    acquired (secondary) 284.89
    congenital 284.09
    idiopathic 284.9
  splenica 289.4
Alexia (congenital) (developmental)
    315.01
  secondary to organic lesion 784.61
Algoneurodystrophy 733.7
Algophobia 300.29
Alibert's disease (mycosis fungoides)
    (M9700/3) 202.1●
Alibert-Bazin disease (M9700/3) 202.1●
Alice in Wonderland syndrome 293.89
Alienation, mental (see also Psychosis)
    298.9
Alkalemia 276.3
Alkalosis 276.3
  metabolic 276.3
    with respiratory acidosis 276.4
  respiratory 276.3
Alkaptonuria 270.2
Allen-Masters syndrome 620.6
Allergic bronchopulmonary aspergillosis
    518.6
Allergy, allergic (reaction) 995.3
  air-borne substance (see also Fever, hay)
    477.9
    specified allergen NEC 477.8
  alveolitis (extrinsic) 495.9
    due to
      Aspergillus clavatus 495.4
      cryptostroma corticale 495.6
      organisms (fungal, thermophilic
        actinomycete, other)
        growing in ventilation
        (air conditioning systems)
        495.7
    specified type NEC 495.8
  anaphylactic shock 999.4
    due to food - see Anaphylactic shock,
      due to, food
  angioneurotic edema 995.1

◀ New   ◀█▌ Revised   ~~deleted~~ Deleted   ● Use Additional Digit(s)   ▓ Omit code

A

Allergy, allergic (*Continued*)
  animal (cat) (dog) (epidermal) 477.8
    dander 477.2
    hair 477.2
  arthritis (*see also* Arthritis, allergic)
      716.2●
  asthma - *see* Asthma
  bee sting (anaphylactic shock) 989.5
  biological - *see* Allergy, drug
  bronchial asthma - *see* Asthma
  conjunctivitis (eczematous) 372.14
  dander, animal (cat) (dog) 477.2
  dandruff 477.8
  dermatitis (venenata) - *see* Dermatitis
  diathesis V15.09
  drug, medicinal substance, and
      biological (any) (correct medicinal
      substance properly administered)
      (external) (internal) 995.27
    wrong substance given or taken
        NEC 977.9
    specified drug or substance - *see*
        Table of Drugs and
        Chemicals
  dust (house) (stock) 477.8
  eczema - *see* Eczema
  endophthalmitis 360.19
  epidermal (animal) 477.8
  existing dental restorative material
      525.66
  feathers 477.8
  food (any) (ingested) 693.1
    atopic 691.8
    in contact with skin 692.5
  gastritis 535.4●
  gastroenteritis 558.3
  gastrointestinal 558.3
  grain 477.0
  grass (pollen) 477.0
    asthma (*see also* Asthma) 493.0●
    hay fever 477.0
  hair, animal (cat) (dog) 477.2
  hay fever (grass) (pollen) (ragweed)
      (tree) (*see also* Fever, hay) 477.9
  history (of) V15.09
    to
        arachnid bite V15.06 ◀
        eggs V15.03
        food additives V15.05
        insect bite V15.06
        latex V15.07
        milk products V15.02
        nuts V15.05
          peanuts V15.01
        radiographic dye V15.08
        seafood V15.04
        specified food NEC V15.05
        spider bite V15.06
  horse serum - *see* Allergy, serum
  inhalant 477.9
    dust 477.8
    pollen 477.0
    specified allergen other than pollen
        477.8
  kapok 477.8
  medicine - *see* Allergy, drug
  migraine 339.00
  milk protein 558.3
  pannus 370.62
  pneumonia 518.3
  pollen (any) (hay fever) 477.0
    asthma (*see also* Asthma) 493.0●
  primrose 477.0
  primula 477.0
  purpura 287.0

Allergy, allergic (*Continued*)
  ragweed (pollen) (Senecio jacobae)
      477.0
    asthma (*see also* Asthma) 493.0●
    hay fever 477.0
  respiratory (*see also* Allergy, inhalant)
      477.9
    due to
        drug - *see* Allergy, drug
        food - *see* Allergy, food
  rhinitis (*see also* Fever, hay) 477.9
    due to food 477.1
  rose 477.0
  Senecio jacobae 477.0
  serum (prophylactic) (therapeutic)
      999.5
    anaphylactic shock 999.4
  shock (anaphylactic) (due to adverse
      effect of correct medicinal
      substance properly administered)
      995.0
    food - *see* Anaphylactic shock, due
        to, food
    from serum or immunization 999.5
        anaphylactic 999.4
  sinusitis (*see also* Fever, hay) 477.9
  skin reaction 692.9
    specified substance - *see* Dermatitis,
        due to
  tree (any) (hay fever) (pollen) 477.0
    asthma (*see also* Asthma) 493.0●
  upper respiratory (*see also* Fever, hay)
      477.9
  urethritis 597.89
  urticaria 708.0
  vaccine - *see* Allergy, serum
Allescheriosis 117.6
Alligator skin disease (ichthyosis
      congenita) 757.1
  acquired 701.1
Allocheiria, allochiria (*see also*
      Disturbance, sensation) 782.0
Almeida's disease (Brazilian
      blastomycosis) 116.1
Alopecia (atrophicans) (pregnancy)
      (premature) (senile) 704.00
  adnata 757.4
  areata 704.01
  celsi 704.01
  cicatrisata 704.09
  circumscripta 704.01
  congenital, congenitalis 757.4
  disseminata 704.01
  effluvium (telogen) 704.02
  febrile 704.09
  generalisata 704.09
  hereditaria 704.09
  marginalis 704.01
  mucinosa 704.09
  postinfectional 704.09
  seborrheica 704.09
  specific 091.82
  syphilitic (secondary) 091.82
  telogen effluvium 704.02
  totalis 704.09
  toxica 704.09
  universalis 704.09
  x-ray 704.09
Alpers' disease 330.8
Alpha-lipoproteinemia 272.4
Alpha thalassemia 282.49
Alphos 696.1
Alpine sickness 993.2
Alport's syndrome (hereditary hematuria-
      nephropathy-deafness) 759.89

ALPS (autoimmune lymphoproliferative
      syndrome) 279.41 ◀
ALTE (apparent life threatening event)
      in newborn and infant 799.82 ◀
Alteration (of), altered
  awareness 780.09
    transient 780.02
  consciousness 780.09
    persistent vegetative state 780.03
    transient 780.02
  mental status 780.97
    amnesia (retrograde) 780.93
    memory loss 780.93
Alternaria (infection) 118
Alternating - *see* condition
Altitude, high (effects) - *see* Effect,
      adverse, high altitude
Aluminosis (of lung) 503
Alvarez syndrome (transient cerebral
      ischemia) 435.9
Alveolar capillary block syndrome 516.3
Alveolitis
  allergic (extrinsic) 495.9
    due to organisms (fungal,
        thermophilic actinomycete,
        other) growing in ventilation
        (air conditioning systems) 495.7
    specified type NEC 495.8
  due to
    Aspergillus clavatus 495.4
    Cryptostroma corticale 495.6
  fibrosing (chronic) (cryptogenic) (lung)
      516.3
    idiopathic 516.3
    rheumatoid 714.81
  jaw 526.5
  sicca dolorosa 526.5
Alveolus, alveolar - *see* condition
Alymphocytosis (pure) 279.2
Alymphoplasia, thymic 279.2
Alzheimer's
  dementia (senile)
    with behavioral disturbance 331.0
        [294.11]
    without behavioral disturbance
        331.0 [294.10]
  disease or sclerosis 331.0
    with dementia - *see* Alzheimer's,
        dementia
Amastia (*see also* Absence, breast) 611.89
Amaurosis (acquired) (congenital) (*see
      also* Blindness) 369.00
  fugax 362.34
  hysterical 300.11
  Leber's (congenital) 362.76
  tobacco 377.34
  uremic - *see* Uremia
Amaurotic familial idiocy (infantile)
      (juvenile) (late) 330.1
Ambisexual 752.7
Amblyopia (acquired) (congenital)
      (partial) 368.00
  color 368.59
    acquired 368.55
  deprivation 368.02
  ex anopsia 368.00
  hysterical 300.11
  nocturnal 368.60
    vitamin A deficiency 264.5
  refractive 368.03
  strabismic 368.01
  suppression 368.01
  tobacco 377.34
  toxic NEC 377.34
  uremic - *see* Uremia

Ameba, amebic (histolytica) - *see also*
    Amebiasis
    abscess 006.3
        bladder 006.8
        brain (with liver and lung abscess)
            006.5
        liver 006.3
            with
                brain abscess (and lung
                    abscess) 006.5
                lung abscess 006.4
            lung (with liver abscess) 006.4
                with brain abscess 006.5
        seminal vesicle 006.8
        spleen 006.8
    carrier (suspected of) V02.2
    meningoencephalitis
        due to Naegleria (gruberi) 136.29
        primary 136.29
Amebiasis NEC 006.9
    with
        brain abscess (with liver or lung
            abscess) 006.5
        liver abscess (without mention of
            brain or lung abscess) 006.3
        lung abscess (with liver abscess)
            006.4
            with brain abscess 006.5
    acute 006.0
    bladder 006.8
    chronic 006.1
    cutaneous 006.6
    cutis 006.6
    due to organism other than Entamoeba
        histolytica 007.8
    hepatic (*see also* Abscess, liver, amebic)
        006.3
    nondysenteric 006.2
    seminal vesicle 006.8
    specified
        organism NEC 007.8
        site NEC 006.8
Ameboma 006.8
Amelia 755.4
    lower limb 755.31
    upper limb 755.21
Ameloblastoma (M9310/0) 213.1
    jaw (bone) (lower) 213.1
        upper 213.0
    long bones (M9261/3) - *see* Neoplasm,
        bone, malignant
    malignant (M9310/3) 170.1
        jaw (bone) (lower) 170.1
            upper 170.0
    mandible 213.1
    tibial (M9261/3) 170.7
Amelogenesis imperfecta 520.5
    nonhereditaria (segmentalis) 520.4
Amenorrhea (primary) (secondary) 626.0
    due to ovarian dysfunction 256.8
    hyperhormonal 256.8
Amentia (*see also* Retardation, mental) 319
    Meynert's (nonalcoholic) 294.0
        alcoholic 291.1
    nevoid 759.6
American
    leishmaniasis 085.5
    mountain tick fever 066.1
    trypanosomiasis - *see* Trypanosomiasis,
        American
Ametropia (*see also* Disorder,
    accommodation) 367.9
Amianthosis 501
Amimia 784.69

Amino acid
    deficiency 270.9
        anemia 281.4
    metabolic disorder (*see also* Disorder,
        amino acid) 270.9
Aminoaciduria 270.9
    imidazole 270.5
Amnesia (retrograde) 780.93
    auditory 784.69
        developmental 315.31
        secondary to organic lesion 784.69
    dissociative 300.12
    hysterical or dissociative type 300.12
    psychogenic 300.12
    transient global 437.7
Amnestic (confabulatory) syndrome 294.0
    alcohol-induced persisting 291.1
    drug-induced persisting 292.83
    posttraumatic 294.0
Amniocentesis screening (for) V28.2
    alphafetoprotein level, raised V28.1
    chromosomal anomalies V28.0
Amnion, amniotic - *see also* condition
    nodosum 658.8●
Amnionitis (complicating pregnancy)
    658.4●
    affecting fetus or newborn 762.7
Amoral trends 301.7
Amotio retinae (*see also* Detachment,
    retina) 361.9
Ampulla
    lower esophagus 530.89
    phrenic 530.89
Amputation
    any part of fetus, to facilitate delivery
        763.89
    cervix (supravaginal) (uteri) 622.8
        in pregnancy or childbirth 654.6●
            affecting fetus or newborn
                763.89
    clitoris - *see* Wound, open, clitoris
    congenital
        lower limb 755.31
        upper limb 755.21
    neuroma (traumatic) - *see also* Injury,
        nerve, by site
        surgical complication (late) 997.61
    penis - *see* Amputation, traumatic,
        penis
    status (without complication) - *see*
        Absence, by site, acquired
    stump (surgical) (posttraumatic)
        abnormal, painful, or with
            complication (late) 997.60
        healed or old NEC - *see also* Absence,
            by site, acquired
            lower V49.70
            upper V49.60
    traumatic (complete) (partial)

+---+
| Note 06 "Complicated" includes |
| traumatic amputation with delayed |
| healing, delayed treatment, foreign |
| body, or infection. |
+---+

        arm 887.4
            at or above elbow 887.2
                complicated 887.3
            below elbow 887.0
                complicated 887.1
            both (bilateral) (any level(s))
                887.6
                complicated 887.7
            complicated 887.5

Amputation (*Continued*)
    traumatic (*Continued*)
        finger(s) (one or both hands) 886.0
            with thumb(s) 885.0
                complicated 885.1
            complicated 886.1
        foot (except toe(s) only) 896.0
            and other leg 897.6
                complicated 897.7
            both (bilateral) 896.2
                complicated 896.3
            complicated 896.1
        toe(s) only (one or both feet) 895.0
            complicated 895.1
        genital organ(s) (external) NEC
            878.8
            complicated 878.9
        hand (except finger(s) only) 887.0
            and other arm 887.6
                complicated 887.7
            both (bilateral) 887.6
                complicated 887.7
            complicated 887.1
            finger(s) (one or both hands)
                886.0
                with thumb(s) 885.0
                    complicated 885.1
                complicated 886.1
            thumb(s) (with fingers of either
                hand) 885.0
                complicated 885.1
        head 874.9
        late effect - *see* Late, effects (of),
            amputation
        leg 897.4
            and other foot 897.6
                complicated 897.7
            at or above knee 897.2
                complicated 897.3
            below knee 897.0
                complicated 897.1
            both (bilateral) 897.6
                complicated 897.7
            complicated 897.5
        lower limb(s) except toe(s) - *see*
            Amputation, traumatic, leg
        nose - *see* Wound, open, nose
        penis 878.0
            complicated 878.1
        sites other than limbs - *see* Wound,
            open, by site
        thumb(s) (with finger(s) of either
            hand) 885.0
            complicated 885.1
        toe(s) (one or both feet) 895.0
            complicated 895.1
        upper limb(s) - *see* Amputation,
            traumatic, arm
Amputee (bilateral) (old) - *see also*
    Absence, by site, acquired V49.70
Amusia 784.69
    developmental 315.39
    secondary to organic lesion 784.69
Amyelencephalus 740.0
Amyelia 742.59
Amygdalitis - *see* Tonsillitis
Amygdalolith 474.8
Amyloid disease or degeneration 277.30
    heart 277.39 [425.7]
Amyloidosis (familial) (general)
    (generalized) (genetic) (primary)
    277.30
    with lung involvement 277.39 [517.8]
    cardiac, hereditary 277.39

◀ New   ◀▥ Revised   ~~deleted~~ Deleted   ● Use Additional Digit(s)   ▨ Omit code

A

Amyloidosis (Continued)
   heart 277.39 [425.7]
   nephropathic 277.39 [583.81]
   neuropathic (Portuguese) (Swiss)
      277.39 [357.4]
   pulmonary 277.39 [517.8]
   secondary 277.39
   systemic, inherited 277.39
Amylopectinosis (brancher enzyme
   deficiency) 271.0
Amylophagia 307.52
Amyoplasia, congenita 756.89
Amyotonia 728.2
   congenita 358.8
Amyotrophia, amyotrophy, amyotrophic
   728.2
   congenita 756.89
   diabetic 250.6 ● [353.5]
      due to secondary diabetes 249.6 ●
         [353.5]
   lateral sclerosis (syndrome)
      335.20
   neuralgic 353.5
   sclerosis (lateral) 335.20
   spinal progressive 335.21
Anacidity, gastric 536.0
   psychogenic 306.4
Anaerosis of newborn 770.88
Analbuminemia 273.8
Analgesia (see also Anesthesia) 782.0
Analphalipoproteinemia 272.5
Anaphylactic shock or reaction (correct
   substance properly administered)
   995.0
   due to
      food 995.60
         additives 995.66
         crustaceans 995.62
         eggs 995.68
         fish 995.65
         fruits 995.63
         milk products 995.67
         nuts (tree) 995.64
         peanuts 995.61
         seeds 995.64
         specified NEC 995.69
         tree nuts 995.64
         vegetables 995.63
      immunization 999.4
      overdose or wrong substance given
         or taken 977.9
      specified drug - see Table of
         Drugs and Chemicals
      serum 999.4
   following sting(s) 989.5
   purpura 287.0
   serum 999.4
Anaphylactoid shock or reaction - see
   Anaphylactic shock
Anaphylaxis - see Anaphylactic shock
Anaplasia, cervix 622.10
Anarthria 784.51
Anarthritic rheumatoid disease
   446.5
Anasarca 782.3
   cardiac (see also Failure, heart)
      428.0
   fetus or newborn 778.0
   lung 514
   nutritional 262
   pulmonary 514
   renal (see also Nephrosis) 581.9
Anaspadias 752.62

Anastomosis
   aneurysmal - see Aneurysm
   arteriovenous, congenital NEC (see also
      Anomaly, arteriovenous) 747.60
      ruptured, of brain (see also
         Hemorrhage, subarachnoid)
         430
   intestinal 569.89
      complicated NEC 997.4
         involving urinary tract 997.5
   retinal and choroidal vessels 743.58
      acquired 362.17
Anatomical narrow angle (glaucoma)
   365.02
Ancylostoma (infection) (infestation)
   126.9
   americanus 126.1
   braziliense 126.2
   caninum 126.8
   ceylanicum 126.3
   duodenale 126.0
   Necator americanus 126.1
Ancylostomiasis (intestinal) 126.9
   ancylostoma
      americanus 126.1
      caninum 126.8
      ceylanicum 126.3
      duodenale 126.0
   braziliense 126.2
   Necator americanus 126.1
Anders' disease or syndrome (adiposis
   tuberosa simplex) 272.8
Andersen's glycogen storage disease
   271.0
Anderson's disease 272.7
Andes disease 993.2
Andrews' disease (bacterid) 686.8
Androblastoma (M8630/1)
   benign (M8630/0)
      specified site - see Neoplasm, by site,
         benign
      unspecified site
         female 220
         male 222.0
   malignant (M8630/3)
      specified site - see Neoplasm, by site,
         malignant
      unspecified site
         female 183.0
         male 186.9
   specified site - see Neoplasm, by site,
      uncertain behavior
   tubular (M8640/0)
      with lipid storage (M8641/0)
         specified site - see Neoplasm, by
          site, benign
         unspecified site
            female 220
            male 222.0
      specified site - see Neoplasm, by site,
         benign
      unspecified site
         female 220
         male 222.0
   unspecified site
      female 236.2
      male 236.4
Android pelvis 755.69
   with disproportion (fetopelvic) 653.3 ●
      affecting fetus or newborn 763.1
      causing obstructed labor 660.1 ●
         affecting fetus or newborn 763.1
Anectasis, pulmonary (newborn or fetus)
   770.5

Anemia 285.9
   with
      disorder of
         anaerobic glycolysis 282.3
         pentose phosphate pathway 282.2
      koilonychia 280.9
   6-phosphogluconic dehydrogenase
      deficiency 282.2
   achlorhydric 280.9
   achrestic 281.8
   Addison's (pernicious) 281.0
   Addison-Biermer (pernicious) 281.0
   agranulocytic 288.09
   amino acid deficiency 281.4
   antineoplastic chemotherapy induced
      285.3 ◄
   aplastic 284.9
      acquired (secondary) 284.89
      congenital 284.01
      constitutional 284.01
      due to
         antineoplastic chemotherapy
          284.89
         chronic systemic disease 284.89
         drugs 284.89
         infection 284.89
         radiation 284.89
      idiopathic 284.9
      myxedema 244.9
      of or complicating pregnancy 648.2 ●
      red cell (acquired) (adult) (with
         thymoma) 284.81
         congenital 284.01
         pure 284.01
      specified type NEC 284.89
      toxic (paralytic) 284.89
   aregenerative 284.9
      congenital 284.01
   asiderotic 280.9
   atypical (primary) 285.9
   autohemolysis of Selwyn and Dacie
      (type I) 282.2
   autoimmune hemolytic 283.0
   Baghdad Spring 282.2
   Balantidium coli 007.0
   Biermer's (pernicious) 281.0
   blood loss (chronic) 280.0
      acute 285.1
   bothriocephalus 123.4
   brickmakers' (see also Ancylostomiasis)
      126.9
   cerebral 437.8
   childhood 282.9
   chlorotic 280.9
   chronica congenita aregenerativa
      284.01
   chronic simple 281.9
   combined system disease NEC 281.0
      [336.2]
      due to dietary deficiency 281.1 [336.2]
   complicating pregnancy or childbirth
      648.2 ●
   congenital (following fetal blood loss)
      776.5
      aplastic 284.01
      due to isoimmunization NEC 773.2
      Heinz-body 282.7
      hereditary hemolytic NEC 282.9
      nonspherocytic
         type I 282.2
         type II 282.3
      pernicious 281.0
      spherocytic (see also Spherocytosis)
         282.0

Anemia *(Continued)*
 Cooley's (erythroblastic) 282.49
 crescent - *see* Disease, sickle-cell
 cytogenic 281.0
 Dacie's (nonspherocytic)
  type I 282.2
  type II 282.3
 Davidson's (refractory) 284.9
 deficiency 281.9
  2, 3 diphosphoglycurate mutase 282.3
  2, 3 PG 282.3
  6-PGD 282.2
  6-phosphogluronic dehydrogenase 282.2
  amino acid 281.4
  combined B_{12} and folate 281.3
  enzyme, drug-induced (hemolytic) 282.2
  erythrocytic glutathione 282.2
  folate 281.2
   dietary 281.2
   drug-induced 281.2
  folic acid 281.2
   dietary 281.2
   drug-induced 281.2
  G-6-PD 282.2
  GGS-R 282.2
  glucose-6-phosphate dehydrogenase (G-6-PD) 282.2
  glucose-phosphate isomerase 282.3
  glutathione peroxidase 282.2
  glutathione reductase 282.2
  glyceraldehyde phosphate dehydrogenase 282.3
  GPI 282.3
  G SH 282.2
  hexokinase 282.3
  iron (Fe) 280.9
   specified NEC 280.8
  nutritional 281.9
   with
    poor iron absorption 280.9
    specified deficiency NEC 281.8
   due to inadequate dietary iron intake 280.1
   specified type NEC 281.8
  of or complicating pregnancy 648.2●
  pentose phosphate pathway 282.2
  PFK 282.3
  phosphofructo-aldolase 282.3
  phosphofructokinase 282.3
  phosphoglycerate kinase 282.3
  PK 282.3
  protein 281.4
  pyruvate kinase (PK) 282.3
  TPI 282.3
  triosephosphate isomerase 282.3
  vitamin B_{12} NEC 281.1
   dietary 281.1
   pernicious 281.0
 Diamond-Blackfan (congenital hypoplastic) 284.01
 dibothriocephalus 123.4
 dimorphic 281.9
 diphasic 281.8
 diphtheritic 032.89
 Diphyllobothrium 123.4
 drepanocytic (*see also* Disease, sickle-cell) 282.60
 due to
  antineoplastic chemotherapy 285.3 ◀
  blood loss (chronic) 280.0
   acute 285.1

Anemia *(Continued)*
 due to *(Continued)*
  chemotherapy, antineoplastic 285.3 ◀
  defect of Embden-Meyerhof pathway glycolysis 282.3
  disorder of glutathione metabolism 282.2
  drug - *see* Anemia, by type (*see also* Table of Drugs and Chemicals)
   chemotherapy, antineoplastic 285.3 ◀
  fetal blood loss 776.5
  fish tapeworm (D. latum) infestation 123.4
  glutathione metabolism disorder 282.2
  hemorrhage (chronic) 280.0
   acute 285.1
  hexose monophosphate (HMP) shunt deficiency 282.2
  impaired absorption 280.9
  loss of blood (chronic) 280.0
   acute 285.1
  myxedema 244.9
  Necator americanus 126.1
  prematurity 776.6
  selective vitamin B_{12} malabsorption with proteinuria 281.1
 Dyke-Young type (secondary) (symptomatic) 283.9
 dyserythropoietic (congenital) (types I, II, III) 285.8
 dyshemopoietic (congenital) 285.8
 Egypt (*see also* Ancylostomiasis) 126.9
 elliptocytosis (*see also* Elliptocytosis) 282.1
 enzyme deficiency, drug-induced 282.2
 epidemic (*see also* Ancylostomiasis) 126.9
 EPO resistant 285.21
 erythroblastic
  familial 282.49
  fetus or newborn (*see also* Disease, hemolytic) 773.2
   late 773.5
 erythrocytic glutathione deficiency 282.2
 erythropoietin-resistant (EPO resistant anemia) 285.21
 essential 285.9
 Faber's (achlorhydric anemia) 280.9
 factitious (self-induced bloodletting) 280.0
 familial erythroblastic (microcytic) 282.49
 Fanconi's (congenital pancytopenia) 284.09
 favism 282.2
 fetal 678.0●
  following blood loss, affecting newborn 776.5
 fetus or newborn
  due to
   ABO
    antibodies 773.1
    incompatibility, maternal/fetal 773.1
    isoimmunization 773.1
   Rh
    antibodies 773.0
    incompatibility, maternal/fetal 773.0
    isoimmunization 773.0
  following fetal blood loss 776.5
 fish tapeworm (D. latum) infestation 123.4

Anemia *(Continued)*
 folate (folic acid) deficiency 281.2
  dietary 281.2
  drug-induced 281.2
 folate malabsorption, congenital 281.2
 folic acid deficiency 281.2
  dietary 281.2
  drug-induced 281.2
 G-6-PD 282.2
 general 285.9
 glucose-6-phosphate dehydrogenase deficiency 282.2
 glutathione-reductase deficiency 282.2
 goat's milk 281.2
 granulocytic 288.09
 Heinz-body, congenital 282.7
 hemoglobin deficiency 285.9
 hemolytic 283.9
  acquired 283.9
   with hemoglobinuria NEC 283.2
   autoimmune (cold type) (idiopathic) (primary) (secondary) (symptomatic) (warm type) 283.0
   due to
    cold reactive antibodies 283.0
    drug exposure 283.0
    warm reactive antibodies 283.0
   fragmentation 283.19
   idiopathic (chronic) 283.9
   infectious 283.19
    autoimmune 283.0
    non-autoimmune 283.10
   toxic 283.19
   traumatic cardiac 283.19
  acute 283.9
   due to enzyme deficiency NEC 282.3
   fetus or newborn (*see also* Disease, hemolytic) 773.2
    late 773.5
   Lederer's (acquired infectious hemolytic anemia) 283.19
  autoimmune (acquired) 283.0
  chronic 282.9
   idiopathic 283.9
  cold type (secondary) (symptomatic) 283.0
  congenital (spherocytic) (*see also* Spherocytosis) 282.0
   nonspherocytic - *see* Anemia, hemolytic, nonspherocytic, congenital
  drug-induced 283.0
   enzyme deficiency 282.2
  due to
   cardiac conditions 283.19
   drugs 283.0
   enzyme deficiency NEC 282.3
    drug-induced 282.2
   presence of shunt or other internal prosthetic device 283.19
   thrombotic thrombocytopenic purpura 446.6
  elliptocytotic (*see also* Elliptocytosis) 282.1
  familial 282.9
  hereditary 282.9
   due to enzyme deficiency NEC 282.3
   specified NEC 282.8
  idiopathic (chronic) 283.9
  infectious (acquired) 283.19

◀ New   ◀▥ Revised   ~~deleted~~ Deleted   ● Use Additional Digit(s)   ▨ Omit code

Anemia *(Continued)*
  hemolytic *(Continued)*
    mechanical 283.19
    microangiopathic 283.19
    nonautoimmune 283.10
    nonspherocytic
      congenital or hereditary NEC
        282.3
        glucose-6-phosphate
          dehydrogenase
          deficiency 282.2
        pyruvate kinase (PK)
          deficiency 282.3
        type I 282.2
        type II 282.3
        type I 282.2
        type II 282.3
    of or complicating pregnancy
      648.2●
    resulting from presence of shunt or
      other internal prosthetic
      device 283.19
    secondary 283.19
      autoimmune 283.0
    sickle-cell - *see* Disease, sickle-cell
    Stransky-Regala type (Hb-E) (*see also*
      Disease, hemoglobin) 282.7
    symptomatic 283.19
      autoimmune 283.0
    toxic (acquired) 283.19
    uremic (adult) (child) 283.11
    warm type (secondary)
      (symptomatic) 283.0
  hemorrhagic (chronic) 280.0
    acute 285.1
  HEMPAS 285.8
  hereditary erythroblast
    multinuclearity-positive acidified
    serum test 285.8
  Herrick's (hemoglobin S disease)
    282.61
  hexokinase deficiency 282.3
  high A_2 282.49
  hookworm (*see also* Ancylostomiasis)
    126.9
  hypochromic (idiopathic) (microcytic)
    (normoblastic) 280.9
    with iron loading 285.0
    due to blood loss (chronic) 280.0
      acute 285.1
    familial sex linked 285.0
    pyridoxine-responsive 285.0
  hypoplasia, red blood cells 284.81
    congenital or familial 284.01
  hypoplastic (idiopathic) 284.9
    congenital 284.01
    familial 284.01
    of childhood 284.09
  idiopathic 285.9
    hemolytic, chronic 283.9
  in (due to) (with) ◀▥
    chronic illness NEC 285.29
    chronic kidney disease 285.21
    end-stage renal disease 285.21
    neoplastic disease 285.22
  infantile 285.9
  infective, infectional 285.9
  intertropical (*see also* Ancylostomiasis)
    126.9
  iron (Fe) deficiency 280.9
    due to blood loss (chronic) 280.0
      acute 285.1
    of or complicating pregnancy 648.2●
    specified NEC 280.8

Anemia *(Continued)*
  Jaksch's (pseudoleukemia infantum)
    285.8
  Joseph-Diamond-Blackfan (congenital
    hypoplastic) 284.01
  labyrinth 386.50
  Lederer's (acquired infectious
    hemolytic anemia) 283.19
  leptocytosis (hereditary) 282.49
  leukoerythroblastic 284.2
  macrocytic 281.9
    nutritional 281.2
    of or complicating pregnancy 648.2●
    tropical 281.2
  malabsorption (familial), selective B_{12}
    with proteinuria 281.1
  malarial (*see also* Malaria) 084.6
  malignant (progressive) 281.0
  malnutrition 281.9
  marsh (*see also* Malaria) 084.6
  Mediterranean (with
    hemoglobinopathy) 282.49
  megaloblastic 281.9
    combined B_{12} and folate deficiency
      281.3
    nutritional (of infancy) 281.2
    of infancy 281.2
    of or complicating pregnancy 648.2●
    refractory 281.3
    specified NEC 281.3
  megalocytic 281.9
  microangiopathic hemolytic 283.19
  microcytic (hypochromic) 280.9
    due to blood loss (chronic) 280.0
      acute 285.1
    familial 282.49
    hypochromic 280.9
  microdrepanocytosis 282.49
  miners' (*see also* Ancylostomiasis) 126.9
  myelopathic 285.8
  myelophthisic (normocytic) 284.2
  newborn (*see also* Disease, hemolytic)
    773.2
    due to isoimmunization (*see also*
      Disease, hemolytic) 773.2
    late, due to isoimmunization 773.5
    posthemorrhagic 776.5
  nonregenerative 284.9
  nonspherocytic hemolytic - *see* Anemia,
    hemolytic, nonspherocytic
  normocytic (infectional) (not due to
    blood loss) 285.9
    due to blood loss (chronic) 280.0
      acute 285.1
    myelophthisic 284.2
  nutritional (deficiency) 281.9
    with
      poor iron absorption 280.9
      specified deficiency NEC 281.8
    due to inadequate dietary iron
      intake 280.1
    megaloblastic (of infancy) 281.2
  of childhood 282.9
  of chronic
    disease NEC 285.29
    illness NEC 285.29
  of or complicating pregnancy 648.2●
    affecting fetus or newborn 760.8
  of prematurity 776.6
  orotic aciduric (congenital) (hereditary)
    281.4
  osteosclerotic 289.89
  ovalocytosis (hereditary) (*see also*
    Elliptocytosis) 282.1

Anemia *(Continued)*
  paludal (*see also* Malaria) 084.6
  pentose phosphate pathway deficiency
    282.2
  pernicious (combined system
    disease) (congenital)
    (dorsolateral spinal
    degeneration) (juvenile)
    (myelopathy) (neuropathy)
    (posterior sclerosis) (primary)
    (progressive) (spleen) 281.0
    of or complicating pregnancy
      648.2●
  pleochromic 285.9
    of sprue 281.8
  portal 285.8
  posthemorrhagic (chronic) 280.0
    acute 285.1
    newborn 776.5
  postoperative
    due to (acute) blood loss 285.1
      chronic blood loss 280.0
    other 285.9
  postpartum 648.2●
  pressure 285.9
  primary 285.9
  profound 285.9
  progressive 285.9
    malignant 281.0
    pernicious 281.0
  protein-deficiency 281.4
  pseudoleukemica infantum 285.8
  puerperal 648.2●
  pure red cell 284.81
    congenital 284.01
  pyridoxine-responsive (hypochromic)
    285.0
  pyruvate kinase (PK) deficiency
    282.3
  refractoria sideroblastica 238.72
  refractory (primary) 238.72
    with
      excess
        blasts-1 (RAEB-1) 238.72 ◀▥
        blasts-2 (RAEB-2) 238.73
      hemochromatosis 238.72
      ringed sideroblasts (RARS)
        238.72
    due to
      drug 285.0
      myelodysplastic syndrome
        238.72
      toxin 285.0
    hereditary 285.0
    idiopathic 238.72
    megaloblastic 281.3
    sideroblastic 238.72
      hereditary 285.0
    sideropenic 280.9
  Rietti-Greppi-Micheli (thalassemia
    minor) 282.49
  scorbutic 281.8
  secondary (to) 285.9
    blood loss (chronic) 280.0
      acute 285.1
    hemorrhage 280.0
      acute 285.1
    inadequate dietary iron intake
      280.1
  semiplastic 284.9
  septic 285.9
  sickle-cell (*see also* Disease, sickle-cell)
    282.60
  sideroachrestic 285.0

Anemia (Continued)
  sideroblastic (acquired) (any type)
    (congenital) (drug-induced) (due
    to disease) (hereditary) (primary)
    (secondary) (sex-linked
    hypochromic) (vitamin B_6
    responsive) 285.0
    refractory 238.72
      congenital 285.0
      drug-induced 285.0
      hereditary 285.0
      sex-linked hypochromic 285.0
      vitamin B_6-responsive 285.0
  sideropenic 280.9
    due to blood loss (chronic) 280.0
      acute 285.1
  simple chronic 281.9
  specified type NEC 285.8
  spherocytic (hereditary) (see also
    Spherocytosis) 282.0
  splenic 285.8
    familial (Gaucher's) 272.7
  splenomegalic 285.8
  stomatocytosis 282.8
  syphilitic 095.8
  target cell (oval) 282.49
  thalassemia 282.49
  thrombocytopenic (see also
    Thrombocytopenia) 287.5
  toxic 284.89
  triosephosphate isomerase deficiency
    282.3
  tropical, macrocytic 281.2
  tuberculous (see also Tuberculosis)
    017.9●
  Vegan's 281.1
  vitamin
    B_6-responsive 285.0
    B_{12} deficiency (dietary) 281.1
      pernicious 281.0
  von Jaksch's (pseudoleukemia
    infantum) 285.8
  Witts' (achlorhydric anemia) 280.9
  Zuelzer (-Ogden) (nutritional
    megaloblastic anemia) 281.2
Anencephalus, anencephaly 740.0
  fetal, affecting management of
    pregnancy 655.0●
Anergasia (see also Psychosis, organic)
  294.9
  senile 290.0
Anesthesia, anesthetic 782.0
  complication or reaction NEC 995.22
    due to
      correct substance properly
        administered 995.22
      overdose or wrong substance
        given 968.4
      specified anesthetic - see Table
        of Drugs and Chemicals
  cornea 371.81
  death from
    correct substance properly
      administered 995.4
    during delivery 668.9●
    overdose or wrong substance given
      968.4
    specified anesthetic - see Table of
      Drugs and Chemicals
  eye 371.81
  functional 300.11
  hyperesthetic, thalamic 338.0
  hysterical 300.11
  local skin lesion 782.0

Anesthesia, anesthetic (Continued)
  olfactory 781.1
  sexual (psychogenic) 302.72
  shock
    due to
      correct substance properly
        administered 995.4
      overdose or wrong substance
        given 968.4
      specified anesthetic - see Table
        of Drugs and Chemicals
  skin 782.0
  tactile 782.0
  testicular 608.9
  thermal 782.0
Anetoderma (maculosum) 701.3
Aneuploidy NEC 758.5
Aneurin deficiency 265.1
Aneurysm (anastomotic) (artery)
  (cirsoid) (diffuse) (false) (fusiform)
  (multiple) (ruptured) (saccular)
  (varicose) 442.9
  abdominal (aorta) 441.4
    ruptured 441.3
    syphilitic 093.0
  aorta, aortic (nonsyphilitic) 441.9
    abdominal 441.4
      dissecting 441.02
      ruptured 441.3
      syphilitic 093.0
    arch 441.2
      ruptured 441.1
    arteriosclerotic NEC 441.9
      ruptured 441.5
    ascending 441.2
      ruptured 441.1
    congenital 747.29
    descending 441.9
      abdominal 441.4
        ruptured 441.3
      ruptured 441.5
      thoracic 441.2
        ruptured 441.1
    dissecting 441.00
      abdominal 441.02
      thoracic 441.01
      thoracoabdominal 441.03
    due to coarctation (aorta) 747.10
    ruptured 441.5
    sinus, right 747.29
    syphilitic 093.0
    thoracoabdominal 441.7
      ruptured 441.6
    thorax, thoracic (arch)
      (nonsyphilitic) 441.2
      dissecting 441.01
      ruptured 441.1
      syphilitic 093.0
    transverse 441.2
      ruptured 441.1
    valve (heart) (see also Endocarditis,
      aortic) 424.1
  arteriosclerotic NEC 442.9
    cerebral 437.3
      ruptured (see also Hemorrhage,
        subarachnoid) 430
  arteriovenous (congenital)
    (peripheral) NEC (see also
    Anomaly, arteriovenous) 747.60
    acquired NEC 447.0
      brain 437.3
        ruptured (see also Hemorrhage,
        subarachnoid) 430

Aneurysm (Continued)
  arteriovenous (Continued)
    acquired NEC (Continued)
      coronary 414.11
      pulmonary 417.0
    brain (cerebral) 747.81
      ruptured (see also Hemorrhage,
        subarachnoid) 430
    coronary 746.85
    pulmonary 747.3
    retina 743.58
    specified site NEC 747.89
      acquired 447.0
    traumatic (see also Injury, blood
      vessel, by site) 904.9
  basal - see Aneurysm, brain
  berry (congenital) (ruptured)
    (see also Hemorrhage,
    subarachnoid) 430
  brain 437.3
    arteriosclerotic 437.3
      ruptured (see also Hemorrhage,
        subarachnoid) 430
    arteriovenous 747.81
      acquired 437.3
        ruptured (see also Hemorrhage,
        subarachnoid) 430
      ruptured (see also Hemorrhage,
        subarachnoid) 430
    berry (congenital) (ruptured) (see
      also Hemorrhage,
      subarachnoid) 430
    congenital 747.81
      ruptured (see also Hemorrhage,
        subarachnoid) 430
    meninges 437.3
      ruptured (see also Hemorrhage,
        subarachnoid) 430
    miliary (congenital) (ruptured) (see
      also Hemorrhage,
      subarachnoid) 430
    mycotic 421.0
      ruptured (see also Hemorrhage,
        subarachnoid) 430
    nonruptured 437.3
    ruptured (see also Hemorrhage,
      subarachnoid) 430
      syphilitic 094.87
    syphilitic (hemorrhage) 094.87
    traumatic - see Injury, intracranial
  cardiac (false) (see also Aneurysm,
    heart) 414.10
  carotid artery (common) (external)
    442.81
    internal (intracranial portion) 437.3
      extracranial portion 442.81
      ruptured into brain (see also
        Hemorrhage, subarachnoid)
        430
    syphilitic 093.89
      intracranial 094.87
  cavernous sinus (see also Aneurysm,
    brain) 437.3
    arteriovenous 747.81
      ruptured (see also Hemorrhage,
        subarachnoid) 430
    congenital 747.81
      ruptured (see also Hemorrhage,
        subarachnoid) 430
  celiac 442.84
  central nervous system, syphilitic
    094.89
  cerebral - see Aneurysm, brain
  chest - see Aneurysm, thorax

◀ New   ◀▦ Revised   ~~deleted~~ Deleted   ● Use Additional Digit(s)   ▦ Omit code

Angiodysgensis spinalis 336.1
Angiodysplasia (intestinalis) (intestine)
    569.84
    with hemorrhage 569.85
    duodenum 537.82
        with hemorrhage 537.83
    stomach 537.82
        with hemorrhage 537.83
Angioedema (allergic) (any site) (with
    urticaria) 995.1
    hereditary 277.6
Angioendothelioma (M9130/1) - see also
        Neoplasm, by site, uncertain
        behavior
    benign (M9130/0) (see also
            Hemangioma, by site) 228.00
    bone (M9260/3) - see Neoplasm, bone,
        malignant
    Ewing's (M9260/3) - see Neoplasm,
        bone, malignant
    nervous system (M9130/0) 228.09
Angiofibroma (M9160/0) - see also
        Neoplasm, by site, benign
    juvenile (M9160/0) 210.7
        specified site - see Neoplasm, by site,
            benign
        unspecified site 210.7
Angiohemophilia (A) (B) 286.4
Angioid streaks (choroid) (retina) 363.43
Angiokeratoma (M9141/0) - see also
        Neoplasm, skin, benign
    corporis diffusum 272.7
Angiokeratosis
    diffuse 272.7
Angioleiomyoma (M8894/0) - see
        Neoplasm, connective tissue,
        benign
Angioleucitis 683
Angiolipoma (M8861/0) (see also Lipoma,
        by site) 214.9
    infiltrating (M8861/1) - see Neoplasm,
        connective tissue, uncertain
        behavior
Angioma (M9120/0) (see also
        Hemangioma, by site) 228.00
    capillary 448.1
    hemorrhagicum hereditaria 448.0
    malignant (M9120/3) - see Neoplasm,
        connective tissue, malignant
    pigmentosum et atrophicum 757.33
    placenta - see Placenta, abnormal
    plexiform (M9131/0) - see
        Hemangioma, by site
    senile 448.1
    serpiginosum 709.1
    spider 448.1
    stellate 448.1
Angiomatosis 757.32
    bacillary 083.8
    corporis diffusum universale 272.7
    cutaneocerebral 759.6
    encephalocutaneous 759.6
    encephalofacial 759.6
    encephalotrigeminal 759.6
    hemorrhagic familial 448.0
    hereditary familial 448.0
    heredofamilial 448.0
    meningo-oculofacial 759.6
    multiple sites 228.09
    neuro-oculocutaneous 759.6
    retina (Hippel's disease) 759.6
    retinocerebellosa 759.6
    retinocerebral 759.6
    systemic 228.09

Angiomyolipoma (M8860/0)
    specified site - see Neoplasm,
        connective tissue, benign
    unspecified site 223.0
Angiomyoliposarcoma (M8860/3) - see
        Neoplasm, connective tissue,
        malignant
Angiomyoma (M8894/0) - see Neoplasm,
        connective tissue, benign
Angiomyosarcoma (M8894/3) - see
        Neoplasm, connective tissue,
        malignant
Angioneurosis 306.2
Angioneurotic edema (allergic) (any site)
        (with urticaria) 995.1
    hereditary 277.6
Angiopathia, angiopathy 459.9
    diabetic (peripheral) 250.7● [443.81]
        due to secondary diabetes 249.7●
            [443.81]
    peripheral 443.9
        diabetic 250.7● [443.81]
            due to secondary diabetes 249.7●
                [443.81]
        specified type NEC 443.89
    retinae syphilitica 093.89
    retinalis (juvenilis) 362.18
        background 362.10
        diabetic 250.5● [362.01]
            due to secondary diabetes 249.5●
                [362.01]
        proliferative 362.29
        tuberculous (see also Tuberculosis)
            017.3● [362.18]
Angiosarcoma (M9120/3) - see Neoplasm,
        connective tissue, malignant
Angiosclerosis - see Arteriosclerosis
Angioscotoma, enlarged 368.42
Angiospasm 443.9
    brachial plexus 353.0
    cerebral 435.9
    cervical plexus 353.2
    nerve
        arm 354.9
            axillary 353.0
            median 354.1
            ulnar 354.2
        autonomic (see also Neuropathy,
            peripheral, autonomic)
            337.9
        axillary 353.0
        leg 355.8
            plantar 355.6
        lower extremity - see Angiospasm,
            nerve, leg
        median 354.1
        peripheral NEC 355.9
        spinal NEC 355.9
        sympathetic (see also Neuropathy,
            peripheral, autonomic) 337.9
        ulnar 354.2
        upper extremity - see Angiospasm,
            nerve, arm
    peripheral NEC 443.9
    traumatic 443.9
        foot 443.9
        leg 443.9
    vessel 443.9
Angiospastic disease or edema 443.9
Angle's
    class I 524.21
    class II 524.22
    class III 524.23
Anguillulosis 127.2

Angulation
    cecum (see also Obstruction, intestine)
        560.9
    coccyx (acquired) 738.6
        congenital 756.19
    femur (acquired) 736.39
        congenital 755.69
    intestine (large) (small) (see also
        Obstruction, intestine) 560.9
    sacrum (acquired) 738.5
        congenital 756.19
    sigmoid (flexure) (see also Obstruction,
        intestine) 560.9
    spine (see also Curvature, spine) 737.9
    tibia (acquired) 736.89
        congenital 755.69
    ureter 593.3
    wrist (acquired) 736.09
        congenital 755.59
Angulus infectiosus 686.8
Anhedonia 780.99
Anhidrosis (lid) (neurogenic)
        (thermogenic) 705.0
Anhydration 276.51
    with
        hypernatremia 276.0
        hyponatremia 276.1
Anhydremia 276.52
    with
        hypernatremia 276.0
        hyponatremia 276.1
Anidrosis 705.0
Aniridia (congenital) 743.45
Anisakiasis (infection) (infestation) 127.1
Anisakis larva infestation 127.1
Aniseikonia 367.32
Anisocoria (pupil) 379.41
    congenital 743.46
Anisocytosis 790.09
Anisometropia (congenital) 367.31
Ankle - see condition
Ankyloblepharon (acquired) (eyelid)
        374.46
    filiforme (adnatum) (congenital) 743.62
    total 743.62
Ankylodactly (see also Syndactylism)
        755.10
Ankyloglossia 750.0
Ankylosis (fibrous) (osseous) 718.50
    ankle 718.57
    any joint, produced by surgical fusion
        V45.4
    cricoarytenoid (cartilage) (joint)
        (larynx) 478.79
    dental 521.6
    ear ossicle NEC 385.22
        malleus 385.21
    elbow 718.52
    finger 718.54
    hip 718.55
    incostapedial joint (infectional) 385.22
    joint, produced by surgical fusion NEC
        V45.4
    knee 718.56
    lumbosacral (joint) 724.6
    malleus 385.21
    multiple sites 718.59
    postoperative (status) V45.4
    sacroiliac (joint) 724.6
    shoulder 718.51
    specified site NEC 718.58
    spine NEC 724.9
    surgical V45.4
    teeth, tooth (hard tissues) 521.6

◀ New   ◀▥ Revised   ~~deleted~~ Deleted   ● Use Additional Digit(s)   ▨ Omit code

Ankylosis *(Continued)*
  temporomandibular joint 524.61
  wrist 718.53
Ankylostoma - *see* Ancylostoma
Ankylostomiasis (intestinal) - *see*
    Ancylostomiasis
Ankylurethria *(see also* Stricture, urethra)
    598.9
Annular - *see also* condition
  detachment, cervix 622.8
  organ or site, congenital NEC - *see*
    Distortion
  pancreas (congenital) 751.7
Anodontia (complete) (partial) (vera) 520.0
  with abnormal spacing 524.30
  acquired 525.10
    causing malocclusion 524.30
    due to
      caries 525.13
      extraction 525.10
      periodontal disease 525.12
      trauma 525.11
Anomaly, anomalous (congenital)
    (unspecified type) 759.9
  abdomen 759.9
  abdominal wall 756.70
  acoustic nerve 742.9
  adrenal (gland) 759.1
  Alder (-Reilly) (leukocyte granulation)
    288.2
  alimentary tract 751.9
    lower 751.5
      specified type NEC 751.8
    upper (any part, except tongue)
      750.9
      tongue 750.10
        specified type NEC 750.19
  alveolar 524.70
    ridge (process) 525.8
    specified NEC 524.79
  ankle (joint) 755.69
  anus, anal (canal) 751.5
  aorta, aortic 747.20
    arch 747.21
    coarctation (postductal) (preductal)
      747.10
    cusp or valve NEC 746.9
    septum 745.0
    specified type NEC 747.29
  aorticopulmonary septum 745.0
  apertures, diaphragm 756.6
  appendix 751.5
  aqueduct of Sylvius 742.3
    with spina bifida *(see also* Spina
      bifida) 741.0●
  arm 755.50
    reduction *(see also* Deformity,
      reduction, upper limb) 755.20
  arteriovenous (congenital) (peripheral)
      NEC 747.60
    brain 747.81
    cerebral 747.81
    coronary 746.85
    gastrointestinal 747.61
      acquired - *see* Angiodysplasia
    lower limb 747.64
    renal 747.62
    specified site NEC 747.69
    spinal 747.82
    upper limb 747.63
  artery *(see also* Anomaly, peripheral
      vascular system) NEC 747.60
    brain 747.81
    cerebral 747.81

Anomaly, anomalous *(Continued)*
  artery NEC *(Continued)*
    coronary 746.85
    eye 743.9
    pulmonary 747.3
    renal 747.62
    retina 743.9
    umbilical 747.5
  arytenoepiglottic folds 748.3
  atrial
    bands 746.9
    folds 746.9
    septa 745.5
  atrioventricular
    canal 745.69
    common 745.69
    conduction 426.7
    excitation 426.7
    septum 745.4
  atrium - *see* Anomaly, atrial
  auditory canal 744.3
    specified type NEC 744.29
      with hearing impairment 744.02
  auricle
    ear 744.3
      causing impairment of hearing
        744.02
    heart 746.9
    septum 745.5
  autosomes, autosomal NEC 758.5
  Axenfeld's 743.44
  back 759.9
  band
    atrial 746.9
    heart 746.9
    ventricular 746.9
  Bartholin's duct 750.9
  biliary duct or passage 751.60
    atresia 751.61
  bladder (neck) (sphincter) (trigone) 753.9
    specified type NEC 753.8
  blood vessel 747.9
    artery - *see* Anomaly, artery
    peripheral vascular - *see* Anomaly,
      peripheral vascular system
    vein - *see* Anomaly, vein
  bone NEC 756.9
    ankle 755.69
    arm 755.50
    chest 756.3
    cranium 756.0
    face 756.0
    finger 755.50
    foot 755.67
    forearm 755.50
    frontal 756.0
    head 756.0
    hip 755.63
    leg 755.60
    lumbosacral 756.10
    nose 748.1
    pelvic girdle 755.60
    rachitic 756.4
    rib 756.3
    shoulder girdle 755.50
    skull 756.0
      with
        anencephalus 740.0
        encephalocele 742.0
        hydrocephalus 742.3
          with spina bifida *(see also*
            Spina bifida) 741.0●
        microcephalus 742.1
  toe 755.66

Anomaly, anomalous *(Continued)*
  brain 742.9
    multiple 742.4
    reduction 742.2
    specified type NEC 742.4
    vessel 747.81
  branchial cleft NEC 744.49
    cyst 744.42
    fistula 744.41
    persistent 744.41
    sinus (external) (internal) 744.41
  breast 757.6   ◀▥
  broad ligament 752.10
    specified type NEC 752.19
  bronchus 748.3
  bulbar septum 745.0
  bulbus cordis 745.9
    persistent (in left ventricle) 745.8
  bursa 756.9
  canal of Nuck 752.9
  canthus 743.9
  capillary NEC *(see also* Anomaly,
      peripheral vascular system)
      747.60
  cardiac 746.9
    septal closure 745.9
      acquired 429.71
    valve NEC 746.9
      pulmonary 746.00
      specified type NEC 746.89
  cardiovascular system 746.9
    complicating pregnancy, childbirth,
      or puerperium 648.5●
  carpus 755.50
  cartilage, trachea 748.3
  cartilaginous 756.9
  caruncle, lacrimal, lachrymal 743.9
  cascade stomach 750.7
  cauda equina 742.59
  cecum 751.5
  cerebral - *see also* Anomaly, brain
    vessels 747.81
  cerebrovascular system 747.81
  cervix (uterus) 752.40
    with doubling of vagina and uterus
      752.2
    in pregnancy or childbirth 654.6●
      affecting fetus or newborn 763.89
      causing obstructed labor 660.2●
        affecting fetus or newborn
          763.1
  Chédiak-Higashi (-Steinbrinck)
      (congenital gigantism of
      peroxidase granules) 288.2
  cheek 744.9
  chest (wall) 756.3
  chin 744.9
    specified type NEC 744.89
  chordae tendineae 746.9
  choroid 743.9
    plexus 742.9
  chromosomes, chromosomal 758.9
    13 (13-15) 758.1
    18 (16-18) 758.2
    21 or 22 758.0
    autosomes NEC *(see also* Abnormal,
      autosomes) 758.5
      deletion 758.39
    Christchurch 758.39
    D_1 758.1
    E_3 758.2
    G 758.0
    mitochondrial 758.9

Anomaly, anomalous *(Continued)*
  chromosomes, chromosomal
      (Continued)
    mosaics 758.89
    sex 758.81
        complement, XO 758.6
        complement, XXX 758.81
        complement, XXY 758.7
        complement, XYY 758.81
        gonadal dysgenesis 758.6
        Klinefelter's 758.7
        Turner's 758.6
      trisomy 21 758.0
  cilia 743.9
  circulatory system 747.9
    specified type NEC 747.89
  clavicle 755.51
  clitoris 752.40
  coccyx 756.10
  colon 751.5
  common duct 751.60
  communication
    coronary artery 746.85
    left ventricle with right atrium
        745.4
  concha (ear) 744.3
  connection
    renal vessels with kidney 747.62
    total pulmonary venous 747.41
  connective tissue 756.9
    specified type NEC 756.89
  cornea 743.9
    shape 743.41
    size 743.41
    specified type NEC 743.49
  coronary
    artery 746.85
    vein 746.89
  cranium - *see* Anomaly, skull
  cricoid cartilage 748.3
  cushion, endocardial 745.60
    specified type NEC 745.69
  cystic duct 751.60
  dental arch 524.20
    specified NEC 524.29
  dental arch relationship 524.20
    angle's class I 524.21
    angle's class II 524.22
    angle's class III 524.23
    articulation
        anterior 524.27
        posterior 524.27
        reverse 524.27
    disto-occlusion 524.22
        division I 524.22
        division II 524.22
    excessive horizontal overlap 524.26
    interarch distance (excessive)
        (inadequate) 524.28
    mesio-occlusion 524.23
    neutro-occlusion 524.21
    open
        anterior occlusal relationship
            524.24
        posterior occlusal relationship
            524.25
    specified NEC 524.29
  dentition 520.6
  dentofacial NEC 524.9
    functional 524.50
    specified type NEC 524.89
  dermatoglyphic 757.2
  Descemet's membrane 743.9
    specified type NEC 743.49

Anomaly, anomalous *(Continued)*
  development
    cervix 752.40
    vagina 752.40
    vulva 752.40
  diaphragm, diaphragmatic (apertures)
      NEC 756.6
  digestive organ(s) or system 751.9
    lower 751.5
    specified type NEC 751.8
    upper 750.9
  distribution, coronary artery 746.85
  ductus
    arteriosus 747.0
    Botalli 747.0
  duodenum 751.5
  dura 742.9
    brain 742.4
    spinal cord 742.59
  ear 744.3
    causing impairment of hearing
        744.00
        specified type NEC 744.09
    external 744.3
        causing impairment of hearing
            744.02
        specified type NEC 744.29
    inner (causing impairment of
        hearing) 744.05
    middle, except ossicles (causing
        impairment of hearing) 744.03
        ossicles 744.04
    ossicles 744.04
    prominent auricle 744.29
    specified type NEC 744.29
        with hearing impairment 744.09
  Ebstein's (heart) 746.2
    tricuspid valve 746.2
  ectodermal 757.9
  Eisenmenger's (ventricular septal
      defect) 745.4
  ejaculatory duct 752.9
    specified type NEC 752.89
  elbow (joint) 755.50
  endocardial cushion 745.60
    specified type NEC 745.69
  endocrine gland NEC 759.2
  epididymis 752.9
  epiglottis 748.3
  esophagus 750.9
    specified type NEC 750.4
  Eustachian tube 744.3
    specified type NEC 744.24
  eye (any part) 743.9
    adnexa 743.9
        specified type NEC 743.69
    anophthalmos 743.00
    anterior
        chamber and related structures
            743.9
        angle 743.9
            specified type NEC 743.44
        specified type NEC 743.44
        segment 743.9
            combined 743.48
            multiple 743.48
            specified type NEC 743.49
    cataract (*see also* Cataract) 743.30
    glaucoma (*see also* Buphthalmia)
        743.20
    lid 743.9
        specified type NEC 743.63
    microphthalmos (*see also*
        Microphthalmos) 743.10

Anomaly, anomalous *(Continued)*
  eye *(Continued)*
    posterior segment 743.9
        specified type NEC 743.59
        vascular 743.58
        vitreous 743.9
            specified type NEC 743.51
    ptosis (eyelid) 743.61
    retina 743.9
        specified type NEC 743.59
    sclera 743.9
        specified type NEC 743.47
    specified type NEC 743.8
  eyebrow 744.89
  eyelid 743.9
    specified type NEC 743.63
  face (any part) 744.9
    bone(s) 756.0
    specified type NEC 744.89
  fallopian tube 752.10
    specified type NEC 752.19
  fascia 756.9
    specified type NEC 756.89
  femur 755.60
  fibula 755.60
  finger 755.50
    supernumerary 755.01
    webbed (*see also* Syndactylism,
        fingers) 755.11
  fixation, intestine 751.4
  flexion (joint) 755.9
    hip or thigh (*see also* Dislocation,
        hip, congenital) 754.30
  folds, heart 746.9
  foot 755.67
  foramen
    Botalli 745.5
    ovale 745.5
  forearm 755.50
  forehead (*see also* Anomaly, skull)
      756.0
  form, teeth 520.2
  fovea centralis 743.9
  frontal bone (*see also* Anomaly, skull)
      756.0
  gallbladder 751.60
  Gartner's duct 752.41
  gastrointestinal tract 751.9
    specified type NEC 751.8
    vessel 747.61
  genitalia, genital organ(s) or system
    female 752.9
        external 752.40
            specified type NEC 752.49
        internal NEC 752.9
    male (external and internal) 752.9
        epispadias 752.62
        hidden penis 752.65
        hydrocele, congenital 778.6
        hypospadias 752.61
        micropenis 752.64
        testis, undescended 752.51
            retractile 752.52
    specified type NEC 752.89
  genitourinary NEC 752.9
  Gerbode 745.4
  globe (eye) 743.9
  glottis 748.3
  granulation or granulocyte, genetic
      288.2
    constitutional 288.2
    leukocyte 288.2
  gum 750.9
  gyri 742.9

◀ New   ◀||| Revised   ~~deleted~~ Deleted   ● Use Additional Digit(s)   ▭ Omit code

Anomaly, anomalous *(Continued)*
  hair 757.9
    specified type NEC 757.4
  hand 755.50
  hard tissue formation in pulp 522.3
  head *(see also Anomaly, skull)* 756.0
  heart 746.9
    auricle 746.9
    bands 746.9
    fibroelastosis cordis 425.3
    folds 746.9
    malposition 746.87
    maternal, affecting fetus or newborn
        760.3
    obstructive NEC 746.84
    patent ductus arteriosus (Botalli)
        747.0
    septum 745.9
      acquired 429.71
      aortic 745.0
      aorticopulmonary 745.0
      atrial 745.5
      auricular 745.5
      between aorta and pulmonary
          artery 745.0
      endocardial cushion type 745.60
        specified type NEC 745.69
      interatrial 745.5
      interventricular 745.4
        with pulmonary stenosis or
            atresia, dextraposition of
            aorta, and hypertrophy of
            right ventricle 745.2
        acquired 429.71
      specified type NEC 745.8
      ventricular 745.4
        with pulmonary stenosis or
            atresia, dextraposition of
            aorta, and hypertrophy
            of right ventricle 745.2
        acquired 429.71
    specified type NEC 746.89
    tetralogy of Fallot 745.2
    valve NEC 746.9
      aortic 746.9
        atresia 746.89
        bicuspid valve 746.4
        insufficiency 746.4
        specified type NEC 746.89
        stenosis 746.3
          subaortic 746.81
          supravalvular 747.22
      mitral 746.9
        atresia 746.89
        insufficiency 746.6
        specified type NEC 746.89
        stenosis 746.5
      pulmonary 746.00
        atresia 746.01
        insufficiency 746.09
        stenosis 746.02
          infundibular 746.83
          subvalvular 746.83
      tricuspid 746.9
        atresia 746.1
        stenosis 746.1
    ventricle 746.9
  heel 755.67
  Hegglin's 288.2
  hemianencephaly 740.0
  hemicephaly 740.0
  hemicrania 740.0
  hepatic duct 751.60
  hip (joint) 755.63

Anomaly, anomalous *(Continued)*
  hourglass
    bladder 753.8
    gallbladder 751.69
    stomach 750.7
  humerus 755.50
  hymen 752.40
  hypersegmentation of neutrophils,
      hereditary 288.2
  hypophyseal 759.2
  ileocecal (coil) (valve) 751.5
  ileum (intestine) 751.5
  ilium 755.60
  integument 757.9
    specified type NEC 757.8
  interarch distance (excessive)
      (inadequate) 524.28
  intervertebral cartilage or disc 756.10
  intestine (large) (small) 751.5
    fixational type 751.4
  iris 743.9
    specified type NEC 743.46
  ischium 755.60
  jaw NEC 524.9
    closure 524.51
    size (major) NEC 524.00
    specified type NEC 524.89
  jaw-cranial base relationship 524.10
    specified NEC 524.19
  jejunum 751.5
  joint 755.9
    hip
      dislocation *(see also Dislocation,*
          hip, congenital) 754.30
      predislocation *(see also*
          Subluxation, congenital,
          hip) 754.32
      preluxation *(see also Subluxation,*
          congenital, hip) 754.32
      subluxation *(see also Subluxation,*
          congenital, hip) 754.32
    lumbosacral 756.10
      spondylolisthesis 756.12
      spondylosis 756.11
    multiple arthrogryposis 754.89
    sacroiliac 755.69
  Jordan's 288.2
  kidney(s) (calyx) (pelvis) 753.9
    vessel 747.62
  Klippel-Feil (brevicollis) 756.16
  knee (joint) 755.64
  labium (majus) (minus) 752.40
  labyrinth, membranous (causing
      impairment of hearing) 744.05
  lacrimal
    apparatus, duct or passage 743.9
      specified type NEC 743.65
    gland 743.9
      specified type NEC 743.64
  Langdon Down (mongolism) 758.0
  larynx, laryngeal (muscle) 748.3
    web, webbed 748.2
  leg (lower) (upper) 755.60
    reduction NEC *(see also Deformity,*
        reduction, lower limb) 755.30
  lens 743.9
    shape 743.36
    specified type NEC 743.39
  leukocytes, genetic 288.2
    granulation (constitutional) 288.2
  lid (fold) 743.9
  ligament 756.9
    broad 752.10
    round 752.9

Anomaly, anomalous *(Continued)*
  limb, except reduction deformity 755.8
    lower 755.60
      reduction deformity *(see also*
          Deformity, reduction, lower
          limb) 755.30
      specified type NEC 755.69
    upper 755.50
      reduction deformity *(see also*
          Deformity, reduction, upper
          limb) 755.20
      specified type NEC 755.59
  lip 750.9
    harelip *(see also Cleft, lip)* 749.10
    specified type NEC 750.26
  liver (duct) 751.60
    atresia 751.69
  lower extremity 755.60
    vessel 747.64
  lumbosacral (joint) (region) 756.10
  lung (fissure) (lobe) NEC 748.60
    agenesis 748.5
    specified type NEC 748.69
  lymphatic system 759.9
  Madelung's (radius) 755.54
  mandible 524.9
    size NEC 524.00
  maxilla 524.90
    size NEC 524.00
  May (-Hegglin) 288.2
  meatus urinarius 753.9
    specified type NEC 753.8
  meningeal bands or folds, constriction
      of 742.8
  meninges 742.9
    brain 742.4
    spinal 742.59
  meningocele *(see also Spina bifida)*
      741.9●
    acquired 349.2
  mesentery 751.9
  metacarpus 755.50
  metatarsus 755.67
  middle ear, except ossicles (causing
      impairment of hearing) 744.03
    ossicles 744.04
  mitral (leaflets) (valve) 746.9
    atresia 746.89
    insufficiency 746.6
    specified type NEC 746.89
    stenosis 746.5
  mouth 750.9
    specified type NEC 750.26
  multiple NEC 759.7
    specified type NEC 759.89
  muscle 756.9
    eye 743.9
      specified type NEC 743.69
    specified type NEC 756.89
  musculoskeletal system, except limbs
      756.9
    specified type NEC 756.9
  nail 757.9
    specified type NEC 757.5
  narrowness, eyelid 743.62
  nasal sinus or septum 748.1
  neck (any part) 744.9
    specified type NEC 744.89
  nerve 742.9
    acoustic 742.9
      specified type NEC 742.8
    optic 742.9
      specified type NEC 742.8
    specified type NEC 742.8

Anomaly, anomalous (Continued)
nervous system NEC 742.9
  brain 742.9
    specified type NEC 742.4
  specified type NEC 742.8
neurological 742.9
nipple 757.6
nonteratogenic NEC 754.89
nose, nasal (bone) (cartilage) (septum)
  (sinus) 748.1
ocular muscle 743.9
omphalomesenteric duct 751.0
opening, pulmonary veins 747.49
optic
  disc 743.9
    specified type NEC 743.57
  nerve 742.9
opticociliary vessels 743.9
orbit (eye) 743.9
  specified type NEC 743.66
organ
  of Corti (causing impairment of
    hearing) 744.05
  or site 759.9
    specified type NEC 759.89
origin
  both great arteries from same
    ventricle 745.11
  coronary artery 746.85
  innominate artery 747.69
  left coronary artery from pulmonary
    artery 746.85
  pulmonary artery 747.3
  renal vessels 747.62
  subclavian artery (left) (right) 747.21
osseous meatus (ear) 744.03
ovary 752.0
oviduct 752.10
palate (hard) (soft) 750.9
  cleft (see also Cleft, palate) 749.00
pancreas (duct) 751.7
papillary muscles 746.9
parathyroid gland 759.2
paraurethral ducts 753.9
parotid (gland) 750.9
patella 755.64
Pelger-Huët (hereditary
  hyposegmentation) 288.2
pelvic girdle 755.60
  specified type NEC 755.69
pelvis (bony) 755.60
  complicating delivery 653.0 ●
  rachitic 268.1
    fetal 756.4
penis (glans) 752.69
pericardium 746.89
peripheral vascular system NEC
  747.60
  gastrointestinal 747.61
  lower limb 747.64
  renal 747.62
  specified site NEC 747.69
  spinal 747.82
  upper limb 747.63
Peter's 743.44
pharynx 750.9
  branchial cleft 744.41
  specified type NEC 750.29
Pierre Robin 756.0
pigmentation 709.00
  congenital 757.33
  specified NEC 709.09
pituitary (gland) 759.2
pleural folds 748.8

Anomaly, anomalous (Continued)
portal vein 747.40
position tooth, teeth 524.30
  crowding 524.31
  displacement 524.30
    horizontal 524.33
    vertical 524.34
  distance
    interocclusal
      excessive 524.37
      insufficient 524.36
  excessive spacing 524.32
  rotation 524.35
  specified NEC 524.39
preauricular sinus 744.46
prepuce 752.9
prostate 752.9
pulmonary 748.60
  artery 747.3
  circulation 747.3
  specified type NEC 748.69
  valve 746.00
    atresia 746.01
    insufficiency 746.09
    specified type NEC 746.09
    stenosis 746.02
      infundibular 746.83
      subvalvular 746.83
  vein 747.40
  venous
    connection 747.49
      partial 747.42
      total 747.41
    return 747.49
      partial 747.42
      total (TAPVR) (complete)
        (subdiaphragmatic)
        (supradiaphragmatic)
        747.41
pupil 743.9
pylorus 750.9
  hypertrophy 750.5
  stenosis 750.5
rachitic, fetal 756.4
radius 755.50
rectovaginal (septum) 752.40
rectum 751.5
refraction 367.9
renal 753.9
  vessel 747.62
respiratory system 748.9
  specified type NEC 748.8
rib 756.3
  cervical 756.2
Rieger's 743.44
rings, trachea 748.3
rotation - see also Malrotation
  hip or thigh (see also Subluxation,
    congenital, hip) 754.32
round ligament 752.9
sacroiliac (joint) 755.69
sacrum 756.10
saddle
  back 754.2
  nose 754.0
    syphilitic 090.5
salivary gland or duct 750.9
  specified type NEC 750.26
scapula 755.50
sclera 743.9
  specified type NEC 743.47
scrotum 752.9
sebaceous gland 757.9

Anomaly, anomalous (Continued)
seminal duct or tract 752.9
sense organs 742.9
  specified type NEC 742.8
septum
  heart - see Anomaly, heart, septum
  nasal 748.1
sex chromosomes NEC (see also
  Anomaly, chromosomes)
  758.81
shoulder (girdle) (joint) 755.50
  specified type NEC 755.59
sigmoid (flexure) 751.5
sinus of Valsalva 747.29
site NEC 759.9
skeleton generalized NEC 756.50
skin (appendage) 757.9
  specified type NEC 757.39
skull (bone) 756.0
  with
    anencephalus 740.0
    encephalocele 742.0
    hydrocephalus 742.3
      with spina bifida (see also
        Spina bifida) 741.0 ●
    microcephalus 742.1
specified type NEC
  adrenal (gland) 759.1
  alimentary tract (complete) (partial)
    751.8
    lower 751.5
    upper 750.8
  ankle 755.69
  anus, anal (canal) 751.5
  aorta, aortic 747.29
    arch 747.21
  appendix 751.5
  arm 755.59
  artery (peripheral) NEC (see also
    Anomaly, peripheral vascular
    system) 747.60
    brain 747.81
    coronary 746.85
    eye 743.58
    pulmonary 747.3
    retinal 743.58
    umbilical 747.5
  auditory canal 744.29
    causing impairment of hearing
      744.02
  bile duct or passage 751.69
  bladder 753.8
    neck 753.8
  bone(s) 756.9
    arm 755.59
    face 756.0
    leg 755.69
    pelvic girdle 755.69
    shoulder girdle 755.59
    skull 756.0
      with
        anencephalus 740.0
        encephalocele 742.0
        hydrocephalus 742.3
          with spina bifida (see
            also Spina bifida)
            741.0 ●
        microcephalus 742.1
  brain 742.4
  breast 757.6
  broad ligament 752.19
  bronchus 748.3
  canal of Nuck 752.89

◀ New   ◀|||| Revised   ~~deleted~~ Deleted   ● Use Additional Digit(s)   ▨ Omit code

Anomaly, anomalous *(Continued)*
  specified type NEC *(Continued)*
    cardiac septal closure 745.8
    carpus 755.59
    cartilaginous 756.9
    cecum 751.5
    cervix 752.49
    chest (wall) 756.3
    chin 744.89
    ciliary body 743.46
    circulatory system 747.89
    clavicle 755.51
    clitoris 752.49
    coccyx 756.19
    colon 751.5
    common duct 751.69
    connective tissue 756.89
    cricoid cartilage 748.3
    cystic duct 751.69
    diaphragm 756.6
    digestive organ(s) or tract 751.8
      lower 751.5
      upper 750.8
    duodenum 751.5
    ear 744.29
      auricle 744.29
        causing impairment of
          hearing 744.02
      causing impairment of hearing
        744.09
      inner (causing impairment of
        hearing) 744.05
      middle, except ossicles 744.03
        ossicles 744.04
    ejaculatory duct 752.89
    endocrine 759.2
    epiglottis 748.3
    esophagus 750.4
    eustachian tube 744.24
    eye 743.8
      lid 743.63
      muscle 743.69
    face 744.89
      bone(s) 756.0
    fallopian tube 752.19
    fascia 756.89
    femur 755.69
    fibula 755.69
    finger 755.59
    foot 755.67
    fovea centralis 743.55
    gallbladder 751.69
    Gartner's duct 752.89
    gastrointestinal tract 751.8
    genitalia, genital organ(s)
      female 752.89
        external 752.49
        internal NEC 752.89
      male 752.89
        penis 752.69
        scrotal transposition
          752.81
    genitourinary tract NEC 752.89
    glottis 748.3
    hair 757.4
    hand 755.59
    heart 746.89
      valve NEC 746.89
        pulmonary 746.09
    hepatic duct 751.69
    hydatid of Morgagni 752.89
    hymen 752.49
    integument 757.8

Anomaly, anomalous *(Continued)*
  specified type NEC *(Continued)*
    intestine (large) (small) 751.5
      fixational type 751.4
    iris 743.46
    jejunum 751.5
    joint 755.8
    kidney 753.3
    knee 755.64
    labium (majus) (minus) 752.49
    labyrinth, membranous 744.05
    larynx 748.3
    leg 755.69
    lens 743.39
    limb, except reduction deformity
      755.8
      lower 755.69
        reduction deformity *(see also*
          Deformity, reduction,
          lower limb) 755.30
      upper 755.59
        reduction deformity *(see also*
          Deformity, reduction,
          upper limb) 755.20
    lip 750.26
    liver 751.69
    lung (fissure) (lobe) 748.69
    meatus urinarius 753.8
    metacarpus 755.59
    mouth 750.26
    muscle 756.89
      eye 743.69
    musculoskeletal system, except
      limbs 756.9
    nail 757.5
    neck 744.89
    nerve 742.8
      acoustic 742.8
      optic 742.8
    nervous system 742.8
    nipple 757.6
    nose 748.1
    organ NEC 759.89
      of Corti 744.05
    osseous meatus (ear) 744.03
    ovary 752.0
    oviduct 752.19
    pancreas 751.7
    parathyroid 759.2
    patella 755.64
    pelvic girdle 755.69
    penis 752.69
    pericardium 746.89
    peripheral vascular system NEC
      (see also Anomaly, peripheral
        vascular system) 747.60
    pharynx 750.29
    pituitary 759.2
    prostate 752.89
    radius 755.59
    rectum 751.5
    respiratory system 748.8
    rib 756.3
    round ligament 752.89
    sacrum 756.19
    salivary duct or gland 750.26
    scapula 755.59
    sclera 743.47
    scrotum 752.89
      transposition 752.81
    seminal duct or tract 752.89
    shoulder girdle 755.59
    site NEC 759.89

Anomaly, anomalous *(Continued)*
  specified type NEC *(Continued)*
    skin 757.39
    skull (bone(s)) 756.0
      with
        anencephalus 740.0
        encephalocele 742.0
        hydrocephalus 742.3
          with spina bifida *(see also*
            Spina bifida) 741.0●
        microcephalus 742.1
    specified organ or site NEC 759.89
    spermatic cord 752.89
    spinal cord 742.59
    spine 756.19
    spleen 759.0
    sternum 756.3
    stomach 750.7
    tarsus 755.67
    tendon 756.89
    testis 752.89
    thorax (wall) 756.3
    thymus 759.2
    thyroid (gland) 759.2
      cartilage 748.3
    tibia 755.69
    toe 755.66
    tongue 750.19
    trachea (cartilage) 748.3
    ulna 755.59
    urachus 753.7
    ureter 753.4
      obstructive 753.29
    urethra 753.8
      obstructive 753.6
    urinary tract 753.8
    uterus 752.3
    uvula 750.26
    vagina 752.49
    vascular NEC *(see also* Anomaly,
      peripheral vascular system)
      747.60
      brain 747.81
    vas deferens 752.89
    vein(s) (peripheral) NEC *(see also*
      Anomaly, peripheral vascular
        system) 747.60
      brain 747.81
      great 747.49
      portal 747.49
      pulmonary 747.49
    vena cava (inferior) (superior) 747.49
    vertebra 756.19
    vulva 752.49
  spermatic cord 752.9
  spine, spinal 756.10
    column 756.10
    cord 742.9
      meningocele *(see also* Spina
        bifida) 741.9●
      specified type NEC 742.59
      spina bifida *(see also* Spina bifida)
        741.9●
      vessel 747.82
    meninges 742.59
    nerve root 742.9
  spleen 759.0
  Sprengel's 755.52
  sternum 756.3
  stomach 750.9
    specified type NEC 750.7
  submaxillary gland 750.9
  superior vena cava 747.40
  talipes - *see* Talipes

Anomaly, anomalous (Continued)
  tarsus 755.67
    with complete absence of distal
      elements 755.31
  teeth, tooth NEC 520.9
    position 524.30
      crowding 524.31
      displacement 524.30
        horizontal 524.33
        vertical 524.34
      distance
        interocclusal
          excessive 524.37
          insufficient 524.36
      excessive spacing 524.32
      rotation 524.35
      specified NEC 524.39
    spacing 524.30
  tendon 756.9
    specified type NEC 756.89
  termination
    coronary artery 746.85
  testis 752.9
  thebesian valve 746.9
  thigh 755.60
    flexion (see also Subluxation,
      congenital, hip) 754.32
  thorax (wall) 756.3
  throat 750.9
  thumb 755.50
    supernumerary 755.01
  thymus gland 759.2
  thyroid (gland) 759.2
    cartilage 748.3
  tibia 755.60
    saber 090.5
  toe 755.66
    supernumerary 755.02
    webbed (see also Syndactylism,
      toes) 755.13
  tongue 750.10
    specified type NEC 750.19
  trachea, tracheal 748.3
    cartilage 748.3
    rings 748.3
  tragus 744.3
  transverse aortic arch 747.21
  trichromata 368.59
  trichromatopsia 368.59
  tricuspid (leaflet) (valve) 746.9
    atresia 746.1
    Ebstein's 746.2
    specified type NEC 746.89
    stenosis 746.1
  trunk 759.9
  Uhl's (hypoplasia of myocardium,
    right ventricle) 746.84
  ulna 755.50
  umbilicus 759.9
    artery 747.5
  union, trachea with larynx 748.3
  unspecified site 759.9
  upper extremity 755.50
    vessel 747.63
  urachus 753.7
    specified type NEC 753.7
  ureter 753.9
    obstructive 753.20
    specified type NEC 753.4
      obstructive 753.29
  urethra (valve) 753.9
    obstructive 753.6
    specified type NEC 753.8

Anomaly, anomalous (Continued)
  urinary tract or system (any part,
    except urachus) 753.9
    specified type NEC 753.8
    urachus 753.7
  uterus 752.3
    with only one functioning horn
      752.3
    in pregnancy or childbirth 654.0●
      affecting fetus or newborn 763.89
      causing obstructed labor 660.2●
        affecting fetus or newborn
          763.1
  uvula 750.9
  vagina 752.40
  valleculae 748.3
  valve (heart) NEC 746.9
    formation, ureter 753.29
    pulmonary 746.00
    specified type NEC 746.89
  vascular NEC (see also Anomaly,
    peripheral vascular system)
    747.60
    ring 747.21
  vas deferens 752.9
  vein(s) (peripheral) NEC (see also
    Anomaly, peripheral vascular
    system) 747.60
    brain 747.81
    cerebral 747.81
    coronary 746.89
    great 747.40
      specified type NEC 747.49
    portal 747.40
    pulmonary 747.40
    retina 743.9
  vena cava (inferior) (superior) 747.40
  venous - see Anomaly, vein
  venous return (pulmonary) 747.49
    partial 747.42
    total 747.41
  ventricle, ventricular (heart) 746.9
    bands 746.9
    folds 746.9
    septa 745.4
  vertebra 756.10
  vesicourethral orifice 753.9
  vessels NEC (see also Anomaly,
    peripheral vascular system)
    747.60
    optic papilla 743.9
  vitelline duct 751.0
  vitreous humor 743.9
    specified type NEC 743.51
  vulva 752.40
  wrist (joint) 755.50
Anomia 784.69
Anonychia 757.5
  acquired 703.8
Anophthalmos, anophthalmus (clinical)
  (congenital) (globe) 743.00
  acquired V45.78
Anopsia (altitudinal) (quadrant) 368.46
Anorchia 752.89
Anorchism, anorchidism 752.89
Anorexia 783.0
  hysterical 300.11
  nervosa 307.1
Anosmia (see also Disturbance, sensation)
  781.1
  hysterical 300.11
  postinfectional 478.9
  psychogenic 306.7
  traumatic 951.8

Anosognosia 780.99
Anosphrasia 781.1
Anosteoplasia 756.50
Anotia 744.09
Anovulatory cycle 628.0
Anoxemia 799.02
  newborn 770.88
Anoxia 799.02
  altitude 993.2
  cerebral 348.1
    with
      abortion - see Abortion, by type,
        with specified complication
        NEC
      ectopic pregnancy (see also
        categories 633.0-633.9) 639.8
      molar pregnancy (see also
        categories 630-632) 639.8
    complicating
      delivery (cesarean) (instrumental)
        669.4●
      ectopic or molar pregnancy 639.8
      obstetric anesthesia or sedation
        668.2●
    during or resulting from a
      procedure 997.01
    following
      abortion 639.8
      ectopic or molar pregnancy
        639.8
    newborn (see also Distress, fetal,
      liveborn infant) 770.88
  due to drowning 994.1
  fetal, affecting newborn 770.88
  heart - see Insufficiency, coronary
  high altitude 993.2
  intrauterine
    fetal death (before onset of labor)
      768.0
      during labor 768.1
    liveborn infant - see Distress, fetal,
      liveborn infant
  myocardial - see Insufficiency, coronary
  newborn 768.9
    mild or moderate 768.6
    severe 768.5
  pathological 799.02
Anteflexion - see Anteversion
Antenatal
  care, normal pregnancy V22.1
    first V22.0
  sampling
    chorionic villus V28.89
  screening of mother (for) V28.9
    based on amniocentesis NEC V28.2
      chromosomal anomalies V28.0
      raised alphafetoprotein levels
        V28.1
    chromosomal anomalies V28.0
    fetal growth retardation using
      ultrasonics V28.4
    genomic V28.89
    isoimmunization V28.5
    malformations using ultrasonics
      V28.3
    proteomic V28.89
    raised alphafetoprotein levels in
      amniotic fluid V28.1
    risk
      pre-term labor V28.82
    specified condition NEC V28.89
    Streptococcus B V28.6
  survey
    fetal anatomic V28.81

◄ New   ◄||| Revised   ~~deleted~~ Deleted   ● Use Additional Digit(s)   ▓ Omit code

Antenatal *(Continued)*
  testing
    nuchal translucency V28.89
Antepartum - *see* condition
Anterior - *see also* condition
  spinal artery compression syndrome 721.1
Antero-occlusion 524.24
Anteversion
  cervix - *see* Anteversion, uterus
  femur (neck), congenital 755.63
  uterus, uterine (cervix) (postinfectional) (postpartal, old) 621.6
    congenital 752.3
    in pregnancy or childbirth 654.4●
      affecting fetus or newborn 763.89
      causing obstructed labor 660.2●
        affecting fetus or newborn 763.1
Anthracosilicosis (occupational) 500
Anthracosis (lung) (occupational) 500
  lingua 529.3
Anthrax 022.9
  with pneumonia 022.1 *[484.5]*
  colitis 022.2
  cutaneous 022.0
  gastrointestinal 022.2
  intestinal 022.2
  pulmonary 022.1
  respiratory 022.1
  septicemia 022.3
  specified manifestation NEC 022.8
Anthropoid pelvis 755.69
  with disproportion (fetopelvic) 653.2●
    affecting fetus or newborn 763.1
    causing obstructed labor 660.1●
      affecting fetus or newborn 763.1
Anthropophobia 300.29
Antibioma, breast 611.0
Antibodies
  maternal (blood group) (*see also* Incompatibility) 656.2●
    anti-D, cord blood 656.1●
      fetus or newborn 773.0
Antibody deficiency syndrome
  agammaglobulinemic 279.00
  congenital 279.04
  hypogammaglobulinemic 279.00
Anticoagulant, intrinsic, circulating, causing hemorrhagic disorder (*see also* Circulating anticoagulants) 286.5 ◀▥
Antimongolism syndrome 758.39
Antimonial cholera 985.4
Antisocial personality 301.7
Antithrombinemia (*see also* Circulating anticoagulants) 286.5
Antithromboplastinemia (*see also* Circulating anticoagulants) 286.5
Antithromboplastinogenemia (*see also* Circulating anticoagulants) 286.5
Antitoxin complication or reaction - *see* Complications, vaccination
Anton (-Babinski) **syndrome** (hemiasomatognosia) 307.9
Antritis (chronic) 473.0
  maxilla 473.0
    acute 461.0
  stomach 535.4●
Antrum, antral - *see* condition
Anuria 788.5
  with
    abortion - *see* Abortion, by type, with renal failure

Anuria *(Continued)*
  with *(Continued)*
    ectopic pregnancy (*see also* categories 633.0-633.9) 639.3
    molar pregnancy (*see also* categories 630-632) 639.3
  calculus (impacted) (recurrent) 592.9
    kidney 592.0
    ureter 592.1
  congenital 753.3
  due to a procedure 997.5
  following
    abortion 639.3
    ectopic or molar pregnancy 639.3
  newborn 753.3
  postrenal 593.4
  puerperal, postpartum, childbirth 669.3●
  specified as due to a procedure 997.5
  sulfonamide
    correct substance properly administered 788.5
    overdose or wrong substance given or taken 961.0
  traumatic (following crushing) 958.5
Anus, anal - *see also* condition
  high risk human papillomavirus (HPV) DNA test positive 796.75
  low risk human papillomavirus (HPV) DNA test positive 796.79
Anusitis 569.49
Anxiety (neurosis) (reaction) (state) 300.00
  alcohol-induced 291.89
  depression 300.4
  drug-induced 292.89
  due to or associated with physical condition 293.84
  generalized 300.02
  hysteria 300.20
  in
    acute stress reaction 308.0
    transient adjustment reaction 309.24
  panic type 300.01
  separation, abnormal 309.21
  syndrome (organic) (transient) 293.84
Aorta, aortic - *see* condition
Aortectasia 441.9
Aortitis (nonsyphilitic) 447.6
  arteriosclerotic 440.0
  calcific 447.6
  Döhle-Heller 093.1
  luetic 093.1
  rheumatic (*see also* Endocarditis, acute, rheumatic) 391.1
  rheumatoid - *see* Arthritis, rheumatoid
  specific 093.1
  syphilitic 093.1
    congenital 090.5
Apathetic ~~thyroid storm (see also Thyrotoxicosis) 242.9~~ 799.25 ◀▥
  thyroid storm (*see also* Thyrotoxicosis) 242.9● ◀
Apathy 799.25 ◀
Apepsia 536.8
  achlorhydric 536.0
  psychogenic 306.4
Aperistalsis, esophagus 530.0
Apert's syndrome (acrocephalosyndactyly) 755.55
Apert-Gallais syndrome (adrenogenital) 255.2
Apertognathia 524.20
Aphagia 787.20
  psychogenic 307.1

Aphakia (acquired) (bilateral) (postoperative) (unilateral) 379.31
  congenital 743.35
Aphalangia (congenital) 755.4
  lower limb (complete) (intercalary) (partial) (terminal) 755.39
    meaning all digits (complete) (partial) 755.31
    transverse 755.31
  upper limb (complete) (intercalary) (partial) (terminal) 755.29
    meaning all digits (complete) (partial) 755.21
    transverse 755.21
Aphasia (amnestic) (ataxic) (auditory) (Broca's) (choreatic) (classic) (expressive) (global) (ideational) (ideokinetic) (ideomotor) (jargon) (motor) (nominal) (receptive) (semantic) (sensory) (syntactic) (verbal) (visual) (Wernicke's) 784.3
  developmental 315.31
  syphilis, tertiary 094.89
  uremic - *see* Uremia
Aphemia 784.3
  uremic - *see* Uremia
Aphonia 784.41
  clericorum 784.49
  hysterical 300.11
  organic 784.41
  psychogenic 306.1
Aphthae, aphthous - *see also* condition
  Bednar's 528.2
  cachectic 529.0
  epizootic 078.4
  fever 078.4
  oral 528.2
  stomatitis 528.2
  thrush 112.0
  ulcer (oral) (recurrent) 528.2
    genital organ(s) NEC
      female 616.50
      male 608.89
    larynx 478.79
Apical - *see* condition
Apical ballooning syndrome 429.83
Aplasia - *see also* Agenesis
  alveolar process (acquired) 525.8
    congenital 750.26
  aorta (congenital) 747.22
  aortic valve (congenital) 746.89
  axialis extracorticalis (congenital) 330.0
  bone marrow (myeloid) 284.9
    acquired (secondary) 284.89
    congenital 284.01
    idiopathic 284.9
  brain 740.0
    specified part 742.2
  breast 757.6
  bronchus 748.3
  cementum 520.4
  cerebellar 742.2
  congenital (pure) red cell 284.01
  corpus callosum 742.2
  erythrocyte 284.81
    congenital 284.01
  extracortical axial 330.0
  eye (congenital) 743.00
  fovea centralis (congenital) 743.55
  germinal (cell) 606.0
  iris 743.45
  labyrinth, membranous 744.05
  limb (congenital) 755.4
    lower NEC 755.30
    upper NEC 755.20

Aplasia *(Continued)*
  lung (bilateral) (congenital) (unilateral) 748.5
  nervous system NEC 742.8
  nuclear 742.8
  ovary 752.0
  Pelizaeus-Merzbacher 330.0
  prostate (congenital) 752.89
  red cell (with thymoma) (adult) 284.81
    acquired (secondary) 284.81
    congenital 284.01
    hereditary 284.01
    of infants 284.01
    primary 284.01
    pure 284.01
  round ligament (congenital) 752.89
  salivary gland 750.21
  skin (congenital) 757.39
  spinal cord 742.59
  spleen 759.0
  testis (congenital) 752.89
  thymic, with immunodeficiency 279.2
  thyroid 243
  uterus 752.3
  ventral horn cell 742.59
Apleuria 756.3
Apnea, apneic (spells) 786.03
  newborn, neonatorum 770.81
    essential 770.81
    obstructive 770.82
    primary 770.81
    sleep 770.81
    specified NEC 770.82
  psychogenic 306.1
  sleep 780.57
    with
      hypersomnia, unspecified 780.53
      hyposomnia, unspecified 780.51
      insomnia, unspecified 780.51
      sleep disturbance 780.57
    central, in conditions classified elsewhere 327.27
    obstructive (adult) (pediatric) 327.23
    organic 327.20
      other 327.29
    primary central 327.21
Apneumatosis newborn 770.4
Apodia 755.31
Apophysitis (bone) *(see also* Osteochondrosis) 732.9
  calcaneus 732.5
  juvenile 732.6
Apoplectiform convulsions *(see also* Disease, cerebrovascular, acute) 436
Apoplexia, apoplexy, apoplectic *(see also* Disease, cerebrovascular, acute) 436
  abdominal 569.89
  adrenal 036.3
  attack 436
  basilar *(see also* Disease, cerebrovascular, acute) 436
  brain *(see also* Disease, cerebrovascular, acute) 436
  bulbar *(see also* Disease, cerebrovascular, acute) 436
  capillary *(see also* Disease, cerebrovascular, acute) 436
  cardiac *(see also* Infarct, myocardium) 410.9●
  cerebral *(see also* Disease, cerebrovascular, acute) 436
  chorea *(see also* Disease, cerebrovascular, acute) 436

Apoplexia, apoplexy, apoplectic *(Continued)*
  congestive *(see also* Disease, cerebrovascular, acute) 436
    newborn 767.4
  embolic *(see also* Embolism, brain) 434.1●
  fetus 767.0
  fit *(see also* Disease, cerebrovascular, acute) 436
  healed or old V12.54
  heart (auricle) (ventricle) *(see also* Infarct, myocardium) 410.9●
  heat 992.0
  hemiplegia *(see also* Disease, cerebrovascular, acute) 436
  hemorrhagic (stroke) *(see also* Hemorrhage, brain) 432.9
  ingravescent *(see also* Disease, cerebrovascular, acute) 436
  late effect - *see* Late effect(s) (of) cerebrovascular disease
  lung - *see* Embolism, pulmonary
  meninges, hemorrhagic *(see also* Hemorrhage, subarachnoid) 430
  neonatorum 767.0
  newborn 767.0
  pancreatitis 577.0
  placenta 641.2●
  progressive *(see also* Disease, cerebrovascular, acute) 436
  pulmonary (artery) (vein) - *see* Embolism, pulmonary
  sanguineous *(see also* Disease, cerebrovascular, acute) 436
  seizure *(see also* Disease, cerebrovascular, acute) 436
  serous *(see also* Disease, cerebrovascular, acute) 436
  spleen 289.59
  stroke *(see also* Disease, cerebrovascular, acute) 436
  thrombotic *(see also* Thrombosis, brain) 434.0●
  uremic - *see* Uremia
  uteroplacental 641.2●
Appendage
  fallopian tube (cyst of Morgagni) 752.11
  intestine (epiploic) 751.5
  preauricular 744.1
  testicular (organ of Morgagni) 752.89
Appendicitis 541
  with
    perforation, peritonitis (generalized), or rupture 540.0
      with peritoneal abscess 540.1
    peritoneal abscess 540.1
  acute (catarrhal) (fulminating) (gangrenous) (inflammatory) (obstructive) (retrocecal) (suppurative) 540.9
    with
      perforation, peritonitis, or rupture 540.0
        with peritoneal abscess 540.1
      peritoneal abscess 540.1
  amebic 006.8
  chronic (recurrent) 542
  exacerbation - *see* Appendicitis, acute
  fulminating - *see* Appendicitis, acute
  gangrenous - *see* Appendicitis, acute
  healed (obliterative) 542
  interval 542
  neurogenic 542

Appendicitis *(Continued)*
  obstructive 542
  pneumococcal 541
  recurrent 542
  relapsing 542
  retrocecal 541
  subacute (adhesive) 542
  subsiding 542
  suppurative - *see* Appendicitis, acute
  tuberculous *(see also* Tuberculosis) 014.8●
Appendiclausis 543.9
Appendicolithiasis 543.9
Appendicopathia oxyurica 127.4
Appendix, appendicular - *see also* condition
  Morgagni (male) 752.89
    fallopian tube 752.11
Appetite
  depraved 307.52
  excessive 783.6
    psychogenic 307.51
  lack or loss *(see also* Anorexia) 783.0
    nonorganic origin 307.59
  perverted 307.52
    hysterical 300.11
Apprehension, apprehensiveness (abnormal) (state) 300.00
  specified type NEC 300.09
Approximal wear 521.10
Apraxia (classic) (ideational) (ideokinetic) (ideomotor) (motor) 784.69
  oculomotor, congenital 379.51
  verbal 784.69
Aptyalism 527.7
Aqueous misdirection 365.83
Arabicum elephantiasis *(see also* Infestation, filarial) 125.9
Arachnidism 989.5
Arachnitis - *see* Meningitis
Arachnodactyly 759.82
Arachnoidism 989.5
Arachnoiditis (acute) (adhesive) (basic) (brain) (cerebrospinal) (chiasmal) (chronic) (spinal) *(see also* Meningitis) 322.9
  meningococcal (chronic) 036.0
  syphilitic 094.2
  tuberculous *(see also* Tuberculosis, meninges) 013.0●
Araneism 989.5
Arboencephalitis, Australian 062.4
Arborization block (heart) 426.6
Arbor virus, arbovirus (infection) NEC 066.9
ARC 042
Arches - *see* condition
Arcuatus uterus 752.3
Arcus (cornea)
  juvenilis 743.43
    interfering with vision 743.42
  senilis 371.41
Arc-welders' lung 503
Arc-welders' syndrome (photokeratitis) 370.24
Areflexia 796.1
Areola - *see* condition
Argentaffinoma (M8241/1) - *see also* Neoplasm, by site, uncertain behavior
  benign (M8241/0) - *see* Neoplasm, by site, benign
  malignant (M8241/3) - *see* Neoplasm, by site, malignant
  syndrome 259.2

Argentinian hemorrhagic fever 078.7
Arginosuccinicaciduria 270.6
Argonz-Del Castillo syndrome
    (nonpuerperal galactorrhea and
    amenorrhea) 253.1
Argyll-Robertson phenomenon, pupil, or
    syndrome (syphilitic) 094.89
    atypical 379.45
    nonluetic 379.45
    nonsyphilitic 379.45
    reversed 379.45
Argyria, argyriasis NEC 985.8
    conjunctiva 372.55
    cornea 371.16
    from drug or medicinal agent
        correct substance properly
            administered 709.09
        overdose or wrong substance given
            or taken 961.2
Arhinencephaly 742.2
Arias-Stella phenomenon 621.30
Ariboflavinosis 266.0
Arizona enteritis 008.1
Arm - *see* condition
Armenian disease 277.31
Arnold-Chiari obstruction or syndrome
    (*see also* Spina bifida) 741.0●
    type I 348.4
    type II (*see also* Spina bifida) 741.0●
    type III 742.0
    type IV 742.2
Arousals
    confusional 327.41
Arrest, arrested
    active phase of labor 661.1●
        affecting fetus or newborn 763.7
    any plane in pelvis
        complicating delivery 660.1●
            affecting fetus or newborn 763.1
    bone marrow (*see also* Anemia, aplastic)
        284.9
    cardiac 427.5
        with
            abortion - *see* Abortion, by type,
                with specified complication
                NEC
            ectopic pregnancy (*see also*
                categories 633.0-633.9) 639.8
            molar pregnancy (*see also*
                categories 630-632) 639.8
        complicating
            anesthesia
                correct substance properly
                    administered 427.5
                obstetric 668.1●
                overdose or wrong substance
                    given 968.4
                specified anesthetic - *see*
                    Table of Drugs and
                    Chemicals
            delivery (cesarean) (instrumental)
                669.4●
            ectopic or molar pregnancy 639.8
            surgery (nontherapeutic)
                (therapeutic) 997.1
        fetus or newborn 779.85
        following
            abortion 639.8
            ectopic or molar pregnancy 639.8
        personal history, successfully
            rescuscitated V12.53
        postoperative (immediate) 997.1
            long-term effect of cardiac
                surgery 429.4

Arrest, arrested (*Continued*)
    cardiorespiratory (*see also* Arrest,
        cardiac) 427.5
    deep transverse 660.3●
        affecting fetus or newborn 763.1
    development or growth
        bone 733.91
        child 783.40
        fetus 764.9●
            affecting management of
                pregnancy 656.5●
        tracheal rings 748.3
    epiphyseal 733.91
    granulopoiesis 288.09
    heart - *see* Arrest, cardiac
    respiratory 799.1
        newborn 770.87
    sinus 426.6
    transverse (deep) 660.3●
        affecting fetus or newborn 763.1
Arrhenoblastoma (M8630/1)
    benign (M8630/0)
        specified site - *see* Neoplasm, by site,
            benign
        unspecified site
            female 220
            male 222.0
    malignant (M8630/3)
        specified site - *see* Neoplasm, by site,
            malignant
        unspecified site
            female 183.0
            male 186.9
    specified site - *see* Neoplasm, by site,
        uncertain behavior
    unspecified site
        female 236.2
        male 236.4
Arrhinencephaly 742.2
    due to
        trisomy 13 (13-15) 758.1
        trisomy 18 (16-18) 758.2
Arrhythmia (auricle) (cardiac) (cordis)
    (gallop rhythm) (juvenile) (nodal)
    (reflex) (sinus) (supraventricular)
    (transitory) (ventricle) 427.9
    bigeminal rhythm 427.89
    block 426.9
    bradycardia 427.89
    contractions, premature 427.60
    coronary sinus 427.89
    ectopic 427.89
    extrasystolic 427.60
    postoperative 997.1
    psychogenic 306.2
    vagal 780.2
Arrillaga-Ayerza syndrome (pulmonary
    artery sclerosis with pulmonary
    hypertension) 416.0
Arsenical
    dermatitis 692.4
    keratosis 692.4
    pigmentation 985.1
        from drug or medicinal agent
            correct substance properly
                administered 709.09
            overdose or wrong substance
                given or taken 961.1
Arsenism 985.1
    from drug or medicinal agent
        correct substance properly
            administered 692.4
        overdose or wrong substance given
            or taken 961.1

Arterial - *see* condition
Arteriectasis 447.8
Arteriofibrosis - *see* Arteriosclerosis
Arteriolar sclerosis - *see* Arteriosclerosis
Arteriolith - *see* Arteriosclerosis
Arteriolitis 447.6
    necrotizing, kidney 447.5
    renal - *see* Hypertension, kidney
Arteriolosclerosis - *see* Arteriosclerosis
Arterionephrosclerosis (*see also*
    Hypertension, kidney) 403.90
Arteriopathy 447.9
Arteriosclerosis, arteriosclerotic (artery)
    (deformans) (diffuse) (disease)
    (endarteritis) (general) (obliterans)
    (obliterative) (occlusive) (senile)
    (with calcification) 440.9
    with
        gangrene 440.24
        psychosis (*see also* Psychosis,
            arteriosclerotic) 290.40
        ulceration 440.23
    aorta 440.0
    arteries of extremities - *see*
        Arteriosclerosis, extremities
    basilar (artery) (*see also* Occlusion,
        artery, basilar) 433.0●
    brain 437.0
    bypass graft
        coronary artery 414.05
            autologous artery
                (gastroepiploic) (internal
                mammary) 414.04
            autologous vein 414.02
            nonautologous biological 414.03
            of transplanted heart 414.07
        extremity 440.30
            autologous vein 440.31
            nonautologous biological 440.32
    cardiac - *see* Arteriosclerosis, coronary
    cardiopathy - *see* Arteriosclerosis,
        coronary
    cardiorenal (*see also* Hypertension,
        cardiorenal) 404.90
    cardiovascular (*see also* Disease,
        cardiovascular) 429.2
    carotid (artery) (common) (internal)
        (*see also* Occlusion, artery, carotid)
        433.1●
    central nervous system 437.0
    cerebral 437.0
        late effect - *see* Late effect(s) (of)
            cerebrovascular disease
    cerebrospinal 437.0
    cerebrovascular 437.0
    coronary (artery) 414.00
        due to lipid rich plaque 414.3
        graft - *see* Arteriosclerosis, bypass
            graft
        native artery 414.01
        of transplanted heart 414.06
    extremities (native artery) NEC 440.20
        bypass graft 440.30
            autologous vein 440.31
            nonautologous biological 440.32
        claudication (intermittent) 440.21
        and
            gangrene 440.24
            rest pain 440.22
                and
                    gangrene 440.24
                    ulceration 440.23
                      and gangrene 440.24
            ulceration 440.23
                and gangrene 440.24

Arteriosclerosis, arteriosclerotic
  (Continued)
  extremities NEC *(Continued)*
    gangrene 440.24
    rest pain 440.22
      and
        gangrene 440.24
        ulceration 440.23
          and gangrene 440.24
    specified site NEC 440.29
    ulceration 440.23
      and gangrene 440.24
  heart (disease) - *see also*
      Arteriosclerosis, coronary
    valve 424.99
      aortic 424.1
      mitral 424.0
      pulmonary 424.3
      tricuspid 424.2
  kidney *(see also* Hypertension, kidney)
      403.90
  labyrinth, labyrinthine 388.00
  medial NEC *(see also* Arteriosclerosis,
      extremities) 440.20
  mesentery (artery) 557.1
  Mönckeberg's *(see also* Arteriosclerosis,
      extremities) 440.20
  myocarditis 429.0
  nephrosclerosis *(see also* Hypertension,
      kidney) 403.90
  peripheral (of extremities) - *see*
      Arteriosclerosis, extremities
  precerebral 433.9●
    specified artery NEC 433.8●
  pulmonary (idiopathic) 416.0
  renal *(see also* Hypertension, kidney)
      403.90
    arterioles *(see also* Hypertension,
        kidney) 403.90
    artery 440.1
  retinal (vascular) 440.8 *[362.13]*
  specified artery NEC 440.8
    with gangrene 440.8 *[785.4]*
  spinal (cord) 437.0
  vertebral (artery) *(see also* Occlusion,
      artery, vertebral) 433.2●
Arteriospasm 443.9
Arteriovenous - *see* condition
Arteritis 447.6
  allergic *(see also* Angiitis,
      hypersensitivity) 446.20
  aorta (nonsyphilitic) 447.6
    syphilitic 093.1
  aortic arch 446.7
  brachiocephalica 446.7
  brain 437.4
    syphilitic 094.89
  branchial 446.7
  cerebral 437.4
    late effect - *see* Late effect(s) (of)
        cerebrovascular disease
    syphilitic 094.89
  coronary (artery) - *see also*
      Arteriosclerosis, coronary
    rheumatic 391.9
      chronic 398.99
    syphilitic 093.89
  cranial (left) (right) 446.5
  deformans - *see* Arteriosclerosis
  giant cell 446.5
  necrosing or necrotizing 446.0
  nodosa 446.0
  obliterans - *see also* Arteriosclerosis
    subclaviocarotica 446.7

Arteritis *(Continued)*
  pulmonary 417.8
  retina 362.18
  rheumatic - *see* Fever, rheumatic
  senile - *see* Arteriosclerosis
  suppurative 447.2
  syphilitic (general) 093.89
    brain 094.89
    coronary 093.89
    spinal 094.89
  temporal 446.5
  young female, syndrome 446.7
Artery, arterial - *see* condition
Arthralgia *(see also* Pain, joint) 719.4●
  allergic *(see also* Pain, joint) 719.4●
  in caisson disease 993.3
  psychogenic 307.89
  rubella 056.71
  Salmonella 003.23
  temporomandibular joint 524.62
Arthritis, arthritic (acute) (chronic)
      (subacute) 716.9●
  meaning Osteoarthritis - *see*
      Osteoarthrosis

Note 08   Use the following fifth-digit
subclassification with categories
711-712, 715-716:

  0   site unspecified
  1   shoulder region
  2   upper arm
  3   forearm
  4   hand
  5   pelvic region and thigh
  6   lower leg
  7   ankle and foot
  8   other specified sites
  9   multiple sites

---

  allergic 716.2●
  ankylosing (crippling) (spine) 720.0
      [713.2]
    sites other than spine 716.9●
  atrophic 714.0
    spine 720.9
  back *(see also* Arthritis, spine) 721.90
  Bechterew's (ankylosing spondylitis)
      720.0
  blennorrhagic 098.50 *[711.6]*●
  cervical, cervicodorsal *(see also*
      Spondylosis, cervical) 721.0
  Charcôt's 094.0 *[713.5]*
    diabetic 250.6● *[713.5]*
      due to secondary diabetes 249.6●
          [713.5]
    syringomyelic 336.0 *[713.5]*
    tabetic 094.0 *[713.5]*
  chylous *(see also* Filariasis) 125.9
      [711.7]●
  climacteric NEC 716.3●
  coccyx 721.8
  cricoarytenoid 478.79
  crystal (-induced) - *see* Arthritis, due to
      crystals
  deformans *(see also* Osteoarthrosis)
      715.9●
    spine 721.90
      with myelopathy 721.91
  degenerative *(see also* Osteoarthrosis)
      715.9●
    idiopathic 715.09
    polyarticular 715.09
    spine 721.90
      with myelopathy 721.91

Arthritis, arthritic *(Continued)*
  dermatoarthritis, lipoid 272.8 *[713.0]*
  due to or associated with
    acromegaly 253.0 *[713.0]*
    actinomycosis 039.8 *[711.4]*●
    amyloidosis 277.39 *[713.7]*
    bacterial disease NEC 040.89
        [711.4]●
    Behçet's syndrome 136.1 *[711.2]*●
    blastomycosis 116.0 *[711.6]*●
    brucellosis *(see also* Brucellosis) 023.9
        [711.4]●
    caisson disease 993.3
    coccidioidomycosis 114.3 *[711.6]*●
    coliform (Escherichia coli) 711.0●
    colitis, ulcerative - *(see also* Colitis,
        ulcerative) 556.9 *[713.1]*
    cowpox 051.01 *[711.5]*●
    crystals -*(see also* Gout)
      dicalcium phosphate 275.49
          [712.1]●
      pyrophosphate 275.49 *[712.2]*●
      specified NEC 275.49 *[712.8]*●
    dermatoarthritis, lipoid 272.8 *[713.0]*
    dermatological disorder NEC 709.9
        [713.3]
    diabetes 250.6● *[713.5]*
      due to secondary diabetes 249.6●
          [713.5]
    diphtheria 032.89 *[711.4]*●
    dracontiasis 125.7 *[711.7]*●
    dysentery 009.0 *[711.3]*●
    endocrine disorder NEC 259.9
        [713.0]
    enteritis NEC 009.1 *[711.3]*●
      infectious *(see also* Enteritis,
          infectious) 009.0 *[711.3]*●
        specified organism NEC 008.8
            [711.3]●
      regional *(see also* Enteritis,
          regional) 555.9 *[713.1]*
        specified organism NEC 008.8
            [711.3]●
    epiphyseal slip, nontraumatic (old)
        716.8●
    erysipelas 035 *[711.4]*●
    erythema
      epidemic 026.1
      multiforme 695.10 *[713.3]*
      nodosum 695.2 *[713.3]*
    Escherichia coli 711.0●
    filariasis NEC 125.9 *[711.7]*●
    gastrointestinal condition NEC 569.9
        [713.1]
    glanders 024 *[711.4]*●
    Gonococcus 098.50
    gout 274.00
    H. influenzae 711.0●
    helminthiasis NEC 128.9 *[711.7]*●
    hematological disorder NEC 289.9
        [713.2]
    hemochromatosis 275.0 *[713.0]*
    hemoglobinopathy NEC *(see also*
        Disease, hemoglobin) 282.7
        [713.2]
    hemophilia *(see also* Hemophilia)
        286.0 *[713.2]*
    Hemophilus influenzae (H.
        influenzae) 711.0●
    Henoch (-Schönlein) purpura 287.0
        [713.6]
    histoplasmosis NEC *(see also*
        Histoplasmosis) 115.99
        [711.6]●

◄ New   ◄▦ Revised   deleted Deleted   ● Use Additional Digit(s)   ▦ Omit code

Arthritis, arthritic *(Continued)*
  due to or associated with *(Continued)*
    human parvovirus 079.83
      [711.5]●
    hyperparathyroidism 252.00
      [713.0]
    hypersensitivity reaction NEC
      995.3 [713.6]
    hypogammaglobulinemia *(see also*
      Hypogammaglobulinemia)
      279.00 [713.0]
    hypothyroidism NEC 244.9
      [713.0]
    infection *(see also* Arthritis,
      infectious) 711.9●
    infectious disease NEC 136.9
      [711.8]●
    leprosy *(see also* Leprosy) 030.9
      [711.4]●
    leukemia NEC (M9800/3) 208.9●
      [713.2]
    lipoid dermatoarthritis 272.8
      [713.0]
    Lyme disease 088.81 [711.8]●
    Mediterranean fever, familial 277.31
      [713.7]
    meningococcal infection 036.82
    metabolic disorder NEC 277.9
      [713.0]
    multiple myelomatosis (M9730/3)
      203.0● [713.2]
    mumps 072.79 [711.5]●
    mycobacteria 031.8 [711.4]●
    mycosis NEC 117.9 [711.6]●
    neurological disorder NEC 349.9
      [713.5]
    ochronosis 270.2 [713.0]
    O'Nyong Nyong 066.3 [711.5]●
    parasitic disease NEC 136.9
      [711.8]●
    paratyphoid fever *(see also* Fever,
      paratyphoid) 002.9 [711.3]●
    parvovirus B19 079.83 [711.5]●
    Pneumococcus 711.0●
    poliomyelitis *(see also* Poliomyelitis)
      045.9● [711.5]●
    Pseudomonas 711.0●
    psoriasis 696.0
    pyogenic organism (E. coli) (H.
      influenzae) (Pseudomonas)
      (Streptococcus) 711.0●
    rat-bite fever 026.1 [711.4]●
    regional enteritis *(see also* Enteritis,
      regional) 555.9 [713.1]
    Reiter's disease 099.3 [711.1]●
    respiratory disorder NEC 519.9
      [713.4]
    reticulosis, malignant (M9720/3)
      202.3● [713.2]
    rubella 056.71
    salmonellosis 003.23
    sarcoidosis 135 [713.7]
    serum sickness 999.5 [713.6]
    Staphylococcus 711.0●
    Streptococcus 711.0●
    syphilis *(see also* Syphilis) 094.0
      [711.4]●
    syringomyelia 336.0 [713.5]
    thalassemia 282.49 [713.2]
    tuberculosis *(see also* Tuberculosis,
      arthritis) 015.9● [711.4]●
    typhoid fever 002.0 [711.3]●
    ulcerative colitis - *(see also* Colitis,
      ulcerative) 556.9 [713.1]

Arthritis, arthritic *(Continued)*
  due to or associated with *(Continued)*
    urethritis
      nongonococcal *(see also* Urethritis,
        nongonococcal) 099.40
        [711.1]●
      nonspecific *(see also* Urethritis,
        nongonococcal) 099.40
        [711.1]●
      Reiter's 099.3 [711.1]●
    viral disease NEC 079.99 [711.5]●
  erythema epidemic 026.1
  gonococcal 098.50
  gouty (acute) 274.00 ◀▥
    acute 274.01 ◀
  hypertrophic *(see also* Osteoarthrosis)
    715.9●
    spine 721.90
      with myelopathy 721.91
  idiopathic, blennorrheal 099.3
  in caisson disease 993.3 [713.8]
  infectious or infective (acute) (chronic)
    (subacute) NEC 711.9●
    nonpyogenic 711.9●
    spine 720.9
  inflammatory NEC 714.9
  juvenile rheumatoid (chronic)
    (polyarticular) 714.30
    acute 714.31
    monoarticular 714.33
    pauciarticular 714.32
  lumbar *(see also* Spondylosis, lumbar)
    721.3
  meningococcal 036.82
  menopausal NEC 716.3●
  migratory - *see* Fever, rheumatic
  neuropathic (Charcôt's) 094.0 [713.5]
    diabetic 250.6● [713.5]
      due to secondary diabetes 249.6●
        [713.5]
    nonsyphilitic NEC 349.9 [713.5]
    syringomyelic 336.0 [713.5]
    tabetic 094.0 [713.5]
  nodosa *(see also* Osteoarthrosis) 715.9●
    spine 721.90
      with myelopathy 721.91
  nonpyogenic NEC 716.9●
    spine 721.90
      with myelopathy 721.91
  ochronotic 270.2 [713.0]
  palindromic *(see also* Rheumatism,
    palindromic) 719.3●
  pneumococcal 711.0●
  postdysenteric 009.0 [711.3]●
  postrheumatic, chronic (Jaccoud's)
    714.4
  primary progressive 714.0
    spine 720.9
  proliferative 714.0
    spine 720.0
  psoriatic 696.0
  purulent 711.0●
  pyogenic or pyemic 711.0●
  rheumatic 714.0
    acute or subacute - *see* Fever,
      rheumatic
    chronic 714.0
    spine 720.9
  rheumatoid (nodular) 714.0
    with
      splenoadenomegaly and
        leukopenia 714.1
      visceral or systemic involvement
        714.2

Arthritis, arthritic *(Continued)*
  rheumatoid *(Continued)*
    aortitis 714.89
    carditis 714.2
    heart disease 714.2
    juvenile (chronic) (polyarticular)
      714.30
      acute 714.31
      monoarticular 714.33
      pauciarticular 714.32
    spine 720.0
    rubella 056.71
    sacral, sacroiliac, sacrococcygeal *(see
      also* Spondylosis, sacral) 721.3
    scorbutic 267
    senile or senescent *(see also*
      Osteoarthrosis) 715.9●
      spine 721.90
        with myelopathy 721.91
    septic 711.0●
    serum (nontherapeutic) (therapeutic)
      999.5 [713.6]
    specified form NEC 716.8●
    spine 721.90
      with myelopathy 721.91
      atrophic 720.9
      degenerative 721.90
        with myelopathy 721.91
      hypertrophic (with deformity) 721.90
        with myelopathy 721.91
      infectious or infective NEC 720.9
      Marie-Strümpell 720.0
      nonpyogenic 721.90
        with myelopathy 721.91
      pyogenic 720.9
      rheumatoid 720.0
      traumatic (old) 721.7
      tuberculous *(see also* Tuberculosis)
        015.0● [720.81]
    staphylococcal 711.0●
    streptococcal 711.0●
    suppurative 711.0●
    syphilitic 094.0 [713.5]
      congenital 090.49 [713.5]
    syphilitica deformans (Charcôt) 094.0
      [713.5]
    temporomandibular joint 524.69
    thoracic *(see also* Spondylosis, thoracic)
      721.2
    toxic of menopause 716.3●
    transient 716.4●
    traumatic (chronic) (old) (post) 716.1●
      current injury - *see* nature of injury
    tuberculous *(see also* Tuberculosis,
      arthritis) 015.9● [711.4]●
    urethritica 099.3 [711.1]●
    urica, uratic 274.00 ◀▥
    venereal 099.3 [711.1]●
    vertebral *(see also* Arthritis, spine)
      721.90
    villous 716.8●
    von Bechterew's 720.0
Arthrocele *(see also* Effusion, joint) 719.0●
Arthrochondritis - *see* Arthritis
Arthrodesis status V45.4
Arthrodynia *(see also* Pain, joint) 719.4●
  psychogenic 307.89
Arthrodysplasia 755.9
Arthrofibrosis, joint *(see also* Ankylosis)
  718.5●
Arthrogryposis 728.3
  multiplex, congenita 754.89
Arthrokatadysis 715.35
Arthrolithiasis 274.00 ◀▥

Arthro-onychodysplasia 756.89
Arthro-osteo-onychodysplasia 756.89
Arthropathy (see also Arthritis) 716.9●

Note 09   Use the following fifth-digit subclassification with categories 711-712, 716:

0   site unspecified
1   shoulder region
2   upper arm
3   forearm
4   hand
5   pelvic region and thigh
6   lower leg
7   ankle and foot
8   other specified sites
9   multiple sites

Behçet's 136.1 [711.2]●
Charcôt's 094.0 [713.5]
    diabetic 250.6● [713.5]
        due to secondary diabetes 249.6● [713.5]
    syringomyelic 336.0 [713.5]
    tabetic 094.0 [713.5]
crystal (-induced) - see Arthritis, due to crystals
gouty 274.00   ◀━▍║║
    acute 274.01   ◀
    chronic (without mention of tophus (tophi)) 274.02   ◀
        with tophus (tophi) 274.03 ◀
neurogenic, neuropathic (Charcôt's) (tabetic) 094.0 [713.5]
    diabetic 250.6● [713.5]
        due to secondary diabetes 249.6● [713.5]
    nonsyphilitic NEC 349.9 [713.5]
    syringomyelic 336.0 [713.5]
postdysenteric NEC 009.0 [711.3]●
postrheumatic, chronic (Jaccoud's) 714.4
psoriatic 696.0
pulmonary 731.2
specified NEC 716.8●
syringomyelia 336.0 [713.5]
tabes dorsalis 094.0 [713.5]
tabetic 094.0 [713.5]
transient 716.4●
traumatic 716.1●
uric acid 274.00   ◀━▍║║
Arthrophyte (see also Loose, body, joint) 718.1●
Arthrophytis 719.80
    ankle 719.87
    elbow 719.82
    foot 719.87
    hand 719.84
    hip 719.85
    knee 719.86
    multiple sites 719.89
    pelvic region 719.85
    shoulder (region) 719.81
    specified site NEC 719.88
    wrist 719.83
Arthropyosis (see also Arthritis, pyogenic) 711.0●
Arthroscopic surgical procedure converted to open procedure V64.43
Arthrosis (deformans) (degenerative) (see also Osteoarthrosis) 715.9●
    Charcôt's 094.0 [713.5]
    polyarticular 715.09
    spine (see also Spondylosis) 721.90

Arthus phenomenon 995.21
    due to
        correct substance properly administered 995.21
        overdose or wrong substance given or taken 977.9
            specified drug - see Table of Drugs and Chemicals
    serum 999.5
Articular - see also condition
    disc disorder (reducing or non-reducing) 524.63
    spondylolisthesis 756.12
Articulation
    anterior 524.27
    posterior 524.27
    reverse 524.27
Artificial
    device (prosthetic) - see Fitting, device
    insemination V26.1
    menopause (states) (symptoms) (syndrome) 627.4
    opening status (functioning) (without complication) V44.9
        anus (colostomy) V44.3
        colostomy V44.3
        cystostomy V44.50
            appendico-vesicostomy V44.52
            cutaneous-vesicostomy V44.51
            specified type NEC V44.59
        enterostomy V44.4
        gastrostomy V44.1
        ileostomy V44.2
        intestinal tract NEC V44.4
        jejunostomy V44.4
        nephrostomy V44.6
        specified site NEC V44.8
    tracheostomy V44.0
    ureterostomy V44.6
    urethrostomy V44.6
    urinary tract NEC V44.6
    vagina V44.7
    vagina status V44.7
ARV (disease) (illness) (infection) - see Human immunodeficiency virus (disease) (illness) (infection)
Arytenoid - see condition
Asbestosis (occupational) 501
Asboe-Hansen's disease (incontinentia pigmenti) 757.33
Ascariasis (intestinal) (lung) 127.0
Ascaridiasis 127.0
Ascaridosis 127.0
Ascaris 127.0
    lumbricoides (infestation) 127.0
    pneumonia 127.0
Ascending - see condition
Aschoff's bodies (see also Myocarditis, rheumatic) 398.0
Ascites 789.59
    abdominal NEC 789.59
    cancerous (M8000/6) 789.51
    cardiac 428.0
    chylous (nonfilarial) 457.8
        filarial (see also Infestation, filarial) 125.9
    congenital 778.0
    due to S. japonicum 120.2
    fetal, causing fetopelvic disproportion 653.7●
    heart 428.0
    joint (see also Effusion, joint) 719.0●
    malignant (M8000/6) 789.51
    pseudochylous 789.59

Ascites (Continued)
    syphilitic 095.2
    tuberculous (see also Tuberculosis) 014.0●
Ascorbic acid (vitamin C) deficiency (scurvy) 267
ASC-H (atypical squamous cells cannot exclude high grade squamous intraepithelial lesion)
    anus 796.72
    cervix 795.02
    vagina 795.12
ASC-US (atypical squamous cells of undetermined significance)
    anus 796.71
    cervix 795.01
    vagina 795.11
ASCVD (arteriosclerotic cardiovascular disease) 429.2
Aseptic - see condition
Asherman's syndrome 621.5
Asialia 527.7
Asiatic cholera (see also Cholera) 001.9
Asocial personality or trends 301.7
Asomatognosia 781.8
Aspergillosis 117.3
    with pneumonia 117.3 [484.6]
    allergic bronchopulmonary 518.6
    nonsyphilitic NEC 117.3
Aspergillus (flavus) (fumigatus) (infection) (terreus) 117.3
Aspermatogenesis 606.0
Aspermia (testis) 606.0
Asphyxia, asphyxiation (by) 799.01
    antenatal - see Distress, fetal
    bedclothes 994.7
    birth (see also Asphyxia, newborn) 768.9
    bunny bag 994.7
    carbon monoxide 986
    caul (see also Asphyxia, newborn) 768.9
    cave-in 994.7
        crushing - see Injury, internal, intrathoracic organs
    constriction 994.7
    crushing - see Injury, internal, intrathoracic organs
    drowning 994.1
    fetal, affecting newborn 768.9
    food or foreign body (in larynx) 933.1
        bronchioles 934.8
        bronchus (main) 934.1
        lung 934.8
        nasopharynx 933.0
        nose, nasal passages 932
        pharynx 933.0
        respiratory tract 934.9
            specified part NEC 934.8
        throat 933.0
        trachea 934.0
    gas, fumes, or vapor NEC 987.9
        specified - see Table of Drugs and Chemicals
    gravitational changes 994.7
    hanging 994.7
    inhalation - see Inhalation
    intrauterine
        fetal death (before onset of labor) 768.0
            during labor 768.1
        liveborn infant - see Distress, fetal, liveborn infant
    local 443.0

◀ New   ◀━▍║║ Revised   ~~deleted~~ Deleted   ● Use Additional Digit(s)   ▨ Omit code

Asphyxia, asphyxiation *(Continued)*
mechanical 994.7
during birth *(see also* Distress, fetal) 768.9
mucus 933.1
bronchus (main) 934.1
larynx 933.1
lung 934.8
nasal passages 932
newborn 770.18
pharynx 933.0
respiratory tract 934.9
specified part NEC 934.8
throat 933.0
trachea 934.0
vaginal (fetus or newborn) 770.18
newborn 768.9
with neurologic involvement 768.5
blue 768.6
livida 768.6
mild or moderate 768.6
pallida 768.5
severe 768.5
white 768.5
pathological 799.01
plastic bag 994.7
postnatal *(see also* Asphyxia, newborn) 768.9
mechanical 994.7
pressure 994.7
reticularis 782.61
strangulation 994.7
submersion 994.1
traumatic NEC - *see* Injury, internal, intrathoracic organs
vomiting, vomitus - *see* Asphyxia, food or foreign body
Aspiration
acid pulmonary (syndrome) 997.39
obstetric 668.0●
amniotic fluid 770.13
with respiratory symptoms 770.14
bronchitis 507.0
clear amniotic fluid 770.13
with
pneumonia 770.14
pneumonitis 770.14
respiratory symptoms 770.14
contents of birth canal 770.17
with respiratory symptoms 770.18
fetal 770.10
blood 770.15
with
pneumonia 770.16
pneumonitis 770.16
pneumonitis 770.18
food, foreign body, or gasoline (with asphyxiation) - *see* Asphyxia, food or foreign body
meconium 770.11
with
pneumonia 770.12
pneumonitis 770.12
respiratory symptoms 770.12
below vocal cords 770.11
with respiratory symptoms 770.12
mucus 933.1
into
bronchus (main) 934.1
lung 934.8
respiratory tract 934.9
specified part NEC 934.8
trachea 934.0

Aspiration *(Continued)*
mucus *(Continued)*
newborn 770.17
vaginal (fetus or newborn) 770.17
newborn 770.10
with respiratory symptoms 770.18
blood 770.15
with
pneumonia 770.16
pneumonitis 770.16
respiratory symptoms 770.16
pneumonia 507.0
fetus or newborn 770.18
meconium 770.12
pneumonitis 507.0
fetus or newborn 770.18
meconium 770.12
obstetric 668.0●
postnatal stomach contents 770.85
with
pneumonia 770.86
pneumonitis 770.86
respiratory symptoms 770.86
syndrome of newborn (massive) 770.18
meconium 770.12
vernix caseosa 770.17
Asplenia 759.0
with mesocardia 746.87
Assam fever 085.0
Assimilation, pelvis
with disproportion 653.2●
affecting fetus or newborn 763.1
causing obstructed labor 660.1●
affecting fetus or newborn 763.1
Assmann's focus *(see also* Tuberculosis) 011.0●
Astasia (-abasia) 307.9
hysterical 300.11
Asteatosis 706.8
cutis 706.8
Astereognosis 780.99
Asterixis 781.3
in liver disease 572.8
Asteroid hyalitis 379.22
Asthenia, asthenic 780.79
cardiac *(see also* Failure, heart) 428.9
psychogenic 306.2
cardiovascular *(see also* Failure, heart) 428.9
psychogenic 306.2
heart *(see also* Failure, heart) 428.9
psychogenic 306.2
hysterical 300.11
myocardial *(see also* Failure, heart) 428.9
psychogenic 306.2
nervous 300.5
neurocirculatory 306.2
neurotic 300.5
psychogenic 300.5
psychoneurotic 300.5
psychophysiologic 300.5
reaction, psychoneurotic 300.5
senile 797
Stiller's 780.79
tropical anhidrotic 705.1
Asthenopia 368.13
accommodative 367.4
hysterical (muscular) 300.11
psychogenic 306.7
Asthenospermia 792.2

Asthma, asthmatic (bronchial) (catarrh) (spasmodic) 493.9●

> Note 10 The following fifth digit subclassification is for use with codes 493.0-493.2, 493.9:
>
> 0 unspecified
> 1 with status asthmaticus
> 2 with (acute) exacerbation

with
chronic obstructive pulmonary disease (COPD) 493.2●
hay fever 493.0●
rhinitis, allergic 493.0●
allergic 493.9●
stated cause (external allergen) 493.0●
atopic 493.0●
cardiac *(see also* Failure, ventricular, left) 428.1
cardiobronchial *(see also* Failure, ventricular, left) 428.1
cardiorenal *(see also* Hypertension, cardiorenal) 404.90
childhood 493.0●
Colliers' 500
cough variant 493.82
croup 493.9●
detergent 507.8
due to
detergent 507.8
inhalation of fumes 506.3
internal immunological process 493.0●
endogenous (intrinsic) 493.1●
eosinophilic 518.3
exercise induced bronchospasm 493.81
exogenous (cosmetics) (dander or dust) (drugs) (dust) (feathers) (food) (hay) (platinum) (pollen) 493.0●
extrinsic 493.0●
grinders' 502
hay 493.0●
heart *(see also* Failure, ventricular, left) 428.1
IgE 493.0●
infective 493.1●
intrinsic 493.1●
Kopp's 254.8
late-onset 493.1●
meat-wrappers' 506.9
Millar's (laryngismus stridulus) 478.75
millstone makers' 502
miners' 500
Monday morning 504
New Orleans (epidemic) 493.0●
platinum 493.0●
pneumoconiotic (occupational) NEC 505
potters' 502
psychogenic 316 [493.9]●
pulmonary eosinophilic 518.3
red cedar 495.8
Rostan's *(see also* Failure, ventricular, left) 428.1
sandblasters' 502
sequoiosis 495.8
stonemasons' 502
thymic 254.8
tuberculous *(see also* Tuberculosis, pulmonary) 011.9●
Wichmann's (laryngismus stridulus) 478.75
wood 495.8

◄ New ◄⫞⫞ Revised ~~deleted~~ Deleted ● Use Additional Digit(s) ▨ Omit code **163**

Astigmatism (compound) (congenital)
  367.20
  irregular 367.22
  regular 367.21
Astroblastoma (M9430/3)
  nose 748.1
  specified site - see Neoplasm, by site,
    malignant
  unspecified site 191.9
Astrocytoma (cystic) (M9400/3)
  anaplastic type (M9401/3)
    specified site - see Neoplasm, by site,
      malignant
    unspecified site 191.9
  fibrillary (M9420/3)
    specified site - see Neoplasm, by site,
      malignant
    unspecified site 191.9
  fibrous (M9420/3)
    specified site - see Neoplasm, by site,
      malignant
    unspecified site 191.9
  gemistocytic (M9411/3)
    specified site - see Neoplasm, by site,
      malignant
    unspecified site 191.9
  juvenile (M9421/3)
    specified site - see Neoplasm, by site,
      malignant
    unspecified site 191.9
  nose 748.1
  pilocytic (M9421/3)
    specified site - see Neoplasm, by site,
      malignant
    unspecified site 191.9
  piloid (M9421/3)
    specified site - see Neoplasm, by site,
      malignant
    unspecified site 191.9
  protoplasmic (M9410/3)
    specified site - see Neoplasm, by site,
      malignant
    unspecified site 191.9
  specified site - see Neoplasm, by site,
    malignant
  subependymal (M9383/1) 237.5
    giant cell (M9384/1) 237.5
  unspecified site 191.9
Astroglioma (M9400/3)
  nose 748.1
  specified site - see Neoplasm, by site,
    malignant
  unspecified site 191.9
Asymbolia 784.60
Asymmetrical breathing 786.09
Asymmetry - see also Distortion
  breast, between native and
    reconstructed 612.1
  chest 786.9
  face 754.0
  jaw NEC 524.12
    maxillary 524.11
  pelvis with disproportion 653.0●
    affecting fetus or newborn
      763.1
    causing obstructed labor 660.1●
      affecting fetus or newborn
        763.1
Asynergia 781.3
Asynergy 781.3
  ventricular 429.89
Asystole (heart) (see also Arrest, cardiac)
  427.5
At risk for falling V15.88

Ataxia, ataxy, ataxic 781.3
  acute 781.3
  brain 331.89
  cerebellar 334.3
    hereditary (Marie's) 334.2
    in
      alcoholism 303.9● [334.4]
      myxedema (see also Myxedema)
        244.9 [334.4]
      neoplastic disease NEC 239.9
        [334.4]
  cerebral 331.89
  family, familial 334.2
    cerebral (Marie's) 334.2
    spinal (Friedreich's) 334.0
  Friedreich's (heredofamilial) (spinal)
    334.0
  frontal lobe 781.3
  gait 781.2
    hysterical 300.11
  general 781.3
  hereditary NEC 334.2
    cerebellar 334.2
    spastic 334.1
    spinal 334.0
  heredofamilial (Marie's) 334.2
  hysterical 300.11
  locomotor (progressive) 094.0
    diabetic 250.6● [337.1]
      due to secondary diabetes 249.6●
        [337.1]
  Marie's (cerebellar) (heredofamilial)
    334.2
  nonorganic origin 307.9
  partial 094.0
  postchickenpox 052.7
  progressive locomotor 094.0
  psychogenic 307.9
  Sanger-Brown's 334.2
  spastic 094.0
    hereditary 334.1
    syphilitic 094.0
  spinal
    hereditary 334.0
    progressive locomotor 094.0
  telangiectasia 334.8
Ataxia-telangiectasia 334.8
Atelectasis (absorption collapse)
    (complete) (compression) (massive)
    (partial) (postinfective) (pressure
    collapse) (pulmonary) (relaxation)
    518.0
  newborn (congenital) (partial) 770.5
    primary 770.4
  primary 770.4
  tuberculous (see also Tuberculosis,
    pulmonary) 011.9●
Ateleiosis, ateliosis 253.3
Atelia - see Distortion
Ateliosis 253.3
Atelocardia 746.9
Atelomyelia 742.59
Athelia 757.6
Atheroembolism
  extremity
    lower 445.02
    upper 445.01
  kidney 445.81
  specified site NEC 445.89
Atheroma, atheromatous (see also
    Arteriosclerosis) 440.9
  aorta, aortic 440.0
    valve (see also Endocarditis, aortic)
      424.1

Atheroma, atheromatous (Continued)
  artery - see Arteriosclerosis
  basilar (artery) (see also Occlusion,
    artery, basilar) 433.0●
  carotid (artery) (common) (internal)
    (see also Occlusion, artery, carotid)
    433.1●
  cerebral (arteries) 437.0
  coronary (artery) - see Arteriosclerosis,
    coronary
  degeneration - see Arteriosclerosis
  heart, cardiac - see Arteriosclerosis,
    coronary
  mitral (valve) 424.0
  myocardium, myocardial - see
    Arteriosclerosis, coronary
  pulmonary valve (heart) (see also
    Endocarditis, pulmonary) 424.3
  skin 706.2
  tricuspid (heart) (valve) 424.2
  valve, valvular - see Endocarditis
  vertebral (artery) (see also Occlusion,
    artery, vertebral) 433.2●
Atheromatosis - see also Arteriosclerosis
  arterial, congenital 272.8
Atherosclerosis - see Arteriosclerosis
Athetosis (acquired) 781.0
  bilateral 333.79
  congenital (bilateral) 333.6
  double 333.71
  unilateral 781.0
Athlete's
  foot 110.4
  heart 429.3
Athletic team examination V70.3
Athrepsia 261
Athyrea (acquired) (see also
    Hypothyroidism) 244.9
  congenital 243
Athyreosis (congenital) 243
  acquired - see Hypothyroidism
Athyroidism (acquired) (see also
    Hypothyroidism) 244.9
  congenital 243
Atmospheric pyrexia 992.0
Atonia, atony, atonic
  abdominal wall 728.2
  bladder (sphincter) 596.4
    neurogenic NEC 596.54
      with cauda equina syndrome
        344.61
  capillary 448.9
  cecum 564.89
    psychogenic 306.4
  colon 564.89
    psychogenic 306.4
  congenital 779.89
  dyspepsia 536.3
    psychogenic 306.4
  intestine 564.89
    psychogenic 306.4
  stomach 536.3
    neurotic or psychogenic 306.4
    psychogenic 306.4
  uterus 661.2●
    with hemorrhage (postpartum)
      666.1●
      affecting fetus or newborn 763.7
    without hemorrhage
      intrapartum 661.2●
      postpartum 669.8●
  vesical 596.4
Atopy NEC V15.09
Atransferrinemia, congenital 273.8

◀ New   ◀▦ Revised   ~~deleted~~ Deleted   ● Use Additional Digit(s)   ▨ Omit code

Atresia, atretic (congenital) 759.89
  alimentary organ or tract NEC
    751.8
    lower 751.2
    upper 750.8
  ani, anus, anal (canal) 751.2
  aorta 747.22
    with hypoplasia of ascending aorta
      and defective development of
      left ventricle (with mitral valve
      atresia) 746.7
    arch 747.11
    ring 747.21
  aortic (orifice) (valve) 746.89
    arch 747.11
  aqueduct of Sylvius 742.3
    with spina bifida (see also Spina
      bifida) 741.0●
  artery NEC (see also Atresia, blood
    vessel) 747.60
    cerebral 747.81
    coronary 746.85
    eye 743.58
    pulmonary 747.3
    umbilical 747.5
  auditory canal (external) 744.02
  bile, biliary duct (common) or passage
    751.61
    acquired (see also Obstruction,
      biliary) 576.2
  bladder (neck) 753.6
  blood vessel (peripheral) NEC
    747.60
    cerebral 747.81
    gastrointestinal 747.61
    lower limb 747.64
    pulmonary artery 747.3
    renal 747.62
    spinal 747.82
    upper limb 747.63
  bronchus 748.3
  canal, ear 744.02
  cardiac
    valve 746.89
      aortic 746.89
      mitral 746.89
      pulmonary 746.01
      tricuspid 746.1
  cecum 751.2
  cervix (acquired) 622.4
    congenital 752.49
    in pregnancy or childbirth 654.6●
      affecting fetus or newborn
        763.89
      causing obstructed labor 660.2●
        affecting fetus or newborn
          763.1
  choana 748.0
  colon 751.2
  cystic duct 751.61
    acquired 575.8
      with obstruction (see also
        Obstruction, gallbladder)
        575.2
  digestive organs NEC 751.8
  duodenum 751.1
  ear canal 744.02
  ejaculatory duct 752.89
  epiglottis 748.3
  esophagus 750.3
  Eustachian tube 744.24
  fallopian tube (acquired) 628.2
    congenital 752.19
  follicular cyst 620.0

Atresia, atretic (Continued)
  foramen of
    Luschka 742.3
      with spina bifida (see also Spina
        bifida) 741.0●
    Magendie 742.3
      with spina bifida (see also Spina
        bifida) 741.0●
  gallbladder 751.69
  genital organ
    external
      female 752.49
      male NEC 752.89
        penis 752.69
    internal
      female 752.89
      male 752.89
  glottis 748.3
  gullet 750.3
  heart
    valve NEC 746.89
      aortic 746.89
      mitral 746.89
      pulmonary 746.01
      tricuspid 746.1
  hymen 752.42
    acquired 623.3
    postinfective 623.3
  ileum 751.1
  intestine (small) 751.1
    large 751.2
  iris, filtration angle (see also
    Buphthalmia) 743.20
  jejunum 751.1
  kidney 753.3
  lacrimal, apparatus 743.65
    acquired - see Stenosis, lacrimal
  larynx 748.3
  ligament, broad 752.19
  lung 748.5
  meatus urinarius 753.6
  mitral valve 746.89
    with atresia or hypoplasia of aortic
      orifice or valve, with
      hypoplasia of ascending aorta
      and defective development of
      left ventricle 746.7
  nares (anterior) (posterior) 748.0
  nasolacrimal duct 743.65
  nasopharynx 748.8
  nose, nostril 748.0
    acquired 738.0
  organ or site NEC - see Anomaly,
    specified type NEC
  osseous meatus (ear) 744.03
  oviduct (acquired) 628.2
    congenital 752.19
  parotid duct 750.23
    acquired 527.8
  pulmonary (artery) 747.3
    valve 746.01
    vein 747.49
  pulmonic 746.01
  pupil 743.46
  rectum 751.2
  salivary duct or gland 750.23
    acquired 527.8
  sublingual duct 750.23
    acquired 527.8
  submaxillary duct or gland 750.23
    acquired 527.8
  trachea 748.3
  tricuspid valve 746.1
  ureter 753.29

Atresia, atretic (Continued)
  ureteropelvic junction 753.21
  ureterovesical orifice 753.22
  urethra (valvular) 753.6
  urinary tract NEC 753.29
  uterus 752.3
    acquired 621.8
  vagina (acquired) 623.2
    congenital 752.49
    postgonococcal (old) 098.2
    postinfectional 623.2
    senile 623.2
  vascular NEC (see also Atresia, blood
    vessel) 747.60
    cerebral 747.81
  vas deferens 752.89
  vein NEC (see also Atresia, blood
    vessel) 747.60
    cardiac 746.89
    great 747.49
    portal 747.49
    pulmonary 747.49
  vena cava (inferior) (superior) 747.49
  vesicourethral orifice 753.6
  vulva 752.49
    acquired 624.8
Atrichia, atrichosis 704.00
  congenital (universal) 757.4
Atrioventricularis commune 745.69
Atrophia - see also Atrophy
  alba 709.09
  cutis 701.8
    idiopathica progressiva 701.8
    senilis 701.8
  dermatological, diffuse (idiopathic)
    701.8
  flava hepatis (acuta) (subacuta) (see also
    Necrosis, liver) 570
  gyrata of choroid and retina (central)
    363.54
    generalized 363.57
  senilis 797
    dermatological 701.8
  unguium 703.8
    congenita 757.5
Atrophoderma, atrophodermia 701.9
  diffusum (idiopathic) 701.8
  maculatum 701.3
    et striatum 701.3
      due to syphilis 095.8
    syphilitic 091.3
  neuriticum 701.8
  pigmentosum 757.33
  reticulatum symmetricum faciei 701.8
  senile 701.8
  symmetrical 701.8
  vermiculata 701.8
Atrophy, atrophic
  adrenal (autoimmune) (capsule)
    (cortex) (gland) 255.41
    with hypofunction 255.41
  alveolar process or ridge (edentulous)
    525.20
    mandible 525.20
      minimal 525.21
      moderate 525.22
      severe 525.23
    maxilla 525.20
      minimal 525.24
      moderate 525.25
      severe 525.26
  appendix 543.9
  Aran-Duchenne muscular 335.21
  arm 728.2

Atrophy, atrophic (Continued)
  arteriosclerotic - see Arteriosclerosis
  arthritis 714.0
    spine 720.9
  bile duct (any) 576.8
  bladder 596.8
  blanche (of Milian) 701.3
  bone (senile) 733.99
    due to
      disuse 733.7
      infection 733.99
      tabes dorsalis (neurogenic)
          094.0
    posttraumatic 733.99
  brain (cortex) (progressive) 331.9
    with dementia 290.10
    Alzheimer's 331.0
      with dementia - see Alzheimer's,
          dementia
    circumscribed (Pick's) 331.11
      with dementia
        with behavioral disturbance
            331.11 [294.11]
        without behavioral
            disturbance 331.11
            [294.10]
    congenital 742.4
    hereditary 331.9
    senile 331.2
  breast 611.4
    puerperal, postpartum 676.3●
  buccal cavity 528.9
  cardiac (brown) (senile) (see also
      Degeneration, myocardial)
      429.1
  cartilage (infectional) (joint) 733.99
  cast, plaster of Paris 728.2
  cerebellar - see Atrophy, brain
  cerebral - see Atrophy, brain
  cervix (endometrium) (mucosa)
      (myometrium) (senile) (uteri)
      622.8
    menopausal 627.8
  Charcôt-Marie-Tooth 356.1
  choroid 363.40
    diffuse secondary 363.42
    hereditary (see also Dystrophy,
        choroid) 363.50
      gyrate
        central 363.54
        diffuse 363.57
        generalized 363.57
    senile 363.41
  ciliary body 364.57
  colloid, degenerative 701.3
  conjunctiva (senile) 372.89
  corpus cavernosum 607.89
  cortical (see also Atrophy, brain) 331.9
  Cruveilhier's 335.21
  cystic duct 576.8
  dacryosialadenopathy 710.2
  degenerative
    colloid 701.3
    senile 701.3
  Déjérine-Thomas 333.0
  diffuse idiopathic, dermatological
      701.8
  disuse
    bone 733.7
    muscle 728.2
    pelvic muscles and anal sphincter
        618.83
  Duchenne-Aran 335.21
  ear 388.9

Atrophy, atrophic (Continued)
  edentulous alveolar ridge 525.20
    mandible 525.20
      minimal 525.21
      moderate 525.22
      severe 525.23
    maxilla 525.20
      minimal 525.24
      moderate 525.25
      severe 525.26
  emphysema, lung 492.8
  endometrium (senile) 621.8
    cervix 622.8
  enteric 569.89
  epididymis 608.3
  eyeball, cause unknown 360.41
  eyelid (senile) 374.50
  facial (skin) 701.9
  facioscapulohumeral (Landouzy-
      Déjérine) 359.1
  fallopian tube (senile), acquired 620.3
  fatty, thymus (gland) 254.8
  gallbladder 575.8
  gastric 537.89
  gastritis (chronic) 535.1●
  gastrointestinal 569.89
  genital organ, male 608.89
  glandular 289.3
  globe (phthisis bulbi) 360.41
  gum (see also Recession, gingival)
      523.20
  hair 704.2
  heart (brown) (senile) (see also
      Degeneration, myocardial) 429.1
  hemifacial 754.0
    Romberg 349.89
  hydronephrosis 591
  infantile 261
    paralysis, acute (see also
        Poliomyelitis, with paralysis)
        045.1●
  intestine 569.89
  iris (generalized) (postinfectional)
      (sector shaped) 364.59
    essential 364.51
    progressive 364.51
    sphincter 364.54
  kidney (senile) (see also Sclerosis, renal)
      587
    with hypertension (see also
        Hypertension, kidney) 403.90
    congenital 753.0
    hydronephrotic 591
    infantile 753.0
  lacrimal apparatus (primary) 375.13
    secondary 375.14
  Landouzy-Déjérine 359.1
  laryngitis, infection 476.0
  larynx 478.79
  Leber's optic 377.16
  lip 528.5
  liver (acute) (subacute) (see also
      Necrosis, liver) 570
    chronic (yellow) 571.8
    yellow (congenital) 570
      with
        abortion - see Abortion, by
            type, with specified
            complication NEC
        ectopic pregnancy (see also
            categories 633.0-633.9)
            639.8
        molar pregnancy (see also
            categories 630-632) 639.8

Atrophy, atrophic (Continued)
  liver (Continued)
    yellow (Continued)
      chronic 571.8
      complicating pregnancy 646.7●
      following
        abortion 639.8
        ectopic or molar pregnancy
            639.8
      from injection, inoculation or
          transfusion (onset within 8
          months after
          administration) - see
          Hepatitis, viral
      healed 571.5
      obstetric 646.7●
      postabortal 639.8
      postimmunization - see Hepatitis,
          viral
      posttransfusion - see Hepatitis,
          viral
      puerperal, postpartum 674.8●
  lung (senile) 518.89
    congenital 748.69
  macular (dermatological) 701.3
    syphilitic, skin 091.3
    striated 095.8
  muscle, muscular 728.2
    disuse 728.2
    Duchenne-Aran 335.21
    extremity (lower) (upper) 728.2
    familial spinal 335.11
    general 728.2
    idiopathic 728.2
    infantile spinal 335.0
    myelopathic (progressive) 335.10
    myotonic 359.21
    neuritic 356.1
    neuropathic (peroneal) (progressive)
        356.1
    peroneal 356.1
    primary (idiopathic) 728.2
    progressive (familial) (hereditary)
        (pure) 335.21
      adult (spinal) 335.19
      infantile (spinal) 335.0
      juvenile (spinal) 335.11
      spinal 335.10
        adult 335.19
        hereditary or familial
            335.11
        infantile 335.0
    pseudohypertrophic 359.1
    spinal (progressive) 335.10
      adult 335.19
      Aran-Duchenne 335.21
      familial 335.11
      hereditary 335.11
      infantile 335.0
      juvenile 335.11
    syphilitic 095.6
  myocardium (see also Degeneration,
      myocardial) 429.1
  myometrium (senile) 621.8
    cervix 622.8
  myotatic 728.2
  myotonia 359.21
  nail 703.8
    congenital 757.5
  nasopharynx 472.2
  nerve - see also Disorder, nerve
    abducens 378.54
    accessory 352.4
    acoustic or auditory 388.5

Atrophy, atrophic *(Continued)*
 nerve *(Continued)*
  cranial 352.9
   first (olfactory) 352.0
   second (optic) *(see also* Atrophy,
     optic nerve) 377.10
   third (oculomotor) (partial)
     378.51
    total 378.52
   fourth (trochlear) 378.53
   fifth (trigeminal) 350.8
   sixth (abducens) 378.54
   seventh (facial) 351.8
   eighth (auditory) 388.5
   ninth (glossopharyngeal) 352.2
   tenth (pneumogastric) (vagus)
     352.3
   eleventh (accessory) 352.4
   twelfth (hypoglossal) 352.5
  facial 351.8
  glossopharyngeal 352.2
  hypoglossal 352.5
  oculomotor (partial) 378.51
   total 378.52
  olfactory 352.0
  peripheral 355.9
  pneumogastric 352.3
  trigeminal 350.8
  trochlear 378.53
  vagus (pneumogastric) 352.3
 nervous system, congenital 742.8
 neuritic *(see also* Disorder, nerve) 355.9
 neurogenic NEC 355.9
  bone
   tabetic 094.0
 nutritional 261
 old age 797
 olivopontocerebellar 333.0
 optic nerve (ascending) (descending)
   (infectional) (nonfamilial)
   (papillomacular bundle)
   (postretinal) (secondary NEC)
   (simple) 377.10
  associated with retinal dystrophy
    377.13
  dominant hereditary 377.16
  glaucomatous 377.14
  hereditary (dominant) (Leber's)
    377.16
  Leber's (hereditary) 377.16
  partial 377.15
  postinflammatory 377.12
  primary 377.11
  syphilitic 094.84
   congenital 090.49
   tabes dorsalis 094.0
 orbit 376.45
 ovary (senile), acquired 620.3
 oviduct (senile), acquired 620.3
 palsy, diffuse 335.20
 pancreas (duct) (senile) 577.8
 papillary muscle 429.81
 paralysis 355.9
 parotid gland 527.0
 patches skin 701.3
  senile 701.8
 penis 607.89
 pharyngitis 472.1
 pharynx 478.29
 pluriglandular 258.8
 polyarthritis 714.0
 prostate 602.2
 pseudohypertrophic 359.1
 renal *(see also* Sclerosis, renal) 587

Atrophy, atrophic *(Continued)*
 reticulata 701.8
 retina *(see also* Degeneration, retina)
   362.60
  hereditary *(see also* Dystrophy,
    retina) 362.70
 rhinitis 472.0
 salivary duct or gland 527.0
 scar NEC 709.2
 sclerosis, lobar (of brain) 331.0
  with dementia
   with behavioral disturbance 331.0
     [294.11]
   without behavioral disturbance
     331.0 *[294.10]*
 scrotum 608.89
 seminal vesicle 608.89
 senile 797
  degenerative, of skin 701.3
 skin (patches) (senile) 701.8
 spermatic cord 608.89
 spinal (cord) 336.8
  acute 336.8
  muscular (chronic) 335.10
   adult 335.19
   familial 335.11
   juvenile 335.10
  paralysis 335.10
   acute *(see also* Poliomyelitis, with
     paralysis) 045.1●
 spine (column) 733.99
 spleen (senile) 289.59
 spots (skin) 701.3
  senile 701.8
 stomach 537.89
 striate and macular 701.3
  syphilitic 095.8
 subcutaneous 701.9
  due to injection 999.9
 sublingual gland 527.0
 submaxillary gland 527.0
 Sudeck's 733.7
 suprarenal (autoimmune) (capsule)
    (gland) 255.41
  with hypofunction 255.41
 tarso-orbital fascia, congenital 743.66
 testis 608.3
 thenar, partial 354.0
 throat 478.29
 thymus (fat) 254.8
 thyroid (gland) 246.8
  with
   cretinism 243
   myxedema 244.9
  congenital 243
 tongue (senile) 529.8
  papillae 529.4
  smooth 529.4
 trachea 519.19
 tunica vaginalis 608.89
 turbinate 733.99
 tympanic membrane (nonflaccid)
    384.82
  flaccid 384.81
 ulcer *(see also* Ulcer, skin) 707.9
 upper respiratory tract 478.9
 uterus, uterine (acquired) (senile) 621.8
  cervix 622.8
  due to radiation (intended effect) 621.8
 vagina (senile) 627.3
 vascular 459.89
 vas deferens 608.89
 vertebra (senile) 733.99
 vulva (primary) (senile) 624.1

Atrophy, atrophic *(Continued)*
 Werdnig-Hoffmann 335.0
 yellow (acute) (congenital) (liver)
   (subacute) *(see also* Necrosis,
   liver) 570
  chronic 571.8
  resulting from administration of
    blood, plasma, serum, or other
    biological substance (within 8
    months of administration) - *see*
    Hepatitis, viral
Attack
 akinetic *(see also* Epilepsy) 345.0●
 angina - *see* Angina
 apoplectic *(see also* Disease,
   cerebrovascular, acute) 436
 benign shuddering 333.93
 bilious - *see* Vomiting
 cataleptic 300.11
 cerebral *(see also* Disease,
   cerebrovascular, acute) 436
 coronary *(see also* Infarct, myocardium)
   410.9●
 cyanotic, newborn 770.83
 epileptic *(see also* Epilepsy) 345.9●
 epileptiform 780.39
 heart *(see also* Infarct, myocardium)
   410.9●
 hemiplegia *(see also* Disease,
   cerebrovascular, acute) 436
 hysterical 300.11
 jacksonian *(see also* Epilepsy) 345.5●
 myocardium, myocardial *(see also*
   Infarct, myocardium) 410.9●
 myoclonic *(see also* Epilepsy) 345.1●
 panic 300.01
 paralysis *(see also* Disease,
   cerebrovascular, acute) 436
 paroxysmal 780.39
 psychomotor *(see also* Epilepsy) 345.4●
 salaam *(see also* Epilepsy) 345.6●
 schizophreniform *(see also*
   Schizophrenia) 295.4●
 sensory and motor 780.39
 syncope 780.2
 toxic, cerebral 780.39
 transient ischemic (TIA) 435.9
 unconsciousness 780.2
  hysterical 300.11
 vasomotor 780.2
 vasovagal (idiopathic) (paroxysmal)
   780.2
Attention to
 artificial
  opening (of) V55.9
   digestive tract NEC V55.4
   specified site NEC V55.8
   urinary tract NEC V55.6
  vagina V55.7
 colostomy V55.3
 cystostomy V55.5
 dressing
  wound V58.30
   nonsurgical V58.30
   surgical V58.31
 gastrostomy V55.1
 ileostomy V55.2
 jejunostomy V55.4
 nephrostomy V55.6
 surgical dressings V58.31
 sutures V58.32
 tracheostomy V55.0
 ureterostomy V55.6
 urethrostomy V55.6

Attrition
  gum (*see also* Recession, gingival) 523.20
  teeth (hard tissues) 521.10
    excessive 521.10
      extending into
        dentine 521.12
        pulp 521.13
      generalized 521.15
      limited to enamel 521.11
      localized 521.14
Atypical - *see also* condition
  cells
    endocervical 795.00
    endometrial 795.00
    glandular
      anus 796.70
      cervical 795.00
      vaginal 795.10
  distribution, vessel (congenital) (peripheral) NEC 747.60
  endometrium 621.9
  kidney 593.89
Atypism, cervix 622.10
Audible tinnitus (*see also* Tinnitus) 388.30
Auditory - *see* condition
Audry's syndrome (acropachyderma) 757.39
Aujeszky's disease 078.89
Aura
  jacksonian (*see also* Epilepsy) 345.5●
  persistent migraine 346.5●
    with cerebral infarction 346.6●
    without cerebral infarction 346.5●
Aurantiasis, cutis 278.3
Auricle, auricular - *see* condition
Auriculotemporal syndrome 350.8
Australian
  Q fever 083.0
  X disease 062.4
Autism, autistic (child) (infantile) 299.0●
Autodigestion 799.89
Autoerythrocyte sensitization 287.2
Autographism 708.3
Autoimmune
  cold sensitivity 283.0
  disease NEC 279.49 ◄▥
  hemolytic anemia 283.0
  lymphoproliferative syndrome (ALPS) 279.41 ◄
  thyroiditis 245.2
Autoinfection, septic - *see* Septicemia
Autointoxication 799.89
Automatism 348.89 ◄▥
  epileptic (*see also* Epilepsy) 345.4●
  paroxysmal, idiopathic (*see also* Epilepsy) 345.4●

Autonomic, autonomous
  bladder 596.54
    neurogenic 596.54
      with cauda equina 344.61
  dysreflexia 337.3
  faciocephalalgia (*see also* Neuropathy, peripheral, autonomic) 337.9
  hysterical seizure 300.11
  imbalance (*see also* Neuropathy, peripheral, autonomic 337.9
Autophony 388.40
Autosensitivity, erythrocyte 287.2
Autotopagnosia 780.99
Autotoxemia 799.89
Autumn - *see* condition
Avellis' syndrome 344.89
Aviators
  disease or sickness (*see also* Effect, adverse, high altitude) 993.2
  ear 993.0
  effort syndrome 306.2
Avitaminosis (multiple NEC) (*see also* Deficiency, vitamin) 269.2
  A 264.9
  B 266.9
    with
      beriberi 265.0
      pellagra 265.2
  B₁ 265.1
  B₂ 266.0
  B₆ 266.1
  B₁₂ 266.2
  C (with scurvy) 267
  D 268.9
    with
      osteomalacia 268.2
      rickets 268.0
  E 269.1
  G 266.0
  H 269.1
  K 269.0
  multiple 269.2
  nicotinic acid 265.2
  P 269.1
Avulsion (traumatic) 879.8
  blood vessel - *see* Injury, blood vessel, by site
  cartilage - *see also* Dislocation, by site
    knee, current (*see also* Tear, meniscus) 836.2
    symphyseal (inner), complicating delivery 665.6●
  complicated 879.9
  diaphragm - *see* Injury, internal, diaphragm

Avulsion (*Continued*)
  ear - *see* Wound, open, ear
  epiphysis of bone - *see* Fracture, by site
  external site other than limb - *see* Wound, open, by site
  eye 871.3
  fingernail - *see* Wound, open, finger
  fracture - *see* Fracture, by site
  genital organs, external - *see* Wound, open, genital organs
  head (intracranial) NEC - *see also* Injury, intracranial, with open intracranial wound
    complete 874.9
    external site NEC 873.8
      complicated 873.9
  internal organ or site - *see* Injury, internal, by site
  joint - *see also* Dislocation, by site
    capsule - *see* Sprain, by site
  ligament - *see* Sprain, by site
  limb - *see also* Amputation, traumatic, by site
    skin and subcutaneous tissue - *see* Wound, open, by site
  muscle - *see* Sprain, by site
  nerve (root) - *see* Injury, nerve, by site
  scalp - *see* Wound, open, scalp
  skin and subcutaneous tissue - *see* Wound, open, by site
  symphyseal cartilage (inner), complicating delivery 665.6●
  tendon - *see also* Sprain, by site
    with open wound - *see* Wound, open, by site
  toenail - *see* Wound, open, toe(s)
  tooth 873.63
    complicated 873.73
Awaiting organ transplant status V49.83
Awareness of heart beat 785.1
Axe grinders' disease 502
Axenfeld's anomaly or syndrome 743.44
Axilla, axillary - *see also* condition
  breast 757.6
Axonotmesis - *see* Injury, nerve, by site
Ayala's disease 756.89
Ayerza's disease or syndrome (pulmonary artery sclerosis with pulmonary hypertension) 416.0
Azoospermia 606.0
Azorean disease (of the nervous system) 334.8
Azotemia 790.6
  meaning uremia (*see also* Uremia) 586
Aztec ear 744.29
Azygos lobe, lung (fissure) 748.69

◄ New ◄▥ Revised ~~deleted~~ Deleted ● Use Additional Digit(s) ▨ Omit code

B

Baader's syndrome (erythema multiforme exudativum) 695.19
Baastrup's syndrome 721.5
Babesiasis 088.82
Babesiosis 088.82
Babington's disease (familial hemorrhagic telangiectasia) 448.0
Babinski's syndrome (cardiovascular syphilis) 093.89
Babinski-Fröhlich syndrome (adiposogenital dystrophy) 253.8
Babinski-Nageotte syndrome 344.89
Bacillary - see condition
Bacilluria 791.9
  asymptomatic, in pregnancy or puerperium 646.5●
  tuberculous (see also Tuberculosis) 016.9●
Bacillus - see also Infection, bacillus
  abortus infection 023.1
  anthracis infection 022.9
  coli
    infection 041.4
      generalized 038.42
      intestinal 008.00
    pyemia 038.42
    septicemia 038.42
  Flexner's 004.1
  fusiformis infestation 101
  mallei infection 024
  Shiga's 004.0
  suipestifer infection (see also Infection, Salmonella) 003.9
Back - see condition
Backache (postural) 724.5
  psychogenic 307.89
  sacroiliac 724.6
Backflow (pyelovenous) (see also Disease, renal) 593.9
Backknee (see also Genu, recurvatum) 736.5
Bacteremia 790.7
  newborn 771.83
Bacteria
  in blood (see also Bacteremia) 790.7
  in urine (see also Bacteriuria) 791.9
Bacterial - see condition
Bactericholia (see also Cholecystitis, acute) 575.0
Bacterid, bacteride (Andrews' pustular) 686.8
Bacteriuria, bacteruria 791.9
  with
    urinary tract infection 599.0
  asymptomatic 791.9
    in pregnancy or puerperium 646.5●
      affecting fetus or newborn 760.1
Bad
  breath 784.99
  heart - see Disease, heart
  trip (see also Abuse, drugs, nondependent) 305.3●
Baehr-Schiffrin disease (thrombotic thrombocytopenic purpura) 446.6
Baelz's disease (cheilitis glandularis apostematosa) 528.5
Baerensprung's disease (eczema marginatum) 110.3
Bagassosis (occupational) 495.1
Baghdad boil 085.1
Bagratuni's syndrome (temporal arteritis) 446.5

Baker's
  cyst (knee) 727.51
    tuberculous (see also Tuberculosis) 015.2●
  itch 692.89
Bakwin-Krida syndrome (craniometa-physeal dysplasia) 756.89
Balanitis (circinata) (gangraenosa) (infectious) (vulgaris) 607.1
  amebic 006.8
  candidal 112.2
  chlamydial 099.53
  due to Ducrey's bacillus 099.0
  erosiva circinata et gangraenosa 607.1
  gangrenous 607.1
  gonococcal (acute) 098.0
    chronic or duration of 2 months or over 098.2
  nongonococcal 607.1
  phagedenic 607.1
  venereal NEC 099.8
  xerotica obliterans 607.81
Balanoposthitis 607.1
  chlamydial 099.53
  gonococcal (acute) 098.0
    chronic or duration of 2 months or over 098.2
  ulcerative NEC 099.8
Balanorrhagia - see Balanitis
Balantidiasis 007.0
Balantidiosis 007.0
Balbuties, balbutio 307.0
Bald
  patches on scalp 704.00
  tongue 529.4
Baldness (see also Alopecia) 704.00
Balfour's disease (chloroma) 205.3●
Balint's syndrome (psychic paralysis of visual fixation) 368.16
Balkan grippe 083.0
Ball
  food 938
  hair 938
Ballantyne (-Runge) syndrome (postmaturity) 766.22
Balloon disease (see also Effect, adverse, high altitude) 993.2
Ballooning posterior leaflet syndrome 424.0
Baló's disease or concentric sclerosis 341.1
Bamberger's disease (hypertrophic pulmonary osteoarthropathy) 731.2
Bamberger-Marie disease (hypertrophic pulmonary osteoarthropathy) 731.2
Bamboo spine 720.0
Bancroft's filariasis 125.0
Band(s)
  adhesive (see also Adhesions, peritoneum) 568.0
  amniotic 658.8●
    affecting fetus or newborn 762.8
  anomalous or congenital - see also Anomaly, specified type NEC
    atrial 746.9
    heart 746.9
    intestine 751.4
    omentum 751.4
    ventricular 746.9
  cervix 622.3
  gallbladder (congenital) 751.69
  intestinal (adhesive) (see also Adhesions, peritoneum) 568.0
  congenital 751.4

Band(s) (Continued)
  obstructive (see also Obstruction, intestine) 560.81
  periappendiceal (congenital) 751.4
  peritoneal (adhesive) (see also Adhesions, peritoneum) 568.0
    with intestinal obstruction 560.81
    congenital 751.4
  uterus 621.5
  vagina 623.2
Bandemia (without diagnosis of specific infection) 288.66
Bandl's ring (contraction)
  complicating delivery 661.4●
  affecting fetus or newborn 763.7
Bang's disease (Brucella abortus) 023.1
Bangkok hemorrhagic fever 065.4
Bannister's disease 995.1
Bantam-Albright-Martin disease (pseudohypoparathyroidism) 275.49
Banti's disease or syndrome (with cirrhosis) (with portal hypertension) - see Cirrhosis, liver
Bar
  calcaneocuboid 755.67
  calcaneonavicular 755.67
  cubonavicular 755.67
  prostate 600.90
    with
      other lower urinary tract symptoms (LUTS) 600.91
      urinary
        obstruction 600.91
        retention 600.91
  talocalcaneal 755.67
Baragnosis 780.99
Barasheh, barashek 266.2
Barcoo disease or rot (see also Ulcer, skin) 707.9
Bard-Pic syndrome (carcinoma, head of pancreas) 157.0
Bärensprung's disease (eczema marginatum) 110.3
Baritosis 503
Barium lung disease 503
Barlow's syndrome (meaning mitral valve prolapse) 424.0
Barlow (-Möller) disease or syndrome (meaning infantile scurvy) 267
Barodontalgia 993.2
Baron Münchausen syndrome 301.51
Barosinusitis 993.1
Barotitis 993.0
Barotrauma 993.2
  odontalgia 993.2
  otitic 993.0
  sinus 993.1
Barraquer's disease or syndrome (progressive lipodystrophy) 272.6
Barré-Guillain syndrome 357.0
Barré-Liéou syndrome (posterior cervical sympathetic) 723.2
Barrel chest 738.3
Barrett's esophagus 530.85
Barrett's syndrome or ulcer (chronic peptic ulcer of esophagus) 530.85
Bársony-Polgár syndrome (corkscrew esophagus) 530.5
Bársony-Teschendorf syndrome (corkscrew esophagus) 530.5
Barth syndrome 759.89
Bartholin's
  adenitis (see also Bartholinitis) 616.89
  gland - see condition

Bartholinitis (suppurating) 616.89
  gonococcal (acute) 098.0
    chronic or duration of 2 months or over 098.2
Bartonellosis 088.0
Bartter's syndrome (secondary hyperaldosteronism with juxtaglomerular hyperplasia) 255.13
Basal - *see* condition
Basan's (hidrotic) ectodermal dysplasia 757.31
Baseball finger 842.13
Basedow's disease or syndrome (exophthalmic goiter) 242.0●
Basic - *see* condition
Basilar - *see* condition
Bason's (hidrotic) ectodermal dysplasia 757.31
Basopenia 288.59
Basophilia 288.65
Basophilism (corticoadrenal) (Cushing's) (pituitary) (thymic) 255.0
Bassen-Kornzweig syndrome (abetalipoproteinemia) 272.5
Bat ear 744.29
Bateman's
  disease 078.0
  purpura (senile) 287.2
Bathing cramp 994.1
Bathophobia 300.23
Batten's disease, retina 330.1 *[362.71]*
Batten-Mayou disease 330.1 *[362.71]*
Batten-Steinert syndrome 359.21
Battered
  adult (syndrome) 995.81
  baby or child (syndrome) 995.54
  spouse (syndrome) 995.81
Battey mycobacterium infection 031.0
Battledore placenta - *see* Placenta, abnormal
Battle exhaustion (*see also* Reaction, stress, acute) 308.9
Baumgarten-Cruveilhier (cirrhosis) disease, or syndrome 571.5
Bauxite
  fibrosis (of lung) 503
  workers' disease 503
Bayle's disease (dementia paralytica) 094.1
Bazin's disease (primary) (*see also* Tuberculosis) 017.1●
Beach ear 380.12
Beaded hair (congenital) 757.4
Beals syndrome 759.82
Beard's disease (neurasthenia) 300.5
Bearn-Kunkel (-Slater) syndrome (lupoid hepatitis) 571.49
Beat
  elbow 727.2
  hand 727.2
  knee 727.2
Beats
  ectopic 427.60
  escaped, heart 427.60
    postoperative 997.1
  premature (nodal) 427.60
    atrial 427.61
    auricular 427.61
    postoperative 997.1
    specified type NEC 427.69
    supraventricular 427.61
    ventricular 427.69

Beau's
  disease or syndrome (*see also* Degeneration, myocardial) 429.1
  lines (transverse furrows on fingernails) 703.8
Bechterew's disease (ankylosing spondylitis) 720.0
Bechterew-Strümpell-Marie syndrome (ankylosing spondylitis) 720.0
Beck's syndrome (anterior spinal artery occlusion) 433.8●
Becker's
  disease
    idiopathic mural endomyocardial disease 425.2
    myotonia congenita, recessive form 359.22
  dystrophy 359.22
Beckwith (-Wiedemann) syndrome 759.89
Bedbugs bite(s) - *see* Injury, superficial, by site
Bedclothes, asphyxiation or suffocation by 994.7
Bed confinement status V49.84
Bednar's aphthae 528.2
Bedsore (*see also* Ulcer, pressure) 707.00
  with gangrene 707.00 *[785.4]*
Bedwetting (*see also* Enuresis) 788.36
Beer-drinkers' heart (disease) 425.5
Bee sting (with allergic or anaphylactic shock) 989.5
Begbie's disease (exophthalmic goiter) 242.0●
Behavior disorder, disturbance - *see also* Disturbance, conduct
  antisocial, without manifest psychiatric disorder
    adolescent V71.02
    adult V71.01
    child V71.02
  dyssocial, without manifest psychiatric disorder
    adolescent V71.02
    adult V71.01
    child V71.02
  high-risk- *see* problem
Behçet's syndrome 136.1
Behr's disease 362.50
Beigel's disease or morbus (white piedra) 111.2
Bejel 104.0
Bekhterev's disease (ankylosing spondylitis) 720.0
Bekhterev-Strümpell-Marie syndrome (ankylosing spondylitis) 720.0
Belching (*see also* Eructation) 787.3
Bell's
  disease (*see also* Psychosis, affective) 296.0●
  mania (*see also* Psychosis, affective) 296.0●
  palsy, paralysis 351.0
    infant 767.5
    newborn 767.5
    syphilitic 094.89
  spasm 351.0
Bence-Jones albuminuria, albuminosuria, or proteinuria 791.0
Bends 993.3
Benedikt's syndrome (paralysis) 344.89

Benign - *see also* condition
  cellular changes, cervix 795.09
  prostate
    hyperplasia 600.20
      with
        other lower urinary tract symptoms (LUTS) 600.21
        urinary
          obstruction 600.21
          retention 600.21
    neoplasm 222.2
Bennett's
  disease (leukemia) 208.9●
  fracture (closed) 815.01
    open 815.11
Benson's disease 379.22
Bent
  back (hysterical) 300.11
  nose 738.0
    congenital 754.0
Bereavement V62.82
  as adjustment reaction 309.0
Berger's paresthesia (lower limb) 782.0
Bergeron's disease (hysteroepilepsy) 300.11
Beriberi (acute) (atrophic) (chronic) (dry) (subacute) (wet) 265.0
  with polyneuropathy 265.0 *[357.4]*
  heart (disease) 265.0 *[425.7]*
  leprosy 030.1
  neuritis 265.0 *[357.4]*
Berlin's disease or edema (traumatic) 921.3
Berloque dermatitis 692.72
Bernard-Horner syndrome (*see also* Neuropathy, peripheral, autonomic) 337.9
Bernard-Sergent syndrome (acute adrenocortical insufficiency) 255.41
Bernard-Soulier disease or thrombopathy 287.1
Bernhardt's disease or paresthesia 355.1
Bernhardt-Roth disease or syndrome (parasthesia) 355.1
Bernheim's syndrome (*see also* Failure, heart) 428.0
Bertielliasis 123.8
Bertolotti's syndrome (sacralization of fifth lumbar vertebra) 756.15
Berylliosis (acute) (chronic) (lung) (occupational) 503
Besnier's
  lupus pernio 135
  prurigo (atopic dermatitis) (infantile eczema) 691.8
Besnier-Boeck disease or sarcoid 135
Besnier-Boeck-Schaumann disease (sarcoidosis) 135
Best's disease 362.76
Bestiality 302.1
Beta-adrenergic hyperdynamic circulatory state 429.82
Beta-aminoisobutyric aciduria 277.2
Beta-mercaptolactate-cysteine disulfiduria 270.0
Beta thalassemia (major) (minor) (mixed) 282.49
Beurmann's disease (sporotrichosis) 117.1

◀ New   ◀▥ Revised   deleted Deleted   ● Use Additional Digit(s)   ▨ Omit code

Bezoar 938
  intestine 936
  stomach 935.2
Bezold's abscess (*see also* Mastoiditis)
  383.01
Bianchi's syndrome (aphasia-apraxia-
  alexia) 784.69
Bicornuate or bicornis uterus 752.3
  in pregnancy or childbirth 654.0●
    with obstructed labor 660.2●
      affecting fetus or newborn 763.1
      affecting fetus or newborn 763.89
Bicuspid aortic valve 746.4
Biedl-Bardet syndrome 759.89
Bielschowsky's disease 330.1
Bielschowsky-Jansky
  amaurotic familial idiocy 330.1
  disease 330.1
Biemond's syndrome (obesity, polydactyly,
  and mental retardation) 759.89
Biermer's anemia or disease (pernicious
  anemia) 281.0
Biett's disease 695.4
Bifid (congenital) - *see also* Imperfect,
  closure
  apex, heart 746.89
  clitoris 752.49
  epiglottis 748.3
  kidney 753.3
  nose 748.1
  patella 755.64
  scrotum 752.89
  toe 755.66
  tongue 750.13
  ureter 753.4
  uterus 752.3
  uvula 749.02
    with cleft lip (*see also* Cleft, palate,
      with cleft lip) 749.20
Biforis uterus (suprasimplex) 752.3
Bifurcation (congenital) - *see also*
  Imperfect, closure
  gallbladder 751.69
  kidney pelvis 753.3
  renal pelvis 753.3
  rib 756.3
  tongue 750.13
  trachea 748.3
  ureter 753.4
  urethra 753.8
  uvula 749.02
    with cleft lip (*see also* Cleft, palate,
      with cleft lip) 749.20
  vertebra 756.19
Bigeminal pulse 427.89
Bigeminy 427.89
Big spleen syndrome 289.4
Bilateral - *see* condition
Bile duct - *see* condition
Bile pigments in urine 791.4
Bilharziasis (*see also* Schistosomiasis)
  120.9
  chyluria 120.0
  cutaneous 120.3
  galacturia 120.0
  hematochyluria 120.0
  intestinal 120.1
  lipemia 120.9
  lipuria 120.0
  Oriental 120.2
  piarhemia 120.9
  pulmonary 120.2
  tropical hematuria 120.0
  vesical 120.0

Biliary - *see* condition
Bilious (attack) - *see also* Vomiting
  fever, hemoglobinuric 084.8
Bilirubinuria 791.4
Biliuria 791.4
Billroth's disease
  meningocele (*see also* Spina bifida)
    741.9●
Bilobate placenta - *see* Placenta, abnormal
Bilocular
  heart 745.7
  stomach 536.8
Bing-Horton syndrome (histamine
  cephalgia) 339.00
Binswanger's disease or dementia
  290.12
Biörck (-Thorson) syndrome (malignant
  carcinoid) 259.2
Biparta, bipartite - *see also* Imperfect,
  closure
  carpal scaphoid 755.59
  patella 755.64
  placenta - *see* Placenta, abnormal
  vagina 752.49
Bird
  face 756.0
  fanciers' lung or disease 495.2
  flu 488.0   ◀
Bird's disease (oxaluria) 271.8
Birth
  abnormal fetus or newborn 763.9
  accident, fetus or newborn - *see* Birth,
    injury
  complications in mother - *see* Delivery,
    complicated
  compression during NEC 767.9
  defect - *see* Anomaly
  delayed, fetus 763.9
  difficult NEC, affecting fetus or
    newborn 763.9
  dry, affecting fetus or newborn 761.1
  forced, NEC, affecting fetus or
    newborn 763.89
  forceps, affecting fetus or newborn
    763.2
  hematoma of sternomastoid 767.8
  immature 765.1●
    extremely 765.0●
  inattention, after or at 995.52
  induced, affecting fetus or newborn
    763.89
  infant - *see* Newborn
  injury NEC 767.9
    adrenal gland 767.8
    basal ganglia 767.0
    brachial plexus (paralysis) 767.6
    brain (compression) (pressure)
      767.0
    cerebellum 767.0
    cerebral hemorrhage 767.0
    conjunctiva 767.8
    eye 767.8
    fracture
      bone, any except clavicle or spine
        767.3
      clavicle 767.2
      femur 767.3
      humerus 767.3
      long bone 767.3
      radius and ulna 767.3
      skeleton NEC 767.3
      skull 767.3
      spine 767.4
      tibia and fibula 767.3

Birth (*Continued*)
  injury NEC (*Continued*)
    hematoma 767.8
      liver (subcapsular) 767.8
      mastoid 767.8
      skull 767.19
      sternomastoid 767.8
      testes 767.8
      vulva 767.8
    intracranial (edema) 767.0
    laceration
      brain 767.0
      by scalpel 767.8
      peripheral nerve 767.7
    liver 767.8
    meninges
      brain 767.0
      spinal cord 767.4
    nerves (cranial, peripheral) 767.7
      brachial plexus 767.6
      facial 767.5
    paralysis 767.7
      brachial plexus 767.6
      Erb (-Duchenne) 767.6
      facial nerve 767.5
      Klumpke (-Déjérine) 767.6
      radial nerve 767.6
      spinal (cord) (hemorrhage)
        (laceration) (rupture) 767.4
    rupture
      intracranial 767.0
      liver 767.8
      spinal cord 767.4
      spleen 767.8
      viscera 767.8
    scalp 767.19
    scalpel wound 767.8
    skeleton NEC 767.3
    specified NEC 767.8
    spinal cord 767.4
    spleen 767.8
    subdural hemorrhage 767.0
    tentorial, tear 767.0
    testes 767.8
    vulva 767.8
  instrumental, NEC, affecting fetus or
    newborn 763.2
  lack of care, after or at 995.52
  multiple
    affected by maternal complications
      of pregnancy 761.5
    healthy liveborn - *see* Newborn,
      multiple
  neglect, after or at 995.52
  newborn - *see* Newborn
  palsy or paralysis NEC 767.7
  precipitate, fetus or newborn 763.6
  premature (infant) 765.1●
  prolonged, affecting fetus or newborn
    763.9
  retarded, fetus or newborn 763.9
  shock, newborn 779.89
  strangulation or suffocation
    due to aspiration of clear amniotic
      fluid 770.13
      with respiratory symptoms
        770.14
    mechanical 767.8
  trauma NEC 767.9
  triplet
    affected by maternal complications
      of pregnancy 761.5
    healthy liveborn - *see* Newborn,
      multiple

Birth *(Continued)*
  twin
    affected by maternal complications
      of pregnancy 761.5
    healthy liveborn - *see* Newborn, twin
  ventouse, affecting fetus or newborn
    763.3
Birthmark 757.32
Birt-Hogg-Dube syndrome 759.89
Bisalbuminemia 273.8
Biskra button 085.1
Bite(s)
  with intact skin surface - *see* Contusion
  animal - *see* Wound, open, by site
    intact skin surface - *see* Contusion
  bedbug - *see* Injury, superficial, by site
  centipede 989.5
  chigger 133.8
  fire ant 989.5
  flea - *see* Injury, superficial, by site
  human (open wound) - *see also* Wound,
    open, by site
    intact skin surface - *see* Contusion
  insect
    nonvenomous - *see* Injury,
      superficial, by site
    venomous 989.5
  mad dog (death from) 071
  open
    anterior 524.24
    posterior 524.25
  poisonous 989.5
  red bug 133.8
  reptile 989.5
    nonvenomous - *see* Wound, open, by
      site
  snake 989.5
    nonvenomous - *see* Wound, open, by
      site
  spider (venomous) 989.5
    nonvenomous - *see* Injury,
      superficial, by site
  venomous 989.5
Biting
  cheek or lip 528.9
  nail 307.9
Black
  death 020.9
  eye NEC 921.0
  hairy tongue 529.3
  heel 924.20
  lung disease 500
  palm 923.20
Blackfan-Diamond anemia or syndrome
  (congenital hypoplastic anemia)
  284.01
Blackhead 706.1
Blackout 780.2
Blackwater fever 084.8
Bladder - *see* condition
Blast
  blindness 921.3
  concussion - *see* Blast, injury
  injury 869.0
    with open wound into cavity 869.1
    abdomen or thorax - *see* Injury,
      internal, by site
    brain (*see also* Concussion, brain)
      850.9
      with skull fracture - *see* Fracture,
        skull
    ear (acoustic nerve trauma) 951.5
      with perforation, tympanic
        membrane - *see* Wound,
        open, ear, drum

Blast *(Continued)*
  injury *(Continued)*
    lung (*see also* Injury, internal, lung)
      861.20
    otitic (explosive) 388.11
Blastomycosis, blastomycotic (chronic)
  (cutaneous) (disseminated) (lung)
  (pulmonary) (systemic) 116.0
  Brazilian 116.1
  European 117.5
  keloidal 116.2
  North American 116.0
  primary pulmonary 116.0
  South American 116.1
Bleb(s) 709.8
  emphysematous (bullous) (diffuse)
    (lung) (ruptured) (solitary) 492.0
  filtering, eye (postglaucoma) (status)
    V45.69
    with complication 997.99
    postcataract extraction
      (complication) 997.99
  lung (ruptured) 492.0
    congenital 770.5
  subpleural (emphysematous) 492.0
Bleeder (familial) (hereditary) (*see also*
  Defect, coagulation) 286.9
  nonfamilial 286.9
Bleeding (*see also* Hemorrhage) 459.0
  anal 569.3
  anovulatory 628.0
  atonic, following delivery 666.1●
  capillary 448.9
  due to subinvolution 621.1
    puerperal 666.2●
  ear 388.69
  excessive, associated with menopausal
    onset 627.0
  familial (*see also* Defect, coagulation)
    286.9
  following intercourse 626.7
  gastrointestinal 578.9
  gums 523.8
  hemorrhoids - *see* Hemorrhoids,
    bleeding
  intermenstrual
    irregular 626.6
    regular 626.5
  intraoperative 998.11
  irregular NEC 626.4
  menopausal 627.0
  mouth 528.9
  nipple 611.79
  nose 784.7
  ovulation 626.5
  postclimacteric 627.1
  postcoital 626.7
  postmenopausal 627.1
    following induced menopause 627.4
  postoperative 998.11
  preclimacteric 627.0
  puberty 626.3
    excessive, with onset of menstrual
      periods 626.3
  rectum, rectal 569.3
  tendencies (*see also* Defect, coagulation)
    286.9
  throat 784.8
  umbilical stump 772.3
  umbilicus 789.9
  unrelated to menstrual cycle 626.6
  uterus, uterine 626.9
    climacteric 627.0
    dysfunctional 626.8

Bleeding *(Continued)*
  uterus, uterine *(Continued)*
    functional 626.8
    unrelated to menstrual cycle
      626.6
  vagina, vaginal 623.8
    functional 626.8
  vicarious 625.8
Blennorrhagia, blennorrhagic - *see*
  Blennorrhea
Blennorrhea (acute) 098.0
  adultorum 098.40
  alveolaris 523.40
  chronic or duration of 2 months or over
    098.2
  gonococcal (neonatorum) 098.40
  inclusion (neonatal) (newborn) 771.6
  neonatorum 098.40
Blepharelosis (*see also* Entropion) 374.00
Blepharitis (eyelid) 373.00
  angularis 373.01
  ciliaris 373.00
    with ulcer 373.01
  marginal 373.00
    with ulcer 373.01
  scrofulous (*see also* Tuberculosis)
    017.3● *[373.00]*
  squamous 373.02
  ulcerative 373.01
Blepharochalasis 374.34
  congenital 743.62
Blepharoclonus 333.81
Blepharoconjunctivitis (*see also*
  Conjunctivitis) 372.20
  angular 372.21
  contact 372.22
Blepharophimosis (eyelid) 374.46
  congenital 743.62
Blepharoplegia 374.89
Blepharoptosis 374.30
  congenital 743.61
Blepharopyorrhea 098.49
Blepharospasm 333.81
  due to drugs 333.85
Blessig's cyst 362.62
Blighted ovum 631
Blind
  bronchus (congenital) 748.3
  eye - *see also* Blindness
    hypertensive 360.42
    hypotensive 360.41
  loop syndrome (postoperative) 579.2
  sac, fallopian tube (congenital) 752.19
  spot, enlarged 368.42
  tract or tube (congenital) NEC - *see*
    Atresia
Blindness (acquired) (congenital) (both
  eyes) 369.00
  with deafness V49.85
  blast 921.3
    with nerve injury - *see* Injury, nerve,
      optic
  Bright's - *see* Uremia
  color (congenital) 368.59
    acquired 368.55
    blue 368.53
    green 368.52
    red 368.51
    total 368.54
  concussion 950.9
  cortical 377.75
  day 368.10
    acquired 368.10
    congenital 368.10

◄ New   ◄▥ Revised   ~~deleted~~ Deleted   ● Use Additional Digit(s)   ▨ Omit code

Blindness *(Continued)*
  day *(Continued)*
    hereditary 368.10
    specified type NEC 368.10
  due to
    injury NEC 950.9
    refractive error - *see* Error, refractive
  eclipse (total) 363.31
  emotional 300.11
  face 368.16
  hysterical 300.11
  legal (both eyes) (USA definition) 369.4
    with impairment of better (less
        impaired) eye
      near-total 369.02
        with
          lesser eye impairment 369.02
            near-total 369.04
            total 369.03
        profound 369.05
          with
            lesser eye impairment
                369.05
            near-total 369.07
            profound 369.08
            total 369.06
        severe 369.21
          with
            lesser eye impairment
                369.21
            blind 369.11
            near-total 369.13
            profound 369.14
            severe 369.22
            total 369.12
      total
        with lesser eye impairment
            total 369.01
  mind 784.69
  moderate
    both eyes 369.25
      with impairment of lesser eye
          (specified as)
        blind, not further specified
            369.15
        low vision, not further
            specified 369.23
        near-total 369.17
        profound 369.18
        severe 369.24
        total 369.16
    one eye 369.74
      with vision of other eye (specified
          as)
        ncar-normal 369.75
        normal 369.76
  near-total
    both eyes 369.04
      with impairment of lesser eye
          (specified as)
        blind, not further specified
            369.02
        total 369.03
    one eye 369.64
      with vision of other eye (specified
          as)
        near-normal 369.65
        normal 369.66
  night 368.60
    acquired 368.62
    congenital (Japanese) 368.61
    hereditary 368.61
    specified type NEC 368.69
    vitamin A deficiency 264.5

Blindness *(Continued)*
  nocturnal - *see* Blindness, night
  one eye 369.60
    with low vision of other eye 369.10
  profound
    both eyes 369.08
      with impairment of lesser eye
          (specified as)
        blind, not further specified
            369.05
        near-total 369.07
        total 369.06
    one eye 369.67
      with vision of other eye (specified
          as)
        near-normal 369.68
        normal 369.69
  psychic 784.69
  severe
    both eyes 369.22
      with impairment of lesser eye
          (specified as)
        blind, not further specified
            369.11
        low vision, not further
            specified 369.21
        near-total 369.13
        profound 369.14
        total 369.12
    one eye 369.71
      with vision of other eye (specified
          as)
        near-normal 369.72
        normal 369.73
  snow 370.24
  sun 363.31
  temporary 368.12
  total
    both eyes 369.01
    one eye 369.61
      with vision of other eye (specified
          as)
        near-normal 369.62
        normal 369.63
  transient 368.12
  traumatic NEC 950.9
  word (developmental) 315.01
    acquired 784.61
    secondary to organic lesion 784.61
Blister - *see also* Injury, superficial,
    by site
  beetle dermatitis 692.89
  due to burn - *see* Burn, by site, second
      degree
  fever 054.9
  multiple, skin, nontraumatic 709.8
Bloating 787.3
Bloch-Siemens syndrome (incontinentia
    pigmenti) 757.33
Bloch-Stauffer dyshormonal dermatosis
    757.33
Bloch-Sulzberger disease or syndrome
    (incontinentia pigmenti)
    (melanoblastosis) 757.33
Block
  alveolar capillary 516.3
  arborization (heart) 426.6
  arrhythmic 426.9
  atrioventricular (AV) (incomplete)
      (partial) 426.10
    with
      2:1 atrioventricular response
          block 426.13
      atrioventricular dissociation 426.0

Block *(Continued)*
  atrioventricular *(Continued)*
    first degree (incomplete) 426.11
    second degree (Mobitz type I)
        426.13
      Mobitz (type II) 426.12
    third degree 426.0
    complete 426.0
      congenital 746.86
    congenital 746.86
    Mobitz (incomplete)
      type I (Wenckebach's) 426.13
      type II 426.12
    partial 426.13
  auriculoventricular *(see also* Block,
      atrioventricular) 426.10
    complete 426.0
      congenital 746.86
    congenital 746.86
  bifascicular (cardiac) 426.53
  bundle branch (complete) (false)
      (incomplete) 426.50
    bilateral 426.53
    left (complete) (main stem) 426.3
      with right bundle branch block
          426.53
      anterior fascicular 426.2
        with
          posterior fascicular block
              426.3
          right bundle branch block
              426.52
      hemiblock 426.2
      incomplete 426.2
        with right bundle branch block
            426.53
      posterior fascicular 426.2
        with
          anterior fascicular block
              426.3
          right bundle branch block
              426.51
    right 426.4
      with
        left bundle branch block
            (incomplete) (main stem)
            426.53
        left fascicular block 426.53
          anterior 426.52
          posterior 426.51
    Wilson's type 426.4
  cardiac 426.9
  conduction 426.9
    complete 426.0
  Eustachian tube *(see also* Obstruction,
      Eustachian tube) 381.60
  fascicular (left anterior) (left posterior)
      426.2
  foramen Magendie (acquired) 331.3
    congenital 742.3
      with spina bifida *(see also* Spina
          bifida) 741.0●
  heart 426.9
    first degree (atrioventricular) 426.11
    second degree (atrioventricular)
        426.13
    third degree (atrioventricular) 426.0
    bundle branch (complete) (false)
        (incomplete) 426.50
      bilateral 426.53
      left *(see also* Block, bundle branch,
          left) 426.3
      right *(see also* Block, bundle
          branch, right) 426.4

Block (*Continued*)
heart (*Continued*)
complete (atrioventricular) 426.0
congenital 746.86
incomplete 426.13
intra-atrial 426.6
intraventricular NEC 426.6
sinoatrial 426.6
specified type NEC 426.6
hepatic vein 453.0
intraventricular (diffuse) (myofibrillar) 426.6
bundle branch (complete) (false) (incomplete) 426.50
bilateral 426.53
left (*see also* Block, bundle branch, left) 426.3
right (*see also* Block, bundle branch, right) 426.4
kidney (*see also* Disease, renal) 593.9
postcystoscopic 997.5
myocardial (*see also* Block, heart) 426.9
nodal 426.10
optic nerve 377.49
organ or site (congenital) NEC - *see* Atresia
parietal 426.6
peri-infarction 426.6
portal (vein) 452
sinoatrial 426.6
sinoauricular 426.6
spinal cord 336.9
trifascicular 426.54
tubal 628.2
vein NEC 453.9
Blocq's disease or syndrome (astasia-abasia) 307.9
Blood
constituents, abnormal NEC 790.6
disease 289.9
specified NEC 289.89
donor V59.01
other blood components V59.09
stem cells V59.02
whole blood V59.01
dyscrasia 289.9
with
abortion - *see* Abortion, by type, with hemorrhage, delayed or excessive
ectopic pregnancy (*see also* categories 633.0–633.9) 639.1
molar pregnancy (*see also* categories 630–632) 639.1
fetus or newborn NEC 776.9
following
abortion 639.1
ectopic or molar pregnancy 639.1
newborn NEC 776.9 ◀
puerperal, postpartum 666.3●
flukes NEC (*see also* Infestation, Schistosoma) 120.9
in
feces (*see also* Melena) 578.1
occult 792.1
urine (*see also* Hematuria) 599.70
mole 631
occult 792.1
poisoning (*see also* Septicemia) 038.9
pressure
decreased, due to shock following injury 958.4
fluctuating 796.4

Blood (*Continued*)
pressure (*Continued*)
high (*see also* Hypertension) 401.9
incidental reading (isolated) (nonspecific), without diagnosis of hypertension 796.2
low (*see also* Hypotension) 458.9
incidental reading (isolated) (nonspecific), without diagnosis of hypotension 796.3
spitting (*see also* Hemoptysis) 786.3
staining cornea 371.12
transfusion
without reported diagnosis V58.2
donor V59.01
stem cells V59.02
reaction or complication - *see* Complications, transfusion
tumor - *see* Hematoma
vessel rupture - *see* Hemorrhage
vomiting (*see also* Hematemesis) 578.0
Blood-forming organ disease 289.9
Bloodgood's disease 610.1
Bloodshot eye 379.93
Bloom (-Machacek) (-Torre) syndrome 757.39
Blotch, palpebral 372.55
Blount's disease (tibia vara) 732.4
Blount-Barber syndrome (tibia vara) 732.4
Blue
baby 746.9
bloater 491.20
with
acute bronchitis 491.22
exacerbation (acute) 491.21
diaper syndrome 270.0
disease 746.9
dome cyst 610.0
drum syndrome 381.02
sclera 743.47
with fragility of bone and deafness 756.51
toe syndrome 445.02
Blueness (*see also* Cyanosis) 782.5
Blurring, visual 368.8
Blushing (abnormal) (excessive) 782.62
BMI (body mass index)
adult
25.0–25.9 V85.21
26.0–26.9 V85.22
27.0–27.9 V85.23
28.0–28.9 V85.24
29.0–29.9 V85.25
30.0–30.9 V85.30
31.0–31.9 V85.31
32.0–32.9 V85.32
33.0–33.9 V85.33
34.0–34.9 V85.34
35.0–35.9 V85.35
36.0–36.9 V85.36
37.0–37.9 V85.37
38.0–38.9 V85.38
39.0–39.9 V85.39
40 and over V85.4
between 19–24 V85.1
less than 19 V85.0
pediatric
5th percentile to less than 85th percentile for age V85.52

BMI (*Continued*)
pediatric (*Continued*)
85th percentile to less than 95th percentile for age V85.53
greater than or equal to 95th percentile for age V85.54
less than 5th percentile for age V85.51
Boarder, hospital V65.0
infant V65.0
Bockhart's impetigo (superficial folliculitis) 704.8
Bodechtel-Guttmann disease (subacute sclerosing panencephalitis) 046.2
Boder-Sedgwick syndrome (ataxia-telangiectasia) 334.8
Body, bodies
Aschoff (*see also* Myocarditis, rheumatic) 398.0
asteroid, vitreous 379.22
choroid, colloid (degenerative) 362.57
hereditary 362.77
cytoid (retina) 362.82
drusen (retina) (*see also* Drusen) 362.57
optic disc 377.21
fibrin, pleura 511.0
foreign - *see* Foreign body
Hassall-Henle 371.41
loose
joint (*see also* Loose, body, joint) 718.1●
knee 717.6
knee 717.6
sheath, tendon 727.82
Mallory's 034.1
mass index (BMI)
adult
25.0–25.9 V85.21
26.0–26.9 V85.22
27.0–27.9 V85.23
28.0–28.9 V85.24
29.0–29.9 V85.25
30.0–30.9 V85.30
31.0–31.9 V85.31
32.0–32.9 V85.32
33.0–33.9 V85.33
34.0–34.9 V85.34
35.0–35.9 V85.35
36.0–36.9 V85.36
37.0–37.9 V85.37
38.0–38.9 V85.38
39.0–39.9 V85.39
40 and over V85.4
between 19–24 V85.1
less than 19 V85.0
pediatric
5th percentile to less than 85th percentile for age V85.52
85th percentile to less than 95th percentile for age V85.53
greater than or equal to 95th percentile for age V85.54
less than 5th percentile for age V85.51
Mooser 081.0
Negri 071
rice (joint) (*see also* Loose, body, joint) 718.1●
knee 717.6
rocking 307.3
Boeck's
disease (sarcoidosis) 135
lupoid (miliary) 135
sarcoid 135

Boerhaave's syndrome (spontaneous esophageal rupture) 530.4
Boggy
   cervix 622.8
   uterus 621.8
Boil (see also Carbuncle) 680.9
   abdominal wall 680.2
   Aleppo 085.1
   ankle 680.6
   anus 680.5
   arm (any part, above wrist) 680.3
   auditory canal, external 680.0
   axilla 680.3
   back (any part) 680.2
   Baghdad 085.1
   breast 680.2
   buttock 680.5
   chest wall 680.2
   corpus cavernosum 607.2
   Delhi 085.1
   ear (any part) 680.0
   eyelid 373.13
   face (any part, except eye) 680.0
   finger (any) 680.4
   flank 680.2
   foot (any part) 680.7
   forearm 680.3
   Gafsa 085.1
   genital organ, male 608.4
   gluteal (region) 680.5
   groin 680.2
   hand (any part) 680.4
   head (any part, except face) 680.8
   heel 680.7
   hip 680.6
   knee 680.6
   labia 616.4
   lacrimal (see also Dacryocystitis) 375.30
      gland (see also Dacryoadenitis) 375.00
      passages (duct) (sac) (see also Dacryocystitis) 375.30
   leg, any part, except foot 680.6
   multiple sites 680.9
   natal 085.1
   neck 680.1
   nose (external) (septum) 680.0
   orbit, orbital 376.01
   partes posteriores 680.5
   pectoral region 680.2
   penis 607.2
   perineum 680.2
   pinna 680.0
   scalp (any part) 680.8
   scrotum 608.4
   seminal vesicle 608.0
   shoulder 680.3
   skin NEC 680.9
   specified site NEC 680.8
   spermatic cord 608.4
   temple (region) 680.0
   testis 608.4
   thigh 680.6
   thumb 680.4
   toe (any) 680.7
   tropical 085.1
   trunk 680.2
   tunica vaginalis 608.4
   umbilicus 680.2
   upper arm 680.3
   vas deferens 608.4
   vulva 616.4
   wrist 680.4

Bold hives (see also Urticaria) 708.9
Bolivian hemorrhagic fever 078.7
Bombé, iris 364.74
Bomford-Rhoads anemia (refractory) 238.72
Bone - see condition
Bonnevie-Ullrich syndrome 758.6
Bonnier's syndrome 386.19
Bonvale Dam fever 780.79
Bony block of joint 718.80
   ankle 718.87
   elbow 718.82
   foot 718.87
   hand 718.84
   hip 718.85
   knee 718.86
   multiple sites 718.89
   pelvic region 718.85
   shoulder (region) 718.81
   specified site NEC 718.88
   wrist 718.83
BOOP (bronchiolitis obliterans organized pneumonia) 516.8
Borderline
   intellectual functioning V62.89
   osteopenia 733.90
   pelvis 653.1●
      with obstruction during labor 660.1●
         affecting fetus or newborn 763.1
   psychosis (see also Schizophrenia) 295.5●
      of childhood (see also Psychosis, childhood) 299.8●
   schizophrenia (see also Schizophrenia) 295.5●
Borna disease 062.9
Bornholm disease (epidemic pleurodynia) 074.1
Borrelia vincentii (mouth) (pharynx) (tonsils) 101
Bostock's catarrh (see also Fever, hay) 477.9
Boston exanthem 048
Botalli, ductus (patent) (persistent) 747.0
Bothriocephalus latus infestation 123.4
Botulism 005.1
   food poisoning 005.1
   infant 040.41
   non-foodborne 040.42
   wound 040.42
Bouba (see also Yaws) 102.9
Bouffée délirante 298.3
Bouillaud's disease or syndrome (rheumatic heart disease) 391.9
Bourneville's disease (tuberous sclerosis) 759.5
Boutonneuse fever 082.1
Boutonniere
   deformity (finger) 736.21
   hand (intrinsic) 736.21
Bouveret (-Hoffmann) disease or syndrome (paroxysmal tachycardia) 427.2
Bovine heart - see Hypertrophy, cardiac
Bowel - see condition
Bowen's
   dermatosis (precancerous) (M8081/2) - see Neoplasm, skin, in situ
   disease (M8081/2) - see Neoplasm, skin, in situ
   epithelioma (M8081/2) - see Neoplasm, skin, in situ

Bowen's (Continued)
   type
      epidermoid carcinoma in situ (M8081/2) - see Neoplasm, skin, in situ
      intraepidermal squamous cell carcinoma (M8081/2) - see Neoplasm, skin, in situ
Bowing
   femur 736.89
      congenital 754.42
   fibula 736.89
      congenital 754.43
   forearm 736.09
      away from midline (cubitus valgus) 736.01
      toward midline (cubitus varus) 736.02
   leg(s), long bones, congenital 754.44
   radius 736.09
      away from midline (cubitus valgus) 736.01
      toward midline (cubitus varus) 736.02
   tibia 736.89
      congenital 754.43
Bowleg(s) 736.42
   congenital 754.44
   rachitic 268.1
Boyd's dysentery 004.2
Brachial - see condition
Brachman-de Lange syndrome (Amsterdam dwarf, mental retardation, and brachycephaly) 759.89
Brachycardia 427.89
Brachycephaly 756.0
Brachymorphism and ectopia lentis 759.89
Bradley's disease (epidemic vomiting) 078.82
Bradycardia 427.89
   chronic (sinus) 427.81
   newborn 779.81
   nodal 427.89
   postoperative 997.1
   reflex 337.09
   sinoatrial 427.89
      with paroxysmal tachyarrhythmia or tachycardia 427.81
      chronic 427.81
   sinus 427.89
      with paroxysmal tachyarrhythmia or tachycardia 427.81
      chronic 427.81
      persistent 427.81
      severe 427.81
   tachycardia syndrome 427.81
   vagal 427.89
Bradykinesia 781.0
Bradypnea 786.09
Brailsford's disease 732.3
   radial head 732.3
   tarsal scaphoid 732.5
Brailsford-Morquio disease or syndrome (mucopolysaccharidosis IV) 277.5
Brain - see also condition
   death 348.89
   syndrome (acute) (chronic) (nonpsychotic) (organic) (with neurotic reaction) (with behavioral reaction) (see also Syndrome, brain) 310.9
      with
         presenile brain disease 290.10
         psychosis, psychotic reaction (see also Psychosis, organic) 294.9

Brain *(Continued)*
  syndrome *(Continued)*
    congenital *(see also* Retardation,
      mental) 319
Branched-chain amino-acid disease 270.3
Branchial - *see* condition
Brandt's syndrome (acrodermatitis
  enteropathica) 686.8
Brash (water) 787.1
Brass-founders' ague 985.8
Bravais-Jacksonian epilepsy *(see also*
  Epilepsy) 345.5●
Braxton Hicks contractions 644.1●
Braziers' disease 985.8
Brazilian
  blastomycosis 116.1
  leishmaniasis 085.5
BRBPR (bright red blood per rectum)
  569.3
Break
  cardiorenal - *see* Hypertension,
    cardiorenal
  retina *(see also* Defect, retina) 361.30
Breakbone fever 061
Breakdown
  device, implant, or graft - *see*
    Complications, mechanical
  nervous *(see also* Disorder, mental,
    nonpsychotic) 300.9
  perineum 674.2●
Breast - *see also* condition
  buds 259.1
    in newborn 779.89
  dense 793.82
  nodule 793.89
Breast feeding difficulties 676.8●
Breath
  foul 784.99
  holder, child 312.81
  holding spells 786.9
  shortness 786.05
Breathing
  asymmetrical 786.09
  bronchial 786.09
  exercises V57.0
  labored 786.09
  mouth 784.99
    causing malocclusion 524.59
  periodic 786.09
    high altitude 327.22
  tic 307.20
Breathlessness 786.09
Breda's disease *(see also* Yaws) 102.9
Breech
  delivery, affecting fetus or newborn
    763.0
  extraction, affecting fetus or newborn
    763.0
  presentation (buttocks) (complete)
    (frank) 652.2●
    with successful version 652.1●
    before labor, affecting fetus or
      newborn 761.7
    during labor, affecting fetus or
      newborn 763.0
Breisky's disease (kraurosis vulvae) 624.09
Brennemann's syndrome (acute
  mesenteric lymphadenitis) 289.2
Brenner's
  tumor (benign) (M9000/0) 220
    borderline malignancy (M9000/1)
      236.2
    malignant (M9000/3) 183.0
    proliferating (M9000/1) 236.2

Bretonneau's disease (diphtheritic
  malignant angina) 032.0
Breus' mole 631
Brevicollis 756.16
Bricklayers' itch 692.89
Brickmakers' anemia 126.9
Bridge
  myocardial 746.85
Bright red blood per rectum (BRBPR) 569.3
Bright's
  blindness - *see* Uremia
  disease *(see also* Nephritis) 583.9
    arteriosclerotic *(see also*
      Hypertension, kidney) 403.90
Brill's disease (recrudescent typhus) 081.1
  flea-borne 081.0
  louse-borne 081.1
Brill-Symmers disease (follicular
  lymphoma) (M9690/3) 202.0●
Brill-Zinsser disease (recrudescent
  typhus) 081.1
Brinton's disease (linitis plastica)
  (M8142/3) 151.9
Brion-Kayser disease *(see also* Fever,
  paratyphoid) 002.9
Briquet's disorder or syndrome 300.81
Brissaud's
  infantilism (infantile myxedema) 244.9
  motor-verbal tic 307.23
Brissaud-Meige syndrome (infantile
  myxedema) 244.9
Brittle
  bones (congenital) 756.51
  nails 703.8
    congenital 757.5
Broad - *see also* condition
  beta disease 272.2
  ligament laceration syndrome 620.6
Brock's syndrome (atelectasis due to
  enlarged lymph nodes) 518.0
Brocq's disease 691.8
  atopic (diffuse) neurodermatitis 691.8
  lichen simplex chronicus 698.3
  parakeratosis psoriasiformis 696.2
  parapsoriasis 696.2
Brocq-Duhring disease (dermatitis
  herpetiformis) 694.0
Brodie's
  abscess (localized) (chronic) *(see also*
    Osteomyelitis) 730.1●
  disease (joint) *(see also* Osteomyelitis)
    730.1●
Broken
  arches 734
    congenital 755.67
  back - *see* Fracture, vertebra, by site
  bone - *see* Fracture, by site
  compensation - *see* Disease, heart
  heart syndrome 429.83
  implant or internal device - *see* listing
    under Complications, mechanical
  neck - *see* Fracture, vertebra, cervical
  nose 802.0
    open 802.1
  tooth, teeth 873.63
    complicated 873.73
Bromhidrosis 705.89
Bromidism, bromism
  acute 967.3
    correct substance properly
      administered 349.82
    overdose or wrong substance given
      or taken 967.3
  chronic *(see also* Dependence) 304.1●

Bromidrosiphobia 300.23
Bromidrosis 705.89
Bronchi, bronchial - *see* condition
Bronchiectasis (cylindrical) (diffuse)
  (fusiform) (localized) (moniliform)
  (postinfectious) (recurrent)
  (saccular) 494.0
  with acute exacerbation 494.1
  congenital 748.61
  tuberculosis *(see also* Tuberculosis)
    011.5●
Bronchiolectasis - *see* Bronchiectasis
Bronchiolitis (acute) (infectious)
  (subacute) 466.19
  with
    bronchospasm or obstruction 466.19
    influenza, flu, or grippe 487.1
  catarrhal (acute) (subacute) 466.19
  chemical 506.0
    chronic 506.4
  chronic (obliterative) 491.8
  due to external agent - *see* Bronchitis,
    acute, due to
  fibrosa obliterans 491.8
  influenzal 487.1
  obliterans 491.8
    with organizing pneumonia (BOOP)
      516.8
    status post lung transplant 996.84
  obliterative (chronic) (diffuse)
    (subacute) 491.8
    due to fumes or vapors 506.4
  respiratory syncytial virus 466.11
  vesicular - *see* Pneumonia, broncho-
Bronchitis (diffuse) (hypostatic)
  (infectious) (inflammatory) (simple)
  490
  with
    emphysema - *see* Emphysema
    influenza, flue, or grippe 487.1
    obstruction airway, chronic 491.20
      with
        acute bronchitis 491.22
        exacerbation (acute) 491.21
    tracheitis 490
      acute or subacute 466.0
        with bronchospasm or
          obstruction 466.0
      chronic 491.8
  acute or subacute 466.0
    with
      bronchiectasis 494.1
      bronchospasm 466.0
      obstruction 466.0
      tracheitis 466.0
    chemical (due to fumes or vapors)
      506.0
    due to
      fumes or vapors 506.0
      radiation 508.8
  allergic (acute) *(see also* Asthma) 493.9●
  arachidic 934.1
  aspiration 507.0
    due to fumes or vapors 506.0
  asthmatic (acute) 493.90
    with
      acute exacerbation 493.92
      status asthmaticus 493.91
    chronic 493.2●
  capillary 466.19
    with bronchospasm or obstruction
      466.19
    chronic 491.8
  caseous *(see also* Tuberculosis) 011.3●

◀ New   ◀▥ Revised   ~~deleted~~ Deleted   ● Use Additional Digit(s)   ▨ Omit code

Bronchitis *(Continued)*
Castellani's 104.8
catarrhal 490
acute - *see* Bronchitis, acute
chronic 491.0
chemical (acute) (subacute) 506.0
chronic 506.4
due to fumes or vapors (acute)
(subacute) 506.0
chronic 506.4
chronic 491.9
with
tracheitis (chronic) 491.8
asthmatic 493.2●
catarrhal 491.0
chemical (due to fumes and vapors)
506.4
due to
fumes or vapors (chemical)
(inhalation) 506.4
radiation 508.8
tobacco smoking 491.0
mucopurulent 491.1
obstructive 491.20
with
acute bronchitis 491.22
exacerbation (acute) 491.21
purulent 491.1
simple 491.0
specified type NEC 491.8
croupous 466.0
with bronchospasm or obstruction
466.0
due to fumes or vapors 506.0
emphysematous 491.20
with
acute bronchitis 491.22
exacerbation (acute) 491.21
exudative 466.0
fetid (chronic) (recurrent) 491.1
fibrinous, acute or subacute 466.0
with bronchospasm or obstruction
466.0
grippal 487.1
influenzal 487.1
membranous, acute or subacute 466.0
with bronchospasm or obstruction
466.0
moulders' 502
mucopurulent (chronic) (recurrent)
491.1
acute or subacute 466.0
obliterans 491.8
obstructive (chronic) 491.20
with
acute bronchitis 491.22
exacerbation (acute) 491.21
pituitous 491.1
plastic (inflammatory) 466.0
pneumococcal, acute or subacute 466.0
with bronchospasm or obstruction
466.0
pseudomembranous 466.0
purulent (chronic) (recurrent) 491.1
acute or subacute 466.0
with bronchospasm or
obstruction 466.0
putrid 491.1
scrofulous (*see also* Tuberculosis)
011.3●
senile 491.9
septic, acute or subacute 466.0
with bronchospasm or obstruction
466.0

Bronchitis *(Continued)*
smokers' 491.0
spirochetal 104.8
suffocative, acute or subacute 466.0
summer (*see also* Asthma) 493.9●
suppurative (chronic) 491.1
acute or subacute 466.0
tuberculous (*see also* Tuberculosis)
011.3●
ulcerative 491.8
Vincent's 101
Vincent's 101
viral, acute or subacute 466.0
Bronchoalveolitis 485
Bronchoaspergillosis 117.3
Bronchocele
meaning
dilatation of bronchus 519.19
goiter 240.9
Bronchogenic carcinoma 162.9
Bronchohemisporosis 117.9
Broncholithiasis 518.89
tuberculous (*see also* Tuberculosis)
011.3●
Bronchomalacia 748.3
Bronchomoniliasis 112.89
Bronchomycosis 112.89
Bronchonocardiosis 039.1
Bronchopleuropneumonia - *see*
Pneumonia, broncho-
Bronchopneumonia - *see* Pneumonia,
broncho-
Bronchopneumonitis - *see* Pneumonia,
broncho-
Bronchopulmonary - *see* condition
Bronchopulmonitis - *see* Pneumonia,
broncho-
Bronchorrhagia 786.3
newborn 770.3
tuberculous (*see also* Tuberculosis)
011.3●
Bronchorrhea (chronic) (purulent)
491.0
acute 466.0
Bronchospasm 519.11
with
asthma - *see* Asthma
bronchiolitis, acute 466.19
due to respiratory syncytial
virus 466.11
bronchitis - *see* Bronchitis
chronic obstructive pulmonary
disease (COPD) 496
emphysema - *see* Emphysema
due to external agent - *see*
Condition, respiratory,
acute, due to
acute 519.11
exercise induced 493.81
Bronchospirochetosis 104.8
Bronchostenosis 519.19
Bronchus - *see* condition
Bronze, bronzed
diabetes 275.0
disease (Addison's) (skin) 255.41
tuberculous (*see also* Tuberculosis)
017.6●
Brooke's disease or tumor (M8100/0) -
see Neoplasm, skin, benign
Brown's tendon sheath syndrome
378.61
Brown enamel of teeth (hereditary)
520.5

Brown-Séquard's paralysis (syndrome)
344.89
Brow presentation complicating delivery
652.4●
Brucella, brucellosis (infection) 023.9
abortus 023.1
canis 023.3
dermatitis, skin 023.9
melitensis 023.0
mixed 023.8
suis 023.2
Bruck's disease 733.99
Bruck-de Lange disease or syndrome
(Amsterdam dwarf, mental
retardation, and brachycephaly)
759.89
Brugada syndrome 746.89
Brug's filariasis 125.1
Brugsch's syndrome (acropachyderma)
757.39
Bruhl's disease (splenic anemia with
fever) 285.8
Bruise (skin surface intact) - *see also*
Contusion
with
fracture - *see* Fracture, by site
open wound - *see* Wound, open, by
site
internal organ (abdomen, chest, or
pelvis) - *see* Injury, internal, by
site
umbilical cord 663.6●
affecting fetus or newborn 762.6
Bruit 785.9
arterial (abdominal) (carotid) 785.9
supraclavicular 785.9
Brushburn - *see* Injury, superficial, by
site
Bruton's X-linked agammaglobulinemia
279.04
Bruxism 306.8
sleep related 327.53
Bubbly lung syndrome 770.7
Bubo 289.3
blennorrhagic 098.89
chancroidal 099.0
climatic 099.1
due to Hemophilus ducreyi 099.0
gonococcal 098.89
indolent NEC 099.8
inguinal NEC 099.8
chancroidal 099.0
climatic 099.1
due to H. ducreyi 099.0
scrofulous (*see also* Tuberculosis)
017.2●
soft chancre 099.0
suppurating 683
syphilitic 091.0
congenital 090.0
tropical 099.1
venereal NEC 099.8
virulent 099.0
Bubonic plague 020.0
Bubonocele - *see* Hernia, inguinal
Buccal - *see* condition
Buchanan's disease (juvenile
osteochondrosis of iliac crest)
732.1
Buchem's syndrome (hyperostosis
corticalis) 733.3
Buchman's disease (osteochondrosis,
juvenile) 732.1

◀ New   ◀▥ Revised   ~~deleted~~ Deleted   ● Use Additional Digit(s)   ▨ Omit code

Bucket handle fracture (semilunar cartilage) (*see also* Tear, meniscus) 836.2

Budd-Chiari syndrome (hepatic vein thrombosis) 453.0

Budgerigar-fanciers' disease or lung 495.2

Büdinger-Ludloff-Läwen disease 717.89

Buds
breast 259.1
in newborn 779.89

Buerger's disease (thromboangiitis obliterans) 443.1

Bulbar - *see* condition

Bulbus cordis 745.9
persistent (in left ventricle) 745.8

Bulging fontanels (congenital) 756.0

Bulimia 783.6
nervosa 307.51
nonorganic origin 307.51

Bulky uterus 621.2

Bulla(e) 709.8
lung (emphysematous) (solitary) 492.0

Bullet wound - *see also* Wound, open, by site
fracture - *see* Fracture, by site, open
internal organ (abdomen, chest, or pelvis) - *see* Injury, internal, by site, with open wound
intracranial - *see* Laceration, brain, with open wound

Bullis fever 082.8

Bullying (*see also* Disturbance, conduct) 312.0●

Bundle
branch block (complete) (false) (incomplete) 426.50
bilateral 426.53
left (*see also* Block, bundle branch, left) 426.3
hemiblock 426.2
right (*see also* Block, bundle branch, right) 426.4
of His - *see* condition
of Kent syndrome (anomalous atrioventricular excitation) 426.7

Bungpagga 040.81

Bunion 727.1

Bunionette 727.1

Bunyamwera fever 066.3

Buphthalmia, buphthalmos (congenital) 743.20
associated with
keratoglobus, congenital 743.22
megalocornea 743.22
ocular anomalies NEC 743.22
isolated 743.21
simple 743.21

Bürger-Grütz disease or syndrome (essential familial hyperlipemia) 272.3

Buried roots 525.3

Burke's syndrome 577.8

Burkitt's
tumor (M9750/3) 200.2●
type malignant, lymphoma, lymphoblastic, or undifferentiated (M9750/3) 200.2●

Burn (acid) (cathode ray) (caustic) (chemical) (electric heating appliance) (electricity) (fire) (flame) (hot liquid or object) (irradiation) (lime) (radiation) (steam) (thermal) (x-ray) 949.0

Note 11   Use the following fifth-digit subclassification with category 948 to indicate the percent of body surface with third degree burn:

0   less than 10 percent or unspecified
1   10–19 percent
2   20–29 percent
3   30–39 percent
4   40–49 percent
5   50–59 percent
6   60–69 percent
7   70–79 percent
8   80–89 percent
9   90 percent or more of body surface
---

with
blisters - *see* Burn, by site, second degree
erythema - *see* Burn, by site, first degree
skin loss (epidermal) - *see also* Burn, by site, second degree
full thickness - *see also* Burn, by site, third degree
with necrosis of underlying tissues - *see* Burn, by site, third degree, deep
first degree - *see* Burn, by site, first degree
second degree - *see* Burn, by site, second degree
third degree - *see also* Burn, by site, third degree
deep - *see* Burn, by site, third degree, deep
abdomen, abdominal (muscle) (wall) 942.03
with
trunk - *see* Burn, trunk, multiple sites
first degree 942.13
second degree 942.23
third degree 942.33
deep 942.43
with loss of body part 942.53
ankle 945.03
with
lower limb(s) - *see* Burn, leg, multiple sites
first degree 945.13
second degree 945.23
third degree 945.33
deep 945.43
with loss of body part 945.53
anus - *see* Burn, trunk, specified site NEC
arm(s) 943.00
first degree 943.10
second degree 943.20
third degree 943.30
deep 943.40
with loss of body part 943.50
lower - *see* Burn, forearm(s)

Burn (*Continued*)
arm(s) (*Continued*)
multiple sites, except hand(s) or wrist(s) 943.09
first degree 943.19
second degree 943.29
third degree 943.39
deep 943.49
with loss of body part 943.59
upper 943.03
first degree 943.13
second degree 943.23
third degree 943.33
deep 943.43
with loss of body part 943.53
auditory canal (external) - *see* Burn, ear
auricle (ear) - *see* Burn, ear
axilla 943.04
with
upper limb(s), except hand(s) or wrist(s) - *see* Burn, arm(s), multiple sites
first degree 943.14
second degree 943.24
third degree 943.34
deep 943.44
with loss of body part 943.54
back 942.04
with
trunk - *see* Burn, trunk, multiple sites
first degree 942.14
second degree 942.24
third degree 942.34
deep 942.44
with loss of body part 942.54
biceps
brachii - *see* Burn, arm(s), upper
femoris - *see* Burn, thigh
breast(s) 942.01
with
trunk - *see* Burn, trunk, multiple sites
first degree 942.11
second degree 942.21
third degree 942.31
deep 942.41
with loss of body part 942.51
brow - *see* Burn, forehead
buttock(s) - *see* Burn, back
canthus (eye) 940.1
chemical 940.0
cervix (uteri) 947.4
cheek (cutaneous) 941.07
with
face or head - *see* Burn, head, multiple sites
first degree 941.17
second degree 941.27
third degree 941.37
deep 941.47
with loss of body part 941.57
chest wall (anterior) 942.02
with
trunk - *see* Burn, trunk, multiple sites
first degree 942.12
second degree 942.22
third degree 942.32
deep 942.42
with loss of body part 942.52

◄ New   ◄ Revised   ~~deleted~~ Deleted   ● Use Additional Digit(s)   Omit code

Burn (Continued)
chin 941.04
with
face or head - see Burn, head,
multiple sites
first degree 941.14
second degree 941.24
third degree 941.34
deep 941.44
with loss of body part 941.54
clitoris - see Burn, genitourinary
organs, external
colon 947.3
conjunctiva (and cornea) 940.4
chemical
acid 940.3
alkaline 940.2
cornea (and conjunctiva) 940.4
chemical
acid 940.3
alkaline 940.2
costal region - see Burn, chest wall
due to ingested chemical agent - see
Burn, internal organs
ear (auricle) (canal) (drum) (external)
941.01
with
face or head - see Burn, head,
multiple sites
first degree 941.11
second degree 941.21
third degree 941.31
deep 941.41
with loss of a body part 941.51
elbow 943.02
with
hand(s) and wrist(s) - see Burn,
multiple specified sites
upper limb(s), except hand(s) or
wrist(s) - see also Burn,
arm(s), multiple sites
first degree 943.12
second degree 943.22
third degree 943.32
deep 943.42
with loss of body part 943.52
electricity, electric current - see Burn, by
site
entire body - see Burn, multiple,
specified sites
epididymis - see Burn, genitourinary
organs, external
epigastric region - see Burn, abdomen
epiglottis 947.1
esophagus 947.2
extent (percent of body surface)
less than 10 percent 948.0 ●
10–19 percent 948.1 ●
20–29 percent 948.2 ●
30–39 percent 948.3 ●
40–49 percent 948.4 ●
50–59 percent 948.5 ●
60–69 percent 948.6 ●
70–79 percent 948.7 ●
80–89 percent 948.8 ●
90 percent or more 948.9 ●
extremity
lower - see Burn, leg
upper - see Burn, arm(s)
eye(s) (and adnexa) (only) 940.9
with
face, head, or neck 941.02
first degree 941.12
second degree 941.22

Burn (Continued)
eye(s) (Continued)
with (Continued)
face, head, or neck (Continued)
third degree 941.32
deep 941.42
with loss of body part
941.52
other sites (classifiable to more
than one category in 940–
945) - see Burn, multiple,
specified sites
resulting rupture and destruction
of eyeball 940.5
specified part - see Burn, by site
eyeball - see also Burn, eye
with resulting rupture and
destruction of eyeball 940.5
eyelid(s) 940.1
chemical 940.0
face - see Burn, head
finger (nail) (subungual) 944.01
with
hand(s) - see Burn, hand(s),
multiple sites
other sites - see Burn, multiple,
specified sites
thumb 944.04
first degree 944.14
second degree 944.24
third degree 944.34
deep 944.44
with loss of body part
944.54
first degree 944.11
second degree 944.21
third degree 944.31
deep 944.41
with loss of body part 944.51
multiple (digits) 944.03
with thumb - see Burn, finger,
with thumb
first degree 944.13
second degree 944.23
third degree 944.33
deep 944.43
with loss of body part
944.53
flank - see Burn, abdomen
foot 945.02
with
lower limb(s) - see Burn, leg,
multiple sites
first degree 945.12
second degree 945.22
third degree 945.32
deep 945.42
with loss of body part 945.52
forearm(s) 943.01
with
upper limb(s), except hand(s) or
wrist(s) - see Burn, arm(s),
multiple sites
first degree 943.11
second degree 943.21
third degree 943.31
deep 943.41
with loss of body part 943.51
forehead 941.07
with
face or head - see Burn, head,
multiple sites
first degree 941.17
second degree 941.27

Burn (Continued)
forehead (Continued)
third degree 941.37
deep 941.47
with loss of body part 941.57
fourth degree - see Burn, by site, third
degree, deep
friction - see Injury, superficial, by site
from swallowing caustic or corrosive
substance NEC - see Burn,
internal organs
full thickness - see Burn, by site, third
degree
gastrointestinal tract 947.3
genitourinary organs
external 942.05
with
trunk - see Burn, trunk,
multiple sites
first degree 942.15
second degree 942.25
third degree 942.35
deep 942.45
with loss of body part
942.55
internal 947.8
globe (eye) - see Burn, eyeball
groin - see Burn, abdomen
gum 947.0
hand(s) (phalanges) (and wrist) 944.00
first degree 944.10
second degree 944.20
third degree 944.30
deep 944.40
with loss of body part 944.50
back (dorsal surface) 944.06
first degree 944.16
second degree 944.26
third degree 944.36
deep 944.46
with loss of body part
944.56
multiple sites 944.08
first degree 944.18
second degree 944.28
third degree 944.38
deep 944.48
with loss of body part
944.58
head (and face) 941.00
eye(s) only 940.9
specified part - see Burn, by site
first degree 941.10
second degree 941.20
third degree 941.30
deep 941.40
with loss of body part 941.50
multiple sites 941.09
with eyes - see Burn, eyes, with
face, head, or neck
first degree 941.19
second degree 941.29
third degree 941.39
deep 941.49
with loss of body part
941.59
heel - see Burn, foot
hip - see Burn, trunk, specified site
NEC
iliac region - see Burn, trunk, specified
site NEC
infected 958.3
inhalation (see also Burn, internal
organs) 947.9

◀ New   ◀◍ Revised   ~~deleted~~ Deleted   ● Use Additional Digit(s)   ▨ Omit code

Burn *(Continued)*
  toe (nail) (subungual) 945.01
    with
      lower limb(s) - *see* Burn, leg,
        multiple sites
    first degree 945.11
    second degree 945.21
    third degree 945.31
      deep 945.41
        with loss of body part 945.51
  tongue 947.0
  tonsil 947.0
  trachea 947.1
  trunk 942.00
    first degree 942.10
    second degree 942.20
    third degree 942.30
      deep 942.40
        with loss of body part 942.50
    multiple sites 942.09
      first degree 942.19
      second degree 942.29
      third degree 942.39
        deep 942.49
          with loss of body part
            942.59
    specified site NEC 942.09
      first degree 942.19
      second degree 942.29
      third degree 942.39
        deep 942.49
          with loss of body part
            942.59
  tunica vaginalis - *see* Burn,
    genitourinary organs, external
  tympanic membrane - *see* Burn, ear
  tympanum - *see* Burn, ear
  ultraviolet 692.82
  unspecified site (multiple) 949.0
    with extent of body surface involved
      specified
      less than 10 percent 948.0●
      10–19 percent 948.1●
      20–29 percent 948.2●
      30–39 percent 948.3●
      40–49 percent 948.4●
      50–59 percent 948.5●
      60–69 percent 948.6●
      70–79 percent 948.7●
      80–89 percent 948.8●
      90 percent or more 948.9●

Burn *(Continued)*
  unspecified site *(Continued)*
    first degree 949.1
    second degree 949.2
    third degree 949.3
      deep 949.4
        with loss of body part 949.5
  uterus 947.4
  uvula 947.0
  vagina 947.4
  vulva - *see* Burn, genitourinary organs,
    external
  wrist(s) 944.07
    with
      hand(s) - *see* Burn, hand(s),
        multiple sites
    first degree 944.17
    second degree 944.27
    third degree 944.37
      deep 944.47
        with loss of body part
          944.57
Burnett's syndrome (milk-alkali)
  275.42
Burnier's syndrome (hypophyseal
  dwarfism) 253.3
Burning
  feet syndrome 266.2
  sensation (*see also* Disturbance,
    sensation) 782.0
  tongue 529.6
Burns' disease (osteochondrosis, lower
  ulna) 732.3
Bursa - *see also* condition
  pharynx 478.29
Bursitis NEC 727.3
  Achilles tendon 726.71
  adhesive 726.90
    shoulder 726.0
  ankle 726.79
  buttock 726.5
  calcaneal 726.79
  collateral ligament
    fibular 726.63
    tibial 726.62
  Duplay's 726.2
  elbow 726.33
  finger 726.8
  foot 726.79
  gonococcal 098.52
  hand 726.4

Bursitis NEC *(Continued)*
  hip 726.5
  infrapatellar 726.69
  ischiogluteal 726.5
  knee 726.60
  occupational NEC 727.2
  olecranon 726.33
  pes anserinus 726.61
  pharyngeal 478.29
  popliteal 727.51
  prepatellar 726.65
  radiohumeral 727.3
  scapulohumeral 726.19
    adhesive 726.0
  shoulder 726.10
    adhesive 726.0
  subacromial 726.19
    adhesive 726.0
  subcoracoid 726.19
  subdeltoid 726.19
    adhesive 726.0
  subpatellar 726.69
  syphilitic 095.7
  Thornwaldt's, Tornwaldt's
    (pharyngeal) 478.29
  toe 726.79
  trochanteric area 726.5
  wrist 726.4
Burst stitches or sutures (complication of
  surgery) (external) (*see also*
  Dehiscence) 998.32
  internal 998.31
Buruli ulcer 031.1
Bury's disease (erythema elevatum
  diutinum) 695.89
Buschke's disease or scleredema
  (adultorum) 710.1
Busquet's disease (osteoperiostitis) (*see
  also* Osteomyelitis) 730.1●
Busse-Buschke disease (cryptococcosis)
  117.5
Buttock - *see* condition
Button
  Biskra 085.1
  Delhi 085.1
  oriental 085.1
Buttonhole hand (intrinsic) 736.21
Bwamba fever (encephalitis) 066.3
Byssinosis (occupational) 504
Bywaters' syndrome 958.5

C

Cacergasia 300.9
Cachexia 799.4
  cancerous - *see also* Neoplasm, by site, malignant 799.4
  cardiac - *see* Disease, heart
  dehydration 276.51
    with
      hypernatremia 276.0
      hyponatremia 276.1
  due to malnutrition 799.4
  exophthalmic 242.0●
  heart - *see* Disease, heart
  hypophyseal 253.2
  hypopituitary 253.2
  lead 984.9
    specified type of lead - *see* Table of Drugs and Chemicals
  malaria 084.9
  malignant *see also* Neoplasm, by site, malignant 799.4
  marsh 084.9
  nervous 300.5
  old age 797
  pachydermic - *see* Hypothyroidism
  paludal 084.9
  pituitary (postpartum) 253.2
  renal (*see also* Disease, renal) 593.9
  saturnine 984.9
    specified type of lead - *see* Table of Drugs and Chemicals
  senile 797
  Simmonds' (pituitary cachexia) 253.2
  splenica 289.59
  strumipriva (*see also* Hypothyroidism) 244.9
  tuberculous NEC (*see also* Tuberculosis) 011.9●
Café au lait spots 709.09
Caffey's disease or syndrome (infantile cortical hyperostosis) 756.59
Caisson disease 993.3
Caked breast (puerperal, postpartum) 676.2●
Cake kidney 753.3
Calabar swelling 125.2
Calcaneal spur 726.73
Calcaneoapophysitis 732.5
Calcaneonavicular bar 755.67
Calcareous - *see* condition
Calcicosis (occupational) 502
Calciferol (vitamin D) deficiency 268.9
  with
    osteomalacia 268.2
    rickets (*see also* Rickets) 268.0
Calcification
  adrenal (capsule) (gland) 255.41
    tuberculous (*see also* Tuberculosis) 017.6●
  aorta 440.0
  artery (annular) - *see* Arteriosclerosis
  auricle (ear) 380.89
  bladder 596.8
    due to S. hematobium 120.0
  brain (cortex) - *see* Calcification, cerebral
  bronchus 519.19
  bursa 727.82
  cardiac (*see also* Degeneration, myocardial) 429.1
  cartilage (postinfectional) 733.99
  cerebral (cortex) 348.89 ◀▥
    artery 437.0

Calcification (*Continued*)
  cervix (uteri) 622.8
  choroid plexus 349.2
  conjunctiva 372.54
  corpora cavernosa (penis) 607.89
  cortex (brain) - *see* Calcification, cerebral
  dental pulp (nodular) 522.2
  dentinal papilla 520.4
  disc, intervertebral 722.90
    cervical, cervicothoracic 722.91
    lumbar, lumbosacral 722.93
    thoracic, thoracolumbar 722.92
  fallopian tube 620.8
  falx cerebri - *see* Calcification, cerebral
  fascia 728.89
  gallbladder 575.8
  general 275.40
  heart (*see also* Degeneration, myocardial) 429.1
    valve - *see* Endocarditis
  intervertebral cartilage or disc (postinfectional) 722.90
    cervical, cervicothoracic 722.91
    lumbar, lumbosacral 722.93
    thoracic, thoracolumbar 722.92
  intracranial - *see* Calcification, cerebral
  intraspinal ligament 728.89
  joint 719.80
    ankle 719.87
    elbow 719.82
    foot 719.87
    hand 719.84
    hip 719.85
    knee 719.86
    multiple sites 719.89
    pelvic region 719.85
    shoulder (region) 719.81
    specified site NEC 719.88
    wrist 719.83
  kidney 593.89
    tuberculous (*see also* Tuberculosis) 016.0●
  larynx (senile) 478.79
  lens 366.8
  ligament 728.89
    intraspinal 728.89
    knee (medial collateral) 717.89
  lung 518.89
    active 518.89
    postinfectional 518.89
    tuberculous (*see also* Tuberculosis, pulmonary) 011.9●
  lymph gland or node (postinfectional) 289.3
    tuberculous (*see also* Tuberculosis, lymph gland) 017.2●
  mammographic 793.89
  massive (paraplegic) 728.10
  medial (*see also* Arteriosclerosis, extremities) 440.20
  meninges (cerebral) 349.2
  metastatic 275.40
  Mönckeberg's - *see* Arteriosclerosis
  muscle 728.10
    heterotopic, postoperative 728.13
  myocardium, myocardial (*see also* Degeneration, myocardial) 429.1
  ovary 620.8
  pancreas 577.8
  penis 607.89
  periarticular 728.89
  pericardium (*see also* Pericarditis) 423.8
  pineal gland 259.8

Calcification (*Continued*)
  pleura 511.0
    postinfectional 518.89
    tuberculous (*see also* Tuberculosis, pleura) 012.0●
  pulp (dental) (nodular) 522.2
  renal 593.89
  Rider's bone 733.99
  sclera 379.16
  semilunar cartilage 717.89
  spleen 289.59
  subcutaneous 709.3
  suprarenal (capsule) (gland) 255.41
  tendon (sheath) 727.82
    with bursitis, synovitis or tenosynovitis 727.82
  trachea 519.19
  ureter 593.89
  uterus 621.8
  vitreous 379.29
Calcified - *see also* Calcification
  hematoma NEC 959.9
Calcinosis (generalized) (interstitial) (tumoral) (universalis) 275.49
  circumscripta 709.3
  cutis 709.3
  intervertebralis 275.49 [722.90]
  Raynaud's phenomenon sclerodactylytelangiectasis (CRST) 710.1
Calciphylaxis (*see also* Calcification, by site) 275.49
Calcium
  blood
    high (*see also* Hypercalcemia) 275.42
    low (*see also* Hypocalcemia) 275.41
  deposits - *see also* Calcification, by site
    in bursa 727.82
    in tendon (sheath) 727.82
      with bursitis, synovitis or tenosynovitis 727.82
  salts or soaps in vitreous 379.22
Calciuria 791.9
Calculi - *see* Calculus
Calculosis, intrahepatic - *see* Choledocholithiasis
Calculus, calculi, calculous 592.9
  ampulla of Vater - *see* Choledocholithiasis
  anuria (impacted) (recurrent) 592.0
  appendix 543.9
  bile duct (any) - *see* Choledocholithiasis
  biliary - *see* Cholelithiasis
  bilirubin, multiple - *see* Cholelithiasis
  bladder (encysted) (impacted) (urinary) 594.1
    diverticulum 594.0
  bronchus 518.89
  calyx (kidney) (renal) 592.0
    congenital 753.3
  cholesterol (pure) (solitary) - *see* Cholelithiasis
  common duct (bile) - *see* Choledocholithiasis
  conjunctiva 372.54
  cystic 594.1
    duct - *see* Cholelithiasis
  dental 523.6
    subgingival 523.6
    supragingival 523.6
  epididymis 608.89
  gallbladder - *see also* Cholelithiasis
    congenital 751.69
  hepatic (duct) - *see* Choledocholithiasis

◀ New ◀▥ Revised ~~deleted~~ Deleted ● Use Additional Digit(s) ▨ Omit code

Calculus, calculi, calculous *(Continued)*
  intestine (impaction) (obstruction) 560.39
  kidney (impacted) (multiple) (pelvis)
    (recurrent) (staghorn) 592.0
    congenital 753.3
  lacrimal (passages) 375.57
  liver (impacted) - *see* Choledocholithiasis
  lung 518.89
  mammographic 793.89
  nephritic (impacted) (recurrent) 592.0
  nose 478.19
  pancreas (duct) 577.8
  parotid gland 527.5
  pelvis, encysted 592.0
  prostate 602.0
  pulmonary 518.89
  renal (impacted) (recurrent) 592.0
    congenital 753.3
  salivary (duct) (gland) 527.5
  seminal vesicle 608.89
  staghorn 592.0
  Stensen's duct 527.5
  sublingual duct or gland 527.5
    congenital 750.26
  submaxillary duct, gland, or region 527.5
  suburethral 594.8
  tonsil 474.8
  tooth, teeth 523.6
  tunica vaginalis 608.89
  ureter (impacted) (recurrent) 592.1
  urethra (impacted) 594.2
  urinary (duct) (impacted) (passage)
    (tract) 592.9
    lower tract NEC 594.9
      specified site 594.8
  vagina 623.8
  vesical (impacted) 594.1
  Wharton's duct 527.5
Caliectasis 593.89
California
  disease 114.0
  encephalitis 062.5
Caligo cornea 371.03
Callositas, callosity (infected) 700
Callus (infected) 700
  bone 726.91
  excessive, following fracture - *see also*
    Late, effect (of), fracture
Calvé (-Perthes) disease (osteochondrosis,
  femoral capital) 732.1
Calvities *(see also* Alopecia) 704.00
Cameroon fever *(see also* Malaria) 084.6
Camptocormia 300.11
Camptodactyly (congenital) 755.59
Camurati-Engelmann disease
  (diaphyseal sclerosis) 756.59
Canal - *see* condition
Canaliculitis (lacrimal) (acute) 375.31
  Actinomyces 039.8
  chronic 375.41
Canavan's disease 330.0
Cancer (M8000/3) - *see also* Neoplasm, by
  site, malignant

Note 12 The term "cancer" when modified by an adjective or adjectival phrase indicating a morphological type should be coded in the same manner as "carcinoma" with that adjective or phrase. Thus, "squamous-cell cancer" should be coded in the same manner as "squamous-cell carcinoma," which appears in the list under "Carcinoma."

Cancer *(Continued)*
  bile duct type (M8160/3), liver 155.1
  hepatocellular (M8170/3) 155.0
Cancerous (M8000/3) - *see* Neoplasm, by
  site, malignant
Cancerphobia 300.29
Cancrum oris 528.1
Candidiasis, candidal 112.9
  with pneumonia 112.4
  balanitis 112.2
  congenital 771.7
  disseminated 112.5
  endocarditis 112.81
  esophagus 112.84
  intertrigo 112.3
  intestine 112.85
  lung 112.4
  meningitis 112.83
  mouth 112.0
  nails 112.3
  neonatal 771.7
  onychia 112.3
  otitis externa 112.82
  otomycosis 112.82
  paronychia 112.3
  perionyxis 112.3
  pneumonia 112.4
  pneumonitis 112.4
  skin 112.3
  specified site NEC 112.89
  systemic 112.5
  urogenital site NEC 112.2
  vagina 112.1
  vulva 112.1
  vulvovaginitis 112.1
Candidiosis - *see* Candidiasis
Candiru infection or infestation 136.8
Canities (premature) 704.3
  congenital 757.4
Canker (mouth) (sore) 528.2
  rash 034.1
Cannabinosis 504
Canton fever 081.9
Cap
  cradle 690.11
Capillariasis 127.5
Capillary - *see* condition
Caplan's syndrome 714.81
Caplan-Colinet syndrome 714.81
Capsule - *see* condition
Capsulitis (joint) 726.90
  adhesive (shoulder) 726.0
  hip 726.5
  knee 726.60
  labyrinthine 387.8
  thyroid 245.9
  wrist 726.4
Caput
  crepitus 756.0
  medusae 456.8
  succedaneum 767.19
Carapata disease 087.1
Carate - *see* Pinta
Carbohydrate-deficient glycoprotein
  syndrome (CDGS) 271.8
Carboxyhemoglobinemia 986
Carbuncle 680.9
  abdominal wall 680.2
  ankle 680.6
  anus 680.5
  arm (any part, above wrist) 680.3
  auditory canal, external 680.0
  axilla 680.3
  back (any part) 680.2

Carbuncle *(Continued)*
  breast 680.2
  buttock 680.5
  chest wall 680.2
  corpus cavernosum 607.2
  ear (any part) (external) 680.0
  eyelid 373.13
  face (any part, except eye) 680.0
  finger (any) 680.4
  flank 680.2
  foot (any part) 680.7
  forearm 680.3
  genital organ (male) 608.4
  gluteal (region) 680.5
  groin 680.2
  hand (any part) 680.4
  head (any part, except face) 680.8
  heel 680.7
  hip 680.6
  kidney *(see also* Abscess, kidney)
    590.2
  knee 680.6
  labia 616.4
  lacrimal
    gland *(see also* Dacryoadenitis)
      375.00
    passages (duct) (sac) *(see also*
      Dacryocystitis) 375.30
  leg, any part except foot 680.6
  lower extremity, any part except foot
    680.6
  malignant 022.0
  multiple sites 680.9
  neck 680.1
  nose (external) (septum) 680.0
  orbit, orbital 376.01
  partes posteriores 680.5
  pectoral region 680.2
  penis 607.2
  perineum 680.2
  pinna 680.0
  scalp (any part) 680.8
  scrotum 608.4
  seminal vesicle 608.0
  shoulder 680.3
  skin NEC 680.9
  specified site NEC 680.8
  spermatic cord 608.4
  temple (region) 680.0
  testis 608.4
  thigh 680.6
  thumb 680.4
  toe (any) 680.7
  trunk 680.2
  tunica vaginalis 608.4
  umbilicus 680.2
  upper arm 680.3
  urethra 597.0
  vas deferens 608.4
  vulva 616.4
  wrist 680.4
Carbunculus *(see also* Carbuncle) 680.9
Carcinoid (tumor) (M8240/1) - *see* Tumor,
  carcinoid
  and struma ovarii (M9091/1) 236.2
  argentaffin (M8241/1) - see Neoplasm,
    by site, uncertain behavior
    malignant (M8241/3) - see
      Neoplasm, by site, malignant
  benign (M9091/0) 220
  composite (M8244/3) - see Neoplasm,
    by site, malignant
  goblet cell (M8243/3) - see Neoplasm,
    by site, malignant

~~Carcinoid (Continued)~~
~~malignant (M8240/3) - see Neoplasm,~~
~~by site, malignant~~
~~nonargentaffin (M8242/1) - see also~~
~~Neoplasm, by site, uncertain~~
~~behavior~~
~~malignant (M8242/3) - see~~
~~Neoplasm, by site, malignant~~
~~strumal (M9091/1) 236.2~~
~~syndrome (intestinal) (metastatic)~~
~~259.2~~
~~type bronchial adenoma (M8240/3) -~~
~~see Neoplasm, lung, malignant~~
Carcinoidosis 259.2
Carcinoma (M8010/3) - see also Neoplasm,
    by site, malignant

> Note 13 Except where otherwise
> indicated, the morphological varieties
> of carcinoma in the list below should
> be coded by site as for "Neoplasm,
> malignant."

with
    apocrine metaplasia (M8573/3)
    cartilaginous (and osseous)
        metaplasia (M8571/3)
    osseous (and cartilaginous)
        metaplasia (M8571/3)
    productive fibrosis (M8141/3)
    spindle cell metaplasia (M8572/3)
    squamous metaplasia (M8570/3)
acidophil (M8280/3)
    specified site - see Neoplasm, by site,
        malignant
    unspecified site 194.3
acidophil-basophil, mixed (M8281/3)
    specified site - see Neoplasm, by site,
        malignant
    unspecified site 194.3
acinar (cell) (M8550/3)
acinic cell (M8550/3)
adenocystic (M8200/3)
adenoid
    cystic (M8200/3)
    squamous cell (M8075/3)
adenosquamous (M8560/3)
adnexal (skin) (M8390/3) - see
    Neoplasm, skin, malignant
adrenal cortical (M8370/3) 194.0
alveolar (M8251/3)
    cell (M8250/3) - see Neoplasm, lung,
        malignant
anaplastic type (M8021/3)
apocrine (M8401/3)
    breast - see Neoplasm, breast,
        malignant
    specified site NEC - see Neoplasm,
        skin, malignant
    unspecified site 173.9
basal cell (pigmented) (M8090/3) -
    see also Neoplasm, skin,
        malignant
    fibro-epithelial type (M8093/3) -
        see Neoplasm, skin,
        malignant
    morphea type (M8092/3) - see
        Neoplasm, skin, malignant
    multicentric (M8091/3) - see
        Neoplasm, skin, malignant
basaloid (M8123/3)
basal-squamous cell, mixed
    (M8094/3) - see Neoplasm, skin,
        malignant

Carcinoma (Continued)
basophil (M8300/3)
    specified site - see Neoplasm, by site,
        malignant
    unspecified site 194.3
basophil-acidophil, mixed (M8281/3)
    specified site - see Neoplasm, by site,
        malignant
    unspecified site 194.3
basosquamous (M8094/3) - see
    Neoplasm, skin, malignant
bile duct type (M8160/3)
    and hepatocellular, mixed
        (M8180/3) 155.0
    liver 155.1
    specified site NEC - see Neoplasm,
        by site, malignant
    unspecified site 155.1
branchial or branchiogenic 146.8
bronchial or bronchogenic - see
    Neoplasm, lung, malignant
bronchiolar (terminal) (M8250/3) -
    see Neoplasm, lung,
        malignant
bronchiolo-alveolar (M8250/3) -
    see Neoplasm, lung,
        malignant
bronchogenic (epidermoid) 162.9
C cell (M8510/3)
    specified site - see Neoplasm, by site,
        malignant
    unspecified site 193
ceruminous (M8420/3) 173.2
chorionic (M9100/3)
    specified site - see Neoplasm, by site,
        malignant
    unspecified site
        female 181
        male 186.9
chromophobe (M8270/3)
    specified site - see Neoplasm, by site,
        malignant
    unspecified site 194.3
clear cell (mesonephroid type)
    (M8310/3)
cloacogenic (M8124/3)
    specified site - see Neoplasm, by site,
        malignant
    unspecified site 154.8
colloid (M8480/3)
cribriform (M8201/3)
cylindroid type (M8200/3)
diffuse type (M8145/3)
    specified site - see Neoplasm, by site,
        malignant
    unspecified site 151.9
duct (cell) (M8500/3)
    with Paget's disease (M8541/3) -
        see Neoplasm, breast,
        malignant
    infiltrating (M8500/3)
        specified site - see Neoplasm, by
            site, malignant
        unspecified site 174.9
ductal (M8500/3)
ductular, infiltrating (M8521/3)
embryonal (M9070/3)
    and teratoma, mixed (M9081/3)
    combined with choriocarcinoma
        (M9101/3) - see Neoplasm, by
        site, malignant
    infantile type (M9071/3)
    liver 155.0
    polyembryonal type (M9072/3)

Carcinoma (Continued)
endometrioid (M8380/3)
eosinophil (M8280/3)
    specified site - see Neoplasm, by site,
        malignant
    unspecified site 194.3
epidermoid (M8070/3) - see also
    Carcinoma, squamous cell
    and adenocarcinoma, mixed
        (M8560/3)
    in situ, Bowen's type (M8081/2) - see
        Neoplasm, skin, in situ
    intradermal - see Neoplasm, skin, in
        situ
fibroepithelial type basal cell
    (M8093/3) - see Neoplasm, skin,
        malignant
follicular (M8330/3)
    and papillary (mixed) (M8340/3) 193
    moderately differentiated type
        (M8332/3) 193
    pure follicle type (M8331/3) 193
    specified site - see Neoplasm, by site,
        malignant
    trabecular type (M8332/3) 193
    unspecified site 193
    well differentiated type (M8331/3)
        193
gelatinous (M8480/3)
giant cell (M8031/3)
    and spindle cell (M8030/3)
granular cell (M8320/3)
granulosa cell (M8620/3) 183.0
hepatic cell (M8170/3) 155.0
hepatocellular (M8170/3) 155.0
    and bile duct, mixed (M8180/3) 155.0
hepatocholangiolitic (M8180/3) 155.0
Hürthle cell (thyroid) 193
hypernephroid (M8311/3)
in
    adenomatous
        polyp (M8210/3)
        polyposis coli (M8220/3) 153.9
    pleomorphic adenoma (M8940/3)
    polypoid adenoma (M8210/3)
    situ (M8010/3) - see Carcinoma, in
        situ
    tubular adenoma (M8210/3)
    villous adenoma (M8261/3)
infiltrating duct (M8500/3)
    with Paget's disease (M8541/3) - see
        Neoplasm, breast, malignant
    specified site - see Neoplasm, by site,
        malignant
    unspecified site 174.9
inflammatory (M8530/3)
    specified site - see Neoplasm, by site,
        malignant
    unspecified site 174.9
in situ (M8010/2) - see also Neoplasm,
    by site, in situ
    epidermoid (M8070/2) - see also
        Neoplasm, by site, in situ
    with questionable stromal
        invasion (M8076/2)
        specified site - see Neoplasm,
            by site, in situ
        unspecified site 233.1
    Bowen's type (M8081/2) - see
        Neoplasm, skin, in situ
    intraductal (M8500/2)
        specified site - see Neoplasm, by
            site, in situ
        unspecified site 233.0

◄ New   ◄▦ Revised   ~~deleted~~ Deleted   ● Use Additional Digit(s)   ▦ Omit code

Carcinoma (Continued)
  in situ (Continued)
    lobular (M8520/2)
      specified site - see Neoplasm, by
        site, in situ
      unspecified site 233.0
    papillary (M8050/2) - see Neoplasm,
      by site, in situ
    squamous cell (M8070/2) - see also
      Neoplasm, by site, in situ
      with questionable stromal
        invasion (M8076/2)
      specified site - see Neoplasm,
        by site, in situ
      unspecified site 233.1
    transitional cell (M8120/2) - see
      Neoplasm, by site, in situ
  intestinal type (M8144/3)
    specified site - see Neoplasm, by site,
      malignant
    unspecified site 151.9
  intraductal (noninfiltrating)
    (M8500/2)
    papillary (M8503/2)
      specified site - see Neoplasm, by
        site, in situ
      unspecified site 233.0
    specified site - see Neoplasm, by site,
      in situ
    unspecified site 233.0
  intraepidermal (M8070/2) - see also
    Neoplasm, skin, in situ
    squamous cell, Bowen's type
      (M8081/2) - see Neoplasm,
      skin, in situ
  intraepithelial (M8010/2) - see also
    Neoplasm, by site, in situ
    squamous cell (M8072/2) - see
      Neoplasm, by site, in situ
  intraosseous (M9270/3) 170.1
    upper jaw (bone) 170.0
  islet cell (M8150/3)
    and exocrine, mixed (M8154/3)
      specified site - see Neoplasm, by
        site, malignant
      unspecified site 157.9
    pancreas 157.4
    specified site NEC - see Neoplasm,
      by site, malignant
    unspecified site 157.4
  juvenile, breast (M8502/3) - see
    Neoplasm, breast, malignant
  Kulchitsky's cell (carcinoid tumor of
    intestine) 259.2
  large cell (M8012/3)
    squamous cell, non-keratinizing
      type (M8072/3)
  Leydig cell (testis) (M8650/3)
    specified site - see Neoplasm, by site,
      malignant
    unspecified site 186.9
      female 183.0
      male 186.9
  liver cell (M8170/3) 155.0
  lobular (infiltrating) (M8520/3)
    noninfiltrating (M8520/3)
      specified site - see Neoplasm, by
        site, in situ
      unspecified site 233.0
    specified site - see Neoplasm, by site,
      malignant
    unspecified site 174.9
  lymphoepithelial (M8082/3)

Carcinoma (Continued)
  medullary (M8510/3)
    with
      amyloid stroma (M8511/3)
        specified site - see Neoplasm,
          by site, malignant
        unspecified site 193
      lymphoid stroma (M8512/3)
        specified site - see Neoplasm,
          by site, malignant
        unspecified site 174.9
    Merkel cell 209.36 ◀
      buttock 209.36 ◀
      ear 209.31 ◀
      eyelid, including canthus 209.31 ◀
      face 209.31 ◀
      genitals 209.36 ◀
      lip 209.31 ◀
      lower limb 209.34 ◀
      neck 209.32 ◀
      nodal presentation 209.75 ◀
      scalp 209.32 ◀
      secondary (any site) 209.75 ◀
      specified site NEC 209.36 ◀
      trunk 209.35 ◀
      unknown primary site 209.75 ◀
      upper limb 209.33 ◀
      visceral metastatic presentation
        209.75 ◀
  mesometanephric (M9110/3)
  mesonephric (M9110/3)
  metastatic (M8010/6) - see Metastasis,
    cancer
  metatypical (M8095/3) - see Neoplasm,
    skin, malignant
  morphea type basal cell (M8092/3) - see
    Neoplasm, skin, malignant
  mucinous (M8480/3)
  mucin-producing (M8481/3)
  mucin-secreting (M8481/3)
  mucoepidermoid (M8430/3)
  mucoid (M8480/3)
    cell (M8300/3)
      specified site - see Neoplasm, by
        site, malignant
      unspecified site 194.3
  mucous (M8480/3)
  neuroendocrine
    high grade (M8240/3) 209.30
    malignant poorly differentiated
      (M8240/3) 209.30
  nonencapsulated sclerosing (M8350/3)
    193
  noninfiltrating
    intracystic (M8504/2) - see
      Neoplasm, by site, in situ
    intraductal (M8500/2)
      papillary (M8503/2)
        specified site - see Neoplasm,
          by site, in situ
        unspecified site 233.0
      specified site - see Neoplasm, by
        site, in situ
      unspecified site 233.0
    lobular (M8520/2)
      specified site - see Neoplasm, by
        site, in situ
      unspecified site 233.0
  oat cell (M8042/3)
    specified site - see Neoplasm, by site,
      malignant
    unspecified site 162.9
  odontogenic (M9270/3) 170.1
    upper jaw (bone) 170.0
  onocytic (M8290/3)

Carcinoma (Continued)
  oxyphilic (M8290/3)
  papillary (M8050/3)
    and follicular (mixed) (M8340/3) 193
    epidermoid (M8052/3)
    intraductal (noninfiltrating)
      (M8503/2)
      specified site - see Neoplasm, by
        site, in situ
      unspecified site 233.0
    serous (M8460/3)
      specified site - see Neoplasm, by
        site, malignant
      surface (M8461/3)
        specified site - see Neoplasm,
          by site, malignant
        unspecified site 183.0
      unspecified site 183.0
    squamous cell (M8052/3)
    transitional cell (M8130/3)
  papillocystic (M8450/3)
    specified site - see Neoplasm, by site,
      malignant
    unspecified site 183.0
  parafollicular cell (M8510/3)
    specified site - see Neoplasm, by site,
      malignant
    unspecified site 193
  pleomorphic (M8022/3)
  polygonal cell (M8034/3)
  prickle cell (M8070/3)
  pseudoglandular, squamous cell
    (M8075/3)
  pseudomucinous (M8470/3)
    specified site - see Neoplasm, by site,
      malignant
    unspecified site 183.0
  pseudosarcomatous (M8033/3)
  regaud type (M8082/3) - see
    Neoplasm, nasopharynx,
    malignant
  renal cell (M8312/3) 189.0
  reserve cell (M8041/3)
  round cell (M8041/3)
  Schmincke (M8082/3) - see
    Neoplasm, nasopharynx,
    malignant
  Schneiderian (M8121/3)
    specified site - see Neoplasm, by site,
      malignant
    unspecified site 160.0
  scirrhous (M8141/3)
  sebaceous (M8410/3) - see Neoplasm,
    skin, malignant
  secondary (M8010/6) - see Neoplasm,
    by site, malignant, secondary
  secretory, breast (M8502/3) - see
    Neoplasm, breast, malignant
  serous (M8441/3)
    papillary (M8460/3)
      specified site - see Neoplasm, by
        site, malignant
      unspecified site 183.0
    surface, papillary (M8461/3)
      specified site - see Neoplasm, by
        site, malignant
      unspecified site 183.0
  Sertoli cell (M8640/3)
    specified site - see Neoplasm, by site,
      malignant
    unspecified site 186.9
  signet ring cell (M8490/3)
    metastatic (M8490/6) - see
      Neoplasm, by site, secondary
  simplex (M8231/3)

Carcinoma (Continued)
  skin appendage (M8390/3) - see
    Neoplasm, skin, malignant
  small cell (M8041/3)
    fusiform cell type (M8043/3)
    squamous cell, nonkeratinizing type
      (M8073/3)
  solid (M8230/3)
    with amyloid stroma (M8511/3)
      specified site - see Neoplasm, by
        site, malignant
      unspecified site 193
  spheroidal cell (M8035/3)
  spindle cell (M8032/3)
    and giant cell (M8030/3)
  spinous cell (M8070/3)
  squamous (cell) (M8070/3)
    adenoid type (M8075/3)
    and adenocarcinoma, mixed
      (M8560/3)
    intraepidermal, Bowen's type - see
      Neoplasm, skin, in situ
    keratinizing type (large cell)
      (M8071/3)
    large cell, nonkeratinizing type
      (M8072/3)
    microinvasive (M8076/3)
      specified site - see Neoplasm, by
        site, malignant
      unspecified site 180.9
    nonkeratinizing type (M8072/3)
    papillary (M8052/3)
    pseudoglandular (M8075/3)
    small cell, nonkeratinizing type
      (M8073/3)
    spindle cell type (M8074/3)
    verrucous (M8051/3)
  superficial spreading (M8143/3)
  sweat gland (M8400/3) - see Neoplasm,
    skin, malignant
  theca cell (M8600/3) 183.0
  thymic (M8580/3) 164.0
  trabecular (M8190/3)
  transitional (cell) (M8120/3)
    papillary (M8130/3)
    spindle cell type (M8122/3)
  tubular (M8211/3)
  undifferentiated type (M8020/3)
  urothelial (M8120/3)
  ventriculi 151.9
  verrucous (epidermoid) (squamous
    cell) (M8051/3)
  villous (M8262/3)
  water-clear cell (M8322/3) 194.1
  wolffian duct (M9110/3)
Carcinomaphobia 300.29
Carcinomatosis
  peritonei (M8010/6) 197.6
  specified site NEC (M8010/3) - see
    Neoplasm, by site, malignant
  unspecified site (M8010/6) 199.0
Carcinosarcoma (M8980/3) - see also
  Neoplasm, by site, malignant
  embryonal type (M8981/3) - see
    Neoplasm, by site, malignant
Cardia, cardial - see condition
Cardiac - see also condition
  death - see Disease, heart
  device
    defibrillator, automatic implantable
      V45.02
    in situ NEC V45.00
    pacemaker
      cardiac
        fitting or adjustment
          V53.31
        in situ V45.01

Cardiac (Continued)
  device (Continued)
    carotid sinus
      fitting or adjustment V53.39
      in situ V45.09
    pacemaker - see Cardiac, device,
      pacemaker
    tamponade 423.3
Cardialgia (see also Pain, precordial)
  786.51
Cardiectasis - see Hypertrophy, cardiac
Cardiochalasia 530.81
Cardiomalacia (see also Degeneration,
  myocardial) 429.1
Cardiomegalia glycogenica diffusa 271.0
Cardiomegaly (see also Hypertrophy,
  cardiac) 429.3
  congenital 746.89
  glycogen 271.0
  hypertensive (see also Hypertension,
    heart) 402.90
  idiopathic 425.4
Cardiomyoliposis (see also Degeneration,
  myocardial) 429.1
Cardiomyopathy (congestive) (constrictive)
  (familial) (infiltrative) (obstructive)
  (restrictive) (sporadic) 425.4
  alcoholic 425.5
  amyloid 277.39 [425.7]
  beriberi 265.0 [425.7]
  cobalt-beer 425.5
  congenital 425.3
  due to
    amyloidosis 277.39 [425.7]
    beriberi 265.0 [425.7]
    cardiac glycogenosis 271.0 [425.7]
    Chagas' disease 086.0
    Friedreich's ataxia 334.0 [425.8]
    hypertension - see Hypertension,
      with, heart involvement
    mucopolysaccharidosis 277.5 [425.7]
    myotonia atrophica 359.21 [425.8]
    progressive muscular dystrophy
      359.1 [425.8]
    sarcoidosis 135 [425.8]
  glycogen storage 271.0 [425.7]
  hypertensive - see Hypertension, with,
    heart involvement
  hypertrophic
    nonobstructive 425.4
    obstructive 425.1
      congenital 746.84
  idiopathic (concentric) 425.4
  in
    Chagas' disease 086.0
    sarcoidosis 135 [425.8]
  ischemic 414.8
  metabolic NEC 277.9 [425.7]
    amyloid 277.39 [425.7]
    thyrotoxic (see also Thyrotoxicosis)
      242.9● [425.7]
    thyrotoxicosis (see also
      Thyrotoxicosis) 242.9● [425.7]
  newborn 425.4
    congenital 425.3
  nutritional 269.9 [425.7]
    beriberi 265.0 [425.7]
  obscure of Africa 425.2
  peripartum 674.5●
  postpartum 674.5●
  primary 425.4
  secondary 425.9
  stress induced 429.83
  takotsubo 429.83
  thyrotoxic (see also Thyrotoxicosis)
    242.9● [425.7]

Cardiomyopathy (Continued)
  toxic NEC 425.9
  tuberculous (see also Tuberculosis)
    017.9● [425.8]
Cardionephritis - see Hypertension,
  cardiorenal
Cardionephropathy - see Hypertension,
  cardiorenal
Cardionephrosis - see Hypertension,
  cardiorenal
Cardioneurosis 306.2
Cardiopathia nigra 416.0
Cardiopathy (see also Disease, heart)
  429.9
  hypertensive (see also Hypertension,
    heart) 402.90
  idiopathic 425.4
  mucopolysaccharidosis 277.5 [425.7]
Cardiopericarditis (see also Pericarditis)
  423.9
Cardiophobia 300.29
Cardioptosis 746.87
Cardiorenal - see condition
Cardiorrhexis (see also Infarct,
  myocardium) 410.9●
Cardiosclerosis - see Arteriosclerosis,
  coronary
Cardiosis - see Disease, heart
Cardiospasm (esophagus) (reflex)
  (stomach) 530.0
  congenital 750.7
Cardiostenosis - see Disease, heart
Cardiosymphysis 423.1
Cardiothyrotoxicosis - see
  Hyperthyroidism
Cardiovascular - see condition
Carditis (acute) (bacterial) (chronic)
  (subacute) 429.89
  Coxsackie 074.20
  hypertensive (see also Hypertension,
    heart) 402.90
  meningococcal 036.40
  rheumatic - see Disease, heart,
    rheumatic
  rheumatoid 714.2
Care (of)
  child (routine) V20.1
  convalescent following V66.9
    chemotherapy V66.2
    medical NEC V66.5
    psychotherapy V66.3
    radiotherapy V66.1
    surgery V66.0
    surgical NEC V66.0
    treatment (for) V66.5
      combined V66.6
      fracture V66.4
      mental disorder NEC V66.3
      specified type NEC V66.5
  end-of-life V66.7
  family member (handicapped) (sick)
    creating problem for family V61.49
    provided away from home for
      holiday relief V60.5
    unavailable, due to
      absence (person rendering care)
        (sufferer) V60.4
      inability (any reason) of person
        rendering care V60.4
  holiday relief V60.5
  hospice V66.7
  lack of (at or after birth) (infant) (child)
    995.52
    adult 995.84
  lactation of mother V24.1
  palliative V66.7

◀ New   ◀▥ Revised   ~~deleted~~ Deleted   ● Use Additional Digit(s)   ▨ Omit code

Care *(Continued)*
  postpartum
    immediately after delivery V24.0
    routine follow-up V24.2
  prenatal V22.1
    first pregnancy V22.0
    high-risk pregnancy V23.9
      specified problem NEC V23.89
  terminal V66.7
  unavailable, due to
    absence of person rendering care
      V60.4
    inability (any reason) of person
      rendering care V60.4
  well baby V20.1
Caries (bone) *(see also* Tuberculosis, bone)
  015.9● *[730.8]*●
  arrested 521.04
  cementum 521.03
  cerebrospinal (tuberculous) 015.0●
    [730.88]
  dental (acute) (chronic) (incipient)
    (infected) 521.00
    with pulp exposure 521.03
    extending to
      dentine 521.02
      pulp 521.03
    other specified NEC 521.09
    pit and fissure 521.06
    primary
      pit and fissure origin 521.06
      root surface 521.08
      smooth surface origin 521.07
    root surface 521.08
    smooth surface 521.07
  dentin (acute) (chronic) 521.02
  enamel (acute) (chronic) (incipient)
    521.01
  external meatus 380.89
  hip *(see also* Tuberculosis) 015.1● *[730.85]*
  initial 521.01
  knee 015.2● *[730.86]*
  labyrinth 386.8
  limb NEC 015.7● *[730.88]*
  mastoid (chronic) (process) 383.1
  middle ear 385.89
  nose 015.7● *[730.88]*
  orbit 015.7● *[730.88]*
  ossicle 385.24
  petrous bone 383.20
  sacrum (tuberculous) 015.0● *[730.88]*
  spine, spinal (column) (tuberculous)
    015.0● *[730.88]*
  syphilitic 095.5
    congenital 090.0 *[730.8]*●
  teeth (internal) 521.00
    initial 521.01
  vertebra (column) (tuberculous) 015.0●
    [730.88]
Carini's syndrome (ichthyosis congenita)
  757.1
Carious teeth 521.00
Carneous mole 631
Carnosinemia 270.5
Carotid body or sinus syndrome 337.01
Carotidynia 337.01
Carotinemia (dietary) 278.3
Carotinosis (cutis) (skin) 278.3
Carpal tunnel syndrome 354.0
Carpenter's syndrome 759.89
Carpopedal spasm *(see also* Tetany) 781.7
Carpoptosis 736.05
Carrier (suspected) of
  amebiasis V02.2
  bacterial disease (meningococcal,
    staphylococcal) NEC V02.59

Carrier *(Continued)*
  cholera V02.0
  cystic fibrosis gene V83.81
  defective gene V83.89
  diphtheria V02.4
  dysentery (bacillary) V02.3
    amebic V02.2
  Endamoeba histolytica V02.2
  gastrointestinal pathogens NEC V02.3
  genetic defect V83.89
  gonorrhea V02.7
  group B streptococcus V02.51
  HAA (hepatitis Australian-antigen)
    V02.61
  hemophilia A (asymptomatic) V83.01
    symptomatic V83.02
  hepatitis V02.60
    Australian-antigen (HAA) V02.61
    B V02.61
    C V02.62
    specified type NEC V02.69
    serum V02.61
    viral V02.60
  infective organism NEC V02.9
  malaria V02.9
  paratyphoid V02.3
  Salmonella V02.3
    typhosa V02.1
  serum hepatitis V02.61
  Shigella V02.3
  Staphylococcus NEC V02.59
    methicillin
      resistant Staphylococcus aureus
        V02.54
      susceptible Staphylococcus
        aureus V02.53
  Streptococcus NEC V02.52
    group B V02.51
  typhoid V02.1
  venereal disease NEC V02.8
Carrión's disease (Bartonellosis) 088.0
Car sickness 994.6
Carter's
  relapsing fever (Asiatic) 087.0
Cartilage - *see* condition
Caruncle (inflamed)
  abscess, lacrimal *(see also*
    Dacryocystitis) 375.30
  conjunctiva 372.00
    acute 372.00
  eyelid 373.00
  labium (majus) (minus) 616.89
  lacrimal 375.30
  urethra (benign) 599.3
  vagina (wall) 616.89
Cascade stomach 537.6
Caseation lymphatic gland *(see also*
  Tuberculosis) 017.2●
Caseous
  bronchitis - *see* Tuberculosis,
    pulmonary
  meningitis 013.0●
  pneumonia - *see* Tuberculosis,
    pulmonary
Cassidy (-Scholte) syndrome (malignant
  carcinoid) 259.2
Castellani's bronchitis 104.8
Castleman's tumor or lymphoma
  (mediastinal lymph node
  hyperplasia) 785.6
Castration, traumatic 878.2
  complicated 878.3
Casts in urine 791.7
Cat's ear 744.29
Catalepsy 300.11
  catatonic (acute) *(see also*
    Schizophrenia) 295.2●

Catalepsy *(Continued)*
  hysterical 300.11
  schizophrenic *(see also* Schizophrenia)
    295.2●
Cataphasia 307.0
Cataplexy (idiopathic) *see also*
  Narcolepsy
Cataract (anterior cortical) (anterior polar)
  (black) (capsular) (central) (cortical)
  (hypermature) (immature)
  (incipient) (mature) 366.9
  anterior
    and posterior axial embryonal
      743.33
    pyramidal 743.31
    subcapsular polar
      infantile, juvenile, or presenile
        366.01
      senile 366.13
  associated with
    calcinosis 275.40 *[366.42]*
    craniofacial dysostosis 756.0 *[366.44]*
    galactosemia 271.1 *[366.44]*
    hypoparathyroidism 252.1 *[366.42]*
    myotonic disorders 359.21 *[366.43]*
    neovascularization 366.33
  blue dot 743.39
  cerulean 743.39
  complicated NEC 366.30
  congenital 743.30
    capsular or subcapsular 743.31
    cortical 743.32
    nuclear 743.33
    specified type NEC 743.39
    total or subtotal 743.34
    zonular 743.32
  coronary (congenital) 743.39
    acquired 366.12
  cupuliform 366.14
  diabetic 250.5● *[366.41]*
    due to secondary diabetes 249.5●
      [366.41]
  drug-induced 366.45
  due to
    chalcosis 360.24 *[366.34]*
    chronic choroiditis *(see also*
      Choroiditis) 363.20 *[366.32]*
    degenerative myopia 360.21 *[366.34]*
    glaucoma *(see also* Glaucoma) 365.9
      [366.31]
    infection, intraocular NEC 366.32
    inflammatory ocular disorder NEC
      366.32
    iridocyclitis, chronic 364.10 *[366.33]*
    pigmentary retinal dystrophy 362.74
      [366.34]
    radiation 366.46
  electric 366.46
  glassblowers' 366.46
  heat ray 366.46
  heterochromic 366.33
  in eye disease NEC 366.30
  infantile *(see also* Cataract, juvenile)
    366.00
  intumescent 366.12
  irradiational 366.46
  juvenile 366.00
    anterior subcapsular polar 366.01
    combined forms 366.09
    cortical 366.03
    lamellar 366.03
    nuclear 366.04
    posterior subcapsular polar 366.02
    specified NEC 366.09
    zonular 366.03

Cataract *(Continued)*
lamellar 743.32
  infantile juvenile, or presenile 366.03
morgagnian 366.18
myotonic 359.21 *[366.43]*
myxedema 244.9 *[366.44]*
  nuclear 366.16
posterior, polar (capsular) 743.31
  infantile, juvenile, or presenile
    366.02
  senile 366.14
presenile *(see also* Cataract, juvenile)
  366.00
punctate
  acquired 366.12
  congenital 743.39
secondary (membrane) 366.50
  obscuring vision 366.53
  specified type, not obscuring vision
    366.52
senile 366.10
  anterior subcapsular polar 366.13
  combined forms 366.19
  cortical 366.15
  hypermature 366.18
  immature 366.12
  incipient 366.12
  mature 366.17
  nuclear 366.16
  posterior subcapsular polar 366.14
  specified NEC 366.19
  total or subtotal 366.17
snowflake 250.5● *[366.41]*
  due to secondary diabetes 249.5●
    [366.41]
specified NEC 366.8
subtotal (senile) 366.17
  congenital 743.34
sunflower 360.24 *[366.34]*
tetanic NEC 252.1 *[366.42]*
total (mature) (senile) 366.17
  congenital 743.34
  localized 366.21
  traumatic 366.22
toxic 366.45
traumatic 366.20
  partially resolved 366.23
  total 366.22
zonular (perinuclear) 743.32
  infantile, juvenile, or presenile
    366.03
Cataracta 366.10
brunescens 366.16
cerulea 743.39
complicata 366.30
congenita 743.30
coralliformis 743.39
coronaria (congenital) 743.39
  acquired 366.12
diabetic 250.5● *[366.41]*
  due to secondary diabetes 249.5●
    [366.41]
floriformis 360.24 *[366.34]*
membranacea
  accreta 366.50
  congenita 743.39
nigra 366.16
Catarrh, catarrhal (inflammation) *(see also* condition) 460
acute 460
asthma, asthmatic *(see also* Asthma)
  493.9●
Bostock's *(see also* Fever, hay) 477.9
bowel - *see* Enteritis

Catarrh, catarrhal *(Continued)*
bronchial 490
  acute 466.0
  chronic 491.0
  subacute 466.0
cervix, cervical (canal) (uteri) - *see*
  Cervicitis
chest *(see also* Bronchitis) 490
chronic 472.0
congestion 472.0
conjunctivitis 372.03
due to syphilis 095.9
  congenital 090.0
enteric - *see* Enteritis
epidemic 487.1
Eustachian 381.50
eye (acute) (vernal) 372.03
fauces *(see also* Pharyngitis) 462
febrile 460
fibrinous acute 466.0
gastroenteric - *see* Enteritis
gastrointestinal - *see* Enteritis
gingivitis 523.00
hay *(see also* Fever, hay) 477.9
infectious 460
intestinal - *see* Enteritis
larynx *(see also* Laryngitis, chronic)
  476.0
liver 070.1
  with hepatic coma 070.0
lung *(see also* Bronchitis) 490
  acute 466.0
  chronic 491.0
middle ear (chronic) - *see* Otitis media,
  chronic
mouth 528.00
nasal (chronic) *(see also* Rhinitis)
  472.0
  acute 460
nasobronchial 472.2
nasopharyngeal (chronic) 472.2
  acute 460
nose - *see* Catarrh, nasal
ophthalmia 372.03
pneumococcal, acute 466.0
pulmonary *(see also* Bronchitis) 490
  acute 466.0
  chronic 491.0
spring (eye) 372.13
suffocating *(see also* Asthma) 493.9●
summer (hay) *(see also* Fever, hay)
  477.9
throat 472.1
tracheitis 464.10
  with obstruction 464.11
tubotympanal 381.4
  acute *(see also* Otitis media, acute,
    nonsuppurative) 381.00
  chronic 381.10
vasomotor *(see also* Fever, hay) 477.9
vesical (bladder) - *see* Cystitis
Catarrhus aestivus *(see also* Fever, hay)
  477.9
Catastrophe, cerebral *(see also* Disease,
  cerebrovascular, acute) 436
Catatonia, catatonic (acute) 781.99
with
  affective psychosis - *see* Psychosis,
    affective
  agitation 295.2●
  dementia (praecox) 295.2●
  due to or associated with physical
    condition 293.89
excitation 295.2●

Catatonia, catatonic *(Continued)*
excited type 295.2●
in conditions classified elsewhere
  293.89
schizophrenia 295.2●
stupor 295.2●
Cat-scratch - *see also* Injury, superficial
disease or fever 078.3
Cauda equina - *see also* condition
syndrome 344.60
Cauliflower ear 738.7
Caul over face 768.9
Causalgia 355.9
lower limb 355.71
upper limb 354.4
Cause
external, general effects NEC 994.9
not stated 799.9
unknown 799.9
Caustic burn - *see also* Burn, by site
from swallowing caustic or corrosive
  substance - *see* Burn, internal
  organs
Cavare's disease (familial periodic
  paralysis) 359.3
Cave-in, injury
crushing (severe) *(see also* Crush, by
  site) 869.1
suffocation 994.7
Cavernitis (penis) 607.2
lymph vessel - *see* Lymphangioma
Cavernositis 607.2
Cavernous - *see* condition
Cavitation of lung *(see also* Tuberculosis)
  011.2●
nontuberculous 518.89
primary, progressive 010.8●
Cavity
lung - *see* Cavitation of lung
optic papilla 743.57
pulmonary - *see* Cavitation of lung
teeth 521.00
vitreous (humor) 379.21
Cavovarus foot, congenital 754.59
Cavus foot (congenital) 754.71
acquired 736.73
Cazenave's
disease (pemphigus) NEC 694.4
lupus (erythematosus) 695.4
CDGS (carbohydrate-deficient
  glycoprotein syndrome) 271.8
Cecitis - *see* Appendicitis
Cecocele - *see* Hernia
Cecum - *see* condition
Celiac
artery compression syndrome 447.4
disease 579.0
infantilism 579.0
Cell, cellular - *see also* condition
anterior chamber (eye) (positive
  aqueous ray) 364.04
Cellulitis (diffuse) (with lymphangitis)
  (see also Abscess) 682.9
abdominal wall 682.2
anaerobic *(see also* Gas gangrene) 040.0
ankle 682.6
anus 566
areola 611.0
arm (any part, above wrist) 682.3
auditory canal (external) 380.10
axilla 682.3
back (any part) 682.2
breast 611.0
  postpartum 675.1●

◀ New   ◀ Revised   ~~deleted~~ Deleted   ● Use Additional Digit(s)   ▬ Omit code

Cellulitis *(Continued)*
  broad ligament *(see also* Disease, pelvis, inflammatory) 614.4
    acute 614.3
  buttock 682.5
  cervical (neck region) 682.1
  cervix (uteri) *(see also* Cervicitis) 616.0
  cheek, external 682.0
    internal 528.3
  chest wall 682.2
  chronic NEC 682.9
  colostomy 569.61
  corpus cavernosum 607.2
  digit 681.9
  Douglas' cul-de-sac or pouch (chronic) *(see also* Disease, pelvis, inflammatory) 614.4
    acute 614.3
  drainage site (following operation) 998.59
  ear, external 380.10
  enterostomy 569.61
  erysipelar *(see also* Erysipelas) 035
  esophagostomy 530.86
  eyelid 373.13
  face (any part, except eye) 682.0
  finger (intrathecal) (periosteal) (subcutaneous) (subcuticular) 681.00
  flank 682.2
  foot (except toe) 682.7
  forearm 682.3
  gangrenous *(see also* Gangrene) 785.4
  genital organ NEC
    female - *see* Abscess, genital organ, female
    male 608.4
  glottis 478.71
  gluteal (region) 682.5
  gonococcal NEC 098.0
  groin 682.2
  hand (except finger or thumb) 682.4
  head (except face) NEC 682.8
  heel 682.7
  hip 682.6
  jaw (region) 682.0
  knee 682.6
  labium (majus) (minus) *(see also* Vulvitis) 616.10
  larynx 478.71
  leg, except foot 682.6
  lip 528.5
  mammary gland 611.0
  mouth (floor) 528.3
  multiple sites NEC 682.9
  nasopharynx 478.21
  navel 682.2
    newborn NEC 771.4
  neck (region) 682.1
  nipple 611.0
  nose 478.19
    external 682.0
  orbit, orbital 376.01
  palate (soft) 528.3
  pectoral (region) 682.2
  pelvis, pelvic
    with
      abortion - *see* Abortion, by type, with sepsis
      ectopic pregnancy *(see also* categories 633.0–633.9) 639.0
      molar pregnancy *(see also* categories 630–632) 639.0

Cellulitis *(Continued)*
  pelvis, pelvic *(Continued)*
    female *(see also* Disease, pelvis, inflammatory) 614.4
      acute 614.3
      following
        abortion 639.0
        ectopic or molar pregnancy 639.0
      male 567.21
      puerperal, postpartum, childbirth 670.8 ◀▥
  penis 607.2
  perineal, perineum 682.2
  perirectal 566
  peritonsillar 475
  periurethral 597.0
  periuterine *(see also* Disease, pelvis, inflammatory) 614.4
    acute 614.3
  pharynx 478.21
  phlegmonous NEC 682.9
  rectum 566
  retromammary 611.0
  retroperitoneal *(see also* Peritonitis) 567.38
  round ligament *(see also* Disease, pelvis, inflammatory) 614.4
    acute 614.3
  scalp (any part) 682.8
    dissecting 704.8
  scrotum 608.4
  seminal vesicle 608.0
  septic NEC 682.9
  shoulder 682.3
  specified sites NEC 682.8
  spermatic cord 608.4
  submandibular (region) (space) (triangle) 682.0
    gland 527.3
  submaxillary 528.3
    gland 527.3
  submental (pyogenic) 682.0
    gland 527.3
  suppurative NEC 682.9
  testis 608.4
  thigh 682.6
  thumb (intrathecal) (periosteal) (subcutaneous) (subcuticular) 681.00
  toe (intrathecal) (periosteal) (subcutaneous) (subcuticular) 681.10
  tonsil 475
  trunk 682.2
  tuberculous (primary) *(see also* Tuberculosis) 017.0 ●
  tunica vaginalis 608.4
  umbilical 682.2
    newborn NEC 771.4
  vaccinal 999.39
  vagina - *see* Vaginitis
  vas deferens 608.4
  vocal cords 478.5
  vulva *(see also* Vulvitis) 616.10
  wrist 682.4
Cementoblastoma, benign (M9273/0) 213.1
  upper jaw (bone) 213.0
Cementoma (M9273/0) 213.1
  gigantiform (M9276/0) 213.1
    upper jaw (bone) 213.0
  upper jaw (bone) 213.0
Cementoperiostitis 523.40
  acute 523.33
  apical 523.40

Cephalgia, cephalagia *(see also* Headache) 784.0
  histamine 339.00
  nonorganic origin 307.81
  other trigeminal autonomic (TACS) 339.09
  psychogenic 307.81
  tension 307.81
Cephalhematocele, cephalematocele
  due to birth injury 767.19
  fetus or newborn 767.19
  traumatic *(see also* Contusion, head) 920
Cephalhematoma, cephalematoma (calcified)
  due to birth injury 767.19
  fetus or newborn 767.19
  traumatic *(see also* Contusion, head) 920
Cephalic - *see* condition
Cephalitis - *see* Encephalitis
Cephalocele 742.0
Cephaloma - *see* Neoplasm, by site, malignant
Cephalomenia 625.8
Cephalopelvic - *see* condition
Cercomoniasis 007.3
Cerebellitis - *see* Encephalitis
Cerebellum (cerebellar) - *see* condition
Cerebral - *see* condition
Cerebritis - *see* Encephalitis
Cerebrohepatorenal syndrome 759.89
Cerebromacular degeneration 330.1
Cerebromalacia *(see also* Softening, brain) 434.9 ●
Cerebrosidosis 272.7
Cerebrospasticity - *see* Palsy, cerebral
Cerebrospinal - *see* condition
Cerebrum - *see* condition
Ceroid storage disease 272.7
Cerumen (accumulation) (impacted) 380.4
Cervical - *see also* condition
  auricle 744.43
  high risk human papillomavirus (HPV) DNA test positive 795.05
  intraepithelial glandular neoplasia 233.1
  low risk human papillomavirus (HPV) DNA test positive 795.09
  rib 756.2
  shortening - *see* Short, cervical
Cervicalgia 723.1
Cervicitis (acute) (chronic) (nonvenereal) (subacute) (with erosion or ectropion) 616.0
  with
    abortion - *see* Abortion, by type, with sepsis
    ectopic pregnancy *(see also* categories 633.0-633.9) 639.0
    molar pregnancy *(see also* categories 630-632) 639.0
    ulceration 616.0
  chlamydial 099.53
  complicating pregnancy or puerperium 646.6 ●
    affecting fetus or newborn 760.8
  following
    abortion 639.0
    ectopic or molar pregnancy 639.0
  gonococcal (acute) 098.15
    chronic or duration of 2 months or more 098.35
  senile (atrophic) 616.0
  syphilitic 095.8

Cervicitis *(Continued)*
trichomonal 131.09
tuberculous *(see also* Tuberculosis)
016.7●
Cervicoaural fistula 744.49
Cervicocolpitis (emphysematosa) *(see also*
Cervicitis) 616.0
Cervix - *see* condition
Cesarean delivery, operation or section
NEC 669.7●
affecting fetus or newborn 763.4
post mortem, affecting fetus or
newborn 761.6
previous, affecting management of
pregnancy 654.2●
Céstan's syndrome 344.89
Céstan-Chenais paralysis 344.89
Céstan-Raymond syndrome 433.8●
Cestode infestation NEC 123.9
specified type NEC 123.8
Cestodiasis 123.9
CGF (congenital generalized fibromatosis)
759.89
Chabert's disease 022.9
Chacaleh 266.2
Chafing 709.8
Chagas' disease *(see also* Trypanosomiasis,
American) 086.2
with heart involvement 086.0
Chagres fever 084.0
Chalasia (cardiac sphincter) 530.81
Chalazion 373.2
Chalazoderma 757.39
Chalcosis 360.24
cornea 371.15
crystalline lens 360.24 *[366.34]*
retina 360.24
Chalicosis (occupational) (pulmonum) 502
Chancre (any genital site) (hard)
(indurated) (infecting) (primary)
(recurrent) 091.0
congenital 090.0
conjunctiva 091.2
Ducrey's 099.0
extragenital 091.2
eyelid 091.2
Hunterian 091.0
lip (syphilis) 091.2
mixed 099.8
nipple 091.2
Nisbet's 099.0
of
carate 103.0
pinta 103.0
yaws 102.0
palate, soft 091.2
phagedenic 099.0
Ricord's 091.0
Rollet's (syphilitic) 091.0
seronegative 091.0
seropositive 091.0
simple 099.0
soft 099.0
bubo 099.0
urethra 091.0
yaws 102.0
Chancriform syndrome 114.1
Chancroid 099.0
anus 099.0
penis (Ducrey's bacillus) 099.0
perineum 099.0
rectum 099.0
scrotum 099.0
urethra 099.0
vulva 099.0

Chandipura fever 066.8
Chandler's disease (osteochondritis
dissecans, hip) 732.7
Change(s) (of) - *see also* Removal of
arteriosclerotic - *see* Arteriosclerosis
battery
cardiac pacemaker V53.31
bone 733.90
diabetic 250.8● *[731.8]*
due to secondary diabetes 249.8●
[731.8]
in disease, unknown cause 733.90
bowel habits 787.99
cardiorenal (vascular) *(see also*
Hypertension, cardiorenal) 404.90
cardiovascular - *see* Disease,
cardiovascular
circulatory 459.9
cognitive or personality change of
other type, nonpsychotic 310.1
color, teeth, tooth
during formation 520.8
extrinsic 523.6
intrinsic posteruptive 521.7
contraceptive device V25.42
cornea, corneal
degenerative NEC 371.40
membrane NEC 371.30
senile 371.41
coronary *(see also* Ischemia, heart) 414.9
degenerative
chamber angle (anterior) (iris) 364.56
ciliary body 364.57
spine or vertebra *(see also*
Spondylosis) 721.90
dental pulp, regressive 522.2
drains V58.49
dressing
wound V58.30
nonsurgical V58.30
surgical V58.31
fixation device V54.89
external V54.89
internal V54.01
heart - *see also* Disease, heart
hip joint 718.95
hyperplastic larynx 478.79
hypertrophic
nasal sinus *(see also* Sinusitis) 473.9
turbinate, nasal 478.0
upper respiratory tract 478.9
inflammatory - *see* Inflammation
joint *(see also* Derangement, joint) 718.90
sacroiliac 724.6
Kirschner wire V54.89
knee 717.9
macular, congenital 743.55
malignant (M----/3) - *see also*
Neoplasm, by site, malignant

> Note 14   For malignant change occur-
> ring in a neoplasm, use the appropriate
> M code with behavior digit/3 e.g.,
> malignant change in uterine fibroid-
> M8890/3. For malignant change occur-
> ring in a nonneoplastic condition (e.g.,
> gastric ulcer) use the M code M8000/3.

mental (status) NEC 780.97
due to or associated with physical
condition - *see* Syndrome, brain
myocardium, myocardial - *see*
Degeneration, myocardial
of life *(see also* Menopause) 627.2
pacemaker battery (cardiac) V53.31

Change(s) *(Continued)*
peripheral nerve 355.9
personality (nonpsychotic) NEC 310.1
plaster cast V54.89
refractive, transient 367.81
regressive, dental pulp 522.2
retina 362.9
myopic (degenerative) (malignant)
360.21
vascular appearance 362.13
sacroiliac joint 724.6
scleral 379.19
degenerative 379.16
senile *(see also* Senility) 797
sensory *(see also* Disturbance,
sensation) 782.0
skin texture 782.8
spinal cord 336.9
splint, external V54.89
subdermal implantable contraceptive
V25.5
suture V58.32
traction device V54.89
trophic 355.9
arm NEC 354.9
leg NEC 355.8
lower extremity NEC 355.8
upper extremity NEC 354.9
vascular 459.9
vasomotor 443.9
voice 784.49
psychogenic 306.1
wound packing V58.30
nonsurgical V58.30
surgical V58.31
Changing sleep-work schedule, affecting
sleep 327.36
Changuinola fever 066.0
Chapping skin 709.8
Character
depressive 301.12
Charcôt's
arthropathy 094.0 *[713.5]*
cirrhosis - *see* Cirrhosis, biliary
disease 094.0
spinal cord 094.0
fever (biliary) (hepatic) (intermittent) -
see Choledocholithiasis
joint (disease) 094.0 *[713.5]*
diabetic 250.6● *[713.5]*
due to secondary diabetes 249.6●
[713.5]
syringomyelic 336.0 *[713.5]*
syndrome (intermittent claudication)
443.9
due to atherosclerosis 440.21
Charcôt-Marie-Tooth disease, paralysis,
or syndrome 356.1
CHARGE association (syndrome) 759.89
Charleyhorse (quadriceps) 843.8
muscle, except quadriceps - *see* Sprain,
by site
Charlouis' disease *(see also* Yaws) 102.9
Chauffeur's fracture - *see* Fracture, ulna,
lower end
Cheadle (-Möller) (-Barlow) disease or
syndrome (infantile scurvy) 267
Checking (of)
contraceptive device (intrauterine)
V25.42
device
fixation V54.89
external V54.89
internal V54.09
traction V54.89

◀ New   ◀▦ Revised   ~~deleted~~ Deleted   ● Use Additional Digit(s)   ▨ Omit code

Checking (Continued)
  Kirschner wire V54.89
  plaster cast V54.89
  splint, external V54.89
Checkup
  following treatment - see Examination
  health V70.0
  infant (over 28 days old) (not sick)
    V20.2 ◄▪▪▪
  newborn, routine
    initial V20.2
    subsequent V20.2
    8 to 28 days old V20.32 ◄
    over 28 days old, routine V20.2 ◄
    under 8 days old V20.31 ◄
    weight V20.32 ◄
  pregnancy (normal) V22.1
    first V22.0
    high-risk pregnancy V23.9
      specified problem NEC V23.89
Chédiak-Higashi (-Steinbrinck) anomaly,
  disease, or syndrome (congenital
  gigantism of peroxidase granules)
  288.2
Cheek - see also condition
  biting 528.9
Cheese itch 133.8
Cheese washers' lung 495.8
Cheilitis 528.5
  actinic (due to sun) 692.72
    chronic NEC 692.74
      due to radiation, except from sun
        692.82
      due to radiation, except from sun
        692.82
  acute 528.5
  angular 528.5
  catarrhal 528.5
  chronic 528.5
  exfoliative 528.5
  gangrenous 528.5
  glandularis apostematosa 528.5
  granulomatosa 351.8
  infectional 528.5
  membranous 528.5
  Miescher's 351.8
  suppurative 528.5
  ulcerative 528.5
  vesicular 528.5
Cheilodynia 528.5
Cheilopalatoschisis (see also Cleft, palate,
  with cleft lip) 749.20
Cheilophagia 528.9
Cheiloschisis (see also Cleft, lip) 749.10
Cheilosis 528.5
  with pellagra 265.2
  angular 528.5
  due to
    dietary deficiency 266.0
    vitamin deficiency 266.0
Cheiromegaly 729.89
Cheiropompholyx 705.81
Cheloid (see also Keloid) 701.4
Chemical burn - see also Burn, by site
  from swallowing chemical - see Burn,
    internal organs
Chemodectoma (M8693/1) - see
  Paraganglioma, nonchromaffin
Chemoprophylaxis NEC V07.39
Chemosis, conjunctiva 372.73
Chemotherapy
  convalescence V66.2
  encounter (for) (oral) (intravenous)
    V58.11 ◄▪▪▪
  maintenance (oral) (intravenous)
    V58.11 ◄▪▪▪

Chemotherapy (Continued)
  prophylactic NEC V07.39
    fluoride V07.31
Cherubism 526.89
Chest - see condition
Cheyne-Stokes respiration (periodic)
  786.04
Chiari's
  disease or syndrome (hepatic vein
    thrombosis) 453.0
  malformation
    type I 348.4
    type II (see also Spina bifida) 741.0●
    type III 742.0
    type IV 742.2
    network 746.89
Chiari-Frommel syndrome 676.6●
Chicago disease (North American
  blastomycosis) 116.0
Chickenpox (see also Varicella) 052.9
  exposure to V01.71
  vaccination and inoculation
    (prophylactic) V05.4
Chiclero ulcer 085.4
Chiggers 133.8
Chignon 111.2
  fetus or newborn (from vacuum
    extraction) 767.19
Chigoe disease 134.1
Chikungunya fever 066.3
Chilaiditi's syndrome (subphrenic
  displacement, colon) 751.4
Chilblains 991.5
  lupus 991.5
Child
  behavior causing concern V61.20
    adopted child V61.24 ◄
    biological child V61.23 ◄
    foster child V61.25 ◄
Childbed fever 670.8 ◄▪▪▪
Childbirth - see also Delivery
  puerperal complications - see Puerperal
Childhood, period of rapid growth V21.0
Chill(s) 780.64
  with fever 780.60
  without fever 780.64
  congestive 780.99
    in malarial regions 084.6
  septic - see Septicemia
  urethral 599.84
Chilomastigiasis 007.8
Chin - see condition
Chinese dysentery 004.9
Chiropractic dislocation (see also Lesion,
  nonallopathic, by site) 739.9
Chitral fever 066.0
Chlamydia, chlamydial - see condition
Chloasma 709.09
  cachecticorum 709.09
  eyelid 374.52
    congenital 757.33
    hyperthyroid 242.0●
  gravidarum 646.8●
  idiopathic 709.09
  skin 709.09
  symptomatic 709.09
Chloroma (M9930/3) 205.3●
Chlorosis 280.9
  Egyptian (see also Ancylostomiasis) 126.9
  miners' (see also Ancylostomiasis) 126.9
Chlorotic anemia 280.9
Chocolate cyst (ovary) 617.1
Choked
  disk or disc - see Papilledema
  on food, phlegm, or vomitus NEC (see
    also Asphyxia, food) 933.1

Choked (Continued)
  phlegm 933.1
  while vomiting NEC (see also Asphyxia,
    food) 933.1
Chokes (resulting from bends) 993.3
Choking sensation 784.99
Cholangiectasis (see also Disease,
  gallbladder) 575.8
Cholangiocarcinoma (M8160/3)
  and hepatocellular carcinoma,
    combined (M8180/3) 155.0
  liver 155.1
  specified site NEC - see Neoplasm, by
    site, malignant
  unspecified site 155.1
Cholangiohepatitis 575.8
  due to fluke infestation 121.1
Cholangiohepatoma (M8180/3) 155.0
Cholangiolitis (acute) (chronic)
  (extrahepatic) (gangrenous) 576.1
  intrahepatic 575.8
  paratyphoidal (see also Fever,
    paratyphoid) 002.9
  typhoidal 002.0
Cholangioma (M8160/0) 211.5
  malignant - see Cholangiocarcinoma
Cholangitis (acute) (ascending)
  (catarrhal) (chronic) (infective)
  (malignant) (primary) (recurrent)
  (sclerosing) (secondary) (stenosing)
  (suppurative) 576.1
  chronic nonsuppurative destructive
    571.6
  nonsuppurative destructive (chronic)
    571.6
Cholecystdocholithiasis - see
  Choledocholithiasis
Cholecystitis 575.10
  with
    calculus, stones in
      bile duct (common) (hepatic) -
        see Choledocholithiasis
      gallbladder - see Cholelithiasis
  acute 575.0
  acute and chronic 575.12
  chronic 575.11
  emphysematous (acute) (see also
    Cholecystitis, acute) 575.0
  gangrenous (see also Cholecystitis,
    acute) 575.0
  paratyphoidal, current (see also Fever,
    paratyphoid) 002.9
  suppurative (see also Cholecystitis,
    acute) 575.0
  typhoidal 002.0
Choledochitis (suppurative) 576.1
Choledocholith - see Choledocholithiasis
Choledocholithiasis 574.5●

Note 15 Use the following fifth-digit
subclassification with category 574:

0 without mention of obstruction
1 with obstruction

with
  cholecystitis 574.4●
    acute 574.3●
    chronic 574.4●
  cholelithiasis 574.9●
    with
      cholecystitis 574.7●
        acute 574.6●
        and chronic 574.8●
      chronic 574.7●

Cholelithiasis (impacted) (multiple) 574.2●

> Note 16   Use the following fifth-digit subclassification with category 574:
>
> 0   without mention of obstruction
> 1   with obstruction

with
 cholecystitis 574.1●
  acute 574.0●
  chronic 574.1●
 choledocholithiasis 574.9●
  with
   cholecystitis 574.7●
    acute 574.6●
     and chronic 574.8●
    chronic cholecystitis 574.7●
Cholemia (see also Jaundice) 782.4
 familial 277.4
 Gilbert's (familial nonhemolytic) 277.4
Cholemic gallstone - see Cholelithiasis
Choleperitoneum, choleperitonitis (see also Disease, gallbladder) 567.81
Cholera (algid) (Asiatic) (asphyctic) (epidemic) (gravis) (Indian) (malignant) (morbus) (pestilential) (spasmodic) 001.9
 antimonial 985.4
 carrier (suspected) of V02.0
 classical 001.0
 contact V01.0
 due to
  Vibrio
   cholerae (Inaba, Ogawa, Hikojima serotypes) 001.0
    el Tor 001.1
  el Tor 001.1
 exposure to V01.0
 vaccination, prophylactic (against) V03.0
Cholerine (see also Cholera) 001.9
Cholestasis 576.8
 due to total parenteral nutrition (TPN) 573.8
Cholesteatoma (ear) 385.30
 attic (primary) 385.31
 diffuse 385.35
 external ear (canal) 380.21
 marginal (middle ear) 385.32
  with involvement of mastoid cavity 385.33
  secondary (with middle ear involvement) 385.33
 mastoid cavity 385.30
 middle ear (secondary) 385.32
  with involvement of mastoid cavity 385.33
 postmastoidectomy cavity (recurrent) 383.32
 primary 385.31
 recurrent, postmastoidectomy cavity 383.32
 secondary (middle ear) 385.32
  with involvement of mastoid cavity 385.33
Cholesteatosis (middle ear) (see also Cholesteatoma) 385.30
 diffuse 385.35
Cholesteremia 272.0
Cholesterin
 granuloma, middle ear 385.82
 in vitreous 379.22

Cholesterol
 deposit
  retina 362.82
  vitreous 379.22
 elevated (high) 272.0
  with elevated (high) triglycerides 272.2
 imbibition of gallbladder (see also Disease, gallbladder) 575.6
Cholesterolemia 272.0
 essential 272.0
 familial 272.0
 hereditary 272.0
Cholesterosis, cholesterolosis (gallbladder) 575.6
 with
  cholecystitis - see Cholecystitis
  cholelithiasis - see Cholelithiasis
 middle ear (see also Cholesteatoma) 385.30
Cholocolic fistula (see also Fistula, gallbladder) 575.5
Choluria 791.4
Chondritis (purulent) 733.99
 auricle 380.03
 costal 733.6
  Tietze's 733.6
 patella, posttraumatic 717.7
 pinna 380.03
 posttraumatica patellae 717.7
 tuberculous (active) (see also Tuberculosis) 015.9●
  intervertebral 015.0● [730.88]
Chondroangiopathia calcarea seu punctate 756.59
Chondroblastoma (M9230/0) - see also Neoplasm, bone, benign
 malignant (M9230/3) - see Neoplasm, bone, malignant
Chondrocalcinosis (articular) (crystal deposition) (dihydrate) (see also Arthritis, due to, crystals) 275.49 [712.3]●
 due to
  calcium pyrophosphate 275.49 [712.2]●
  dicalcium phosphate crystals 275.49 [712.1]●
  pyrophosphate crystals 275.49 [712.2]●
Chondrodermatitis nodularis helicis 380.00
Chondrodysplasia 756.4
 angiomatose 756.4
 calcificans congenita 756.59
 epiphysialis punctata 756.59
 hereditary deforming 756.4
 rhizomelic punctata 277.86
Chondrodystrophia (fetalis) 756.4
 calcarea 756.4
 calcificans congenita 756.59
 fetalis hypoplastica 756.59
 hypoplastica calcinosa 756.59
 punctata 756.59
 tarda 277.5
Chondrodystrophy (familial) (hypoplastic) 756.4
 myotonic (congenital) 359.23
Chondroectodermal dysplasia 756.55
Chondrolysis 733.99
Chondroma (M9220/0) - see also Neoplasm, cartilage, benign
 juxtacortical (M9221/0) - see Neoplasm, bone, benign

Chondroma (Continued)
 periosteal (M9221/0) - see Neoplasm, bone, benign
Chondromalacia 733.92
 epiglottis (congenital) 748.3
 generalized 733.92
 knee 717.7
 larynx (congenital) 748.3
 localized, except patella 733.92
 patella, patellae 717.7
 systemic 733.92
 tibial plateau 733.92
 trachea (congenital) 748.3
Chondromatosis (M9220/1) - see Neoplasm, cartilage, uncertain behavior
Chondromyxosarcoma (M9220/3) - see Neoplasm, cartilage, malignant
Chondro-osteodysplasia (Morquio-Brailsford type) 277.5
Chondro-osteodystrophy 277.5
Chondro-osteoma (M9210/0) - see Neoplasm, bone, benign
Chondropathia tuberosa 733.6
Chondrosarcoma (M9220/3) - see also Neoplasm, cartilage, malignant
 juxtacortical (M9221/3) - see Neoplasm, bone, malignant
 mesenchymal (M9240/3) - see Neoplasm, connective tissue, malignant
Chordae tendineae rupture (chronic) 429.5
Chordee (nonvenereal) 607.89
 congenital 752.63
 gonococcal 098.2
Chorditis (fibrinous) (nodosa) (tuberosa) 478.5
Chordoma (M9370/3) - see Neoplasm, by site, malignant
Chorea (gravis) (minor) (spasmodic) 333.5
 with
  heart involvement - see Chorea with rheumatic heart disease
  rheumatic heart disease (chronic, inactive, or quiescent) (conditions classifiable to 393–398) - see- rheumatic heart condition involved,
  active or acute (conditions classifiable to 391) 392.0
 acute - see Chorea, Sydenham's
 apoplectic (see also Disease, cerebrovascular, acute) 436
 chronic 333.4
 electric 049.8
 gravidarum - see Eclampsia, pregnancy
 habit 307.22
 hereditary 333.4
 Huntington's 333.4
 posthemiplegic 344.89
 pregnancy - see Eclampsia, pregnancy
 progressive 333.4
  chronic 333.4
  hereditary 333.4
 rheumatic (chronic) 392.9
  with heart disease or involvement - see Chorea, with rheumatic heart disease
 senile 333.5
 Sydenham's 392.9
  with heart involvement - see Chorea, with rheumatic heart disease
  nonrheumatic 333.5
 variabilis 307.23

◀ New   ◀ Revised   deleted Deleted   ● Use Additional Digit(s)   Omit code

Choreoathetosis (paroxysmal) 333.5
Chorioadenoma (destruens) (M9100/1) 236.1
Chorioamnionitis 658.4●
  affecting fetus or newborn 762.7
Chorioangioma (M9120/0) 219.8
Choriocarcinoma (M9100/3)
  combined with
    embryonal carcinoma (M9101/3) - see Neoplasm, by site, malignant
    teratoma (M9101/3) - see Neoplasm, by site, malignant
  specified site - see Neoplasm, by site, malignant
  unspecified site
    female 181
    male 186.9
Chorioencephalitis, lymphocytic (acute) (serous) 049.0
Chorioepithelioma (M9100/3) - see Choriocarcinoma
Choriomeningitis (acute) (benign) (lymphocytic) (serous) 049.0
Chorionepithelioma (M9100/3) - see Choriocarcinoma
Chorionitis (see also Scleroderma) 710.1
Chorioretinitis 363.20
  disseminated 363.10
    generalized 363.13
    in
      neurosyphilis 094.83
      secondary syphilis 091.51
    peripheral 363.12
    posterior pole 363.11
    tuberculous (see also Tuberculosis) 017.3● [363.13]
  due to
    histoplasmosis (see also Histoplasmosis) 115.92
    toxoplasmosis (acquired) 130.2
      congenital (active) 771.2
  focal 363.00
    juxtapapillary 363.01
    peripheral 363.04
    posterior pole NEC 363.03
  juxtapapillaris, juxtapapillary 363.01
  progressive myopia (degeneration) 360.21
  syphilitic (secondary) 091.51
    congenital (early) 090.0 [363.13]
      late 090.5 [363.13]
    late 095.8 [363.13]
  tuberculous (see also Tuberculosis) 017.3● [363.13]
Choristoma - see Neoplasm, by site, benign
Choroid - see condition
Choroideremia, choroidermia (initial stage) (late stage) (partial or total atrophy) 363.55
Choroiditis (see also Chorioretinitis) 363.20
  leprous 030.9 [363.13]
  senile guttate 363.41
  sympathetic 360.11
  syphilitic (secondary) 091.51
    congenital (early) 090.0 [363.13]
      late 090.5 [363.13]
    late 095.8 [363.13]
  Tay's 363.41
  tuberculous (see also Tuberculosis) 017.3 ● [363.13]

Choroidopathy NEC 363.9
  degenerative (see also Degeneration, choroid) 363.40
  hereditary (see also Dystrophy, choroid) 363.50
  specified type NEC 363.8
Choroidoretinitis - see Chorioretinitis
Choroidosis, central serous 362.41
Choroidretinopathy, serous 362.41
Christian's syndrome (chronic histiocytosis X) 277.89
Christian-Weber disease (nodular nonsuppurative panniculitis) 729.30
Christmas disease 286.1
Chromaffinoma (M8700/0) - see also Neoplasm, by site, benign
  malignant (M8700/3) - see Neoplasm, by site, malignant
Chromatopsia 368.59
Chromhidrosis, chromidrosis 705.89
Chromoblastomycosis 117.2
Chromomycosis 117.2
Chromophytosis 111.0
Chromotrichomycosis 111.8
Chronic - see condition
Churg-Strauss syndrome 446.4
Chyle cyst, mesentery 457.8
Chylocele (nonfilarial) 457.8
  filarial (see also Infestation, filarial) 125.9
  tunica vaginalis (nonfilarial) 608.84
    filarial (see also Infestation, filarial) 125.9
Chylomicronemia (fasting) (with hyperprebetalipoproteinemia) 272.3
Chylopericardium (acute) 420.90
Chylothorax (nonfilarial) 457.8
  filarial (see also Infestation, filarial) 125.9
Chylous
  ascites 457.8
  cyst of peritoneum 457.8
  hydrocele 603.9
  hydrothorax (nonfilarial) 457.8
    filarial (see also Infestation, filarial) 125.9
Chyluria 791.1
  bilharziasis 120.0
  due to
    Brugia (malayi) 125.1
    Wuchereria (bancrofti) 125.0
      malayi 125.1
  filarial (see also Infestation, filarial) 125.9
  filariasis (see also Infestation, filarial) 125.9
  nonfilarial 791.1
Cicatricial (deformity) - see Cicatrix
Cicatrix (adherent) (contracted) (painful) (vicious) 709.2
  adenoid 474.8
  alveolar process 525.8
  anus 569.49
  auricle 380.89
  bile duct (see also Disease, biliary) 576.8
  bladder 596.8
  bone 733.99
  brain 348.89 ◀▥
  cervix (postoperative) (postpartal) 622.3
    in pregnancy or childbirth 654.6●
      causing obstructed labor 660.2●

Cicatrix (Continued)
  chorioretinal 363.30
    disseminated 363.35
    macular 363.32
    peripheral 363.34
    posterior pole NEC 363.33
  choroid - see Cicatrix, chorioretinal
  common duct (see also Disease, biliary) 576.8
  congenital 757.39
  conjunctiva 372.64
  cornea 371.00
    tuberculous (see also Tuberculosis) 017.3● [371.05]
  duodenum (bulb) 537.3
  esophagus 530.3
  eyelid 374.46
    with
      ectropion - see Ectropion
      entropion - see Entropion
  hypopharynx 478.29
  knee, semilunar cartilage 717.5
  lacrimal
    canaliculi 375.53
    duct
      acquired 375.56
      neonatal 375.55
    punctum 375.52
    sac 375.54
  larynx 478.79
  limbus (cystoid) 372.64
  lung 518.89
  macular 363.32
    disseminated 363.35
    peripheral 363.34
  middle ear 385.89
  mouth 528.9
  muscle 728.89
  nasolacrimal duct
    acquired 375.56
    neonatal 375.55
  nasopharynx 478.29
  palate (soft) 528.9
  penis 607.89
  prostate 602.8
  rectum 569.49
  retina 363.30
    disseminated 363.35
    macular 363.32
    peripheral 363.34
    posterior pole NEC 363.33
  semilunar cartilage - see Derangement, meniscus
  seminal vesicle 608.89
  skin 709.2
    infected 686.8
    postinfectional 709.2
    tuberculous (see also Tuberculosis) 017.0●
  specified site NEC 709.2
  throat 478.29
  tongue 529.8
  tonsil (and adenoid) 474.8
  trachea 478.9
  tuberculous NEC (see also Tuberculosis) 011.9●
  ureter 593.89
  urethra 599.84
  uterus 621.8
  vagina 623.4
    in pregnancy or childbirth 654.7●
      causing obstructed labor 660.2●
  vocal cord 478.5
  wrist, constricting (annular) 709.2

CIDP (chronic inflammatory demyelinating polyneuropathy) 357.81
CIN I [cervical intraepithelial neoplasia I] 622.11
CIN II [cervical intraepithelial neoplasia II] 622.12
CIN III [cervical intraepithelial neoplasia III] 233.1
Cinchonism
    correct substance properly administered 386.9
    overdose or wrong substance given or taken 961.4
Circine herpes 110.5
Circle of Willis - see condition
Circular - see also condition
    hymen 752.49
Circulating, intrinsic anticoagulants causing hemorrhagic disorder 286.5 ◀▦
    following childbirth 666.3●
    postpartum 666.3●
Circulation
    collateral (venous), any site 459.89
    defective 459.9
        congenital 747.9
        lower extremity 459.89
    embryonic 747.9
    failure 799.89
        fetus or newborn 779.89
        peripheral 785.59
    fetal, persistent 747.83
    heart, incomplete 747.9
Circulatory system - see condition
Circulus senilis 371.41
Circumcision
    in absence of medical indication V50.2
    ritual V50.2
    routine V50.2
Circumscribed - see condition
Circumvallata placenta - see Placenta, abnormal
Cirrhosis, cirrhotic 571.5
    with alcoholism 571.2
    alcoholic (liver) 571.2
    atrophic (of liver) - see Cirrhosis, portal
    Baumgarten-Cruveilhier 571.5
    biliary (cholangiolitic) (cholangitic) (cholestatic) (extrahepatic) (hypertrophic) (intrahepatic) (nonobstructive) (obstructive) (pericholangiolitic) (posthepatic) (primary) (secondary) (xanthomatous) 571.6
        due to
            clonorchiasis 121.1
            flukes 121.3
    brain 331.9
    capsular - see Cirrhosis, portal
    cardiac 571.5
        alcoholic 571.2
    central (liver) - see Cirrhosis, liver
    Charcôt's 571.6
    cholangiolitic - see Cirrhosis, biliary
    cholangitic - see Cirrhosis, biliary
    cholestatic - see Cirrhosis, biliary
    clitoris (hypertrophic) 624.2
    coarsely nodular 571.5
    congestive (liver) - see Cirrhosis, cardiac
    Cruveilhier-Baumgarten 571.5
    cryptogenic (of liver) 571.5
        alcoholic 571.2
    dietary (see also Cirrhosis, portal) 571.5

Cirrhosis, cirrhotic (Continued)
    due to
        bronzed diabetes 275.0
        congestive hepatomegaly - see Cirrhosis, cardiac
        cystic fibrosis 277.00
        hemochromatosis 275.0
        hepatolenticular degeneration 275.1
        passive congestion (chronic) - see Cirrhosis, cardiac
        Wilson's disease 275.1
        xanthomatosis 272.2
    extrahepatic (obstructive) - see Cirrhosis, biliary
    fatty 571.8
        alcoholic 571.0
    florid 571.2
    Glisson's - see Cirrhosis, portal
    Hanot's (hypertrophic) - see Cirrhosis, biliary
    hepatic - see Cirrhosis, liver
    hepatolienal - see Cirrhosis, liver
    hobnail - see Cirrhosis, portal
    hypertrophic - see also Cirrhosis, liver
        biliary - see Cirrhosis, biliary
        Hanot's - see Cirrhosis, biliary
    infectious NEC - see Cirrhosis, portal
    insular - see Cirrhosis, portal
    intrahepatic (obstructive) (primary) (secondary) - see Cirrhosis, biliary
    juvenile (see also Cirrhosis, portal) 571.5
    kidney (see also Sclerosis, renal) 587
    Laennec's (of liver) 571.2
        nonalcoholic 571.5
    liver (chronic) (hepatolienal) (hypertrophic) (nodular) (splenomegalic) (unilobar) 571.5
        with alcoholism 571.2
        alcoholic 571.2
        congenital (due to failure of obliteration of umbilical vein) 777.8
        cryptogenic 571.5
            alcoholic 571.2
        fatty 571.8
            alcoholic 571.0
        macronodular 571.5
            alcoholic 571.2
        micronodular 571.5
            alcoholic 571.2
        nodular, diffuse 571.5
            alcoholic 571.2
        pigmentary 275.0
        portal 571.5
            alcoholic 571.2
        postnecrotic 571.5
            alcoholic 571.2
        syphilitic 095.3
    lung (chronic) (see also Fibrosis, lung) 515
    macronodular (of liver) 571.5
        alcoholic 571.2
    malarial 084.9
    metabolic NEC 571.5
    micronodular (of liver) 571.5
        alcoholic 571.2
    monolobular - see Cirrhosis, portal
    multilobular - see Cirrhosis, portal
    nephritis (see also Sclerosis, renal) 587
    nodular - see Cirrhosis, liver
    nutritional (fatty) 571.5
    obstructive (biliary) (extrahepatic) (intrahepatic) - see Cirrhosis, biliary

Cirrhosis, cirrhotic (Continued)
    ovarian 620.8
    paludal 084.9
    pancreas (duct) 577.8
    pericholangiolitic - see Cirrhosis, biliary
    periportal - see Cirrhosis, portal
    pigment, pigmentary (of liver) 275.0
    portal (of liver) 571.5
        alcoholic 571.2
    posthepatitic (see also Cirrhosis, postnecrotic) 571.5
    postnecrotic (of liver) 571.5
        alcoholic 571.2
    primary (intrahepatic) - see Cirrhosis, biliary
    pulmonary (see also Fibrosis, lung) 515
    renal (see also Sclerosis, renal) 587
    septal (see also Cirrhosis, postnecrotic) 571.5
    spleen 289.51
    splenomegalic (of liver) - see Cirrhosis, liver
    stasis (liver) - see Cirrhosis, liver
    stomach 535.4●
    Todd's (see also Cirrhosis, biliary) 571.6
    toxic (nodular) - see Cirrhosis, postnecrotic
    trabecular - see Cirrhosis, postnecrotic
    unilobar - see Cirrhosis, liver
    vascular (of liver) - see Cirrhosis, liver
    xanthomatous (biliary) (see also Cirrhosis, biliary) 571.6
        due to xanthomatosis (familial) (metabolic) (primary) 272.2
Cistern, subarachnoid 793.0
Citrullinemia 270.6
Citrullinuria 270.6
Ciuffini-Pancoast tumor (M8010/3) (carcinoma, pulmonary apex) 162.3
Civatte's disease or poikiloderma 709.09
CJD (Creutzfeldt-Jakob disease) 046.19
    variant (vCJD) 046.11
Clam diggers' itch 120.3
Clap - see Gonorrhea
Clark's paralysis 343.9
Clarke-Hadfield syndrome (pancreatic infantilism) 577.8
Clastothrix 704.2
Claude's syndrome 352.6
Claude Bernard-Horner syndrome (see also Neuropathy, peripheral, autonomic) 337.9
Claudication, intermittent 443.9
    cerebral (artery) (see also Ischemia, cerebral, transient) 435.9
    due to atherosclerosis 440.21
    spinal cord (arteriosclerotic) 435.1
        syphilitic 094.89
    spinalis 435.1
    venous (axillary) 453.89 ◀▦
Claudicatio venosa intermittens 453.89 ◀▦
Claustrophobia 300.29
Clavus (infected) 700
Clawfoot (congenital) 754.71
    acquired 736.74
Clawhand (acquired) 736.06
    congenital 755.59
Clawtoe (congenital) 754.71
    acquired 735.5
Clay eating 307.52
Clay shovelers' fracture - see Fracture, vertebra, cervical
Cleansing of artificial opening (see also Attention to artificial opening) V55.9

◀ New   ◀▦ Revised   ~~deleted~~ Deleted   ● Use Additional Digit(s)   ▦ Omit code

Cleft (congenital) - see also Imperfect, closure
  alveolar process 525.8
  branchial (persistent) 744.41
    cyst 744.42
  clitoris 752.49
  cricoid cartilage, posterior 748.3
  facial (see also Cleft, lip) 749.10
  lip 749.10
    with cleft palate 749.20
      bilateral (lip and palate) 749.24
        with unilateral lip or palate 749.25
        complete 749.23
        incomplete 749.24
      unilateral (lip and palate) 749.22
        with bilateral lip or palate 749.25
        complete 749.21
        incomplete 749.22
    bilateral 749.14
      with cleft palate, unilateral 749.25
      complete 749.13
      incomplete 749.14
    unilateral 749.12
      with cleft palate, bilateral 749.25
      complete 749.11
      incomplete 749.12
  nose 748.1
  palate 749.00
    with cleft lip 749.20
      bilateral (lip and palate) 749.24
        with unilateral lip or palate 749.25
        complete 749.23
        incomplete 749.24
      unilateral (lip and palate) 749.22
        with bilateral lip or palate 749.25
        complete 749.21
        incomplete 749.22
    bilateral 749.04
      with cleft lip, unilateral 749.25
      complete 749.03
      incomplete 749.04
    unilateral 749.02
      with cleft lip, bilateral 749.25
      complete 749.01
      incomplete 749.02
  penis 752.69
  posterior, cricoid cartilage 748.3
  scrotum 752.89
  sternum (congenital) 756.3
  thyroid cartilage (congenital) 748.3
  tongue 750.13
  uvula 749.02
    with cleft lip (see also Cleft, lip, with cleft palate) 749.20
  water 366.12
Cleft hand (congenital) 755.58
Cleidocranial dysostosis 755.59
Cleidotomy, fetal 763.89
Cleptomania 312.32
Clérambault's syndrome 297.8
  erotomania 302.89
Clergyman's sore throat 784.49
Click, clicking
  systolic syndrome 785.2
Clifford's syndrome (postmaturity) 766.22
Climacteric (see also Menopause) 627.2
  arthritis NEC (see also Arthritis, climacteric) 716.3●

Climacteric (Continued)
  depression (see also Psychosis, affective) 296.2●
  disease 627.2
    recurrent episode 296.3●
    single episode 296.2●
  female (symptoms) 627.2
  male (symptoms) (syndrome) 608.89
  melancholia (see also Psychosis, affective) 296.2●
    recurrent episode 296.3●
    single episode 296.2●
  paranoid state 297.2
  paraphrenia 297.2
  polyarthritis NEC 716.39
    male 608.89
  symptoms (female) 627.2
Clinical research investigation (control) (participant) V70.7
Clinodactyly 755.59
Clitoris - see condition
Cloaca, persistent 751.5
Clonorchiasis 121.1
Clonorchiosis 121.1
Clonorchis infection, liver 121.1
Clonus 781.0
Closed bite 524.20
Closed surgical procedure converted to open procedure
  arthroscopic V64.43
  laparoscopic V64.41
  thoracoscopic V64.42
Closure
  artificial opening (see also Attention to artificial opening) V55.9
  congenital, nose 748.0
  cranial sutures, premature 756.0
  defective or imperfect NEC - see Imperfect, closure
  fistula, delayed - see Fistula
  fontanelle, delayed 756.0
  foramen ovale, imperfect 745.5
  hymen 623.3
  interauricular septum, defective 745.5
  interventricular septum, defective 745.4
  lacrimal duct 375.56
    congenital 743.65
    neonatal 375.55
  nose (congenital) 748.0
    acquired 738.0
  vagina 623.2
  valve - see Endocarditis
  vulva 624.8
Clot (blood)
  artery (obstruction) (occlusion) (see also Embolism) 444.9
  atrial appendage 429.89
  bladder 596.7
  brain (extradural or intradural) (see also Thrombosis, brain) 434.0●
    late effect - see Late effect(s) (of) cerebrovascular disease
  circulation 444.9
  heart (see also Infarct, myocardium) 410.9●
    without myocardial infarction 429.89
  vein (see also Thrombosis) 453.9
Clotting defect NEC (see also Defect, coagulation) 286.9
Clouded state 780.09
  epileptic (see also Epilepsy) 345.9●
  paroxysmal (idiopathic) (see also Epilepsy) 345.9●

Clouding
  corneal graft 996.51
Cloudy
  antrum, antra 473.0
  dialysis effluent 792.5
Clouston's (hidrotic) ectodermal dysplasia 757.31
Clubbing of fingers 781.5
Clubfinger 736.29
  acquired 736.29
  congenital 754.89
Clubfoot (congenital) 754.70
  acquired 736.71
  equinovarus 754.51
  paralytic 736.71
Club hand (congenital) 754.89
  acquired 736.07
Clubnail (acquired) 703.8
  congenital 757.5
Clump kidney 753.3
Clumsiness 781.3
  syndrome 315.4
Cluttering 307.0
Clutton's joints 090.5
Coagulation, intravascular (diffuse) (disseminated) (see also Fibrinolysis) 286.6
  newborn 776.2
Coagulopathy (see also Defect, coagulation) 286.9
  consumption 286.6
  intravascular (disseminated) NEC 286.6
  newborn 776.2
Coalition
  calcaneoscaphoid 755.67
  calcaneus 755.67
  tarsal 755.67
Coal miners'
  elbow 727.2
  lung 500
Coal workers' lung or pneumoconiosis 500
Coarctation
  aorta (postductal) (preductal) 747.10
  pulmonary artery 747.3
Coated tongue 529.3
Coats' disease 362.12
Cocainism (see also Dependence) 304.2●
Coccidioidal granuloma 114.3
Coccidioidomycosis 114.9
  with pneumonia 114.0
  cutaneous (primary) 114.1
  disseminated 114.3
  extrapulmonary (primary) 114.1
  lung 114.5
    acute 114.0
    chronic 114.4
    primary 114.0
  meninges 114.2
  primary (pulmonary) 114.0
    acute 114.0
  prostate 114.3
  pulmonary 114.5
    acute 114.0
    chronic 114.4
    primary 114.0
  specified site NEC 114.3
Coccidioidosis 114.9
  lung 114.5
    acute 114.0
    chronic 114.4
    primary 114.0
  meninges 114.2

Coccidiosis (colitis) (diarrhea) (dysentery) 007.2
Cocciuria 791.9
Coccus in urine 791.9
Coccydynia 724.79
Coccygodynia 724.79
Coccyx - *see* condition
Cochin-China
   diarrhea 579.1
      anguilluliasis 127.2
   ulcer 085.1
Cock's peculiar tumor 706.2
Cockayne's disease or syndrome
      (microcephaly and dwarfism) 759.89
Cockayne-Weber syndrome
      (epidermolysis bullosa) 757.39
Cocked-up toe 735.2
Codman's tumor (benign
      chondroblastoma) (M9230/0) - *see*
      Neoplasm, bone, benign
Coenurosis 123.8
Coffee workers' lung 495.8
Cogan's syndrome 370.52
   congenital oculomotor apraxia 379.51
   nonsyphilitic interstitial keratitis 370.52
Coiling, umbilical cord - *see*
      Complications, umbilical cord
Coitus, painful (female) 625.0
   male 608.89
   psychogenic 302.76
Cold 460
   with influenza, flu, or grippe 487.1
   abscess - *see also* Tuberculosis, abscess
   articular - *see* Tuberculosis, joint
   agglutinin
      disease (chronic) or syndrome 283.0
      hemoglobinuria 283.0
         paroxysmal (cold) (nocturnal) 283.2
   allergic (*see also* Fever, hay) 477.9
   bronchus or chest - *see* Bronchitis
      with grippe or influenza 487.1
   common (head) 460
      vaccination, prophylactic (against) V04.7
   deep 464.10
   effects of 991.9
      specified effect NEC 991.8
   excessive 991.9
      specified effect NEC 991.8
   exhaustion from 991.8
   exposure to 991.9
      specified effect NEC 991.8
   grippy 487.1
   head 460
   injury syndrome (newborn) 778.2
   intolerance 780.99
   on lung - *see* Bronchitis
   rose 477.0
   sensitivity, autoimmune 283.0
   virus 460
Coldsore (*see also* Herpes, simplex) 054.9
Colibacillosis 041.4
   generalized 038.42
Colibacilluria 791.9
Colic (recurrent) 789.7 ◄▥
   abdomen 789.7 ◄▥
      psychogenic 307.89
   appendicular 543.9
   appendix 543.9
   bile duct - *see* Choledocholithiasis
   biliary - *see* Cholelithiasis
   bilious - *see* Cholelithiasis
   common duct - *see* Choledocholithiasis

Colic (*Continued*)
   Devonshire NEC 984.9
      specified type of lead - *see* Table of Drugs and Chemicals
   flatulent 787.3
   gallbladder or gallstone - *see* Cholelithiasis
   gastric 536.8
   hepatic (duct) - *see* Choledocholithiasis
   hysterical 300.11
   in ◄
      adult 789.0 ◄
      child over 12 months old 789.0 ◄
      infant 789.7 ◄
   infantile 789.7 ◄▥
   intestinal 789.7 ◄▥
   kidney 788.0
   lead NEC 984.9
      specified type of lead - *see* Table of Drugs and Chemicals
   liver (duct) - *see* Choledocholithiasis
   mucous 564.9
      psychogenic 316 [564.9]
   nephritic 788.0
   Painter's NEC 984.9
   pancreas 577.8
   psychogenic 306.4
   renal 788.0
   saturnine NEC 984.9
      specified type of lead - *see* Table of Drugs and Chemicals
   spasmodic 789.7 ◄▥
   ureter 788.0
   urethral 599.84
      due to calculus 594.2
   uterus 625.8
      menstrual 625.3
   vermicular 543.9
   virus 460
   worm NEC 128.9
Colicystitis (*see also* Cystitis) 595.9
Colitis (acute) (catarrhal) (croupous) (cystica superficialis) (exudative) (hemorrhagic) (noninfectious) (phlegmonous) (presumed noninfectious) 558.9
   adaptive 564.9
   allergic 558.3
   amebic (*see also* Amebiasis) 006.9
      nondysenteric 006.2
   anthrax 022.2
   bacillary (*see also* Infection, Shigella) 004.9
   balantidial 007.0
   chronic 558.9
      ulcerative (*see also* Colitis, ulcerative) 556.9
   coccidial 007.2
   dietetic 558.9
   due to radiation 558.1
   eosinophilic 558.42 ◄▥
   functional 558.9
   gangrenous 009.0
   giardial 007.1
   granulomatous 555.1
   gravis (*see also* Colitis, ulcerative) 556.9
   infectious (*see also* Enteritis, due to, specific organism) 009.0
      presumed 009.1
   ischemic 557.9
      acute 557.0
      chronic 557.1
      due to mesenteric artery insufficiency 557.1

Colitis (*Continued*)
   membranous 564.9
      psychogenic 316 [564.9]
   mucous 564.9
      psychogenic 316 [564.9]
   necrotic 009.0
   polyposa (*see also* Colitis, ulcerative) 556.9
   protozoal NEC 007.9
   pseudomembranous 008.45
   pseudomucinous 564.9
   regional 555.1
   segmental 555.1
   septic (*see also* Enteritis, due to, specific organism) 009.0
   spastic 564.9
      psychogenic 316 [564.9]
   Staphylococcus 008.41
      food 005.0
   thromboulcerative 557.0
   toxic 558.2
   transmural 555.1
   trichomonal 007.3
   tuberculous (ulcerative) 014.8●
   ulcerative (chronic) (idiopathic) (nonspecific) 556.9
      entero- 556.0
      fulminant 557.0
      ileo- 556.1
      left-sided 556.5
      procto- 556.2
      proctosigmoid 556.3
      psychogenic 316 [556]
      specified NEC 556.8
      universal 556.6
Collagen disease NEC 710.9
   nonvascular 710.9
   vascular (allergic) (*see also* Angiitis, hypersensitivity) 446.20
Collagenosis (*see also* Collagen disease) 710.9
   cardiovascular 425.4
   mediastinal 519.3
Collapse 780.2
   adrenal 255.8
   cardiorenal (*see also* Hypertension, cardiorenal) 404.90
   cardiorespiratory 785.51
      fetus or newborn 779.85
   cardiovascular (*see also* Disease, heart) 785.51
      fetus or newborn 779.85
   circulatory (peripheral) 785.59
      with
         abortion - *see* Abortion, by type, with shock
         ectopic pregnancy (*see also* categories 633.0–633.9) 639.5
         molar pregnancy (*see also* categories 630–632) 639.5
      during or after labor and delivery 669.1●
      fetus or newborn 779.85
      following
         abortion 639.5
         ectopic or molar pregnancy 639.5
   during or after labor and delivery 669.1●
   fetus or newborn 779.89
   external ear canal 380.50
      secondary to
         inflammation 380.53
         surgery 380.52
         trauma 380.51
   general 780.2

◄ New   ◄▥ Revised   ~~deleted~~ Deleted   ● Use Additional Digit(s)   ▨ Omit code

Collapse *(Continued)*
  heart - *see* Disease, heart
  heat 992.1
  hysterical 300.11
  labyrinth, membranous (congenital)
    744.05
  lung (massive) *(see also* Atelectasis) 518.0
    pressure, during labor 668.0●
  myocardial - *see* Disease, heart
  nervous *(see also* Disorder, mental,
    nonpsychotic) 300.9
  neurocirculatory 306.2
  nose 738.0
  postoperative (cardiovascular) 998.0
  pulmonary *(see also* Atelectasis) 518.0
    fetus or newborn 770.5
      partial 770.5
      primary 770.4
  thorax 512.8
    iatrogenic 512.1
    postoperative 512.1
  trachea 519.19
  valvular - *see* Endocarditis
  vascular (peripheral) 785.59
    with
      abortion - *see* Abortion, by type,
        with shock
      ectopic pregnancy *(see also*
        categories 633.0–633.9) 639.5
      molar pregnancy *(see also*
        categories 630–632) 639.5
    cerebral *(see also* Disease,
      cerebrovascular, acute) 436
    during or after labor and delivery
      669.1●
    fetus or newborn 779.89
    following
      abortion 639.5
      ectopic or molar pregnancy 639.5
  vasomotor 785.59
  vertebra 733.13
Collateral - *see also* condition
  circulation (venous) 459.89
  dilation, veins 459.89
Colles' fracture (closed) (reversed)
    (separation) 813.41
  open 813.51
Collet's syndrome 352.6
Collet-Sicard syndrome 352.6
Colliculitis urethralis *(see also* Urethritis)
    597.89
Colliers'
  asthma 500
  lung 500
  phthisis *(see also* Tuberculosis) 011.4●
Collodion baby (ichthyosis congenita)
    757.1
Colloid milium 709.3
Coloboma NEC 743.49
  choroid 743.59
  fundus 743.52
  iris 743.46
  lens 743.36
  lids 743.62
  optic disc (congenital) 743.57
    acquired 377.23
  retina 743.56
  sclera 743.47
Coloenteritis - *see* Enteritis
Colon - *see* condition
Colonization
  MRSA (methicillin resistant
    Staphylococcus aureus) V02.54
  MSSA (methicillin susceptible
    Staphylococcus aureus) V02.53

Coloptosis 569.89
Color
  amblyopia NEC 368.59
    acquired 368.55
  blindness NEC (congenital) 368.59
    acquired 368.55
Colostomy
  attention to V55.3
  fitting or adjustment V55.3
  malfunctioning 569.62
  status V44.3
Colpitis *(see also* Vaginitis) 616.10
Colpocele 618.6
Colpocystitis *(see also* Vaginitis) 616.10
Colporrhexis 665.4●
Colpospasm 625.1
Column, spinal, vertebral - *see* condition
Coma 780.01
  apoplectic *(see also* Disease,
    cerebrovascular, acute) 436
  diabetic (with ketoacidosis) 250.3●
    due to secondary diabetes 249.3●
    hyperosmolar 250.2●
      due to secondary diabetes
        249.2●
  eclamptic *(see also* Eclampsia) 780.39
  epileptic 345.3
  hepatic 572.2
  hyperglycemic 250.2●
    due to secondary diabetes 249.2●
  hyperosmolar (diabetic) (nonketotic)
    250.2●
    due to secondary diabetes 249.2●
  hypoglycemic 251.0
    diabetic 250.3●
      due to secondary diabetes
        249.3●
  insulin 250.3●
    due to secondary diabetes 249.3●
    hyperosmolar 250.2●
      due to secondary diabetes
        249.2●
    nondiabetic 251.0
    organic hyperinsulinism 251.0
  Kussmaul's (diabetic) 250.3●
    due to secondary diabetes 249.3●
  liver 572.2
  newborn 779.2
  prediabetic 250.2●
    due to secondary diabetes 249.2●
  uremic - *see* Uremia
Combat fatigue *(see also* Reaction, stress,
    acute) 308.9
Combined - *see* condition
Comedo 706.1
Comedocarcinoma (M8501/3) - *see also*
    Neoplasm, breast, malignant
  noninfiltrating (M8501/2)
    specified site - *see* Neoplasm, by site,
      in situ
    unspecified site 233.0
Comedomastitis 610.4
Comedones 706.1
  lanugo 757.4
Comma bacillus, carrier (suspected) of
    V02.3
Comminuted fracture - *see* Fracture, by
    site
Common
  aortopulmonary trunk 745.0
  atrioventricular canal (defect) 745.69
  atrium 745.69
  cold (head) 460
    vaccination, prophylactic (against)
      V04.7

Common *(Continued)*
  truncus (arteriosus) 745.0
  ventricle 745.3
Commotio (current)
  cerebri *(see also* Concussion, brain) 850.9
    with skull fracture - *see* Fracture,
      skull, by site
  retinae 921.3
  spinalis - *see* Injury, spinal, by site
Commotion (current)
  brain (without skull fracture) *(see also*
    Concussion, brain) 850.9
    with skull fracture - *see* Fracture,
      skull, by site
  spinal cord - *see* Injury, spinal, by site
Communication
  abnormal - *see also* Fistula
    between
      base of aorta and pulmonary
        artery 745.0
      left ventricle and right atrium
        745.4
      pericardial sac and pleural sac
        748.8
      pulmonary artery and pulmonary
        vein 747.3
    congenital, between uterus and
      anterior abdominal wall 752.3
      bladder 752.3
      intestine 752.3
      rectum 752.3
    left ventricular-right atrial 745.4
    pulmonary artery-pulmonary vein
      747.3
Compartment syndrome - *see* Syndrome,
    compartment
Compensation
  broken - *see* Failure, heart
  failure - *see* Failure, heart
  neurosis, psychoneurosis 300.11
Complaint - *see also* Disease
  bowel, functional 564.9
    psychogenic 306.4
  intestine, functional 564.9
    psychogenic 306.4
  kidney *(see also* Disease, renal) 593.9
  liver 573.9
  miners' 500
Complete - *see* condition
Complex
  cardiorenal *(see also* Hypertension,
    cardiorenal) 404.90
  castration 300.9
  Costen's 524.60
  ego-dystonic homosexuality 302.0
  Eisenmenger's (ventricular septal
    defect) 745.4
  homosexual, ego-dystonic 302.0
  hypersexual 302.89
  inferiority 301.9
  jumped process
    spine - *see* Dislocation, vertebra
  primary, tuberculosis *(see also*
    Tuberculosis) 010.0●
  regional pain syndrome 355.9
    type I 337.20
      lower limb 337.22
      specified site NEC 337.29
      upper limb 337.21
    type II
      lower limb 355.71
      upper limb 354.4
  Taussig-Bing (transposition, aorta and
    overriding pulmonary artery)
    745.11

Complications

abortion NEC - *see* categories 634–639
accidental puncture or laceration
    during a procedure 998.2
amniocentesis, fetal 679.1●
amputation stump (late) (surgical)
    997.60
    traumatic - *see* Amputation,
      traumatic
anastomosis (and bypass) - *see also*
    Complications, due to (presence
    of) any device, implant, or graft
    classified to 996.0–996.5 NEC
    hemorrhage NEC 998.11
    intestinal (internal) NEC 997.4
      involving urinary tract 997.5
    mechanical - *see* Complications,
      mechanical, graft
    urinary tract (involving intestinal
      tract) 997.5
anesthesia, anesthetic NEC (*see also*
    Anesthesia, complication)
    995.22
    in labor and delivery 668.9●
      affecting fetus or newborn 763.5
      cardiac 668.1●
      central nervous system 668.2●
      pulmonary 668.0●
      specified type NEC 668.8●
aortocoronary (bypass) graft 996.03
    atherosclerosis - *see* Arteriosclerosis,
      coronary
    embolism 996.72
    occlusion NEC 996.72
    thrombus 996.72
arthroplasty (*see also* Complications,
    prosthetic joint) 996.49
artificial opening
    cecostomy 569.60
    colostomy 569.60
    cystostomy 997.5
    enterostomy 569.60
    esophagostomy 530.87
      infection 530.86
      mechanical 530.87
    gastrostomy 536.40
    ileostomy 569.60
    jejunostomy 569.60
    nephrostomy 997.5
    tracheostomy 519.00
    ureterostomy 997.5
    urethrostomy 997.5
bariatric surgery 997.4
bile duct implant (prosthetic) NEC
    996.79
    infection or inflammation 996.69
    mechanical 996.59
bleeding (intraoperative)
    (postoperative) 998.11
blood vessel graft 996.1
    aortocoronary 996.03
      atherosclerosis - *see*
        Arteriosclerosis, coronary
      embolism 996.72
      occlusion NEC 996.72
      thrombus 996.72
    atherosclerosis - *see* Arteriosclerosis,
      extremities
    embolism 996.74
    occlusion NEC 996.74
    thrombus 996.74
bone growth stimulator NEC 996.78
    infection or inflammation 996.67
bone marrow transplant 996.85

Complications (*Continued*)

breast implant (prosthetic) NEC
    996.79
    infection or inflammation 996.69
    mechanical 996.54
bypass - *see also* Complications,
    anastomosis
    aortocoronary 996.03
      atherosclerosis - *see*
        Arteriosclerosis, coronary
      embolism 996.72
      occlusion NEC 996.72
      thrombus 996.72
    carotid artery 996.1
      atherosclerosis - *see*
        Arteriosclerosis, coronary
      embolism 996.74
      occlusion NEC 996.74
      thrombus 996.74
cardiac (*see also* Disease, heart) 429.9
    device, implant, or graft NEC 996.72
      infection or inflammation 996.61
      long-term effect 429.4
      mechanical (*see also*
        Complications, mechanical,
        by type) 996.00
      valve prosthesis 996.71
        infection or inflammation
          996.61
    postoperative NEC 997.1
      long-term effect 429.4
cardiorenal (*see also* Hypertension,
    cardiorenal) 404.90
carotid artery bypass graft 996.1
    atherosclerosis - *see* Arteriosclerosis,
      coronary
    embolism 996.74
    occlusion NEC 996.74
    thrombus 996.74
cataract fragments in eye 998.82
catheter device NEC - *see also*
    Complications, due to (presence
    of) any device, implant, or graft
    classified to 996.0-996.5 NEC
    mechanical - *see* Complications,
      mechanical, catheter
cecostomy 569.60
cesarean section wound 674.3●
chemotherapy (antineoplastic) 995.29
chin implant (prosthetic) NEC 996.79
    infection or inflammation 996.69
    mechanical 996.59
colostomy (enterostomy) 569.60
    specified type NEC 569.69
contraceptive device, intrauterine NEC
    996.76
    infection 996.65
    inflammation 996.65
    mechanical 996.32
cord (umbilical) - *see* Complications,
    umbilical cord
cornea
    due to
      contact lens 371.82
coronary (artery) bypass (graft) NEC
    996.03
    atherosclerosis - *see* Arteriosclerosis,
      coronary
    embolism 996.72
    infection or inflammation 996.61
    mechanical 996.03
    occlusion NEC 996.72
    specified type NEC 996.72
    thrombus 996.72

Complications (*Continued*)

cystostomy 997.5
delivery 669.9●
    procedure (instrumental) (manual)
      (surgical) 669.4●
    specified type NEC 669.8●
dialysis (hemodialysis) (peritoneal)
    (renal) NEC 999.9
    catheter NEC - *see also*
      Complications, due to
      (presence of) any device,
      implant, or graft classified to
      996.0–996.5 NEC
      infection or inflammation 996.62
        peritoneal 996.68
      mechanical 996.1
        peritoneal 996.56
drug NEC 995.29
due to (presence of) any device,
    implant, or graft classified to
    996.0–996.5 NEC 996.70
    with infection or inflammation - *see*
      Complications, infection or
      inflammation, due to (presence
      of) any device, implant, or
      graft classified to 996.0–996.5
      NEC
    arterial NEC 996.74
      coronary NEC 996.03
        atherosclerosis - *see*
          Arteriosclerosis,
          coronary
        embolism 996.72
        occlusion NEC 996.72
        specified type NEC 996.72
        thrombus 996.72
      renal dialysis 996.73
    arteriovenous fistula or shunt NEC
      996.74
    bone growth stimulator 996.78
    breast NEC 996.79
    cardiac NEC 996.72
      defibrillator 996.72
      pacemaker 996.72
      valve prosthesis 996.71
    catheter NEC 996.79
      spinal 996.75
      urinary, indwelling 996.76
      vascular NEC 996.74
        renal dialysis 996.73
      ventricular shunt 996.75
    coronary (artery) bypass (graft) NEC
      996.03
      atherosclerosis - *see*
        Arteriosclerosis, coronary
      embolism 996.72
      occlusion NEC 996.72
      thrombus 996.72
    electrodes
      brain 996.75
      heart 996.72
    esophagostomy 530.87
    gastrointestinal NEC 996.79
    genitourinary NEC 996.76
    heart valve prosthesis NEC
      996.71
    infusion pump 996.74
    insulin pump 996.57
    internal
      joint prosthesis 996.77
      orthopedic NEC 996.78
      specified type NEC 996.79
    intrauterine contraceptive device
      NEC 996.76

◀ New   ◀▥ Revised   ~~deleted~~ Deleted   ● Use Additional Digit(s)   ▨ Omit code

Complications *(Continued)*
  due to any device, implant, or graft
    classified to 996.0–996.5 NEC
    (Continued)
    joint prosthesis, internal NEC 996.77
    mechanical - *see* Complications,
      mechanical
    nervous system NEC 996.75
    ocular lens NEC 996.79
    orbital NEC 996.79
    orthopedic NEC 996.78
      joint, internal 996.77
    renal dialysis 996.73
    specified type NEC 996.79
    urinary catheter, indwelling 996.76
    vascular NEC 996.74
    ventricular shunt 996.75
  during dialysis NEC 999.9
  ectopic or molar pregnancy NEC 639.9
  electroshock therapy NEC 999.9
  enterostomy 569.60
    specified type NEC 569.69
  esophagostomy 530.87
    infection 530.86
    mechanical 530.87
  external (fixation) device with internal
    component(s) NEC 996.78
    infection or inflammation 996.67
    mechanical 996.49
  extracorporeal circulation NEC 999.9
  eye implant (prosthetic) NEC 996.79
    infection or inflammation 996.69
    mechanical
      ocular lens 996.53
      orbital globe 996.59
  fetal, from amniocentesis 679.1 ●
  gastrointestinal, postoperative NEC
    (*see also* Complications, surgical
    procedures) 997.4
  gastrostomy 536.40
    specified type NEC 536.49
  genitourinary device, implant or graft
    NEC 996.76
    infection or inflammation 996.65
      urinary catheter, indwelling 996.64
    mechanical (*see also* Complications,
      mechanical, by type) 996.30
      specified NEC 996.39
  graft (bypass) (patch) - *see also*
    Complications, due to (presence
    of) any device, implant, or graft
    classified to 996.0–996.5 NEC
    bone marrow 996.85
    corneal NEC 996.79
      infection or inflammation 996.69
      rejection or reaction 996.51
    mechanical - *see* Complications,
      mechanical, graft
    organ (immune or nonimmune
      cause) (partial) (total) 996.80
      bone marrow 996.85
      heart 996.83
      intestines 996.87
      kidney 996.81
      liver 996.82
      lung 996.84
      pancreas 996.86
      specified NEC 996.89
    skin NEC 996.79
      infection or inflammation 996.69
      rejection 996.52
        artificial 996.55
        decellularized allodermis
          996.55

Complications *(Continued)*
  heart - *see also* Disease, heart transplant
    (immune or nonimmune cause)
    996.83
  hematoma (intraoperative)
    (postoperative) 998.12
  hemorrhage (intraoperative)
    (postoperative) 998.11
  hyperalimentation therapy NEC 999.9
  immunization (procedure) - *see*
    Complications, vaccination
  implant - *see also* Complications, due to
    (presence of) any device, implant,
    or graft classified to 996.0–996.5
    NEC
    dental placement, hemorrhagic
      525.71
    mechanical, - *see* Complications,
      mechanical, implant
  infection and inflammation
    due to (presence of) any device,
      implant or graft classified to
      996.0–996.5 NEC 996.60
      arterial NEC 996.62
        coronary 996.61
        renal dialysis 996.62
      arteriovenous fistula or shunt
        996.62
      artificial heart 996.61
      bone growth stimulator 996.67
      breast 996.69
      cardiac 996.61
      catheter NEC 996.69
        central venous 999.31
        Hickman 999.31
        peripherally inserted central
          (PICC) 999.31
        peritoneal 996.68
        portacath (port-a-cath) 999.31
        spinal 996.63
        triple lumen 999.31
        umbilical venous 999.31
        urinary, indwelling 996.64
        vascular (arterial) (dialysis)
          (peripheral venous) NEC
          996.62
        ventricular shunt 996.63
      central venous catheter 999.31
      coronary artery bypass 996.61
      electrodes
        brain 996.63
        heart 996.61
      gastrointestinal NEC 996.69
      genitourinary NEC 996.65
        indwelling urinary catheter
          996.64
      heart assist device 996.61
      heart valve 996.61
      Hickman catheter 999.31
      infusion pump 996.62
      insulin pump 996.69
      intrauterine contraceptive device
        996.65
      joint prosthesis, internal 996.66
      ocular lens 996.69
      orbital (implant) 996.69
      orthopedic NEC 996.67
        joint, internal 996.66
      peripherally inserted central
        catheter (PICC) 999.31
      portacath (port-a-cath) 999.31
      specified type NEC 996.69
      triple lumen catheter 999.31
      umbilical venous catheter 999.31

Complications *(Continued)*
  infection and inflammation *(Continued)*
    due to any device *(Continued)*
      urinary catheter, indwelling 996.64
      ventricular shunt 996.63
  infusion (procedure) 999.88
    blood - *see* Complications,
      transfusion
    infection NEC 999.39
    sepsis NEC 999.39
  inhalation therapy NEC 999.9
  injection (procedure) 999.9
    drug reaction (*see also* Reaction,
      drug) 995.27
    infection NEC 999.39
    sepsis NEC 999.39
    serum (prophylactic) (therapeutic) -
      see Complications, vaccination
    vaccine (any) - *see* Complications,
      vaccination
  inoculation (any) - *see* Complications,
    vaccination
  insulin pump 996.57
  internal device (catheter) (electronic)
    (fixation) (prosthetic) - *see also*
    Complications, due to (presence
    of) any device, implant, or graft
    classified to 996.0–996.5 NEC
    mechanical - *see* Complications,
      mechanical
  intestinal pouch, specified NEC ◄
    569.79
  intestinal transplant (immune or
    nonimmune cause) 996.87
  intraoperative bleeding or hemorrhage
    998.11
  intrauterine contraceptive device (*see*
    also Complications, contraceptive
    device) 996.76
    with fetal damage affecting
      management of pregnancy
      655.8 ●
    infection or inflammation 996.65
  in utero procedure
    fetal 679.1 ●
    maternal 679.0 ●
  jejunostomy 569.60
  kidney transplant (immune or
    nonimmune cause) 996.81
  labor 669.9 ●
    specified condition NEC 669.8 ●
  liver transplant (immune or
    nonimmune cause) 996.82
  lumbar puncture 349.0
  mechanical
    anastomosis - *see* Complications,
      mechanical, graft
    artificial heart 996.09
    bypass - *see* Complications,
      mechanical, graft
    catheter NEC 996.59
      cardiac 996.09
      cystostomy 996.39
      dialysis (hemodialysis) 996.1
        peritoneal 996.56
      during a procedure 998.2
      urethral, indwelling 996.31
    colostomy 569.62
    device NEC 996.59
      balloon (counterpulsation),
        intra-aortic 996.1
      cardiac 996.00
        automatic implantable
          defibrillator 996.04
        long-term effect 429.4
        specified NEC 996.09

Complications *(Continued)*
  mechanical *(Continued)*
    device NEC *(Continued)*
      contraceptive, intrauterine 996.32
      counterpulsation, intra-aortic 996.1
      fixation, external, with internal components 996.49
      fixation, internal (nail, rod, plate) 996.40
      genitourinary 996.30
        specified NEC 996.39
      insulin pump 996.57
      nervous system 996.2
      orthopedic, internal 996.40
        prosthetic joint *(see also* Complications, mechanical, device, orthopedic, prosthetic, joint) 996.47
      prosthetic NEC 996.59
        joint *(see also Complications, prosthetic joint)* 996.47
          articular bearing surface wear 996.46
          aseptic loosening 996.41
          breakage 996.43
          dislocation 996.42
          failure 996.47
          fracture 996.43
            around prosthetic 996.44
            peri-prosthetic 996.44
          instability 996.42
          loosening 996.41
          peri-prosthetic osteolysis 996.45
          subluxation 996.42
          wear 996.46
      umbrella, vena cava 996.1
      vascular 996.1
    dorsal column stimulator 996.2
    electrode NEC 996.59
      brain 996.2
      cardiac 996.01
      spinal column 996.2
    enterostomy 569.62
    esophagostomy 530.87
    fistula, arteriovenous, surgically created 996.1
    gastrostomy 536.42
    graft NEC 996.52
      aortic (bifurcation) 996.1
      aortocoronary bypass 996.03
      blood vessel NEC 996.1
      bone 996.49
      cardiac 996.00
      carotid artery bypass 996.1
      cartilage 996.49
      corneal 996.51
      coronary bypass 996.03
      decellularized allodermis 996.55
      genitourinary 996.30
        specified NEC 996.39
      muscle 996.49
      nervous system 996.2
      organ (immune or nonimmune cause) 996.80
        heart 996.83
        intestines 996.87
        kidney 996.81
        liver 996.82
        lung 996.84
        pancreas 996.86
        specified NEC 996.89

Complications *(Continued)*
  mechanical *(Continued)*
    graft NEC *(Continued)*
      orthopedic, internal 996.49
      peripheral nerve 996.2
      prosthetic NEC 996.59
      skin 996.52
        artificial 996.55
      specified NEC 996.59
      tendon 996.49
      tissue NEC 996.52
      tooth 996.59
      ureter, without mention of resection 996.39
      vascular 996.1
    heart valve prosthesis 996.02
      long-term effect 429.4
    implant NEC 996.59
      cardiac 996.00
        automatic implantable defibrillator 996.04
        long-term effect 429.4
        specified NEC 996.09
      electrode NEC 996.59
        brain 996.2
        cardiac 996.01
        spinal column 996.2
      genitourinary 996.30
      nervous system 996.2
      orthopedic, internal 996.49
      prosthetic NEC 996.59
        in
          bile duct 996.59
          breast 996.54
          chin 996.59
          eye
            ocular lens 996.53
            orbital globe 996.59
      vascular 996.1
    insulin pump 996.57
    nonabsorbable surgical material 996.59
    pacemaker NEC 996.59
      brain 996.2
      cardiac 996.01
      nerve (phrenic) 996.2
    patch - *see* Complications, mechanical, graft
    prosthesis NEC 996.59
      bile duct 996.59
      breast 996.54
      chin 996.59
      ocular lens 996.53
      reconstruction, vas deferens 996.39
    reimplant NEC 996.59
      extremity *(see also* Complications, reattached, extremity) 996.90
      organ *(see also* Complications, transplant, organ, by site) 996.80
    repair - *see* Complications, mechanical, graft
    respirator [ventilator] V46.14
    shunt NEC 996.59
      arteriovenous, surgically created 996.1
      ventricular (communicating) 996.2
    stent NEC 996.59
    tracheostomy 519.02
    vas deferens reconstruction 996.39
    ventilator [respirator] V46.14

Complications *(Continued)*
  medical care NEC 999.9
    cardiac NEC 997.1
    gastrointestinal NEC 997.4
    nervous system NEC 997.00
    peripheral vascular NEC 997.2
    respiratory NEC 997.39
    urinary NEC 997.5
    vascular
      mesenteric artery 997.71
      other vessels 997.79
      peripheral vessels 997.2
      renal artery 997.72
  nephrostomy 997.5
  nervous system
    device, implant, or graft NEC 349.1
      mechanical 996.2
    postoperative NEC 997.00
  obstetric 669.9●
    procedure (instrumental) (manual) (surgical) 669.4●
    specified NEC 669.8●
    surgical wound 674.3●
  ocular lens implant NEC 996.79
    infection or inflammation 996.69
    mechanical 996.53
  organ transplant - *see* Complications, transplant, organ, by site
  orthopedic device, implant, or graft
    internal (fixation) (nail) (plate) (rod) NEC 996.78
      infection or inflammation 996.67
      joint prosthesis 996.77
        infection or inflammation 996.66
        mechanical 996.40
  pacemaker (cardiac) 996.72
    infection or inflammation 996.61
    mechanical 996.01
  pancreas transplant (immune or nonimmune cause) 996.86
  perfusion NEC 999.9
  perineal repair (obstetrical) 674.3●
    disruption 674.2●
  pessary (uterus) (vagina) - *see* Complications, contraceptive device
  phototherapy 990
  postcystoscopic 997.5
  postmastoidectomy NEC 383.30
  postoperative - *see* Complications, surgical procedures
  pregnancy NEC 646.9●
    affecting fetus or newborn 761.9
  prosthetic device, internal - *see also* Complications, due to (presence of) any device, implant or graft classified to 996.0–996.5 NEC
    mechanical NEC *(see also* Complications, mechanical) 996.59
  puerperium NEC *(see also* Puerperal) 674.9●
  puncture, spinal 349.0
  pyelogram 997.5
  radiation 990
  radiotherapy 990
  reattached
    body part, except extremity 996.99
    extremity (infection) (rejection) 996.90
      arm(s) 996.94
      digit(s) (hand) 996.93
        foot 996.95

◀ New   ◀▦ Revised   ~~deleted~~ Deleted   ● Use Additional Digit(s)   ▦ Omit code

Complications *(Continued)*
  reattached *(Continued)*
    extremity *(Continued)*
      finger(s) 996.93
      foot 996.95
      forearm 996.91
      hand 996.92
      leg 996.96
      lower NEC 996.96
      toe(s) 996.95
      upper NEC 996.94
    reimplant NEC - *see also* Complications,
      due to (presence of) any device,
      implant, or graft classified to
      996.0–996.5 NEC
      bone marrow 996.85
      extremity *(see also* Complications,
        reattached, extremity) 996.90
        due to infection 996.90
      mechanical - *see* Complications,
        mechanical, reimplant
      organ (immune or nonimmune
        cause) (partial) (total) *(see also*
        Complications, transplant,
        organ, by site) 996.80
    renal allograft 996.81
    renal dialysis - *see* Complications,
      dialysis
    respirator [ventilator], mechanical
      V46.14
    respiratory 519.9
      device, implant or graft NEC
        996.79
        infection or inflammation 996.69
        mechanical 996.59
      distress syndrome, adult, following
        trauma or surgery 518.5
      insufficiency, acute, postoperative
        518.5
      postoperative NEC 997.39
      therapy NEC 999.9
    sedation during labor and delivery
      668.9●
      affecting fetus or newborn 763.5
      cardiac 668.1●
      central nervous system 668.2●
      pulmonary 668.0●
      specified type NEC 668.8●
    seroma (intraoperative) (postoperative)
      (noninfected) 998.13
      infected 998.51
    shunt - *see also* Complications, due to
      (presence of) any device, implant,
      or graft classified to 996.0–996.5
      NEC
      mechanical - *see* Complications,
        mechanical, shunt
    specified body system NEC
      device, implant, or graft - *see*
        Complications, due to
        (presence of) any device,
        implant, or graft classified to
        996.0–996.5 NEC
      postoperative NEC 997.99
    spinal puncture or tap 349.0
    stoma, external
      gastrointestinal tract
        colostomy 569.60
        enterostomy 569.60
        esophagostomy 530.87
          infection 530.86
          mechanical 530.87
        gastrostomy 536.40
      urinary tract 997.5

Complications *(Continued)*
  stomach banding 997.4
  stomach stapling 997.4
  surgical procedures 998.9
    accidental puncture or laceration
      998.2
    amputation stump (late) 997.60
    anastomosis - *see* Complications,
      anastomosis
    burst stitches or sutures (external)
      (see also Dehiscence) 998.32
      internal 998.31
    cardiac 997.1
      long-term effect following cardiac
        surgery 429.4
    catheter device - *see* Complications,
      catheter device
    cataract fragments in eye 998.82
    cecostomy malfunction 569.62
    colostomy malfunction 569.62
    cystostomy malfunction 997.5
    dehiscence (of incision) (external)
      (see also Dehiscence) 998.32
      internal 998.31
    dialysis NEC *(see also* Complications,
      dialysis) 999.9
    disruption *(see also* Dehiscence)
      anastomosis (internal) - *see*
        Complications, mechanical,
        graft
      internal suture (line) 998.31
      wound (external) 998.32
        internal 998.31
    dumping syndrome
      (postgastrectomy) 564.2
    elephantiasis or lymphedema 997.99
      postmastectomy 457.0
    emphysema (surgical) 998.81
    enterostomy malfunction 569.62
    esophagostomy malfunction 530.87
    evisceration 998.32
    fistula (persistent postoperative)
      998.6
    foreign body inadvertently left in
      wound (sponge) (suture)
      (swab) 998.4
    from nonabsorbable surgical
      material (Dacron) (mesh)
      (permanent suture)
      (reinforcing) (Teflon) - *see*
      Complications due to
      (presence of) any device,
      implant, or graft classified to
      996.0–996.5 NEC
    gastrointestinal NEC 997.4
    gastrostomy malfunction 536.42
    hematoma 998.12
    hemorrhage 998.11
    ileostomy malfunction 569.62
    internal prosthetic device NEC *(see
      also* Complications, internal
      device) 996.70
      hemolytic anemia 283.19
      infection or inflammation 996.60
      malfunction - *see* Complications,
        mechanical
      mechanical complication - *see*
        Complications, mechanical
      thrombus 996.70
    jejunostomy malfunction 569.62
    nervous system NEC 997.00
    obstruction, internal anastomosis -
      see Complications, mechanical,
      graft

Complications *(Continued)*
  surgical procedures *(Continued)*
    other body system NEC 997.99
    peripheral vascular NEC 997.2
    postcardiotomy syndrome 429.4
    postcholecystectomy syndrome 576.0
    postcommissurotomy syndrome
      429.4
    postgastrectomy dumping
      syndrome 564.2
    postmastectomy lymphedema
      syndrome 457.0
    postmastoidectomy 383.30
      cholesteatoma, recurrent 383.32
      cyst, mucosal 383.31
      granulation 383.33
      inflammation, chronic 383.33
    postvagotomy syndrome 564.2
    postvalvulotomy syndrome 429.4
    reattached extremity (infection)
      (rejection) *(see also*
      Complications, reattached,
      extremity) 996.90
    respiratory NEC 997.39
    seroma 998.13
    shock (endotoxic) (hypovolemic)
      (septic) 998.0
    shunt, prosthetic (thrombus) - *see
      also* Complications, due to
      (presence of) any device,
      implant, or graft classified to
      996.0–996.5 NEC
      hemolytic anemia 283.19
    specified complication NEC 998.89
    stitch abscess 998.59
    transplant - *see* Complications, graft
    ureterostomy malfunction 997.5
    urethrostomy malfunction 997.5
    urinary NEC 997.5
    vascular
      mesenteric artery 997.71
      other vessels 997.79
      peripheral vessels 997.2
      renal artery 997.72
    wound infection 998.59
  therapeutic misadventure NEC 999.9
    surgical treatment 998.9
  tracheostomy 519.00
  transfusion (blood) (lymphocytes)
    (plasma) NEC 999.89
    acute lung injury (TRALI) 518.7
    atrophy, liver, yellow, subacute
      (within 8 months of
      administration) - *see* Hepatitis,
      viral
    bone marrow 996.85
    embolism
      air 999.1
      thrombus 999.2
    hemolysis NEC 999.89
      bone marrow 996.85
    hepatitis (serum) (type B) (within 8
      months after administration) -
      see Hepatitis, viral
    incompatibility reaction ~~(ABO)~~
      ~~(blood group) 999.6~~ ◀▥
      ABO 999.6 ◀
      minor blood group 999.89 ◀
      Rh (factor) 999.7
    infection 999.39
    jaundice (serum) (within 8 months
      after administration) - *see*
      Hepatitis, viral
    sepsis 999.39

Complications (Continued)
  transfusion NEC (Continued)
    shock or reaction NEC 999.89
      bone marrow 996.85
    subacute yellow atrophy of liver
      (within 8 months after
      administration) - see Hepatitis,
      viral
    thromboembolism 999.2
  transplant NEC - see also
      Complications, due to (presence
      of) any device, implant, or graft
      classified to 996.0–996.5 NEC
    bone marrow 996.85
    organ (immune or nonimmune
      cause) (partial) (total) 996.80
      bone marrow 996.85
      heart 996.83
      intestines 996.87
      kidney 996.81
      liver 996.82
      lung 996.84
      pancreas 996.86
      specified NEC 996.89
  trauma NEC (early) 958.8
  ultrasound therapy NEC 999.9
  umbilical cord
    affecting fetus or newborn 762.6
    complicating delivery 663.9●
      affecting fetus or newborn 762.6
      specified type NEC 663.8●
  urethral catheter NEC 996.76
    infection or inflammation 996.64
    mechanical 996.31
  urinary, postoperative NEC 997.5
  vaccination 999.9
    anaphylaxis NEC 999.4
    cellulitis 999.39
    encephalitis or encephalomyelitis
      323.51
    hepatitis (serum) (type B) (within 8
      months after administration) -
      see Hepatitis, viral
    infection (general) (local) NEC
      999.39
    jaundice (serum) (within 8 months
      after administration) - see
      Hepatitis, viral
    meningitis 997.09 [321.8]
    myelitis 323.52
    protein sickness 999.5
    reaction (allergic) 999.5
      Herxheimer's 995.0
      serum 999.5
    sepsis 999.39
    serum intoxication, sickness, rash, or
      other serum reaction NEC
      999.5
    shock (allergic) (anaphylactic) 999.4
    subacute yellow atrophy of liver
      (within 8 months after
      administration) - see Hepatitis,
      viral
    vaccinia (generalized) 999.0
      localized 999.39
  vascular
    device, implant, or graft NEC 996.74
      infection or inflammation 996.62
      mechanical NEC 996.1
        cardiac (see also Complications,
          mechanical, by type)
          996.00
    following infusion, perfusion, or
      transfusion 999.2

Complications (Continued)
  vascular (Continued)
    postoperative NEC 997.2
      mesenteric artery 997.71
      other vessels 997.79
      peripheral vessels 997.2
      renal artery 997.72
    ventilation therapy NEC 999.9
    ventilator [respirator], mechanical
      V46.14
Compound presentation, complicating
    delivery 652.8●
  causing obstructed labor 660.0●
Compressed air disease 993.3
Compression
  with injury - see specific injury
  arm NEC 354.9
  artery 447.1
    celiac, syndrome 447.4
  brachial plexus 353.0
  brain (stem) 348.4
    due to
      contusion, brain - see Contusion,
        brain
      injury NEC - see also Hemorrhage,
        brain, traumatic
        birth - see Birth, injury, brain
      laceration, brain - see Laceration,
        brain
    osteopathic 739.0
  bronchus 519.19
  by cicatrix - see Cicatrix
  cardiac 423.9
  cauda equina 344.60
    with neurogenic bladder 344.61
  celiac (artery) (axis) 447.4
  cerebral - see Compression, brain
  cervical plexus 353.2
  cord (umbilical) - see Compression,
    umbilical cord
  cranial nerve 352.9
    second 377.49
    third (partial) 378.51
      total 378.52
    fourth 378.53
    fifth 350.8
    sixth 378.54
    seventh 351.8
  divers' squeeze 993.3
  duodenum (external) (see also
    Obstruction, duodenum) 537.3
  during birth 767.9
  esophagus 530.3
    congenital, external 750.3
  Eustachian tube 381.63
  facies (congenital) 754.0
  fracture - see Fracture, by site
  heart - see Disease, heart
  intestine (see also Obstruction, intestine)
    560.9
    with hernia - see Hernia, by site,
      with obstruction
  laryngeal nerve, recurrent 478.79
  leg NEC 355.8
  lower extremity NEC 355.8
  lumbosacral plexus 353.1
  lung 518.89
  lymphatic vessel 457.1
  medulla - see Compression, brain
  nerve NEC - see also Disorder, nerve
    arm NEC 354.9
    autonomic nervous system (see also
      Neuropathy, peripheral,
      autonomic) 337.9

Compression (Continued)
  nerve NEC (Continued)
    axillary 353.0
    cranial NEC 352.9
    due to displacement of
      intervertebral disc 722.2
      with myelopathy 722.70
      cervical 722.0
        with myelopathy 722.71
      lumbar, lumbosacral 722.10
        with myelopathy 722.73
      thoracic, thoracolumbar 722.11
        with myelopathy 722.72
    iliohypogastric 355.79
    ilioinguinal 355.79
    leg NEC 355.8
    lower extremity NEC 355.8
    median (in carpal tunnel) 354.0
    obturator 355.79
    optic 377.49
    plantar 355.6
    posterior tibial (in tarsal tunnel)
      355.5
    root (by scar tissue) NEC 724.9
      cervical NEC 723.4
      lumbar NEC 724.4
      lumbosacral 724.4
      thoracic 724.4
    saphenous 355.79
    sciatic (acute) 355.0
    sympathetic 337.9
    traumatic - see Injury, nerve
    ulnar 354.2
    upper extremity NEC 354.9
  peripheral - see Compression, nerve
  spinal (cord) (old or nontraumatic)
    336.9
    by displacement of intervertebral
      disc - see Displacement,
      intervertebral disc
    nerve
      root NEC 724.9
        postoperative 722.80
          cervical region 722.81
          lumbar region 722.83
          thoracic region 722.82
        traumatic - see Injury, nerve,
          spinal
      traumatic - see Injury, nerve,
        spinal
    spondylogenic 721.91
      cervical 721.1
      lumbar, lumbosacral 721.42
      thoracic 721.41
    traumatic - see also Injury, spinal, by
      site
      with fracture, vertebra - see
        Fracture, vertebra, by site,
        with spinal cord injury
    spondylogenic - see Compression,
      spinal cord, spondylogenic
  subcostal nerve (syndrome) 354.8
  sympathetic nerve NEC 337.9
  syndrome 958.5
  thorax 512.8
    iatrogenic 512.1
    postoperative 512.1
  trachea 519.19
    congenital 748.3
  ulnar nerve (by scar tissue) 354.2
  umbilical cord
    affecting fetus or newborn
      762.5
    cord prolapsed 762.4

◄ New ◄▥ Revised ~~deleted~~ Deleted ● Use Additional Digit(s) ▨ Omit code

Compression *(Continued)*
　umbilical cord *(Continued)*
　　complicating delivery 663.2●
　　　cord around neck 663.1●
　　　cord prolapsed 663.0●
　upper extremity NEC 354.9
　ureter 593.3
　urethra - *see* Stricture, urethra
　vein 459.2
　vena cava (inferior) (superior) 459.2
　vertebral NEC - *see* Compression,
　　spinal (cord)
Compulsion, compulsive
　eating 307.51
　neurosis (obsessive) 300.3
　personality 301.4
　states (mixed) 300.3
　swearing 300.3
　　in Gilles de la Tourette's syndrome
　　　307.23
　tics and spasms 307.22
　water drinking NEC (syndrome) 307.9
Concato's disease (pericardial
　　polyserositis) 423.2
　peritoneal 568.82
　pleural - *see* Pleurisy
Concavity, chest wall 738.3
Concealed
　hemorrhage NEC 459.0
　penis 752.65
Concentric fading 368.12
Concern (normal) about sick person in
　　family V61.49
Concrescence (teeth) 520.2
Concretio cordis 423.1
　rheumatic 393
Concretion - *see also* Calculus
　appendicular 543.9
　canaliculus 375.57
　clitoris 624.8
　conjunctiva 372.54
　eyelid 374.56
　intestine (impaction) (obstruction)
　　560.39
　lacrimal (passages) 375.57
　prepuce (male) 605
　　female (clitoris) 624.8
　salivary gland (any) 527.5
　seminal vesicle 608.89
　stomach 537.89
　tonsil 474.8
Concussion (current) 850.9
　with
　　loss of consciousness 850.5
　　　brief (less than one hour)
　　　　30 minutes or less 850.11
　　　　31–59 minutes 850.12
　　　moderate (1–24 hours) 850.2
　　　prolonged (more than 24 hours)
　　　　(with complete recovery)
　　　　(with return to pre-existing
　　　　conscious level) 850.3
　　　　without return to pre-existing
　　　　　conscious level 850.4
　　mental confusion or disorientation
　　　(without loss of consciousness)
　　　850.0
　　　with loss of consciousness - *see*
　　　　Concussion, with, loss of
　　　　consciousness
　without loss of consciousness 850.0
　blast (air) (hydraulic) (immersion)
　　(underwater) 869.0
　　with open wound into cavity 869.1

Concussion *(Continued)*
　blast *(Continued)*
　　abdomen or thorax - *see* Injury,
　　　internal, by site
　　brain - *see* Concussion, brain
　　ear (acoustic nerve trauma) 951.5
　　　with perforation, tympanic
　　　　membrane - *see* Wound,
　　　　open, ear drum
　　thorax - *see* Injury, internal,
　　　intrathoracic organs NEC
　brain or cerebral (without skull
　　fracture) 850.9
　　with
　　　loss of consciousness 850.5
　　　　brief (less than one hour)
　　　　　30 minutes or less 850.11
　　　　　31–59 minutes 850.12
　　　　moderate (1–24 hours) 850.2
　　　　prolonged (more than 24
　　　　　hours) (with complete
　　　　　recovery) (with return to
　　　　　pre-existing conscious
　　　　　level) 850.3
　　　　　without return to pre-
　　　　　　existing conscious
　　　　　　level 850.4
　　　mental confusion or
　　　　disorientation (without loss
　　　　of consciousness) 850.0
　　　with loss of consciousness - *see*
　　　　Concussion, brain, with,
　　　　loss of consciousness
　　skull fracture - *see* Fracture, skull,
　　　by site
　　without loss of consciousness 850.0
　cauda equina 952.4
　cerebral - *see* Concussion, brain
　conus medullaris (spine) 952.4
　hydraulic - *see* Concussion, blast
　internal organs - *see* Injury, internal, by
　　site
　labyrinth - *see* Injury, intracranial
　ocular 921.3
　osseous labyrinth - *see* Injury,
　　intracranial
　spinal (cord) - *see also* Injury, spinal, by
　　site
　　due to
　　　broken
　　　　back - *see* Fracture, vertebra,
　　　　　by site, with spinal cord
　　　　　injury
　　　　neck - *see* Fracture, vertebra,
　　　　　cervical, with spinal cord
　　　　　injury
　　　fracture, fracture dislocation, or
　　　　compression fracture of
　　　　spine or vertebra - *see*
　　　　Fracture, vertebra, by site,
　　　　with spinal cord injury
　syndrome 310.2
　underwater blast - *see* Concussion, blast
Condition - *see also* Disease
　fetal hematologic 678.0●
　psychiatric 298.9
　respiratory NEC 519.9
　　acute or subacute NEC 519.9
　　　due to
　　　　external agent 508.9
　　　　　specified type NEC 508.8
　　　　fumes or vapors (chemical)
　　　　　(inhalation) 506.3
　　　　radiation 508.0

Condition *(Continued)*
　respiratory NEC *(Continued)*
　　chronic NEC 519.9
　　　due to
　　　　external agent 508.9
　　　　　specified type NEC 508.8
　　　　fumes or vapors (chemical)
　　　　　(inhalation) 506.4
　　　　radiation 508.1
　　　due to
　　　　external agent 508.9
　　　　　specified type NEC 508.8
　　　　fumes or vapors (chemical)
　　　　　inhalation 506.9
Conduct disturbance (*see also*
　　Disturbance, conduct) 312.9
　adjustment reaction 309.3
　hyperkinetic 314.2
Condyloma NEC 078.11
　acuminatum 078.11
　gonorrheal 098.0
　latum 091.3
　syphilitic 091.3
　　congenital 090.0
　venereal, syphilitic 091.3
Confinement - *see* Delivery
Conflagration - *see also* Burn, by site
　asphyxia (by inhalation of smoke,
　　gases, fumes, or vapors) 987.9
　　specified agent - *see* Table of Drugs
　　　and Chemicals
Conflict
　family V61.9
　　specified circumstance NEC V61.8
　interpersonal NEC V62.81
　marital V61.10
　　involving
　　　divorce V61.03
　　　estrangement V61.09
　parent (guardian)-child V61.20　　◀▥
　　adopted child V61.24　　◀
　　biological child V61.23　　◀
　　foster child V61.25　　◀
　partner V61.10
Confluent - *see* condition
Confusion, confused (mental) (state) (*see*
　　also State, confusional) 298.9
　acute 293.0
　epileptic 293.0
　postoperative 293.9
　psychogenic 298.2
　reactive (from emotional stress,
　　psychological trauma) 298.2
　subacute 293.1
Confusional arousals 327.41
Congelation 991.9
Congenital - *see also* condition
　aortic septum 747.29
　generalized fibromatosis (CGF) 759.89
　intrinsic factor deficiency 281.0
　malformation - *see* Anomaly
Congestion, congestive
　asphyxia, newborn 768.9
　bladder 596.8
　bowel 569.89
　brain (*see also* Disease, cerebrovascular
　　NEC) 437.8
　　malarial 084.9
　breast 611.79
　bronchi 519.19
　bronchial tube 519.19
　catarrhal 472.0
　cerebral - *see* Congestion, brain
　cerebrospinal - *see* Congestion, brain
　chest 786.9

Congestion, congestive *(Continued)*
  chill 780.99
    malarial *(see also* Malaria) 084.6
  circulatory NEC 459.9
  conjunctiva 372.71
  due to disturbance of circulation 459.9
  duodenum 537.3
  enteritis - *see* Enteritis
  eye 372.71
  fibrosis syndrome (pelvic) 625.5
  gastroenteritis - *see* Enteritis
  general 799.89
  glottis 476.0
  heart *(see also* Failure, heart) 428.0
  hepatic 573.0
  hypostatic (lung) 514
  intestine 569.89
  intracranial - *see* Congestion, brain
  kidney 593.89
  labyrinth 386.50
  larynx 476.0
  liver 573.0
  lung 786.9
    active or acute *(see also* Pneumonia) 486
      congenital 770.0
    chronic 514
    hypostatic 514
    idiopathic, acute 518.5
    passive 514
  malaria, malarial (brain) (fever) *(see also* Malaria) 084.6
  medulla - *see* Congestion, brain
  nasal 478.19
  nose 478.19
  orbit, orbital 376.33
    inflammatory (chronic) 376.10
      acute 376.00
  ovary 620.8
  pancreas 577.8
  pelvic, female 625.5
  pleural 511.0
  prostate (active) 602.1
  pulmonary - *see* Congestion, lung
  renal 593.89
  retina 362.89
  seminal vesicle 608.89
  spinal cord 336.1
  spleen 289.51
    chronic 289.51
  stomach 537.89
  trachea 464.11
  urethra 599.84
  uterus 625.5
    with subinvolution 621.1
  viscera 799.89
Congestive - *see* Congestion
Conical
  cervix 622.6
  cornea 371.60
  teeth 520.2
Conjoined twins 759.4
  causing disproportion (fetopelvic) 678.1 ●
  fetal 678.1 ●
Conjugal maladjustment V61.10
  involving
    divorce V61.03
    estrangement V61.09
Conjunctiva - *see* condition
Conjunctivitis (exposure) (infectious) (nondiphtheritic) (pneumococcal) (pustular) (staphylococcal) (streptococcal) NEC 372.30
  actinic 370.24

Conjunctivitis *(Continued)*
  acute 372.00
    atopic 372.05
    chemical 372.06 ◄
    contagious 372.03
    follicular 372.02
    hemorrhagic (viral) 077.4
    toxic 372.06 ◄
  adenoviral (acute) 077.3
  allergic (chronic) 372.14
    with hay fever 372.05
  anaphylactic 372.05
  angular 372.03
  Apollo (viral) 077.4
  atopic 372.05
  blennorrhagic (neonatorum) 098.40
  catarrhal 372.03
  chemical 372.06 ◄⫴
    allergic 372.05
    meaning corrosion - *see* Burn, conjunctiva
  chlamydial 077.98
    due to
      Chlamydia trachomatis - *see* Trachoma
      paratrachoma 077.0
  chronic 372.10
    allergic 372.14
    follicular 372.12
    simple 372.11
    specified type NEC 372.14
    vernal 372.13
  diphtheritic 032.81
  due to
    dust 372.05
    enterovirus type 70 077.4
    erythema multiforme 695.10 *[372.33]*
    filariasis *(see also* Filariasis) 125.9 *[372.15]*
    mucocutaneous
      disease NEC 372.33
      leishmaniasis 085.5 *[372.15]*
    Reiter's disease 099.3 *[372.33]*
    syphilis 095.8 *[372.10]*
    toxoplasmosis (acquired) 130.1
      congenital (active) 771.2
    trachoma - *see* Trachoma
  dust 372.05
  eczematous 370.31
  epidemic 077.1
    hemorrhagic 077.4
  follicular (acute) 372.02
    adenoviral (acute) 077.3
    chronic 372.12
  glare 370.24
  gonococcal (neonatorum) 098.40
  granular (trachomatous) 076.1
    late effect 139.1
  hemorrhagic (acute) (epidemic) 077.4
  herpetic (simplex) 054.43
    zoster 053.21
  inclusion 077.0
  infantile 771.6
  influenzal 372.03
  Koch-Weeks 372.03
  light 372.05
  medicamentosa 372.05
  membranous 372.04
  meningococcic 036.89
  Morax-Axenfeld 372.02
  mucopurulent NEC 372.03
  neonatal 771.6
    gonococcal 098.40
  Newcastle's 077.8

Conjunctivitis *(Continued)*
  nodosa 360.14
  of Beal 077.3
  parasitic 372.15
    filariasis *(see also* Filariasis) 125.9 *[372.15]*
    mucocutaneous leishmaniasis 085.5 *[372.15]*
  Parinaud's 372.02
  petrificans 372.39
  phlyctenular 370.31
  pseudomembranous 372.04
    diphtheritic 032.81
  purulent 372.03
  Reiter's 099.3 *[372.33]*
  rosacea 695.3 *[372.31]*
  serous 372.01
    viral 077.99
  simple chronic 372.11
  specified NEC 372.39
  sunlamp 372.04
  swimming pool 077.0
  toxic 372.06 ◄
  trachomatous (follicular) 076.1
    acute 076.0
    late effect 139.1
  traumatic NEC 372.39
  tuberculous *(see also* Tuberculosis) 017.3 ● *[370.31]*
  tularemic 021.3
  tularensis 021.3
  vernal 372.13
    limbar 372.13 *[370.32]*
  viral 077.99
    acute hemorrhagic 077.4
    specified NEC 077.8
Conjunctivochalasis 372.81
Conjunctoblepharitis - *see* Conjunctivitis
Conn (-Louis) syndrome (primary aldosteronism) 255.12
Connective tissue - *see* condition
Conradi (-Hünermann) syndrome or disease (chondrodysplasia calcificans congenita) 756.59
Consanguinity V19.7
Consecutive - *see* condition
Consolidated lung (base) - *see* Pneumonia, lobar
Constipation 564.00
  atonic 564.09
  drug induced
    correct substance properly administered 564.09
    overdose or wrong substance given or taken 977.9
    specified drug - *see* Table of Drugs and Chemicals
  neurogenic 564.09
  other specified NEC 564.09
  outlet dysfunction 564.02
  psychogenic 306.4
  simple 564.00
  slow transit 564.01
  spastic 564.09
Constitutional - *see also* condition
  arterial hypotension *(see also* Hypotension) 458.9
  obesity 278.00
    morbid 278.01
  psychopathic state 301.9
  short stature in childhood 783.43
  state, developmental V21.9
    specified development NEC V21.8
  substandard 301.6

◄ New   ◄⫴ Revised   ~~deleted~~ Deleted   ● Use Additional Digit(s)   ▨ Omit code

Constitutionally substandard 301.6
Constriction
  anomalous, meningeal bands or folds
    742.8
  aortic arch (congenital) 747.10
  asphyxiation or suffocation by 994.7
  bronchus 519.19
  canal, ear (see also Stricture, ear canal,
    acquired) 380.50
  duodenum 537.3
  gallbladder (see also Obstruction,
    gallbladder) 575.2
    congenital 751.69
  intestine (see also Obstruction, intestine)
    560.9
  larynx 478.74
    congenital 748.3
  meningeal bands or folds, anomalous
    742.8
  organ or site, congenital NEC - see
    Atresia
  prepuce (congenital) 605
  pylorus 537.0
    adult hypertrophic 537.0
    congenital or infantile 750.5
    newborn 750.5
  ring (uterus) 661.4●
    affecting fetus or newborn 763.7
  spastic - see also Spasm
    ureter 593.3
    urethra - see Stricture, urethra
  stomach 537.89
  ureter 593.3
  urethra - see Stricture, urethra
  visual field (functional) (peripheral)
    368.45
Constrictive - see condition
Consultation V65.9
  medical - see also Counseling, medical
  specified reason NEC V65.8
  without complaint or sickness V65.9
    feared complaint unfounded V65.5
    specified reason NEC V65.8
Consumption - see Tuberculosis
Contact
  with
    AIDS virus V01.79
    anthrax V01.81
    asbestos V15.84 ◄
    cholera V01.0
    communicable disease V01.9
      specified type NEC V01.89
      viral NEC V01.79
    Escherichia coli (E. coli) V01.83
    German measles V01.4
    gonorrhea V01.6
    HIV V01.79
    human immunodeficiency virus
      V01.79
    lead V15.86 ◄
    meningococcus V01.84
    parasitic disease NEC V01.89
    poliomyelitis V01.2
    potentially hazardous body fluids
      V15.85 ◄
    rabies V01.5
    rubella V01.4
    SARS-associated coronavirus V01.82
    smallpox V01.3
    syphilis V01.6
    tuberculosis V01.1
    varicella V01.71
    venereal disease V01.6
    viral disease NEC V01.79
  dermatitis - see Dermatitis

Contamination, food (see also Poisoning,
    food) 005.9
Contraception, contraceptive
  advice NEC V25.09
    family planning V25.09
    fitting of diaphragm V25.02
    prescribing or use of
      oral contraceptive agent V25.01
      specified agent NEC V25.02
  counseling NEC V25.09
    emergency V25.03
    family planning V25.09
    fitting of diaphragm V25.02
    prescribing or use of
      oral contraceptive agent V25.01
        emergency V25.03
        postcoital V25.03
      specified agent NEC V25.02
  device (in situ) V45.59
    causing menorrhagia 996.76
    checking V25.42
    complications 996.32
    insertion V25.1
    intrauterine V45.51
    reinsertion V25.42
    removal V25.42
    subdermal V45.52
  fitting of diaphragm V25.02
  insertion
    intrauterine contraceptive device
      V25.1
    subdermal implantable V25.5
  maintenance V25.40
    examination V25.40
      intrauterine device V25.42
      oral contraceptive V25.41
      specified method NEC V25.49
      subdermal implantable V25.43
    intrauterine device V25.42
    oral contraceptive V25.41
    specified method NEC V25.49
    subdermal implantable V25.43
  management NEC V25.49
  prescription
    oral contraceptive agent V25.01
      emergency V25.03
      postcoital V25.03
      repeat V25.41
    specified agent NEC V25.02
      repeat V25.49
  sterilization V25.2
  surveillance V25.40
    intrauterine device V25.42
    oral contraceptive agent V25.41
    specified method NEC V25.49
    subdermal implantable V25.43
Contraction, contracture, contracted
  Achilles tendon (see also Short, tendon,
    Achilles) 727.81
  anus 564.89
  axilla 729.90
  bile duct (see also Disease, biliary) 576.8
  bladder 596.8
    neck or sphincter 596.0
  bowel (see also Obstruction, intestine)
    560.9
  Braxton Hicks 644.1●
  breast implant, capsular 611.83
  bronchus 519.19
  burn (old) - see Cicatrix
  capsular, of breast implant 611.83
  cecum (see also Obstruction, intestine)
    560.9
  cervix (see also Stricture, cervix) 622.4
    congenital 752.49

Contraction, contracture, contracted
    (Continued)
  cicatricial - see Cicatrix
  colon (see also Obstruction, intestine)
    560.9
  conjunctiva, trachomatous, active
    076.1
    late effect 139.1
  Dupuytren's 728.6
  eyelid 374.41
  eye socket (after enucleation) 372.64
  face 729.90
  fascia (lata) (postural) 728.89
    Dupuytren's 728.6
    palmar 728.6
    plantar 728.71
  finger NEC 736.29
    congenital 755.59
    joint (see also Contraction, joint)
      718.44
  flaccid, paralytic
    joint (see also Contraction, joint)
      718.4●
    muscle 728.85
      ocular 378.50
  gallbladder (see also Obstruction,
    gallbladder) 575.2
  hamstring 728.89
    tendon 727.81
  heart valve - see Endocarditis
  Hicks' 644.1●
  hip (see also Contraction, joint) 718.4●
  hourglass
    bladder 596.8
      congenital 753.8
    gallbladder (see also Obstruction,
      gallbladder) 575.2
      congenital 751.69
    stomach 536.8
      congenital 750.7
      psychogenic 306.4
    uterus 661.4●
      affecting fetus or newborn 763.7
  hysterical 300.11
  infantile (see also Epilepsy) 345.6●
  internal os (see also Stricture, cervix)
    622.4
  intestine (see also Obstruction, intestine)
    560.9
  joint (abduction) (acquired)
    (adduction) (flexion) (rotation)
    718.40
    ankle 718.47
    congenital NEC 755.8
      generalized or multiple 754.89
        lower limb joints 754.89
      hip (see also Subluxation,
        congenital, hip) 754.32
      lower limb (including pelvic
        girdle) not involving hip
        754.89
      upper limb (including shoulder
        girdle) 755.59
    elbow 718.42
    foot 718.47
    hand 718.44
    hip 718.45
    hysterical 300.11
    knee 718.46
    multiple sites 718.49
    pelvic region 718.45
    shoulder (region) 718.41
    specified site NEC 718.48
    wrist 718.43

Contraction, contracture, contracted
  (Continued)
    kidney (granular) (secondary) *(see also*
        Sclerosis, renal) 587
      congenital 753.3
      hydronephritic 591
      pyelonephritic *(see also* Pyelitis,
          chronic) 590.00
      tuberculous *(see also* Tuberculosis)
          016.0●
    ligament 728.89
      congenital 756.89
    liver - *see* Cirrhosis, liver
    muscle (postinfectional) (postural)
        NEC 728.85
      congenital 756.89
        sternocleidomastoid 754.1
      extraocular 378.60
      eye (extrinsic) *(see also* Strabismus)
          378.9
        paralytic *(see also* Strabismus,
            paralytic) 378.50
      flaccid 728.85
      hysterical 300.11
      ischemic (Volkmann's) 958.6
      paralytic 728.85
      posttraumatic 958.6
      psychogenic 306.0
        specified as conversion reaction
            300.11
    myotonic 728.85
    neck *(see also* Torticollis) 723.5
      congenital 754.1
      psychogenic 306.0
    ocular muscle *(see also* Strabismus)
        378.9
      paralytic *(see also* Strabismus,
          paralytic) 378.50
    organ or site, congenital NEC - *see*
        Atresia
    outlet (pelvis) - *see* Contraction, pelvis
    palmar fascia 728.6
    paralytic
      joint *(see also* Contraction, joint)
          718.4●
      muscle 728.85
        ocular *(see also* Strabismus,
            paralytic) 378.50
    pelvis (acquired) (general) 738.6
      affecting fetus or newborn 763.1
      complicating delivery 653.1●
        causing obstructed labor
            660.1●
      generally contracted 653.1●
        causing obstructed labor
            660.1●
      inlet 653.2●
        causing obstructed labor
            660.1●
      midpelvic 653.8●
        causing obstructed labor
            660.1●
      midplane 653.8●
        causing obstructed labor
            660.1●
      outlet 653.3●
        causing obstructed labor
            660.1●
    plantar fascia 728.71
    premature
      atrial 427.61
      auricular 427.61
      auriculoventricular 427.61
      heart (junctional) (nodal) 427.60

Contraction, contracture, contracted
  (Continued)
    premature *(Continued)*
      supraventricular 427.61
      ventricular 427.69
    prostate 602.8
    pylorus *(see also* Pylorospasm) 537.81
    rectosigmoid *(see also* Obstruction,
        intestine) 560.9
    rectum, rectal (sphincter) 564.89
      psychogenic 306.4
    ring (Bandl's) 661.4●
      affecting fetus or newborn 763.7
    scar - *see* Cicatrix
    sigmoid *(see also* Obstruction, intestine)
        560.9
    socket, eye 372.64
    spine *(see also* Curvature, spine) 737.9
    stomach 536.8
      hourglass 536.8
        congenital 750.7
        psychogenic 306.4
      psychogenic 306.4
    tendon (sheath) *(see also* Short, tendon)
        727.81
    toe 735.8
    ureterovesical orifice (postinfectional)
        593.3
    urethra 599.84
    uterus 621.8
      abnormal 661.9●
        affecting fetus or newborn 763.7
      clonic, hourglass or tetanic 661.4●
        affecting fetus or newborn 763.7
      dyscoordinate 661.4●
        affecting fetus or newborn 763.7
      hourglass 661.4●
        affecting fetus or newborn 763.7
      hypotonic NEC 661.2●
        affecting fetus or newborn 763.7
      incoordinate 661.4●
        affecting fetus or newborn 763.7
      inefficient or poor 661.2●
        affecting fetus or newborn 763.7
      irregular 661.2●
        affecting fetus or newborn 763.7
      tetanic 661.4●
        affecting fetus or newborn 763.7
    vagina (outlet) 623.2
    vesical 596.8
      neck or urethral orifice 596.0
    visual field, generalized 368.45
    Volkmann's (ischemic) 958.6
Contusion (skin surface intact) 924.9
  with
    crush injury - *see* Crush
    dislocation - *see* Dislocation, by site
    fracture - *see* Fracture, by site
    internal injury - *see also* Injury,
        internal, by site
      heart - *see* Contusion, cardiac
      kidney - *see* Contusion, kidney
      liver - *see* Contusion, liver
      lung - *see* Contusion, lung
      spleen - *see* Contusion, spleen
    intracranial injury - *see* Injury,
        intracranial
    nerve injury - *see* Injury, nerve
    open wound - *see* Wound, open, by
        site
  abdomen, abdominal (muscle) (wall)
      922.2
    organ(s) NEC 868.00
  adnexa, eye NEC 921.9

Contusion *(Continued)*
  ankle 924.21
    with other parts of foot 924.20
  arm 923.9
    lower (with elbow) 923.10
    upper 923.03
      with shoulder or axillary region
          923.09
  auditory canal (external) (meatus) (and
      other part(s) of neck, scalp, or
      face, except eye) 920
  auricle, ear (and other part(s) of neck,
      scalp, or face except eye) 920
  axilla 923.02
    with shoulder or upper arm 923.09
  back 922.31
  bone NEC 924.9
  brain (cerebral) (membrane) (with
      hemorrhage) 851.8●

Note 17   Use the following fifth-
digit subclassification with categories
851–854:

  0   unspecified state of
        consciousness
  1   with no loss of consciousness
  2   with brief [less than one hour]
        loss of consciousness
  3   with moderate [1-24 hours] loss
        of consciousness
  4   with prolonged [more than 24
        hours] loss of consciousness
        and return to pre-existing
        conscious level
  5   with prolonged [more than 24
        hours] loss of
        consciousness, without
        return to pre-existing
        conscious level

Use fifth-digit 5 to designate when a
patient is unconscious and dies before
regaining consciousness, regardless of
the duration of the loss of consciousness

  6   with loss of consciousness of
        unspecified duration
  9   with concussion, unspecified

---

  with
    open intracranial wound 851.9●
    skull fracture - *see* Fracture, skull,
        by site
  cerebellum 851.4●
    with open intracranial wound
        851.5●
  cortex 851.0●
    with open intracranial wound
        851.1●
  occipital lobe 851.4●
    with open intracranial wound
        851.5●
  stem 851.4●
    with open intracranial wound
        851.5●
  breast 922.0
  brow (and other part(s) of neck, scalp,
      or face, except eye) 920
  buttock 922.32
  canthus 921.1
  cardiac 861.01
    with open wound into thorax 861.11
  cauda equina (spine) 952.4
  cerebellum - *see* Contusion, brain,
      cerebellum

Contusion (*Continued*)
  cerebral - *see* Contusion, brain
  cheek(s) (and other part(s) of neck, scalp, or face, except eye) 920
  chest (wall) 922.1
  chin (and other part(s) of neck, scalp, or face, except eye) 920
  clitoris 922.4
  conjunctiva 921.1
  conus medullaris (spine) 952.4
  cornea 921.3
  corpus cavernosum 922.4
  cortex (brain) (cerebral) - *see* Contusion, brain, cortex
  costal region 922.1
  ear (and other part(s) of neck, scalp, or face except eye) 920
  elbow 923.11
    with forearm 923.10
  epididymis 922.4
  epigastric region 922.2
  eye NEC 921.9
  eyeball 921.3
  eyelid(s) (and periocular area) 921.1
  face (and neck, or scalp, any part, except eye) 920
  femoral triangle 922.2
  fetus or newborn 772.6
  finger(s) (nail) (subungual) 923.3
  flank 922.2
  foot (with ankle) (excluding toe(s)) 924.20
  forearm (and elbow) 923.10
  forehead (and other part(s) of neck, scalp, or face, except eye) 920
  genital organs, external 922.4
  globe (eye) 921.3
  groin 922.2
  gum(s) (and other part(s) of neck, scalp, or face, except eye) 920
  hand(s) (except fingers alone) 923.20
  head (any part, except eye) (and face) (and neck) 920
  heart - *see* Contusion, cardiac
  heel 924.20
  hip 924.01
    with thigh 924.00
  iliac region 922.2
  inguinal region 922.2
  internal organs (abdomen, chest, or pelvis) NEC - *see* Injury, internal, by site
  interscapular region 922.33
  iris (eye) 921.3
  kidney 866.01
    with open wound into cavity 866.11
  knee 924.11
    with lower leg 924.10
  labium (majus) (minus) 922.4
  lacrimal apparatus, gland, or sac 921.1
  larynx (and other part(s) of neck, scalp, or face, except eye) 920
  late effect - *see* Late, effects (of), contusion
  leg 924.5
    lower (with knee) 924.10
  lens 921.3
  lingual (and other part(s) of neck, scalp, or face, except eye) 920
  lip(s) (and other part(s) of neck, scalp, or face, except eye) 920

Contusion (*Continued*)
  liver 864.01
    with
      laceration - *see* Laceration, liver
      open wound into cavity 864.11
  lower extremity 924.5
    multiple sites 924.4
  lumbar region 922.31
  lung 861.21
    with open wound into thorax 861.31
  malar region (and other part(s) of neck, scalp, or face, except eye) 920
  mandibular joint (and other part(s) of neck, scalp, or face, except eye) 920
  mastoid region (and other part(s) of neck, scalp, or face, except eye) 920
  membrane, brain - *see* Contusion, brain
  midthoracic region 922.1
  mouth (and other part(s) of neck, scalp, or face, except eye) 920
  multiple sites (not classifiable to same three-digit category) 924.8
    lower limb 924.4
    trunk 922.8
    upper limb 923.8
  muscle NEC 924.9
  myocardium - *see* Contusion, cardiac
  nasal (septum) (and other part(s) of neck, scalp, or face, except eye) 920
  neck (and scalp, or face, any part, except eye) 920
  nerve - *see* Injury, nerve, by site
  nose (and other part(s) of neck, scalp, or face, except eye) 920
  occipital region (scalp) (and neck or face, except eye) 920
    lobe - *see* Contusion, brain, occipital lobe
  orbit (region) (tissues) 921.2
  palate (soft) (and other part(s) of neck, scalp, or face, except eye) 920
  parietal region (scalp) (and neck, or face, except eye) 920
    lobe - *see* Contusion, brain
  penis 922.4
  pericardium - *see* Contusion, cardiac
  perineum 922.4
  periocular area 921.1
  pharynx (and other part(s) of neck, scalp, or face, except eye) 920
  popliteal space (*see also* Contusion, knee) 924.11
  prepuce 922.4
  pubic region 922.4
  pudenda 922.4
  pulmonary - *see* Contusion, lung
  quadriceps femoralis 924.00
  rib cage 922.1
  sacral region 922.32
  salivary ducts or glands (and other part(s) of neck, scalp, or face, except eye) 920
  scalp (and neck, or face, any part, except eye) 920
  scapular region 923.01
    with shoulder or upper arm 923.09
  sclera (eye) 921.3
  scrotum 922.4
  shoulder 923.00
    with upper arm or axillar regions 923.09

Contusion (*Continued*)
  skin NEC 924.9
  skull 920
  spermatic cord 922.4
  spinal cord - *see also* Injury, spinal, by site
    cauda equina 952.4
    conus medullaris 952.4
  spleen 865.01
    with open wound into cavity 865.11
  sternal region 922.1
  stomach - *see* Injury, internal, stomach
  subconjunctival 921.1
  subcutaneous NEC 924.9
  submaxillary region (and other part(s) of neck, scalp, or face, except eye) 920
  submental region (and other part(s) of neck, scalp, or face, except eye) 920
  subperiosteal NEC 924.9
  supraclavicular fossa (and other part(s) of neck, scalp, or face, except eye) 920
  supraorbital (and other part(s) of neck, scalp, or face, except eye) 920
  temple (region) (and other part(s) of neck, scalp, or face, except eye) 920
  testis 922.4
  thigh (and hip) 924.00
  thorax 922.1
    organ - *see* Injury, internal, intrathoracic
  throat (and other part(s) of neck, scalp, or face, except eye) 920
  thumb(s) (nail) (subungual) 923.3
  toe(s) (nail) (subungual) 924.3
  tongue (and other part(s) of neck, scalp, or face, except eye) 920
  trunk 922.9
    multiple sites 922.8
    specified site - *see* Contusion, by site
  tunica vaginalis 922.4
  tympanum (membrane) (and other part(s) of neck, scalp, or face, except eye) 920
  upper extremity 923.9
    multiple sites 923.8
  uvula (and other part(s) of neck, scalp, or face, except eye) 920
  vagina 922.4
  vocal cord(s) (and other part(s) of neck, scalp, or face, except eye) 920
  vulva 922.4
  wrist 923.21
    with hand(s), except finger(s) alone 923.20
Conus (any type) (congenital) 743.57
  acquired 371.60
  medullaris syndrome 336.8
Convalescence (following) V66.9
  chemotherapy V66.2
  medical NEC V66.5
  psychotherapy V66.3
  radiotherapy V66.1
  surgery NEC V66.0
  treatment (for) NEC V66.5
    combined V66.6
    fracture V66.4
    mental disorder NEC V66.3
    specified disorder NEC V66.5

◀ New ◀▥ Revised ~~deleted~~ Deleted ● Use Additional Digit(s) ▧ Omit code

Counseling NEC *(Continued)*
  injury prevention V65.43
  insulin pump training V65.46
  marital V61.10
  medical (for) V65.9
    boarding school resident V60.6
    condition not demonstrated V65.5
    feared complaint and no disease
      found V65.5
    institutional resident V60.6
    on behalf of another V65.19
    person living alone V60.3
  natural family planning
    procreative V26.41
    to avoid pregnancy V25.04
  parent (guardian)-child conflict
    V61.20 ◄▐▐▐
    adopted child V61.24 ◄
    biological child V61.23 ◄
    foster child V61.25 ◄
    specified problem NEC V61.29
  partner abuse
    perpetrator V61.12
    victim V61.11
  pediatric pre-birth visit for expectant
    mother V65.11 ◄▐▐▐
    pre-adoption visit for adoptive
      parent(s) V65.11 ◄
    pre-birth visit for expectant parents
      V65.11 ◄
  perpetrator of
    child abuse V62.83
      parental V61.22
    partner abuse V61.12
    spouse abuse V61.12
  procreative V65.49
  sex NEC V65.49
  transmitted disease NEC V65.45
    HIV V65.44
  specified reason NEC V65.49
  spousal abuse
    perpetrator V61.12
    victim V61.11
  substance use and abuse V65.42
  syphilis V65.45
  victim (of)
    abuse NEC V62.89
    child abuse V61.21
    partner abuse V61.11
    spousal abuse V61.11
Coupled rhythm 427.89
Couvelaire uterus (complicating
  delivery) - *see* Placenta, separation
Cowper's gland - *see* condition
Cowperitis *(see also* Urethritis) 597.89
  gonorrheal (acute) 098.0
    chronic or duration of 2 months or
      over 098.2
Cowpox (abortive) 051.01
  due to vaccination 999.0
  eyelid 051.01 *[373.5]*
    postvaccination 999.0 *[373.5]*
Coxa
  plana 732.1
  valga (acquired) 736.31
    congenital 755.61
    late effect of rickets 268.1
  vara (acquired) 736.32
    congenital 755.62
    late effect of rickets 268.1
Coxae malum senilis 715.25
Coxalgia (nontuberculous) 719.45
  tuberculous *(see also* Tuberculosis)
    015.1● *[730.85]*
Coxalgic pelvis 736.30

Coxitis 716.65
Coxsackie (infection) (virus) 079.2
  central nervous system NEC 048
  endocarditis 074.22
  enteritis 008.67
  meningitis (aseptic) 047.0
  myocarditis 074.23
  pericarditis 074.21
  pharyngitis 074.0
  pleurodynia 074.1
  specific disease NEC 074.8
Crabs, meaning pubic lice 132.2
Crack baby 760.75
Cracked
  nipple 611.2
    puerperal, postpartum 676.1●
  tooth 521.81
Cradle cap 690.11
Craft neurosis 300.89
Craigiasis 007.8
Cramp(s) 729.82
  abdominal 789.0●
  bathing 994.1
  colic 789.7 ◄▐▐▐
    infantile 789.7
    psychogenic 306.4
  due to immersion 994.1
  extremity (lower) (upper) NEC
    729.82
  fireman 992.2
  heat 992.2
  hysterical 300.11
  immersion 994.1
  intestinal 789.0●
    psychogenic 306.4
  linotypist's 300.89
    organic 333.84
  muscle (extremity) (general) 729.82
    due to immersion 994.1
    hysterical 300.11
  occupational (hand) 300.89
    organic 333.84
  psychogenic 307.89
  salt depletion 276.1
  sleep related leg 327.52
  stoker 992.2
  stomach 789.0●
  telegraphers' 300.89
    organic 333.84
  typists' 300.89
    organic 333.84
  uterus 625.8
    menstrual 625.3
  writers' 333.84
    organic 333.84
    psychogenic 300.89
Cranial - *see* condition
Cranioclasis, fetal 763.89
Craniocleidodysostosis 755.59
Craniofenestria (skull) 756.0
Craniolacunia (skull) 756.0
Craniopagus 759.4
Craniopathy, metabolic 733.3
Craniopharyngeal - *see* condition
Craniopharyngioma (M9350/1) 237.0
Craniorachischisis (totalis) 740.1
Cranioschisis 756.0
Craniostenosis 756.0
Craniosynostosis 756.0
Craniotabes (cause unknown) 733.3
  rachitic 268.1
  syphilitic 090.5
Craniotomy, fetal 763.89
Cranium - *see* condition
Craw-craw 125.3

CRBSI (catheter-related bloodstream
  infection) 999.31
Creaking joint 719.60
  ankle 719.67
  elbow 719.62
  foot 719.67
  hand 719.64
  hip 719.65
  knee 719.66
  multiple sites 719.69
  pelvic region 719.65
  shoulder (region) 719.61
  specified site NEC 719.68
  wrist 719.63
Creeping
  eruption 126.9
  palsy 335.21
  paralysis 335.21
Crenated tongue 529.8
Creotoxism 005.9
Crepitus
  caput 756.0
  joint 719.60
    ankle 719.67
    elbow 719.62
    foot 719.67
    hand 719.64
    hip 719.65
    knee 719.66
    multiple sites 719.69
    pelvic region 719.65
    shoulder (region) 719.61
    specified site NEC 719.68
    wrist 719.63
Crescent or conus choroid, congenital
  743.57
Cretin, cretinism (athyrotic) (congenital)
  (endemic) (metabolic) (nongoitrous)
  (sporadic) 243
  goitrous (sporadic) 246.1
  pelvis (dwarf type) (male type) 243
    with disproportion (fetopelvic)
      653.1●
      affecting fetus or newborn
        763.1
      causing obstructed labor 660.1●
        affecting fetus or newborn
          763.1
  pituitary 253.3
Cretinoid degeneration 243
Creutzfeldt-Jakob disease (CJD)
  (syndrome) 046.19
  with dementia
    with behavioral disturbance 046.19
      [294.11]
    without behavioral disturbance
      046.19 *[294.10]*
  familial 046.19
  iatrogenic 046.19
  specified NEC 046.19
  sporadic 046.19
  variant (vCJD) 046.11
    with dementia
      with behavioral disturbance
        046.11 *[294.11]*
      without behavioral disturbance
        046.11 *[294.10]*
Crib death 798.0
Cribriform hymen 752.49
Cri-du-chat syndrome 758.31
Crigler-Najjar disease or syndrome
  (congenital hyperbilirubinemia)
  277.4
Crimean hemorrhagic fever 065.0
Criminalism 301.7

◄ New   ◄▐▐▐ Revised   ~~deleted~~ Deleted   ● Use Additional Digit(s)   ▨ Omit code

Crisis
  abdomen 789.0●
  addisonian (acute adrenocortical
      insufficiency) 255.41
  adrenal (cortical) 255.41
  asthmatic - *see* Asthma
  brain, cerebral (*see also* Disease,
      cerebrovascular, acute) 436
  celiac 579.0
  Dietl's 593.4
  emotional NEC 309.29
      acute reaction to stress 308.0
      adjustment reaction 309.9
      specific to childhood or adolescence
          313.9
  gastric (tabetic) 094.0
  glaucomatocyclitic 364.22
  heart (*see also* Failure, heart) 428.9
  hypertensive - *see* Hypertension
  nitritoid
      correct substance properly
          administered 458.29
      overdose or wrong substance given
          or taken 961.1
  oculogyric 378.87
      psychogenic 306.7
  Pel's 094.0
  psychosexual identity 302.6
  rectum 094.0
  renal 593.81
  sickle cell 282.62
  stomach (tabetic) 094.0
  tabetic 094.0
  thyroid (*see also* Thyrotoxicosis) 242.9●
  thyrotoxic (*see also* Thyrotoxicosis)
      242.9●
  vascular - *see* Disease, cerebrovascular,
      acute
Crocq's disease (acrocyanosis) 443.89
Crohn's disease (*see also* Enteritis,
    regional) 555.9
Cronkhite-Canada syndrome 211.3
Crooked septum, nasal 470
Cross
  birth (of fetus) complicating delivery
      652.3●
      with successful version 652.1●
      causing obstructed labor 660.0●
  bite, anterior or posterior 524.27
  eye (*see also* Esotropia) 378.00
Crossed ectopia of kidney 753.3
Crossfoot 754.50
Croup, croupous (acute) (angina)
    (catarrhal) (infective)
    (inflammatory) (laryngeal)
    (membranous) (nondiphtheritic)
    (pseudomembranous) 464.4
  asthmatic (*see also* Asthma) 493.9●
  bronchial 466.0
  diphtheritic (membranous) 032.3
  false 478.75
  spasmodic 478.75
      diphtheritic 032.3
  stridulous 478.75
      diphtheritic 032.3
Crouzon's disease (craniofacial
    dysostosis) 756.0
Crowding, teeth 524.31
CRST syndrome (cutaneous systemic
    sclerosis) 710.1
Cruchet's disease (encephalitis lethargica)
    049.8
Cruelty in children (*see also* Disturbance,
    conduct) 312.9

Crural ulcer (*see also* Ulcer, lower
    extremity) 707.10
Crush, crushed, crushing (injury) 929.9
  abdomen 926.19
      internal - *see* Injury, internal,
          abdomen
  ankle 928.21
      with other parts of foot 928.20
  arm 927.9
      lower (and elbow) 927.10
      upper 927.03
          with shoulder or axillary region
              927.09
  axilla 927.02
      with shoulder or upper arm 927.09
  back 926.11
  breast 926.19
  buttock 926.12
  cheek 925.1
  chest - *see* Injury, internal, chest
  ear 925.1
  elbow 927.11
      with forearm 927.10
  face 925.1
  finger(s) 927.3
      with hand(s) 927.20
      and wrist(s) 927.21
  flank 926.19
  foot, excluding toe(s) alone (with
      ankle) 928.20
  forearm (and elbow) 927.10
  genitalia, external (female) (male) 926.0
      internal - *see* Injury, internal, genital
          organ NEC
  hand, except finger(s) alone (and wrist)
      927.20
  head - *see* Fracture, skull, by site
  heel 928.20
  hip 928.01
      with thigh 928.00
  internal organ (abdomen, chest, or
      pelvis) - *see* Injury, internal, by
      site
  knee 928.11
      with leg, lower 928.10
  labium (majus) (minus) 926.0
  larynx 925.2
  late effect - *see* Late, effects (of), crushing
  leg 928.9
      lower 928.10
          and knee 928.11
      upper 928.00
  limb
      lower 928.9
          multiple sites 928.8
      upper 927.9
          multiple sites 927.8
  multiple sites NEC 929.0
  neck 925.2
  nerve - *see* Injury, nerve, by site
  nose 802.0
      open 802.1
  penis 926.0
  pharynx 925.2
  scalp 925.1
  scapular region 927.01
      with shoulder or upper arm 927.09
  scrotum 926.0
  shoulder 927.00
      with upper arm or axillary region
          927.09
  skull or cranium - *see* Fracture, skull, by
      site
  spinal cord - *see* Injury, spinal, by site

Crush, crushed, crushing (*Continued*)
  syndrome (complication of trauma)
      958.5
  testis 926.0
  thigh (with hip) 928.00
  throat 925.2
  thumb(s) (and fingers) 927.3
  toe(s) 928.3
      with foot 928.20
      and ankle 928.21
  tonsil 925.2
  trunk 926.9
      chest - *see* Injury, internal,
          intrathoracic organs NEC
      internal organ - *see* Injury, internal,
          by site
      multiple sites 926.8
      specified site NEC 926.19
  vulva 926.0
  wrist 927.21
      with hand(s), except fingers alone
          927.20
Crusta lactea 690.11
Crusts 782.8
Crutch paralysis 953.4
Cruveilhier's disease 335.21
**Cruveilhier-Baumgarten cirrhosis,
    disease, or syndrome** 571.5
Cruz-Chagas disease (*see also*
    Trypanosomiasis) 086.2
Crying
  constant, continuous
      adolescent 780.95
      adult 780.95
      baby 780.92
      child 780.95
      infant 780.92
      newborn 780.92
  excessive
      adolescent 780.95
      adult 780.95
      baby 780.92
      child 780.95
      infant 780.92
      newborn 780.92
Cryofibrinogenemia 273.2
Cryoglobulinemia (mixed) 273.2
Crypt (anal) (rectal) 569.49
Cryptitis (anal) (rectal) 569.49
Cryptococcosis (European) (pulmonary)
    (systemic) 117.5
Cryptococcus 117.5
  epidermicus 117.5
  neoformans, infection by 117.5
Cryptopapillitis (anus) 569.49
Cryptophthalmos (eyelid) 743.06
**Cryptorchid, cryptorchism,
    cryptorchidism** 752.51
Cryptosporidiosis 007.4
  hepatobiliary 136.8 ◀
  respiratory 136.8 ◀
Cryptotia 744.29
Crystallopathy
  calcium pyrophosphate (*see also*
      Arthritis) 275.49 [712.2]●
  dicalcium phosphate (*see also* Arthritis)
      275.49 [712.1]●
  gouty 274.00 ◀▥
  pyrophosphate NEC (*see also* Arthritis)
      275.49 [712.2]●
  uric acid 274.00 ◀▥
Crystalluria 791.9
Csillag's disease (lichen sclerosus et
    atrophicus) 701.0
Cuban itch 050.1

Cubitus
    valgus (acquired) 736.01
        congenital 755.59
        late effect of rickets 268.1
    varus (acquired) 736.02
        congenital 755.59
        late effect of rickets 268.1
Cultural deprivation V62.4
Cupping of optic disc 377.14
Curling's ulcer - *see* Ulcer, duodenum
Curling esophagus 530.5
Curschmann (-Batten) (-Steinert) disease
        or syndrome 359.21
Curvature
    organ or site, congenital NEC - *see*
        Distortion
    penis (lateral) 752.69
    Pott's (spinal) (*see also* Tuberculosis)
        015.0● [737.43]
    radius, idiopathic, progressive
        (congenital) 755.54
    spine (acquired) (angular) (idiopathic)
        (incorrect) (postural) 737.9
        congenital 754.2
        due to or associated with
            Charcôt-Marie-Tooth disease
                356.1 [737.40]
            mucopolysaccharidosis 277.5
                [737.40]
            neurofibromatosis 237.71 [737.40]
            osteitis
                deformans 731.0 [737.40]
                fibrosa cystica 252.01 [737.40]
            osteoporosis (*see also*
                Osteoporosis) 733.00
                [737.40]
            poliomyelitis (*see also*
                Poliomyelitis) 138 [737.40]
            tuberculosis (Pott's curvature) (*see*
                also Tuberculosis) 015.0●
                [737.43]
        kyphoscoliotic (*see also*
            Kyphoscoliosis) 737.30
        kyphotic (*see also* Kyphosis) 737.10
        late effect of rickets 268.1 [737.40]
        Pott's 015.0● [737.40]
        scoliotic (*see also* Scoliosis) 737.30
        specified NEC 737.8
        tuberculous 015.0● [737.40]
Cushing's
    basophilism, disease, or syndrome
        (iatrogenic) (idiopathic) (pituitary
        basophilism) (pituitary
        dependent) 255.0
    ulcer - *see* Ulcer, peptic
Cushingoid due to steroid therapy
    correct substance properly
        administered 255.0
    overdose or wrong substance given or
        taken 962.0
Cut (external) - *see* Wound, open, by site
Cutaneous - *see also* condition
    hemorrhage 782.7
    horn (cheek) (eyelid) (mouth) 702.8
    larva migrans 126.9
Cutis - *see also* condition
    hyperelastic 756.83
        acquired 701.8
    laxa 756.83
        senilis 701.8
    marmorata 782.61
    osteosis 709.3
    pendula 756.83
        acquired 701.8

Cutis (*Continued*)
    rhomboidalis nuchae 701.8
    verticis gyrata 757.39
        acquired 701.8
Cyanopathy, newborn 770.83
Cyanosis 782.5
    autotoxic 289.7
    common atrioventricular canal
        745.69
    congenital 770.83
    conjunctiva 372.71
    due to
        endocardial cushion defect
            745.60
        nonclosure, foramen botalli 745.5
        patent foramen botalli 745.5
        persistent foramen ovale 745.5
    enterogenous 289.7
    fetus or newborn 770.83
    ostium primum defect 745.61
    paroxysmal digital 443.0
    retina, retinal 362.10
Cycle
    anovulatory 628.0
    menstrual, irregular 626.4
Cyclencephaly 759.89
Cyclical vomiting 536.2
    associated with migraine 346.2●
    psychogenic 306.4
Cyclitic membrane 364.74
Cyclitis (*see also* Iridocyclitis) 364.3
    acute 364.00
        primary 364.01
        recurrent 364.02
    chronic 364.10
        in
            sarcoidosis 135 [364.11]
            tuberculosis (*see also* Tuberculosis)
                017.3● [364.11]
    Fuchs' heterochromic 364.21
    granulomatous 364.10
    lens induced 364.23
    nongranulomatous 364.00
    posterior 363.21
    primary 364.01
    recurrent 364.02
    secondary (noninfectious) 364.04
        infectious 364.03
    subacute 364.00
        primary 364.01
        recurrent 364.02
Cyclokeratitis - *see* Keratitis
Cyclophoria 378.44
Cyclopia, cyclops 759.89
Cycloplegia 367.51
Cyclospasm 367.53
Cyclosporiasis 007.5
Cyclothymia 301.13
Cyclothymic personality 301.13
Cyclotropia 378.33
Cyesis - *see* Pregnancy
Cylindroma (M8200/3) - *see also*
        Neoplasm, by site, malignant
    eccrine dermal (M8200/0) - *see*
        Neoplasm, skin, benign
    skin (M8200/0) - *see* Neoplasm, skin,
        benign
Cylindruria 791.7
Cyllosoma 759.89
Cynanche
    diphtheritic 032.3
    tonsillaris 475
Cynorexia 783.6
Cyphosis - *see* Kyphosis

Cyprus fever (*see also* Brucellosis) 023.9
Cyriax's syndrome (slipping rib) 733.99
Cyst (mucus) (retention) (serous) (simple)

Note 18 In general, cysts are not
neoplastic and are classified to the
appropriate category for disease of
the specified anatomical site. This
generalization does not apply to certain
types of cysts which are neoplastic in
nature, for example, dermoid, nor does
it apply to cysts of certain structures,
for example, branchial cleft, which are
classified as developmental anomalies.

The following listing includes some
of the most frequently reported sites
of cysts as well as qualifiers which
indicate the type of cyst. The latter
qualifiers usually are not repeated
under the anatomical sites. Since the
code assignment for a given site may
vary depending upon the type of cyst,
the coder should refer to the listings
under the specified type of cyst before
consideration is given to the site.

---

    accessory, fallopian tube 752.11
    adenoid (infected) 474.8
    adrenal gland 255.8
        congenital 759.1
    air, lung 518.89
    allantoic 753.7
    alveolar process (jaw bone) 526.2
    amnion, amniotic 658.8●
    anterior chamber (eye) 364.60
        exudative 364.62
        implantation (surgical) (traumatic)
            364.61
        parasitic 360.13
    anterior nasopalatine 526.1
    antrum 478.19
    anus 569.49
    apical (periodontal) (tooth) 522.8
    appendix 543.9
    arachnoid, brain 348.0
    arytenoid 478.79
    auricle 706.2
    Baker's (knee) 727.51
        tuberculous (*see also* Tuberculosis)
            015.2●
    Bartholin's gland or duct 616.2
    bile duct (*see also* Disease, biliary)
        576.8
    bladder (multiple) (trigone) 596.8
    Blessig's 362.62
    blood, endocardial (*see also*
        Endocarditis) 424.90
    blue dome 610.0
    bone (local) 733.20
        aneurysmal 733.22
        jaw 526.2
            developmental (odontogenic)
                526.0
            fissural 526.1
            latent 526.89
        solitary 733.21
        unicameral 733.21
    brain 348.0
        congenital 742.4
        hydatid (*see also* Echinococcus)
            122.9
        third ventricle (colloid) 742.4
    branchial (cleft) 744.42
    branchiogenic 744.42

Cyst (Continued)
  breast (benign) (blue dome)
      (pedunculated) (solitary)
      (traumatic) 610.0
    involution 610.4
    sebaceous 610.8
  broad ligament (benign) 620.8
    embryonic 752.11
  bronchogenic (mediastinal)
      (sequestration) 518.89
    congenital 748.4
  buccal 528.4
  bulbourethral gland (Cowper's) 599.89
  bursa, bursal 727.49
    pharyngeal 478.26
  calcifying odontogenic (M9301/0) 213.1
    upper jaw (bone) 213.0
  canal of Nuck (acquired) (serous) 629.1
    congenital 752.41
  canthus 372.75
  carcinomatous (M8010/3) - see
      Neoplasm, by site, malignant
  cartilage (joint) - see Derangement, joint
  cauda equina 336.8
  cavum septi pellucidi NEC 348.0
  celomic (pericardium) 746.89
  cerebellopontine (angle) - see Cyst,
      brain
  cerebellum - see Cyst, brain
  cerebral - see Cyst, brain
  cervical lateral 744.42
  cervix 622.8
    embryonal 752.41
    nabothian (gland) 616.0
  chamber, anterior (eye) 364.60
    exudative 364.62
    implantation (surgical) (traumatic)
        364.61
    parasitic 360.13
  chiasmal, optic NEC (see also Lesion,
      chiasmal) 377.54
  chocolate (ovary) 617.1
  choledochal (congenital) 751.69
    acquired 576.8
  choledochus 751.69
  chorion 658.8●
  choroid plexus 348.0
  chyle, mesentery 457.8
  ciliary body 364.60
    exudative 364.64
    implantation 364.61
    primary 364.63
  clitoris 624.8
  coccyx (see also Cyst, bone) 733.20
  colloid
    third ventricle (brain) 742.4
    thyroid gland - see Goiter
  colon 569.89
  common (bile) duct (see also Disease,
      biliary) 576.8
  congenital NEC 759.89
    adrenal glands 759.1
    epiglottis 748.3
    esophagus 750.4
    fallopian tube 752.11
    kidney 753.10
      multiple 753.19
      single 753.11
    larynx 748.3
    liver 751.62
    lung 748.4
    mediastinum 748.8
    ovary 752.0
    oviduct 752.11

Cyst (Continued)
  congenital NEC (Continued)
    pancreas 751.7
    periurethral (tissue) 753.8
    prepuce NEC 752.69
      penis 752.69
    sublingual 750.26
    submaxillary gland 750.26
    thymus (gland) 759.2
    tongue 750.19
    ureterovesical orifice 753.4
    vulva 752.41
  conjunctiva 372.75
  cornea 371.23
  corpora quadrigemina 348.0
  corpus
    albicans (ovary) 620.2
    luteum (ruptured) 620.1
  Cowper's gland (benign) (infected)
      599.89
  cranial meninges 348.0
  craniobuccal pouch 253.8
  craniopharyngeal pouch 253.8
  cystic duct (see also Disease,
      gallbladder) 575.8
  Cysticercus (any site) 123.1
  Dandy-Walker 742.3
    with spina bifida (see also Spina
        bifida) 741.0●
  dental 522.8
    developmental 526.0
    eruption 526.0
    lateral periodontal 526.0
    primordial (keratocyst) 526.0
    root 522.8
  dentigerous 526.0
    mandible 526.0
    maxilla 526.0
  dermoid (M9084/0) - see also
      Neoplasm, by site, benign
    with malignant transformation
        (M9084/3) 183.0
    implantation
      external area or site (skin) NEC
          709.8
      iris 364.61
      skin 709.8
      vagina 623.8
      vulva 624.8
    mouth 528.4
    oral soft tissue 528.4
    sacrococcygeal 685.1
      with abscess 685.0
  developmental of ovary, ovarian
      752.0
  dura (cerebral) 348.0
    spinal 349.2
  ear (external) 706.2
  echinococcal (see also Echinococcus)
      122.9
  embryonal
    cervix uteri 752.41
    genitalia, female external 752.41
    uterus 752.3
    vagina 752.41
  endometrial 621.8
    ectopic 617.9
  endometrium (uterus) 621.8
    ectopic - see Endometriosis
  enteric 751.5
  enterogenous 751.5
  epidermal (inclusion) (see also Cyst,
      skin) 706.2

Cyst (Continued)
  epidermoid (inclusion) (see also Cyst,
      skin) 706.2
    mouth 528.4
    not of skin - see Cyst, by site
    oral soft tissue 528.4
  epididymis 608.89
  epiglottis 478.79
  epiphysis cerebri 259.8
  epithelial (inclusion) (see also Cyst,
      skin) 706.2
  epoophoron 752.11
  eruption 526.0
  esophagus 530.89
  ethmoid sinus 478.19
  eye (retention) 379.8
    congenital 743.03
    posterior segment, congenital 743.54
  eyebrow 706.2
  eyelid (sebaceous) 374.84
    infected 373.13
    sweat glands or ducts 374.84
  falciform ligament (inflammatory)
      573.8
  fallopian tube 620.8
    congenital 752.11
  female genital organs NEC 629.89
  fimbrial (congenital) 752.11
  fissural (oral region) 526.1
  follicle (atretic) (graafian) (ovarian)
      620.0
    nabothian (gland) 616.0
  follicular (atretic) (ovarian) 620.0
    dentigerous 526.0
  frontal sinus 478.19
  gallbladder or duct 575.8
  ganglion 727.43
  Gartner's duct 752.41
  gas, of mesentery 568.89
  gingiva 523.8
  gland of moll 374.84
  globulomaxillary 526.1
  graafian follicle 620.0
  granulosal lutein 620.2
  hemangiomatous (M9121/0) (see also
      Hemangioma) 228.00
  hydatid (see also Echinococcus) 122.9
    fallopian tube (Morgagni) 752.11
    liver NEC 122.8
    lung NEC 122.9
    Morgagni 752.89
      fallopian tube 752.11
    specified site NEC 122.9
  hymen 623.8
    embryonal 752.41
  hypopharynx 478.26
  hypophysis, hypophyseal (duct)
      (recurrent) 253.8
    cerebri 253.8
  implantation (dermoid)
    anterior chamber (eye) 364.61
    external area or site (skin) NEC
        709.8
    iris 364.61
    vagina 623.8
    vulva 624.8
  incisor, incisive canal 526.1
  inclusion (epidermal) (epithelial)
      (epidermoid) (mucous)
      (squamous) (see also Cyst, skin)
      706.2
    not of skin - see Neoplasm, by site,
        benign
  intestine (large) (small) 569.89

◄ New   ◄▥ Revised   ~~deleted~~ Deleted   ● Use Additional Digit(s)   ▨ Omit code

Cyst *(Continued)*
  intracranial - *see* Cyst, brain
  intraligamentous 728.89
    knee 717.89
  intrasellar 253.8
  iris (idiopathic) 364.60
    exudative 364.62
    implantation (surgical) (traumatic) 364.61
    miotic pupillary 364.55
    parasitic 360.13
  Iwanoff's 362.62
  jaw (bone) (aneurysmal) (extravasation) (hemorrhagic) (traumatic) 526.2
    developmental (odontogenic) 526.0
    fissural 526.1
  keratin 706.2
  kidney (congenital) 753.10
    acquired 593.2
    calyceal (*see also* Hydronephrosis) 591
    multiple 753.19
    pyelogenic (*see also* Hydronephrosis) 591
    simple 593.2
    single 753.11
    solitary (not congenital) 593.2
  labium (majus) (minus) 624.8
    sebaceous 624.8
  lacrimal
    apparatus 375.43
    gland or sac 375.12
  larynx 478.79
  lens 379.39
    congenital 743.39
  lip (gland) 528.5
  liver 573.8
    congenital 751.62
    hydatid (*see also* Echinococcus) 122.8
      granulosis 122.0
      multilocularis 122.5
  lung 518.89
    congenital 748.4
    giant bullous 492.0
  lutein 620.1
  lymphangiomatous (M9173/0) 228.1
  lymphoepithelial
    mouth 528.4
    oral soft tissue 528.4
  macula 362.54
  malignant (M8000/3) - *see* Neoplasm, by site, malignant
  mammary gland (sweat gland) (*see also* Cyst, breast) 610.0
  mandible 526.2
    dentigerous 526.0
    radicular 522.8
  maxilla 526.2
    dentigerous 526.0
    radicular 522.8
  median
    anterior maxillary 526.1
    palatal 526.1
  mediastinum (congenital) 748.8
  meibomian (gland) (retention) 373.2
    infected 373.12
  membrane, brain 348.0
  meninges (cerebral) 348.0
    spinal 349.2
  meniscus knee 717.5
  mesentery, mesenteric (gas) 568.89
    chyle 457.8
    gas 568.89

Cyst *(Continued)*
  mesonephric duct 752.89
  mesothelial
    peritoneum 568.89
    pleura (peritoneal) 568.89
  milk 611.5
  miotic pupillary (iris) 364.55
  Morgagni (hydatid) 752.89
    fallopian tube 752.11
  mouth 528.4
  Müllerian duct 752.89
    appendix testis 608.89
    cervix (embryonal) 752.41
    fallopian tube 752.11
    prostatic utricle 599.89
    vagina (embryonal) 752.41
  multilocular (ovary) (M8000/1) 239.5
  myometrium 621.8
  nabothian (follicle) (ruptured) 616.0
  nasal sinus 478.19
  nasoalveolar 528.4
  nasolabial 528.4
  nasopalatine (duct) 526.1
    anterior 526.1
  nasopharynx 478.26
  neoplastic (M8000/1) - *see also* Neoplasm, by site, unspecified nature
    benign (M8000/0) - *see* Neoplasm, by site, benign
    uterus 621.8
  nervous system - *see* Cyst, brain
  neuroenteric 742.59
  neuroepithelial ventricle 348.0
  nipple 610.0
  nose 478.19
    skin of 706.2
  odontogenic, developmental 526.0
  omentum (lesser) 568.89
    congenital 751.8
  oral soft tissue (dermoid) (epidermoid) (lymphoepithelial) 528.4
  ora serrata 361.19
  orbit 376.81
  ovary, ovarian (twisted) 620.2
    adherent 620.2
    chocolate 617.1
    corpus
      albicans 620.2
      luteum 620.1
    dermoid (M9084/0) 220
    developmental 752.0
    due to failure of involution NEC 620.2
    endometrial 617.1
    follicular (atretic) (graafian) (hemorrhagic) 620.0
    hemorrhagic 620.2
    in pregnancy or childbirth 654.4●
      affecting fetus or newborn 763.89
      causing obstructed labor 660.2●
        affecting fetus or newborn 763.1
    multilocular (M8000/1) 239.5
    pseudomucinous (M8470/0) 220
    retention 620.2
    serous 620.2
    theca lutein 620.2
    tuberculous (*see also* Tuberculosis) 016.6●
    unspecified 620.2
  oviduct 620.8
  palatal papilla (jaw) 526.1

Cyst *(Continued)*
  palate 526.1
    fissural 526.1
      median (fissural) 526.1
  palatine, of papilla 526.1
  pancreas, pancreatic 577.2
    congenital 751.7
    false 577.2
    hemorrhagic 577.2
    true 577.2
  paralabral
    hip 718.85
    shoulder 840.7
  paramesonephric duct - *see* Cyst, Müllerian duct
  paranephric 593.2
  paraoovarian 752.11
  paraphysis, cerebri 742.4
  parasitic NEC 136.9
  parathyroid (gland) 252.8
  paratubal (fallopian) 620.8
  paraurethral duct 599.89
  paroophoron 752.11
  parotid gland 527.6
    mucous extravasation or retention 527.6
  parovarian 752.11
  pars planus 364.60
    exudative 364.64
    primary 364.63
  pelvis, female
    in pregnancy or childbirth 654.4●
      affecting fetus or newborn 763.89
      causing obstructed labor 660.2●
        affecting fetus or newborn 763.1
  penis (sebaceous) 607.89
  periapical 522.8
  pericardial (congenital) 746.89
    acquired (secondary) 423.8
  pericoronal 526.0
  perineural (Tarlov's) 355.9
  periodontal 522.8
    lateral 526.0
  peripancreatic 577.2
  peripelvic (lymphatic) 593.2
  peritoneum 568.89
    chylous 457.8
  pharynx (wall) 478.26
  pilonidal (infected) (rectum) 685.1
    with abscess 685.0
    malignant (M9084/3) 173.5
  pituitary (duct) (gland) 253.8
  placenta (amniotic) - *see* Placenta, abnormal
  pleura 519.8
  popliteal 727.51
  porencephalic 742.4
    acquired 348.0
  postanal (infected) 685.1
    with abscess 685.0
  posterior segment of eye, congenital 743.54
  postmastoidectomy cavity 383.31
  preauricular 744.47
  prepuce 607.89
    congenital 752.69
  primordial (jaw) 526.0
  prostate 600.3
  pseudomucinous (ovary) (M8470/0) 220
  pudenda (sweat glands) 624.8
  pupillary, miotic 364.55
    sebaceous 624.8
  radicular (residual) 522.8

Cyst (Continued)
  radiculodental 522.8
  ranular 527.6
  Rathke's pouch 253.8
  rectum (epithelium) (mucous) 569.49
  renal - see Cyst, kidney
  residual (radicular) 522.8
  retention (ovary) 620.2
  retina 361.19
    macular 362.54
    parasitic 360.13
    primary 361.13
    secondary 361.14
  retroperitoneal 568.89
  sacrococcygeal (dermoid) 685.1
    with abscess 685.0
  salivary gland or duct 527.6
    mucous extravasation or retention
      527.6
  Sampson's 617.1
  sclera 379.19
  scrotum (sebaceous) 706.2
    sweat glands 706.2
  sebaceous (duct) (gland) 706.2
    breast 610.8
    eyelid 374.84
    genital organ NEC
      female 629.89
      male 608.89
    scrotum 706.2
  semilunar cartilage (knee) (multiple)
    717.5
  seminal vesicle 608.89
  serous (ovary) 620.2
  sinus (antral) (ethmoidal) (frontal)
      (maxillary) (nasal) (sphenoidal)
      478.19
  Skene's gland 599.89
  skin (epidermal) (epidermoid,
      inclusion) (epithelial) (inclusion)
      (retention) (sebaceous) 706.2
    breast 610.8
    eyelid 374.84
    genital organ NEC
      female 629.89
      male 608.89
    neoplastic 216.3
    scrotum 706.2
    sweat gland or duct 705.89
  solitary
    bone 733.21
    kidney 593.2
  spermatic cord 608.89
  sphenoid sinus 478.19
  spinal meninges 349.2
  spine (see also Cyst, bone) 733.20
  spleen NEC 289.59
    congenital 759.0
    hydatid (see also Echinococcus) 122.9
  spring water (pericardium) 746.89
  subarachnoid 348.0
    intrasellar 793.0
  subdural (cerebral) 348.0
    spinal cord 349.2
  sublingual gland 527.6
    mucous extravasation or retention
      527.6
  submaxillary gland 527.6
    mucous extravasation or retention
      527.6
  suburethral 599.89
  suprarenal gland 255.8
  suprasellar - see Cyst, brain
  sweat gland or duct 705.89

Cyst (Continued)
  sympathetic nervous system 337.9
  synovial 727.40
    popliteal space 727.51
  Tarlov's 355.9
  tarsal 373.2
  tendon (sheath) 727.42
  testis 608.89
  theca-lutein (ovary) 620.2
  Thornwaldt's, Tornwaldt's 478.26
  thymus (gland) 254.8
  thyroglossal (duct) (infected)
      (persistent) 759.2
  thyroid (gland) 246.2
    adenomatous - see Goiter, nodular
    colloid (see also Goiter) 240.9
  thyrolingual duct (infected) (persistent)
      759.2
  tongue (mucous) 529.8
  tonsil 474.8
  tooth (dental root) 522.8
  tubo-ovarian 620.8
    inflammatory 614.1
  tunica vaginalis 608.89
  turbinate (nose) (see also Cyst, bone)
      733.20
  Tyson's gland (benign) (infected)
      607.89
  umbilicus 759.89
  urachus 753.7
  ureter 593.89
  ureterovesical orifice 593.89
    congenital 753.4
  urethra 599.84
  urethral gland (Cowper's) 599.89
  uterine
    ligament 620.8
      embryonic 752.11
    tube 620.8
  uterus (body) (corpus) (recurrent) 621.8
    embryonal 752.3
  utricle (ear) 386.8
    prostatic 599.89
  utriculus masculinus 599.89
  vagina, vaginal (squamous cell) (wall)
      623.8
    embryonal 752.41
    implantation 623.8
    inclusion 623.8
  vallecula, vallecular 478.79
  ventricle, neuroepithelial 348.0
  verumontanum 599.89
  vesical (orifice) 596.8
  vitreous humor 379.29
  vulva (sweat glands) 624.8
    congenital 752.41
    implantation 624.8
    inclusion 624.8
    sebaceous gland 624.8
  vulvovaginal gland 624.8
  wolffian 752.89
Cystadenocarcinoma (M8440/3) - see also
    Neoplasm, by site, malignant
  bile duct type (M8161/3) 155.1
  endometrioid (M8380/3) - see
    Neoplasm, by site, malignant
  mucinous (M8470/3)
    papillary (M8471/3)
      specified site - see Neoplasm, by
        site, malignant
      unspecified site 183.0
    specified site - see Neoplasm, by site,
      malignant
    unspecified site 183.0

Cystadenocarcinoma (Continued)
  papillary (M8450/3)
    mucinous (M8471/3)
      specified site - see Neoplasm, by
        site, malignant
      unspecified site 183.0
    pseudomucinous (M8471/3)
      specified site - see Neoplasm, by
        site, malignant
      unspecified site 183.0
    serous (M8460/3)
      specified site - see Neoplasm, by
        site, malignant
      unspecified site 183.0
    specified site - see Neoplasm, by site,
      malignant
    unspecified 183.0
  pseudomucinous (M8470/3)
    papillary (M8471/3)
      specified site - see Neoplasm, by
        site, malignant
      unspecified site 183.0
    specified site - see Neoplasm, by site,
      malignant
    unspecified site 183.0
  serous (M8441/3)
    papillary (M8460/3)
      specified site - see Neoplasm, by
        site, malignant
      unspecified site 183.0
    specified site - see Neoplasm, by site,
      malignant
    unspecified site 183.0
Cystadenofibroma (M9013/0)
  clear cell (M8313/0) - see Neoplasm, by
    site, benign
  endometrioid (M8381/0) 220
    borderline malignancy (M8381/1)
      236.2
    malignant (M8381/3) 183.0
  mucinous (M9015/0)
    specified site - see Neoplasm, by site,
      benign
    unspecified site 220
  serous (M9014/0)
    specified site - see Neoplasm, by site,
      benign
    unspecified site 220
  specified site - see Neoplasm, by site,
    benign
  unspecified site 220
Cystadenoma (M8440/0) - see also
    Neoplasm, by site, benign
  bile duct (M8161/0) 211.5
  endometrioid (M8380/0) - see also
    Neoplasm, by site, benign
    borderline malignancy (M8380/1) -
      see Neoplasm, by site,
      uncertain behavior
    malignant (M8440/3) - see Neoplasm,
      by site, malignant
  mucinous (M8470/0)
    borderline malignancy
      (M8470/1)
      specified site - see Neoplasm,
        uncertain behavior
      unspecified site 236.2
    papillary (M8471/0)
      borderline malignancy
        (M8471/1)
        specified site - see Neoplasm,
          by site, uncertain
          behavior
        unspecified site 236.2

Cystadenoma (Continued)
  mucinous (Continued)
    papillary (Continued)
      specified site - see Neoplasm, by
        site, benign
      unspecified site 220
    specified site - see Neoplasm, by site,
      benign
    unspecified site 220
  papillary (M8450/0)
    borderline malignancy (M8450/1)
      specified site - see Neoplasm, by
        site, uncertain behavior
      unspecified site 236.2
    lymphomatosum (M8561/0) 210.2
    mucinous (M8471/0)
      borderline malignancy (M8471/1)
        specified site - see Neoplasm, by
          site, uncertain behavior
        unspecified site 236.2
      specified site - see Neoplasm, by
        site, benign
      unspecified site 220
    pseudomucinous (M8471/0)
      borderline malignancy (M8471/1)
        specified site - see Neoplasm,
          by site uncertain
          behavior
        unspecified site 236.2
      specified site - see Neoplasm, by
        site, benign
      unspecified site 220
  serous (M8460/0)
    borderline malignancy (M8460/1)
      specified site - see Neoplasm,
        by site, uncertain
        behavior
      unspecified site 236.2
    specified site - see Neoplasm, by
      site, benign
    unspecified site 220
    specified site - see Neoplasm, by site,
      benign
    unspecified site 220
  pseudomucinous (M8470/0)
    borderline malignancy (M8470/1)
      specified site - see Neoplasm, by
        site uncertain behavior
      unspecified site 236.2
    papillary (M8471/0)
      borderline malignancy (M8471/1)
        specified site - see Neoplasm,
          by site uncertain
          behavior
        unspecified site 236.2
      specified site - see Neoplasm, by
        site, benign
      unspecified site 220
    specified site - see Neoplasm, by site,
      benign
    unspecified site 220
  serous (M8441/0)
    borderline malignancy (M8441/1)
      specified site - see Neoplasm, by
        site, uncertain behavior
      unspecified site 236.2
    papillary (M8460/0)
      borderline malignancy (M8460/1)
        specified site - see Neoplasm,
          by site, uncertain
          behavior
        unspecified site 236.2
      specified site - see Neoplasm, by
        site, benign
      unspecified site 220

Cystadenoma (Continued)
  serous (Continued)
    specified site - see Neoplasm, by site,
      benign
    unspecified site 220
  thyroid 226
Cystathioninemia 270.4
Cystathioninuria 270.4
Cystic - see also condition
  breast, chronic 610.1
  corpora lutea 620.1
  degeneration, congenital
    brain 742.4
    kidney (see also Cystic, disease,
      kidney) 753.10
  disease
    breast, chronic 610.1
    kidney, congenital 753.10
      medullary 753.16
      multiple 753.19
      polycystic - see Polycystic, kidney
      single 753.11
      specified NEC 753.19
    liver, congenital 751.62
    lung 518.89
      congenital 748.4
    pancreas, congenital 751.7
    semilunar cartilage 717.5
  duct - see condition
  eyeball, congenital 743.03
  fibrosis (pancreas) 277.00
    with
      manifestations
        gastrointestinal 277.03
        pulmonary 277.02
        specified NEC 277.09
      meconium ileus 277.01
      pulmonary exacerbation 277.02
  hygroma (M9173/0) 228.1
  kidney, congenital 753.10
    medullary 753.16
    multiple 753.19
    polycystic - see Polycystic, kidney
    single 753.11
    specified NEC 753.19
  liver, congenital 751.62
  lung 518.89
    congenital 748.4
  mass - see Cyst
  mastitis, chronic 610.1
  ovary 620.2
  pancreas, congenital 751.7
Cysticerciasis 123.1
Cysticercosis (mammary) (subretinal)
  123.1
Cysticercus 123.1
  cellulosae infestation 123.1
Cystinosis (malignant) 270.0
Cystinuria 270.0
Cystitis (bacillary) (colli) (diffuse)
  (exudative) (hemorrhagic)
  (purulent) (recurrent) (septic)
  (suppurative) (ulcerative) 595.9
  with
    abortion - see Abortion, by type,
      with urinary tract infection
    ectopic pregnancy (see also
      categories 633.0–633.9) 639.8
    fibrosis 595.1
    leukoplakia 595.1
    malakoplakia 595.1
    metaplasia 595.1
    molar pregnancy (see also categories
      630–632) 639.8

Cystitis (Continued)
  actinomycotic 039.8 [595.4]
  acute 595.0
    of trigone 595.3
  allergic 595.89
  amebic 006.8 [595.4]
  bilharzial 120.9 [595.4]
  blennorrhagic (acute) 098.11
    chronic or duration of 2 months or
      more 098.31
  bullous 595.89
  calculous 594.1
  chlamydial 099.53
  chronic 595.2
    interstitial 595.1
    of trigone 595.3
  complicating pregnancy, childbirth, or
    puerperium 646.6●
    affecting fetus or newborn 760.1
  cystic(a) 595.81
  diphtheritic 032.84
  echinococcal
    glanulosus 122.3 [595.4]
    multilocularis 122.6 [595.4]
  emphysematous 595.89
  encysted 595.81
  follicular 595.3
  following
    abortion 639.8
    ectopic or molar pregnancy 639.8
  gangrenous 595.89
  glandularis 595.89
  gonococcal (acute) 098.11
    chronic or duration of 2 months or
      more 098.31
  incrusted 595.89
  interstitial 595.1
  irradiation 595.82
  irritation 595.89
  malignant 595.89
  monilial 112.2
  of trigone 595.3
  panmural 595.1
  polyposa 595.89
  prostatic 601.3
  radiation 595.82
  Reiter's (abacterial) 099.3
  specified NEC 595.89
  subacute 595.2
  submucous 595.1
  syphilitic 095.8
  trichomoniasis 131.09
  tuberculous (see also Tuberculosis)
    016.1●
  ulcerative 595.1
Cystocele
  female (without uterine prolapse)
    618.01
    with uterine prolapse 618.4
      complete 618.3
      incomplete 618.2
    lateral 618.02
    midline 618.01
    paravaginal 618.02
  in pregnancy or childbirth 654.4●
    affecting fetus or newborn 763.89
    causing obstructed labor 660.2●
      affecting fetus or newborn 763.1
  male 596.8
Cystoid
  cicatrix limbus 372.64
  degeneration macula 362.53
Cystolithiasis 594.1

Cystoma (M8440/0) - *see also* Neoplasm,
    by site, benign
  endometrial, ovary 617.1
  mucinous (M8470/0)
    specified site - *see* Neoplasm, by site,
      benign
    unspecified site 220
  serous (M8441/0)
    specified site - *see* Neoplasm, by site,
      benign
    unspecified site 220
  simple (ovary) 620.2
Cystoplegia 596.53
Cystoptosis 596.8
Cystopyelitis (*see also* Pyelitis) 590.80
Cystorrhagia 596.8

Cystosarcoma phyllodes (M9020/1) 238.3
  benign (M9020/0) 217
  malignant (M9020/3) - *see* Neoplasm,
    breast, malignant
Cystostomy status V44.50
  with complication 997.5
  appendico-vesicostomy V44.52
  cutaneous-vesicostomy V44.51
  specified type NEC V44.59
Cystourethritis (*see also* Urethritis) 597.89
Cystourethrocele (*see also* Cystocele)
  female (without uterine prolapse) 618.09
    with uterine prolapse 618.4
      complete 618.3
      incomplete 618.2
  male 596.8

Cytomegalic inclusion disease 078.5
  congenital 771.1
Cytomycosis, reticuloendothelial (*see also*
  Histoplasmosis, American) 115.00
Cytopenia 289.9
  refractory
    with
      multilineage dysplasia (RCMD)
        238.72
      and ringed sideroblasts
        (RCMD-RS) 238.72

◄ New   ◄▥ Revised   ~~deleted~~ Deleted   ● Use Additional Digit(s)   ▨ Omit code

D

Daae (-Finsen) disease (epidemic pleurodynia) 074.1
Dabney's grip 074.1
Da Costa's syndrome (neurocirculatory asthenia) 306.2
Dacryoadenitis, dacryadenitis 375.00
  acute 375.01
  chronic 375.02
Dacryocystitis 375.30
  acute 375.32
  chronic 375.42
  neonatal 771.6
  phlegmonous 375.33
  syphilitic 095.8
    congenital 090.0
  trachomatous, active 076.1
    late effect 139.1
  tuberculous (*see also* Tuberculosis) 017.3●
Dacryocystoblennorrhea 375.42
Dacryocystocele 375.43
Dacryolith, dacryolithiasis 375.57
Dacryoma 375.43
Dacryopericystitis (acute) (subacute) 375.32
  chronic 375.42
Dacryops 375.11
Dacryosialadenopathy, atrophic 710.2
Dacryostenosis 375.56
  congenital 743.65
Dactylitis
  bone (*see also* Osteomyelitis) 730.2●
  sickle-cell 282.62
    Hb-C 282.64
    Hb-SS 282.62
    specified NEC 282.69
  syphilitic 095.5
  tuberculous (*see also* Tuberculosis) 015.5●
Dactylolysis spontanea 136.0
Dactylosymphysis (*see also* Syndactylism) 755.10
Damage
  arteriosclerotic - *see* Arteriosclerosis
  brain 348.9
    anoxic, hypoxic 348.1
      during or resulting from a procedure 997.01
      ischemic, in newborn 768.70 ◀▥
        mild 768.71 ◀
        moderate 768.72 ◀
        severe 768.73 ◀
    child NEC 343.9
    due to birth injury 767.0
    minimal (child) (*see also* Hyperkinesia) 314.9
    newborn 767.0
  cardiac - *see also* Disease, heart
  cardiorenal (vascular) (*see also* Hypertension, cardiorenal) 404.90
  central nervous system - *see* Damage, brain
  cerebral NEC - *see* Damage, brain
  coccyx, complicating delivery 665.6●
  coronary (*see also* Ischemia, heart) 414.9
  eye, birth injury 767.8
  heart - *see also* Disease, heart
    valve - *see* Endocarditis
  hypothalamus NEC 348.9
  liver 571.9
    alcoholic 571.3
  medication 995.20
  myocardium (*see also* Degeneration, myocardial) 429.1
  pelvic

Damage *(Continued)*
  pelvic *(Continued)*
    joint or ligament, during delivery 665.6●
    organ NEC
      with
        abortion - *see* Abortion, by type, with damage to pelvic organs
        ectopic pregnancy (*see also* categories 633.0–633.9) 639.2
        molar pregnancy (*see also* categories 630–632) 639.2
      during delivery 665.5●
      following
        abortion 639.2
        ectopic or molar pregnancy 639.2
  renal (*see also* Disease, renal) 593.9
  skin, solar 692.79
    acute 692.72
    chronic 692.74
  subendocardium, subendocardial (*see also* Degeneration, myocardial) 429.1
  vascular 459.9
Dameshek's syndrome (erythroblastic anemia) 282.49
Dana-Putnam syndrome (subacute combined sclerosis with pernicious anemia) 281.0 [336.2]
Danbolt (-Closs) syndrome (acrodermatitis enteropathica) 686.8
Dandruff 690.18
Dandy fever 061
Dandy-Walker deformity or syndrome (atresia, foramen of Magendie) 742.3
  with spina bifida (*see also* Spina bifida) 741.0●
Dangle foot 736.79
Danielssen's disease (anesthetic leprosy) 030.1
Danlos' syndrome 756.83
Darier's disease (congenital) (keratosis follicularis) 757.39
  due to vitamin A deficiency 264.8
  meaning erythema annulare centrifugum 695.0
Darier-Roussy sarcoid 135
Dark area on retina 239.81 ◀
Darling's
  disease (*see also* Histoplasmosis, American) 115.00
  histoplasmosis (*see also* Histoplasmosis, American) 115.00
Dartre 054.9
Darwin's tubercle 744.29
Davidson's anemia (refractory) 284.9
Davies' disease 425.0
Davies-Colley syndrome (slipping rib) 733.99
Dawson's encephalitis 046.2
Day blindness (*see also* Blindness, day) 368.60
Dead
  fetus
    retained (in utero) 656.4●
      early pregnancy (death before 22 completed weeks' gestation) 632
      late (death after 22 completed weeks' gestation) 656.4●
    syndrome 641.3●

Dead *(Continued)*
  labyrinth 386.50
  ovum, retained 631
Deaf and dumb NEC 389.7
Deaf mutism (acquired) (congenital) NEC 389.7
  endemic 243
  hysterical 300.11
  syphilitic, congenital 090.0
Deafness (acquired) (complete) (congenital) (hereditary) (middle ear) (partial) 389.9
  with
    blindness V49.85
    blue sclera and fragility of bone 756.51
  auditory fatigue 389.9
  aviation 993.0
    nerve injury 951.5
  boilermakers' 951.5
  central 389.14
    with conductive hearing loss 389.20
      bilateral 389.22
      unilateral 389.21
  conductive (air) 389.00
    with sensorineural hearing loss 389.20
      bilateral 389.22
      unilateral 389.21
    bilateral 389.06
    combined types 389.08
    external ear 389.01
    inner ear 389.04
    middle ear 389.03
    multiple types 389.08
    tympanic membrane 389.02
    unilateral 389.05
  emotional (complete) 300.11
  functional (complete) 300.11
  high frequency 389.8
  hysterical (complete) 300.11
  injury 951.5
  low frequency 389.8
  mental 784.69
  mixed conductive and sensorineural 389.20
    bilateral 389.22
    unilateral 389.21
  nerve
    with conductive hearing loss 389.20
      bilateral 389.22
      unilateral 389.21
    bilateral 389.12
    unilateral 389.13
  neural
    with conductive hearing loss 389.20
      bilateral 389.22
      unilateral 389.21
    bilateral 389.12
    unilateral 389.13
  noise-induced 388.12
    nerve injury 951.5
  nonspeaking 389.7
  perceptive 389.10
    with conductive hearing loss 389.20
      bilateral 389.22
      unilateral 389.21
    central 389.14
    neural
      bilateral 389.12
      unilateral 389.13

Deafness (Continued)
  perceptive (Continued)
    sensorineural 389.10
      asymmetrical 389.16
      bilateral 389.18
      unilateral 389.15
    sensory
      bilateral 389.11
      unilateral 389.17
  psychogenic (complete) 306.7
  sensorineural (see also Deafness,
      perceptive) 389.10
    asymmetrical 389.16
    bilateral 389.18
    unilateral 389.15
  sensory
    with conductive hearing loss 389.20
      bilateral 389.22
      unilateral 389.21
    bilateral 389.11
    unilateral 389.17
  specified type NEC 389.8
  sudden NEC 388.2
  syphilitic 094.89
  transient ischemic 388.02
  transmission - see Deafness, conductive
  traumatic 951.5
  word (secondary to organic lesion)
      784.69
    developmental 315.31
Death
  after delivery (cause not stated)
      (sudden) 674.9●
  anesthetic
    due to
      correct substance properly
          administered 995.4
      overdose or wrong substance
          given 968.4
        specified anesthetic - see Table
            of Drugs and Chemicals
    during delivery 668.9●
  brain 348.89   ◄▮▮▮
  cardiac (sudden) (SCD) - code to
      underlying condition
    family history of V17.41
    personal history of, successfully
        resuscitated V12.53
  cause unknown 798.2
  cot (infant) 798.0
  crib (infant) 798.0
  fetus, fetal (cause not stated)
      (intrauterine) 779.9
    early, with retention (before 22
        completed weeks' gestation)
        632
    from asphyxia or anoxia (before
        labor) 768.0
      during labor 768.1
    late, affecting management of
        pregnancy (after 22 completed
        weeks' gestation) 656.4●
  from pregnancy NEC 646.9●
  instantaneous 798.1
  intrauterine (see also Death, fetus)
      779.9
    complicating pregnancy 656.4●
  maternal, affecting fetus or newborn
      761.6
  neonatal NEC 779.9
  sudden (cause unknown) 798.1
    cardiac (SCD)
      family history of V17.41
      personal history of, successfully
          resuscitated V12.53

Death (Continued)
  sudden (Continued)
    during delivery 669.9●
      under anesthesia NEC 668.9●
    infant, syndrome (SIDS) 798.0
    puerperal, during puerperium
        674.9●
  unattended (cause unknown) 798.9
  under anesthesia NEC
    due to
      correct substance properly
          administered 995.4
      overdose or wrong substance
          given 968.4
        specified anesthetic - see
            Table of Drugs and
            Chemicals
    during delivery 668.9●
  violent 798.1
de Beurmann-Gougerot disease
    (sporotrichosis) 117.1
Debility (general) (infantile)
    (postinfectional) 799.3
  with nutritional difficulty 269.9
  congenital or neonatal NEC 779.9
  nervous 300.5
  old age 797
  senile 797
Débove's disease (splenomegaly) 789.2
Decalcification
  bone (see also Osteoporosis) 733.00
  teeth 521.89
Decapitation 874.9
  fetal (to facilitate delivery) 763.89
Decapsulation, kidney 593.89
Decay
  dental 521.00
  senile 797
  tooth, teeth 521.00
Decensus, uterus - see Prolapse, uterus
Deciduitis (acute)
  with
    abortion - see Abortion, by type,
        with sepsis
    ectopic pregnancy (see also
        categories 633.0–633.9)
        639.0
    molar pregnancy (see also categories
        630–632) 639.0
  affecting fetus or newborn 760.8
  following
    abortion 639.0
    ectopic or molar pregnancy 639.0
  in pregnancy 646.6●
  puerperal, postpartum 670.1   ◄▮▮▮
Deciduoma malignum (M9100/3) 181
Deciduous tooth (retained) 520.6
Decline (general) (see also Debility)
    799.3
Decompensation
  cardiac (acute) (chronic) (see also
      Disease, heart) 429.9
    failure - see Failure, heart
  cardiorenal (see also Hypertension,
      cardiorenal) 404.90
  cardiovascular (see also Disease,
      cardiovascular) 429.2
  heart (see also Disease, heart) 429.9
    failure - see Failure, heart
  hepatic 572.2
  myocardial (acute) (chronic) (see also
      Disease, heart) 429.9
    failure - see Failure, heart
  respiratory 519.9
Decompression sickness 993.3

Decrease, decreased
  blood
    platelets (see also Thrombocytopenia)
        287.5
    pressure 796.3
      due to shock following
          injury 958.4
          operation 998.0
    white cell count 288.50
      specified NEC 288.59
  cardiac reserve - see Disease, heart
  estrogen 256.39
    postablative 256.2
  fetal movements 655.7●
  fragility of erythrocytes 289.89
  function
    adrenal (cortex) 255.41
      medulla 255.5
    ovary in hypopituitarism 253.4
    parenchyma of pancreas 577.8
    pituitary (gland) (lobe) (anterior)
        253.2
      posterior (lobe) 253.8
  functional activity 780.99
  glucose 790.29
  haptoglobin (serum) NEC 273.8
  leukocytes 288.50
  libido 799.81
  lymphocytes 288.51
  platelets (see also Thrombocytopenia)
      287.5
  pulse pressure 785.9
  respiration due to shock following
      injury 958.4
  sexual desire 799.81
  tear secretion NEC 375.15
  tolerance
    fat 579.8
    salt and water 276.9
  vision NEC 369.9
  white blood cell count 288.50
Decubital gangrene (see also Ulcer,
    pressure) 707.00 [785.4]
Decubiti (see also Ulcer, pressure)
    707.00
Decubitus (ulcer) (see also Ulcer, pressure)
    707.00
  with gangrene 707.00 [785.4]
  ankle 707.06
  back
    lower 707.03
    upper 707.02
  buttock 707.05
  coccyx 707.03   ◄▮▮▮
  elbow 707.01
  head 707.09
  heel 707.07
  hip 707.04
  other site 707.09
  sacrum 707.03
  shoulder blades 707.02
Deepening acetabulum 718.85
Defect, defective 759.9
  3-beta-hydroxysteroid dehydrogenase
      255.2
  11-hydroxylase 255.2
  21-hydroxylase 255.2
  abdominal wall, congenital 756.70
  aorticopulmonary septum 745.0
  aortic septal 745.0
  atrial septal (ostium secundum type)
      745.5
    acquired 429.71
    ostium primum type 745.61
    sinus venosus 745.8

◄ New   ◄▮▮▮ Revised   deleted Deleted   ● Use Additional Digit(s)   Omit code

Defect, defective (Continued)

atrioventricular

canal 745.69

septum 745.4

acquired 429.71

atrium secundum 745.5

acquired 429.71

auricular septal 745.5

acquired 429.71

bilirubin excretion 277.4

biosynthesis, testicular androgen 257.2

bridge 525.60

bulbar septum 745.0

butanol-insoluble iodide 246.1

chromosome - see Anomaly, chromosome

circulation (acquired) 459.9

congenital 747.9

newborn 747.9

clotting NEC (see also Defect, coagulation) 286.9

coagulation (factor) (see also Deficiency, coagulation factor) 286.9

with

abortion - see Abortion, by type, with hemorrhage

ectopic pregnancy (see also categories 634–638) 639.1

molar pregnancy (see also categories 630–632) 639.1

acquired (any) 286.7

antepartum or intrapartum 641.3●

affecting fetus or newborn 762.1

causing hemorrhage of pregnancy or delivery 641.3●

complicating pregnancy, childbirth, or puerperium 649.3●

due to

liver disease 286.7

vitamin K deficiency 286.7

newborn, transient 776.3

postpartum 666.3●

specified type NEC 286.9

conduction (heart) 426.9

bone (see also Deafness, conductive) 389.00

congenital, organ or site NEC - see also Anomaly

circulation 747.9

Descemet's membrane 743.9

specified type NEC 743.49

diaphragm 756.6

ectodermal 757.9

esophagus 750.9

pulmonic cusps - see Anomaly, heart valve

respiratory system 748.9

specified type NEC 748.8

crown 525.60

cushion endocardial 745.60

dental restoration 525.60

dentin (hereditary) 520.5

Descemet's membrane (congenital) 743.9

acquired 371.30

specific type NEC 743.49

deutan 368.52

Defect, defective (Continued)

developmental - see also Anomaly, by site

cauda equina 742.59

left ventricle 746.9

with atresia or hypoplasia of aortic orifice or valve, with hypoplasia of ascending aorta 746.7

in hypoplastic left heart syndrome 746.7

testis 752.9

vessel 747.9

diaphragm

with elevation, eventration, or hernia - see Hernia, diaphragm

congenital 756.6

with elevation, eventration, or hernia 756.6

gross (with elevation, eventration, or hernia) 756.6

ectodermal, congenital 757.9

Eisenmenger's (ventricular septal defect) 745.4

endocardial cushion 745.60

specified type NEC 745.69

esophagus, congenital 750.9

extensor retinaculum 728.9

fibrin polymerization (see also Defect, coagulation) 286.3

filling

biliary tract 793.3

bladder 793.5

dental 525.60

gallbladder 793.3

kidney 793.5

stomach 793.4

ureter 793.5

fossa ovalis 745.5

gene, carrier (suspected) of V83.89

Gerbode 745.4

glaucomatous, without elevated tension 365.89

Hageman (factor) (see also Defect, coagulation) 286.3

hearing (see also Deafness) 389.9

high grade 317

homogentisic acid 270.2

interatrial septal 745.5

acquired 429.71

interauricular septal 745.5

acquired 429.71

interventricular septal 745.4

with pulmonary stenosis or atresia, dextraposition of aorta, and hypertrophy of right ventricle 745.2

acquired 429.71

in tetralogy of Fallot 745.2

iodide trapping 246.1

iodotyrosine dehalogenase 246.1

kynureninase 270.2

learning, specific 315.2

major osseous 731.3

mental (see also Retardation, mental) 319

osseous, major 731.3

osteochondral NEC 738.8

ostium

primum 745.61

secundum 745.5

pericardium 746.89

peroxidase-binding 246.1

placental blood supply - see Placenta, insufficiency

platelet (qualitative) 287.1

constitutional 286.4

Defect, defective (Continued)

postural, spine 737.9

protan 368.51

pulmonic cusps, congenital 746.00

renal pelvis 753.9

obstructive 753.29

specified type NEC 753.3

respiratory system, congenital 748.9

specified type NEC 748.8

retina, retinal 361.30

with detachment (see also Detachment, retina, with retinal defect) 361.00

multiple 361.33

with detachment 361.02

nerve fiber bundle 362.85

single 361.30

with detachment 361.01

septal (closure) (heart) NEC 745.9

acquired 429.71

atrial 745.5

specified type NEC 745.8

speech NEC 784.59   ◄▪▪▪

developmental 315.39

late effect of cerebrovascular disease - see Late effect(s) (of) cerebrovascular disease, speech and language deficit   ◄

secondary to organic lesion 784.59   ◄▪▪▪

Taussig-Bing (transposition, aorta and overriding pulmonary artery) 745.11

teeth, wedge 521.20

thyroid hormone synthesis 246.1

tritan 368.53

ureter 753.9

obstructive 753.29

vascular (acquired) (local) 459.9

congenital (peripheral) NEC 747.60

gastrointestinal 747.61

lower limb 747.64

renal 747.62

specified NEC 747.69

spinal 747.82

upper limb 747.63

ventricular septal 745.4

with pulmonary stenosis or atresia, dextraposition of aorta, and hypertrophy of right ventricle 745.2

acquired 429.71

atrioventricular canal type 745.69

between infundibulum and anterior portion 745.4

in tetralogy of Fallot 745.2

isolated anterior 745.4

vision NEC 369.9

visual field 368.40

arcuate 368.43

heteronymous, bilateral 368.47

homonymous, bilateral 368.46

localized NEC 368.44

nasal step 368.44

peripheral 368.44

sector 368.43

voice and resonance 784.40   ◄▪▪▪

wedge, teeth (abrasion) 521.20

Defeminization syndrome 255.2

Deferentitis 608.4

gonorrheal (acute) 098.14

chronic or duration of 2 months or over 098.34

Defibrination syndrome (see also Fibrinolysis) 286.6

◄ New   ◄▪▪▪ Revised   ~~deleted~~ Deleted   ● Use Additional Digit(s)   ▓▓▓ Omit code   **219**

Deficiency, deficient
  3-beta-hydroxysteroid dehydrogenase
    255.2
  6-phosphogluconic dehydrogenase
    (anemia) 282.2
  11-beta-hydroxylase 255.2
  17-alpha-hydroxylase 255.2
  18-hydroxysteroid dehydrogenase
    255.2
  20-alpha-hydroxylase 255.2
  21-hydroxylase 255.2
  AAT (alpha-1 antitrypsin) 273.4
  abdominal muscle syndrome 756.79
  accelerator globulin (Ac G) (blood) (*see
    also* Defect, coagulation) 286.3
  AC globulin (congenital) (*see also*
    Defect, coagulation) 286.3
    acquired 286.7
  activating factor (blood) (*see also* Defect,
    coagulation) 286.3
  adenohypophyseal 253.2
  adenosine deaminase 277.2
  aldolase (hereditary) 271.2
  alpha-1-antitrypsin 273.4
  alpha-1-trypsin inhibitor 273.4
  alpha-fucosidase 271.8
  alpha-lipoprotein 272.5
  alpha-mannosidase 271.8
  amino acid 270.9
  anemia - *see* Anemia, deficiency
  aneurin 265.1
    with beriberi 265.0
  antibody NEC 279.00
  antidiuretic hormone 253.5
  antihemophilic
    factor (A) 286.0
      B 286.1
      C 286.2
    globulin (AHG) NEC 286.0
  antithrombin III 289.81
  antitrypsin 273.4
  argininosuccinate synthetase or lyase
    270.6
  ascorbic acid (with scurvy) 267
  autoprothrombin
    I (*see also* Defect, coagulation) 286.3
    II 286.1
    C (*see also* Defect, coagulation)
      286.3
  bile salt 579.8
  biotin 266.2
  biotinidase 277.6
  bradykinase-1 277.6
  brancher enzyme (amylopectinosis)
    271.0
  calciferol 268.9
    with
      osteomalacia 268.2
      rickets (*see also* Rickets) 268.0
  calcium 275.40
    dietary 269.3
  calorie, severe 261
  carbamyl phosphate synthetase 270.6
  cardiac (*see also* Insufficiency,
    myocardial) 428.0
  carnitine 277.81
    due to
      hemodialysis 277.83
      inborn errors of metabolism
        277.82
      valproic acid therapy 277.83
    iatrogenic 277.83
    palmitoyltransferase (CPT1, CPT2)
      277.85

Deficiency, deficient (*Continued*)
  carnitine (*Continued*)
    palmityl transferase (CPT1, CPT2)
      277.85
    primary 277.81
    secondary 277.84
  carotene 264.9
  Carr factor (*see also* Defect, coagulation)
    286.9
  central nervous system 349.9
  ceruloplasmin 275.1
  cevitamic acid (with scurvy) 267
  choline 266.2
  Christmas factor 286.1
  chromium 269.3
  citrin 269.1
  clotting (blood) (*see also* Defect,
    coagulation) 286.9
  coagulation factor NEC 286.9
    with
      abortion - *see* Abortion, by type,
        with hemorrhage
      ectopic pregnancy (*see also*
        categories 634–638) 639.1
      molar pregnancy (*see also*
        categories 630–632) 639.1
    acquired (any) 286.7
    antepartum or intrapartum 641.3●
      affecting fetus or newborn
        762.1
    complicating pregnancy,
      childbirth, or puerperium
      649.3●
    due to
      liver disease 286.7
      vitamin K deficiency 286.7
    newborn, transient 776.3
    postpartum 666.3●
    specified type NEC 286.3
  color vision (congenital) 368.59
    acquired 368.55
  combined glucocorticoid and
    mineralocorticoid 255.41
  combined, two or more coagulation
    factors (*see also* Defect,
    coagulation) 286.9
  complement factor NEC 279.8
  contact factor (*see also* Defect,
    coagulation) 286.3
  copper NEC 275.1
  corticoadrenal 255.41
  craniofacial axis 756.0
  cyanocobalamin (vitamin B_{12}) 266.2
  debrancher enzyme (limit dextrinosis)
    271.0
  desmolase 255.2
  diet 269.9
  dihydrofolate reductase 281.2
  dihydropteridine reductase 270.1
  disaccharidase (intestinal) 271.3
  disease NEC 269.9
  ear(s) V48.8
  edema 262
  endocrine 259.9
  enzymes, circulating NEC (*see also*
    Deficiency, by specific enzyme)
    277.6
  ergosterol 268.9
    with
      osteomalacia 268.2
      rickets (*see also* Rickets) 268.0
  erythrocytic glutathione (anemia)
    282.2
  eyelid(s) V48.8

Deficiency, deficient (*Continued*)
  factor (*see also* Defect, coagulation)
    286.9
    I (congenital) (fibrinogen) 286.3
      antepartum or intrapartum
        641.3●
        affecting fetus or newborn
          762.1
      newborn, transient 776.3
      postpartum 666.3●
    II (congenital) (prothrombin) 286.3
    V (congenital) (labile) 286.3
    VII (congenital) (stable) 286.3
    VIII (congenital) (functional) 286.0
      with
        functional defect 286.0
        vascular defect 286.4
    IX (Christmas) (congenital)
      (functional) 286.1
    X (congenital) (Stuart-Prower) 286.3
    XI (congenital) (plasma
      thromboplastin antecedent)
      286.2
    XII (congenital) (Hageman) 286.3
    XIII (congenital) (fibrin stabilizing)
      286.3
    Hageman 286.3
    multiple (congenital) 286.9
      acquired 286.7
  fibrinase (*see also* Defect, coagulation)
    286.3
  fibrinogen (congenital) (*see also* Defect,
    coagulation) 286.3
    acquired 286.6
  fibrin-stabilizing factor (congenital) (*see
    also* Defect, coagulation) 286.3
    acquired 286.7
  finger - *see* Absence, finger
  fletcher factor (*see also* Defect,
    coagulation) 286.9
  fluorine 269.3
  folate, anemia 281.2
  folic acid (vitamin B_C) 266.2
    anemia 281.2
  follicle-stimulating hormone (FSH)
    253.4
  fructokinase 271.2
  fructose-1, 6-diphosphate 271.2
  fructose-1-phosphate aldolase 271.2
  FSH (follicle-stimulating hormone)
    253.4
  fucosidase 271.8
  galactokinase 271.1
  galactose-1-phosphate uridyl
    transferase 271.1
  gamma globulin in blood 279.00
  glass factor (*see also* Defect,
    coagulation) 286.3
  glucocorticoid 255.41
  glucose-6-phosphatase 271.0
  glucose-6-phosphate dehydrogenase
    anemia 282.2
  glucuronyl transferase 277.4
  glutathione-reductase (anemia) 282.2
  glycogen synthetase 271.0
  growth hormone 253.3
  Hageman factor (congenital) (*see also*
    Defect, coagulation) 286.3
  head V48.0
  hemoglobin (*see also* Anemia) 285.9
  hepatophosphorylase 271.0
  hexose monophosphate (HMP) shunt
    282.2
  HGH (human growth hormone) 253.3

◀ New   ◀▥ Revised   ~~deleted~~ Deleted   ● Use Additional Digit(s)   ▦ Omit code

Deficiency, deficient *(Continued)*
  HG-PRT 277.2
  homogentisic acid oxidase 270.2
  hormone - *see also* Deficiency, by
        specific hormone
     anterior pituitary (isolated) (partial)
        NEC 253.4
        growth (human) 253.3
     follicle-stimulating 253.4
     growth (human) (isolated) 253.3
     human growth 253.3
     interstitial cell-stimulating 253.4
     luteinizing 253.4
     melanocyte-stimulating 253.4
     testicular 257.2
  human growth hormone 253.3
  humoral 279.00
     with
        hyper-IgM 279.05
           autosomal recessive 279.05
           X-linked 279.05
        increased IgM 279.05
        congenital hypogammaglobulinemia
           279.04
        non-sex-linked 279.06
        selective immunoglobulin NEC
           279.03
           IgA 279.01
           IgG 279.03
           IgM 279.02
              increased 279.05
        specified NEC 279.09
  hydroxylase 255.2
  hypoxanthine-guanine
        phosphoribosyltransferase
        (HG-PRT) 277.2
  ICSH (interstitial cell-stimulating
        hormone) 253.4
  immunity NEC 279.3
     cell-mediated 279.10
        with
           hyperimmunoglobulinemia
              279.2
           thrombocytopenia and eczema
              279.12
        specified NEC 279.19
     combined (severe) 279.2
        syndrome 279.2
     common variable 279.06
     humoral NEC 279.00
     IgA (secretory) 279.01
     IgG 279.03
     IgM 279.02
  immunoglobulin, selective NEC 279.03
     IgA 279.01
     IgG 279.03
     IgM 279.02
  inositol (B complex) 266.2
  interferon 279.49   ◀▥
  internal organ V47.0
  interstitial cell-stimulating hormone
        (ICSH) 253.4
  intrinsic factor (Castle's) (congenital)
        281.0
  intrinsic (urethral) sphincter (ISD)
        599.82
  invertase 271.3
  iodine 269.3
  iron, anemia 280.9
  labile factor (congenital) (*see also*
        Defect, coagulation) 286.3
     acquired 286.7
  lacrimal fluid (acquired) 375.15
     congenital 743.64

Deficiency, deficient *(Continued)*
  lactase 271.3
  Laki-Lorand factor (*see also* Defect,
        coagulation) 286.3
  lecithin-cholesterol acyltranferase
        272.5
  LH (luteinizing hormone) 253.4
  limb V49.0
     lower V49.0
        congenital (*see also* Deficiency,
           lower limb, congenital)
           755.30
     upper V49.0
        congenital (*see also* Deficiency,
           upper limb, congenital)
           755.20
  lipocaic 577.8
  lipoid (high-density) 272.5
  lipoprotein (familial) (high-density)
        272.5
  liver phosphorylase 271.0
  long chain 3-hydroxyacyl CoA
        dehydrogenase (LCHAD) 277.85
  long chain/very long chain acyl CoA
        dehydrogenase (LCAD, VLCAD)
        277.85
  lower limb V49.0
     congenital 755.30
        with complete absence of distal
           elements 755.31
        longitudinal (complete) (partial)
           (with distal deficiencies,
           incomplete) 755.32
           with complete absence of
              distal elements 755.31
           combined femoral, tibial,
              fibular (incomplete)
              755.33
           femoral 755.34
           fibular 755.37
           metatarsal(s) 755.38
           phalange(s) 755.39
              meaning all digits 755.31
           tarsal(s) 755.38
           tibia 755.36
           tibiofibular 755.35
        transverse 755.31
  luteinizing hormone (LH) 253.4
  lysosomal alpha-1, 4 glucosidase
        271.0
  magnesium 275.2
  mannosidase 271.8
  medium chain acyl CoA
        dehydrogenase (MCAD) 277.85
  melanocyte stimulating hormone
        (MSH) 253.4
  menadione (vitamin K) 269.0
     newborn 776.0
  mental (familial) (hereditary) (*see also*
        Retardation, mental) 319
  methylenetetrahydrofolate reductase
        (MTHFR) 270.4
  mineral NEC 269.3
  mineralocorticoid 255.42
  molybdenum 269.3
  moral 301.7
  multiple, syndrome 260
  myocardial (*see also* Insufficiency,
        myocardial) 428.0
  myophosphorylase 271.0
  NADH (DPNH)-methemoglobin-
        reductase (congenital) 289.7
  NADH diaphorase or reductase
        (congenital) 289.7

Deficiency, deficient *(Continued)*
  neck V48.1
  niacin (amide) (-tryptophan) 265.2
  nicotinamide 265.2
  nicotinic acid (amide) 265.2
  nose V48.8
  number of teeth (*see also* Anodontia)
        520.0
  nutrition, nutritional 269.9
     specified NEC 269.8
  ornithine transcarbamylase 270.6
  ovarian 256.39
  oxygen (*see also* Anoxia) 799.02
  pantothenic acid 266.2
  parathyroid (gland) 252.1
  phenylalanine hydroxylase 270.1
  phosphoenolpyruvate carboxykinase
        271.8
  phosphofructokinase 271.2
  phosphoglucomutase 271.0
  phosphohexosisomerase 271.0
  phosphomannomutase 271.8
  phosphomannose isomerase 271.8
  phosphomannosyl mutase 271.8
  phosphorylase kinase, liver 271.0
  pituitary (anterior) 253.2
     posterior 253.5
  placenta - *see* Placenta, insufficiency
  plasma
     cell 279.00
     protein (paraproteinemia)
           (pyroglobulinemia) 273.8
        gamma globulin 279.00
     thromboplastin
        antecedent (PTA) 286.2
        component (PTC) 286.1
  platelet NEC 287.1
     constitutional 286.4
  polyglandular 258.9
  potassium (K) 276.8
  proaccelerin (congenital) (*see also*
        Defect, congenital) 286.3
     acquired 286.7
  proconvertin factor (congenital) (*see
        also* Defect, coagulation) 286.3
     acquired 286.7
  prolactin 253.4
  protein 260
     anemia 281.4
     C 289.81
     plasma - *see* Deficiency, plasma,
           protein
     S 289.81
  prothrombin (congenital) (*see also*
        Defect, coagulation) 286.3
     acquired 286.7
  Prower factor (*see also* Defect,
        coagulation) 286.3
  PRT 277.2
  pseudocholinesterase 289.89
  psychobiological 301.6
  PTA 286.2
  PTC 286.1
  purine nucleoside phosphorylase 277.2
  pyracin (alpha) (beta) 266.1
  pyridoxal 266.1
  pyridoxamine 266.1
  pyridoxine (derivatives) 266.1
  pyruvate carboxylase 271.8
  pyruvate dehydrogenase 271.8
  pyruvate kinase (PK) 282.3
  riboflavin (vitamin B_2) 266.0
  saccadic eye movements 379.57
  salivation 527.7

Deficiency, deficient (Continued)
salt 276.1
secretion
ovary 256.39
salivary gland (any) 527.7
urine 788.5
selenium 269.3
serum
antitrypsin, familial 273.4
protein (congenital) 273.8
short chain acyl CoA dehydrogenase (SCAD) 277.85
short stature homeobox gene (SHOX)
with
dyschondrosteosis 756.89
short stature (idiopathic) 783.43
Turner's syndrome 758.6
smooth pursuit movements (eye) 379.58
sodium (Na) 276.1
SPCA (see also Defect, coagulation) 286.3
specified NEC 269.8
stable factor (congenital) (see also Defect, coagulation) 286.3
acquired 286.7
Stuart (-Prower) factor (see also Defect, coagulation) 286.3
sucrase 271.3
sucrase-isomaltase 271.3
sulfite oxidase 270.0
syndrome, multiple 260
thiamine, thiaminic (chloride) 265.1
thrombokinase (see also Defect, coagulation) 286.3
newborn 776.0
thrombopoieten 287.39
thymolymphatic 279.2
thyroid (gland) 244.9
tocopherol 269.1
toe - see Absence, toe
tooth bud (see also Anodontia) 520.0
trunk V48.1
UDPG-glycogen transferase 271.0
upper limb V49.0
congenital 755.20
with complete absence of distal elements 755.21
longitudinal (complete) (partial) (with distal deficiencies, incomplete) 755.22
carpal(s) 755.28
combined humeral, radial, ulnar (incomplete) 755.23
humeral 755.24
metacarpal(s) 755.28
phalange(s) 755.29
meaning all digits 755.21
radial 755.26
radioulnar 755.25
ulnar 755.27
transverse (complete) (partial) 755.21
vascular 459.9
vasopressin 253.5
viosterol (see also Deficiency, calciferol) 268.9
vitamin (multiple) NEC 269.2
A 264.9
with
Bitôt's spot 264.1
corneal 264.2
with corneal ulceration 264.3

Deficiency, deficient (Continued)
vitamin (Continued)
A (Continued)
with (Continued)
keratomalacia 264.4
keratosis, follicular 264.8
night blindness 264.5
scar of cornea, xerophthalmic 264.6
specified manifestation NEC 264.8
ocular 264.7
xeroderma 264.8
xerophthalmia 264.7
xerosis
conjunctival 264.0
with Bitôt's spot 264.1
corneal 264.2
with corneal ulceration 264.3
B (complex) NEC 266.9
with
beriberi 265.0
pellagra 265.2
specified type NEC 266.2
B₁ NEC 265.1
beriberi 265.0
B₂ 266.0
B₆ 266.1
B₁₂ 266.2
B_C (folic acid) 266.2
C (ascorbic acid) (with scurvy) 267
D (calciferol) (ergosterol) 268.9
with
osteomalacia 268.2
rickets (see also Rickets) 268.0
E 269.1
folic acid 266.2
G 266.0
H 266.2
K 269.0
of newborn 776.0
nicotinic acid 265.2
P 269.1
PP 265.2
specified NEC 269.1
zinc 269.3
Deficient - see also Deficiency
blink reflex 374.45
craniofacial axis 756.0
number of teeth (see also Anodontia) 520.0
secretion of urine 788.5
Deficit
neurologic NEC 781.99
due to
cerebrovascular lesion (see also Disease, cerebrovascular, acute) 436
late effect - see Late effect(s) (of) cerebrovascular disease
transient ischemic attack 435.9
ischemic
reversible (RIND) 434.91
history of (personal) V12.54
prolonged (PRIND) 434.91
history of (personal) V12.54
oxygen 799.02
Deflection
radius 736.09
septum (acquired) (nasal) (nose) 470
spine - see Curvature, spine
turbinate (nose) 470

Defluvium
capillorum (see also Alopecia) 704.00
ciliorum 374.55
unguium 703.8
Deformity 738.9
abdomen, congenital 759.9
abdominal wall
acquired 738.8
congenital 756.70
muscle deficiency syndrome 756.79
acquired (unspecified site) 738.9
specified site NEC 738.8
adrenal gland (congenital) 759.1
alimentary tract, congenital 751.9
lower 751.5
specified type NEC 751.8
upper (any part, except tongue) 750.9
specified type NEC 750.8
tongue 750.10
specified type NEC 750.19
ankle (joint) (acquired) 736.70
abduction 718.47
congenital 755.69
contraction 718.47
specified NEC 736.79
anus (congenital) 751.5
acquired 569.49
aorta (congenital) 747.20
acquired 447.8
arch 747.21
acquired 447.8
coarctation 747.10
aortic
arch 747.21
acquired 447.8
cusp or valve (congenital) 746.9
acquired (see also Endocarditis, aortic) 424.1
ring 747.21
appendix 751.5
arm (acquired) 736.89
congenital 755.50
arteriovenous (congenital) (peripheral) NEC 747.60
gastrointestinal 747.61
lower limb 747.64
renal 747.62
specified NEC 747.69
spinal 747.82
upper limb 747.63
artery (congenital) (peripheral) NEC (see also Deformity, vascular) 747.60
acquired 447.8
cerebral 747.81
coronary (congenital) 746.85
acquired (see also Ischemia, heart) 414.9
retinal 743.9
umbilical 747.5
atrial septal (congenital) (heart) 745.5
auditory canal (congenital) (external) (see also Deformity, ear) 744.3
acquired 380.50
auricle
ear (congenital) (see also Deformity, ear) 744.3
acquired 380.32
heart (congenital) 746.9
back (acquired) - see Deformity, spine
Bartholin's duct (congenital) 750.9

◄ New   ◄◖ Revised   ~~deleted~~ Deleted   ● Use Additional Digit(s)   ▨ Omit code

Deformity (Continued)
bile duct (congenital) 751.60
   acquired 576.8
      with calculus, choledocholithiasis,
        or stones - see
        Choledocholithiasis
biliary duct or passage (congenital)
   751.60
   acquired 576.8
      with calculus, choledocholithiasis,
        or stones - see
        Choledocholithiasis
bladder (neck) (sphincter) (trigone)
   (acquired) 596.8
   congenital 753.9
bone (acquired) NEC 738.9
   congenital 756.9
   turbinate 738.0
boutonniere (finger) 736.21
brain (congenital) 742.9
   acquired 348.89
   multiple 742.4
   reduction 742.2
   vessel (congenital) 747.81
breast (acquired) 611.89
   congenital 757.6
   reconstructed 612.0
bronchus (congenital) 748.3
   acquired 519.19
bursa, congenital 756.9
canal of Nuck 752.9
canthus (congenital) 743.9
   acquired 374.89
capillary (acquired) 448.9
   congenital NEC (see also Deformity,
      vascular) 747.60
cardiac - see Deformity, heart
cardiovascular system (congenital)
   746.9
caruncle, lacrimal (congenital)
   743.9
   acquired 375.69
cascade, stomach 537.6
cecum (congenital) 751.5
   acquired 569.89
cerebral (congenital) 742.9
   acquired 348.89
cervix (acquired) (uterus) 622.8
   congenital 752.40
cheek (acquired) 738.19
   congenital 744.9
chest (wall) (acquired) 738.3
   congenital 754.89
   late effect of rickets 268.1
chin (acquired) 738.19
   congenital 744.9
choroid (congenital) 743.9
   acquired 363.8
   plexus (congenital) 742.9
      acquired 349.2
cicatricial - see Cicatrix
cilia (congenital) 743.9
   acquired 374.89
circulatory system (congenital)
   747.9
clavicle (acquired) 738.8
   congenital 755.51
clitoris (congenital) 752.40
   acquired 624.8
clubfoot - see Clubfoot
coccyx (acquired) 738.6
   congenital 756.10
colon (congenital) 751.5
   acquired 569.89

Deformity (Continued)
concha (ear) (congenital) (see also
   Deformity, ear) 744.3
   acquired 380.32
congenital, organ or site not listed (see
   also Anomaly) 759.9
cornea (congenital) 743.9
   acquired 371.70
coronary artery (congenital) 746.85
   acquired (see also Ischemia, heart)
      414.9
cranium (acquired) 738.19
   congenital (see also Deformity, skull,
      congenital) 756.0
cricoid cartilage (congenital) 748.3
   acquired 478.79
cystic duct (congenital) 751.60
   acquired 575.8
Dandy-Walker 742.3
   with spina bifida (see also Spina
      bifida) 741.0●
diaphragm (congenital) 756.6
   acquired 738.8
digestive organ(s) or system
   (congenital) NEC 751.9
   specified type NEC 751.8
ductus arteriosus 747.0
duodenal bulb 537.89
duodenum (congenital) 751.5
   acquired 537.89
dura (congenital) 742.9
   brain 742.4
      acquired 349.2
   spinal 742.59
      acquired 349.2
ear (congenital) 744.3
   acquired 380.32
   auricle 744.3
      causing impairment of hearing
        744.02
   causing impairment of hearing
      744.00
   external 744.3
      causing impairment of hearing
        744.02
   internal 744.05
   lobule 744.3
   middle 744.03
      ossicles 744.04
   ossicles 744.04
ectodermal (congenital) NEC 757.9
   specified type NEC 757.8
ejaculatory duct (congenital) 752.9
   acquired 608.89
elbow (joint) (acquired) 736.00
   congenital 755.50
   contraction 718.42
endocrine gland NEC 759.2
epididymis (congenital) 752.9
   acquired 608.89
   torsion 608.24
epiglottis (congenital) 748.3
   acquired 478.79
esophagus (congenital) 750.9
   acquired 530.89
Eustachian tube (congenital) NEC
   744.3
   specified type NEC 744.24
extremity (acquired) 736.9
   congenital, except reduction
      deformity 755.9
      lower 755.60
      upper 755.50
   reduction - see Deformity, reduction

Deformity (Continued)
eye (congenital) 743.9
   acquired 379.8
   muscle 743.9
eyebrow (congenital) 744.89
eyelid (congenital) 743.9
   acquired 374.89
   specified type NEC 743.62
face (acquired) 738.19
   congenital (any part) 744.9
      due to intrauterine malposition
        and pressure 754.0
fallopian tube (congenital) 752.10
   acquired 620.8
femur (acquired) 736.89
   congenital 755.60
fetal
   with fetopelvic disproportion
      653.7●
      affecting fetus or newborn 763.1
   causing obstructed labor 660.1●
      affecting fetus or newborn 763.1
   known or suspected, affecting
      management of pregnancy
      655.9●
finger (acquired) 736.20
   boutonniere type 736.21
   congenital 755.50
   flexion contracture 718.44
   swan neck 736.22
flexion (joint) (acquired) 736.9
   congenital NEC 755.9
   hip or thigh (acquired) 736.39
      congenital (see also Subluxation,
        congenital, hip) 754.32
foot (acquired) 736.70
   cavovarus 736.75
      congenital 754.59
   congenital NEC 754.70
      specified type NEC 754.79
   valgus (acquired) 736.79
      congenital 754.60
        specified type NEC 754.69
   varus (acquired) 736.79
      congenital 754.50
        specified type NEC 754.59
forearm (acquired) 736.00
   congenital 755.50
forehead (acquired) 738.19
   congenital (see also Deformity, skull,
      congenital) 756.0
frontal bone (acquired) 738.19
   congenital (see also Deformity, skull,
      congenital) 756.0
gallbladder (congenital) 751.60
   acquired 575.8
gastrointestinal tract (congenital) NEC
   751.9
   acquired 569.89
   specified type NEC 751.8
genitalia, genital organ(s) or system
   NEC
   congenital 752.9
   female (congenital) 752.9
      acquired 629.89
      external 752.40
      internal 752.9
   male (congenital) 752.9
      acquired 608.89
globe (eye) (congenital) 743.9
   acquired 360.89
gum (congenital) 750.9
   acquired 523.9
gunstock 736.02

Deformity (Continued)
  hand (acquired) 736.00
    claw 736.06
    congenital 755.50
    minus (and plus) (intrinsic) 736.09
    pill roller (intrinsic) 736.09
    plus (and minus) (intrinsic) 736.09
    swan neck (intrinsic) 736.09
  head (acquired) 738.10
    congenital (see also Deformity, skull,
        congenital) 756.0
    specified NEC 738.19
  heart (congenital) 746.9
    auricle (congenital) 746.9
    septum 745.9
      auricular 745.5
      specified type NEC 745.8
      ventricular 745.4
    valve (congenital) NEC 746.9
      acquired - see Endocarditis
      pulmonary (congenital) 746.00
      specified type NEC 746.89
    ventricle (congenital) 746.9
  heel (acquired) 736.76
    congenital 755.67
  hepatic duct (congenital) 751.60
    acquired 576.8
      with calculus, choledocholithiasis,
          or stones - see
          Choledocholithiasis
  hip (joint) (acquired) 736.30
    congenital NEC 755.63
    flexion 718.45
      congenital (see also Subluxation,
          congenital, hip) 754.32
  hourglass - see Contraction, hourglass
  humerus (acquired) 736.89
    congenital 755.50
  hymen (congenital) 752.40
  hypophyseal (congenital) 759.2
  ileocecal (coil) (valve) (congenital)
      751.5
    acquired 569.89
  ileum (intestine) (congenital) 751.5
    acquired 569.89
  ilium (acquired) 738.6
    congenital 755.60
  integument (congenital) 757.9
  intervertebral cartilage or disc
      (acquired) - see also Displacement,
      intervertebral disc
    congenital 756.10
  intestine (large) (small) (congenital)
      751.5
    acquired 569.89
  iris (acquired) 364.75
    congenital 743.9
    prolapse 364.89
  ischium (acquired) 738.6
    congenital 755.60
  jaw (acquired) (congenital) NEC 524.9
    due to intrauterine malposition and
        pressure 754.0
  joint (acquired) NEC 738.8
    congenital 755.9
    contraction (abduction) (adduction)
        (extension) (flexion) - see
        Contraction, joint
  kidney(s) (calyx) (pelvis) (congenital)
      753.9
    acquired 593.89
    vessel 747.62
      acquired 459.9
  Klippel-Feil (brevicollis) 756.16

Deformity (Continued)
  knee (acquired) NEC 736.6
    congenital 755.64
  labium (majus) (minus) (congenital)
      752.40
    acquired 624.8
  lacrimal apparatus or duct (congenital)
      743.9
    acquired 375.69
  larynx (muscle) (congenital)
      748.3
    acquired 478.79
    web (glottic) (subglottic) 748.2
  leg (lower) (upper) (acquired) NEC
      736.89
    congenital 755.60
      reduction - see Deformity,
          reduction, lower limb
  lens (congenital) 743.9
    acquired 379.39
  lid (fold) (congenital) 743.9
    acquired 374.89
  ligament (acquired) 728.9
    congenital 756.9
  limb (acquired) 736.9
    congenital, except reduction
        deformity 755.9
    lower 755.60
      reduction (see also
          Deformity, reduction,
          lower limb) 755.30
    upper 755.50
      reduction (see also
          Deformity, reduction,
          lower limb) 755.20
    specified NEC 736.89
  lip (congenital) NEC 750.9
    acquired 528.5
    specified type NEC 750.26
  liver (congenital) 751.60
    acquired 573.8
    duct (congenital) 751.60
      acquired 576.8
        with calculus,
            choledocholithiasis,
            or stones - see
            Choledocholithiasis
  lower extremity - see Deformity, leg
  lumbosacral (joint) (region)
      (congenital) 756.10
    acquired 738.5
  lung (congenital) 748.60
    acquired 518.89
    specified type NEC 748.69
  lymphatic system, congenital
      759.9
  Madelung's (radius) 755.54
  maxilla (acquired) (congenital)
      524.9
  meninges or membrane (congenital)
      742.9
    brain 742.4
      acquired 349.2
    spinal (cord) 742.59
      acquired 349.2
  mesentery (congenital) 751.9
    acquired 568.89
  metacarpus (acquired) 736.00
    congenital 755.50
  metatarsus (acquired) 736.70
    congenital 754.70
  middle ear, except ossicles (congenital)
      744.03
    ossicles 744.04

Deformity (Continued)
  mitral (leaflets) (valve) (congenital)
      746.9
    acquired - see Endocarditis, mitral
    Ebstein's 746.89
    parachute 746.5
    specified type NEC 746.89
    stenosis, congenital 746.5
  mouth (acquired) 528.9
    congenital NEC 750.9
      specified type NEC 750.26
  multiple, congenital NEC 759.7
    specified type NEC 759.89
  muscle (acquired) 728.9
    congenital 756.9
      specified type NEC 756.89
    sternocleidomastoid (due to
        intrauterine malposition
        and pressure) 754.1
  musculoskeletal system, congenital
      NEC 756.9
    specified type NEC 756.9
  nail (acquired) 703.9
    congenital 757.9
  nasal - see Deformity, nose
  neck (acquired) NEC 738.2
    congenital (any part) 744.9
      sternocleidomastoid 754.1
  nervous system (congenital) 742.9
  nipple (congenital) 757.6   ◀▦▦
    acquired 611.89
  nose, nasal (cartilage) (acquired) 738.0
    bone (turbinate) 738.0
    congenital 748.1
      bent 754.0
      squashed 754.0
      saddle 738.0
        syphilitic 090.5
    septum 470
      congenital 748.1
    sinus (wall) (congenital) 748.1
      acquired 738.0
    syphilitic (congenital) 090.5
      late 095.8
  ocular muscle (congenital) 743.9
    acquired 378.60
  opticociliary vessels (congenital) 743.9
  orbit (congenital) (eye) 743.9
    acquired NEC 376.40
      associated with craniofacial
          deformities 376.44
      due to
        bone disease 376.43
        surgery 376.47
        trauma 376.47
  organ of Corti (congenital) 744.05
  ovary (congenital) 752.0
    acquired 620.8
  oviduct (congenital) 752.10
    acquired 620.8
  palate (congenital) 750.9
    acquired 526.89
    cleft (congenital) (see also Cleft,
        palate) 749.00
    hard, acquired 526.89
    soft, acquired 528.9
  pancreas (congenital) 751.7
    acquired 577.8
  parachute, mitral valve 746.5
  parathyroid (gland) 759.2
  parotid (gland) (congenital) 750.9
    acquired 527.8
  patella (acquired) 736.6
    congenital 755.64

◀ New   ◀▦▦ Revised   ~~deleted~~ Deleted   ● Use Additional Digit(s)   ▦▦ Omit code

Deformity (Continued)
pelvis, pelvic (acquired) (bony) 738.6
　with disproportion (fetopelvic) 653.0●
　　affecting fetus or newborn 763.1
　　causing obstructed labor 660.1●
　　　affecting fetus or newborn 763.1
　congenital 755.60
　rachitic (late effect) 268.1
penis (glans) (congenital) 752.9
　acquired 607.89
pericardium (congenital) 746.9
　acquired - see Pericarditis
pharynx (congenital) 750.9
　acquired 478.29
Pierre Robin (congenital) 756.0
pinna (acquired) 380.32
　congenital 744.3
pituitary (congenital) 759.2
pleural folds (congenital) 748.8
portal vein (congenital) 747.40
posture - see Curvature, spine
prepuce (congenital) 752.9
　acquired 607.89
prostate (congenital) 752.9
　acquired 602.8
pulmonary valve - see Endocarditis, pulmonary
pupil (congenital) 743.9
　acquired 364.75
pylorus (congenital) 750.9
　acquired 537.89
rachitic (acquired), healed or old 268.1
radius (acquired) 736.00
　congenital 755.50
　　reduction - see Deformity, reduction, upper limb
rectovaginal septum (congenital) 752.40
　acquired 623.8
rectum (congenital) 751.5
　acquired 569.49
reduction (extremity) (limb) 755.4
　brain 742.2
　lower limb 755.30
　　with complete absence of distal elements 755.31
　　longitudinal (complete) (partial) (with distal deficiencies, incomplete) 755.32
　　　with complete absence of distal elements 755.31
　　combined femoral, tibial, fibular (incomplete) 755.33
　　femoral 755.34
　　fibular 755.37
　　metatarsal(s) 755.38
　　phalange(s) 755.39
　　　meaning all digits 755.31
　　tarsal(s) 755.38
　　tibia 755.36
　　tibiofibular 755.35
　　transverse 755.31
　upper limb 755.20
　　with complete absence of distal elements 755.21
　　longitudinal (complete) (partial) (with distal deficiencies, incomplete) 755.22
　　　with complete absence of distal elements 755.21
　　carpal(s) 755.28

Deformity (Continued)
reduction (Continued)
　upper limb (Continued)
　　longitudinal (Continued)
　　　combined humeral, radial, ulnar (incomplete) 755.23
　　　humeral 755.24
　　　metacarpal(s) 755.28
　　　phalange(s) 755.29
　　　　meaning all digits 755.21
　　　radial 755.26
　　　radioulnar 755.25
　　　ulnar 755.27
　　transverse (complete) (partial) 755.21
renal - see Deformity, kidney
respiratory system (congenital) 748.9
　specified type NEC 748.8
rib (acquired) 738.3
　congenital 756.3
　　cervical 756.2
rotation (joint) (acquired) 736.9
　congenital 755.9
　hip or thigh 736.39
　　congenital (see also Subluxation, congenital, hip) 754.32
sacroiliac joint (congenital) 755.69
　acquired 738.5
sacrum (acquired) 738.5
　congenital 756.10
saddle
　back 737.8
　nose 738.0
　　syphilitic 090.5
salivary gland or duct (congenital) 750.9
　acquired 527.8
scapula (acquired) 736.89
　congenital 755.50
scrotum (congenital) 752.9
　acquired 608.89
sebaceous gland, acquired 706.8
seminal tract or duct (congenital) 752.9
　acquired 608.89
septum (nasal) (acquired) 470
　congenital 748.1
shoulder (joint) (acquired) 736.89
　congenital 755.50
　　specified type NEC 755.59
　contraction 718.41
sigmoid (flexure) (congenital) 751.5
　acquired 569.89
sinus of Valsalva 747.29
skin (congenital) 757.9
　acquired NEC 709.8
skull (acquired) 738.19
　congenital 756.0
　　with
　　　anencephalus 740.0
　　　encephalocele 742.0
　　　hydrocephalus 742.3
　　　　with spina bifida (see also Spina bifida) 741.0●
　　　microcephalus 742.1
　　due to intrauterine malposition and pressure 754.0
soft parts, organs or tissues (of pelvis) in pregnancy or childbirth NEC 654.9●
　affecting fetus or newborn 763.89
　causing obstructed labor 660.2●
　　affecting fetus or newborn 763.1

Deformity (Continued)
spermatic cord (congenital) 752.9
　acquired 608.89
　　torsion 608.22
　　　extravaginal 608.21
　　　intravaginal 608.22
spinal
　column - see Deformity, spine
　cord (congenital) 742.9
　　acquired 336.8
　　vessel (congenital) 747.82
　nerve root (congenital) 742.9
　　acquired 724.9
spine (acquired) NEC 738.5
　congenital 756.10
　　due to intrauterine malposition and pressure 754.2
　kyphoscoliotic (see also Kyphoscoliosis) 737.30
　kyphotic (see also Kyphosis) 737.10
　lordotic (see also Lordosis) 737.20
　rachitic 268.1
　scoliotic (see also Scoliosis) 737.30
spleen
　acquired 289.59
　congenital 759.0
Sprengel's (congenital) 755.52
sternum (acquired) 738.3
　congenital 756.3
stomach (congenital) 750.9
　acquired 537.89
submaxillary gland (congenital) 750.9
　acquired 527.8
swan neck (acquired)
　finger 736.22
　hand 736.09
talipes - see Talipes
teeth, tooth NEC 520.9
testis (congenital) 752.9
　acquired 608.89
　　torsion 608.20
thigh (acquired) 736.89
　congenital 755.60
thorax (acquired) (wall) 738.3
　congenital 754.89
　late effect of rickets 268.1
thumb (acquired) 736.20
　congenital 755.50
thymus (tissue) (congenital) 759.2
thyroid (gland) (congenital) 759.2
　cartilage 748.3
　　acquired 478.79
tibia (acquired) 736.89
　congenital 755.60
　saber 090.5
toe (acquired) 735.9
　congenital 755.66
　specified NEC 735.8
tongue (congenital) 750.10
　acquired 529.8
tooth, teeth NEC 520.9
trachea (rings) (congenital) 748.3
　acquired 519.19
transverse aortic arch (congenital) 747.21
tricuspid (leaflets) (valve) (congenital) 746.9
　acquired - see Endocarditis, tricuspid
　atresia or stenosis 746.1
　specified type NEC 746.89
trunk (acquired) 738.3
　congenital 759.9
ulna (acquired) 736.00
　congenital 755.50

Deformity *(Continued)*
  upper extremity - *see* Deformity, arm
  urachus (congenital) 753.7
  ureter (opening) (congenital) 753.9
    acquired 593.89
  urethra (valve) (congenital) 753.9
    acquired 599.84
  urinary tract or system (congenital) 753.9
    urachus 753.7
  uterus (congenital) 752.3
    acquired 621.8
  uvula (congenital) 750.9
    acquired 528.9
  vagina (congenital) 752.40
    acquired 623.8
  valve, valvular (heart) (congenital) 746.9
    acquired - *see* Endocarditis
    pulmonary 746.00
    specified type NEC 746.89
  vascular (congenital) (peripheral) NEC 747.60
    acquired 459.9
    gastrointestinal 747.61
    lower limb 747.64
    renal 747.62
    specified site NEC 747.69
    spinal 747.82
    upper limb 747.63
  vas deferens (congenital) 752.9
    acquired 608.89
  vein (congenital) NEC (*see also* Deformity, vascular) 747.60
    brain 747.81
    coronary 746.9
    great 747.40
  vena cava (inferior) (superior) (congenital) 747.40
  vertebra - *see* Deformity, spine
  vesicourethral orifice (acquired) 596.8
    congenital NEC 753.9
      specified type NEC 753.8
  vessels of optic papilla (congenital) 743.9
  visual field (contraction) 368.45
  vitreous humor (congenital) 743.9
    acquired 379.29
  vulva (congenital) 752.40
    acquired 624.8
  wrist (joint) (acquired) 736.00
    congenital 755.50
    contraction 718.43
    valgus 736.03
      congenital 755.59
    varus 736.04
      congenital 755.59

Degeneration, degenerative
  adrenal (capsule) (gland) 255.8
    with hypofunction 255.41
    fatty 255.8
    hyaline 255.8
    infectional 255.8
    lardaceous 277.39
  amyloid (any site) (general) 277.39
  anterior cornua, spinal cord 336.8
  anterior labral 840.8
  aorta, aortic 440.0
    fatty 447.8
    valve (heart) (*see also* Endocarditis, aortic) 424.1
  arteriovascular - *see* Arteriosclerosis

Degeneration, degenerative *(Continued)*
  artery, arterial (atheromatous) (calcareous) - *see also* Arteriosclerosis
    amyloid 277.39
    lardaceous 277.39
    medial NEC (*see also* Arteriosclerosis, extremities) 440.20
  articular cartilage NEC (*see also* Disorder, cartilage, articular) 718.0●
    elbow 718.02
    knee 717.5
    patella 717.7
    shoulder 718.01
    spine (*see also* Spondylosis) 721.90
  atheromatous - *see* Arteriosclerosis
  bacony (any site) 277.39
  basal nuclei or ganglia NEC 333.0
  bone 733.90
  brachial plexus 353.0
  brain (cortical) (progressive) 331.9
    arteriosclerotic 437.0
    childhood 330.9
      specified type NEC 330.8
    congenital 742.4
    cystic 348.0
      congenital 742.4
    familial NEC 331.89
    grey matter 330.8
    heredofamilial NEC 331.89
    in
      alcoholism 303.9● [331.7]
      beriberi 265.0 [331.7]
      cerebrovascular disease 437.9 [331.7]
      congenital hydrocephalus 742.3 [331.7]
        with spina bifida (*see also* Spina bifida) 741.0● [331.7]
      Babry's disease 272.7 [330.2]
      Gaucher's disease 272.7 [330.2]
      Hunter's disease or syndrome 277.5 [330.3]
      lipidosis
        cerebral 330.1
        generalized 272.7 [330.2]
      mucopolysaccharidosis 277.5 [330.3]
      myxedema (*see also* Myxedema) 244.9 [331.7]
      neoplastic disease NEC (M8000/1) 239.9 [331.7]
      Niemann-Pick disease 272.7 [330.2]
      sphingolipidosis 272.7 [330.2]
      vitamin B$_{12}$ deficiency 266.2 [331.7]
    motor centers 331.89
    senile 331.2
    specified type NEC 331.89
  breast - *see* Disease, breast
  Bruch's membrane 363.40
  bundle of His 426.50
    left 426.3
    right 426.4
  calcareous NEC 275.49
  capillaries 448.9
    amyloid 277.39
    fatty 448.9
    lardaceous 277.39

Degeneration, degenerative *(Continued)*
  cardiac (brown) (calcareous) (fatty) (fibrous) (hyaline) (mural) (muscular) (pigmentary) (senile) (with arteriosclerosis) (*see also* Degeneration, myocardial) 429.1
    valve, valvular - *see* Endocarditis
  cardiorenal (*see also* Hypertension, cardiorenal) 404.90
  cardiovascular (*see also* Disease, cardiovascular) 429.2
    renal (*see also* Hypertension, cardiorenal) 404.90
  cartilage (joint) - *see* Derangement, joint
  cerebellar NEC 334.9
    primary (hereditary) (sporadic) 334.2
  cerebral - *see* Degeneration, brain
  cerebromacular 330.1
  cerebrovascular 437.1
    due to hypertension 437.2
    late effect - *see* Late effect(s) (of) cerebrovascular disease
  cervical plexus 353.2
  cervix 622.8
    due to radiation (intended effect) 622.8
      adverse effect or misadventure 622.8
  changes, spine or vertebra (*see also* Spondylosis) 721.90
  chitinous 277.39
  chorioretinal 363.40
    congenital 743.53
    hereditary 363.50
  choroid (colloid) (drusen) 363.40
    hereditary 363.50
    senile 363.41
      diffuse secondary 363.42
  cochlear 386.8
  collateral ligament (knee) (medial) 717.82
    lateral 717.81
  combined (spinal cord) (subacute) 266.2 [336.2]
    with anemia (pernicious) 281.0 [336.2]
      due to dietary deficiency 281.1 [336.2]
    due to vitamin B$_{12}$ deficiency anemia (dietary) 281.1 [336.2]
  conjunctiva 372.50
    amyloid 277.39 [372.50]
  cornea 371.40
    calcerous 371.44
    familial (hereditary) (*see also* Dystrophy, cornea) 371.50
      macular 371.55
      reticular 371.54
    hyaline (of old scars) 371.41
    marginal (Terrien's) 371.48
    mosaic (shagreen) 371.41
    nodular 371.46
    peripheral 371.48
    senile 371.41
  cortical (cerebellar) (parenchymatous) 334.2
    alcoholic 303.9● [334.4]
    diffuse, due to arteriopathy 437.0
  corticostriatal-spinal 334.8
  cretinoid 243
  cruciate ligament (knee) (posterior) 717.84
    anterior 717.83

◀ New   ◀═ Revised   ~~deleted~~ Deleted   ● Use Additional Digit(s)   ▨ Omit code

Degeneration, degenerative *(Continued)*
  cutis 709.3
    amyloid 277.39
  dental pulp 522.2
  disc disease - *see* Degeneration,
      intervertebral disc
  dorsolateral (spinal cord) - *see*
      Degeneration, combined
  endocardial 424.90
  extrapyramidal NEC 333.90
  eye NEC 360.40
    macular (*see also* Degeneration,
        macula) 362.50
      congenital 362.75
      hereditary 362.76
  fatty (diffuse) (general) 272.8
    liver 571.8
      alcoholic 571.0
    localized site - *see* Degeneration, by
        site, fatty
    placenta - *see* Placenta, abnormal
  globe (eye) NEC 360.40
    macular - *see* Degeneration,
        macula
  grey matter 330.8
  heart (brown) (calcareous) (fatty)
      (fibrous) (hyaline) (mural)
      (muscular) (pigmentary) (senile)
      (with arteriosclerosis) (*see also*
      Degeneration, myocardial)
      429.1
    amyloid 277.39 [*425.7*]
    atheromatous - *see* Arteriosclerosis,
        coronary
    gouty 274.82
    hypertensive (*see also* Hypertension,
        heart) 402.90
    ischemic 414.9
    valve, valvular - *see* Endocarditis
  hepatolenticular (Wilson's) 275.1
  hepatorenal 572.4
  heredofamilial
    brain NEC 331.89
    spinal cord NEC 336.8
  hyaline (diffuse) (generalized) 728.9
    localized - *see also* Degeneration, by
        site
      cornea 371.41
      keratitis 371.41
  hypertensive vascular - *see*
      Hypertension
  infrapatellar fat pad 729.31
  internal semilunar cartilage 717.3
  intervertebral disc 722.6
    with myelopathy 722.70
    cervical, cervicothoracic 722.4
      with myelopathy 722.71
    lumbar, lumbosacral 722.52
      with myelopathy 722.73
    thoracic, thoracolumbar 722.51
      with myelopathy 722.72
  intestine 569.89
    amyloid 277.39
    lardaceous 277.39
  iris (generalized) (*see also* Atrophy, iris)
      364.59
    pigmentary 364.53
    pupillary margin 364.54
  ischemic - *see* Ischemia
  joint disease (*see also* Osteoarthrosis)
      715.9●
    multiple sites 715.09
    spine (*see also* Spondylosis)
      721.90

Degeneration, degenerative *(Continued)*
  kidney (*see also* Sclerosis, renal) 587
    amyloid 277.39 [*583.81*]
    cyst, cystic (multiple) (solitary) 593.2
      congenital (*see also* Cystic,
          disease, kidney) 753.10
    fatty 593.89
    fibrocystic (congenital) 753.19
    lardaceous 277.39 [*583.81*]
    polycystic (congenital) 753.12
      adult type (APKD) 753.13
      autosomal dominant 753.13
      autosomal recessive 753.14
      childhood type (CPKD) 753.14
      infantile type 753.14
    waxy 277.39 [*583.81*]
  Kuhnt-Junius (retina) 362.52
  labyrinth, osseous 386.8
  lacrimal passages, cystic 375.12
  lardaceous (any site) 277.39
  lateral column (posterior), spinal cord
      (*see also* Degeneration, combined)
      266.2 [*336.2*]
  lattice 362.63
  lens 366.9
    infantile, juvenile, or presenile
        366.00
    senile 366.10
  lenticular (familial) (progressive)
      (Wilson's) (with cirrhosis of liver)
      275.1
    striate artery 437.0
  lethal ball, prosthetic heart valve 996.02
  ligament
    collateral (knee) (medial) 717.82
      lateral 717.81
    cruciate (knee) (posterior) 717.84
      anterior 717.83
  liver (diffuse) 572.8
    amyloid 277.39
    congenital (cystic) 751.62
    cystic 572.8
      congenital 751.62
    fatty 571.8
      alcoholic 571.0
    hypertrophic 572.8
    lardaceous 277.39
    parenchymatous, acute or subacute
        (*see also* Necrosis, liver) 570
    pigmentary 572.8
    toxic (acute) 573.8
    waxy 277.39
  lung 518.89
  lymph gland 289.3
    hyaline 289.3
    lardaceous 277.39
  macula (acquired) (senile) 362.50
    atrophic 362.51
    Best's 362.76
    congenital 362.75
    cystic 362.54
    cystoid 362.53
    disciform 362.52
    dry 362.51
    exudative 362.52
    familial pseudoinflammatory
        362.77
    hereditary 362.76
    hole 362.54
    juvenile (Stargardt's) 362.75
    nonexudative 362.51
    pseudohole 362.54
    wet 362.52
  medullary - *see* Degeneration, brain

Degeneration, degenerative *(Continued)*
  membranous labyrinth, congenital
      (causing impairment of hearing)
      744.05
  meniscus - *see* Derangement, joint
  microcystoid 362.62
  mitral - *see* Insufficiency, mitral
  Mönckeberg's (*see also* Arteriosclerosis,
      extremities) 440.20
  moral 301.7
  motor centers, senile 331.2
  mural (*see also* Degeneration,
      myocardial) 429.1
    heart, cardiac (*see also* Degeneration,
        myocardial) 429.1
    myocardium, myocardial (*see also*
        Degeneration, myocardial)
        429.1
  muscle 728.9
    fatty 728.9
    fibrous 728.9
    heart (*see also* Degeneration,
        myocardial) 429.1
    hyaline 728.9
  muscular progressive 728.2
  myelin, central nervous system NEC
      341.9
  myocardium, myocardial (brown)
      (calcareous) (fatty) (fibrous)
      (hyaline) (mural) (muscular)
      (pigmentary) (senile) (with
      arteriosclerosis) 429.1
    with rheumatic fever (conditions
        classifiable to 390) 398.0
      active, acute, or subacute 391.2
        with chorea 392.0
      inactive or quiescent (with
          chorea) 398.0
    amyloid 277.39 [*425.7*]
    congenital 746.89
    fetus or newborn 779.89
    gouty 274.82
    hypertensive (*see also* Hypertension,
        heart) 402.90
    ischemic 414.8
    rheumatic (*see also* Degeneration,
        myocardium, with rheumatic
        fever) 398.0
    syphilitic 093.82
  nasal sinus (mucosa) (*see also* Sinusitis)
      473.9
    frontal 473.1
    maxillary 473.0
  nerve - *see* Disorder, nerve
  nervous system 349.89
    amyloid 277.39 [*357.4*]
    autonomic (*see also* Neuropathy,
        peripheral, autonomic) 337.9
    fatty 349.89
    peripheral autonomic NEC (*see also*
        Neuropathy, peripheral,
        autonomic) 337.9
  nipple 611.9
  nose 478.19
  oculoacousticocerebral, congenital
      (progressive) 743.8
  olivopontocerebellar (familial)
      (hereditary) 333.0
  osseous labyrinth 386.8
  ovary 620.8
    cystic 620.2
    microcystic 620.2
  pallidal, pigmentary (progressive)
      333.0

Degeneration, degenerative *(Continued)*
pancreas 577.8
  tuberculous *(see also* Tuberculosis) 017.9●
papillary muscle 429.81
paving stone 362.61
penis 607.89
peritoneum 568.89
pigmentary (diffuse) (general)
  localized - *see* Degeneration, by site
  pallidal (progressive) 333.0
  secondary 362.65
pineal gland 259.8
pituitary (gland) 253.8
placenta (fatty) (fibrinoid) (fibroid) -
  see Placenta, abnormal
popliteal fat pad 729.31
posterolateral (spinal cord) *(see also* Degeneration, combined) 266.2 *[336.2]*
pulmonary valve (heart) *(see also* Endocarditis, pulmonary) 424.3
pulp (tooth) 522.2
pupillary margin 364.54
renal *(see also* Sclerosis, renal) 587
  fibrocystic 753.19
  polycystic 753.12
    adult type (APKD) 753.13
    autosomal dominant 753.13
    autosomal recessive 753.14
    childhood type (CPKD) 753.14
    infantile type 753.14
reticuloendothelial system 289.89
retina (peripheral) 362.60
  with retinal defect *(see also* Detachment, retina, with retinal defect) 361.00
  cystic (senile) 362.50
  cystoid 362.53
  hereditary *(see also* Dystrophy, retina) 362.70
    cerebroretinal 362.71
    congenital 362.75
    juvenile (Stargardt's) 362.75
    macula 362.76
  Kuhnt-Junius 362.52
  lattice 362.63
  macular *(see also* Degeneration, macula) 362.50
  microcystoid 362.62
  palisade 362.63
  paving stone 362.61
  pigmentary (primary) 362.74
    secondary 362.65
  posterior pole *(see also* Degeneration, macula) 362.50
  secondary 362.66
  senile 362.60
    cystic 362.53
    reticular 362.64
saccule, congenital (causing impairment of hearing) 744.05
sacculocochlear 386.8
senile 797
  brain 331.2
  cardiac, heart, or myocardium *(see also* Degeneration, myocardial) 429.1
  motor centers 331.2
  reticule 362.64
  retina, cystic 362.50
  vascular - *see* Arteriosclerosis
silicone rubber poppet (prosthetic valve) 996.02

Degeneration, degenerative *(Continued)*
sinus (cystic) *(see also* Sinusitis) 473.9
  polypoid 471.1
skin 709.3
  amyloid 277.39
  colloid 709.3
spinal (cord) 336.8
  amyloid 277.39
  column 733.90
  combined (subacute) *(see also* Degeneration, combined) 266.2 *[336.2]*
    with anemia (pernicious) 281.0 *[336.2]*
  dorsolateral *(see also* Degeneration, combined) 266.2 *[336.2]*
  familial NEC 336.8
  fatty 336.8
  funicular *(see also* Degeneration, combined) 266.2 *[336.2]*
  heredofamilial NEC 336.8
  posterolateral *(see also* Degeneration, combined) 266.2 *[336.2]*
  subacute combined - *see* Degeneration, combined
  tuberculous *(see also* Tuberculosis) 013.8
spine 733.90
spleen 289.59
  amyloid 277.39
  lardaceous 277.39
stomach 537.89
  lardaceous 277.39
strionigral 333.0
sudoriparous (cystic) 705.89
suprarenal (capsule) (gland) 255.8
  with hypofunction 255.41
sweat gland 705.89
synovial membrane (pulpy) 727.9
tapetoretinal 362.74
  adult or presenile form 362.50
testis (postinfectional) 608.89
thymus (gland) 254.8
  fatty 254.8
  lardaceous 277.39
thyroid (gland) 246.8
tricuspid (heart) (valve) - *see* Endocarditis, tricuspid
tuberculous NEC *(see also* Tuberculosis) 011.9●
turbinate 733.90
uterus 621.8
  cystic 621.8
vascular (senile) - *see also* Arteriosclerosis
  hypertensive - *see* Hypertension
vitreoretinal (primary) 362.73
  secondary 362.66
vitreous humor (with infiltration) 379.21
wallerian NEC - *see* Disorder, nerve
waxy (any site) 277.39
Wilson's hepatolenticular 275.1
Deglutition
paralysis 784.99
  hysterical 300.11
pneumonia 507.0
Degos' disease or syndrome 447.8
Degradation disorder, branched-chain amino-acid 270.3
Dehiscence
anastomosis - *see* Complications, anastomosis
cesarean wound 674.1●

Dehiscence *(Continued)*
closure of
  cornea 998.32
  fascia, superficial or muscular 998.31
  internal organ 998.31
  mucosa 998.32
  muscle or muscle flap 998.31
  ribs or rib cage 998.31
  skin 998.32
  skull or craniotomy 998.31
  sternum or sternotomy 998.31
  subcutaneous tissue 998.32
  tendon or ligament 998.31
  traumatic laceration (external) (internal) 998.33
episiotomy 674.2●
operation wound 998.32
  deep 998.31
  external 998.32
  internal 998.31
  superficial 998.32
perineal wound (postpartum) 674.2●
postoperative 998.32
  abdomen 998.32
    internal 998.31
  internal 998.31
traumatic injury wound repair 998.33
uterine wound 674.1●
Dehydration (cachexia) 276.51
with
  hypernatremia 276.0
  hyponatremia 276.1
newborn 775.5
Deiters' nucleus syndrome 386.19
Déjérine's disease 356.0
Déjérine-Klumpke paralysis 767.6
Déjérine-Roussy syndrome 338.0
Déjérine-Sottas disease or neuropathy (hypertrophic) 356.0
Déjérine-Thomas atrophy or syndrome 333.0
de Lange's syndrome (Amsterdam dwarf, mental retardation, and brachycephaly) 759.89
Delay, delayed
adaptation, cones or rods 368.63
any plane in pelvis
  affecting fetus or newborn 763.1
  complicating delivery 660.1●
birth or delivery NEC 662.1●
  affecting fetus or newborn 763.9
  second twin, triplet, or multiple mate 662.3●
closure - *see also* Fistula
  cranial suture 756.0
  fontanel 756.0
coagulation NEC 790.92
conduction (cardiac) (ventricular) 426.9
delivery NEC 662.1●
  second twin, triplet, etc. 662.3●
  affecting fetus or newborn 763.89
development
  in childhood 783.40
    physiological 783.40
  intellectual NEC 315.9
  learning NEC 315.2
  reading 315.00
  sexual 259.0
  speech 315.39
    and language due to hearing loss 315.34
    associated with hyperkinesis 314.1
  spelling 315.09

◀ New ◀ Revised deleted Deleted ● Use Additional Digit(s) Omit code

Delay, delayed *(Continued)*
gastric emptying 536.8
menarche 256.39
due to pituitary hypofunction 253.4
menstruation (cause unknown) 626.8
milestone in childhood 783.42
motility - *see* Hypomotility
passage of meconium (newborn) 777.1
primary respiration 768.9
puberty 259.0
separation of umbilical cord 779.83
sexual maturation, female 259.0
vaccination V64.00
Del Castillo's syndrome (germinal aplasia) 606.0
Deleage's disease 359.89
Deletion syndrome
5p 758.31
22q11.2 758.32
autosomal NEC 758.39
constitutional 5q deletion 758.39
Delhi (boil) (button) (sore) 085.1
Delinquency (juvenile) 312.9
group (*see also* Disturbance, conduct) 312.2●
neurotic 312.4
Delirium, delirious 780.09
acute (psychotic) 293.0
alcoholic 291.0
acute 291.0
chronic 291.1
alcoholicum 291.0
chronic (*see also* Psychosis) 293.89
due to or associated with physical condition - *see* Psychosis, organic
drug-induced 292.81
due to conditions classified elsewhere 293.0
eclamptic (*see also* Eclampsia) 780.39
exhaustion (*see also* Reaction, stress, acute) 308.9
hysterical 300.11
in
presenile dementia 290.11
senile dementia 290.3
induced by drug 292.81
manic, maniacal (acute) (*see also* Psychosis, affective) 296.0●
recurrent episode 296.1●
single episode 296.0●
puerperal 293.9
senile 290.3
subacute (psychotic) 293.1
thyroid (*see also* Thyrotoxicosis) 242.9●
traumatic - *see also* Injury, intracranial
with
lesion, spinal cord - *see* Injury, spinal, by site
shock, spinal - *see* Injury, spinal, by site
tremens (impending) 291.0
uremic - *see* Uremia
withdrawal
alcoholic (acute) 291.0
chronic 291.1
drug 292.0

Delivery

> **Note 19** Use the following fifth-digit subclassification with categories 640–649, 651–676:
>
> 0 unspecified as to episode of care
> 1 delivered, with or without mention of antepartum condition
> 2 delivered, with mention of postpartum complication
> 3 antepartum condition or complication
> 4 postpartum condition or complication

breech (assisted) (buttocks) (complete) (frank) (spontaneous) 652.2●
affecting fetus or newborn 763.0
extraction NEC 669.6●
cesarean (for) 669.7●
abnormal
cervix 654.6●
pelvic organs of tissues 654.9●
pelvis (bony) (major) NEC 653.0●
presentation or position 652.9●
in multiple gestation 652.6●
size, fetus 653.5●
soft parts (of pelvis) 654.9●
uterus, congenital 654.0●
vagina 654.7●
vulva 654.8●
abruptio placentae 641.2●
acromion presentation 652.8●
affecting fetus or newborn 763.4
anteversion, cervix or uterus 654.4●
atony, uterus 661.2●
with hemorrhage 666.1●
bicornis or bicornuate uterus 654.0●
breech presentation (buttocks) (complete) (frank) 652.2●
brow presentation 652.4●
cephalopelvic disproportion (normally formed fetus) 653.4●
chin presentation 652.4●
cicatrix of cervix 654.6●
contracted pelvis (general) 653.1●
inlet 653.2●
outlet 653.3●
cord presentation or prolapse 663.0●
cystocele 654.4●
deformity (acquired) (congenital)
pelvic organs or tissues NEC 654.9●
pelvis (bony) NEC 653.0●
displacement, uterus NEC 654.4●
disproportion NEC 653.9●
distress
fetal 656.8●
maternal 669.0●
eclampsia 642.6●
face presentation 652.4●
failed
forceps 660.7●
trial of labor NEC 660.6●
vacuum extraction 660.7●
ventouse 660.7●
fetal deformity 653.7●
fetal-maternal hemorrhage 656.0●
fetus, fetal
distress 656.8●
prematurity 656.8●
fibroid (tumor) (uterus) 654.1●

Delivery *(Continued)*
cesarean *(Continued)*
footling 652.8●
with successful version 652.1●
hemorrhage (antepartum) (intrapartum) NEC 641.9●
hydrocephalic fetus 653.6●
incarceration of uterus 654.3●
incoordinate uterine action 661.4●
inertia, uterus 661.2●
primary 661.0●
secondary 661.1●
lateroversion, uterus or cervix 654.4●
mal lie 652.9●
malposition
fetus 652.9●
in multiple gestation 652.6●
pelvic organs or tissues NEC 654.9●
uterus NEC or cervix 654.4●
malpresentation NEC 652.9●
in multiple gestation 652.6●
maternal
diabetes mellitus (conditions classifiable to 249 and 250) 648.0●
heart disease NEC 648.6●
meconium in liquor 656.8●
staining only 792.3
oblique presentation 652.3●
oversize fetus 653.5●
pelvic tumor NEC 654.9●
placental insufficiency 656.5●
placenta previa 641.0●
with hemorrhage 641.1●
poor dilation, cervix 661.0●
pre-eclampsia 642.4●
severe 642.5●
previous
cesarean delivery, section 654.2●
surgery (to)
cervix 654.6●
gynecological NEC 654.9●
rectum 654.8●
uterus NEC 654.9●
previous cesarean delivery, section 654.2●
vagina 654.7●
prolapse
arm or hand 652.7●
uterus 654.4●
prolonged labor 662.1●
rectocele 654.4●
retroversion, uterus or cervix 654.3●
rigid
cervix 654.6●
pelvic floor 654.4●
perineum 654.8●
vagina 654.7●
vulva 654.8●
sacculation, pregnant uterus 654.4●
scar(s)
cervix 654.6●
cesarean delivery, section 654.2●
uterus NEC 654.9●
due to previous cesarean delivery, section 654.2●
Shirodkar suture in situ 654.5●
shoulder presentation 652.8●
stenosis or stricture, cervix 654.6●
transverse presentation or lie 652.3●

Delivery *(Continued)*
  cesarean *(Continued)*
    tumor, pelvic organs or tissues NEC 654.4●
    umbilical cord presentation or prolapse 663.0●
  completely normal case - *see* category 650
  complicated (by) NEC 669.9●
    abdominal tumor, fetal 653.7●
      causing obstructed labor 660.1●
    abnormal, abnormality of
      cervix 654.6●
        causing obstructed labor 660.2●
      forces of labor 661.9●
      formation of uterus 654.0●
      pelvic organs or tissues 654.9●
        causing obstructed labor 660.2●
      pelvis (bony) (major) NEC 653.0●
        causing obstructed labor 660.1●
      presentation or position NEC 652.9●
        causing obstructed labor 660.0●
      size, fetus 653.5●
        causing obstructed labor 660.1●
      soft parts (of pelvis) 654.9●
        causing obstructed labor 660.2●
      uterine contractions NEC 661.9●
      uterus (formation) 654.0●
        causing obstructed labor 660.2●
      vagina 654.7●
        causing obstructed labor 660.2●
    abnormally formed uterus (any type) (congenital) 654.0●
      causing obstructed labor 660.2●
    acromion presentation 652.8●
      causing obstructed labor 660.0●
    adherent placenta 667.0●
      with hemorrhage 666.0●
    adhesions, uterus (to abdominal wall) 654.4●
    advanced maternal age NEC 659.6●
      multigravida 659.6●
      primigravida 659.5●
    air embolism 673.0●
    amnionitis 658.4●
    amniotic fluid embolism 673.1●
    anesthetic death 668.9●
    annular detachment, cervix 665.3●
    antepartum hemorrhage - *see* Delivery, complicated, hemorrhage
    anteversion, cervix or uterus 654.4●
      causing obstructed labor 660.2●
    apoplexy 674.0●
      placenta 641.2●
    arrested active phase 661.1●
    asymmetrical pelvis bone 653.0●
      causing obstructed labor 660.1●
    atony, uterus with hemorrhage (hypotonic) (inertia) 666.1●
      hypertonic 661.4●
    Bandl's ring 661.4●
    Battledore placenta - *see* Placenta, abnormal

Delivery *(Continued)*
  complicated (by) NEC *(Continued)*
    bicornis or bicornuate uterus 654.0●
      causing obstructed labor 660.2●
    birth injury to mother NEC 665.9●
    bleeding (*see also* Delivery, complicated, hemorrhage) 641.9●
    breech presentation (assisted) (buttocks) (complete) (frank) (spontaneous) 652.2●
      with successful version 652.1●
    brow presentation 652.4●
    cephalopelvic disproportion (normally formed fetus) 653.4●
      causing obstructed labor 660.1●
    cerebral hemorrhage 674.0●
    cervical dystocia 661.2●
    chin presentation 652.4●
      causing obstructed labor 660.0●
    cicatrix
      cervix 654.6●
        causing obstructed labor 660.2●
      vagina 654.7●
        causing obstructed labor 660.2●
    coagulation defect 649.3●
    colporrhexis 665.4●
      with perineal laceration 664.0●
    compound presentation 652.8●
      causing obstructed labor 660.0●
    compression of cord (umbilical) 663.2●
      around neck 663.1●
      cord prolapsed 663.0●
    contraction, contracted pelvis 653.1●
      causing obstructed labor 660.1●
      general 653.1●
        causing obstructed labor 660.1●
      inlet 653.2●
        causing obstructed labor 660.1●
      midpelvic 653.8●
        causing obstructed labor 660.1●
      midplane 653.8●
        causing obstructed labor 660.1●
      outlet 653.3●
        causing obstructed labor 660.1●
    contraction ring 661.4●
    cord (umbilical) 663.9●
      around neck, tightly or with compression 663.1●
        without compression 663.3●
      bruising 663.6●
      complication NEC 663.9●
        specified type NEC 663.8●
      compression NEC 663.2●
      entanglement NEC 663.3●
        with compression 663.2●
      forelying 663.0●
      hematoma 663.6●
      marginal attachment 663.8●
      presentation 663.0●
      prolapse (complete) (occult) (partial) 663.0●
      short 663.4●

Delivery *(Continued)*
  complicated (by) NEC *(Continued)*
    cord *(Continued)*
      specified complication NEC 663.8●
      thrombosis (vessels) 663.6●
      vascular lesion 663.6●
      velamentous insertion 663.8●
    Couvelaire uterus 641.2●
    cretin pelvis (dwarf type) (male type) 653.1●
      causing obstructed labor 660.1●
    crossbirth 652.3●
      with successful version 652.1●
      causing obstructed labor 660.0●
    cyst (Gartner's duct) 654.7●
    cystocele 654.4●
      causing obstructed labor 660.2●
    death of fetus (near term) 656.4●
      early (before 22 completed weeks' gestation) 632
    deformity (acquired) (congenital)
      fetus 653.7●
        causing obstructed labor 660.1●
      pelvic organs or tissues NEC 654.9●
        causing obstructed labor 660.2●
      pelvis (bony) NEC 653.0●
        causing obstructed labor 660.1●
    delay, delayed
      delivery in multiple pregnancy 662.3●
        due to locked mates 660.5●
      following rupture of membranes (spontaneous) 658.2●
        artificial 658.3●
    depressed fetal heart tones 659.7●
    diastasis recti 665.8●
    dilatation
      bladder 654.4●
        causing obstructed labor 660.2●
      cervix, incomplete, poor or slow 661.0●
    diseased placenta 656.7●
    displacement uterus NEC 654.4●
      causing obstructed labor 660.2●
    disproportion NEC 653.9●
      causing obstructed labor 660.1●
    disruptio uteri - *see* Delivery, complicated, rupture, uterus
    distress
      fetal 656.8●
      maternal 669.0●
    double uterus (congenital) 654.0●
      causing obstructed labor 660.2●
    dropsy amnion 657●
    dysfunction, uterus 661.9●
      hypertonic 661.4●
      hypotonic 661.2●
        primary 661.0●
        secondary 661.1●
      incoordinate 661.4●
    dystocia
      cervical 661.2●
      fetal - *see* Delivery, complicated, abnormal, presentation
      maternal - *see* Delivery, complicated, prolonged labor

◀ New   ◀▥ Revised   ~~deleted~~ Deleted   ● Use Additional Digit(s)   ▨ Omit code

Delivery *(Continued)*
  complicated (by) NEC *(Continued)*
    dystocia *(Continued)*
      pelvic - *see* Delivery, complicated,
        contraction pelvis
      positional 652.8●
      shoulder girdle 660.4●
    eclampsia 642.6●
    ectopic kidney 654.4●
      causing obstructed labor 660.2●
    edema, cervix 654.6●
      causing obstructed labor 660.2●
    effusion, amniotic fluid 658.1●
    elderly multigravida 659.6●
    elderly primigravida 659.5●
    embolism (pulmonary) 673.2●
      air 673.0●
      amniotic fluid 673.1●
      blood-clot 673.2●
      cerebral 674.0●
      fat 673.8●
      pyemic 673.3●
      septic 673.3●
    entanglement, umbilical cord 663.3●
      with compression 663.2●
      around neck (with compression)
        663.1●
    eversion, cervix or uterus 665.2●
    excessive
      fetal growth 653.5●
        causing obstructed labor
          660.1●
      size of fetus 653.5●
        causing obstructed labor
          660.1●
    face presentation 652.4●
      causing obstructed labor 660.0●
      to pubes 660.3●
    failure, fetal head to enter pelvic
      brim 652.5●
      causing obstructed labor 660.0●
    female genital mutilation 660.8●
    fetal
      acid-base balance 656.8●
      death (near term) NEC 656.4●
        early (before 22 completed
          weeks' gestation) 632
      deformity 653.7●
        causing obstructed labor
          660.1●
      distress 656.8●
      heart rate or rhythm 659.7●
      reduction of multiple fetuses
        reduced to single fetus
        651.7●
    fetopelvic disproportion 653.4●
      causing obstructed labor 660.1●
    fever during labor 659.2●
    fibroid (tumor) (uterus) 654.1●
      causing obstructed labor 660.2●
    fibromyomata 654.1●
      causing obstructed labor 660.2●
    forelying umbilical cord 663.0●
    fracture of coccyx 665.6●
    hematoma 664.5●
      broad ligament 665.7●
      ischial spine 665.7●
      pelvic 665.7●
      perineum 664.5●
      soft tissues 665.7●
      subdural 674.0●
      umbilical cord 663.6●
      vagina 665.7●
      vulva or perineum 664.5●

Delivery *(Continued)*
  complicated (by) NEC *(Continued)*
    hemorrhage (uterine) (antepartum)
      (intrapartum) (pregnancy)
      641.9●
      accidental 641.2●
      associated with
        afibrinogenemia 641.3●
        coagulation defect 641.3●
          hyperfibrinolysis 641.3●
          hypofibrinogenemia
            641.3●
      cerebral 674.0●
      due to
        low-lying placenta 641.1●
        placenta previa 641.1●
        premature separation of
          placenta (normally
          implanted) 641.2●
        retained placenta 666.0●
        trauma 641.8●
        uterine leiomyoma 641.8●
      marginal sinus rupture 641.2●
      placenta NEC 641.9●
      postpartum (atonic) (immediate)
        (within 24 hours) 666.1●
      with retained or trapped
        placenta 666.0●
      delayed 666.2●
      secondary 666.2●
      third stage 666.0●
    hourglass contraction, uterus 661.4●
    hydramnios 657
    hydrocephalic fetus 653.6●
      causing obstructed labor 660.1●
    hydrops fetalis 653.7●
      causing obstructed labor 660.1●
    hypertension - *see* Hypertension,
      complicating pregnancy
    hypertonic uterine dysfunction
      661.4●
    hypotonic uterine dysfunction
      661.2●
    impacted shoulders 660.4●
    incarceration, uterus 654.3●
      causing obstructed labor 660.2●
    incomplete dilation (cervix) 661.0●
    incoordinate uterus 661.4●
    indication NEC 659.9●
      specified type NEC 659.8●
    inertia, uterus 661.2●
      hypertonic 661.4●
      hypotonic 661.2●
      primary 661.0●
      secondary 661.1●
    infantile
      genitalia 654.4●
        causing obstructed labor
          660.2●
      uterus (os) 654.4●
        causing obstructed labor
          660.2●
    injury (to mother) NEC 665.9●
    intrauterine fetal death (near term)
      NEC 656.4●
      early (before 22 completed weeks'
        gestation) 632
    inversion, uterus 665.2●
    kidney, ectopic 654.4●
      causing obstructed labor 660.2●
    knot (true), umbilical cord 663.2●
    labor, premature (before 37
      completed weeks' gestation)
      644.2●

Delivery *(Continued)*
  complicated (by) NEC *(Continued)*
    laceration 664.9●
      anus (sphincter) (healed) (old)
        654.8●
        with mucosa 664.3●
        not associated with third-
          degree perineal
          laceration 664.6●
      bladder (urinary) 665.5●
      bowel 665.5●
      central 664.4●
      cervix (uteri) 665.3●
      fourchette 664.0●
      hymen 664.0●
      labia (majora) (minora) 664.0●
      pelvic
        floor 664.1●
        organ NEC 665.5●
      perineum, perineal 664.4●
        first degree 664.0●
        second degree 664.1●
        third degree 664.2●
        fourth degree 664.3●
        central 664.4●
        extensive NEC 664.4●
        muscles 664.1●
        skin 664.0●
        slight 664.0●
      peritoneum 665.5●
      periurethral tissue 664.8●
      rectovaginal (septum) (without
        perineal laceration) 665.4●
        with perineum 664.2●
          with anal or rectal mucosa
            664.3●
      skin (perineum) 664.0●
      specified site or type NEC 664.8●
      sphincter ani (healed) (old)
        654.8●
        with mucosa 664.3●
        not associated with third-
          degree perineal
          laceration 664.6●
      urethra 665.5●
      uterus 665.1●
        before labor 665.0●
      vagina, vaginal (deep) (high)
        (sulcus) (wall) (without
        perineal laceration)
        665.4●
        with perineum 664.0●
        muscles, with perineum
          664.1●
      vulva 664.0●
    lateroversion, uterus or cervix
      654.4●
      causing obstructed labor
        660.2●
    locked mates 660.5●
    low implantation of placenta - *see*
      Delivery, complicated,
      placenta, previa
    mal lie 652.9●
    malposition
      fetus NEC 652.9●
        causing obstructed labor
          660.0●
      pelvic organs or tissues NEC
        654.9●
        causing obstructed labor
          660.2●
      placenta 641.1●
        without hemorrhage 641.0●

Delivery *(Continued)*
  complicated (by) NEC *(Continued)*
    malposition *(Continued)*
      uterus NEC or cervix 654.4●
        causing obstructed labor
          660.2●
    malpresentation 652.9●
      causing obstructed labor 660.0●
    marginal sinus (bleeding) (rupture)
      641.2●
    maternal hypotension syndrome
      669.2●
    meconium in liquor 656.8●
    membranes, retained - *see* Delivery,
      complicated, placenta,
      retained
    mentum presentation 652.4●
      causing obstructed labor 660.0●
    metrorrhagia (myopathia) - *see*
      Delivery, complicated,
      hemorrhage
    metrorrhexis - *see* Delivery,
      complicated, rupture, uterus
    multiparity (grand) 659.4●
    myelomeningocele, fetus 653.7●
      causing obstructed labor 660.1●
    Nägele's pelvis 653.0●
      causing obstructed labor 660.1●
    nonengagement, fetal head 652.5●
      causing obstructed labor 660.0●
    oblique presentation 652.3●
      causing obstructed labor
        660.0●
    obstetric
      shock 669.1●
      trauma NEC 665.9●
    obstructed labor 660.9●
      due to
        abnormality of pelvic organs
          or tissues (conditions
          classifiable to 654.0–
          654.9) 660.2●
        deep transverse arrest 660.3●
        impacted shoulders 660.4●
        locked twins 660.5●
        malposition and
          malpresentation of fetus
          (conditions classifiable to
          652.0–652.9) 660.0●
        persistent occipitoposterior
          660.3●
        shoulder dystocia 660.4●
    occult prolapse of umbilical cord
      663.0●
    oversize fetus 653.5●
      causing obstructed labor 660.1●
    pathological retraction ring, uterus
      661.4●
    pelvic
      arrest (deep) (high) (of fetal head)
        (transverse) 660.3●
      deformity (bone) - *see also*
        Deformity, pelvis, with
        disproportion
        soft tissue 654.9●
          causing obstructed labor
            660.2●
      tumor NEC 654.9●
        causing obstructed labor
          660.2●
    penetration, pregnant uterus by
      instrument 665.1●
    perforation - *see* Delivery,
      complicated, laceration

Delivery *(Continued)*
  complicated (by) NEC *(Continued)*
    persistent
      hymen 654.8●
        causing obstructed labor
          660.2●
      occipitoposterior 660.3●
    placenta, placental
      ablatio 641.2●
      abnormality 656.7●
        with hemorrhage 641.2●
      abruptio 641.2●
      accreta 667.0●
        with hemorrhage 666.0●
      adherent (without hemorrhage)
        667.0●
        with hemorrhage 666.0●
      apoplexy 641.2●
      Battledore - *see* Placenta,
        abnormal
      detachment (premature)
        641.2●
      disease 656.7●
      hemorrhage NEC 641.9●
      increta (without hemorrhage)
        667.0●
        with hemorrhage 666.0●
      low (implantation) 641.1●
        without hemorrhage 641.0●
      malformation 656.7●
        with hemorrhage 641.2●
      malposition 641.1●
        without hemorrhage 641.0●
      marginal sinus rupture 641.2●
      percreta 667.0●
        with hemorrhage 666.0●
      premature separation 641.2●
      previa (central) (lateral)
        (marginal) (partial) 641.1●
        without hemorrhage 641.0●
      retained (with hemorrhage)
        666.0●
        without hemorrhage 667.0●
      rupture of marginal sinus 641.2●
      separation (premature) 641.2●
      trapped 666.0●
        without hemorrhage 667.0●
      vicious insertion 641.1●
    polyhydramnios 657●
    polyp, cervix 654.6●
      causing obstructed labor 660.2●
    precipitate labor 661.3●
    premature
      labor (before 37 completed
        weeks' gestation) 644.2●
      rupture, membranes 658.1●
        delayed delivery following
          658.2●
    presenting umbilical cord 663.0●
    previous
      cesarean delivery, section 654.2●
      surgery
        cervix 654.6●
          causing obstructed labor
            660.2●
        gynecological NEC 654.9●
          causing obstructed labor
            660.2●
        perineum 654.8●
        rectum 654.8●
        uterus NEC 654.9●
          due to previous cesarean
            delivery, section
            654.2●

Delivery *(Continued)*
  complicated (by) NEC *(Continued)*
    previous *(Continued)*
      surgery *(Continued)*
        vagina 654.7●
          causing obstructed labor
            660.2●
        vulva 654.8●
    primary uterine inertia 661.0●
    primipara, elderly or old 659.5●
    prolapse
      arm or hand 652.7●
        causing obstructed labor
          660.0●
      cord (umbilical) 663.0●
      fetal extremity 652.8●
      foot or leg 652.8●
        causing obstructed labor
          660.0●
      umbilical cord (complete) (occult)
        (partial) 663.0●
      uterus 654.4●
        causing obstructed labor
          660.2●
    prolonged labor 662.1●
      first stage 662.0●
      second stage 662.2●
      active phase 661.2●
      due to
        cervical dystocia 661.2●
        contraction ring 661.4●
        tetanic uterus 661.4●
        uterine inertia 661.2●
          primary 661.0●
          secondary 661.1●
      latent phase 661.0●
    pyrexia during labor 659.2●
    rachitic pelvis 653.2●
      causing obstructed labor 660.1●
    rectocele 654.4●
      causing obstructed labor 660.2●
    retained membranes or portions of
      placenta 666.2●
      without hemorrhage 667.1●
    retarded (prolonged) birth 662.1●
    retention secundines (with
      hemorrhage) 666.2●
      without hemorrhage 667.1●
    retroversion, uterus or cervix
      654.3●
      causing obstructed labor 660.2●
    rigid
      cervix 654.6●
        causing obstructed labor
          660.2●
      pelvic floor 654.4●
        causing obstructed labor
          660.2●
      perineum or vulva 654.8●
        causing obstructed labor
          660.2●
      vagina 654.7●
        causing obstructed labor
          660.2●
    Robert's pelvis 653.0●
      causing obstructed labor
        660.1●
    rupture - *see also* Delivery,
      complicated, laceration
      bladder (urinary) 665.5●
      cervix 665.3●
      marginal sinus 641.2●
      membranes, premature 658.1●
      pelvic organ NEC 665.5●

◀ New   ◀|||| Revised   ~~deleted~~ Deleted   ● Use Additional Digit(s)   ▨ Omit code

Delivery *(Continued)*
  complicated (by) NEC *(Continued)*
    rupture *(Continued)*
      perineum (without mention of
        other laceration) - *see*
        Delivery, complicated,
        laceration, perineum
      peritoneum 665.5●
      urethra 665.5●
      uterus (during labor) 665.1●
        before labor 665.0●
    sacculation, pregnant uterus 654.4●
    sacral teratomas, fetal 653.7●
      causing obstructed labor 660.1●
    scar(s)
      cervix 654.6●
        causing obstructed labor
          660.2●
      cesarean delivery, section 654.2●
        causing obstructed labor
          660.2●
      perineum 654.8●
        causing obstructed labor
          660.2●
      uterus NEC 654.9●
        causing obstructed labor
          660.2●
        due to previous cesarean
          delivery, section 654.2●
      vagina 654.7●
        causing obstructed labor
          660.2●
      vulva 654.8●
        causing obstructed labor
          660.2●
    scoliotic pelvis 653.0●
      causing obstructed labor 660.1●
    secondary uterine inertia 661.1●
    secundines, retained - *see* Delivery,
      complicated, placenta,
      retained
    separation
      placenta (premature) 641.2●
      pubic bone 665.6●
      symphysis pubis 665.6●
    septate vagina 654.7●
      causing obstructed labor 660.2●
    shock (birth) (obstetric) (puerperal)
      669.1●
    short cord syndrome 663.4●
    shoulder
      girdle dystocia 660.4●
      presentation 652.8●
        causing obstructed labor
          660.0●
    Siamese twins 678.1●
      ~~causing obstructed labor 660.1●~~
    slow slope active phase 661.2●
    spasm
      cervix 661.4●
      uterus 661.4●
    spondylolisthesis, pelvis 653.3●
      causing obstructed labor 660.1●
    spondylolysis (lumbosacral) 653.3●
      causing obstructed labor 660.1●
    spondylosis 653.0●
      causing obstructed labor 660.1●
    stenosis or stricture
      cervix 654.6●
        causing obstructed labor
          660.2●
      vagina 654.7●
        causing obstructed labor
          660.2●

Delivery *(Continued)*
  complicated (by) NEC *(Continued)*
    sudden death, unknown cause
      669.9●
    tear (pelvic organ) *(see also* Delivery,
      complicated, laceration)
      664.9●
      anal sphincter (healed) (old)
        654.8●
        not associated with third-
          degree perineal
          laceration 664.6●
    teratomas, sacral, fetal 653.7●
      causing obstructed labor 660.1●
    tetanic uterus 661.4●
    tipping pelvis 653.0●
      causing obstructed labor 660.1●
    transverse
      arrest (deep) 660.3●
      presentation or lie 652.3●
        with successful version
          652.1●
        causing obstructed labor
          660.0●
    trauma (obstetrical) NEC 665.9●
    tumor
      abdominal, fetal 653.7●
        causing obstructed labor
          660.1●
      pelvic organs or tissues NEC
        654.9●
        causing obstructed labor
          660.2●
    umbilical cord *(see also* Delivery,
      complicated, cord) 663.9●
      around neck tightly, or with
        compression 663.1●
      entanglement NEC 663.3●
        with compression 663.2●
      prolapse (complete) (occult)
        (partial) 663.0●
    unstable lie 652.0●
      causing obstructed labor
        660.0●
    uterine
      inertia *(see also* Delivery,
        complicated, inertia,
        uterus) 661.2●
      spasm 661.4●
    vasa previa 663.5●
    velamentous insertion of cord
      663.8●
    young maternal age 659.8●
  delayed NEC 662.1●
    following rupture of membranes
      (spontaneous) 658.2●
      artificial 658.3●
    second twin, triplet, etc. 662.3●
  difficult NEC 669.9●
    previous, affecting management of
      pregnancy or childbirth
      V23.49
    specified type NEC 669.8●
  early onset (spontaneous) 644.2●
  footling 652.8●
    with successful version 652.1●
  forceps NEC 669.5●
    affecting fetus or newborn 763.2
  missed (at or near term) 656.4●
  multiple gestation NEC 651.9●
    with fetal loss and retention of one
      or more fetus(es) 651.6●
    following (elective) fetal reduction
      651.7●

Delivery *(Continued)*
  multiple gestation NEC *(Continued)*
    specified type NEC 651.8●
      with fetal loss and retention of
        one or more fetus(es)
        651.6●
      following (elective) fetal
        reduction 651.7●
  nonviable infant 656.4●
  normal - *see* category 650
  precipitate 661.3●
    affecting fetus or newborn 763.6
  premature NEC (before 37 completed
    weeks' gestation) 644.2●
  previous, affecting management of
    pregnancy V23.41
  quadruplet NEC 651.2●
    with fetal loss and retention of one
      or more fetus(es) 651.5●
    following (elective) fetal reduction
      651.7●
  quintuplet NEC 651.8●
    with fetal loss and retention of one
      or more fetus(es) 651.6●
    following (elective) fetal reduction
      651.7●
  sextuplet NEC 651.8●
    with fetal loss and retention of one
      or more fetus(es) 651.6●
    following (elective) fetal reduction
      651.7●
  specified complication NEC
    669.8●
  stillbirth (near term) NEC 656.4●
    early (before 22 completed weeks'
      gestation) 632
  term pregnancy (live birth) NEC - *see*
    category 650
    stillbirth NEC 656.4●
  threatened premature 644.2●
  triplets NEC 651.1●
    with fetal loss and retention of one
      or more fetus(es) 651.4●
    delayed delivery (one or more
      mates) 662.3●
    following (elective) fetal reduction
      651.7●
    locked mates 660.5●
  twins NEC 651.0●
    with fetal loss and retention of one
      fetus 651.3●
    delayed delivery (one or more
      mates) 662.3●
    following (elective) fetal reduction
      651.7●
    locked mates 660.5●
  uncomplicated - *see* category 650
  vacuum extractor NEC 669.5●
    affecting fetus or newborn
      763.3
  ventouse NEC 669.5●
    affecting fetus or newborn
      763.3
Dellen, cornea 371.41
Delusions (paranoid) 297.9
  grandiose 297.1
  parasitosis 300.29
  systematized 297.1
Dementia 294.8
  alcohol-induced persisting *(see
    also* Psychosis, alcoholic)
    291.2
  Alzheimer's - *see* Alzheimer's,
    dementia

◀ New   ◀▥ Revised   ~~deleted~~ Deleted   ● Use Additional Digit(s)   ▨ Omit code   **233**

Dementia *(Continued)*
  arteriosclerotic (simple type)
      (uncomplicated) 290.40
    with
      acute confusional state 290.41
      delirium 290.41
      delusions 290.42
      depressed mood 290.43
    depressed type 290.43
    paranoid type 290.42
  Binswanger's 290.12
  catatonic (acute) *(see also*
      Schizophrenia) 295.2●
  congenital *(see also* Retardation, mental)
      319
  degenerative 290.9
    presenile-onset - *see* Dementia,
        presenile
    senile-onset - *see* Dementia, senile
  developmental *(see also* Schizophrenia)
      295.9●
  dialysis 294.8
    transient 293.9
  drug-induced persisting *(see also*
      Psychosis, drug) 292.82
  due to or associated with condition(s)
      classified elsewhere
    Alzheimer's
      with behavioral disturbance 331.0
          [294.11]
      without behavioral disturbance
          331.0 [294.10]
    cerebral lipidoses
      with behavioral disturbance 330.1
          [294.11]
      without behavioral disturbance
          330.1 [294.10]
    epilepsy
      with behavioral disturbance
          345.9● [294.11]
      without behavioral disturbance
          345.9● [294.10]
    hepatolenticular degeneration
      with behavioral disturbance 275.1
          [294.11]
      without behavioral disturbance
          275.1 [294.10]
    HIV
      with behavioral disturbance 042
          [294.11]
      without behavioral disturbance
          042 [294.10]
    Huntington's chorea
      with behavioral disturbance 333.4
          [294.11]
      without behavioral disturbance
          333.4 [294.10]
    Jakob-Creutzfeldt disease (CJD)
      with behavioral disturbance
          046.19 [294.11]
      without behavioral disturbance
          046.19 [294.10]
      variant (vCJD) 046.11
        with dementia
          with behavioral disturbance
              046.11 [294.11]
          without behavioral
              disturbance 046.11
              [294.10]
    Lewy bodies
      with behavioral disturbance
          331.82 [294.11]
      without behavioral disturbance
          331.82 [294.10]

Dementia *(Continued)*
  due to or associated with condition(s)
      classified elsewhere *(Continued)*
    multiple sclerosis
      with behavioral disturbance 340
          [294.11]
      without behavioral disturbance
          340 [294.10]
    neurosyphilis
      with behavioral disturbance 094.9
          [294.11]
      without behavioral disturbance
          094.9 [294.10]
    Parkinsonism
      with behavioral disturbance
          331.82 [294.11]
      without behavioral disturbance
          331.82 [294.10]
    Pelizaeus-Merzbacher disease
      with behavioral disturbance 333.0
          [294.11]
      without behavioral disturbance
          333.0 [294.10]
    Pick's disease
      with behavioral disturbance
          331.11 [294.11]
      without behavioral disturbance
          331.11 [294.10]
    polyarteritis nodosa
      with behavioral disturbance 446.0
          [294.11]
      without behavioral disturbance
          446.0 [294.10]
    syphilis
      with behavioral disturbance 094.1
          [294.11]
      without behavioral disturbance
          094.1 [294.10]
    Wilson's disease
      with behavioral disturbance 275.1
          [294.11]
      without behavioral disturbance
          275.1 [294.10]
  frontal 331.19
    with behavioral disturbance 331.19
        [294.11]
    without behavioral disturbance
        331.19 [294.10]
  frontotemporal 331.19
    with behavioral disturbance 331.19
        [294.11]
    without behavioral disturbance
        331.19 [294.10]
  hebephrenic (acute) 295.1●
  Heller's (infantile psychosis) *(see also*
      Psychosis, childhood) 299.1●
  idiopathic 290.9
    presenile-onset - *see* Dementia,
        presenile
    senile-onset - *see* Dementia, senile
  in
    arteriosclerotic brain disease 290.40
    senility 290.0
  induced by drug 292.82
  infantile, infantilia *(see also* Psychosis,
      childhood) 299.0●
  Lewy body 331.82
    with behavioral disturbance 331.82
        [294.11]
    without behavioral disturbance
        331.82 [294.10]
  multi-infarct (cerebrovascular) *(see also*
      Dementia, arteriosclerotic) 290.40
  old age 290.0

Dementia *(Continued)*
  paralytica, paralytic 094.1
    juvenilis 090.40
      syphilitic 094.1
        congenital 090.40
    tabetic form 094.1
  paranoid *(see also* Schizophrenia)
      295.3●
  paraphrenic *(see also* Schizophrenia)
      295.3●
  paretic 094.1
  praecox *(see also* Schizophrenia) 295.9●
  presenile 290.10
    with
      acute confusional state 290.11
      delirium 290.11
      delusional features 290.12
      depressive features 290.13
    depressed type 290.13
    paranoid type 290.12
    simple type 290.10
    uncomplicated 290.10
  primary (acute) *(see also* Schizophrenia)
      295.0●
  progressive, syphilitic 094.1
  puerperal - *see* Psychosis, puerperal
  schizophrenic *(see also* Schizophrenia)
      295.9●
  senile 290.0
    with
      acute confusional state 290.3
      delirium 290.3
      delusional features 290.20
      depressive features 290.21
    depressed type 290.21
    exhaustion 290.0
    paranoid type 290.20
  simple type (acute) *(see also*
      Schizophrenia) 295.0●
  simplex (acute) *(see also* Schizophrenia)
      295.0●
  syphilitic 094.1
  uremic - *see* Uremia
  vascular 290.40
    with
      delirium 290.41
      delusions 290.42
      depressed mood 290.43
Demerol dependence *(see also*
    Dependence) 304.0●
Demineralization, ankle *(see also*
    Osteoporosis) 733.00
Demodex folliculorum (infestation) 133.8
Demoralization 799.25 ◀
de Morgan's spots (senile angiomas) 448.1
Demyelinating
  polyneuritis, chronic inflammatory
      357.81
Demyelination, demyelinization
  central nervous system 341.9
    specified NEC 341.8
  corpus callosum (central) 341.8
  global 340
Dengue (fever) 061
  sandfly 061
  vaccination, prophylactic (against)
      V05.1
  virus hemorrhagic fever 065.4
Dens
  evaginatus 520.2
  in dente 520.2
  invaginatus 520.2
Dense
  breast(s) - *omit code*

◀ New   ◀▥ Revised   ~~deleted~~ Deleted   ● Use Additional Digit(s)   ▨ Omit code

Density
 increased, bone (disseminated)
  (generalized) (spotted) 733.99
 lung (nodular) 518.89
Dental - *see also* condition
 examination only V72.2
Dentia praecox 520.6
Denticles (in pulp) 522.2
Dentigerous cyst 526.0
Dentin
 irregular (in pulp) 522.3
 opalescent 520.5
 secondary (in pulp) 522.3
 sensitive 521.89
Dentinogenesis imperfecta 520.5
Dentinoma (M9271/0) 213.1
 upper jaw (bone) 213.0
Dentition 520.7
 abnormal 520.6
 anomaly 520.6
 delayed 520.6
 difficult 520.7
 disorder of 520.6
 precocious 520.6
 retarded 520.6
Denture sore (mouth) 528.9
Dependence

┌─────────────────────────────────────┐
│ Note 20 Use the following fifth-digit │
│ subclassification with category 304: │
│   │
│ 0 unspecified   │
│ 1 continuous   │
│ 2 episodic   │
│ 3 in remission   │
└─────────────────────────────────────┘

with
 withdrawal symptoms
  alcohol 291.81
  drug 292.0
 14-hydroxy-dihydromorphinone
  304.0 ●
 absinthe 304.6 ●
 acemorphan 304.0 ●
 acetanilid(e) 304.6 ●
 acetophenetidin 304.6 ●
 acetorphine 304.0 ●
 acetyldihydrocodeine 304.0 ●
 acetyldihydrocodeinone 304.0 ●
 Adalin 304.1 ●
 Afghanistan black 304.3 ●
 agrypnal 304.1 ●
 alcohol, alcoholic (ethyl) (methyl)
  (wood) 303.9 ●
  maternal, with suspected fetal
   damage affecting management
   of pregnancy 655.4 ●
 allobarbitone 304.1 ●
 allonal 304.1 ●
 allylisopropylacetylurea 304.1 ●
 alphaprodine (hydrochloride) 304.0 ●
 Alurate 304.1 ●
 Alvodine 304.0 ●
 amethocaine 304.6 ●
 amidone 304.0 ●
 amidopyrine 304.6 ●
 aminopyrine 304.6 ●
 amobarbital 304.1 ●
 amphetamine(s) (type) (drugs
  classifiable to 969.7) 304.4 ●
 amylene hydrate 304.6 ●
 amylobarbitone 304.1 ●
 amylocaine 304.6 ●
 Amytal (sodium) 304.1 ●

Dependence *(Continued)*
 analgesic (drug) NEC 304.6 ●
  synthetic with morphine-like effect
   304.0 ●
 anesthetic (agent) (drug) (gas) (general)
  (local) NEC 304.6 ●
 Angel dust 304.6 ●
 anileridine 304.0 ●
 antipyrine 304.6 ●
 anxiolytic 304.1 ●
 aprobarbital 304.1 ●
 aprobarbitone 304.1 ●
 atropine 304.6 ●
 Avertin (bromide) 304.6 ●
 barbenyl 304.1 ●
 barbital(s) 304.1 ●
 barbitone 304.1 ●
 barbiturate(s) (compounds) (drugs
  classifiable to 967.0) 304.1 ●
 barbituric acid (and compounds)
  304.1 ●
 benzedrine 304.4 ●
 benzylmorphine 304.0 ●
 Beta-chlor 304.1 ●
 bhang 304.3 ●
 blue velvet 304.0 ●
 Brevital 304.1 ●
 bromal (hydrate) 304.1 ●
 bromide(s) NEC 304.1 ●
 bromine compounds NEC 304.1 ●
 bromisovalum 304.1 ●
 bromoform 304.1 ●
 Bromo-seltzer 304.1 ●
 bromural 304.1 ●
 butabarbital (sodium) 304.1 ●
 butabarpal 304.1 ●
 butallylonal 304.1 ●
 butethal 304.1 ●
 buthalitone (sodium) 304.1 ●
 Butisol 304.1 ●
 butobarbitone 304.1 ●
 butyl chloral (hydrate) 304.1 ●
 caffeine 304.4 ●
 cannabis (indica) (sativa) (resin)
  (derivatives) (type) 304.3 ●
 carbamazepine 304.6 ●
 Carbrital 304.1 ●
 carbromal 304.1 ●
 carisoprodol 304.6 ●
 Catha (edulis) 304.4 ●
 chloral (betaine) (hydrate) 304.1 ●
 chloralamide 304.1 ●
 chloralformamide 304.1 ●
 chloralose 304.1 ●
 chlordiazepoxide 304.1 ●
 Chloretone 304.1 ●
 chlorobutanol 304.1 ●
 chlorodyne 304.1 ●
 chloroform 304.6 ●
 Cliradon 304.0 ●
 coca (leaf) and derivatives 304.2 ●
 cocaine 304.2 ●
  hydrochloride 304.2 ●
  salt (any) 304.2 ●
 codeine 304.0 ●
 combination of drugs (excluding
  morphine or opioid type drug)
  NEC 304.8 ●
  morphine or opioid type drug with
   any other drug 304.7 ●
 croton-chloral 304.1 ●
 cyclobarbital 304.1 ●
 cyclobarbitone 304.1 ●
 dagga 304.3 ●

Dependence *(Continued)*
 Delvinal 304.1 ●
 Demerol 304.0 ●
 desocodeine 304.0 ●
 desomorphine 304.0 ●
 desoxyephedrine 304.4 ●
 DET 304.5 ●
 dexamphetamine 304.4 ●
 dexedrine 304.4 ●
 dextromethorphan 304.0 ●
 dextromoramide 304.0 ●
 dextronorpseudoephedrine 304.4 ●
 dextrorphan 304.0 ●
 diacetylmorphine 304.0 ●
 Dial 304.1 ●
 diallylbarbituric acid 304.1 ●
 diamorphine 304.0 ●
 diazepam 304.1 ●
 dibucaine 304.6 ●
 dichloroethane 304.6 ●
 diethyl barbituric acid 304.1 ●
 diethylsulfone-diethylmethane 304.1 ●
 difencloxazine 304.0 ●
 dihydrocodeine 304.0 ●
 dihydrocodeinone 304.0 ●
 dihydrohydroxycodeinone 304.0 ●
 dihydroisocodeine 304.0 ●
 dihydromorphine 304.0 ●
 dihydromorphinone 304.0 ●
 dihydroxcodeinone 304.0 ●
 Dilaudid 304.0 ●
 dimenhydrinate 304.6 ●
 dimethylmeperidine 304.0 ●
 dimethyltriptamine 304.5 ●
 Dionin 304.0 ●
 diphenoxylate 304.6 ●
 dipipanone 304.0 ●
 d-lysergic acid diethylamide 304.5 ●
 DMT 304.5 ●
 Dolophine 304.0 ●
 DOM 304.2 ●
 doriden 304.1 ●
 dormiral 304.1 ●
 Dormison 304.1 ●
 Dromoran 304.0 ●
 drug NEC 304.9 ●
  analgesic NEC 304.6 ●
  combination (excluding morphine
   or opioid type drug) NEC
   304.8 ●
  morphine or opioid type drug
   with any other drug 304.7 ●
  complicating pregnancy, childbirth,
   or puerperium 648.3 ●
   affecting fetus or newborn 779.5
  hallucinogenic 304.5 ●
  hypnotic NEC 304.1 ●
  narcotic NEC 304.9
  psychostimulant NEC 304.4 ●
  sedative 304.1 ●
  soporific NEC 304.1 ●
  specified type NEC 304.6 ●
  suspected damage to fetus affecting
   management of pregnancy
   655.5 ●
  synthetic, with morphine-like effect
   304.0 ●
  tranquilizing 304.1 ●
 duboisine 304.6 ●
 ectylurea 304.1 ●
 Endocaine 304.6 ●
 Equanil 304.1 ●
 Eskabarb 304.1 ●
 ethchlorvynol 304.1 ●

Dependence *(Continued)*

ether (ethyl) (liquid) (vapor) (vinyl) 304.6●
ethidene 304.6●
ethinamate 304.1●
ethoheptazine 304.6●
ethyl
    alcohol 303.9●
    bromide 304.6●
    carbamate 304.6●
    chloride 304.6●
    morphine 304.0●
ethylene (gas) 304.6●
    dichloride 304.6●
ethylidene chloride 304.6●
etilfen 304.1●
etorphine 304.0●
etoval 304.1●
eucodal 304.0●
euneryl 304.1●
Evipal 304.1●
Evipan 304.1●
fentanyl 304.0●
ganja 304.3●
gardenal 304.1●
gardenpanyl 304.1●
gelsemine 304.6●
Gelsemium 304.6●
Gemonil 304.1●
glucochloral 304.1●
glue (airplane) (sniffing) 304.6●
glutethimide 304.1●
hallucinogenics 304.5●
hashish 304.3●
headache powder NEC 304.6●
Heavenly Blue 304.5●
hedonal 304.1●
hemp 304.3●
heptabarbital 304.1●
Heptalgin 304.0●
heptobarbitone 304.1●
heroin 304.0●
    salt (any) 304.0●
hexethal (sodium) 304.1●
hexobarbital 304.1●
Hycodan 304.0●
hydrocodone 304.0●
hydromorphinol 304.0●
hydromorphinone 304.0●
hydromorphone 304.0●
hydroxycodeine 304.0●
hypnotic NEC 304.1●
Indian hemp 304.3●
inhalant 304.6●
intranarcon 304.1●
Kemithal 304.1●
ketobemidone 304.0●
khat 304.4●
kif 304.3●
Lactuca (virosa) extract 304.1●
lactucarium 304.1●
laudanum 304.0●
Lebanese red 304.3●
Leritine 304.0●
lettuce opium 304.1●
Levanil 304.1●
Levo-Dromoran 304.0●
levo-iso-methadone 304.0●
levorphanol 304.0●
Librium 304.1●
Lomotil 304.6●
Lotusate 304.1●
LSD (-25) (and derivatives) 304.5●
Luminal 304.1●

Dependence *(Continued)*

lysergic acid 304.5●
    amide 304.5●
maconha 304.3●
magic mushroom 304.5●
marihuana 304.3●
MDA (methylene dioxyamphetamine) 304.4●
Mebaral 304.1●
Medinal 304.1●
Medomin 304.1●
megahallucinogenics 304.5●
meperidine 304.0●
mephobarbital 304.1●
meprobamate 304.1●
mescaline 304.5●
methadone 304.0●
methamphetamine(s) 304.4●
methaqualone 304.1●
metharbital 304.1●
methitural 304.1●
methobarbitone 304.1●
methohexital 304.1●
methopholine 304.6●
methyl●
    alcohol 303.9●
    bromide 304.6●
    morphine 304.0●
    sulfonal 304.1●
methylated spirit 303.9●
methylbutinol 304.6●
methyldihydromorphinone 304.0●
methylene
    chloride 304.6●
    dichloride 304.6●
    dioxyamphetamine (MDA) 304.4●
methylparafynol 304.1●
methylphenidate 304.4●
methyprylone 304.1●
metopon 304.0●
Miltown 304.1●
morning glory seeds 304.5●
morphinan(s) 304.0●
morphine (sulfate) (sulfite) (type) (drugs classifiable to 965.00–965.09) 304.0●
morphine or opioid type drug (drugs classifiable to 965.00–965.09) with any other drug 304.7●
morphinol(s) 304.0●
morphinon 304.0●
morpholinylethylmorphine 304.0●
mylomide 304.1●
myristicin 304.5●
narcotic (drug) NEC 304.9●
nealbarbital 304.1●
nealbarbitone 304.1●
Nembutal 304.1●
Neonal 304.1●
Neraval 304.1●
Neravan 304.1●
neurobarb 304.1●
nicotine 305.1
Nisentil 304.0●
nitrous oxide 304.6●
Noctec 304.1●
Noludar 304.1●
nonbarbiturate sedatives and tranquilizers with similar effect 304.1●
noptil 304.1●
normorphine 304.0●
noscapine 304.0●
Novocaine 304.6●
Numorphan 304.0●

Dependence *(Continued)*

nunol 304.1●
Nupercaine 304.6●
Oblivon 304.1●
on
    aspirator V46.0
    hemodialysis V45.11
    hyperbaric chamber V46.8
    iron lung V46.11
    machine (enabling) V46.9
        specified type NEC V46.8
    peritoneal dialysis V45.11
    Possum (patient-operated-selector-mechanism) V46.8
    renal dialysis machine V45.11
    respirator [ventilator] V46.11
        encounter
            during
                power failure V46.12
                mechanical failure V46.14
            for weaning V46.13
    supplemental oxygen V46.2
    wheelchair V46.3
opiate 304.0●
opioids 304.0●
opioid type drug 304.0●
    with any other drug 304.7●
opium (alkaloids) (derivatives) (tincture) 304.0●
ortal 304.1●
oxazepam 304.1●
oxycodone 304.0●
oxymorphone 304.0●
Palfium 304.0●
Panadol 304.6●
pantopium 304.0●
pantopon 304.0●
papaverine 304.0●
paracetamol 304.6●
paracodin 304.0●
paraldehyde 304.1●
paregoric 304.0●
Parzone 304.0●
PCP (phencyclidine) 304.6●
Pearly Gates 304.5●
pentazocine 304.0●
pentobarbital 304.1●
pentobarbitone (sodium) 304.1●
Pentothal 304.1●
Percaine 304.6●
Percodan 304.0●
Perichlor 304.1●
Pernocton 304.1●
Pernoston 304.1●
peronine 304.0●
pethidine (hydrochloride) 304.0●
petrichloral 304.1●
peyote 304.5●
Phanodorn 304.1●
phenacetin 304.6●
phenadoxone 304.0●
phenaglycodol 304.1●
phenazocine 304.0●
phencyclidine 304.6●
phenmetrazine 304.4●
phenobal 304.1●
phenobarbital 304.1●
phenobarbitone 304.1●
phenomorphan 304.0●
phenonyl 304.1●
phenoperidine 304.0●
pholcodine 304.0●
piminodine 304.0●
Pipadone 304.0●
Pitkin's solution 304.6●

◄ New   ◄▥ Revised   ~~deleted~~ Deleted   ● Use Additional Digit(s)   ▨ Omit code

Dependence *(Continued)*
 Placidyl 304.1 ●
 polysubstance 304.8 ●
 Pontocaine 304.6 ●
 pot 304.3 ●
 potassium bromide 304.1 ●
 Preludin 304.4 ●
 Prinadol 304.0 ●
 probarbital 304.1 ●
 procaine 304.6 ●
 propanal 304.1 ●
 propoxyphene 304.6 ●
 psilocibin 304.5 ●
 psilocin 304.5 ●
 psilocybin 304.5 ●
 psilocyline 304.5 ●
 psilocyn 304.5 ●
 psychedelic agents 304.5 ●
 psychostimulant NEC 304.4 ●
 psychotomimetic agents 304.5 ●
 pyrahexyl 304.3 ●
 Pyramidon 304.6 ●
 quinalbarbitone 304.1 ●
 racemoramide 304.0 ●
 racemorphan 304.0 ●
 Rela 304.6 ●
 scopolamine 304.6 ●
 secobarbital 304.1 ●
 seconal 304.1 ●
 sedative NEC 304.1 ●
  nonbarbiturate with barbiturate
    effect 304.1 ●
 Sedormid 304.1 ●
 sernyl 304.1 ●
 sodium bromide 304.1 ●
 Soma 304.6 ●
 Somnal 304.1 ●
 Somnos 304.1 ●
 Soneryl 304.1 ●
 soporific (drug) NEC 304.1 ●
 specified drug NEC 304.6 ●
 speed 304.4 ●
 spinocaine 304.6 ●
 stovaine 304.6 ●
 STP 304.5 ●
 stramonium 304.6 ●
 Sulfonal 304.1 ●
 sulfonethylmethane 304.1 ●
 sulfonmethane 304.1 ●
 Surital 304.1 ●
 synthetic drug with morphine-like
    effect 304.0 ●
 talbutal 304.1 ●
 tetracaine 304.6 ●
 tetrahydrocannabinol 304.3 ●
 tetronal 304.1 ●
 THC 304.3 ●
 thebacon 304.0 ●
 thebaine 304.0 ●
 thiamil 304.1 ●
 thiamylal 304.1 ●
 thiopental 304.1 ●
 tobacco 305.1 ●
 toluene, toluol 304.6 ●
 tranquilizer NEC 304.1 ●
  nonbarbiturate with barbiturate
    effect 304.1 ●
 tribromacetaldehyde 304.6 ●
 tribromethanol 304.6 ●
 tribromomethane 304.6 ●
 trichloroethanol 304.6 ●
 trichoroethyl phosphate 304.1 ●
 triclofos 304.1 ●
 Trional 304.1 ●
 Tuinal 304.1 ●

Dependence *(Continued)*
 Turkish green 304.3 ●
 urethan(e) 304.6 ●
 Valium 304.1 ●
 Valmid 304.1 ●
 veganin 304.0 ●
 veramon 304.1 ●
 Veronal 304.1 ●
 versidyne 304.6 ●
 vinbarbital 304.1 ●
 vinbarbitone 304.1 ●
 vinyl bitone 304.1 ●
 vitamin B$_6$ 266.1
 wine 303.9 ●
 Zactane 304.6 ●
Dependency
 passive 301.6
 reactions 301.6
Depersonalization (episode, in neurotic
   state) (neurotic) (syndrome) 300.6
Depletion
 carbohydrates 271.9
 complement factor 279.8
 extracellular fluid 276.52
 plasma 276.52
 potassium 276.8
  nephropathy 588.89
 salt or sodium 276.1
  causing heat exhaustion or
    prostration 992.4
  nephropathy 593.9
 volume 276.50
  extracellular fluid 276.52
  plasma 276.52
Deployment (military) ◄
 personal history of V62.22 ◄
 returned from V62.22 ◄
 status V62.21 ◄
Deposit
 argentous, cornea 371.16
 bone, in Boeck's sarcoid 135
 calcareous, calcium - *see*
    Calcification
 cholesterol
  retina 362.82
  skin 709.3
  vitreous (humor) 379.22
 conjunctival 372.56
 cornea, corneal NEC 371.10
  argentous 371.16
  in
   cystinosis 270.0 *[371.15]*
   mucopolysaccharidosis 277.5
    [371.15]
 crystalline, vitreous (humor) 379.22
 hemosiderin, in old scars of cornea
    371.11
 metallic, in lens 366.45
 skin 709.3
 teeth, tooth (betel) (black) (green)
    (materia alba) (orange) (soft)
    (tobacco) 523.6
 urate, in kidney (*see also* Disease, renal)
    593.9
Depraved appetite 307.52
Depression 311
 acute (*see also* Psychosis, affective)
    296.2 ●
  recurrent episode 296.3 ●
  single episode 296.2 ●
 agitated (*see also* Psychosis, affective)
    296.2 ●
  recurrent episode 296.3 ●
  single episode 296.2 ●
 anaclitic 309.21

Depression *(Continued)*
 anxiety 300.4
 arches 734
  congenital 754.61
 autogenous (*see also* Psychosis,
    affective) 296.2 ●
  recurrent episode 296.3 ●
  single episode 296.2 ●
 basal metabolic rate (BMR) 794.7
 bone marrow 289.9
 central nervous system 799.1
  newborn 779.2
 cerebral 331.9
  newborn 779.2
 cerebrovascular 437.8
  newborn 779.2
 chest wall 738.3
 endogenous (*see also* Psychosis,
    affective) 296.2 ●
  recurrent episode 296.3 ●
  single episode 296.2 ●
 functional activity 780.99
 hysterical 300.11
 involutional, climacteric, or
    menopausal (*see also* Psychosis,
    affective) 296.2 ●
  recurrent episode 296.3 ●
  single episode 296.2 ●
 manic (*see also* Psychosis, affective)
    296.80
 medullary 348.89   ◄▥
  newborn 779.2
 mental 300.4
 metatarsal heads - *see* Depression,
    arches
 metatarsus - *see* Depression, arches
 monopolar (*see also* Psychosis,
    affective) 296.2 ●
  recurrent episode 296.3 ●
  single episode 296.2 ●
 nervous 300.4
 neurotic 300.4
 nose 738.0
 postpartum 648.4 ●
 psychogenic 300.4
  reactive 298.0
 psychoneurotic 300.4
 psychotic (*see also* Psychosis, affective)
    296.2 ●
  reactive 298.0
  recurrent episode 296.3 ●
  single episode 296.2 ●
 reactive 300.4
  neurotic 300.4
  psychogenic 298.0
  psychoneurotic 300.4
  psychotic 298.0
 recurrent 296.3 ●
 respiratory center 348.89   ◄▥
  newborn 770.89
 scapula 736.89
 senile 290.21
 situational (acute) (brief) 309.0
  prolonged 309.1
 skull 754.0
 sternum 738.3
 visual field 368.40
Depressive reaction - *see also* Reaction,
   depressive
 acute (transient) 309.0
  with anxiety 309.28
 prolonged 309.1
 situational (acute) 309.0
  prolonged 309.1

Deprivation
  cultural V62.4
  emotional V62.89
    affecting
      adult 995.82
      infant or child 995.51
  food 994.2
    specific substance NEC 269.8
  protein (familial) (kwashiorkor)
      260
  sleep V69.4
  social V62.4
    affecting
      adult 995.82
      infant or child 995.51
  symptoms, syndrome
    alcohol 291.81
    drug 292.0
  vitamins (*see also* Deficiency, vitamin)
      269.2
  water 994.3
de Quervain's
  disease (tendon sheath) 727.04
  syndrome 259.51
  thyroiditis (subacute granulomatous
      thyroiditis) 245.1
Derangement
  ankle (internal) 718.97
    current injury (*see also* Dislocation,
        ankle) 837.0
    recurrent 718.37
  cartilage (articular) NEC (*see also*
      Disorder, cartilage, articular)
      718.0●
    knee 717.9
      recurrent 718.36
    recurrent 718.3●
  collateral ligament (knee) (medial)
      (tibial) 717.82
    current injury 844.1
      lateral (fibular) 844.0
    lateral (fibular) 717.81
      current injury 844.0
  cruciate ligament (knee) (posterior)
      717.84
    anterior 717.83
      current injury 844.2
    current injury 844.2
  elbow (internal) 718.92
    current injury (*see also* Dislocation,
        elbow) 832.00
    recurrent 718.32
  gastrointestinal 536.9
  heart - *see* Disease, heart
  hip (joint) (internal) (old) 718.95
    current injury (*see also* Dislocation,
        hip) 835.00
    recurrent 718.35
  intervertebral disc - *see* Displacement,
      intervertebral disc
  joint (internal) 718.90
    ankle 718.97
    current injury - *see also* Dislocation,
        by site
      knee, meniscus or cartilage
          (*see also* Tear, meniscus)
          836.2
    elbow 718.92
    foot 718.97
    hand 718.94
    hip 718.95
    knee 717.9
    multiple sites 718.99
    pelvic region 718.95

Derangement (*Continued*)
  joint (*Continued*)
    recurrent 718.30
      ankle 718.37
      elbow 718.32
      foot 718.37
      hand 718.34
      hip 718.35
      knee 718.36
      multiple sites 718.39
      pelvic region 718.35
      shoulder (region) 718.31
      specified site NEC 718.38
      temporomandibular (old) 524.69
      wrist 718.33
    shoulder (region) 718.91
    specified site NEC 718.98
    spine NEC 724.9
    temporomandibular 524.69
    wrist 718.93
  knee (cartilage) (internal) 717.9
    current injury (*see also* Tear,
        meniscus) 836.2
    ligament 717.89
      capsular 717.85
      collateral - *see* Derangement,
          collateral ligament
      cruciate - *see* Derangement,
          cruciate ligament
      specified NEC 717.85
    recurrent 718.36
  low back NEC 724.9
  meniscus NEC (knee) 717.5
    current injury (*see also* Tear,
        meniscus) 836.2
    lateral 717.40
      anterior horn 717.42
      posterior horn 717.43
      specified NEC 717.49
    medial 717.3
      anterior horn 717.1
      posterior horn 717.2
    recurrent 718.3●
    site other than knee - *see* Disorder,
        cartilage, articular
  mental (*see also* Psychosis) 298.9
  rotator cuff (recurrent) (tear) 726.10
    current 840.4
  sacroiliac (old) 724.6
    current - *see* Dislocation, sacroiliac
  semilunar cartilage (knee) 717.5
    current injury 836.2
      lateral 836.1
      medial 836.0
    recurrent 718.3●
  shoulder (internal) 718.91
    current injury (*see also* Dislocation,
        shoulder) 831.00
    recurrent 718.31
  spine (recurrent) NEC 724.9
    current - *see* Dislocation, spine
  temporomandibular (internal) (joint)
      (old) 524.69
    current - *see* Dislocation, jaw
Dercum's disease or syndrome (adiposis
      dolorosa) 272.8
Derealization (neurotic) 300.6
Dermal - *see* condition
Dermaphytid - *see* Dermatophytosis
Dermatergosis - *see* Dermatitis
Dermatitis (allergic) (contact)
      (occupational) (venenata) 692.9
  ab igne 692.82
  acneiform 692.9

Dermatitis (*Continued*)
  actinic (due to sun) 692.70
    acute 692.72
    chronic NEC 692.74
    other than from sun NEC 692.82
  ambustionis
    due to
      burn or scald - *see* Burn, by site
      sunburn (*see also* Sunburn)
          692.71
  amebic 006.6
  ammonia 691.0
  anaphylactoid NEC 692.9
  arsenical 692.4
  artefacta 698.4
    psychogenic 316 [*698.4*]
  asthmatic 691.8
  atopic (allergic) (intrinsic) 691.8
    psychogenic 316 [*691.8*]
  atrophicans 701.8
    diffusa 701.8
    maculosa 701.3
  autoimmune progesterone 279.49 ◄
  berlock, berloque 692.72
  blastomycetic 116.0
  blister beetle 692.89
  Brucella NEC 023.9
  bullosa 694.9
    striata pratensis 692.6
  bullous 694.9
    mucosynechial, atrophic 694.60
      with ocular involvement 694.61
    seasonal 694.8
  calorica
    due to
      burn or scald - *see* Burn, by site
      cold 692.89
      sunburn (*see also* Sunburn) 692.71
  caterpillar 692.89
  cercarial 120.3
  combustionis
    due to
      burn or scald - *see* Burn, by
          site
      sunburn (*see also* Sunburn)
          692.71
  congelationis 991.5
  contusiformis 695.2
  diabetic 250.8●
  diaper 691.0
  diphtheritica 032.85
  due to
    acetone 692.2
    acids 692.4
    adhesive plaster 692.4
    alcohol (skin contact) (substances
        classifiable to 980.0–980.9)
        692.4
      taken internally 693.8
    alkalis 692.4
    allergy NEC 692.9
    ammonia (household) (liquid)
        692.4
    animal
      dander (cat) (dog) 692.84
      hair (cat) (dog) 692.84
    arnica 692.3
    arsenic 692.4
      taken internally 693.8
    blister beetle 692.89
    cantharides 692.3
    carbon disulphide 692.2
    caterpillar 692.89
    caustics 692.4

Dermatitis *(Continued)*
  due to *(Continued)*
    cereal (ingested) 693.1
      contact with skin 692.5
    chemical(s) NEC 692.4
      internal 693.8
      irritant NEC 692.4
      taken internally 693.8
    chlorocompounds 692.2
    coffee (ingested) 693.1
      contact with skin 692.5
    cold weather 692.89
    cosmetics 692.81
    cyclohexanes 692.2
    dander, animal (cat) (dog) 692.84
    deodorant 692.81
    detergents 692.0
    dichromate 692.4
    drugs and medicinals (correct substance properly administered) (internal use) 693.0
      external (in contact with skin) 692.3
        wrong substance given or taken 976.9
        specified substance - *see* Table of Drugs and Chemicals
      wrong substance given or taken 977.9
      specified substance - *see* Table of Drugs and Chemicals
    dyes 692.89
      hair 692.89
    epidermophytosis - *see* Dermatophytosis
    esters 692.2
    external irritant NEC 692.9
      specified agent NEC 692.89
    eye shadow 692.81
    fish (ingested) 693.1
      contact with skin 692.5
    flour (ingested) 693.1
      contact with skin 692.5
    food (ingested) 693.1
      in contact with skin 692.5
    fruit (ingested) 693.1
      contact with skin 692.5
    fungicides 692.3
    furs 692.84
    glycols 692.2
    greases NEC 692.1
    hair, animal (cat) (dog) 692.84
    hair dyes 692.89
    hot
      objects and materials - *see* Burn, by site
      weather or places 692.89
    hydrocarbons 692.2
    infrared rays, except from sun 692.82
    solar NEC (*see also* Dermatitis, due to, sun) 692.70
    ingested substance 693.9
      drugs and medicinals (*see also* Dermatitis, due to, drugs and medicinals) 693.0
      food 693.1
      specified substance NEC 693.8

Dermatitis *(Continued)*
  due to *(Continued)*
    ingestion or injection of
      chemical 693.8
      drug (correct substance properly administered) 693.0
        wrong substance given or taken 977.9
        specified substance - *see* Table of Drugs and Chemicals
    insecticides 692.4
    internal agent 693.9
      drugs and medicinals (*see also* Dermatitis, due to, drugs and medicinals) 693.0
      food (ingested) 693.1
        in contact with skin 692.5
      specified agent NEC 693.8
    iodine 692.3
    iodoform 692.3
    irradiation 692.82
    jewelry 692.83
    keratolytics 692.3
    ketones 692.2
    lacquer tree (Rhus verniciflua) 692.6
    light (sun) NEC (*see also* Dermatitis, due to, sun) 692.70
      other 692.82
    low temperature 692.89
    mascara 692.81
    meat (ingested) 693.1
      contact with skin 692.5
    mercury, mercurials 692.3
    metals 692.83
    milk (ingested) 693.1
      contact with skin 692.5
    Neomycin 692.3
    nylon 692.4
    oils NEC 692.1
    paint solvent 692.2
    pediculocides 692.3
    petroleum products (substances classifiable to 981) 692.4
    phenol 692.3
    photosensitiveness, photosensitivity (sun) 692.72
      other light 692.82
    plants NEC 692.6
    plasters, medicated (any) 692.3
    plastic 692.4
    poison
      ivy (Rhus toxicodendron) 692.6
      oak (Rhus diversiloba) 692.6
      plant or vine 692.6
      sumac (Rhus venenata) 692.6
      vine (Rhus radicans) 692.6
    preservatives 692.89
    primrose (primula) 692.6
    primula 692.6
    radiation 692.82
      sun NEC (*see also* Dermatitis, due to, sun) 692.70
      tanning bed 692.82
    radioactive substance 692.82
    radium 692.82
    ragweed (Senecio jacobae) 692.6
    Rhus (diversiloba) (radicans) (toxicodendron) (venenata) (verniciflua) 692.6
    rubber 692.4
    scabicides 692.3
    Senecio jacobae 692.6

Dermatitis *(Continued)*
  due to *(Continued)*
    solar radiation - *see* Dermatitis, due to, sun
    solvents (any) (substances classifiable to 982.0–982.8) 692.2
      chlorocompound group 692.2
      cyclohexane group 692.2
      ester group 692.2
      glycol group 692.2
      hydrocarbon group 692.2
      ketone group 692.2
      paint 692.2
    specified agent NEC 692.89
    sun 692.70
      acute 692.72
      chronic NEC 692.74
      specified NEC 692.79
    sunburn (*see also* Sunburn) 692.71
    sunshine NEC (*see also* Dermatitis, due to, sun) 692.70
    tanning bed 692.82
    tetrachlorethylene 692.2
    toluene 692.2
    topical medications 692.3
    turpentine 692.2
    ultraviolet rays, except from sun 692.82
      sun NEC (*see also* Dermatitis, due to, sun) 692.70
    vaccine or vaccination (correct substance properly administered) 693.0
      wrong substance given or taken bacterial vaccine 978.8
        specified - *see* Table of Drugs and Chemicals
        other vaccines NEC 979.9
        specified - *see* Table of Drugs and Chemicals
    varicose veins (*see also* Varicose, vein, inflamed or infected) 454.1
    x-rays 692.82
  dyshydrotic 705.81
  dysmenorrheica 625.8
  eczematoid NEC 692.9
    infectious 690.8
  eczematous NEC 692.9
  epidemica 695.89
  erysipelatosa 695.81
  escharotica - *see* Burn, by site
  exfoliativa, exfoliative 695.89
    generalized 695.89
    infantum 695.81
    neonatorum 695.81
  eyelid 373.31
    allergic 373.32
    contact 373.32
    eczematous 373.31
    herpes (zoster) 053.20
      simplex 054.41
    infective 373.5
      due to
        actinomycosis 039.3 *[373.5]*
        herpes
          simplex 054.41
          zoster 053.20
        impetigo 684 *[373.5]*
        leprosy (*see also* Leprosy) 030.0 *[373.4]*

Dermatitis *(Continued)*
  eyelid *(Continued)*
    infective *(Continued)*
      due to *(Continued)*
        lupus vulgaris (tuberculous)
            (*see also* Tuberculosis)
            017.0 ● *[373.4]*
        mycotic dermatitis (*see also*
            Dermatomycosis) 111.9
            [373.5]
        vaccinia 051.02 *[373.5]*
            postvaccination 999.0
                [373.5]
        yaws (*see also* Yaws) 102.9 *[373.4]*
  facta, factitia 698.4
    psychogenic 316 *[698.4]*
  ficta 698.4
    psychogenic 316 *[698.4]*
  flexural 691.8
  follicularis 704.8
  friction 709.8
  fungus 111.9
    specified type NEC 111.8
  gangrenosa, gangrenous (infantum)
      (*see also* Gangrene) 785.4
  gestationis 646.8●
  gonococcal 098.89
  gouty 274.89
  harvest mite 133.8
  heat 692.89
  herpetiformis (bullous) (erythematous)
      (pustular) (vesicular) 694.0
    juvenile 694.2
    senile 694.5
  hiemalis 692.89
  hypostatic, hypostatica 454.1
    with ulcer 454.2
  impetiginous 684
  infantile (acute) (chronic)
      (intertriginous) (intrinsic)
      (seborrheic) 690.12
  infectiosa eczematoides 690.8
  infectious (staphylococcal)
      (streptococcal) 686.9
    eczematoid 690.8
  infective eczematoid 690.8
  Jacquet's (diaper dermatitis) 691.0
  leptus 133.8
  lichenified NEC 692.9
  lichenoid, chronic 701.0
  lichenoides purpurica pigmentosa
      709.1
  meadow 692.6
  medicamentosa (correct substance
      properly administered) (internal
      use) (*see also* Dermatitis, due to,
      drugs or medicinals) 693.0
    due to contact with skin 692.3
  mite 133.8
  multiformis 694.0
    juvenile 694.2
    senile 694.5
  napkin 691.0
  neuro 698.3
  neurotica 694.0
  nummular NEC 692.9
  osteatosis, osteatotic 706.8
  papillaris capillitii 706.1
  pellagrous 265.2
  perioral 695.3
  perstans 696.1
  photosensitivity (sun) 692.72
    other light 692.82
  pigmented purpuric lichenoid 709.1

Dermatitis *(Continued)*
  polymorpha dolorosa 694.0
  primary irritant 692.9
  pruriginosa 694.0
  pruritic NEC 692.9
  psoriasiform nodularis 696.2
  psychogenic 316
  purulent 686.00
  pustular contagious 051.2
  pyococcal 686.00
  pyocyaneus 686.09
  pyogenica 686.00
  radiation 692.82
  repens 696.1
  Ritter's (exfoliativa) 695.81
  Schamberg's (progressive pigmentary
      dermatosis) 709.09
  schistosome 120.3
  seasonal bullous 694.8
  seborrheic 690.10
    infantile 690.12
  sensitization NEC 692.9
  septic (*see also* Septicemia) 686.00
    gonococcal 098.89
  solar, solare NEC (*see also* Dermatitis,
      due to, sun) 692.70
  stasis 454.1
    due to
      postphlebitic syndrome 459.12
          with ulcer 459.13
      varicose veins - *see* Varicose
    ulcerated or with ulcer (varicose)
        454.2
  sunburn (*see also* Sunburn) 692.71
  suppurative 686.00
  traumatic NEC 709.8
  trophoneurotica 694.0
  ultraviolet, except from sun 692.82
    due to sun NEC (*see also* Dermatitis,
        due to, sun) 692.70
  varicose 454.1
    with ulcer 454.2
  vegetans 686.8
  verrucosa 117.2
  xerotic 706.8
Dermatoarthritis, lipoid 272.8 *[713.0]*
Dermatochalasia, dermatochalasis 374.87
Dermatofibroma (lenticulare) (M8832/0) -
    see also Neoplasm, skin, benign
  protuberans (M8832/1) - *see* Neoplasm,
      skin, uncertain behavior
Dermatofibrosarcoma (protuberans)
    (M8832/3) - *see* Neoplasm, skin,
    malignant
Dermatographia 708.3
Dermatolysis (congenital) (exfoliativa)
    757.39
  acquired 701.8
  eyelids 374.34
  palpebrarum 374.34
  senile 701.8
Dermatomegaly NEC 701.8
Dermatomucomyositis 710.3
Dermatomycosis 111.9
  furfuracea 111.0
  specified type NEC 111.8
Dermatomyositis (acute) (chronic) 710.3
Dermatoneuritis of children 985.0
Dermatophiliasis 134.1
Dermatophytide - *see* Dermatophytosis
Dermatophytosis (Epidermophyton)
    (infection) (microsporum) (tinea)
    (Trichophyton) 110.9
  beard 110.0

Dermatophytosis *(Continued)*
  body 110.5
  deep seated 110.6
  fingernails 110.1
  foot 110.4
  groin 110.3
  hand 110.2
  nail 110.1
  perianal (area) 110.3
  scalp 110.0
  scrotal 110.8
  specified site NEC 110.8
  toenails 110.1
  vulva 110.8
Dermatopolyneuritis 985.0
Dermatorrhexis 756.83
  acquired 701.8
Dermatosclerosis (*see also* Scleroderma)
    710.1
  localized 701.0
Dermatosis 709.9
  Andrews' 686.8
  atopic 691.8
  Bowen's (M8081/2) - *see* Neoplasm,
      skin, in situ
  bullous 694.9
    specified type NEC 694.8
  erythematosquamous 690.8
  exfoliativa 695.89
  factitial 698.4
  gonococcal 098.89
  herpetiformis 694.0
    juvenile 694.2
    senile 694.5
  hysterical 300.11
  linear IgA 694.8
  menstrual NEC 709.8
  neutrophilic, acute febrile 695.89
  occupational (*see also* Dermatitis)
      692.9
  papulosa nigra 709.8
  pigmentary NEC 709.00
    progressive 709.09
    Schamberg's 709.09
    Siemens-Bloch 757.33
  progressive pigmentary 709.09
  psychogenic 316
  pustular subcorneal 694.1
  Schamberg's (progressive pigmentary)
      709.09
  senile NEC 709.3
  specified NEC 702.8
  Unna's (seborrheic dermatitis) 690.10
Dermographia 708.3
Dermographism 708.3
Dermoid (cyst) (M9084/0) - *see also*
    Neoplasm, by site, benign
  with malignant transformation
      (M9084/3) 183.0
Dermopathy
  infiltrative, with thyrotoxicosis
      242.0●
  nephrogenic fibrosing 701.8
  senile NEC 709.3
Dermophytosis - *see* Dermatophytosis
Descemet's membrane - *see* condition
Descemetocele 371.72
Descending - *see* condition
Descensus uteri (complete) (incomplete)
    (partial) (without vaginal wall
    prolapse) 618.1
  with mention of vaginal wall prolapse -
      see Prolapse, uterovaginal
Desensitization to allergens V07.1

◄ New   ◄▥ Revised   ~~deleted~~ Deleted   ● Use Additional Digit(s)   ▨ Omit code

Desert
rheumatism 114.0
sore (see also Ulcer, skin) 707.9
Desertion (child) (newborn) 995.52
adult 995.84
Desmoid (extra-abdominal) (tumor)
(M8821/1) - see also Neoplasm,
connective tissue, uncertain
behavior
abdominal (M8822/1) - see Neoplasm,
connective tissue, uncertain
behavior
Despondency 300.4
Desquamative dermatitis NEC 695.89
Destruction
articular facet (see also Derangement,
joint) 718.9 ●
vertebra 724.9
bone 733.90
syphilitic 095.5
joint (see also Derangement, joint)
718.9 ●
sacroiliac 724.6
kidney 593.89
live fetus to facilitate birth NEC 763.89
ossicles (ear) 385.24
rectal sphincter 569.49
septum (nasal) 478.19
tuberculous NEC (see also Tuberculosis)
011.9 ●
tympanic membrane 384.82
tympanum 385.89
vertebral disc - see Degeneration,
intervertebral disc
Destructiveness (see also Disturbance,
conduct) 312.9
adjustment reaction 309.3
Detachment
cartilage - see also Sprain, by site
knee - see Tear, meniscus
cervix, annular 622.8
complicating delivery 665.3 ●
choroid (old) (postinfectional)
(simple) (spontaneous)
363.70
hemorrhagic 363.72
serous 363.71
knee, medial meniscus (old) 717.3
current injury 836.0
ligament - see Sprain, by site
placenta (premature) - see Placenta,
separation
retina (recent) 361.9
with retinal defect
(rhegmatogenous) 361.00
giant tear 361.03
multiple 361.02
partial
with
giant tear 361.03
multiple defects 361.02
retinal dialysis (juvenile)
361.04
single defect 361.01
retinal dialysis (juvenile)
361.04
single 361.01
subtotal 361.05
total 361.05
delimited (old) (partial) 361.06
old
delimited 361.06
partial 361.06
total or subtotal 361.07

Detachment (Continued)
retina (Continued)
pigment epithelium (RPE) (serous)
362.42
exudative 362.42
hemorrhagic 362.43
rhegmatogenous (see also
Detachment, retina, with retinal
defect) 361.00
serous (without retinal defect)
361.2
specified type NEC 361.89
traction (with vitreoretinal
organization) 361.81
vitreous humor 379.21
Detergent asthma 507.8
Deterioration
epileptic
with behavioral disturbance 345.9 ●
[294.11]
without behavioral disturbance
345.9 ● [294.10]
heart, cardiac (see also Degeneration,
myocardial) 429.1
mental (see also Psychosis) 298.9
myocardium, myocardial (see also
Degeneration, myocardial)
429.1
senile (simple) 797
transplanted organ - see
Complications, transplant,
organ, by site
de Toni-Fanconi syndrome (cystinosis)
270.0
Deuteranomaly 368.52
Deuteranopia (anomalous trichromat)
(complete) (incomplete) 368.52
Deutschländer's disease - see Fracture,
foot
Development
abnormal, bone 756.9
arrested 783.40
bone 733.91
child 783.40
due to malnutrition (protein-calorie)
263.2
fetus or newborn 764.9 ●
tracheal rings (congenital) 748.3
defective, congenital - see also Anomaly
cauda equina 742.59
left ventricle 746.9
with atresia or hypoplasia of
aortic orifice or valve with
hypoplasia of ascending
aorta 746.7
in hypoplastic left heart
syndrome 746.7
delayed (see also Delay, development)
783.40
arithmetical skills 315.1
language (skills) 315.31
and speech due to hearing loss
315.34
expressive 315.31
mixed receptive-expressive
315.32
learning skill, specified NEC 315.2
mixed skills 315.5
motor coordination 315.4
reading 315.00
specified
learning skill NEC 315.2
type NEC, except learning
315.8

Development (Continued)
delayed (Continued)
speech 315.39
and language due to hearing loss
315.34
associated with hyperkinesia
314.1
phonological 315.39
spelling 315.09
written expression 315.2
imperfect, congenital - see also Anomaly
heart 746.9
lungs 748.60
improper (fetus or newborn) 764.9 ●
incomplete (fetus or newborn) 764.9 ●
affecting management of pregnancy
656.5 ●
bronchial tree 748.3
organ or site not listed - see
Hypoplasia
respiratory system 748.9
sexual, precocious NEC 259.1
tardy, mental (see also Retardation,
mental) 319
Developmental - see condition
Devergie's disease (pityriasis rubra
pilaris) 696.4
Deviation
conjugate (eye) 378.87
palsy 378.81
spasm, spastic 378.82
esophagus 530.89
eye, skew 378.87
mandible, opening and closing 524.53
midline (jaw) (teeth) 524.29
specified site NEC - see Malposition
occlusal plane 524.76
organ or site, congenital NEC - see
Malposition, congenital
septum (acquired) (nasal) 470
congenital 754.0
sexual 302.9
bestiality 302.1
coprophilia 302.89
ego-dystonic
homosexuality 302.0
lesbianism 302.0
erotomania 302.89
Clérambault's 297.8
exhibitionism (sexual) 302.4
fetishism 302.81
transvestic 302.3
frotteurism 302.89
homosexuality, ego-dystonic 302.0
pedophilic 302.2
lesbianism, ego-dystonic 302.0
masochism 302.83
narcissism 302.89
necrophilia 302.89
nymphomania 302.89
pederosis 302.2
pedophilia 302.2
sadism 302.84
sadomasochism 302.84
satyriasis 302.89
specified type NEC 302.89
transvestic fetishism 302.3
transvestism 302.3
voyeurism 302.82
zoophilia (erotica) 302.1
teeth, midline 524.29
trachea 519.19
ureter (congenital) 753.4
Devic's disease 341.0

Device
cerebral ventricle (communicating) in situ V45.2
contraceptive - *see* Contraceptive, device
drainage, cerebrospinal fluid V45.2
Devil's
grip 074.1
pinches (purpura simplex) 287.2
Devitalized tooth 522.9
Devonshire colic 984.9
specified type of lead - *see* Table of Drugs and Chemicals
Dextraposition, aorta 747.21
with ventricular septal defect, pulmonary stenosis or atresia, and hypertrophy of right ventricle 745.2
in tetralogy of Fallot 745.2
Dextratransposition, aorta 745.11
Dextrinosis, limit (debrancher enzyme deficiency) 271.0
Dextrocardia (corrected) (false) (isolated) (secondary) (true) 746.87
with
complete transposition of viscera 759.3
situs inversus 759.3
Dextroversion, kidney (left) 753.3
Dhobie itch 110.3
Diabetes, diabetic (brittle) (congenital) (familial) (mellitus) (poorly controlled) (severe) (slight) (without complication) 250.0●

Note 21 Use the following fifth-digit subclassification with category 250:

0 type II or unspecified type, not stated as uncontrolled
Fifth-digit 0 is for use for type II patients, even if the patient requires insulin
1 type I [juvenile type], not stated as uncontrolled
2 type II or unspecified type, uncontrolled
Fifth-digit 2 is for use for type II patients, even if the patient requires insulin
3 type I [juvenile type], uncontrolled

---

with
coma (with ketoacidosis) 250.3●
due to secondary diabetes 249.3●
hyperosmolar (nonketotic) 250.2●
due to secondary diabetes 249.2●
complication NEC 250.9●
due to secondary diabetes 249.9●
specified NEC 250.8●
due to secondary diabetes 249.8●
gangrene 250.7● [785.4]
due to secondary diabetes 249.7● [785.4]
hyperglycemia - *code to* Diabetes, by type, with 5th digit for not stated as uncontrolled

Diabetes, diabetic *(Continued)*
with *(Continued)*
hyperosmolarity 250.2●
due to secondary diabetes 249.2●
ketosis, ketoacidosis 250.1●
due to secondary diabetes 249.1●
osteomyelitis 250.8● [731.8]
due to secondary diabetes 249.8● [731.8]
specified manifestations NEC 250.8●
due to secondary diabetes 249.8●
acetonemia 250.1●
due to secondary diabetes 249.1●
acidosis 250.1●
due to secondary diabetes 249.1●
amyotrophy 250.6● [353.5]
due to secondary diabetes 249.6● [353.5]
angiopathy, peripheral 250.7● [443.81]
due to secondary diabetes 249.7● [443.81]
asymptomatic 790.29
autonomic neuropathy (peripheral) 250.6● [337.1]
due to secondary diabetes 249.6● [337.1]
bone change 250.8● [731.8]
due to secondary diabetes 249.8● [731.8]
bronze, bronzed 275.0
cataract 250.5● [366.41]
due to secondary diabetes 249.5● [366.41]
chemical induced - *see* Diabetes, secondary
complicating pregnancy, childbirth, or puerperium 648.0●
coma (with ketoacidosis) 250.3●
due to secondary diabetes 249.3●
hyperglycemic 250.3●
due to secondary diabetes 249.3●
hyperosmolar (nonketotic) 250.2●
due to secondary diabetes 249.2●
hypoglycemic 250.3●
due to secondary diabetes 249.3●
insulin 250.3●
due to secondary diabetes 249.3●
complicating pregnancy, childbirth, or puerperium (maternal) (conditions classifiable to 249 and 250) 648.0●
affecting fetus or newborn 775.0
complication NEC 250.9●
due to secondary diabetes 249.9●
specified NEC 250.8●
due to secondary diabetes 249.8●
dorsal sclerosis 250.6● [340]
due to secondary diabetes 249.6● [340]
drug-induced - *see also* Diabetes, secondary
overdose or wrong substance given or taken - *see* Table of Drugs and Chemicals
due to
cystic fibrosis - *see* Diabetes, secondary
infection - *see* Diabetes, secondary
dwarfism-obesity syndrome 258.1
gangrene 250.7● [785.4]
due to secondary diabetes 249.7● [785.4]
gastroparesis 250.6● [536.3]
due to secondary diabetes 249.6● [536.3]

Diabetes, diabetic *(Continued)*
gestational 648.8●
complicating pregnancy, childbirth, or puerperium 648.8●
glaucoma 250.5● [365.44]
due to secondary diabetes 249.5● [365.44]
glomerulosclerosis (intercapillary) 250.4● [581.81]
due to secondary diabetes 249.4● [581.81]
glycogenosis, secondary 250.8● [259.8]
due to secondary diabetes 249.8● [259.8]
hemochromatosis 275.0
hyperosmolar coma 250.2●
due to secondary diabetes 249.2●
hyperosmolarity 250.2●
due to secondary diabetes 249.2●
hypertension-nephrosis syndrome 250.4● [581.81]
due to secondary diabetes 249.4● [581.81]
hypoglycemia 250.8●
due to secondary diabetes 249.8●
hypoglycemic shock 250.8●
due to secondary diabetes 249.8●
inadequately controlled - *code to* Diabetes, by type, with 5th digit for not stated as uncontrolled
insipidus 253.5
nephrogenic 588.1
pituitary 253.5
vasopression-resistant 588.1
intercapillary glomerulosclerosis 250.4● [581.81]
due to secondary diabetes 249.4● [581.81]
iritis 250.5● [364.42]
due to secondary diabetes 249.5● [364.42]
ketosis, ketoacidosis 250.1●
due to secondary diabetes 249.1●
Kimmelstiel (-Wilson) disease or syndrome (intercapillary glomerulosclerosis) 250.4● [581.81]
due to secondary diabetes 249.4● [581.81]
Lancereaux's (diabetes mellitus with marked emaciation) 250.8● [261]
due to secondary diabetes 249.8● [261]
latent (chemical) - *see* Diabetes, secondary
complicating pregnancy, childbirth, or puerperium 648.0●
lipoidosis 250.8● [272.7]
due to secondary diabetes 249.8● [272.7]
macular edema 250.5● [362.07]
due to secondary diabetes 249.5● [362.07]
maternal
with manifest disease in the infant 775.1
affecting fetus or newborn 775.0
microaneurysms, retinal 250.5● [362.01]
due to secondary diabetes 249.5● [362.01]
mononeuropathy 250.6● [355.9]
due to secondary diabetes 249.6● [355.9]
neonatal, transient 775.1

◀ New   ◀▥ Revised   ~~deleted~~ Deleted   ● Use Additional Digit(s)   ▨ Omit code

Diabetes, diabetic *(Continued)*
  nephropathy 250.4● *[583.81]*
    due to secondary diabetes 249.4● *[583.81]* ◀▥
  nephrosis (syndrome) 250.4● *[581.81]*
    due to secondary diabetes 249.4● *[583.81]*
  neuralgia 250.6● *[357.2]*
    due to secondary diabetes 249.6● *[357.2]*
  neuritis 250.6● *[357.2]*
    due to secondary diabetes 249.6● *[357.2]*
  neurogenic arthropathy 250.6● *[713.5]*
    due to secondary diabetes 249.6● *[713.5]*
  neuropathy 250.6● *[357.2]*
    autonomic (peripheral) 250.6 *[337.1]* ◀
      due to secondary diabetes 249.6 *[337.1]* ◀
    due to secondary diabetes 249.6● *[357.2]*
  nonclinical 790.29
  osteomyelitis 250.8● *[731.8]*
    due to secondary diabetes 249.8● *[731.8]*
  out of control - *code to* Diabetes, by type, with 5th digit for uncontrolled
  peripheral autonomic neuropathy 250.6● *[337.1]*
    due to secondary diabetes 249.6● *[337.1]*
  phosphate 275.3
  polyneuropathy 250.6● *[357.2]*
    due to secondary diabetes 249.6● *[357.2]*
  poorly controlled - *code to* Diabetes, by type, with 5th digit for not stated as uncontrolled
  renal (true) 271.4
  retinal
    edema 250.5● *[362.07]*
      due to secondary diabetes 249.5● *[362.07]*
    hemorrhage 250.5● *[362.01]*
      due to secondary diabetes 249.5● *[362.01]*
    microaneurysms 250.5● *[362.01]*
      due to secondary diabetes 249.5● *[362.01]*
    retinitis 250.5● *[362.01]*
      due to secondary diabetes 249.5● *[362.01]*
    retinopathy 250.5● *[362.01]*
      due to secondary diabetes 249.5● *[362.01]*
      background 250.5● *[362.01]*
        due to secondary diabetes 249.5● *[362.01]*
      nonproliferative 250.5● *[362.03]*
        due to secondary diabetes 249.5● *[362.03]*
        mild 250.5● *[362.04]*
          due to secondary diabetes 249.5● *[362.04]*
        moderate 250.5● *[362.05]*
          due to secondary diabetes 249.5● *[362.05]*
        severe 250.5● *[362.06]*
          due to secondary diabetes 249.5● *[362.06]*

Diabetes, diabetic *(Continued)*
  retinopathy *(Continued)*
    proliferative 250.5● *[362.02]*
      due to secondary diabetes 249.5● *[362.02]*
  secondary (chemical-induced) (due to chronic condition) (due to infection) (drug-induced) 249.0●
    with
      coma (with ketoacidosis) 249.3●
        hyperosmolar (nonketotic) 249.2●
      complication NEC 249.9●
        specified NEC 249.8●
      gangrene 249.7● *[785.4]*
      hyperosmolarity 249.2●
      ketosis, ketoacidosis 249.1●
      osteomyelitis 249.8● *[731.8]*
      specified manifestations NEC 249.8●
    acetonemia 249.1●
    acidosis 249.1●
    amyotrophy 249.6 ● *[353.5]*
    angiopathy, peripheral 249.7● *[443.81]*
    autonomic neuropathy (peripheral) 249.6● *[337.1]*
    bone change 249.8● *[731.8]*
    cataract 249.5● *[366.41]*
    coma (with ketoacidosis) 249.3●
      hyperglycemic 249.3●
      hyperosmolar (nonketotic) 249.2●
      hypoglycemic 249.3●
      insulin 249.3●
    complicating pregnancy, childbirth, or puerperium (maternal) 648.0●
      affecting fetus or newborn 775.0
    complication NEC 249.9●
      specified NEC 249.8●
    dorsal sclerosis 249.6● *[340]*
    due to overdose or wrong substance given or taken - *see* Table of Drugs and Chemicals
    gangrene 249.7● *[785.4]*
    gastroparesis 249.6● *[536.3]*
    glaucoma 249.5● *[365.44]*
    glomerulosclerosis (intercapillary) 249.4● *[581.81]*
    glycogenosis, secondary 249.8● *[259.8]*
    hyperosmolar coma 249.2●
    hyperosmolarity 249.2●
    hypertension-nephrosis syndrome 249.4● *[581.81]*
    hypoglycemia 249.8●
    hypoglycemic shock 249.8●
    intercapillary glomerulosclerosis 249.4● *[581.81]*
    iritis 249.5● *[364.42]*
    ketosis, ketoacidosis 249.1●
    Kimmelstiel (-Wilson) disease or syndrome (intercapillary glomerulosclerosis) 249.4● *[581.81]*
    Lancereaux's (diabetes mellitus with marked emaciation) 249.8● *[261]*
    lipoidosis 249.8● *[272.7]*
    macular edema 249.5● *[362.07]*

Diabetes, diabetic *(Continued)*
  secondary *(Continued)*
    maternal
      with manifest disease in the infant 775.1
      affecting fetus or newborn 775.0
    microaneurysms, retinal 249.5● *[362.01]*
    mononeuropathy 249.6● *[355.9]*
    nephropathy 249.4● *[583.81]* ◀▥
    nephrosis (syndrome) 249.4● *[581.81]*
    neuralgia 249.6● *[357.2]*
    neuritis 249.6● *[357.2]*
    neurogenic arthropathy 249.6● *[713.5]*
    neuropathy 249.6● *[357.2]*
      autonomic (peripheral) 249.6 *[337.1]* ◀
    osteomyelitis 249.8● *[731.8]*
    peripheral autonomic neuropathy 249.6● *[337.1]*
    polyneuropathy 249.6● *[357.2]*
    retinal
      edema 249.5● *[362.07]*
      hemorrhage 249.5● *[362.01]*
      microaneurysms 249.5● *[362.01]*
    retinitis 249.5● *[362.01]*
    retinopathy 249.5● *[362.01]*
      background 249.5● *[362.01]*
      nonproliferative 249.5● *[362.03]*
        mild 249.5● *[362.04]*
        moderate 249.5● *[362.05]*
        severe 249.5● *[362.06]*
      proliferative 249.5● *[362.02]*
    ulcer (skin) 249.8● *[707.9]*
      lower extremity 249.8● *[707.10]*
        ankle 249.8● *[707.13]*
        calf 249.8● *[707.12]*
        foot 249.8● *[707.15]*
        heel 249.8● *[707.14]*
        knee 249.8● *[707.19]*
        specified site NEC 249.8● *[707.19]*
        thigh 249.8● *[707.11]*
        toes 249.8● *[707.15]*
      specified site NEC 249.8● *[707.8]*
    xanthoma 249.8● *[272.2]*
  steroid induced - *see also* Diabetes, secondary
    overdose or wrong substance given or taken 962.0
  stress 790.29
  subclinical 790.29
  subliminal 790.29
  sugar 250.0●
  ulcer (skin) 250.8● *[707.9]*
    due to secondary diabetes 249.8● *[707.9]*
    lower extremity 250.8● *[707.10]*
      due to secondary diabetes 249.8● *[707.10]*
      ankle 250.8● *[707.13]*
        due to secondary diabetes 249.8● *[707.13]*
      calf 250.8● *[707.12]*
        due to secondary diabetes 249.8● *[707.12]*
      foot 250.8● *[707.15]*
        due to secondary diabetes 249.8● *[707.15]*
      heel 250.8● *[707.14]*
        due to secondary diabetes 249.8● *[707.14]*
      knee 250.8● *[707.19]*
        due to secondary diabetes 249.8● *[707.19]*

Diabetes, diabetic (Continued)
  ulcer (Continued)
    lower extremity (Continued)
      specified site NEC 250.8●
        [707.19]
        due to secondary diabetes
          249.8● [707.19]
      thigh 250.8● [707.11]
        due to secondary diabetes
          249.8● [707.11]
      toes 250.8● [707.15]
        due to secondary diabetes
          249.8● [707.15]
      specified site NEC 250.8● [707.8]
        due to secondary diabetes 249.8●
        [707.8]
    xanthoma 250.8● [272.2]
      due to secondary diabetes 249.8●
      [272.2]
Diacyclothrombopathia 287.1
Diagnosis deferred 799.9
Dialysis (intermittent) (treatment)
  anterior retinal (juvenile) (with
    detachment) 361.04
  extracorporeal V56.0
  hemodialysis V56.0
    status only V45.11
  peritoneal V56.8
    status only V45.11
  renal V56.0
    status only V45.11
  specified type NEC V56.8
Diamond-Blackfan anemia or syndrome
  (congenital hypoplastic anemia)
  284.01
Diamond-Gardener syndrome
  (autoerythrocyte sensitization)
  287.2
Diaper rash 691.0
Diaphoresis (excessive) NEC (see also
  Hyperhidrosis) 780.8
Diaphragm - see condition
Diaphragmalgia 786.52
Diaphragmitis 519.4
Diaphyseal aclasis 756.4
Diaphysitis 733.99
Diarrhea, diarrheal (acute) (autumn)
  (bilious) (bloody) (catarrhal)
  (choleraic) (chronic) (gravis) (green)
  (infantile) (lienteric) (noninfectious)
  (presumed noninfectious)
  (putrefactive) (secondary) (sporadic)
  (summer) (symptomatic) (thermic)
  787.91
  achlorhydric 536.0
  allergic 558.3
  amebic (see also Amebiasis) 006.9
    with abscess - see Abscess, amebic
    acute 006.0
    chronic 006.1
    nondysenteric 006.2
  bacillary - see Dysentery, bacillary
  bacterial NEC 008.5
  balantidial 007.0
  bile salt-induced 579.8
  cachectic NEC 787.91
  chilomastix 007.8
  choleriformis 001.1
  coccidial 007.2
  Cochin-China 579.1
    anguilluliasis 127.2
    psilosis 579.1
  Dientamoeba 007.8
  dietetic 787.91

Diarrhea, diarrheal (Continued)
  due to
    achylia gastrica 536.8
    Aerobacter aerogenes 008.2
    Bacillus coli - see Enteritis, E. coli
    bacteria NEC 008.5
    bile salts 579.8
    Capillaria
      hepatica 128.8
      philippinensis 127.5
    Clostridium perfringens (C) (F)
      008.46
    Enterobacter aerogenes 008.2
    enterococci 008.49
    Escherichia coli - see Enteritis, E. coli
    Giardia lamblia 007.1
    Heterophyes heterophyes 121.6
    irritating foods 787.91
    Metagonimus yokogawai 121.5
    Necator americanus 126.1
    Paracolobactrum arizonae 008.1
    Paracolon bacillus NEC 008.47
      Arizona 008.1
    Proteus (bacillus) (mirabilis)
      (Morganii) 008.3
    Pseudomonas aeruginosa 008.42
    S. japonicum 120.2
    specified organism NEC 008.8
      bacterial 008.49
      viral NEC 008.69
    Staphylococcus 008.41
    Streptococcus 008.49
      anaerobic 008.46
    Strongyloides stercoralis 127.2
    Trichuris trichiuria 127.3
    virus NEC (see also Enteritis, viral)
      008.69
  dysenteric 009.2
    due to specified organism NEC
      008.8
  dyspeptic 787.91
  endemic 009.3
    due to specified organism NEC
      008.8
  epidemic 009.2
    due to specified organism NEC
      008.8
  fermentative 787.91
  flagellate 007.9
  Flexner's (ulcerative) 004.1
  functional 564.5
    following gastrointestinal surgery
      564.4
    psychogenic 306.4
  giardial 007.1
  Giardia lamblia 007.1
  hill 579.1
  hyperperistalsis (nervous) 306.4
  infectious 009.2
    due to specified organism NEC
      008.8
    presumed 009.3
  inflammatory 787.91
    due to specified organism NEC
      008.8
  malarial (see also Malaria) 084.6
  mite 133.8
  mycotic 117.9
  nervous 306.4
  neurogenic 564.5
  parenteral NEC 009.2
  postgastrectomy 564.4
  postvagotomy 564.4
  prostaglandin induced 579.8

Diarrhea, diarrheal (Continued)
  protozoal NEC 007.9
  psychogenic 306.4
  septic 009.2
    due to specified organism NEC
      008.8
  specified organism NEC 008.8
    bacterial 008.49
    viral NEC 008.69
  Staphylococcus 008.41
  Streptococcus 008.49
    anaerobic 008.46
  toxic 558.2
  travelers' 009.2
    due to specified organism NEC
      008.8
  trichomonal 007.3
  tropical 579.1
  tuberculous 014.8●
  ulcerative (chronic) (see also Colitis,
    ulcerative) 556.9
  viral (see also Enteritis, viral) 008.8
  zymotic NEC 009.2
Diastasis
  cranial bones 733.99
    congenital 756.0
  joint (traumatic) - see Dislocation, by
    site
  muscle 728.84
    congenital 756.89
  recti (abdomen) 728.84
    complicating delivery 665.8●
    congenital 756.79
Diastema, teeth, tooth 524.30
Diastematomyelia 742.51
Diataxia, cerebral, infantile 343.0
Diathesis
  allergic V15.09
  bleeding (familial) 287.9
  cystine (familial) 270.0
  gouty 274.9
  hemorrhagic (familial) 287.9
    newborn NEC 776.0
  oxalic 271.8
  scrofulous (see also Tuberculosis)
    017.2●
  spasmophilic (see also Tetany) 781.7
  ulcer 536.9
  uric acid 274.9
Diaz's disease or osteochondrosis 732.5
Dibothriocephaliasis 123.4
  larval 123.5
Dibothriocephalus (infection)
  (infestation) (latus) 123.4
  larval 123.5
Dicephalus 759.4
Dichotomy, teeth 520.2
Dichromat, dichromata (congenital)
  368.59
Dichromatopsia (congenital) 368.59
Dichuchwa 104.0
Dicroceliasis 121.8
Didelphys, didelphic (see also Double
  uterus) 752.2
Didymitis (see also Epididymitis) 604.90
Died - see also Death
  without
    medical attention (cause unknown)
      798.9
    sign of disease 798.2
Dientamoeba diarrhea 007.8
Dietary
  inadequacy or deficiency 269.9
  surveillance and counseling V65.3

◀ New   ◀▥ Revised   ~~deleted~~ Deleted   ● Use Additional Digit(s)   ▭ Omit code

Dietl's crisis 593.4
Dieulafoy lesion (hemorrhagic)
   of
      duodenum 537.84
      esophagus 530.82
      intestine 569.86
      stomach 537.84
Difficult
   birth, affecting fetus or newborn
      763.9
   delivery NEC 669.9●
Difficulty
   feeding 783.3
      adult 783.3
      breast 676.8●
      child 783.3
      elderly 783.3
      infant 783.3
      newborn 779.31 ◄▥
      nonorganic (infant) NEC 307.59
   mechanical, gastroduodenal stoma
      537.89
   reading 315.00
   specific, spelling 315.09
   swallowing (see also Dysphagia)
      787.20
   walking 719.7
Diffuse - see condition
Diffused ganglion 727.42
Di George's syndrome (thymic
   hypoplasia) 279.11
Digestive - see condition
Di Guglielmo's disease or syndrome
   (M9841/3) 207.0●
Diktyoma (M9051/3) - see Neoplasm, by
   site, malignant
Dilaceration, tooth 520.4
Dilatation
   anus 564.89
      venule - see Hemorrhoids
   aorta (focal) (general) (see also
      Aneurysm, aorta) 441.9
      congenital 747.29
      infectional 093.0
      ruptured 441.5
      syphilitic 093.0
   appendix (cystic) 543.9
   artery 447.8
   bile duct (common) (cystic)
      (congenital) 751.69
      acquired 576.8
   bladder (sphincter) 596.8
      congenital 753.8
      in pregnancy or childbirth
         654.4●
         causing obstructed labor
            660.2●
            affecting fetus or newborn
               763.1
   blood vessel 459.89
   bronchus, bronchi 494.0
      with acute exacerbation 494.1
   calyx (due to obstruction) 593.89
   capillaries 448.9
   cardiac (acute) (chronic) (see also
      Hypertrophy, cardiac) 429.3
      congenital 746.89
         valve NEC 746.89
            pulmonary 746.09
      hypertensive (see also Hypertension,
         heart) 402.90
   cavum septi pellucidi 742.4
   cecum 564.89
      psychogenic 306.4

Dilatation (Continued)
   cervix (uteri) - see also Incompetency,
      cervix
      incomplete, poor, slow
         affecting fetus or newborn 763.7
         complicating delivery 661.0●
            affecting fetus or newborn
               763.7
   colon 564.7
      congenital 751.3
      due to mechanical obstruction
         560.89
      psychogenic 306.4
   common bile duct (congenital) 751.69
      acquired 576.8
         with calculus,
            choledocholithiasis, or
            stones - see
            Choledocholithiasis
   cystic duct 751.69
      acquired (any bile duct) 575.8
   duct, mammary 610.4
   duodenum 564.89
   esophagus 530.89
      congenital 750.4
      due to
         achalasia 530.0
         cardiospasm 530.0
   Eustachian tube, congenital 744.24
   fontanel 756.0
   gallbladder 575.8
      congenital 751.69
   gastric 536.8
      acute 536.1
      psychogenic 306.4
   heart (acute) (chronic) (see also
      Hypertrophy, cardiac) 429.3
      congenital 746.89
      hypertensive (see also Hypertension,
         heart) 402.90
      valve - see also Endocarditis
         congenital 746.89
   ileum 564.89
      psychogenic 306.4
   inguinal rings - see Hernia, inguinal
   jejunum 564.89
      psychogenic 306.4
   kidney (calyx) (collecting structures)
      (cystic) (parenchyma) (pelvis)
      593.89
   lacrimal passages 375.69
   lymphatic vessel 457.1
   mammary duct 610.4
   Meckel's diverticulum (congenital)
      751.0
   meningeal vessels, congenital 742.8
   myocardium (acute) (chronic) (see also
      Hypertrophy, cardiac) 429.3
   organ or site, congenital NEC - see
      Distortion
   pancreatic duct 577.8
   pelvis, kidney 593.89
   pericardium - see Pericarditis
   pharynx 478.29
   prostate 602.8
   pulmonary
      artery (idiopathic) 417.8
         congenital 747.3
      valve, congenital 746.09
   pupil 379.43
   rectum 564.89
   renal 593.89
   saccule vestibularis, congenital 744.05
   salivary gland (duct) 527.8

Dilatation (Continued)
   sphincter ani 564.89
   stomach 536.8
      acute 536.1
      psychogenic 306.4
   submaxillary duct 527.8
   trachea, congenital 748.3
   ureter (idiopathic) 593.89
      congenital 753.20
      due to obstruction 593.5
   urethra (acquired) 599.84
   vasomotor 443.9
   vein 459.89
   ventricular, ventricle (acute) (chronic)
      (see also Hypertrophy, cardiac)
      429.3
      cerebral, congenital 742.4
      hypertensive (see also Hypertension,
         heart) 402.90
   venule 459.89
      anus - see Hemorrhoids
   vesical orifice 596.8
Dilated, dilation - see Dilatation
Diminished
   hearing (acuity) (see also Deafness)
      389.9
   pulse pressure 785.9
   vision NEC 369.9
   vital capacity 794.2
Diminuta taenia 123.6
Diminution, sense or sensation (cold)
   (heat) (tactile) (vibratory) (see also
   Disturbance, sensation) 782.0
Dimitri-Sturge-Weber disease
   (encephalocutaneous angiomatosis)
   759.6
Dimple
   parasacral 685.1
      with abscess 685.0
   pilonidal 685.1
      with abscess 685.0
   postanal 685.1
      with abscess 685.0
Dioctophyma renale (infection)
   (infestation) 128.8
Dipetalonemiasis 125.4
Diphallus 752.69
Diphtheria, diphtheritic (gangrenous)
   (hemorrhagic) 032.9
   carrier (suspected) of V02.4
   cutaneous 032.85
   cystitis 032.84
   faucial 032.0
   infection of wound 032.85
   inoculation (anti) (not sick) V03.5
   laryngeal 032.3
   myocarditis 032.82
   nasal anterior 032.2
   nasopharyngeal 032.1
   neurological complication 032.89
   peritonitis 032.83
   specified site NEC 032.89
Diphyllobothriasis (intestine) 123.4
   larval 123.5
Diplacusis 388.41
Diplegia (upper limbs) 344.2
   brain or cerebral 437.8
   congenital 343.0
   facial 351.0
      congenital 352.6
   infantile or congenital (cerebral)
      (spastic) (spinal) 343.0
   lower limbs 344.1
   syphilitic, congenital 090.49

Diplococcus, diplococcal - *see* condition
Diplomyelia 742.59
Diplopia 368.2
  refractive 368.15
Dipsomania (*see also* Alcoholism) 303.9●
  with psychosis (*see also* Psychosis,
    alcoholic) 291.9
Dipylidiasis 123.8
  intestine 123.8
Direction, teeth, abnormal 524.30
Dirt-eating child 307.52
Disability
  heart - *see* Disease, heart
  learning NEC 315.2
  special spelling 315.09
Disarticulation (*see also* Derangement,
    joint) 718.9●
  meaning
    amputation
      status - *see* Absence, by site
      traumatic - *see* Amputation,
        traumatic
    dislocation, traumatic or congenital -
      see Dislocation
Disaster, cerebrovascular (*see also*
    Disease, cerebrovascular, acute) 436
Discharge
  anal NEC 787.99
  breast (female) (male) 611.79
  conjunctiva 372.89
  continued locomotor idiopathic (*see
    also* Epilepsy) 345.5●
  diencephalic autonomic idiopathic (*see
    also* Epilepsy) 345.5●
  ear 388.60
    blood 388.69
    cerebrospinal fluid 388.61
  excessive urine 788.42
  eye 379.93
  nasal 478.19
  nipple 611.79
  patterned motor idiopathic (*see also*
    Epilepsy) 345.5●
  penile 788.7
  postnasal - *see* Sinusitis
  sinus, from mediastinum 510.0
  umbilicus 789.9
  urethral 788.7
    bloody 599.84
  vaginal 623.5
Discitis 722.90
  cervical, cervicothoracic 722.91
  lumbar, lumbosacral 722.93
  thoracic, thoracolumbar 722.92
Discogenic syndrome - *see* Displacement,
    intervertebral disc
Discoid
  kidney 753.3
  meniscus, congenital 717.5
  semilunar cartilage 717.5
Discoloration
  mouth 528.9
  nails 703.8
  teeth 521.7
    due to
      drugs 521.7
      metals (copper) (silver) 521.7
      pulpal bleeding 521.7
    during formation 520.8
    extrinsic 523.6
    intrinsic posteruptive 521.7
Discomfort
  chest 786.59
  visual 368.13

Discomycosis - *see* Actinomycosis
Discontinuity, ossicles, ossicular chain
  385.23
Discrepancy
  centric occlusion
    maximum intercuspation 524.55
    of teeth 524.55
  leg length (acquired) 736.81
    congenital 755.30
  uterine size-date 649.6●
Discrimination
  political V62.4
  racial V62.4
  religious V62.4
  sex V62.4
Disease, diseased - *see also* Syndrome
  Abrami's (acquired hemolytic jaundice)
    283.9
  absorbent system 459.89
  accumulation - *see* Thesaurismosis
  acid-peptic 536.8
  Acosta's 993.2
  Adams-Stokes (-Morgagni) (syncope
    with heart block) 426.9
  Addison's (bronze) (primary adrenal
    insufficiency) 255.41
    anemia (pernicious) 281.0
    tuberculous (*see also* Tuberculosis)
      017.6●
  Addison-Gull - *see* Xanthoma
  adenoids (and tonsils) (chronic) 474.9
  adrenal (gland) (capsule) (cortex)
    255.9
    hyperfunction 255.3
    hypofunction 255.41
    specified type NEC 255.8
  ainhum (dactylolysis spontanea)
    136.0
  akamushi (scrub typhus) 081.2
  Akureyri (epidemic neuromyasthenia)
    049.8
  Albarrán's (colibacilluria) 791.9
  Albers-Schönberg's (marble bones)
    756.52
  Albert's 726.71
  Albright (-Martin) (-Bantam) 275.49
  Alibert's (mycosis fungoides)
    (M9700/3) 202.1●
  Alibert-Bazin (M9700/3) 202.1●
  alimentary canal 569.9
  alligator skin (ichthyosis congenita)
    757.1
    acquired 701.1
  Almeida's (Brazilian blastomycosis)
    116.1
  Alpers' 330.8
  alpine 993.2
  altitude 993.2
  alveoli, teeth 525.9
  Alzheimer's - *see* Alzheimer's
  amyloid (any site) 277.30
  anarthritic rheumatoid 446.5
  Anders' (adiposis tuberosa simplex)
    272.8
  Andersen's (glycogenosis IV) 271.0
  Anderson's (angiokeratoma corporis
    diffusum) 272.7
  Andes 993.2
  Andrews' (bacterid) 686.8
  angiopastic, angiospasmodic 443.9
    cerebral 435.9
      with transient neurologic deficit
        435.9
    vein 459.89

Disease, diseased (*Continued*)
  anterior
    chamber 364.9
    horn cell 335.9
      specified type NEC 335.8
  antral (chronic) 473.0
    acute 461.0
  anus NEC 569.49
  aorta (nonsyphilitic) 447.9
    syphilitic NEC 093.89
  aortic (heart) (valve) (*see also*
    Endocarditis, aortic) 424.1
  apollo 077.4
  aponeurosis 726.90
  appendix 543.9
  aqueous (chamber) 364.9
  arc-welders' lung 503
  Armenian 277.31
  Arnold-Chiari (*see also* Spina bifida)
    741.0●
  arterial 447.9
    occlusive (*see also* Occlusion, by site)
      444.22
      with embolus or thrombus - *see*
        Occlusion, by site
      due to stricture or stenosis 447.1
    specified type NEC 447.8
  arteriocardiorenal (*see also*
    Hypertension, cardiorenal) 404.90
  arteriolar (generalized) (obliterative)
    447.90
    specified type NEC 447.8
  arteriorenal - *see* Hypertension, kidney
  arteriosclerotic - *see also* Arteriosclerosis
    cardiovascular 429.2
    coronary - *see* Arteriosclerosis,
      coronary
    heart - *see* Arteriosclerosis, coronary
    vascular - *see* Arteriosclerosis
  artery 447.9
    cerebral 437.9
    coronary - *see* Arteriosclerosis,
      coronary
    specified type NEC 447.8
  arthropod-borne NEC 088.9
    specified type NEC 088.89
  Asboe-Hansen's (incontinentia
    pigmenti) 757.33
  atticoantral, chronic (with posterior or
    superior marginal perforation of
    ear drum) 382.2
  auditory canal, ear 380.9
  Aujeszky's 078.89
  auricle, ear NEC 380.30
  Australian X 062.4
  autoimmune NEC 279.49
    hemolytic (cold type) (warm type)
      283.0
    parathyroid 252.1
    thyroid 245.2
  aviators' (*see also* Effect, adverse, high
    altitude) 993.2
  ax(e)-grinders' 502
  Ayala's 756.89
  Ayerza's (pulmonary artery sclerosis
    with pulmonary hypertension)
    416.0
  Azorean (of the nervous system) 334.8
  Babington's (familial hemorrhagic
    telangiectasia) 448.0
  back bone NEC 733.90
  bacterial NEC 040.89
    zoonotic NEC 027.9
      specified type NEC 027.8

◀ New   ⬅ Revised   ~~deleted~~ Deleted   ● Use Additional Digit(s)   ▨ Omit code

Disease, diseased (*Continued*)
  Baehr-Schiffrin (thrombotic thrombocytopenic purpura) 446.6
  Baelz's (cheilitis glandularis apostematosa) 528.5
  Baerensprung's (eczema marginatum) 110.3
  Balfour's (chloroma) 205.3●
  balloon (*see also* Effect, adverse, high altitude) 993.2
  Baló's 341.1
  Bamberger (-Marie) (hypertrophic pulmonary osteoarthropathy) 731.2
  Bang's (Brucella abortus) 023.1
  Bannister's 995.1
  Banti's (with cirrhosis) (with portal hypertension) - *see* Cirrhosis, liver
  Barcoo (*see also* Ulcer, skin) 707.9
  barium lung 503
  Barlow (-Möller) (infantile scurvy) 267
  barometer makers' 985.0
  Barraquer (-Simons) (progressive lipodystrophy) 272.6
  basal ganglia 333.90
    degenerative NEC 333.0
    specified NEC 333.89
  Basedow's (exophthalmic goiter) 242.0●
  basement membrane NEC 583.89
    with
      pulmonary hemorrhage (Goodpasture's syndrome) 446.21 [583.81]
  Bateman's 078.0
    purpura (senile) 287.2
  Batten's 330.1 [362.71]
  Batten-Mayou (retina) 330.1 [362.71]
  Batten-Steinert 359.21
  Battey 031.0
  Baumgarten-Cruveilhier (cirrhosis of liver) 571.5
  bauxite-workers' 503
  Bayle's (dementia paralytica) 094.1
  Bazin's (primary) (*see also* Tuberculosis) 017.1●
  Beard's (neurasthenia) 300.5
  Beau's (*see also* Degeneration, myocardial) 429.1
  Bechterew's (ankylosing spondylitis) 720.0
  Becker's
    idiopathic mural endomyocardial disease 425.2
    myotonia congenita, recessive form 359.22
  Begbie's (exophthalmic goiter) 242.0●
  Behr's 362.50
  Beigel's (white piedra) 111.2
  Bekhterev's (ankylosing spondylitis) 720.0
  Bell's (*see also* Psychosis, affective) 296.0●
  Bennett's (leukemia) 208.9●
  Benson's 379.22
  Bergeron's (hysteroepilepsy) 300.11
  Berlin's 921.3
  Bernard-Soulier (thrombopathy) 287.1
  Bernhardt (-Roth) 355.1
  beryllium 503
  Besnier-Boeck (-Schaumann) (sarcoidosis) 135
  Best's 362.76

Disease, diseased (*Continued*)
  Beurmann's (sporotrichosis) 117.1
  Bielschowsky (-Jansky) 330.1
  Biermer's (pernicious anemia) 281.0
  Biett's (discoid lupus erythematosus) 695.4
  bile duct (*see also* Disease, biliary) 576.9
  biliary (duct) (tract) 576.9
    with calculus, choledocholithiasis, or stones - *see* Choledocholithiasis
  Billroth's (meningocele) (*see also* Spina bifida) 741.9●
  Binswanger's 290.12
  Bird's (oxaluria) 271.8
  bird fanciers' 495.2
  black lung 500
  bladder 596.9
    specified NEC 596.8
  bleeder's 286.0
  Bloch-Sulzberger (incontinentia pigmenti) 757.33
  Blocq's (astasia-abasia) 307.9
  blood (-forming organs) 289.9
    specified NEC 289.89
    vessel 459.9
  Bloodgood's 610.1
  Blount's (tibia vara) 732.4
  blue 746.9
  Bodechtel-Guttmann (subacute sclerosing panencephalitis) 046.2
  Boeck's (sarcoidosis) 135
  bone 733.90
    fibrocystic NEC 733.29
      jaw 526.2
    marrow 289.9
    Paget's (osteitis deformans) 731.0
    specified type NEC 733.99
    von Recklinghausen's (osteitis fibrosa cystica) 252.01
  Bonfils' - *see* Disease, Hodgkin's
  Borna 062.9
  Bornholm (epidemic pleurodynia) 074.1
  Bostock's (*see also* Fever, hay) 477.9
  Bouchard's (myopathic dilatation of the stomach) 536.1
  Bouillaud's (rheumatic heart disease) 391.9
  Bourneville (-Brissaud) (tuberous sclerosis) 759.5
  Bouveret (-Hoffmann) (paroxysmal tachycardia) 427.2
  bowel 569.9
    functional 564.9
      psychogenic 306.4
  Bowen's (M8081/2) - *see* Neoplasm, skin, in situ
  Bozzolo's (multiple myeloma) (M9730/3) 203.0●
  Bradley's (epidemic vomiting) 078.82
  Brailsford's 732.3
    radius, head 732.3
    tarsal, scaphoid 732.5
  Brailsford-Morquio (mucopolysaccharidosis IV) 277.5
  brain 348.9
    Alzheimer's 331.0
      with dementia - *see* Alzheimer's, dementia
    arterial, artery 437.9
    arteriosclerotic 437.0

Disease, diseased (*Continued*)
  brain (*Continued*)
    congenital 742.9
    degenerative - *see* Degeneration, brain
    inflammatory - *see also* Encephalitis
      late effect - *see* category 326
    organic 348.9
      arteriosclerotic 437.0
    parasitic NEC 123.9
    Pick's 331.11
      with dementia
        with behavioral disturbance 331.11 [294.11]
        without behavioral disturbance 331.11 [294.10]
    senile 331.2
  braziers' 985.8
  breast 611.9
    cystic (chronic) 610.1
    fibrocystic 610.1
    inflammatory 611.0
    Paget's (M8540/3) 174.0
    puerperal, postpartum NEC 676.3●
    specified NEC 611.89
  Breda's (*see also* Yaws) 102.9
  Breisky's (kraurosis vulvae) 624.09
  Bretonneau's (diphtheritic malignant angina) 032.0
  Bright's (*see also* Nephritis) 583.9
    arteriosclerotic (*see also* Hypertension, kidney) 403.90
  Brill's (recrudescent typhus) 081.1
    flea-borne 081.0
    louse-borne 081.1
  Brill-Symmers (follicular lymphoma) (M9690/3) 202.0●
  Brill-Zinsser (recrudescent typhus) 081.1
  Brinton's (leather bottle stomach) (M8142/3) 151.9
  Brion-Kayser (*see also* Fever, paratyphoid) 002.9
  broad
    beta 272.2
    ligament, noninflammatory 620.9
      specified NEC 620.8
  Brocq's 691.8
    meaning
      atopic (diffuse) neurodermatitis 691.8
      dermatitis herpetiformis 694.0
      lichen simplex chronicus 698.3
      parapsoriasis 696.2
      prurigo 698.2
  Brocq-Duhring (dermatitis herpetiformis) 694.0
  Brodie's (joint) (*see also* Osteomyelitis) 730.1●
  bronchi 519.19
  bronchopulmonary 519.19
  bronze (Addison's) 255.41
    tuberculous (*see also* Tuberculosis) 017.6●
  Brown-Séquard 344.89
  Bruck's 733.99
  Bruck-de Lange (Amsterdam dwarf, mental retardation, and brachycephaly) 759.89
  Bruhl's (splenic anemia with fever) 285.8
  Bruton's (X-linked agammaglobulinemia) 279.04

Disease, diseased *(Continued)*
  buccal cavity 528.9
  Buchanan's (juvenile osteochondrosis,
      iliac crest) 732.1
  Buchman's (osteochondrosis juvenile)
      732.1
  Budgerigar-Fanciers' 495.2
  Budinger-Ludloff-Läwen 717.89
  Büerger's (thromboangiitis obliterans)
      443.1
  Burger-Grütz (essential familial
      hyperlipemia) 272.1
  Burns' (lower ulna) 732.3
  bursa 727.9
  Bury's (erythema elevatum diutinum)
      695.89
  Buschke's 710.1
  Busquet's (*see also* Osteomyelitis)
      730.1●
  Busse-Buschke (cryptococcosis) 117.5
  C₂ (*see also* Alcoholism) 303.9●
  Caffey's (infantile cortical hyperostosis)
      756.59
  caisson 993.3
  calculous 592.9
  California 114.0
  Calvé (-Perthes) (osteochondrosis,
      femoral capital) 732.1
  Camurati-Engelmann (diaphyseal
      sclerosis) 756.59
  Canavan's 330.0
  capillaries 448.9
  Carapata 087.1
  cardiac - *see* Disease, heart
  cardiopulmonary, chronic 416.9
  cardiorenal (arteriosclerotic) (hepatic)
      (hypertensive) (vascular) (*see also*
      Hypertension, cardiorenal)
      404.90
  cardiovascular (arteriosclerotic) 429.2
    congenital 746.9
    hypertensive (*see also* Hypertension,
        heart) 402.90
      benign 402.10
      malignant 402.00
    renal (*see also* Hypertension,
        cardiorenal) 404.90
    syphilitic (asymptomatic) 093.9
  carotid gland 259.8
  Carrión's (Bartonellosis) 088.0
  cartilage NEC 733.90
    specified NEC 733.99
  Castellani's 104.8
  cat-scratch 078.3
  Cavare's (familial periodic paralysis)
      359.3
  Cazenave's (pemphigus) 694.4
  cecum 569.9
  celiac (adult) 579.0
    infantile 579.0
  cellular tissue NEC 709.9
  central core 359.0
  cerebellar, cerebellum - *see* Disease,
      brain
  cerebral (*see also* Disease, brain) 348.9
    arterial, artery 437.9
    degenerative - *see* Degeneration,
        brain
  cerebrospinal 349.9
  cerebrovascular NEC 437.9
    acute 436
      embolic - *see* Embolism, brain
      late effect - *see* Late effect(s) (of)
          cerebrovascular disease

Disease, diseased *(Continued)*
  cerebrovascular NEC *(Continued)*
    acute *(Continued)*
      puerperal, postpartum, childbirth
          674.0●
      thrombotic - *see* Thrombosis,
          brain
    arteriosclerotic 437.0
    embolic - *see* Embolism, brain
    ischemic, generalized NEC 437.1
    late effect - *see* Late effect(s) (of)
        cerebrovascular disease
    occlusive 437.1
    puerperal, postpartum, childbirth
        674.0●
    specified type NEC 437.8
    thrombotic - *see* Thrombosis, brain
  ceroid storage 272.7
  cervix (uteri)
    inflammatory 616.0
    noninflammatory 622.9
      specified NEC 622.8
  Chabert's 022.9
  Chagas' (*see also* Trypanosomiasis,
      American) 086.2
  Chandler's (osteochondritis dissecans,
      hip) 732.7
  Charcôt's (joint) 094.0 [713.5]
    spinal cord 094.0
  Charcôt-Marie-Tooth 356.1
  Charlouis' (*see also* Yaws) 102.9
  Cheadle (-Möller) (-Barlow) (infantile
      scurvy) 267
  Chédiak-Steinbrinck (-Higashi)
      (congenital gigantism of
      peroxidase granules) 288.2
  cheek, inner 528.9
  chest 519.9
  Chiari's (hepatic vein thrombosis) 453.0
  Chicago (North American
      blastomycosis) 116.0
  chignon (white piedra) 111.2
  chigoe, chigo (jigger) 134.1
  childhood granulomatous 288.1
  Chinese liver fluke 121.1
  chlamydial NEC 078.88
  cholecystic (*see also* Disease,
      gallbladder) 575.9
  choroid 363.9
    degenerative (*see also* Degeneration,
        choroid) 363.40
    hereditary (*see also* Dystrophy,
        choroid) 363.50
    specified type NEC 363.8
  Christian's (chronic histiocytosis X)
      277.89
  Christian-Weber (nodular
      nonsuppurative panniculitis)
      729.30
  Christmas 286.1
  ciliary body 364.9
    specified NEC 364.89
  circulatory (system) NEC 459.9
    chronic, maternal, affecting fetus or
        newborn 760.3
    specified NEC 459.89
    syphilitic 093.9
      congenital 090.5
  Civatte's (poikiloderma) 709.09
  climacteric 627.2
    male 608.89
  coagulation factor deficiency
      (congenital) (*see also* Defect,
      coagulation) 286.9

Disease, diseased *(Continued)*
  Coats' 362.12
  coccidioidal pulmonary 114.5
    acute 114.0
    chronic 114.4
    primary 114.0
    residual 114.4
  Cockayne's (microcephaly and
      dwarfism) 759.89
  Cogan's 370.52
  cold
    agglutinin 283.0
      or hemoglobinuria 283.0
        paroxysmal (cold) (nocturnal)
            283.2
    hemagglutinin (chronic) 283.0
  collagen NEC 710.9
    nonvascular 710.9
    specified NEC 710.8
    vascular (allergic) (*see also* Angiitis,
        hypersensitivity) 446.20
  colon 569.9
    functional 564.9
      congenital 751.3
    ischemic 557.0
  combined system (of spinal cord) 266.2
      [336.2]
    with anemia (pernicious) 281.0
        [336.2]
  compressed air 993.3
  Concato's (pericardial polyserositis)
      423.2
    peritoneal 568.82
    pleural - *see* Pleurisy
  congenital NEC 799.89
  conjunctiva 372.9
    chlamydial 077.98
      specified NEC 077.8
    specified type NEC 372.89
    viral 077.99
      specified NEC 077.8
  connective tissue, diffuse (*see also*
      Disease, collagen) 710.9
  Conor and Bruch's (boutonneuse fever)
      082.1
  Conradi (-Hünermann) 756.59
  Cooley's (erythroblastic anemia)
      282.49
  Cooper's 610.1
  Corbus' 607.1
  cork-handlers' 495.3
  cornea (*see also* Keratopathy) 371.9
  coronary (*see also* Ischemia, heart)
      414.9
    congenital 746.85
    ostial, syphilitic 093.20
      aortic 093.22
      mitral 093.21
      pulmonary 093.24
      tricuspid 093.23
  Corrigan's - *see* Insufficiency, aortic
  Cotugno's 724.3
  Coxsackie (virus) NEC 074.8
  cranial nerve NEC 352.9
  Creutzfeldt-Jakob (CJD) 046.19
    with dementia
      with behavioral disturbance
          046.19 [294.11]
      without behavioral disturbance
          046.19 [294.10]
    familial 046.19
    iatrogenic 046.19
    specified NEC 046.19
    sporadic 046.19

◀ New   ◀|||| Revised   ~~deleted~~ Deleted   ● Use Additional Digit(s)   ▨ Omit code

Disease, diseased *(Continued)*
Creutzfeldt-Jakob *(Continued)*
variant (vCJD) 046.11
with dementia
with behavioral disturbance
046.11 *[294.11]*
without behavioral
disturbance 046.11
[294.10]
Crigler-Najjar (congenital
hyperbilirubinemia) 277.4
Crocq's (acrocyanosis) 443.89
Crohn's (intestine) *(see also* Enteritis,
regional) 555.9
Crouzon's (craniofacial dysostosis)
756.0
Cruchet's (encephalitis lethargica)
049.8
Cruveilhier's 335.21
Cruz-Chagas *(see also*
Trypanosomiasis,
American) 086.2
crystal deposition *(see also* Arthritis,
due to, crystals) 712.9●
Csillag's (lichen sclerosus et
atrophicus) 701.0
Curschmann's 359.21
Cushing's (pituitary basophilism)
255.0
cystic
breast (chronic) 610.1
kidney, congenital *(see also* Cystic,
disease, kidney) 753.10
liver, congenital 751.62
lung 518.89
congenital 748.4
pancreas 577.2
congenital 751.7
renal, congenital *(see also* Cystic,
disease, kidney) 753.10
semilunar cartilage 717.5
cysticercus 123.1
cystine storage (with renal sclerosis)
270.0
cytomegalic inclusion (generalized)
078.5
with
pneumonia 078.5 *[484.1]*
congenital 771.1
Daae (-Finsen) (epidemic pleurodynia)
074.1
dancing 297.8
Danielssen's (anesthetic leprosy)
030.1
Darier's (congenital) (keratosis
follicularis) 757.39
erythema annulare centrifugum
695.0
vitamin A deficiency 264.8
Darling's (histoplasmosis) *(see also*
Histoplasmosis, American)
115.00
Davies' 425.0
de Beurmann-Gougerot
(sporotrichosis) 117.1
Débove's (splenomegaly) 789.2
deer fly *(see also* Tularemia) 021.9
deficiency 269.9
degenerative - *see also* Degeneration
disc - *see* Degeneration,
intervertebral disc
Degos' 447.8
Déjérine (-Sottas) 356.0
Déleage's 359.89

Disease, diseased *(Continued)*
demyelinating, demyelinizating (brain
stem) (central nervous system)
341.9
multiple sclerosis 340
specified NEC 341.8
de Quervain's (tendon sheath) 727.04
thyroid (subacute granulomatous
thyroiditis) 245.1
Dercum's (adiposis dolorosa) 272.8
Deutschländer's - *see* Fracture, foot
Devergie's (pityriasis rubra pilaris)
696.4
Devic's 341.0
diaphorase deficiency 289.7
diaphragm 519.4
diarrheal, infectious 009.2
diatomaceous earth 502
Diaz's (osteochondrosis astragalus)
732.5
digestive system 569.9
Di Guglielmo's (erythemic myelosis)
(M9841/3) 207.0●
Dimitri-Sturge-Weber
(encephalocutaneous
angiomatosis) 759.6
disc, degenerative - *see* Degeneration,
intervertebral disc
discogenic *(see also* Disease,
intervertebral disc) 722.90
diverticular - *see* Diverticula
Down's (mongolism) 758.0
Dubini's (electric chorea) 049.8
Dubois' (thymus gland) 090.5
Duchenne's 094.0
locomotor ataxia 094.0
muscular dystrophy 359.1
paralysis 335.22
pseudohypertrophy, muscles 359.1
Duchenne-Griesinger 359.1
ductless glands 259.9
Duhring's (dermatitis herpetiformis)
694.0
Dukes (-Filatov) 057.8
duodenum NEC 537.9
specified NEC 537.89
Duplay's 726.2
Dupré's (meningism) 781.6
Dupuytren's (muscle contracture) 728.6
Durand-Nicolas-Favre (climatic bubo)
099.1
Duroziez's (congenital mitral stenosis)
746.5
Dutton's (trypanosomiasis) 086.9
Eales' 362.18
ear (chronic) (inner) NEC 388.9
middle 385.9
adhesive *(see also* Adhesions,
middle ear) 385.10
specified NEC 385.89
Eberth's (typhoid fever) 002.0
Ebstein's
heart 746.2
meaning diabetes 250.4● *[581.81]*
due to secondary diabetes 249.4●
[581.81]
Echinococcus *(see also* Echinococcus)
122.9
ECHO virus NEC 078.89
Economo's (encephalitis lethargica)
049.8
Eddowes' (brittle bones and blue
sclera) 756.51
Edsall's 992.2

Disease, diseased *(Continued)*
Eichstedt's (pityriasis versicolor) 111.0
Ellis-van Creveld (chondroectodermal
dysplasia) 756.55
endocardium - *see* Endocarditis
endocrine glands or system NEC 259.9
specified NEC 259.8
endomyocardial, idiopathic mural 425.2
Engel-von Recklinghausen (osteitis
fibrosa cystica) 252.01
Engelmann's (diaphyseal sclerosis)
756.59
English (rickets) 268.0
Engman's (infectious eczematoid
dermatitis) 690.8
enteroviral, enterovirus NEC 078.89
central nervous system NEC 048
epidemic NEC 136.9
epididymis 608.9
epigastric, functional 536.9
psychogenic 306.4
Erb (-Landouzy) 359.1
Erb-Goldflam 358.00
Erdheim-Chester (ECD) 277.89   ◄
Erichsen's (railway spine) 300.16
esophagus 530.9
functional 530.5
psychogenic 306.4
Eulenburg's (congenital paramyotonia)
359.29
Eustachian tube 381.9
Evans' (thrombocytopenic purpura)
287.32
external auditory canal 380.9
extrapyramidal NEC 333.90
eye 379.90
anterior chamber 364.9
inflammatory NEC 364.3
muscle 378.9
eyeball 360.9
eyelid 374.9
eyeworm of Africa 125.2
Fabry's (angiokeratoma corporis
diffusum) 272.7
facial nerve (seventh) 351.9
newborn 767.5
Fahr-Volhard (malignant
nephrosclerosis) 403.00
fallopian tube, noninflammatory 620.9
specified NEC 620.8
familial periodic 277.31
paralysis 359.3
Fanconi's (congenital pancytopenia)
284.09
Farber's (disseminated
lipogranulomatosis) 272.8
fascia 728.9
inflammatory 728.9
Fauchard's (periodontitis) 523.40
Favre-Durand-Nicolas (climatic bubo)
099.1
Favre-Racouchot (elastoidosis cutanea
nodularis) 701.8
Fede's 529.0
Feer's 985.0
Felix's (juvenile osteochondrosis, hip)
732.1
Fenwick's (gastric atrophy) 537.89
Fernels' (aortic aneurysm) 441.9
fibrocaseous, of lung *(see also*
Tuberculosis, pulmonary) 011.9●
fibrocystic - *see also* Fibrocystic, disease
newborn 277.01
Fiedler's (leptospiral jaundice) 100.0

Disease, diseased *(Continued)*
fifth 057.0
Filatoff's (infectious mononucleosis)
075
Filatov's (infectious mononucleosis)
075
file-cutters' 984.9
specified type of lead - *see* Table of
Drugs and Chemicals
filterable virus NEC 078.89
fish skin 757.1
acquired 701.1
Flajani (-Basedow) (exophthalmic
goiter) 242.0●
Flatau-Schilder 341.1
flax-dressers' 504
Fleischner's 732.3
flint 502
fluke - *see* Infestation, fluke
Følling's (phenylketonuria) 270.1
foot and mouth 078.4
foot process 581.3
Forbes' (glycogenosis III) 271.0
Fordyce's (ectopic sebaceous glands)
(mouth) 750.26
Fordyce-Fox (apocrine miliaria) 705.82
Fothergill's
meaning scarlatina anginosa 034.1
neuralgia (*see also* Neuralgia,
trigeminal) 350.1
Fournier's 608.83
fourth 057.8
Fox (-Fordyce) (apocrine miliaria)
705.82
Francis' (*see also* Tularemia) 021.9
Franklin's (heavy chain) 273.2
Frei's (climatic bubo) 099.1
Freiberg's (flattening metatarsal) 732.5
Friedländer's (endarteritis obliterans) -
see Arteriosclerosis
Friedreich's
combined systemic or ataxia 334.0
facial hemihypertrophy 756.0
myoclonia 333.2
Fröhlich's (adiposogenital dystrophy)
253.8
Frommel's 676.6●
frontal sinus (chronic) 473.1
acute 461.1
Fuller's earth 502
fungus, fungous NEC 117.9
Gaisböck's (polycythemia hypertonica)
289.0
gallbladder 575.9
congenital 751.60
Gamna's (siderotic splenomegaly)
289.51
Gamstorp's (adynamia episodica
hereditaria) 359.3
Gandy-Nanta (siderotic splenomegaly)
289.51
Gannister (occupational) 502
Garré's (*see also* Osteomyelitis) 730.1●
gastric (*see also* Disease, stomach) 537.9
gastroesophageal reflux (GERD)
530.81
gastrointestinal (tract) 569.9
amyloid 277.39
functional 536.9
psychogenic 306.4
Gaucher's (adult) (cerebroside
lipidosis) (infantile) 272.7
Gayet's (superior hemorrhagic
polioencephalitis) 265.1

Disease, diseased *(Continued)*
Gee (-Herter) (-Heubner) (-Thaysen)
(nontropical sprue) 579.0
generalized neoplastic (M8000/6) 199.0
genital organs NEC
female 629.9
specified NEC 629.89
male 608.9
Gerhardt's (erythromelalgia) 443.82
Gerlier's (epidemic vertigo) 078.81
Gibert's (pityriasis rosea) 696.3
Gibney's (perispondylitis) 720.9
Gierke's (glycogenosis I) 271.0
Gilbert's (familial nonhemolytic
jaundice) 277.4
Gilchrist's (North American
blastomycosis) 116.0
Gilford (-Hutchinson) (progeria) 259.8
Gilles de la Tourette's (motor-verbal
tic) 307.23
Giovannini's 117.9
gland (lymph) 289.9
Glanzmann's (hereditary hemorrhagic
thrombasthenia) 287.1
glassblowers' 527.1
Glénard's (enteroptosis) 569.89
Glisson's (*see also* Rickets) 268.0
glomerular
membranous, idiopathic 581.1
minimal change 581.3
glycogen storage (Andersen's) (Cori
types 1-7) (Forbes') (McArdle-
Schmid-Pearson) (Pompe's)
(types I-VII) 271.0
cardiac 271.0 *[425.7]*
generalized 271.0
glucose-6-phosphatase deficiency
271.0
heart 271.0 *[425.7]*
hepatorenal 271.0
liver and kidneys 271.0
myocardium 271.0 *[425.7]*
von Gierke's (glycogenosis I)
271.0
Goldflam-Erb 358.00
Goldscheider's (epidermolysis bullosa)
757.39
Goldstein's (familial hemorrhagic
telangiectasia) 448.0
gonococcal NEC 098.0
Goodall's (epidemic vomiting) 078.82
Gordon's (exudative enteropathy)
579.8
Gougerot's (trisymptomatic) 709.1
Gougerot-Carteaud (confluent
reticulate papillomatosis) 701.8
Gougerot-Hailey-Hailey (benign
familial chronic pemphigus)
757.39
graft-versus-host 279.50
acute 279.51
on chronic 279.53
chronic 279.52
grain-handlers' 495.8
Grancher's (splenopneumonia) - *see*
Pneumonia
granulomatous (childhood) (chronic)
288.1
graphite lung 503
Graves' (exophthalmic goiter) 242.0●
Greenfield's 330.0
green monkey 078.89
Griesinger's (*see also* Ancylostomiasis)
126.9

Disease, diseased *(Continued)*
grinders' 502
Grisel's 723.5
Gruby's (tinea tonsurans) 110.0
Guertin's (electric chorea) 049.8
Guillain-Barré 357.0
Guinon's (motor-verbal tic) 307.23
Gull's (thyroid atrophy with
myxedema) 244.8
Gull and Sutton's - *see* Hypertension,
kidney
gum NEC 523.9
Günther's (congenital erythropoietic
porphyria) 277.1
gynecological 629.9
specified NEC 629.89
H 270.0
Haas' 732.3
Habermann's (acute parapsoriasis
varioliformis) 696.2
Haff 985.1
Hageman (congenital factor XII
deficiency) (*see also* Defect,
congenital) 286.3
Haglund's (osteochondrosis os tibiale
externum) 732.5
Hagner's (hypertrophic pulmonary
osteoarthropathy) 731.2
Hailey-Hailey (benign familial chronic
pemphigus) 757.39
hair (follicles) NEC 704.9
specified type NEC 704.8
Hallervorden-Spatz 333.0
Hallopeau's (lichen sclerosus et
atrophicus) 701.0
Hamman's (spontaneous mediastinal
emphysema) 518.1
hand, foot, and mouth 074.3
Hand-Schüller-Christian (chronic
histiocytosis X) 277.89
Hanot's - *see* Cirrhosis, biliary
Hansen's (leprosy) 030.9
benign form 030.1
malignant form 030.0
Harada's 363.22
Harley's (intermittent hemoglobinuria)
283.2
Hart's (pellagra-cerebellar ataxia-renal
aminoaciduria) 270.0
Hartnup (pellagra-cerebellar ataxia-
renal aminoaciduria) 270.0
Hashimoto's (struma lymphomatosa)
245.2
Hb - *see* Disease, hemoglobin
heart (organic) 429.9
with
acute pulmonary edema (*see also*
Failure, ventricular, left)
428.1
hypertensive 402.91
with renal failure 404.92
benign 402.11
with renal failure 404.12
malignant 402.01
with renal failure 404.02
kidney disease - *see*
Hypertension,
cardiorenal
rheumatic fever (conditions
classifiable to 390)
active 391.9
with chorea 392.0
inactive or quiescent (with
chorea) 398.90

◀ New   ◀▥ Revised   ~~deleted~~ Deleted   ● Use Additional Digit(s)   ▨ Omit code

Disease, diseased *(Continued)*
  heart *(Continued)*
    amyloid 277.39 *[425.7]*
    aortic (valve) *(see also* Endocarditis, aortic) 424.1
    arteriosclerotic or sclerotic (minimal) (senile) - *see* Arteriosclerosis, coronary
    artery, arterial - *see* Arteriosclerosis, coronary
    atherosclerotic - *see* Arteriosclerosis, coronary
    beer drinkers' 425.5
    beriberi 265.0 *[425.7]*
    black 416.0
    congenital NEC 746.9
      cyanotic 746.9
      maternal, affecting fetus or newborn 760.3
      specified type NEC 746.89
    congestive *(see also* Failure, heart) 428.0
    coronary 414.9
    cryptogenic 429.9
    due to
      amyloidosis 277.39 *[425.7]*
      beriberi 265.0 *[425.7]*
      cardiac glycogenosis 271.0 *[425.7]*
      Friedreich's ataxia 334.0 *[425.8]*
      gout 274.82
      mucopolysaccharidosis 277.5 *[425.7]*
      myotonia atrophica 359.21 *[425.8]*
      progressive muscular dystrophy 359.1 *[425.8]*
      sarcoidosis 135 *[425.8]*
    fetal 746.9
      inflammatory 746.89
    fibroid *(see also* Myocarditis) 429.0
    functional 427.9
      postoperative 997.1
      psychogenic 306.2
    glycogen storage 271.0 *[425.7]*
    gonococcal NEC 098.85
    gouty 274.82
    hypertensive *(see also* Hypertension, heart) 402.90
      benign 402.10
      malignant 402.00
    hyperthyroid *(see also* Hyperthyroidism) 242.9● *[425.7]*
    incompletely diagnosed - *see* Disease, heart
    ischemic (chronic) *(see also* Ischemia, heart) 414.9
      acute *(see also* Infarct, myocardium) 410.9●
        without myocardial infarction 411.89
          with coronary (artery) occlusion 411.81
      asymptomatic 412
      diagnosed on ECG or other special investigation but currently presenting no symptoms 412
    kyphoscoliotic 416.1
    mitral *(see also* Endocarditis, mitral) 394.9
    muscular *(see also* Degeneration, myocardial) 429.1
    postpartum 674.8●
    psychogenic (functional) 306.2

Disease, diseased *(Continued)*
  heart *(Continued)*
    pulmonary (chronic) 416.9
      acute 415.0
      specified NEC 416.8
    rheumatic (chronic) (inactive) (old) (quiescent) (with chorea) 398.90
      active or acute 391.9
        with chorea (active) (rheumatic) (Sydenham's) 392.0
        specified type NEC 391.8
      maternal, affecting fetus or newborn 760.3
    rheumatoid - *see* Arthritis, rheumatoid
    sclerotic - *see* Arteriosclerosis, coronary
    senile *(see also* Myocarditis) 429.0
    specified type NEC 429.89
    syphilitic 093.89
      aortic 093.1
        aneurysm 093.0
      asymptomatic 093.89
      congenital 090.5
    thyroid (gland) *(see also* Hyperthyroidism) 242.9● *[425.7]*
    thyrotoxic *(see also* Thyrotoxicosis) 242.9● *[425.7]*
    tuberculous *(see also* Tuberculosis) 017.9● *[425.8]*
    valve, valvular (obstructive) (regurgitant) - *see also* Endocarditis
      congenital NEC *(see also* Anomaly, heart, valve) 746.9
      pulmonary 746.00
      specified type NEC 746.89
    vascular - *see* Disease, cardiovascular
  heavy-chain (gamma G) 273.2
  Heberden's 715.04
  Hebra's
    dermatitis exfoliativa 695.89
    erythema multiforme exudativum 695.19
    pityriasis
      maculata et circinata 696.3
      rubra 695.89
      pilaris 696.4
    prurigo 698.2
  Heerfordt's (uveoparotitis) 135
  Heidenhain's 290.10
    with dementia 290.10
  Heilmeyer-Schöner (M9842/3) 207.1●
  Heine-Medin *(see also* Poliomyelitis) 045.9●
  Heller's *(see also* Psychosis, childhood) 299.1●
  Heller-Döhle (syphilitic aortitis) 093.1
  hematopoietic organs 289.9
  hemoglobin (Hb) 282.7
    with thalassemia 282.49
    abnormal (mixed) NEC 282.7
      with thalassemia 282.49
    AS genotype 282.5
    Bart's 282.49
    C (Hb-C) 282.7
      with other abnormal hemoglobin NEC 282.7
      elliptocytosis 282.7

Disease, diseased *(Continued)*
  hemoglobin (Hb) *(Continued)*
    C (Hb-C) *(Continued)*
      Hb-S (without crisis) 282.63
        with
          crisis 282.64
          vaso-occlusive pain 282.64
      sickle-cell (without crisis) 282.63
        with
          crisis 282.64
          vaso-occlusive pain 282.64
      thalassemia 282.49
    constant spring 282.7
    D (Hb-D) 282.7
      with other abnormal hemoglobin NEC 282.7
      Hb-S (without crisis) 282.68
        with crisis 282.69
      sickle-cell (without crisis) 282.68
        with crisis 282.69
      thalassemia 282.49
    E (Hb-E) 282.7
      with other abnormal hemoglobin NEC 282.7
      Hb-S (without crisis) 282.68
        with crisis 282.69
      sickle-cell (without crisis) 282.68
        with crisis 282.69
      thalassemia 282.49
    elliptocytosis 282.7
    F (Hb-F) 282.7
    G (Hb-G) 282.7
    H (Hb-H) 282.49
    hereditary persistence, fetal (HPFH) ("Swiss variety") 282.7
    high fetal gene 282.7
    I thalassemia 282.49
    M 289.7
    S - *see also* Disease, sickle-cell, Hb-S
      thalassemia (without crisis) 282.41
        with
          crisis 282.42
          vaso-occlusive pain 282.42
    spherocytosis 282.7
    unstable, hemolytic 282.7
    Zurich (Hb-Zurich) 282.7
  hemolytic (fetus) (newborn) 773.2
    autoimmune (cold type) (warm type) 283.0
    due to or with
      incompatibility
        ABO (blood group) 773.1
        blood (group) (Duffy) (Kell) (Kidd) (Lewis) (M) (S) NEC 773.2
        Rh (blood group) (factor) 773.0
        Rh negative mother 773.0
    unstable hemoglobin 282.7
  hemorrhagic 287.9
    newborn 776.0
  Henoch (-Schönlein) (purpura nervosa) 287.0
  hepatic - *see* Disease, liver
  hepatolenticular 275.1
  heredodegenerative NEC
    brain 331.89
    spinal cord 336.8
  Hers' (glycogenosis VI) 271.0
  Herter (-Gee) (-Heubner) (nontropical sprue) 579.0
  Herxheimer's (diffuse idiopathic cutaneous atrophy) 701.8
  Heubner's 094.89

Disease, diseased *(Continued)*
  Heubner-Herter (nontropical sprue) 579.0
  high fetal gene or hemoglobin thalassemia 282.49
  Hildenbrand's (typhus) 081.9
  hip (joint) NEC 719.95
    congenital 755.63
    suppurative 711.05
    tuberculous *(see also* Tuberculosis) 015.1● *[730.85]*
  Hippel's (retinocerebral angiomatosis) 759.6
  Hirschfeld's (acute diabetes mellitus) *(see also* Diabetes) 250.0●
    due to secondary diabetes 249.0●
  Hirschsprung's (congenital megacolon) 751.3
  His (-Werner) (trench fever) 083.1
  HIV 042
  Hodgkin's (M9650/3) 201.9●

Note 22   Use the following fifth-digit subclassification with category 201:

  0   unspecified site
  1   lymph nodes of head, face, and neck
  2   intrathoracic lymph nodes
  3   intra-abdominal lymph nodes
  4   lymph nodes of axilla and upper limb
  5   lymph nodes of inguinal region and lower limb
  6   intrapelvic lymph nodes
  7   spleen
  8   lymph nodes of multiple sites

---

  lymphocytic
    depletion (M9653/3) 201.7●
      diffuse fibrosis (M9654/3) 201.7●
      reticular type (M9655/3) 201.7●
    predominance (M9651/3) 201.4●
  lymphocytic-histiocytic
    predominance (M9651/3) 201.4●
  mixed cellularity (M9652/3) 201.6●
  nodular sclerosis (M9656/3) 201.5●
    cellular phase (M9657/3) 201.5●
  Hodgson's 441.9
    ruptured 441.5
  Hoffa (-Kastert) (liposynovitis prepatellaris) 272.8
  Holla *(see also* Spherocytosis) 282.0
  homozygous-Hb-S 282.61
  hoof and mouth 078.4
  hookworm *(see also* Ancylostomiasis) 126.9
  Horton's (temporal arteritis) 446.5
  host-versus-graft (immune or nonimmune cause) 279.50
  HPFH (hereditary persistence of fetal hemoglobin) ("Swiss variety") 282.7
  Huchard's (continued arterial hypertension) 401.9
  Huguier's (uterine fibroma) 218.9

Disease, diseased *(Continued)*
  human immunodeficiency (virus) 042
  hunger 251.1
  Hunt's
    dyssynergia cerebellaris myoclonica 334.2
    herpetic geniculate ganglionitis 053.11
  Huntington's 333.4
  Huppert's (multiple myeloma) (M9730/3) 203.0●
  Hurler's (mucopolysaccharidosis I) 277.5
  Hutchinson's, meaning
    angioma serpiginosum 709.1
    cheiropompholyx 705.81
    prurigo estivalis 692.72
  Hutchinson-Boeck (sarcoidosis) 135
  Hutchinson-Gilford (progeria) 259.8
  hyaline (diffuse) (generalized) 728.9
    membrane (lung) (newborn) 769
  hydatid *(see also* Echinococcus) 122.9
  Hyde's (prurigo nodularis) 698.3
  hyperkinetic *(see also* Hyperkinesia) 314.9
    heart 429.82
  hypertensive *(see also* Hypertension) 401.9
  hypophysis 253.9
    hyperfunction 253.1
    hypofunction 253.2
  Iceland (epidemic neuromyasthenia) 049.8
  I cell 272.7
  ill-defined 799.89
  immunologic NEC 279.9
  immunoproliferative 203.8●
  inclusion 078.5
    salivary gland 078.5
  infancy, early NEC 779.9
  infective NEC 136.9
  inguinal gland 289.9
  internal semilunar cartilage, cystic 717.5
  intervertebral disc 722.90
    with myelopathy 722.70
    cervical, cervicothoracic 722.91
      with myelopathy 722.71
    lumbar, lumbosacral 722.93
      with myelopathy 722.73
    thoracic, thoracolumbar 722.92
      with myelopathy 722.72
  intestine 569.9
    functional 564.9
      congenital 751.3
      psychogenic 306.4
    lardaceous 277.39
    organic 569.9
    protozoal NEC 007.9
  iris 364.9
    specified NEC 364.89
  iron
    metabolism 275.0
    storage 275.0
  Isambert's *(see also* Tuberculosis, larynx) 012.3●
  Iselin's (osteochondrosis, fifth metatarsal) 732.5
  island (scrub typhus) 081.2
  itai-itai 985.5
  Jadassohn's (maculopapular erythroderma) 696.2
  Jadassohn-Pellizari's (anetoderma) 701.3

Disease, diseased *(Continued)*
  Jakob-Creutzfeldt (CJD) 046.19
    with dementia
      with behavioral disturbance 046.19 *[294.11]*
      without behavioral disturbance 046.19 *[294.10]*
    familial 046.19
    iatrogenic 046.19
    specified NEC 046.19
    sporadic 046.19
    variant (vCJD) 046.11
      with dementia
        with behavioral disturbance 046.11 *[294.11]*
        without behavioral disturbance 046.11 *[294.10]*
  Jaksch (-Luzet) (pseudoleukemia infantum) 285.8
  Janet's 300.89
  Jansky-Bielschowsky 330.1
  jaw NEC 526.9
    fibrocystic 526.2
  Jensen's 363.05
  Jeune's (asphyxiating thoracic dystrophy) 756.4
  Jigger 134.1
  Johnson-Stevens (erythema multiforme exudativum) 695.13
  joint NEC 719.9●
    ankle 719.97
    Charcôt 094.0 *[713.5]*
    degenerative *(see also* Osteoarthrosis) 715.9●
      multiple 715.09
      spine *(see also* Spondylosis) 721.90
    elbow 719.92
    foot 719.97
    hand 719.94
    hip 719.95
    hypertrophic (chronic) (degenerative) *(see also* Osteoarthrosis) 715.9●
      spine *(see also* Spondylosis) 721.90
    knee 719.96
    Luschka 721.90
    multiple sites 719.99
    pelvic region 719.95
    sacroiliac 724.6
    shoulder (region) 719.91
    specified site NEC 719.98
    spine NEC 724.9
      pseudarthrosis following fusion 733.82
      sacroiliac 724.6
    wrist 719.93
  Jourdain's (acute gingivitis) 523.00
  Jüngling's (sarcoidosis) 135
  Kahler (-Bozzolo) (multiple myeloma) (M9730/3) 203.0●
  Kalischer's 759.6
  Kaposi's 757.33
    lichen ruber 697.8
      acuminatus 696.4
      moniliformis 697.8
    xeroderma pigmentosum 757.33
  Kaschin-Beck (endemic polyarthritis) 716.00
    ankle 716.07
    arm 716.02
      lower (and wrist) 716.03
      upper (and elbow) 716.02
    foot (and ankle) 716.07

◀ New   ◀▥ Revised   ~~deleted~~ Deleted   ● Use Additional Digit(s)   ▨ Omit code

Disease, diseased *(Continued)*
  Kaschin-Beck *(Continued)*
    forearm (and wrist) 716.03
    hand 716.04
    leg 716.06
      lower 716.06
      upper 716.05
    multiple sites 716.09
    pelvic region (hip) (thigh) 716.05
    shoulder region 716.01
    specified site NEC 716.08
  Katayama 120.2
  Kawasaki 446.1
  Kedani (scrub typhus) 081.2
  kidney (functional) (pelvis) *(see also*
      Disease, renal) 593.9
    chronic 585.9
      requiring chronic dialysis 585.6
      stage
        I 585.1
        II (mild) 585.2
        III (moderate) 585.3
        IV (severe) 585.4
        V 585.5
    cystic (congenital) 753.10
      multiple 753.19
      single 753.11
      specified NEC 753.19
    fibrocystic (congenital) 753.19
    in gout 274.10
    polycystic (congenital) 753.12
      adult type (APKD) 753.13
      autosomal dominant 753.13
      autosomal recessive 753.14
      childhood type (CPKD) 753.14
      infantile type 753.14
  Kienböck's (carpal lunate) (wrist) 732.3
  Kimmelstiel (-Wilson) (intercapillary
      glomerulosclerosis) 250.4●
      [581.81]
    due to secondary diabetes 249.4●
      [581.81]
  Kinnier Wilson's (hepatolenticular
      degeneration) 275.1
  kissing 075
  Kleb's *(see also* Nephritis) 583.9
  Klinger's 446.4
  Klippel's 723.8
  Klippel-Feil (brevicollis) 756.16
  Knight's 911.1
  Köbner's (epidermolysis bullosa)
      757.39
  Koenig-Wichmann (pemphigus) 694.4
  Köhler's
    first (osteoarthrosis juvenilis) 732.5
    second (Freiberg's infraction,
        metatarsal head) 732.5
    patellar 732.4
    tarsal navicular (bone)
        (osteoarthrosis juvenilis) 732.5
  Köhler-Freiberg (infraction, metatarsal
      head) 732.5
  Köhler-Mouchet (osteoarthrosis
      juvenilis) 732.5
  Köhler-Pellegrini-Stieda (calcification,
      knee joint) 726.62
  Kok 759.89
  König's (osteochondritis dissecans)
      732.7
  Korsakoff's (nonalcoholic) 294.0
    alcoholic 291.1
  Kostmann's (infantile genetic
      agranulocytosis) 288.01
  Krabbe's 330.0

Disease, diseased *(Continued)*
  Kraepelin-Morel *(see also*
      Schizophrenia) 295.9●
  Kraft-Weber-Dimitri 759.6
  Kufs' 330.1
  Kugelberg-Welander 335.11
  Kuhnt-Junius 362.52
  Kümmell's (-Verneuil) (spondylitis)
      721.7
  Kundrat's (lymphosarcoma) 200.1●
  kuru 046.0
  Kussmaul (-Meier) (polyarteritis
      nodosa) 446.0
  Kyasanur Forest 065.2
  Kyrle's (hyperkeratosis follicularis in
      cutem penetrans) 701.1
  labia
    inflammatory 616.10
    noninflammatory 624.9
      specified NEC 624.8
  labyrinth, ear 386.8
  lacrimal system (apparatus) (passages)
      375.9
    gland 375.00
    specified NEC 375.89
  Lafora's 333.2
  Lagleyze-von Hippel (retinocerebral
      angiomatosis) 759.6
  Lancereaux-Mathieu (leptospiral
      jaundice) 100.0
  Landry's 357.0
  Lane's 569.89
  lardaceous (any site) 277.39
  Larrey-Weil (leptospiral jaundice)
      100.0
  Larsen (-Johansson) (juvenile
      osteopathia patellae) 732.4
  larynx 478.70
  Lasègue's (persecution mania) 297.9
  Leber's 377.16
  Lederer's (acquired infectious
      hemolytic anemia) 283.19
  Legg's (capital femoral
      osteochondrosis) 732.1
  Legg-Calvé-Perthes (capital femoral
      osteochondrosis) 732.1
  Legg-Calvé-Waldenström (femoral
      capital osteochondrosis) 732.1
  Legg-Perthes (femoral capital
      osteochrondosis) 732.1
  Legionnaires' 482.84
  Leigh's 330.8
  Leiner's (exfoliative dermatitis)
      695.89
  Leloir's (lupus erythematosus) 695.4
  Lenegre's 426.0
  lens (eye) 379.39
  Leriche's (osteoporosis, posttraumatic)
      733.7
  Letterer-Siwe (acute histiocytosis X)
      (M9722/3) 202.5●
  Lev's (acquired complete heart block)
      426.0
  Lewandowski's *(see also* Tuberculosis)
      017.0●
  Lewandowski-Lutz
      (epidermodysplasia
      verruciformis) 078.19
  Lewy body 331.82
    with dementia
      with behavioral disturbance
          331.82 *[294.11]*
      without behavioral disturbance
          331.82 *[294.10]*

Disease, diseased *(Continued)*
  Leyden's (periodic vomiting) 536.2
  Libman-Sacks (verrucous endocarditis)
      710.0 *[424.91]*
  Lichtheim's (subacute combined
      sclerosis with pernicious anemia)
      281.0 *[336.2]*
  ligament 728.9
  light chain 203.0●
  Lightwood's (renal tubular acidosis)
      588.89
  Lignac's (cystinosis) 270.0
  Lindau's (retinocerebral angiomatosis)
      759.6
  Lindau-von Hippel (angiomatosis
      retinocerebellosa) 759.6
  lip NEC 528.5
  lipidosis 272.7
  lipoid storage NEC 272.7
  Lipschütz's 616.50
  Little's - *see* Palsy, cerebral
  liver 573.9
    alcoholic 571.3
      acute 571.1
      chronic 571.3
    chronic 571.9
      alcoholic 571.3
    cystic, congenital 751.62
    drug-induced 573.3
    due to
      chemicals 573.3
      fluorinated agents 573.3
      hypersensitivity drugs 573.3
      isoniazids 573.3
    end stage NEC 572.8
      due to hepatitis - *see* Hepatitis
    fibrocystic (congenital) 751.62
    glycogen storage 271.0
    organic 573.9
    polycystic (congenital) 751.62
  Lobo's (keloid blastomycosis) 116.2
  Lobstein's (brittle bones and blue
      sclera) 756.51
  locomotor system 334.9
  Lorain's (pituitary dwarfism) 253.3
  Lou Gehrig's 335.20
  Lucas-Championnière (fibrinous
      bronchitis) 466.0
  Ludwig's (submaxillary cellulitis)
      528.3
  luetic - *see* Syphilis
  lumbosacral region 724.6
  lung NEC 518.89
    black 500
    congenital 748.60
    cystic 518.89
      congenital 748.4
    fibroid (chronic) *(see also* Fibrosis,
        lung) 515
    fluke 121.2
      oriental 121.2
    in
      amyloidosis 277.39 *[517.8]*
      polymyositis 710.4 *[517.8]*
      sarcoidosis 135 *[517.8]*
      Sjögren's syndrome 710.2
          [517.8]
      syphilis 095.1
      systemic lupus erythematosus
          710.0 *[517.8]*
      systemic sclerosis 710.1 *[517.2]*
    interstitial (chronic) 515
      acute 136.3
    nonspecific, chronic 496

Disease, diseased (Continued)
  lung NEC (Continued)
    obstructive (chronic) (COPD) 496
      with
        acute
          bronchitis 491.22
          exacerbation NEC 491.21
        alveolitis, allergic (see also
          Alveolitis, allergic) 495.9
        asthma (chronic) (obstructive)
          493.2●
        bronchiectasis 494.0
          with acute exacerbation
            494.1
        bronchitis (chronic) 491.20
          with
            acute bronchitis 491.22
            exacerbation (acute)
              491.21
        decompensated 491.21
          with exacerbation 491.21
        emphysema NEC 492.8
      diffuse (with fibrosis) 496
    polycystic 518.89
      asthma (chronic) (obstructive)
        493.2●
      congenital 748.4
      purulent (cavitary) 513.0
      restrictive 518.89
      rheumatoid 714.81
        diffuse interstitial 714.81
      specified NEC 518.89
  Lutembacher's (atrial septal defect
    with mitral stenosis) 745.5
  Lutz-Miescher (elastosis perforans
    serpiginosa) 701.1
  Lutz-Splendore-de Almeida (Brazilian
    blastomycosis) 116.1
  Lyell's (toxic epidermal necrolysis)
    695.15
    due to drug
      correct substance properly
        administered 695.15
      overdose or wrong substance
        given or taken 977.9
      specific drug - see Table of
        Drugs and Chemicals
  Lyme 088.81
  lymphatic (gland) (system) 289.9
    channel (noninfective) 457.9
    vessel (noninfective) 457.9
      specified NEC 457.8
  lymphoproliferative (chronic)
    (M9970/1) 238.79
  Machado-Joseph 334.8
  Madelung's (lipomatosis) 272.8
  Madura (actinomycotic) 039.9
    mycotic 117.4
  Magitot's 526.4
  Majocchi's (purpura annularis
    telangiectodes) 709.1
  malarial (see also Malaria) 084.6
  Malassez's (cystic) 608.89
  Malibu 919.8
    infected 919.9
  malignant (M8000/3) - see also
    Neoplasm, by site, malignant
    previous, affecting management of
      pregnancy V23.89
  Manson's 120.1
  maple bark 495.6
  maple syrup (urine) 270.3
  Marburg (virus) 078.89
  Marchiafava (-Bignami) 341.8

Disease, diseased (Continued)
  Marfan's 090.49
    congenital syphilis 090.49
    meaning Marfan's syndrome 759.82
  Marie-Bamberger (hypertrophic
    pulmonary osteoarthropathy)
    (secondary) 731.2
    primary or idiopathic
      (acropachyderma) 757.39
    pulmonary (hypertrophic
      osteoarthropathy) 731.2
  Marie-Strümpell (ankylosing
    spondylitis) 720.0
  Marion's (bladder neck obstruction)
    596.0
  Marsh's (exophthalmic goiter) 242.0●
  Martin's 715.27
  mast cell 757.33
    systemic (M9741/3) 202.6●
  mastoid (see also Mastoiditis) 383.9
    process 385.9
  maternal, unrelated to pregnancy NEC,
    affecting fetus or newborn 760.9
  Mathieu's (leptospiral jaundice) 100.0
  Mauclaire's 732.3
  Mauriac's (erythema nodosum
    syphiliticum) 091.3
  Maxcy's 081.0
  McArdle (-Schmid-Pearson)
    (glycogenosis V) 271.0
  mediastinum NEC 519.3
  Medin's (see also Poliomyelitis) 045.9●
  Mediterranean (with
    hemoglobinopathy) 282.49
  medullary center (idiopathic)
    (respiratory) 348.89 ◄▥
  Meige's (chronic hereditary edema)
    757.0
  Meleda 757.39
  Ménétrier's (hypertrophic gastritis)
    535.2●
  Ménière's (active) 386.00
    cochlear 386.02
    cochleovestibular 386.01
    inactive 386.04
    in remission 386.04
    vestibular 386.03
  meningeal - see Meningitis
  mental (see also Psychosis) 298.9
  Merzbacher-Pelizaeus 330.0
  mesenchymal 710.9
  mesenteric embolic 557.0
  metabolic NEC 277.9
  metal polishers' 502
  metastatic - see Metastasis
  Mibelli's 757.39
  microdrepanocytic 282.49
  microvascular - code to condition
  Miescher's 709.3
  Mikulicz's (dryness of mouth, absent
    or decreased lacrimation) 527.1
  Milkman (-Looser) (osteomalacia with
    pseudofractures) 268.2
  Miller's (osteomalacia) 268.2
  Mills' 335.29
  Milroy's (chronic hereditary edema)
    757.0
  Minamata 985.0
  Minor's 336.1
  Minot's (hemorrhagic disease,
    newborn) 776.0
  Minot-von Willebrand-Jürgens
    (angiohemophilia) 286.4
  Mitchell's (erythromelalgia) 443.82

Disease, diseased (Continued)
  mitral - see Endocarditis, mitral
  Mljet (mal de Meleda) 757.39
  Möbius', Moebius' 346.2●
  Möeller's 267
  Möller (-Barlow) (infantile scurvy)
    267
  Mönckeberg's (see also Arteriosclerosis,
    extremities) 440.20
  Mondor's (thrombophlebitis of breast)
    451.89
  Monge's 993.2
  Morel-Kraepelin (see also
    Schizophrenia) 295.9●
  Morgagni's (syndrome) (hyperostosis
    frontalis interna) 733.3
  Morgagni-Adams-Stokes (syncope
    with heart block) 426.9
  Morquio (-Brailsford) (-Ullrich)
    (mucopolysaccharidosis IV) 277.5
  Morton's (with metatarsalgia) 355.6
  Morvan's 336.0
  motor neuron (bulbar) (mixed type)
    335.20
  Mouchet's (juvenile osteochondrosis,
    foot) 732.5
  mouth 528.9
  Moyamoya 437.5
  Mucha's (acute parapsoriasis
    varioliformis) 696.2
  mu-chain 273.2
  mucolipidosis (I) (II) (III) 272.7
  Münchmeyer's (exostosis luxurians)
    728.11
  Murri's (intermittent hemoglobinuria)
    283.2
  muscle 359.9
    inflammatory 728.9
    ocular 378.9
  musculoskeletal system 729.90
  mushroom workers' 495.5
  Myà's (congenital dilation, colon) 751.3
  mycotic 117.9
  myeloproliferative (chronic) (M9960/1)
    238.79
  myocardium, myocardial (see also
    Degeneration, myocardial) 429.1
    hypertensive (see also Hypertension,
      heart) 402.90
    primary (idiopathic) 425.4
  myoneural 358.9
  Naegeli's 287.1
  nail 703.9
    specified type NEC 703.8
  Nairobi sheep 066.1
  nasal 478.19
    cavity NEC 478.19
    sinus (chronic) - see Sinusitis
  navel (newborn) NEC 779.89
    delayed separation of umbilical cord
      779.83
  nemaline body 359.0
  neoplastic, generalized (M8000/6)
    199.0
  nerve - see Disorder, nerve
  nervous system (central) 349.9
    autonomic, peripheral (see also
      Neuropathy, peripheral,
      autonomic) 337.9
    congenital 742.9
    inflammatory - see Encephalitis
    parasympathetic (see also
      Neuropathy, peripheral,
      autonomic) 337.9

◄ New   ◄▥ Revised   deleted Deleted   ● Use Additional Digit(s)   ▨ Omit code

Disease, diseased *(Continued)*
  nervous system *(Continued)*
    peripheral NEC 355.9
    prion NEC 046.79
    specified NEC 349.89
    sympathetic *(see also* Neuropathy,
        peripheral, autonomic) 337.9
    vegetative *(see also* Neuropathy,
        peripheral, autonomic) 337.9
  Nettleship's (urticaria pigmentosa)
      757.33
  Neumann's (pemphigus vegetans)
      694.4
  neurologic (central) NEC *(see also*
      Disease, nervous system) 349.9
    peripheral NEC 355.9
  neuromuscular system NEC 358.9
  Newcastle 077.8
  Nicolas (-Durand) -Favre (climatic
      bubo) 099.1
  Niemann-Pick (lipid histiocytosis)
      272.7
  nipple 611.9
    Paget's (M8540/3) 174.0
  Nishimoto (-Takeuchi) 437.5
  nonarthropod-borne NEC 078.89
    central nervous system NEC 049.9
    enterovirus NEC 078.89
  nonautoimmune hemolytic NEC 283.10
  Nonne-Milroy-Meige (chronic
      hereditary edema) 757.0
  Norrie's (congenital progressive
      oculoacousticocerebral
      degeneration) 743.8
  nose 478.19
  nucleus pulposus - *see* Disease,
      intervertebral disc
  nutritional 269.9
    maternal, affecting fetus or newborn
        760.4
  oasthouse, urine 270.2
  obliterative vascular 447.1
  Odelberg's (juvenile osteochondrosis)
      732.1
  Oguchi's (retina) 368.61
  Ohara's *(see also* Tularemia) 021.9
  Ollier's (chondrodysplasia) 756.4
  Opitz's (congestive splenomegaly)
      289.51
  Oppenheim's 358.8
  Oppenheim-Urbach (necrobiosis
      lipoidica diabeticorum) 250.8●
      [709.3]
    due to secondary diabetes 249.8●
      [709.3]
  optic nerve NEC 377.49
  orbit 376.9
    specified NEC 376.89
  Oriental liver fluke 121.1
  Oriental lung fluke 121.2
  Ormond's 593.4
  Osgood's tibia (tubercle) 732.4
  Osgood-Schlatter 732.4
  Osler (-Vaquez) (polycythemia vera)
      (M9950/1) 238.4
  Osler-Rendu (familial hemorrhagic
      telangiectasia) 448.0
  osteofibrocystic 252.01
  Otto's 715.35
  outer ear 380.9
  ovary (noninflammatory) NEC 620.9
    cystic 620.2
    polycystic 256.4
    specified NEC 620.8

Disease, diseased *(Continued)*
  Owren's (congenital) *(see also* Defect,
      coagulation) 286.3
  Paas' 756.59
  Paget's (osteitis deformans) 731.0
    with infiltrating duct carcinoma of
        the breast (M8541/3) - *see*
        Neoplasm, breast, malignant
    bone 731.0
      osteosarcoma in (M9184/3) - *see*
          Neoplasm, bone, malignant
    breast (M8540/3) 174.0
    extramammary (M8542/3) - *see also*
        Neoplasm, skin, malignant
      anus 154.3
      skin 173.5
    malignant (M8540/3)
      breast 174.0
      specified site NEC (M8542/3) -
          see Neoplasm, skin,
          malignant
      unspecified site 174.0
    mammary (M8540/3) 174.0
    nipple (M8540/3) 174.0
  palate (soft) 528.9
  Paltauf-Sternberg 201.9●
  pancreas 577.9
    cystic 577.2
      congenital 751.7
    fibrocystic 277.00
  Panner's 732.3
    capitellum humeri 732.3
    head of humerus 732.3
    tarsal navicular (bone)
        (osteochondrosis) 732.5
  panvalvular - *see* Endocarditis, mitral
  parametrium 629.9
  parasitic NEC 136.9
    cerebral NEC 123.9
    intestinal NEC 129
    mouth 112.0
    skin NEC 134.9
    specified type - *see* Infestation
    tongue 112.0
  parathyroid (gland) 252.9
    specified NEC 252.8
  Parkinson's 332.0
  parodontal 523.9
  Parrot's (syphilitic osteochondritis)
      090.0
  Parry's (exophthalmic goiter) 242.0●
  Parson's (exophthalmic goiter)
      242.0●
  Pavy's 593.6
  Paxton's (white piedra) 111.2
  Payr's (splenic flexure syndrome)
      569.89
  pearl-workers' (chronic osteomyelitis)
      (see also Osteomyelitis) 730.1●
  Pel-Ebstein - *see* Disease, Hodgkin's
  Pelizaeus-Merzbacher 330.0
    with dementia
      with behavioral disturbance 330.0
          [294.11]
      without behavioral disturbance
          330.0 *[294.10]*
  Pellegrini-Stieda (calcification, knee
      joint) 726.62
  pelvis, pelvic
    female NEC 629.9
      specified NEC 629.89
    gonococcal (acute) 098.19
      chronic or duration of 2 months
          or over 098.39

Disease, diseased *(Continued)*
  pelvis, pelvic *(Continued)*
    infection *(see also* Disease, pelvis,
        inflammatory) 614.9
    inflammatory (female) (PID) 614.9
      with
        abortion - *see* Abortion, by
            type, with sepsis
        ectopic pregnancy *(see also*
            categories 633.0–633.9)
            639.0
        molar pregnancy *(see also*
            categories 630–632) 639.0
      acute 614.3
      chronic 614.4
      complicating pregnancy 646.6●
        affecting fetus or newborn
            760.8
      following
        abortion 639.0
        ectopic or molar pregnancy
            639.0
      peritonitis (acute) 614.5
        chronic NEC 614.7
      puerperal, postpartum, childbirth
          670.8   ◀▥▥
      specified NEC 614.8
    organ, female NEC 629.9
      specified NEC 629.89
    peritoneum, female NEC 629.9
      specified NEC 629.89
  penis 607.9
    inflammatory 607.2
  peptic NEC 536.9
    acid 536.8
  periapical tissues NEC 522.9
  pericardium 423.9
    specified type NEC 423.8
  perineum
    female
      inflammatory 616.9
        specified NEC 616.89
      noninflammatory 624.9
        specified NEC 624.8
    male (inflammatory) 682.2
  periodic (familial) (Reimann's) NEC
      277.31
    paralysis 359.3
  periodontal NEC 523.9
    specified NEC 523.8
  periosteum 733.90
  peripheral
    arterial 443.9
    autonomic nervous system *(see also*
        Neuropathy, autonomic) 337.9
    nerve NEC *(see also* Neuropathy)
        356.9
      multiple - *see* Polyneuropathy
    vascular 443.9
      specified type NEC 443.89
  peritoneum 568.9
    pelvic, female 629.9
      specified NEC 629.89
  Perrin-Ferraton (snapping hip) 719.65
  persistent mucosal (middle ear) (with
      posterior or superior marginal
      perforation of ear drum) 382.2
  Perthes' (capital femoral
      osteochondrosis) 732.1
  Petit's *(see also* Hernia, lumbar) 553.8
  Peutz-Jeghers 759.6
  Peyronie's 607.85
  Pfeiffer's (infectious mononucleosis)
      075

Disease, diseased *(Continued)*
  pharynx 478.20
  Phocas' 610.1
  photochromogenic (acid-fast bacilli)
    (pulmonary) 031.0
    nonpulmonary 031.9
  Pick's
    brain 331.11
      with dementia
        with behavioral disturbance
          331.11 *[294.11]*
        without behavioral
          disturbance 331.11
          [294.10]
    cerebral atrophy 331.11
      with dementia
        with behavioral disturbance
          331.11 *[294.11]*
        without behavioral
          disturbance 331.11
          [294.10]
    lipid histiocytosis 272.7
    liver (pericardial pseudocirrhosis of
      liver) 423.2
    pericardium (pericardial
      pseudocirrhosis of liver) 423.2
    polyserositis (pericardial
      pseudocirrhosis of liver)
      423.2
  Pierson's (osteochondrosis) 732.1
  pigeon fanciers' or breeders' 495.2
  pineal gland 259.8
  pink 985.0
  Pinkus' (lichen nitidus) 697.1
  pinworm 127.4
  pituitary (gland) 253.9
    hyperfunction 253.1
    hypofunction 253.2
  pituitary snuff-takers' 495.8
  placenta
    affecting fetus or newborn 762.2
    complicating pregnancy or
      childbirth 656.7●
  pleura (cavity) *(see also* Pleurisy)
    511.0
  Plummer's (toxic nodular goiter)
    242.3●
  pneumatic
    drill 994.9
    hammer 994.9
  policeman's 729.2
  Pollitzer's (hidradenitis suppurativa)
    705.83
  polycystic (congenital) 759.89
    kidney or renal 753.12
      adult type (APKD) 753.13
      autosomal dominant 753.13
      autosomal recessive 753.14
      childhood type (CPKD) 753.14
      infantile type 753.14
    liver or hepatic 751.62
    lung or pulmonary 518.89
      congenital 748.4
    ovary, ovaries 256.4
    spleen 759.0
  Pompe's (glycogenosis II) 271.0
  Poncet's (tuberculous rheumatism) *(see
    also* Tuberculosis) 015.9●
  Posada-Wernicke 114.9
  Potain's (pulmonary edema) 514
  Pott's *(see also* Tuberculosis) 015.0 ●
    [730.88]
    osteomyelitis 015.0 ● *[730.88]*
    paraplegia 015.0 ● *[730.88]*

Disease, diseased *(Continued)*
  Pott's *(Continued)*
    spinal curvature 015.0● *[737.43]*
    spondylitis 015.0● *[720.81]*
  Potter's 753.0
  Poulet's 714.2
  pregnancy NEC *(see also* Pregnancy)
    646.9●
  Preiser's (osteoporosis) 733.09
  Pringle's (tuberous sclerosis) 759.5
  Profichet's 729.90
  prostate 602.9
    specified type NEC 602.8
  protozoal NEC 136.8
    intestine, intestinal NEC 007.9
  pseudo-Hurler's (mucolipidosis III)
    272.7
  psychiatric *(see also* Psychosis) 298.9
  psychotic *(see also* Psychosis) 298.9
  Puente's (simple glandular cheilitis)
    528.5
  puerperal NEC *(see also* Puerperal)
    674.9●
  pulmonary - *see also* Disease, lung
    amyloid 277.39 *[517.8]*
    artery 417.9
    circulation, circulatory 417.9
      specified NEC 417.8
    diffuse obstructive (chronic) 496
      with
        acute bronchitis 491.22
        asthma (chronic) (obstructive)
          493.2●
        exacerbation NEC (acute)
          491.21
    heart (chronic) 416.9
      specified NEC 416.8
    hypertensive (vascular) 416.0
      cardiovascular 416.0
    obstructive diffuse (chronic) 496
      with
        acute bronchitis 491.22
        asthma (chronic) (obstructive)
          493.2●
        bronchitis (chronic) 491.20
          with
            exacerbation (acute)
              491.21
          acute 491.22
        exacerbation NEC (acute)
          491.21
        decompensated 491.21
          with exacerbation 491.21
    valve *(see also* Endocarditis,
      pulmonary) 424.3
  pulp (dental) NEC 522.9
  pulseless 446.7
  Putnam's (subacute combined sclerosis
    with pernicious anemia) 281.0
    [336.2]
  Pyle (-Cohn) (craniometaphyseal
    dysplasia) 756.89
  pyramidal tract 333.90
  Quervain's
    tendon sheath 727.04
    thyroid (subacute granulomatous
      thyroiditis) 245.1
  Quincke's - *see* Edema,
    angioneurotic
  Quinquaud (acne decalvans)
    704.09
  rag sorters' 022.1
  Raynaud's (paroxysmal digital
    cyanosis) 443.0

Disease, diseased *(Continued)*
  reactive airway - *see* Asthma
  Recklinghausen's (M9540/1) 237.71
    bone (osteitis fibrosa cystica) 252.01
  Recklinghausen-Applebaum
    (hemochromatosis) 275.0
  Reclus' (cystic) 610.1
  rectum NEC 569.49
  Refsum's (heredopathia atactica
    polyneuritiformis) 356.3
  Reichmann's (gastrosuccorrhea) 536.8
  Reimann's (periodic) 277.31
  Reiter's 099.3
  renal (functional) (pelvis) *(see also*
    Disease, kidney) 593.9
    with
      edema *(see also* Nephrosis) 581.9
      exudative nephritis 583.89
      lesion of interstitial nephritis
        583.89
      stated generalized cause - *see*
        Nephritis
    acute 593.9
    basement membrane NEC 583.89
      with
        pulmonary hemorrhage
          (Goodpasture's
          syndrome) 446.21
          [583.81]
    chronic *(see also* Disease, kidney,
      chronic) 585.9
    complicating pregnancy or
      puerperium NEC 646.2●
      with hypertension - *see* Toxemia,
        of pregnancy
      affecting fetus or newborn 760.1
    cystic, congenital *(see also* Cystic,
      disease, kidney) 753.10
    diabetic 250.4● *[583.81]*
      due to secondary diabetes 249.4●
        [581.81]
    due to
      amyloidosis 277.39 *[583.81]*
      diabetes mellitus 250.4 ●
        [583.81]
        due to secondary diabetes
          249.4 ● *[581.81]*
      systemic lupus erythematosis
        710.0 *[583.81]*
    end-stage 585.6
    exudative 583.89
    fibrocystic (congenital) 753.19
    gonococcal 098.19 *[583.81]*
    gouty 274.10
    hypertensive *(see also* Hypertension,
      kidney) 403.90
    immune complex NEC 583.89
    interstitial (diffuse) (focal) 583.89
    lupus 710.0 *[583.81]*
    maternal, affecting fetus or newborn
      760.1
      hypertensive 760.0
    phosphate-losing (tubular) 588.0
    polycystic (congenital) 753.12
      adult type (APKD) 753.13
      autosomal dominant 753.13
      autosomal recessive 753.14
      childhood type (CPKD) 753.14
      infantile type 753.14
    specified lesion or cause NEC *(see
      also* Glomerulonephritis)
      583.89
    subacute 581.9
    syphilitic 095.4

Disease, diseased *(Continued)*
  renal *(Continued)*
    tuberculous *(see also* Tuberculosis)
      016.0● *[583.81]*
    tubular *(see also* Nephrosis, tubular)
      584.5
  Rendu-Osler-Weber (familial
    hemorrhagic telangiectasia) 448.0
  renovascular (arteriosclerotic) *(see also*
    Hypertension, kidney) 403.90
  respiratory (tract) 519.9
    acute or subacute (upper) NEC
      465.9
      due to fumes or vapors 506.3
      multiple sites NEC 465.8
      noninfectious 478.9
      streptococcal 034.0
    chronic 519.9
      arising in the perinatal period
        770.7
      due to fumes or vapors 506.4
    due to
      aspiration of liquids or solids
        508.9
      external agents NEC 508.9
        specified NEC 508.8
      fumes or vapors 506.9
        acute or subacute NEC 506.3
        chronic 506.4
    fetus or newborn NEC 770.9
    obstructive 496
    specified type NEC 519.8
    upper (acute) (infectious) NEC
      465.9
      multiple sites NEC 465.8
      noninfectious NEC 478.9
      streptococcal 034.0
  retina, retinal NEC 362.9
    Batten's or Batten-Mayou 330.1
      [362.71]
    degeneration 362.89
    vascular lesion 362.17
  rheumatic *(see also* Arthritis) 716.8●
    heart - *see* Disease, heart, rheumatic
  rheumatoid (heart) - *see* Arthritis,
    rheumatoid
  rickettsial NEC 083.9
    specified type NEC 083.8
  Riedel's (ligneous thyroiditis) 245.3
  Riga (-Fede) (cachectic aphthae) 529.0
  Riggs' (compound periodontitis)
    523.40
  Ritter's 695.81
  Rivalta's (cervicofacial actinomycosis)
    039.3
  Robles' (onchocerciasis) 125.3 *[360.13]*
  Roger's (congenital interventricular
    septal defect) 745.4
  Rokitansky's *(see also* Necrosis, liver)
    570
  Romberg's 349.89
  Rosenthal's (factor XI deficiency) 286.2
  Rossbach's (hyperchlorhydria) 536.8
    psychogenic 306.4
  Roth (-Bernhardt) 355.1
  Runeberg's (progressive pernicious
    anemia) 281.0
  Rust's (tuberculous spondylitis) *(see
    also* Tuberculosis) 015.0 ● *[720.81]*
  Rustitskii's (multiple myeloma)
    (M9730/3) 203.0●
  Ruysch's (Hirschsprung's disease) 751.3
  Sachs (-Tay) 330.1
  sacroiliac NEC 724.6

Disease, diseased *(Continued)*
  salivary gland or duct NEC 527.9
    inclusion 078.5
      streptococcal 034.0
    virus 078.5
  Sander's (paranoia) 297.1
  Sandhoff's 330.1
  sandworm 126.9
  Savill's (epidemic exfoliative
    dermatitis) 695.89
  Schamberg's (progressive pigmentary
    dermatosis) 709.09
  Schaumann's (sarcoidosis) 135
  Schenck's (sporotrichosis) 117.1
  Scheuermann's (osteochondrosis) 732.0
  Schilder (-Flatau) 341.1
  Schimmelbusch's 610.1
  Schlatter's tibia (tubercle) 732.4
  Schlatter-Osgood 732.4
  Schmorl's 722.30
    cervical 722.39
    lumbar, lumbosacral 722.32
    specified region NEC 722.39
    thoracic, thoracolumbar 722.31
  Scholz's 330.0
  Schönlein (-Henoch) (purpura
    rheumatica) 287.0
  Schottmüller's *(see also* Fever,
    paratyphoid) 002.9
  Schüller-Christian (chronic
    histiocytosis X) 277.89
  Schultz's (agranulocytosis) 288.09
  Schwalbe-Ziehen-Oppenheimer 333.6
  Schwartz-Jampel 359.23
  Schweninger-Buzzi (macular atrophy)
    701.3
  sclera 379.19
  scrofulous *(see also* Tuberculosis)
    017.2●
  scrotum 608.9
  sebaceous glands NEC 706.9
  Secretan's (posttraumatic edema) 782.3
  semilunar cartilage, cystic 717.5
  seminal vesicle 608.9
  Senear-Usher (pemphigus
    erythematosus) 694.4
  serum NEC 999.5
  Sever's (osteochondrosis calcaneum)
    732.5
  sexually transmitted - *see* Disease,
    venereal
  Sézary's (reticulosis) (M9701/3)
    202.2●
  Shaver's (bauxite pneumoconiosis)
    503
  Sheehan's (postpartum pituitary
    necrosis) 253.2
  shimamushi (scrub typhus) 081.2
  shipyard 077.1
  sickle-cell 282.60
    with
      crisis 282.62
      Hb-S disease 282.61
      other abnormal hemoglobin
        (Hb-D) (Hb-E) (Hb-G)
        (Hb-J) (Hb-K) (Hb-O)
        (Hb-P) (high fetal gene)
        (without crisis) 282.68
        with crisis 282.69
    elliptocytosis 282.60
    Hb-C (without crisis) 282.63
      with
        crisis 282.64
        vaso-occlusive pain 282.64

Disease, diseased *(Continued)*
  sickle-cell *(Continued)*
    Hb-S 282.61
      with
        crisis 282.62
        Hb-C (without crisis) 282.63
          with
            crisis 282.64
            vaso-occlusive pain
              282.64
        other abnormal hemoglobin
          (Hb-D) (Hb-E) (Hb-G)
          (Hb-J) (Hb-K) (Hb-O)
          (Hb-P) (high fetal gene)
          (without crisis) 282.68
        with crisis 282.69
    spherocytosis 282.60
    thalassemia (without crisis) 282.41
      with
        crisis 282.42
        vaso-occlusive pain 282.42
  Siegal-Cattan-Mamou (periodic) 277.31
  silo fillers' 506.9
  Simian B 054.3
  Simmonds' (pituitary cachexia) 253.2
  Simons' (progressive lipodystrophy)
    272.6
  Sinding-Larsen (juvenile osteopathia
    patellae) 732.4
  sinus - *see also* Sinusitis
    brain 437.9
    specified NEC 478.19
  Sirkari's 085.0
  sixth *(see also* Exanthem subitum)
    058.10
  Sjögren (-Gougerot) 710.2
    with lung involvement 710.2 *[517.8]*
  Skevas-Zerfus 989.5
  skin NEC 709.9
    due to metabolic disorder 277.9
    specified type NEC 709.8
  sleeping *(see also* Narcolepsy) 347.00
    meaning sleeping sickness *(see also*
      Trypanosomiasis) 086.5
  small vessel 443.9
  Smith-Strang (oasthouse urine) 270.2
  Sneddon-Wilkinson (subcorneal
    pustular dermatosis) 694.1
  South African creeping 133.8
  Spencer's (epidemic vomiting) 078.82
  Spielmeyer-Stock 330.1
  Spielmeyer-Vogt 330.1
  spine, spinal 733.90
    combined system *(see also*
      Degeneration, combined) 266.2
      [336.2]
      with pernicious anemia 281.0
        [336.2]
    cord NEC 336.9
      congenital 742.9
    demyelinating NEC 341.8
    joint *(see also* Disease, joint, spine)
      724.9
      tuberculous 015.0● *[730.8]*●
  spinocerebellar 334.9
    specified NEC 334.8
  spleen (organic) (postinfectional)
    289.50
    amyloid 277.39
    lardaceous 277.39
    polycystic 759.0
    specified NEC 289.59
  sponge divers' 989.5
  Stanton's (melioidosis) 025

Disease, diseased *(Continued)*
Stargardt's 362.75
Startle 759.89
Steinert's 359.21
Sternberg's - *see* Disease, Hodgkin's
Stevens-Johnson (erythema multiforme
  exudativum) 695.13
Sticker's (erythema infectiosum) 057.0
Stieda's (calcification, knee joint) 726.62
Still's (juvenile rheumatoid arthritis)
  714.30
  adult onset 714.2
Stiller's (asthenia) 780.79
Stokes' (exophthalmic goiter) 242.0●
Stokes-Adams (syncope with heart
  block) 426.9
Stokvis (-Talma) (enterogenous
  cyanosis) 289.7
stomach NEC (organic) 537.9
  functional 536.9
    psychogenic 306.4
  lardaceous 277.39
stonemasons' 502
storage
  glycogen (*see also* Disease, glycogen
    storage) 271.0
  lipid 272.7
  mucopolysaccharide 277.5
striatopallidal system 333.90
  specified NEC 333.89
Strümpell-Marie (ankylosing
  spondylitis) 720.0
Stuart's (congenital factor X deficiency)
  (*see also* Defect, coagulation) 286.3
Stuart-Prower (congenital factor X
  deficiency) (*see also* Defect,
  coagulation) 286.3
Sturge (-Weber) (-Dimitri)
  (encephalocutaneous
  angiomatosis) 759.6
Stuttgart 100.89
Sudeck's 733.7
supporting structures of teeth NEC
  525.9
suprarenal (gland) (capsule) 255.9
  hyperfunction 255.3
  hypofunction 255.41
Sutton's 709.09
Sutton and Gull's - *see* Hypertension,
  kidney
sweat glands NEC 705.9
  specified type NEC 705.89
sweating 078.2
Sweeley-Klionsky 272.4
Swift (-Feer) 985.0
swimming pool (bacillus) 031.1
swineherd's 100.89
Sylvest's (epidemic pleurodynia) 074.1
Symmers (follicular lymphoma)
  (M9690/3) 202.0●
sympathetic nervous system (*see also*
  Neuropathy, peripheral,
  autonomic) 337.9
synovium 727.9
syphilitic - *see* Syphilis
systemic tissue mast cell (M9741/3)
  202.6●
Taenzer's 757.4
Takayasu's (pulseless) 446.7
Talma's 728.85
Tangier (familial high-density
  lipoprotein deficiency) 272.5
Tarral-Besnier (pityriasis rubra pilaris)
  696.4

Disease, diseased *(Continued)*
Tay-Sachs 330.1
Taylor's 701.8
tear duct 375.69
teeth, tooth 525.9
  hard tissues 521.9
    specified NEC 521.89
  pulp NEC 522.9
tendon 727.9
  inflammatory NEC 727.9
terminal vessel 443.9
testis 608.9
Thaysen-Gee (nontropical sprue) 579.0
Thomsen's 359.22
Thomson's (congenital poikiloderma)
  757.33
Thornwaldt's, Tornwaldt's (pharyngeal
  bursitis) 478.29
throat 478.20
  septic 034.0
thromboembolic (*see also* Embolism)
  444.9
thymus (gland) 254.9
  specified NEC 254.8
thyroid (gland) NEC 246.9
  heart (*see also* Hyperthyroidism)
    242.9 ● [425.7]
  lardaceous 277.39
  specified NEC 246.8
Tietze's 733.6
Tommaselli's
  correct substance properly
    administered 599.70
  overdose or wrong substance given
    or taken 961.4
tongue 529.9
tonsils, tonsillar (and adenoids)
  (chronic) 474.9
  specified NEC 474.8
tooth, teeth 525.9
  hard tissues 521.9
    specified NEC 521.89
  pulp NEC 522.9
Tornwaldt's (pharyngeal bursitis)
  478.29
Tourette's 307.23
trachea 519.19
tricuspid - *see* Endocarditis, tricuspid
triglyceride-storage, type I, II, III
  272.7
triple vessel - *see* Arteriosclerosis,
  coronary
trisymptomatic, Gougerot's 709.1
trophoblastic (*see also* Hydatidiform
  mole) 630
  previous, affecting management of
    pregnancy V23.1
tsutsugamushi (scrub typhus) 081.2
tube (fallopian), noninflammatory
  620.9
  specified NEC 620.8
tuberculous NEC (*see also* Tuberculosis)
  011.9●
tubo-ovarian
  inflammatory (*see also* Salpingo-
    oophoritis) 614.2
  noninflammatory 620.9
    specified NEC 620.8
tubotympanic, chronic (with anterior
  perforation of ear drum) 382.1
tympanum 385.9
Uhl's 746.84
umbilicus (newborn) NEC 779.89
  delayed separation 779.83

Disease, diseased *(Continued)*
Underwood's (sclerema neonatorum)
  778.1
undiagnosed 799.9
Unna's (seborrheic dermatitis) 690.18
unstable hemoglobin hemolytic
  282.7
Unverricht (-Lundborg) 345.1 ◄▥
Urbach-Oppenheim (necrobiosis
  lipoidica diabeticorum) 250.8●
  [709.3]
  due to secondary diabetes 249.8●
  [709.3]
Urbach-Wiethe (lipoid proteinosis)
  272.8
ureter 593.9
urethra 599.9
  specified type NEC 599.84
urinary (tract) 599.9
  bladder 596.9
    specified NEC 596.8
  maternal, affecting fetus or newborn
    760.1
Usher-Senear (pemphigus
  erythematosus) 694.4
uterus (organic) 621.9
  infective (*see also* Endometritis) 615.9
  inflammatory (*see also* Endometritis)
    615.9
  noninflammatory 621.9
    specified type NEC 621.8
uveal tract
  anterior 364.9
  posterior 363.9
vagabonds' 132.1
vagina, vaginal
  inflammatory 616.10
  noninflammatory 623.9
    specified NEC 623.8
Valsuani's (progressive pernicious
  anemia, puerperal) 648.2●
  complicating pregnancy or
    puerperium 648.2●
valve, valvular - *see also* Endocarditis
  congenital NEC (*see also* Anomaly,
    heart, valve) 746.9
  pulmonary 746.00
    specified type NEC 746.89
van Bogaert-Nijssen (-Peiffer) 330.0
van Creveld-von Gierke (glycogenosis
  I) 271.0
van den Bergh's (enterogenous
  cyanosis) 289.7
van Neck's (juvenile osteochondrosis)
  732.1
Vaquez (-Osler) (polycythemia vera)
  (M9950/1) 238.4
vascular 459.9
  arteriosclerotic - *see* Arteriosclerosis
  hypertensive - *see* Hypertension
  obliterative 447.1
    peripheral 443.9
  occlusive 459.9
  peripheral (occlusive) 443.9
    in (due to) (with) diabetes
      mellitus 250.7● [443.81] ◄▥
    in (due to) (with) secondary
      diabetes 249.7●
      [443.81] ◄▥
    specified type NEC 443.89
vas deferens 608.9
vasomotor 443.9
vasospastic 443.9
vein 459.9

◄ New   ◄▥ Revised   ~~deleted~~ Deleted   ● Use Additional Digit(s)   ▨ Omit code

Disease, diseased *(Continued)*
  venereal 099.9
    chlamydial NEC 099.50
      anus 099.52
      bladder 099.53
      cervix 099.53
      epididymis 099.54
      genitourinary NEC 099.55
        lower 099.53
          specified NEC 099.54
      pelvic inflammatory disease 099.54
      perihepatic 099.56
      peritoneum 099.56
      pharynx 099.51
      rectum 099.52
      specified site NEC 099.59
      testis 099.54
      vagina 099.53
      vulva 099.53
    fifth 099.1
    sixth 099.1
    complicating pregnancy, childbirth, or puerperium 647.2●
    specified nature or type NEC 099.8
      chlamydial - *see* Disease, venereal, chlamydial
  Verneuil's (syphilitic bursitis) 095.7
  Verse's (calcinosis intervertebralis) 275.49 *[722.90]*
  vertebra, vertebral NEC 733.90
    disc - *see* Disease, Intervertebral disc
  vibration NEC 994.9
  Vidal's (lichen simplex chronicus) 698.3
  Vincent's (trench mouth) 101
  Virchow's 733.99
  virus (filterable) NEC 078.89
    arbovirus NEC 066.9
    arthropod-borne NEC 066.9
    central nervous system NEC 049.9
      specified type NEC 049.8
    complicating pregnancy, childbirth, or puerperium 647.6●
    contact (with) V01.79
      varicella V01.71
    exposure to V01.79
      varicella V01.71
    Marburg 078.89
    maternal
      with fetal damage affecting management of pregnancy 655.3●
    nonarthropod-borne NEC 078.89
      central nervous system NEC 049.9
        specified NEC 049.8
    vaccination, prophylactic (against) V04.89
  vitreous 379.29
  vocal cords NEC 478.5
  Vogt's (Cecile) 333.71
  Vogt-Spielmeyer 330.1
  Volhard-Fahr (malignant nephrosclerosis) 403.00
  Volkmann's
    acquired 958.6
  von Bechterew's (ankylosing spondylitis) 720.0
  von Economo's (encephalitis lethargica) 049.8
  von Eulenburg's (congenital paramyotonia) 359.29

Disease, diseased *(Continued)*
  von Gierke's (glycogenosis I) 271.0
  von Graefe's 378.72
  von Hippel's (retinocerebral angiomatosis) 759.6
  von Hippel-Lindau (angiomatosis retinocerebellosa) 759.6
  von Jaksch's (pseudoleukemia infantum) 285.8
  von Recklinghausen's (M9540/1) 237.71
    bone (osteitis fibrosa cystica) 252.01
  von Recklinghausen-Applebaum (hemochromatosis) 275.0
  von Willebrand (-Jürgens) (angiohemophilia) 286.4
  von Zambusch's (lichen sclerosus et atrophicus) 701.0
  Voorhoeve's (dyschondroplasia) 756.4
  Vrolik's (osteogenesis imperfecta) 756.51
  vulva
    inflammatory 616.10
    noninflammatory 624.9
      specified NEC 624.8
  Wagner's (colloid milium) 709.3
  Waldenström's (osteochondrosis capital femoral) 732.1
  Wallgren's (obstruction of splenic vein with collateral circulation) 459.89
  Wardrop's (with lymphangitis) 681.9
    finger 681.02
    toe 681.11
  Wassilieff's (leptospiral jaundice) 100.0
  wasting NEC 799.4
    due to malnutrition 261
    paralysis 335.21
  Waterhouse-Friderichsen 036.3
  waxy (any site) 277.39
  Weber-Christian (nodular nonsuppurative panniculitis) 729.30
  Wegner's (syphilitic osteochondritis) 090.0
  Weil's (leptospiral jaundice) 100.0
    of lung 100.0
  Weir Mitchell's (erythromelalgia) 443.82
  Werdnig-Hoffmann 335.0
  Werlhof's (*see also* Purpura, thrombocytopenic) 287.39
  Wermer's 258.01
  Werner's (progeria adultorum) 259.8
  Werner-His (trench fever) 083.1
  Werner-Schultz (agranulocytosis) 288.09
  Wernicke's (superior hemorrhagic polioencephalitis) 265.1
  Wernicke-Posadas 114.9
  Whipple's (intestinal lipodystrophy) 040.2
  whipworm 127.3
  white
    blood cell 288.9
      specified NEC 288.8
    spot 701.0
  White's (congenital) (keratosis follicularis) 757.39
  Whitmore's (melioidosis) 025
  Widal-Abrami (acquired hemolytic jaundice) 283.9
  Wilkie's 557.1
  Wilkinson-Sneddon (subcorneal pustular dermatosis) 694.1

Disease, diseased *(Continued)*
  Willis' (diabetes mellitus) (*see also* Diabetes) 250.0●
    due to secondary diabetes 249.0●
  Wilson's (hepatolenticular degeneration) 275.1
  Wilson-Brocq (dermatitis exfoliativa) 695.89
  winter vomiting 078.82
  Wise's 696.2
  Wohlfart-Kugelberg-Welander 335.11
  Woillez's (acute idiopathic pulmonary congestion) 518.5
  Wolman's (primary familial xanthomatosis) 272.7
  wool-sorters' 022.1
  Zagari's (xerostomia) 527.7
  Zahorsky's (exanthem subitum) 058.10
  Ziehen-Oppenheim 333.6
  zoonotic, bacterial NEC 027.9
    specified type NEC 027.8
Disfigurement (due to scar) 709.2
  head V48.6
  limb V49.4
  neck V48.7
  trunk V48.7
Disgerminoma - *see* Dysgerminoma
Disinsertion, retina 361.04
Disintegration, complete, of the body 799.89
  traumatic 869.1
Disk kidney 753.3
Dislocatable hip, congenital (*see also* Dislocation, hip, congenital) 754.30
Dislocation (articulation) (closed) (displacement) (simple) (subluxation) 839.8

Note 23

"Closed" includes simple, complete, partial, uncomplicated, and unspecified dislocation.

"Open" includes dislocation specified as infected or compound and dislocation with foreign body.

"Chronic," "habitual," "old," or "recurrent" dislocations should be coded as indicated under the entry "Dislocation, recurrent"; and "pathological" as indicated under the entry "Dislocation, pathological."

For late effect of dislocation *see* Late, effect, dislocation.

---

  with fracture - *see* Fracture, by site
  acromioclavicular (joint) (closed) 831.04
    open 831.14
  anatomical site (closed)
    specified NEC 839.69
      open 839.79
    unspecified or ill-defined 839.8
      open 839.9
  ankle (scaphoid bone) (closed) 837.0
    open 837.1
  arm (closed) 839.8
    open 839.9
  astragalus (closed) 837.0
    open 837.1
  atlanto-axial (closed) 839.01
    open 839.11

Dislocation (Continued)
  atlas (closed) 839.01
    open 839.11
  axis (closed) 839.02
    open 839.12
  back (closed) 839.8
    open 839.9
  Bell-Daly 723.8
  breast bone (closed) 839.61
    open 839.71
  capsule, joint - see Dislocation, by site
  carpal (bone) - see Dislocation, wrist
  carpometacarpal (joint) (closed) 833.04
    open 833.14
  cartilage (joint) - see also Dislocation, by
      site
    knee - see Tear, meniscus
  cervical, cervicodorsal, or
      cervicothoracic (spine)
      (vertebra) - see Dislocation,
      vertebra, cervical
  chiropractic (see also Lesion,
      nonallopathic) 739.9
  chondrocostal - see Dislocation,
      costochondral
  chronic - see Dislocation, recurrent
  clavicle (closed) 831.04
    open 831.14
  coccyx (closed) 839.41
    open 839.51
  collar bone (closed) 831.04
    open 831.14
  compound (open) NEC 839.9
  congenital NEC 755.8
    hip (see also Dislocation, hip,
        congenital) 754.30
    lens 743.37
    rib 756.3
    sacroiliac 755.69
    spine NEC 756.19
    vertebra 756.19
  coracoid (closed) 831.09
    open 831.19
  costal cartilage (closed) 839.69
    open 839.79
  costochondral (closed) 839.69
    open 839.79
  cricoarytenoid articulation (closed)
      839.69
    open 839.79
  cricothyroid (cartilage) articulation
      (closed) 839.69
    open 839.79
  dorsal vertebrae (closed) 839.21
    open 839.31
  ear ossicle 385.23
  elbow (closed) 832.00
    anterior (closed) 832.01
      open 832.11
    congenital 754.89
    divergent (closed) 832.09
      open 832.19
    lateral (closed) 832.04
      open 832.14
    medial (closed) 832.03
      open 832.13
    open 832.10
    posterior (closed) 832.02
      open 832.12
    recurrent 718.32
    specified type NEC 832.09
      open 832.19
  eye 360.81
    lateral 376.36

Dislocation (Continued)
  eyeball 360.81
    lateral 376.36
  femur
    distal end (closed) 836.50
      anterior 836.52
        open 836.62
      lateral 836.54   ◀▬
        open 836.64   ◀▬
      medial 836.53   ◀▬
        open 836.63   ◀▬
      open 836.60
      posterior 836.51
        open 836.61
    proximal end (closed) 835.00
      anterior (pubic) 835.03
        open 835.13
      obturator 835.02
        open 835.12
      open 835.10
      posterior 835.01
        open 835.11
  fibula
    distal end (closed) 837.0
      open 837.1
    proximal end (closed) 836.59
      open 836.69
  finger(s) (phalanx) (thumb) (closed)
      834.00
    interphalangeal (joint) 834.02
      open 834.12
    metacarpal (bone), distal end
        834.01
      open 834.11
    metacarpophalangeal (joint) 834.01
      open 834.11
    open 834.10
    recurrent 718.34
  foot (closed) 838.00
    open 838.10
    recurrent 718.37
  forearm (closed) 839.8
    open 839.9
  fracture - see Fracture, by site
  glenoid (closed) 831.09
    open 831.19
  habitual - see Dislocation, recurrent
  hand (closed) 839.8
    open 839.9
  hip (closed) 835.00
    anterior 835.03
      obturator 835.02
        open 835.12
      open 835.13
    congenital (unilateral) 754.30
      with subluxation of other hip
          754.35
      bilateral 754.31
    developmental 718.75
    open 835.10
    posterior 835.01
      open 835.11
    recurrent 718.35
  humerus (closed) 831.00
    distal end (see also Dislocation,
        elbow) 832.00
    open 831.10
    proximal end (closed) 831.00
      anterior (subclavicular)
          (subcoracoid) (subglenoid)
          (closed) 831.01
        open 831.11
      inferior (closed) 831.03
        open 831.13

Dislocation (Continued)
  humerus (Continued)
    proximal end (Continued)
      open 831.10
      posterior (closed) 831.02
        open 831.12
    implant - see Complications,
        mechanical
    incus 385.23
    infracoracoid (closed) 831.01
      open 831.11
    innominate (pubic junction) (sacral
        junction) (closed) 839.69
      acetabulum (see also Dislocation,
          hip) 835.00
      open 839.79
    interphalangeal (joint)
      finger or hand (closed) 834.02
        open 834.12
      foot or toe (closed) 838.06
        open 838.16
    jaw (cartilage) (meniscus) (closed)
        830.0
      open 830.1
      recurrent 524.69
    joint NEC (closed) 839.8
      developmental 718.7●
      open 839.9
      pathological - see Dislocation,
          pathological
      recurrent - see Dislocation,
          recurrent
    knee (closed) 836.50
      anterior 836.51
        open 836.61
      congenital (with genu recurvatum)
          754.41
      habitual 718.36
      lateral 836.54
        open 836.64
      medial 836.53
        open 836.63
      old 718.36
      open 836.60
      posterior 836.52
        open 836.62
      recurrent 718.36
      rotatory 836.59
        open 836.69
    lacrimal gland 375.16
    leg (closed) 839.8
      open 839.9
    lens (crystalline) (complete) (partial)
        379.32
      anterior 379.33
      congenital 743.37
      ocular implant 996.53
      posterior 379.34
      traumatic 921.3
    ligament - see Dislocation, by site
    lumbar (vertebrae) (closed) 839.20
      open 839.30
    lumbosacral (vertebrae) (closed)
        839.20
      congenital 756.19
      open 839.30
    mandible (closed) 830.0
      open 830.1
    maxilla (inferior) (closed) 830.0
      open 830.1
    meniscus (knee) - see also Tear,
        meniscus
      other sites - see Dislocation, by
          site

◀ New   ◀▬ Revised   ~~deleted~~ Deleted   ● Use Additional Digit(s)   ▨ Omit code

Dislocation (Continued)
  metacarpal (bone)
    distal end (closed) 834.01
      open 834.11
    proximal end (closed) 833.05
      open 833.15
  metacarpophalangeal (joint) (closed)
    834.01
    open 834.11
  metatarsal (bone) (closed) 838.04
    open 838.14
  metatarsophalangeal (joint) (closed)
    838.05
    open 838.15
  midcarpal (joint) (closed) 833.03
    open 833.13
  midtarsal (joint) (closed) 838.02
    open 838.12
  Monteggia's - see Dislocation, hip
  multiple locations (except fingers only
    or toes only) (closed) 839.8
    open 839.9
  navicular (bone) foot (closed) 837.0
    open 837.1
  neck (see also Dislocation, vertebra,
    cervical) 839.00
  Nélaton's - see Dislocation, ankle
  nontraumatic (joint) - see Dislocation,
    pathological
  nose (closed) 839.69
    open 839.79
  not recurrent, not current injury - see
    Dislocation, pathological
  occiput from atlas (closed) 839.01
    open 839.11
  old - see Dislocation, recurrent
  open (compound) NEC 839.9
  ossicle, ear 385.23
  paralytic (flaccid) (spastic) - see
    Dislocation, pathological
  patella (closed) 836.3
    congenital 755.64
    open 836.4
  pathological NEC 718.20
    ankle 718.27
    elbow 718.22
    foot 718.27
    hand 718.24
    hip 718.25
    knee 718.26
    lumbosacral joint 724.6
    multiple sites 718.29
    pelvic region 718.25
    sacroiliac 724.6
    shoulder (region) 718.21
    specified site NEC 718.28
    spine 724.8
      sacroiliac 724.6
    wrist 718.23
  pelvis (closed) 839.69
    acetabulum (see also Dislocation,
      hip) 835.00
    open 839.79
  phalanx
    foot or toe (closed) 838.09
      open 838.19
    hand or finger (see also Dislocation,
      finger) 834.00
  postpoliomyelitic - see Dislocation,
    pathological
  prosthesis, internal - see Complications,
    mechanical
  radiocarpal (joint) (closed) 833.02
    open 833.12

Dislocation (Continued)
  radioulnar (joint)
    distal end (closed) 833.01
      open 833.11
    proximal end (see also Dislocation,
      elbow) 832.00
  radius
    distal end (closed) 833.00
      open 833.10
    proximal end (closed) 832.01
      open 832.11
  recurrent (see also Derangement, joint,
    recurrent) 718.3●
    elbow 718.32
    hip 718.35
    joint NEC 718.38
    knee 718.36
    lumbosacral (joint) 724.6
    patella 718.36
    sacroiliac 724.6
    shoulder 718.31
    temporomandibular 524.69
  rib (cartilage) (closed) 839.69
    congenital 756.3
    open 839.79
  sacrococcygeal (closed) 839.42
    open 839.52
  sacroiliac (joint) (ligament) (closed)
    839.42
    congenital 755.69
    open 839.52
    recurrent 724.6
  sacrum (closed) 839.42
    open 839.52
  scaphoid (bone)
    ankle or foot (closed) 837.0
      open 837.1
    wrist (closed) (see also Dislocation,
      wrist) 833.00
      open 833.10
  scapula (closed) 831.09
    open 831.19
  semilunar cartilage, knee - see Tear,
    meniscus
  septal cartilage (nose) (closed) 839.69
    open 839.79
  septum (nasal) (old) 470
  sesamoid bone - see Dislocation, by site
  shoulder (blade) (ligament) (closed)
    831.00
    anterior (subclavicular) (subcoracoid)
      (subglenoid) (closed) 831.01
      open 831.11
    chronic 718.31
    inferior 831.03
      open 831.13
    open 831.10
    posterior (closed) 831.02
      open 831.12
    recurrent 718.31
  skull - see Injury, intracranial
  Smith's - see Dislocation, foot
  spine (articular process) (see also
    Dislocation, vertebra) (closed)
    839.40
    atlanto-axial (closed) 839.01
      open 839.11
      recurrent 723.8
    cervical, cervicodorsal,
      cervicothoracic (closed) (see
      also Dislocation, vertebrae,
      cervical) 839.00
      open 839.10
      recurrent 723.8

Dislocation (Continued)
  spine (Continued)
    coccyx 839.41
      open 839.51
    congenital 756.19
    due to birth trauma 767.4
    open 839.50
    recurrent 724.9
    sacroiliac 839.42
      recurrent 724.6
    sacrum (sacrococcygeal) (sacroiliac)
      839.42
      open 839.52
  spontaneous - see Dislocation,
    pathological
  sternoclavicular (joint) (closed)
    839.61
    open 839.71
  sternum (closed) 839.61
    open 839.71
  subastragalar - see Dislocation, foot
  subglenoid (closed) 831.01
    open 831.11
  symphysis
    jaw (closed) 830.0
      open 830.1
    mandibular (closed) 830.0
      open 830.1
    pubis (closed) 839.69
      open 839.79
  tarsal (bone) (joint) 838.01
    open 838.11
  tarsometatarsal (joint) 838.03
    open 838.13
  temporomandibular (joint) (closed)
    830.0
    open 830.1
    recurrent 524.69
  thigh
    distal end (see also Dislocation,
      femur, distal end) 836.50
    proximal end (see also Dislocation,
      hip) 835.00
  thoracic (vertebrae) (closed) 839.21
    open 839.31
  thumb(s) (see also Dislocation, finger)
    834.00
  thyroid cartilage (closed) 839.69
    open 839.79
  tibia
    distal end (closed) 837.0
      open 837.1
    proximal end (closed) 836.50
      anterior 836.51
        open 836.61
      lateral 836.54
        open 836.64
      medial 836.53
        open 836.63
      open 836.60
      posterior 836.52
        open 836.62
      rotatory 836.59
        open 836.69
  tibiofibular
    distal (closed) 837.0
      open 837.1
    superior (closed) 836.59
      open 836.69
  toe(s) (closed) 838.09
    open 838.19
  trachea (closed) 839.69
    open 839.79

Dislocation *(Continued)*
  ulna
    distal end (closed) 833.09
      open 833.19
    proximal end - *see* Dislocation,
      elbow
    vertebra (articular process) (body)
      (closed) (traumatic) 839.40
    cervical, cervicodorsal or
        cervicothoracic (closed) 839.00
      first (atlas) 839.01
        open 839.11
      second (axis) 839.02
        open 839.12
      third 839.03
        open 839.13
      fourth 839.04
        open 839.14
      fifth 839.05
        open 839.15
      sixth 839.06
        open 839.16
      seventh 839.07
        open 839.17
      congenital 756.19
      multiple sites 839.08
        open 839.18
      open 839.10
    congenital 756.19
    dorsal 839.21
      open 839.31
      recurrent 724.9
    lumbar, lumbosacral 839.20
      open 839.30
    non-traumatic - *see* Displacement,
      intervertebral disc
    open NEC 839.50
    recurrent 724.9
    specified region NEC 839.49
      open 839.59
    thoracic 839.21
      open 839.31
  wrist (carpal bone) (scaphoid)
      (semilunar) (closed) 833.00
    carpometacarpal (joint) 833.04
      open 833.14
    metacarpal bone, proximal end
      833.05
      open 833.15
    midcarpal (joint) 833.03
      open 833.13
    open 833.10
    radiocarpal (joint) 833.02
      open 833.12
    radioulnar (joint) 833.01
      open 833.11
    recurrent 718.33
    specified site NEC 833.09
      open 833.19
  xiphoid cartilage (closed) 839.61
    open 839.71
Dislodgement
  artificial skin graft 996.55
  decellularized allodermis graft
    996.55
Disobedience, hostile (covert) (overt)
    (*see also* Disturbance, conduct)
    312.0●
Disorder - *see also* Disease
  academic underachievement,
    childhood and adolescence 313.83
  accommodation 367.51
    drug-induced 367.89
    toxic 367.89

Disorder *(Continued)*
  adjustment (*see also* Reaction,
    adjustment) 309.9
    with
      anxiety 309.24
      anxiety and depressed mood
        309.28
      depressed mood 309.0
      disturbance of conduct 309.3
      disturbance of emotions and
        conduct 309.4
  adrenal (capsule) (cortex) (gland) 255.9
    specified type NEC 255.8
  adrenogenital 255.2
  affective (*see also* Psychosis, affective)
    296.90
    atypical 296.81
  aggressive, unsocialized (*see also*
    Disturbance, conduct) 312.0●
  alcohol, alcoholic (*see also* Alcohol)
    291.9
  allergic - *see* Allergy
  amino acid (metabolic) (*see also*
    Disturbance, metabolism, amino
    acid) 270.9
    albinism 270.2
    alkaptonuria 270.2
    argininosuccinicaciduria 270.6
    beta-amino-isobutyricaciduria 277.2
    cystathioninuria 270.4
    cystinosis 270.0
    cystinuria 270.0
    glycinuria 270.0
    homocystinuria 270.4
    imidazole 270.5
    maple syrup (urine) disease 270.3
    neonatal, transitory 775.89
    oasthouse urine disease 270.2
    ochronosis 270.2
    phenylketonuria 270.1
    phenylpyruvic oligophrenia 270.1
    purine NEC 277.2
    pyrimidine NEC 277.2
    renal transport NEC 270.0
    specified type NEC 270.8
    transport NEC 270.0
      renal 270.0
    xanthinuria 277.2
  amnestic (*see also* Amnestic syndrome)
    294.8
    alcohol-induced persisting 291.1
    drug-induced persisting 292.83
    in conditions classified elsewhere
      294.0
  anaerobic glycolysis with anemia 282.3
  anxiety (*see also* Anxiety) 300.00
    due to or associated with physical
      condition 293.84
  arteriole 447.9
    specified type NEC 447.8
  artery 447.9
    specified type NEC 447.8
  articulation - *see* Disorder, joint
  Asperger's 299.8●
  attachment of infancy or early
    childhood 313.89
  attention deficit 314.00
    with hyperactivity 314.01
    predominantly
    combined hyperactive/inattentive
      314.01
      hyperactive/impulsive 314.01
      inattentive 314.00
    residual type 314.8

Disorder *(Continued)*
  auditory processing disorder 388.45
    acquired 388.45
    developmental 315.32
  autistic 299.0●
  autoimmune NEC 279.49   ◀▥
    hemolytic (cold type) (warm type)
      283.0
    parathyroid 252.1
    thyroid 245.2
  avoidant, childhood or adolescence
    313.21
  balance
    acid-base 276.9
      mixed (with hypercapnia)
        276.4
    electrolyte 276.9
    fluid 276.9
  behavior NEC (*see also* Disturbance,
    conduct) 312.9
    disruptive 312.9
  bilirubin excretion 277.4
  bipolar (affective) (alternating)
    296.80

  Note 63   Use the following fifth-digit
  subclassification with categories 296.0–
  296.6:

  0   unspecified
  1   mild
  2   moderate
  3   severe, without mention of
          psychotic behavior
  4   severe, specified as with
          psychotic behavior
  5   in partial or unspecified
          remission
  6   in full remission

    atypical 296.7
    specified type NEC 296.89
    type I 296.7
      most recent episode (or current)
        depressed 296.5●
        hypomanic 296.4●
        manic 296.4●
        mixed 296.6●
        unspecified 296.7
      single manic episode 296.0●
    type II (recurrent major depressive
      episodes with hypomania)
      296.89
  bladder 596.9
    functional NEC 596.59
    specified NEC 596.8
  bleeding 286.9
  bone NEC 733.90
    specified NEC 733.99
  brachial plexus 353.0
  branched-chain amino-acid
    degradation 270.3
  breast 611.9
    puerperal, postpartum 676.3●
    specified NEC 611.89
  Briquet's 300.81
  bursa 727.9
    shoulder region 726.10
  carbohydrate metabolism, congenital
    271.9
  cardiac, functional 427.9
    postoperative 997.1
    psychogenic 306.2
  cardiovascular, psychogenic 306.2

Disorder *(Continued)*
    cartilage NEC 733.90
        articular 718.00
            ankle 718.07
            elbow 718.02
            foot 718.07
            hand 718.04
            hip 718.05
            knee 717.9
            multiple sites 718.09
            pelvic region 718.05
            shoulder region 718.01
            specified
                site NEC 718.08
                type NEC 733.99
            wrist 718.03
    catatonic - *see* Catatonia
    central auditory processing 315.32
        acquired 388.45
        developmental 315.32
    cervical region NEC 723.9
    cervical root (nerve) NEC 353.2
    character NEC *(see also* Disorder,
            personality) 301.9
    ciliary body 364.9
        specified NEC 364.89
    coagulation (factor) *(see also* Defect,
            coagulation) 286.9
        factor VIII (congenital) (functional)
            286.0
        factor IX (congenital) (functional)
            286.1
        neonatal, transitory 776.3
    coccyx 724.70
        specified NEC 724.79
    cognitive 294.9
    colon 569.9
        functional 564.9
            congenital 751.3
    communication 307.9
    conduct *(see also* Disturbance, conduct)
            312.9
        adjustment reaction 309.3
        adolescent onset type 312.82
        childhood onset type 312.81
        compulsive 312.30
            specified type NEC 312.39
        hyperkinetic 314.2
        onset unspecified 312.89
        socialized (type) 312.20
            aggressive 312.23
            unaggressive 312.21
        specified NEC 312.89
    conduction, heart 426.9
        specified NEC 426.89
    conflict
        sexual orientation 302.0
    congenital
        glycosylation (CDG) 271.8
    convulsive (secondary) *(see also*
            Convulsions) 780.39
        due to injury at birth 767.0
        idiopathic 780.39
    coordination 781.3
    cornea NEC 371.89
        due to contact lens 371.82
    corticosteroid metabolism NEC
            255.2
    cranial nerve - *see* Disorder, nerve,
            cranial
    cyclothymic 301.13
    degradation, branched-chain amino
            acid 270.3
    delusional 297.1

Disorder *(Continued)*
    dentition 520.6
    depersonalization 300.6
    depressive NEC 311
        atypical 296.82
        major *(see also* Psychosis, affective)
            296.2●
            recurrent episode 296.3●
            single episode 296.2●
    development, specific 315.9
        associated with hyperkinesia
            314.1
        coordination 315.4
        language 315.31
            and speech due to hearing loss
                315.34
        learning 315.2
            arithmetical 315.1
            reading 315.00
        mixed 315.5
        motor coordination 315.4
        specified type NEC 315.8
        speech 315.39
            and language due to hearing loss
                315.34
    diaphragm 519.4
    digestive 536.9
        fetus or newborn 777.9
            specified NEC 777.8
        psychogenic 306.4
    disintegrative childhood 299.1●
    dissociative 300.15
        identity 300.14
        nocturnal 307.47
    drug-related 292.9
    dysmorphic body 300.7
    dysthymic 300.4
    ear 388.9
        degenerative NEC 388.00
        external 380.9
            specified 380.89
        pinna 380.30
        specified type NEC 388.8
        vascular NEC 388.00
    eating NEC 307.50
    electrolyte NEC 276.9
        with
            abortion - *see* Abortion, by type,
                with metabolic disorder
            ectopic pregnancy *(see also*
                categories 633.0–633.9)
                639.4
            molar pregnancy *(see also*
                categories 630–632) 639.4
        acidosis 276.2
            metabolic 276.2
            respiratory 276.2
        alkalosis 276.3
            metabolic 276.3
            respiratory 276.3
        following
            abortion 639.4
            ectopic or molar pregnancy
                639.4
        neonatal, transitory NEC 775.5
    emancipation as adjustment reaction
            309.22
    emotional *(see also* Disorder, mental,
            nonpsychotic) V40.9
    endocrine 259.9
        specified type NEC 259.8
    esophagus 530.9
        functional 530.5
        psychogenic 306.4

Disorder *(Continued)*
    explosive
        intermittent 312.34
        isolated 312.35
    expressive language 315.31
    eye 379.90
        globe - *see* Disorder, globe
        ill-defined NEC 379.99
        limited duction NEC 378.63
        specified NEC 379.8
    eyelid 374.9
        degenerative 374.50
        sensory 374.44
        specified type NEC 374.89
        vascular 374.85
    factitious (with combined
            psychological and physical
            signs and symptoms) (with
            predominantly physical signs
            and symptoms) 300.19
        with predominantly psychological
            signs and symptoms 300.16
    factor, coagulation *(see also* Defect,
            coagulation) 286.9
        VIII (congenital) (functional)
            286.0
        IX (congenital) (functional) 286.1
    fascia 728.9
    fatty acid oxidation 277.85
    feeding - *see* Feeding
    female sexual arousal 302.72
    fluid NEC 276.9
    gastric (functional) 536.9
        motility 536.8
        psychogenic 306.4
        secretion 536.8
    gastrointestinal (functional) NEC
            536.9
        newborn (neonatal) 777.9
            specified NEC 777.8
        psychogenic 306.4
    gender (child) 302.6
        adult 302.85
    gender identity (childhood) 302.6
        adolescents 302.85
        adults (-life) 302.85
    genitourinary system, psychogenic
            306.50
    globe 360.9
        degenerative 360.20
            specified NEC 360.29
        specified type NEC 360.89
    hearing - *see also* Deafness
        conductive type (air) *(see also*
                Deafness, conductive)
                389.00
        mixed conductive and
                sensorineural 389.20
            bilateral 389.22
            unilateral 389.21
        nerve
            bilateral 389.12
            unilateral 389.13
        perceptive *(see also* Deafness,
                perceptive) 389.10
        sensorineural type NEC *(see also*
                Deafness, sensorineural)
                389.10
    heart action 427.9
        postoperative 997.1
    hematological, transient neonatal
            776.9
        specified type NEC 776.8
    hematopoietic organs 289.9

Disorder *(Continued)*
  hemorrhagic NEC 287.9
    due to intrinsic circulating
      anticoagulants 286.5
    specified type NEC 287.8
  hemostasis *(see also* Defect, coagulation)
    286.9
  homosexual conflict 302.0
  hypomanic (chronic) 301.11
  identity
    childhood and adolescence 313.82
      gender 302.6
  immune mechanism (immunity) 279.9
    single complement (C_1–C_9) 279.8
    specified type NEC 279.8
  impulse control *(see also* Disturbance,
    conduct, compulsive) 312.30
  infant sialic acid storage 271.8
  integument, fetus or newborn 778.9
    specified type NEC 778.8
  interactional psychotic (childhood) *(see*
    also Psychosis, childhood)
    299.1●
  intermittent explosive 312.34
  intervertebral disc 722.90
    cervical, cervicothoracic 722.91
    lumbar, lumbosacral 722.93
    thoracic, thoracolumbar 722.92
  intestinal 569.9
    functional NEC 564.9
      congenital 751.3
      postoperative 564.4
    psychogenic 306.4
  introverted, of childhood and
    adolescence 313.22
  involuntary emotional expression
    (IEED) 310.8
  iris 364.9
    specified NEC 364.89
  iron, metabolism 275.0
  isolated explosive 312.35
  joint NEC 719.90
    ankle 719.97
    elbow 719.92
    foot 719.97
    hand 719.94
    hip 719.95
    knee 719.96
    multiple sites 719.99
    pelvic region 719.95
    psychogenic 306.0
    shoulder (region) 719.91
    specified site NEC 719.98
    temporomandibular 524.60
      sounds on opening or closing
        524.64
      specified NEC 524.69
    wrist 719.93
  kidney 593.9
    functional 588.9
      specified NEC 588.89
  labyrinth, labyrinthine 386.9
    specified type NEC 386.8
  lactation 676.9●
  language (developmental) (expressive)
    315.31
    mixed receptive-expressive 315.32
  learning 315.9
  ligament 728.9
  ligamentous attachments, peripheral -
    see also Enthesopathy
    spine 720.1
  limb NEC 729.90
    psychogenic 306.0

Disorder *(Continued)*
  lipid
    metabolism, congenital 272.9
    storage 272.7
  lipoprotein deficiency (familial) 272.5
  low back NEC 724.9
    psychogenic 306.0
  lumbosacral
    plexus 353.1
    root (nerve) NEC 353.4
  lymphoproliferative (chronic) NEC
    (M9970/1) 238.79
    post-transplant (PTLD) 238.77
  major depressive *(see also* Psychosis,
    affective) 296.2●
    recurrent episode 296.3●
    single episode 296.2●
  male erectile 607.84
    nonorganic origin 302.72
  manic *(see also* Psychosis, affective)
    296.0●
    atypical 296.81
  mathematics 315.1
  meniscus NEC *(see also* Disorder,
    cartilage, articular) 718.0●
  menopausal 627.9
    specified NEC 627.8
  menstrual 626.9
    psychogenic 306.52
    specified NEC 626.8
  mental (nonpsychotic) 300.9
    affecting management of pregnancy,
      childbirth, or puerperium
      648.4●
    drug-induced 292.9
      hallucinogen persisting
        perception 292.89
      specified type NEC 292.89
    due to or associated with
      alcoholism 291.9
      drug consumption NEC 292.9
        specified type NEC 292.89
      physical condition NEC 293.9
    induced by drug 292.9
      specified type NEC 292.89
    neurotic *(see also* Neurosis) 300.9
    of infancy, childhood or adolescence
      313.9
    persistent
      other
        due to conditions classified
          elsewhere 294.8
      unspecified
        due to conditions classified
          elsewhere 294.9
    presenile 310.1
      psychotic NEC 290.10
    previous, affecting management of
      pregnancy V23.89
    psychoneurotic *(see also* Neurosis)
      300.9
    psychotic *(see also* Psychosis) 298.9
      brief 298.8
      senile 290.20
    specific, following organic brain
      damage 310.9
      cognitive or personality change
        of other type 310.1
      frontal lobe syndrome 310.0
      postconcussional syndrome 310.2
      specified type NEC 310.8
    transient
      in conditions classified elsewhere
      293.9

Disorder *(Continued)*
  metabolism NEC 277.9
    with
      abortion - *see* Abortion, by type,
        with metabolic disorder
      ectopic pregnancy *(see also*
        categories 633.0–633.9)
        639.4
      molar pregnancy *(see also*
        categories 630–632) 639.4
    alkaptonuria 270.2
    amino acid *(see also* Disorder, amino
      acid) 270.9
      specified type NEC 270.8
    ammonia 270.6
    arginine 270.6
    argininosuccinic acid 270.6
    basal 794.7
    bilirubin 277.4
    calcium 275.40
    carbohydrate 271.9
      specified type NEC 271.8
    cholesterol 272.9
    citrulline 270.6
    copper 275.1
    corticosteroid 255.2
    cystine storage 270.0
    cystinuria 270.0
    fat 272.9
      fatty acid oxidation 277.85
    following
      abortion 639.4
      ectopic or molar pregnancy
        639.4
    fructosemia 271.2
    fructosuria 271.2
    fucosidosis 271.8
    galactose-1-phosphate uridyl
      transferase 271.1
    glutamine 270.7
    glycine 270.7
    glycogen storage NEC 271.0
      hepatorenal 271.0
    hemochromatosis 275.0
    in labor and delivery 669.0●
    iron 275.0
    lactose 271.3
    lipid 272.9
      specified type NEC 272.8
      storage 272.7
    lipoprotein - *see also* Hyperlipemia
      deficiency (familial) 272.5
    lysine 270.7
    magnesium 275.2
    mannosidosis 271.8
    mineral 275.9
      specified type NEC 275.8
      mitochondrial 277.87
    mucopolysaccharide 277.5
    nitrogen 270.9
    ornithine 270.6
    oxalosis 271.8
    pentosuria 271.8
    phenylketonuria 270.1
    phosphate 275.3
    phosphorus 275.3
    plasma protein 273.9
      specified type NEC 273.8
    porphyrin 277.1
    purine 277.2
    pyrimidine 277.2
    serine 270.7
    sodium 276.9
    specified type NEC 277.89

◀ New   ◀▐ Revised   ~~deleted~~ Deleted   ● Use Additional Digit(s)   ▓ Omit code

Disorder *(Continued)*
  metabolism NEC *(Continued)*
    steroid 255.2
    threonine 270.7
    urea cycle 270.6
    xylose 271.8
  micturition NEC 788.69
    psychogenic 306.53
  misery and unhappiness, of childhood
    and adolescence 313.1
  mitochondrial metabolism 277.87
  mitral valve 424.0
  mood (*see also* Disorder, bipolar) 296.90
    episodic 296.90
      specified NEC 296.99
    in conditions classified elsewhere
      293.83
  motor tic 307.20
    chronic 307.22
    transient (childhood) 307.21
  movement NEC 333.90
    hysterical 300.11
    medication-induced 333.90
    periodic limb 327.51
    sleep related unspecified 780.58
      other organic 327.59
    specified type NEC 333.99
    stereotypic 307.3
  mucopolysaccharide 277.5
  muscle 728.9
    psychogenic 306.0
    specified type NEC 728.3
  muscular attachments, peripheral - *see
    also* Enthesopathy
    spine 720.1
  musculoskeletal system NEC 729.90
    psychogenic 306.0
  myeloproliferative (chronic) NEC
    (M9960/1) 238.79
  myoneural 358.9
    due to lead 358.2
    specified type NEC 358.8
    toxic 358.2
  myotonic 359.29
  neck region NEC 723.9
  nerve 349.9
    abducens NEC 378.54
    accessory 352.4
    acoustic 388.5
    auditory 388.5
    auriculotemporal 350.8
    axillary 353.0
    cerebral - *see* Disorder, nerve, cranial
    cranial 352.9
      first 352.0
      second 377.49
      third
        partial 378.51
        total 378.52
      fourth 378.53
      fifth 350.9
      sixth 378.54
      seventh NEC 351.9
      eighth 388.5
      ninth 352.2
      tenth 352.3
      eleventh 352.4
      twelfth 352.5
      multiple 352.6
    entrapment - *see* Neuropathy,
      entrapment
    facial 351.9
      specified NEC 351.8
    femoral 355.2

Disorder *(Continued)*
  nerve *(Continued)*
    glossopharyngeal NEC 352.2
    hypoglossal 352.5
    iliohypogastric 355.79
    ilioinguinal 355.79
    intercostal 353.8
    lateral
      cutaneous of thigh 355.1
      popliteal 355.3
    lower limb NEC 355.8
    medial, popliteal 355.4
    median NEC 354.1
    obturator 355.79
    oculomotor
      partial 378.51
      total 378.52
    olfactory 352.0
    optic 377.49
      hypoplasia 377.43
      ischemic 377.41
      nutritional 377.33
      toxic 377.34
    peroneal 355.3
    phrenic 354.8
    plantar 355.6
    pneumogastric 352.3
    posterior tibial 355.5
    radial 354.3
    recurrent laryngeal 352.3
    root 353.9
      specified NEC 353.8
    saphenous 355.79
    sciatic NEC 355.0
    specified NEC 355.9
      lower limb 355.79
      upper limb 354.8
    spinal 355.9
    sympathetic NEC 337.9
    trigeminal 350.9
      specified NEC 350.8
    trochlear 378.53
    ulnar 354.2
    upper limb NEC 354.9
    vagus 352.3
  nervous system NEC 349.9
    autonomic (peripheral) (*see also*
      Neuropathy, peripheral,
      autonomic) 337.9
    cranial 352.9
    parasympathetic (*see also*
      Neuropathy, peripheral,
      autonomic) 337.9
    specified type NEC 349.89
    sympathetic (*see also* Neuropathy,
      peripheral, autonomic) 337.9
    vegetative (*see also* Neuropathy,
      peripheral, autonomic) 337.9
  neurohypophysis NEC 253.6
  neurological NEC 781.99
    peripheral NEC 355.9
  neuromuscular NEC 358.9
    hereditary NEC 359.1
    specified NEC 358.8
    toxic 358.2
  neurotic 300.9
    specified type NEC 300.89
  neutrophil, polymorphonuclear
    (functional) 288.1
  nightmare 307.47
  night terror 307.46
  obsessive-compulsive 300.3
  oppositional defiant, childhood and
    adolescence 313.81

Disorder *(Continued)*
  optic
    chiasm 377.54
      associated with
        inflammatory disorders 377.54
        neoplasm NEC 377.52
          pituitary 377.51
        pituitary disorders 377.51
        vascular disorders 377.53
    nerve 377.49
    radiations 377.63
    tracts 377.63
  orbit 376.9
    specified NEC 376.89
  orgasmic
    female 302.73
    male 302.74
  overanxious, of childhood and
    adolescence 313.0
  oxidation, fatty acid 277.85
  pancreas, internal secretion (other than
    diabetes mellitus) 251.9
    specified type NEC 251.8
  panic 300.01
    with agoraphobia 300.21
  papillary muscle NEC 429.81
  paranoid 297.9
    induced 297.3
    shared 297.3
  parathyroid 252.9
    specified type NEC 252.8
  paroxysmal, mixed 780.39
  pentose phosphate pathway with
    anemia 282.2
  periodic limb movement 327.51
  peroxisomal 277.86
  personality 301.9
    affective 301.10
    aggressive 301.3
    amoral 301.7
    anancastic, anankastic 301.4
    antisocial 301.7
    asocial 301.7
    asthenic 301.6
    avoidant 301.82
    borderline 301.83
    compulsive 301.4
    cyclothymic 301.13
    dependent-passive 301.6
    dyssocial 301.7
    emotional instability 301.59
    epileptoid 301.3
    explosive 301.3
    following organic brain damage
      310.1
    histrionic 301.50
    hyperthymic 301.11
    hypomanic (chronic) 301.11
    hypothymic 301.12
    hysterical 301.50
    immature 301.89
    inadequate 301.6
    introverted 301.21
    labile 301.59
    moral deficiency 301.7
    narcissistic 301.81
    obsessional 301.4
    obsessive-compulsive 301.4
    overconscientious 301.4
    paranoid 301.0
    passive (-dependent) 301.6
    passive-aggressive 301.84
    pathological NEC 301.9
    pseudosocial 301.7

Disorder *(Continued)*
  personality *(Continued)*
    psychopathic 301.9
    schizoid 301.20
      introverted 301.21
      schizotypal 301.22
    schizotypal 301.22
    seductive 301.59
    type A 301.4
    unstable 301.59
  pervasive developmental 299.9●
    childhood-onset 299.8●
    specified NEC 299.8●
  phonological 315.39
  pigmentation, choroid (congenital) 743.53
  pinna 380.30
    specified type NEC 380.39
  pituitary, thalamic 253.9
    anterior NEC 253.4
    iatrogenic 253.7
    postablative 253.7
    specified NEC 253.8
  pityriasis-like NEC 696.8
  platelets (blood) 287.1
  polymorphonuclear neutrophils (functional) 288.1
  porphyrin metabolism 277.1
  postmenopausal 627.9
    specified type NEC 627.8
  post-transplant lymphoproliferative (PTLD) 238.77
  post-traumatic stress (PTSD) 309.81
  posttraumatic stress 309.81
    acute 309.81
    brief 309.81
    chronic 309.81
  premenstrual dysphoric (PMDD) 625.4
  psoriatic-like NEC 696.8
  psychic, with diseases classified elsewhere 316
  psychogenic NEC *(see also* condition) 300.9
    allergic NEC
      respiratory 306.1
    anxiety 300.00
      atypical 300.00
      generalized 300.02
    appetite 307.59
    articulation, joint 306.0
    asthenic 300.5
    blood 306.8
    cardiovascular (system) 306.2
    compulsive 300.3
    cutaneous 306.3
    depressive 300.4
    digestive (system) 306.4
    dysmenorrheic 306.52
    dyspneic 306.1
    eczematous 306.3
    endocrine (system) 306.6
    eye 306.7
    feeding 307.59
    functional NEC 306.9
    gastric 306.4
    gastrointestinal (system) 306.4
    genitourinary (system) 306.50
    heart (function) (rhythm) 306.2
    hemic 306.8
    hyperventilatory 306.1
    hypochondriacal 300.7
    hysterical 300.10
    intestinal 306.4

Disorder *(Continued)*
  psychogenic NEC *(Continued)*
    joint 306.0
    learning 315.2
    limb 306.0
    lymphatic (system) 306.8
    menstrual 306.52
    micturition 306.53
    monoplegic NEC 306.0
    motor 307.9
    muscle 306.0
    musculoskeletal 306.0
    neurocirculatory 306.2
    obsessive 300.3
    occupational 300.89
    organ or part of body NEC 306.9
    organs of special sense 306.7
    paralytic NEC 306.0
    phobic 300.20
    physical NEC 306.9
    pruritic 306.3
    rectal 306.4
    respiratory (system) 306.1
    rheumatic 306.0
    sexual (function) 302.70
      specified type NEC 302.79
    sexual orientation conflict 302.0
    skin (allergic) (eczematous) (pruritic) 306.3
    sleep 307.40
      initiation or maintenance 307.41
        persistent 307.42
        transient 307.41
      movement 780.58
      sleep terror 307.46
      specified type NEC 307.49
    specified part of body NEC 306.8
    stomach 306.4
  psychomotor NEC 307.9
    hysterical 300.11
  psychoneurotic *(see also* Neurosis) 300.9
    mixed NEC 300.89
  psychophysiologic *(see also* Disorder, psychosomatic) 306.9
  psychosexual identity (childhood) 302.6
    adult-life 302.85
  psychosomatic NEC 306.9
    allergic NEC
      respiratory 306.1
    articulation, joint 306.0
    cardiovascular (system) 306.2
    cutaneous 306.3
    digestive (system) 306.4
    dysmenorrheic 306.52
    dyspneic 306.1
    endocrine (system) 306.6
    eye 306.7
    gastric 306.4
    gastrointestinal (system) 306.4
    genitourinary (system) 306.50
    heart (functional) (rhythm) 306.2
    hyperventilatory 306.1
    intestinal 306.4
    joint 306.0
    limb 306.0
    lymphatic (system) 306.8
    menstrual 306.52
    micturition 306.53
    monoplegic NEC 306.0
    muscle 306.0
    musculoskeletal 306.0
    neurocirculatory 306.2
    organs of special sense 306.7

Disorder *(Continued)*
  psychosomatic NEC *(Continued)*
    paralytic NEC 306.0
    pruritic 306.3
    rectal 306.4
    respiratory (system) 306.1
    rheumatic 306.0
    sexual (function) 302.70
      specified type NEC 302.79
    skin 306.3
    specified part of body NEC 306.8
    stomach 306.4
  psychotic *(see also* Psychosis) 298.9
    brief 298.8
  purine metabolism NEC 277.2
  pyrimidine metabolism NEC 277.2
  reactive attachment of infancy or early childhood 313.89
  reading, developmental 315.00
  reflex 796.1
  REM sleep behavior 327.42
  renal function, impaired 588.9
    specified type NEC 588.89
  renal transport NEC 588.89
  respiration, respiratory NEC 519.9
    due to
      aspiration of liquids or solids 508.9
      inhalation of fumes or vapors 506.9
    psychogenic 306.1
  retina 362.9
    specified type NEC 362.89
  rumination 307.53
  sacroiliac joint NEC 724.6
  sacrum 724.6
  schizo-affective *(see also* Schizophrenia) 295.7●
  schizoid, childhood or adolescence 313.22
  schizophreniform 295.4●
  schizotypal personality 301.22
  secretion, thyrocalcitonin 246.0
  seizure 345.9●
    recurrent 345.9●
      epileptic - *see* Epilepsy
  semantic pragmatic 315.39
    with autism 299.0●
  sense of smell 781.1
    psychogenic 306.7
  separation anxiety 309.21
  sexual *(see also* Deviation, sexual) 302.9
    aversion 302.79
    desire, hypoactive 302.71
    function, psychogenic 302.70
  shyness, of childhood and adolescence 313.21
  single complement (C_1–C_9) 279.8
  skin NEC 709.9
    fetus or newborn 778.9
      specified type 778.8
    psychogenic (allergic) (eczematous) (pruritic) 306.3
    specified type NEC 709.8
    vascular 709.1
  sleep 780.50
    with apnea - *see* Apnea, sleep
    alcohol induced 291.82
    arousal 307.46
      confusional 327.41
    circadian rhythm 327.30
      advanced sleep phase type 327.32
      alcohol induced 291.82
      delayed sleep phase type 327.31

◀ New   ◀▥ Revised   ~~deleted~~ Deleted   ● Use Additional Digit(s)   ▨ Omit code

Disorder *(Continued)*
  sleep *(Continued)*
    circadian rhythm *(Continued)*
      drug induced 292.85
      free running type 327.34
      in conditions classified elsewhere
        327.37
      irregular sleep-wake type
        327.33
      jet lag type 327.35
      other 327.39
      shift work type 327.36
    drug induced 292.85
    initiation or maintenance *(see also*
      Insomnia) 780.52
    nonorganic origin (transient)
      307.41
      persistent 307.42
    nonorganic origin 307.40
      specified type NEC 307.49
    organic specified type NEC 327.8
    periodic limb movement 327.51
    specified NEC 780.59
    wake
      cycle - *see* Disorder, sleep,
        circadian rhythm
      schedule - *see* Disorder, sleep,
        circadian rhythm
  social, of childhood and adolescence
    313.22
  soft tissue 729.90
    specified type NEC 729.99
  somatization 300.81
  somatoform (atypical)
    (undifferentiated) 300.82
    severe 300.81
    specified type NEC 300.89
  speech NEC 784.59 ◀▥
    nonorganic origin 307.9
  spine NEC 724.9
    ligamentous or muscular
      attachments, peripheral 720.1
  steroid metabolism NEC 255.2
  stomach (functional) *(see also* Disorder,
    gastric) 536.9
    psychogenic 306.4
  storage, iron 275.0
  stress *(see also* Reaction, stress, acute)
    308.3
    posttraumatic
      acute 309.81
      brief 309.81
      chronic (motor or vocal)
        309.81
  substitution 300.11
  suspected - *see* Observation
  synovium 727.9
  temperature regulation, fetus or
    newborn 778.4
  temporomandibular joint NEC 524.60
    sounds on opening or closing
      524.64
    specified NEC 524.69
  tendon 727.9
    shoulder region 726.10
  thoracic root (nerve) NEC 353.3
  thyrocalcitonin secretion 246.0
  thyroid (gland) NEC 246.9
    specified type NEC 246.8
  tic 307.20
    chronic (motor or vocal) 307.22
    motor-verbal 307.23
    organic origin 333.1
    transient (of childhood) 307.21

Disorder *(Continued)*
  tooth NEC 525.9
    development NEC 520.9
      specified type NEC 520.8
    eruption 520.6
    specified type NEC 525.8
  Tourette's 307.23
  transport, carbohydrate 271.9
    specified type NEC 271.8
  tubular, phosphate-losing 588.0
  tympanic membrane 384.9
  unaggressive, unsocialized *(see also*
    Disturbance, conduct) 312.1●
  undersocialized, unsocialized *(see also*
    Disturbance, conduct)
    aggressive (type) 312.0●
    unaggressive (type) 312.1●
  vision, visual NEC 368.9
    binocular NEC 368.30
    cortex 377.73
      associated with
        inflammatory disorders 377.73
        neoplasms 377.71
        vascular disorders 377.72
    pathway NEC 377.63
      associated with
        inflammatory disorders 377.63
        neoplasms 377.61
        vascular disorders 377.62
  vocal tic
    chronic 307.22
  wakefulness *(see also* Hypersomnia)
    780.54
    nonorganic origin (transient) 307.43
      persistent 307.44
  written expression 315.2
Disorganized globe 360.29
Displacement, displaced

Note 24 For acquired displacement of
bones, cartilage, joints, tendons, due to
injury, *see also* Dislocation.

Displacements at ages under one year
should be considered congenital,
provided there is no indication the
condition was acquired after birth.

----

  acquired traumatic of bone, cartilage,
    joint, tendon NEC (without
    fracture) *(see also* Dislocation)
    839.8
    with fracture - *see* Fracture, by site
  adrenal gland (congenital) 759.1
  alveolus and teeth, vertical 524.75
  appendix, retrocecal (congenital) 751.5
  auricle (congenital) 744.29
  bladder (acquired) 596.8
    congenital 753.8
  brachial plexus (congenital) 742.8
  brain stem, caudal 742.4
  canaliculus lacrimalis 743.65
  cardia, through esophageal hiatus 750.6
  cerebellum, caudal 742.4
  cervix - *see* Displacement, uterus
  colon (congenital) 751.4
  device, implant, or graft - *see*
    Complications, mechanical
  epithelium
    columnar of cervix 622.10
    cuboidal, beyond limits of external
      os (uterus) 752.49
  esophageal mucosa into cardia of
    stomach, congenital 750.4

Displacement, displaced *(Continued)*
  esophagus (acquired) 530.89
    congenital 750.4
  eyeball (acquired) (old) 376.36
    congenital 743.8
    current injury 871.3
    lateral 376.36
  fallopian tube (acquired) 620.4
    congenital 752.19
    opening (congenital) 752.19
  gallbladder (congenital) 751.69
  gastric mucosa 750.7
    into
      duodenum 750.7
      esophagus 750.7
      Meckel's diverticulum, congenital
        750.7
  globe (acquired) (lateral) (old) 376.36
    current injury 871.3
  graft
    artificial skin graft 996.55
    decellularized allodermis graft
      996.55
  heart (congenital) 746.87
    acquired 429.89
  hymen (congenital) (upward) 752.49
  internal prosthesis NEC - *see*
    Complications, mechanical
  intervertebral disc (with neuritis,
    radiculitis, sciatica, or other pain)
    722.2
    with myelopathy 722.70
    cervical, cervicodorsal,
      cervicothoracic 722.0
      with myelopathy 722.71
      due to major trauma - *see*
        Dislocation, vertebra,
        cervical
    due to trauma - *see* Dislocation,
      vertebra
    lumbar, lumbosacral 722.10
      with myelopathy 722.73
      due to major trauma - *see*
        Dislocation, vertebra,
        lumbar
    thoracic, thoracolumbar 722.11
      with myelopathy 722.72
      due to major trauma - *see*
        Dislocation, vertebra,
        thoracic
  intrauterine device 996.32
  kidney (acquired) 593.0
    congenital 753.3
  lacrimal apparatus or duct (congenital)
    743.65
  macula (congenital) 743.55
  Meckel's diverticulum (congenital)
    751.0
  nail (congenital) 757.5
    acquired 703.8
  opening of Wharton's duct in mouth
    750.26
  organ or site, congenital NEC - *see*
    Malposition, congenital
  ovary (acquired) 620.4
    congenital 752.0
    free in peritoneal cavity (congenital)
      752.0
    into hernial sac 620.4
  oviduct (acquired) 620.4
    congenital 752.19
  parathyroid (gland) 252.8
  parotid gland (congenital) 750.26
  punctum lacrimale (congenital) 743.65

Displacement, displaced *(Continued)*
  sacroiliac (congenital) (joint) 755.69
    current injury - *see* Dislocation,
      sacroiliac
    old 724.6
  spine (congenital) 756.19
  spleen, congenital 759.0
  stomach (congenital) 750.7
    acquired 537.89
  subglenoid (closed) 831.01
  sublingual duct (congenital) 750.26
  teeth, tooth 524.30
    horizontal 524.33
    vertical 524.34
  tongue (congenital) (downward)
    750.19
  trachea (congenital) 748.3
  ureter or ureteric opening or orifice
    (congenital) 753.4
  uterine opening of oviducts or
    fallopian tubes 752.19
  uterus, uterine *(see also* Malposition,
    uterus) 621.6
    congenital 752.3
  ventricular septum 746.89
    with rudimentary ventricle 746.89
  xyphoid bone (process) 738.3
Disproportion 653.9●
  affecting fetus or newborn 763.1
  breast, reconstructed 612.1
    between native and reconstructed
      612.1
  caused by
    conjoined twins 678.1●
    contraction, pelvis (general) 653.1●
      inlet 653.2●
      midpelvic 653.8●
      midplane 653.8●
      outlet 653.3●
    fetal
      ascites 653.7●
      hydrocephalus 653.6●
      hydrops 653.7●
      meningomyelocele 653.7●
      sacral teratoma 653.7●
      tumor 653.7●
    hydrocephalic fetus 653.6●
    pelvis, pelvic, abnormality (bony)
      NEC 653.0●
    unusually large fetus 653.5●
  causing obstructed labor 660.1●
  cephalopelvic, normally formed fetus
    653.4●
    causing obstructed labor 660.1●
  fetal NEC 653.5●
    causing obstructed labor 660.1●
  fetopelvic, normally formed fetus
    653.4●
    causing obstructed labor 660.1●
  mixed maternal and fetal origin,
    normally, formed fetus 653.4●
  pelvis, pelvic (bony) NEC 653.1●
    causing obstructed labor 660.1●
  specified type NEC 653.8●
Disruption
  cesarean wound 674.1●
  family V61.09
    due to
      child in
        care of non-parental family
          member V61.06
        foster care V61.06
        welfare custody V61.05
      death of family member V61.07 ◄
      divorce V61.03

Disruption *(Continued)*
  family *(Continued)*
    due to *(Continued)*
      estrangement V61.09
        parent-child V61.04
      extended absence of family
        member NEC V61.08 ◄
      family member
        on military deployment V61.01
        return from military
          deployment V61.02
      legal separation V61.03
  gastrointestinal anastomosis 997.4
  ligament(s) - *see also* Sprain
    knee
      current injury - *see* Dislocation,
        knee
      old 717.89
        capsular 717.85
        collateral (medial) 717.82
          lateral 717.81
        cruciate (posterior) 717.84
          anterior 717.83
        specified site NEC 717.85
  marital V61.10
    involving
      divorce V61.03
      estrangement V61.09
  operation wound (external) *(see also*
    Dehiscence) 998.32
    internal 998.31
  organ transplant, anastomosis site - *see*
    Complications, transplant, organ,
    by site
  ossicles, ossicular chain 385.23
    traumatic - *see* Fracture, skull, base
  parenchyma
    liver (hepatic) - *see* Laceration, liver,
      major
    spleen - *see* Laceration, spleen,
      parenchyma, massive
  phase-shift, of 24 hour sleep-wake
    cycle, unspecified 780.55
    nonorganic origin 307.45
  sleep-wake cycle (24 hour), unspecified
    780.55
    circadian rhythm 327.33
    nonorganic origin 307.45
  suture line (external) *(see also*
    Dehiscence) 998.32
    internal 998.31
  wound 998.30
    cesarean operation 674.1●
    episiotomy 674.2●
    operation (surgical) 998.32
      cesarean 674.1●
      internal 998.31
    perineal (obstetric) 674.2●
    uterine 674.1●
Disruptio uteri - *see also* Rupture, uterus
  complicating delivery - *see* Delivery,
    complicated, rupture, uterus
Dissatisfaction with
  employment V62.29
  school environment V62.3
Dissecting - *see* condition
Dissection
  aorta 441.00
    abdominal 441.02
    thoracic 441.01
    thoracoabdominal 441.03
  artery, arterial
    carotid 443.21
    coronary 414.12
    iliac 443.22

Dissection *(Continued)*
  artery, arterial *(Continued)*
    renal 443.23
    specified NEC 443.29
    vertebral 443.24
    vascular 459.9
    wound - *see* Wound, open, by site
Disseminated - *see* condition
Dissociated personality NEC 300.15
Dissociation
  auriculoventricular or atrioventricular
    (any degree) (AV) 426.89
    with heart block 426.0
  interference 426.89
  isorhythmic 426.89
  rhythm
    atrioventricular (AV) 426.89
    interference 426.89
Dissociative
  identity disorder 300.14
  reaction NEC 300.15
Dissolution, vertebra *(see also*
    Osteoporosis) 733.00
Distention
  abdomen (gaseous) 787.3
  bladder 596.8
  cecum 569.89
  colon 569.89
  gallbladder 575.8
  gaseous (abdomen) 787.3
  intestine 569.89
  kidney 593.89
  liver 573.9
  seminal vesicle 608.89
  stomach 536.8
    acute 536.1
    psychogenic 306.4
  ureter 593.5
  uterus 621.8
Distichia, distichiasis (eyelid) 743.63
Distoma hepaticum infestation 121.3
Distomiasis 121.9
  bile passages 121.3
    due to Clonorchis sinensis 121.1
  hemic 120.9
  hepatic (liver) 121.3
    due to Clonorchis sinensis
      (clonorchiasis) 121.1
  intestinal 121.4
  liver 121.3
    due to Clonorchis sinensis 121.1
  lung 121.2
  pulmonary 121.2
Distomolar (fourth molar) 520.1
  causing crowding 524.31
Disto-occlusion (division I) (division II)
  524.22
Distortion (congenital)
  adrenal (gland) 759.1
  ankle (joint) 755.69
  anus 751.5
  aorta 747.29
  appendix 751.5
  arm 755.59
  artery (peripheral) NEC *(see also*
    Distortion, peripheral vascular
    system) 747.60
    cerebral 747.81
    coronary 746.85
    pulmonary 747.3
    retinal 743.58
    umbilical 747.5
  auditory canal 744.29
    causing impairment of hearing
      744.02

◄ New   ◄III Revised   ~~deleted~~ Deleted   ● Use Additional Digit(s)   ▨ Omit code

Distortion (Continued)
  bile duct or passage 751.69
  bladder 753.8
  brain 742.4
  bronchus 748.3
  cecum 751.5
  cervix (uteri) 752.49
  chest (wall) 756.3
  clavicle 755.51
  clitoris 752.49
  coccyx 756.19
  colon 751.5
  common duct 751.69
  cornea 743.41
  cricoid cartilage 748.3
  cystic duct 751.69
  duodenum 751.5
  ear 744.29
    auricle 744.29
      causing impairment of hearing
        744.02
    causing impairment of hearing
      744.09
    external 744.29
      causing impairment of hearing
        744.02
    inner 744.05
    middle, except ossicles 744.03
      ossicles 744.04
    ossicles 744.04
  endocrine (gland) NEC 759.2
  epiglottis 748.3
  Eustachian tube 744.24
  eye 743.8
    adnexa 743.69
  face bone(s) 756.0
  fallopian tube 752.19
  femur 755.69
  fibula 755.69
  finger(s) 755.59
  foot 755.67
  gallbladder 751.69
  genitalia, genital organ(s)
    female 752.89
      external 752.49
      internal NEC 752.89
    male 752.89
      penis 752.69
  glottis 748.3
  gyri 742.4
  hand bone(s) 755.59
  heart (auricle) (ventricle) 746.89
    valve (cusp) 746.89
  hepatic duct 751.69
  humerus 755.59
  hymen 752.49
  ileum 751.5
  intestine (large) (small) 751.5
    with anomalous adhesions, fixation
      or malrotation 751.4
  jaw NEC 524.89
  jejunum 751.5
  kidney 753.3
  knee (joint) 755.64
  labium (majus) (minus) 752.49
  larynx 748.3
  leg 755.69
  lens 743.36
  liver 751.69
  lumbar spine 756.19
    with disproportion (fetopelvic)
      653.0●
      affecting fetus or newborn
        763.1
      causing obstructed labor 660.1●

Distortion (Continued)
  lumbosacral (joint) (region) 756.19
  lung (fissures) (lobe) 748.69
  nerve 742.8
  nose 748.1
  organ
    of Corti 744.05
    of site not listed - see Anomaly,
      specified type NEC
  ossicles, ear 744.04
  ovary 752.0
  oviduct 752.19
  pancreas 751.7
  parathyroid (gland) 759.2
  patella 755.64
  peripheral vascular system NEC
    747.60
    gastrointestinal 747.61
    lower limb 747.64
    renal 747.62
    spinal 747.82
    upper limb 747.63
  pituitary (gland) 759.2
  radius 755.59
  rectum 751.5
  rib 756.3
  sacroiliac joint 755.69
  sacrum 756.19
  scapula 755.59
  shoulder girdle 755.59
  site not listed - see Anomaly, specified
    type NEC
  skull bone(s) 756.0
    with
      anencephalus 740.0
      encephalocele 742.0
      hydrocephalus 742.3
        with spina bifida (see also
          Spina bifida) 741.0●
      microcephalus 742.1
  spinal cord 742.59
  spine 756.19
  spleen 759.0
  sternum 756.3
  thorax (wall) 756.3
  thymus (gland) 759.2
  thyroid (gland) 759.2
    cartilage 748.3
  tibia 755.69
  toe(s) 755.66
  tongue 750.19
  trachea (cartilage) 748.3
  ulna 755.59
  ureter 753.4
    causing obstruction 753.20
  urethra 753.8
    causing obstruction 753.6
  uterus 752.3
  vagina 752.49
  vein (peripheral) NEC (see also
    Distortion, peripheral vascular
    system) 747.60
    great 747.49
    portal 747.49
    pulmonary 747.49
  vena cava (inferior) (superior)
    747.49
  vertebra 756.19
  visual NEC 368.15
    shape or size 368.14
  vulva 752.49
  wrist (bones) (joint) 755.59
Distress
  abdomen 789.0●
  colon 564.9

Distress (Continued)
  emotional V40.9
  epigastric 789.0●
  fetal (syndrome) 768.4
    affecting management of
      pregnancy or childbirth
      656.8●
    liveborn infant 768.4
      first noted
        before onset of labor 768.2
        during labor and delivery
          768.3
      stillborn infant (death before onset
        of labor) 768.0
      death during labor 768.1
  gastrointestinal (functional) 536.9
    psychogenic 306.4
  intestinal (functional) NEC 564.9
    psychogenic 306.4
  intrauterine - see Distress, fetal
  leg 729.5
  maternal 669.0●
  mental V40.9
  respiratory 786.09
    acute (adult) 518.82
    adult syndrome (following
      shock, surgery, or trauma)
      518.5
      specified NEC 518.82
    fetus or newborn 770.89
    syndrome (idiopathic) (newborn)
      769
  stomach 536.9
    psychogenic 306.4
Distribution vessel, atypical NEC
  747.60
  coronary artery 746.85
  spinal 747.82
Districhiasis 704.2
Disturbance - see also Disease
  absorption NEC 579.9
    calcium 269.3
    carbohydrate 579.8
    fat 579.8
    protein 579.8
    specified type NEC 579.8
    vitamin (see also Deficiency,
      vitamin) 269.2
  acid-base equilibrium 276.9
  activity and attention, simple, with
    hyperkinesis 314.01
  amino acid (metabolic) (see also
    Disorder, amino acid) 270.9
    imidazole 270.5
    maple syrup (urine) disease
      270.3
    transport 270.0
  assimilation, food 579.9
  attention, simple 314.00
    with hyperactivity 314.01
  auditory, nerve, except deafness
    388.5
  behavior (see also Disturbance, conduct)
    312.9
  blood clotting (hypoproteinemia)
    (mechanism) (see also Defect,
    coagulation) 286.9
  central nervous system NEC
    349.9
  cerebral nerve NEC 352.9
  circulatory 459.9
  conduct 312.9
    adjustment reaction 309.3
    adolescent onset type 312.82

Disturbance (*Continued*)
 conduct (*Continued*)
  childhood onset type 312.81

> Note 25   Use the following fifth-digit subclassification with categories 312.0–312.2:
>
> 0   unspecified
> 1   mild
> 2   moderate
> 3   severe

   compulsive 312.30
    intermittent explosive disorder 312.34
    isolated explosive disorder 312.35
    kleptomania 312.32
    pathological gambling 312.31
    pyromania 312.33
   hyperkinetic 314.2
   intermittent explosive 312.34
   isolated explosive 312.35
   mixed with emotions 312.4
   socialized (type) 312.20
    aggressive 312.23
    unaggressive 312.21
   specified type NEC 312.89
   undersocialized, unsocialized
    aggressive (type) 312.0●
    unaggressive (type) 312.1●
  coordination 781.3
  cranial nerve NEC 352.9
  deep sensibility - *see* Disturbance, sensation
  digestive 536.9
   psychogenic 306.4
  electrolyte - *see* Imbalance, electrolyte
  emotions specific to childhood or adolescence 313.9
   with
    academic underachievement 313.83
    anxiety and fearfulness 313.0
    elective mutism 313.23
    identity disorder 313.82
    jealousy 313.3
    misery and unhappiness 313.1
    oppositional defiant disorder 313.81
    overanxiousness 313.0
    sensitivity 313.21
    shyness 313.21
    social withdrawal 313.22
    withdrawal reaction 313.22
   involving relationship problems 313.3
   mixed 313.89
   specified type NEC 313.89
  endocrine (gland) 259.9
   neonatal, transitory 775.9
    specified NEC 775.89
  equilibrium 780.4
  feeding (elderly) (infant) 783.3
   newborn 779.31 ◀▥
   nonorganic origin NEC 307.59
   psychogenic NEC 307.59
  fructose metabolism 271.2
  gait 781.2
   hysterical 300.11
  gastric (functional) 536.9
   motility 536.8
   psychogenic 306.4
   secretion 536.8

Disturbance (*Continued*)
 gastrointestinal (functional) 536.9
  psychogenic 306.4
 habit, child 307.9
 hearing, except deafness 388.40
 heart, functional (conditions classifiable to 426, 427, 428)
  due to presence of (cardiac) prosthesis 429.4
  postoperative (immediate) 997.1
   long-term effect of cardiac surgery 429.4
  psychogenic 306.2
 hormone 259.9
 innervation uterus, sympathetic, parasympathetic 621.8
 keratinization NEC
  gingiva 523.10
  lip 528.5
  oral (mucosa) (soft tissue) 528.79
   residual ridge mucosa
    excessive 528.72
    minimal 528.71
  tongue 528.79
 labyrinth, labyrinthine (vestibule) 386.9
 learning, specific NEC 315.2
 memory (*see also* Amnesia) 780.93
  mild, following organic brain damage 310.8
 mental (*see also* Disorder, mental) 300.9
  associated with diseases classified elsewhere 316
 metabolism (acquired) (congenital) (*see also* Disorder, metabolism) 277.9
  with
   abortion - *see* Abortion, by type, with metabolic disorder
   ectopic pregnancy (*see also* categories 633.0–633.9) 639.4
   molar pregnancy (*see also* categories 630–632) 639.4
  amino acid (*see also* Disorder, amino acid) 270.9
   aromatic NEC 270.2
   branched-chain 270.3
   specified type NEC 270.8
   straight-chain NEC 270.7
   sulfur-bearing 270.4
   transport 270.0
  ammonia 270.6
  arginine 270.6
  argininosuccinic acid 270.6
  carbohydrate NEC 271.9
  cholesterol 272.9
  citrulline 270.6
  cystathionine 270.4
  fat 272.9
  following
   abortion 639.4
   ectopic or molar pregnancy 639.4
  general 277.9
   carbohydrate 271.9
   iron 275.0
   phosphate 275.3
   sodium 276.9
  glutamine 270.7
  glycine 270.7
  histidine 270.5
  homocystine 270.4
  in labor or delivery 669.0●
  iron 275.0
  isoleucine 270.3

Disturbance (*Continued*)
 metabolism (*Continued*)
  leucine 270.3
  lipoid 272.9
   specified type NEC 272.8
  lysine 270.7
  methionine 270.4
  neonatal, transitory 775.9
   specified type NEC 775.89
  nitrogen 788.99
  ornithine 270.6
  phosphate 275.3
  phosphatides 272.7
  serine 270.7
  sodium NEC 276.9
  threonine 270.7
  tryptophan 270.2
  tyrosine 270.2
  urea cycle 270.6
  valine 270.3
 motor 796.1
 nervous functional 799.21 ◀▥
 neuromuscular mechanism (eye) due to syphilis 094.84
 nutritional 269.9
  nail 703.8
 ocular motion 378.87
  psychogenic 306.7
 oculogyric 378.87
  psychogenic 306.7
 oculomotor NEC 378.87
  psychogenic 306.7
 olfactory nerve 781.1
 optic nerve NEC 377.49
 oral epithelium, including tongue 528.79
  residual ridge mucosa
   excessive 528.72
   minimal 528.71
 personality (pattern) (trait) (*see also* Disorder, personality) 301.9
  following organic brain damage 310.1
 polyglandular 258.9
 psychomotor 307.9
 pupillary 379.49
 reflex 796.1
 rhythm, heart 427.9
  postoperative (immediate) 997.1
   long-term effect of cardiac surgery 429.4
  psychogenic 306.2
 salivary secretion 527.7
 sensation (cold) (heat) (localization) (tactile discrimination localization) (texture) (vibratory) NEC 782.0
  hysterical 300.11
  skin 782.0
  smell 781.1
  taste 781.1
 sensory (*see also* Disturbance, sensation) 782.0
  innervation 782.0
 situational (transient) (*see also* Reaction, adjustment) 309.9
  acute 308.3
 sleep 780.50
  with apnea - *see* Apnea, sleep
  initiation or maintenance (*see also* Insomnia) 780.52
   nonorganic origin 307.41
  nonorganic origin 307.40
   specified type NEC 307.49

◀ New   ◀▥ Revised   ~~deleted~~ Deleted   ● Use Additional Digit(s)   ▥ Omit code

Disturbance (Continued)
  sleep (Continued)
    specified NEC 780.59
      nonorganic origin 307.49
    wakefulness (see also Hypersomnia)
      780.54
      nonorganic origin 307.43
  sociopathic 301.7
  speech NEC 784.59 ◀▥
    developmental 315.39
      associated with hyperkinesis
        314.1
    secondary to organic lesion 784.59 ◀▥
  stomach (functional) (see also
    Disturbance, gastric) 536.9
  sympathetic (nerve) (see also
    Neuropathy, peripheral,
    autonomic) 337.9
  temperature sense 782.0
    hysterical 300.11
  tooth
    eruption 520.6
    formation 520.4
    structure, hereditary NEC 520.5
  touch (see also Disturbance, sensation)
    782.0
  vascular 459.9
    arteriosclerotic - see Arteriosclerosis
  vasomotor 443.9
  vasospastic 443.9
  vestibular labyrinth 386.9
  vision, visual NEC 368.9
    psychophysical 368.16
    specified NEC 368.8
    subjective 368.10
  voice and resonance 784.40 ◀▥
  wakefulness (initiation or
    maintenance) (see also
    Hypersomnia) 780.54
    nonorganic origin 307.43
Disulfiduria, beta-mercaptolactate-
  cysteine 270.0
Disuse atrophy, bone 733.7
Ditthomska syndrome 307.81
Diuresis 788.42
Divers'
  palsy or paralysis 993.3
  squeeze 993.3
Diverticula, diverticulosis, diverticulum
  (acute) (multiple) (perforated)
  (ruptured) 562.10
  with diverticulitis 562.11
  aorta (Kommerell's) 747.21
  appendix (noninflammatory) 543.9
  bladder (acquired) (sphincter) 596.3
    congenital 753.8
  broad ligament 620.8
  bronchus (congenital) 748.3
    acquired 494.0
      with acute exacerbation 494.1
  calyx, calyceal (kidney) 593.89
  cardia (stomach) 537.1
  cecum 562.10
    with
      diverticulitis 562.11
        with hemorrhage 562.13
      hemorrhage 562.12
    congenital 751.5
  colon (acquired) 562.10
    with
      diverticulitis 562.11
        with hemorrhage 562.13
      hemorrhage 562.12
    congenital 751.5

Diverticula, diverticulosis, diverticulum (Continued)
  duodenum 562.00
    with
      diverticulitis 562.01
        with hemorrhage 562.03
      hemorrhage 562.02
    congenital 751.5
  epiphrenic (esophagus) 530.6
  esophagus (congenital) 750.4
    acquired 530.6
    epiphrenic 530.6
    pulsion 530.6
    traction 530.6
    Zenker's 530.6
  Eustachian tube 381.89
  fallopian tube 620.8
  gallbladder (congenital) 751.69
  gastric 537.1
  heart (congenital) 746.89
  ileum 562.00
    with
      diverticulitis 562.01
        with hemorrhage 562.03
      hemorrhage 562.03
  intestine (large) 562.10
    with
      diverticulitis 562.11
        with hemorrhage 562.13
      hemorrhage 562.12
    congenital 751.5
    small 562.00
      with
        diverticulitis 562.01
          with hemorrhage 562.03
        hemorrhage 562.02
      congenital 751.5
  jejunum 562.00
    with
      diverticulitis 562.01
        with hemorrhage 562.03
      hemorrhage 562.02
  kidney (calyx) (pelvis) 593.89
    with calculus 592.0
  Kommerell's 747.21
  laryngeal ventricle (congenital)
    748.3
  Meckel's (displaced) (hypertrophic)
    751.0
  midthoracic 530.6
  organ or site, congenital NEC - see
    Distortion
  pericardium (congenital) (cyst)
    746.89
    acquired (true) 423.8
  pharyngoesophageal (pulsion)
    530.6
  pharynx (congenital) 750.27
  pulsion (esophagus) 530.6
  rectosigmoid 562.10
    with
      diverticulitis 562.11
        with hemorrhage 562.13
      hemorrhage 562.12
    congenital 751.5
  rectum 562.10
    with
      diverticulitis 562.11
        with hemorrhage 562.13
      hemorrhage 562.12
  renal (calyces) (pelvis) 593.89
    with calculus 592.0
  Rokitansky's 530.6
  seminal vesicle 608.0

Diverticula, diverticulosis, diverticulum (Continued)
  sigmoid 562.10
    with
      diverticulitis 562.11
        with hemorrhage 562.13
      hemorrhage 562.12
    congenital 751.5
  small intestine 562.00
    with
      diverticulitis 562.01
        with hemorrhage 562.03
      hemorrhage 562.02
  stomach (cardia) (juxtacardia)
    (juxtapyloric) (acquired) 537.1
    congenital 750.7
  subdiaphragmatic 530.6
  trachea (congenital) 748.3
    acquired 519.19
  traction (esophagus) 530.6
  ureter (acquired) 593.89
    congenital 753.4
  ureterovesical orifice 593.89
  urethra (acquired) 599.2
    congenital 753.8
  ventricle, left (congenital) 746.89
  vesical (urinary) 596.3
    congenital 753.8
  Zenker's (esophagus) 530.6
Diverticulitis (acute) (see also Diverticula)
  562.11
  with hemorrhage 562.13
  bladder (urinary) 596.3
  cecum (perforated) 562.11
    with hemorrhage 562.13
  colon (perforated) 562.11
    with hemorrhage 562.13
  duodenum 562.01
    with hemorrhage 562.03
  esophagus 530.6
  ileum (perforated) 562.01
    with hemorrhage 562.03
  intestine (large) (perforated) 562.11
    with hemorrhage 562.13
    small 562.01
      with hemorrhage 562.03
  jejunum (perforated) 562.01
    with hemorrhage 562.03
  Meckel's (perforated) 751.0
  pharyngoesophageal 530.6
  rectosigmoid (perforated) 562.11
    with hemorrhage 562.13
  rectum 562.11
    with hemorrhage 562.13
  sigmoid (old) (perforated) 562.11
    with hemorrhage 562.13
  small intestine (perforated) 562.01
    with hemorrhage 562.03
  vesical (urinary) 596.3
Diverticulosis - see Diverticula
Division
  cervix uteri 622.8
    external os into two openings by
      frenum 752.49
  external (cervical) into two openings
    by frenum 752.49
  glans penis 752.69
  hymen 752.49
  labia minora (congenital) 752.49
  ligament (partial or complete)
    (current) - see also Sprain, by
    site
    with open wound - see Wound,
      open, by site

Division (*Continued*)
  muscle (partial or complete) (current) -
    see also Sprain, by site
      with open wound - *see* Wound,
        open, by site
  nerve - *see* Injury, nerve, by site
  penis glans 752.69
  spinal cord - *see* Injury, spinal, by site
  vein 459.9
      traumatic - *see* Injury, vascular, by
        site
Divorce V61.03
Dix-Hallpike neurolabyrinthitis
    386.12
Dizziness 780.4
  hysterical 300.11
  psychogenic 306.9
Doan-Wiseman syndrome (primary
    splenic neutropenia) 289.53
Dog bite - *see* Wound, open, by site
Döhle-Heller aortitis 093.1
Döhle body-panmyelopathic syndrome
    288.2
Dolichocephaly, dolichocephalus
    754.0
Dolichocolon 751.5
Dolichostenomelia 759.82
Donohue's syndrome (leprechaunism)
    259.8
Donor
  blood V59.01
    other blood components V59.09
    stem cells V59.02
    whole blood V59.01
  bone V59.2
    marrow V59.3
  cornea V59.5
  egg (oocyte) (ovum) V59.70
    over age 35 V59.73
      anonymous recipient V59.73
      designated recipient V59.74
    under age 35 V59.71
      anonymous recipient V59.71
      designated recipient V59.72
  heart V59.8
  kidney V59.4
  liver V59.6
  lung V59.8
  lymphocyte V59.8
  organ V59.9
    specified NEC V59.8
  potential, examination of V70.8
  skin V59.1
  specified organ or tissue NEC V59.8
  sperm V59.8
  stem cells V59.02
  tissue V59.9
    specified type NEC V59.8
Donovanosis (granuloma venereum)
    099.2
DOPS (diffuse obstructive pulmonary
    syndrome) 496
Double
  albumin 273.8
  aortic arch 747.21
  auditory canal 744.29
  auricle (heart) 746.82
  bladder 753.8
  external (cervical) os 752.49
  kidney with double pelvis (renal)
    753.3
  larynx 748.3
  meatus urinarius 753.8
  organ or site NEC - *see* Accessory

Double (*Continued*)
  orifice
    heart valve NEC 746.89
      pulmonary 746.09
  outlet, right ventricle 745.11
  pelvis (renal) with double ureter 753.4
  penis 752.69
  tongue 750.13
  ureter (one or both sides) 753.4
    with double pelvis (renal) 753.4
  urethra 753.8
  urinary meatus 753.8
  uterus (any degree) 752.2
      with doubling of cervix and vagina
        752.2
      in pregnancy or childbirth 654.0●
        affecting fetus or newborn
          763.89
  vagina 752.49
      with doubling of cervix and uterus
        752.2
  vision 368.2
  vocal cords 748.3
  vulva 752.49
  whammy (syndrome) 360.81
Douglas' pouch, cul-de-sac - *see* condition
Down's disease or syndrome
    (mongolism) 758.0
Down-growth, epithelial (anterior
    chamber) 364.61
Dracontiasis 125.7
Dracunculiasis 125.7
Dracunculosis 125.7
Drainage
  abscess (spontaneous) - *see* Abscess
  anomalous pulmonary veins to hepatic
    veins or right atrium 747.41
  stump (amputation) (surgical) 997.62
  suprapubic, bladder 596.8
Dream state, hysterical 300.13
Drepanocytic anemia (*see also* Disease,
    sickle cell) 282.60
Dresbach's syndrome (elliptocytosis)
    282.1
Dreschlera (infection) 118
  hawaiiensis 117.8
Dressler's syndrome (postmyocardial
    infarction) 411.0
Dribbling (post-void) 788.35
Drift, ulnar 736.09
Drinking (alcohol) - *see also* Alcoholism
  excessive, to excess NEC (*see also*
    Abuse, drugs, nondependent)
    305.0●
      bouts, periodic 305.0●
      continual 303.9●
      episodic 305.0●
      habitual 303.9●
      periodic 305.0●
Drip, postnasal (chronic) 784.91
  due to:
    allergic rhinitis - *see* Rhinitis, allergic
    common cold 460
    gastroesophageal reflux - *see* Reflux,
      gastroesophageal
    nasopharyngitis - *see*
      Nasopharyngitis
    other known condition - *code to*
      condition
    sinusitis - *see* Sinusitis
Drivers' license examination V70.3
Droop
  Cooper's 611.81
  facial 781.94

Drop
  finger 736.29
  foot 736.79
  hematocrit (precipitous) 790.01
  hemoglobin 790.01
  toe 735.8
  wrist 736.05 ◀
Dropped
  dead 798.1
  heart beats 426.6
Dropsy, dropsical (*see also* Edema) 782.3
  abdomen 789.59
  amnion (*see also* Hydramnios) 657●
  brain - *see* Hydrocephalus
  cardiac (*see also* Failure, heart) 428.0
  cardiorenal (*see also* Hypertension,
    cardiorenal) 404.90
  chest 511.9
  fetus or newborn 778.0
    due to isoimmunization 773.3
  gangrenous (*see also* Gangrene) 785.4
  heart (*see also* Failure, heart) 428.0
  hepatic - *see* Cirrhosis, liver
  infantile - *see* Hydrops, fetalis
  kidney (*see also* Nephrosis) 581.9
  liver - *see* Cirrhosis, liver
  lung 514
  malarial (*see also* Malaria) 084.9
  neonatorum - *see* Hydrops, fetalis
  nephritic 581.9
  newborn - *see* Hydrops, fetalis
  nutritional 269.9
  ovary 620.8
  pericardium (*see also* Pericarditis) 423.9
  renal (*see also* Nephrosis) 581.9
  uremic - *see* Uremia
Drowned, drowning (near) 994.1
  lung 518.5
Drowsiness 780.09
Drug - *see also* condition
  addiction (*see also* Dependence)
    304.9●
  adverse effect NEC, correct substance
    properly administered 995.20
  allergy 995.27
  dependence (*see also* Dependence)
    304.9●
  habit (*see also* Dependence) 304.9●
  hypersensitivity 995.27
  induced
    circadian rhythm sleep disorder
      292.85
    hypersomnia 292.85
    insomnia 292.85
    mental disorder 292.9
      anxiety 292.89
      mood 292.84
      sexual 292.89
      sleep 292.85
      specified type 292.89
    parasomnia 292.85
    persisting
      amnestic disorder 292.83
      dementia 292.82
    psychotic disorder
      with
        delusions 292.11
        hallucinations 292.12
    sleep disorder 292.85
  intoxication 292.89
  overdose - *see* Table of Drugs and
    Chemicals
  poisoning - *see* Table of Drugs and
    Chemicals

◀ New   ◀▥ Revised   ~~deleted~~ Deleted   ● Use Additional Digit(s)   ▨ Omit code

Drug *(Continued)*
  therapy (maintenance) status NEC
    chemotherapy, antineoplastic
      V58.11
    immunotherapy, antineoplastic
      V58.12
    long-term (current) use V58.69
      antibiotics V58.62
      anticoagulants V58.61
      anti-inflammatories, non-
        steroidal (NSAID) V58.64
      antiplatelets V58.63
      antithrombotics V58.63
      aspirin V58.66
      high-risk medications NEC
        V58.69
      insulin V58.67
      methadone V58.69
      opiate analgesic V58.69
      steroids V58.65
    wrong substance given or taken in
      error - *see* Table of Drugs and
      Chemicals
Drunkenness (*see also* Abuse, drugs,
    nondependent) 305.0●
  acute in alcoholism (*see also*
    Alcoholism) 303.0●
  chronic (*see also* Alcoholism) 303.9●
  pathologic 291.4
  simple (acute) 305.0●
    in alcoholism 303.0●
  sleep 307.47
Drusen
  optic disc or papilla 377.21
  retina (colloid) (hyaloid degeneration)
    362.57
    hereditary 362.77
Drusenfieber 075
Dry, dryness - *see also* condition
  eye 375.15
    syndrome 375.15
  larynx 478.79
  mouth 527.7
  nose 478.19
  skin syndrome 701.1
  socket (teeth) 526.5
  throat 478.29
DSAP (disseminated superficial actinic
    porokeratosis) 692.75
Duane's retraction syndrome 378.71
Duane-Stilling-Türk syndrome (ocular
    retraction syndrome) 378.71
Dubin-Johnson disease or syndrome
    277.4
Dubini's disease (electric chorea) 049.8
Dubois' abscess or disease 090.5
Duchenne's
  disease 094.0
    locomotor ataxia 094.0
    muscular dystrophy 359.1
    pseudohypertrophy, muscles
      359.1
  paralysis 335.22
  syndrome 335.22
Duchenne-Aran myelopathic, muscular
    atrophy (nonprogressive)
    (progressive) 335.21
Duchenne-Griesinger disease 359.1
Ducrey's
  bacillus 099.0
  chancre 099.0
  disease (chancroid) 099.0
Duct, ductus - *see* condition
Duengero 061

Duhring's disease (dermatitis
    herpetiformis) 694.0
Dukes (-Filatov) disease 057.8
Dullness
  cardiac (decreased) (increased) 785.3
Dumb ague (*see also* Malaria) 084.6
Dumbness (*see also* Aphasia) 784.3
Dumdum fever 085.0
Dumping syndrome (postgastrectomy)
    564.2
  nonsurgical 536.8
Duodenitis (nonspecific) (peptic)
    535.60
  with hemorrhage 535.61
  due to
    strongyloides stercoralis 127.2
Duodenocholangitis 575.8
Duodenum, duodenal - *see* condition
Duplay's disease, periarthritis, or
    syndrome 726.2
Duplex - *see also* Accessory
  kidney 753.3
  placenta - *see* Placenta, abnormal
  uterus 752.2
Duplication - *see also* Accessory
  anus 751.5
  aortic arch 747.21
  appendix 751.5
  biliary duct (any) 751.69
  bladder 753.8
  cecum 751.5
    and appendix 751.5
  clitoris 752.49
  cystic duct 751.69
  digestive organs 751.8
  duodenum 751.5
  esophagus 750.4
  fallopian tube 752.19
  frontonasal process 756.0
  gallbladder 751.69
  ileum 751.5
  intestine (large) (small) 751.5
  jejunum 751.5
  kidney 753.3
  liver 751.69
  nose 748.1
  pancreas 751.7
  penis 752.69
  respiratory organs NEC 748.9
  salivary duct 750.22
  spinal cord (incomplete) 742.51
  stomach 750.7
  ureter 753.4
  vagina 752.49
  vas deferens 752.89
  vocal cords 748.3
Dupré's disease or syndrome
    (meningism) 781.6
Dupuytren's
  contraction 728.6
  disease (muscle contracture) 728.6
  fracture (closed) 824.4
    ankle (closed) 824.4
      open 824.5
    fibula (closed) 824.4
      open 824.5
    open 824.5
    radius (closed) 813.42
      open 813.52
  muscle contracture 728.6
Durand-Nicolas-Favre disease (climatic
    bubo) 099.1
Durotomy, incidental (inadvertent) (*see
    also* Tear, dural) 349.31

Duroziez's disease (congenital mitral
    stenosis) 746.5
Dust
  conjunctivitis 372.05
  reticulation (occupational) 504
Dutton's
  disease (trypanosomiasis) 086.9
  relapsing fever (West African) 087.1
Dwarf, dwarfism 259.4
  with infantilism (hypophyseal) 253.3
  achondroplastic 756.4
  Amsterdam 759.89
  bird-headed 759.89
  congenital 259.4
  constitutional 259.4
  hypophyseal 253.3
  infantile 259.4
  Levi type 253.3
  Lorain-Levi (pituitary) 253.3
  Lorain type (pituitary) 253.3
  metatropic 756.4
  nephrotic-glycosuric, with
    hypophosphatemic rickets
      270.0
  nutritional 263.2
  ovarian 758.6
  pancreatic 577.8
  pituitary 253.3
  polydystrophic 277.5
  primordial 253.3
  psychosocial 259.4
  renal 588.0
    with hypertension - *see*
      Hypertension, kidney
  Russell's (uterine dwarfism and
    craniofacial dysostosis) 759.89
Dyke-Young anemia or syndrome
    (acquired macrocytic hemolytic
    anemia) (secondary) (symptomatic)
    283.9
Dynia abnormality (*see also* Defect,
    coagulation) 286.9
Dysacousis 388.40
Dysadrenocortism 255.9
  hyperfunction 255.3
  hypofunction 255.41
Dysarthria 784.51 ◄▥
  due to late effect of cerebrovascular
    disease (*see also* Late effect(s) (of)
    cerebrovascular disease) 438.13 ◄
Dysautonomia (*see also* Neuropathy,
    peripheral, autonomic) 337.9
  familial 742.8
Dysbarism 993.3
Dysbasia 719.7
  angiosclerotica intermittens 443.9
    due to atherosclerosis 440.21
  hysterical 300.11
  lordotica (progressiva) 333.6
  nonorganic origin 307.9
  psychogenic 307.9
Dysbetalipoproteinemia (familial)
    272.2
Dyscalculia 315.1
Dyschezia (*see also* Constipation) 564.00
Dyschondroplasia (with hemangiomata)
    756.4
  Voorhoeve's 756.4
Dyschondrosteosis 756.59
Dyschromia 709.00
Dyscollagenosis 710.9
Dyscoria 743.41
Dyscraniopyophalangy 759.89

Dyscrasia
   blood 289.9
      with antepartum hemorrhage 641.3●
      ~~fetus or newborn NEC 76.9~~
      hemorrhage, subungual 287.8
      puerperal, postpartum 666.3●
   ovary 256.8
   plasma cell 273.9
   pluriglandular 258.9
   polyglandular 258.9
Dysdiadochokinesia 781.3
Dysectasia, vesical neck 596.8
Dysendocrinism 259.9
Dysentery, dysenteric (bilious)
      (catarrhal) (diarrhea) (epidemic)
      (gangrenous) (hemorrhagic)
      (infectious) (sporadic) (tropical)
      (ulcerative) 009.0
   abscess, liver (*see also* Abscess, amebic)
      006.3
   amebic (*see also* Amebiasis) 006.9
      with abscess - *see* Abscess, amebic
      acute 006.0
      carrier (suspected) of V02.2
      chronic 006.1
   arthritis (*see also* Arthritis, due to,
      dysentery) 009.0 [711.3]●
      bacillary 004.9 [711.3]●
   asylum 004.9
   bacillary 004.9
      arthritis 004.9 [711.3]●
      Boyd 004.2
      Flexner 004.1
      Schmitz (-Stutzer) 004.0
      Shiga 004.0
      Shigella 004.9
         group A 004.0
         group B 004.1
         group C 004.2
         group D 004.3
         specified type NEC 004.8
      Sonne 004.3
      specified type NEC 004.8
   bacterium 004.9
   balantidial 007.0
   Balantidium coli 007.0
   Boyd's 004.2
   Chilomastix 007.8
   Chinese 004.9
   choleriform 001.1
   coccidial 007.2
   Dientamoeba fragilis 007.8
   due to specified organism NEC - *see*
      Enteritis, due to, by organism
   Embadomonas 007.8
   Endolimax nana - *see* Dysentery,
      amebic
   Entamoba, entamebic - *see* Dysentery,
      amebic
   Flexner's 004.1
   Flexner-Boyd 004.2
   giardial 007.1
   Giardia lamblia 007.1
   Hiss-Russell 004.1
   lamblia 007.1
   leishmanial 085.0
   malarial (*see also* Malaria) 084.6
   metazoal 127.9
   Monilia 112.89
   protozoal NEC 007.9
   Russell's 004.8
   salmonella 003.0
   schistosomal 120.1
   Schmitz (-Stutzer) 004.0

Dysentery, dysenteric (*Continued*)
   Shiga 004.0
   Shigella NEC (*see also* Dysentery,
      bacillary) 004.9
      boydii 004.2
      dysenteriae 004.0
         Schmitz 004.0
         Shiga 004.0
      flexneri 004.1
      group A 004.0
      group B 004.1
      group C 004.2
      group D 004.3
      Schmitz 004.0
      Shiga 004.0
      Sonnei 004.3
   Sonne 004.3
   strongyloidiasis 127.2
   trichomonal 007.3
   tuberculous (*see also* Tuberculosis)
      014.8●
   viral (*see also* Enteritis, viral) 008.8
Dysequilibrium 780.4
Dysesthesia 782.0
   hysterical 300.11
Dysfibrinogenemia (congenital) (*see also*
      Defect, coagulation) 286.3
Dysfunction
   adrenal (cortical) 255.9
      hyperfunction 255.3
      hypofunction 255.41
   associated with sleep stages or arousal
      from sleep 780.56
      nonorganic origin 307.47
   bladder NEC 596.59
   bleeding, uterus 626.8
   brain, minimal (*see also* Hyperkinesia)
      314.9
   cerebral 348.30
   colon 564.9
      psychogenic 306.4
   colostomy or enterostomy 569.62
   cystic duct 575.8
   diastolic 429.9
      with heart failure - *see* Failure, heart
      due to
         cardiomyopathy - *see*
            Cardiomyopathy
         hypertension - *see* Hypertension,
            heart
   endocrine NEC 259.9
   endometrium 621.8
   enteric stoma 569.62
   enterostomy 569.62
   erectile 607.84
      nonorganic origin 302.72
   esophagostomy 530.87
   Eustachian tube 381.81
   gallbladder 575.8
   gastrointestinal 536.9
   gland, glandular NEC 259.9
   heart 427.9
      postoperative (immediate) 997.1
         long-term effect of cardiac
            surgery 429.4
   hemoglobin 289.89
   hepatic 573.9
   hepatocellular NEC 573.9
   hypophysis 253.9
      hyperfunction 253.1
      hypofunction 253.2
      posterior lobe 253.6
         hypofunction 253.5
   kidney (*see also* Disease, renal) 593.9

Dysfunction (*Continued*)
   labyrinthine 386.50
      specified NEC 386.58
   liver 573.9
      constitutional 277.4
   minimal brain (child) (*see also*
      Hyperkinesia) 314.9
   ovary, ovarian 256.9
      hyperfunction 256.1
         estrogen 256.0
      hypofunction 256.39
         postablative 256.2
      postablative 256.2
      specified NEC 256.8
   papillary muscle 429.81
      with myocardial infarction 410.8●
   parathyroid 252.8
      hyperfunction 252.00
      hypofunction 252.1
   pineal gland 259.8
   pituitary (gland) 253.9
      hyperfunction 253.1
      hypofunction 253.2
      posterior 253.6
         hypofunction 253.5
   placental - *see* Placenta, insufficiency
   platelets (blood) 287.1
   polyglandular 258.9
      specified NEC 258.8
   psychosexual 302.70
      with
         dyspareunia (functional)
            (psychogenic) 302.76
         frigidity 302.72
         impotence 302.72
         inhibition
            orgasm
               female 302.73
               male 302.74
            sexual
               desire 302.71
               excitement 302.72
         premature ejaculation 302.75
         sexual aversion 302.79
         specified disorder NEC 302.79
         vaginismus 306.51
   pylorus 537.9
   rectum 564.9
      psychogenic 306.4
   segmental (*see also* Dysfunction,
      somatic) 739.9
   senile 797
   sexual 302.70
   sinoatrial node 427.81
   somatic 739.9
      abdomen 739.9
      acromioclavicular 739.7
      cervical 739.1
      cervicothoracic 739.1
      costochondral 739.8
      costovertebral 739.8
      extremities
         lower 739.6
         upper 739.7
      head 739.0
      hip 739.5
      lumbar, lumbosacral 739.3
      occipitocervical 739.0
      pelvic 739.5
      pubic 739.5
      rib cage 739.8
      sacral 739.4
      sacrococcygeal 739.4
      sacroiliac 739.4

◄ New   ◄▐▐ Revised   ~~deleted~~ Deleted   ● Use Additional Digit(s)   ▨ Omit code

Dysfunction (Continued)
  somatic (Continued)
    specified site NEC 739.9
    sternochondral 739.8
    sternoclavicular 739.7
    temporomandibular 739.0
    thoracic, thoracolumbar 739.2
  stomach 536.9
    psychogenic 306.4
  suprarenal 255.9
    hyperfunction 255.3
    hypofunction 255.41
  symbolic NEC 784.60
    specified type NEC 784.69
  systolic 429.9
    with heart failure - see Failure,
      heart
  temporomandibular (joint) (joint-pain-
      syndrome) NEC 524.60
    sounds on opening or closing
      524.64
    specified NEC 524.69
  testicular 257.9
    hyperfunction 257.0
    hypofunction 257.2
    specified type NEC 257.8
  thymus 254.9
  thyroid 246.9
    complicating pregnancy, childbirth,
      or puerperium 648.1●
    hyperfunction - see Hyperthyroidism
    hypofunction - see Hypothyroidism
  uterus, complicating delivery 661.9●
    affecting fetus or newborn 763.7
    hypertonic 661.4●
    hypotonic 661.2●
      primary 661.0●
      secondary 661.1●
  velopharyngeal (acquired) 528.9
    congenital 750.29
  ventricular 429.9
    with congestive heart failure (see also
      Failure, heart) 428.0
    due to
      cardiomyopathy - see
        Cardiomyopathy
      hypertension - see Hypertension,
        heart
    left, reversible following sudden
      emotional stress 429.83
  vesicourethral NEC 596.59
  vestibular 386.50
    specified type NEC 386.58
Dysgammaglobulinemia 279.06
Dysgenesis
  gonadal (due to chromosomal
      anomaly) 758.6
    pure 752.7
  kidney(s) 753.0
  ovarian 758.6
  renal 753.0
  reticular 279.2
  seminiferous tubules 758.6
  tidal platelet 287.31
Dysgerminoma (M9060/3)
  specified site - see Neoplasm, by site,
      malignant
  unspecified site
    female 183.0
    male 186.9
Dysgeusia 781.1
Dysgraphia 781.3
Dyshidrosis 705.81
Dysidrosis 705.81

Dysinsulinism 251.8
Dyskaryotic cervical smear 795.09
Dyskeratosis (see also Keratosis) 701.1
  bullosa hereditaria 757.39
  cervix 622.10
  congenital 757.39
  follicularis 757.39
    vitamin A deficiency 264.8
  gingiva 523.8
  oral soft tissue NEC 528.79
  tongue 528.79
  uterus NEC 621.8
Dyskinesia 781.3
  biliary 575.8
  esophagus 530.5
  hysterical 300.11
  intestinal 564.89
  neuroleptic-induced tardive 333.85
  nonorganic origin 307.9
  orofacial 333.82
    due to drugs 333.85
  psychogenic 307.9
  subacute, due to drugs 333.85
  tardive (oral) 333.85
Dyslalia 784.59   ◀▥
  developmental 315.39
Dyslexia 784.61
  developmental 315.02
  secondary to organic lesion 784.61
Dyslipidemia 272.4
Dysmaturity (see also Immaturity)
    765.1●
  lung 770.4
  pulmonary 770.4
Dysmenorrhea (essential) (exfoliative)
    (functional) (intrinsic)
    (membranous) (primary)
    (secondary) 625.3
  psychogenic 306.52
Dysmetabolic syndrome X 277.7
Dysmetria 781.3
Dysmorodystrophia mesodermalis
    congenita 759.82
Dysnomia 784.3
Dysorexia 783.0
  hysterical 300.11
Dysostosis
  cleidocranial, cleidocranialis 755.59
  craniofacial 756.0
  Fairbank's (idiopathic familial
      generalized osteophytosis)
      756.50
  mandibularis 756.0
  mandibulofacial, incomplete 756.0
  multiplex 277.5
  orodigitofacial 759.89
Dyspareunia (female) 625.0
  male 608.89
  psychogenic 302.76
Dyspepsia (allergic) (congenital)
    (fermentative) (flatulent)
    (functional) (gastric)
    (gastrointestinal) (neurogenic)
    (occupational) (reflex) 536.8
  acid 536.8
  atonic 536.3
    psychogenic 306.4
  diarrhea 787.91
    psychogenic 306.4
  intestinal 564.89
    psychogenic 306.4
  nervous 306.4
  neurotic 306.4
  psychogenic 306.4

Dysphagia 787.20
  cervical 787.29
  functional 300.11
  hysterical 300.11
  nervous 300.11
  neurogenic 787.29
  oral phase 787.21
  oropharyngeal phase 787.22
  pharyngeal phase 787.23
  pharyngoesophageal phase 787.24
  psychogenic 306.4
  sideropenic 280.8
  spastica 530.5
  specified NEC 787.29
Dysphagocytosis, congenital 288.1
Dysphasia 784.59   ◀▥
Dysphonia 784.42   ◀▥
  clericorum 784.49
  functional 300.11
  hysterical 300.11
  psychogenic 306.1
  spastica 478.79
Dyspigmentation - see also Pigmentation
  eyelid (acquired) 374.52
Dyspituitarism 253.9
  hyperfunction 253.1
  hypofunction 253.2
  posterior lobe 253.6
Dysplasia - see also Anomaly
  anus 569.44
    intraepithelial neoplasia I [AIN I]
      (histologically confirmed)
      569.44
    intraepithelial neoplasia II [AIN II]
      (histologically confirmed)
      569.44
    intraepithelial neoplasia III [AIN III]
      230.6
    anal canal 230.5
    mild (histologically confirmed)
      569.44
    moderate (histologically confirmed)
      569.44
    severe 230.6
    anal canal 230.5
  artery
    fibromuscular NEC 447.8
      carotid 447.8
      renal 447.3
  bladder 596.8
  bone (fibrous) NEC 733.29
    diaphyseal, progressive 756.59
    jaw 526.89
    monostotic 733.29
    polyostotic 756.54
    solitary 733.29
  brain 742.9
  bronchopulmonary, fetus or newborn
      770.7
  cervix (uteri) 622.10
    cervical intraepithelial neoplasia I
      [CIN I] 622.11
    cervical intraepithelial neoplasia II
      [CIN II] 622.12
    cervical intraepithelial neoplasia III
      [CIN III] 233.1
    CIN I 622.11
    CIN II 622.12
    CIN III 233.1
    mild 622.11
    moderate 622.12
    severe 233.1
  chondroectodermal 756.55
  chondromatose 756.4

Dysplasia (*Continued*)
colon 211.3
craniocarpotarsal 759.89
craniometaphyseal 756.89
dentinal 520.5
diaphyseal, progressive 756.59
ectodermal (anhidrotic) (Bason)
    (Clouston's) (congenital)
    (Feinmesser) (hereditary)
    (hidrotic) (Marshall)
    (Robinson's) 757.31
epiphysealis 756.9
    multiplex 756.56
    punctata 756.59
epiphysis 756.9
    multiple 756.56
epithelial
    epiglottis 478.79
    uterine cervix 622.10
erythroid NEC 289.89
eye (*see also* Microphthalmos)
    743.10
familial metaphyseal 756.89
fibromuscular, artery NEC 447.8
    carotid 447.8
    renal 447.3
fibrous
    bone NEC 733.29
    diaphyseal, progressive 756.59
    jaw 526.89
    monostotic 733.29
    polyostotic 756.54
    solitary 733.29
high grade, focal - *see* Neoplasm, by
    site, benign
hip (congenital) 755.63
    with dislocation (*see also* Dislocation,
        hip, congenital) 754.30
hypohidrotic ectodermal 757.31
joint 755.8
kidney 753.15
leg 755.69
linguofacialis 759.89
lung 748.5
macular 743.55
mammary (benign) (gland) 610.9
    cystic 610.1
    specified type NEC 610.8
metaphyseal 756.9
    familial 756.89
monostotic fibrous 733.29
muscle 756.89
myeloid NEC 289.89
nervous system (general) 742.9
neuroectodermal 759.6
oculoauriculovertebral 756.0
oculodentodigital 759.89
olfactogenital 253.4
osteo-onycho-arthro (hereditary) 756.89
periosteum 733.99
polyostotic fibrous 756.54
progressive diaphyseal 756.59
prostate 602.3
    intraepithelial neoplasia I
        [PIN I] 602.3
    intraepithelial neoplasia II
        [PIN II] 602.3
    intraepithelial neoplasia III
        [PIN III] 233.4
renal 753.15
renofacialis 753.0
retinal NEC 743.56
retrolental (*see also* Retinopathy of
    prematurity) 362.21

Dysplasia (*Continued*)
skin 709.8
spinal cord 742.9
thymic, with immunodeficiency
    279.2
vagina 623.0
    mild 623.0
    moderate 623.0
    severe 233.31
vocal cord 478.5
vulva 624.8
    intraepithelial neoplasia I [VIN I]
        624.01
    intraepithelial neoplasia II [VIN II]
        624.02
    intraepithelial neoplasia III [VIN III]
        233.32
    mild 624.01
    moderate 624.02
    severe 233.32
    VIN I 624.01
    VIN II 624.02
    VIN III 233.32
Dyspnea (nocturnal) (paroxysmal) 786.09
asthmatic (bronchial) (*see also* Asthma)
    493.9●
    with bronchitis (*see also* Asthma)
        493.9●
    chronic 493.2●
cardiac (*see also* Failure, ventricular,
    left) 428.1
cardiac (*see also* Failure, ventricular,
    left) 428.1
functional 300.11
hyperventilation 786.01
hysterical 300.11
Monday morning 504
newborn 770.89
psychogenic 306.1
uremic - *see* Uremia
Dyspraxia 781.3
syndrome 315.4
Dysproteinemia 273.8
transient with copper deficiency
    281.4
Dysprothrombinemia (constitutional)
    (*see also* Defect, coagulation) 286.3
Dysreflexia, autonomic 337.3
Dysrhythmia
cardiac 427.9
    postoperative (immediate) 997.1
        long-term effect of cardiac
            surgery 429.4
    specified type NEC 427.89
    cerebral or cortical 348.30
Dyssecretosis, mucoserous 710.2
**Dyssocial reaction, without manifest
    psychiatric disorder**
adolescent V71.02
adult V71.01
child V71.02
Dyssomnia NEC 780.56
nonorganic origin 307.47
Dyssplenism 289.4
Dyssynergia
biliary (*see also* Disease, biliary)
    576.8
cerebellaris myoclonica 334.2
detrusor sphincter (bladder) 596.55
ventricular 429.89
Dystasia, hereditary areflexic 334.3
Dysthymia 300.4
Dysthymic disorder 300.4
Dysthyroidism 246.9

Dystocia 660.9●
affecting fetus or newborn 763.1
cervical 661.2●
    affecting fetus or newborn 763.7
contraction ring 661.4●
    affecting fetus or newborn 763.7
fetal 660.9●
    abnormal size 653.5●
        affecting fetus or newborn 763.1
    deformity 653.7●
maternal 660.9●
    affecting fetus or newborn 763.1
positional 660.0●
    affecting fetus or newborn 763.1
shoulder (girdle) 660.4●
    affecting fetus or newborn 763.1
uterine NEC 661.4●
    affecting fetus or newborn 763.7
Dystonia
acute
    due to drugs 333.72
    neuroleptic-induced acute 333.72
deformans progressiva 333.6
lenticularis 333.6
musculorum deformans 333.6
torsion (idiopathic) 333.6
    acquired 333.79
    fragments (of) 333.89
    genetic 333.6
    symptomatic 333.79
Dystonic
movements 781.0
Dystopia kidney 753.3
Dystrophy, dystrophia 783.9
adiposogenital 253.8
asphyxiating thoracic 756.4
Becker's type 359.22
brevicollis 756.16
Bruch's membrane 362.77
cervical (sympathetic) NEC 337.09
chondro-osseus with punctate
    epiphyseal dysplasia 756.59
choroid (hereditary) 363.50
    central (areolar) (partial) 363.53
        total (gyrate) 363.54
    circinate 363.53
    circumpapillary (partial) 363.51
        total 363.52
    diffuse
        partial 363.56
        total 363.57
    generalized
        partial 363.56
        total 363.57
    gyrate
        central 363.54
        generalized 363.57
    helicoid 363.52
    peripapillary - *see* Dystrophy,
        choroid, circumpapillary
    serpiginous 363.54
cornea (hereditary) 371.50
    anterior NEC 371.52
    Cogan's 371.52
    combined 371.57
    crystalline 371.56
    endothelial (Fuchs') 371.57
    epithelial 371.50
        juvenile 371.51
        microscopic cystic 371.52
    granular 371.53
    lattice 371.54
    macular 371.55
    marginal (Terrien's) 371.48

◀ New   ◀▥ Revised   ~~deleted~~ Deleted   ● Use Additional Digit(s)   ▨ Omit code

Dystrophy, dystrophia *(Continued)*
  cornea *(Continued)*
    Meesman's 371.51
    microscopic cystic (epithelial)
      371.52
    nodular, Salzmann's 371.46
    polymorphous 371.58
    posterior NEC 371.58
    ring-like 371.52
    Salzmann's nodular 371.46
    stromal NEC 371.56
  dermatochondrocorneal 371.50
  Duchenne's 359.1
  due to malnutrition 263.9
  Erb's 359.1
  familial
    hyperplastic periosteal 756.59
    osseous 277.5
  foveal 362.77
  Fuchs', cornea 371.57
  Gowers' muscular 359.1
  hair 704.2
  hereditary, progressive muscular
    359.1
  hypogenital, with diabetic tendency
    759.81
  Landouzy-Déjérine 359.1
  Leyden-Möbius 359.1
  mesodermalis congenita 759.82
  muscular 359.1
    congenital (hereditary) 359.0
      myotonic 359.22
    distal 359.1
    Duchenne's 359.1
    Erb's 359.1
    fascioscapulohumeral 359.1
    Gowers' 359.1
    hereditary (progressive) 359.1

Dystrophy, dystrophia *(Continued)*
  muscular *(Continued)*
    Landouzy-Déjérine 359.1
    limb-girdle 359.1
    myotonic 359.21
    progressive (hereditary) 359.1
      Charcôt-Marie-Tooth 356.1
    pseudohypertrophic (infantile)
      359.1
  myocardium, myocardial *(see also*
    Degeneration, myocardial)
    429.1
  myotonic 359.21
  myotonica 359.21
  nail 703.8
    congenital 757.5
  neurovascular (traumatic) *(see also*
    Neuropathy, peripheral,
    autonomic) 337.9
  nutritional 263.9
  ocular 359.1
  oculocerebrorenal 270.8
  oculopharyngeal 359.1
  ovarian 620.8
  papillary (and pigmentary) 701.1
  pelvicrural atrophic 359.1
  pigmentary *(see also* Acanthosis)
    701.2
  pituitary (gland) 253.8
  polyglandular 258.8
  posttraumatic sympathetic - *see*
    Dystrophy, symphatic
  progressive ophthalmoplegic 359.1
  reflex neuromuscular - *see* Dystrophy,
    sympathetic
  retina, retinal (hereditary) 362.70
    albipunctate 362.74
    Bruch's membrane 362.77

Dystrophy, dystrophia *(Continued)*
  retina, retinal *(Continued)*
    cone, progressive 362.75
    hyaline 362.77
    in
      Bassen-Kornzweig syndrome
        272.5 *[362.72]*
      cerebroretinal lipidosis 330.1
        [362.71]
      Refsum's disease 356.3 *[362.72]*
      systemic lipidosis 272.7 *[362.71]*
    juvenile (Stargardt's) 362.75
    pigmentary 362.74
    pigment epithelium 362.76
    progressive cone (-rod) 362.75
    pseudoinflammatory foveal
      362.77
    rod, progressive 362.75
    sensory 362.75
    vitelliform 362.76
  Salzmann's nodular 371.46
  scapuloperoneal 359.1
  skin NEC 709.9
  sympathetic (posttraumatic) (reflex)
    337.20
    lower limb 337.22
    specified site NEC 337.29
    upper limb 337.21
  tapetoretinal NEC 362.74
  thoracic asphyxiating 756.4
  unguium 703.8
    congenital 757.5
  vitreoretinal (primary) 362.73
    secondary 362.66
  vulva 624.09
Dysuria 788.1
  psychogenic 306.53

E

Eagle-Barrett syndrome 756.71
Eales' disease (syndrome) 362.18
Ear - *see also* condition
  ache 388.70
    otogenic 388.71
    referred 388.72
  lop 744.29
  piercing V50.3
  swimmers' acute 380.12
  tank 380.12
  tropical 111.8 *[380.15]*
  wax 380.4
Earache 388.70
  otogenic 388.71
  referred 388.72
Early satiety 780.94
Eaton-Lambert syndrome (*see also*
  Neoplasm, by site, malignant)
  199.1 *[358.1]*
Eberth's disease (typhoid fever) 002.0
Ebstein's
  anomaly or syndrome (downward
    displacement, tricuspid valve
    into right ventricle) 746.2
  disease (diabetes) 250.4● *[581.81]*
    due to secondary diabetes 249.4●
    [581.81]
Eccentro-osteochondrodysplasia
  277.5
Ecchondroma (M9210/0) - *see* Neoplasm,
  bone, benign
Ecchondrosis (M9210/1) 238.0
Ecchordosis physaliphora 756.0
Ecchymosis (multiple) 459.89
  conjunctiva 372.72
  eye (traumatic) 921.0
  eyelids (traumatic) 921.1
  newborn 772.6
  spontaneous 782.7
  traumatic - *see* Contusion
ECD (Erdheim-Chester disease) 277.89 ◄
Echinocociasis - *see* Echinococcus
Echinococcosis - *see* Echinococcus
Echinococcus (infection) 122.9
  granulosus 122.4
    liver 122.0
    lung 122.1
    orbit 122.3 *[376.13]*
    specified site NEC 122.3
    thyroid 122.2
  liver NEC 122.8
    granulosus 122.0
    multilocularis 122.5
  lung NEC 122.9
    granulosus 122.1
    multilocularis 122.6
  multilocularis 122.7
    liver 122.5
    specified site NEC 122.6
  orbit 122.9 *[376.13]*
    granulosus 122.3 *[376.13]*
    multilocularis 122.6 *[376.13]*
  specified site NEC 122.9
    granulosus 122.3
    multilocularis 122.6 *[376.13]*
  thyroid NEC 122.9
    granulosus 122.2
    multilocularis 122.6
Echinorhynchiasis 127.7
Echinostomiasis 121.8
Echolalia 784.69
ECHO virus infection NEC 079.1

Eclampsia, eclamptic (coma)
  (convulsions) (delirium) 780.39
  female, child-bearing age NEC - *see*
    Eclampsia, pregnancy
  gravidarum - *see* Eclampsia, pregnancy
  male 780.39
  not associated with pregnancy or
    childbirth 780.39
  pregnancy, childbirth, or puerperium
    642.6●
    with pre-existing hypertension
      642.7●
    affecting fetus or newborn 760.0
  uremic 586
Eclipse blindness (total) 363.31
Economic circumstance affecting care
  V60.9
  specified type NEC V60.89   ◄▥
Economo's disease (encephalitis
  lethargica) 049.8
Ectasia, ectasis
  aorta (*see also* Aneurysm, aorta) 441.9
    ruptured 441.5
  breast 610.4
  capillary 448.9
  cornea (marginal) (postinfectional)
    371.71
  duct (mammary) 610.4
  gastric antral vascular (GAVE) 537.82
    with hemorrhage 537.83
    without hemorrhage 537.82
  kidney 593.89
  mammary duct (gland) 610.4
  papillary 448.9
  renal 593.89
  salivary gland (duct) 527.8
  scar, cornea 371.71
  sclera 379.11
Ecthyma 686.8
  contagiosum 051.2
  gangrenosum 686.09
  infectiosum 051.2
Ectocardia 746.87
Ectodermal dysplasia, congenital 757.31
Ectodermosis erosiva pluriorificialis
  695.19
Ectopic, ectopia (congenital) 759.89
  abdominal viscera 751.8
    due to defect in anterior abdominal
      wall 756.79
  ACTH syndrome 255.0
  adrenal gland 759.1
  anus 751.5
  auricular beats 427.61
  beats 427.60
  bladder 753.5
  bone and cartilage in lung 748.69
  brain 742.4
  breast tissue 757.6
  cardiac 746.87
  cerebral 742.4
  cordis 746.87
  endometrium 617.9
  gallbladder 751.69
  gastric mucosa 750.7
  gestation - *see* Pregnancy, ectopic
  heart 746.87
  hormone secretion NEC 259.3
  hyperparathyroidism 259.3
  kidney (crossed) (intrathoracic) (pelvis)
    753.3
    in pregnancy or childbirth 654.4●
      causing obstructed labor 660.2●
  lens 743.37

Ectopic, ectopia (*Continued*)
  lentis 743.37
  mole - *see* Pregnancy, ectopic
  organ or site NEC - *see* Malposition,
    congenital
  ovary 752.0
  pancreas, pancreatic tissue 751.7
  pregnancy - *see* Pregnancy, ectopic
  pupil 364.75
  renal 753.3
  sebaceous glands of mouth 750.26
  secretion
    ACTH 255.0
    adrenal hormone 259.3
    adrenalin 259.3
    adrenocorticotropin 255.0
    antidiuretic hormone (ADH) 259.3
    epinephrine 259.3
    hormone NEC 259.3
    norepinephrine 259.3
    pituitary (posterior) 259.3
  spleen 759.0
  testis 752.51
  thyroid 759.2
  ureter 753.4
  ventricular beats 427.69
  vesicae 753.5
Ectrodactyly 755.4
  finger (*see also* Absence, finger,
    congenital) 755.29
  toe (*see also* Absence, toe, congenital)
    755.39
Ectromelia 755.4
  lower limb 755.30
  upper limb 755.20
Ectropion 374.10
  anus 569.49
  cervix 622.0
    with mention of cervicitis 616.0
  cicatricial 374.14
  congenital 743.62
  eyelid 374.10
    cicatricial 374.14
    congenital 743.62
    mechanical 374.12
    paralytic 374.12
    senile 374.11
    spastic 374.13
  iris (pigment epithelium) 364.54
  lip (congenital) 750.26
    acquired 528.5
  mechanical 374.12
  paralytic 374.12
  rectum 569.49
  senile 374.11
  spastic 374.13
  urethra 599.84
  uvea 364.54
Eczema (acute) (allergic) (chronic)
  (erythematous) (fissum)
  (occupational) (rubrum) (squamous)
  692.9
  asteatotic 706.8
  atopic 691.8
  contact NEC 692.9
  dermatitis NEC 692.9
  due to specified cause - *see* Dermatitis,
    due to
  dyshidrotic 705.81
  external ear 380.22
  flexural 691.8
  gouty 274.89
  herpeticum 054.0
  hypertrophicum 701.8

◄ New   ◄▥ Revised   ~~deleted~~ Deleted   ● Use Additional Digit(s)   ▥ Omit code

Eczema *(Continued)*
  hypostatic - *see* Varicose, vein
  impetiginous 684
  infantile (acute) (chronic) (due to any
     substance) (intertriginous)
     (seborrheic) 690.12
  intertriginous NEC 692.9
    infantile 690.12
  intrinsic 691.8
  lichenified NEC 692.9
  marginatum 110.3
  nummular 692.9
  pustular 686.8
  seborrheic 690.18
    infantile 690.12
  solare 692.72
  stasis (lower extremity) 454.1
    ulcerated 454.2
  vaccination, vaccinatum 999.0
  varicose (lower extremity) - *see*
     Varicose, vein
  verrucosum callosum 698.3
Eczematoid, exudative 691.8
Eddowes' syndrome (brittle bones and
    blue sclera) 756.51
Edema, edematous 782.3
  with nephritis (*see also* Nephrosis)
    581.9
  allergic 995.1
  angioneurotic (allergic) (any site)
    (with urticaria) 995.1
    hereditary 277.6
  angiospastic 443.9
  Berlin's (traumatic) 921.3
  brain 348.5
    due to birth injury 767.8
    fetus or newborn 767.8
  cardiac (*see also* Failure, heart) 428.0
  cardiovascular (*see also* Failure, heart)
    428.0
  cerebral - *see* Edema, brain
  cerebrospinal vessel - *see* Edema,
    brain
  cervix (acute) (uteri) 622.8
    puerperal, postpartum 674.8●
  chronic hereditary 757.0
  circumscribed, acute 995.1
    hereditary 277.6
  complicating pregnancy (gestational)
    646.1●
    with hypertension - *see* Toxemia, of
     pregnancy
  conjunctiva 372.73
  connective tissue 782.3
  cornea 371.20
    due to contact lenses 371.24
    idiopathic 371.21
    secondary 371.22
  cystoid macular 362.53
  due to
    lymphatic obstruction - *see* Edema,
     lymphatic
    salt retention 276.0
  epiglottis - *see* Edema, glottis
  essential, acute 995.1
    hereditary 277.6
  extremities, lower - *see* Edema, legs
  eyelid NEC 374.82
  familial, hereditary (legs) 757.0
  famine 262
  fetus or newborn 778.5
  genital organs
    female 629.89
    male 608.86

Edema, edematous *(Continued)*
  gestational 646.1●
    with hypertension - *see* Toxemia, of
     pregnancy
  glottis, glottic, glottides (obstructive)
    (passive) 478.6
    allergic 995.1
     hereditary 277.6
    due to external agent - *see*
     Condition, respiratory, acute,
     due to specified agent
  heart (*see also* Failure, heart) 428.0
    newborn 779.89
  heat 992.7
  hereditary (legs) 757.0
  inanition 262
  infectious 782.3
  intracranial 348.5
    due to injury at birth 767.8
  iris 364.89
  joint (*see also* Effusion, joint) 719.0●
  larynx (*see also* Edema, glottis) 478.6
  legs 782.3
    due to venous obstruction 459.2
    hereditary 757.0
  localized 782.3
    due to venous obstruction 459.2
    lower extremity 459.2
  lower extremities - *see* Edema, legs
  lung 514
    acute 518.4
     with heart disease or failure (*see*
      also Failure, ventricular, left)
      428.1
      congestive 428.0
     chemical (due to fumes or
      vapors) 506.1
     due to
      external agent(s) NEC 508.9
       specified NEC 508.8
      fumes and vapors (chemical)
       (inhalation) 506.1
      radiation 508.0
    chemical (acute) 506.1
     chronic 506.4
    chronic 514
     chemical (due to fumes or
      vapors) 506.4
     due to
      external agent(s) NEC 508.9
       specified NEC 508.8
      fumes or vapors (chemical)
       (inhalation) 506.4
      radiation 508.1
    due to
     external agent 508.9
      specified NEC 508.8
     high altitude 993.2
     near drowning 994.1
    postoperative 518.4
    terminal 514
  lymphatic 457.1
    due to mastectomy operation
     457.0
  macula 362.83
    cystoid 362.53
    diabetic 250.5● *[362.07]*
     due to secondary diabetes 249.5●
      [362.07]
  malignant (*see also* Gangrene, gas)
    040.0
  Milroy's 757.0
  nasopharynx 478.25
  neonatorum 778.5

Edema, edematous *(Continued)*
  nutritional (newborn) 262
    with dyspigmentation, skin and hair
     260
  optic disc or nerve - *see* Papilledema
  orbit 376.33
    circulatory 459.89
  palate (soft) (hard) 528.9
  pancreas 577.8
  penis 607.83
  periodic 995.1
    hereditary 277.6
  pharynx 478.25
  pitting 782.3
  pulmonary - *see* Edema, lung
  Quincke's 995.1
    hereditary 277.6
  renal (*see also* Nephrosis) 581.9
  retina (localized) (macular) (peripheral)
    362.83
    cystoid 362.53
    diabetic 250.5● *[362.07]*
     due to secondary diabetes 249.5●
      [362.07]
  salt 276.0
  scrotum 608.86
  seminal vesicle 608.86
  spermatic cord 608.86
  spinal cord 336.1
  starvation 262
  stasis - *see also* Hypertension, venous
    459.30
  subconjunctival 372.73
  subglottic (*see also* Edema, glottis) 478.6
  supraglottic (*see also* Edema, glottis)
    478.6
  testis 608.86
  toxic NEC 782.3
  traumatic NEC 782.3
  tunica vaginalis 608.86
  vas deferens 608.86
  vocal cord - *see* Edema, glottis
  vulva (acute) 624.8
Edentia (complete) (partial) (*see also*
    Absence, tooth) 520.0
  acquired (*see also* Edentulism) 525.40
    due to
     caries 525.13
     extraction 525.10
     periodontal disease 525.12
     specified NEC 525.19
     trauma 525.11
  causing malocclusion 524.30
  congenital (deficiency of tooth buds)
    520.0
Edentulism 525.40
  complete 525.40
    class I 525.41
    class II 525.42
    class III 525.43
    class IV 525.44
  partial 525.50
    class I 525.51
    class II 525.52
    class III 525.53
    class IV 525.54
Edsall's disease 992.2
Educational handicap V62.3
Edwards' syndrome 758.2
Effect, adverse NEC
  abnormal gravitational (G) forces or
    states 994.9
  air pressure - *see* Effect, adverse,
    atmospheric pressure

Effect, adverse NEC (*Continued*)
altitude (high) - *see* Effect, adverse,
    high altitude
anesthetic
    in labor and delivery NEC 668.9●
        affecting fetus or newborn 763.5
antitoxin - *see* Complications,
    vaccination
atmospheric pressure 993.9
    due to explosion 993.4
    high 993.3
    low - *see* Effect, adverse, high
        altitude
    specified effect NEC 993.8
biological, correct substance properly
    administered (*see also* Effect,
    adverse, drug) 995.20
blood (derivatives) (serum)
    (transfusion) - *see* Complications,
    transfusion
chemical substance NEC 989.9
    specified - *see* Table of Drugs and
        Chemicals
cobalt, radioactive (*see also* Effect,
    adverse, radioactive substance)
    990
cold (temperature) (weather) 991.9
    chilblains 991.5
    frostbite - *see* Frostbite
    specified effect NEC 991.8
drugs and medicinals 995.20
    correct substance properly
        administered 995.20
    overdose or wrong substance given
        or taken 977.9
        specified drug - *see* Table of
            Drugs and Chemicals
electric current (shock) 994.8
    burn - *see* Burn, by site
electricity (electrocution) (shock) 994.8
    burn - *see* Burn, by site
exertion (excessive) 994.5
exposure 994.9
    exhaustion 994.4
external cause NEC 994.9
fallout (radioactive) NEC 990
fluoroscopy NEC 990
foodstuffs
    allergic reaction (*see also* Allergy,
        food) 693.1
        anaphylactic shock due to food
            NEC 995.60
    noxious 988.9
        specified type NEC (*see also*
            Poisoning, by name of
            noxious foodstuff) 988.8
gases, fumes, or vapors - *see* Table of
    Drugs and Chemicals
glue (airplane) sniffing 304.6●
heat - *see* Heat
high altitude NEC 993.2
    anoxia 993.2
    on
        ears 993.0
        sinuses 993.1
    polycythemia 289.0
hot weather - *see* Heat
hunger 994.2
immersion, foot 991.4
immunization - *see* Complications,
    vaccination
immunological agents - *see*
    Complications, vaccination
implantation (removable) of isotope or
    radium NEC 990

Effect, adverse NEC (*Continued*)
infrared (radiation) (rays) NEC 990
    burn - *see* Burn, by site
    dermatitis or eczema 692.82
infusion - *see* Complications, infusion
ingestion or injection of isotope
    (therapeutic) NEC 990
irradiation NEC (*see also* Effect,
    adverse, radiation) 990
isotope (radioactive) NEC 990
lack of care (child) (infant) (newborn)
    995.52
    adult 995.84
lightning 994.0
    burn - *see* Burn, by site
Lirugin - *see* Complications,
    vaccination
medicinal substance, correct, properly
    administered (*see also* Effect,
    adverse, drugs) 995.20
mesothorium NEC 990
motion 994.6
noise, inner ear 388.10
other drug, medicinal and biological
    substance 995.29
overheated places - *see* Heat
polonium NEC 990
psychosocial, of work environment
    V62.1
radiation (diagnostic) (fallout)
    (infrared) (natural source)
    (therapeutic) (tracer) (ultraviolet)
    (x-ray) NEC 990
    with pulmonary manifestations
        acute 508.0
        chronic 508.1
    dermatitis or eczema 692.82
        due to sun NEC (*see also*
            Dermatitis, due to, sun)
            692.70
    fibrosis of lungs 508.1
    maternal with suspected damage to
        fetus affecting management of
        pregnancy 655.6●
    pneumonitis 508.0
radioactive substance NEC 990
    dermatitis or eczema 692.82
radioactivity NEC 990
radiotherapy NEC 990
    dermatitis or eczema 692.82
radium NEC 990
reduced temperature 991.9
    frostbite - *see* Frostbite
    immersion, foot (hand) 991.4
    specified effect NEC 991.8
roentgenography NEC 990
roentgenoscopy NEC 990
roentgen rays NEC 990
serum (prophylactic) (therapeutic)
    NEC 999.5
specified NEC 995.89
    external cause NEC 994.9
strangulation 994.7
submersion 994.1
teletherapy NEC 990
thirst 994.3
transfusion - *see* Complications,
    transfusion
ultraviolet (radiation) (rays) NEC 990
    burn - *see also* Burn, by site
        from sun (*see also* Sunburn) 692.71
    dermatitis or eczema 692.82
        due to sun NEC (*see also*
            Dermatitis, due to, sun)
            692.70

Effect, adverse NEC (*Continued*)
uranium NEC 990
vaccine (any) - *see* Complications,
    vaccination
weightlessness 994.9
whole blood - *see also* Complications,
    transfusion
    overdose or wrong substance given
        (*see also* Table of Drugs and
        Chemicals) 964.7
working environment V62.1
x-rays NEC 990
    dermatitis or eczema 692.82
Effect, remote
of cancer - *see* condition
Effects, late - *see* Late, effect (of)
Effluvium, telogen 704.02
Effort
intolerance 306.2
syndrome (aviators) (psychogenic)
    306.2
Effusion
amniotic fluid (*see also* Rupture,
    membranes, premature) 658.1●
brain (serous) 348.5
bronchial (*see also* Bronchitis) 490
cerebral 348.5
cerebrospinal (*see also* Meningitis) 322.9
    vessel 348.5
chest - *see* Effusion, pleura
intracranial 348.5
joint 719.00
    ankle 719.07
    elbow 719.02
    foot 719.07
    hand 719.04
    hip 719.05
    knee 719.06
    multiple sites 719.09
    pelvic region 719.05
    shoulder (region) 719.01
    specified site NEC 719.08
    wrist 719.03
meninges (*see also* Meningitis) 322.9
pericardium, pericardial (*see also*
    Pericarditis) 423.9
    acute 420.90
peritoneal (chronic) 568.82
pleura, pleurisy, pleuritic,
    pleuropericardial 511.9
    bacterial, nontuberculous 511.1
    fetus or newborn 511.9
    malignant 511.81
    nontuberculous 511.9
        bacterial 511.1
    pneumococcal 511.1
    staphylococcal 511.1
    streptococcal 511.1
    traumatic 862.29
        with open wound 862.39
    tuberculous (*see also* Tuberculosis,
        pleura) 012.0●
        primary progressive 010.1●
pulmonary - *see* Effusion, pleura
spinal (*see also* Meningitis) 322.9
thorax, thoracic - *see* Effusion, pleura
Egg (oocyte) (ovum)
donor V59.70
    over age 35 V59.73
        anonymous recipient V59.73
        designated recipient V59.74
    under age 35 V59.71
        anonymous recipient V59.71
        designated recipient V59.72
Eggshell nails 703.8
congenital 757.5

◀ New   ◀▥ Revised   ~~deleted~~ Deleted   ● Use Additional Digit(s)   ▨ Omit code

Ego-dystonic
  homosexuality 302.0
  lesbianism 302.0
  sexual orientation 302.0
Egyptian splenomegaly 120.1
Ehlers-Danlos syndrome 756.83
Ehrlichiosis 082.40
  chaffeensis 082.41
  specified type NEC 082.49
Eichstedt's disease (pityriasis versicolor)
    111.0
EIN (endometrial intraepithelial
    neoplasia) 621.35 ◄
Eisenmenger's complex or syndrome
    (ventricular septal defect) 745.4
Ejaculation, semen
  painful 608.89
    psychogenic 306.59
  premature 302.75
  retrograde 608.87
Ekbom syndrome (restless legs) 333.94
Ekman's syndrome (brittle bones and
    blue sclera) 756.51
Elastic skin 756.83
  acquired 701.8
Elastofibroma (M8820/0) - see Neoplasm,
    connective tissue, benign
Elastoidosis
  cutanea nodularis 701.8
  cutis cystica et comedonica 701.8
Elastoma 757.39
  juvenile 757.39
  Miescher's (elastosis perforans
    serpiginosa) 701.1
Elastomyofibrosis 425.3
Elastosis 701.8
  atrophicans 701.8
  perforans serpiginosa 701.1
  reactive perforating 701.1
  senilis 701.8
  solar (actinic) 692.74
Elbow - see condition
Electric
  current, electricity, effects (concussion)
      (fatal) (nonfatal) (shock) 994.8
    burn - see Burn, by site
  feet (foot) syndrome 266.2
  shock from electroshock gun (taser)
      994.8
Electrocution 994.8
Electrolyte imbalance 276.9
  with
    abortion - see Abortion, by type,
      with metabolic disorder
    ectopic pregnancy (see also
        categories 633.0–633.9) 639.4
    hyperemesis gravidarum (before 22
        completed weeks' gestation)
        643.1●
    molar pregnancy (see also categories
        630–632) 639.4
  following
    abortion 639.4
    ectopic or molar pregnancy 639.4
Elephant man syndrome 237.71
Elephantiasis (nonfilarial) 457.1
  arabicum (see also Infestation, filarial)
      125.9
  congenita hereditaria 757.0
  congenital (any site) 757.0
  due to
    Brugia (malayi) 125.1
    mastectomy operation 457.0
    Wuchereria (bancrofti) 125.0
      malayi 125.1

Elephantiasis (Continued)
  eyelid 374.83
  filarial (see also Infestation, filarial)
      125.9
  filariensis (see also Infestation, filarial)
      125.9
  gingival 523.8
  glandular 457.1
  graecorum 030.9
  lymphangiectatic 457.1
  lymphatic vessel 457.1
    due to mastectomy operation 457.0
  neuromatosa 237.71
  postmastectomy 457.0
  scrotum 457.1
  streptococcal 457.1
  surgical 997.99
    postmastectomy 457.0
  telangiectodes 457.1
  vulva (nonfilarial) 624.8
Elevated - see Elevation
  findings on laboratory examination -
      see Findings, abnormal, without
      diagnosis (examination)
      (laboratory test) ◄
  GFR (glomerular filtration rate) -
      see Findings, abnormal, without
      diagnosis (examination)
      (laboratory test) ◄
Elevation
  17-ketosteroids 791.9
  acid phosphatase 790.5
  alkaline phosphatase 790.5
  amylase 790.5
  antibody titers 795.79
  basal metabolic rate (BMR) 794.7
  blood pressure (see also Hypertension)
      401.9
    reading (incidental) (isolated)
        (nonspecific), no diagnosis of
        hypertension 796.2
  blood sugar 790.29
  body temperature (of unknown origin)
      (see also Pyrexia) 780.60
  cancer antigen 125 [CA 125] 795.82
  carcinoembryonic antigen [CEA]
      795.81
  cholesterol 272.0
    with high triglycerides 272.2
  conjugate, eye 378.81
  C-reactive protein (CRP) 790.95
  CRP (C-reactive protein) 790.95
  diaphragm, congenital 756.6
  GFR (glomerular filtration rate) - see
      Findings, abnormal, without
      diagnosis (examination)
      (laboratory test) ◄
  glucose
    fasting 790.21
    tolerance test 790.22
  immunoglobulin level 795.79
  indolacetic acid 791.9
  lactic acid dehydrogenase (LDH) level
      790.4
  leukocytes 288.60
  lipase 790.5
  lipoprotein a level 272.8
  liver function test (LFT) 790.6
    alkaline phosphatase 790.5
    aminotransferase 790.4
    bilirubin 782.4
    hepatic enzyme NEC 790.5
    lactate dehydrogenase 790.4
  lymphocytes 288.61
  prostate specific antigen (PSA)
      790.93

Elevation (Continued)
  renin 790.99
    in hypertension (see also
        Hypertension, renovascular)
        405.91
  Rh titer 999.7
  scapula, congenital 755.52
  sedimentation rate 790.1
  SGOT 790.4
  SGPT 790.4
  transaminase 790.4
  triglycerides 272.1
    with high cholesterol 272.2
  vanillylmandelic acid 791.9
  venous pressure 459.89
  VMA 791.9
  white blood cell count 288.60
    specified NEC 288.69
Elliptocytosis (congenital) (hereditary)
    282.1
  Hb-C (disease) 282.7
  hemoglobin disease 282.7
  sickle-cell (disease) 282.60
    trait 282.5
Ellis-van Creveld disease or syndrome
    (chondroectodermal dysplasia)
    756.55
Ellison-Zollinger syndrome
    (gastric hypersecretion with pancreatic
        islet cell tumor) 251.5
Elongation, elongated (congenital) - see
    also Distortion
  bone 756.9
  cervix (uteri) 752.49
    acquired 622.6
    hypertrophic 622.6
  colon 751.5
  common bile duct 751.69
  cystic duct 751.69
  frenulum, penis 752.69
  labia minora, acquired 624.8
  ligamentum patellae 756.89
  petiolus (epiglottidis) 748.3
  styloid bone (process) 733.99
  tooth, teeth 520.2
  uvula 750.26
    acquired 528.9
Elschnig bodies or pearls 366.51
El Tor cholera 001.1
Emaciation (due to malnutrition) 261
Emancipation disorder 309.22
Embadomoniasis 007.8
Embarrassment heart, cardiac - see
    Disease, heart
Embedded tooth, teeth 520.6
  root only 525.3
Embolic - see condition
Embolism 444.9
  with
    abortion - see Abortion, by type,
      with embolism
    ectopic pregnancy (see also
        categories 633.0–633.9) 639.6
    molar pregnancy (see also categories
        630–632) 639.6
  air (any site) 958.0
    with
      abortion - see Abortion, by type,
        with embolism
      ectopic pregnancy (see also
          categories 633.0–633.9)
          639.6
      molar pregnancy (see also
          categories 630–632)
          639.6

Embolism (*Continued*)
  air (*Continued*)
    due to implanted device - *see*
      Complications, due to
      (presence of) any device,
      implant, or graft classified to
      996.0–996.5 NEC
    following
      abortion 639.6
      ectopic or molar pregnancy 639.6
      infusion, perfusion, or
        transfusion 999.1
    in pregnancy, childbirth, or
      puerperium 673.0●
    traumatic 958.0
  amniotic fluid (pulmonary) 673.1●
    with
      abortion - *see* Abortion, by type,
        with embolism
      ectopic pregnancy (*see also*
        categories 633.0–633.9) 639.6
      molar pregnancy (*see also*
        categories 630–632) 639.6
    following
      abortion 639.6
      ectopic or molar pregnancy 639.6
  aorta, aortic 444.1
    abdominal 444.0
    bifurcation 444.0
    saddle 444.0
    thoracic 444.1
  artery 444.9
    auditory, internal 433.8●
    basilar (*see also* Occlusion, artery,
      basilar) 433.0●
    bladder 444.89
    carotid (common) (internal) (*see also*
      Occlusion, artery, carotid)
      433.1●
    cerebellar (anterior inferior)
      (posterior inferior) (superior)
      433.8●
    cerebral (*see also* Embolism, brain)
      434.1●
    choroidal (anterior) 433.8●
    communicating posterior 433.8●
    coronary (*see also* Infarct,
      myocardium) 410.9●
      without myocardial infarction
        411.81
    extremity 444.22
      lower 444.22
      upper 444.21
    hypophyseal 433.8●
    mesenteric (with gangrene)
      557.0
    ophthalmic (*see also* Occlusion,
      retina) 362.30
    peripheral 444.22
    pontine 433.8●
    precerebral NEC - *see* Occlusion,
      artery, precerebral
    pulmonary - *see* Embolism,
      pulmonary
    pyemic 449
      pulmonary 415.12
    renal 593.81
    retinal (*see also* Occlusion, retina)
      362.30
    septic 449
      pulmonary 415.12
    specified site NEC 444.89
    vertebral (*see also* Occlusion, artery,
      vertebral) 433.2●
  auditory, internal 433.8●
  basilar (artery) (*see also* Occlusion,
    artery, basilar) 433.0●

Embolism (*Continued*)
  birth, mother - *see* Embolism,
    obstetrical
  blood-clot
    with
      abortion - *see* Abortion, by type,
        with embolism
      ectopic pregnancy (*see also*
        categories 633.0–633.9) 639.6
      molar pregnancy (*see also*
        categories 630–632) 639.6
    following
      abortion 639.6
      ectopic or molar pregnancy 639.6
    in pregnancy, childbirth, or
      puerperium 673.2●
  brain 434.1●
    with
      abortion - *see* Abortion, by type,
        with embolism
      ectopic pregnancy (*see also*
        categories 633.0–633.9)
        639.6
      molar pregnancy (*see also*
        categories 630–632) 639.6
    following
      abortion 639.6
      ectopic or molar pregnancy 639.6
    late effect - *see* Late effect(s) (of)
      cerebrovascular disease
    puerperal, postpartum, childbirth
      674.0●
  capillary 448.9
  cardiac (*see also* Infarct, myocardium)
    410.9●
  carotid (artery) (common) (internal)
    (*see also* Occlusion, artery, carotid)
    433.1●
  cavernous sinus (venous) - *see*
    Embolism, intracranial venous
    sinus
  cerebral (*see also* Embolism, brain)
    434.1●
  cholesterol - *see* Atheroembolism
  choroidal (anterior) (artery) 433.8●
  coronary (artery or vein) (systemic) (*see
    also* Infarct, myocardium) 410.9●
    without myocardial infarction 411.81
  due to (presence of) any device,
    implant, or graft classifiable to
    996.0–996.5 - *see* Complications,
    due to (presence of) any device,
    implant, or graft classified to
    996.0–996.5 NEC
  encephalomalacia (*see also* Embolism,
    brain) 434.1●
  extremities 444.22
    lower 444.22
    upper 444.21
  eye 362.30
  fat (cerebral) (pulmonary) (systemic)
    958.1
    with
      abortion - *see* Abortion, by type,
        with embolism
      ectopic pregnancy (*see also*
        categories 633.0–633.9) 639.6
      molar pregnancy (*see also*
        categories 630–632) 639.6
    complicating delivery or
      puerperium 673.8●
    following
      abortion 639.6
      ectopic or molar pregnancy
        639.6
    in pregnancy, childbirth, or the
      puerperium 673.8●

Embolism (*Continued*)
  femoral (artery) 444.22
    vein 453.6 ⬅▥
      deep 453.41
    following
      abortion 639.6
      ectopic or molar pregnancy
        639.6
    infusion, perfusion, or transfusion
      air 999.1
      thrombus 999.2
  heart (fatty) (*see also* Infarct,
    myocardium) 410.9●
  hepatic (vein) 453.0
  iliac (artery) 444.81
  iliofemoral 444.81
  in pregnancy, childbirth, or
    puerperium (pulmonary) - *see*
    Embolism, obstetrical
  intestine (artery) (vein) (with gangrene)
    557.0
  intracranial (*see also* Embolism, brain)
    434.1●
    venous sinus (any) 325
      late effect - *see* category 326
      nonpyogenic 437.6
        in pregnancy or puerperium
          671.5●
  kidney (artery) 593.81
  lateral sinus (venous) - *see*
    Embolism, intracranial venous
    sinus
  longitudinal sinus (venous) - *see*
    Embolism, intracranial venous
    sinus
  lower extremity 444.22
  lung (massive) - *see* Embolism,
    pulmonary
  meninges (*see also* Embolism, brain)
    434.1●
  mesenteric (artery) (with gangrene)
    557.0
  multiple NEC 444.9
  obstetrical (pulmonary) 673.2●
    air 673.0●
    amniotic fluid (pulmonary) 673.1●
    blood-clot 673.2●
    cardiac 674.8●
    fat 673.8●
    heart 674.8●
    pyemic 673.3●
    septic 673.3●
    specified NEC 674.8●
  ophthalmic (*see also* Occlusion, retina)
    362.30
  paradoxical NEC 444.9
  penis 607.82
  peripheral arteries NEC 444.22
    lower 444.22
    upper 444.21
  pituitary 253.8
  popliteal (artery) 444.22
  portal (vein) 452
  postoperative NEC 997.2
    cerebral 997.02
    mesenteric artery 997.71
    other vessels 997.79
    peripheral vascular 997.2
    pulmonary 415.11
      septic 415.11
    renal artery 997.72
  precerebral artery (*see also*
    Occlusion, artery, precerebral)
    433.9●
  puerperal - *see* Embolism,
    obstetrical

◀ New   ◀▥ Revised   ~~deleted~~ Deleted   ● Use Additional Digit(s)   ▨ Omit code

Embolism *(Continued)*
  pulmonary (acute) (artery) (vein)
    415.19 ◀▥
    with
      abortion - *see* Abortion, by type,
        with embolism
      ectopic pregnancy (*see also*
        categories 633.0–633.9) 639.6
      molar pregnancy (*see also*
        categories 630–632) 639.6
    chronic 416.2 ◀
    following
      abortion 639.6
      ectopic or molar pregnancy 639.6
    healed or old V12.51 ◀
    iatrogenic 415.11
    in pregnancy, childbirth, or
      puerperium - *see* Embolism,
      obstetrical
    personal history of V12.51 ◀
    postoperative 415.11
    septic 415.12
  pyemic (multiple) (*see also* Septicemia)
    415.12
    with
      abortion - *see* Abortion, by type,
        with embolism
      ectopic pregnancy (*see also*
        categories 633.0–633.9) 639.6
      molar pregnancy (*see also*
        categories 630–632) 639.6
    Aerobacter aerogenes 415.12
    enteric gram-negative bacilli 415.12

    Enterobacter aerogenes 415.12
    Escherichia coli 415.12
    following
      abortion 639.6
      ectopic or molar pregnancy 639.6
    Hemophilus influenzae 415.12
    pneumococcal 415.12
    Proteus vulgaris 415.12
    Pseudomonas (aeruginosa) 415.12
    puerperal, postpartum, childbirth
      (any organism) 673.3●
    Serratia 415.12
    specified organism NEC 415.12
    staphylococcal 415.12
      aureus 415.12
      specified organism NEC 415.12
    streptococcal 415.12
  renal (artery) 593.81
    vein 453.3
  retina, retinal (*see also* Occlusion, retina)
    362.30
  saddle (aorta) 444.0
  septic 415.12
    arterial 449
  septicemic - *see* Embolism, pyemic
  sinus - *see* Embolism, intracranial
    venous sinus
  soap
    with
      abortion - *see* Abortion, by type,
        with embolism
      ectopic pregnancy (*see also*
        categories 633.0–633.9) 639.6
      molar pregnancy (*see also*
        categories 630–632) 639.6
    following
      abortion 639.6
      ectopic or molar pregnancy 639.6
  spinal cord (nonpyogenic) 336.1
    in pregnancy or puerperium 671.5●
    pyogenic origin 324.1
      late effect - *see* category 326
  spleen, splenic (artery) 444.89

Embolism *(Continued)*
  thrombus (thromboembolism)
    following infusion, perfusion, or
      transfusion 999.2
  upper extremity 444.21
  vein 453.9
    with inflammation or phlebitis - *see*
      Thrombophlebitis
    antecubital ◀
      acute 453.81 ◀
      chronic 453.71 ◀
    axillary ◀
      acute 453.84 ◀
      chronic 453.74 ◀
    basilic ◀
      acute 453.81 ◀
      chronic 453.71 ◀
    brachial ◀
      acute 453.82 ◀
      chronic 453.72 ◀
    brachiocephalic (innominate) ◀
      acute 453.87 ◀
      chronic 453.77 ◀
    cephalic ◀
      acute 453.81 ◀
      chronic 453.71 ◀
    cerebral (*see also* Embolism, brain)
      434.1●
    coronary (*see also* Infarct,
      myocardium) 410.9●
      without myocardial infarction
        411.81
    hepatic 453.0
    internal jugular ◀
      acute 453.86 ◀
      chronic 453.76 ◀
    lower extremity (superficial)
      453.6 ◀▥
      deep 453.40
        acute 453.40 ◀
          calf 453.42 ◀
          distal (lower leg) 453.42 ◀
          femoral 453.41 ◀
          iliac 453.41 ◀
          lower leg 453.42 ◀
          peroneal 453.42 ◀
          popliteal 453.41 ◀
          proximal (upper leg)
            453.41 ◀
          thigh 453.41 ◀
          tibial 453.42 ◀
        calf 453.42
        chronic 453.50 ◀
          calf 453.52 ◀
          distal (lower leg) 453.52 ◀
          femoral 453.51 ◀
          iliac 453.51 ◀
          lower leg 453.52 ◀
          peroneal 453.52 ◀
          popliteal 453.51 ◀
          proximal (upper leg)
            453.51 ◀
          thigh 453.51 ◀
          tibial 453.52 ◀
        distal (lower leg) 453.42
        femoral 453.41
        iliac 453.41
        lower leg 453.42
        peroneal 453.42
        popliteal 453.41
        proximal (upper leg) 453.41
        thigh 453.41
        tibial 453.42
      saphenous (greater) (lesser)
        453.6 ◀
      superficial 453.6 ◀

Embolism *(Continued)*
  vein *(Continued)*
    mesenteric (with gangrene) 557.0
    portal 452
    pulmonary - *see* Embolism, pulmonary
    radial
      acute 453.82 ◀
      chronic 453.72 ◀
    renal 453.3
    saphenous (greater) (lesser) 453.6 ◀
    specified NEC (acute) 453.89 ◀▥
      chronic 453.79 ◀
      with inflammation or phlebitis -
        see Thrombophlebitis
    subclavian ◀
      acute 453.85 ◀
      chronic 453.75 ◀
    superior vena cava ◀
      acute 453.87 ◀
      chronic 453.77 ◀
    thoracic ◀
      acute 453.87 ◀
      chronic 453.77 ◀
    ulnar ◀
      acute 453.82 ◀
      chronic 453.72 ◀
    upper extremity 453.83 ◀
      acute 453.83 ◀
        deep 453.82 ◀
        superficial 453.81 ◀
      chronic 453.73 ◀
        deep 453.72 ◀
        superficial 453.71 ◀
    vena cava (inferior) (superior) 453.2 ◀▥
      inferior 453.2 ◀
      superior ◀
        acute 453.87 ◀
        chronic 453.77 ◀
  vessels of brain (*see also* Embolism,
    brain) 434.1●
Embolization - *see* Embolism
Embolus - *see* Embolism
Embryoma (M9080/1) - *see also*
  Neoplasm, by site, uncertain
  behavior
  benign (M9080/0) - *see* Neoplasm, by
    site, benign
  kidney (M8960/3) 189.0
  liver (M8970/3) 155.0
  malignant (M9080/3) - *see also*
    Neoplasm, by site, malignant
    kidney (M8960/3) 189.0
    liver (M8970/3) 155.0
    testis (M9070/3) 186.9
      undescended 186.0
  testis (M9070/3) 186.9
    undescended 186.0
Embryonic
  circulation 747.9
  heart 747.9
  vas deferens 752.89
Embryopathia NEC 759.9
Embryotomy, fetal 763.89
Embryotoxon 743.43
  interfering with vision 743.42
Emesis - *see also* Vomiting
  bilious 787.04 ◀
  gravidarum - *see* Hyperemesis,
    gravidarum
Emissions, nocturnal (semen) 608.89
Emotional
  crisis - *see* Crisis, emotional
  disorder (*see also* Disorder, mental) 300.9
  instability (excessive) 301.3
  lability 799.24 ◀
  overlay - *see* Reaction, adjustment
  upset 300.9

Emotionality, pathological 301.3
Emotogenic disease (see also Disorder, psychogenic) 306.9
Emphysema (atrophic) (centriacinar) (centrilobular) (chronic) (diffuse) (essential) (hypertrophic) (interlobular) (lung) (obstructive) (panlobular) (paracicatricial) (paracinar) (postural) (pulmonary) (senile) (subpleural) (traction) (unilateral) (unilobular) (vesicular) 492.8
  with bronchitis
    chronic 491.20
      with
        acute bronchitis 491.22
        exacerbation (acute) 491.21
  bullous (giant) 492.0
  cellular tissue 958.7
    surgical 998.81
  compensatory 518.2
  congenital 770.2
  conjunctiva 372.89
  connective tissue 958.7
    surgical 998.81
  due to fumes or vapors 506.4
  eye 376.89
  eyelid 374.85
    surgical 998.81
    traumatic 958.7
  fetus or newborn (interstitial) (mediastinal) (unilobular) 770.2
  heart 416.9
  interstitial 518.1
    congenital 770.2
    fetus or newborn 770.2
  laminated tissue 958.7
    surgical 998.81
  mediastinal 518.1
    fetus or newborn 770.2
  newborn (interstitial) (mediastinal) (unilobular) 770.2
  obstructive diffuse with fibrosis 492.8
  orbit 376.89
  subcutaneous 958.7
    due to trauma 958.7
    nontraumatic 518.1
    surgical 998.81
  surgical 998.81
  thymus (gland) (congenital)254.8
  traumatic 958.7
  tuberculous (see also Tuberculosis, pulmonary) 011.9●
Employment examination (certification) V70.5
Empty sella (turcica) syndrome 253.8
Empyema (chest) (diaphragmatic) (double) (encapsulated) (general) (interlobar) (lung) (medial) (necessitatis) (perforating chest wall) (pleura) (pneumococcal) (residual) (sacculated) (streptococcal) (supradiaphragmatic) 510.9
  with fistula 510.0
  accessory sinus (chronic) (see also Sinusitis) 473.9
  acute 510.9
    with fistula 510.0
  antrum (chronic) (see also Sinusitis, maxillary) 473.0
  brain (any part) (see also Abscess, brain) 324.0
  ethmoidal (sinus) (chronic) (see also Sinusitis, ethmoidal) 473.2
  extradural (see also Abscess, extradural) 324.9

Empyema (Continued)
  frontal (sinus) (chronic) (see also Sinusitis, frontal) 473.1
  gallbladder (see also Cholecystitis, acute) 575.0
  mastoid (process) (acute) (see also Mastoiditis, acute) 383.00
  maxilla, maxillary 526.4
    sinus (chronic) (see also Sinusitis, maxillary) 473.0
  nasal sinus (chronic) (see also Sinusitis) 473.9
  sinus (accessory) (nasal) (see also Sinusitis) 473.9
  sphenoidal (chronic) (sinus) (see also Sinusitis, sphenoidal) 473.3
  subarachnoid (see also Abscess, extradural) 324.9
  subdural (see also Abscess, extradural) 324.9
  tuberculous (see also Tuberculosis, pleura) 012.0●
  ureter (see also Ureteritis) 593.89
  ventricular (see also Abscess, brain) 324.0
Enameloma 520.2
Encephalitis (bacterial) (chronic) (hemorrhagic) (idiopathic) (nonepidemic) (spurious) (subacute) 323.9
  acute - see also Encephalitis, viral
    disseminated (postinfectious) NEC 136.9 [323.61]
      postimmunization or postvaccination 323.51
    inclusional 049.8
    inclusion body 049.8
    necrotizing 049.8
  arboviral, arbovirus NEC 064
  arthropod-borne (see also Encephalitis, viral, arthropod-borne) 064
  Australian X 062.4
  Bwamba fever 066.3
  California (virus) 062.5
  Central European 063.2
  Czechoslovakian 063.2
  Dawson's (inclusion body) 046.2
  diffuse sclerosing 046.2
  due to
    actinomycosis 039.8 [323.41]
    cat-scratch disease 078.3 [323.01]
    human herpesvirus 6 058.21
    human herpesvirus 7 058.29
    human herpesvirus NEC 058.29
    infection classified elsewhere 136.9 [323.41]
    infectious mononucleosis 075 [323.01]
    malaria (see also Malaria) 084.6 [323.2]
    Negishi virus 064
    ornithosis 073.7 [323.01]
    prophylactic inoculation against smallpox 323.51
    rickettsiosis (see also Rickettsiosis) 083.9 [323.1]
    rubella 056.01
    toxoplasmosis (acquired) 130.0
      congenital (active) 771.2 [323.41]
    typhus (fever) (see also Typhus) 081.9 [323.1]
    vaccination (smallpox) 323.51
  Eastern equine 062.2
  endemic 049.8
  epidemic 049.8
  equine (acute) (infectious) (viral) 062.9
    eastern 062.2
    Venezuelan 066.2
    western 062.1

Encephalitis (Continued)
  Far Eastern 063.0
  following vaccination or other immunization procedure 323.51
  herpes 054.3
  human herpesvirus 6 058.21
  human herpesvirus 7 058.29
  human herpesvirus NEC 058.29
  Ilheus (virus) 062.8
  inclusion body 046.2
  infectious (acute) (virus) NEC 049.8
  influenzal 487.8 [323.41]
    lethargic 049.8
  Japanese (B type) 062.0
  La Crosse 062.5
  Langat 063.8
  late effect - see Late, effect, encephalitis
  lead 984.9 [323.71]
  lethargic (acute) (infectious) (influenzal) 049.8
  lethargica 049.8
  louping ill 063.1
  lupus 710.0 [323.81]
  lymphatica 049.0
  Mengo 049.8
  meningococcal 036.1
  mumps 072.2
  Murray Valley 062.4
  myoclonic 049.8
  Negishi virus 064
  otitic NEC 382.4 [323.41]
  parasitic NEC 123.9 [323.41]
  periaxialis (concentrica) (diffusa) 341.1
  postchickenpox 052.0
  postexanthematous NEC 057.9 [323.62]
  postimmunization 323.51
  postinfectious NEC 136.9 [323.62]
  postmeasles 055.0
  posttraumatic 323.81
  postvaccinal (smallpox) 323.51
  postvaricella 052.0
  postviral NEC 079.99 [323.62]
    postexanthematous 057.9 [323.62]
    specified NEC 057.8 [323.62]
  Powassan 063.8
  progressive subcortical (Binswanger's) 290.12
  Rasmussen 323.81
  Rio Bravo 049.8
  rubella 056.01
  Russian
    autumnal 062.0
    spring-summer type (taiga) 063.0
  saturnine 984.9 [323.71]
  Semliki Forest 062.8
  serous 048
  slow-acting virus NEC 046.8
  specified cause NEC 323.81
  St. Louis type 062.3
  subacute sclerosing 046.2
  subcorticalis chronica 290.12
  summer 062.0
  suppurative 324.0
  syphilitic 094.81
    congenital 090.41
  tick-borne 063.9
  torula, torular 117.5 [323.41]
  toxic NEC 989.9 [323.71]
  toxoplasmic (acquired) 130.0
    congenital (active) 771.2 [323.41]
  trichinosis 124 [323.41]
  Trypanosomiasis (see also Trypanosomiasis) 086.9 [323.2]
  tuberculous (see also Tuberculosis) 013.6●
  type B (Japanese) 062.0

◀ New　◀█ Revised　~~deleted~~ Deleted　● Use Additional Digit(s)　▨ Omit code

Encephalitis *(Continued)*
   type C 062.3
   van Bogaert's 046.2
   Venezuelan 066.2
   Vienna type 049.8
   viral, virus 049.9
     arthropod-borne NEC 064
       mosquito-borne 062.9
         Australian X disease 062.4
         California virus 062.5
         Eastern equine 062.2
         Ilheus virus 062.8
         Japanese (B type) 062.0
         Murray Valley 062.4
         specified type NEC 062.8
         St. Louis 062.3
         type B 062.0
         type C 062.3
         Western equine 062.1
       tick-borne 063.9
         biundulant 063.2
         Central European 063.2
         Czechoslovakian 063.2
         diphasic meningoencephalitis 063.2
         Far Eastern 063.0
         Langat 063.8
         louping ill 063.1
         Powassan 063.8
         Russian spring-summer (taiga) 063.0
         specified type NEC 063.8
       vector unknown 064
     slow acting NEC 046.8
     specified type NEC 049.8
     vaccination, prophylactic (against) V05.0
   von Economo's 049.8
   Western equine 062.1
   West Nile type 066.41
Encephalocele 742.0
   orbit 376.81
Encephalocystocele 742.0
Encephalomalacia (brain) (cerebellar) (cerebral) (cerebrospinal) *(see also* Softening, brain) 434.9●
   due to
     hemorrhage *(see also* Hemorrhage, brain) 431
     recurrent spasm of artery 435.9
   embolic (cerebral) *(see also* Embolism, brain) 434.1●
   subcorticalis chronicus arteriosclerotica 290.12
   thrombotic *(see also* Thrombosis, brain) 434.0●
Encephalomeningitis - *see* Meningoencephalitis
Encephalomeningocele 742.0
Encephalomeningomyelitis - *see* Meningoencephalitis
Encephalomeningopathy *(see also* Meningoencephalitis) 349.9
Encephalomyelitis (chronic) (granulomatous) (myalgic, benign) *(see also* Encephalitis) 323.9
   abortive disseminated 049.8
   acute disseminated (ADEM) (postinfectious) 136.9 *[323.61]*
     infectious 136.9 *[323.61]*
     noninfectious 323.81
     postimmunization 323.51
   due to
     cat-scratch disease 078.3 *[323.01]*
     infectious mononucleosis 075 *[323.01]*

Encephalitis *(Continued)*
   due to *(Continued)*
     ornithosis 073.7 *[323.01]*
     vaccination (any) 323.51
   equine (acute) (infectious) 062.9
     eastern 062.2
     Venezuelan 066.2
     western 062.1
   funicularis infectiosa 049.8
   late effect - *see* Late, effect, encephalitis
   Munch-Peterson's 049.8
   postchickenpox 052.0
   postimmunization 323.51
   postmeasles 055.0
   postvaccinal (smallpox) 323.51
   rubella 056.01
   specified cause NEC 323.81
   syphilitic 094.81
   West Nile 066.41
Encephalomyelocele 742.0
Encephalomyelomeningitis - *see* Meningoencephalitis
Encephalomyeloneuropathy 349.9
Encephalomyelopathy 349.9
   subacute necrotizing (infantile) 330.8
Encephalomyeloradiculitis (acute) 357.0
Encephalomyeloradiculoneuritis (acute) 357.0
Encephalomyeloradiculopathy 349.9
Encephalomyocarditis 074.23
Encephalopathia hyperbilirubinemica, newborn 774.7
   due to isoimmunization (conditions classifiable to 773.0–773.2) 773.4
Encephalopathy (acute) 348.30
   alcoholic 291.2
   anoxic - *see* Damage, brain, anoxic
   arteriosclerotic 437.0
     late effect - *see* Late effect(s) (of) cerebrovascular disease
   bilirubin, newborn 774.7
     due to isoimmunization 773.4
   congenital 742.9
   demyelinating (callosal) 341.8
   due to
     birth injury (intracranial) 767.8
     dialysis 294.8
       transient 293.9
     drugs - *(see also* Table of Drugs and Chemicals) 348.39
     hyperinsulinism - *see* Hyperinsulinism
     influenza (virus) 487.8
     lack of vitamin *(see also* Deficiency, vitamin) 269.2
     nicotinic acid deficiency 291.2
     serum (nontherapeutic) (therapeutic) 999.5
     syphilis 094.81
     trauma (postconcussional) 310.2
       current *(see also* Concussion, brain) 850.9
         with skull fracture - *see* Fracture, skull, by site, with intracranial injury
     vaccination 323.51
   hepatic 572.2
   hyperbilirubinemic, newborn 774.7
     due to isoimmunization (conditions classifiable to 773.0–773.2) 773.4
   hypertensive 437.2
   hypoglycemic 251.2
   hypoxic - *see also* Damage, brain, anoxic
     ischemic (HIE) 768.70
       mild 768.71
       moderate 768.72
       severe 768.73

Encephalopathy *(Continued)*
   infantile cystic necrotizing (congenital) 341.8
   lead 984.9 *[323.71]*
   leukopolio 330.0
   metabolic *(see also* Delirium) 348.31
     toxic 349.82
   necrotizing
     hemorrhagic (acute) 323.61
     subacute 330.8
   other specified type NEC 348.39
   pellagrous 265.2
   portal-systemic 572.2
   postcontusional 310.2
   posttraumatic 310.2
   saturnine 984.9 *[323.71]*
   septic 348.31
   spongioform, subacute (viral) 046.19
   subacute
     necrotizing 330.8
     spongioform 046.19
     viral, spongioform 046.19
   subcortical progressive (Schilder) 341.1
     chronic (Binswanger's) 290.12
   toxic 349.82
     metabolic 349.82
   traumatic (postconcussional) 310.2
     current *(see also* Concussion, brain) 850.9
       with skull fracture - *see* Fracture, skull, by site, with intracranial injury
   vitamin B deficiency NEC 266.9
   Wernicke's (superior hemorrhagic polioencephalitis) 265.1
Encephalorrhagia *(see also* Hemorrhage, brain) 432.9
   healed or old V12.54
   late effect - *see* Late effect(s) (of) cerebrovascular disease
Encephalosis, posttraumatic 310.2
Enchondroma (M9220/0) - *see also* Neoplasm, bone, benign
   multiple, congenital 756.4
Enchondromatosis (cartilaginous) (congenital) (multiple) 756.4
Enchondroses, multiple (cartilaginous) (congenital) 756.4
Encopresis *(see also* Incontinence, feces) 787.6
   nonorganic origin 307.7
Encounter for - *see also* Admission for administrative purpose only V68.9
   referral of patient without examination or treatment V68.81
   specified purpose NEC V68.89
   chemotherapy, (oral) (intravenous), antineoplastic V58.11 ◀▥
   dialysis
     extracorporeal (renal) V56.0
     peritoneal V56.8
   disability examination V68.01
   end-of-life care V66.7
   hospice care V66.7
   immunizations (childhood)
     appropriate for age V20.2 ◀
   immunotherapy, antineoplastic V58.12
   palliative care V66.7
   paternity testing V70.4
   radiotherapy V58.0
   respirator [ventilator] dependence during
     mechanical failure V46.14
     power failure V46.12
     for weaning V46.13
   routine infant and child vision and hearing testing V20.2 ◀
   school examination V70.3 ◀
     following surgery V67.09 ◀

◀ New   ◀▥ Revised   ~~deleted~~ Deleted   ● Use Additional Digit(s)   ▨ Omit code

Encounter for (Continued)
  screening mammogram NEC V76.12
    for high-risk patient V76.11
  terminal care V66.7
  weaning from respirator [ventilator]
    V46.13
Encystment - see Cyst
End-of-life care V66.7
Endamebiasis - see Amebiasis
Endamoeba - see Amebiasis
Endarteritis (bacterial, subacute)
    (infective) (septic) 447.6
  brain, cerebral or cerebrospinal 437.4
    late effect - see Late effect(s) (of)
      cerebrovascular disease
  coronary (artery) - see Arteriosclerosis,
    coronary
  deformans - see Arteriosclerosis
  embolic (see also Embolism) 444.9
  obliterans - see also Arteriosclerosis
    pulmonary 417.8
  pulmonary 417.8
  retina 362.18
  senile - see Arteriosclerosis
  syphilitic 093.89
    brain or cerebral 094.89
    congenital 090.5
    spinal 094.89
  tuberculous (see also Tuberculosis)
    017.9●
Endemic - see condition
Endocarditis (chronic) (indeterminate)
    (interstitial) (marantic) (nonbacterial
    thrombotic) (residual) (sclerotic)
    (sclerous) (senile) (valvular) 424.90
  with
    rheumatic fever (conditions
      classifiable to 390)
      active - see Endocarditis, acute,
        rheumatic
      inactive or quiescent (with
        chorea) 397.9
  acute or subacute 421.9
    rheumatic (aortic) (mitral)
      (pulmonary) (tricuspid) 391.1
      with chorea (acute) (rheumatic)
        (Sydenham's) 392.0
  aortic (heart) (nonrheumatic) (valve)
    424.1
    with
      mitral (valve) disease 396.9
        active or acute 391.1
          with chorea (acute)
            (rheumatic)
            (Sydenham's) 392.0
        bacterial 421.0
      rheumatic fever (conditions
        classifiable to 390)
        active - see Endocarditis, acute,
          rheumatic
        inactive or quiescent (with
          chorea) 395.9
          with mitral disease 396.9
    acute or subacute 421.9
    arteriosclerotic 424.1
    congenital 746.89
    hypertensive 424.1
    rheumatic (chronic) (inactive) 395.9
      with mitral (valve) disease 396.9
        active or acute 391.1
          with chorea (acute)
            (rheumatic)
            (Sydenham's) 392.0
      active or acute 391.1
        with chorea (acute)
          (rheumatic)
          (Sydenham's) 392.0

Endocarditis (Continued)
  aortic (Continued)
    specified cause, except rheumatic
      424.1
    syphilitic 093.22
  arteriosclerotic or due to
    arteriosclerosis 424.99
  atypical verrucous (Libman-Sacks)
    710.0 [424.91]
  bacterial (acute) (any valve) (chronic)
    (subacute) 421.0
  blastomycotic 116.0 [421.1]
  candidal 112.81
  congenital 425.3
  constrictive 421.0
  Coxsackie 074.22
  due to
    blastomycosis 116.0 [421.1]
    candidiasis 112.81
    Coxsackie (virus) 074.22
    disseminated lupus erythematosus
      710.0 [424.91]
    histoplasmosis (see also
      Histoplasmosis) 115.94
    hypertension (benign) 424.99
    moniliasis 112.81
    prosthetic cardiac valve 996.61
    Q fever 083.0 [421.1]
    serratia marcescens 421.0
    typhoid (fever) 002.0 [421.1]
  fetal 425.3
  gonococcal 098.84
  hypertensive 424.99
  infectious or infective (acute) (any
    valve) (chronic) (subacute)
    421.0
  lenta (acute) (any valve) (chronic)
    (subacute) 421.0
  Libman-Sacks 710.0 [424.91]
  Loeffler's (parietal fibroplastic)
    421.0
  malignant (acute) (any valve) (chronic)
    (subacute) 421.0
  meningococcal 036.42
  mitral (chronic) (double) (fibroid)
    (heart) (inactive) (valve) (with
    chorea) 394.9
    with
      aortic (valve) disease 396.9
        active or acute 391.1
          with chorea (acute)
            (rheumatic)
            (Sydenham's) 392.0
      rheumatic fever (conditions
        classifiable to 390)
        active - see Endocarditis,
          acute, rheumatic
        inactive or quiescent (with
          chorea) 394.9
          with aortic valve disease
            396.9
    active or acute 391.1
      with chorea (acute) (rheumatic)
        (Sydenham's) 392.0
    bacterial 421.0
    arteriosclerotic 424.0
    congenital 746.89
    hypertensive 424.0
    nonrheumatic 424.0
      acute or subacute 421.9
    syphilitic 093.21
  monilial 112.81
  mycotic (acute) (any valve) (chronic)
    (subacute) 421.0
  pneumococcic (acute) (any valve)
    (chronic) (subacute)
    421.0

Endocarditis (Continued)
  pulmonary (chronic) (heart) (valve) 424.3
    with
      rheumatic fever (conditions
        classifiable to 390)
        active - see Endocarditis, acute,
          rheumatic
        inactive or quiescent (with
          chorea) 397.1
    acute or subacute 421.9
      rheumatic 391.1
        with chorea (acute)
          (rheumatic)
          (Sydenham's) 392.0
    arteriosclerotic or due to
      arteriosclerosis 424.3
    congenital 746.09
    hypertensive or due to hypertension
      (benign) 424.3
    rheumatic (chronic) (inactive) (with
      chorea) 397.1
      active or acute 391.1
        with chorea (acute)
          (rheumatic)
          (Sydenham's) 392.0
    syphilitic 093.24
  purulent (acute) (any valve) (chronic)
    (subacute) 421.0
  rheumatic (chronic) (inactive) (with
    chorea) 397.9
    active or acute (aortic) (mitral)
      (pulmonary) (tricuspid) 391.1
      with chorea (acute) (rheumatic)
        (Sydenham's) 392.0
  septic (acute) (any valve) (chronic)
    (subacute) 421.0
  specified cause, except rheumatic
    424.99
  streptococcal (acute) (any valve)
    (chronic) (subacute) 421.0
  subacute - see Endocarditis, acute
  suppurative (any valve) (acute)
    (chronic) (subacute) 421.0
  syphilitic NEC 093.20
  toxic (see also Endocarditis, acute) 421.9
  tricuspid (chronic) (heart) (inactive)
    (rheumatic) (valve) (with chorea)
    397.0
    with
      rheumatic fever (conditions
        classifiable to 390)
        active - see Endocarditis, acute,
          rheumatic
        inactive or quiescent (with
          chorea) 397.0
    active or acute 391.1
      with chorea (acute) (rheumatic)
        (Sydenham's) 392.0
    arteriosclerotic 424.2
    congenital 746.89
    hypertensive 424.2
    nonrheumatic 424.2
      acute or subacute 421.9
    specified cause, except rheumatic
      424.2
    syphilitic 093.23
  tuberculous (see also Tuberculosis)
    017.9● [424.91]
  typhoid 002.0 [421.1]
  ulcerative (acute) (any valve) (chronic)
    (subacute) 421.0
  vegetative (acute) (any valve) (chronic)
    (subacute) 421.0
  verrucous (acute) (any valve) (chronic)
    (subacute) NEC 710.0 [424.91]
    nonbacterial 710.0 [424.91]
    nonrheumatic 710.0 [424.91]

◀ New ◀ Revised deleted Deleted ● Use Additional Digit(s) ▨ Omit code

Endocardium, endocardial - *see also*
    condition
    cushion defect 745.60
        specified type NEC 745.69
Endocervicitis (*see also* Cervicitis) 616.0
    due to
        intrauterine (contraceptive) device
            996.65
    gonorrheal (acute) 098.15
        chronic or duration of 2 months or
            over 098.35
    hyperplastic 616.0
    syphilitic 095.8
    trichomonal 131.09
    tuberculous (*see also* Tuberculosis) 016.7●
Endocrine - *see* condition
Endocrinopathy, pluriglandular 258.9
Endodontitis 522.0
Endomastoiditis (*see also* Mastoiditis)
    383.9
Endometrioma 617.9
Endometriosis 617.9
    appendix 617.5
    bladder 617.8
    bowel 617.5
    broad ligament 617.3
    cervix 617.0
    colon 617.5
    cul-de-sac (Douglas') 617.3
    exocervix 617.0
    fallopian tube 617.2
    female genital organ NEC 617.8
    gallbladder 617.8
    in scar of skin 617.6
    internal 617.0
    intestine 617.5
    lung 617.8
    myometrium 617.0
    ovary 617.1
    parametrium 617.3
    pelvic peritoneum 617.3
    peritoneal (pelvic) 617.3
    rectovaginal septum 617.4
    rectum 617.5
    round ligament 617.3
    skin 617.6
    specified site NEC 617.8
    stromal (M8931/1) 236.0
    umbilicus 617.8
    uterus 617.0
        internal 617.0
    vagina 617.4
    vulva 617.8
Endometritis (nonspecific) (purulent)
    (septic) (suppurative) 615.9
    with
        abortion - *see* Abortion, by type,
            with sepsis
        ectopic pregnancy (*see also*
            categories 633.0-633.9) 639.0
        molar pregnancy (*see also* categories
            630-632) 639.0
    acute 615.0
    blennorrhagic 098.16
        acute 098.16
        chronic or duration of 2 months or
            over 098.36
    cervix, cervical (*see also* Cervicitis) 616.0
        hyperplastic 616.0
    chronic 615.1
    complicating pregnancy 670.1 ◀▦
        affecting fetus or newborn 760.8
        septic 670.2 ◀
    decidual 615.9
    following
        abortion 639.0
        ectopic or molar pregnancy 639.0

Endometritis (*Continued*)
    gonorrheal (acute) 098.16
        chronic or duration of 2 months or
            over 098.36
    hyperplastic (*see also* Hyperplasia,
        endometrium) 621.30
        cervix 616.0
    polypoid - *see* Endometritis,
        hyperplastic
    puerperal, postpartum, childbirth
        670.1 ◀▦
        septic 670.2 ◀
    senile (atrophic) 615.9
    subacute 615.0
    tuberculous (*see also* Tuberculosis)
        016.7●
Endometrium - *see* condition
Endomyocardiopathy, South African
    425.2
Endomyocarditis - *see* Endocarditis
Endomyofibrosis 425.0
Endomyometritis (*see also* Endometritis)
    615.9
Endopericarditis - *see* Endocarditis
Endoperineuritis - *see* Disorder, nerve
Endophlebitis (*see also* Phlebitis) 451.9
    leg 451.2
        deep (vessels) 451.19
        superficial (vessels) 451.0
    portal (vein) 572.1
    retina 362.18
    specified site NEC 451.89
    syphilitic 093.89
Endophthalmia (*see also* Endophthalmitis)
    360.00
    gonorrheal 098.42
Endophthalmitis (globe) (infective)
    (metastatic) (purulent) (subacute)
    360.00
    acute 360.01
    bleb associated 379.63
    chronic 360.03
    parasitic 360.13
    phacoanaphylactic 360.19
    specified type NEC 360.19
    sympathetic 360.11
Endosalpingioma (M9111/1) 236.2
Endosalpingiosis 629.89
Endosteitis - *see* Osteomyelitis
Endothelioma, bone (M9260/3) - *see*
    Neoplasm, bone, malignant
Endotheliosis 287.8
    hemorrhagic infectional 287.8
Endotoxemia - *code to* condition
Endotoxic shock 785.52
Endotrachelitis (*see also* Cervicitis) 616.0
Enema rash 692.89
Engel-von Recklinghausen disease or
    syndrome (osteitis fibrosa cystica)
    252.01
Engelmann's disease (diaphyseal
    sclerosis) 756.59
English disease (*see also* Rickets) 268.0
Engman's disease (infectious eczematoid
    dermatitis) 690.8
Engorgement
    breast 611.79
        newborn 778.7
        puerperal, postpartum 676.2●
    liver 573.9
    lung 514
    pulmonary 514
    retina, venous 362.37
    stomach 536.8
    venous, retina 362.37
Enlargement, enlarged - *see also*
    Hypertrophy

Enlargement, enlarged (*Continued*)
    abdomen 789.3●
    adenoids 474.12
        and tonsils 474.10
    alveolar process or ridge 525.8
    apertures of diaphragm (congenital)
        756.6
    blind spot, visual field 368.42
    gingival 523.8
    heart, cardiac (*see also* Hypertrophy,
        cardiac) 429.3
    lacrimal gland, chronic 375.03
    liver (*see also* Hypertrophy, liver) 789.1
    lymph gland or node 785.6
    orbit 376.46
    organ or site, congenital NEC - *see*
        Anomaly, specified type NEC
    parathyroid (gland) 252.01
    pituitary fossa 793.0
    prostate (simple) (soft) 600.00
        with
            other lower urinary tract
                symptoms (LUTS) 600.01
            urinary
                obstruction 600.01
                retention 600.01
    sella turcica 793.0
    spleen (*see also* Splenomegaly) 789.2
        congenital 759.0
    thymus (congenital) (gland) 254.0
    thyroid (gland) (*see also* Goiter) 240.9
    tongue 529.8
    tonsils 474.11
        and adenoids 474.10
    uterus 621.2
Enophthalmos 376.50
    due to
        atrophy of orbital tissue 376.51
        surgery 376.52
        trauma 376.52
Enostosis 526.89
Entamebiasis - *see* Amebiasis
Entamebic - *see* Amebiasis
Entanglement, umbilical cord(s)
    663.3●
    with compression 663.2●
    affecting fetus or newborn 762.5
    around neck with compression 663.1●
    twins in monoamniotic sac 663.2●
Enteralgia 789.0●
Enteric - *see* condition
Enteritis (acute) (catarrhal) (choleraic)
    (chronic) (congestive) (diarrheal)
    (exudative) (follicular)
    (hemorrhagic) (infantile) (lienteric)
    (noninfectious) (perforative)
    (phlegmonous) (presumed
    noninfectious)
    (pseudomembranous) 558.9
    adaptive 564.9
    aertrycke infection 003.0
    allergic 558.3
    amebic (*see also* Amebiasis) 006.9
        with abscess - *see* Abscess, amebic
        acute 006.0
            with abscess - *see* Abscess, amebic
            nondysenteric 006.2
        chronic 006.1
            with abscess - *see* Abscess, amebic
            nondysenteric 006.2
        nondysenteric 006.2
    anaerobic (cocci) (gram-negative)
        (gram-positive) (mixed) NEC
        008.46
    bacillary NEC 004.9
    bacterial NEC 008.5
        specified NEC 008.49

Enteritis (Continued)
  Bacteroides (fragilis)
      (melaninogeniscus) (oralis) 008.46
  Butyrivibrio (fibrisolvens) 008.46
  Campylobacter 008.43
  Candida 112.85
  Chilomastix 007.8
  choleriformis 001.1
  chronic 558.9
    ulcerative (see also Colitis, ulcerative)
        556.9
  cicatrizing (chronic) 555.0
  Clostridium
    botulinum 005.1
    difficile 008.45
    haemolyticum 008.46
    novyi 008.46
    perfringens (C) (F) 008.46
    specified type NEC 008.46
  coccidial 007.2
  dietetic 558.9
  due to
    achylia gastrica 536.8
    adenovirus 008.62
    Aerobacter aerogenes 008.2
    anaerobes (see also Enteritis,
        anaerobic) 008.46
    Arizona (bacillus) 008.1
    astrovirus 008.66
    Bacillus coli - see Enteritis, E. coli
    bacteria NEC 008.5
      specified NEC 008.49
    Bacteroides (see also Enteritis,
        Bacteroides) 008.46
    Butyrivibrio (fibrisolvens)
        008.46
    calicivirus 008.65   ◀▥▥
    Campylobacter 008.43
    Clostridium - see Enteritis,
        Clostridium
    Cockle agent 008.64
    Coxsackie (virus) 008.67
    Ditchling agent 008.64
    ECHO virus 008.67
    Enterobacter aerogenes 008.2
    enterococci 008.49
    enterovirus NEC 008.67
    Escherichia coli - see Enteritis, E. coli
    Eubacterium 008.46
    Fusobacterium (nucleatum) 008.46
    gram-negative bacteria NEC 008.47
        anaerobic NEC 008.46
    Hawaii agent 008.63
    irritating foods 558.9
    Klebsiella aerogenes 008.47
    Marin County agent 008.66
    Montgomery County agent 008.63
    noroviris 008.63   ◀
    Norwalk-like agent 008.63
    Norwalk virus 008.63
    Otofuke agent 008.63
    Paracolobactrum arizonae 008.1
    paracolon bacillus NEC 008.47
        Arizona 008.1
    Paramatta agent 008.64
    Peptococcus 008.46
    Peptostreptococcus 008.46
    Proprionibacterium 008.46
    Proteus (bacillus) (mirabilis)
        (morganii) 008.3
    Pseudomonas aeruginosa 008.42
    Rotavirus 008.61
    Sapporo agent 008.63
    small round virus (SRV) NEC
        008.64
      featureless NEC 008.63
      structured NEC 008.63

Enteritis (Continued)
  due to (Continued)
    Snow Mountain (SM) agent 008.63
    specified
      bacteria NEC 008.49
      organism, nonbacterial NEC 008.8
      virus NEC 008.69
    Staphylococcus 008.41
    Streptococcus 008.49
      anaerobic 008.46
    Taunton agent 008.63
    Torovirus 008.69
    Treponema 008.46
    Veillonella 008.46
    virus 008.8
      specified type NEC 008.69
    Wollan (W) agent 008.64
    Yersinia enterocolitica 008.44
  dysentery - see Dysentery
  E. coli 008.00
    enterohemorrhagic 008.04
    enteroinvasive 008.03
    enteropathogenic 008.01
    enterotoxigenic 008.02
    specified type NEC 008.09
  El Tor 001.1
  embadomonial 007.8
  eosinophilic 558.41
  epidemic 009.0
  Eubacterium 008.46
  fermentative 558.9
  fulminant 557.0
  Fusobacterium (nucleatum) 008.46
  gangrenous (see also Enteritis, due to,
      by organism) 009.0
  giardial 007.1
  gram-negative bacteria NEC 008.47
      anaerobic NEC 008.46
  infectious NEC (see also Enteritis, due
      to, by organism) 009.0
      presumed 009.1
  influenzal 487.8
  ischemic 557.9
    acute 557.0
    chronic 557.1
    due to mesenteric artery
        insufficiency 557.1
  membranous 564.9
  mucous 564.9
  myxomembranous 564.9
  necrotic (see also Enteritis, due to, by
      organism) 009.0
  necroticans 005.2
  necrotizing of fetus or newborn (see also
      Enterocolitis, necrotizing,
      newborn) 777.50
  neurogenic 564.9
  newborn 777.8
    necrotizing (see also Enterocolitis,
        necrotizing, newborn)
        777.50
  parasitic NEC 129
  paratyphoid (fever) (see also Fever,
      paratyphoid) 002.9
  Peptococcus 008.46
  Peptostreptococcus 008.46
  Proprionibacterium 008.46
  protozoal NEC 007.9
  radiation 558.1
  regional (of) 555.9
    intestine
      large (bowel, colon, or rectum)
          555.1
        with small intestine 555.2
      small (duodenum, ileum, or
          jejunum) 555.0
        with large intestine 555.2

Enteritis (Continued)
  Salmonella infection 003.0
  salmonellosis 003.0
  segmental (see also Enteritis, regional)
      555.9
  septic (see also Enteritis, due to, by
      organism) 009.0
  Shigella 004.9
  simple 558.9
  spasmodic 564.9
  spastic 564.9
  staphylococcal 008.41
    due to food 005.0
  streptococcal 008.49
    anaerobic 008.46
  toxic 558.2
  Treponema (denticola) (macrodentium)
      008.46
  trichomonal 007.3
  tuberculous (see also Tuberculosis) 014.8●
  typhosa 002.0
  ulcerative (chronic) (see also Colitis,
      ulcerative) 556.9
  Veillonella 008.46
  viral 008.8
    adenovirus 008.62
    enterovirus 008.67
    specified virus NEC 008.69
  Yersinia enterocolitica 008.44
  zymotic 009.0
Enteroarticular syndrome 099.3
Enterobiasis 127.4
Enterobius vermicularis 127.4
Enterocele (see also Hernia) 553.9
  pelvis, pelvic (acquired) (congenital)
      618.6
  vagina, vaginal (acquired) (congenital)
      618.6
Enterocolitis - see also Enteritis
  fetus or newborn (see also Enterocolitis,
      necrotizing, newborn) 777.8
    necrotizing 777.50
  fulminant 557.0
  granulomatous 555.2
  hemorrhagic (acute) 557.0
    chronic 557.1
  necrotizing (acute) (membranous) 557.0
    newborn 777.50
      with
        perforation 777.53
        pneumatosis without
            perforation 777.52
        pneumatosis and perforation
            777.53
      without pneumatosis, without
          perforation 777.51   ◀
      stage I 777.51
      stage II 777.52
      stage III 777.53
    primary necrotizing (see also
        Enterocolitis, necrotizing,
        newborn) 777.50
  pseudomembranous 008.45
    newborn 008.45   ◀
  radiation 558.1
    newborn (see also Enterocolitis,
        necrotizing, newborn) 777.50
  ulcerative 556.0
Enterocystoma 751.5
Enterogastritis - see Enteritis
Enterogenous cyanosis 289.7
Enterolith, enterolithiasis (impaction)
    560.39
  with hernia - see also Hernia, by site,
      with obstruction
    gangrenous - see Hernia, by site,
        with gangrene

◀ New   ◀▥▥ Revised   ~~deleted~~ Deleted   ● Use Additional Digit(s)   ▥▥ Omit code

Enteropathy 569.9
  exudative (of Gordon) 579.8
  gluten 579.0
  hemorrhagic, terminal 557.0
  protein-losing 579.8
Enteroperitonitis (see also Peritonitis)
    567.9
Enteroptosis 569.89
Enterorrhagia 578.9
Enterospasm 564.9
  psychogenic 306.4
Enterostenosis (see also Obstruction,
    intestine) 560.9
Enterostomy status V44.4
  with complication 569.60
Enthesopathy 726.90
  ankle and tarsus 726.70
  elbow region 726.30
    specified NEC 726.39
  hip 726.5
  knee 726.60
  peripheral NEC 726.8
  shoulder region 726.10
    adhesive 726.0
  spinal 720.1
  wrist and carpus 726.4
Entrance, air into vein - see Embolism,
    air
Entrapment, nerve - see Neuropathy,
    entrapment
Entropion (eyelid) 374.00
  cicatricial 374.04
  congenital 743.62
  late effect of trachoma (healed)
      139.1
  mechanical 374.02
  paralytic 374.02
  senile 374.01
  spastic 374.03
Enucleation of eye (current) (traumatic)
    871.3
Enuresis 788.30
  habit disturbance 307.6
  nocturnal 788.36
    psychogenic 307.6
  nonorganic origin 307.6
  psychogenic 307.6
Enzymopathy 277.9
Eosinopenia 288.59
Eosinophilia 288.3
  allergic 288.3
  hereditary 288.3
  idiopathic 288.3
  infiltrative 518.3
  Loeffler's 518.3
  myalgia syndrome 710.5
  pulmonary (tropical) 518.3
  secondary 288.3
  tropical 518.3
Eosinophilic - see also condition
  fasciitis 728.89
  granuloma (bone) 277.89
  infiltration lung 518.3
Ependymitis (acute) (cerebral) (chronic)
    (granular) (see also Meningitis)
    322.9
Ependymoblastoma (M9392/3)
  specified site - see Neoplasm, by site,
    malignant
  unspecified site 191.9
Ependymoma (epithelial) (malignant)
    (M9391/3)
  anaplastic type (M9392/3)
    specified site - see Neoplasm, by site,
      malignant
    unspecified site 191.9

Ependymoma (Continued)
  benign (M9391/0)
    specified site - see Neoplasm, by site,
      benign
    unspecified site 225.0
  myxopapillary (M9394/1) 237.5
  papillary (M9393/1) 237.5
    specified site - see Neoplasm, by site,
      malignant
    unspecified site 191.9
Ependymopathy 349.2
  spinal cord 349.2
Ephelides, ephelis 709.09
Ephemeral fever (see also Pyrexia)
    780.60
Epiblepharon (congenital) 743.62
Epicanthus, epicanthic fold (congenital)
    (eyelid) 743.63
Epicondylitis (elbow) (lateral) 726.32
  medial 726.31
Epicystitis (see also Cystitis) 595.9
Epidemic - see condition
Epidermidalization, cervix - see condition
Epidermidization, cervix - see condition
Epidermis, epidermal - see condition
Epidermization, cervix - see condition
Epidermodysplasia verruciformis
    078.19
Epidermoid
  cholesteatoma - see Cholesteatoma
  inclusion (see also Cyst, skin) 706.2
Epidermolysis
  acuta (combustiformis) (toxica)
      695.15
  bullosa 757.39
  necroticans combustiformis 695.15
    due to drug
      correct substance properly
        administered 695.15
      overdose or wrong substance
        given or taken 977.9
      specified drug - see Table of
        Drugs and Chemicals
Epidermophytid - see Dermatophytosis
Epidermophytosis (infected) - see
    Dermatophytosis
Epidermosis, ear (middle) (see also
    Cholesteatoma) 385.30
Epididymis - see condition
Epididymitis (nonvenereal) 604.90
  with abscess 604.0
  acute 604.99
  blennorrhagic (acute) 098.0
    chronic or duration of 2 months or
      over 098.2
  caseous (see also Tuberculosis) 016.4●
  chlamydial 099.54
  diphtheritic 032.89 [604.91]
  filarial 125.9 [604.91]
  gonococcal (acute) 098.0
    chronic or duration of 2 months or
      over 098.2
  recurrent 604.99
  residual 604.99
  syphilitic 095.8 [604.91]
  tuberculous (see also Tuberculosis)
      016.4●
Epididymo-orchitis (see also Epididymitis)
    604.90
  with abscess 604.0
  chlamydial 099.54
  gonococcal (acute) 098.13
    chronic or duration of 2 months or
      over 098.33
Epidural - see condition
Epigastritis (see also Gastritis) 535.5●
Epigastrium, epigastric - see condition

Epigastrocele (see also Hernia, epigastric)
    553.29
Epiglottiditis (acute) 464.30
  with obstruction 464.31
  chronic 476.1
  viral 464.30
    with obstruction 464.31
Epiglottis - see condition
Epiglottitis (acute) 464.30
  with obstruction 464.31
  chronic 476.1
  viral 464.30
    with obstruction 464.31
Epignathus 759.4
Epilepsia
  partialis continua (see also Epilepsy)
      345.7●
  procursiva (see also Epilepsy)
      345.8●
Epilepsy, epileptic (idiopathic)
    345.9●

Note 26   use the following fifth-digit
subclassifications with categories 345.0,
345.1, 345.4–345.9

  0   without mention of intractable
        epilepsy
  1   with intractable epilepsy
        pharmacoresistant
          (pharmacologically
          resistant)   ◄
        poorly controlled   ◄
        refractory (medically)   ◄
        treatment resistant   ◄

  abdominal 345.5●
  absence (attack) 345.0●
  akinetic 345.0●
    psychomotor 345.4●
  automatism 345.4●
  autonomic diencephalic 345.5●
  brain 345.9●
  Bravais-Jacksonian 345.5●
  cerebral 345.9●
  climacteric 345.9●
  clonic 345.1●
  clouded state 345.9●
  coma 345.3●
  communicating 345.4●
  complicating pregnancy, childbirth, or
      the puerperium 649.4●
  congenital 345.9●
  convulsions 345.9●
  cortical (focal) (motor) 345.5●
  cursive (running) 345.8●
  cysticercosis 123.1
  deterioration
    with behavioral disturbance 345.9●
      [294.11]
    without behavioral disturbance
      345.9● [294.10]
  due to syphilis 094.89
  equivalent 345.5●
  fit 345.9●
  focal (motor) 345.5●
  gelastic 345.8●
  generalized 345.9●
    convulsive 345.1●
    flexion 345.1●
    nonconvulsive 345.0●
  grand mal (idiopathic) 345.1●
  Jacksonian (motor) (sensory)
      345.5●
  Kojevnikoff's, Kojevnikov's,
      Kojewnikoff's 345.7●
  laryngeal 786.2
  limbic system 345.4●

Epilepsy, epileptic *(Continued)*
  localization related (focal) (partial) and
      epileptic syndromes
    with
        complex partial seizures 345.4●
        simple partial seizures 345.5●
  major (motor) 345.1●
  minor 345.0●
  mixed (type) 345.9●
  motor partial 345.5●
  musicogenic 345.1●
  myoclonus, myoclonic 345.1●
    progressive (familial) 345.1 ◀▥
  nonconvulsive, generalized
      345.0●
  parasitic NEC 123.9
  partial (focalized) 345.5●
    with
        impairment of consciousness
            345.4●
        memory and ideational
            disturbances 345.4●
        without impairment of
            consciousness 345.5●
    abdominal type 345.5●
    motor type 345.5●
    psychomotor type 345.4●
    psychosensory type 345.4●
    secondarily generalized
        345.4●
    sensory type 345.5●
    somatomotor type 345.5●
    somatosensory type 345.5●
    temporal lobe type 345.4●
    visceral type 345.5●
    visual type 345.5●
  peripheral 345.9●
  petit mal 345.0●
  photokinetic 345.8●
  progressive myoclonic (familial)
      345.1 ◀▥
  psychic equivalent 345.5●
  psychomotor 345.4●
  psychosensory 345.4●
  reflex 345.1●
  seizure 345.9●
  senile 345.9●
  sensory-induced 345.5●
  sleep (see also Narcolepsy) 347.00
  somatomotor type 345.5●
  somatosensory 345.5●
  specified type NEC 345.8●
  status (grand mal) 345.3
    focal motor 345.7●
    petit mal 345.2●
    psychomotor 345.7●
    temporal lobe 345.7●
  symptomatic 345.9●
  temporal lobe 345.4●
  tonic (-clonic) 345.1●
  traumatic (injury unspecified)
      907.0
    injury specified - see Late, effect (of)
        specified injury
  twilight 293.0
  uncinate (gyrus) 345.4●
  Unverricht (-Lundborg) (familial
      myoclonic) 345.1 ◀▥
  visceral 345.5●
  visual 345.5●
Epileptiform
  convulsions 780.39
  seizure 780.39
Epiloia 759.5
Epimenorrhea 626.2
Epipharyngitis (see also Nasopharyngitis)
    460

Epiphora 375.20
  due to
      excess lacrimation 375.21
      insufficient drainage 375.22
Epiphyseal arrest 733.91
  femoral head 732.2
Epiphyseolysis, epiphysiolysis (see also
    Osteochondrosis) 732.9
Epiphysitis (see also Osteochondrosis)
    732.9
  juvenile 732.6
  marginal (Scheuermann's) 732.0
  os calcis 732.5
  syphilitic (congenital) 090.0
  vertebral (Scheuermann's) 732.0
Epiplocele (see also Hernia)553.9
Epiploitis (see also Peritonitis) 567.9
Epiplosarcomphalocele (see also Hernia,
    umbilicus) 553.1
Episcleritis 379.00
  gouty 274.89 [379.09]
  nodular 379.02
  periodica fugax 379.01
    angioneurotic - see Edema,
        angioneurotic
  specified NEC 379.09
  staphylococcal 379.00
  suppurative 379.00
  syphilitic 095.0
  tuberculous (see also Tuberculosis)
      017.3● [379.09]
Episode
  brain (see also Disease, cerebrovascular,
      acute) 436
  cerebral (see also Disease,
      cerebrovascular, acute) 436
  depersonalization (in neurotic
      state) 300.6
  hyporesponsive 780.09
  psychotic (see also Psychosis) 298.9
    organic, transient 293.9
  schizophrenic (acute) NEC (see also
      Schizophrenia) 295.4●
Epispadias
  female 753.8
  male 752.62
Episplenitis 289.59
Epistaxis (multiple) 784.7
  hereditary 448.0
  vicarious menstruation 625.8
Epithelioma (malignant) (M8011/3) - see
    also Neoplasm, by site, malignant
  adenoides cysticum (M8100/0) - see
      Neoplasm, skin, benign
  basal cell (M8090/3) - see Neoplasm,
      skin, malignant
  benign (M8011/0) - see Neoplasm, by
      site, benign
  Bowen's (M8081/2) - see Neoplasm,
      skin, in situ
  calcifying (benign) (Malherbe's)
      (M8110/0) - see Neoplasm, skin,
      benign
  external site - see Neoplasm, skin,
      malignant
  intraepidermal, Jadassohn (M8096/0) -
      see Neoplasm, skin, benign
  squamous cell (M8070/3) - see
      Neoplasm, by site, malignant
Epitheliopathy
  pigment, retina 363.15
  posterior multifocal placoid (acute)
      363.15
Epithelium, epithelial - see condition
Epituberculosis (allergic) (with
    atelectasis) (see also Tuberculosis)
    010.8●

Eponychia 757.5
Epstein's
  nephrosis or syndrome (see also
      Nephrosis) 581.9
  pearl (mouth) 528.4
Epstein-Barr infection (viral) 075
  chronic 780.79 [139.8]
Epulis (giant cell) (gingiva) 523.8
Equinia 024
Equinovarus (congenital) 754.51
  acquired 736.71
Equivalent ◀
  angina 413.9
  convulsive (abdominal) (see also
      Epilepsy) 345.5●
  epileptic (psychic) (see also Epilepsy)
      345.5●
Erb's
  disease 359.1
  palsy, paralysis (birth) (brachial)
      (newborn) 767.6
    spinal (spastic) syphilitic 094.89
  pseudohypertrophic muscular
      dystrophy 359.1
Erb (-Duchenne) paralysis (birth injury)
    (newborn) 767.6
Erb-Goldflam disease or syndrome
    358.00
Erdheim-Chester disease (ECD) 277.89 ◀
Erdheim's syndrome (acromegalic
    macrospondylitis) 253.0
Erection, painful (persistent) 607.3
Ergosterol deficiency (vitamin D) 268.9
  with
      osteomalacia 268.2
      rickets (see also Rickets) 268.0
Ergotism (ergotized grain) 988.2
  from ergot used as drug (migraine
      therapy)
    correct substance properly
        administered 349.82
    overdose or wrong substance given
        or taken 975.0
Erichsen's disease (railway spine) 300.16
Erlacher-Blount syndrome (tibia vara)
    732.4
Erosio interdigitalis blastomycetica 112.3
Erosion
  arteriosclerotic plaque - see
      Arteriosclerosis, by site
  artery NEC 447.2
    without rupture 447.8
  bone 733.99
  bronchus 519.19
  cartilage (joint) 733.99
  cervix (uteri) (acquired) (chronic)
      (congenital) 622.0
    with mention of cervicitis 616.0
  cornea (recurrent) (see also Keratitis)
      371.42
    traumatic 918.1
  dental (idiopathic) (occupational)
      521.30
    extending into
        dentine 521.32
        pulp 521.33
    generalized 521.35
    limited to enamel 521.31
    localized 521.34
  duodenum, postpyloric - see Ulcer,
      duodenum
  esophagus 530.89
  gastric 535.4●
  intestine 569.89
  lymphatic vessel 457.8
  pylorus, pyloric (ulcer) 535.4●
  sclera 379.16

◀ New   ◀▥ Revised   ~~deleted~~ Deleted   ● Use Additional Digit(s)   ▨ Omit code

Erosion (*Continued*)
  spine, aneurysmal 094.89
  spleen 289.59 ●
  stomach 535.4 ●
  teeth (idiopathic) (occupational) (*see also* Erosion, dental) 521.30
    due to
      medicine 521.30
      persistent vomiting 521.30
  urethra 599.84
  uterus 621.8
  vertebra 733.99
Erotomania 302.89
  Clerambault's 297.8
Error
  in diet 269.9
  refractive 367.9
    astigmatism (*see also* Astigmatism) 367.20
    drug-induced 367.89
    hypermetropia 367.0
    hyperopia 367.0
    myopia 367.1
    presbyopia 367.4
    toxic 367.89
Eructation 787.3
  nervous 306.4
  psychogenic 306.4
Eruption
  creeping 126.9
  drug - *see* Dermatitis, due to, drug
  Hutchinson, summer 692.72
  Kaposi's varicelliform 054.0
  napkin (psoriasiform) 691.0
  polymorphous
    light (sun) 692.72
      other source 692.82
  psoriasiform, napkin 691.0
  recalcitrant pustular 694.8
  ringed 695.89
  skin (*see also* Dermatitis) 782.1
    creeping (meaning hookworm) 126.9
    due to
      chemical(s) NEC 692.4
        internal use 693.8
      drug - *see* Dermatitis, due to, drug
      prophylactic inoculation or vaccination against
        disease - *see* Dermatitis, due to, vaccine
      smallpox vaccination NEC - *see* Dermatitis, due to, vaccine
    erysipeloid 027.1
    feigned 698.4
    Hutchinson, summer 692.72
    Kaposi's, varicelliform 054.0
      vaccinia 999.0
    lichenoid, axilla 698.3
    polymorphous, due to light 692.72
    toxic NEC 695.0
    vesicular 709.8
  teeth, tooth
    accelerated 520.6
    delayed 520.6
    difficult 520.6
    disturbance of 520.6
    in abnormal sequence 520.6
    incomplete 520.6
    late 520.6
    natal 520.6
    neonatal 520.6
    obstructed 520.6
    partial 520.6
    persistent primary 520.6
    premature 520.6
    prenatal 520.6
  vesicular 709.8

Erysipelas (gangrenous) (infantile) (newborn) (phlegmonous) (suppurative) 035
  external ear 035 [*380.13*]
  puerperal, postpartum, childbirth 670.8 ◀‖‖
Erysipelatoid (Rosenbach's) 027.1
Erysipeloid (Rosenbach's) 027.1
Erythema, erythematous (generalized) 695.9
  ab igne - *see* Burn, by site, first degree
  annulare (centrifugum) (rheumaticum) 695.0
  arthriticum epidemicum 026.1
  brucellum (*see also* Brucellosis) 023.9
  bullosum 695.19
  caloricum - *see* Burn, by site, first degree
  chronicum migrans 088.81
  circinatum 695.19
  diaper 691.0
  due to
    chemical (contact) NEC 692.4
      internal 693.8
    drug (internal use) 693.0
      contact 692.3
  elevatum diutinum 695.89
  endemic 265.2
  epidemic, arthritic 026.1
  figuratum perstans 695.0
  gluteal 691.0
  gyratum (perstans) (repens) 695.19
  heat - *see* Burn, by site, first degree
  ichthyosiforme congenitum 757.1
  induratum (primary) (scrofulosorum) (*see also* Tuberculosis) 017.1 ●
    nontuberculous 695.2
  infantum febrile 057.8
  infectional NEC 695.9
  infectiosum 057.0
  inflammation NEC 695.9
  intertrigo 695.89
  iris 695.10
  lupus (discoid) (localized) (*see also* Lupus, erythematosus) 695.4
  marginatum 695.0
    rheumaticum - *see* Fever, rheumatic
  medicamentosum - *see* Dermatitis, due to, drug
  migrans 529.1
    chronicum 088.81
  multiforme 695.10
    bullosum 695.19
    conjunctiva 695.19
    exudativum (Hebra) 695.19
    major 695.12
    minor 695.11
    pemphigoides 694.5
  napkin 691.0
  neonatorum 778.8
  nodosum 695.2
    tuberculous (*see also* Tuberculosis) 017.1 ●
  nummular, nummulare 695.19
  palmar 695.0
  palmaris hereditarium 695.0
  pernio 991.5
  perstans solare 692.72
  rash, newborn 778.8
  scarlatiniform (exfoliative) (recurrent) 695.0
  simplex marginatum 057.8
  solare (*see also* Sunburn) 692.71
  streptogenes 696.5
  toxic, toxicum NEC 695.0
    newborn 778.8

Erythema, erythematous (*Continued*)
  tuberculous (primary) (*see also* Tuberculosis) 017.0 ●
  venenatum 695.0
Erythematosus - *see* condition
Erythematosus - *see* condition
Erythermalgia (primary) 443.82
Erythralgia 443.82
Erythrasma 039.0
Erythredema 985.0
  polyneuritica 985.0
  polyneuropathy 985.0
Erythremia (acute) (M9841/3) 207.0 ●
  chronic (M9842/3) 207.1 ●
  secondary 289.0
Erythroblastopenia (acquired) 284.89
  congenital 284.01
Erythroblastophthisis 284.01
Erythroblastosis (fetalis) (newborn) 773.2
  due to
    ABO
      antibodies 773.1
      incompatibility, maternal/fetal 773.1
      isoimmunization 773.1
    Rh
      antibodies 773.0
      incompatibility, maternal/fetal 773.0
      isoimmunization 773.0
Erythrocyanosis (crurum) 443.89
Erythrocythemia - *see* Erythremia
Erythrocytopenia 285.9
Erythrocytosis (megalosplenic)
  familial 289.6
  oval, hereditary (*see also* Elliptocytosis) 282.1
  secondary 289.0
  stress 289.0
Erythroderma (*see also* Erythema) 695.9
  desquamativa (in infants) 695.89
  exfoliative 695.89
  ichthyosiform, congenital 757.1
  infantum 695.89
  maculopapular 696.2
  neonatorum 778.8
  psoriaticum 696.1
  secondary 695.9
Erythrodysesthesia, palmar plantar (PPE) 693.0
Erythrogenesis imperfecta 284.09
Erythroleukemia (M9840/3) 207.0 ●
Erythromelalgia 443.82
Erythromelia 701.8
Erythropenia 285.9
Erythrophagocytosis 289.9
Erythrophobia 300.23
Erythroplakia
  oral mucosa 528.79
  tongue 528.79
Erythroplasia (Queyrat) (M8080/2)
  specified site - *see* Neoplasm, skin, in situ
  unspecified site 233.5
Erythropoiesis, idiopathic ineffective 285.0
Escaped beats, heart 427.60
  postoperative 997.1
Esoenteritis - *see* Enteritis
Esophagalgia 530.89
Esophagectasis 530.89
  due to cardiospasm 530.0
Esophagismus 530.5
Esophagitis (alkaline) (chemical) (chronic) (infectional) (necrotic) (peptic) (postoperative) (regurgitant) 530.10

Esophagitis (Continued)
  acute 530.12
  candidal 112.84
  eosinophilic 530.13
  reflux 530.11
  specified NEC 530.19
  tuberculous (see also Tuberculosis)
    017.8●
  ulcerative 530.19
Esophagocele 530.6
Esophagodynia 530.89
Esophagomalacia 530.89
Esophagoptosis 530.89
Esophagospasm 530.5
Esophagostenosis 530.3
Esophagostomiasis 127.7
Esophagostomy
  complication 530.87
    infection 530.86
    malfunctioning 530.87
    mechanical 530.87
Esophagotracheal - see condition
Esophagus - see condition
Esophoria 378.41
  convergence, excess 378.84
  divergence, insufficiency 378.85
Esotropia (nonaccommodative) 378.00
  accommodative 378.35
  alternating 378.05
    with
      A pattern 378.06
      specified noncomitancy NEC
        378.08
      V pattern 378.07
      X pattern 378.08
      Y pattern 378.08
    intermittent 378.22
  intermittent 378.20
    alternating 378.22
    monocular 378.21
  monocular 378.01
    with
      A pattern 378.02
      specified noncomitancy NEC
        378.04
      V pattern 378.03
      X pattern 378.04
      Y pattern 378.04
    intermittent 378.21
Espundia 085.5
Essential - see condition
Esterapenia 289.89
Esthesioneuroblastoma (M9522/3) 160.0
Esthesioneurocytoma (M9521/3) 160.0
Esthesioneuroepithelioma (M9523/3)
  160.0
Esthiomene 099.1
Estivo-autumnal
  fever 084.0
  malaria 084.0
Estrangement V61.09
Estriasis 134.0
Ethanolaminuria 270.8
Ethanolism (see also Alcoholism) 303.9●
Ether dependence, dependency (see also
  Dependence) 304.6●
Etherism (see also Dependence) 304.6●
Ethmoid, ethmoidal - see condition
Ethmoiditis (chronic) (nonpurulent)
  (purulent) (see also Sinusitis,
  ethmoidal) 473.2
  influenzal 487.1
  Woakes' 471.1
Ethylism (see also Alcoholism) 303.9●

Eulenburg's disease (congenital
  paramyotonia) 359.29
Eunuchism 257.2
Eunuchoidism 257.2
  hypogonadotropic 257.2
European blastomycosis 117.5
Eustachian - see condition
Euthyroid sick syndrome 790.94
Euthyroidism 244.9
Evaluation
  fetal lung maturity 659.8●
  for suspected condition (see also
    Observation) V71.9
    abuse V71.81
    exposure
      anthrax V71.82
      biologic agent NEC V71.83
      SARS V71.83
    neglect V71.81
    newborn - see Observation,
      suspected, condition, newborn
    specified condition NEC V71.89
  mental health V70.2
    requested by authority V70.1
  nursing care V63.8
  social service V63.8
Evans' syndrome (thrombocytopenic
  purpura) 287.32
Event, apparent life threatening in
  newborn and infant (ALTE) 799.82 ◀
Eventration
  colon into chest - see Hernia,
    diaphragm
  diaphragm (congenital) 756.6
Eversion
  bladder 596.8
  cervix (uteri) 622.0
    with mention of cervicitis 616.0
  foot NEC 736.79
    congenital 755.67
  lacrimal punctum 375.51
  punctum lacrimale (postinfectional)
    (senile) 375.51
  ureter (meatus) 593.89
  urethra (meatus) 599.84
  uterus 618.1
    complicating delivery 665.2●
      affecting fetus or newborn 763.89
    puerperal, postpartum 674.8●
Evidence
  of malignancy
    cytologic
      without histologic confirmation
        anus 796.76
        cervix 795.06
        vagina 795.16
Evisceration
  birth injury 767.8
  bowel (congenital) - see Hernia, ventral
  congenital (see also Hernia, ventral)
    553.29
  operative wound 998.32
  traumatic NEC 869.1
    eye 871.3
Evulsion - see Avulsion
Ewing's
  angioendothelioma (M9260/3) - see
    Neoplasm, bone, malignant
  sarcoma (M9260/3) - see Neoplasm,
    bone, malignant
  tumor (M9260/3) - see Neoplasm, bone,
    malignant
Exaggerated lumbosacral angle (with
  impinging spine) 756.12

Examination (general) (routine) (of) (for)
  V70.9
  allergy V72.7
  annual V70.0
  cardiovascular preoperative V72.81
  cervical Papanicolaou smear V76.2
    as a part of routine gynecological
      examination V72.31
    to confirm findings of recent normal
      smear following initial
      abnormal smear V72.32
  child care (routine) V20.2
  clinical research investigation (normal
    control patient) (participant)
    V70.7
  dental V72.2
  developmental testing (child) (infant)
    V20.2
  donor (potential) V70.8
  ear V72.19
  eye V72.0
  following
    accident (motor vehicle) V71.4
    alleged rape or seduction (victim or
      culprit) V71.5
    inflicted injury (victim or culprit)
      NEC V71.6
    rape or seduction, alleged (victim or
      culprit) V71.5
    treatment (for) V67.9
      combined V67.6
      fracture V67.4
      involving high-risk medication
        NEC V67.51
      mental disorder V67.3
      specified condition NEC V67.59
  follow-up (routine) (following) V67.9
    cancer chemotherapy V67.2
    chemotherapy V67.2
    disease NEC V67.59
    high-risk medication NEC V67.51
    injury NEC V67.59
    population survey V70.6
    postpartum V24.2
    psychiatric V67.3
    psychotherapy V67.3
    radiotherapy V67.1
    specified surgery NEC V67.09
    surgery V67.00
      vaginal pap smear V67.01
  gynecological V72.31
    for contraceptive maintenance V25.40
      intrauterine device V25.42
      pill V25.41
      specified method NEC V25.49
  health (of)
    armed forces personnel V70.5
    checkup V70.0
    child, routine V20.2
    defined subpopulation NEC V70.5
    inhabitants of institutions V70.5
    occupational V70.5
    pre-employment screening V70.5
    preschool children V70.5
      for admission to school V70.3
    prisoners V70.5
      for entrance into prison V70.3
    prostitutes V70.5
    refugees V70.5
    school children V70.5
    students V70.5
  hearing V72.19
    following failed hearing screening
      V72.11

◀ New   ◀▥ Revised   ~~deleted~~ Deleted   ● Use Additional Digit(s)   ▦ Omit code

Examination (*Continued*)
  infant ~~V20.2~~ ◀▥
    8 to 28 days old V20.32 ◀
    over 28 days old, routine V20.2 ◀
    under 8 days old V20.31 ◀
  laboratory V72.60 ◀▥
    ordered as part of a routine general
      medical examination V72.62 ◀
    pre-operative V72.63 ◀
    pre-procedural V72.63 ◀
    specified NEC V72.69 ◀
  lactating mother V24.1
  medical (for) (of) V70.9
    administrative purpose NEC
      V70.3
    admission to
      old age home V70.3
      prison V70.3
      school V70.3
    adoption V70.3
    armed forces personnel V70.5
    at health care facility V70.0
    camp V70.3
    child, routine V20.2
    clinical research (control) (normal
      comparison) (participant)
      V70.7
    defined subpopulation NEC V70.5
    donor (potential) V70.8
    driving license V70.3
    general V70.9
      routine V70.0
      specified reason NEC V70.8
    immigration V70.3
    inhabitants of institutions V70.5
    insurance certification V70.3
    marriage V70.3
    medicolegal reasons V70.4
    naturalization V70.3
    occupational V70.5
    population survey V70.6
    pre-employment V70.5
    preschool children V70.5
      for admission to school V70.3
    prison V70.3
    prisoners V70.5
      for entrance into prison V70.3
    prostitutes V70.5
    refugees V70.5
    school children V70.5
    specified reason NEC V70.8
    sport competition V70.3
    students V70.5
  medicolegal reason V70.4
  pelvic (annual) (periodic) V72.31
  periodic (annual) (routine) V70.0
  postpartum
    immediately after delivery V24.0
    routine follow-up V24.2
  pregnancy (unconfirmed) (possible)
    V72.40
    negative result V72.41
    positive result V72.42
  prenatal V22.1
    first pregnancy V22.0
    high-risk pregnancy V23.9
      specified problem NEC V23.89
  preoperative V72.84
    cardiovascular V72.81
    respiratory V72.82
    specified NEC V72.83
  preprocedural V72.84
    cardiovascular V72.81
    general physical V72.83
    respiratory V72.82
    specified NEC V72.83

Examination (*Continued*)
  prior to chemotherapy V72.83 ◀
  psychiatric V70.2
    follow-up not needing further care
      V67.3
    requested by authority V70.1
  radiological NEC V72.5
  respiratory preoperative V72.82
  screening - *see* Screening
  sensitization V72.7
  skin V72.7
    hypersensitivity V72.7
  special V72.9
  specified type or reason NEC V72.85
    preoperative V72.83
      specified NEC V72.83
  teeth V72.2
  vaginal Papanicolaou smear V76.47
    following hysterectomy for
      malignant condition V67.01
  victim or culprit following
    alleged rape or seduction V71.5
    inflicted injury NEC V71.6
  vision V72.0
  well baby V20.2
Exanthem, exanthema (*see also* Rash) 782.1
  Boston 048
  epidemic, with meningitis 048
  lichenoid psoriasiform 696.2
  subitum 058.10
    due to
      human herpesvirus 6 058.11
      human herpesvirus 7 058.12
  viral, virus NEC 057.9
    specified type NEC 057.8
Excess, excessive, excessively
  alcohol level in blood 790.3
  carbohydrate tissue, localized 278.1
  carotene (dietary) 278.3
  cold 991.9
    specified effect NEC 991.8
  convergence 378.84
  crying 780.95
    of
      adolescent 780.95
      adult 780.95
      baby 780.92
      child 780.95
      infant (baby) 780.92
      newborn 780.92
  development, breast 611.1
  diaphoresis (*see also* Hyperhidrosis)
    780.8
  distance, interarch 524.28
  divergence 378.85
  drinking (alcohol) NEC (*see also*
    Abuse, drugs, nondependent)
    305.0●
    continual (*see also* Alcoholism)
      303.9●
    habitual (*see also* Alcoholism) 303.9●
  eating 783.6
  eyelid fold (congenital) 743.62
  fat 278.02
    in heart (*see also* Degeneration,
      myocardial) 429.1
    tissue, localized 278.1
  foreskin 605
  gas 787.3
  gastrin 251.5
  glucagon 251.4
  heat (*see also* Heat) 992.9
  horizontal
    overjet 524.26
    overlap 524.26
  interarch distance 524.28

Excess, excessive, excessively (*Continued*)
  intermaxillary vertical dimension
    524.37
  interocclusal distance of teeth 524.37
  large
    colon 564.7
      congenital 751.3
    fetus or infant 766.0
      with obstructed labor 660.1●
      affecting management of
        pregnancy 656.6●
      causing disproportion 653.5●
    newborn (weight of 4500 grams or
      more) 766.0
    organ or site, congenital NEC - *see*
      Anomaly, specified type NEC
  lid fold (congenital) 743.62
  long
    colon 751.5
    organ or site, congenital NEC - *see*
      Anomaly, specified type NEC
    umbilical cord (entangled)
      affecting fetus or newborn 762.5
      in pregnancy or childbirth 663.3●
        with compression 663.2●
  menstruation 626.2
  number of teeth 520.1
    causing crowding 524.31
  nutrients (dietary) NEC 783.6
  potassium (K) 276.7
  salivation (*see also* Ptyalism) 527.7
  secretion - *see also* Hypersecretion
    milk 676.6●
    sputum 786.4
    sweat (*see also* Hyperhidrosis)
      780.8
  short
    organ or site, congenital NEC - *see*
      Anomaly, specified type NEC
    umbilical cord
      affecting fetus or newborn 762.6
      in pregnancy or childbirth
        663.4●
  skin NEC 701.9
    eyelid 743.62
      acquired 374.30
  sodium (Na) 276.0
  spacing of teeth 524.32
  sputum 786.4
  sweating (*see also* Hyperhidrosis)
    780.8
  tearing (ducts) (eye) (*see also* Epiphora)
    375.20
  thirst 783.5
    due to deprivation of water 994.3
  tissue in reconstructed breast 612.0
  tuberosity 524.07
  vitamin
    A (dietary) 278.2
      administered as drug (chronic)
        (prolonged excessive
        intake) 278.2
      reaction to sudden overdose
        963.5
    D (dietary) 278.4
      administered as drug (chronic)
        (prolonged excessive
        intake) 278.4
      reaction to sudden overdose
        963.5
  weight 278.02
    gain 783.1
      of pregnancy 646.1●
    loss 783.21
Excitability, abnormal, under minor
  stress 309.29

Excitation
catatonic (*see also* Schizophrenia)
295.2●
psychogenic 298.1
reactive (from emotional stress,
psychological trauma) 298.1
Excitement
manic (*see also* Psychosis, affective)
296.0●
recurrent episode 296.1●
single episode 296.0●
mental, reactive (from emotional stress,
psychological trauma) 298.1
state, reactive (from emotional stress,
psychological trauma) 298.1
Excluded pupils 364.76
Excoriation (traumatic) (*see also* Injury,
superficial, by site) 919.8
neurotic 698.4
Excyclophoria 378.44
Excyclotropia 378.33
Exencephalus, exencephaly 742.0
Exercise
breathing V57.0
remedial NEC V57.1
therapeutic NEC V57.1
Exfoliation
skin
due to erythematous condition
695.50
involving (percent of body
surface)
less than 10 percent 695.50
10-19 percent 695.51
20-29 percent 695.52
30-39 percent 695.53
40-49 percent 695.54
50-59 percent 695.55
60-69 percent 695.56
70-79 percent 695.57
80-89 percent 695.58
90 percent or more 695.59
teeth
due to systemic causes 525.0
Exfoliative - *see also* condition
dermatitis 695.89
Exhaustion, exhaustive (physical NEC)
780.79
battle (*see also* Reaction, stress, acute)
308.9
cardiac (*see also* Failure, heart) 428.9
delirium (*see also* Reaction, stress,
acute) 308.9
due to
cold 991.8
excessive exertion 994.5
exposure 994.4
overexertion 994.5
fetus or newborn 779.89
heart (*see also* Failure, heart) 428.9
heat 992.5
due to
salt depletion 992.4
water depletion 992.3
manic (*see also* Psychosis, affective)
296.0●
recurrent episode 296.1●
single episode 296.0●
maternal, complicating delivery 669.8●
affecting fetus or newborn 763.89
mental 300.5
myocardium, myocardial (*see also*
Failure, heart) 428.9
nervous 300.5

Exhaustion, exhaustive (*Continued*)
old age 797
postinfectional NEC 780.79
psychogenic 300.5
psychosis (*see also* Reaction, stress,
acute) 308.9
senile 797
dementia 290.0
Exhibitionism (sexual) 302.4
Exomphalos 756.72
Exophoria 378.42
convergence, insufficiency 378.83
divergence, excess 378.85
Exophthalmic
cachexia 242.0●
goiter 242.0●
ophthalmoplegia 242.0● [376.22]
Exophthalmos 376.30
congenital 743.66
constant 376.31
endocrine NEC 259.9 [376.22]
hyperthyroidism 242.0● [376.21]
intermittent NEC 376.34
malignant 242.0● [376.21]
pulsating 376.35
endocrine NEC 259.9 [376.22]
thyrotoxic 242.0● [376.21]
Exostosis 726.91
cartilaginous (M9210/0) - *see*
Neoplasm, bone, benign
congenital 756.4
ear canal, external 380.81
gonococcal 098.89
hip 726.5
intracranial 733.3
jaw (bone) 526.81
luxurians 728.11
multiple (cancellous) (congenital)
(hereditary) 756.4
nasal bones 726.91
orbit, orbital 376.42
osteocartilaginous (M9210/0) - *see*
Neoplasm, bone, benign
spine 721.8
with spondylosis - *see*
Spondylosis
syphilitic 095.5
wrist 726.4
Exotropia 378.10
alternating 378.15
with
A pattern 378.16
specified noncomitancy NEC
378.18
V pattern 378.17
X pattern 378.18
Y pattern 378.18
intermittent 378.24
intermittent 378.20
alternating 378.24
monocular 378.23
monocular 378.11
with
A pattern 378.12
specified noncomitancy NEC
378.14
V pattern 378.13
X pattern 378.14
Y pattern 378.14
intermittent 378.23
Explanation of
investigation finding V65.4
medication V65.4

Exposure (suspected) 994.9
algae bloom V87.32
cold 991.9
specified effect NEC 991.8
effects of 994.9
exhaustion due to 994.4
to
AIDS virus V01.79
anthrax V01.81
aromatic
amines V87.11
dyes V87.19
arsenic V87.01
asbestos V15.84
benzene V87.12
body fluids (hazardous) V15.85
cholera V01.0
chromium compounds V87.09
communicable disease V01.9
specified type NEC V01.89
dyes V87.2
aromatic V87.19
Escherichia coli (E. coli) V01.83
German measles V01.4
gonorrhea V01.6
hazardous
aromatic compounds NEC
V87.19
body fluids V15.85
chemicals NEC V87.2
metals V87.09
substances V87.39
HIV V01.79
human immunodeficiency virus
V01.79
lead V15.86
meningococcus V01.84
mold V87.31
nickel dust V87.09
parasitic disease V01.89
poliomyelitis V01.2
polycyclic aromatic hydrocarbons
V87.19
potentially hazardous body fluids
V15.85
rabies V01.5
rubella V01.4
SARS-associated coronavirus V01.82
smallpox V01.3
syphilis V01.6
tuberculosis V01.1
varicella V01.71
venereal disease V01.6
viral disease NEC V01.79
varicella V01.71
Exsanguination, fetal 772.0
Exstrophy
abdominal content 751.8
bladder (urinary) 753.5
Extensive - *see* condition
Extra - *see also* Accessory
rib 756.3
cervical 756.2
Extraction
with hook 763.89
breech NEC 669.6●
affecting fetus or newborn 763.0
cataract postsurgical V45.61
manual NEC 669.8●
affecting fetus or newborn 763.89
Extrasystole 427.60
atrial 427.61
postoperative 997.1
ventricular 427.69

◄ New ◄▯ Revised ~~deleted~~ Deleted ● Use Additional Digit(s) ▮ Omit code

Extrauterine gestation or pregnancy - *see*
    Pregnancy, ectopic
Extravasation
  blood 459.0
    lower extremity 459.0
  chemotherapy, vesicant 999.81
  chyle into mesentery 457.8
  pelvicalyceal 593.4
  pyelosinus 593.4
  urine 788.8
    from ureter 788.8
  vesicant
    agent NEC 999.82
    chemotherapy 999.81
Extremity - *see* condition

Extrophy - *see* Exstrophy
Extroversion
  bladder 753.5
  uterus 618.1
    complicating delivery 665.2●
      affecting fetus or newborn
        763.89
    postpartal (old) 618.1
Extruded tooth 524.34
Extrusion
  alveolus and teeth 524.75
  breast implant (prosthetic) 996.54
  device, implant, or graft - *see*
    Complications, mechanical
  eye implant (ball) (globe) 996.59

Extrusion (*Continued*)
  intervertebral disc - *see* Displacement,
    intervertebral disc
  lacrimal gland 375.43
  mesh (reinforcing) 996.59
  ocular lens implant 996.53
  prosthetic device NEC - *see*
    Complications, mechanical
  vitreous 379.26
Exudate, pleura - *see* Effusion, pleura
Exudates, retina 362.82
Exudative - *see* condition
Eye, eyeball, eyelid - *see* condition
Eyestrain 368.13
Eyeworm disease of Africa 125.2

F

Faber's anemia or syndrome
(achlorhydric anemia) 280.9
Fabry's disease (angiokeratoma corporis
diffusum) 272.7
Face, facial - *see* condition
Facet of cornea 371.44
Faciocephalalgia, autonomic (*see also*
Neuropathy, peripheral, autonomic)
337.9
Facioscapulohumeral myopathy 359.1
Factitious disorder, illness - *see* Illness,
factitious
Factor
deficiency - *see* Deficiency, factor
psychic, associated with diseases
classified elsewhere 316
risk-see problem
Fahr-Volhard disease (malignant
nephrosclerosis) 403.00
Failure, failed
adenohypophyseal 253.2
attempted abortion (legal) (*see also*
Abortion, failed) 638.9
bone marrow (anemia) 284.9
acquired (secondary) 284.89
congenital 284.09
idiopathic 284.9
cardiac (*see also* Failure, heart) 428.9
newborn 779.89
cardiorenal (chronic) 428.9
hypertensive (*see also* Hypertension,
cardiorenal) 404.93
cardiorespiratory 799.1
specified during or due to a
procedure 997.1
long-term effect of cardiac
surgery 429.4
cardiovascular (chronic) 428.9
cerebrovascular 437.8
cervical dilatation in labor 661.0●
affecting fetus or newborn 763.7
circulation, circulatory 799.89
fetus or newborn 779.89
peripheral 785.50
compensation - *see* Disease, heart
congestive (*see also* Failure, heart) 428.0
conscious sedation, during
procedure 995.24
coronary (*see also* Insufficiency,
coronary) 411.89
dental implant 525.79
due to
infection 525.71
lack of attached gingiva
525.72
occlusal trauma (caused by poor
prosthetic design) 525.72
parafunctional habits 525.72
periodontal infection
(periimplantitis) 525.72
poor oral hygiene 525.72
unintentional loading 525.71
endosseous NEC 525.79
mechanical 525.73
osseointegration 525.71
due to
complications of systemic
disease 525.71
poor bone quality 525.71
premature loading 525.71
following intentional prosthetic
loading 525.72
iatrogenic 525.71
prior to intentional prosthetic
loading 525.71

Failure, failed (*Continued*)
dental implant (*Continued*)
post-osseointegration
biological 525.72
iatrogenic 525.72
due to complications of systemic
disease 525.72
mechanical 525.73
pre-integration 525.71
pre-osseointegration 525.71
dental prosthesis causing loss of dental
implant 525.73
dental restoration
marginal integrity 525.61
periodontal anatomical integrity
525.65
descent of head (at term) 652.5●
affecting fetus or newborn 763.1
in labor 660.0●
affecting fetus or newborn
763.1
device, implant, or graft - *see*
Complications, mechanical
engagement of head NEC 652.5●
in labor 660.0●
extrarenal 788.99
fetal head to enter pelvic brim
652.5●
affecting fetus or newborn 763.1
in labor 660.0●
affecting fetus or newborn 763.1
forceps NEC 660.7●
affecting fetus or newborn 763.1
fusion (joint) (spinal) 996.49
growth in childhood 783.43
heart (acute) (sudden) 428.9
with
abortion - *see* Abortion, by type,
with specified complication
NEC
acute pulmonary edema (*see also*
Failure, ventricular, left)
428.1
with congestion (*see also*
Failure, heart) 428.0
decompensation (*see also* Failure,
heart) 428.0
dilation - *see* Disease, heart
ectopic pregnancy (*see also*
categories 633.0–633.9)
639.8
molar pregnancy (*see also*
categories 630–632) 639.8
arteriosclerotic 440.9
combined left-right sided 428.0
combined systolic and diastolic
428.40
acute 428.41
acute on chronic 428.43
chronic 428.42
compensated (*see also* Failure, heart)
428.0
complicating
abortion - *see* Abortion, by type,
with specified complication
NEC
delivery (cesarean) (instrumental)
669.4●
ectopic pregnancy (*see also*
categories 633.0–633.9) 639.8
molar pregnancy (*see also*
categories 630–632) 639.8
obstetric anesthesia or sedation
668.1●
surgery 997.1

Failure, failed (*Continued*)
heart (*Continued*)
congestive (compensated)
(decompensated) (*see also*
Failure, heart) 428.0
with rheumatic fever (conditions
classifiable to 390)
active 391.8
inactive or quiescent (with
chorea) 398.91
fetus or newborn 779.89
hypertensive (*see also*
Hypertension, heart)
402.91
with renal disease (*see also*
Hypertension,
cardiorenal) 404.91
with renal failure 404.93
benign 402.11
malignant 402.01
rheumatic (chronic) (inactive)
(with chorea) 398.91
active or acute 391.8
with chorea (Sydenham's)
392.0
decompensated (*see also* Failure,
heart) 428.0
degenerative (*see also* Degeneration,
myocardial) 429.1
diastolic 428.30
acute 428.31
acute on chronic 428.33
chronic 428.32
due to presence of (cardiac)
prosthesis 429.4
fetus or newborn 779.89
following
abortion 639.8
cardiac surgery 429.4
ectopic or molar pregnancy
639.8
high output NEC 428.9
hypertensive (*see also* Hypertension,
heart) 402.91
with renal disease (*see also*
Hypertension, cardiorenal)
404.91
with renal failure 404.93
benign 402.11
malignant 402.01
left (ventricular) (*see also* Failure,
ventricular, left) 428.1
with right-sided failure (*see also*
Failure, heart) 428.0
low output (syndrome) NEC
428.9
organic - *see* Disease, heart
postoperative (immediate) 997.1
long term effect of cardiac
surgery 429.4
rheumatic (chronic) (congestive)
(inactive) 398.91
right (secondary to left heart failure,
conditions classifiable to 428.1)
(ventricular) (*see also* Failure,
heart) 428.0
senile 797
specified during or due to a
procedure 997.1
long-term effect of cardiac
surgery 429.4
systolic 428.20
acute 428.21
acute on chronic 428.23
chronic 428.22

◀ New   ◀▥ Revised   ~~deleted~~ Deleted   ● Use Additional Digit(s)   ▨ Omit code

Failure, failed (Continued)
  heart (Continued)
    thyrotoxic (see also Thyrotoxicosis)
      242.9● [425.7]
    valvular - see Endocarditis
  hepatic 572.8
    acute 570
    due to a procedure 997.4
  hepatorenal 572.4
  hypertensive heart (see also
      Hypertension, heart) 402.91
    benign 402.11
    malignant 402.01
  induction (of labor) 659.1●
    abortion (legal) (see also Abortion,
        failed) 638.9
    affecting fetus or newborn 763.89
    by oxytocic drugs 659.1●
    instrumental 659.0●
    mechanical 659.0●
    medical 659.1●
    surgical 659.0●
  initial alveolar expansion, newborn
      770.4
  involution, thymus (gland) 254.8
  kidney - see Failure, renal
  lactation 676.4●
  Leydig's cell, adult 257.2
  liver 572.8
    acute 570
  medullary 799.89
  mitral - see Endocarditis, mitral
  moderate sedation, during
      procedure 995.24
  myocardium, myocardial (see also
      Failure, heart) 428.9
    chronic (see also Failure, heart)
        428.0
    congestive (see also Failure, heart)
        428.0
  ovarian (primary) 256.39
    iatrogenic 256.2
    postablative 256.2
    postirradiation 256.2
    postsurgical 256.2
  ovulation 628.0
  prerenal 788.99
  renal (kidney) 586   ◄▐▐▐
    with
      abortion - see Abortion, by type,
          with renal failure
      ectopic pregnancy (see also
          categories 633.0–633.9) 639.3
      edema (see also Nephrosis) 581.9
      hypertension (see also
          Hypertension, kidney)
          403.91
      hypertensive heart disease
          (conditions classifiable to
          402) 404.92
        with heart failure 404.93
        benign 404.12
          with heart failure 404.13
        malignant 404.02
          with heart failure 404.03
      molar pregnancy (see also
          categories 630–632) 639.3
    tubular necrosis (acute) 584.5
    acute 584.9
      with lesion of
        necrosis
          cortical (renal) 584.6
          medullary (renal)
              (papillary) 584.7
          tubular 584.5
        specified pathology NEC
            584.8

Failure, failed (Continued)
  renal (Continued)
    chronic 585.9
      hypertensive or with
          hypertension (see also
          Hypertension, kidney)
          403.91
      due to a procedure 997.5
    following
      abortion 639.3
      crushing 958.5
      ectopic or molar pregnancy
          639.3
      labor and delivery (acute)
          669.3●
    hypertensive (see also Hypertension,
        kidney) 403.91
    puerperal, postpartum 669.3●
  respiration, respiratory 518.81
    acute 518.81
    acute and chronic 518.84
    center 348.89   ◄▐▐▐
      newborn 770.84
    chronic 518.83
    due to trauma, surgery or shock
        518.5
    newborn 770.84
  rotation
    cecum 751.4
    colon 751.4
    intestine 751.4
    kidney 753.3
  sedation, during procedure   ◄
    conscious 995.24   ◄
    moderate 995.24   ◄
  segmentation - see also Fusion
    fingers (see also Syndactylism,
        fingers) 755.11
    toes (see also Syndactylism, toes)
        755.13
  seminiferous tubule, adult 257.2
  senile (general) 797
    with psychosis 290.20
  testis, primary (seminal) 257.2
  to progress 661.2●
  to thrive
    adult 783.7
    child 783.41
    newborn 779.34   ◄
  transplant 996.80
    bone marrow 996.85
    organ (immune or nonimmune
        cause) 996.80
      bone marrow 996.85
      heart 996.83
      intestines 996.87
      kidney 996.81
      liver 996.82
      lung 996.84
      pancreas 996.86
      specified NEC 996.89
    skin 996.52
      artificial 996.55
      decellularized allodermis
          996.55
      temporary allograft or pigskin
          graft - omit code
  trial of labor NEC 660.6●
    affecting fetus or newborn 763.1
  tubal ligation 998.89
  urinary 586
  vacuum extraction
    abortion - see Abortion, failed
    delivery NEC 660.7●
      affecting fetus or newborn
          763.1
  vasectomy 998.89

Failure, failed (Continued)
  ventouse NEC 660.7●
    affecting fetus or newborn 763.1
  ventricular (see also Failure, heart) 428.9
    left 428.1
      with rheumatic fever (conditions
          classifiable to 390)
        active 391.8
          with chorea 392.0
        inactive or quiescent (with
            chorea) 398.91
      hypertensive (see also
          Hypertension, heart)
          402.91
        benign 402.11
        malignant 402.01
      rheumatic (chronic) (inactive)
          (with chorea) 398.91
        active or acute 391.8
          with chorea 392.0
    right (see also Failure, heart) 428.0
  vital centers, fetus or newborn
      779.89
  weight gain in childhood 783.41
Fainting (fit) (spell) 780.2
Falciform hymen 752.49
Fall, maternal, affecting fetus or
    newborn 760.5
Fallen arches 734
Falling, any organ or part - see Prolapse
Fallopian
  insufflation
    fertility testing V26.21
    following sterilization reversal
        V26.22
  tube - see condition
Fallot's
  pentalogy 745.2
  tetrad or tetralogy 745.2
  triad or trilogy 746.09
Fallout, radioactive (adverse effect) NEC
    990
False - see also condition
  bundle branch block 426.50
  bursa 727.89
  croup 478.75
  joint 733.82
  labor (pains) 644.1●
  opening, urinary, male 752.69
  passage, urethra (prostatic) 599.4
  positive
    serological test for syphilis 795.6
    Wassermann reaction 795.6
  pregnancy 300.11
Family, familial - see also condition
  affected by
    family member
      currently on deployment
          (military) V61.01
      returned from deployment
          (military) (current or past
          conflict) V61.02
  disruption (see also Disruption, family)
      V61.09
  estrangement V61.09
  hemophagocytic
    lymphohistiocytosis 288.4
    reticulosis 288.4
  Li-Fraumeni (syndrome) V84.01
  planning advice V25.09
    natural
      procreative V26.41
      to avoid pregnancy V25.04
  problem V61.9
    specified circumstance NEC
        V61.8
  retinoblastoma (syndrome) 190.5

Famine 994.2
  edema 262
Fanconi's anemia (congenital
  pancytopenia) 284.09
Fanconi (-de Toni) (-Debré) syndrome
  (cystinosis) 270.0
Farber (-Uzman) syndrome or disease
  (disseminated lipogranulomatosis)
  272.8
Farcin 024
Farcy 024
Farmers'
  lung 495.0
  skin 692.74
Farsightedness 367.0
Fascia - see condition
Fasciculation 781.0
Fasciculitis optica 377.32
Fasciitis 729.4
  eosinophilic 728.89
  necrotizing 728.86
  nodular 728.79
  perirenal 593.4
  plantar 728.71
  pseudosarcomatous 728.79
  traumatic (old) NEC 728.79
    current - see Sprain, by site
Fasciola hepatica infestation 121.3
Fascioliasis 121.3
Fasciolopsiasis (small intestine) 121.4
Fasciolopsis (small intestine) 121.4
Fast pulse 785.0
Fat
  embolism (cerebral) (pulmonary)
    (systemic) 958.1
    with
      abortion - see Abortion, by type,
        with embolism
      ectopic pregnancy (see also
        categories 633.0–633.9) 639.6
      molar pregnancy (see also
        categories 630–632) 639.6
      complicating delivery or
        puerperium 673.8●
      following
        abortion 639.6
        ectopic or molar pregnancy
          639.6
      in pregnancy, childbirth, or the
        puerperium 673.8●
  excessive 278.02
    in heart (see also Degeneration,
      myocardial) 429.1
  general 278.02
  hernia, herniation 729.30
    eyelid 374.34
    knee 729.31
    orbit 374.34
    retro-orbital 374.34
    retropatellar 729.31
    specified site NEC 729.39
  indigestion 579.8
  in stool 792.1
  localized (pad) 278.1
    heart (see also Degeneration,
      myocardial) 429.1
    knee 729.31
    retropatellar 729.31
  necrosis - see also Fatty, degeneration
    breast (aseptic) (segmental) 611.3
    mesentery 567.82
    omentum 567.82
    peritoneum 567.82
  pad 278.1

Fatal familial insomnia (FFI) 046.72
Fatal syncope 798.1
Fatigue 780.79
  auditory deafness (see also Deafness)
    389.9
  chronic, syndrome 780.71
  combat (see also Reaction, stress, acute)
    308.9
  during pregnancy 646.8●
  general 780.79
    psychogenic 300.5
  heat (transient) 992.6
  muscle 729.89
  myocardium (see also Failure, heart)
    428.9
  nervous 300.5
  neurosis 300.5
  operational 300.89
  postural 729.89
  posture 729.89
  psychogenic (general) 300.5
  senile 797
  syndrome NEC 300.5
    chronic 780.71
  undue 780.79
  voice 784.49
Fatness 278.02
Fatty - see also condition
  apron 278.1
  degeneration (diffuse) (general) NEC
    272.8
    localized - see Degeneration, by site,
      fatty
    placenta - see Placenta, abnormal
  heart (enlarged) (see also Degeneration,
    myocardial) 429.1
  infiltration (diffuse) (general) (see also
    Degeneration, by site, fatty) 272.8
    heart (enlarged) (see also
      Degeneration, myocardial)
      429.1
  liver 571.8
    alcoholic 571.0
  necrosis - see Degeneration, fatty
  phanerosis 272.8
Fauces - see condition
Fauchard's disease (periodontitis) 523.40
Faucitis 478.29
Faulty - see also condition
  position of teeth 524.30
Favism (anemia) 282.2
Favre-Racouchot disease (elastoidosis
  cutanea nodularis) 701.8
Favus 110.9
  beard 110.0
  capitis 110.0
  corporis 110.5
  eyelid 110.8
  foot 110.4
  hand 110.2
  scalp 110.0
  specified site NEC 110.8
Fear, fearfulness (complex) (reaction)
  300.20
  child 313.0
  of
    animals 300.29
    closed spaces 300.29
    crowds 300.29
    eating in public 300.23
    heights 300.29
    open spaces 300.22
      with panic attacks 300.21
    public speaking 300.23

Fear, fearfulness (Continued)
  of (Continued)
    streets 300.22
      with panic attacks 300.21
    travel 300.22
      with panic attacks 300.21
    washing in public 300.23
    transient 308.0
Feared complaint unfounded V65.5
Febricula (continued) (simple) (see also
  Pyrexia) 780.60
Febrile (see also Pyrexia) 780.60
  convulsion (simple) 780.31
    complex 780.32
    seizure (simple) 780.31
      atypical 780.32
      complex 780.32
      complicated 780.32
Febris (see also Fever) 780.60
  aestiva (see also Fever, hay) 477.9
  flava (see also Fever, yellow) 060.9
  melitensis 023.0
  pestis (see also Plague) 020.9
  puerperalis 672●
  recurrens (see also Fever, relapsing)
    087.9
    pediculo vestimenti 087.0
  rubra 034.1
  typhoidea 002.0
  typhosa 002.0
Fecal - see condition
Fecalith (impaction) 560.39
  with hernia - see also Hernia, by site,
    with obstruction
      gangrenous - see Hernia, by site,
        with gangrene
  appendix 543.9
  congenital 777.1
Fede's disease 529.0
Feeble-minded 317
Feeble rapid pulse due to shock
  following injury 958.4
Feeding
  faulty (elderly) (infant) 783.3
    newborn 779.31 ◀▥
  formula check V20.2
  improper (elderly) (infant) 783.3
    newborn 779.31 ◀▥
  problem (elderly) (infant) 783.3
    newborn 779.31 ◀▥
    nonorganic origin 307.59
Feeling of foreign body in throat
  784.99
Feer's disease 985.0
Feet - see condition
Feigned illness V65.2
Feil-Klippel syndrome (brevicollis) 756.16
Feinmesser's (hidrotic) ectodermal
  dysplasia 757.31
Felix's disease (juvenile osteochondrosis,
  hip) 732.1
Felon (any digit) (with lymphangitis)
  681.01
  herpetic 054.6
Felty's syndrome (rheumatoid arthritis
  with splenomegaly and leukopenia)
  714.1
Feminism in boys 302.6
Feminization, testicular 259.51
  with pseudohermaphroditism, male
    259.51
Femoral hernia - see Hernia, femoral
Femora vara 736.32
Femur, femoral - see condition

◀ New   ◀▥ Revised   ~~deleted~~ Deleted   ● Use Additional Digit(s)   ▨ Omit code

Fenestrata placenta - *see* Placenta, abnormal
Fenestration, fenestrated - *see also*
    Imperfect, closure
    aorta-pulmonary 745.0
    aorticopulmonary 745.0
    aortopulmonary 745.0
    cusps, heart valve NEC 746.89
        pulmonary 746.09
    hymen 752.49
    pulmonic cusps 746.09
Fenwick's disease 537.89
Fermentation (gastric) (gastrointestinal)
    (stomach) 536.8
    intestine 564.89
        psychogenic 306.4
    psychogenic 306.4
Fernell's disease (aortic aneurysm) 441.9
Fertile eunuch syndrome 257.2
Fertility, meaning multiparity - *see*
    Multiparity
Fetal
    alcohol syndrome 760.71
    anemia 678.0●
    thrombocytopenia 678.0●
    twin to twin transfusion 678.0●
Fetalis uterus 752.3
Fetid
    breath 784.99
    sweat 705.89
Fetishism 302.81
    transvestic 302.3
Fetomaternal hemorrhage
    affecting management of pregnancy
        656.0●
    fetus or newborn 772.0
Fetus, fetal - *see also* condition
    papyraceous 779.89
    type lung tissue 770.4
Fever 780.60
    with chills 780.60
        in malarial regions (*see also* Malaria)
        084.6
    abortus NEC 023.9
    aden 061
    African tick-borne 087.1
    American
        mountain tick 066.1
        spotted 082.0
    and ague (*see also* Malaria) 084.6
    aphthous 078.4
    arbovirus hemorrhagic 065.9
    Assam 085.0
    Australian A or Q 083.0
    Bangkok hemorrhagic 065.4
    biliary, Charcôt's intermittent - *see*
        Choledocholithiasis
    bilious, hemoglobinuric 084.8
    blackwater 084.8
    blister 054.9
    Bonvale Dam 780.79
    boutonneuse 082.1
    brain 323.9
        late effect - *see* category 326
    breakbone 061
    Bullis 082.8
    Bunyamwera 066.3
    Burdwan 085.0
    Bwamba (encephalitis) 066.3
    Cameroon (*see also* Malaria) 084.6
    Canton 081.9
    catarrhal (acute) 460
        chronic 472.0
    cat-scratch 078.3
    cerebral 323.9
        late effect - *see* category 326

Fever (*Continued*)
    cerebrospinal (meningococcal) (*see also*
        Meningitis, cerebrospinal) 036.0
    Chagres 084.0
    Chandipura 066.8
    changuinola 066.0
    Charcôt's (biliary) (hepatic)
        (intermittent) *see*
        Choledocholithiasis
    Chikungunya (viral) 066.3
        hemorrhagic 065.4
    childbed 670.8 ◀▥
    Chitral 066.0
    Colombo (*see also* Fever, paratyphoid)
        002.9
    Colorado tick (virus) 066.1
    congestive
        malarial (*see also* Malaria) 084.6
        remittent (*see also* Malaria) 084.6
    Congo virus 065.0
    continued 780.60
        malarial 084.0
    Corsican (*see also* Malaria) 084.6
    Crimean hemorrhagic 065.0
    Cyprus (*see also* Brucellosis) 023.9
    dandy 061
    deer fly (*see also* Tularemia) 021.9
    dehydration, newborn 778.4
    dengue (virus) 061
        hemorrhagic 065.4
    desert 114.0
    due to heat 992.0
    Dumdum 085.0
    enteric 002.0
    ephemeral (of unknown origin) (*see also*
        Pyrexia) 780.60
    epidemic, hemorrhagic of the Far East
        065.0
    erysipelatous (*see also* Erysipelas) 035
    estivo-autumnal (malarial) 084.0
    etiocholanolone 277.31
    famine - *see also* Fever, relapsing
        meaning typhus - *see* Typhus
    Far Eastern hemorrhagic 065.0
    five day 083.1
    Fort Bragg 100.89
    gastroenteric 002.0
    gastromalarial (*see also* Malaria) 084.6
    Gibraltar (*see also* Brucellosis) 023.9
    glandular 075
    Guama (viral) 066.3
    Haverhill 026.1
    hay (allergic) (with rhinitis) 477.9
        with
            asthma (bronchial) (*see also*
                Asthma) 493.0●
        due to
            dander, animal (cat) (dog) 477.2
            dust 477.8
            fowl 477.8
            hair, animal (cat) (dog) 477.2
            pollen, any plant or tree 477.0
            specified allergen other than
                pollen 477.8
    heat (effects) 992.0
    hematuric, bilious 084.8
    hemoglobinuric (malarial) 084.8
        bilious 084.8
    hemorrhagic (arthropod-borne) NEC
        065.9
        with renal syndrome 078.6
        arenaviral 078.7
        Argentine 078.7
        Bangkok 065.4

Fever (*Continued*)
    hemorrhagic NEC (*Continued*)
        Bolivian 078.7
        Central Asian 065.0
        chikungunya 065.4
        Crimean 065.0
        dengue (virus) 065.4
        Ebola 065.8
        epidemic 078.6
            of Far East 065.0
        Far Eastern 065.0
        Junin virus 078.7
        Korean 078.6
        Kyasanur forest 065.2
        Machupo virus 078.7
        mite-borne NEC 065.8
        mosquito-borne 065.4
        Omsk 065.1
        Philippine 065.4
        Russian (Yaroslav) 078.6
        Singapore 065.4
        Southeast Asia 065.4
        Thailand 065.4
        tick-borne NEC 065.3
    hepatic (*see also* Cholecystitis) 575.8
        intermittent (Charcôt's) - *see*
            Choledocholithiasis
    herpetic (*see also* Herpes) 054.9
    hyalomma tick 065.0
    icterohemorrhagic 100.0
    inanition 780.60
        newborn 778.4
    in conditions classified elsewhere
        780.61
    infective NEC 136.9
    intermittent (bilious) (*see also* Malaria)
        084.6
        hepatic (Charcôt) - *see*
            Choledocholithiasis
        of unknown origin (*see also* Pyrexia)
            780.60
        pernicious 084.0
    iodide
        correct substance properly
            administered 780.60
        overdose or wrong substance given
            or taken 975.5
    Japanese river 081.2
    jungle yellow 060.0
    Junin virus, hemorrhagic 078.7
    Katayama 120.2
    Kedani 081.2
    Kenya 082.1
    Korean hemorrhagic 078.6
    Lassa 078.89
    Lone Star 082.8
    lung - *see* Pneumonia
    Machupo virus, hemorrhagic 078.7
    malaria, malarial (*see also* Malaria)
        084.6
    Malta (*see also* Brucellosis) 023.9
    Marseilles 082.1
    marsh (*see also* Malaria) 084.6
    Mayaro (viral) 066.3
    Mediterranean (*see also* Brucellosis)
        023.9
        familial 277.31
        tick 082.1
    meningeal - *see* Meningitis
    metal fumes NEC 985.8
    Meuse 083.1
    Mexican - *see* Typhus, Mexican
    Mianeh 087.1
    miasmatic (*see also* Malaria) 084.6

Fever *(Continued)*
  miliary 078.2
  milk, female 672●
  mill 504
  mite-borne hemorrhagic 065.8
  Monday 504
  mosquito-borne NEC 066.3
    hemorrhagic NEC 065.4
  mountain 066.1
    meaning
      Rocky Mountain spotted 082.0
      undulant fever *(see also*
        Brucellosis) 023.9
    tick (American) 066.1
  Mucambo (viral) 066.3
  mud 100.89
  Neapolitan *(see also* Brucellosis) 023.9
  neutropenic 288.00
  newborn (environmentally-induced)
    778.4
  nine-mile 083.0
  nonexanthematous tick 066.1
  North Asian tick-borne typhus 082.2
  Omsk hemorrhagic 065.1
  O'nyong nyong (viral) 066.3
  Oropouche (viral) 066.3
  Oroya 088.0
  paludal *(see also* Malaria) 084.6
  Panama 084.0
  pappataci 066.0
  paratyphoid 002.9
    A 002.1
    B (Schottmüller's) 002.2
    C (Hirschfeld) 002.3
  parrot 073.9
  periodic 277.31
  pernicious, acute 084.0
  persistent (of unknown origin) *(see also*
    Pyrexia) 780.60
  petechial 036.0
  pharyngoconjunctival 077.2
    adenoviral type 3 077.2
  Philippine hemorrhagic 065.4
  phlebotomus 066.0
  Piry 066.8
  Pixuna (viral) 066.3
  Plasmodium ovale 084.3
  pleural *(see also* Pleurisy) 511.0
  pneumonic - *see* Pneumonia
  polymer fume 987.8
  postimmunization 780.63
  postoperative 780.62
    due to infection 998.59
  postvaccination 780.63
  pretibial 100.89
  puerperal, postpartum 672●
  putrid - *see* Septicemia
  pyemic - *see* Septicemia
  Q 083.0
    with pneumonia 083.0 *[484.8]*
  quadrilateral 083.0
  quartan (malaria) 084.2
  Queensland (coastal) 083.0
    seven-day 100.89
  Quintan (A) 083.1
  quotidian 084.0
  rabbit *(see also* Tularemia) 021.9
  rat-bite 026.9
    due to
      Spirillum minor or minus 026.0
      Spirochaeta morsus muris 026.0
      Streptobacillus moniliformis
        026.1
  recurrent - *see* Fever, relapsing

Fever *(Continued)*
  relapsing 087.9
    Carter's (Asiatic) 087.0
    Dutton's (West African) 087.1
    Koch's 087.9
    louse-borne (epidemic) 087.0
    Novy's (American) 087.1
    Obermeyer's (European) 087.0
    spirillum NEC 087.9
    tick-borne (endemic) 087.1
  remittent (bilious) (congestive) (gastric)
    (see also Malaria) 084.6
  rheumatic (active) (acute) (chronic)
    (subacute) 390
    with heart involvement 391.9
      carditis 391.9
      endocarditis (aortic) (mitral)
        (pulmonary) (tricuspid)
        391.1
      multiple sites 391.8
      myocarditis 391.2
      pancarditis, acute 391.8
      pericarditis 391.0
      specified type NEC 391.8
      valvulitis 391.1
    inactive or quiescent with
      cardiac hypertrophy 398.99
      carditis 398.90
      endocarditis 397.9
        aortic (valve) 395.9
          with mitral (valve) disease
            396.9
        mitral (valve) 394.9
          with aortic (valve) disease
            396.9
        pulmonary (valve) 397.1
        tricuspid (valve) 397.0
      heart conditions (classifiable to
        429.3, 429.6, 429.9) 398.99
      failure (congestive) (conditions
        classifiable to 428.0,
        428.9) 398.91
      left ventricular failure
        (conditions classifiable
        to 428.1) 398.91
      myocardial degeneration
        (conditions classifiable to
        429.1) 398.0
      myocarditis (conditions
        classifiable to 429.0) 398.0
      pancarditis 398.99
      pericarditis 393
  Rift Valley (viral) 066.3
  Rocky Mountain spotted 082.0
  rose 477.0
  Ross river (viral) 066.3
  Russian hemorrhagic 078.6
  sandfly 066.0
  San Joaquin (valley) 114.0
  Sao Paulo 082.0
  scarlet 034.1
  septic - *see* Septicemia
  seven-day 061
    Japan 100.89
    Queensland 100.89
  shin bone 083.1
  Singapore hemorrhagic 065.4
  solar 061
  sore 054.9
  South African tick-bite 087.1
  Southeast Asia hemorrhagic 065.4
  spinal - *see* Meningitis
  spirillary 026.0
  splenic *(see also* Anthrax) 022.9

Fever *(Continued)*
  spotted (Rocky Mountain) 082.0
    American 082.0
    Brazilian 082.0
    Colombian 082.0
    meaning
      cerebrospinal meningitis 036.0
      typhus 082.9
  spring 309.23
  steroid
    correct substance properly
      administered 780.60
    overdose or wrong substance given
      or taken 962.0
  streptobacillary 026.1
  subtertian 084.0
  Sumatran mite 081.2
  sun 061
  swamp 100.89
  sweating 078.2
  swine 003.8
  sylvatic yellow 060.0
  Tahyna 062.5
  tertian - *see* Malaria, tertian
  Thailand hemorrhagic 065.4
  thermic 992.0
  three day 066.0
    with Coxsackie exanthem 074.8
  tick
    American mountain 066.1
    Colorado 066.1
    Kemerovo 066.1
    Mediterranean 082.1
    mountain 066.1
    nonexanthematous 066.1
    Quaranfil 066.1
  tick-bite NEC 066.1
  tick-borne NEC 066.1
    hemorrhagic NEC 065.3
  transitory of newborn 778.4
  trench 083.1
  tsutsugamushi 081.2
  typhogastric 002.0
  typhoid (abortive) (ambulant) (any
    site) (hemorrhagic) (infection)
    (intermittent) (malignant)
    (rheumatic) 002.0
  typhomalarial *(see also* Malaria) 084.6
  typhus - *see* Typhus
  undulant *(see also* Brucellosis) 023.9
  unknown origin *(see also* Pyrexia)
    780.60
  uremic - *see* Uremia
  uveoparotid 135
  valley (Coccidioidomycosis) 114.0
  Venezuelan equine 066.2
  Volhynian 083.1
  Wesselsbron (viral) 066.3
  West
    African 084.8
    Nile (viral) 066.40
      with
        cranial nerve disorders
          066.42
        encephalitis 066.41
        optic neuritis 066.42
        other complications 066.49
        other neurologic manifestations
          066.42
        polyradiculitis 066.42
  Whitmore's 025
  Wolhynian 083.1
  worm 128.9
  Yaroslav hemorrhagic 078.6

Fever *(Continued)*
yellow 060.9
jungle 060.0
sylvatic 060.0
urban 060.1
vaccination, prophylactic (against)
V04.4
Zika (viral) 066.3
Fibrillation
atrial (established) (paroxysmal) 427.31
auricular (atrial) (established) 427.31
cardiac (ventricular) 427.41
coronary *(see also* Infarct, myocardium)
410.9●
heart (ventricular) 427.41
muscular 728.9
postoperative 997.1
ventricular 427.41
Fibrin
ball or bodies, pleural (sac) 511.0
chamber, anterior (eye) (gelatinous
exudate) 364.04
Fibrinogenolysis (hemorrhagic) - *see*
Fibrinolysis
Fibrinogenopenia (congenital) (hereditary)
(see also Defect, coagulation) 286.3
acquired 286.6
Fibrinolysis (acquired) (hemorrhagic)
(pathologic) 286.6
with
abortion - *see* Abortion, by type, with
hemorrhage, delayed or
excessive
ectopic pregnancy *(see also*
categories 633.0–633.9) 639.1
molar pregnancy *(see also* categories
630–632) 639.1
antepartum or intrapartum 641.3●
affecting fetus or newborn 762.1
following
abortion 639.1
ectopic or molar pregnancy 639.1
newborn, transient 776.2
postpartum 666.3●
Fibrinopenia (hereditary) *(see also* Defect,
coagulation) 286.3
acquired 286.6
Fibrinopurulent - *see* condition
Fibrinous - *see* condition
Fibroadenoma (M9010/0)
cellular intracanalicular (M9020/0) 217
giant (intracanalicular) (M9020/0) 217
intracanalicular (M9011/0)
cellular (M9020/0) 217
giant (M9020/0) 217
specified site - *see* Neoplasm, by site,
benign
unspecified site 217
juvenile (M9030/0) 217
pericanicular (M9012/0)
specified site - *see* Neoplasm, by site,
benign
unspecified site 217
phyllodes (M9020/0) 217
prostate 600.20
with
other lower urinary tract
symptoms (LUTS) 600.21
urinary
obstruction 600.21
retention 600.21
specified site - *see* Neoplasm, by site,
benign
unspecified site 217

Fibroadenosis, breast (chronic) (cystic)
(diffuse) (periodic) (segmental) 610.2
Fibroangioma (M9160/0) - *see also*
Neoplasm, by site, benign
juvenile (M9160/0)
specified site - *see* Neoplasm, by site,
benign
unspecified site 210.7
Fibrocellulitis progressiva ossificans
728.11
Fibrochondrosarcoma (M9220/3) - *see*
Neoplasm, cartilage, malignant
Fibrocystic
disease 277.00
bone NEC 733.29
breast 610.1
jaw 526.2
kidney (congenital) 753.19
liver 751.62
lung 518.89
congenital 748.4
pancreas 277.00
kidney (congenital) 753.19
Fibrodysplasia ossificans multiplex
(progressiva) 728.11
Fibroelastosis (cordis) (endocardial)
(endomyocardial) 425.3
Fibroid (tumor) (M8890/0) - *see also*
Neoplasm, connective tissue, benign
disease, lung (chronic) *(see also* Fibrosis,
lung) 515
heart (disease) *(see also* Myocarditis)
429.0
induration, lung (chronic) *(see also*
Fibrosis, lung) 515
in pregnancy or childbirth 654.1●
affecting fetus or newborn 763.89
causing obstructed labor 660.2●
affecting fetus or newborn
763.1
liver - *see* Cirrhosis, liver
lung *(see also* Fibrosis, lung) 515
pneumonia (chronic) *(see also* Fibrosis,
lung) 515
uterus (M8890/0) *(see also* Leiomyoma,
uterus) 218.9
Fibrolipoma (M8851/0) *(see also* Lipoma,
by site) 214.9
Fibroliposarcoma (M8850/3) - *see*
Neoplasm, connective tissue,
malignant
Fibroma (M8810/0) - *see also* Neoplasm,
connective tissue, benign
ameloblastic (M9330/0) 213.1
upper jaw (bone) 213.0
bone (nonossifying) 733.99
ossifying (M9262/0) - *see* Neoplasm,
bone, benign
cementifying (M9274/0) - *see*
Neoplasm, bone, benign
chondromyxoid (M9241/0) - *see*
Neoplasm, bone, benign
desmoplastic (M8823/1) - *see*
Neoplasm, connective tissue,
uncertain behavior
facial (M8813/0) - *see* Neoplasm,
connective tissue, benign
invasive (M8821/1) - *see* Neoplasm,
connective tissue, uncertain
behavior
molle (M8851/0) *(see also* Lipoma, by
site) 214.9
myxoid (M8811/0) - *see* Neoplasm,
connective tissue, benign

Fibroma *(Continued)*
nasopharynx, nasopharyngeal
(juvenile) (M9160/0) 210.7
nonosteogenic (nonossifying) - *see*
Dysplasia, fibrous
odontogenic (M9321/0) 213.1
upper jaw (bone) 213.0
ossifying (M9262/0) - *see* Neoplasm,
bone, benign
periosteal (M8812/0) - *see* Neoplasm,
bone, benign
prostate 600.20
with
other lower urinary tract
symptoms (LUTS) 600.21
urinary
obstruction 600.21
retention 600.21
soft (M8851/0) *(see also* Lipoma, by
site) 214.9
Fibromatosis 728.79
abdominal (M8822/1) - *see* Neoplasm,
connective tissue, uncertain
behavior
aggressive (M8821/1) - *see* Neoplasm,
connective tissue, uncertain
behavior
congenital generalized (CGF) 759.89
Dupuytren's 728.6
gingival 523.8
plantar fascia 728.71
proliferative 728.79
pseudosarcomatous (proliferative)
(subcutaneous) 728.79
subcutaneous pseudosarcomatous
(proliferative) 728.79
Fibromyalgia 729.1
Fibromyoma (M8890/0) - *see also*
Neoplasm, connective tissue, benign
uterus (corpus) *(see also* Leiomyoma,
uterus) 218.9
in pregnancy or childbirth 654.1●
affecting fetus or newborn 763.89
causing obstructed labor 660.2●
affecting fetus or newborn
763.1
Fibromyositis *(see also* Myositis) 729.1
scapulohumeral 726.2
Fibromyxolipoma (M8852/0) *(see also*
Lipoma, by site) 214.9
Fibromyxoma (M8811/0) - *see* Neoplasm,
connective tissue, benign
Fibromyxosarcoma (M8811/3) - *see*
Neoplasm, connective tissue,
malignant
Fibro-odontoma, ameloblastic (M9290/0)
213.1
upper jaw (bone) 213.0
Fibro-osteoma (M9262/0) - *see* Neoplasm,
bone, benign
Fibroplasia, retrolental *(see also*
Retinopathy of prematurity) 362.21
Fibropurulent - *see* condition
Fibrosarcoma (M8810/3) - *see also*
Neoplasm, connective tissue,
malignant
ameloblastic (M9330/3) 170.1
upper jaw (bone) 170.0
congenital (M8814/3) - *see* Neoplasm,
connective tissue, malignant
fascial (M8813/3) - *see* Neoplasm,
connective tissue, malignant
infantile (M8814/3) - *see* Neoplasm,
connective tissue, malignant

◄ New   ◀▥ Revised   ~~deleted~~ Deleted   ● Use Additional Digit(s)   ▨ Omit code   **301**

Fibrosarcoma *(Continued)*
  odontogenic (M9330/3) 170.1
    upper jaw (bone) 170.0
  periosteal (M8812/3) - *see* Neoplasm,
    bone, malignant
Fibrosclerosis
  breast 610.3
  corpora cavernosa (penis) 607.89
  familial multifocal NEC 710.8
  multifocal (idiopathic) NEC 710.8
  penis (corpora cavernosa) 607.89
Fibrosis, fibrotic
  adrenal (gland) 255.8
  alveolar (diffuse) 516.3
  amnion 658.8●
  anal papillae 569.49
  anus 569.49
  appendix, appendiceal,
    noninflammatory 543.9
  arteriocapillary - *see* Arteriosclerosis
  bauxite (of lung) 503
  biliary 576.8
    due to Clonorchis sinensis 121.1
  bladder 596.8
    interstitial 595.1
    localized submucosal 595.1
    panmural 595.1
  bone, diffuse 756.59
  breast 610.3
  capillary - *see also* Arteriosclerosis
    lung (chronic) (*see also* Fibrosis,
      lung) 515
  cardiac (*see also* Myocarditis) 429.0
  cervix 622.8
  chorion 658.8●
  corpus cavernosum 607.89
  cystic (of pancreas) 277.00
    with
      manifestations
        gastrointestinal 277.03
        pulmonary 277.02
        specified NEC 277.09
      meconium ileus 277.01
      pulmonary exacerbation 277.02
  due to (presence of) any device,
    implant, or graft - *see*
    Complications, due to
    (presence of) any device, implant,
    or graft classified to 996.0–996.5
    NEC
  ejaculatory duct 608.89
  endocardium (*see also* Endocarditis)
    424.90
  endomyocardial (African) 425.0
  epididymis 608.89
  eye muscle 378.62
  graphite (of lung) 503
  heart (*see also* Myocarditis) 429.0
  hepatic - *see also* Cirrhosis, liver
    due to Clonorchis sinensis 121.1
  hepatolienal - *see* Cirrhosis, liver
  hepatosplenic - *see* Cirrhosis, liver
  infrapatellar fat pad 729.31
  interstitial pulmonary, newborn
    770.7
  intrascrotal 608.89
  kidney (*see also* Sclerosis, renal) 587
  liver - *see* Cirrhosis, liver
  lung (atrophic) (capillary) (chronic)
    (confluent) (massive)
    (perialveolar) (peribronchial)
    515
    with
      anthracosilicosis (occupational)
        500

Fibrosis, fibrotic *(Continued)*
  lung *(Continued)*
    with *(Continued)*
      anthracosis (occupational) 500
      asbestosis (occupational) 501
      bagassosis (occupational) 495.1
      bauxite 503
      berylliosis (occupational) 503
      byssinosis (occupational) 504
      calcicosis (occupational) 502
      chalicosis (occupational) 502
      dust reticulation (occupational)
        504
      farmers' lung 495.0
      gannister disease (occupational)
        502
      graphite 503
      pneumoconiosis (occupational)
        505
      pneumosiderosis (occupational)
        503
      siderosis (occupational) 503
      silicosis (occupational) 502
      tuberculosis (*see also* Tuberculosis)
        011.4●
    diffuse (idiopathic) (interstitial)
      516.3
    due to
      bauxite 503
      fumes or vapors (chemical)
        (inhalation) 506.4
      graphite 503
    following radiation 508.1
    postinflammatory 515
    silicotic (massive) (occupational)
      502
    tuberculous (*see also* Tuberculosis)
      011.4●
  lymphatic gland 289.3
  median bar 600.90
    with
      other lower urinary tract
        symptoms (LUTS) 600.91
      urinary
        obstruction 600.91
        retention 600.91
  mediastinum (idiopathic) 519.3
  meninges 349.2
  muscle NEC 728.2
    iatrogenic (from injection) 999.9
  myocardium, myocardial (*see also*
    Myocarditis) 429.0
  oral submucous 528.8
  ovary 620.8
  oviduct 620.8
  pancreas 577.8
    cystic 277.00
      with
        manifestations
          gastrointestinal 277.03
          pulmonary 277.02
          specified NEC 277.09
        meconium ileus 277.01
        pulmonary exacerbation
          277.02
  penis 607.89
  periappendiceal 543.9
  periarticular (*see also* Ankylosis)
    718.5●
  pericardium 423.1
  perineum, in pregnancy or childbirth
    654.8●
    affecting fetus or newborn 763.89
    causing obstructed labor 660.2●
      affecting fetus or newborn 763.1

Fibrosis, fibrotic *(Continued)*
  perineural NEC 355.9
    foot 355.6
  periureteral 593.89
  placenta - *see* Placenta, abnormal
  pleura 511.0
  popliteal fat pad 729.31
  preretinal 362.56
  prostate (chronic) 600.90
    with
      other lower urinary tract
        symptoms (LUTS) 600.91
      urinary
        obstruction 600.91
        retention 600.91
  pulmonary (chronic) (*see also* Fibrosis,
    lung) 515
    alveolar capillary block 516.3
    interstitial
      diffuse (idiopathic) 516.3
      newborn 770.7
  radiation - *see* Effect, adverse, radiation
  rectal sphincter 569.49
  retroperitoneal, idiopathic 593.4
  sclerosing mesenteric (idiopathic)
    567.82
  scrotum 608.89
  seminal vesicle 608.89
  senile 797
  skin NEC 709.2
  spermatic cord 608.89
  spleen 289.59
    bilharzial (*see also* Schistosomiasis)
      120.9
  subepidermal nodular (M8832/0) - *see*
    Neoplasm, skin, benign
  submucous NEC 709.2
    oral 528.8
    tongue 528.8
  syncytium - *see* Placenta, abnormal
  testis 608.89
    chronic, due to syphilis 095.8
  thymus (gland) 254.8
  tunica vaginalis 608.89
  ureter 593.89
  urethra 599.84
  uterus (nonneoplastic) 621.8
    bilharzial (*see also* Schistosomiasis)
      120.9
    neoplastic (*see also* Leiomyoma,
      uterus) 218.9
  vagina 623.8
  valve, heart (*see also* Endocarditis)
    424.90
  vas deferens 608.89
  vein 459.89
    lower extremities 459.89
  vesical 595.1
Fibrositis (periarticular) (rheumatoid)
  729.0
  humeroscapular region 726.2
  nodular, chronic
    Jaccoud's 714.4
    rheumatoid 714.4
  ossificans 728.11
  scapulohumeral 726.2
Fibrothorax 511.0
Fibrotic - *see* Fibrosis
Fibrous - *see* condition
Fibroxanthoma (M8831/0) - *see also*
  Neoplasm, connective tissue,
  benign
  atypical (M8831/1) - *see* Neoplasm,
    connective tissue, uncertain
    behavior

◀ New   ◀‖‖ Revised   ~~deleted~~ Deleted   ● Use Additional Digit(s)   ▨ Omit code

Fibroxanthoma (Continued)
  malignant (M8831/3) - see Neoplasm,
    connective tissue, malignant
Fibroxanthosarcoma (M8831/3) - see
  Neoplasm, connective tissue,
    malignant
Fiedler's
  disease (leptospiral jaundice) 100.0
  myocarditis or syndrome (acute
    isolated myocarditis) 422.91
Fiessinger-Leroy (-Reiter) syndrome 099.3
Fiessinger-Rendu syndrome (erythema
  muliforme exudativum) 695.19
Fifth disease (eruptive) 057.0
  venereal 099.1
Filaria, filarial - see Infestation, filarial
Filariasis (see also Infestation, filarial) 125.9
  bancroftian 125.0
  Brug's 125.1
  due to
    bancrofti 125.0
    Brugia (Wuchereria) (malayi) 125.1
    Loa loa 125.2
    malayi 125.1
    organism NEC 125.6
    Wuchereria (bancrofti) 125.0
      malayi 125.1
  Malayan 125.1
  ozzardi 125.5
  specified type NEC 125.6
Filatoff's, Filatov's, Filatow's disease
  (infectious mononucleosis) 075
File-cutters' disease 984.9
  specified type of lead - see Table of
    Drugs and Chemicals
Filling defect
  biliary tract 793.3
  bladder 793.5
  duodenum 793.4
  gallbladder 793.3
  gastrointestinal tract 793.4
  intestine 793.4
  kidney 793.5
  stomach 793.4
  ureter 793.5
Filtering bleb, eye (postglaucoma)
  (status) V45.69
  with complication or rupture 997.99
  postcataract extraction (complication)
    997.99
Fimbrial cyst (congenital) 752.11
Fimbriated hymen 752.49
Financial problem affecting care V60.2
Findings, (abnormal), without diagnosis
  (examination) (laboratory
    test) 796.4 ◀║║
  17-ketosteroids, elevated 791.9
  acetonuria 791.6
  acid phosphatase 790.5
  albumin-globulin ratio 790.99
  albuminuria 791.0
  alcohol in blood 790.3
  alkaline phosphatase 790.5
  amniotic fluid 792.3
  amylase 790.5
  antenatal screening 796.5
  anisocytosis 790.09
  anthrax, positive 795.31
  antibody titers, elevated 795.79
  anticardiolipin antibody 795.79
  antigen-antibody reaction 795.79
  antiphospholipid antibody 795.79
  bacteriuria 791.9
  ballistocardiogram 794.39
  bicarbonate 276.9
  bile in urine 791.4
  bilirubin 277.4

Findings, abnormal, without diagnosis
  (Continued)
  bleeding time (prolonged) 790.92
  blood culture, positive 790.7
  blood gas level (arterial) 790.91
  blood sugar level 790.29
    high 790.29
      fasting glucose 790.21
      glucose tolerance test 790.22
    low 251.2
  C-reactive protein (CRP) 790.95
  calcium 275.40
  cancer antigen 125 [CA 125] 795.82
  carbonate 276.9
  carcinoembryonic antigen [CEA] 795.81
  casts, urine 791.7
  catecholamines 791.9
  cells, urine 791.7
  cerebrospinal fluid (color) (content)
    (pressure) 792.0
  cervical
    high risk human papillomavirus
      (HPV) DNA test positive
      795.05
    low risk human papillomavirus
      (HPV) DNA test positive
      795.09
  chloride 276.9
  cholesterol 272.9
    high 272.0
      with high triglycerides 272.2
  chromosome analysis 795.2
  chyluria 791.1
  circulation time 794.39
  cloudy dialysis effluent 792.5
  cloudy urine 791.9
  coagulation study 790.92
  cobalt, blood 790.6
  color of urine (unusual) NEC 791.9
  copper, blood 790.6
  creatinine clearance 794.4
  crystals, urine 791.9
  culture, positive NEC 795.39
    blood 790.7
    HIV V08
    human immunodeficiency virus
      V08
    nose 795.39
      Staphylococcus - see Carrier
        (suspected) of,
        Staphylococcus
    skin lesion NEC 795.39
    spinal fluid 792.0
    sputum 795.39
    stool 792.1
    throat 795.39
    urine 791.9
    viral
      human immunodeficiency V08
    wound 795.39
  cytology specified site NEC 796.9 ◀
  echocardiogram 793.2
  echoencephalogram 794.01
  echogram NEC - see Findings,
    abnormal, structure
  electrocardiogram (ECG) (EKG)
    794.31
  electroencephalogram (EEG) 794.02
  electrolyte level, urinary 791.9
  electromyogram (EMG) 794.17
    ocular 794.14
  electro-oculogram (EOG) 794.12
  electroretinogram (ERG) 794.11
  enzymes, serum NEC 790.5
  fibrinogen titer coagulation study
    790.92
  filling defect - see Filling defect

Findings, abnormal, without diagnosis
  (Continued)
  function study NEC 794.9
    auditory 794.15
    bladder 794.9
    brain 794.00
    cardiac 794.30
    endocrine NEC 794.6
      thyroid 794.5
    kidney 794.4
    liver 794.8
    nervous system
      central 794.00
      peripheral 794.19
    oculomotor 794.14
    pancreas 794.9
    placenta 794.9
    pulmonary 794.2
    retina 794.11
    special senses 794.19
    spleen 794.9
    vestibular 794.16
  gallbladder, nonvisualization 793.3
  glucose 790.29
    elevated
      fasting 790.21
      tolerance test 790.22
  glycosuria 791.5
  heart
    shadow 793.2
    sounds 785.3
  hematinuria 791.2
  hematocrit
    drop (precipitous) 790.01
    elevated 282.7
    low 285.9
  hematologic NEC 790.99
  hematuria 599.70
  hemoglobin
    drop 790.01   ◀
    elevated 282.7
    low 285.9
  hemoglobinuria 791.2
  histological NEC 795.4
  hormones 259.9
  immunoglobulins, elevated 795.79
  indolacetic acid, elevated 791.9
  iron 790.6
  karyotype 795.2
  ketonuria 791.6
  lactic acid dehydrogenase
    (LDH) 790.4
  lead 790.6
  lipase 790.5
  lipids NEC 272.9
  lithium, blood 790.6
  liver function test 790.6
  lung field (coin lesion) (shadow)
    793.1
  magnesium, blood 790.6
  mammogram 793.80
    calcification 793.89
    calculus 793.89
    dense breasts 793.82   ◀
    inconclusive 793.82   ◀
      due to dense breasts 793.82 ◀
    microcalcification 793.81
  mediastinal shift 793.2
  melanin, urine 791.9
  microbiologic NEC 795.39
  mineral, blood NEC 790.6
  myoglobinuria 791.3
  nasal swab, anthrax 795.31
  neonatal screening 796.6
  nitrogen derivatives, blood 790.6
  nonvisualization of gallbladder 793.3
  nose culture, positive 795.39

Findings, abnormal, without diagnosis
(Continued)
odor of urine (unusual) NEC 791.9
oxygen saturation 790.91
Papanicolaou (smear) 796.9
anus 796.70
with
atypical squamous cells
cannot exclude high
grade squamous
intraepithelial
lesion (ASC-H)
796.72
of undetermined
significance
(ASC-US) 796.71
cytologic evidence of
malignancy 796.76
high grade squamous
intraepithelial lesion
(HGSIL) 796.74
low grade squamous
intraepithelial lesion
(LGSIL) 796.73
glandular 796.70
specified finding NEC 796.79
cervix 795.00
with
atypical squamous cells
cannot exclude high grade
squamous
intraepithelial lesion
(ASC-H) 795.02
of undetermined
significance
(ASC-US) 795.01
cytologic evidence of
malignancy 795.06
high grade squamous
intraepithelial lesion
(HGSIL) 795.04
low grade squamous
intraepithelial lesion
(LGSIL) 795.03
dyskaryotic 795.09
nonspecific finding NEC
795.09
other site 796.9
vagina 795.10
with
atypical squamous cells
cannot exclude high grade
squamous
intraepithelial lesion
(ASC-H) 795.12
of undetermined
significance
(ASC-US) 795.11
cytologic evidence of
malignancy 795.16
high grade squamous
intraepithelial lesion
(HGSIL) 795.14
low grade squamous
intraepithelial lesion
(LGSIL) 795.13
glandular 795.10
specified NEC 795.19
peritoneal fluid 792.9
phonocardiogram 794.39
phosphorus 275.3
pleural fluid 792.9
pneumoencephalogram 793.0
PO₂-oxygen ratio 790.91
poikilocytosis 790.09

Findings, abnormal, without diagnosis
(Continued)
potassium
deficiency 276.8
excess 276.7
PPD 795.5
prostate specific antigen (PSA)
790.93
protein, serum NEC 790.99
proteinuria 791.0
prothrombin time (prolonged) (partial)
(PT) (PTT) 790.92
pyuria 791.9
radiologic (x-ray) 793.99
abdomen 793.6
biliary tract 793.3
breast 793.89
abnormal mammogram NOS
793.80
mammographic
calcification 793.89
calculus 793.89
microcalcification 793.81
gastrointestinal tract 793.4
genitourinary organs 793.5
head 793.0
image test inconclusive due to
excess body fat 793.91
intrathoracic organs NEC 793.2
lung 793.1
musculoskeletal 793.7
placenta 793.99
retroperitoneum 793.6
skin 793.99
skull 793.0
subcutaneous tissue 793.99
red blood cell 790.09
count 790.09
morphology 790.09
sickling 790.09
volume 790.09
saliva 792.4
scan NEC 794.9
bladder 794.9
bone 794.9
brain 794.09
kidney 794.4
liver 794.8
lung 794.2
pancreas 794.9
placental 794.9
spleen 794.9
thyroid 794.5
sedimentation rate, elevated 790.1
semen 792.2
serological (for)
human immunodeficiency virus
(HIV)
inconclusive 795.71
positive V08
syphilis - see Findings, serology for
syphilis
serology for syphilis
false positive 795.6
positive 097.1
false 795.6
follow-up of latent syphilis - see
Syphilis, latent
only finding - see Syphilis, latent
serum 790.99
blood NEC 790.99
enzymes NEC 790.5
proteins 790.99
SGOT 790.4
SGPT 790.4

Findings, abnormal, without diagnosis
(Continued)
sickling of red blood cells 790.09
skin test, positive 795.79
tuberculin (without active
tuberculosis) 795.5
sodium 790.6
deficiency 276.1
excess 276.0
specified NEC 796.9 ◄
spermatozoa 792.2
spinal fluid 792.0
culture, positive 792.0
sputum culture, positive 795.39
for acid-fast bacilli 795.39
stool NEC 792.1
bloody 578.1
occult 792.1
color 792.1
culture, positive 792.1
occult blood 792.1
stress test 794.39
structure, body (echogram)
(thermogram) (ultrasound) (x-ray)
NEC 793.99
abdomen 793.6
breast 793.89
abnormal mammogram 793.80
mammographic
calcification 793.89
calculus 793.89
microcalcification 793.81
gastrointestinal tract 793.4
genitourinary organs 793.5
head 793.0
echogram (ultrasound) 794.01
intrathoracic organs NEC 793.2
lung 793.1
musculoskeletal 793.7
placenta 793.99
retroperitoneum 793.6
skin 793.99
subcutaneous tissue NEC 793.99
synovial fluid 792.9
thermogram - see Findings, abnormal,
structure
throat culture, positive 795.39
thyroid (function) 794.5
metabolism (rate) 794.5
scan 794.5
uptake 794.5
total proteins 790.99
toxicology (drugs) (heavy metals) 796.0
transaminase (level) 790.4
triglycerides 272.9
high 272.1
with high cholesterol 272.2
tuberculin skin test (without active
tuberculosis) 795.5
tumor markers NEC 795.89
ultrasound - see also Findings,
abnormal, structure
cardiogram 793.2
uric acid, blood 790.6
urine, urinary constituents 791.9
acetone 791.6
albumin 791.0
bacteria 791.9
bile 791.4
blood 599.70
casts or cells 791.7
chyle 791.1
culture, positive 791.9
glucose 791.5
hemoglobin 791.2

◄ New   ◄▥ Revised   ~~deleted~~ Deleted   ● Use Additional Digit(s)   ▨ Omit code

Findings, abnormal, without diagnosis
(Continued)
  urine, urinary constituents (Continued)
    ketone 791.6
    protein 791.0
    pus 791.9
    sugar 791.5
  vaginal
    fluid 792.9
    high risk human papillomavirus
        (HPV) DNA test positive
        795.15
    low risk human papillomavirus
        (HPV) DNA test positive
        795.19
  vanillylmandelic acid, elevated 791.9
  vectorcardiogram (VCG) 794.39
  ventriculogram (cerebral) 793.0
  VMA, elevated 791.9
  Wassermann reaction
    false positive 795.6
    positive 097.1
      follow-up of latent syphilis - see
          Syphilis, latent
      only finding - see Syphilis, latent
  white blood cell 288.9
    count 288.9
      elevated 288.60
      low 288.50
    differential 288.9
    morphology 288.9
  wound culture 795.39
  xerography 793.89
  zinc, blood 790.6
Finger - see condition
Finnish type nephrosis (congenital)
    759.89
Fire, St. Anthony's (see also Erysipelas) 035
Fish
  hook stomach 537.89
  meal workers' lung 495.8
Fisher's syndrome 357.0
Fissure, fissured
  abdominal wall (congenital) 756.79
  anus, anal 565.0
    congenital 751.5
  buccal cavity 528.9
  clitoris (congenital) 752.49
  ear, lobule (congenital) 744.29
  epiglottis (congenital) 748.3
  larynx 478.79
    congenital 748.3
  lip 528.5
    congenital (see also Cleft, lip) 749.10
  nipple 611.2
    puerperal, postpartum 676.1●
  palate (congenital) (see also Cleft,
      palate) 749.00
  postanal 565.0
  rectum 565.0
  skin 709.8
    streptococcal 686.9
  spine (congenital) (see also Spina bifida)
      741.9●
  sternum (congenital) 756.3
  tongue (acquired) 529.5
    congenital 750.13
Fistula (sinus) 686.9
  abdomen (wall) 569.81
    bladder 596.2
    intestine 569.81
    ureter 593.82
    uterus 619.2
  abdominorectal 569.81
  abdominosigmoidal 569.81

Fistula (Continued)
  abdominothoracic 510.0
  abdominouterine 619.2
    congenital 752.3
  abdominovesical 596.2
  accessory sinuses (see also Sinusitis)
      473.9
  actinomycotic - see Actinomycosis
  alveolar
    antrum (see also Sinusitis, maxillary)
        473.0
    process 522.7
  anorectal 565.1
  antrobuccal (see also Sinusitis,
      maxillary) 473.0
  antrum (see also Sinusitis, maxillary)
      473.0
  anus, anal (infectional) (recurrent)
      565.1
    congenital 751.5
    tuberculous (see also Tuberculosis)
        014.8●
  aortic sinus 747.29
  aortoduodenal 447.2
  appendix, appendicular 543.9
  arteriovenous (acquired) 447.0
    brain 437.3
      congenital 747.81
        ruptured (see also
            Hemorrhage,
            subarachnoid) 430
      ruptured (see also Hemorrhage,
          subarachnoid) 430
    cerebral 437.3
      congenital 747.81
    congenital (peripheral) 747.60
      brain - see Fistula,
          arteriovenous,
          brain, congenital
      coronary 746.85
      gastrointestinal 747.61
      lower limb 747.64
      pulmonary 747.3
      renal 747.62
      specified site NEC 747.69
      upper limb 747.63
    coronary 414.19
      congenital 746.85
    heart 414.19
    pulmonary (vessels) 417.0
      congenital 747.3
    surgically created (for dialysis)
        V45.11
      complication NEC 996.73
        atherosclerosis - see
            Arteriosclerosis,
            extremities
        embolism 996.74
        infection or inflammation
            996.62
        mechanical 996.1
        occlusion NEC 996.74
        thrombus 996.74
    traumatic - see Injury, blood vessel,
        by site
  artery 447.2
  aural 383.81
    congenital 744.49
  auricle 383.81
    congenital 744.49
  Bartholin's gland 619.8
  bile duct (see also Fistula, biliary)
      576.4
  biliary (duct) (tract) 576.4
    congenital 751.69

Fistula (Continued)
  bladder (neck) (sphincter) 596.2
    into seminal vesicle 596.2
  bone 733.99
  brain 348.89   ◀▥▥
    arteriovenous - see Fistula,
        arteriovenous, brain
  branchial (cleft) 744.41
  branchiogenous 744.41
  breast 611.0
    puerperal, postpartum 675.1●
  bronchial 510.0
  bronchocutaneous,
      bronchomediastinal,
      bronchopleural,
      bronchopleuromediastinal
      (infective) 510.0
    tuberculous (see also Tuberculosis)
        011.3●
  bronchoesophageal 530.84
    congenital 750.3
  buccal cavity (infective) 528.3
  canal, ear 380.89
  carotid-cavernous
    congenital 747.81
      with hemorrhage 430
    traumatic 900.82
      with hemorrhage (see also
          Hemorrhage, brain,
          traumatic) 853.0●
      late effect 908.3
  cecosigmoidal 569.81
  cecum 569.81
  cerebrospinal (fluid) 349.81
  cervical, lateral (congenital)
      744.41
  cervicoaural (congenital) 744.49
  cervicosigmoidal 619.1
  cervicovesical 619.0
  cervix 619.8
  chest (wall) 510.0
  cholecystocolic (see also Fistula,
      gallbladder) 575.5
  cholecystocolonic (see also Fistula,
      gallbladder) 575.5
  cholecystoduodenal (see also Fistula,
      gallbladder) 575.5
  cholecystoenteric (see also Fistula,
      gallbladder) 575.5
  cholecystogastric (see also Fistula,
      gallbladder) 575.5
  cholecystointestinal (see also Fistula,
      gallbladder) 575.5
  choledochoduodenal 576.4
  cholocolic (see also Fistula, gallbladder)
      575.5
  coccyx 685.1
    with abscess 685.0
  colon 569.81
  colostomy 569.69
  colovaginal (acquired) 619.1
  common duct (bile duct) 576.4
  congenital, NEC - see Anomaly,
      specified type NEC
  cornea, causing hypotony
      360.32
  coronary, arteriovenous 414.19
    congenital 746.85
  costal region 510.0
  cul-de-sac, Douglas' 619.8
  cutaneous 686.9
  cystic duct (see also Fistula, gallbladder)
      575.5
    congenital 751.69
  dental 522.7

Fistula *(Continued)*
  diaphragm 510.0
    bronchovisceral 510.0
    pleuroperitoneal 510.0
    pulmonoperitoneal 510.0
  duodenum 537.4
  ear (canal) (external) 380.89
  enterocolic 569.81
  enterocutaneous 569.81
  enteroenteric 569.81
  entero-uterine 619.1
    congenital 752.3
  enterovaginal 619.1
    congenital 752.49
  enterovesical 596.1
  epididymis 608.89
    tuberculous *(see also* Tuberculosis)
      016.4●
  esophagobronchial 530.89
    congenital 750.3
  esophagocutaneous 530.89
  esophagopleurocutaneous 530.89
  esophagotracheal 530.84
    congenital 750.3
  esophagus 530.89
    congenital 750.4
  ethmoid *(see also* Sinusitis, ethmoidal)
    473.2
  eyeball (cornea) (sclera) 360.32
  eyelid 373.11
  fallopian tube (external) 619.2
  fecal 569.81
    congenital 751.5
  from periapical lesion 522.7
  frontal sinus *(see also* Sinusitis, frontal)
    473.1
  gallbladder 575.5
    with calculus, cholelithiasis, stones
      (see also Cholelithiasis) 574.2●
    congenital 751.69
  gastric 537.4
  gastrocolic 537.4
    congenital 750.7
    tuberculous *(see also* Tuberculosis)
      014.8●
  gastroenterocolic 537.4
  gastroesophageal 537.4
  gastrojejunal 537.4
  gastrojejunocolic 537.4
  genital
    organs
      female 619.9
        specified site NEC 619.8
      male 608.89
    tract-skin (female) 619.2
  hepatopleural 510.0
  hepatopulmonary 510.0
  horseshoe 565.1
  ileorectal 569.81
  ileosigmoidal 569.81
  ileostomy 569.69
  ileovesical 596.1
  ileum 569.81
  in ano 565.1
    tuberculous *(see also* Tuberculosis)
      014.8●
  inner ear *(see also* Fistula, labyrinth)
    386.40
  intestine 569.81
  intestinocolonic (abdominal) 569.81
  intestinoureteral 593.82
  intestinouterine 619.1
  intestinovaginal 619.1
    congenital 752.49

Fistula *(Continued)*
  intestinovesical 596.1
  involving female genital tract 619.9
    digestive-genital 619.1
    genital tract-skin 619.2
    specified site NEC 619.8
    urinary-genital 619.0
  ischiorectal (fossa) 566
  jejunostomy 569.69
  jejunum 569.81
  joint 719.80
    ankle 719.87
    elbow 719.82
    foot 719.87
    hand 719.84
    hip 719.85
    knee 719.86
    multiple sites 719.89
    pelvic region 719.85
    shoulder (region) 719.81
    specified site NEC 719.88
    tuberculous - *see* Tuberculosis, joint
    wrist 719.83
  kidney 593.89
  labium (majus) (minus) 619.8
  labyrinth, labyrinthine NEC 386.40
    combined sites 386.48
    multiple sites 386.48
    oval window 386.42
    round window 386.41
    semicircular canal 386.43
  lacrimal, lachrymal (duct) (gland) (sac)
    375.61
  lacrimonasal duct 375.61
  laryngotracheal 748.3
  larynx 478.79
  lip 528.5
    congenital 750.25
  lumbar, tuberculous *(see also*
    Tuberculosis) 015.0● *[730.8]●*
  lung 510.0
  lymphatic (node) (vessel) 457.8
  mamillary 611.0
  mammary (gland) 611.0
    puerperal, postpartum 675.1●
  mastoid (process) (region) 383.1
  maxillary *(see also* Sinusitis, maxillary)
    473.0
  mediastinal 510.0
  mediastinobronchial 510.0
  mediastinocutaneous 510.0
  middle ear 385.89
  mouth 528.3
  nasal 478.19
    sinus *(see also* Sinusitis) 473.9
  nasopharynx 478.29
  nipple - *see* Fistula, breast
  nose 478.19
  oral (cutaneous) 528.3
    maxillary *(see also* Sinusitis,
      maxillary) 473.0
    nasal (with cleft palate) *(see also*
      Cleft, palate) 749.00
  orbit, orbital 376.10
  oro-antral *(see also* Sinusitis, maxillary)
    473.0
  oval window (internal ear) 386.42
  oviduct (external) 619.2
  palate (hard) 526.89
    soft 528.9
  pancreatic 577.8
  pancreaticoduodenal 577.8
  parotid (gland) 527.4
    region 528.3

Fistula *(Continued)*
  pelvoabdominointestinal 569.81
  penis 607.89
  perianal 565.1
  pericardium (pleura) (sac) *(see also*
    Pericarditis) 423.8
  pericecal 569.81
  perineal - *see* Fistula, perineum
  perineorectal 569.81
  perineosigmoidal 569.81
  perineo-urethroscrotal 608.89
  perineum, perineal (with urethral
    involvement) NEC 599.1
    tuberculous *(see also* Tuberculosis)
      017.9●
    ureter 593.82
  perirectal 565.1
    tuberculous *(see also* Tuberculosis)
      014.8●
  peritoneum *(see also* Peritonitis) 567.22
  periurethral 599.1
  pharyngo-esophageal 478.29
  pharynx 478.29
    branchial cleft (congenital) 744.41
  pilonidal (infected) (rectum) 685.1
    with abscess 685.0
  pleura, pleural, pleurocutaneous,
    pleuroperitoneal 510.0
    stomach 510.0
    tuberculous *(see also* Tuberculosis)
      012.0●
  pleuropericardial 423.8
  postauricular 383.81
  postoperative, persistent 998.6
  preauricular (congenital) 744.46
  prostate 602.8
  pulmonary 510.0
    arteriovenous 417.0
      congenital 747.3
    tuberculous *(see also* Tuberculosis,
      pulmonary) 011.9●
  pulmonoperitoneal 510.0
  rectolabial 619.1
  rectosigmoid (intercommunicating)
    569.81
  rectoureteral 593.82
  rectourethral 599.1
    congenital 753.8
  rectouterine 619.1
    congenital 752.3
  rectovaginal 619.1
    congenital 752.49
    old, postpartal 619.1
    tuberculous *(see also* Tuberculosis)
      014.8●
  rectovesical 596.1
    congenital 753.8
  rectovesicovaginal 619.1
  rectovulvar 619.1
    congenital 752.49
  rectum (to skin) 565.1
    tuberculous *(see also* Tuberculosis)
      014.8●
  renal 593.89
  retroauricular 383.81
  round window (internal ear) 386.41
  salivary duct or gland 527.4
    congenital 750.24
  sclera 360.32
  scrotum (urinary) 608.89
    tuberculous *(see also* Tuberculosis)
      016.5●
  semicircular canals (internal ear)
    386.43

◀ New   ◀||||| Revised   ~~deleted~~ Deleted   ● Use Additional Digit(s)   ▨ Omit code

Fistula *(Continued)*
  sigmoid 569.81
    vesicoabdominal 596.1
  sigmoidovaginal 619.1
    congenital 752.49
  skin 686.9
    ureter 593.82
    vagina 619.2
  sphenoidal sinus *(see also* Sinusitis,
      sphenoidal) 473.3
  splenocolic 289.59
  stercoral 569.81
  stomach 537.4
  sublingual gland 527.4
    congenital 750.24
  submaxillary
    gland 527.4
      congenital 750.24
    region 528.3
  thoracic 510.0
    duct 457.8
  thoracicoabdominal 510.0
  thoracicogastric 510.0
  thoracicointestinal 510.0
  thoracoabdominal 510.0
  thoracogastric 510.0
  thorax 510.0
  thyroglossal duct 759.2
  thyroid 246.8
  trachea (congenital) (external)
      (internal) 748.3
  tracheoesophageal 530.84
    congenital 750.3
    following tracheostomy 519.09
  traumatic
    arteriovenous *(see also* Injury, blood
        vessel, by site) 904.9
    brain - *see* Injury, intracranial
  tuberculous - *see* Tuberculosis, by site
  typhoid 002.0
  umbilical 759.89
  umbilico-urinary 753.8
  urachal, urachus 753.7
  ureter (persistent) 593.82
  ureteroabdominal 593.82
  ureterocervical 593.82
  ureterorectal 593.82
  ureterosigmoido-abdominal 593.82
  ureterovaginal 619.0
  ureterovesical 596.2
  urethra 599.1
    congenital 753.8
    tuberculous *(see also* Tuberculosis)
        016.3●
  urethroperineal 599.1
  urethroperineovesical 596.2
  urethrorectal 599.1
    congenital 753.8
  urethroscrotal 608.89
  urethrovaginal 619.0
  urethrovesical 596.2
  urethrovesicovaginal 619.0
  urinary (persistent) (recurrent) 599.1
  uteroabdominal (anterior wall)
      619.2
    congenital 752.3
  uteroenteric 619.1
  uterofecal 619.1
  uterointestinal 619.1
    congenital 752.3
  uterorectal 619.1
    congenital 752.3
  uteroureteric 619.0
  uterovaginal 619.8

Fistula *(Continued)*
  uterovesical 619.0
    congenital 752.3
  uterus 619.8
  vagina (wall) 619.8
    postpartal, old 619.8
  vaginocutaneous (postpartal) 619.2
  vaginoileal (acquired) 619.1
  vaginoperineal 619.2
  vesical NEC 596.2
  vesicoabdominal 596.2
  vesicocervicovaginal 619.0
  vesicocolic 596.1
  vesicocutaneous 596.2
  vesicoenteric 596.1
  vesicointestinal 596.1
  vesicometrorectal 619.1
  vesicoperineal 596.2
  vesicorectal 596.1
    congenital 753.8
  vesicosigmoidal 596.1
  vesicosigmoidovaginal 619.1
  vesicoureteral 596.2
  vesicoureterovaginal 619.0
  vesicourethral 596.2
  vesicourethrorectal 596.1
  vesicouterine 619.0
    congenital 752.3
  vesicovaginal 619.0
  vulvorectal 619.1
    congenital 752.49
Fit 780.39
  apoplectic *(see also* Disease,
      cerebrovascular, acute) 436
    late effect - *see* Late effect(s) (of)
        cerebrovascular disease
  epileptic *(see also* Epilepsy) 345.9●
  fainting 780.2
  hysterical 300.11
  newborn 779.0
Fitting (of)
  artificial
    arm (complete) (partial) V52.0
    breast V52.4
      implant exchange (different
          material) (different size)
          V52.4
    eye(s) V52.2
    leg(s) (complete) (partial) V52.1
  brain neuropacemaker V53.02
  cardiac pacemaker V53.31
  carotid sinus pacemaker V53.39
  cerebral ventricle (communicating)
      shunt V53.01
  colostomy belt V55.3
  contact lenses V53.1
  cystostomy device V53.6
  defibrillator, automatic implantable
      cardiac V53.32
  dentures V52.3
  device, unspecified type V53.90
    abdominal V53.59   ◀▥●
    cardiac
      defibrillator, automatic
          implantable V53.32
      pacemaker V53.31
      specified NEC V53.39
    cerebral ventricle (communicating)
        shunt V53.01
    gastrointestinal NEC V53.59   ◀
    insulin pump V53.91
    intestinal V53.50   ◀
    intrauterine contraceptive V25.1
    nervous system V53.09

Fitting *(Continued)*
  device, unspecified type *(Continued)*
    orthodontic V53.4
    orthoptic V53.1
    other device V53.99
    prosthetic V52.9
      breast V52.4
      dental V52.3
      eye V52.2
      specified type NEC V52.8
    special senses V53.09
    substitution
      auditory V53.09
      nervous system V53.09
      visual V53.09
    urinary V53.6
  diaphragm (contraceptive) V25.02
  gastric lap band V53.51   ◀
  gastrointestinal appliance and device
      NEC V53.59   ◀
  glasses (reading) V53.1
  growth rod V54.02
  hearing aid V53.2
  ileostomy device V55.2
  intestinal appliance and ~~or~~ device ~~NEC~~
      V53.50   ◀▥
  intrauterine contraceptive device V25.1
  neuropacemaker (brain) (peripheral
      nerve) (spinal cord) V53.02
  orthodontic device V53.4
  orthopedic (device) V53.7
    brace V53.7
    cast V53.7
    corset V53.7
    shoes V53.7
  pacemaker (cardiac) V53.31
    brain V53.02
    carotid sinus V53.39
    peripheral nerve V53.02
    spinal cord V53.02
  prosthesis V52.9
    arm (complete) (partial) V52.0
    breast V52.4
      implant exchange (different
          material) (different size)
          V52.4
    dental V52.3
    eye V52.2
    leg (complete) (partial) V52.1
    specified type NEC V52.8
  spectacles V53.1
  wheelchair V53.8
Fitz's syndrome (acute hemorrhagic
    pancreatitis) 577.0
Fitz-Hugh and Curtis syndrome 098.86
  due to
    Chlamydia trachomatis 099.56
    Neisseria gonorrhoeae (gonococcal
        peritonitis) 098.86
Fixation
  joint - *see* Ankylosis
  larynx 478.79
  pupil 364.76
  stapes 385.22
    deafness *(see also* Deafness,
        conductive) 389.04
  uterus (acquired) - *see* Malposition,
      uterus
  vocal cord 478.5
Flaccid - *see also* condition
  foot 736.79
  forearm 736.09
  palate, congenital 750.26
Flail
  chest 807.4
    newborn 767.3

Flail *(Continued)*
  joint (paralytic) 718.80
    ankle 718.87
    elbow 718.82
    foot 718.87
    hand 718.84
    hip 718.85
    knee 718.86
    multiple sites 718.89
    pelvic region 718.85
    shoulder (region) 718.81
    specified site NEC 718.88
    wrist 718.83
Flajani (-Basedow) syndrome or disease
    (exophthalmic goiter) 242.0●
Flap, liver 572.8
Flare, anterior chamber (aqueous) (eye)
    364.04
Flashback phenomena (drug)
    (hallucinogenic) 292.89
Flat
  chamber (anterior) (eye) 360.34
  chest, congenital 754.89
  electroencephalogram (EEG) 348.89 ◀▥
  foot (acquired) (fixed type) (painful)
    (postural) (spastic) 734
    congenital 754.61
      rocker bottom 754.61
      vertical talus 754.61
    rachitic 268.1
    rocker bottom (congenital) 754.61
    vertical talus, congenital 754.61
  organ or site, congenital NEC - *see*
    Anomaly, specified type NEC
  pelvis 738.6
    with disproportion (fetopelvic)
      653.2●
      affecting fetus or newborn 763.1
      causing obstructed labor 660.1●
        affecting fetus or newborn
          763.1
    congenital 755.69
Flatau-Schilder disease 341.1
Flattening
  head, femur 736.39
  hip 736.39
  lip (congenital) 744.89
  nose (congenital) 754.0
    acquired 738.0
Flatulence 787.3
Flatus 787.3
  vaginalis 629.89
Flax dressers' disease 504
Flea bite - *see* Injury, superficial, by site
Fleischer (-Kayser) ring (corneal
    pigmentation) 275.1 *[371.14]*
Fleischner's disease 732.3
Fleshy mole 631
Flexibilitas cerea (*see also* Catalepsy) 300.11
Flexion
  cervix - *see* Flexion, uterus
  contracture, joint (*see also* Contraction,
    joint) 718.4●
  deformity, joint (*see also* Contraction,
    joint) 736.9
    hip, congenital (*see also* Subluxation,
      congenital, hip) 754.32
  uterus (*see also* Malposition, uterus)
    621.6
Flexner's
  bacillus 004.1
  diarrhea (ulcerative) 004.1
  dysentery 004.1
Flexner-Boyd dysentery 004.2

Flexure - *see* condition
Floater, vitreous 379.24
Floating
  cartilage (joint) (*see also* Disorder,
    cartilage, articular) 718.0●
    knee 717.6
  gallbladder (congenital) 751.69
  kidney 593.0
    congenital 753.3
  liver (congenital) 751.69
  rib 756.3
  spleen 289.59
Flooding 626.2
Floor - *see* condition
Floppy
  infant NEC 781.99
  iris syndrome 364.81
  valve syndrome (mitral) 424.0
Flu - *see also* Influenza
  bird 488.0   ◀
  gastric NEC 008.8
  swine 488.1   ◀
Fluctuating blood pressure 796.4
Fluid
  abdomen 789.59
  chest (*see also* Pleurisy, with effusion)
    511.9
  heart (*see also* Failure, heart) 428.0
  joint (*see also* Effusion, joint) 719.0●
  loss (acute) 276.50
    with
      hypernatremia 276.0
      hyponatremia 276.1
  lung - *see also* Edema, lung
    encysted 511.89
  peritoneal cavity 789.59
    malignant 789.51
  pleural cavity (*see also* Pleurisy, with
    effusion) 511.9
  retention 276.6
Flukes NEC (*see also* Infestation, fluke)
    121.9
  blood NEC (*see also* Infestation,
    Schistosoma) 120.9
  liver 121.3
Fluor (albus) (vaginalis) 623.5
  trichomonal (Trichomonas vaginalis)
    131.00
Fluorosis (dental) (chronic) 520.3
Flushing 782.62
  menopausal 627.2
Flush syndrome 259.2
Flutter
  atrial or auricular 427.32
  heart (ventricular) 427.42
    atrial 427.32
  impure 427.32
  postoperative 997.1
  ventricular 427.42
Flux (bloody) (serosanguineous) 009.0
Focal - *see* condition
Fochier's abscess - *see* Abscess, by site
Focus, Assmann's (*see also* Tuberculosis)
    011.0●
Fogo selvagem 694.4
Foix-Alajouanine syndrome 336.1
Folds, anomalous - *see also* Anomaly,
    specified type NEC
  Bowman's membrane 371.31
  Descemet's membrane 371.32
  epicanthic 743.63
  heart 746.89
  posterior segment of eye, congenital
    743.54

Folie a deux 297.3
Follicle
  cervix (nabothian) (ruptured) 616.0
  graafian, ruptured, with hemorrhage
    620.0
  nabothian 616.0
Folliclis (primary) (*see also* Tuberculosis)
    017.0●
Follicular - *see also* condition
  cyst (atretic) 620.0
Folliculitis 704.8
  abscedens et suffodiens 704.8
  decalvans 704.09
  gonorrheal (acute) 098.0
    chronic or duration of 2 months or
      more 098.2
  keloid, keloidalis 706.1
  pustular 704.8
  ulerythematosa reticulata 701.8
Folliculosis, conjunctival 372.02
Følling's disease (phenylketonuria) 270.1
Follow-up (examination) (routine)
    (following) V67.9
  cancer chemotherapy V67.2
  chemotherapy V67.2
  fracture V67.4
  high-risk medication V67.51
  injury NEC V67.59
  postpartum
    immediately after delivery V24.0
    routine V24.2
  psychiatric V67.3
  psychotherapy V67.3
  radiotherapy V67.1
  specified condition NEC V67.59
  specified surgery NEC V67.09
  surgery V67.00
    vaginal pap smear V67.01
  treatment V67.9
    combined NEC V67.6
    fracture V67.4
    involving high-risk medication NEC
      V67.51
    mental disorder V67.3
    specified NEC V67.59
Fong's syndrome (hereditary
    osteoonychodysplasia) 756.89
Food
  allergy 693.1
  anaphylactic shock - *see* Anaphylactic
    shock, due to food
  asphyxia (from aspiration or
    inhalation) (*see also* Asphyxia,
    food) 933.1
  choked on (*see also* Asphyxia, food) 933.1
  deprivation 994.2
    specified kind of food NEC 269.8
  intoxication (*see also* Poisoning, food)
    005.9
  lack of 994.2
  poisoning (*see also* Poisoning, food)
    005.9
  refusal or rejection NEC 307.59
  strangulation or suffocation (*see also*
    Asphyxia, food) 933.1
  toxemia (*see also* Poisoning, food) 005.9
Foot - *see also* condition
  and mouth disease 078.4
  process disease 581.3
Foramen ovale (nonclosure) (patent)
    (persistent) 745.5
Forbes' (glycogen storage) disease 271.0
Forbes-Albright syndrome (nonpuerperal
    amenorrhea and lactation associated
    with pituitary tumor) 253.1

Forced birth or delivery NEC 669.8●
   affecting fetus or newborn NEC 763.89
Forceps
   delivery NEC 669.5●
      affecting fetus or newborn 763.2
Fordyce's disease (ectopic sebaceous
   glands) (mouth) 750.26
Fordyce-Fox disease (apocrine miliaria)
   705.82
Forearm - *see* condition
Foreign body

> **Note 27** For foreign body with open
> wound or other injury, see Wound,
> open, or the type of injury specified.

   accidentally left during a procedure
      998.4
   anterior chamber (eye) 871.6
      magnetic 871.5
         retained or old 360.51
      retained or old 360.61
   ciliary body (eye) 871.6
      magnetic 871.5
         retained or old 360.52
      retained or old 360.62
   entering through orifice (current) (old)
      accessory sinus 932
      air passage (upper) 933.0
         lower 934.8
      alimentary canal 938
      alveolar process 935.0
      antrum (Highmore) 932
      anus 937
      appendix 936
      asphyxia due to (*see also* Asphyxia,
         food) 933.1
      auditory canal 931
      auricle 931
      bladder 939.0
      bronchioles 934.8
      bronchus (main) 934.1
      buccal cavity 935.0
      canthus (inner) 930.1
      cecum 936
      cervix (canal) uterine 939.1
      coil, ileocecal 936
      colon 936
      conjunctiva 930.1
      conjunctival sac 930.1
      cornea 930.0
      digestive organ or tract NEC 938
      duodenum 936
      ear (external) 931
      esophagus 935.1
      eye (external) 930.9
         combined sites 930.8
         intraocular - *see* Foreign body, by
            site
         specified site NEC 930.8
      eyeball 930.8
         intraocular - *see* Foreign body,
            intraocular
      eyelid 930.1
         retained or old 374.86
      frontal sinus 932
      gastrointestinal tract 938
      genitourinary tract 939.9
      globe 930.8
         penetrating 871.6
            magnetic 871.5
               retained or old 360.50
            retained or old 360.60
      gum 935.0

Foreign body (*Continued*)
   entering through orifice (*Continued*)
      Highmore's antrum 932
      hypopharynx 933.0
      ileocecal coil 936
      ileum 936
      inspiration (of) 933.1
      intestine (large) (small) 936
      lacrimal apparatus, duct, gland, or
         sac 930.2
      larynx 933.1
      lung 934.8
      maxillary sinus 932
      mouth 935.0
      nasal sinus 932
      nasopharynx 933.0
      nose (passage) 932
      nostril 932
      oral cavity 935.0
      palate 935.0
      penis 939.3
      pharynx 933.0
      pyriform sinus 933.0
      rectosigmoid 937
         junction 937
      rectum 937
      respiratory tract 934.9
         specified part NEC 934.8
      sclera 930.1
      sinus 932
         accessory 932
         frontal 932
         maxillary 932
         nasal 932
         pyriform 933.0
      small intestine 936
      stomach (hairball) 935.2
      suffocation by (*see also* Asphyxia,
         food) 933.1
      swallowed 938
         tongue 933.0
      tear ducts or glands 930.2
      throat 933.0
      tongue 935.0
         swallowed 933.0
      tonsil, tonsillar 933.0
         fossa 933.0
      trachea 934.0
      ureter 939.0
      urethra 939.0
      uterus (any part) 939.1
      vagina 939.2
      vulva 939.2
      wind pipe 934.0
   feeling of, in throat 784.99
   granuloma (old) 728.82
      bone 733.99
      in operative wound (inadvertently
         left) 998.4
         due to surgical material
            intentionally left - *see*
            Complications, due to
            (presence of) any device,
            implant, or graft classified
            to 996.0–996.5 NEC
      muscle 728.82
      skin 709.4
      soft tissue NEC 709.4
      subcutaneous tissue 709.4
   in
      bone (residual) 733.99
      open wound - *see* Wound, open, by
         site complicated
      soft tissue (residual) 729.6

Foreign body (*Continued*)
   inadvertently left in operation
      wound (causing adhesions,
      obstruction, or perforation)
      998.4
   ingestion, ingested NEC 938
   inhalation or inspiration (*see also*
      Asphyxia, food) 933.1
   internal organ, not entering
      through an orifice - *see* Injury,
      internal, by site, with open
      wound
   intraocular (nonmagnetic) 871.6
      combined sites 871.6
         magnetic 871.5
            retained or old 360.59
         retained or old 360.69
      magnetic 871.5
         retained or old 360.50
      retained or old 360.60
      specified site NEC 871.6
         magnetic 871.5
            retained or old 360.59
         retained or old 360.69
   iris (nonmagnetic) 871.6
      magnetic 871.5
         retained or old 360.52
      retained or old 360.62
   lens (nonmagnetic) 871.6
      magnetic 871.5
         retained or old 360.53
      retained or old 360.63
   lid, eye 930.1
   ocular muscle 870.4
      retained or old 376.6
   old or residual
      bone 733.99
      eyelid 374.86
      middle ear 385.83
      muscle 729.6
         ocular 376.6
         retrobulbar 376.6
      skin 729.6
         with granuloma 709.4
      soft tissue 729.6
         with granuloma 709.4
      subcutaneous tissue 729.6
         with granuloma 709.4
   operation wound, left accidentally
      998.4
   orbit 870.4
      retained or old 376.6
   posterior wall, eye 871.6
      magnetic 871.5
         retained or old 360.55
      retained or old 360.65
   respiratory tree 934.9
      specified site NEC 934.8
   retained (old) (nonmagnetic) (in)
      anterior chamber (eye) 360.61
         magnetic 360.51
      ciliary body 360.62
         magnetic 360.52
      eyelid 374.86
      globe 360.60
         magnetic 360.50
      intraocular 360.60
         magnetic 360.50
         specified site NEC 360.69
            magnetic 360.59
      iris 360.62
         magnetic 360.52
      lens 360.63
         magnetic 360.53

Foreign body (*Continued*)
  retained (*Continued*)
    muscle 729.6
    orbit 376.6
    posterior wall of globe 360.65
      magnetic 360.55
    retina 360.65
      magnetic 360.55
    retrobulbar 376.6
    skin 729.6
      with granuloma 709.4
    soft tissue 729.6
      with granuloma 709.4
    subcutaneous tissue 729.6
      with granuloma 709.4
    vitreous 360.64
      magnetic 360.54
  retina 871.6
    magnetic 871.5
      retained or old 360.55
    retained or old 360.65
  superficial, without major open wound
    (*see also* Injury, superficial, by site)
    919.6
  swallowed NEC 938
  throat, feeling of 784.99
  vitreous (humor) 871.6
    magnetic 871.5
      retained or old 360.54
    retained or old 360.64
Forking, aqueduct of Sylvius
  742.3
  with spina bifida (*see also*
    Spina bifida) 741.0●
Formation
  bone in scar tissue (skin) 709.3
  connective tissue in vitreous
    379.25
  Elschnig pearls (postcataract
    extraction) 366.51
  hyaline in cornea 371.49
  sequestrum in bone (due to infection)
    (*see also* Osteomyelitis)
    730.1●
  valve
    colon, congenital 751.5
    ureter (congenital) 753.29
Formication 782.0
Fort Bragg fever 100.89
Fossa - *see also* condition
  pyriform - *see* condition
Foster care (status) V60.81 ◀
Foster-Kennedy syndrome 377.04
Fothergill's
  disease, meaning scarlatina anginosa
    034.1
  neuralgia (*see also* Neuralgia,
    trigeminal) 350.1
Foul breath 784.99
Found dead (cause unknown)
  798.9
Foundling V20.0
Fournier's disease (idiopathic gangrene)
  608.83
Fourth
  cranial nerve - *see* condition
  disease 057.8
  molar 520.1
Foville's syndrome 344.89
Fox's
  disease (apocrine miliaria) 705.82
  impetigo (contagiosa) 684
Fox-Fordyce disease (apocrine miliaria)
  705.82

Fracture (abduction) (adduction)
  (avulsion) (compression) (crush)
  (dislocation) (oblique) (separation)
  (closed) 829.0

Note 28   For fracture of any of the following sites with fracture of other bones - *see* Fracture, multiple.

"Closed" includes the following descriptions of fractures, with or without delayed healing, unless they are specified as open or compound:

  comminuted
  depressed
  elevated
  fissured
  greenstick
  impacted
  linear
  simple
  slipped epiphysis
  spiral
  unspecified

"Open" includes the following descriptions of fractures, with or without delayed healing:

  compound
  infected
  missile
  puncture
  with foreign body

For late effect of fracture, *see* Late, effect, fracture, by site.

---

  with
    internal injuries in same region
      (conditions classifiable to
      860–869) - *see also* Injury,
      internal, by site
      pelvic region - *see* Fracture,
        pelvis
  acetabulum (with visceral injury)
    (closed) 808.0
    open 808.1
  acromion (process) (closed) 811.01
    open 811.11
  alveolus (closed) 802.8
    open 802.9
  ankle (malleolus) (closed) 824.8
    bimalleolar (Dupuytren's) (Pott's)
      824.4
      open 824.5
    bone 825.21
      open 825.31
    lateral malleolus only (fibular)
      824.2
      open 824.3
    medial malleolus only (tibial) 824.0
      open 824.1
    open 824.9
    pathologic 733.16
    talus 825.21
      open 825.31
    trimalleolar 824.6
      open 824.7
  antrum - *see* Fracture, skull, base
  arm (closed) 818.0
    and leg(s) (any bones) 828.0
      open 828.1
    both (any bones) (with rib(s)) (with
      sternum) 819.0
      open 819.1

Fracture (*Continued*)
  arm (*Continued*)
    lower 813.80
      open 813.90
      open 818.1
    upper - *see* Fracture, humerus
  astragalus (closed) 825.21
    open 825.31
  atlas - *see* Fracture, vertebra, cervical,
    first
  axis - *see* Fracture, vertebra, cervical,
    second
  back - *see* Fracture, vertebra, by site
  Barton's - *see* Fracture, radius, lower end
  basal (skull) - *see* Fracture, skull, base
  Bennett's (closed) 815.01
    open 815.11
  bimalleolar (closed) 824.4
    open 824.5
  bone (closed) NEC 829.0
    birth injury NEC 767.3
    open 829.1
    pathological NEC (*see also* Fracture,
      pathologic) 733.10
    stress NEC (*see also* Fracture, stress)
      733.95
  boot top - *see* Fracture, fibula
  boxers' - *see* Fracture, metacarpal
    bone(s)
  breast bone - *see* Fracture, sternum
  buckle - *see* Fracture, torus   ◀
  bucket handle (semilunar cartilage) -
    see Tear, meniscus
  burst - *see* Fracture, traumatic, by site
  bursting - *see* Fracture, phalanx, hand,
    distal
  calcaneus (closed) 825.0
    open 825.1
  capitate (bone) (closed) 814.07
    open 814.17
  capitellum (humerus) (closed) 812.49
    open 812.59
  carpal bone(s) (wrist NEC) (closed)
    814.00
    open 814.10
    specified site NEC 814.09
      open 814.19
  cartilage, knee (semilunar) - *see* Tear,
    meniscus
  cervical - *see* Fracture, vertebra, cervical
  chauffeur's - *see* Fracture, ulna, lower
    end
  chisel - *see* Fracture, radius, upper end
  chronic - *see* Fracture, pathologic   ◀
  clavicle (interligamentous part)
    (closed) 810.00
    acromial end 810.03
      open 810.13
    due to birth trauma 767.2
    open 810.10
    shaft (middle third) 810.02
      open 810.12
    sternal end 810.01
      open 810.11
  clayshovelers' - *see* Fracture, vertebra,
    cervical
  coccyx - *see also* Fracture, vertebra,
    coccyx
    complicating delivery 665.6●
  collar bone - *see* Fracture, clavicle
  Colles' (reversed) (closed) 813.41
    open 813.51
  comminuted - *see* Fracture, by site
  compression - *see also* Fracture, by site
    nontraumatic - *see* Fracture,
      pathologic

◀ New   ◀▥ Revised   ~~deleted~~ Deleted   ● Use Additional Digit(s)   ▨ Omit code

Fracture (Continued)
  congenital 756.9
  coracoid process (closed) 811.02
    open 811.12
  coronoid process (ulna) (closed) 813.02
    mandible (closed) 802.23
      open 802.33
    open 813.12
  corpus cavernosum penis 959.13
  costochondral junction - see Fracture, rib
  costosternal junction - see Fracture, rib
  cranium - see Fracture, skull, by site
  cricoid cartilage (closed) 807.5
    open 807.6
  cuboid (ankle) (closed) 825.23
    open 825.33
  cuneiform
    foot (closed) 825.24
      open 825.34
    wrist (closed) 814.03
      open 814.13
  dental implant 525.73
  dental restorative material
    with loss of material 525.64
    without loss of material 525.63
  due to
    birth injury - see Birth injury, fracture
    gunshot - see Fracture, by site, open
    neoplasm - see Fracture, pathologic
    osteoporosis - see Fracture, pathologic
  Dupuytren's (ankle) (fibula) (closed) 824.4
    open 824.5
    radius 813.42
      open 813.52
  Duverney's - see Fracture, ilium
  elbow - see also Fracture, humerus, lower end
    olecranon (process) (closed) 813.01
      open 813.11
    supracondylar (closed) 812.41
      open 812.51
  ethmoid (bone) (sinus) - see Fracture, skull, base
  face bone(s) (closed) NEC 802.8
    with
      other bone(s) - see Fracture, multiple, skull
      skull - see also Fracture, skull
        involving other bones - see Fracture, multiple, skull
    open 802.9
  fatigue - see Fracture, march
  femur, femoral (closed) 821.00
    cervicotrochanteric 820.03
      open 820.13
    condyles, epicondyles 821.21
      open 821.31
    distal end - see Fracture, femur, lower end
    epiphysis (separation)
      capital 820.01
        open 820.11
      head 820.01
        open 820.11
      lower 821.22
        open 821.32
      trochanteric 820.01
        open 820.11
      upper 820.01
        open 820.11

Fracture (Continued)
  femur, femoral (Continued)
    head 820.09
      open 820.19
    lower end or extremity (distal end) (closed) 821.20
      condyles, epicondyles 821.21
        open 821.31
      epiphysis (separation) 821.22
        open 821.32
      multiple sites 821.29
        open 821.39
      open 821.30
      specified site NEC 821.29
        open 821.39
      supracondylar 821.23
        open 821.33
      T-shaped 821.21
        open 821.31
    neck (closed) 820.8
      base (cervicotrochanteric) 820.03
        open 820.13
      extracapsular 820.20
        open 820.30
      intertrochanteric (section) 820.21
        open 820.31
      intracapsular 820.00
        open 820.10
      intratrochanteric 820.21
        open 820.31
      midcervical 820.02
        open 820.12
      open 820.9
      pathologic 733.14
        specified part NEC 733.15
      specified site NEC 820.09
        open 820.19
      transcervical 820.02
        open 820.12
      transtrochanteric 820.20
        open 820.30
    open 821.10
    pathologic 733.14
      specified part NEC 733.15
    peritrochanteric (section) 820.20
      open 820.30
    shaft (lower third) (middle third) (upper third) 821.01
      open 821.11
    subcapital 820.09
      open 820.19
    subtrochanteric (region) (section) 820.22
      open 820.32
    supracondylar 821.23
      open 821.33
    transepiphyseal 820.01
      open 820.11
    trochanter (greater) (lesser) (see also Fracture, femur, neck, by site) 820.20
      open 820.30
    T-shaped, into knee joint 821.21
      open 821.31
    upper end 820.8
      open 820.9
  fibula (closed) 823.81
    with tibia 823.82
      open 823.92
    distal end 824.8
      open 824.9

Fracture (Continued)
  fibula (Continued)
    epiphysis
      lower 824.8
        open 824.9
      upper - see Fracture, fibula, upper end
    head - see Fracture, fibula, upper end
    involving ankle 824.2
      open 824.3
    lower end or extremity 824.8
      open 824.9
    malleolus (external) (lateral) 824.2
      open 824.3
    open NEC 823.91
    pathologic 733.16
    proximal end - see Fracture, fibula, upper end
    shaft 823.21
      with tibia 823.22
        open 823.32
      open 823.31
    stress 733.93
    torus 823.41
      with tibia 823.42
    upper end or extremity (epiphysis) (head) (proximal end) (styloid) 823.01
      with tibia 823.02
        open 823.12
      open 823.11
  finger(s), of one hand (closed) (see also Fracture, phalanx, hand) 816.00
    with
      metacarpal bone(s), of same hand 817.0
        open 817.1
      thumb of same hand 816.03
        open 816.13
    open 816.10
  foot, except toe(s) alone (closed) 825.20
    open 825.30
  forearm (closed) NEC 813.80
    lower end (distal end) (lower epiphysis) 813.40
      open 813.50
    open 813.90
    shaft 813.20
      open 813.30
    upper end (proximal end) (upper epiphysis) 813.00
      open 813.10
  fossa, anterior, middle, or posterior - see Fracture, skull, base
  frontal (bone) - see also Fracture, skull, vault
    sinus - see Fracture, skull, base
  Galeazzi's - see Fracture, radius, lower end
  glenoid (cavity) (fossa) (scapula) (closed) 811.03
    open 811.13
  Gosselin's - see Fracture, ankle
  greenstick - see Fracture, by site
  grenade-throwers' - see Fracture, humerus, shaft
  gutter - see Fracture, skull, vault
  hamate (closed) 814.08
    open 814.18
  hand, one (closed) 815.00
    carpals 814.00
      open 814.10
      specified site NEC 814.09
        open 814.19

Fracture (Continued)
  hand, one (Continued)
    metacarpals 815.00
      open 815.10
    multiple, bones of one hand
      817.0
      open 817.1
    open 815.10
    phalanges (see also Fracture,
      phalanx, hand) 816.00
      open 816.10
  healing
    aftercare (see also Aftercare, fracture)
      V54.89
    change of cast V54.89
    complications - see condition
    convalescence V66.4
    removal of
      cast V54.89
      fixation device
        external V54.89
        internal V54.01
  heel bone (closed) 825.0
    open 825.1
  Hill-Sachs 812.09
  hip (closed) (see also Fracture, femur,
    neck) 820.8
    open 820.9
    pathologic 733.14
  humerus (closed) 812.20
    anatomical neck 812.02
      open 812.12
    articular process (see also Fracture
      humerus, condyle(s)) 812.44
      open 812.54
    capitellum 812.49
      open 812.59
    condyle(s) 812.44
      lateral (external) 812.42
        open 812.52
      medial (internal epicondyle)
        812.43
        open 812.53
      open 812.54
    distal end - see Fracture, humerus,
      lower end
    epiphysis
      lower (see also Fracture, humerus,
        condyle(s)) 812.44
        open 812.54
      upper 812.09
        open 812.19
    external condyle 812.42
      open 812.52
    great tuberosity 812.03
      open 812.13
    head 812.09
      open 812.19
    internal epicondyle 812.43
      open 812.53
    lesser tuberosity 812.09
      open 812.19
    lower end or extremity (distal end)
      (see also Fracture, humerus, by
      site) 812.40
      multiple sites NEC 812.49
        open 812.59
      open 812.50
      specified site NEC 812.49
        open 812.59
    neck 812.01
      open 812.11
    open 812.30
    pathologic 733.11

Fracture (Continued)
  humerus (Continued)
    proximal end - see Fracture,
      humerus, upper end
    shaft 812.21
      open 812.31
    supracondylar 812.41
      open 812.51
    surgical neck 812.01
      open 812.11
    trochlea 812.49
      open 812.59
    T-shaped 812.44
      open 812.54
    tuberosity - see Fracture, humerus,
      upper end
    upper end or extremity (proximal
      end) (see also Fracture,
      humerus, by site) 812.00
      open 812.10
      specified site NEC 812.09
        open 812.19
  hyoid bone (closed) 807.5
    open 807.6
  hyperextension - see Fracture, radius,
    lower end
  ilium (with visceral injury) (closed)
    808.41
    open 808.51
  impaction, impacted - see Fracture, by
    site
  incus - see Fracture, skull, base
  innominate bone (with visceral injury)
    (closed) 808.49
    open 808.59
  instep, of one foot (closed) 825.20
    with toe(s) of same foot 827.0
      open 827.1
    open 825.30
  insufficiency - see Fracture, pathologic,
    by site
  internal
    ear - see Fracture, skull, base
    semilunar cartilage, knee - see Tear,
      meniscus, medial
  intertrochanteric - see Fracture, femur,
    neck, intertrochanteric
  ischium (with visceral injury) (closed)
    808.42
    open 808.52
  jaw (bone) (lower) (closed) (see also
    Fracture, mandible) 802.20
    angle 802.25
      open 802.35
    open 802.30
    upper - see Fracture, maxilla
  knee
    cap (closed) 822.0
      open 822.1
    cartilage (semilunar) - see Tear,
      meniscus
  labyrinth (osseous) - see Fracture, skull,
    base
  larynx (closed) 807.5
    open 807.6
  late effect - see Late, effects (of),
    fracture
  Le Fort's - see Fracture, maxilla
  leg (closed) 827.0
    with rib(s) or sternum 828.0
      open 828.1
    both (any bones) 828.0
      open 828.1
    lower - see Fracture, tibia

Fracture (Continued)
  leg (Continued)
    open 827.1
    upper - see Fracture, femur
  limb
    lower (multiple) (closed) NEC
      827.0
      open 827.1
    upper (multiple) (closed) NEC
      818.0
      open 818.1
  long bones, due to birth trauma - see
    Birth injury, fracture
  lumbar - see Fracture, vertebra,
    lumbar
  lunate bone (closed) 814.02
    open 814.12
  malar bone (closed) 802.4
    open 802.5
  Malgaigne's (closed) 808.43
    open 808.53
  malleolus (closed) 824.8
    bimalleolar 824.4
      open 824.5
    lateral 824.2
      and medial - see also Fracture,
        malleolus, bimalleolar
        with lip of tibia - see
          Fracture, malleolus,
          trimalleolar
      open 824.3
    medial (closed) 824.0
      and lateral - see also Fracture,
        malleolus, bimalleolar
        with lip of tibia - see
          Fracture, malleolus,
          trimalleolar
      open 824.1
    open 824.9
    trimalleolar (closed) 824.6
      open 824.7
  malleus - see Fracture, skull, base
  malunion 733.81
  mandible (closed) 802.20
    angle 802.25
      open 802.35
    body 802.28
      alveolar border 802.27
        open 802.37
      open 802.38
      symphysis 802.26
        open 802.36
    condylar process 802.21
      open 802.31
    coronoid process 802.23
      open 802.33
    multiple sites 802.29
      open 802.39
    open 802.30
    ramus NEC 802.24
      open 802.34
    subcondylar 802.22
      open 802.32
  manubrium - see Fracture, sternum
  march 733.95
    fibula 733.93
    metatarsals 733.94
    tibia 733.93
  maxilla, maxillary (superior) (upper
    jaw) (closed) 802.4
    inferior - see Fracture, mandible
    open 802.5
  meniscus, knee - see Tear, meniscus

Fracture *(Continued)*
  metacarpus, metacarpal (bone(s)), of
    one hand (closed) 815.00
    with phalanx, phalanges, hand
      (finger(s)) (thumb) of same
      hand 817.0
      open 817.1
    base 815.02
      first metacarpal 815.01
        open 815.11
        open 815.12
      thumb 815.01
        open 815.11
    multiple sites 815.09
      open 815.19
    neck 815.04
      open 815.14
    open 815.10
    shaft 815.03
      open 815.13
  metatarsus, metatarsal (bone(s)), of one
    foot (closed) 825.25
    with tarsal bone(s) 825.29
      open 825.39
    open 825.35
  Monteggia's (closed) 813.03
    open 813.13
  Moore's - *see* Fracture, radius, lower
    end
  multangular bone (closed)
    larger 814.05
      open 814.15
    smaller 814.06
      open 814.16
  multiple (closed) 829.0

Note 29 Multiple fractures of sites classifiable to the same three- or four-digit category are coded to that category, except for sites classifiable to 810–818 or 820–827 in different limbs.

Multiple fractures of sites classifiable to different fourth-digit subdivisions within the same three-digit category should be dealt with according to coding rules.

Multiple fractures of sites classifiable to different three-digit categories (identifiable from the listing under "Fracture"), and of sites classifiable to 810–818 or 820–827 in different limbs should be coded according to the following list, which should be referred to in the following priority order: skull or face bones, pelvis or vertebral column, legs, arms.

---

  arm (multiple bones in same arm
    except in hand alone) (sites
    classifiable to 810–817 with
    sites classifiable to a different
    three-digit category in
    810–817 in same arm) (closed)
    818.0
    open 818.1
  arms, both or arm(s) with rib(s) or
    sternum (sites classifiable to
    810–818 with sites classifiable
    to same range of categories in
    other limb or to 807) (closed)
    819.0
    open 819.1

Fracture *(Continued)*
  multiple *(Continued)*
    bones of trunk NEC (closed) 809.0
      open 809.1
    hand, metacarpal bone(s) with
      phalanx or phalanges of same
      hand (sites classifiable to 815
      with sites classifiable to 816 in
      same hand) (closed) 817.0
      open 817.1
    leg (multiple bones in same leg)
      (sites classifiable to 820–826
      with sites classifiable to a
      different three-digit category
      in that range in same leg)
      (closed) 827.0
      open 827.1
    legs, both or leg(s) with arm(s),
      rib(s), or sternum (sites
      classifiable to 820–827 with
      sites classifiable to same range
      of categories in other leg or to
      807 or 810–819) (closed) 828.0
      open 828.1
    open 829.1
    pelvis with other bones except skull
      or face bones (sites classifiable
      to 808 with sites classifiable to
      805–807 or 810–829) (closed)
      809.0
      open 809.1
    skull, specified or unspecified bones,
      or face bone(s) with any other
      bone(s) (sites classifiable to
      800–803 with sites classifiable
      to 805–829) (closed) 804.0●

Note 30 Use the following fifth-digit subclassification with categories 800, 801, 803, and 804:

0 unspecified state of
     consciousness
1 with no loss of consciousness
2 with brief [less than one hour]
     loss of consciousness
3 with moderate [1–24 hours] loss
     of consciousness
4 with prolonged [more than 24
     hours] loss of
     consciousness and return
     to pre-existing conscious
     level
5 with prolonged [more than 24
     hours] loss of
     consciousness, without
     return to pre-existing
     conscious level

Use fifth-digit 5 to designate when a patient is unconscious and dies before regaining consciousness, regardless of the duration of the loss of consciousness

6 with loss of consciousness of
     unspecified duration
9 with concussion, unspecified

---

  with
    contusion, cerebral 804.1●
    epidural hemorrhage 804.2●
    extradural hemorrhage 804.2●
    hemorrhage (intracranial) NEC
      804.3●
    intracranial injury NEC 804.4●
    laceration, cerebral 804.1●

Fracture *(Continued)*
  multiple *(Continued)*
    with *(Continued)*
      subarachnoid hemorrhage 804.2●
      subdural hemorrhage 804.2●
    open 804.5●
      with
        contusion, cerebral 804.6●
        epidural hemorrhage 804.7●
        extradural hemorrhage 804.7●
        hemorrhage (intracranial)
          NEC 804.8●
        intracranial injury NEC 804.9●
        laceration, cerebral 804.6●
        subarachnoid hemorrhage
          804.7●
        subdural hemorrhage 804.7●
  vertebral column with other bones,
    except skull or face bones (sites
    classifiable to 805 or 806 with
    sites classifiable to 807–808 or
    810–829) (closed) 809.0
    open 809.1
  nasal (bone(s)) (closed) 802.0
    open 802.1
    sinus - *see* Fracture, skull, base
  navicular
    carpal (wrist) (closed) 814.01
      open 814.11
    tarsal (ankle) (closed) 825.22
      open 825.32
  neck - *see* Fracture, vertebra, cervical
  neural arch - *see* Fracture, vertebra, by
    site
  nonunion 733.82
  nose, nasal, (bone) (septum) (closed)
    802.0
    open 802.1
  occiput - *see* Fracture, skull, base
  odontoid process - *see* Fracture,
    vertebra, cervical
  olecranon (process) (ulna) (closed)
    813.01
    open 813.11
  open 829.1
  orbit, orbital (bone) (region) (closed)
    802.8
    floor (blow-out) 802.6
      open 802.7
    open 802.9
    roof - *see* Fracture, skull, base
    specified part NEC 802.8
      open 802.9
  os
    calcis (closed) 825.0
      open 825.1
    magnum (closed) 814.07
      open 814.17
    pubis (with visceral injury) (closed)
      808.2
      open 808.3
    triquetrum (closed) 814.03
      open 814.13
  osseous
    auditory meatus - *see* Fracture, skull,
      base
    labyrinth - *see* Fracture, skull, base
  ossicles, auditory (incus) (malleus)
    (stapes) - *see* Fracture, skull, base
  osteoporotic - *see* Fracture, pathologic
  palate (closed) 802.8
    open 802.9
  paratrooper - *see* Fracture, tibia, lower
    end

Fracture *(Continued)*
  parietal bone - *see* Fracture, skull, vault
  parry - *see* Fracture, Monteggia's
  patella (closed) 822.0
    open 822.1
  pathologic (cause unknown)
        733.10
    ankle 733.16
    femur (neck) 733.14
      specified NEC 733.15
    fibula 733.16
    hip 733.14
    humerus 733.11
    radius (distal) 733.12
    specified site NEC 733.19
    tibia 733.16
    ulna 733.12
    vertebrae (collapse) 733.13
    wrist 733.12
  pedicle (of vertebral arch) - *see*
      Fracture, vertebra, by site
  pelvis, pelvic (bone(s)) (with visceral
      injury) (closed) 808.8
    multiple (with disruption of pelvic
        circle) 808.43
      open 808.53
    open 808.9
    rim (closed) 808.49
      open 808.59
  peritrochanteric (closed) 820.20
    open 820.30
  phalanx, phalanges, of one
    foot (closed) 826.0
      with bone(s) of same lower limb
          827.0
        open 827.1
      open 826.1
    hand (closed) 816.00
      with metacarpal bone(s) of same
          hand 817.0
        open 817.1
      distal 816.02
        open 816.12
      middle 816.01
        open 816.11
      multiple sites NEC 816.03
        open 816.13
      open 816.10
      proximal 816.01
        open 816.11
  pisiform (closed) 814.04
    open 814.14
  pond - *see* Fracture, skull, vault
  Pott's (closed) 824.4
    open 824.5
  prosthetic device, internal - *see*
      Complications, mechanical
  pubis (with visceral injury) (closed)
      808.2
    open 808.3
  Quervain's (closed) 814.01
    open 814.11
  radius (alone) (closed) 813.81
    with ulna NEC 813.83
      open 813.93
    distal end - *see* Fracture, radius,
        lower end
    epiphysis
      lower - *see* Fracture, radius, lower
          end
      upper - *see* Fracture, radius,
          upper end
    head - *see* Fracture, radius, upper
        end

Fracture *(Continued)*
  radius *(Continued)*
    lower end or extremity (distal end)
        (lower epiphysis) 813.42
      with ulna (lower end) 813.44
        open 813.54
      open 813.52
      torus 813.45
        with ulna 813.47   ◄
    neck - *see* Fracture, radius, upper
        end
    open NEC 813.91
    pathologic 733.12
    proximal end - *see* Fracture, radius,
        upper end
    shaft (closed) 813.21
      with ulna (shaft) 813.23
        open 813.33
      open 813.31
    upper end 813.07
      with ulna (upper end) 813.08
        open 813.18
      epiphysis 813.05
        open 813.15
      head 813.05
        open 813.15
      multiple sites 813.07
        open 813.17
      neck 813.06
        open 813.16
      open 813.17
      specified site NEC 813.07
        open 813.17
  ramus
    inferior or superior (with visceral
        injury) (closed) 808.2
      open 808.3
    ischium - *see* Fracture, ischium
    mandible 802.24
      open 802.34
  rib(s) (closed) 807.0 ●

┌─────────────────────────────────────┐
Note 31   Use the following fifth-digit
subclassification with categories 807.0–
807.1:

  0   rib(s), unspecified
  1   one rib
  2   two ribs
  3   three ribs
  4   four ribs
  5   five ribs
  6   six ribs
  7   seven ribs
  8   eight or more ribs
  9   multiple ribs, unspecified
└─────────────────────────────────────┘

    with flail chest (open) 807.4
      open 807.1 ●
  root, tooth 873.63
    complicated 873.73
  sacrum - *see* Fracture, vertebra, sacrum
  scaphoid
    ankle (closed) 825.22
      open 825.32
    wrist (closed) 814.01
      open 814.11
  scapula (closed) 811.00
    acromial, acromion (process) 811.01
      open 811.11
    body 811.09
      open 811.19
    coracoid process 811.02
      open 811.12

Fracture *(Continued)*
  scapula *(Continued)*
    glenoid (cavity) (fossa) 811.03
      open 811.13
    neck 811.03
      open 811.13
    open 811.10
  semilunar
    bone, wrist (closed) 814.02
      open 814.12
    cartilage (interior) (knee) - *see* Tear,
        meniscus
  sesamoid bone - *see* Fracture, by site
  Shepherd's (closed) 825.21
    open 825.31
  shoulder - *see also* Fracture, humerus,
      upper end
    blade - *see* Fracture, scapula
  silverfork - *see* Fracture, radius, lower
      end
  sinus (ethmoid) (frontal) (maxillary)
      (nasal) (sphenoidal) - *see* Fracture,
      skull, base
  Skillern's - *see* Fracture, radius, shaft
  skull (multiple NEC) (with face bones)
      (closed) 803.0 ●

┌──┐
Note 32   Use the following fifth-digit
subclassification with categories 800,
801, 803, and 804:

  0   unspecified state of
          consciousness
  1   with no loss of consciousness
  2   with brief [less than one hour]
          loss of consciousness
  3   with moderate [1-24 hours] loss
          of consciousness
  4   with prolonged [more than 24
          hours] loss of
          consciousness and return
          to pre-existing conscious
          level
  5   with prolonged [more than 24
          hours] loss of
          consciousness, without
          return to pre-existing
          conscious level

Use fifth-digit 5 to designate when a
patient is unconscious and dies before
regaining consciousness, regardless of
the duration of the loss of consciousness

  6   with loss of consciousness of
          unspecified duration
  9   with concussion, unspecified
└──┘

    with
      contusion, cerebral 803.1 ●
      epidural hemorrhage 803.2 ●
      extradural hemorrhage 803.2 ●
      hemorrhage (intracranial) NEC
          803.3 ●
      intracranial injury NEC 803.4 ●
      laceration, cerebral 803.1 ●
      other bones - *see* Fracture,
          multiple, skull
      subarachnoid hemorrhage 803.2 ●
      subdural hemorrhage 803.2 ●
    base (antrum) (ethmoid bone) (fossa)
        (internal ear) (nasal sinus)
        (occiput) (sphenoid) (temporal
        bone) (closed) 801.0 ●
      with
        contusion, cerebral 801.1 ●
        epidural hemorrhage 801.2 ●

Fracture *(Continued)*
  skull *(Continued)*
    base *(Continued)*
      with *(Continued)*
        extradural hemorrhage 801.2●
        hemorrhage (intracranial) NEC 801.3●
        intracranial injury NEC 801.4●
        laceration, cerebral 801.1●
        subarachnoid hemorrhage 801.2●
        subdural hemorrhage 801.2●
      open 801.5●
        with
          contusion, cerebral 801.6●
          epidural hemorrhage 801.7●
          extradural hemorrhage 801.7●
          hemorrhage (intracranial) NEC 801.8●
          intracranial injury NEC 801.9●
          laceration, cerebral 801.6●
          subarachnoid hemorrhage 801.7●
          subdural hemorrhage 801.7●
  birth injury 767.3
  face bones - *see* Fracture, face bones
  open 803.5●
    with
      contusion, cerebral 803.6●
      epidural hemorrhage 803.7●
      extradural hemorrhage 803.7●
      hemorrhage (intracranial) NEC 803.8●
      intracranial injury NEC 803.9●
      laceration, cerebral 803.6●
      subarachnoid hemorrhage 803.7●
      subdural hemorrhage 803.7●
  vault (frontal bone) (parietal bone) (vertex) (closed) 800.0●
    with
      contusion, cerebral 800.1●
      epidural hemorrhage 800.2●
      extradural hemorrhage 800.2●
      hemorrhage (intracranial) NEC 800.3●
      intracranial injury NEC 800.4●
      laceration, cerebral 800.1●
      subarachnoid hemorrhage 800.2●
      subdural hemorrhage 800.2●
    open 800.5●
      with
        contusion, cerebral 800.6●
        epidural hemorrhage 800.7●
        extradural hemorrhage 800.7●
        hemorrhage (intracranial) NEC 800.8●
        intracranial injury NEC 800.9●
        laceration, cerebral 800.6●
        subarachnoid hemorrhage 800.7●
        subdural hemorrhage 800.7●

Fracture *(Continued)*
  Smith's 813.41
    open 813.51
  sphenoid (bone) (sinus) - *see* Fracture, skull, base
  spine - *see also* Fracture, vertebra, by site due to birth trauma 767.4
  spinous process - *see* Fracture, vertebra, by site
  spontaneous - *see* Fracture, pathologic
  sprinters' - *see* Fracture, ilium
  stapes - *see* Fracture, skull, base
  stave - *see also* Fracture, metacarpus, metacarpal bone(s)
    spine - *see* Fracture, tibia, upper end
  sternum (closed) 807.2
    with flail chest (open) 807.4
    open 807.3
  Stieda's - *see* Fracture, femur, lower end
  stress 733.95
    fibula 733.93
    metatarsals 733.94
    specified site NEC 733.95
    tibia 733.93
  styloid process
    metacarpal (closed) 815.02
      open 815.12
    radius - *see* Fracture, radius, lower end
    temporal bone - *see* Fracture, skull, base
    ulna - *see* Fracture, ulna, lower end
  supracondylar, elbow 812.41
    open 812.51
  symphysis pubis (with visceral injury) (closed) 808.2
    open 808.3
  talus (ankle bone) (closed) 825.21
    open 825.31
  tarsus, tarsal bone(s) (with metatarsus) of one foot (closed) NEC 825.29
    open 825.39
  temporal bone (styloid) - *see* Fracture, skull, base
  tendon - *see* Sprain, by site
  thigh - *see* Fracture, femur, shaft
  thumb (and finger(s)) of one hand (closed) (*see also* Fracture, phalanx, hand) 816.00
    with metacarpal bone(s) of same hand 817.0
      open 817.1
    metacarpal(s) - *see* Fracture, metacarpus
    open 816.10
  thyroid cartilage (closed) 807.5
    open 807.6
  tibia (closed) 823.80
    with fibula 823.82
      open 823.92
    condyles - *see* Fracture, tibia, upper end
    distal end 824.8
      open 824.9
    epiphysis
      lower 824.8
        open 824.9
      upper - *see* Fracture, tibia, upper end

Fracture *(Continued)*
  tibia *(Continued)*
    head (involving knee joint) - *see* Fracture, tibia, upper end
    intercondyloid eminence - *see* Fracture, tibia, upper end
    involving ankle 824.0
      open 824.1
    lower end or extremity (anterior lip) (posterior lip) 824.8
      open 824.9
    malleolus (internal) (medial) 824.0
      open 824.1
    open NEC 823.90
    pathologic 733.16
    proximal end - *see* Fracture, tibia, upper end
    shaft 823.20
      with fibula 823.22
        open 823.32
      open 823.30
    spine - *see* Fracture, tibia, upper end
    stress 733.93
    torus 823.40
      with fibula 823.42
    tuberosity - *see* Fracture, tibia, upper end
    upper end or extremity (condyle) (epiphysis) (head) (spine) (proximal end) (tuberosity) 823.00
      with fibula 823.02
        open 823.12
      open 823.10
  toe(s), of one foot (closed) 826.0
    with bone(s) of same lower limb 827.0
      open 827.1
    open 826.1
  tooth (root) 873.63
    complicated 873.73
  torus
    fibula 823.41
      with tibia 823.42
    humerus 812.49 ◄
    radius (alone) 813.45 ◄▥
      with ulna 813.47 ◄
    tibia 823.40
      with fibula 823.42
    ulna (alone) 813.46 ◄
      with radius 813.47 ◄
  trachea (closed) 807.5
    open 807.6
  transverse process - *see* Fracture, vertebra, by site
  trapezium (closed) 814.05
    open 814.15
  trapezoid bone (closed) 814.06
    open 814.16
  trimalleolar (closed) 824.6
    open 824.7
  triquetral (bone) (closed) 814.03
    open 814.13
  trochanter (greater) (lesser) (closed) (*see also* Fracture, femur, neck, by site) 820.20
    open 820.30
  trunk (bones) (closed) 809.0
    open 809.1
  tuberosity (external) - *see* Fracture, by site
  ulna (alone) (closed) 813.82
    with radius NEC 813.83
      open 813.93

Fracture *(Continued)*
  ulna *(Continued)*
    coronoid process (closed) 813.02
      open 813.12
    distal end - *see* Fracture, ulna, lower
        end
    epiphysis
      lower - *see* Fracture, ulna, lower
          end
      upper - *see* Fracture, ulna, upper,
          end
    head - *see* Fracture, ulna, lower
        end
    lower end (distal end) (head)
        (lower epiphysis) (styloid
        process) 813.43
      with radius (lower end) 813.44
        open 813.54
      open 813.53
    olecranon process (closed) 813.01
      open 813.11
    open NEC 813.92
    pathologic 733.12
    proximal end - *see* Fracture, ulna,
        upper end
    shaft 813.22
      with radius (shaft) 813.23
        open 813.33
      open 813.32
    styloid process - *see* Fracture, ulna,
        lower end
    torus 813.46 ◄
      with radius 813.47 ◄
    transverse - *see* Fracture, ulna, by
        site
    upper end (epiphysis) 813.04
      with radius (upper end)
          813.08
        open 813.18
      multiple sites 813.04
        open 813.14
      open 813.14
      specified site NEC 813.04
        open 813.14
  unciform (closed) 814.08
    open 814.18
  vertebra, vertebral (back) (body)
      (column) (neural arch) (pedicle)
      (spine) (spinous process)
      (transverse process) (closed)
      805.8
    with
      hematomyelia - *see* Fracture,
          vertebra, by site, with
          spinal cord injury
      injury to
        cauda equina - *see* Fracture,
            vertebra, sacrum, with
            spinal cord injury
        nerve - *see* Fracture, vertebra,
            by site, with spinal cord
            injury
      paralysis - *see* Fracture, vertebra,
          by site, with spinal cord
          injury
      paraplegia - *see* Fracture,
          vertebra, by site, with
          spinal cord injury
      quadriplegia - *see* Fracture,
          vertebra, by site, with
          spinal cord injury
      spinal concussion - *see* Fracture,
          vertebra, by site, with
          spinal cord injury

Fracture *(Continued)*
  vertebra, vertebral *(Continued)*
    with *(Continued)*
      spinal cord injury (closed) NEC
          806.8

> Note 33   Use the following fifth-digit
> subclassification with categories 806.0–
> 806.3:
>
> C_1–C_4 or unspecified level and D_1–D_6
> (T_1–T_6) or unspecified level with:
>
> 0   unspecified spinal cord injury
> 1   complete lesion of cord
> 2   anterior cord syndrome
> 3   central cord syndrome
> 4   specified injury NEC
>
> level and D_1–D_{12} level with:
>
> 5   unspecified spinal cord injury
> 6   complete lesion of cord
> 7   anterior cord syndrome
> 8   central cord syndrome
> 9   specified injury NEC

    cervical 806.0●
      open 806.1●
    chronic 733.13
    dorsal, dorsolumbar 806.2●
      open 806.3●
    open 806.9
    thoracic, thoracolumbar
        806.2●
      open 806.3●
    atlanto-axial - *see* Fracture,
        vertebra, cervical
    cervical (hangman) (teardrop)
        (closed) 805.00
      with spinal cord injury -
          see Fracture, vertebra,
          with spinal cord injury,
          cervical
      first (atlas) 805.01
        open 805.11
      second (axis) 805.02
        open 805.12
      third 805.03
        open 805.13
      fourth 805.04
        open 805.14
      fifth 805.05
        open 805.15
      sixth 805.06
        open 805.16
      seventh 805.07
        open 805.17
      multiple sites 805.08
        open 805.18
      open 805.10
    coccyx (closed) 805.6
      with spinal cord injury (closed)
          806.60
        cauda equina injury 806.62
          complete lesion 806.61
            open 806.71
          open 806.72
        open 806.70
          specified type NEC
              806.69
        open 806.79
      open 805.7
    collapsed 733.13
    compression, not due to trauma
        733.13

Fracture *(Continued)*
  dorsal (closed) 805.2
    with spinal cord injury - *see* Fracture,
        vertebra, with spinal cord
        injury, dorsal
    open 805.3
  dorsolumbar (closed) 805.2
    with spinal cord injury - *see* Fracture,
        vertebra, with spinal cord
        injury, dorsal
    open 805.3
  due to osteoporosis 733.13
  fetus or newborn 767.4
  lumbar (closed) 805.4
    with spinal cord injury (closed)
        806.4
      open 806.5
    open 805.5
  nontraumatic 733.13
  open NEC 805.9
  pathologic (any site) 733.13
  sacrum (closed) 805.6
    with spinal cord injury 806.60
      cauda equina injury 806.62
        complete lesion 806.61
          open 806.71
        open 806.72
      open 806.70
        specified type NEC 806.69
          open 806.79
    open 805.7
  site unspecified (closed) 805.8
    with spinal cord injury (closed)
        806.8
      open 806.9
    open 805.9
  stress (any site) 733.95
  thoracic (closed) 805.2
    with spinal cord injury - *see* Fracture,
        vertebra, with spinal cord
        injury, thoracic
    open 805.3
  vertex - *see* Fracture, skull, vault
  vomer (bone) 802.0
    open 802.1
  Wagstaffe's - *see* Fracture, ankle
  wrist (closed) 814.00
    open 814.10
    pathologic 733.12
  xiphoid (process) - *see* Fracture,
      sternum
  zygoma (zygomatic arch) (closed) 802.4
    open 802.5
Fragile X syndrome 759.83
Fragilitas
  crinium 704.2
  hair 704.2
  ossium 756.51
    with blue sclera 756.51
  unguium 703.8
    congenital 757.5
Fragility
  bone 756.51
    with deafness and blue sclera
        756.51
  capillary (hereditary) 287.8
  hair 704.2
  nails 703.8
Fragmentation - *see* Fracture, by site
Frailty 797
Frambesia, frambesial (tropica) (*see also*
    Yaws) 102.9
  initial lesion or ulcer 102.0
  primary 102.0

Frambeside
  gummatous 102.4
  of early yaws 102.2
Frambesioma 102.1
Franceschetti's syndrome
    (mandibulofacial dysostosis)
    756.0
Francis' disease (see also Tularemia)
    021.9
Frank's essential thrombocytopenia (see
    also Purpura, thrombocytopenic)
    287.39
Franklin's disease (heavy chain) 273.2
Fraser's syndrome 759.89
Freckle 709.09
  malignant melanoma in (M8742/3) - see
    Melanoma
  melanotic (of Hutchinson) (M8742/2) -
    see Neoplasm, skin, in situ
  retinal 239.81 ◄
Freeman-Sheldon syndrome 759.89
Freezing 991.9
  specified effect NEC 991.8
Frei's disease (climatic bubo) 099.1
Freiberg's
  disease (osteochondrosis, second
    metatarsal) 732.5
  infraction of metatarsal head 732.5
  osteochondrosis 732.5
Fremitus, friction, cardiac 785.3
Frenulum linguae 750.0
Frenum
  external os 752.49
  tongue 750.0
Frequency (urinary) NEC 788.41
  micturition 788.41
  nocturnal 788.43
  polyuria 788.42
  psychogenic 306.53
Frey's syndrome (auriculotemporal
    syndrome) 705.22
Friction
  burn (see also Injury, superficial, by site)
    919.0
  fremitus, cardiac 785.3
  precordial 785.3
  sounds, chest 786.7
Friderichsen-Waterhouse syndrome or
    disease 036.3
Friedländer's
  B (bacillus) NEC (see also condition)
    041.3
    sepsis or septicemia 038.49
  disease (endarteritis obliterans) - see
    Arteriosclerosis
Friedreich's
  ataxia 334.0
  combined systemic disease 334.0
  disease 333.2
    combined systemic 334.0
  myoclonia 333.2
  sclerosis (spinal cord) 334.0
Friedrich-Erb-Arnold syndrome
    (acropachyderma) 757.39
Frigidity 302.72
  psychic or psychogenic 302.72
Fröhlich's disease or syndrome
    (adiposogenital dystrophy) 253.8
Froin's syndrome 336.8
Frommel's disease 676.6●
Frommel-Chiari syndrome 676.6●
Frontal - see also condition
  lobe syndrome 310.0

Frostbite 991.3
  face 991.0
  foot 991.2
  hand 991.1
  specified site NEC 991.3
Frotteurism 302.89
Frozen 991.9
  pelvis 620.8
  shoulder 726.0
Fructosemia 271.2
Fructosuria (benign) (essential) 271.2
Fuchs'
  black spot (myopic) 360.21
  corneal dystrophy (endothelial)
    371.57
  heterochromic cyclitis 364.21
Fucosidosis 271.8
Fugue 780.99
  dissociative 300.13
  hysterical (dissociative) 300.13
  reaction to exceptional stress (transient)
    308.1
Fukuhara syndrome 277.87
Fuller Albright's syndrome (osteitis
    fibrosa disseminata) 756.59
Fuller's earth disease 502
Fulminant, fulminating - see condition
Functional - see condition
Functioning
  borderline intellectual V62.89
Fundus - see also condition
  flavimaculatus 362.76
Fungemia 117.9
Fungus, fungous
  cerebral 348.89 ◄▪▪
  disease NEC 117.9
  infection - see Infection, fungus
  testis (see also Tuberculosis) 016.5●
    [608.81]
Funiculitis (acute) 608.4
  chronic 608.4
  endemic 608.4
  gonococcal (acute) 098.14
    chronic or duration of 2 months or
      over 098.34
  tuberculous (see also Tuberculosis)
    016.5●
FUO (see also Pyrexia) 780.60
Funnel
  breast (acquired) 738.3
    congenital 754.81
    late effect of rickets 268.1
  chest (acquired) 738.3
    congenital 754.81
    late effect of rickets 268.1
  pelvis (acquired) 738.6
    with disproportion (fetopelvic)
      653.3●
    affecting fetus or newborn
      763.1
    causing obstructed labor
      660.1●
    affecting fetus or newborn
      763.1
    congenital 755.69
    tuberculous (see also Tuberculosis)
      016.9●
Furfur 690.18
  microsporon 111.0
Furor, paroxysmal (idiopathic) (see also
    Epilepsy) 345.8●
Furriers' lung 495.8
Furrowed tongue 529.5
  congenital 750.13

Furrowing nail(s) (transverse) 703.8
  congenital 757.5
Furuncle 680.9
  abdominal wall 680.2
  ankle 680.6
  anus 680.5
  arm (any part, above wrist) 680.3
  auditory canal, external 680.0
  axilla 680.3
  back (any part) 680.2
  breast 680.2
  buttock 680.5
  chest wall 680.2
  corpus cavernosum 607.2
  ear (any part) 680.0
  eyelid 373.13
  face (any part, except eye) 680.0
  finger (any) 680.4
  flank 680.2
  foot (any part) 680.7
  forearm 680.3
  gluteal (region) 680.5
  groin 680.2
  hand (any part) 680.4
  head (any part, except face) 680.8
  heel 680.7
  hip 680.6
  kidney (see also Abscess, kidney) 590.2
  knee 680.6
  labium (majus) (minus) 616.4
  lacrimal
    gland (see also Dacryoadenitis)
      375.00
    passages (duct) (sac) (see also
      Dacryocystitis) 375.30
  leg, any part except foot 680.6
  malignant 022.0
  multiple sites 680.9
  neck 680.1
  nose (external) (septum) 680.0
  orbit 376.01
  partes posteriores 680.5
  pectoral region 680.2
  penis 607.2
  perineum 680.2
  pinna 680.0
  scalp (any part) 680.8
  scrotum 608.4
  seminal vesicle 608.0
  shoulder 680.3
  skin NEC 680.9
  specified site NEC 680.8
  spermatic cord 608.4
  temple (region) 680.0
  testis 604.90
  thigh 680.6
  thumb 680.4
  toe (any) 680.7
  trunk 680.2
  tunica vaginalis 608.4
  umbilicus 680.2
  upper arm 680.3
  vas deferens 608.4
  vulva 616.4
  wrist 680.4
Furunculosis (see also Furuncle) 680.9
  external auditory meatus 680.0 [380.13]
Fusarium (infection) 118
Fusion, fused (congenital)
  anal (with urogenital canal) 751.5
  aorta and pulmonary artery 745.0
  astragaloscaphoid 755.67
  atria 745.5
  atrium and ventricle 745.69

Fusion, fused (*Continued*)
auditory canal 744.02
auricles, heart 745.5
binocular, with defective stereopsis
368.33
bone 756.9
cervical spine - *see* Fusion, spine
choanal 748.0
commissure, mitral valve 746.5
cranial sutures, premature 756.0
cusps, heart valve NEC 746.89
mitral 746.5
tricuspid 746.89
ear ossicles 744.04
fingers (*see also* Syndactylism, fingers)
755.11
hymen 752.42
hymeno-urethral 599.89
causing obstructed labor 660.1●
affecting fetus or newborn
763.1
joint (acquired) - *see also* Ankylosis
congenital 755.8
kidneys (incomplete) 753.3

Fusion, fused (*Continued*)
labium (majus) (minus) 752.49
larynx and trachea 748.3
limb 755.8
lower 755.69
upper 755.59
lobe, lung 748.5
lumbosacral (acquired) 724.6
congenital 756.15
surgical V45.4
nares (anterior) (posterior) 748.0
nose, nasal 748.0
nostril(s) 748.0
organ or site NEC - *see* Anomaly,
specified type NEC
ossicles 756.9
auditory 744.04
pulmonary valve segment 746.02
pulmonic cusps 746.02
ribs 756.3
sacroiliac (acquired) (joint) 724.6
congenital 755.69
surgical V45.4
skull, imperfect 756.0

Fusion, fused (*Continued*)
spine (acquired) 724.9
arthrodesis status V45.4
congenital (vertebra) 756.15
postoperative status V45.4
sublingual duct with submaxillary duct
at opening in mouth 750.26
talonavicular (bar) 755.67
teeth, tooth 520.2
testes 752.89
toes (*see also* Syndactylism, toes) 755.13
trachea and esophagus 750.3
twins 759.4
urethral-hymenal 599.89
vagina 752.49
valve cusps - *see* Fusion, cusps, heart
valve
ventricles, heart 745.4
vertebra (arch) - *see* Fusion, spine
vulva 752.49
Fusospirillosis (mouth) (tongue) (tonsil)
101
Fussy infant (baby) 780.91

◀ New   ◀▥ Revised   ~~deleted~~ Deleted   ● Use Additional Digit(s)   ▨ Omit code

G

Gafsa boil 085.1
Gain, weight (abnormal) (excessive) (*see also* Weight, gain) 783.1
Gaisböck's disease or syndrome (polycythemia hypertonica) 289.0
Gait
  abnormality 781.2
    hysterical 300.11
  ataxic 781.2
    hysterical 300.11
  disturbance 781.2
    hysterical 300.11
  paralytic 781.2
  scissor 781.2
  spastic 781.2
  staggering 781.2
    hysterical 300.11
Galactocele (breast) (infected) 611.5
  puerperal, postpartum 676.8●
Galactophoritis 611.0
  puerperal, postpartum 675.2●
Galactorrhea 676.6●
  not associated with childbirth 611.6
Galactosemia (classic) (congenital) 271.1
Galactosuria 271.1
Galacturia 791.1
  bilharziasis 120.0
Galen's vein - *see* condition
Gallbladder - *see also* condition
  acute (*see also* Disease, gallbladder) 575.0
Gall duct - *see* condition
Gallop rhythm 427.89
Gallstone (cholemic) (colic) (impacted) - *see also* Cholelithiasis
  causing intestinal obstruction 560.31
Gambling, pathological 312.31
Gammaloidosis 277.39
Gammopathy 273.9
  macroglobulinemia 273.3
  monoclonal (benign) (essential) (idiopathic) (with lymphoplasmacytic dyscrasia) 273.1
Gamna's disease (siderotic splenomegaly) 289.51
Gampsodactylia (congenital) 754.71
Gamstorp's disease (adynamia episodica hereditaria) 359.3
Gandy-Nanta disease (siderotic splenomegaly) 289.51
Gang activity, without manifest psychiatric disorder V71.09
  adolescent V71.02
  adult V71.01
  child V71.02
Gangliocytoma (M9490/0) - *see* Neoplasm, connective tissue, benign
Ganglioglioma (M9505/1) - *see* Neoplasm, by site, uncertain behavior
Ganglion 727.43
  joint 727.41
  of yaws (early) (late) 102.6
  periosteal (*see also* Periostitis) 730.3●
  tendon sheath (compound) (diffuse) 727.42
  tuberculous (*see also* Tuberculosis) 015.9●
Ganglioneuroblastoma (M9490/3) - *see* Neoplasm, connective tissue, malignant

Ganglioneuroma (M9490/0) - *see also* Neoplasm, connective tissue, benign
  malignant (M9490/3) - *see* Neoplasm, connective tissue, malignant
Ganglioneuromatosis (M9491/0) - *see* Neoplasm, connective tissue, benign
Ganglionitis
  fifth nerve (*see also* Neuralgia, trigeminal) 350.1
  gasserian 350.1
  geniculate 351.1
    herpetic 053.11
    newborn 767.5
  herpes zoster 053.11
  herpetic geniculate (Hunt's syndrome) 053.11
Gangliosidosis 330.1
Gangosa 102.5
Gangrene, gangrenous (anemia) (artery) (cellulitis) (dermatitis) (dry) (infective) (moist) (pemphigus) (septic) (skin) (stasis) (ulcer) 785.4
  with
    arteriosclerosis (native artery) 440.24
      bypass graft 440.30
        autologous vein 440.31
        nonautologous biological 440.32
    diabetes (mellitus) 250.7● [*785.4*]
      due to secondary diabetes 249.7● [*785.4*]
  abdomen (wall) 785.4
  adenitis 683
  alveolar 526.5
  angina 462
    diphtheritic 032.0
  anus 569.49
  appendices epiploicae - *see* Gangrene, mesentery
  appendix - *see* Appendicitis, acute
  arteriosclerotic - *see* Arteriosclerosis, with, gangrene
  auricle 785.4
  Bacillus welchii (*see also* Gangrene, gas) 040.0
  bile duct (*see also* Cholangitis) 576.8
  bladder 595.89
  bowel - *see* Gangrene, intestine
  cecum - *see* Gangrene, intestine
  Clostridium perfringens or welchii (*see also* Gangrene, gas) 040.0
  colon - *see* Gangrene, intestine
  connective tissue 785.4
  cornea 371.40
  corpora cavernosa (infective) 607.2
    noninfective 607.89
  cutaneous, spreading 785.4
  decubital (*see also* Ulcer, pressure) 707.00 [*785.4*]
  diabetic (any site) 250.7● [*785.4*]
    due to secondary diabetes 249.7● [*785.4*]
  dropsical 785.4
  emphysematous (*see also* Gangrene, gas) 040.0
  epidemic (ergotized grain) 988.2
  epididymis (infectional) (*see also* Epididymitis) 604.99
  erysipelas (*see also* Erysipelas) 035
  extremity (lower) (upper) 785.4
  gallbladder or duct (*see also* Cholecystitis, acute) 575.0

Gangrene, gangrenous (*Continued*)
  gas (bacillus) 040.0
    with
      abortion - *see* Abortion, by type, with sepsis
      ectopic pregnancy (*see also* categories 633.0–633.9) 639.0
      molar pregnancy (*see also* categories 630–632) 639.0
    following
      abortion 639.0
      ectopic or molar pregnancy 639.0
    puerperal, postpartum, childbirth 670.8 ◀█
  glossitis 529.0
  gum 523.8
  hernia - *see* Hernia, by site, with gangrene
  hospital noma 528.1
  intestine, intestinal (acute) (hemorrhagic) (massive) 557.0
    with
      hernia - *see* Hernia, by site, with gangrene
      mesenteric embolism or infarction 557.0
      obstruction (*see also* Obstruction, intestine) 560.9
  laryngitis 464.00
    with obstruction 464.01
  liver 573.8
  lung 513.0
    spirochetal 104.8
  lymphangitis 457.2
  Meleney's (cutaneous) 686.09
  mesentery 557.0
    with
      embolism or infarction 557.0
      intestinal obstruction (*see also* Obstruction, intestine) 560.9
  mouth 528.1
  noma 528.1
  orchitis 604.90
  ovary (*see also* Salpingo-oophoritis) 614.2
  pancreas 577.0
  penis (infectional) 607.2
    noninfective 607.89
  perineum 785.4
  pharynx 462
    septic 034.0
  pneumonia 513.0
  Pott's 440.24
  presenile 443.1
  pulmonary 513.0
  pulp, tooth 522.1
  quinsy 475
  Raynaud's (symmetric gangrene) 443.0 [*785.4*]
  rectum 569.49
  retropharyngeal 478.24
  rupture - *see* Hernia, by site, with gangrene
  scrotum 608.4
    noninfective 608.83
  senile 440.24
  sore throat 462
  spermatic cord 608.4
    noninfective 608.89
  spine 785.4
  spirochetal NEC 104.8
  spreading cutaneous 785.4
  stomach 537.89
  stomatitis 528.1

Gangrene, gangrenous *(Continued)*
    symmetrical 443.0 [785.4]
    testis (infectional) *(see also* Orchitis)
        604.99
        noninfective 608.89
    throat 462
        diphtheritic 032.0
    thyroid (gland) 246.8
    tonsillitis (acute) 463
    tooth (pulp) 522.1
    tuberculous NEC *(see also* Tuberculosis)
        011.9●
    tunica vaginalis 608.4
        noninfective 608.89
    umbilicus 785.4
    uterus *(see also* Endometritis) 615.9
    uvulitis 528.3
    vas deferens 608.4
        noninfective 608.89
    vulva *(see also* Vulvitis) 616.10
Gannister disease (occupational) 502
    with tuberculosis - *see* Tuberculosis,
        pulmonary
Ganser's syndrome, hysterical 300.16
Gardner-Diamond syndrome
        (autoerythrocyte sensitization) 287.2
Gargoylism 277.5
Garré's
    disease *(see also* Osteomyelitis) 730.1●
    osteitis (sclerosing) *(see also*
        Osteomyelitis) 730.1●
    osteomyelitis *(see also* Osteomyelitis)
        730.1●
Garrod's pads, knuckle 728.79
Gartner's duct
    cyst 752.41
    persistent 752.41
Gas 787.3
    asphyxia, asphyxiation, inhalation,
        poisoning, suffocation NEC 987.9
        specified gas - *see* Table of Drugs
            and Chemicals
    bacillus gangrene or infection - *see* Gas,
        gangrene
    cyst, mesentery 568.89
    excessive 787.3
    gangrene 040.0
        with
            abortion - *see* Abortion, by type,
                with sepsis
            ectopic pregnancy *(see also*
                categories 633.0–633.9) 639.0
            molar pregnancy *(see also*
                categories 630–632) 639.0
        following
            abortion 639.0
            ectopic or molar pregnancy
                639.0
        puerperal, postpartum,
            childbirth 670.8 ◀▥
    on stomach 787.3
    pains 787.3
Gastradenitis 535.0●
Gastralgia 536.8
    psychogenic 307.89
Gastrectasis, gastrectasia 536.1
    psychogenic 306.4
Gastric - *see* condition
Gastrinoma (M8153/1)
    malignant (M8153/3)
        pancreas 157.4
        specified site NEC - *see* Neoplasm,
            by site, malignant
        unspecified site 157.4

Gastrinoma *(Continued)*
    specified site - *see* Neoplasm, by site,
        uncertain behavior
    unspecified site 235.5
Gastritis 535.5●

Note 34	Use the following fifth-digit

subclassification for category 535:

    0   without mention of hemorrhage
    1   with hemorrhage

---

    acute 535.0●
    alcoholic 535.3●
    allergic 535.4●
    antral 535.4●
    atrophic 535.1●
    atrophic-hyperplastic 535.1●
    bile-induced 535.4●
    catarrhal 535.0●
    chronic (atrophic) 535.1●
    cirrhotic 535.4●
    corrosive (acute) 535.4●
    dietetic 535.4●
    due to diet deficiency 269.9 [535.4]●
    eosinophilic 535.7●
    erosive 535.4●
    follicular 535.4●
        chronic 535.1●
    giant hypertrophic 535.2●
    glandular 535.4●
        chronic 535.1●
    hypertrophic (mucosa) 535.2●
        chronic giant 211.1
    irritant 535.4●
    nervous 306.4
    phlegmonous 535.0●
    psychogenic 306.4
    sclerotic 535.4●
    spastic 536.8
    subacute 535.0●
    superficial 535.4●
    suppurative 535.0●
    toxic 535.4●
    tuberculous *(see also* Tuberculosis)
        017.9●
Gastrocarcinoma (M8010/3) 151.9
Gastrocolic - *see* condition
Gastrocolitis - *see* Enteritis
Gastrodisciasis 121.8
Gastroduodenitis *(see also* Gastritis)
        535.5●
    catarrhal 535.0●
    infectional 535.0●
    virus, viral 008.8
        specified type NEC 008.69
Gastrodynia 536.8
Gastroenteritis (acute) (catarrhal)
        (congestive) (hemorrhagic)
        (noninfectious) *(see also* Enteritis)
        558.9
    aertrycke infection 003.0
    allergic 558.3
    chronic 558.9
        ulcerative *(see also* Colitis, ulcerative)
            556.9
    dietetic 558.9
    due to
        antineoplastic chemotherapy 558.9
        food poisoning *(see also* Poisoning,
            food) 005.9
        radiation 558.1
    eosinophilic 558.41
    epidemic 009.0

Gastroenteritis *(Continued)*
    functional 558.9
    infectious *(see also* Enteritis, due to, by
        organism) 009.0
        presumed 009.1
    salmonella 003.0
    septic *(see also* Enteritis, due to, by
        organism) 009.0
    toxic 558.2
    tuberculous *(see also* Tuberculosis)
        014.8●
    ulcerative *(see also* Colitis, ulcerative)
        556.9
    viral NEC 008.8
        specified type NEC 008.69
    zymotic 009.0
Gastroenterocolitis - *see* Enteritis
Gastroenteropathy, protein-losing 579.8
Gastroenteroptosis 569.89
Gastroesophageal laceration-hemorrhage
        syndrome 530.7
Gastroesophagitis 530.19
Gastrohepatitis *(see also* Gastritis) 535.5●
Gastrointestinal - *see* condition
Gastrojejunal - *see* condition
Gastrojejunitis *(see also* Gastritis) 535.5●
Gastrojejunocolic - *see* condition
Gastroliths 537.89
Gastromalacia 537.89
Gastroparalysis 536.3
    diabetic 250.6● [536.3]
        due to secondary diabetes 249.6●
            [536.3]
Gastroparesis 536.3
    diabetic 250.6● [536.3]
        due to secondary diabetes 249.6●
            [536.3]
Gastropathy 537.9
    congestive portal 537.89
    erythematous 535.5●
    exudative 579.8
    portal hypertensive 537.89
Gastroptosis 537.5
Gastrorrhagia 578.0
Gastrorrhea 536.8
    psychogenic 306.4
Gastroschisis (congenital) 756.73   ◀▥
    acquired 569.89
Gastrospasm (neurogenic) (reflex) 536.8
    neurotic 306.4
    psychogenic 306.4
Gastrostaxis 578.0
Gastrostenosis 537.89
Gastrostomy
    attention to V55.1
    complication 536.40
        specified type 536.49
    infection 536.41
    malfunctioning 536.42
    status V44.1
Gastrosuccorrhea (continuous)
        (intermittent) 536.8
    neurotic 306.4
    psychogenic 306.4
Gaucher's
    disease (adult) (cerebroside lipidosis)
        (infantile) 272.7
    hepatomegaly 272.7
    splenomegaly (cerebroside lipidosis)
        272.7
GAVE (gastric antral vascular ectasia)
        537.82
    with hemorrhage 537.83
    without hemorrhage 537.82

Gayet's disease (superior hemorrhagic polioencephalitis) 265.1
Gayet-Wernicke's syndrome (superior hemorrhagic polioencephalitis) 265.1
Gee (-Herter) (-Heubner) (-Thaysen) disease or syndrome (nontropical sprue) 579.0
Gélineau's syndrome (see also Narcolepsy) 347.00
Gemination, teeth 520.2
Gemistocytoma (M9411/3)
  specified site - see Neoplasm, by site, malignant
  unspecified site 191.9
General, generalized - see condition
Genetic
  susceptibility to
    MEN (multiple endocrine neoplasia) V84.81
    neoplasia
      multiple endocrine [MEN] V84.81
    neoplasm
      malignant, of
        breast V84.01
        endometrium V84.04
        other V84.09
        ovary V84.02
        prostate V84.03
      specified disease NEC V84.89
Genital - see condition
  warts 078.11
Genito-anorectal syndrome 099.1
Genitourinary system - see condition
Genu
  congenital 755.64
  extrorsum (acquired) 736.42
    congenital 755.64
    late effects of rickets 268.1
  introrsum (acquired) 736.41
    congenital 755.64
    late effects of rickets 268.1
  rachitic (old) 268.1
  recurvatum (acquired) 736.5
    congenital 754.40
      with dislocation of knee 754.41
    late effects of rickets 268.1
  valgum (acquired) (knock-knee) 736.41
    congenital 755.64
    late effects of rickets 268.1
  varum (acquired) (bowleg) 736.42
    congenital 755.64
    late effect of rickets 268.1
Geographic tongue 529.1
Geophagia 307.52
Geotrichosis 117.9
  intestine 117.9
  lung 117.9
  mouth 117.9
Gephyrophobia 300.29
Gerbode defect 745.4
GERD (gastroesophageal reflux disease) 530.81
Gerhardt's
  disease (erythromelalgia) 443.82
  syndrome (vocal cord paralysis) 478.30
Gerlier's disease (epidemic vertigo) 078.81
German measles 056.9
  exposure to V01.4
Germinoblastoma (diffuse) (M9614/3) 202.8●
  follicular (M9692/3) 202.0●
Germinoma (M9064/3) - see Neoplasm, by site, malignant

Gerontoxon 371.41
Gerstmann-Sträussler-Scheinker syndrome (GSS) 046.71
Gerstmann's syndrome (finger agnosia) 784.69
Gestation (period) - see also Pregnancy
  ectopic NEC (see also Pregnancy, ectopic) 633.90
    with intrauterine pregnancy 633.91
Gestational proteinuria 646.2●
  with hypertension - see Toxemia, of pregnancy
Ghon tubercle primary infection (see also Tuberculosis) 010.0●
Ghost
  teeth 520.4
  vessels, cornea 370.64
Ghoul hand 102.3
Gianotti Crosti syndrome 057.8
  due to known virus - see Infection, virus
  due to unknown virus 057.8
Giant
  cell
    epulis 523.8
    peripheral (gingiva) 523.8
    tumor, tendon sheath 727.02
  colon (congenital) 751.3
  esophagus (congenital) 750.4
  kidney 753.3
  urticaria 995.1
    hereditary 277.6
Giardia lamblia infestation 007.1
Giardiasis 007.1
Gibert's disease (pityriasis rosea) 696.3
Gibraltar fever - see Brucellosis
Giddiness 780.4
  hysterical 300.11
  psychogenic 306.9
Gierke's disease (glycogenosis I) 271.0
Gigantism (cerebral) (hypophyseal) (pituitary) 253.0
Gilbert's disease or cholemia (familial nonhemolytic jaundice) 277.4
Gilchrist's disease (North American blastomycosis) 116.0
Gilford (-Hutchinson) disease or syndrome (progeria) 259.8
Gilles de la Tourette's disease (motor-verbal tic) 307.23
Gillespie's syndrome (dysplasia oculodentodigitalis) 759.89
Gingivitis 523.10
  acute 523.00
    necrotizing 101
    non-plaque induced 523.01
    plaque induced 523.00
  catarrhal 523.00
  chronic 523.10
    non-plaque induced 523.11
  desquamative 523.10
  expulsiva 523.40
  hyperplastic 523.10
  marginal, simple 523.10
  necrotizing, acute 101
  non-plaque induced 523.11
  pellagrous 265.2
  plaque induced 523.10
  ulcerative 523.10
    acute necrotizing 101
  Vincent's 101
Gingivoglossitis 529.0
Gingivopericementitis 523.40
Gingivosis 523.10

Gingivostomatitis 523.10
  herpetic 054.2
Giovannini's disease 117.9
GISA (glycopeptide intermediate staphylococcus aureus) V09.8
Gland, glandular - see condition
Glanders 024
Glanzmann (-Naegeli) disease or thrombasthenia 287.1
Glassblowers' disease 527.1
Glaucoma (capsular) (inflammatory) (noninflammatory) (primary) 365.9
  with increased episcleral venous pressure 365.82
  absolute 360.42
  acute 365.22
    narrow angle 365.22
    secondary 365.60
  angle closure 365.20
    acute 365.22
    chronic 365.23
    intermittent 365.21
    interval 365.21
    residual stage 365.24
    subacute 365.21
  borderline 365.00
  chronic 365.11
    noncongestive 365.11
    open angle 365.11
    simple 365.11
  closed angle - see Glaucoma, angle closure
  congenital 743.20
    associated with other eye anomalies 743.22
    simple 743.21
  congestive - see Glaucoma, narrow angle
  corticosteroid-induced (glaucomatous stage) 365.31
    residual stage 365.32
  hemorrhagic 365.60
  hypersecretion 365.81
  in or with
    aniridia 365.42
    Axenfeld's anomaly 365.41
    congenital syndromes NEC 759.89 [365.44]
    disorder of lens NEC 365.59
    inflammation, ocular 365.62
    iris
      anomalies NEC 365.42
      atrophy, essential 365.42
      bombé 365.61
    microcornea 365.43
    neurofibromatosis 237.71 [365.44]
    ocular
      cysts NEC 365.64
      disorders NEC 365.60
      trauma 365.65
      tumors NEC 365.64
    pupillary block or seclusion 365.61
    Rieger's anomaly or syndrome 365.41
    seclusion of pupil 365.61
    Sturge-Weber (-Dimitri) syndrome 759.6 [365.44]
    systemic syndrome NEC 365.44
    tumor of globe 365.64
    vascular disorders NEC 365.63
  infantile 365.14
    congenital 743.20
      associated with other eye anomalies 743.22
      simple 743.21

Glaucoma (Continued)
  juvenile 365.14
  low tension 365.12
  malignant 365.83
  narrow angle (primary) 365.20
    acute 365.22
    chronic 365.23
    intermittent 365.21
    interval 365.21
    residual stage 365.24
    subacute 365.21
  newborn 743.20
    associated with other eye anomalies 743.22
    simple 743.21
  noncongestive (chronic) 365.11
  nonobstructive (chronic) 365.11
  obstructive 365.60
    due to lens changes 365.59
  open angle 365.10
    with
        borderline intraocular pressure 365.01
        cupping of optic discs 365.01
      primary 365.11
      residual stage 365.15
  phacolytic 365.51
  pigmentary 365.13
  postinfectious 365.60
  pseudoexfoliation 365.52
  secondary NEC 365.60
  simple (chronic) 365.11
  simplex 365.11
  steroid responders 365.03
  suspect 365.00
  syphilitic 095.8
  traumatic NEC 365.65
    newborn 767.8
  wide angle (see also Glaucoma, open angle) 365.10
Glaucomatous flecks (subcapsular) 366.31
Glazed tongue 529.4
Gleet 098.2
Glénard's disease or syndrome (enteroptosis) 569.89
Glinski-Simmonds syndrome (pituitary cachexia) 253.2
Glioblastoma (multiforme) (M9440/3)
  with sarcomatous component (M9442/3)
    specified site - see Neoplasm, by site, malignant
    unspecified site 191.9
  giant cell (M9441/3)
    specified site - see Neoplasm, by site, malignant
    unspecified site 191.9
  specified site - see Neoplasm, by site, malignant
  unspecified site 191.9
Glioma (malignant) (M9380/3)
  astrocytic (M9400/3)
    specified site - see Neoplasm, by site, malignant
    unspecified site 191.9
  mixed (M9382/3)
    specified site - see Neoplasm, by site, malignant
    unspecified site 191.9
  nose 748.1
  specified site NEC - see Neoplasm, by site, malignant
  subependymal (M9383/1) 237.5
  unspecified site 191.9

Gliomatosis cerebri (M9381/3) 191.0
Glioneuroma (M9505/1) - see Neoplasm, by site, uncertain behavior
Gliosarcoma (M9380/3)
  specified site - see Neoplasm, by site, malignant
  unspecified site 191.9
Gliosis (cerebral) 349.89
  spinal 336.0
Glisson's
  cirrhosis - see Cirrhosis, portal
  disease (see also Rickets) 268.0
Glissonitis 573.3
Globinuria 791.2
Globus 306.4
  hystericus 300.11
Glomangioma (M8712/0) (see also Hemangioma) 228.00
Glomangiosarcoma (M8710/3) - see Neoplasm, connective tissue, malignant
Glomerular nephritis (see also Nephritis) 583.9
Glomerulitis (see also Nephritis) 583.9
Glomerulonephritis (see also Nephritis) 583.9
  with
    edema (see also Nephrosis) 581.9
    lesion of
      exudative nephritis 583.89
      interstitial nephritis (diffuse) (focal) 583.89
      necrotizing glomerulitis 583.4
        acute 580.4
        chronic 582.4
      renal necrosis 583.9
        cortical 583.6
        medullary 583.7
      specified pathology NEC 583.89
        acute 580.89
        chronic 582.89
    necrosis, renal 583.9
      cortical 583.6
      medullary (papillary) 583.7
    specified pathology or lesion NEC 583.89
  acute 580.9
    with
      exudative nephritis 580.89
      interstitial nephritis (diffuse) (focal) 580.89
      necrotizing glomerulitis 580.4
    extracapillary with epithelial crescents 580.4
    poststreptococcal 580.0
    proliferative (diffuse) 580.0
    rapidly progressive 580.4
    specified pathology NEC 580.89
  arteriolar (see also Hypertension, kidney) 403.90
  arteriosclerotic (see also Hypertension, kidney) 403.90
  ascending (see also Pyelitis) 590.80
  basement membrane NEC 583.89
    with
      pulmonary hemorrhage (Goodpasture's syndrome) 446.21 [583.81]
  chronic 582.9
    with
      exudative nephritis 582.89
      interstitial nephritis (diffuse) (focal) 582.89
      necrotizing glomerulitis 582.4

Glomerulonephritis (Continued)
  chronic (Continued)
    with (Continued)
        specified pathology or lesion NEC 582.89
      endothelial 582.2
      extracapillary with epithelial crescents 582.4
      hypocomplementemic persistent 582.2
      lobular 582.2
      membranoproliferative 582.2
      membranous 582.1
        and proliferative (mixed) 582.2
        sclerosing 582.1
      mesangiocapillary 582.2
      mixed membranous and proliferative 582.2
      proliferative (diffuse) 582.0
      rapidly progressive 582.4
      sclerosing 582.1
  cirrhotic - see Sclerosis, renal
  desquamative - see Nephrosis
  due to or associated with
    amyloidosis 277.39 [583.81]
      with nephrotic syndrome 277.39 [581.81]
      chronic 277.39 [582.81]
    diabetes mellitus 250.4● [583.81]
      due to secondary diabetes 249.4● [581.81]
      with nephrotic syndrome 250.4● [581.81]
        due to secondary diabetes 249.4● [581.81]
    diphtheria 032.89 [580.81]
    gonococcal infection (acute) 098.19 [583.81]
      chronic or duration of 2 months or over 098.39 [583.81]
    infectious hepatitis 070.9 [580.81]
    malaria (with nephrotic syndrome) 084.9 [581.81]
    mumps 072.79 [580.81]
    polyarteritis (nodosa) (with nephrotic syndrome) 446.0 [581.81]
    specified pathology NEC 583.89
      acute 580.89
      chronic 582.89
    streptotrichosis 039.8 [583.81]
    subacute bacterial endocarditis 421.0 [580.81]
    syphilis (late) 095.4
      congenital 090.5 [583.81]
      early 091.69 [583.81]
    systemic lupus erythematosus 710.0 [583.81]
      with nephrotic syndrome 710.0 [581.81]
      chronic 710.0 [582.81]
    tuberculosis (see also Tuberculosis) 016.0● [583.81]
    typhoid fever 002.0 [580.81]
  extracapillary with epithelial crescents 583.4
    acute 580.4
    chronic 582.4
  exudative 583.89
    acute 580.89
    chronic 582.89
  focal (see also Nephritis) 583.9
    embolic 580.4
  granular 582.89

◀ New   ◀▦ Revised   ~~deleted~~ Deleted   ● Use Additional Digit(s)   ▦ Omit code

Glomerulonephritis *(Continued)*
  granulomatous 582.89
  hydremic *(see also* Nephrosis) 581.9
  hypocomplementemic persistent 583.2
    with nephrotic syndrome 581.2
    chronic 582.2
  immune complex NEC 583.89
  infective *(see also* Pyelitis) 590.80
  interstitial (diffuse) (focal) 583.89
    with nephrotic syndrome 581.89
    acute 580.89
    chronic 582.89
  latent or quiescent 582.9
  lobular 583.2
    with nephrotic syndrome 581.2
    chronic 582.2
  membranoproliferative 583.2
    with nephrotic syndrome 581.2
    chronic 582.2
  membranous 583.1
    with nephrotic syndrome 581.1
    and proliferative (mixed) 583.2
      with nephrotic syndrome 581.2
      chronic 582.2
    chronic 582.1
    sclerosing 582.1
      with nephrotic syndrome 581.1
  mesangiocapillary 583.2
    with nephrotic syndrome 581.2
    chronic 582.2
  minimal change 581.3
  mixed membranous and proliferative
    583.2
    with nephrotic syndrome 581.2
    chronic 582.2
  necrotizing 583.4
    acute 580.4
    chronic 582.4
  nephrotic *(see also* Nephrosis) 581.9
  old - *see* Glomerulonephritis, chronic
  parenchymatous 581.89
  poststreptococcal 580.0
  proliferative (diffuse) 583.0
    with nephrotic syndrome 581.0
    acute 580.0
    chronic 582.0
  purulent *(see also* Pyelitis) 590.80
  quiescent - *see* Nephritis, chronic
  rapidly progressive 583.4
    acute 580.4
    chronic 582.4
  sclerosing membranous (chronic)
    582.1
    with nephrotic syndrome 581.1
  septic *(see also* Pyelitis) 590.80
  specified pathology or lesion NEC
    583.89
    with nephrotic syndrome 581.89
    acute 580.89
    chronic 582.89
  suppurative (acute) (disseminated) *(see
    also* Pyelitis) 590.80
  toxic - *see* Nephritis, acute
  tubal, tubular - *see* Nephrosis, tubular
  type II (Ellis) - *see* Nephrosis
  vascular - *see* Hypertension, kidney
Glomerulosclerosis *(see also* Sclerosis,
    renal) 587
  focal 582.1
    with nephrotic syndrome 581.1
  intercapillary (nodular) (with diabetes)
    250.4 ● *[581.81]*
    due to secondary diabetes 249.4 ●
      [581.81]

Glossagra 529.6
Glossalgia 529.6
Glossitis 529.0
  areata exfoliativa 529.1
  atrophic 529.4
  benign migratory 529.1
  gangrenous 529.0
  Hunter's 529.4
  median rhomboid 529.2
  Moeller's 529.4
  pellagrous 265.2
Glossocele 529.8
Glossodynia 529.6
  exfoliativa 529.4
Glossoncus 529.8
Glossophytia 529.3
Glossoplegia 529.8
Glossoptosis 529.8
Glossopyrosis 529.6
Glossotrichia 529.3
Glossy skin 701.9
Glottis - *see* condition
Glottitis - *see* Glossitis
Glucagonoma (M8152/0)
  malignant (M8152/3)
    pancreas 157.4
    specified site NEC - *see* Neoplasm,
      by site, malignant
    unspecified site 157.4
  pancreas 211.7
  specified site NEC - *see* Neoplasm, by
    site, benign
  unspecified site 211.7
Glucoglycinuria 270.7
Glue ear syndrome 381.20
Glue sniffing (airplane glue) *(see also*
    Dependence) 304.6 ●
Glycinemia (with methylmalonic
    acidemia) 270.7
Glycinuria (renal) (with ketosis) 270.0
Glycogen
  infiltration *(see also* Disease, glycogen
    storage) 271.0
  storage disease *(see also* Disease,
    glycogen storage) 271.0
Glycogenosis *(see also* Disease, glycogen
    storage) 271.0
  cardiac 271.0 *[425.7]*
  Cori, types I-VII 271.0
  diabetic, secondary 250.8 ● *[259.8]*
    due to secondary diabetes 249.8 ●
      [259.8]
  diffuse (with hepatic cirrhosis) 271.0
  generalized 271.0
  glucose-6-phosphatase deficiency
    271.0
  hepatophosphorylase deficiency
    271.0
  hepatorenal 271.0
  myophosphorylase deficiency 271.0
Glycopenia 251.2
Glycopeptide
  intermediate staphylococcus aureus
    (GISA) V09.8
  resistant
    enterococcus V09.8
    staphylococcus aureus (GRSA)
      V09.8
Glycoprolinuria 270.8
Glycosuria 791.5
  renal 271.4
Gnathostoma (spinigerum) (infection)
    (infestation) 128.1
  wandering swellings from 128.1

Gnathostomiasis 128.1
Goiter (adolescent) (colloid) (diffuse)
    (dipping) (due to iodine deficiency)
    (endemic) (euthyroid) (heart)
    (hyperplastic) (internal)
    (intrathoracic) (juvenile) (mixed
    type) (nonendemic)
    (parenchymatous) (plunging)
    (sporadic) (subclavicular)
    (substernal) 240.9
  with
    hyperthyroidism (recurrent) *(see also*
      Goiter, toxic) 242.0 ●
    thyrotoxicosis *(see also* Goiter, toxic)
      242.0 ●
  adenomatous *(see also* Goiter, nodular)
    241.9
  cancerous (M8000/3) 193
  complicating pregnancy, childbirth, or
    puerperium 648.1 ●
  congenital 246.1
  cystic *(see also* Goiter, nodular) 241.9
  due to enzyme defect in synthesis of
    thyroid hormone (butane-
    insoluble iodine) (coupling)
    (deiodinase) (iodide trapping or
    organification) (iodotyrosine
    dehalogenase) (peroxidase) 246.1
  dyshormonogenic 246.1
  exophthalmic *(see also* Goiter, toxic)
    242.0 ●
  familial (with deaf-mutism) 243
  fibrous 245.3
  lingual 759.2
  lymphadenoid 245.2
  malignant (M8000/3) 193
  multinodular (nontoxic) 241.1
    toxic or with hyperthyroidism *(see
      also* Goiter, toxic) 242.2 ●
  nodular (nontoxic) 241.9
    with
      hyperthyroidism *(see also* Goiter,
        toxic) 242.3 ●
      thyrotoxicosis *(see also* Goiter,
        toxic) 242.3 ●
    endemic 241.9
    exophthalmic (diffuse) *(see also*
      Goiter, toxic) 242.0 ●
    multinodular (nontoxic) 241.1
    sporadic 241.9
    toxic *(see also* Goiter, toxic) 242.3 ●
    uninodular (nontoxic) 241.0
  nontoxic (nodular) 241.9
    multinodular 241.1
    uninodular 241.0
  pulsating *(see also* Goiter, toxic) 242.0 ●
  simple 240.0
  toxic 242.0 ●

Note 35   Use the following fifth-digit
subclassification with category 242:

  0   without mention of thyrotoxic
      crisis or storm
  1   with mention of thyrotoxic crisis
      or storm

  adenomatous 242.3 ●
    multinodular 242.2 ●
    uninodular 242.1 ●
  multinodular 242.2 ●
  nodular 242.3 ●
    multinodular 242.2 ●
    uninodular 242.1 ●
  uninodular 242.1 ●

Goiter *(Continued)*
 uninodular (nontoxic) 241.0
  toxic or with hyperthyroidism *(see also* Goiter, toxic) 242.1●
Goldberg (-Maxwell) (-Morris) syndrome (testicular feminization) 259.51
Goldblatt's
 hypertension 440.1
 kidney 440.1
Goldenhar's syndrome (oculoauriculovertebral dysplasia) 756.0
Goldflam-Erb disease or syndrome 358.00
Goldscheider's disease (epidermolysis bullosa) 757.39
Goldstein's disease (familial hemorrhagic telangiectasia) 448.0
Golfer's elbow 726.32
Goltz-Gorlin syndrome (dermal hypoplasia) 757.39
Gonadoblastoma (M9073/1)
 specified site - *see* Neoplasm, by site, uncertain behavior
 unspecified site
  female 236.2
  male 236.4
Gonecystitis *(see also* Vesiculitis) 608.0
Gongylonemiasis 125.6
 mouth 125.6
Goniosynechiae 364.73
Gonococcemia 098.89
Gonococcus, gonococcal (disease) (infection) *(see also* condition) 098.0
 anus 098.7
 bursa 098.52
 chronic NEC 098.2
 complicating pregnancy, childbirth, or puerperium 647.1●
  affecting fetus or newborn 760.2
 conjunctiva, conjunctivitis (neonatorum) 098.40
 dermatosis 098.89
 endocardium 098.84
 epididymo-orchitis 098.13
  chronic or duration of 2 months or over 098.33
 eye (newborn) 098.40
 fallopian tube (chronic) 098.37
  acute 098.17
 genitourinary (acute) (organ) (system) (tract) *(see also* Gonorrhea) 098.0
  lower 098.0
   chronic 098.2
  upper 098.10
   chronic 098.30
 heart NEC 098.85
 joint 098.50
 keratoderma 098.81
 keratosis (blennorrhagica) 098.81
 lymphatic (gland) (node) 098.89
 meninges 098.82
 orchitis (acute) 098.13
  chronic or duration of 2 months or over 098.33
 pelvis (acute) 098.19
  chronic or duration of 2 months or over 098.39
 pericarditis 098.83
 peritonitis 098.86
 pharyngitis 098.6
 pharynx 098.6
 proctitis 098.7

Gonococcus, gonococcal *(Continued)*
 pyosalpinx (chronic) 098.37
  acute 098.17
 rectum 098.7
 septicemia 098.89
 skin 098.89
 specified site NEC 098.89
 synovitis 098.51
 tendon sheath 098.51
 throat 098.6
 urethra (acute) 098.0
  chronic or duration of 2 months or over 098.2
 vulva (acute) 098.0
  chronic or duration of 2 months or over 098.2
Gonocytoma (M9073/1)
 specified site - *see* Neoplasm, by site, uncertain behavior
 unspecified site
  female 236.2
  male 236.4
Gonorrhea 098.0
 acute 098.0
 Bartholin's gland (acute) 098.0
  chronic or duration of 2 months or over 098.2
 bladder (acute) 098.11
  chronic or duration of 2 months or over 098.31
 carrier (suspected of) V02.7
 cervix (acute) 098.15
  chronic or duration of 2 months or over 098.35
 chronic 098.2
 complicating pregnancy, childbirth, or puerperium 647.1●
  affecting fetus or newborn 760.2
 conjunctiva, conjunctivitis (neonatorum) 098.40
 contact V01.6
 Cowper's gland (acute) 098.0
  chronic or duration of 2 months or over 098.2
 duration of 2 months or over 098.2
 exposure to V01.6
 fallopian tube (chronic) 098.37
  acute 098.17
 genitourinary (acute) (organ) (system) (tract) 098.0
  chronic 098.2
  duration of 2 months or over 098.2
 kidney (acute) 098.19
  chronic or duration of 2 months or over 098.39
 ovary (acute) 098.19
  chronic or duration of 2 months or over 098.39
 pelvis (acute) 098.19
  chronic or duration of 2 months or over 098.39
 penis (acute) 098.0
  chronic or duration of 2 months or over 098.2
 prostate (acute) 098.12
  chronic or duration of 2 months or over 098.32
 seminal vesicle (acute) 098.14
  chronic or duration of 2 months or over 098.34
 specified site NEC - *see* Gonococcus
 spermatic cord (acute) 098.14
  chronic or duration of 2 months or over 098.34

Gonorrhea *(Continued)*
 urethra (acute) 098.0
  chronic or duration of 2 months or over 098.2
 vagina (acute) 098.0
  chronic or duration of 2 months or over 098.2
 vas deferens (acute) 098.14
  chronic or duration of 2 months or over 098.34
 vulva (acute) 098.0
  chronic or duration of 2 months or over 098.2
Goodpasture's syndrome (pneumorenal) 446.21
Good's syndrome 279.06
Gopalan's syndrome (burning feet) 266.2
Gordon's disease (exudative enteropathy) 579.8
Gorlin-Chaudhry-Moss syndrome 759.89
Gougerot's syndrome (trisymptomatic) 709.1
Gougerot-Blum syndrome (pigmented purpuric lichenoid dermatitis) 709.1
Gougerot-Carteaud disease or syndrome (confluent reticulate papillomatosis) 701.8
Gougerot-Hailey-Hailey disease (benign familial chronic pemphigus) 757.39
Gougerot (-Houwer)-Sjögren syndrome (keratoconjunctivitis sicca) 710.2
Gouley's syndrome (constrictive pericarditis) 423.2
Goundou 102.6
Gout, gouty 274.9
 with ~~specified manifestations NEC 274.89~~ ◀▥
  specified manifestations NEC 274.89 ◀
  tophi (tophus) 274.03 ◀
 acute 274.01 ◀
 arthritis ~~(acute)~~ 274.00 ◀▥
  acute 274.01 ◀
 arthropathy 274.00 ◀▥
  acute 274.01 ◀
  chronic (without mention of tophus (tophi)) 274.02 ◀
   with tophus (tophi) 274.03 ◀
 attack 274.01 ◀
 chronic 274.02 ◀
  tophaceous 274.03 ◀
 degeneration, heart 274.82
 diathesis 274.9
 eczema 274.89
 episcleritis 274.89 *[379.09]*
 external ear (tophus) 274.81
 flare 274.01 ◀
 glomerulonephritis 274.10
 iritis 274.89 *[364.11]*
 joint 274.00 ◀▥
 kidney 274.10
 lead 984.9
  specified type of lead - *see* Table of Drugs and Chemicals
 nephritis 274.10
 neuritis 274.89 *[357.4]*
 phlebitis 274.89 *[451.9]*
 rheumatic 714.0
 saturnine 984.9
  specified type of lead - *see* Table of Drugs and Chemicals
 spondylitis 274.00 ◀▥

Gout, gouty (*Continued*)
  synovitis 274.00 ◀▥
  syphilitic 095.8 ◀▥
  tophi 274.03 ◀▥
    ear 274.81
    heart 274.82
    specified site NEC 274.82
Gowers'
  muscular dystrophy 359.1
  syndrome (vasovagal attack) 780.2
Gowers-Paton-Kennedy syndrome
    377.04
Gradenigo's syndrome 383.02
Graft-versus-host disease 279.50
~~bone marrow 996.85~~
  due to organ transplant NEC - *see*
    Complications, transplant, organ
Graham Steell's murmur (pulmonic
    regurgitation) (*see also* Endocarditis,
    pulmonary) 424.3
Grain-handlers' disease or lung 495.8
Grain mite (itch) 133.8
Grand
  mal (idiopathic) (*see also* Epilepsy)
    345.1●
    hysteria of Charcôt 300.11
    nonrecurrent or isolated 780.39
  multipara
    affecting management of labor and
      delivery 659.4●
    status only (not pregnant) V61.5
Granite workers' lung 502
Granular - *see also* condition
  inflammation, pharynx 472.1
  kidney (contracting) (*see also* Sclerosis,
    renal) 587
  liver - *see* Cirrhosis, liver
  nephritis - *see* Nephritis
Granulation tissue, abnormal - *see also*
    Granuloma
  abnormal or excessive 701.5
  postmastoidectomy cavity 383.33
  postoperative 701.5
  skin 701.5
Granulocytopenia, granulocytopenic
    (primary) 288.00
  malignant 288.09
Granuloma NEC 686.1
  abdomen (wall) 568.89
    skin (pyogenicum) 686.1
      from residual foreign body 709.4
  annulare 695.89
  anus 569.49
  apical 522.6
  appendix 543.9
  aural 380.23
  beryllium (skin) 709.4
    lung 503
  bone (*see also* Osteomyelitis) 730.1●
    eosinophilic 277.89
    from residual foreign body
      733.99
  canaliculus lacrimalis 375.81
  cerebral 348.89 ◀▥
  cholesterin, middle ear 385.82
  coccidioidal (progressive) 114.3
    lung 114.4
    meninges 114.2
    primary (lung) 114.0
  colon 569.89
  conjunctiva 372.61
  dental 522.6
  ear, middle (cholesterin) 385.82
    with otitis media - *see* Otitis media

Granuloma NEC (*Continued*)
  eosinophilic 277.89
    bone 277.89
    lung 277.89
    oral mucosa 528.9
  exuberant 701.5
  eyelid 374.89
  facial
    lethal midline 446.3
    malignant 446.3
  faciale 701.8
  fissuratum (gum) 523.8
  foot NEC 686.1
  foreign body (in soft tissue) NEC
    728.82
    bone 733.99
    in operative wound 998.4
    muscle 728.82
    skin 709.4
    subcutaneous tissue 709.4
  fungoides 202.1●
  gangraenescens 446.3
  giant cell (central) (jaw) (reparative)
    526.3
    gingiva 523.8
    peripheral (gingiva) 523.8
  gland (lymph) 289.3
  Hodgkin's (M9661/3) 201.1●
  ileum 569.89
  infectious NEC 136.9
  inguinale (Donovan) 099.2
    venereal 099.2
  intestine 569.89
  iridocyclitis 364.10
  jaw (bone) 526.3
    reparative giant cell 526.3
  kidney (*see also* Infection, kidney) 590.9
  lacrimal sac 375.81
  larynx 478.79
  lethal midline 446.3
  lipid 277.89
  lipoid 277.89
  liver 572.8
  lung (infectious) (*see also* Fibrosis, lung)
    515
    coccidioidal 114.4
    eosinophilic 277.89
  lymph gland 289.3
  Majocchi's 110.6
  malignant, face 446.3
  mandible 526.3
  mediastinum 519.3
  midline 446.3
  monilial 112.3
  muscle 728.82
    from residual foreign body 728.82
  nasal sinus (*see also* Sinusitis) 473.9
  operation wound 998.59
    foreign body 998.4
    stitch (external) 998.89
      internal wound 998.89
    talc 998.7
  oral mucosa, eosinophilic or pyogenic
    528.9
  orbit, orbital 376.11
  paracoccidioidal 116.1
  penis, venereal 099.2
  periapical 522.6
  peritoneum 568.89
    due to ova of helminths NEC (*see*
      also Helminthiasis) 128.9
  postmastoidectomy cavity 383.33
  postoperative - *see* Granuloma,
    operation wound

Granuloma NEC (*Continued*)
  prostate 601.8
  pudendi (ulcerating) 099.2
  pudendorum (ulcerative) 099.2
  pulp, internal (tooth) 521.49
  pyogenic, pyogenicum (skin) 686.1
    maxillary alveolar ridge 522.6
    oral mucosa 528.9
  rectum 569.49
  reticulohistiocytic 277.89
  rubrum nasi 705.89
  sarcoid 135
  Schistosoma 120.9
  septic (skin) 686.1
  silica (skin) 709.4
  sinus (accessory) (infectional) (nasal)
    (*see also* Sinusitis) 473.9
  skin (pyogenicum) 686.1
    from foreign body or material 709.4
  sperm 608.89
  spine
    syphilitic (epidural) 094.89
    tuberculous (*see also* Tuberculosis)
      015.0● [730.88]
  stitch (postoperative) 998.89
    internal wound 998.89
  suppurative (skin) 686.1
  suture (postoperative) 998.89
    internal wound 998.89
  swimming pool 031.1
  talc 728.82
    in operation wound 998.7
  telangiectaticum (skin) 686.1
  tracheostomy 519.09
  trichophyticum 110.6
  tropicum 102.4
  umbilicus 686.1
    newborn 771.4
  urethra 599.84
  uveitis 364.10
  vagina 099.2
  venereum 099.2
  vocal cords 478.5
  Wegener's (necrotizing respiratory
    granulomatosis) 446.4
Granulomatosis NEC 686.1
  disciformis chronica et progressiva 709.3
  infantiseptica 771.2
  lipoid 277.89
  lipophagic, intestinal 040.2
  miliary 027.0
  necrotizing, respiratory 446.4
  progressive, septic 288.1
  Wegener's (necrotizing respiratory)
    446.4
Granulomatous tissue - *see* Granuloma
Granulosis rubra nasi 705.89
Graphite fibrosis (of lung) 503
Graphospasm 300.89
  organic 333.84
Grating scapula 733.99
Gravel (urinary) (*see also* Calculus) 592.9
Graves' disease (exophthalmic goiter) (*see*
    also Goiter, toxic) 242.0●
Gravis - *see* condition
Grawitz's tumor (hypernephroma)
    (M8312/3) 189.0
Grayness, hair (premature) 704.3
  congenital 757.4
Gray or grey syndrome
    (chloramphenicol) (newborn)
    779.4
Greenfield's disease 330.0
Green sickness 280.9

Greenstick fracture - *see* Fracture,
  by site
Greig's syndrome (hypertelorism)
  756.0
Grief 309.0
Griesinger's disease (*see also*
  Ancylostomiasis) 126.9
Grinders'
  asthma 502
  lung 502
  phthisis (*see also* Tuberculosis) 011.4●
Grinding, teeth 306.8
Grip
  Dabney's 074.1
  devil's 074.1
Grippe, grippal - *see also* Influenza
  Balkan 083.0
  intestinal 487.8
  summer 074.8
Grippy cold 487.1
Grisel's disease 723.5
Groin - *see* condition
Grooved
  nails (transverse) 703.8
  tongue 529.5
    congenital 750.13
Ground itch 126.9
Growing pains, children 781.99
Growth (fungoid) (neoplastic) (new)
  (M8000/1) - *see also* Neoplasm, by
  site, unspecified nature
  adenoid (vegetative) 474.12
  benign (M8000/0) - *see* Neoplasm, by
    site, benign
  fetal, poor 764.9●
    affecting management of pregnancy
      656.5●
  malignant (M8000/3) - *see* Neoplasm,
    by site, malignant
  rapid, childhood V21.0
  secondary (M8000/6) - *see* Neoplasm,
    by site, malignant, secondary
GRSA (glycopeptide resistant
  staphylococcus aureus) V09.8
Gruber's hernia - *see* Hernia, Gruber's
Gruby's disease (tinea tonsurans) 110.0
GSS (Gerstmann-Sträussler-Scheinker
  syndrome) 046.71

G-trisomy 758.0
Guama fever 066.3
Gubler (-Millard) paralysis or syndrome
  344.89
Guérin-Stern syndrome (arthrogryposis
  multiplex congenita) 754.89
Guertin's disease (electric chorea) 049.8
Guillain-Barré disease or syndrome 357.0
Guinea worms (infection) (infestation)
  125.7
Guinon's disease (motor-verbal tic)
  307.23
Gull's disease (thyroid atrophy with
  myxedema) 244.8
Gull and Sutton's disease - *see*
  Hypertension, kidney
Gum - *see* condition
Gumboil 522.7
Gumma (syphilitic) 095.9
  artery 093.89
    cerebral or spinal 094.89
  bone 095.5
    of yaws (late) 102.6
  brain 094.89
  cauda equina 094.89
  central nervous system NEC 094.9
  ciliary body 095.8 [364.11]
  congenital 090.5
    testis 090.5
  eyelid 095.8 [373.5]
  heart 093.89
  intracranial 094.89
  iris 095.8 [364.11]
  kidney 095.4
  larynx 095.8
  leptomeninges 094.2
  liver 095.3
  meninges 094.2
  myocardium 093.82
  nasopharynx 095.8
  neurosyphilitic 094.9
  nose 095.8
  orbit 095.8
  palate (soft) 095.8
  penis 095.8
  pericardium 093.81
  pharynx 095.8

Gumma(*Continued*)
  pituitary 095.8
  scrofulous (*see also* Tuberculosis)
    017.0●
Gumma (*Continued*)
  skin 095.8
  specified site NEC 095.8
  spinal cord 094.89
  tongue 095.8
  tonsil 095.8
  trachea 095.8
  tuberculous (*see also* Tuberculosis)
    017.0●
  ulcerative due to yaws 102.4
  ureter 095.8
  yaws 102.4
    bone 102.6
Gunn's syndrome (jaw-winking
  syndrome) 742.8
Gunshot wound - *see also* Wound, open,
  by site
  fracture - *see* Fracture, by site, open
  internal organs (abdomen, chest, or
    pelvis) - *see* Injury, internal, by
    site, with open wound
  intracranial - *see* Laceration, brain,
    with open intracranial wound
Günther's disease or syndrome
  (congenital erythropoietic
  porphyria) 277.1
Gustatory hallucination 780.1
Gynandrism 752.7
Gynandroblastoma (M8632/1)
  specified site - *see* Neoplasm, by site,
    uncertain behavior
  unspecified site
    female 236.2
    male 236.4
Gynandromorphism 752.7
Gynatresia (congenital) 752.49
Gynecoid pelvis, male 738.6
Gynecological examination V72.31
  for contraceptive maintenance
    V25.40
Gynecomastia 611.1
Gynephobia 300.29
Gyrate scalp 757.39

◀ New ◀▥ Revised ~~deleted~~ Deleted ● Use Additional Digit(s) ▧ Omit code

H

Haas' disease (osteochondrosis head of humerus) 732.3
Habermann's disease (acute parapsoriasis varioliformis) 696.2
Habit, habituation
  chorea 307.22
  disturbance, child 307.9
  drug (see also Dependence) 304.9●
  laxative (see also Abuse, drugs, nondependent) 305.9●
  spasm 307.20
    chronic 307.22
    transient (of childhood) 307.21
  tic 307.20
    chronic 307.22
    transient (of childhood) 307.21
  use of
    nonprescribed drugs (see also Abuse, drugs, nondependent) 305.9●
    patent medicines (see also Abuse, drugs, nondependent) 305.9●
  vomiting 536.2
Hadfield-Clarke syndrome (pancreatic infantilism) 577.8
Haff disease 985.1
Hag teeth, tooth 524.39
Hageman factor defect, deficiency, or disease (see also Defect, coagulation) 286.3
Haglund's disease (osteochondrosis os tibiale externum) 732.5
Haglund-Läwen-Fründ syndrome 717.89
Hagner's disease (hypertrophic pulmonary osteoarthropathy) 731.2
Hailey-Hailey disease (benign familial chronic pemphigus) 757.39
Hair - see also condition
  plucking 307.9
Hairball in stomach 935.2
Hairy black tongue 529.3
Half vertebra 756.14
Halitosis 784.99
Hallermann-Streiff syndrome 756.0
Hallervorden-Spatz disease or syndrome 333.0
Hallopeau's
  acrodermatitis (continua) 696.1
  disease (lichen sclerosis et atrophicus) 701.0
Hallucination (auditory) (gustatory) (olfactory) (tactile) 780.1
  alcohol-induced 291.3
  drug-induced 292.12
  visual 368.16
Hallucinosis 298.9
  alcohol-induced (acute) 291.3
  drug-induced 292.12
Hallus - see Hallux
Hallux 735.9
  limitus 735.8
  malleus (acquired) 735.3
  rigidus (acquired) 735.2
    congenital 755.66
    late effects of rickets 268.1
  valgus (acquired) 735.0
    congenital 755.66
  varus (acquired) 735.1
    congenital 755.66
Halo, visual 368.15
Hamartoblastoma 759.6

Hamartoma 759.6
  epithelial (gingival), odontogenic, central, or peripheral (M9321/0) 213.1
  upper jaw (bone) 213.0
  vascular 757.32
Hamartosis, hamartoses NEC 759.6
Hamman's disease or syndrome (spontaneous mediastinal emphysema) 518.1
Hamman-Rich syndrome (diffuse interstitial pulmonary fibrosis) 516.3
Hammer toe (acquired) 735.4
  congenital 755.66
  late effects of rickets 268.1
Hand - see condition
Hand-Schüller-Christian disease or syndrome (chronic histiocytosis x) 277.89
Hand-foot syndrome 693.0
Hanging (asphyxia) (strangulation) (suffocation) 994.7
Hangnail (finger) (with lymphangitis) 681.02
Hangover (alcohol) (see also Abuse, drugs, nondependent) 305.0●
Hanot's cirrhosis or disease - see Cirrhosis, biliary
Hanot-Chauffard (-Troisier) syndrome (bronze diabetes) 275.0
Hansen's disease (leprosy) 030.9
  benign form 030.1
  malignant form 030.0
Harada's disease or syndrome 363.22
Hard chancre 091.0
Hard firm prostate 600.10
  with
    urinary
      obstruction 600.11
      retention 600.11
Hardening
  artery - see Arteriosclerosis
  brain 348.89
  liver 571.8
Hare's syndrome (M8010/3) (carcinoma, pulmonary apex) 162.3
Harelip (see also Cleft, lip) 749.10
Harkavy's syndrome 446.0
Harlequin (fetus) 757.1
  color change syndrome 779.89
Harley's disease (intermittent hemoglobinuria) 283.2
Harris'
  lines 733.91
  syndrome (organic hyperinsulinism) 251.1
Hart's disease or syndrome (pellagra-cerebellar ataxia-renal aminoaciduria) 270.0
Hartmann's pouch (abnormal sacculation of gallbladder neck) 575.8
  of intestine V44.3
  attention to V55.3
Hartnup disease (pellagra-cerebellar ataxia-renal aminoaciduria) 270.0
Harvester lung 495.0
Hashimoto's disease or struma (struma lymphomatosa) 245.2
Hassall-Henle bodies (corneal warts) 371.41
Haut mal (see also Epilepsy) 345.1●
Haverhill fever 026.1
Hawaiian wood rose dependence 304.5●
Hawkins' keloid 701.4

Hay
  asthma (see also Asthma) 493.0●
  fever (allergic) (with rhinitis) 477.9
    with asthma (bronchial) (see also Asthma) 493.0●
    allergic, due to grass, pollen, ragweed, or tree 477.0
    conjunctivitis 372.05
    due to
      dander, animal (cat) (dog) 477.2
      dust 477.8
      fowl 477.8
      hair, animal (cat) (dog) 477.2
      pollen 477.0
      specified allergen other than pollen 477.8
Hayem-Faber syndrome (achlorhydric anemia) 280.9
Hayem-Widal syndrome (acquired hemolytic jaundice) 283.9
Haygarth's nodosities 715.04
Hazard-Crile tumor (M8350/3) 193
Hb (abnormal)
  disease - see Disease, hemoglobin
  trait - see Trait
H disease 270.0
Head - see also condition
  banging 307.3
Headache 784.0
  allergic 339.00
  associated with sexual activity 339.82
  cluster 339.00
    chronic 339.02
    episodic 339.01
  daily
    chronic 784.0
    new persistent (NPDH) 339.42
  drug induced 339.3
  due to
    loss, spinal fluid 349.0
    lumbar puncture 349.0
    saddle block 349.0
  emotional 307.81
  histamine 339.00
  hypnic 339.81
  lumbar puncture 349.0
  medication overuse 339.3
  menopausal 627.2
  menstrual 346.4●
  migraine 346.9●
  nasal septum 784.0
  nonorganic origin 307.81
  orgasmic 339.82
  postspinal 349.0
  post-traumatic 339.20
    acute 339.21
    chronic 339.22
  premenstrual 346.4●
  preorgasmic 339.82
  primary
    cough 339.83
    exertional 339.84
    stabbing 339.85
    thunderclap 339.43
  psychogenic 307.81
  psychophysiologic 307.81
  rebound 339.3
  short lasting unilateral neuralgiform with conjunctival injection and tearing (SUNCT) 339.05
  sick 346.9●

Headache *(Continued)*
  spinal 349.0
    complicating labor and delivery
      668.8●
      postpartum 668.8●
  spinal fluid loss 349.0
  syndrome
    cluster 339.00
    complicated NEC 339.44
    periodic in child or adolescent
      346.2●
    specified NEC 339.89
  tension 307.81
    type 339.10
      chronic 339.12
      episodic 339.11
  vascular 784.0
    migraine type 346.9●
  vasomotor 346.9●
Health
  advice V65.4
  audit V70.0
  checkup V70.0
  education V65.4
  hazard *(see also* History of) V15.9
    falling V15.88
    specified cause NEC V15.89
  instruction V65.4
  services provided because (of)
    boarding school residence V60.6
    holiday relief for person providing
      home care V60.5
    inadequate
      housing V60.1
      resources V60.2
    lack of housing V60.0
    no care available in home V60.4
    person living alone V60.3
    poverty V60.3
    residence in institution V60.6
    specified cause NEC V60.89 ◀▥
    vacation relief for person providing
      home care V60.5
Healthy
  donor *(see also* Donor) V59.9
  infant or child
    accompanying sick mother V65.0
    receiving care V20.1
  person
    accompanying sick relative V65.0
    admitted for sterilization V25.2
    receiving prophylactic inoculation
      or vaccination *(see also*
      Vaccination, prophylactic)
      V05.9
Hearing
  conservation and treatment V72.12
  examination V72.19
    following failed hearing screening
      V72.11
Heart - *see* condition
Heartburn 787.1
  psychogenic 306.4
Heat (effects) 992.9
  apoplexy 992.0
  burn - *see also* Burn, by site
    from sun *(see also* Sunburn) 692.71
  collapse 992.1
  cramps 992.2
  dermatitis or eczema 692.89
  edema 992.7
  erythema - *see* Burn, by site
  excessive 992.9
    specified effect NEC 992.8

Heat *(Continued)*
  exhaustion 992.5
    anhydrotic 992.3
    due to
      salt (and water) depletion
        992.4
      water depletion 992.3
  fatigue (transient) 992.6
  fever 992.0
  hyperpyrexia 992.0
  prickly 705.1
  prostration - *see* Heat, exhaustion
  pyrexia 992.0
  rash 705.1
  specified effect NEC 992.8
  stroke 992.0
  sunburn *(see also* Sunburn) 692.71
  syncope 992.1
Heavy-chain disease 273.2
Heavy-for-dates (fetus or infant) 766.1
  4500 grams or more 766.0
  exceptionally 766.0
Hebephrenia, hebephrenic (acute) *(see*
    also Schizophrenia) 295.1●
  dementia (praecox) *(see also*
    Schizophrenia) 295.1●
  schizophrenia *(see also* Schizophrenia)
    295.1●
Heberden's
  disease or nodes 715.04
  syndrome (angina pectoris) 413.9
Hebra's disease
  dermatitis exfoliativa 695.89
  erythema multiforme exudativum
    695.19
  pityriasis 695.89
    maculata et circinata 696.3
    rubra 695.89
      pilaris 696.4
  prurigo 698.2
Hebra, nose 040.1
Hedinger's syndrome (malignant
    carcinoid) 259.2
Heel - *see* condition
Heerfordt's disease or syndrome
    (uveoparotitis) 135
Hegglin's anomaly or syndrome 288.2
Heidenhain's disease 290.10
  with dementia 290.10
Heilmeyer-Schoner disease (M9842/3)
    207.1●
Heine-Medin disease *(see also*
    Poliomyelitis) 045.9●
Heinz-body anemia, congenital 282.7
Heller's disease or syndrome (infantile
    psychosis) *(see also* Psychosis,
    childhood) 299.1●
H.E.L.L.P. 642.5●
Helminthiasis *(see also* Infestation, by
    specific parasite) 128.9
  Ancylostoma *(see also* Ancylostoma)
    126.9
  intestinal 127.9
    mixed types (types classifiable to
      more than one of the
      categories 120.0–127.7) 127.8
    specified type 127.7
  mixed types (intestinal) (types
    classifiable to more than one
    of the categories 120.0–127.7)
    127.8
  Necator americanus 126.1
  specified type NEC 128.8
  Trichinella 124

Heloma 700
Hemangioblastoma (M9161/1) - *see also*
    Neoplasm, connective tissue,
    uncertain behavior
  malignant (M9161/3) - *see* Neoplasm,
    connective tissue, malignant
Hemangioblastomatosis, cerebelloretinal
    759.6
Hemangioendothelioma (M9130/1) - *see*
    also Neoplasm, by site, uncertain
    behavior
  benign (M9130/0) 228.00
  bone (diffuse) (M9130/3) - *see*
    Neoplasm, bone, malignant
  malignant (M9130/3) - *see* Neoplasm,
    connective tissue, malignant
  nervous system (M9130/0) 228.09
Hemangioendotheliosarcoma
    (M9130/3) - *see* Neoplasm,
    connective tissue, malignant
Hemangiofibroma (M9160/0) - *see*
    Neoplasm, by site, benign
Hemangiolipoma (M8861/0) - *see*
    Lipoma
Hemangioma (M9120/0) 228.00
  arteriovenous (M9123/0) - *see*
    Hemangioma, by site
  brain 228.02
  capillary (M9131/0) - *see* Hemangioma,
    by site
  cavernous (M9121/0) - *see*
    Hemangioma, by site
  central nervous system NEC
    228.09
  choroid 228.09
  heart 228.09
  infantile (M9131/0) - *see* Hemangioma,
    by site
  intra-abdominal structures 228.04
  intracranial structures 228.02
  intramuscular (M9132/0) - *see*
    Hemangioma, by site
  iris 228.09
  juvenile (M9131/0) - *see* Hemangioma,
    by site
  malignant (M9120/3) - *see*
    Neoplasm, connective
    tissue, malignant
  meninges 228.09
    brain 228.02
    spinal cord 228.09
  peritoneum 228.04
  placenta - *see* Placenta, abnormal
  plexiform (M9131/0) - *see*
    Hemangioma, by site
  racemose (M9123/0) - *see*
    Hemangioma, by site
  retina 228.03
  retroperitoneal tissue 228.04
  sclerosing (M8832/0) - *see* Neoplasm,
    skin, benign
  simplex (M9131/0) - *see*
    Hemangioma, by site
  skin and subcutaneous tissue
    228.01
  specified site NEC 228.09
  spinal cord 228.09
  venous (M9122/0) - *see* Hemangioma,
    by site
  verrucous keratotic (M9142/0) - *see*
    Hemangioma, by site
Hemangiomatosis (systemic) 757.32
  involving single site - *see*
    Hemangioma

◀ New   ◀▥ Revised   ~~deleted~~ Deleted   ● Use Additional Digit(s)   ▥ Omit code

Hemangiopericytoma (M9150/1) - *see also*
 Neoplasm, connective tissue,
 uncertain behavior
 benign (M9150/0) - *see* Neoplasm,
  connective tissue, benign
 malignant (M9150/3) - *see* Neoplasm,
  connective tissue, malignant
Hemangiosarcoma (M9120/3) - *see*
 Neoplasm, connective tissue,
 malignant
Hemarthrosis (nontraumatic) 719.10
 ankle 719.17
 elbow 719.12
 foot 719.17
 hand 719.14
 hip 719.15
 knee 719.16
 multiple sites 719.19
 pelvic region 719.15
 shoulder (region) 719.11
 specified site NEC 719.18
 traumatic - *see* Sprain, by site
 wrist 719.13
Hematemesis 578.0
 with ulcer - *see* Ulcer, by site, with
  hemorrhage
 due to S. japonicum 120.2
 Goldstein's (familial hemorrhagic
  telangiectasia) 448.0
 newborn 772.4
  due to swallowed maternal blood
   777.3
Hematidrosis 705.89
Hematinuria (*see also* Hemoglobinuria)
 791.2
 malarial 084.8
 paroxysmal 283.2
Hematite miners' lung 503
Hematobilia 576.8
Hematocele (congenital) (diffuse)
 (idiopathic) 608.83
 broad ligament 620.7
 canal of Nuck 629.0
 cord, male 608.83
 fallopian tube 620.8
 female NEC 629.0
 ischiorectal 569.89
 male NEC 608.83
 ovary 629.0
 pelvis, pelvic
  female 629.0
   with ectopic pregnancy (*see also*
    Pregnancy, ectopic) 633.90
    with intrauterine pregnancy
     633.91
  male 608.83
 periuterine 629.0
 retrouterine 629.0
 scrotum 608.83
 spermatic cord (diffuse) 608.83
 testis 608.84
 traumatic - *see* Injury, internal, pelvis
 tunica vaginalis 608.83
 uterine ligament 629.0
 uterus 621.4
 vagina 623.6
 vulva 624.5
Hematocephalus 742.4
Hematochezia (*see also* Melena) 578.1
Hematochyluria (*see also* Infestation,
 filarial) 125.9
Hematocolpos 626.8
Hematocornea 371.12
Hematogenous - *see* condition

Hematoma (skin surface intact)
 (traumatic) - *see also* Contusion

Note 36   Hematomas are coded
according to origin and the nature and
site of the hematoma or the
accompanying injury. Hematomas of
unspecified origin are coded as injuries
of the sites involved, except:

(a) hematomas of genital organs
 which are coded as
 diseases of the organ
 involved unless they
 complicate pregnancy or
 delivery
(b) hematomas of the eye which are
 coded as diseases of the
 eye.

For late effect of hematoma classifiable
to 920–924 *see* Late, effect, contusion.

---

 with
  crush injury - *see* Crush
  fracture - *see* Fracture, by site
  injury of internal organs - *see also*
   Injury, internal, by site
   kidney - *see* Hematoma, kidney,
    traumatic
   liver - *see* Hematoma, liver,
    traumatic
   spleen - *see* Hematoma, spleen
  nerve injury - *see* Injury, nerve
  open wound - *see* Wound, open, by
   site
  skin surface intact - *see* Contusion
 abdomen (wall) - *see* Contusion,
  abdomen
 amnion 658.8●
 aorta, dissecting 441.00
  abdominal 441.02
  thoracic 441.01
  thoracoabdominal 441.03
 arterial (complicating trauma) 904.9
  specified site - *see* Injury, blood
   vessel, by site
 auricle (ear) 380.31
 birth injury 767.8
  skull 767.19
 brain (traumatic) 853.0●

Note 37   Use the following fifth-digit
subclassification with categories 851–854:

0   unspecified state of
  consciousness
1   with no loss of consciousness
2   with brief [less than one hour]
  loss of consciousness
3   with moderate [1–24 hours] loss
  of consciousness
4   with prolonged [more than 24
  hours] loss of consciousness
  and return to pre-existing
  conscious level
5   with prolonged [more than 24
  hours] loss of
  consciousness, without
  return to pre-existing
  conscious level

Use fifth-digit 5 to designate when a
patient is unconscious and dies before
regaining consciousness, regardless of
the duration of the loss of consciousness

6   with loss of consciousness of
  unspecified duration
9   with concussion, unspecified

Hematoma (*Continued*)
 brain (*Continued*)
  with
   cerebral
    contusion - *see* Contusion,
     brain
    laceration - *see* Laceration,
     brain
    open intracranial wound
     853.1●
    skull fracture - *see* Fracture,
     skull, by site
   extradural or epidural 852.4●
    with open intracranial wound
     852.5●
   fetus or newborn 767.0
   nontraumatic 432.0
  fetus or newborn NEC 767.0
  nontraumatic (*see also* Hemorrhage,
   brain) 431
   epidural or extradural 432.0
   newborn NEC 772.8
   subarachnoid, arachnoid, or
    meningeal (*see also*
    Hemorrhage, subarachnoid)
    430
   subdural (*see also* Hemorrhage,
    subdural) 432.1
  subarachnoid, arachnoid, or
   meningeal 852.0●
   with open intracranial wound
    852.1●
   fetus or newborn 772.2
   nontraumatic (*see also*
    Hemorrhage,
    subarachnoid) 430
  subdural 852.2●
   with open intracranial wound
    852.3●
   fetus or newborn (localized)
    767.0
   nontraumatic (*see also*
    Hemorrhage, subdural)
    432.1
 breast (nontraumatic) 611.89
 broad ligament (nontraumatic)
  620.7
  complicating delivery 665.7●
  traumatic - *see* Injury, internal,
   broad ligament
 calcified NEC 959.9
 capitis 920
  due to birth injury 767.19
  newborn 767.19
 cerebral - *see* Hematoma, brain
 cesarean section wound 674.3●
 chorion - *see* Placenta, abnormal
 complicating delivery (perineum)
  (vulva) 664.5●
  pelvic 665.7●
  vagina 665.7●
 corpus
  cavernosum (nontraumatic)
   607.82
  luteum (nontraumatic) (ruptured)
   620.1
 dura (mater) - *see* Hematoma, brain,
  subdural
 epididymis (nontraumatic) 608.83
 epidural (traumatic) - *see also*
  Hematoma, brain, extradural
  spinal - *see* Injury, spinal, by site
 episiotomy 674.3●
 external ear 380.31

Hematoma (*Continued*)
  extradural - *see also* Hematoma, brain, extradural
    fetus or newborn 767.0
    nontraumatic 432.0
      fetus or newborn 767.0
  fallopian tube 620.8
  genital organ (nontraumatic)
    female NEC 629.89
    male NEC 608.83
    traumatic (external site) 922.4
      internal - *see* Injury, internal, genital organ
  graafian follicle (ruptured) 620.0
  internal organs (abdomen, chest, or pelvis) - *see also* Injury, internal, by site
    kidney - *see* Hematoma, kidney, traumatic
    liver - *see* Hematoma, liver, traumatic
    spleen - *see* Hematoma, spleen
  intracranial - *see* Hematoma, brain
  kidney, cystic 593.81
    traumatic 866.01
      with open wound into cavity 866.11
  labia (nontraumatic) 624.5
  lingual (and other parts of neck, scalp, or face, except eye) 920
  liver (subcapsular) 573.8
    birth injury 767.8
    fetus or newborn 767.8
    traumatic NEC 864.01
      with
        laceration - *see* Laceration, liver
        open wound into cavity 864.11
  mediastinum - *see* Injury, internal, mediastinum
  meninges, meningeal (brain) - *see also* Hematoma, brain, subarachnoid
  spinal - *see* Injury, spinal, by site
  mesosalpinx (nontraumatic) 620.8
    traumatic - *see* Injury, internal, pelvis
  muscle (traumatic) - *see* Contusion, by site
    nontraumatic 729.92
  nasal (septum) (and other part(s) of neck, scalp, or face, except eye) 920
  obstetrical surgical wound 674.3●
  orbit, orbital (nontraumatic) 376.32
    traumatic 921.2
  ovary (corpus luteum) (nontraumatic) 620.1
    traumatic - *see* Injury, internal, ovary
  pelvis (female) (nontraumatic) 629.89
    complicating delivery 665.7●
    male 608.83
    traumatic - *see also* Injury, internal, pelvis
      specified organ NEC (*see also* Injury, internal, pelvis) 867.6
  penis (nontraumatic) 607.82
  pericranial (and neck, or face any part, except eye) 920
    due to injury at birth 767.19
  perineal wound (obstetrical) 674.3●
    complicating delivery 664.5●
  perirenal, cystic 593.81
  pinna 380.31

Hematoma (*Continued*)
  placenta - *see* Placenta, abnormal
  postoperative 998.12
  retroperitoneal (nontraumatic) 568.81
    traumatic - *see* Injury, internal, retroperitoneum
  retropubic, male 568.81
  scalp (and neck, or face any part, except eye) 920
    fetus or newborn 767.19
  scrotum (nontraumatic) 608.83
    traumatic 922.4
  seminal vesicle (nontraumatic) 608.83
    traumatic - *see* Injury, internal, seminal, vesicle
  soft tissue, nontraumatic 729.92
  spermatic cord - *see also* Injury, internal, spermatic cord
    nontraumatic 608.83
  spinal (cord) (meninges) - *see also* Injury, spinal, by site
    fetus or newborn 767.4
    nontraumatic 336.1
  spleen 865.01
    with
      laceration - *see* Laceration, spleen
      open wound into cavity 865.11
  sternocleidomastoid, birth injury 767.8
  sternomastoid, birth injury 767.8
  subarachnoid - *see also* Hematoma, brain, subarachnoid
    fetus or newborn 772.2
    nontraumatic (*see also* Hemorrhage, subarachnoid) 430
      newborn 772.2
  subdural - *see also* Hematoma, brain, subdural
    fetus or newborn (localized) 767.0
    nontraumatic (*see also* Hemorrhage, subdural) 432.1
  subperiosteal (syndrome) 267
    traumatic - *see* Hematoma, by site
  superficial, fetus or newborn 772.6
  syncytium - *see* Placenta, abnormal
  testis (nontraumatic) 608.83
    birth injury 767.8
    traumatic 922.4
  tunica vaginalis (nontraumatic) 608.83
  umbilical cord 663.6●
    affecting fetus or newborn 762.6
  uterine ligament (nontraumatic) 620.7
    traumatic - *see* Injury, internal, pelvis
  uterus 621.4
    traumatic - *see* Injury, internal, pelvis
  vagina (nontraumatic) (ruptured) 623.6
    complicating delivery 665.7●
    traumatic 922.4
  vas deferens (nontraumatic) 608.83
    traumatic - *see* Injury, internal, vas deferens
  vitreous 379.23
  vocal cord 920
  vulva (nontraumatic) 624.5
    complicating delivery 664.5●
    fetus or newborn 767.8
    traumatic 922.4
Hematometra 621.4
Hematomyelia 336.1
  with fracture of vertebra (*see also* Fracture, vertebra, by site, with spinal cord injury) 806.8
  fetus or newborn 767.4
Hematomyelitis 323.9
  late effect - *see* category 326

Hematoperitoneum (*see also* Hemoperitoneum) 568.81
Hematopneumothorax (*see also* Hemothorax) 511.89
Hematopoiesis, cyclic 288.02
Hematoporphyria (acquired) (congenital) 277.1
Hematoporphyrinuria (acquired) (congenital) 277.1
Hematorachis, hematorrhachis 336.1
  fetus or newborn 767.4
Hematosalpinx 620.8
  with
    ectopic pregnancy (*see also* categories 633.0–633.9) 639.2
    molar pregnancy (*see also* categories 630–632) 639.2
    infectional (*see also* Salpingo-oophoritis) 614.2
Hematospermia 608.82
Hematothorax (*see also* Hemothorax) 511.89
Hematotympanum 381.03
Hematuria (benign) (essential) (idiopathic) 599.70
  due to S. hematobium 120.0
  endemic 120.0
  gross 599.71
  intermittent 599.70
  malarial 084.8
  microscopic 599.72
  paroxysmal 599.70
  sulfonamide
    correct substance properly administered 599.70
    overdose or wrong substance given or taken 961.0
  tropical (bilharziasis) 120.0
  tuberculous (*see also* Tuberculosis) 016.9●
Hematuric bilious fever 084.8
Hemeralopia 368.10
Hemiabiotrophy 799.89
Hemi-akinesia 781.8
Hemianalgesia (*see also* Disturbance, sensation) 782.0
Hemianencephaly 740.0
Hemianesthesia (*see also* Disturbance, sensation) 782.0
Hemianopia, hemianopsia (altitudinal) (homonymous) 368.46
  binasal 368.47
  bitemporal 368.47
  heteronymous 368.47
  syphilitic 095.8
Hemiasomatognosia 307.9
Hemiathetosis 781.0
Hemiatrophy 799.89
  cerebellar 334.8
  face 349.89
    progressive 349.89
  fascia 728.9
  leg 728.2
  tongue 529.8
Hemiballism (us) 333.5
Hemiblock (cardiac) (heart) (left) 426.2
Hemicardia 746.89
Hemicephalus, hemicephaly 740.0
Hemichorea 333.5
Hemicrania 346.9●
  congenital malformation 740.0
  continua 339.41
  paroxysmal 339.03
    chronic 339.04
    episodic 339.03

Hemidystrophy - *see* Hemiatrophy
Hemiectromelia 755.4
Hemihypalgesia (*see also* Disturbance, sensation) 782.0
Hemihypertrophy (congenital) 759.89
  cranial 756.0
Hemihypesthesia (*see also* Disturbance, sensation) 782.0
Hemi-inattention 781.8
Hemimelia 755.4
  lower limb 755.30
    paraxial (complete) (incomplete) (intercalary) (terminal) 755.32
      fibula 755.37
      tibia 755.36
    transverse (complete) (partial) 755.31
  upper limb 755.20
    paraxial (complete) (incomplete) (intercalary) (terminal) 755.22
      radial 755.26
      ulnar 755.27
    transverse (complete) (partial) 755.21
Hemiparalysis (*see also* Hemiplegia) 342.9●
Hemiparesis (*see also* Hemiplegia) 342.9●
Hemiparesthesia (*see also* Disturbance, sensation) 782.0
Hemiplegia 342.9●
  acute (*see also* Disease, cerebrovascular, acute) 436
  alternans facialis 344.89
  apoplectic (*see also* Disease, cerebrovascular, acute) 436
    late effect or residual
      affecting
        dominant side 438.21
        nondominant side 438.22
        unspecified side 438.20
  arteriosclerotic 437.0
    late effect or residual
      affecting
        dominant side 438.21
        nondominant side 438.22
        unspecified side 438.20
  ascending (spinal) NEC 344.89
  attack (*see also* Disease, cerebrovascular, acute) 436
  brain, cerebral (current episode) 437.8
    congenital 343.1
  cerebral - *see* Hemiplegia, brain
  congenital (cerebral) (spastic) (spinal) 343.1
  conversion neurosis (hysterical) 300.11
  cortical - *see* Hemiplegia, brain
  due to
    arteriosclerosis 437.0
      late effect or residual
        affecting
          dominant side 438.21
          nondominant side 438.22
          unspecified side 438.20
    cerebrovascular lesion (*see also* Disease, cerebrovascular, acute) 436
      late effect
        affecting
          dominant side 438.21
          nondominant side 438.22
          unspecified side 438.20

Hemiplegia (*Continued*)
  embolic (current) (*see also* Embolism, brain) 434.1●
    late effect
      affecting
        dominant side 438.21
        nondominant side 438.22
        unspecified side 438.20
  flaccid 342.0●
  hypertensive (current episode) 437.8
  infantile (postnatal) 343.4
  late effect
    birth injury, intracranial or spinal 343.4
    cerebrovascular lesion - *see* Late effect(s) (of) cerebrovascular disease
    viral encephalitis 139.0
  middle alternating NEC 344.89
  newborn NEC 767.0
  seizure (current episode) (*see also* Disease, cerebrovascular, acute) 436
  spastic 342.1●
    congenital or infantile 343.1
  specified NEC 342.8●
  thrombotic (current) (*see also* Thrombosis, brain) 434.0●
    late effect - *see* Late effect(s) (of) cerebrovascular disease
Hemisection, spinal cord - *see* Fracture, vertebra, by site, with spinal cord injury
Hemispasm 781.0
  facial 781.0
Hemispatial neglect 781.8
Hemisporosis 117.9
Hemitremor 781.0
Hemivertebra 756.14
Hemobilia 576.8
Hemocholecyst 575.8
Hemochromatosis (acquired) (diabetic) (hereditary) (liver) (myocardium) (primary idiopathic) (secondary) 275.0
  with refractory anemia 238.72
Hemodialysis V56.0
Hemoglobin - *see also* condition
  abnormal (disease) - *see* Disease, hemoglobin
  AS genotype 282.5
  fetal, hereditary persistence 282.7
  high-oxygen-affinity 289.0
  low NEC 285.9
  S (Hb-S), heterozygous 282.5
Hemoglobinemia 283.2
  due to blood transfusion NEC 999.89
    bone marrow 996.85
  paroxysmal 283.2
Hemoglobinopathy (mixed) (*see also* Disease, hemoglobin) 282.7
  with thalassemia 282.49
  sickle-cell 282.60
    with thalassemia (without crisis) 282.41
      with
        crisis 282.42
        vaso-occlusive pain 282.42
Hemoglobinuria, hemoglobinuric 791.2
  with anemia, hemolytic, acquired (chronic) NEC 283.2
  cold (agglutinin) (paroxysmal) (with Raynaud's syndrome) 283.2

Hemoglobinuria, hemoglobinuric (*Continued*)
  due to
    exertion 283.2
    hemolysis (from external causes) NEC 283.2
  exercise 283.2
  fever (malaria) 084.8
  infantile 791.2
  intermittent 283.2
  malarial 084.8
  march 283.2
  nocturnal (paroxysmal) 283.2
  paroxysmal (cold) (nocturnal) 283.2
Hemolymphangioma (M9175/0) 228.1
Hemolysis
  fetal - *see* Jaundice, fetus or newborn
  intravascular (disseminated) NEC 286.6
    with
      abortion - *see* Abortion, by type, with hemorrhage, delayed or excessive
      ectopic pregnancy (*see also* categories 633.0–633.9) 639.1
      hemorrhage of pregnancy 641.3●
        affecting fetus or newborn 762.1
      molar pregnancy (*see also* categories 630–632) 639.1
    acute 283.2
    following
      abortion 639.1
      ectopic or molar pregnancy 639.1
  neonatal - *see* Jaundice, fetus or newborn
  transfusion NEC 999.89
    bone marrow 996.85
Hemolytic - *see also* condition
  anemia - *see* Anemia, hemolytic
  uremic syndrome 283.11
Hemometra 621.4
Hemopericardium (with effusion) 423.0
  newborn 772.8
  traumatic (*see also* Hemothorax, traumatic) 860.2
    with open wound into thorax 860.3
Hemoperitoneum 568.81
  infectional (*see also* Peritonitis) 567.29
  traumatic - *see* Injury, internal, peritoneum
Hemophagocytic syndrome 288.4
  infection-associated 288.4
Hemophilia (familial) (hereditary) 286.0
  A 286.0
    carrier (asymptomatic) V83.01
      symptomatic V83.02
  acquired 286.5
  B (Leyden) 286.1
  C 286.2
  calcipriva (*see also* Fibrinolysis) 286.7
  classical 286.0
  nonfamilial 286.7
  secondary 286.5
  vascular 286.4
Hemophilus influenzae NEC 041.5
  arachnoiditis (basic) (brain) (spinal) 320.0
    late effect - *see* category 326
  bronchopneumonia 482.2
  cerebral ventriculitis 320.0
    late effect - *see* category 326
  cerebrospinal inflammation 320.0
    late effect - *see* category 326

Hemophilus influenzae NEC (*Continued*)
  infection NEC 041.5
  leptomeningitis 320.0
    late effect - *see* category 326
  meningitis (cerebral) (cerebrospinal)
      (spinal) 320.0
    late effect - *see* category 326
  meningomyelitis 320.0
    late effect - *see* category 326
  pachymeningitis (adhesive) (fibrous)
      (hemorrhagic) (hypertrophic)
      (spinal) 320.0
    late effect - *see* category 326
  pneumonia (broncho-) 482.2
Hemophthalmos 360.43
Hemopneumothorax (*see also*
    Hemothorax) 511.89
  traumatic 860.4
    with open wound into thorax
        860.5
Hemoptysis 786.3
  due to Paragonimus (westermani)
      121.2
  newborn 770.3
  tuberculous (*see also* Tuberculosis,
      pulmonary) 011.9●
Hemorrhage, hemorrhagic
    (nontraumatic) 459.0
  abdomen 459.0
  accidental (antepartum) 641.2●
    affecting fetus or newborn 762.1
  adenoid 474.8
  adrenal (capsule) (gland) (medulla)
      255.41
    newborn 772.5
  after labor - *see* Hemorrhage,
      postpartum
  alveolar
    lung, newborn 770.3
    process 525.8
  alveolus 525.8
  amputation stump (surgical) 998.11
    secondary, delayed 997.69
  anemia (chronic) 280.0
    acute 285.1
  antepartum - *see* Hemorrhage,
      pregnancy
  anus (sphincter) 569.3
  apoplexy (stroke) 432.9
  arachnoid - *see* Hemorrhage,
      subarachnoid
  artery NEC 459.0
    brain (*see also* Hemorrhage, brain)
        431
    middle meningeal - *see* Hemorrhage,
        subarachnoid
  basilar (ganglion) (*see also* Hemorrhage,
      brain) 431
  bladder 596.8
  blood dyscrasia 289.9
  bowel 578.9
    newborn 772.4
  brain (miliary) (nontraumatic) 431
    with
      birth injury 767.0
      arachnoid - *see* Hemorrhage,
          subarachnoid
      due to
        birth injury 767.0
        rupture of aneurysm (congenital)
            (*see also* Hemorrhage,
            subarachnoid) 430
          mycotic 431
        syphilis 094.89

Hemorrhage, hemorrhagic (*Continued*)
  brain (*Continued*)
    epidural or extradural - *see*
        Hemorrhage, extradural
    fetus or newborn (anoxic) (hypoxic)
        (due to birth trauma)
        (nontraumatic) 767.0
      intraventricular 772.10
        grade I 772.11
        grade II 772.12
        grade III 772.13
        grade IV 772.14
      iatrogenic 997.02
      postoperative 997.02
    puerperal, postpartum, childbirth
        674.0●
    stem 431
    subarachnoid, arachnoid, or
        meningeal - *see* Hemorrhage,
        subarachnoid
    subdural - *see* Hemorrhage,
        subdural
    traumatic NEC 853.0●

Note 38   Use the following fifth-digit
subclassification with categories 851–854:

  0   unspecified state of
        consciousness
  1   with no loss of consciousness
  2   with brief [less than one hour]
        loss of consciousness
  3   with moderate [1–24 hours] loss
        of consciousness
  4   with prolonged [more than 24
        hours] loss of
        consciousness and return
        to pre-existing conscious
        level
  5   with prolonged [more than 24
        hours] loss of
        consciousness, without
        return to pre-existing
        conscious level

Use fifth-digit 5 to designate when a
patient is unconscious and dies before
regaining consciousness, regardless of
the duration of the loss of consciousness

  6   with loss of consciousness of
        unspecified duration
  9   with concussion, unspecified

---

    with
      cerebral
        contusion - *see* Contusion,
            brain
        laceration - *see* Laceration,
            brain
      open intracranial wound
          853.1●
      skull fracture - *see* Fracture,
          skull, by site
    extradural or epidural 852.4●
      with open intracranial wound
          852.5●
    subarachnoid 852.0●
      with open intracranial wound
          852.1●
    subdural 852.2●
      with open intracranial wound
          852.3●
  breast 611.79
  bronchial tube - *see* Hemorrhage, lung
  bronchopulmonary - *see* Hemorrhage,
      lung

Hemorrhage, hemorrhagic (*Continued*)
  bronchus (cause unknown) (*see also*
      Hemorrhage, lung) 786.3
  bulbar (*see also* Hemorrhage, brain) 431
  bursa 727.89
  capillary 448.9
    primary 287.8
  capsular - *see* Hemorrhage, brain
  cardiovascular 429.89
  cecum 578.9
  cephalic (*see also* Hemorrhage, brain)
      431
  cerebellar (*see also* Hemorrhage, brain)
      431
  cerebellum (*see also* Hemorrhage, brain)
      431
  cerebral (*see also* Hemorrhage, brain)
      431
    fetus or newborn (anoxic)
        (traumatic) 767.0
  cerebromeningeal (*see also*
      Hemorrhage, brain) 431
  cerebrospinal (*see also* Hemorrhage,
      brain) 431
  cerebrovascular accident - *see*
      Hemorrhage, brain
  cerebrum (*see also* Hemorrhage, brain)
      431
  cervix (stump) (uteri) 622.8
  cesarean section wound 674.3●
  chamber, anterior (eye) 364.41
  childbirth - *see* Hemorrhage,
      complicating, delivery
  choroid 363.61
    expulsive 363.62
  ciliary body 364.41
  cochlea 386.8
  colon - *see* Hemorrhage, intestine
  complicating
    delivery 641.9●
      affecting fetus or newborn 762.1
      associated with
        afibrinogenemia 641.3●
          affecting fetus or newborn
              763.89
        coagulation defect 641.3●
          affecting fetus or newborn
              763.89
        hyperfibrinolysis 641.3●
          affecting fetus or newborn
              763.89
        hypofibrinogenemia 641.3●
          affecting fetus or newborn
              763.89
      due to
        low-lying placenta 641.1●
          affecting fetus or newborn
              762.0
        placenta previa 641.1●
          affecting fetus or newborn
              762.0
        premature separation of
            placenta 641.2●
          affecting fetus or newborn
              762.1
        retained
          placenta 666.0●
          secundines 666.2●
        trauma 641.8●
          affecting fetus or newborn
              763.89
        uterine leiomyoma 641.8●
          affecting fetus or newborn
              763.89

◄ New   ◄▥ Revised   ~~deleted~~ Deleted   ● Use Additional Digit(s)   ▨ Omit code

Hemorrhage, hemorrhagic *(Continued)*
  complication(s)
    of dental implant placement 525.71
    surgical procedure 998.11
  concealed NEC 459.0
  congenital 772.9
  conjunctiva 372.72
    newborn 772.8
  cord, newborn 772.0
    slipped ligature 772.3
    stump 772.3
  corpus luteum (ruptured) 620.1
  cortical *(see also* Hemorrhage, brain)
    431
  cranial 432.9
  cutaneous 782.7
    newborn 772.6
  cyst, pancreas 577.2
  cystitis - *see* Cystitis
  delayed
    with
      abortion - *see* Abortion, by type,
        with hemorrhage, delayed
        or excessive
      ectopic pregnancy *(see also*
        categories 633.0–633.9) 639.1
      molar pregnancy *(see also*
        categories 630–632) 639.1
    following
      abortion 639.1
      ectopic or molar pregnancy
        639.1
    postpartum 666.2●
  diathesis (familial) 287.9
    newborn 776.0
  disease 287.9
    newborn 776.0
    specified type NEC 287.8
  disorder 287.9
    due to intrinsic circulating
      anticoagulants 286.5
    specified type NEC 287.8
  due to
    any device, implant, or graft
      (presence of) classifiable to
      996.0–996.5 - *see*
      Complications, due to
      (presence of) any device,
      implant, or graft classified to
      996.0–996.5 NEC
    intrinsic circulating anticoagulant
      286.5
  duodenum, duodenal 537.89
    ulcer - *see* Ulcer, duodenum, with
      hemorrhage
  dura mater - *see* Hemorrhage, subdural
  endotracheal - *see* Hemorrhage, lung
  epicranial subaponeurotic (massive)
    767.11
  epidural - *see* Hemorrhage, extradural
  episiotomy 674.3●
  esophagus 530.82
    varix *(see also* Varix, esophagus,
      bleeding) 456.0
  excessive
    with
      abortion - *see* Abortion, by type,
        with hemorrhage, delayed
        or excessive
      ectopic pregnancy *(see also*
        categories 633.0–633.9)
        639.1
      molar pregnancy *(see also*
        categories 630–632) 639.1

Hemorrhage, hemorrhagic *(Continued)*
  excessive *(Continued)*
    following
      abortion 639.1
      ectopic or molar pregnancy 639.1
  external 459.0
  extradural (traumatic) - *see also*
    Hemorrhage, brain, traumatic,
    extradural
    birth injury 767.0
    fetus or newborn (anoxic)
      (traumatic) 767.0
    nontraumatic 432.0
  eye 360.43
    chamber (anterior) (aqueous) 364.41
    fundus 362.81
  eyelid 374.81
  fallopian tube 620.8
  fetomaternal 772.0
    affecting management of pregnancy
      or puerperium 656.0●
  fetus, fetal, affecting newborn 772.0 ◄▬
    from
      cut end of co-twin's cord 772.0
      placenta 772.0
      ruptured cord 772.0
      vasa previa 772.0
    into
      co-twin 772.0
      mother's circulation 772.0
        affecting management of
        pregnancy or
        puerperium 656.0●
  fever *(see also* Fever, hemorrhagic) 065.9
    with renal syndrome 078.6
    arthropod-borne NEC 065.9
    Bangkok 065.4
    Crimean 065.0
    dengue virus 065.4
    epidemic 078.6
    Junin virus 078.7
    Korean 078.6
    Machupo virus 078.7
    mite-borne 065.8
    mosquito-borne 065.4
    Philippine 065.4
    Russian (Yaroslav) 078.6
    Singapore 065.4
    Southeast Asia 065.4
    Thailand 065.4
    tick-borne NEC 065.3
  fibrinogenolysis *(see also* Fibrinolysis)
    286.6
  fibrinolytic (acquired) *(see also*
    Fibrinolysis) 286.6
  fontanel 767.19
  from tracheostomy stoma 519.09
  fundus, eye 362.81
  funis
    affecting fetus or newborn 772.0
    complicating delivery 663.8●
  gastric *(see also* Hemorrhage, stomach)
    578.9
  gastroenteric 578.9
    newborn 772.4
  gastrointestinal (tract) 578.9
    newborn 772.4
  genitourinary (tract) NEC 599.89
  gingiva 523.8
  globe 360.43
  gravidarum - *see* Hemorrhage,
    pregnancy
  gum 523.8
  heart 429.89

Hemorrhage, hemorrhagic *(Continued)*
  hypopharyngeal (throat) 784.8
  intermenstrual 626.6
    irregular 626.6
    regular 626.5
  internal (organs) 459.0
    capsule *(see also* Hemorrhage brain)
      431
    ear 386.8
    newborn 772.8
  intestine 578.9
    congenital 772.4
    newborn 772.4
  into
    bladder wall 596.7
    bursa 727.89
    corpus luysii *(see also* Hemorrhage,
      brain) 431
  intra-abdominal 459.0
    during or following surgery 998.11
  intra-alveolar, newborn (lung) 770.3
  intracerebral *(see also* Hemorrhage,
    brain) 431
  intracranial NEC 432.9
    puerperal, postpartum, childbirth
      674.0●
    traumatic - *see* Hemorrhage, brain,
      traumatic
  intramedullary NEC 336.1
  intraocular 360.43
  intraoperative 998.11
  intrapartum - *see* Hemorrhage,
    complicating, delivery
  intrapelvic
    female 629.89
    male 459.0
  intraperitoneal 459.0
  intrapontine *(see also* Hemorrhage,
    brain) 431
  intrauterine 621.4
    complicating delivery - *see*
      Hemorrhage, complicating,
      delivery
    in pregnancy or childbirth - *see*
      Hemorrhage, pregnancy
    postpartum *(see also* Hemorrhage,
      postpartum) 666.1●
  intraventricular *(see also* Hemorrhage,
    brain) 431
    fetus or newborn (anoxic)
      (traumatic) 772.10
      grade I 772.11
      grade II 772.12
      grade III 772.13
      grade IV 772.14
  intravesical 596.7
  iris (postinfectional)
    (postinflammatory) (toxic) 364.41
  joint (nontraumatic) 719.10
    ankle 719.17
    elbow 719.12
    foot 719.17
    forearm 719.13
    hand 719.14
    hip 719.15
    knee 719.16
    lower leg 719.16
    multiple sites 719.19
    pelvic region 719.15
    shoulder (region) 719.11
    specified site NEC 719.18
    thigh 719.15
    upper arm 719.12
    wrist 719.13

Hemorrhage, hemorrhagic *(Continued)*
  kidney 593.81
  knee (joint) 719.16
  labyrinth 386.8
  leg NEC 459.0
  lenticular striate artery *(see also* Hemorrhage, brain) 431
  ligature, vessel 998.11
  liver 573.8
  lower extremity NEC 459.0
  lung 786.3
    newborn 770.3
    tuberculous *(see also* Tuberculosis, pulmonary) 011.9●
  malaria 084.8
  marginal sinus 641.2●
  massive subaponeurotic, birth injury 767.11
  maternal, affecting fetus or newborn 762.1
  mediastinum 786.3
  medulla *(see also* Hemorrhage, brain) 431
  membrane (brain) *(see also* Hemorrhage, subarachnoid) 430
    spinal cord - *see* Hemorrhage, spinal cord
  meninges, meningeal (brain) (middle) *(see also* Hemorrhage, subarachnoid) 430
    spinal cord - *see* Hemorrhage, spinal cord
  mesentery 568.81
  metritis 626.8
  midbrain *(see also* Hemorrhage, brain) 431
  mole 631
  mouth 528.9
  mucous membrane NEC 459.0
    newborn 772.8
  muscle 728.89
  nail (subungual) 703.8
  nasal turbinate 784.7
    newborn 772.8
  nasopharynx 478.29
  navel, newborn 772.3
  newborn 772.9
    adrenal 772.5
    alveolar (lung) 770.3
    brain (anoxic) (hypoxic) (due to birth trauma) 767.0
    cerebral (anoxic) (hypoxic) (due to birth trauma) 767.0
    conjunctiva 772.8
    cutaneous 772.6
    diathesis 776.0
    due to vitamin K deficiency 776.0
    epicranial subaponeurotic (massive) 767.11
    gastrointestinal 772.4
    internal (organs) 772.8
    intestines 772.4
    intra-alveolar (lung) 770.3
    intracranial (from any perinatal cause) 767.0
    intraventricular (from any perinatal cause) 772.10
      grade I 772.11
      grade II 772.12
      grade III 772.13
      grade IV 772.14
    lung 770.3

Hemorrhage, hemorrhagic *(Continued)*
  newborn *(Continued)*
    pulmonary (massive) 770.3
    spinal cord, traumatic 767.4
    stomach 772.4
    subaponeurotic (massive) 767.11
    subarachnoid (from any perinatal cause) 772.2
    subconjunctival 772.8
    subgaleal 767.11
    umbilicus 772.0
      slipped ligature 772.3
      vasa previa 772.0
  nipple 611.79
  nose 784.7
    newborn 772.8
  obstetrical surgical wound 674.3●
  omentum 568.89
    newborn 772.4
  optic nerve (sheath) 377.42
  orbit 376.32
  ovary 620.1
  oviduct 620.8
  pancreas 577.8
  parathyroid (gland) (spontaneous) 252.8
  parturition - *see* Hemorrhage, complicating, delivery
  penis 607.82
  pericardium, pericarditis 423.0
  perineal wound (obstetrical) 674.3●
  peritoneum, peritoneal 459.0
  peritonsillar tissue 474.8
    after operation on tonsils 998.11
    due to infection 475
  petechial 782.7
  pituitary (gland) 253.8
  placenta NEC 641.9●
    affecting fetus or newborn 762.1
    from surgical or instrumental damage 641.8●
      affecting fetus or newborn 762.1
    previa 641.1●
      affecting fetus or newborn 762.0
  pleura - *see* Hemorrhage, lung
  polioencephalitis, superior 265.1
  polymyositis - *see* Polymyositis
  pons *(see also* Hemorrhage, brain) 431
  pontine *(see also* Hemorrhage, brain) 431
  popliteal 459.0
  postcoital 626.7
  postextraction (dental) 998.11
  postmenopausal 627.1
  postnasal 784.7
  postoperative 998.11
  postpartum (atonic) (following delivery of placenta) 666.1●
    delayed or secondary (after 24 hours) 666.2●
    retained placenta 666.0●
    third stage 666.0●
  pregnancy (concealed) 641.9●
    accidental 641.2●
      affecting fetus or newborn 762.1
    affecting fetus or newborn 762.1
    before 22 completed weeks' gestation 640.9●
      affecting fetus or newborn 762.1

Hemorrhage, hemorrhagic *(Continued)*
  pregnancy *(Continued)*
    due to
      abruptio placenta 641.2●
        affecting fetus or newborn 762.1
      afibrinogenemia or other coagulation defect (conditions classifiable to 286.0–286.9) 641.3●
        affecting fetus or newborn 762.1
      coagulation defect 641.3●
        affecting fetus or newborn 762.1
      hyperfibrinolysis 641.3●
        affecting fetus or newborn 762.1
      hypofibrinogenemia 641.3●
        affecting fetus or newborn 762.1
      leiomyoma, uterus 641.8●
        affecting fetus or newborn 762.1
      low-lying placenta 641.1●
        affecting fetus or newborn 762.1
      marginal sinus (rupture) 641.2●
        affecting fetus or newborn 762.1
      placenta previa 641.1●
        affecting fetus or newborn 762.0
      premature separation of placenta (normally implanted) 641.2●
        affecting fetus or newborn 762.1
      threatened abortion 640.0●
        affecting fetus or newborn 762.1
      trauma 641.8●
        affecting fetus or newborn 762.1
    early (before 22 completed weeks' gestation) 640.9●
      affecting fetus or newborn 762.1
    previous, affecting management of pregnancy or childbirth V23.49
    unavoidable - *see* Hemorrhage, pregnancy, due to placenta previa
  prepartum (mother) - *see* Hemorrhage, pregnancy
  preretinal, cause unspecified 362.81
  prostate 602.1
  puerperal *(see also* Hemorrhage, postpartum) 666.1●
  pulmonary - *see also* Hemorrhage, lung
    newborn (massive) 770.3
    renal syndrome 446.21
  purpura (primary) *(see also* Purpura, thrombocytopenic) 287.39
  rectum (sphincter) 569.3
  recurring, following initial hemorrhage at time of injury 958.2
  renal 593.81
    pulmonary syndrome 446.21
  respiratory tract *(see also* Hemorrhage, lung) 786.3

◀ New   ◀▥ Revised   ~~deleted~~ Deleted   ● Use Additional Digit(s)   ▨ Omit code

Hemorrhage, hemorrhagic *(Continued)*
retina, retinal (deep) (superficial)
  (vessels) 362.81
  diabetic 250.5● *[362.01]*
    due to secondary diabetes 249.5●
      [362.01]
  due to birth injury 772.8
retrobulbar 376.89
retroperitoneal 459.0
retroplacental *(see also* Placenta,
  separation) 641.2●
scalp 459.0
  due to injury at birth 767.19
scrotum 608.83
secondary (nontraumatic) 459.0
  following initial hemorrhage at time
    of injury 958.2
seminal vesicle 608.83
skin 782.7
  newborn 772.6
spermatic cord 608.83
spinal (cord) 336.1
  aneurysm (ruptured) 336.1
    syphilitic 094.89
  due to birth injury 767.4
  fetus or newborn 767.4
spleen 289.59
spontaneous NEC 459.0
  petechial 782.7
stomach 578.9
  newborn 772.4
  ulcer - *see* Ulcer, stomach, with
    hemorrhage
subaponeurotic, newborn 767.11
  massive (birth injury) 767.11
subarachnoid (nontraumatic) 430
  fetus or newborn (anoxic)
    (traumatic) 772.2
  puerperal, postpartum, childbirth
    674.0●
  traumatic - *see* Hemorrhage, brain,
    traumatic, subarachnoid
subconjunctival 372.72
  due to birth injury 772.8
  newborn 772.8
subcortical *(see also* Hemorrhage, brain)
  431
subcutaneous 782.7
subdiaphragmatic 459.0
subdural (nontraumatic) 432.1
  due to birth injury 767.0
  fetus or newborn (anoxic) (hypoxic)
    (due to birth trauma) 767.0
  puerperal, postpartum, childbirth
    674.0●
  spinal 336.1
  traumatic - *see* Hemorrhage, brain,
    traumatic, subdural
subgaleal 767.11
subhyaloid 362.81
subperiosteal 733.99
subretinal 362.81
subtentorial *(see also* Hemorrhage,
  subdural) 432.1
subungual 703.8
  due to blood dyscrasia 287.8
suprarenal (capsule) (gland) 255.41
  fetus or newborn 772.5
tentorium (traumatic) - *see also*
  Hemorrhage, brain, traumatic
  fetus or newborn 767.0
  nontraumatic - *see* Hemorrhage,
    subdural
testis 608.83

Hemorrhage, hemorrhagic *(Continued)*
thigh 459.0
third stage 666.0●
thorax - *see* Hemorrhage, lung
throat 784.8
thrombocythemia 238.71
thymus (gland) 254.8
thyroid (gland) 246.3
  cyst 246.3
tongue 529.8
tonsil 474.8
  postoperative 998.11
tooth socket (postextraction) 998.11
trachea - *see* Hemorrhage, lung
traumatic - *see also* nature of injury
  brain - *see* Hemorrhage, brain,
    traumatic
  recurring or secondary (following
    initial hemorrhage at time of
    injury) 958.2
tuberculous NEC *(see also* Tuberculosis,
  pulmonary) 011.9●
tunica vaginalis 608.83
ulcer - *see* Ulcer, by site, with
  hemorrhage
umbilicus, umbilical cord 772.0
  after birth, newborn 772.3
  complicating delivery 663.8●
    affecting fetus or newborn
      772.0
  slipped ligature 772.3
  stump 772.3
unavoidable (due to placenta previa)
  641.1●
  affecting fetus or newborn
    762.0
upper extremity 459.0
urethra (idiopathic) 599.84
uterus, uterine (abnormal) 626.9
  climacteric 627.0
  complicating delivery - *see*
    Hemorrhage, complicating,
    delivery
  due to
    intrauterine contraceptive device
      996.76
    perforating uterus 996.32
  functional or dysfunctional
    626.8
  in pregnancy - *see* Hemorrhage,
    pregnancy
  intermenstrual 626.6
    irregular 626.6
    regular 626.5
  postmenopausal 627.1
  postpartum *(see also* Hemorrhage,
    postpartum) 666.1●
  prepubertal 626.8
  pubertal 626.3
  puerperal (immediate) 666.1●
vagina 623.8
vasa previa 663.5●
  affecting fetus or newborn
    772.0
vas deferens 608.83
ventricular *(see also* Hemorrhage,
  brain) 431
vesical 596.8
viscera 459.0
  newborn 772.8
vitreous (humor) (intraocular)
  379.23
vocal cord 478.5
vulva 624.8

Hemorrhoids (anus) (rectum) (without
  complication) 455.6
  bleeding, prolapsed, strangulated, or
    ulcerated NEC 455.8
  external 455.5
  internal 455.2
  complicated NEC 455.8
  complicating pregnancy and
    puerperium 671.8●
  external 455.3
    with complication NEC 455.5
    bleeding, prolapsed, strangulated,
      or ulcerated 455.5
    thrombosed 455.4
  internal 455.0
    with complication NEC 455.2
    bleeding, prolapsed, strangulated,
      or ulcerated 455.2
    thrombosed 455.1
  residual skin tag 455.9
  sentinel pile 455.9
  thrombosed NEC 455.7
    external 455.4
    internal 455.1
Hemosalpinx 620.8
Hemosiderosis 275.0
  dietary 275.0
  pulmonary (idiopathic) 275.0 *[516.1]*
  transfusion NEC 999.89
    bone marrow 996.85
Hemospermia 608.82
Hemothorax 511.89
  bacterial, nontuberculous 511.1
  newborn 772.8
  nontuberculous 511.89
    bacterial 511.1
  pneumococcal 511.1
  postoperative 998.11
  staphylococcal 511.1
  streptococcal 511.1
  traumatic 860.2
    with
      open wound into thorax 860.3
      pneumothorax 860.4
        with open wound into thorax
          860.5
  tuberculous *(see also* Tuberculosis,
    pleura) 012.0●
Hemotympanum 385.89
Hench-Rosenberg syndrome
  (palindromic arthritis) *(see also*
  Rheumatism, palindromic)
  719.3●
Henle's warts 371.41
Henoch (-Schönlein)
  disease or syndrome (allergic purpura)
    287.0
  purpura (allergic) 287.0
Henpue, henpuye 102.6
Heparin-induced thrombocytopenia
  (HIT) 289.84
Heparitinuria 277.5
Hepar lobatum 095.3
Hepatalgia 573.8
Hepatic - *see also* condition
  flexure syndrome 569.89
Hepatitis 573.3
  acute *(see also* Necrosis, liver) 570
    alcoholic 571.1
    infective 070.1
      with hepatic coma 070.0
  alcoholic 571.1
  amebic - *see* Abscess, liver, amebic
  anicteric (acute) - *see* Hepatitis, viral

Hepatitis (Continued)
  antigen-associated (HAA) - see
    Hepatitis, viral, type B
  Australian antigen (positive) - see
    Hepatitis, viral, type B
  autoimmune 571.42
  catarrhal (acute) 070.1
    with hepatic coma 070.0
    chronic 571.40
    newborn 070.1
      with hepatic coma 070.0
  chemical 573.3
  cholangiolitic 573.8
  cholestatic 573.8
  chronic 571.40
    active 571.49
      viral - see Hepatitis, viral
    aggressive 571.49
    persistent 571.41
    viral - see Hepatitis, viral
  cytomegalic inclusion virus 078.5 [573.1]
  diffuse 573.3
  "dirty needle" - see Hepatitis, viral
  drug-induced 573.3
  due to
    Coxsackie 074.8 [573.1]
    cytomegalic inclusion virus 078.5
      [573.1]
    infectious mononucleosis 075 [573.1]
    malaria 084.9 [573.2]
    mumps 072.71
    secondary syphilis 091.62
    toxoplasmosis (acquired) 130.5
      congenital (active) 771.2
  epidemic - see Hepatitis, viral, type A
  fetus or newborn 774.4
  fibrous (chronic) 571.49
    acute 570
  from injection, inoculation, or
    transfusion (blood) (other
    substance) (plasma) (serum)
    (onset within 8 months after
    administration) - see Hepatitis,
    viral
  fulminant (viral) (see also Hepatitis,
    viral) 070.9
    with hepatic coma 070.6
    type A 070.1
      with hepatic coma 070.0
    type B - see Hepatitis, viral, type B
  giant cell (neonatal) 774.4
  hemorrhagic 573.8
  history of
    B V12.09
    C V12.09
  homologous serum - see Hepatitis, viral
  hypertrophic (chronic) 571.49
    acute 570
  infectious, infective (acute) (chronic)
    (subacute) 070.1
    with hepatic coma 070.0
  inoculation - see Hepatitis, viral
  interstitial (chronic) 571.49
    acute 570
  lupoid 571.49
  malarial 084.9 [573.2]
  malignant (see also Necrosis, liver) 570
  neonatal (toxic) 774.4
  newborn 774.4
  parenchymatous (acute) (see also
    Necrosis, liver) 570
  peliosis 573.3
  persistent, chronic 571.41
  plasma cell 571.49

Hepatitis (Continued)
  postimmunization - see Hepatitis, viral
  postnecrotic 571.49
  posttransfusion - see Hepatitis, viral
  recurrent 571.49
  septic 573.3
  serum - see Hepatitis, viral
    carrier (suspected of) V02.61
  subacute (see also Necrosis, liver) 570
  suppurative (diffuse) 572.0
  syphilitic (late) 095.3
    congenital (early) 090.0 [573.2]
      late 090.5 [573.2]
    secondary 091.62
  toxic (noninfectious) 573.3
    fetus or newborn 774.4
  tuberculous (see also Tuberculosis)
    017.9●
  viral (acute) (anicteric) (cholangiolitic)
    (cholestatic) (chronic) (subacute)
    070.9
    with hepatic coma 070.6
    AU-SH type virus - see Hepatitis,
      viral, type B
    Australian antigen - see Hepatitis,
      viral, type B
    B-antigen - see Hepatitis, viral, type B
    Coxsackie 074.8 [573.1]
    cytomegalic inclusion 078.5 [573.1]
    IH (virus) - see Hepatitis, viral, type A
    infectious hepatitis virus - see
      Hepatitis, viral, type A
    serum hepatitis virus - see Hepatitis,
      viral, type B
    SH - see Hepatitis, viral, type B
    specified type NEC 070.59
      with hepatic coma 070.49
    type A 070.1
      with hepatic coma 070.0
    type B (acute) 070.30
      with
        hepatic coma 070.20
      carrier status V02.61
      chronic 070.32
        with
          hepatic coma 070.22
            with hepatitis delta
              070.23
          hepatitis delta 070.33
            with hepatic coma 070.23
      with hepatitis delta 070.21
      hepatitis delta 070.31
        with hepatic coma 070.21
    type C
      acute 070.51
        with hepatic coma 070.41
      carrier status V02.62
      chronic 070.54
        with hepatic coma 070.44
      in remission 070.54
      unspecified 070.70
        with hepatic coma 070.71
    type delta (with hepatitis B carrier
      state) 070.52
      with
        active hepatitis B disease - see
          Hepatitis, viral, type B
        hepatic coma 070.42
    type E 070.53
      with hepatic coma 070.43
    vaccination and inoculation
      (prophylactic) V05.3
  Waldenström's (lupoid hepatitis)
    571.49

Hepatization, lung (acute) - see also
  Pneumonia, lobar
  chronic (see also Fibrosis, lung) 515
Hepatoblastoma (M8970/3) 155.0
Hepatocarcinoma (M8170/3) 155.0
Hepatocholangiocarcinoma (M8180/3)
  155.0
Hepatocholangioma, benign (M8180/0)
  211.5
Hepatocholangitis 573.8
Hepatocystitis (see also Cholecystitis)
  575.10
Hepatodystrophy 570
Hepatolenticular degeneration 275.1
Hepatolithiasis - see Choledocholithiasis
Hepatoma (malignant) (M8170/3) 155.0
  benign (M8170/0) 211.5
  congenital (M8970/3) 155.0
  embryonal (M8970/3) 155.0
Hepatomegalia glycogenica diffusa 271.0
Hepatomegaly (see also Hypertrophy,
  liver) 789.1
  congenital 751.69
    syphilitic 090.0
  due to Clonorchis sinensis 121.1
  Gaucher's 272.7
  syphilitic (congenital) 090.0
Hepatoptosis 573.8
Hepatorrhexis 573.8
Hepatosis, toxic 573.8
Hepatosplenomegaly 571.8
  due to S. japonicum 120.2
  hyperlipemic (Bürger-Grutz type)
    272.3
Herald patch 696.3
Hereditary - see condition
Heredodegeneration 330.9
  macular 362.70
Heredopathia atactica polyneuritiformis
  356.3
Heredosyphilis (see also Syphilis,
  congenital) 090.9
Hermaphroditism (true) 752.7
  with specified chromosomal anomaly -
    see Anomaly, chromosomes, sex
Hernia, hernial (acquired) (recurrent)
  553.9
  with
    gangrene (obstructed) NEC 551.9
    obstruction NEC 552.9
      and gangrene 551.9
  abdomen (wall) - see Hernia, ventral
  abdominal, specified site NEC 553.8
    with
      gangrene (obstructed) 551.8
      obstruction 552.8
        and gangrene 551.8
  appendix 553.8
    with
      gangrene (obstructed) 551.8
      obstruction 552.8
        and gangrene 551.8
  bilateral (inguinal) - see Hernia,
    inguinal
  bladder (sphincter)
    congenital (female) (male) 756.71
    female (see also Cystocele, female)
      618.01
    male 596.8
  brain 348.4
    congenital 742.0
  broad ligament 553.8
  cartilage, vertebral - see Displacement,
    intervertebral disc

◄ New   ◄▥ Revised   deleted Deleted   ● Use Additional Digit(s)   ▨ Omit code

Hernia, hernial *(Continued)*
cerebral 348.4
  congenital 742.0
  endaural 742.0
ciliary body 364.89
  traumatic 871.1
colic 553.9
  with
    gangrene (obstructed) 551.9
    obstruction 552.9
      and gangrene 551.9
colon 553.9
  with
    gangrene (obstructed) 551.9
    obstruction 552.9
      and gangrene 551.9
colostomy (stoma) 569.69
Cooper's (retroperitoneal) 553.8
  with
    gangrene (obstructed) 551.8
    obstruction 552.8
      and gangrene 551.8
crural - *see* Hernia, femoral
diaphragm, diaphragmatic 553.3
  with
    gangrene (obstructed) 551.3
    obstruction 552.3
      and gangrene 551.3
  congenital 756.6
  due to gross defect of diaphragm
    756.6
  traumatic 862.0
    with open wound into cavity
      862.1
direct (inguinal) - *see* Hernia, inguinal
disc, intervertebral - *see* Displacement,
  intervertebral disc
diverticulum, intestine 553.9
  with
    gangrene (obstructed) 551.9
    obstruction 552.9
      and gangrene 551.9
double (inguinal) - *see* Hernia,
  inguinal
due to adhesion with obstruction
  560.81
duodenojejunal 553.8
  with
    gangrene (obstructed) 551.8
    obstruction 552.8
      and gangrene 551.8
en glissade - *see* Hernia, inguinal
enterostomy (stoma) 569.69
epigastric 553.29
  with
    gangrene (obstruction) 551.29
    obstruction 552.29
      and gangrene 551.29
  recurrent 553.21
    with
      gangrene (obstructed)
        551.21
      obstruction 552.21
        and gangrene 551.21
esophageal hiatus (sliding) 553.3
  with
    gangrene (obstructed) 551.3
    obstruction 552.3
      and gangrene 551.3
  congenital 750.6
external (inguinal) - *see* Hernia,
  inguinal
fallopian tube 620.4
fascia 728.89

Hernia, hernial *(Continued)*
fat 729.30
  eyelid 374.34
  orbital 374.34
  pad 729.30
    eye, eyelid 374.34
    knee 729.31
    orbit 374.34
    popliteal (space) 729.31
    specified site NEC 729.39
femoral (unilateral) 553.00
  with
    gangrene (obstructed) 551.00
    obstruction 552.00
      with gangrene 551.00
  bilateral 553.02
    gangrenous (obstructed)
      551.02
    obstructed 552.02
      with gangrene 551.02
    recurrent 553.03
      gangrenous (obstructed)
        551.03
      obstructed 552.03
        with gangrene 551.03
  recurrent (unilateral) 553.01
    bilateral 553.03
      gangrenous (obstructed)
        551.03
      obstructed 552.03
        with gangrene 551.03
    gangrenous (obstructed)
      551.01
    obstructed 552.01
      with gangrene 551.01
foramen
  Bochdalek 553.3
    with
      gangrene (obstructed) 551.3
      obstruction 552.3
        and gangrene 551.3
    congenital 756.6
  magnum 348.4
  Morgagni, Morgagnian 553.3
    with
      gangrene 551.3
      obstruction 552.3
        and gangrene 551.3
    congenital 756.6
funicular (umbilical) 553.1
  with
    gangrene (obstructed) 551.1
    obstruction 552.1
      and gangrene 551.1
  spermatic cord - *see* Hernia, inguinal
gangrenous - *see* Hernia, by site, with
  gangrene
gastrointestinal tract 553.9
  with
    gangrene (obstructed) 551.9
    obstruction 552.9
      and gangrene 551.9
gluteal - *see* Hernia, femoral
Gruber's (internal mesogastric)
  553.8
  with
    gangrene (obstructed) 551.8
    obstruction 552.8
      and gangrene 551.8
Hesselbach's 553.8
  with
    gangrene (obstructed) 551.8
    obstruction 552.8
      and gangrene 551.8

Hernia, hernial *(Continued)*
hiatal (esophageal) (sliding) 553.3
  with
    gangrene (obstructed) 551.3
    obstruction 552.3
      and gangrene 551.3
  congenital 750.6
incarcerated (*see also* Hernia, by site,
  with obstruction) 552.9
  gangrenous (*see also* Hernia, by site,
    with gangrene) 551.9
incisional 553.21
  with
    gangrene (obstructed) 551.21
    obstruction 552.21
      and gangrene 551.21
  lumbar - *see* Hernia, lumbar
  recurrent 553.21
    with
      gangrene (obstructed) 551.21
      obstruction 552.21
        and gangrene 551.21
indirect (inguinal) - *see* Hernia, inguinal
infantile - *see* Hernia, inguinal
infrapatellar fat pad 729.31
inguinal (direct) (double) (encysted)
  (external) (funicular) (indirect)
  (infantile) (internal) (interstitial)
  (oblique) (scrotal) (sliding)
  550.9●

┌─────────────────────────────────────┐
│ Note 41 Use the following fifth-digit │
│ subclassification with category 550:   │
│   │
│ 0   unilateral or unspecified (not   │
│   specified as recurrent)   │
│ 1   unilateral or unspecified,   │
│   recurrent   │
│ 2   bilateral (not specified as   │
│   recurrent)   │
│ 3   bilateral, recurrent   │
└─────────────────────────────────────┘

  with
    gangrene (obstructed) 550.0●
    obstruction 550.1●
      and gangrene 550.0●
internal 553.8
  with
    gangrene (obstructed) 551.8
    obstruction 552.8
      and gangrene 551.8
  inguinal - *see* Hernia, inguinal
interstitial 553.9
  with
    gangrene (obstructed) 551.9
    obstruction 552.9
      and gangrene 551.9
  inguinal - *see* Hernia, inguinal
intervertebral cartilage or disc - *see*
  Displacement, intervertebral disc
intestine, intestinal 553.9
  with
    gangrene (obstructed) 551.9
    obstruction 552.9
      and gangrene 551.9
intra-abdominal 553.9
  with
    gangrene (obstructed) 551.9
    obstruction 552.9
      and gangrene 551.9
intraparietal 553.9
  with
    gangrene (obstructed) 551.9
    obstruction 552.9
      and gangrene 551.9

Hernia, hernial *(Continued)*
  iris 364.89
    traumatic 871.1
  irreducible (*see also* Hernia, by site,
      with obstruction) 552.9
    gangrenous (with obstruction) (*see
      also* Hernia, by site, with
      gangrene) 551.9
  ischiatic 553.8
    with
      gangrene (obstructed) 551.8
      obstruction 552.8
        and gangrene 551.8
  ischiorectal 553.8
    with
      gangrene (obstructed) 551.8
      obstruction 552.8
        and gangrene 551.8
  lens 379.32
    traumatic 871.1
  linea
    alba - *see* Hernia, epigastric
    semilunaris - *see* Hernia,
        spigelian
  Littre's (diverticular) 553.9
    with
      gangrene (obstructed) 551.9
      obstruction 552.9
        and gangrene 551.9
  lumbar 553.8
    with
      gangrene (obstructed) 551.8
      obstruction 552.8
        and gangrene 551.8
    intervertebral disc 722.10
  lung (subcutaneous) 518.89
    congenital 748.69
  mediastinum 519.3
  mesenteric (internal) 553.8
    with
      gangrene (obstructed) 551.8
      obstruction 552.8
        and gangrene 551.8
  mesocolon 553.8
    with
      gangrene (obstructed) 551.8
      obstruction 552.8
        and gangrene 551.8
  muscle (sheath) 728.89
  nucleus pulposus - *see* Displacement,
      intervertebral disc
  oblique (inguinal) - *see* Hernia,
      inguinal
  obstructive (*see also* Hernia, by site,
      with obstruction) 552.9
    gangrenous (with obstruction)
        (*see also* Hernia, by site,
        with gangrene) 551.9
  obturator 553.8
    with
      gangrene (obstructed)
          551.8
      obstruction 552.8
        and gangrene 551.8
  omental 553.8
    with
      gangrene (obstructed)
          551.8
      obstruction 552.8
        and gangrene 551.8
  orbital fat (pad) 374.34
  ovary 620.4
  oviduct 620.4
  paracolostomy (stoma) 569.69

Hernia, hernial *(Continued)*
  paraduodenal 553.8
    with
      gangrene (obstructed) 551.8
      obstruction 552.8
        and gangrene 551.8
  paraesophageal 553.3
    with
      gangrene (obstructed) 551.3
      obstruction 552.3
        and gangrene 551.3
    congenital 750.6
  parahiatal 553.3
    with
      gangrene (obstructed) 551.3
      obstruction 552.3
        and gangrene 551.3
  paraumbilical 553.1
    with
      gangrene (obstructed) 551.1
      obstruction 552.1
        and gangrene 551.1
  parietal 553.9
    with
      gangrene (obstructed) 551.9
      obstruction 552.9
        and gangrene 551.9
  perineal 553.8
    with
      gangrene (obstructed) 551.8
      obstruction 552.8
        and gangrene 551.8
  peritoneal sac, lesser 553.8
    with
      gangrene (obstructed) 551.8
      obstruction 552.8
        and gangrene 551.8
  popliteal fat pad 729.31
  postoperative 553.21
    with
      gangrene (obstructed) 551.21
      obstruction 552.21
        and gangrene 551.21
  pregnant uterus 654.4●
  prevesical 596.8
  properitoneal 553.8
    with
      gangrene (obstructed) 551.8
      obstruction 552.8
        and gangrene 551.8
  pudendal 553.8
    with
      gangrene (obstructed) 551.8
      obstruction 552.8
        and gangrene 551.8
  rectovaginal 618.6
  retroperitoneal 553.8
    with
      gangrene (obstructed)
          551.8
      obstruction 552.8
        and gangrene 551.8
  Richter's (parietal) 553.9
    with
      gangrene (obstructed)
          551.9
      obstruction 552.9
        and gangrene 551.9
  Rieux's, Riex's (retrocecal) 553.8
    with
      gangrene (obstructed)
          551.8
      obstruction 552.8
        and gangrene 551.8

Hernia, hernial *(Continued)*
  sciatic 553.8
    with
      gangrene (obstructed) 551.8
      obstruction 552.8
        and gangrene 551.8
  scrotum, scrotal - *see* Hernia, inguinal
  sliding (inguinal) - *see also* Hernia,
      inguinal
    hiatus - *see* Hernia, hiatal
  spigelian 553.29
    with
      gangrene (obstructed) 551.29
      obstruction 552.29
        and gangrene 551.29
  spinal (*see also* Spina bifida) 741.9●
    with hydrocephalus 741.0●
  strangulated (*see also* Hernia, by site,
      with obstruction) 552.9
    gangrenous (with obstruction) (*see
      also* Hernia, by site, with
      gangrene) 551.9
  supraumbilicus (linea alba) - *see*
      Hernia, epigastric
  tendon 727.9
  testis (nontraumatic) 550.9●
    meaning
      scrotal hernia 550.9●
      symptomatic late syphilis 095.8
  Treitz's (fossa) 553.8
    with
      gangrene (obstructed) 551.8
      obstruction 552.8
        and gangrene 551.8
  tunica
    albuginea 608.89
    vaginalis 752.89
  umbilicus, umbilical 553.1
    with
      gangrene (obstructed) 551.1
      obstruction 552.1
        and gangrene 551.1
  ureter 593.89
    with obstruction 593.4
  uterus 621.8
    pregnant 654.4●
  vaginal (posterior) 618.6
  Velpeau's (femoral) (*see also* Hernia,
      femoral) 553.00
  ventral 553.20
    with
      gangrene (obstructed) 551.20
      obstruction 552.20
        and gangrene 551.20
    incisional 553.21
    recurrent 553.21
      with
        gangrene (obstructed) 551.21
        obstruction 552.21
          and gangrene 551.21
  vesical
    congenital (female) (male) 756.71
    female (*see also* Cystocele, female)
        618.01
    male 596.8
  vitreous (into anterior chamber)
      379.21
    traumatic 871.1
Herniation - *see also* Hernia
  brain (stem) 348.4
  cerebral 348.4
  gastric mucosa (into duodenal bulb)
      537.89
  mediastinum 519.3

◀ New   ◀▦ Revised   ~~deleted~~ Deleted   ● Use Additional Digit(s)   ▨ Omit code

Herniation *(Continued)*
nucleus pulposus - *see* Displacement, intervertebral disc
Herpangina 074.0
Herpes, herpetic 054.9
auricularis (zoster) 053.71
simplex 054.73
blepharitis (zoster) 053.20
simplex 054.41
circinate 110.5
circinatus 110.5
bullous 694.5
conjunctiva (simplex) 054.43
zoster 053.21
cornea (simplex) 054.43
disciform (simplex) 054.43
zoster 053.21
encephalitis 054.3
eye (zoster) 053.29
simplex 054.40
eyelid (zoster) 053.20
simplex 054.41
febrilis 054.9
fever 054.9
geniculate ganglionitis 053.11
genital, genitalis 054.10
specified site NEC 054.19
gestationis 646.8●
gingivostomatitis 054.2
iridocyclitis (simplex) 054.44
zoster 053.22
iris (any site) 695.10
iritis (simplex) 054.44
keratitis (simplex) 054.43
dendritic 054.42
disciform 054.43
interstitial 054.43
zoster 053.21
keratoconjunctivitis (simplex) 054.43
zoster 053.21
labialis 054.9
meningococcal 036.89
lip 054.9
meningitis (simplex) 054.72
zoster 053.0
ophthalmicus (zoster) 053.20
simplex 054.40
otitis externa (zoster) 053.71
simplex 054.73
penis 054.13
perianal 054.10
pharyngitis 054.79
progenitalis 054.10
scrotum 054.19
septicemia 054.5
simplex 054.9
complicated 054.8
ophthalmic 054.40
specified NEC 054.49
specified NEC 054.79
congenital 771.2
external ear 054.73
keratitis 054.43
dendritic 054.42
meningitis 054.72
myelitis 054.74
neuritis 054.79
specified complication NEC 054.79
ophthalmic 054.49
visceral 054.71
stomatitis 054.2
tonsurans 110.0
maculosus (of Hebra) 696.3
visceral 054.71
vulva 054.12

Herpes, herpetic *(Continued)*
vulvovaginitis 054.11
whitlow 054.6
zoster 053.9
auricularis 053.71
complicated 053.8
specified NEC 053.79
conjunctiva 053.21
cornea 053.21
ear 053.71
eye 053.29
geniculate 053.11
keratitis 053.21
interstitial 053.21
myelitis 053.14
neuritis 053.10
ophthalmicus(a) 053.20
oticus 053.71
otitis externa 053.71
specified complication NEC 053.79
specified site NEC 053.9
zosteriform, intermediate type 053.9
Herrick's
anemia (hemoglobin S disease) 282.61
syndrome (hemoglobin S disease) 282.61
Hers' disease (glycogenosis VI) 271.0
Herter's infantilism (nontropical sprue) 579.0
Herter (-Gee) disease or syndrome (nontropical sprue) 579.0
Herxheimer's disease (diffuse idiopathic cutaneous atrophy) 701.8
Herxheimer's reaction 995.0
Hesitancy, urinary 788.64
Hesselbach's hernia - *see* Hernia, Hesselbach's
Heterochromia (congenital) 743.46
acquired 364.53
cataract 366.33
cyclitis 364.21
hair 704.3
iritis 364.21
retained metallic foreign body 360.62
magnetic 360.52
uveitis 364.21
Heterophoria 378.40
alternating 378.45
vertical 378.43
Heterophyes, small intestine 121.6
Heterophyiasis 121.6
Heteropsia 368.8
Heterotopia, heterotopic - *see also* Malposition, congenital
cerebralis 742.4
pancreas, pancreatic 751.7
spinalis 742.59
Heterotropia 378.30
intermittent 378.20
vertical 378.31
vertical (constant) (intermittent) 378.31
Heubner's disease 094.89
Heubner-Herter disease or syndrome (nontropical sprue) 579.0
Hexadactylism 755.00
Heyd's syndrome (hepatorenal) 572.4
HGSIL (high grade squamous intraepithelial lesion) (cytologic finding) (Pap smear finding)
anus 796.74
cervix 795.04
biopsy finding - *code to* CIN II or CIN III
vagina 795.14
Hibernoma (M8880/0) - *see* Lipoma

Hiccough 786.8
epidemic 078.89
psychogenic 306.1
Hiccup (*see also* Hiccough) 786.8
Hicks (-Braxton) contractures 644.1●
Hidden penis 752.65
Hidradenitis (axillaris) (suppurative) 705.83
Hidradenoma (nodular) (M8400/0) - *see also* Neoplasm, skin, benign
clear cell (M8402/0) - *see* Neoplasm, skin, benign
papillary (M8405/0) - *see* Neoplasm, skin, benign
Hidrocystoma (M8404/0) - *see* Neoplasm, skin, benign
HIE (hypoxic-ischemic encephalopathy) 768.70
mild 768.71
moderate 768.72
severe 768.73
High
A₂ anemia 282.49
altitude effects 993.2
anoxia 993.2
on
ears 993.0
sinuses 993.1
polycythemia 289.0
arch
foot 755.67
palate 750.26
artery (arterial) tension (*see also* Hypertension) 401.9
without diagnosis of hypertension 796.2
basal metabolic rate (BMR) 794.7
blood pressure (*see also* Hypertension) 401.9
incidental reading (isolated) (nonspecific), no diagnosis of hypertension 796.2
cholesterol 272.0
with high triglycerides 272.2
compliance bladder 596.4
diaphragm (congenital) 756.6
frequency deafness (congenital) (regional) 389.8
head at term 652.5●
affecting fetus or newborn 763.1
output failure (cardiac) (*see also* Failure, heart) 428.9
oxygen-affinity hemoglobin 289.0
palate 750.26
risk
behavior - *see* problem
family situation V61.9
specified circumstance NEC V61.8
human papillomavirus (HPV) DNA test positive
anal 796.75
cervical 795.05
vaginal 795.15
individual NEC V62.89
infant NEC V20.1
patient taking drugs (prescribed) V67.51
nonprescribed (*see also* Abuse, drugs, nondependent) 305.9●
pregnancy V23.9
inadequate prenatal care V23.7
specified problem NEC V23.89
temperature (of unknown origin) (*see also* Pyrexia) 780.60

High *(Continued)*
  thoracic rib 756.3
  triglycerides 272.1
    with high cholesterol 272.2
Hildenbrand's disease (typhus) 081.9
Hilger's syndrome 337.09
Hill diarrhea 579.1
Hilliard's lupus *(see also* Tuberculosis)
  017.0●
Hilum - *see* condition
Hip - *see* condition
Hippel's disease (retinocerebral
  angiomatosis) 759.6
Hippus 379.49
Hirschfeld's disease (acute diabetes
  mellitus) *(see also* Diabetes) 250.0●
  due to secondary diabetes 249.0●
Hirschsprung's disease or megacolon
  (congenital) 751.3
Hirsuties *(see also* Hypertrichosis)
  704.1
Hirsutism *(see also* Hypertrichosis)
  704.1
Hirudiniasis (external) (internal)
  134.2
His-Werner disease (trench fever)
  083.1
Hiss-Russell dysentery 004.1
Histamine cephalgia 339.00
Histidinemia 270.5
Histidinuria 270.5
Histiocytic syndromes 288.4
Histiocytoma (M8832/0) - *see also*
  Neoplasm, skin, benign
  fibrous (M8830/0) - *see also* Neoplasm,
    skin, benign
    atypical (M8830/1) - *see* Neoplasm,
      connective tissue, uncertain
      behavior
    malignant (M8830/3) - *see*
      Neoplasm, connective tissue,
      malignant
Histiocytosis (acute) (chronic) (subacute)
  277.89
  acute differentiated progressive
    (M9722/3) 202.5●
  cholesterol 277.89
  essential 277.89
  lipid, lipoid (essential) 272.7
  lipochrome (familial) 288.1
  malignant (M9720/3) 202.3●
  non-Langerhans cell 277.89 ◄
  polyostotic sclerosing 277.89 ◄
  X (chronic) 277.89
    acute (progressive) (M9722/3)
      202.5●
Histoplasmosis 115.90
  with
    endocarditis 115.94
    meningitis 115.91
    pericarditis 115.93
    pneumonia 115.95
    retinitis 115.92
    specified manifestation NEC
      115.99
  African (due to Histoplasma duboisii)
    115.10
    with
      endocarditis 115.14
      meningitis 115.11
      pericarditis 115.13
      pneumonia 115.15
      retinitis 115.12
      specified manifestation NEC
        115.19

Histoplasmosis *(Continued)*
  American (due to Histoplasma
    capsulatum) 115.00
    with
      endocarditis 115.04
      meningitis 115.01
      pericarditis 115.03
      pneumonia 115.05
      retinitis 115.02
      specified manifestation NEC
        115.09
  Darling's - *see* Histoplasmosis,
    American
  large form *(see also* Histoplasmosis,
    African) 115.10
  lung 115.05
  small form *(see also* Histoplasmosis,
    American) 115.00
History (personal) of
  abuse
    emotional V15.42
    neglect V15.42
    physical V15.41
    sexual V15.41
  affective psychosis V11.1
  alcoholism V11.3
    specified as drinking problem *(see*
      also Abuse, drugs,
      nondependent) 305.0●
  allergy to
    analgesic agent NEC V14.6
    anesthetic NEC V14.4
    antibiotic agent NEC V14.1
      penicillin V14.0
    anti-infective agent NEC V14.3
    arachnid bite V15.06 ◄
    diathesis V15.09
    drug V14.9
      specified type NEC V14.8
    eggs V15.03
    food additives V15.05
    insect bite V15.06
    latex V15.07
    medicinal agents V14.9
      specified type NEC V14.8
    milk products V15.02
    narcotic agent NEC V14.5
    nuts V15.05
      peanuts V15.01
    penicillin V14.0
    radiographic dye V15.08
    seafood V15.04
    serum V14.7
    specified food NEC V15.05
    specified nonmedicinal agents NEC
      V15.09
    spider bite V15.06
    sulfa V14.2
    sulfonamides V14.2
    therapeutic agent NEC V15.09
    vaccine V14.7
  anemia V12.3
  arrest, sudden cardiac V12.53
  arthritis V13.4
  attack, transient ischemic (TIA)
    V12.54
  benign neoplasm of brain V12.41
  blood disease V12.3
  calculi, urinary V13.01
  cardiovascular disease V12.50
    myocardial infarction 412
  chemotherapy, antineoplastic
    V87.41
  child abuse V15.41
  cigarette smoking V15.82

History (personal) *(Continued)*
  circulatory system disease
    V12.50
    myocardial infarction 412
  congenital malformation
    V13.69
  contraception V15.7
  death, sudden, successfully
    resuscitated V12.53
  deficit
    prolonged reversible ischemic
      neurologic (PRIND)
      V12.54
    reversible ischemic neurologic
      (RIND) V12.54
  diathesis, allergic V15.09
  digestive system disease V12.70
    peptic ulcer V12.71
    polyps, colonic V12.72
    specified NEC V12.79
  disease (of) V13.9
    blood V12.3
    blood-forming organs V12.3
    cardiovascular system V12.50
    circulatory system V12.50
      specified NEC V12.59
    digestive system V12.70
      peptic ulcer V12.71
      polyps, colonic V12.72
      specified NEC V12.79
    infectious V12.00
      malaria V12.03
      methicillin resistant
        Staphylococcus aureus
        (MRSA) V12.04
      MRSA (methicillin resistant
        Staphylococcus aureus)
        V12.04
      poliomyelitis V12.02
      specified NEC V12.09
      tuberculosis V12.01
    parasitic V12.00
      specified NEC V12.09
    respiratory system V12.60
      pneumonia V12.61
      specified NEC V12.69
    skin V13.3
    specified site NEC V13.8
    subcutaneous tissue V13.3
    trophoblastic V13.1
      affecting management of
        pregnancy V23.1
  disorder (of) V13.9
    endocrine V12.2
    genital system V13.29
    hematological V12.3
    immunity V12.2
    mental V11.9
      affective type V11.1
      manic-depressive V11.1
      neurosis V11.2
      schizophrenia V11.0
      specified type NEC V11.8
    metabolic V12.2
    musculoskeletal NEC V13.59
    nervous system V12.40
      specified type NEC V12.49
    obstetric V13.29
      affecting management of current
        pregnancy V23.49
        pre-term labor V23.41
      pre-term labor V13.21
    sense organs V12.40
      specified type NEC V12.49
    specified site NEC V13.8

◄ New   ◄▥ Revised   ~~deleted~~ Deleted   ● Use Additional Digit(s)   ▨ Omit code

History (personal) *(Continued)*
  disorder *(Continued)*
    urinary system V13.00
      calculi V13.01
      infection V13.02
      nephrotic syndrome V13.03
      specified NEC V13.09
  drug use
    nonprescribed *(see also* Abuse,
      drugs, nondependent) 305.9●
    patent *(see also* Abuse, drugs,
      nondependent) 305.9●
  dysplasia
    cervical (conditions classifiable to
      622.10–622.12) V13.22
  effect NEC of external cause V15.89
  embolism (pulmonary) V12.51
  emotional abuse V15.42
  encephalitis V12.42
  endocrine disorder V12.2
  estrogen therapy V87.43 ◄
  extracorporeal membrane oxygenation
    (ECMO) V15.87
  failed ◄
    conscious sedation V15.80 ◄
    moderate sedation V15.80 ◄
  falling V15.88
  family
    allergy V19.6
    anemia V18.2
    arteriosclerosis V17.49
    arthritis V17.7
    asthma V17.5
    blindness V19.0
    blood disorder NEC V18.3
    cardiovascular disease V17.49
    carrier, genetic disease V18.9
    cerebrovascular disease V17.1
    chronic respiratory condition NEC
      V17.6
    colonic polyps V18.51
    congenital anomalies V19.5
    consanguinity V19.7
    coronary artery disease V17.3
    cystic fibrosis V18.19
    deafness V19.2
    diabetes mellitus V18.0
    digestive disorders V18.59
    disease or disorder (of)
      allergic V19.6
      blood NEC V18.3
      cardiovascular NEC V17.49
      cerebrovascular V17.1
      colonic polyps V18.51
      coronary artery V17.3
      death, sudden cardiac (SCD)
        V17.41
      digestive V18.59
      ear NEC V19.3
      endocrine V18.19
        multiple neoplasia [MEN]
          syndrome V18.11
      eye NEC V19.1
      genitourinary NEC V18.7
      hypertensive V17.49
      infectious V18.8
      ischemic heart V17.3
      kidney V18.69
        polycystic V18.61
      mental V17.0
      metabolic V18.19
      musculoskeletal NEC V17.89
        osteoporosis V17.81
      neurological NEC V17.2
      parasitic V18.8
      psychiatric condition V17.0
      skin condition V19.4

History *(Continued)*
  family *(Continued)*
    ear disorder NEC V19.3
    endocrine disease V18.19
      multiple neoplasia [MEN]
        syndrome V18.11
    epilepsy V17.2
    eye disorder NEC V19.1
    genetic disease carrier V18.9
    genitourinary disease NEC V18.7
    glomerulonephritis V18.69
    gout V18.19
    hay fever V17.6
    hearing loss V19.2
    hematopoietic neoplasia V16.7
    Hodgkin's disease V16.7
    Huntington's chorea V17.2
    hydrocephalus V19.5
    hypertension V17.49
    infarction, myocardial V17.3
    infectious disease V18.8
    ischemic heart disease V17.3
    kidney disease V18.69
      polycystic V18.61
    leukemia V16.6
    lymphatic malignant neoplasia
      NEC V16.7
    malignant neoplasm (of) NEC
      V16.9
      anorectal V16.0
      anus V16.0
      appendix V16.0
      bladder V16.52
      bone V16.8
      brain V16.8
      breast V16.3
        male V16.8
      bronchus V16.1
      cecum V16.0
      cervix V16.49
      colon V16.0
      duodenum V16.0
      esophagus V16.0
      eye V16.8
      gallbladder V16.0
      gastrointestinal tract V16.0
      genital organs V16.40
      hemopoietic NEC V16.7
      ileum V16.0
      ilium V16.8
      intestine V16.0
      intrathoracic organs NEC V16.2
      kidney V16.51
      larynx V16.2
      liver V16.0
      lung V16.1
      lymphatic NEC V16.7
      ovary V16.41
      oviduct V16.41
      pancreas V16.0
      penis V16.49
      prostate V16.42
      rectum V16.0
      respiratory organs NEC V16.2
      skin V16.8
      specified site NEC V16.8
      stomach V16.0
      testis V16.43
      trachea V16.1
      ureter V16.59
      urethra V16.59
      urinary organs V16.59
      uterus V16.49
      vagina V16.49
      vulva V16.49

History *(Continued)*
  family *(Continued)*
    MEN (multiple endocrine neoplasia
      syndrome) V18.11
    mental retardation V18.4
    metabolic disease NEC V18.19
    mongolism V19.5
    ~~monoclonal drug therapy V87.42~~
    multiple
      endocrine neoplasia [MEN]
        syndrome V18.11
      myeloma V16.7
    musculoskeletal disease NEC
      V17.89
      osteoporosis V17.81
    myocardial infarction V17.3
    nephritis V18.69
    nephrosis V18.69
      osteoporosis V17.81
    parasitic disease V18.8
    polycystic kidney disease V18.61
    psychiatric disorder V17.0
    psychosis V17.0
    retardation, mental V18.4
    retinitis pigmentosa V19.1
    schizophrenia V17.0
    skin conditions V19.4
    specified condition NEC V19.8
    stroke (cerebrovascular) V17.1
    sudden cardiac death (SCD)
      V17.41
    visual loss V19.0
  fracture, healed
    pathologic V13.51
    stress V13.52
    traumatic V15.51
  genital system disorder V13.29
    pre-term labor V13.21
  health hazard V15.9
    falling V15.88
    specified cause NEC V15.89
  hepatitis
    B V12.09
    C V12.09
  Hodgkin's disease V10.72
  hypospadias V13.61
  immunity disorder V12.2
  immunosuppression therapy V87.46 ◄
  infarction, cerebral, without residual
    deficits V12.54
  infection
    central nervous system V12.42
    urinary (tract) V13.02
  infectious disease V12.00
    malaria V12.03
    methicillin resistant Staphylococcus
      aureus (MRSA) V12.04
    MRSA (methicillin resistant
      Staphylococcus aureus)
      V12.04 poliomyelitis
      V12.02
    specified NEC V12.09
    tuberculosis V12.01
  injury NEC V15.59
    traumatic brain V15.52 ◄
  insufficient prenatal care V23.7
  in utero procedure
    during pregnancy V15.21
    while a fetus V15.22
  irradiation V15.3
  leukemia V10.60
    lymphoid V10.61
    monocytic V10.63
    myeloid V10.62
    specified type NEC V10.69

History (personal) *(Continued)*
  little or no prenatal care V23.7
  low birth weight (*see also* Status, low
    birth weight) V21.30
  lymphosarcoma V10.71
  malaria V12.03
  malignant carcinoid tumor V10.91 ◄
  malignant neoplasm (of) V10.90 ◄═
    accessory sinus V10.22
    adrenal V10.88
    anus V10.06
    bile duct V10.09
    bladder V10.51
    bone V10.81
    brain V10.85
    breast V10.3
    bronchus V10.11
    cervix uteri V10.41
    colon V10.05
    connective tissue NEC V10.89
    corpus uteri V10.42
    digestive system V10.00
      specified part NEC V10.09
    duodenum V10.09
    endocrine gland NEC V10.88
    epididymis V10.48
    esophagus V10.03
    eye V10.84
    fallopian tube V10.44
    female genital organ V10.40
      specified site NEC V10.44
    gallbladder V10.09
    gastrointestinal tract V10.00
    gum V10.02
    hematopoietic NEC V10.79
    hypopharynx V10.02
    ileum V10.09
    intrathoracic organs NEC
      V10.20
    jejunum V10.09
    kidney V10.52
    large intestine V10.05
    larynx V10.21
    lip V10.02
    liver V10.07
    lung V10.11
    lymphatic NEC V10.79
    lymph glands or nodes NEC
      V10.79
    male genital organ V10.45
      specified site NEC V10.49
    mediastinum V10.29
    melanoma (of skin) V10.82
    middle ear V10.22
    mouth V10.02
      specified part NEC V10.02
    nasal cavities V10.22
    nasopharynx V10.02
    nervous system NEC V10.86
    nose V10.22
    oropharynx V10.02
    ovary V10.43
    pancreas V10.09
    parathyroid V10.88
    penis V10.49
    pharynx V10.02
    pineal V10.88
    pituitary V10.88
    placenta V10.44
    pleura V10.29
    prostate V10.46
    rectosigmoid junction V10.06
    rectum V10.06
    renal pelvis V10.53

History (personal) *(Continued)*
  malignant neoplasm *(Continued)*
    respiratory organs NEC V10.20
    salivary gland V10.02
    skin V10.83
      melanoma V10.82
    small intestine NEC V10.09
    soft tissue NEC V10.89
    specified site NEC V10.89
    stomach V10.04
    testis V10.47
    thymus V10.29
    thyroid V10.87
    tongue V10.01
    trachea V10.12
    ureter V10.59
    urethra V10.59
    urinary organ V10.50
    uterine adnexa V10.44
    uterus V10.42
    vagina V10.44
    vulva V10.44
  malignant neuroendocrine
    tumor V10.91 ◄
  manic-depressive psychosis V11.1
  meningitis V12.42
  mental disorder V11.9
    affective type V11.1
    manic-depressive V11.1
    neurosis V11.2
    schizophrenia V11.0
    specified type NEC V11.8
  Merkel cell carcinoma V10.91 ◄
  metabolic disorder V12.2
  methicillin resistant Staphylococcus
    aureus (MRSA) V12.04
  MRSA (methicillin resistant
    Staphylococcus aureus)
    V12.04
  musculoskeletal disorder NEC
    V13.59
  myocardial infarction 412
  neglect (emotional) V15.42
  nephrotic syndrome V13.03
  nervous system disorder V12.40
    specified type NEC V12.49
  neurosis V11.2
  noncompliance with medical treatment
    V15.81
  nutritional deficiency V12.1
  obstetric disorder V13.29
    affecting management of current
      pregnancy V23.49
      pre-term labor V23.41
    pre-term labor V13.21
  parasitic disease V12.00
    specified NEC V12.09
  perinatal problems V13.7
    low birth weight (*see also* Status,
      low birth weight) V21.30
  physical abuse V15.41
  poisoning V15.6
  poliomyelitis V12.02
  polyps, colonic V12.72
  poor obstetric V13.29
    affecting management of current
      pregnancy V23.49
      pre-term labor V23.41
    pre-term labor V13.21
  prolonged reversible ischemic
    neurologic deficit (PRIND)
    V12.54
  psychiatric disorder V11.9
    affective type V11.1
    manic-depressive V11.1
    neurosis V11.2

History (personal) *(Continued)*
  psychiatric disorder *(Continued)*
    schizophrenia V11.0
    specified type NEC V11.8
  psychological trauma V15.49
    emotional abuse V15.42
    neglect V15.42
    physical abuse V15.41
    rape V15.41
  psychoneurosis V11.2
  radiation therapy V15.3
  rape V15.41
  respiratory system disease V12.60
    pneumonia V12.61
    specified NEC V12.69
  reticulosarcoma V10.71
  return from military deployment
    V62.22
  reversible ischemic neurologic deficit
    (RIND) V12.54
  schizophrenia V11.0
  skin disease V13.3
  smoking (tobacco) V15.82
  steroid therapy V87.45 ◄
    inhaled V87.44 ◄
    systemic V87.45 ◄
  stroke without residual deficits
    V12.54
  subcutaneous tissue disease V13.3
  sudden
    cardiac
      arrest V12.53
      death (successfully resuscitated)
        V12.53
  surgery to
    great vessels V15.1
    heart V15.1
    in utero
      during pregnancy V15.21
      while a fetus V15.22
    organs NEC V15.29
  syndrome, nephrotic V13.03
  therapy
    antineoplastic drug V87.41
    drug NEC V87.49
    estrogen V87.43 ◄
    immunosuppression V87.46 ◄
    monoclonal drug V87.42
    steroid V87.45 ◄
      inhaled V87.44 ◄
      systemic V87.45 ◄
  thrombophlebitis V12.52
  thrombosis V12.51
  tobacco use V15.82
  trophoblastic disease V13.1
    affecting management of pregnancy
      V23.1
  tuberculosis V12.01
  ulcer, peptic V12.71
  urinary system disorder V13.00
    calculi V13.01
    infection V13.02
    nephrotic syndrome V13.03
    specified NEC V13.09
HIT (heparin-induced thrombocytopenia)
  289.84
HIV infection (disease) (illness) - *see*
  Human immunodeficiency virus
  (disease) (illness) (infection)
Hives (bold) (*see also* Urticaria)
  708.9
Hoarseness 784.42 ◄═
Hobnail liver - *see* Cirrhosis, portal
Hobo, hoboism V60.0

◄ New   ◄═ Revised   ~~deleted~~ Deleted   ● Use Additional Digit(s)   � Omit code

Hodgkin's
  disease (M9650/3) 201.9●
    lymphocytic
      depletion (M9653/3) 201.7●
        diffuse fibrosis (M9654/3)
          201.7●
        reticular type (M9655/3)
          201.7●
      predominance (M9651/3) 201.4●
    lymphocytic-histiocytic
      predominance (M9651/3)
        201.4●
Hodgkin's (Continued)
  disease (Continued)
    mixed cellularity (M9652/3) 201.6●
    nodular sclerosis (M9656/3) 201.5●
      cellular phase (M9657/3) 201.5●
    granuloma (M9661/3) 201.1●
    lymphogranulomatosis (M9650/3)
      201.9●
    lymphoma (M9650/3) 201.9●
    lymphosarcoma (M9650/3) 201.9●
    paragranuloma (M9660/3) 201.0●
    sarcoma (M9662/3) 201.2●
Hodgson's disease (aneurysmal dilatation
    of aorta) 441.9
  ruptured 441.5
Hodi-potsy 111.0
Hoffa (-Kastert) disease or syndrome
    (liposynovitis prepatellaris) 272.8
Hoffmann's syndrome 244.9 [359.5]
Hoffmann-Bouveret syndrome
    (paroxysmal tachycardia) 427.2
Hole
  macula 362.54
  optic disc, crater-like 377.22
  retina (macula) 362.54
    round 361.31
      with detachment 361.01
Holla disease (see also Spherocytosis) 282.0
Holländer-Simons syndrome
    (progressive lipodystrophy) 272.6
Hollow foot (congenital) 754.71
  acquired 736.73
Holmes' syndrome (visual disorientation)
    368.16
Holoprosencephaly 742.2
  due to
    trisomy 13 758.1
    trisomy 18 758.2
Holthouse's hernia - see Hernia,
    inguinal
Homesickness 309.89
Homocystinemia 270.4
Homocystinuria 270.4
Homologous serum jaundice
    (prophylactic) (therapeutic) - see
    Hepatitis, viral
Homosexuality - omit code
  ego-dystonic 302.0
  pedophilic 302.2
  problems with 302.0
Homozygous Hb-S disease 282.61
Honeycomb lung 518.89
  congenital 748.4
Hong Kong ear 117.3
HOOD (hereditary osteo-
    onychodysplasia) 756.89
Hooded
  clitoris 752.49
  penis 752.69
Hookworm (anemia) (disease)
    (infestation) - see Ancylostomiasis
Hoppe-Goldflam syndrome 358.00

Hordeolum (external) (eyelid) 373.11
  internal 373.12
Horn
  cutaneous 702.8
    cheek 702.8
    eyelid 702.8
    penis 702.8
  iliac 756.89
  nail 703.8
    congenital 757.5
  papillary 700
Horner's
  syndrome (see also Neuropathy,
      peripheral, autonomic) 337.9
    traumatic 954.0
  teeth 520.4
Horseshoe kidney (congenital) 753.3
Horton's
  disease (temporal arteritis) 446.5
  headache or neuralgia 339.00
Hospice care V66.7
Hospitalism (in children) NEC 309.83
Hourglass contraction, contracture
  bladder 596.8
  gallbladder 575.2
    congenital 751.69
  stomach 536.8
    congenital 750.7
    psychogenic 306.4
  uterus 661.4●
    affecting fetus or newborn 763.7
Household circumstance affecting care
    V60.9
  specified type NEC V60.89   ◀▭▭▭
Housemaid's knee 727.2
Housing circumstance affecting care V60.9
  specified type NEC V60.89   ◀▭▭▭
Huchard's disease (continued arterial
    hypertension) 401.9
Hudson-Stähli lines 371.11
Huguier's disease (uterine fibroma) 218.9
Hum, venous - omit code
Human bite (open wound) - (see also
    Wound, open, by site)
  intact skin surface - see Contusion
Human immunodeficiency virus
    (disease) (illness) 042
  infection V08
    with symptoms, symptomatic 042
Human immunodeficiency virus-2
    infection 079.53
Human immunovirus (disease) (illness)
    (infection) - see Human
    immunodeficiency virus (disease)
    (illness) (infection)
Human papillomavirus 079.4
  high risk, DNA test positive
    anal 796.75
    cervical 795.05
    vaginal 795.15
  low risk, DNA test positive
    anal 796.79
    cervical 795.09
    vaginal 795.19
Human parvovirus 079.83
Human T-cell lymphotrophic virus I
    infection 079.51
Human T-cell lymphotrophic virus II
    infection 079.52
Human T-cell lymphotropic virus-III
    (disease) (illness) (infection) - see
    Human immunodeficiency virus
    (disease) (illness) (infection)
HTLV-I infection 079.51

HTLV-II infection 079.52
HTLV-III (disease) (illness) (infection) -
    see Human immunodeficiency
    virus (disease) (illness)
    (infection)
HTLV-III/LAV (disease) (illness)
    (infection) - see Human
    immunodeficiency virus (disease)
    (illness) (infection)
Humpback (acquired) 737.9
  congenital 756.19
Hunchback (acquired) 737.9
  congenital 756.19
Hunger 994.2
  air, psychogenic 306.1
  disease 251.1
Hungry bone syndrome 275.5
Hunner's ulcer (see also Cystitis) 595.1
Hunt's
  neuralgia 053.11
  syndrome (herpetic geniculate
      ganglionitis) 053.11
    dyssynergia cerebellaris myoclonica
      334.2
Hunter's glossitis 529.4
Hunter (-Hurler) syndrome
    (mucopolysaccharidosis II) 277.5
Hunterian chancre 091.0
Huntington's
  chorea 333.4
  disease 333.4
Huppert's disease (multiple myeloma)
    (M9730/3) 203.0●
Hurler (-Hunter) disease or syndrome
    (mucopolysaccharidosis II) 277.5
Hürthle cell
  adenocarcinoma (M8290/3) 193
  adenoma (M8290/0) 226
  carcinoma (M8290/3) 193
  tumor (M8290/0) 226
Hutchinson's
  disease meaning
    angioma serpiginosum 709.1
    cheiropompholyx 705.81
    prurigo estivalis 692.72
    summer eruption, or summer
      prurigo 692.72
  incisors 090.5
  melanotic freckle (M8742/2) - see also
    Neoplasm, skin, in situ
    malignant melanoma in (M8742/3) -
      see Melanoma
  teeth or incisors (congenital syphilis)
    090.5
Hutchinson-Boeck disease or syndrome
    (sarcoidosis) 135
Hutchinson-Gilford disease or syndrome
    (progeria) 259.8
Hyaline
  degeneration (diffuse) (generalized)
    728.9
    localized - see Degeneration, by site
  membrane (disease) (lung) (newborn)
    769
Hyalinosis cutis et mucosae 272.8
Hyalin plaque, sclera, senile 379.16
Hyalitis (asteroid) 379.22
  syphilitic 095.8
Hydatid
  cyst or tumor - see also Echinococcus
    fallopian tube 752.11
  mole - see Hydatidiform mole
  Morgagni (congenital) 752.89
    fallopian tube 752.11

Hydatidiform mole (benign) (complicating pregnancy) (delivered) (undelivered) 630
  invasive (M9100/1) 236.1
  malignant (M9100/1) 236.1
  previous, affecting management of pregnancy V23.1
Hydatidosis - see Echinococcus
Hyde's disease (prurigo nodularis) 698.3
Hydradenitis 705.83
Hydradenoma (M8400/0) - see Hidradenoma
Hydralazine lupus or syndrome
  correct substance properly administered 695.4
  overdose or wrong substance given or taken 972.6
Hydramnios 657●
  affecting fetus or newborn 761.3
Hydrancephaly 742.3
  with spina bifida (see also Spina bifida) 741.0●
Hydranencephaly 742.3
  with spina bifida (see also Spina bifida) 741.0●
Hydrargyrism NEC 985.0
Hydrarthrosis (see also Effusion, joint) 719.0●
  gonococcal 098.50
  intermittent (see also Rheumatism, palindromic) 719.3●
  of yaws (early) (late) 102.6
  syphilitic 095.8
    congenital 090.5
Hydremia 285.9
Hydrencephalocele (congenital) 742.0
Hydrencephalomeningocele (congenital) 742.0
Hydroa 694.0
  aestivale 692.72
  gestationis 646.8●
  herpetiformis 694.0
  pruriginosa 694.0
  vacciniforme 692.72
Hydroadenitis 705.83
Hydrocalycosis (see also Hydronephrosis) 591
  congenital 753.29
Hydrocalyx (see also Hydronephrosis) 591
Hydrocele (calcified) (chylous) (idiopathic) (infantile) (inguinal canal) (recurrent) (senile) (spermatic cord) (testis) (tunica vaginalis) 603.9
  canal of Nuck (female) 629.1
    male 603.9
  congenital 778.6
  encysted 603.0
    congenital 778.6
  female NEC 629.89
  infected 603.1
  round ligament 629.89
  specified type NEC 603.8
    congenital 778.6
  spinalis (see also Spina bifida) 741.9●
  vulva 624.8
Hydrocephalic fetus
  affecting management or pregnancy 655.0●
  causing disproportion 653.6●
    with obstructed labor 660.1●
      affecting fetus or newborn 763.1

Hydrocephalus (acquired) (external) (internal) (malignant) (noncommunicating) (obstructive) (recurrent) 331.4
  aqueduct of Sylvius stricture 742.3
    with spina bifida (see also Spina bifida) 741.0●
  chronic 742.3
    with spina bifida (see also Spina bifida) 741.0●
Hydrocephalus (Continued)
  communicating 331.3
  congenital (external) (internal) 742.3
    with spina bifida (see also Spina bifida) 741.0●
  due to
    stricture of aqueduct of Sylvius 742.3
      with spina bifida (see also Spina bifida) 741.0●
    toxoplasmosis (congenital) 771.2
  fetal affecting management of pregnancy 655.0●
  foramen Magendie block (acquired) 331.3
    congenital 742.3
      with spina bifida (see also Spina bifida) 741.0●
  newborn 742.3
    with spina bifida (see also Spina bifida) 741.0●
  normal pressure 331.5
    idiopathic (INPH) 331.5
    secondary 331.3
  otitic 348.2
  syphilitic, congenital 090.49
  tuberculous (see also Tuberculosis) 013.8●
Hydrocolpos (congenital) 623.8
Hydrocystoma (M8404/0) - see Neoplasm, skin, benign
Hydroencephalocele (congenital) 742.0
Hydroencephalomeningocele (congenital) 742.0
Hydrohematopneumothorax (see also Hemothorax) 511.89
Hydromeningitis - see Meningitis
Hydromeningocele (spinal) (see also Spina bifida) 741.9●
  cranial 742.0
Hydrometra 621.8
Hydrometrocolpos 623.8
Hydromicrocephaly 742.1
Hydromphalus (congenital) (since birth) 757.39
Hydromyelia 742.53
Hydromyelocele (see also Spina bifida) 741.9●
Hydronephrosis 591
  atrophic 591
  congenital 753.29
  due to S. hematobium 120.0
  early 591
  functionless (infected) 591
  infected 591
  intermittent 591
  primary 591
  secondary 591
  tuberculous (see also Tuberculosis) 016.0●
Hydropericarditis (see also Pericarditis) 423.9
Hydropericardium (see also Pericarditis) 423.9
Hydroperitoneum 789.59
Hydrophobia 071

Hydrophthalmos (see also Buphthalmia) 743.20
Hydropneumohemothorax (see also Hemothorax) 511.89
Hydropneumopericarditis (see also Pericarditis) 423.9
Hydropneumopericardium (see also Pericarditis) 423.9
Hydropneumothorax 511.89
  nontuberculous 511.89
    bacterial 511.1
    pneumococcal 511.1
    staphylococcal 511.1
    streptococcal 511.1
  traumatic 860.0
    with open wound into thorax 860.1
  tuberculous (see also Tuberculosis, pleura) 012.0●
Hydrops 782.3
  abdominis 789.59
  amnii (complicating pregnancy) (see also Hydramnios) 657●
  articulorum intermittens (see also Rheumatism, palindromic) 719.3●
  cardiac (see also Failure, heart) 428.0
  congenital - see Hydrops, fetalis
  endolymphatic (see also Disease, Ménière's) 386.00
  fetal(is) or newborn 778.0
    due to isoimmunization 773.3
    not due to isoimmunization 778.0
  gallbladder 575.3
  idiopathic (fetus or newborn) 778.0
  joint (see also Effusion, joint) 719.0●
  labyrinth (see also Disease, Ménière's) 386.00
  meningeal NEC 331.4
  nutritional 262
  pericardium - see Pericarditis
  pleura (see also Hydrothorax) 511.89
  renal (see also Nephrosis) 581.9
  spermatic cord (see also Hydrocele) 603.9
Hydropyonephrosis (see also Pyelitis) 590.80
  chronic 590.00
Hydrorachis 742.53
Hydrorrhea (nasal) 478.19
  gravidarum 658.1●
  pregnancy 658.1●
Hydrosadenitis 705.83
Hydrosalpinx (fallopian tube) (follicularis) 614.1
Hydrothorax (double) (pleural) 511.89
  chylous (nonfilarial) 457.8
    filaria (see also Infestation, filarial) 125.9
  nontuberculous 511.89
    bacterial 511.1
    pneumococcal 511.1
    staphylococcal 511.1
    streptococcal 511.1
  traumatic 862.29
    with open wound into thorax 862.39
  tuberculous (see also Tuberculosis, pleura) 012.0●
Hydroureter 593.5
  congenital 753.22
Hydroureteronephrosis (see also Hydronephrosis) 591
Hydrourethra 599.84
Hydroxykynureninuria 270.2
Hydroxyprolinemia 270.8
Hydroxyprolinuria 270.8

◀ New   ◀▦ Revised   ~~deleted~~ Deleted   ● Use Additional Digit(s)   ▨ Omit code

Hygroma (congenital) (cystic) (M9173/0)
228.1
  prepatellar 727.3
  subdural - *see* Hematoma, subdural
Hymen - *see* condition
Hymenolepiasis (diminuta) (infection)
  (infestation) (nana) 123.6
Hymenolepsis (diminuta) (infection)
  (infestation) (nana) 123.6
Hypalgesia (*see also* Disturbance,
  sensation) 782.0
Hyperabduction syndrome 447.8
Hyperacidity, gastric 536.8
  psychogenic 306.4
Hyperactive, hyperactivity 314.01
  basal cell, uterine cervix 622.10
  bladder 596.51
  bowel (syndrome) 564.9
    sounds 787.5
  cervix epithelial (basal) 622.10
  child 314.01
  colon 564.9
  gastrointestinal 536.8
    psychogenic 306.4
  intestine 564.9
  labyrinth (unilateral) 386.51
    with loss of labyrinthine reactivity
      386.58
    bilateral 386.52
  nasal mucous membrane 478.19
  stomach 536.8
  thyroid (gland) (*see also* Thyrotoxicosis)
    242.9●
Hyperacusis 388.42
Hyperadrenalism (cortical) 255.3
  medullary 255.6
Hyperadrenocorticism 255.3
  congenital 255.2
  iatrogenic
    correct substance properly
      administered 255.3
    overdose or wrong substance given
      or taken 962.0
Hyperaffectivity 301.11
Hyperaldosteronism (atypical)
  (hyperplastic) (normoaldosteronal)
  (nor-motensive) (primary) 255.10
  secondary 255.14
Hyperalgesia (*see also* Disturbance,
  sensation) 782.0
Hyperalimentation 783.6
  carotene 278.3
  specified NEC 278.8
  vitamin A 278.2
  vitamin D 278.4
Hyperaminoaciduria 270.9
  arginine 270.6
  citrulline 270.6
  cystine 270.0
  glycine 270.0
  lysine 270.7
  ornithine 270.6
  renal (types I, II, III) 270.0
Hyperammonemia (congenital) 270.6
Hyperamnesia 780.99
Hyperamylasemia 790.5
Hyperaphia 782.0
Hyperazotemia 791.9
Hyperbetalipoproteinemia (acquired)
  (essential) (familial) (hereditary)
  (primary) (secondary) 272.0
  with prebetalipoproteinemia 272.2
Hyperbilirubinemia 782.4
  congenital 277.4
  constitutional 277.4
  neonatal (transient) (*see also* Jaundice,
    fetus or newborn) 774.6
    of prematurity 774.2

Hyperbilirubinemica encephalopathia,
  newborn 774.7
  due to isoimmunization 773.4
Hypercalcemia, hypercalcemic
  (idiopathic) 275.42
  nephropathy 588.89
Hypercalcinuria 275.40
Hypercapnia 786.09
  with mixed acid-based disorder
    276.4
  fetal, affecting newborn 770.89
Hypercarotinemia 278.3
Hypercementosis 521.5
Hyperchloremia 276.9
Hyperchlorhydria 536.8
  neurotic 306.4
  psychogenic 306.4
Hypercholesterinemia - *see*
  Hypercholesterolemia
Hypercholesterolemia 272.0
  with hyperglyceridemia, endogenous
    272.2
  essential 272.0
  familial 272.0
  hereditary 272.0
  primary 272.0
  pure 272.0
Hypercholesterolosis 272.0
Hyperchylia gastrica 536.8
  psychogenic 306.4
Hyperchylomicronemia (familial) (with
  hyperbetalipoproteinemia) 272.3
Hypercoagulation syndrome (primary)
  289.81
  secondary 289.82
Hypercorticosteronism
  correct substance properly
    administered 255.3
  overdose or wrong substance given or
    taken 962.0
Hypercortisonism
  correct substance properly
    administered 255.3
  overdose or wrong substance given or
    taken 962.0
Hyperdynamic beta-adrenergic state or
  syndrome (circulatory) 429.82
Hyperekplexia 759.89
Hyperelectrolytemia 276.9
Hyperemesis 536.2
  arising during pregnancy - *see*
    Hyperemesis, gravidarum
  gravidarum (mild) (before 22
    completed weeks' gestation)
    643.0●
    with
      carbohydrate depletion 643.1●
      dehydration 643.1●
      electrolyte imbalance 643.1●
      metabolic disturbance 643.1●
    affecting fetus or newborn 761.8
    severe (with metabolic disturbance)
      643.1●
  psychogenic 306.4
Hyperemia (acute) 780.99
  anal mucosa 569.49
  bladder 596.7
  cerebral 437.8
  conjunctiva 372.71
  ear, internal, acute 386.30
  enteric 564.89
  eye 372.71
  eyelid (active) (passive) 374.82
  intestine 564.89
  iris 364.41
  kidney 593.81

Hyperemia (*Continued*)
  labyrinth 386.30
  liver (active) (passive) 573.8
  lung 514
  ovary 620.8
  passive 780.99
  pulmonary 514
  renal 593.81
  retina 362.89
  spleen 289.59
  stomach 537.89
Hyperesthesia (body surface) (*see also*
  Disturbance, sensation) 782.0
  larynx (reflex) 478.79
    hysterical 300.11
  pharynx (reflex) 478.29
Hyperestrinism 256.0
Hyperestrogenism 256.0
Hyperestrogenosis 256.0
Hyperexplexia 759.89
Hyperextension, joint 718.80
  ankle 718.87
  elbow 718.82
  foot 718.87
  hand 718.84
  hip 718.85
  knee 718.86
  multiple sites 718.89
  pelvic region 718.85
  shoulder (region) 718.81
  specified site NEC 718.88
  wrist 718.83
Hyperfibrinolysis - *see* Fibrinolysis
Hyperfolliculinism 256.0
Hyperfructosemia 271.2
Hyperfunction
  adrenal (cortex) 255.3
    androgenic, acquired benign 255.3
    medulla 255.6
    virilism 255.2
  corticoadrenal NEC 255.3
  labyrinth - *see* Hyperactive, labyrinth
  medulloadrenal 255.6
  ovary 256.1
    estrogen 256.0
  pancreas 577.8
  parathyroid (gland) 252.00
  pituitary (anterior) (gland) (lobe) 253.1
  testicular 257.0
Hypergammaglobulinemia 289.89
  monoclonal, benign (BMH) 273.1
  polyclonal 273.0
  Waldenström's 273.0
Hyperglobulinemia 273.8
Hyperglycemia 790.29
  maternal
    affecting fetus or newborn 775.0
    manifest diabetes in infant 775.1
  postpancreatectomy (complete)
    (partial) 251.3
Hyperglyceridemia 272.1
  endogenous 272.1
  essential 272.1
  familial 272.1
  hereditary 272.1
  mixed 272.3
  pure 272.1
Hyperglycinemia 270.7
Hypergonadism
  ovarian 256.1
  testicular (infantile) (primary) 257.0
Hyperheparinemia (*see also* Circulating
  anticoagulants) 286.5
Hyperhidrosis, hyperidrosis 705.21
  axilla 705.21
  face 705.21

Hyperhidrosis, hyperidrosis (Continued)
  focal (localized) 705.21
    primary 705.21
      axilla 705.21
      face 705.21
      palms 705.21
      soles 705.21
    secondary 705.22
      axilla 705.22
      face 705.22
      palms 705.22
      soles 705.22
  generalized 780.8
  palms 705.21
  psychogenic 306.3
  secondary 780.8
  soles 705.21
Hyperhistidinemia 270.5
Hyperinsulinism (ectopic) (functional)
    (organic) NEC 251.1
  iatrogenic 251.0
  reactive 251.2
  spontaneous 251.2
  therapeutic misadventure (from
    administration of insulin) 962.3
Hyperiodemia 276.9
Hyperirritability (cerebral), in newborn
    779.1
Hyperkalemia 276.7
Hyperkeratosis (see also Keratosis) 701.1
  cervix 622.2
  congenital 757.39
  cornea 371.89
  due to yaws (early) (late) (palmar or
    plantar) 102.3
  eccentrica 757.39
  figurata centrifuga atrophica 757.39
  follicularis 757.39
    in cutem penetrans 701.1
  limbic (cornea) 371.89
  palmoplantaris climacterica 701.1
  pinta (carate) 103.1
  senile (with pruritus) 702.0
  tongue 528.79
  universalis congenita 757.1
  vagina 623.1
  vocal cord 478.5
  vulva 624.09
Hyperkinesia, hyperkinetic (disease)
    (reaction) (syndrome) 314.9
  with
    attention deficit - see Disorder,
      attention deficit
    conduct disorder 314.2
    developmental delay 314.1
    simple disturbance of activity and
      attention 314.01
    specified manifestation NEC 314.8
  heart (disease) 429.82
  of childhood or adolescence NEC 314.9
Hyperlacrimation (see also Epiphora)
    375.20
Hyperlipemia (see also Hyperlipidemia)
    272.4
Hyperlipidemia 272.4
  carbohydrate-induced 272.1
  combined 272.2
  endogenous 272.1
  exogenous 272.3
  fat-induced 272.3
  group
    A 272.0
    B 272.1
    C 272.2
    D 272.3
  mixed 272.2
  specified type NEC 272.4

Hyperlipidosis 272.7
  hereditary 272.7
Hyperlipoproteinemia (acquired)
    (essential) (familial) (hereditary)
    (primary) (secondary) 272.4
  Fredrickson type
    I 272.3
    IIA 272.0
    IIB 272.2
    III 272.2
    IV 272.1
    V 272.3
  low-density-lipoid-type (LDL) 272.0
  very-low-density-lipoid-type [VLDL]
    272.1
Hyperlucent lung, unilateral 492.8
Hyperluteinization 256.1
Hyperlysinemia 270.7
Hypermagnesemia 275.2
  neonatal 775.5
Hypermaturity (fetus or newborn)
  post-term infant 766.21
  prolonged gestation infant 766.22
Hypermenorrhea 626.2
Hypermetabolism 794.7
Hypermethioninemia 270.4
Hypermetropia (congenital) 367.0
Hypermobility
  cecum 564.9
  coccyx 724.71
  colon 564.9
    psychogenic 306.4
  ileum 564.89
  joint (acquired) 718.80
    ankle 718.87
    elbow 718.82
    foot 718.87
    hand 718.84
    hip 718.85
    knee 718.86
    multiple sites 718.89
    pelvic region 718.85
    shoulder (region) 718.81
    specified site NEC 718.88
    wrist 718.83
  kidney, congenital 753.3
  meniscus (knee) 717.5
  scapula 718.81
  stomach 536.8
    psychogenic 306.4
  syndrome 728.5
  testis, congenital 752.52
  urethral 599.81
Hypermotility
  gastrointestinal 536.8
  intestine 564.9
    psychogenic 306.4
  stomach 536.8
Hypernasality 784.43
Hypernatremia 276.0
  with water depletion 276.0
Hypernephroma (M8312/3) 189.0
Hyperopia 367.0
Hyperorexia 783.6
Hyperornithinemia 270.6
Hyperosmia (see also Disturbance,
    sensation) 781.1
Hyperosmolality 276.0
Hyperosteogenesis 733.99
Hyperostosis 733.99
  calvarial 733.3
  cortical 733.3
    infantile 756.59
  frontal, internal of skull 733.3

Hyperostosis (Continued)
  interna frontalis 733.3
  monomelic 733.99
  skull 733.3
    congenital 756.0
  vertebral 721.8
    with spondylosis - see Spondylosis
    ankylosing 721.6
Hyperovarianism 256.1
Hyperovarism, hyperovaria 256.1
Hyperoxaluria (primary) 271.8
Hyperoxia 987.8
Hyperparathyroidism 252.00
  ectopic 259.3
  other 252.08
  primary 252.01
  secondary (of renal origin) 588.81
    non-renal 252.02
  tertiary 252.08
Hyperpathia (see also Disturbance,
    sensation) 782.0
  psychogenic 307.80
Hyperperistalsis 787.4
  psychogenic 306.4
Hyperpermeability, capillary 448.9
Hyperphagia 783.6
Hyperphenylalaninemia 270.1
Hyperphoria 378.40
  alternating 378.45
Hyperphosphatemia 275.3
Hyperpiesia (see also Hypertension) 401.9
Hyperpiesis (see also Hypertension) 401.9
Hyperpigmentation - see Pigmentation
Hyperpinealism 259.8
Hyperpipecolatemia 270.7
Hyperpituitarism 253.1
Hyperplasia, hyperplastic
  adenoids (lymphoid tissue) 474.12
    and tonsils 474.10
  adrenal (capsule) (cortex) (gland) 255.8
    with
      sexual precocity (male) 255.2
      virilism, adrenal 255.2
      virilization (female) 255.2
    congenital 255.2
    due to excess ACTH (ectopic)
      (pituitary) 255.0
    medulla 255.8
  alpha cells (pancreatic)
    with
      gastrin excess 251.5
      glucagon excess 251.4
  appendix (lymphoid) 543.0
  artery, fibromuscular NEC 447.8
    carotid 447.8
    renal 447.3
  bone 733.99
    marrow 289.9
  breast (see also Hypertrophy, breast)
    611.1
    ductal 610.8
      atypical 610.8
  carotid artery 447.8
  cementation, cementum (teeth) (tooth)
    521.5
  cervical gland 785.6
  cervix (uteri) 622.10
    basal cell 622.10
    congenital 752.49
    endometrium 622.10
    polypoid 622.10
  chin 524.05
  clitoris, congenital 752.49
  dentin 521.5
  endocervicitis 616.0

  ◀ New ◀▦ Revised ~~deleted~~ Deleted ● Use Additional Digit(s) ▦ Omit code

Hyperplasia, hyperplastic *(Continued)*
  endometrium, endometrial
        (adenomatous) (atypical) (cystic)
        (glandular) (polypoid) (uterus)
        621.30
      with atypia 621.33
      without atypia
        complex 621.32
        simple 621.31
      benign 621.34
      cervix 622.10
  epithelial 709.8
      focal, oral, including tongue 528.79
      mouth (focal) 528.79
      nipple 611.89
      skin 709.8
      tongue (focal) 528.79
      vaginal wall 623.0
  erythroid 289.9
  fascialis ossificans (progressiva) 728.11
  fibromuscular, artery NEC 447.8
      carotid 447.8
      renal 447.3
  genital
      female 629.89
      male 608.89
  gingiva 523.8
  glandularis
      cystica uteri 621.30
      endometrium (uterus) 621.30
      interstitialis uteri 621.30
  granulocytic 288.69
  gum 523.8
  hymen, congenital 752.49
  islands of Langerhans 251.1
  islet cell (pancreatic) 251.9
      alpha cells
        with excess
            gastrin 251.5
            glucagon 251.4
      beta cells 251.1
  juxtaglomerular (complex) (kidney)
        593.89
  kidney (congenital) 753.3
  liver (congenital) 751.69
  lymph node (gland) 785.6
  lymphoid (diffuse) (nodular) 785.6
      appendix 543.0
      intestine 569.89
  mandibular 524.02
      alveolar 524.72
      unilateral condylar 526.89
  Marchand multiple nodular (liver) -
        see Cirrhosis, postnecrotic
  maxillary 524.01
      alveolar 524.71
  medulla, adrenal 255.8
  myometrium, myometrial 621.2
  nose (lymphoid) (polypoid) 478.19
  oral soft tissue (inflammatory)
        (irritative) (mucosa) NEC 528.9
      gingiva 523.8
      tongue 529.8
  organ or site, congenital NEC - *see*
        Anomaly, specified type NEC
  ovary 620.8
  palate, papillary 528.9
  pancreatic islet cells 251.9
      alpha
        with excess
            gastrin 251.5
            glucagon 251.4
      beta 251.1
  parathyroid (gland) 252.01
  persistent, vitreous (primary) 743.51

Hyperplasia, hyperplastic *(Continued)*
  pharynx (lymphoid) 478.29
  prostate 600.90
      with
        other lower urinary tract
            symptoms (LUTS) 600.91
        urinary
            obstruction 600.91
            retention 600.91
      adenofibromatous 600.20
        with
            other lower urinary tract
                symptoms (LUTS)
                600.21
            urinary
                obstruction 600.21
                retention 600.21
      nodular 600.10
        with
            urinary
                obstruction 600.11
                retention 600.11
  renal artery (fibromuscular) 447.3
  reticuloendothelial (cell) 289.9
  salivary gland (any) 527.1
  Schimmelbusch's 610.1
  suprarenal (capsule) (gland) 255.8
  thymus (gland) (persistent) 254.0
  thyroid *(see also* Goiter) 240.9
      primary 242.0●
      secondary 242.2●
  tonsil (lymphoid tissue) 474.11
      and adenoids 474.10
  urethrovaginal 599.89
  uterus, uterine (myometrium) 621.2
      endometrium *(see also* Hyperplasia,
            endometrium) 621.30
  vitreous (humor), primary persistent
        743.51
  vulva 624.3
  zygoma 738.11
Hyperpnea *(see also* Hyperventilation)
      786.01
Hyperpotassemia 276.7
Hyperprebetalipoproteinemia 272.1
  with chylomicronemia 272.3
  familial 272.1
Hyperprolactinemia 253.1
Hyperprolinemia 270.8
Hyperproteinemia 273.8
Hyperprothrombinemia 289.89
Hyperpselaphesia 782.0
Hyperpyrexia 780.60
  heat (effects of) 992.0
  malarial *(see also* Malaria) 084.6
  malignant, due to anesthetic 995.86
  rheumatic - *see* Fever, rheumatic
  unknown origin *(see also* Pyrexia)
        780.60
Hyperreactor, vascular 780.2
Hyperreflexia 796.1
  bladder, autonomic 596.54
      with cauda equina 344.61
  detrusor 344.61
Hypersalivation *(see also* Ptyalism)
      527.7
Hypersarcosinemia 270.8
Hypersecretion
  ACTH 255.3
  androgens (ovarian) 256.1
  calcitonin 246.0
  corticoadrenal 255.3
  cortisol 255.0
  estrogen 256.0
  gastric 536.8
      psychogenic 306.4

Hypersecretion *(Continued)*
  gastrin 251.5
  glucagon 251.4
  hormone
      ACTH 255.3
      anterior pituitary 253.1
      growth NEC 253.0
      ovarian androgen 256.1
      testicular 257.0
      thyroid stimulating 242.8●
  insulin - *see* Hyperinsulinism
  lacrimal glands *(see also* Epiphora) 375.20
  medulloadrenal 255.6
  milk 676.6●
  ovarian androgens 256.1
  pituitary (anterior) 253.1
  salivary gland (any) 527.7
  testicular hormones 257.0
  thyrocalcitonin 246.0
  upper respiratory 478.9
Hypersegmentation, hereditary 288.2
  eosinophils 288.2
  neutrophil nuclei 288.2
Hypersensitive, hypersensitiveness,
      hypersensitivity - *see also* Allergy
  angiitis 446.20
      specified NEC 446.29
  carotid sinus 337.01
  colon 564.9
      psychogenic 306.4
  DNA (deoxyribonucleic acid)
      NEC 287.2
  drug *(see also* Allergy, drug) 995.27
  esophagus 530.89
  insect bites - *see* Injury, superficial, by
      site
  labyrinth 386.58
  pain *(see also* Disturbance, sensation)
      782.0
  pneumonitis NEC 495.9
  reaction *(see also* Allergy) 995.3
      upper respiratory tract NEC 478.8
  stomach (allergic) (nonallergic) 536.8
      psychogenic 306.4
Hypersomatotropism (classic) 253.0
Hypersomnia, unspecified 780.54
  with sleep apnea, unspecified 780.53
  alcohol induced 291.82
  drug induced 292.85
  due to
      medical condition classified
            elsewhere 327.14
      mental disorder 327.15
  idiopathic
      with long sleep time 327.11
      without long sleep time 327.12
  menstrual related 327.13
  nonorganic origin 307.43
      persistent (primary) 307.44
      transient 307.43
  organic 327.10
      other 327.19
  primary 307.44
  recurrent 327.13
Hypersplenia 289.4
Hypersplenism 289.4
Hypersteatosis 706.3
Hyperstimulation, ovarian 256.1
Hypersuprarenalism 255.3
Hypersusceptibility - *see* Allergy
Hyper-TBG-nemia 246.8
Hypertelorism 756.0
  orbit, orbital 376.41
Hypertension, hypertensive - *see* table
      on pg. 348–351

	Malignant	Benign	Unspecified
Hypertension, hypertensive (arterial) (arteriolar) (crisis) (degeneration) (disease) (essential) (fluctuating) (idiopathic) (intermittent) (labile) (low renin) (orthostatic) (paroxysmal) (primary) (systemic) (uncontrolled) (vascular)	401.0	401.1	401.9
with			
chronic kidney disease	—	—	—
stage I through stage IV, or unspecified	403.00	403.10	403.90
stage V or end stage renal disease	403.01	403.11	403.91
heart involvement (conditions classifiable to 429.0–429.3, 429.8, 429.9 due to hypertension) (*see also* Hypertension, heart)	402.00	402.10	402.90
with kidney involvement - *see* Hypertension, cardiorenal			
renal (kidney) involvement (only conditions classifiable to 585, ~~586, 587~~) (excludes conditions classifiable to 584) (*see also* Hypertension, kidney)	403.00	403.10	403.90
with heart involvement - *see* Hypertension, cardiorenal failure (and sclerosis) (*see also* Hypertension, kidney)	403.01	403.11	403.91
sclerosis without failure (*see also* Hypertension, kidney)	403.00	403.10	403.90
accelerated (*see also* Hypertension, by type, malignant)	401.0	—	—
antepartum - *see* Hypertension, complicating pregnancy, childbirth, or the puerperium			
cardiorenal (disease)	404.00	404.10	404.90
with			
chronic kidney disease	—	—	—
stage I through stage IV, or unspecified	404.00	404.10	404.90
and heart failure	404.01	404.11	404.91
stage V or end stage renal disease	404.02	404.12	404.92
and heart failure	404.03	404.13	404.93
heart failure	404.01	404.11	404.91
and chronic kidney disease	404.01	404.11	404.91
stage I through stage IV or unspecified	404.01	404.11	404.91
stage V or end stage renal disease	404.03	404.13	404.93
cardiovascular disease (arteriosclerotic) (sclerotic)	402.00	402.10	402.90
with			
heart failure	402.01	402.11	402.91
renal involvement (conditions classifiable to 403) (*see also* Hypertension, cardiorenal)	404.00	404.10	404.90
cardiovascular renal (disease) (sclerosis) (*see also* Hypertension, cardiorenal)	404.00	404.10	404.90
cerebrovascular disease NEC	437.2	437.2	437.2
complicating pregnancy, childbirth, or the puerperium	642.2●	642.0●	642.9●
with			
albuminuria (and edema) (mild)	—	—	642.4●
severe	—	—	642.5●
chronic kidney disease	642.2●	642.2●	642.2●
and heart disease	642.2●	642.2●	642.2●
edema (mild)	—	—	642.4●
severe	—	—	642.5●
heart disease	642.2●	642.2●	642.2●
and chronic kidney disease	642.2●	642.2●	642.2●
renal disease	642.2●	642.2●	642.2●
and heart disease	642.2●	642.2●	642.2●

◄ New   ◄▥ Revised   ~~deleted~~ Deleted   ● Use Additional Digit(s)   ▨ Omit code

	Malignant	Benign	Unspecified
Hypertension, hypertensive *(Continued)*			
complicating pregnancy, childbirth, or the puerperium *(Continued)*			
chronic	642.2●	642.0●	642.0●
with pre-eclampsia or eclampsia	642.7●	642.7●	642.7●
fetus or newborn	760.0	760.0	760.0
essential	—	642.0●	642.0●
with pre-eclampsia or eclampsia	—	642.7●	642.7●
fetus or newborn	760.0	760.0	760.0
fetus or newborn	760.0	760.0	760.0
gestational	—	—	642.3●
pre-existing	642.2●	642.0●	642.0●
with pre-eclampsia or eclampsia	642.7●	642.7●	642.7●
fetus or newborn	760.0	760.0	760.0
secondary to renal disease	642.1●	642.1●	642.1●
with pre-eclampsia or eclampsia	642.7●	642.7●	642.7●
fetus or newborn	760.0	760.0	760.0
transient	—	—	642.3●
due to			
aldosteronism, primary	405.09	405.19	405.99
brain tumor	405.09	405.19	405.99
bulbar poliomyelitis	405.09	405.19	405.99
calculus			
kidney	405.09	405.19	405.99
ureter	405.09	405.19	405.99
coarctation, aorta	405.09	405.19	405.99
Cushing's disease	405.09	405.19	405.99
glomerulosclerosis (*see also* Hypertension, kidney)	403.00	403.10	403.90
periarteritis nodosa	405.09	405.19	405.99
pheochromocytoma	405.09	405.19	405.99
polycystic kidney(s)	405.09	405.19	405.99
polycythemia	405.09	405.19	405.99
porphyria	405.09	405.19	405.99
pyelonephritis	405.09	405.19	405.99
renal (artery)			
aneurysm	405.01	405.11	405.91
anomaly	405.01	405.11	405.91
embolism	405.01	405.11	405.91
fibromuscular hyperplasia	405.01	405.11	405.91
occlusion	405.01	405.11	405.91
stenosis	405.01	405.11	405.91
thrombosis	405.01	405.11	405.91
encephalopathy	437.2	437.2	437.2
gestational (transient) NEC	—	—	642.3●
Goldblatt's	440.1	440.1	440.1

◀ New   ◀▥ Revised   ~~deleted~~ Deleted   ● Use Additional Digit(s)   ▨ Omit code

	Malignant	Benign	Unspecified
Hypertension, hypertensive *(Continued)*			
heart (disease) (conditions classifiable to 429.0–429.3, 429.8, 429.9 due to hypertension)	402.00	402.10	402.90
with			
heart failure	402.01	402.11	402.91
hypertensive kidney disease (conditions classifiable to 403) (*see also* Hypertension, cardiorenal)	404.00	404.10	404.90
renal sclerosis (*see also* Hypertension, cardiorenal)	404.00	404.10	404.90
intracranial, benign	—	348.2	—
intraocular	—	—	365.04
kidney	403.00	403.10	403.90
with			
chronic kidney disease	—	—	—
stage I through stage IV, or unspecified	403.00	403.10	403.90
stage V or end stage renal disease	403.01	403.11	403.91
heart involvement (conditions classifiable to 429.0–429.3, 429.8, 429.9 due to hypertension) (*see also* Hypertension, cardiorenal)	404.00	404.10	404.90
hypertensive heart (disease) (conditions classifiable to 402) (*see also* Hypertension, cardiorenal)	404.00	404.10	404.90
lesser circulation	—	—	416.0
necrotizing	401.0	—	—
pancreatic duct - *code to* underlying condition			
with			
chronic pancreatitis	—	—	577.11
ocular			365.04
portal (due to chronic liver disease)	—	—	572.3
postoperative			997.91
psychogenic	—	—	306.2
puerperal, postpartum - *see* Hypertension, complicating pregnancy, childbirth, or the puerperium			
pulmonary (artery)	—	—	416.8
with cor pulmonale (chronic)	—	—	416.8
acute	—	—	415.0
idiopathic	—	—	416.0
primary	—	—	416.0
of newborn	—	—	747.83
secondary	—	—	416.8
renal (disease) (*see also* Hypertension, kidney)	403.00	403.10	403.90
renovascular NEC	405.01	405.11	405.91

◀ New   ◀▥ Revised   ~~deleted~~ Deleted   ● Use Additional Digit(s)   ▥ Omit code

	Malignant	Benign	Unspecified
Hypertension, hypertensive *(Continued)*			
secondary NEC	405.09	405.19	405.99
due to			
aldosteronism, primary	405.09	405.19	405.99
brain tumor	405.09	405.19	405.99
bulbar poliomyelitis	405.09	405.19	405.99
calculus			
kidney	405.09	405.19	405.99
ureter	405.09	405.19	405.99
coarctation, aorta	405.09	405.19	405.99
Cushing's disease	405.09	405.19	405.99
glomerulosclerosis (*see also* Hypertension, kidney)	403.00	403.10	403.90
periarteritis nodosa	405.09	405.19	405.99
pheochromocytoma	405.09	405.19	405.99
polycystic kidney(s)	405.09	405.19	405.99
polycythemia	405.09	405.19	405.99
porphyria	405.09	405.19	405.99
pyelonephritis	405.09	405.19	405.99
renal (artery)			
aneurysm	405.01	405.11	405.91
anomaly	405.01	405.11	405.91
embolism	405.01	405.11	405.91
fibromuscular hyperplasia	405.01	405.11	405.91
occlusion	405.01	405.11	405.91
stenosis	405.01	405.11	405.91
thrombosis	405.01	405.11	405.91
transient	—	—	796.2
of pregnancy	—	—	642.3●
venous, chronic (asymptomatic) (idiopathic)	—	—	459.30
with			
complication, NEC	—	—	459.39
inflammation	—	—	459.32
with ulcer	—	—	459.33
ulcer	—	—	459.31
with inflammation	—	—	459.33
due to			
deep vein thrombosis (*see also* Syndrome, postphlebitic)	—	—	459.10

Hyperthecosis, ovary 256.8
Hyperthermia (of unknown origin) (see also Pyrexia) 780.60
    malignant (due to anesthesia) 995.86
    newborn 778.4
Hyperthymergasia (see also Psychosis, affective) 296.0●
    reactive (from emotional stress, psychological trauma) 298.1
    recurrent episode 296.1●
    single episode 296.0●
Hyperthymism 254.8
Hyperthyroid (recurrent) - see Hyperthyroidism
Hyperthyroidism (latent) (preadult) (recurrent) (without goiter) 242.9●

> Note 43   Use the following fifth-digit subclassification with category 242:
>
> 0   without mention of thyrotoxic crisis or storm
> 1   with mention of thyrotoxic crisis or storm

    with
        goiter (diffuse) 242.0●
            adenomatous 242.3●
                multinodular 242.2●
                uninodular 242.1●
            nodular 242.3●
                multinodular 242.2●
                uninodular 242.1●
            thyroid nodule 242.1●
        complicating pregnancy, childbirth, or puerperium 648.1●
        neonatal (transient) 775.3
Hypertonia - see Hypertonicity
Hypertonicity
    bladder 596.51
    fetus or newborn 779.89
    gastrointestinal (tract) 536.8
    infancy 779.89
        due to electrolyte imbalance 779.89
    muscle 728.85
    stomach 536.8
        psychogenic 306.4
    uterus, uterine (contractions) 661.4●
        affecting fetus or newborn 763.7
Hypertony - see Hypertonicity
Hypertransaminemia 790.4
Hypertrichosis 704.1
    congenital 757.4
    eyelid 374.54
    lanuginosa 757.4
        acquired 704.1
Hypertriglyceridemia, essential 272.1
Hypertrophy, hypertrophic
    adenoids (infectional) 474.12
        and tonsils (faucial) (infective) (lingual) (lymphoid) 474.10
    adrenal 255.8
    alveolar process or ridge 525.8
    anal papillae 569.49
    apocrine gland 705.82
    artery NEC 447.8
        carotid 447.8
        congenital (peripheral) NEC 747.60
            gastrointestinal 747.61
            lower limb 747.64
            renal 747.62
            specified NEC 747.69
            spinal 747.82
            upper limb 747.63
        renal 447.3

Hypertrophy, hypertrophic (Continued)
    arthritis (chronic) (see also Osteoarthrosis) 715.9●
        spine (see also Spondylosis) 721.90
    arytenoid 478.79
    asymmetrical (heart) 429.9
    auricular - see Hypertrophy, cardiac
    Bartholin's gland 624.8
    bile duct 576.8
    bladder (sphincter) (trigone) 596.8
    blind spot, visual field 368.42
    bone 733.99
    brain 348.89
    breast 611.1
        cystic 610.1
        fetus or newborn 778.7
        fibrocystic 610.1
        massive pubertal 611.1
        puerperal, postpartum 676.3●
        senile (parenchymatous) 611.1
    cardiac (chronic) (idiopathic) 429.3
        with
            rheumatic fever (conditions classifiable to 390)
                active 391.8
                    with chorea 392.0
                inactive or quiescent (with chorea) 398.99
        congenital NEC 746.89
        fatty (see also Degeneration, myocardial) 429.1
        hypertensive (see also Hypertension, heart) 402.90
        rheumatic (with chorea) 398.99
            active or acute 391.8
                with chorea 392.0
        valve (see also Endocarditis) 424.90
            congenital NEC 746.89
    cartilage 733.99
    cecum 569.89
    cervix (uteri) 622.6
        congenital 752.49
        elongation 622.6
    clitoris (cirrhotic) 624.2
        congenital 752.49
    colon 569.89
        congenital 751.3
    conjunctiva, lymphoid 372.73
    cornea 371.89
    corpora cavernosa 607.89
    duodenum 537.89
    endometrium (uterus) (see also Hyperplasia, endometrium) 621.30
        cervix 622.6
    epididymis 608.89
    esophageal hiatus (congenital) 756.6
        with hernia - see Hernia, diaphragm
    eyelid 374.30
    falx, skull 733.99
    fat pad 729.30
        infrapatellar 729.31
        knee 729.31
        orbital 374.34
        popliteal 729.31
        prepatellar 729.31
        retropatellar 729.31
        specified site NEC 729.39
    foot (congenital) 755.67
    frenum, frenulum (tongue) 529.8
        linguae 529.8
        lip 528.5
    gallbladder or cystic duct 575.8

Hypertrophy, hypertrophic (Continued)
    gastric mucosa 535.2●
    gingiva 523.8
    gland, glandular (general) NEC 785.6
    gum (mucous membrane) 523.8
    heart (idiopathic) - see also Hypertrophy, cardiac
        valve - see also Endocarditis
            congenital NEC 746.89
    hemifacial 754.0
    hepatic - see Hypertrophy, liver
    hiatus (esophageal) 756.6
    hilus gland 785.6
    hymen, congenital 752.49
    ileum 569.89
    infrapatellar fat pad 729.31
    intestine 569.89
    jejunum 569.89
    kidney (compensatory) 593.1
        congenital 753.3
    labial frenulum 528.5
    labium (majus) (minus) 624.3
    lacrimal gland, chronic 375.03
    ligament 728.9
        spinal 724.8
    linguae frenulum 529.8
    lingual tonsil (infectional) 474.11
    lip (frenum) 528.5
        congenital 744.81
    liver 789.1
        acute 573.8
        cirrhotic - see Cirrhosis, liver
        congenital 751.69
        fatty - see Fatty, liver
    lymph gland 785.6
        tuberculous - see Tuberculosis, lymph gland
    mammary gland - see Hypertrophy, breast
    maxillary frenulum 528.5
    Meckel's diverticulum (congenital) 751.0
    medial meniscus, acquired 717.3
    median bar 600.90
        with
            other lower urinary tract symptoms (LUTS) 600.91
            urinary
                obstruction 600.91
                retention 600.91
    mediastinum 519.3
    meibomian gland 373.2
    meniscus, knee, congenital 755.64
    metatarsal head 733.99
    metatarsus 733.99
    mouth 528.9
    mucous membrane
        alveolar process 523.8
        nose 478.19
        turbinate (nasal) 478.0
    muscle 728.9
    muscular coat, artery NEC 447.8
        carotid 447.8
        renal 447.3
    myocardium (see also Hypertrophy, cardiac) 429.3
        idiopathic 425.4
    myometrium 621.2
    nail 703.8
        congenital 757.5
    nasal 478.19
        alae 478.19
        bone 738.0
        cartilage 478.19

◄ New   ◄▥ Revised   ~~deleted~~ Deleted   ● Use Additional Digit(s)   ▨ Omit code

Hypertrophy, hypertrophic *(Continued)*
  nasal *(Continued)*
    mucous membrane (septum)
      478.19
    sinus *(see also* Sinusitis) 473.9
    turbinate 478.0
  nasopharynx, lymphoid (infectional)
    (tissue) (wall) 478.29
  neck, uterus 622.6
  nipple 611.1
  normal aperture diaphragm
    (congenital) 756.6
  nose *(see also* Hypertrophy, nasal)
    478.19
  orbit 376.46
  organ or site, congenital NEC - *see*
    Anomaly, specified type NEC
  osteoarthropathy (pulmonary) 731.2
  ovary 620.8
  palate (hard) 526.89
    soft 528.9
  pancreas (congenital) 751.7
  papillae
    anal 569.49
    tongue 529.3
  parathyroid (gland) 252.01
  parotid gland 527.1
  penis 607.89
  phallus 607.89
    female (clitoris) 624.2
  pharyngeal tonsil 474.12
  pharyngitis 472.1
  pharynx 478.29
    lymphoid (infectional) (tissue) (wall)
      478.29
  pituitary (fossa) (gland) 253.8
  popliteal fat pad 729.31
  preauricular (lymph) gland
    (Hampstead) 785.6
  prepuce (congenital) 605
    female 624.2
  prostate (asymptomatic) (early)
    (recurrent) 600.90
    with
      other lower urinary tract
        symptoms (LUTS) 600.91
      urinary
        obstruction 600.91
        retention 600.91
    adenofibromatous 600.20
      with
        other lower urinary tract
          symptoms (LUTS)
          600.21
        urinary
          obstruction 600.21
          retention 600.21
    benign 600.00
      with
        other lower urinary tract
          symptoms (LUTS)
          600.01
        urinary
          obstruction 600.01
          retention 600.01
    congenital 752.89
  pseudoedematous hypodermal 757.0
  pseudomuscular 359.1
  pylorus (muscle) (sphincter) 537.0
    congenital 750.5
    infantile 750.5
  rectal sphincter 569.49
  rectum 569.49
  renal 593.1

Hypertrophy, hypertrophic *(Continued)*
  rhinitis (turbinate) 472.0
  salivary duct or gland 527.1
    congenital 750.26
  scaphoid (tarsal) 733.99
  scar 701.4
  scrotum 608.89
  sella turcica 253.8
  seminal vesicle 608.89
  sigmoid 569.89
  skin condition NEC 701.9
  spermatic cord 608.89
  spinal ligament 724.8
  spleen - *see* Splenomegaly
  spondylitis (spine) *(see also*
    Spondylosis) 721.90
  stomach 537.89
  subaortic stenosis (idiopathic) 425.1
  sublingual gland 527.1
    congenital 750.26
  submaxillary gland 527.1
  suprarenal (gland) 255.8
  tendon 727.9
  testis 608.89
    congenital 752.89
  thymic, thymus (congenital) (gland)
    254.0
  thyroid (gland) *(see also* Goiter) 240.9
    primary 242.0●
    secondary 242.2●
  toe (congenital) 755.65
    acquired 735.8
  tongue 529.8
    congenital 750.15
    frenum 529.8
    papillae (foliate) 529.3
  tonsil (faucial) (infective) (lingual)
    (lymphoid) 474.11
    with
      adenoiditis 474.01
      tonsillitis 474.00
        and adenoiditis 474.02
    and adenoids 474.10
  tunica vaginalis 608.89
  turbinate (mucous membrane) 478.0
  ureter 593.89
  urethra 599.84
  uterus 621.2
    puerperal, postpartum 674.8●
  uvula 528.9
  vagina 623.8
  vas deferens 608.89
  vein 459.89
  ventricle, ventricular (heart) (left)
    (right) - *see also* Hypertrophy,
    cardiac
    congenital 746.89
    due to hypertension (left) (right) *(see
      also* Hypertension, heart)
      402.90
      benign 402.10
      malignant 402.00
    right with ventricular septal defect,
      pulmonary stenosis or atresia,
      and dextraposition of aorta
      745.2
  verumontanum 599.89
  vesical 596.8
  vocal cord 478.5
  vulva 624.3
    stasis (nonfilarial) 624.3
Hypertropia (intermittent) (periodic)
  378.31
Hypertyrosinemia 270.2

Hyperuricemia 790.6
Hypervalinemia 270.3
Hyperventilation (tetany) 786.01
  hysterical 300.11
  psychogenic 306.1
  syndrome 306.1
Hyperviscidosis 277.00
Hyperviscosity (of serum) (syndrome)
  NEC 273.3
  polycythemic 289.0
  sclerocythemic 282.8
Hypervitaminosis (dietary) NEC 278.8
  A (dietary) 278.2
  D (dietary) 278.4
  from excessive administration or use of
    vitamin preparations (chronic)
    278.8
    reaction to sudden overdose 963.5
  vitamin A 278.2
    reaction to sudden overdose 963.5
  vitamin D 278.4
    reaction to sudden overdose 963.5
  vitamin K
    correct substance properly
      administered 278.8
    overdose or wrong substance
      given or taken 964.3
Hypervolemia 276.6
Hypesthesia *(see also* Disturbance,
  sensation) 782.0
  cornea 371.81
Hyphema (anterior chamber) (ciliary
  body) (iris) 364.41
  traumatic 921.3
Hyphemia - *see* Hyphema
Hypoacidity, gastric 536.8
  psychogenic 306.4
Hypoactive labyrinth (function) - *see*
  Hypofunction, labyrinth
Hypoadrenalism 255.41
  tuberculous *(see also* Tuberculosis)
    017.6●
Hypoadrenocorticism 255.41
  pituitary 253.4
Hypoalbuminemia 273.8
Hypoaldosteronism 255.42
Hypoalphalipoproteinemia 272.5
Hypobarism 993.2
Hypobaropathy 993.2
Hypobetalipoproteinemia (familial) 272.5
Hypocalcemia 275.41
  cow's milk 775.4
  dietary 269.3
  neonatal 775.4
  phosphate-loading 775.4
Hypocalcification, teeth 520.4
Hypochloremia 276.9
Hypochlorhydria 536.8
  neurotic 306.4
  psychogenic 306.4
Hypocholesteremia 272.5
Hypochondria (reaction) 300.7
Hypochondriac 300.7
Hypochondriasis 300.7
Hypochromasia blood cells 280.9
Hypochromic anemia 280.9
  due to blood loss (chronic) 280.0
    acute 285.1
  microcytic 280.9
Hypocoagulability *(see also* Defect,
  coagulation) 286.9
Hypocomplementemia 279.8
Hypocythemia (progressive) 284.9
Hypodontia *(see also* Anodontia) 520.0

Hypoeosinophilia 288.59
Hypoesthesia (see also Disturbance, sensation) 782.0
   cornea 371.81
   tactile 782.0
Hypoestrinism 256.39
Hypoestrogenism 256.39
Hypoferremia 280.9
   due to blood loss (chronic) 280.0
Hypofertility
   female 628.9
   male 606.1
Hypofibrinogenemia 286.3
   acquired 286.6
   congenital 286.3
Hypofunction
   adrenal (gland) 255.41
      cortex 255.41
      medulla 255.5
      specified NEC 255.5
   cerebral 331.9
   corticoadrenal NEC 255.41
   intestinal 564.89
   labyrinth (unilateral) 386.53
      with loss of labyrinthine reactivity 386.55
      bilateral 386.54
         with loss of labyrinthine reactivity 386.56
   Leydig cell 257.2
   ovary 256.39
      postablative 256.2
   pituitary (anterior) (gland) (lobe) 253.2
      posterior 253.5
   testicular 257.2
      iatrogenic 257.1
      postablative 257.1
      postirradiation 257.1
      postsurgical 257.1
Hypogammaglobulinemia 279.00
   acquired primary 279.06
   non-sex-linked, congenital 279.06
   sporadic 279.06
   transient of infancy 279.09
Hypogenitalism (congenital) (female) (male) 752.89
   penis 752.69
Hypoglycemia (spontaneous) 251.2
   coma 251.0
      diabetic 250.3●
         due to secondary diabetes 249.3●
      diabetic 250.8●
         due to secondary diabetes 249.8●
      due to insulin 251.0
         therapeutic misadventure 962.3
   familial (idiopathic) 251.2
   following gastrointestinal surgery 579.3
   infantile (idiopathic) 251.2
   in infant of diabetic mother 775.0
   leucine-induced 270.3
   neonatal 775.6
   reactive 251.2
   specified NEC 251.1
Hypoglycemic shock 251.0
   diabetic 250.8●
      due to secondary diabetes 249.8●
   due to insulin 251.0
   functional (syndrome) 251.1

Hypogonadism
   female 256.39
   gonadotrophic (isolated) 253.4
   hypogonadotropic (isolated) (with anosmia) 253.4
   isolated 253.4
   male 257.2
      hereditary familial (Reifenstein's syndrome) 259.52
   ovarian (primary) 256.39
   pituitary (secondary) 253.4
   testicular (primary) (secondary) 257.2
Hypohidrosis 705.0
Hypohidrotic ectodermal dysplasia 757.31
Hypoidrosis 705.0
Hypoinsulinemia, postsurgical 251.3
   postpancreatectomy (complete) (partial) 251.3
Hypokalemia 276.8
Hypokinesia 780.99
Hypoleukia splenica 289.4
Hypoleukocytosis 288.50
Hypolipidemia 272.5
Hypolipoproteinemia 272.5
Hypomagnesemia 275.2
   neonatal 775.4
Hypomania, hypomanic reaction (see also Psychosis, affective) 296.0●
   recurrent episode 296.1●
   single episode 296.0●
Hypomastia (congenital) 611.82
Hypomenorrhea 626.1
Hypometabolism 783.9
Hypomotility
   gastrointestinal tract 536.8
      psychogenic 306.4
   intestine 564.89
      psychogenic 306.4
   stomach 536.8
      psychogenic 306.4
Hyponasality 784.44 ◀▥
Hyponatremia 276.1
Hypo-ovarianism 256.39
Hypo-ovarism 256.39
Hypoparathyroidism (idiopathic) (surgically induced) 252.1
   neonatal 775.4
Hypopharyngitis 462
Hypophoria 378.40
Hypophosphatasia 275.3
Hypophosphatemia (acquired) (congenital) (familial) 275.3
   renal 275.3
Hypophyseal, hypophysis - see also condition
   dwarfism 253.3
   gigantism 253.0
   syndrome 253.8
Hypophyseothalamic syndrome 253.8
Hypopiesis - see Hypotension
Hypopigmentation 709.00
   eyelid 374.53
Hypopinealism 259.8
Hypopituitarism (juvenile) (syndrome) 253.2
   due to
      hormone therapy 253.7
      hypophysectomy 253.7
      radiotherapy 253.7
   postablative 253.7
   postpartum hemorrhage 253.2

Hypoplasia, hypoplasis 759.89
   adrenal (gland) 759.1
   alimentary tract 751.8
      lower 751.2
      upper 750.8
   anus, anal (canal) 751.2
   aorta 747.22
   aortic
      arch (tubular) 747.10
      orifice or valve with hypoplasia of ascending aorta and defective development of left ventricle (with mitral valve atresia) 746.7
   appendix 751.2
   areola 757.6
   arm (see also Absence, arm, congenital) 755.20
   artery (congenital) (peripheral) 747.60
      brain 747.81
      cerebral 747.81
      coronary 746.85
      gastrointestinal 747.61
      lower limb 747.64
      pulmonary 747.3
      renal 747.62
      retinal 743.58
      specified NEC 747.69
      spinal 747.82
      umbilical 747.5
      upper limb 747.63
   auditory canal 744.29
      causing impairment of hearing 744.02
   biliary duct (common) or passage 751.61
   bladder 753.8
   bone NEC 756.9
      face 756.0
      malar 756.0
      mandible 524.04
         alveolar 524.74
      marrow 284.9
         acquired (secondary) 284.89
         congenital 284.09
         idiopathic 284.9
      maxilla 524.03
         alveolar 524.73
      skull (see also Hypoplasia, skull) 756.0
   brain 742.1
      gyri 742.2
      specified part 742.2
   breast (areola) 611.82
   bronchus (tree) 748.3
   cardiac 746.89
      valve - see Hypoplasia, heart, valve
      vein 746.89
   carpus (see also Absence, carpal, congenital) 755.28
   cartilaginous 756.9
   cecum 751.2
   cementum 520.4
      hereditary 520.5
   cephalic 742.1
   cerebellum 742.2
   cervix (uteri) 752.49
   chin 524.06
   clavicle 755.51
   coccyx 756.19
   colon 751.2
   corpus callosum 742.2
   cricoid cartilage 748.3
   dermal, focal (Goltz) 757.39

◀ New   ◀▥ Revised   ~~deleted~~ Deleted   ● Use Additional Digit(s)   ▨ Omit code

Hypoplasia, hypoplasis *(Continued)*
  digestive organ(s) or tract NEC 751.8
    lower 751.2
    upper 750.8
  ear 744.29
    auricle 744.23
    lobe 744.29
    middle, except ossicles 744.03
      ossicles 744.04
    ossicles 744.04
  enamel of teeth (neonatal) (postnatal)
      (prenatal) 520.4
    hereditary 520.5
  endocrine (gland) NEC 759.2
  endometrium 621.8
  epididymis 752.89
  epiglottis 748.3
  erythroid, congenital 284.01
  erythropoietic, chronic acquired 284.81
  esophagus 750.3
  Eustachian tube 744.24
  eye *(see also* Microphthalmos) 743.10
    lid 743.62
  face 744.89
    bone(s) 756.0
  fallopian tube 752.19
  femur *(see also* Absence, femur,
      congenital) 755.34
  fibula *(see also* Absence, fibula,
      congenital) 755.37
  finger *(see also* Absence, finger,
      congenital) 755.29
  focal dermal 757.39
  foot 755.31
  gallbladder 751.69
  genitalia, genital organ(s)
    female 752.89
      external 752.49
      internal NEC 752.89
    in adiposogenital dystrophy 253.8
    male 752.89
      penis 752.69
  glottis 748.3
  hair 757.4
  hand 755.21
  heart 746.89
    left (complex) (syndrome) 746.7
    valve NEC 746.89
      pulmonary 746.01
  humerus *(see also* Absence, humerus,
      congenital) 755.24
  hymen 752.49
  intestine (small) 751.1
    large 751.2
  iris 743.46
  jaw 524.09
  kidney(s) 753.0
  labium (majus) (minus) 752.49
  labyrinth, membranous 744.05
  lacrimal duct (apparatus) 743.65
  larynx 748.3
  leg *(see also* Absence, limb, congenital,
      lower) 755.30
  limb 755.4
    lower *(see also* Absence, limb,
        congenital, lower) 755.30
    upper *(see also* Absence, limb,
        congenital, upper) 755.20
  liver 751.69
  lung (lobe) 748.5
  mammary (areolar) 611.82
  mandibular 524.04
    alveolar 524.74
    unilateral condylar 526.89

Hypoplasia, hypoplasis *(Continued)*
  maxillary 524.03
    alveolar 524.73
  medullary 284.9
  megakaryocytic 287.30
  metacarpus *(see also* Absence,
      metacarpal, congenital) 755.28
  metatarsus *(see also* Absence,
      metatarsal, congenital) 755.38
  muscle 756.89
    eye 743.69
  myocardium (congenital) (Uhl's
      anomaly) 746.84
  nail(s) 757.5
  nasolacrimal duct 743.65
  nervous system NEC 742.8
  neural 742.8
  nose, nasal 748.1
  ophthalmic *(see also* Microphthalmos)
      743.10
  optic nerve 377.43
  organ
    of Corti 744.05
    or site NEC - *see* Anomaly, by site
  osseous meatus (ear) 744.03
  ovary 752.0
  oviduct 752.19
  pancreas 751.7
  parathyroid (gland) 759.2
  parotid gland 750.26
  patella 755.64
  pelvis, pelvic girdle 755.69
  penis 752.69
  peripheral vascular system (congenital)
      NEC 747.60
    gastrointestinal 747.61
    lower limb 747.64
    renal 747.62
    specified NEC 747.69
    spinal 747.82
    upper limb 747.63
  pituitary (gland) 759.2
  pulmonary 748.5
    arteriovenous 747.3
    artery 747.3
    valve 746.01
  punctum lacrimale 743.65
  radioulnar *(see also* Absence, radius,
      congenital, with ulna) 755.25
  radius *(see also* Absence, radius,
      congenital) 755.26
  rectum 751.2
  respiratory system NEC 748.9
  rib 756.3
  sacrum 756.19
  scapula 755.59
  shoulder girdle 755.59
  skin 757.39
  skull (bone) 756.0
    with
      anencephalus 740.0
      encephalocele 742.0
      hydrocephalus 742.3
        with spina bifida *(see also*
            Spina bifida) 741.0●
      microcephalus 742.1
  spinal (cord) (ventral horn cell) 742.59
    vessel 747.82
  spine 756.19
  spleen 759.0
  sternum 756.3
  tarsus *(see also* Absence, tarsal,
      congenital) 755.38
  testis, testicle 752.89

Hypoplasia, hypoplasis *(Continued)*
  thymus (gland) 279.11
  thyroid (gland) 243
    cartilage 748.3
  tibiofibular *(see also* Absence, tibia,
      congenital, with fibula) 755.35
  toe *(see also* Absence, toe, congenital)
      755.39
  tongue 750.16
  trachea (cartilage) (rings) 748.3
  Turner's (tooth) 520.4
  ulna *(see also* Absence, ulna, congenital)
      755.27
  umbilical artery 747.5
  ureter 753.29
  uterus 752.3
  vagina 752.49
  vascular (peripheral) NEC *(see also*
      Hypoplasia, peripheral vascular
      system) 747.60
    brain 747.81
  vein(s) (peripheral) NEC *(see also*
      Hypoplasia, peripheral vascular
      system) 747.60
    brain 747.81
    cardiac 746.89
    great 747.49
    portal 747.49
    pulmonary 747.49
  vena cava (inferior) (superior) 747.49
  vertebra 756.19
  vulva 752.49
  zonule (ciliary) 743.39
  zygoma 738.12
Hypopotassemia 276.8
Hypoproaccelerinemia *(see also* Defect,
    coagulation) 286.3
Hypoproconvertinemia (congenital) *(see
    also* Defect, coagulation) 286.3
Hypoproteinemia (essential)
    (hypermetabolic) (idiopathic) 273.8
Hypoproteinosis 260
Hypoprothrombinemia (congenital)
    (hereditary) (idiopathic) *(see also*
    Defect, coagulation) 286.3
  acquired 286.7
  newborn 776.3
Hypopselaphesia 782.0
Hypopyon (anterior chamber) (eye)
    364.05
  iritis 364.05
  ulcer (cornea) 370.04
Hypopyrexia 780.99
Hyporeflex 796.1
Hyporeninemia, extreme 790.99
  in primary aldosteronism 255.10
Hyporesponsive episode 780.09
Hyposecretion
  ACTH 253.4
  ovary 256.39
    postablative 256.2
  salivary gland (any) 527.7
Hyposegmentation of neutrophils,
    hereditary 288.2
Hyposiderinemia 280.9
Hyposmolality 276.1
  syndrome 276.1
Hyposomatotropism 253.3
Hyposomnia, unspecified *(see also*
    Insomnia) 780.52
  with sleep apnea, unspecified 780.51
Hypospadias (male) 752.61
  female 753.8
Hypospermatogenesis 606.1

Hyposphagma 372.72
Hyposplenism 289.59
Hypostasis, pulmonary 514
Hypostatic - *see* condition
Hyposthenuria 593.89
Hyposuprarenalism 255.41
Hypo-TBG-nemia 246.8
Hypotension (arterial) (constitutional)
458.9
  chronic 458.1
  iatrogenic 458.29
  maternal, syndrome (following labor
    and delivery) 669.2 ●
  of hemodialysis 458.21
  orthostatic (chronic) 458.0
    dysautonomic-dyskinetic syndrome
      333.0
  permanent idiopathic 458.1
  postoperative 458.29
  postural 458.0
  specified type NEC 458.8
  transient 796.3
Hypothermia (accidental) 991.6
  anesthetic 995.89
  associated with low environmental
    temperature 991.6
  newborn NEC 778.3
  not associated with low environmental
    temperature 780.65
Hypothymergasia (*see also* Psychosis,
    affective) 296.2 ●
  recurrent episode 296.3 ●
  single episode 296.2 ●
Hypothyroidism (acquired) 244.9
  complicating pregnancy, childbirth, or
    puerperium 648.1 ●
  congenital 243
  due to
    ablation 244.1
      radioactive iodine 244.1
      surgical 244.0
    iodine (administration) (ingestion)
      244.2
      radioactive 244.1

Hypothyroidism (*Continued*)
  due to (*Continued*)
    irradiation therapy 244.1
    p-aminosalicylic acid (PAS) 244.3
    phenylbutazone 244.3
    resorcinol 244.3
    specified cause NEC 244.8
    surgery 244.0
  goitrous (sporadic) 246.1
  iatrogenic NEC 244.3
  iodine 244.2
  pituitary 244.8
  postablative NEC 244.1
  postsurgical 244.0
  primary 244.9
  secondary NEC 244.8
  specified cause NEC 244.8
  sporadic goitrous 246.1
Hypotonia, hypotonicity, hypotony
    781.3
  benign congenital 358.8
  bladder 596.4
  congenital 779.89
    benign 358.8
  eye 360.30
    due to
      fistula 360.32
      ocular disorder NEC 360.33
    following loss of aqueous or
      vitreous 360.33
    primary 360.31
  infantile muscular (benign) 359.0
  muscle 728.9
  uterus, uterine (contractions) - *see*
    Inertia, uterus
Hypotrichosis 704.09
  congenital 757.4
  lid (congenital) 757.4
    acquired 374.55
  postinfectional NEC 704.09
Hypotropia 378.32
Hypoventilation 786.09
  congenital central alveolar syndrome
    327.25

Hypoventilation (*Continued*)
  idiopathic sleep related nonobstructive
    alveolar 327.24
  sleep related, in conditions classifiable
    elsewhere 327.26
Hypovitaminosis (*see also* Deficiency,
    vitamin) 269.2
Hypovolemia 276.52
  surgical shock 998.0
  traumatic (shock) 958.4
Hypoxemia (*see also* Anoxia) 799.02
  sleep related, in conditions classifiable
    elsewhere 327.26
Hypoxia (*see also* Anoxia) 799.02
  cerebral 348.1
    during or resulting from a
      procedure 997.01
    newborn 770.88
      mild or moderate 768.6
      severe 768.5
  fetal, affecting newborn 770.88
  intrauterine - *see* Distress, fetal
  myocardial (*see also* Insufficiency,
      coronary) 411.89
    arteriosclerotic - *see* Arteriosclerosis,
      coronary
  newborn 770.88
  sleep related 327.24
Hypoxic-ischemic encephalopathy
    (HIE) 768.70   ◀▥
  mild 768.71   ◀
  moderate 768.72   ◀
  severe 768.73   ◀
Hypsarrhythmia (*see also* Epilepsy)
    345.6 ●
Hysteralgia, pregnant uterus 646.8 ●
Hysteria, hysterical 300.10
  anxiety 300.20
  Charcôt's gland 300.11
  conversion (any manifestation)
    300.11
  dissociative type NEC 300.15
  psychosis, acute 298.1
Hysteroepilepsy 300.11
Hysterotomy, affecting fetus or newborn
    763.89

◀ New   ◀▥ Revised   ~~deleted~~ Deleted   ● Use Additional Digit(s)   ▩ Omit code

I

Iatrogenic syndrome of excess cortisol 255.0
IBM (inclusion body myositis) 359.71 ◀
Iceland disease (epidemic neuromyasthenia) 049.8
Ichthyosis (congenita) 757.1
  acquired 701.1
  fetalis gravior 757.1
  follicularis 757.1
  hystrix 757.39
  lamellar 757.1
  lingual 528.6
  palmaris and plantaris 757.39
  simplex 757.1
  vera 757.1
  vulgaris 757.1
Ichthyotoxism 988.0
  bacterial (see also Poisoning, food) 005.9
Icteroanemia, hemolytic (acquired) 283.9
  congenital (see also Spherocytosis) 282.0
Icterus (see also Jaundice) 782.4
  catarrhal - see Icterus, infectious
  conjunctiva 782.4
    newborn 774.6
  epidemic - see Icterus, infectious
  febrilis - see Icterus, infectious
  fetus or newborn - see Jaundice, fetus or newborn
  gravis (see also Necrosis, liver) 570
    complicating pregnancy 646.7●
      affecting fetus or newborn 760.8
    fetus or newborn NEC 773.0
    obstetrical 646.7●
      affecting fetus or newborn 760.8
  hematogenous (acquired) 283.9
  hemolytic (acquired) 283.9
    congenital (see also Spherocytosis) 282.0
  hemorrhagic (acute) 100.0
    leptospiral 100.0
    newborn 776.0
    spirochetal 100.0
  infectious 070.1
    with hepatic coma 070.0
    leptospiral 100.0
    spirochetal 100.0
  intermittens juvenilis 277.4
  malignant (see also Necrosis, liver) 570
  neonatorum (see also Jaundice, fetus or newborn) 774.6
  pernicious (see also Necrosis, liver) 570
  spirochetal 100.0
Ictus solaris, solis 992.0
Id reaction (due to bacteria) 692.89
Ideation
  suicidal V62.84
Identity disorder 313.82
  dissociative 300.14
  gender role (child) 302.6
    adult 302.85
  psychosexual (child) 302.6
    adult 302.85
Idioglossia 307.9
Idiopathic - see condition
Idiosyncrasy (see also Allergy) 995.3
  drug, medicinal substance, and biological - see Allergy, drug
Idiot, idiocy (congenital) 318.2
  amaurotic (Bielschowsky) (-Jansky) (family) (infantile (late)) (juvenile (late)) (Vogt-Spielmeyer) 330.1
  microcephalic 742.1
  Mongolian 758.0
  oxycephalic 756.0

IEED (involuntary emotional expression disorder) 310.8
IFIS (intraoperative floppy iris syndrome) 364.81
IgE asthma 493.0●
Ileitis (chronic) (see also Enteritis) 558.9
  infectious 009.0
  noninfectious 558.9
  regional (ulcerative) 555.0
    with large intestine 555.2
  segmental 555.0
    with large intestine 555.2
  terminal (ulcerative) 555.0
    with large intestine 555.2
Ileocolitis (see also Enteritis) 558.9
  infectious 009.0
  regional 555.2
  ulcerative 556.1
Ileostomy status V44.2
  with complication 569.60
Ileotyphus 002.0
Ileum - see condition
Ileus (adynamic) (bowel) (colon) (inhibitory) (intestine) (neurogenic) (paralytic) 560.1
  arteriomesenteric duodenal 537.2
  due to gallstone (in intestine) 560.31
  duodenal, chronic 537.2
  following gastrointestinal surgery 997.4
  gallstone 560.31
  mechanical (see also Obstruction, intestine) 560.9
  meconium 777.1
    due to cystic fibrosis 277.01
  myxedema 564.89
  postoperative 997.4
  transitory, newborn 777.4
Iliac - see condition
Iliotibial band friction syndrome 728.89
Ill, louping 063.1
Illegitimacy V61.6
Illness - see also Disease
  factitious 300.19
    with
      combined psychological and physical signs and symptoms 300.19
      physical symptoms 300.19
      predominantly
        physical signs and symptoms 300.19
        psychological symptoms 300.16
    chronic (with physical symptoms) 301.51
  heart - see Disease, heart
  manic-depressive (see also Psychosis, affective) 296.80
  mental (see also Disorder, mental) 300.9
Imbalance 781.2
  autonomic (see also Neuropathy, peripheral, autonomic) 337.9
  electrolyte 276.9
    with
      abortion - see Abortion, by type, with metabolic disorder
      ectopic pregnancy (see also categories 633.0–633.9) 639.4
      hyperemesis gravidarum (before 22 completed weeks' gestation) 643.1●
      molar pregnancy (see also categories 630–632) 639.4

Imbalance (Continued)
  electrolyte (Continued)
    following
      abortion 639.4
      ectopic or molar pregnancy 639.4
    neonatal, transitory NEC 775.5
  endocrine 259.9
  eye muscle NEC 378.9
    heterophoria - see Heterophoria
  glomerulotubular NEC 593.89
  hormone 259.9
  hysterical (see also Hysteria) 300.10
  labyrinth NEC 386.50
  posture 729.90
  sympathetic (see also Neuropathy, peripheral, autonomic) 337.9
Imbecile, imbecility 318.0
  moral 301.7
  old age 290.9
  senile 290.9
  specified IQ - see IQ
  unspecified IQ 318.0
Imbedding, intrauterine device 996.32
Imbibition, cholesterol (gallbladder) 575.6
Imerslund (-Gräsbeck) syndrome (anemia due to familial selective vitamin B_{12} malabsorption) 281.1
Iminoacidopathy 270.8
Iminoglycinuria, familial 270.8
Immature - see also Immaturity
  personality 301.89
Immaturity 765.1●
  extreme 765.0●
  fetus or infant light-for-dates - see Light-for-dates
  lung, fetus or newborn 770.4
  organ or site NEC - see Hypoplasia
  pulmonary, fetus or newborn 770.4
  reaction 301.89
  sexual (female) (male) 259.0
Immersion 994.1
  foot 991.4
  hand 991.4
Immobile, immobility
  complete
    due to severe physical disability or frality 780.72
  intestine 564.89
  joint - see Ankylosis
  syndrome (paraplegic) 728.3
Immunization
  ABO
    affecting management of pregnancy 656.2●
    fetus or newborn 773.1
  complication - see Complications, vaccination
  Rh factor
    affecting management of pregnancy 656.1●
    fetus or newborn 773.0
    from transfusion 999.7
Immunodeficiency 279.3
  with
    adenosine-deaminase deficiency 279.2
    defect, predominant
      B-cell 279.00
      T-cell 279.10
    hyperimmunoglobulinemia 279.2
    lymphopenia, hereditary 279.2
    thrombocytopenia and eczema 279.12

Immunodeficiency *(Continued)*
  with *(Continued)*
    thymic
      aplasia 279.2
      dysplasia 279.2
    autosomal recessive, Swiss-type 279.2
    common variable 279.06
    severe combined (SCID) 279.2
    to Rh factor
      affecting management of pregnancy 656.1●
      fetus or newborn 773.0
    X-linked, with increased IgM 279.05
Immunotherapy, prophylactic V07.2
  antineoplastic V58.12
Impaction, impacted
  bowel, colon, rectum 560.30
    with hernia - *see also* Hernia, by site, with, obstruction
      gangrenous - *see* Hernia, by site, with gangrene
    by
      calculus 560.39
      gallstone 560.31
    fecal 560.39
    specified type NEC 560.39
  calculus - *see* Calculus
  cerumen (ear) (external) 380.4
  cuspid 520.6
  dental 520.6
  fecal, feces 560.39
    with hernia - *see also* Hernia, by site, with obstruction
      gangrenous - *see* Hernia, by site, with gangrene
  fracture - *see* Fracture, by site
  gallbladder - *see* Cholelithiasis
  gallstone(s) - *see* Cholelithiasis
    in intestine (any part) 560.31
  intestine(s) 560.30
    with hernia - *see also* Hernia, by site, with obstruction
      gangrenous - *see* Hernia, by site, with gangrene
    by
      calculus 560.39
      gallstone 560.31
    fecal 560.39
    specified type NEC 560.39
  intrauterine device (IUD) 996.32
  molar 520.6
  shoulder 660.4●
    affecting fetus or newborn 763.1
  tooth, teeth 520.6
  turbinate 733.99
Impaired, impairment (function)
  arm V49.1
    movement, involving
      musculoskeletal system V49.1
      nervous system V49.2
  auditory discrimination 388.43
  back V48.3
  body (entire) V49.89
  cognitive, mild, so stated 331.83
  combined visual hearing V49.85
  dual sensory V49.85
  glucose
    fasting 790.21
    tolerance test (oral) 790.22
  hearing (*see also* Deafness) 389.9
    combined with visual impairment V49.85
  heart - *see* Disease, heart

Impaired, impairment *(Continued)*
  kidney (*see also* Disease, renal) 593.9
    disorder resulting from 588.9
      specified NEC 588.89
  leg V49.1
    movement, involving
      musculoskeletal system V49.1
      nervous system V49.2
  limb V49.1
    movement, involving
      musculoskeletal system V49.1
      nervous system V49.2
  liver 573.8
  mastication 524.9
  mild cognitive, so stated 331.83
  mobility
    ear ossicles NEC 385.22
    incostapedial joint 385.22
    malleus 385.21
  myocardium, myocardial (*see also* Insufficiency, myocardial) 428.0
  neuromusculoskeletal NEC V49.89
    back V48.3
    head V48.2
    limb V49.2
    neck V48.3
    spine V48.3
    trunk V48.3
  rectal sphincter 787.99
  renal (*see also* Disease, renal) 593.9
    disorder resulting from 588.9
      specified NEC 588.89
  spine V48.3
  vision NEC 369.9
    both eyes NEC 369.3
    combined with hearing impairment V49.85
    moderate 369.74
      both eyes 369.25
        with impairment of lesser eye (specified as)
          blind, not further specified 369.15
          low vision, not further specified 369.23
          near-total 369.17
          profound 369.18
          severe 369.24
          total 369.16
      one eye 369.74
        with vision of other eye (specified as)
          near-normal 369.75
          normal 369.76
    near-total 369.64
      both eyes 369.04
        with impairment of lesser eye (specified as)
          blind, not further specified 369.02
          total 369.03
      one eye 369.64
        with vision of other eye (specified as)
          near-normal 369.65
          normal 369.66
    one eye 369.60
      with low vision of other eye 369.10

Impaired, impairment *(Continued)*
  vision NEC *(Continued)*
    profound 369.67
      both eyes 369.08
        with impairment of lesser eye (specified as)
          blind, not further specified 369.05
          near-total 369.07
          total 369.06
      one eye 369.67
        with vision of other eye (specified as)
          near-normal 369.68
          normal 369.69
    severe 369.71
      both eyes 369.22
        with impairment of lesser eye (specified as)
          blind, not further specified 369.11
          low vision, not further specified 369.21
          near-total 369.13
          profound 369.14
          total 369.12
      one eye 369.71
        with vision of other eye (specified as)
          near-normal 369.72
          normal 369.73
    total
      both eyes 369.01
      one eye 369.61
        with vision of other eye (specified as)
          near-normal 369.62
          normal 369.63
Impaludism - *see* Malaria
Impediment, speech NEC 784.59 ◀▥
  psychogenic 307.9
  secondary to organic lesion 784.59 ◀▥
Impending
  cerebrovascular accident or attack 435.9
  coronary syndrome 411.1
  delirium tremens 291.0
  myocardial infarction 411.1
Imperception, auditory (acquired) (congenital) 389.9
Imperfect
  aeration, lung (newborn) 770.5
  closure (congenital)
    alimentary tract NEC 751.8
      lower 751.5
      upper 750.8
    atrioventricular ostium 745.69
    atrium (secundum) 745.5
      primum 745.61
    branchial cleft or sinus 744.41
    choroid 743.59
    cricoid cartilage 748.3
    cusps, heart valve NEC 746.89
      pulmonary 746.09
    ductus
      arteriosus 747.0
      Botalli 747.0
    ear drum 744.29
      causing impairment of hearing 744.03
    endocardial cushion 745.60
    epiglottis 748.3
    esophagus with communication to bronchus or trachea 750.3
    Eustachian valve 746.89

◀ New　◀▥ Revised　~~deleted~~ Deleted　● Use Additional Digit(s)　▦ Omit code

Imperfect *(Continued)*
closure *(Continued)*
eyelid 743.62
face, facial *(see also* Cleft, lip) 749.10
foramen
Botalli 745.5
ovale 745.5
genitalia, genital organ(s) or system
female 752.89
external 752.49
internal NEC 752.89
uterus 752.3
male 752.89
penis 752.69
glottis 748.3
heart valve (cusps) NEC 746.89
interatrial ostium or septum 745.5
interauricular ostium or septum 745.5
interventricular ostium or septum 745.4
iris 743.46
kidney 753.3
larynx 748.3
lens 743.36
lip *(see also* Cleft, lip) 749.10
nasal septum or sinus 748.1
nose 748.1
omphalomesenteric duct 751.0
optic nerve entry 743.57
organ or site NEC - *see* Anomaly, specified type, by site
ostium
interatrial 745.5
interauricular 745.5
interventricular 745.4
palate *(see also* Cleft, palate) 749.00
preauricular sinus 744.46
retina 743.56
roof of orbit 742.0
sclera 743.47
septum
aortic 745.0
aorticopulmonary 745.0
atrial (secundum) 745.5
primum 745.61
between aorta and pulmonary artery 745.0
heart 745.9
interatrial (secundum) 745.5
primum 745.61
interauricular (secundum) 745.5
primum 745.61
interventricular 745.4
with pulmonary stenosis or atresia, dextraposition of aorta, and hypertrophy of right ventricle 745.2
in tetralogy of Fallot 745.2
nasal 748.1
ventricular 745.4
with pulmonary stenosis or atresia, dextraposition of aorta, and hypertrophy of right ventricle 745.2
in tetralogy of Fallot 745.2
skull 756.0
with
anencephalus 740.0
encephalocele 742.0
hydrocephalus 742.3
with spina bifida *(see also* Spina bifida) 741.0 ●
microcephalus 742.1

Imperfect *(Continued)*
closure *(Continued)*
spine (with meningocele) *(see also* Spina bifida) 741.90
thyroid cartilage 748.3
trachea 748.3
tympanic membrane 744.29
causing impairment of hearing 744.03
uterus (with communication to bladder, intestine, or rectum) 752.3
uvula 749.02
with cleft lip *(see also* Cleft, palate, with cleft lip) 749.20
vitelline duct 751.0
development - *see* Anomaly, by site
erection 607.84
fusion - *see* Imperfect, closure
inflation lung (newborn) 770.5
intestinal canal 751.5
poise 729.90
rotation - *see* Malrotation
septum, ventricular 745.4
Imperfectly descended testis 752.51
Imperforate (congenital) - *see also* Atresia
anus 751.2
bile duct 751.61
cervix (uteri) 752.49
esophagus 750.3
hymen 752.42
intestine (small) 751.1
large 751.2
jejunum 751.1
pharynx 750.29
rectum 751.2
salivary duct 750.23
urethra 753.6
urinary meatus 753.6
vagina 752.49
Impervious (congenital) - *see also* Atresia
anus 751.2
bile duct 751.61
esophagus 750.3
intestine (small) 751.1
large 751.5
rectum 751.2
urethra 753.6
Impetiginization of other dermatoses 684
Impetigo (any organism) (any site) (bullous) (circinate) (contagiosa) (neonatorum) (simplex) 684
Bockhart's (superficial folliculitis) 704.8
external ear 684 [380.13]
eyelid 684 [373.5]
Fox's (contagiosa) 684
furfuracea 696.5
herpetiformis 694.3
nonobstetrical 694.3
staphylococcal infection 684
ulcerative 686.8
vulgaris 684
Impingement, soft tissue between teeth 524.89
anterior 524.81
posterior 524.82
Implant, endometrial 617.9
Implantation
anomalous - *see also* Anomaly, specified type, by site
ureter 753.4

Implantation *(Continued)*
cyst
external area or site (skin) NEC 709.8
iris 364.61
vagina 623.8
vulva 624.8
dermoid (cyst)
external area or site (skin) NEC 709.8
iris 364.61
vagina 623.8
vulva 624.8
placenta, low or marginal - *see* Placenta previa
Impotence (sexual) 607.84
organic origin NEC 607.84
psychogenic 302.72
Impoverished blood 285.9
Impression, basilar 756.0
Imprisonment V62.5
Improper
development, infant 764.9 ●
Improperly tied umbilical cord (causing hemorrhage) 772.3
Impulses, obsessional 300.3
Impulsive neurosis 300.3 799.23 ◀||||
neurosis 300.3 ◀
Impulsiveness 799.23 ◀
Inaction, kidney *(see also* Disease, renal) 593.9
Inactive - *see* condition
Inadequate, inadequacy
aesthetics of dental restoration 525.67
biologic 301.6
cardiac and renal - *see* Hypertension, cardiorenal
constitutional 301.6
development
child 783.40
fetus 764.9 ●
affecting management of pregnancy 656.5 ●
genitalia
after puberty NEC 259.0
congenital - *see* Hypoplasia, genitalia
lungs 748.5
organ or site NEC - *see* Hypoplasia, by site
dietary 269.9
distance, interarch 524.28
education V62.3
environment
economic problem V60.2
household condition NEC V60.1
poverty V60.2
unemployment V62.0
functional 301.6
household care, due to
family member
handicapped or ill V60.4
temporarily away from home V60.4
on vacation V60.5
technical defects in home V60.1
temporary absence from home of person rendering care V60.4
housing (heating) (space) V60.1
interarch distance 524.28
material resources V60.2
mental *(see also* Retardation, mental) 319
nervous system 799.29 ◀||||
personality 301.6

Inadequate, inadequacy *(Continued)*
  prenatal care in current pregnancy
      V23.7
  pulmonary
      function 786.09
          newborn 770.89
      ventilation, newborn 770.89
  respiration 786.09
      newborn 770.89
  sample
      cytology
          anal 796.78
          cervical 795.08
          vaginal 795.18
  social 301.6
Inanition 263.9
  with edema 262
  due to
      deprivation of food 994.2
      malnutrition 263.9
  fever 780.60
Inappropriate secretion
  ACTH 255.0
  antidiuretic hormone (ADH)
      (excessive) 253.6
      deficiency 253.5
  ectopic hormone NEC 259.3
  pituitary (posterior) 253.6
Inattention after or at birth 995.52
Inborn errors of metabolism - *see*
      Disorder, metabolism
Incarceration, incarcerated
  bubonocele - *see also* Hernia, inguinal,
      with obstruction
      gangrenous - *see* Hernia, inguinal,
          with gangrene
  colon (by hernia) - *see also* Hernia, by
      site with obstruction
      gangrenous - *see* Hernia, by site,
          with gangrene
  enterocele 552.9
      gangrenous 551.9
  epigastrocele 552.29
      gangrenous 551.29
  epiplocele 552.9
      gangrenous 551.9
  exomphalos 552.1
      gangrenous 551.1
  fallopian tube 620.8
  hernia - *see also* Hernia, by site, with
      obstruction
      gangrenous - *see* Hernia, by site,
          with gangrene
  iris, in wound 871.1
  lens, in wound 871.1
  merocele (*see also* Hernia, femoral, with
      obstruction) 552.00
  omentum (by hernia) - *see also* Hernia,
      by site, with obstruction
      gangrenous - *see* Hernia, by site,
          with gangrene
  omphalocele 756.72   ◀▥
  rupture (meaning hernia) (*see also*
      Hernia, by site, with obstruction)
      552.9
      gangrenous (*see also* Hernia, by site,
          with gangrene) 551.9
  sarcoepiplocele 552.9
      gangrenous 551.9
  sarcoepiplomphalocele 552.1
      with gangrene 551.1
  uterus 621.8
      gravid 654.3●
          causing obstructed labor 660.2●
              affecting fetus or newborn
                  763.1

Incident, cerebrovascular (*see also*
      Disease, cerebrovascular, acute) 436
Incineration (entire body) (from fire,
      conflagration, electricity, or
      lightning) - *see* Burn, multiple,
      specified sites
Incised wound
  external - *see* Wound, open, by site
  internal organs (abdomen, chest, or
      pelvis) - *see* Injury, internal, by
      site, with open wound
Incision, incisional
  hernia - *see* Hernia, incisional
  surgical, complication - *see*
      Complications, surgical
      procedures
  traumatic
      external - *see* Wound, open, by site
      internal organs (abdomen, chest, or
          pelvis) - *see* Injury, internal, by
          site, with open wound
Inclusion
  azurophilic leukocytic 288.2
  blennorrhea (neonatal) (newborn)
      771.6
  cyst - *see* Cyst, skin
  gallbladder in liver (congenital) 751.69
Incompatibility
  ABO
      affecting management of pregnancy
          656.2●
      fetus or newborn 773.1
      infusion or transfusion reaction
          999.6
  blood (group) (Duffy) (E) (K(ell))
      (Kidd) (Lewis) (M) (N) (P) (S)
      NEC
      affecting management of pregnancy
          656.2●
      fetus or newborn 773.2
      infusion or transfusion reaction
          999.89   ◀▥
  contour of existing restoration of
      tooth
      with oral health 525.65
  marital V61.10
      involving
          divorce V61.03
          estrangement V61.09
  Rh (blood group) (factor)
      affecting management of pregnancy
          656.1●
      fetus or newborn 773.0
      infusion or transfusion reaction
          999.7
  Rhesus - *see* Incompatibility, Rh
**Incompetency, incompetence,
      incompetent**
  annular
      aortic (valve) (*see also* Insufficiency,
          aortic) 424.1
      mitral (valve) - (*see also* Insufficiency,
          mitral) 424.0
      pulmonary valve (heart) (*see also*
          Endocarditis, pulmonary)
          424.3
  aortic (valve) (*see also* Insufficiency,
      aortic) 424.1
      syphilitic 093.22
  cardiac (orifice) 530.0
      valve - *see* Endocarditis
  cervix, cervical (os) 622.5
      in pregnancy 654.5●
          affecting fetus or newborn
              761.0

Incompetency, incompetence, incompetent
      (Continued)
  chronotropic 426.89
      with
          autonomic dysfunction 337.9
          ischemic heart disease 414.9
          left ventricular dysfunction
              429.89   ◀▥
          sinus node dysfunction 427.81
  esophagogastric (junction) (sphincter)
      530.0
  heart valve, congenital 746.89
  mitral (valve) - *see* Insufficiency, mitral
  papillary muscle (heart) 429.81
  pelvic fundus
      pubocervical tissue 618.81
      rectovaginal tissue 618.82
  pulmonary valve (heart) (*see also*
      Endocarditis, pulmonary) 424.3
      congenital 746.09
  tricuspid (annular) (rheumatic) (valve)
      (*see also* Endocarditis, tricuspid)
      397.0
  valvular - *see* Endocarditis
  vein, venous (saphenous) (varicose)
      (*see also* Varicose, vein) 454.9
  velopharyngeal (closure)
      acquired 528.9
      congenital 750.29
Incomplete - *see also* condition
  bladder emptying 788.21
  expansion lungs (newborn) 770.5
  gestation (liveborn) - *see* Immaturity
  rotation - *see* Malrotation
Inconclusive   ◀
  image test due to excess body
      fat 793.91   ◀
  mammogram, mammography 793.82 ◀
      due to dense breasts 793.82   ◀
Incontinence 788.30
  without sensory awareness 788.34
  anal sphincter 787.6
  continuous leakage 788.37
  feces 787.6
      due to hysteria 300.11
      nonorganic origin 307.7
  hysterical 300.11
  mixed (male) (female) (urge and stress)
      788.33
  overflow 788.38
  paradoxical 788.39
  rectal 787.6
  specified NEC 788.39
  stress (female) 625.6
      male NEC 788.32
  urethral sphincter 599.84
  urge 788.31
      and stress (male) (female) 788.33
  urine 788.30
      active 788.30
      due to
          cognitive impairment 788.91
          severe physical disability 788.91
          immobility 788.91
      functional 788.91
      male 788.30
          stress 788.32
              and urge 788.33
      neurogenic 788.39
      nonorganic origin 307.6
      stress (female) 625.6
          male NEC 788.32
      urge 788.31
          and stress 788.33
Incontinentia pigmenti 757.33

Incoordinate
  uterus (action) (contractions) 661.4●
    affecting fetus or newborn 763.7
Incoordination
  esophageal-pharyngeal (newborn)
    787.24
  muscular 781.3
  papillary muscle 429.81
Increase, increased
  abnormal, in development 783.9
  androgens (ovarian) 256.1
  anticoagulants (antithrombin) (anti-
    VIIIa) (anti-IXa) (anti-Xa) (anti-
    XIa) 286.5
    postpartum 666.3●
  cold sense (see also Disturbance,
    sensation) 782.0
  estrogen 256.0
  function
    adrenal (cortex) 255.3
      medulla 255.6
    pituitary (anterior) (gland) (lobe)
      253.1
      posterior 253.6
  heat sense (see also Disturbance,
    sensation) 782.0
  intracranial pressure 781.99
    injury at birth 767.8
  light reflex of retina 362.13
  permeability, capillary 448.9
  pressure
    intracranial 781.99
      injury at birth 767.8
    intraocular 365.00
  pulsations 785.9
  pulse pressure 785.9
  sphericity, lens 743.36
  splenic activity 289.4
  venous pressure 459.89
    portal 572.3
Incrustation, cornea, lead, or zinc
  930.0
Incyclophoria 378.44
Incyclotropia 378.33
Indeterminate sex 752.7
India rubber skin 756.83
Indicanuria 270.2
Indigestion (bilious) (functional) 536.8
  acid 536.8
  catarrhal 536.8
  due to decomposed food NEC 005.9
  fat 579.8
  nervous 306.4
  psychogenic 306.4
Indirect - see condition
Indolent bubo NEC 099.8
Induced
  abortion - see Abortion, induced
  birth, affecting fetus or newborn
    763.89
  delivery - see Delivery
  labor - see Delivery
Induration, indurated
  brain 348.89
  breast (fibrous) 611.79
    puerperal, postpartum 676.3●
  broad ligament 620.8
  chancre 091.0
    anus 091.1
    congenital 090.0
    extragenital NEC 091.2
  corpora cavernosa (penis) (plastic)
    607.89
  liver (chronic) 573.8
    acute 573.8

Induration, indurated (Continued)
  lung (black) (brown) (chronic) (fibroid)
    (see also Fibrosis, lung) 515
    essential brown 275.0 [516.1]
  penile 607.89
  phlebitic - see Phlebitis
  skin 782.8
  stomach 537.89
Induratio penis plastica 607.89
Industrial - see condition
Inebriety (see also Abuse, drugs,
  nondependent) 305.0●
Inefficiency
  kidney (see also Disease, renal) 593.9
  thyroid (acquired) (gland) 244.9
Inelasticity, skin 782.8
Inequality, leg (acquired) (length) 736.81
  congenital 755.30
Inertia
  bladder 596.4
    neurogenic 596.54
      with cauda equina syndrome
        344.61
  stomach 536.8
    psychogenic 306.4
  uterus, uterine 661.2●
    affecting fetus or newborn 763.7
    primary 661.0●
    secondary 661.1●
  vesical 596.4
    neurogenic 596.54
      with cauda equina 344.61
Infant - see also condition
  excessive crying of 780.92
  fussy (baby) 780.91
  held for adoption V68.89
  newborn - see Newborn
  post-term (gestation period over 40
    completed weeks to 42 completed
    weeks) 766.21
  prolonged gestation of (period over 42
    completed weeks) 766.22
  syndrome of diabetic mother 775.0
"Infant Hercules" syndrome 255.2
Infantile - see also condition
  genitalia, genitals 259.0
    in pregnancy or childbirth NEC
      654.4●
      affecting fetus or newborn
        763.89
      causing obstructed labor 660.2●
        affecting fetus or newborn
          763.1
  heart 746.9
  kidney 753.3
  lack of care 995.52
  macula degeneration 362.75
  melanodontia 521.05
  os, uterus (see also Infantile, genitalia)
    259.0
  pelvis 738.6
    with disproportion (fetopelvic)
      653.1●
      affecting fetus or newborn 763.1
      causing obstructed labor 660.1●
        affecting fetus or newborn
          763.1
  penis 259.0
  testis 257.2
  uterus (see also Infantile, genitalia) 259.0
  vulva 752.49
Infantilism 259.9
  with dwarfism (hypophyseal) 253.3
  Brissaud's (infantile myxedema) 244.9
  celiac 579.0

Infantilism (Continued)
  Herter's (nontropical sprue)
    579.0
  hypophyseal 253.3
  hypothalamic (with obesity) 253.8
  idiopathic 259.9
  intestinal 579.0
  pancreatic 577.8
  pituitary 253.3
  renal 588.0
  sexual (with obesity) 259.0
Infants, healthy liveborn - see Newborn
Infarct, infarction
  adrenal (capsule) (gland) 255.41
  amnion 658.8●
  anterior (with contiguous portion of
    intraventricular septum) NEC
    (see also Infarct, myocardium)
    410.1●
  appendices epiploicae 557.0
  bowel 557.0
  brain (stem) 434.91
    embolic (see also Embolism, brain)
      434.11
    healed or old without residuals
      V12.54
    iatrogenic 997.02
    lacunar 434.91
    late effect - see Late effect(s) (of)
      cerebrovascular disease
    postoperative 997.02
    puerperal, postpartum, childbirth
      674.0●
    thrombotic (see also Thrombosis,
      brain) 434.01
  breast 611.89
  Brewer's (kidney) 593.81
  cardiac (see also Infarct, myocardium)
    410.9●
  cerebellar (see also Infarct, brain)
    434.91
    embolic (see also Embolism, brain)
      434.11
  cerebral (see also Infarct, brain)
    434.91
    aborted 434.91
    embolic (see also Embolism, brain)
      434.11
    thrombotic (see also Infarct, brain)
      434.01
  chorion 658.8●
  colon (acute) (agnogenic) (embolic)
    (hemorrhagic) (nonocclusive)
    (nonthrombotic) (occlusive)
    (segmental) (thrombotic) (with
    gangrene) 557.0
  coronary artery (see also Infarct,
    myocardium) 410.9●
  cortical 434.91
  embolic (see also Embolism) 444.9
  fallopian tube 620.8
  gallbladder 575.8
  heart (see also Infarct, myocardium)
    410.9●
  hepatic 573.4
  hypophysis (anterior lobe) 253.8
  impending (myocardium) 411.1
  intestine (acute) (agnogenic) (embolic)
    (hemorrhagic) (nonocclusive)
    (nonthrombotic) (occlusive)
    (thrombotic) (with gangrene)
    557.0
  kidney 593.81
  lacunar 434.91
  liver 573.4

Infarct, infarction (Continued)
  lung (embolic) (thrombotic) 415.19
    with
      abortion - see Abortion, by type,
        with, embolism
      ectopic pregnancy (see also
        categories 633.0–633.9) 639.6
      molar pregnancy (see also
        categories 630–632) 639.6
    following
      abortion 639.6
      ectopic or molar pregnancy 639.6
    iatrogenic 415.11
    in pregnancy, childbirth, or
      puerperium - see Embolism,
      obstetrical
    postoperative 415.11
    septic 415.12
  lymph node or vessel 457.8
  medullary (brain) - see Infarct, brain
  meibomian gland (eyelid) 374.85
  mesentery, mesenteric (embolic)
    (thrombotic) (with gangrene)
    557.0
  midbrain - see Infarct, brain
  myocardium, myocardial (acute or
    with a stated duration of 8 weeks
    or less) (with hypertension)
    410.9●

> Note 44 Use the following fifth-digit
> subclassification with category 410:
>
> 0 episode unspecified
> 1 initial episode
> 2 subsequent episode without
>   recurrence

    with symptoms after 8 weeks from
      date of infarction 414.8
    anterior (wall) (with contiguous
      portion of intraventricular
      septum) NEC 410.1●
    anteroapical (with contiguous
      portion of intraventricular
      septum) 410.1●
    anterolateral (wall) 410.0●
    anteroseptal (with contiguous
      portion of intraventricular
      septum) 410.1●
    apical-lateral 410.5●
    atrial 410.8●
    basal-lateral 410.5●
    chronic (with symptoms after 8
      weeks from date of infarction)
      414.8
    diagnosed on ECG, but presenting
      no symptoms 412
    diaphragmatic wall (with
      contiguous portion of
      intraventricular septum)
      410.4●
    healed or old, currently presenting
      no symptoms 412
    high lateral 410.5●
    impending 411.1
    inferior (wall) (with contiguous
      portion of intraventricular
      septum) 410.4●
    inferolateral (wall) 410.2●
    inferoposterior wall 410.3●
    intraoperative 997.1
    lateral wall 410.5●
    non-Q wave 410.7●

Infarct, infarction (Continued)
  myocardium, myocardial (Continued)
    non-ST elevation (NSTEMI) 410.7●
    nontransmural 410.7●
    papillary muscle 410.8●
    past (diagnosed on ECG or other
      special investigation, but
      currently presenting no
      symptoms) 412
      with symptoms NEC 414.8
    posterior (strictly) (true) (wall)
      410.6●
    posterobasal 410.6●
    posteroinferior 410.3●
    posterolateral 410.5●
    postprocedural 997.1
    previous, currently presenting no
      symptoms 412
    Q wave (see also Infarct,
      myocardium, by site) 410.9●
    septal 410.8●
    specified site NEC 410.8●
    ST elevation (STEMI) 410.9●
      anterior (wall) 410.1●
      anterolateral (wall) 410.0●
      inferior (wall) 410.4●
      inferolateral (wall) 410.2●
      inferoposterior wall 410.3●
      lateral wall 410.5●
      posterior (strictly) (true) (wall)
        410.6●
      specified site NEC 410.8●
    subendocardial 410.7●
    syphilitic 093.82
  non-ST elevation myocardial infarction
    (NSTEMI) 410.7●
  nontransmural 410.7●
  omentum 557.0
  ovary 620.8
  pancreas 577.8
  papillary muscle (see also Infarct,
    myocardium) 410.8●
  parathyroid gland 252.8
  pituitary (gland) 253.8
  placenta (complicating pregnancy)
    656.7●
    affecting fetus or newborn 762.2
  pontine - see Infarct, brain
  posterior NEC (see also Infarct,
    myocardium) 410.6●
  prostate 602.8
  pulmonary (artery) (hemorrhagic)
    (vein) 415.19
    with
      abortion - see Abortion, by type,
        with embolism
      ectopic pregnancy (see also
        categories 633.0–633.9)
        639.6
      molar pregnancy (see also
        categories 630–632) 639.6
    following
      abortion 639.6
      ectopic or molar pregnancy 639.6
    iatrogenic 415.11
    in pregnancy, childbirth, or
      puerperium - see Embolism,
      obstetrical
    postoperative 415.11
    septic 415.12
  renal 593.81
    embolic or thrombotic 593.81
  retina, retinal 362.84
    with occlusion - see Occlusion, retina

Infarct, infarction (Continued)
  spinal (acute) (cord) (embolic)
    (nonembolic) 336.1
  spleen 289.59
    embolic or thrombotic 444.89
  subchorionic - see Infarct, placenta
  subendocardial (see also Infarct,
    myocardium) 410.7●
  suprarenal (capsule) (gland) 255.41
  syncytium - see Infarct, placenta
  testis 608.83
  thrombotic (see also Thrombosis)
    453.9
    artery, arterial - see Embolism
  thyroid (gland) 246.3
  ventricle (heart) (see also Infarct,
    myocardium) 410.9●
Infecting - see condition
Infection, infected, infective
    (opportunistic) 136.9
  with lymphangitis - see Lymphangitis
  abortion - see Abortion, by type, with,
    sepsis
  abscess (skin) - see Abscess, by site
  Absidia 117.7
  acanthamoeba 136.21
  Acanthocheilonema (perstans) 125.4
    streptocerca 125.6
  accessory sinus (chronic) (see also
    Sinusitis) 473.9
  Achorion - see Dermatophytosis
  Acremonium falciforme 117.4
  acromioclavicular (joint) 711.91
  Actinobacillus
    lignieresii 027.8
    mallei 024
    muris 026.1
  Actinomadura - see Actinomycosis
  Actinomyces (israelii) - see also
    Actinomycosis
    muris-ratti 026.1
  Actinomycetales (Actinomadura)
    (Actinomyces) (Nocardia)
    (Streptomyces) - see
    Actinomycosis
  actinomycotic NEC (see also
    Actinomycosis) 039.9
  adenoid (chronic) 474.01
    acute 463
    and tonsil (chronic) 474.02
    acute or subacute 463
  adenovirus NEC 079.0
    in diseases classified elsewhere - see
      category 079
    unspecified nature or site 079.0
  Aerobacter aerogenes NEC 041.85
    enteritis 008.2
  Aerogenes capsulatus (see also
    Gangrene, gas) 040.0
  aertrycke (see also Infection,
    Salmonella) 003.9
  Ajellomyces dermatitidis 116.0
  alimentary canal NEC (see also
    Enteritis, due to, by organism)
    009.0
  Allescheria boydii 117.6
  Alternaria 118
  alveolus, alveolar (process) (pulpal
    origin) 522.4
  ameba, amebic (histolytica) (see also
    Amebiasis) 006.9
    acute 006.0
    chronic 006.1
    free-living 136.29

◄ New   ◄▥ Revised   deleted Deleted   ● Use Additional Digit(s)   ▥ Omit code

Infection, infected, infective *(Continued)*
  ameba, amebic *(Continued)*
    hartmanni 007.8
    specified
      site NEC 006.8
      type NEC 007.8
  amniotic fluid or cavity 658.4●
    affecting fetus or newborn 762.7
  anaerobes (cocci) (gram-negative)
    (gram-positive) (mixed) NEC
    041.84
  anal canal 569.49
  Ancylostoma braziliense 126.2
  Angiostrongylus cantonensis 128.8
  anisakiasis 127.1
  Anisakis larva 127.1
  anthrax *(see also* Anthrax) 022.9
  antrum (chronic) *(see also* Sinusitis,
    maxillary) 473.0
  anus (papillae) (sphincter) 569.49
  arbor virus NEC 066.9
  arbovirus NEC 066.9
  argentophil-rod 027.0
  Ascaris lumbricoides 127.0
  ascomycetes 117.4
  Aspergillus (flavus) (fumigatus)
    (terreus) 117.3
  atypical
    acid-fast (bacilli) *(see also*
      Mycobacterium, atypical)
      031.9
    mycobacteria *(see also*
      Mycobacterium, atypical)
      031.9
  auditory meatus (circumscribed)
    (diffuse) (external) *(see also* Otitis,
    externa) 380.10
  auricle (ear) *(see also* Otitis, externa)
    380.10
  axillary gland 683
  Babesiasis 088.82
  Babesiosis 088.82
  Bacillus NEC 041.89
    abortus 023.1
    anthracis *(see also* Anthrax) 022.9
    cereus (food poisoning) 005.89
    coli - *see* Infection, Escherichia coli
    coliform NEC 041.85
    Ducrey's (any location) 099.0
    Flexner's 004.1
    Friedländer's NEC 041.3
    fusiformis 101
    gas (gangrene) *(see also* Gangrene,
      gas) 040.0
    mallei 024
    melitensis 023.0
    paratyphoid, paratyphosus 002.9
      A 002.1
      B 002.2
      C 002.3
    Schmorl's 040.3
    Shiga 004.0
    suipestifer *(see also* Infection,
      Salmonella) 003.9
    swimming pool 031.1
    typhosa 002.0
    welchii *(see also* Gangrene, gas)
      040.0
    Whitmore's 025
  bacterial NEC 041.9
    specified NEC 041.89
      anaerobic NEC 041.84
      gram-negative NEC 041.85
        anaerobic NEC 041.84

Infection, infected, infective *(Continued)*
  Bacterium
    paratyphosum 002.9
      A 002.1
      B 002.2
      C 002.3
    typhosum 002.9
  Bacteroides (fragilis) (melaninogenicus)
    (oralis) NEC 041.82
  Balantidium coli 007.0
  Bartholin's gland 616.89
  Basidiobolus 117.7
  Bedsonia 079.98
    specified NEC 079.88
  bile duct 576.1
  bladder *(see also* Cystitis) 595.9
  Blastomyces, blastomycotic 116.0
    brasiliensis 116.1
    dermatitidis 116.0
    European 117.5
    loboi 116.2
    North American 116.0
    South American 116.1
  bleb
    postprocedural 379.60
      stage 1 379.61
      stage 2 379.62
      stage 3 379.63
  blood stream - *see also* Septicemia
    catheter-related (CRBSI) 999.31
  bone 730.9●
    specified - *see* Osteomyelitis
  Bordetella 033.9
    bronchiseptica 033.8
    parapertussis 033.1
    pertussis 033.0
  Borrelia
    bergdorfi 088.81
    vincentii (mouth) (pharynx) (tonsil)
      101
  bovine stomatitis 059.11
  brain *(see also* Encephalitis) 323.9
    late effect - *see* category 326
    membranes - *(see also* Meningitis)
      322.9
    septic 324.0
      late effect - *see* category 326
      meninges *(see also* Meningitis)
        320.9
  branchial cyst 744.42
  breast 611.0
    puerperal, postpartum 675.2●
      with nipple 675.9●
        specified type NEC 675.8●
      nonpurulent 675.2●
      purulent 675.1●
  bronchus *(see also* Bronchitis) 490
    fungus NEC 117.9
  Brucella 023.9
    abortus 023.1
    canis 023.3
    melitensis 023.0
    mixed 023.8
    suis 023.2
  Brugia (Wuchereria) malayi 125.1
  bursa - *see* Bursitis
  buttocks (skin) 686.9
  Candida (albicans) (tropicalis) *(see also*
    Candidiasis) 112.9
    congenital 771.7
  Candiru 136.8
  Capillaria
    hepatica 128.8
    philippinensis 127.5

Infection, infected, infective *(Continued)*
  cartilage 733.99
  cat liver fluke 121.0
  catheter-related bloodstream (CRBSI)
    999.31
  cellulitis - *see* Cellulitis, by site
  Cephalosporum falciforme 117.4
  Cercomonas hominis (intestinal) 007.3
  cerebrospinal *(see also* Meningitis) 322.9
    late effect - *see* category 326
  cervical gland 683
  cervix *(see also* Cervicitis) 616.0
  cesarean section wound 674.3●
  Chilomastix (intestinal) 007.8
  Chlamydia 079.98
    specified NEC 079.88
  Cholera *(see also* Cholera) 001.9
  chorionic plate 658.8●
  Cladosporium
    bantianum 117.8
    carrionii 117.2
    mansoni 111.1
    trichoides 117.8
    wernecki 111.1
  Clonorchis (sinensis) (liver) 121.1
  Clostridium (haemolyticum) (novyi)
    NEC 041.84
    botulinum 005.1
    histolyticum *(see also* Gangrene, gas)
      040.0
    oedematiens *(see also* Gangrene, gas)
      040.0
    perfringens 041.83
      due to food 005.2
    septicum *(see also* Gangrene, gas)
      040.0
    sordellii *(see also* Gangrene, gas)
      040.0
    welchii *(see also* Gangrene, gas)
      040.0
      due to food 005.2
  Coccidioides (immitis) *(see also*
    Coccidioidomycosis) 114.9
  coccus NEC 041.89
  colon *(see also* Enteritis, due to, by
    organism) 009.0
    bacillus - *see* Infection, Escherichia
      coli
  colostomy or enterostomy 569.61
  common duct 576.1
  complicating pregnancy, childbirth, or
    puerperium NEC 647.9●
    affecting fetus or newborn 760.2
  Condiobolus 117.7
  congenital NEC 771.89
    Candida albicans 771.7
    chronic 771.2
    Cytomegalovirus 771.1
    hepatitis, viral 771.2
    herpes simplex 771.2
    listeriosis 771.2
    malaria 771.2
    poliomyelitis 771.2
    rubella 771.0
    toxoplasmosis 771.2
    tuberculosis 771.2
    urinary (tract) 771.82
    vaccinia 771.2
  coronavirus 079.89
    SARS-associated 079.82
  corpus luteum *(see also* Salpingo-
    oophoritis) 614.2
  Corynebacterium diphtheriae - *see*
    Diphtheria

Infection, infected, infective *(Continued)*
  cotia virus 059.8
  Coxsackie *(see also* Coxsackie) 079.2
    endocardium 074.22
    heart NEC 074.20
    in diseases classified elsewhere - *see*
      category 079
    meninges 047.0
    myocardium 074.23
    pericardium 074.21
    pharynx 074.0
    specified disease NEC 074.8
    unspecified nature or site 079.2
  Cryptococcus neoformans 117.5
  Cryptosporidia 007.4
  Cunninghamella 117.7
  cyst - *see* Cyst
  Cysticercus cellulosae 123.1
  cytomegalovirus 078.5
    congenital 771.1
  dental (pulpal origin) 522.4
  deuteromycetes 117.4
  Dicrocoelium dendriticum 121.8
  Dipetalonema (perstans) 125.4
    streptocerca 125.6
  diphtherial - *see* Diphtheria
  Diphyllobothrium (adult) (latum)
    (pacificum) 123.4
    larval 123.5
  Diplogonoporus (grandis) 123.8
  Dipylidium (caninum) 123.8
  Dirofilaria 125.6
  dog tapeworm 123.8
  Dracunculus medinensis 125.7
  Dreschlera 118
    hawaiiensis 117.8
  Ducrey's bacillus (any site) 099.0
  due to or resulting from
    central venous catheter 999.31
    device, implant, or graft (any)
      (presence of) - *see*
      Complications, infection and
      inflammation, due to (presence
      of) any device, implant, or
      graft classified to 996.0–996.5
      NEC
    injection, inoculation, infusion,
      transfusion, or vaccination
      (prophylactic) (therapeutic)
      999.39
    injury NEC - *see* Wound, open, by
      site, complicated
    surgery 998.59
  duodenum 535.6●
  ear - *see also* Otitis
    external *(see also* Otitis, externa)
      380.10
    inner *(see also* Labyrinthitis) 386.30
    middle - *see* Otitis, media
  Eaton's agent NEC 041.81
  Eberthella typhosa 002.0
  Ebola 078.89
  echinococcosis 122.9
  Echinococcus *(see also* Echinococcus)
    122.9
  Echinostoma 121.8
  ECHO virus 079.1
    in diseases classified elsewhere - *see*
      category 079
    unspecified nature or site 079.1
  Ehrlichiosis 082.40
    chaffeensis 082.41
    specified type NEC 082.49
  Endamoeba - *see* Infection, ameba

Infection, infected, infective *(Continued)*
  endocardium *(see also* Endocarditis)
    421.0
  endocervix *(see also* Cervicitis) 616.0
  Entamoeba - *see* Infection, ameba
  enteric *(see also* Enteritis, due to, by
    organism) 009.0
  Enterobacter aerogenes NEC 041.85
  Enterobacter sakazakii 041.85
  Enterobius vermicularis 127.4
  enterococcus NEC 041.04
  enterovirus NEC 079.89
    central nervous system NEC 048
    enteritis 008.67
    meningitis 047.9
  Entomophthora 117.7
  Epidermophyton - *see* Dermatophytosis
  epidermophytosis - *see*
    Dermatophytosis
  episiotomy 674.3●
  Epstein-Barr virus 075
    chronic 780.79 [139.8]
  erysipeloid 027.1
  Erysipelothrix (insidiosa)
    (rhusiopathiae) 027.1
  erythema infectiosum 057.0
  Escherichia coli NEC 041.4
    enteritis - *see* Enteritis, E. coli
    generalized 038.42
    intestinal - *see* Enteritis, E. coli
  esophagostomy 530.86
  ethmoidal (chronic) (sinus) *(see also*
    Sinusitis, ethmoidal) 473.2
  Eubacterium 041.84
  Eustachian tube (ear) 381.50
    acute 381.51
    chronic 381.52
  exanthema subitum *(see also* Exanthem
    subitum) 058.10
  external auditory canal (meatus) *(see
    also* Otitis, externa) 380.10
  eye NEC 360.00
  eyelid 373.9
    specified NEC 373.8
  fallopian tube *(see also* Salpingo-
    oophoritis) 614.2
  fascia 728.89
  Fasciola
    gigantica 121.3
    hepatica 121.3
  Fasciolopsis (buski) 121.4
  fetus (intra-amniotic) - *see* Infection,
    congenital
  filarial - *see* Infestation, filarial
  finger (skin) 686.9
    abscess (with lymphangitis) 681.00
      pulp 681.01
    cellulitis (with lymphangitis)
      681.00
    distal closed space (with
      lymphangitis) 681.00
    nail 681.02
      fungus 110.1
  fish tapeworm 123.4
    larval 123.5
  flagellate, intestinal 007.9
  fluke - *see* Infestation, fluke
  focal
    teeth (pulpal origin) 522.4
    tonsils 474.00
      and adenoids 474.02
  Fonsecaea
    compactum 117.2
    pedrosoi 117.2

Infection, infected, infective *(Continued)*
  food *(see also* Poisoning, food) 005.9
  foot (skin) 686.9
    fungus 110.4
  Francisella tularensis *(see also*
    Tularemia) 021.9
  frontal sinus (chronic) *(see also* Sinusitis,
    frontal) 473.1
  fungus NEC 117.9
    beard 110.0
    body 110.5
    dermatiacious NEC 117.8
    foot 110.4
    groin 110.3
    hand 110.2
    nail 110.1
    pathogenic to compromised host
      only 118
    perianal (area) 110.3
    scalp 110.0
    scrotum 110.8
    skin 111.9
      foot 110.4
      hand 110.2
      toenails 110.1
      trachea 117.9
  Fusarium 118
  Fusobacterium 041.84
  gallbladder *(see also* Cholecystitis,
    acute) 575.0
  Gardnerella vaginalis 041.89
  gas bacillus *(see also* Gas, gangrene)
    040.0
  gastric *(see also* Gastritis) 535.5●
  Gastrodiscoides hominis 121.8
  gastroenteric *(see also* Enteritis, due to,
    by organism) 009.0
  gastrointestinal *(see also* Enteritis, due
    to, by organism) 009.0
  gastrostomy 536.41
  generalized NEC *(see also* Septicemia)
    038.9
  genital organ or tract NEC
    female 614.9
      with
        abortion - *see* Abortion, by
          type, with sepsis
        ectopic pregnancy *(see also*
          categories 633.0–633.9)
          639.0
        molar pregnancy *(see also*
          categories 630–632)
          639.0
      complicating pregnancy 646.6●
        affecting fetus or newborn
          760.8
      following
        abortion 639.0
        ectopic or molar pregnancy
          639.0
      puerperal, postpartum, childbirth
        670.8   ◄▥
        minor or localized 646.6●
          affecting fetus or newborn
            760.8
    male 608.4
  genitourinary tract NEC 599.0
  Ghon tubercle, primary *(see also*
    Tuberculosis) 010.0●
  Giardia lamblia 007.1
  gingival (chronic) 523.10
    acute 523.00
    Vincent's 101
  glanders 024

◄ New   ◄▥ Revised   ~~deleted~~ Deleted   ● Use Additional Digit(s)   ▥ Omit code

Infection, infected, infective *(Continued)*
  Glenosporopsis amazonica 116.2
  Gnathostoma spinigerum 128.1
  Gongylonema 125.6
  gonococcal NEC *(see also* Gonococcus) 098.0
  gram-negative bacilli NEC 041.85
    anaerobic 041.84
  guinea worm 125.7
  gum *(see also* Infection, gingival) 523.10
  Hantavirus 079.81
  heart 429.89
  Helicobactor pylori [H. pylori] 041.86 ◀▦
  helminths NEC 128.9
    intestinal 127.9
      mixed (types classifiable to more than one category in 120.0–127.7) 127.8
      specified type NEC 127.7
    specified type NEC 128.8
  Hemophilus influenzae NEC 041.5
    generalized 038.41
  Herpes (simplex) *(see also* Herpes, simplex) 054.9
    congenital 771.2
    zoster *(see also* Herpes, zoster) 053.9
      eye NEC 053.29
  Heterophyes heterophyes 121.6
  Histoplasma *(see also* Histoplasmosis) 115.90
    capsulatum *(see also* Histoplasmosis, American) 115.00
    duboisii *(see also* Histoplasmosis, African) 115.10
  HIV V08
    with symptoms, symptomatic 042
  hookworm *(see also* Ancylostomiasis) 126.9
  human herpesvirus 6 058.81
  human herpesvirus 7 058.82
  human herpesvirus 8 058.89
  human herpesvirus NEC 058.89
  human immunodeficiency virus V08
    with symptoms, symptomatic 042
  human papillomavirus 079.4
  hydrocele 603.1
  hydronephrosis 591
  Hymenolepis 123.6
  hypopharynx 478.29
  inguinal glands 683
    due to soft chancre 099.0
  intestine, intestinal *(see also* Enteritis, due to, by organism) 009.0
  intrauterine *(see also* Endometritis) 615.9
    complicating delivery 646.6●
  isospora belli or hominis 007.2
  Japanese B encephalitis 062.0
  jaw (bone) (acute) (chronic) (lower) (subacute) (upper) 526.4
  joint - *see* Arthritis, infectious or infective
  Kaposi's sarcoma-associated herpesvirus 058.89
  kidney (cortex) (hematogenous) 590.9
    with
      abortion - *see* Abortion, by type, with urinary tract infection
      calculus 592.0
      ectopic pregnancy *(see also* categories 633.0–633.9) 639.8
      molar pregnancy *(see also* categories 630–632) 639.8

Infection, infected, infective *(Continued)*
  kidney *(Continued)*
    complicating pregnancy or puerperium 646.6●
      affecting fetus or newborn 760.1
    following
      abortion 639.8
      ectopic or molar pregnancy 639.8
    pelvis and ureter 590.3
  Klebsiella pneumoniae NEC 041.3
  knee (skin) NEC 686.9
    joint - *see* Arthritis, infectious
  Koch's *(see also* Tuberculosis, pulmonary) 011.9●
  labia (majora) (minora) *(see also* Vulvitis) 616.10
  lacrimal
    gland *(see also* Dacryoadenitis) 375.00
    passages (duct) (sac) *(see also* Dacryocystitis) 375.30
  larynx NEC 478.79
  leg (skin) NEC 686.9
  Leishmania *(see also* Leishmaniasis) 085.9
    braziliensis 085.5
    donovani 085.0
    Ethiopica 085.3
    furunculosa 085.1
    infantum 085.0
    Mexicana 085.4
    tropica (minor) 085.1
      major 085.2
  Leptosphaeria senegalensis 117.4
  Leptospira *(see also* Leptospirosis) 100.9
    australis 100.89
    bataviae 100.89
    pyrogenes 100.89
    specified type NEC 100.89
  leptospirochetal NEC *(see also* Leptospirosis) 100.9
  Leptothrix - *see* Actinomycosis
  Listeria monocytogenes (listeriosis) 027.0
    congenital 771.2
  liver fluke - *see* Infestation, fluke, liver
  Loa loa 125.2
    eyelid 125.2 [373.6]
  Loboa loboi 116.2
  local, skin (staphylococcal) (streptococcal) NEC 686.9
    abscess - *see* Abscess, by site
    cellulitis - *see* Cellulitis, by site
    ulcer *(see also* Ulcer, skin) 707.9
  Loefflerella
    mallei 024
    whitmori 025
  lung 518.89
    atypical Mycobacterium 031.0
    tuberculous *(see also* Tuberculosis, pulmonary) 011.9●
    basilar 518.89
    chronic 518.89
    fungus NEC 117.9
    spirochetal 104.8
    virus - *see* Pneumonia, virus
  lymph gland (axillary) (cervical) (inguinal) 683
    mesenteric 289.2
  lymphoid tissue, base of tongue or posterior pharynx, NEC 474.00

Infection, infected, infective *(Continued)*
  Madurella
    grisea 117.4
    mycetomii 117.4
  major
    with
      abortion - *see* Abortion, by type, with sepsis
      ectopic pregnancy *(see also* categories 633.0–633.9) 639.0
      molar pregnancy *(see also* categories 630–632) 639.0
    following
      abortion 639.0
      ectopic or molar pregnancy 639.0
    puerperal, postpartum, childbirth 670.0 ◀▦
  malarial - *see* Malaria
  Malassezia furfur 111.0
  Malleomyces
    mallei 024
    pseudomallei 025
  mammary gland 611.0
    puerperal, postpartum 675.2●
  Mansonella (ozzardi) 125.5
  mastoid (suppurative) - *see* Mastoiditis
  maxilla, maxillary 526.4
    sinus (chronic) *(see also* Sinusitis, maxillary) 473.0
  mediastinum 519.2
  medina 125.7
  meibomian
    cyst 373.12
    gland 373.12
  melioidosis 025
  meninges *(see also* Meningitis) 320.9
  meningococcal *(see also* condition) 036.9
    brain 036.1
    cerebrospinal 036.0
    endocardium 036.42
    generalized 036.2
    meninges 036.0
    meningococcemia 036.2
    specified site NEC 036.89
  mesenteric lymph nodes or glands NEC 289.2
  Metagonimus 121.5
  metatarsophalangeal 711.97
  methicillin
    resistant Staphylococcus aureus (MRSA) 041.12
    susceptible Staphylococcus aureus (MSSA) 041.11
  microorganism resistant to drugs - *see* Resistance (to), drugs by microorganisms
  Microsporidia 136.8
  microsporum, microsporic - *see* Dermatophytosis
  mima polymorpha NEC 041.85
  mixed flora NEC 041.89
  Monilia *(see also* Candidiasis) 112.9
    neonatal 771.7
  monkeypox 059.01
  Monosporium apiospermum 117.6
  mouth (focus) NEC 528.9
    parasitic 136.9
  MRSA (methicillin resistant Staphylococcus aureus) 041.12
  MSSA (methicillin susceptible Staphylococcus aureus) 041.11

Infection, infected, infective *(Continued)*
  Mucor 117.7
  muscle NEC 728.89
  mycelium NEC 117.9
  mycetoma
    actinomycotic NEC *(see also*
      Actinomycosis)* 039.9
    mycotic NEC 117.4
  Mycobacterium, mycobacterial *(see also*
    Mycobacterium)* 031.9
  Mycoplasma NEC 041.81
  mycotic NEC 117.9
    pathogenic to compromised host
      only 118
    skin NEC 111.9
    systemic 117.9
  myocardium NEC 422.90
  nail (chronic) (with lymphangitis)
    681.9
    finger 681.02
      fungus 110.1
    ingrowing 703.0
    toe 681.11
      fungus 110.1
  nasal sinus (chronic *(see also* Sinusitis)
    473.9
  nasopharynx (chronic) 478.29
    acute 460
  navel 686.9
    newborn 771.4
  Neisserian - *see* Gonococcus
  Neotestudina rosatii 117.4
  newborn, generalized 771.89
  nipple 611.0
    puerperal, postpartum 675.0●
      with breast 675.9●
        specified type NEC 675.8●
  Nocardia - *see* Actinomycosis
  nose 478.19
  nostril 478.19
  obstetrical surgical wound 674.3●
  Oesophagostomum (apiostomum)
    127.7
  Oestrus ovis 134.0
  Oidium albicans *(see also* Candidiasis)
    112.9
  Onchocerca (volvulus) 125.3
    eye 125.3 *[360.13]*
    eyelid 125.3 *[373.6]*
  operation wound 998.59
  Opisthorchis (felineus) (tenuicollis)
    (viverrini) 121.0
  orbit 376.00
    chronic 376.10
  orthopoxvirus 059.00
    specified NEC 059.09
  ovary *(see also* Salpingo-oophoritis)
    614.2
  Oxyuris vermicularis 127.4
  pancreas 577.0
  Paracoccidioides brasiliensis 116.1
  Paragonimus (westermani) 121.2
  parainfluenza virus 079.89
  parameningococcus NEC 036.9
    with meningitis 036.0
  parapoxvirus 059.10
    specified NEC 059.19
  parasitic NEC 136.9
  paratyphoid 002.9
    type A 002.1
    type B 002.2
    type C 002.3
  paraurethral ducts 597.89
  parotid gland 527.2

Infection, infected, infective *(Continued)*
  Pasteurella NEC 027.2
    multocida (cat-bite) (dog-bite)
      027.2
    pestis *(see also* Plague) 020.9
    pseudotuberculosis 027.2
    septica (cat-bite) (dog-bite) 027.2
    tularensis *(see also* Tularemia) 021.9
  pelvic, female *(see also* Disease, pelvis,
    inflammatory) 614.9
  penis (glans) (retention) NEC 607.2
    herpetic 054.13
  Peptococcus 041.84
  Peptostreptococcus 041.84
  periapical (pulpal origin) 522.4
  peridental 523.30
  perineal wound (obstetrical) 674.3●
  periodontal 523.31
  periorbital 376.00
    chronic 376.10
  perirectal 569.49
  perirenal *(see also* Infection, kidney)
    590.9
  peritoneal *(see also* Peritonitis) 567.9
  periureteral 593.89
  periurethral 597.89
  Petriellidium boydii 117.6
  pharynx 478.29
    Coxsackie virus 074.0
    phlegmonous 462
    posterior, lymphoid 474.00
  Phialophora
    gougerotii 117.8
    jeanselmei 117.8
    verrucosa 117.2
  Piedraia hortai 111.3
  pinna, acute 380.11
  pinta 103.9
    intermediate 103.1
    late 103.2
    mixed 103.3
    primary 103.0
  pinworm 127.4
  pityrosporum furfur 111.0
  pleuropneumonia-like organisms NEC
    (PPLO) 041.81
  pneumococcal NEC 041.2
    generalized (purulent) 038.2
  Pneumococcus NEC 041.2
  postoperative wound 998.59
  posttraumatic NEC 958.3
  postvaccinal 999.39
  poxvirus 059.9
    specified NEC 059.8
  prepuce NEC 607.1
  Proprionibacterium 041.84
  prostate (capsule) *(see also* Prostatitis)
    601.9
  Proteus (mirabilis) (morganii)
    (vulgaris) NEC 041.6
    enteritis 008.3
  protozoal NEC 136.8
    intestinal NEC 007.9
  Pseudomonas NEC 041.7
    mallei 024
    pneumonia 482.1
    pseudomallei 025
  psittacosis 073.9
  puerperal, postpartum (major) 670.0 ◀▦
    minor 646.6●
  pulmonary - *see* Infection, lung
  purulent - *see* Abscess
  putrid, generalized - *see* Septicemia
  pyemic - *see* Septicemia

Infection, infected, infective *(Continued)*
  Pyrenochaeta romeroi 117.4
  Q fever 083.0
  rabies 071
  rectum (sphincter) 569.49
  renal *(see also* Infection, kidney) 590.9
    pelvis and ureter 590.3
  resistant to drugs - *see* Resistance (to),
    drugs by microorganisms
  respiratory 519.8
    chronic 519.8
    influenzal (acute) (upper) 487.1
    lung 518.89
    rhinovirus 460
    syncytial virus 079.6
    upper (acute) (infectious) NEC
      465.9
      with flu, grippe, or influenza
        487.1
      influenzal 487.1
      multiple sites NEC 465.8
      streptococcal 034.0
      viral NEC 465.9
  respiratory syncytial virus (RSV)
    079.6
  resulting from presence of shunt or
    other internal prosthetic device -
    see Complications, infection and
    inflammation, due to (presence
    of) any device, implant, or graft
    classified to 996.0–996.5 NEC
  retroperitoneal 567.39
  retrovirus 079.50
    human immunodeficiency virus
      type 2 [HIV 2] 079.53
    human T-cell lymphotrophic virus
      type I [HTLV-I] 079.51
    human T-cell lymphotrophic virus
      type II [HTLV-II] 079.52
    specified NEC 079.59
  Rhinocladium 117.1
  Rhinosporidium (seeberi) 117.0
  rhinovirus
    in diseases classified elsewhere - *see*
      category 079
    unspecified nature or site 079.3
  Rhizopus 117.7
  rickettsial 083.9
  rickettsialpox 083.2
  rubella *(see also* Rubella) 056.9
    congenital 771.0
  Saccharomyces *(see also* Candidiasis)
    112.9
  Saksenaea 117.7
  salivary duct or gland (any) 527.2
  Salmonella (aertrycke) (callinarum)
    (choleraesuis) (enteritidis)
    (suipestifer) (typhimurium)
    003.9
    with
      arthritis 003.23
      gastroenteritis 003.0
      localized infection 003.20
        specified type NEC 003.29
      meningitis 003.21
      osteomyelitis 003.24
      pneumonia 003.22
      septicemia 003.1
      specified manifestation NEC
        003.8
    due to food (poisoning) (any
      serotype) *(see also* Poisoning,
      food, due to, Salmonella)
    hirschfeldii 002.3

Infection, infected, infective (Continued)
  Salmonella (Continued)
    localized 003.20
      specified type NEC 003.29
    paratyphi 002.9
      A 002.1
      B 002.2
      C 002.3
    schottmuelleri 002.2
    specified type NEC 003.8
    typhi 002.0
    typhosa 002.0
  saprophytic 136.8
  Sarcocystis, lindemanni 136.5
  SARS-associated coronavirus 079.82
  scabies 133.0
  Schistosoma - see Infestation,
      Schistosoma
  Schmorl's bacillus 040.3
  scratch or other superficial injury - see
      Injury, superficial, by site
  scrotum (acute) NEC 608.4
  sealpox 059.12
  secondary, burn or open wound
      (dislocation) (fracture) 958.3
  seminal vesicle (see also Vesiculitis)
      608.0
  septic
    generalized - see Septicemia
    localized, skin (see also Abscess)
      682.9
  septicemic - see Septicemia
  seroma 998.51
  Serratia (marcescens) 041.85
    generalized 038.44
  sheep liver fluke 121.3
  Shigella 004.9
    boydii 004.2
    dysenteriae 004.0
    Flexneri 004.1
    group
      A 004.0
      B 004.1
      C 004.2
      D 004.3
    Schmitz (-Stutzer) 004.0
    Schmitzii 004.0
    Shiga 004.0
    Sonnei 004.3
    specified type NEC 004.8
  Sin Nombre virus 079.81
  sinus (see also Sinusitis) 473.9
    pilonidal 685.1
      with abscess 685.0
    skin NEC 686.9
  Skene's duct or gland (see also
      Urethritis) 597.89
  skin (local) (staphylococcal)
      (streptococcal) NEC 686.9
    abscess - see Abscess, by site
    cellulitis - see Cellulitis, by site
    due to fungus 111.9
      specified type NEC 111.8
    mycotic 111.9
      specified type NEC 111.8
    ulcer (see also Ulcer, skin) 707.9
  slow virus 046.9
    specified condition NEC 046.8
  Sparganum (mansoni) (proliferum)
      123.5
  spermatic cord NEC 608.4
  sphenoidal (chronic) (sinus) (see also
      Sinusitis, sphenoidal) 473.3
  Spherophorus necrophorus 040.3

Infection, infected, infective (Continued)
  spinal cord NEC (see also Encephalitis)
      323.9
    abscess 324.1
      late effect - see category 326
    late effect - see category 326
    meninges - see Meningitis
    streptococcal 320.2
  Spirillum
    minus or minor 026.0
    morsus muris 026.0
    obermeieri 087.0
  spirochetal NEC 104.9
    lung 104.8
    specified nature or site NEC
      104.8
  spleen 289.59
  Sporothrix schenckii 117.1
  Sporotrichum (schenckii) 117.1
  Sporozoa 136.8
  staphylococcal NEC 041.10
    aureus 041.11
      methicillin
        resistant (MRSA) 041.12
        susceptible MSSA) 041.11
    food poisoning 005.0
    generalized (purulent) 038.10
      aureus 038.11
        methicillin
          resistant 038.12
          susceptible 038.11
      specified organism NEC 038.19
    pneumonia 482.40
      aureus 482.41
        methicillin
          resistant (MRSA) 482.42
          susceptible (MSSA)
            482.41
        MRSA (methicillin resistant
          staphylococcus aureus)
          482.42
        MSSA (methicillin susceptible
          staphylococcus aureus)
          482.41
      specified type NEC 482.49
    septicemia 038.10
      aureus 038.11
        methicillin
          resistant (MRSA) 038.12
          susceptible (MSSA) 038.11
        MRSA (methicillin resistant
          staphylococcus aureus)
          038.12
        MSSA (methicillin susceptible
          staphylococcus aureus)
          038.11
      specified organism NEC 038.19
    specified NEC 041.19
  steatoma 706.2
  Stellantchasmus falcatus 121.6
  Streptobacillus moniliformis 026.1
  streptococcal NEC 041.00
    generalized (purulent) 038.0
    group
      A 041.01
      B 041.02
      C 041.03
      D [enterococcus] 041.04
      G 041.05
    pneumonia - see Pneumonia,
      streptococcal
    septicemia 038.0
    sore throat 034.0
    specified NEC 041.09

Infection, infected, infective (Continued)
  Streptomyces - see Actinomycosis
  streptotrichosis - see Actinomycosis
  Strongyloides (stercoralis) 127.2
  stump (amputation) (posttraumatic)
      (surgical) 997.62
    traumatic - see Amputation,
      traumatic, by site, complicated
  subcutaneous tissue, local NEC 686.9
  submaxillary region 528.9
  suipestifer (see also Infection,
      Salmonella) 003.9
  swimming pool bacillus 031.1
  syphilitic - see Syphilis
  systemic - see Septicemia
  Taenia - see Infestation, Taenia
  Taeniarhynchus saginatus 123.2
  tanapox 059.21
  tapeworm - see Infestation, tapeworm
  tendon (sheath) 727.89
  Ternidens diminutus 127.7
  testis (see also Orchitis) 604.90
  thigh (skin) 686.9
  threadworm 127.4
  throat 478.29
    pneumococcal 462
    staphylococcal 462
    streptococcal 034.0
    viral NEC (see also Pharyngitis) 462
  thumb (skin) 686.9
    abscess (with lymphangitis)
      681.00
      pulp 681.01
    cellulitis (with lymphangitis)
      681.00
    nail 681.02
  thyroglossal duct 529.8
  toe (skin) 686.9
    abscess (with lymphangitis)
      681.10
    cellulitis (with lymphangitis)
      681.10
    nail 681.11
      fungus 110.1
  tongue NEC 529.0
    parasitic 112.0
  tonsil (faucial) (lingual) (pharyngeal)
      474.00
    acute or subacute 463
    and adenoid 474.02
    tag 474.00
  tooth, teeth 522.4
    periapical (pulpal origin) 522.4
    peridental 523.30
    periodontal 523.31
    pulp 522.0
    socket 526.5
  TORCH - see Infection, congenital
      NEC
    without active infection 760.2
  Torula histolytica 117.5
  Toxocara (cani) (cati) (felis) 128.0
  Toxoplasma gondii (see also
      Toxoplasmosis) 130.9
  trachea, chronic 491.8
    fungus 117.9
  traumatic NEC 958.3
  trematode NEC 121.9
  trench fever 083.1
  Treponema
    denticola 041.84
    macrodenticum 041.84
    pallidum (see also Syphilis) 097.9
  Trichinella (spiralis) 124

Infection, infected, infective *(Continued)*
  Trichomonas 131.9
    bladder 131.09
    cervix 131.09
    hominis 007.3
    intestine 007.3
    prostate 131.03
    specified site NEC 131.8
    urethra 131.02
    urogenitalis 131.00
    vagina 131.01
    vulva 131.01
  Trichophyton, trichophytid - *see*
    Dermatophytosis
  Trichosporon (beigelii) cutaneum 111.2
  Trichostrongylus 127.6
  Trichuris (trichiuria) 127.3
  Trombicula (irritans) 133.8
  Trypanosoma *(see also*
    Trypanosomiasis) 086.9
    cruzi 086.2
  tubal *(see also* Salpingo-oophoritis)
    614.2
  tuberculous NEC *(see also* Tuberculosis)
    011.9●
  tubo-ovarian *(see also* Salpingo-
    oophoritis) 614.2
  tunica vaginalis 608.4
  tympanic membrane - *see* Myringitis
  typhoid (abortive) (ambulant)
    (bacillus) 002.0
  typhus 081.9
    flea-borne (endemic) 081.0
    louse-borne (epidemic) 080
    mite-borne 081.2
    recrudescent 081.1
    tick-borne 082.9
      African 082.1
      North Asian 082.2
  umbilicus (septic) 686.9
    newborn NEC 771.4
  ureter 593.89
  urethra *(see also* Urethritis) 597.80
  urinary (tract) NEC 599.0
    with
      abortion - *see* Abortion, by type,
        with urinary tract infection
      ectopic pregnancy *(see also*
        categories 633.0–633.9) 639.8
      molar pregnancy *(see also*
        categories 630–632) 639.8
    candidal 112.2
    complicating pregnancy, childbirth,
      or puerperium 646.6●
      affecting fetus or newborn 760.1
      asymptomatic 646.5●
        affecting fetus or newborn
          760.1
    diplococcal (acute) 098.0
      chronic 098.2
    due to Trichomonas (vaginalis)
      131.00
    following
      abortion 639.8
      ectopic or molar pregnancy 639.8
    gonococcal (acute) 098.0
      chronic or duration of 2 months
        or over 098.2
    newborn 771.82
    trichomonal 131.00
    tuberculous *(see also* Tuberculosis)
      016.3●
  uterus, uterine *(see also* Endometritis)
    615.9

Infection, infected, infective *(Continued)*
  utriculus masculinus NEC 597.89
  vaccination 999.39
  vagina (granulation tissue) (wall) *(see*
    also Vaginitis) 616.10
  varicella 052.9
  varicose veins - *see* Varicose, veins
  variola 050.9
    major 050.0
    minor 050.1
  vas deferens NEC 608.4
  Veillonella 041.84
  verumontanum 597.89
  vesical *(see also* Cystitis) 595.9
  Vibrio
    cholerae 001.0
      El Tor 001.1
    parahaemolyticus (food poisoning)
      005.4
    vulnificus 041.85
  Vincent's (gums) (mouth) (tonsil) 101
  virus, viral 079.99
    adenovirus
      in diseases classified elsewhere -
        see category 079
      unspecified nature or site 079.0
    central nervous system NEC 049.9
      enterovirus 048
        meningitis 047.9
          specified type NEC 047.8
      slow virus 046.9
        specified condition NEC 046.8
    chest 519.8
    conjunctivitis 077.99
      specified type NEC 077.89
    coronavirus 079.89
      SARS-associated 079.82
    Coxsackie *(see also* Infection,
      Coxsackie) 079.2
    Ebola 065.8
    ECHO
      in diseases classified elsewhere -
        see category 079
      unspecified nature or site 079.1
    encephalitis 049.9
      arthropod-borne NEC 064
      tick-borne 063.9
        specified type NEC 063.8
    enteritis NEC *(see also* Enteritis,
      viral) 008.8
    exanthem NEC 057.9
    Hantavirus 079.81
    human papilloma 079.4
    in diseases classified elsewhere - *see*
      category 079
    intestine *(see also* Enteritis, viral)
      008.8
    lung - *see* Pneumonia, viral
    respiratory syncytial (RSV) 079.6
    Retrovirus 079.50
    rhinovirus
      in diseases classified elsewhere -
        see category 079
      unspecified nature or site 079.3
    salivary gland disease 078.5
    slow 046.9
      specified condition NEC 046.8
    specified type NEC 079.89
      in diseases classified elsewhere -
        see category 079
    unspecified nature or site 079.99
    warts 078.10
      specified NEC 078.19
    yaba monkey tumor 059.22

Infection, infected, infective *(Continued)*
  vulva *(see also* Vulvitis) 616.10
  whipworm 127.3
  Whitmore's bacillus 025
  wound (local) (posttraumatic) NEC
    958.3
    with
      dislocation - *see* Dislocation, by
        site, open
      fracture - *see* Fracture, by site,
        open
      open wound - *see* Wound, open,
        by site, complicated
    postoperative 998.59
    surgical 998.59
  Wuchereria 125.0
    bancrofti 125.0
    malayi 125.1
  yaba monkey tumor virus 059.22
  yatapoxvirus 059.20
  yaws - *see* Yaws
  yeast *(see also* Candidiasis) 112.9
  yellow fever *(see also* Fever, yellow)
    060.9
  Yersinia pestis *(see also* Plague) 020.9
  Zeis' gland 373.12
  zoonotic bacterial NEC 027.9
  Zopfia senegalensis 117.4
Infective, infectious - *see* condition
Inferiority complex 301.9
  constitutional psychopathic 301.9
Infertility
  female 628.9
    age related 628.8
    associated with
      adhesions, peritubal 614.6 *[628.2]*
      anomaly
        cervical mucus 628.4
        congenital
          cervix 628.4
          fallopian tube 628.2
          uterus 628.3
          vagina 628.4
      anovulation 628.0
      dysmucorrhea 628.4
      endometritis, tuberculous *(see also*
        Tuberculosis) 016.7● *[628.3]*
      Stein-Leventhal syndrome 256.4
        [628.0]
    due to
      adiposogenital dystrophy 253.8
        [628.1]
      anterior pituitary disorder NEC
        253.4 *[628.1]*
        hyperfunction 253.1 *[628.1]*
      cervical anomaly 628.4
      fallopian tube anomaly 628.2
      ovarian failure 256.39 *[628.0]*
      Stein-Leventhal syndrome 256.4
        [628.0]
      uterine anomaly 628.3
      vaginal anomaly 628.4
    nonimplantation 628.3
    origin
      cervical 628.4
      pituitary-hypothalamus NEC
        253.8 *[628.1]*
        anterior pituitary NEC 253.4
          [628.1]
          hyperfunction NEC 253.1
            [628.1]
        dwarfism 253.3 *[628.1]*
        panhypopituitarism 253.2
          [628.1]

◀ New   ◀▥ Revised   ~~deleted~~ Deleted   ● Use Additional Digit(s)   ▨ Omit code

Infertility *(Continued)*
   female *(Continued)*
      origin *(Continued)*
         specified NEC 628.8
         tubal (block) (occlusion)
            (stenosis) 628.2
            adhesions 614.6 *[628.2]*
         uterine 628.3
         vaginal 628.4
      previous, requiring supervision of
         pregnancy V23.0
   male 606.9
      absolute 606.0
      due to
         azoospermia 606.0
         drug therapy 606.8
         extratesticular cause NEC
            606.8
         germinal cell
            aplasia 606.0
            desquamation 606.1
         hypospermatogenesis 606.1
         infection 606.8
         obstruction, afferent ducts 606.8
         oligospermia 606.1
         radiation 606.8
         spermatogenic arrest (complete)
            606.0
            incomplete 606.1
         systemic disease 606.8
Infestation 134.9
   Acanthocheilonema (perstans)
      125.4
      streptocerca 125.6
   Acariasis 133.9
      demodex folliculorum 133.8
      sarcoptes scabiei 133.0
      trombiculae 133.8
   Agamofilaria streptocerca 125.6
   Ancylostoma, Ankylostoma 126.9
      americanum 126.1
      braziliense 126.2
      canium 126.8
      ceylanicum 126.3
      duodenale 126.0
      new world 126.1
      old world 126.0
   Angiostrongylus cantonensis 128.8
   anisakiasis 127.1
   Anisakis larva 127.1
   arthropod NEC 134.1
   Ascaris lumbricoides 127.0
   Bacillus fusiformis 101
   Balantidium coli 007.0
   beef tapeworm 123.2
   Bothriocephalus (latus) 123.4
      larval 123.5
   broad tapeworm 123.4
      larval 123.5
   Brugia malayi 125.1
   Candiru 136.8
   Capillaria
      hepatica 128.8
      philippinensis 127.5
   cat liver fluke 121.0
   Cercomonas hominis (intestinal)
      007.3
   cestodes 123.9
      specified type NEC 123.8
   chigger 133.8
   chigoe 134.1
   Chilomastix 007.8
   Clonorchis (sinensis) (liver) 121.1
   coccidia 007.2

Infestation *(Continued)*
   complicating pregnancy, childbirth, or
      puerperium 647.9●
      affecting fetus or newborn 760.8
   Cysticercus cellulosae 123.1
   Demodex folliculorum 133.8
   Dermatobia (hominis) 134.0
   Dibothriocephalus (latus) 123.4
      larval 123.5
   Dicrocoelium dendriticum 121.8
   Diphyllobothrium (adult) (intestinal)
      (latum) (pacificum) 123.4
      larval 123.5
   Diplogonoporus (grandis) 123.8
   Dipylidium (caninum) 123.8
   Distoma hepaticum 121.3
   dog tapeworm 123.8
   Dracunculus medinensis 125.7
   dragon worm 125.7
   dwarf tapeworm 123.6
   Echinococcus (*see also* Echinococcus)
      122.9
   Echinostoma ilocanum 121.8
   Embadomonas 007.8
   Endamoeba (histolytica) - *see* Infection,
      ameba
   Entamoeba (histolytica) - *see* Infection,
      ameba
   Enterobius vermicularis 127.4
   Epidermophyton - *see*
      Dermatophytosis
   eyeworm 125.2
   Fasciola
      gigantica 121.3
      hepatica 121.3
   Fasciolopsis (buski) (small intestine)
      121.4
   filarial 125.9
      due to
         acanthocheilonema (perstans)
            125.4
            streptocerca 125.6
         Brugia (Wuchereria) malayi
            125.1
         Dracunculus medinensis 125.7
         guinea worms 125.7
         Mansonella (ozzardi) 125.5
         Onchocerca volvulus 125.3
            eye 125.3 *[360.13]*
            eyelid 125.3 *[373.6]*
         Wuchereria (bancrofti) 125.0
            malayi 125.1
      specified type NEC 125.6
   fish tapeworm 123.4
      larval 123.5
   fluke 121.9
      blood NEC (*see also* Schistosomiasis)
         120.9
      cat liver 121.0
      intestinal (giant) 121.4
      liver (sheep) 121.3
         cat 121.0
         Chinese 121.1
         clonorchiasis 121.1
         fascioliasis 121.3
         Oriental 121.1
      lung (oriental) 121.2
      sheep liver 121.3
   fly larva 134.0
   Gasterophilus (intestinalis) 134.0
   Gastrodiscoides hominis 121.8
   Giardia lamblia 007.1
   Gnathostoma (spinigerum) 128.1
   Gongylonema 125.6

Infestation *(Continued)*
   guinea worm 125.7
   helminth NEC 128.9
      intestinal 127.9
         mixed (types classifiable to more
            than one category in 120.0–
            127.7) 127.8
         specified type NEC 127.7
      specified type NEC 128.8
   Heterophyes heterophyes (small
      intestine) 121.6
   hookworm (*see also* Infestation,
      ancylostoma) 126.9
   Hymenolepis (diminuta) (nana) 123.6
   intestinal NEC 129
   leeches (aquatic) (land) 134.2
   Leishmania - *see* Leishmaniasis
   lice (*see also* Infestation, pediculus)
      132.9
   Linguatulidae, linguatula (pentastoma)
      (serrata) 134.1
   Loa loa 125.2
      eyelid 125.2 *[373.6]*
   louse (*see also* Infestation, pediculus)
      132.9
      body 132.1
      head 132.0
      pubic 132.2
   maggots 134.0
   Mansonella (ozzardi) 125.5
   medina 125.7
   Metagonimus yokogawai (small
      intestine) 121.5
   Microfilaria streptocerca 125.3
      eye 125.3 *[360.13]*
      eyelid 125.3 *[373.6]*
   Microsporon furfur 111.0
   microsporum - *see* Dermatophytosis
   mites 133.9
      scabic 133.0
      specified type NEC 133.8
   Monilia (albicans) (*see also* Candidiasis)
      112.9
      vagina 112.1
      vulva 112.1
   mouth 112.0
   Necator americanus 126.1
   nematode (intestinal) 127.9
      Ancylostoma (*see also* Ancylostoma)
         126.9
      Ascaris lumbricoides 127.0
      conjunctiva NEC 128.9
      Dioctophyma 128.8
      Enterobius vermicularis 127.4
      Gnathostoma spinigerum 128.1
      Oesophagostomum (apiostomum)
         127.7
      Physaloptera 127.4
      specified type NEC 127.7
      Strongyloides stercoralis 127.2
      Ternidens diminutus 127.7
      Trichinella spiralis 124
      Trichostrongylus 127.6
      Trichuris (trichiuria) 127.3
   Oesophagostomum (apiostomum)
      127.7
   Oestrus ovis 134.0
   Onchocerca (volvulus) 125.3
      eye 125.3 *[360.13]*
      eyelid 125.3 *[373.6]*
   Opisthorchis (felineus) (tenuicollis)
      (viverrini) 121.0
   Oxyuris vermicularis 127.4
   Paragonimus (westermani) 121.2

Infestation (Continued)
    parasite, parasitic NEC 136.9
        eyelid 134.9 [373.6]
        intestinal 129
        mouth 112.0
        orbit 376.13
        skin 134.9
        tongue 112.0
    pediculus 132.9
        capitis (humanus) (any site) 132.0
        corporis (humanus) (any site) 132.1
        eyelid 132.0 [373.6]
        mixed (classifiable to more than
            one category in 132.0–132.2)
            132.3
        pubis (any site) 132.2
    phthirus (pubis) (any site) 132.2
        with any infestation classifiable to
            132.0 and 132.1 132.3
    pinworm 127.4
    pork tapeworm (adult) 123.0
    protozoal NEC 136.8
    pubic louse 132.2
    rat tapeworm 123.6
    red bug 133.8
    roundworm (large) NEC 127.0
    sand flea 134.1
    saprophytic NEC 136.8
    Sarcoptes scabiei 133.0
    scabies 133.0
    Schistosoma 120.9
        bovis 120.8
        cercariae 120.3
        hematobium 120.0
        intercalatum 120.8
        japonicum 120.2
        mansoni 120.1
        mattheii 120.8
        specified
            site - see Schistosomiasis
            type NEC 120.8
        spindale 120.8
    screw worms 134.0
    skin NEC 134.9
    Sparganum (mansoni) (proliferum)
        123.5
        larval 123.5
    specified type NEC 134.8
    Spirometra larvae 123.5
    Sporozoa NEC 136.8
    Stellantchasmus falcatus 121.6
    Strongyloides 127.2
    Strongylus (gibsoni) 127.7
    Taenia 123.3
        diminuta 123.6
        Echinococcus (see also Echinococcus)
            122.9
        mediocanellata 123.2
        nana 123.6
        saginata (mediocanellata) 123.2
        solium (intestinal form) 123.0
            larval form 123.1
    Taeniarhynchus saginatus 123.2
    tapeworm 123.9
        beef 123.2
        broad 123.4
            larval 123.5
        dog 123.8
        dwarf 123.6
        fish 123.4
            larval 123.5
        pork 123.0
        rat 123.6
    Ternidens diminutus 127.7

Infestation (Continued)
    Tetranychus molestissimus 133.8
    threadworm 127.4
    tongue 112.0
    Toxocara (cani) (cati) (felis) 128.0
    trematode(s) NEC 121.9
    Trichina spiralis 124
    Trichinella spiralis 124
    Trichocephalus 127.3
    Trichomonas 131.9
        bladder 131.09
        cervix 131.09
        intestine 007.3
        prostate 131.03
        specified site NEC 131.8
        urethra (female) (male) 131.02
        urogenital 131.00
        vagina 131.01
        vulva 131.01
    Trichophyton - see Dermatophytosis
    Trichostrongylus instabilis 127.6
    Trichuris (trichiuria) 127.3
    Trombicula (irritans) 133.8
    Trypanosoma - see Trypanosomiasis
    Tunga penetrans 134.1
    Uncinaria americana 126.1
    whipworm 127.3
    worms NEC 128.9
        intestinal 127.9
    Wuchereria 125.0
        bancrofti 125.0
        malayi 125.1
Infiltrate, infiltration
    with an iron compound 275.0
    amyloid (any site) (generalized)
        277.39
    calcareous (muscle) NEC 275.49
        localized - see Degeneration, by
            site
    calcium salt (muscle) 275.49
    chemotherapy, vesicant 999.81 ◀▥
    corneal (see also Edema, cornea)
        371.20
    eyelid 373.9
    fatty (diffuse) (generalized) 272.8
        localized - see Degeneration, by site,
            fatty
    glycogen, glycogenic (see also Disease,
        glycogen storage) 271.0
    heart, cardiac
        fatty (see also Degeneration,
            myocardial) 429.1
        glycogenic 271.0 [425.7]
    inflammatory in vitreous 379.29
    kidney (see also Disease, renal) 593.9
    leukemic (M9800/3) - see Leukemia
    liver 573.8
        fatty - see Fatty, liver
        glycogen (see also Disease, glycogen
            storage) 271.0
    lung (see also Infiltrate, pulmonary)
        518.3
        eosinophilic 518.3
        x-ray finding only 793.1
    lymphatic (see also Leukemia,
        lymphatic) 204.9 ●
        gland, pigmentary 289.3
    muscle, fatty 728.9
    myelogenous (see also Leukemia,
        myeloid) 205.9 ●
    myocardium, myocardial
        fatty (see also Degeneration,
            myocardial) 429.1
        glycogenic 271.0 [425.7]

Infiltrate, infiltration (Continued)
    pulmonary 518.3
        with
            eosinophilia 518.3
            pneumonia - see Pneumonia, by
                type
        x-ray finding only 793.1
    Ranke's primary (see also Tuberculosis)
        010.0 ●
    skin, lymphocytic (benign) 709.8
    thymus (gland) (fatty) 254.8
    urine 788.8
    vesicant
        agent NEC 999.82 ◀▥
        chemotherapy 999.81 ◀▥
    vitreous humor 379.29
Infirmity 799.89
    senile 797
Inflammation, inflamed, inflammatory
    (with exudation)
    abducens (nerve) 378.54
    accessory sinus (chronic) (see also
        Sinusitis) 473.9
    adrenal (gland) 255.8
    alimentary canal - see Enteritis
    alveoli (teeth) 526.5
        scorbutic 267
    amnion - see Amnionitis
    anal canal 569.49
    antrum (chronic) (see also Sinusitis,
        maxillary) 473.0
    anus 569.49
    appendix (see also Appendicitis) 541
    arachnoid - see Meningitis
    areola 611.0
        puerperal, postpartum 675.0 ●
    areolar tissue NEC 686.9
    artery - see Arteritis
    auditory meatus (external) (see also
        Otitis, externa) 380.10
    Bartholin's gland 616.89
    bile duct or passage 576.1
    bladder (see also Cystitis) 595.9
    bleb
        postprocedural 379.60
            stage 1 379.61
            stage 2 379.62
            stage 3 379.63
    bone - see Osteomyelitis
    bowel (see also Enteritis) 558.9
    brain (see also Encephalitis) 323.9
        late effect - see category 326
        membrane - see Meningitis
    breast 611.0
        puerperal, postpartum 675.2 ●
    broad ligament (see also Disease, pelvis,
        inflammatory) 614.4
        acute 614.3
    bronchus - see Bronchitis
    bursa - see Bursitis
    capsule
        liver 573.3
        spleen 289.59
    catarrhal (see also Catarrh) 460
        vagina 616.10
    cecum (see also Appendicitis) 541
    cerebral (see also Encephalitis) 323.9
        late effect - see category 326
        membrane - see Meningitis
    cerebrospinal (see also Meningitis) 322.9
        late effect - see category 326
        meningococcal 036.0
        tuberculous (see also Tuberculosis)
            013.6 ●

◀ New   ◀▥ Revised   ~~deleted~~ Deleted   ● Use Additional Digit(s)   ▨ Omit code

Inflammation, inflamed, inflammatory
(*Continued*)
cervix (uteri) (*see also* Cervicitis) 616.0
chest 519.9
choroid NEC (*see also* Choroiditis) 363.20
cicatrix (tissue) - *see* Cicatrix
colon (*see also* Enteritis) 558.9
　granulomatous 555.1
　newborn 558.9
connective tissue (diffuse) NEC 728.9
cornea (*see also* Keratitis) 370.9
　with ulcer (*see also* Ulcer, cornea) 370.00
corpora cavernosa (penis) 607.2
cranial nerve - *see* Disorder, nerve, cranial
diarrhea - *see* Diarrhea
disc (intervertebral) (space) 722.90
　cervical, cervicothoracic 722.91
　lumbar, lumbosacral 722.93
　thoracic, thoracolumbar 722.92
Douglas' cul-de-sac or pouch (chronic) (*see also* Disease, pelvis, inflammatory) 614.4
　acute 614.3
due to (presence of) any device, implant, or graft classifiable to 996.0–996.5 - *see* Complications, infection and inflammation, due to (presence of) any device, implant, or graft classified to 996.0–996.5 NEC
duodenum 535.6●
dura mater - *see* Meningitis
ear - *see also* Otitis
　external (*see also* Otitis, externa) 380.10
　inner (*see also* Labyrinthitis) 386.30
　middle - *see* Otitis media
esophagus 530.10
ethmoidal (chronic) (sinus) (*see also* Sinusitis, ethmoidal) 473.2
Eustachian tube (catarrhal) 381.50
　acute 381.51
　chronic 381.52
extrarectal 569.49
eye 379.99
eyelid 373.9
　specified NEC 373.8
fallopian tube (*see also* Salpingo-oophoritis) 614.2
fascia 728.9
fetal membranes (acute) 658.4●
　affecting fetus or newborn 762.7
follicular, pharynx 472.1
frontal (chronic) (sinus) (*see also* Sinusitis, frontal) 473.1
gallbladder (*see also* Cholecystitis, acute) 575.0
gall duct (*see also* Cholecystitis) 575.10
gastrointestinal (*see also* Enteritis) 558.9
genital organ (diffuse) (internal)
　female 614.9
　　with
　　　abortion - *see* Abortion, by type, with sepsis
　　　ectopic pregnancy (*see also* categories 633.0–633.9) 639.0
　　　molar pregnancy (*see also* categories 630–632) 639.0

Inflammation, inflamed, inflammatory
(*Continued*)
genital organ (*Continued*)
　female (*Continued*)
　　complicating pregnancy, childbirth, or puerperium 646.6●
　　　affecting fetus or newborn 760.8
　　following
　　　abortion 639.0
　　　ectopic or molar pregnancy 639.0
　male 608.4
gland (lymph) (*see also* Lymphadenitis) 289.3
glottis (*see also* Laryngitis) 464.00
　with obstruction 464.01
granular, pharynx 472.1
gum 523.10
heart (*see also* Carditis) 429.89
hepatic duct 576.8
hernial sac - *see* Hernia, by site
ileum (*see also* Enteritis) 558.9
　terminal or regional 555.0
　　with large intestine 555.2
intervertebral disc 722.90
　cervical, cervicothoracic 722.91
　lumbar, lumbosacral 722.93
　thoracic, thoracolumbar 722.92
intestine (*see also* Enteritis) 558.9
jaw (acute) (bone) (chronic) (lower) (suppurative) (upper) 526.4
jejunum - *see* Enteritis
joint NEC (*see also* Arthritis) 716.9●
　sacroiliac 720.2
kidney (*see also* Nephritis) 583.9
knee (joint) 716.66
　tuberculous (active) (*see also* Tuberculosis) 015.2●
labium (majus) (minus) (*see also* Vulvitis) 616.10
lacrimal
　gland (*see also* Dacryoadenitis) 375.00
　passages (duct) (sac) (*see also* Dacryocystitis) 375.30
larynx (*see also* Laryngitis) 464.00
　with obstruction 464.01
　diphtheritic 032.3
leg NEC 686.9
lip 528.5
liver (capsule) (*see also* Hepatitis) 573.3
　acute 570
　chronic 571.40
　suppurative 572.0
lung (acute) (*see also* Pneumonia) 486
　chronic (interstitial) 518.89
lymphatic vessel (*see also* Lymphangitis) 457.2
lymph node or gland (*see also* Lymphadenitis) 289.3
mammary gland 611.0
　puerperal, postpartum 675.2●
maxilla, maxillary 526.4
　sinus (chronic) (*see also* Sinusitis, maxillary) 473.0
membranes of brain or spinal cord - *see* Meningitis
meninges - *see* Meningitis
mouth 528.00
muscle 728.9
myocardium (*see also* Myocarditis) 429.0

Inflammation, inflamed, inflammatory
(*Continued*)
nasal sinus (chronic) (*see also* Sinusitis) 473.9
nasopharynx - *see* Nasopharyngitis
navel 686.9
　newborn NEC 771.4
nerve NEC 729.2
nipple 611.0
　puerperal, postpartum 675.0●
nose 478.19
　suppurative 472.0
oculomotor nerve 378.51
optic nerve 377.30
orbit (chronic) 376.10
　acute 376.00
　chronic 376.10
ovary (*see also* Salpingo-oophoritis) 614.2
oviduct (*see also* Salpingo-oophoritis) 614.2
pancreas - *see* Pancreatitis
parametrium (chronic) (*see also* Disease, pelvis, inflammatory) 614.4
　acute 614.3
parotid region 686.9
　gland 527.2
pelvis, female (*see also* Disease, pelvis, inflammatory) 614.9
penis (corpora cavernosa) 607.2
perianal 569.49
pericardium (*see also* Pericarditis) 423.9
perineum (female) (male) 686.9
perirectal 569.49
peritoneum (*see also* Peritonitis) 567.9
periuterine (*see also* Disease, pelvis, inflammatory) 614.9
perivesical (*see also* Cystitis) 595.9
petrous bone (*see also* Petrositis) 383.20
pharynx (*see also* Pharyngitis) 462
　follicular 472.1
　granular 472.1
pia mater - *see* Meningitis
pleura - *see* Pleurisy
postmastoidectomy cavity 383.30
　chronic 383.33
pouch, internal ileoanal 569.71　◀
prostate (*see also* Prostatitis) 601.9
rectosigmoid - *see* Rectosigmoiditis
rectum (*see also* Proctitis) 569.49
respiratory, upper (*see also* Infection, respiratory, upper) 465.9
　chronic, due to external agent - *see* Condition, respiratory, chronic, due to, external agent
　due to
　　fumes or vapors (chemical) (inhalation) 506.2
　　radiation 508.1
retina (*see also* Retinitis) 363.20
retrocecal (*see also* Appendicitis) 541
retroperitoneal (*see also* Peritonitis) 567.9
salivary duct or gland (any) (suppurative) 527.2
scorbutic, alveoli, teeth 267
scrotum 608.4
sigmoid - *see* Enteritis
sinus (*see also* Sinusitis) 473.9
Skene's duct or gland (*see also* Urethritis) 597.89
skin 686.9
spermatic cord 608.4
sphenoidal (sinus) (*see also* Sinusitis, sphenoidal) 473.3

Inflammation, inflamed, inflammatory (Continued)

spinal
  cord (see also Encephalitis) 323.9
    late effect - see category 326
  membrane - see Meningitis
  nerve - see Disorder, nerve
spine (see also Spondylitis) 720.9
spleen (capsule) 289.59
stomach - see Gastritis
stricture, rectum 569.49
subcutaneous tissue NEC 686.9
suprarenal (gland) 255.8
synovial (fringe) (membrane) - see Bursitis
tendon (sheath) NEC 726.90
testis (see also Orchitis) 604.90
thigh 686.9
throat (see also Sore throat) 462
thymus (gland) 254.8
thyroid (gland) (see also Thyroiditis) 245.9
tongue 529.0
tonsil - see Tonsillitis
trachea - see Tracheitis
trochlear nerve 378.53
tubal (see also Salpingo-oophoritis) 614.2
tuberculous NEC (see also Tuberculosis) 011.9●
tubo-ovarian (see also Salpingo-oophoritis) 614.2
tunica vaginalis 608.4
tympanic membrane - see Myringitis
umbilicus, umbilical 686.9
  newborn NEC 771.4
uterine ligament (see also Disease, pelvis, inflammatory) 614.4
  acute 614.3
uterus (catarrhal) (see also Endometritis) 615.9
uveal tract (anterior) (see also Iridocyclitis) 364.3
  posterior - see Chorioretinitis
  sympathetic 360.11
vagina (see also Vaginitis) 616.10
vas deferens 608.4
vein (see also Phlebitis) 451.9
  thrombotic 451.9
    cerebral (see also Thrombosis, brain) 434.0●
    leg 451.2
      deep (vessels) NEC 451.19
      superficial (vessels) 451.0
    lower extremity 451.2
      deep (vessels) NEC 451.19
      superficial (vessels) 451.0
vocal cord 478.5
vulva (see also Vulvitis) 616.10
Inflation, lung imperfect (newborn) 770.5
Influenza, influenzal 487.1
with
  bronchitis 487.1
  bronchopneumonia 487.0
  cold (any type) 487.1
  digestive manifestations 487.8
  hemoptysis 487.1
  involvement of
    gastrointestinal tract 487.8
    nervous system 487.8
  laryngitis 487.1
  manifestations NEC 487.8
    respiratory 487.1
      pneumonia 487.0

Influenza, influenzal (Continued)
with (Continued)
  pharyngitis 487.1
  pneumonia (any form classifiable to 480–483, 485–486) 487.0
  respiratory manifestations NEC 487.1
  sinusitis 487.1
  sore throat 487.1
  tonsillitis 487.1
  tracheitis 487.1
  upper respiratory infection (acute) 487.1
A/H5N1 488.0 ◀
abdominal 487.8
Asian 487.1
avian 488.0 ◀
bronchial 487.1
bronchopneumonia 487.0
catarrhal 487.1
due to identified ~~avian influenza virus 488~~ ◀▮
  avian influenza virus 488.0 ◀
  novel H1N1 influenza virus 488.1 ◀
epidemic 487.1
gastric 487.8
intestinal 487.8
laryngitis 487.1
maternal affecting fetus or newborn 760.2
  manifest influenza in infant 771.2 ◀
novel (2009) H1N1 488.1 ◀
novel A/H1N1 488.1 ◀
pharyngitis 487.1
pneumonia (any form) 487.0
respiratory (upper) 487.1
specified NEC 487.1 ◀
stomach 487.8
vaccination, prophylactic (against) V04.81
Influenza-like disease 487.1
Infraction, Freiberg's (metatarsal head) 732.5
Infraeruption, teeth 524.34
Infusion complication, misadventure, or reaction - see Complication, infusion
Ingestion
chemical - see Table of Drugs and Chemicals
drug or medicinal substance
  overdose or wrong substance given or taken 977.9
    specified drug - see Table of Drugs and Chemicals
foreign body NEC (see also Foreign body) 938
Ingrowing
hair 704.8
nail (finger) (toe) (infected) 703.0
Inguinal - see also condition
testis 752.51
Inhalation
carbon monoxide 986
flame
  mouth 947.0
  lung 947.1
food or foreign body (see also Asphyxia, food or foreign body) 933.1
gas, fumes, or vapor (noxious) 987.9
  specified agent - see Table of Drugs and Chemicals
liquid or vomitus (see also Asphyxia, food or foreign body) 933.1
  lower respiratory tract NEC 934.9

Inhalation (Continued)
meconium (fetus or newborn) 770.11
  with respiratory symptoms 770.12
mucus (see also Asphyxia, mucus) 933.1
oil (causing suffocation) (see also Asphyxia, food or foreign body) 933.1
pneumonia - see Pneumonia, aspiration
smoke 987.9
steam 987.9
stomach contents or secretions (see also Asphyxia, food or foreign body) 933.1
  in labor and delivery 668.0●
Inhibition, inhibited
academic as adjustment reaction 309.23
orgasm
  female 302.73
  male 302.74
sexual
  desire 302.71
  excitement 302.72
work as adjustment reaction 309.23
Inhibitor, systemic lupus erythematosus (presence of) 286.5
Iniencephalus, iniencephaly 740.2
Injected eye 372.74
Injury 959.9

> **Note 45** For abrasion, insect bite (nonvenomous), blister, or scratch, see Injury, superficial.
>
> For laceration, traumatic rupture, tear, or penetrating wound of internal organs, such as heart, lung, liver, kidney, pelvic organs, whether or not accompanied by open wound in the same region, see Injury, internal.
>
> For nerve injury, see Injury, nerve.
>
> For late effect of injuries classifiable to 850–854, 860–869, 900–919, 950–959, see Late, effect, injury, by type.

abdomen, abdominal (viscera) - see also Injury, internal, abdomen
  muscle or wall 959.12
acoustic, resulting in deafness 951.5
adenoid 959.09
adrenal (gland) - see Injury, internal, adrenal
alveolar (process) 959.09
ankle (and foot) (and knee) (and leg, except thigh) 959.7
anterior chamber, eye 921.3
anus 959.19
aorta (thoracic) 901.0
  abdominal 902.0
appendix - see Injury, internal, appendix
arm, upper (and shoulder) 959.2
artery (complicating trauma) (see also Injury, blood vessel, by site) 904.9
  cerebral or meningeal (see also Hemorrhage, brain, traumatic, subarachnoid) 852.0●
auditory canal (external) (meatus) 959.09
auricle, auris, ear 959.09
axilla 959.2
back 959.19

◀ New   ◀▮ Revised   ~~deleted~~ Deleted   ● Use Additional Digit(s)   ▮ Omit code

Injury (Continued)
  bile duct - see Injury, internal, bile duct
  birth - see also Birth, injury
    canal NEC, complicating delivery
      665.9●
  bladder (sphincter) - see Injury, internal,
    bladder
  blast (air) (hydraulic) (immersion)
      (underwater) NEC 869.0
    with open wound into cavity NEC
      869.1
    abdomen or thorax - see Injury,
      internal, by site
    brain - see Concussion, brain
    ear (acoustic nerve trauma) 951.5
      with perforation of tympanic
        membrane - see Wound,
        open, ear, drum
  blood vessel NEC 904.9
    abdomen 902.9
      multiple 902.87
      specified NEC 902.89
    aorta (thoracic) 901.0
      abdominal 902.0
    arm NEC 903.9
    axillary 903.00
      artery 903.1
      vein 903.02
    azygos vein 901.89
    basilic vein 903.1
    brachial (artery) (vein) 903.1
    bronchial 901.89
    carotid artery 900.00
      common 900.01
      external 900.02
      internal 900.03
    celiac artery 902.20
      specified branch NEC 902.24
    cephalic vein (arm) 903.1
    colica dextra 902.26
    cystic
      artery 902.24
      vein 902.39
    deep plantar 904.6
    digital (artery) (vein) 903.5
    due to accidental puncture or
      laceration during procedure
      998.2
    extremity
      lower 904.8
        multiple 904.7
        specified NEC 904.7
      upper 903.9
        multiple 903.8
        specified NEC 903.8
    femoral
      artery (superficial) 904.1
        above profunda origin 904.0
        common 904.0
      vein 904.2
    gastric
      artery 902.21
      vein 902.39
    head 900.9
      intracranial - see Injury,
        intracranial
      multiple 900.82
      specified NEC 900.89
    hemiazygos vein 901.89
    hepatic
      artery 902.22
      vein 902.11
    hypogastric 902.59
      artery 902.51
      vein 902.52

Injury (Continued)
  blood vessel (Continued)
    ileocolic
      artery 902.26
      vein 902.31
    iliac 902.50
      artery 902.53
      specified branch NEC 902.59
      vein 902.54
    innominate
      artery 901.1
      vein 901.3
    intercostal (artery) (vein) 901.81
    jugular vein (external) 900.81
      internal 900.1
    leg NEC 904.8
    mammary (artery) (vein) 901.82
    mesenteric
      artery 902.20
        inferior 902.27
        specified branch NEC 902.29
        superior (trunk) 902.25
          branches, primary 902.26
      vein 902.39
        inferior 902.32
        superior (and primary
          subdivisions) 902.31
    neck 900.9
      multiple 900.82
      specified NEC 900.89
    ovarian 902.89
      artery 902.81
      vein 902.82
    palmar artery 903.4
    pelvis 902.9
      multiple 902.87
      specified NEC 902.89
    plantar (deep) (artery) (vein)
      904.6
    popliteal 904.40
      artery 904.41
      vein 904.42
    portal 902.33
    pulmonary 901.40
      artery 901.41
      vein 901.42
    radial (artery) (vein) 903.2
    renal 902.40
      artery 902.41
      specified NEC 902.49
      vein 902.42
    saphenous
      artery 904.7
      vein (greater) (lesser) 904.3
    splenic
      artery 902.23
      vein 902.34
    subclavian
      artery 901.1
      vein 901.3
    suprarenal 902.49
    thoracic 901.9
      multiple 901.83
      specified NEC 901.89
    tibial 904.50
      artery 904.50
        anterior 904.51
        posterior 904.53
      vein 904.50
        anterior 904.52
        posterior 904.54
    ulnar (artery) (vein) 903.3
    uterine 902.59
      artery 902.55
      vein 902.56

Injury (Continued)
  blood vessel (Continued)
    vena cava
      inferior 902.10
        specified branches NEC 902.19
      superior 901.2
  brachial plexus 953.4
    newborn 767.6
  brain (traumatic) NEC (see also Injury,
    intracranial) 854.0●   ◀▥
    due to fracture of skull -
      see Fracture, skull, by site   ◀
  breast 959.19
  broad ligament - see Injury, internal,
    broad ligament
  bronchus, bronchi - see Injury, internal,
    bronchus
  brow 959.09
  buttock 959.19
  canthus, eye 921.1
  cathode ray 990
  cauda equina 952.4
    with fracture, vertebra - see Fracture,
      vertebra, sacrum
  cavernous sinus (see also Injury,
    intracranial) 854.0●
  cecum - see Injury, internal, cecum
  celiac ganglion or plexus 954.1
  cerebellum (see also Injury, intracranial)
    854.0●
  cervix (uteri) - see Injury, internal,
    cervix
  cheek 959.09
  chest - see Injury, internal, chest
    wall 959.11
  childbirth - see also Birth, injury
    maternal NEC 665.9●
  chin 959.09
  choroid (eye) 921.3
  clitoris 959.14
  coccyx 959.19
    complicating delivery 665.6●
  colon - see Injury, internal, colon
  common duct - see Injury, internal,
    common duct
  conjunctiva 921.1
    superficial 918.2
    cord
      spermatic - see Injury, internal,
        spermatic cord
      spinal - see Injury, spinal, by site
  cornea 921.3
    abrasion 918.1
    due to contact lens 371.82
    penetrating - see Injury, eyeball,
      penetrating
    superficial 918.1
    due to contact lens 371.82
  cortex (cerebral) (see also Injury,
    intracranial) 854.0●
    visual 950.3
  costal region 959.11
  costochondral 959.11
  cranial
    bones - see Fracture, skull, by site
    cavity (see also Injury, intracranial)
      854.0●
    nerve - see Injury, nerve, cranial
  crushing - see Crush
  cutaneous sensory nerve
    lower limb 956.4
    upper limb 955.5
  deep tissue - see Contusion, by site
    meaning pressure ulcer 707.25
  delivery - see also Birth, injury
    maternal NEC 665.9●

Injury (Continued)
Descemet's membrane - see Injury, eyeball, penetrating
diaphragm - see Injury, internal, diaphragm
diffuse axonal - see Injury, intracranial
duodenum - see Injury, internal, duodenum
ear (auricle) (canal) (drum) (external) 959.09
elbow (and forearm) (and wrist) 959.3
epididymis 959.14
epigastric region 959.12
epiglottis 959.09
epiphyseal, current - see Fracture, by site
esophagus - see Injury, internal, esophagus
Eustachian tube 959.09
extremity (lower) (upper) NEC 959.8
eye 921.9
  penetrating eyeball - see Injury, eyeball, penetrating
  superficial 918.9
eyeball 921.3
  penetrating 871.7
    with
      partial loss (of intraocular tissue) 871.2
      prolapse or exposure (of intraocular tissue) 871.1
      without prolapse 871.0
      foreign body (nonmagnetic) 871.6
        magnetic 871.5
  superficial 918.9
eyebrow 959.09
eyelid(s) 921.1
  laceration - see Laceration, eyelid
  superficial 918.0
face (and neck) 959.09
fallopian tube - see Injury, internal, fallopian tube
fingers(s) (nail) 959.5
flank 959.19
foot (and ankle) (and knee) (and leg, except thigh) 959.7
forceps NEC 767.9
  scalp 767.19
forearm (and elbow) (and wrist) 959.3
forehead 959.09
gallbladder - see Injury, internal, gallbladder
gasserian ganglion 951.2
gastrointestinal tract - see Injury, internal, gastrointestinal tract
genital organ(s)
  with
    abortion - see Abortion, by type, with, damage to pelvic organs
    ectopic pregnancy (see also categories 633.0–633.9) 639.2
    molar pregnancy (see also categories 630–632) 639.2
  external 959.14
  fracture of corpus cavernosum penis 959.13
  following
    abortion 639.2
    ectopic or molar pregnancy 639.2

Injury (Continued)
  genital organ(s) (Continued)
    internal - see Injury, internal, genital organs
    obstetrical trauma NEC 665.9●
      affecting fetus or newborn 763.89
  gland
    lacrimal 921.1
      laceration 870.8
    parathyroid 959.09
    salivary 959.09
    thyroid 959.09
  globe (eye) (see also Injury, eyeball) 921.3
  grease gun - see Wound, open, by site, complicated
  groin 959.19
  gum 959.09
  hand(s) (except fingers) 959.4
  head NEC 959.01
    with
      loss of consciousness 850.5
      skull fracture - see Fracture, skull, by site
  heart - see Injury, internal, heart
  heel 959.7
  hip (and thigh) 959.6
  hymen 959.14
  hyperextension (cervical) (vertebra) 847.0
  ileum - see Injury, internal, ileum
  iliac region 959.19
  infrared rays NEC 990
  instrumental (during surgery) 998.2
    birth injury - see Birth, injury
    nonsurgical (see also Injury, by site) 959.9
    obstetrical 665.9●
      affecting fetus or newborn 763.89
      bladder 665.5●
      cervix 665.3●
      high vaginal 665.4●●
      perineal NEC 664.9●●
      urethra 665.5●
      uterus 665.5●
  internal 869.0

Note 46   For injury of internal organ(s) by foreign body entering through a natural orifice (e.g., inhaled, ingested, or swallowed)-see Foreign body, entering through orifice.

For internal injury of any of the following sites with internal injury of any other of the sites-see Injury, internal, multiple.

  with
    fracture
      pelvis - see Fracture, pelvis
      specified site, except pelvis - see Injury, internal, by site
    open wound into cavity 869.1
  abdomen, abdominal (viscera) NEC 868.00
    with
      fracture, pelvis - see Fracture, pelvis
      open wound into cavity 868.10
    specified site NEC 868.09
      with open wound into cavity 868.19

Injury (Continued)
  internal (Continued)
    adrenal (gland) 868.01
      with open wound into cavity 868.11
    aorta (thoracic) 901.0
      abdominal 902.0
    appendix 863.85
      with open wound into cavity 863.95
    bile duct 868.02
      with open wound into cavity 868.12
    bladder (sphincter) 867.0
      with
        abortion - see Abortion, by type, with, damage to pelvic organs
        ectopic pregnancy (see also categories 633.0–633.9) 639.2
        molar pregnancy (see also categories 630–632) 639.2
        open wound into cavity 867.1
      following
        abortion 639.2
        ectopic or molar pregnancy 639.2
      obstetrical trauma 665.5●
        affecting fetus or newborn 763.89
    blood vessel - see Injury, blood vessel, by site
    broad ligament 867.6
      with open wound into cavity 867.7
    bronchus, bronchi 862.21
      with open wound into cavity 862.31
    cecum 863.89
      with open wound into cavity 863.99
    cervix (uteri) 867.4
      with
        abortion - see Abortion, by type, with, damage to pelvic organs
        ectopic pregnancy (see also categories 633.0–633.9) 639.2
        molar pregnancy (see also categories 630–632) 639.2
        open wound into cavity 867.5
      following
        abortion 639.2
        ectopic or molar pregnancy 639.2
      obstetrical trauma 665.3●
        affecting fetus or newborn 763.89
    chest (see also Injury, internal, intrathoracic organs) 862.8
      with open wound into cavity 862.9
    colon 863.40
      with
        open wound into cavity 863.50
        rectum 863.46
          with open wound into cavity 863.56
      ascending (right) 863.41
        with open wound into cavity 863.51

Injury (Continued)
  internal (Continued)
    colon (Continued)
      descending (left) 863.43
        with open wound into cavity
        863.53
      multiple sites 863.46
        with open wound into cavity
        863.56
      sigmoid 863.44
        with open wound into cavity
        863.54
      specified site NEC 863.49
        with open wound into cavity
        863.59
      transverse 863.42
        with open wound into cavity
        863.52
    common duct 868.02
      with open wound into cavity
      868.12
    complicating delivery 665.9 ●
      affecting fetus or newborn 763.89
    diaphragm 862.0
      with open wound into cavity
      862.1
    duodenum 863.21
      with open wound into cavity
      863.31
    esophagus (intrathoracic) 862.22
      with open wound into cavity
      862.32
      cervical region 874.4
        complicated 874.5
    fallopian tube 867.6
      with open wound into cavity
      867.7
    gallbladder 868.02
      with open wound into cavity
      868.12
    gastrointestinal tract NEC 863.80
      with open wound into cavity
      863.90
    genital organ NEC 867.6
      with open wound into cavity
      867.7
    heart 861.00
      with open wound into thorax
      861.10
    ileum 863.29
      with open wound into cavity
      863.39
    intestine NEC 863.89
      with open wound into cavity
      863.99
      large NEC 863.40
        with open wound into cavity
        863.50
      small NEC 863.20
        with open wound into cavity
        863.30
    intra-abdominal (organ) 868.00
      with open wound into cavity
      868.10
      multiple sites 868.09
        with open wound into cavity
        868.19
      specified site NEC 868.09
        with open wound into cavity
        868.19
    intrathoracic organs (multiple)
      862.8
      with open wound into cavity
      862.9

Injury (Continued)
  internal (Continued)
    intrathoracic organs (Continued)
      diaphragm (only) - see Injury,
        internal, diaphragm
      heart (only) - see Injury, internal,
        heart
      lung (only) - see Injury, internal,
        lung
      specified site NEC 862.29
        with open wound into cavity
        862.39
    intrauterine (see also Injury, internal,
      uterus) 867.4
      with open wound into cavity
      867.5
    jejunum 863.29
      with open wound into cavity
      863.39
    kidney (subcapsular) 866.00
      with
        disruption of parenchyma
          (complete) 866.03
          with open wound into
          cavity 866.13
        hematoma (without rupture of
          capsule) 866.01
          with open wound into
          cavity 866.11
        laceration 866.02
          with open wound into
          cavity 866.12
        open wound into cavity
          866.10
    liver 864.00
      with
        contusion 864.01
          with open wound into
          cavity 864.11
        hematoma 864.01
          with open wound into
          cavity 864.11
        laceration 864.05
          with open wound into
          cavity 864.15
        major (disruption of hepatic
          parenchyma) 864.04
          with open wound into
          cavity 864.14
        minor (capsule only)
          864.02
          with open wound into
          cavity 864.12
        moderate (involving
          parenchyma) 864.03
          with open wound into
          cavity 864.13
        multiple 864.04
        stellate 864.04
          with open wound into
          cavity 864.14
        open wound into cavity
          864.10
    lung 861.20
      with open wound into thorax
      861.30
      hemopneumothorax - see
        Hemopneumothorax,
        traumatic
      hemothorax - see Hemothorax,
        traumatic
      pneumohemothorax - see
        Pneumohemothorax,
        traumatic

Injury (Continued)
  internal (Continued)
    lung (Continued)
      pneumothorax - see
        Pneumothorax,
        traumatic
      transfusion related, acute
        (TRALI) 518.7
    mediastinum 862.29
      with open wound into cavity
      862.39
    mesentery 863.89
      with open wound into cavity
      863.99
    mesosalpinx 867.6
      with open wound into cavity
      867.7
    multiple 869.0

> **Note 47**   Multiple internal injuries of sites classifiable to the same three- or four-digit category should be classified to that category.
>
> Multiple injuries classifiable to different fourth-digit subdivisions of 861.-(heart and lung injuries) should be dealt with according to coding rules.

      internal 869.0
        with open wound into cavity
        869.1
      intra-abdominal organ (sites
        classifiable to 863–868)
        with
          intrathoracic organ(s) (sites
            classifiable to 861–862)
            869.0
            with open wound into
            cavity 869.1
          other intra-abdominal
            organ(s) (sites
            classifiable to
            863–868, except
            where classifiable
            to the same three-
            digit category)
            868.09
            with open wound into
            cavity 868.19
      intrathoracic organ (sites
        classifiable to 861–862)
        with
          intra-abdominal organ(s)
            (sites classifiable to
            863–868) 869.0
            with open wound into
            cavity 869.1
          other intrathoracic organs(s)
            (sites classifiable to
            861–862, except where
            classifiable to the same
            three-digit category)
            862.8
            with open wound into cavity
            862.9
    myocardium - see Injury, internal,
      heart
    ovary 867.6
      with open wound into cavity
      867.7
    pancreas (multiple sites) 863.84
      with open wound into cavity
      863.94

Injury (Continued)
   internal (Continued)
      pancreas (Continued)
         body 863.82
            with open wound into cavity
               863.92
         head 863.81
            with open wound into cavity
               863.91
         tail 863.83
         with open wound into cavity
            863.93
      pelvis, pelvic (organs) (viscera) 867.8
         with
            fracture, pelvis - see Fracture,
               pelvis
            open wound into cavity 867.9
         specified site NEC 867.6
            with open wound into cavity
               867.7
      peritoneum 868.03
         with open wound into cavity
            868.13
      pleura 862.29
         with open wound into cavity
            862.39
      prostate 867.6
         with open wound into cavity
            867.7
      rectum 863.45
         with
            colon 863.46
               with open wound into
                  cavity 863.56
            open wound into cavity
               863.55
      retroperitoneum 868.04
         with open wound into cavity
            868.14
      round ligament 867.6
         with open wound into cavity
            867.7
      seminal vesicle 867.6
         with open wound into cavity
            867.7
      spermatic cord 867.6
         with open wound into cavity
            867.7
      scrotal - see Wound, open,
         spermatic cord
      spleen 865.00
         with
            disruption of parenchyma
               (massive) 865.04
               with open wound into
                  cavity 865.14
            hematoma (without rupture of
               capsule) 865.01
               with open wound into
                  cavity 865.11
            open wound into cavity 865.10
            tear, capsular 865.02
               with open wound into
                  cavity 865.12
               extending into parenchyma
                  865.03
                  with open wound into
                      cavity 865.13
      stomach 863.0
         with open wound into cavity
            863.1
      suprarenal gland (multiple) 868.01
         with open wound into cavity
            868.11

Injury (Continued)
   internal (Continued)
      thorax, thoracic (cavity) (organs)
         (multiple) (see also Injury,
         internal, intrathoracic organs)
         862.8
         with open wound into cavity
            862.9
      thymus (gland) 862.29
         with open wound into cavity
            862.39
      trachea (intrathoracic) 862.29
         with open wound into cavity
            862.39
         cervical region (see also Wound,
            open, trachea) 874.02
      ureter 867.2
         with open wound into cavity
            867.3
      urethra (sphincter) 867.0
         with
            abortion - see Abortion, by
               type, with, damage to
               pelvic organs
            ectopic pregnancy (see also
               categories 633.0–633.9)
               639.2
            molar pregnancy (see also
               categories 630–632)
               639.2
            open wound into cavity 867.1
         following
            abortion 639.2
            ectopic or molar pregnancy
               639.2
         obstetrical trauma 665.5●
            affecting fetus or newborn
               763.89
      uterus 867.4
         with
            abortion - see Abortion, by
               type, with, damage to
               pelvic organs
            ectopic pregnancy (see also
               categories 633.0–633.9)
               639.2
            molar pregnancy (see also
               categories 630–632)
               639.2
            open wound into cavity 867.5
         following
            abortion 639.2
            ectopic or molar pregnancy
               639.2
         obstetrical trauma NEC 665.5●
            affecting fetus or newborn
               763.89
      vas deferens 867.6
         with open wound into cavity
            867.7
      vesical (sphincter) 867.0
         with open wound into cavity
            867.1
      viscera (abdominal) (see also Injury,
         internal, multiple) 868.00
         with
            fracture, pelvis - see Fracture,
               pelvis
            open wound into cavity 868.10
         thoracic NEC (see also Injury,
            internal, intrathoracic
            organs) 862.8
            with open wound into cavity
               862.9

Injury (Continued)
   interscapular region 959.19
   intervertebral disc 959.19
   intestine - see Injury, internal, intestine
   intra-abdominal (organs) NEC - see
      Injury, internal, intra-abdominal
   intracranial (traumatic) 854.0 ◄▥

Note 48	Use the following fifth-digit subclassification with categories 851–854:
0	unspecified state of consciousness
1	with no loss of consciousness
2	with brief [less than one hour] loss of consciousness
3	with moderate [1–24 hours] loss of consciousness
4	with prolonged [more than 24 hours] loss of consciousness and return to pre-existing conscious level
5	with prolonged [more than 24 hours] loss of consciousness, without return to pre-existing conscious level

Use fifth-digit 5 to designate when a patient is unconscious and dies before regaining consciousness, regardless of the duration of the loss of consciousness

| 6 | with loss of consciousness of unspecified duration |
| 9 | with concussion, unspecified |

      with
         open intracranial wound
            854.1●
         skull fracture - see Fracture,
            skull, by site
      contusion 851.8●
         with open intracranial wound
            851.9●
         brain stem 851.4●
            with open intracranial wound
               851.5●
         cerebellum 851.4●
            with open intracranial wound
               851.5●
         cortex (cerebral) 851.0●
            with open intracranial wound
               851.2●
         hematoma - see Injury,
            intracranial, hemorrhage
         hemorrhage 853.0●
            with
               laceration - see Injury,
                 intracranial,
                 laceration
              open intracranial wound
                 853.1●
            extradural 852.4●
               with open intracranial
                 wound 852.5●
            subarachnoid 852.0●
               with open intracranial
                 wound 852.1●
            subdural 852.2●
               with open intracranial
                 wound 852.3●
         laceration 851.8●
            with open intracranial wound
            851.9●

◄ New   ◄▥ Revised   deleted Deleted   ● Use Additional Digit(s)   ▨ Omit code

Injury *(Continued)*
  intracranial *(Continued)*
    contusion *(Continued)*
      laceration *(Continued)*
        brain stem 851.6 ●
          with open intracranial
            wound 851.7 ●
        cerebellum 851.6 ●
          with open intracranial
            wound 851.7 ●
        cortex (cerebral) 851.2 ●
          with open intracranial
            wound 851.3 ●
  intraocular - *see* Injury, eyeball,
    penetrating
  intrathoracic organs (multiple) - *see*
    Injury, internal, intrathoracic
    organs
  intrauterine - *see* Injury, internal,
    intrauterine
  iris 921.3
    penetrating - *see* Injury, eyeball,
      penetrating
  jaw 959.09
  jejunum - *see* Injury, internal, jejunum
  joint NEC 959.9
    old or residual 718.80
      ankle 718.87
      elbow 718.82
      foot 718.87
      hand 718.84
      hip 718.85
      knee 718.86
      multiple sites 718.89
      pelvic region 718.85
      shoulder (region) 718.81
      specified site NEC 718.88
      wrist 718.83
  kidney - *see* Injury, internal, kidney
    acute (nontraumatic) 584.9
  knee (and ankle) (and foot) (and leg,
    except thigh) 959.7
  labium (majus) (minus) 959.14
  labyrinth, ear 959.09
  lacrimal apparatus, gland, or sac 921.1
    laceration 870.8
  larynx 959.09
  late effect - *see* Late, effects (of), injury
  leg, except thigh (and ankle) (and foot)
    (and knee) 959.7
    upper or thigh 959.6
  lens, eye 921.3
    penetrating - *see* Injury, eyeball,
      penetrating
  lid, eye - *see* Injury, eyelid
  lip 959.09
  liver - *see* Injury, internal, liver
  lobe, parietal - *see* Injury, intracranial
  lumbar (region) 959.19
    plexus 953.5
  lumbosacral (region) 959.19
    plexus 953.5
  lung - *see* Injury, internal, lung
  malar region 959.09
  mastoid region 959.09
  maternal, during pregnancy, affecting
    fetus or newborn 760.5
  maxilla 959.09
  mediastinum - *see* Injury, internal,
    mediastinum
  membrane
    brain (*see also* Injury, intracranial)
      854.0 ●
    tympanic 959.09

Injury *(Continued)*
  meningeal artery - *see* Hemorrhage,
    brain, traumatic, subarachnoid
  meninges (cerebral) - *see* Injury,
    intracranial
  mesenteric
    artery - *see* Injury, blood vessel,
      mesenteric, artery
    plexus, inferior 954.1
    vein - *see* Injury, blood vessel,
      mesenteric, vein
  mesentery - *see* Injury, internal,
    mesentery
  mesosalpinx - *see* Injury, internal,
    mesosalpinx
  middle ear 959.09
  midthoracic region 959.11
  mouth 959.09
  multiple (sites not classifiable to the
    same four-digit category in 959.0–
    959.7) 959.8
    internal 869.0
      with open wound into cavity
        869.1
  musculocutaneous nerve 955.4
  nail
    finger 959.5
    toe 959.7
  nasal (septum) (sinus) 959.09
  nasopharynx 959.09
  neck (and face) 959.09
  nerve 957.9
    abducens 951.3
    abducent 951.3
    accessory 951.6
    acoustic 951.5
    ankle and foot 956.9
    anterior crural, femoral 956.1
    arm (*see also* Injury, nerve, upper
      limb) 955.9
    auditory 951.5
    axillary 955.0
    brachial plexus 953.4
    cervical sympathetic 954.0
    cranial 951.9
      first or olfactory 951.8
      second or optic 950.0
      third or oculomotor 951.0
      fourth or trochlear 951.1
      fifth or trigeminal 951.2
      sixth or abducens 951.3
      seventh or facial 951.4
      eighth, acoustic, or auditory
        951.5
      ninth or glossopharyngeal 951.8
      tenth, pneumogastric, or vagus
        951.8
      eleventh or accessory 951.6
      twelfth or hypoglossal 951.7
      newborn 767.7
    cutaneous sensory
      lower limb 956.4
      upper limb 955.5
    digital (finger) 955.6
      toe 956.5
    facial 951.4
      newborn 767.5
    femoral 956.1
    finger 955.9
    foot and ankle 956.9
    forearm 955.9
    glossopharyngeal 951.8
    hand and wrist 955.9
    head and neck, superficial 957.0

Injury *(Continued)*
  nerve *(Continued)*
    hypoglossal 951.7
    involving several parts of body
      957.8
    leg (*see also* Injury, nerve, lower
      limb) 956.9
    lower limb 956.9
      multiple 956.8
      specified site NEC 956.5
    lumbar plexus 953.5
    lumbosacral plexus 953.5
    median 955.1
      forearm 955.1
      wrist and hand 955.1
    multiple (in several parts of body)
      (sites not classifiable to the
      same three-digit category)
      957.8
    musculocutaneous 955.4
    musculospiral 955.3
      upper arm 955.3
    oculomotor 951.0
    olfactory 951.8
    optic 950.0
    pelvic girdle 956.9
      multiple sites 956.8
      specified site NEC 956.5
    peripheral 957.9
      multiple (in several regions)
        (sites not classifiable to the
        same three-digit category)
        957.8
      specified site NEC 957.1
    peroneal 956.3
      ankle and foot 956.3
      lower leg 956.3
    plantar 956.5
    plexus 957.9
      celiac 954.1
      mesenteric, inferior 954.1
      spinal 953.9
        brachial 953.4
        lumbosacral 953.5
        multiple sites 953.8
      sympathetic NEC 954.1
    pneumogastric 951.8
    radial 955.3
      wrist and hand 955.3
    sacral plexus 953.5
    sciatic 956.0
      thigh 956.0
    shoulder girdle 955.9
      multiple 955.8
      specified site NEC 955.7
    specified site NEC 957.1
    spinal 953.9
      plexus - *see* Injury, nerve, plexus,
        spinal
      root 953.9
        cervical 953.0
        dorsal 953.1
        lumbar 953.2
        multiple sites 953.8
        sacral 953.3
    splanchnic 954.1
    sympathetic NEC 954.1
      cervical 954.0
    thigh 956.9
    tibial 956.5
      ankle and foot 956.2
      lower leg 956.5
      posterior 956.2
    toe 956.9

Injury (Continued)
  nerve (Continued)
    trigeminal 951.2
    trochlear 951.1
    trunk, excluding shoulder and
        pelvic girdles 954.9
      specified site NEC 954.8
      sympathetic NEC 954.1
    ulnar 955.2
      forearm 955.2
      wrist (and hand) 955.2
    upper limb 955.9
      multiple 955.8
      specified site NEC 955.7
    vagus 951.8
    wrist and hand 955.9
  nervous system, diffuse 957.8
  nose (septum) 959.09
  obstetrical NEC 665.9●
    affecting fetus or newborn 763.89
  occipital (region) (scalp) 959.09
    lobe (see also Injury, intracranial)
        854.0●
  optic 950.9
    chiasm 950.1
    cortex 950.3
    nerve 950.0
    pathways 950.2
  orbit, orbital (region) 921.2
    penetrating 870.3
      with foreign body 870.4
  ovary - see Injury, internal, ovary
  paint-gun - see Wound, open, by site,
      complicated
  palate (soft) 959.09
  pancreas - see Injury, internal, pancreas
  parathyroid (gland) 959.09
  parietal (region) (scalp) 959.09
    lobe - see Injury, intracranial
  pelvic
    floor 959.19
      complicating delivery 664.1●
        affecting fetus or newborn
            763.89
    joint or ligament, complicating
        delivery 665.6●
      affecting fetus or newborn
          763.89
    organs - see also Injury, internal,
        pelvis
      with
        abortion - see Abortion, by
            type, with damage to
            pelvic organs
        ectopic pregnancy (see also
            categories 633.0–633.9)
            639.2
        molar pregnancy (see also
            categories 633.0–633.9)
            639.2
      following
        abortion 639.2
        ectopic or molar pregnancy
            639.2
      obstetrical trauma 665.5●
        affecting fetus or newborn
            763.89
  pelvis 959.19
  penis 959.14
    fracture of corpus cavernosum
        959.13
  perineum 959.14
  peritoneum - see Injury, internal,
      peritoneum

Injury (Continued)
  periurethral tissue
    with
      abortion - see Abortion, by type,
          with damage to pelvic
          organs
      ectopic pregnancy (see also
          categories 633.0–633.9) 639.2
      molar pregnancy (see also
          categories 630–632) 639.2
    complicating delivery 665.5●
      affecting fetus or newborn 763.89
    following
      abortion 639.2
      ectopic or molar pregnancy
          639.2
  phalanges
    foot 959.7
    hand 959.5
  pharynx 959.09
  pleura - see Injury, internal, pleura
  popliteal space 959.7
  post-cardiac surgery (syndrome)
      429.4
  prepuce 959.14
  prostate - see Injury, internal, prostate
  pubic region 959.19
  pudenda 959.14
  radiation NEC 990
  radioactive substance or radium NEC
      990
  rectovaginal septum 959.14
  rectum - see Injury, internal, rectum
  retina 921.3
    penetrating - see Injury, eyeball,
        penetrating
  retroperitoneal - see Injury, internal,
      retroperitoneum
  roentgen rays NEC 990
  round ligament - see Injury, internal,
      round ligament
  sacral (region) 959.19
    plexus 953.5
  sacroiliac ligament NEC 959.19
  sacrum 959.19
  salivary ducts or glands 959.09
  scalp 959.09
    due to birth trauma 767.19
    fetus or newborn 767.19
  scapular region 959.2
  sclera 921.3
    penetrating - see Injury, eyeball,
        penetrating
    superficial 918.2
  scrotum 959.14
  seminal vesicle - see Injury, internal,
      seminal vesicle
  shoulder (and upper arm) 959.2
  sinus
    cavernous (see also Injury,
        intracranial) 854.0●
    nasal 959.09
  skeleton NEC, birth injury 767.3
  skin NEC 959.9
  skull - see Fracture, skull, by site
  soft tissue (of external sites) (severe) -
      see Wound, open, by site
  specified site NEC 959.8
  spermatic cord - see Injury, internal,
      spermatic cord
  spinal (cord) 952.9
    with fracture, vertebra - see Fracture,
        vertebra, by site, with spinal
        cord injury

Injury (Continued)
  spinal (Continued)
    cervical (C₁–C₄) 952.00
      with
        anterior cord syndrome 952.02
        central cord syndrome 952.03
        complete lesion of cord 952.01
        incomplete lesion NEC 952.04
        posterior cord syndrome
            952.04
      C₅–C₇ level 952.05
        with
          anterior cord syndrome
              952.07
          central cord syndrome
              952.08
          complete lesion of cord
              952.06
          incomplete lesion NEC
              952.09
          posterior cord syndrome
              952.09
        specified type NEC 952.09
      specified type NEC 952.04
    dorsal (D₁–D₆) (T₁–T₆) (thoracic)
        952.10
      with
        anterior cord syndrome
            952.12
        central cord syndrome
            952.13
        complete lesion of cord
            952.11
        incomplete lesion NEC
            952.14
        posterior cord syndrome
            952.14
      D₇–D₁₂ level (T₇–T₁₂) 952.15
        with
          anterior cord syndrome
              952.17
          central cord syndrome
              952.18
          complete lesion of cord
              952.16
          incomplete lesion NEC
              952.19
          posterior cord syndrome
              952.19
        specified type NEC 952.19
      specified type NEC 952.14
    lumbar 952.2
    multiple sites 952.8
    nerve (root) NEC - see Injury, nerve,
        spinal, root
    plexus 953.9
      brachial 953.4
      lumbosacral 953.5
      multiple sites 953.8
    sacral 952.3
    thoracic (see also Injury, spinal,
        dorsal) 952.10
  spleen - see Injury, internal, spleen
  stellate ganglion 954.1
  sternal region 959.11
  stomach - see Injury, internal, stomach
  subconjunctival 921.1
  subcutaneous 959.9
  subdural - see Injury, intracranial
  submaxillary region 959.09
  submental region 959.09
  subungual
    fingers 959.5
    toes 959.7

◄ New   ◄▥ Revised   deleted Deleted   ● Use Additional Digit(s)   ▧ Omit code

Injury *(Continued)*
  superficial 919

> **Note 49** Use the following fourth-digit subdivisions with categories 910–919:
>
> .0 abrasion or friction burn without mention of infection
> .1 abrasion or friction burn, infected
> .2 blister without mention of infection
> .3 blister, infected
> .4 insect bite, nonvenomous, without mention of infection
> .5 insect bite, nonvenomous, infected
> .6 superficial foreign body (splinter) without major open wound and without mention of infection
> .7 superficial foreign body (splinter) without major open wound, infected
> .8 other and unspecified superficial injury without mention of infection
> .9 other and unspecified superficial injury, infected
>
> For late effects of superficial injury, *see* category 906.2.

    abdomen, abdominal (muscle) (wall) (and other part(s) of trunk) 911
    ankle (and hip, knee, leg, or thigh) 916
    anus (and other part(s) of trunk) 911
    arm 913
      upper (and shoulder) 912
    auditory canal (external) (meatus) (and other part(s) of face, neck, or scalp, except eye) 910
    axilla (and upper arm) 912
    back (and other part(s) of trunk) 911
    breast (and other part(s) of trunk) 911
    brow (and other part(s) of face, neck, or scalp, except eye) 910
    buttock (and other part(s) of trunk) 911
    canthus, eye 918.0
    cheek(s) (and other part(s) of face, neck, or scalp, except eye) 910
    chest wall (and other part(s) of trunk) 911
    chin (and other part(s) of face, neck, or scalp, except eye) 910
    clitoris (and other part(s) of trunk) 911
    conjunctiva 918.2
    cornea 918.1
      due to contact lens 371.82
    costal region (and other part(s) of trunk) 911
    ear(s) (auricle) (canal) (drum) (external) (and other part(s) of face, neck, or scalp, except eye) 910
    elbow (and forearm) (and wrist) 913

Injury *(Continued)*
  superficial *(Continued)*
    epididymis (and other part(s) of trunk) 911
    epigastric region (and other part(s) of trunk) 911
    epiglottis (and other part(s) of face, neck, or scalp, except eye) 910
    eye(s) (and adnexa) NEC 918.9
    eyelid(s) (and periocular area) 918.0
    face (any part(s), except eye) (and neck or scalp) 910
    finger(s) (nail) (any) 915
    flank (and other part(s) of trunk) 911
    foot (phalanges) (and toe(s)) 917
    forearm (and elbow) (and wrist) 913
    forehead (and other part(s) of face, neck, or scalp, except eye) 910
    globe (eye) 918.9
    groin (and other part(s) of trunk) 911
    gum(s) (and other part(s) of face, neck, or scalp, except eye) 910
    hand(s) (except fingers alone) 914
    head (and other part(s) of face, neck, or scalp, except eye) 910
    heel (and foot or toe) 917
    hip (and ankle, knee, leg, or thigh) 916
    iliac region (and other part(s) of trunk) 911
    interscapular region (and other part(s) of trunk) 911
    iris 918.9
    knee (and ankle, hip, leg, or thigh) 916
    labium (majus) (minus) (and other part(s) of trunk) 911
    lacrimal (apparatus) (gland) (sac) 918.0
    leg (lower) (upper) (and ankle, hip, knee, or thigh) 916
    lip(s) (and other part(s) of face, neck, or scalp, except eye) 910
    lower extremity (except foot) 916
    lumbar region (and other part(s) of trunk) 911
    malar region (and other part(s) of face, neck, or scalp, except eye) 910
    mastoid region (and other part(s) of face, neck, or scalp, except eye) 910
    midthoracic region (and other part(s) of trunk) 911
    mouth (and other part(s) of face, neck, or scalp, except eye) 910
    multiple sites (not classifiable to the same three-digit category) 919
    nasal (septum) (and other part(s) of face, neck, or scalp, except eye) 910
    neck (and face or scalp, any part(s), except eye) 910
    nose (septum) (and other part(s) of face, neck, or scalp, except eye) 910
    occipital region (and other part(s) of face, neck, or scalp, except eye) 910
    orbital region 918.0
    palate (soft) (and other part(s) of face, neck, or scalp, except eye) 910

Injury *(Continued)*
  superficial *(Continued)*
    parietal region (and other part(s) of face, neck, or scalp, except eye) 910
    penis (and other part(s) of trunk) 911
    perineum (and other part(s) of trunk) 911
    periocular area 918.0
    pharynx (and other part(s) of face, neck, or scalp, except eye) 910
    popliteal space (and ankle, hip, leg, or thigh) 916
    prepuce (and other part(s) of trunk) 911
    pubic region (and other part(s) of trunk) 911
    pudenda (and other part(s) of trunk) 911
    sacral region (and other part(s) of trunk) 911
    salivary (ducts) (glands) (and other part(s) of face, neck, or scalp, except eye) 910
    scalp (and other part(s) of face or neck, except eye) 910
    scapular region (and upper arm) 912
    sclera 918.2
    scrotum (and other part(s) of trunk) 911
    shoulder (and upper arm) 912
    skin NEC 919
    specified site(s) NEC 919
    sternal region (and other part(s) of trunk) 911
    subconjunctival 918.2
    subcutaneous NEC 919
    submaxillary region (and other part(s) of face, neck, or scalp, except eye) 910
    submental region (and other part(s) of face, neck, or scalp, except eye) 910
    supraclavicular fossa (and other part(s) of face, neck, or scalp, except eye) 910
    supraorbital 918.0
    temple (and other part(s) of face, neck, or scalp, except eye) 910
    temporal region (and other part(s) of face, neck, or scalp, except eye) 910
    testis (and other part(s) of trunk) 911
    thigh (and ankle, hip, knee, or leg) 916
    thorax, thoracic (external) (and other part(s) of trunk) 911
    throat (and other part(s) of face, neck, or scalp, except eye) 910
    thumb(s) (nail) 915
    toe(s) (nail) (subungual) (and foot) 917
    tongue (and other part(s) of face, neck, or scalp, except eye) 910
    tooth, teeth (*see also* Abrasion, dental) 521.20
    trunk (any part(s)) 911
    tunica vaginalis (and other part(s) of trunk) 911
    tympanum, tympanic membrane (and other part(s) of face, neck, or scalp, except eye) 910
    upper extremity NEC 913

Injury *(Continued)*
 superficial *(Continued)*
  uvula (and other part(s) of face, neck, or scalp, except eye) 910
  vagina (and other part(s) of trunk) 911
  vulva (and other part(s) of trunk) 911
  wrist (and elbow) (and forearm) 913
 supraclavicular fossa 959.19
 supraorbital 959.09
 surgical complication (external or internal site) 998.2
 symphysis pubis 959.19
  complicating delivery 665.6●
   affecting fetus or newborn 763.89
 temple 959.09
 temporal region 959.09
 testis 959.14
 thigh (and hip) 959.6
 thorax, thoracic (external) 959.11
  cavity - *see* Injury, internal, thorax
  internal - *see* Injury, internal, intrathoracic organs
 throat 959.09
 thumb(s) (nail) 959.5
 thymus - *see* Injury, internal, thymus
 thyroid (gland) 959.09
 toe (nail) (any) 959.7
 tongue 959.09
 tonsil 959.09
 tooth NEC 873.63
  complicated 873.73
 trachea - *see* Injury, internal, trachea
 trunk 959.19
 tunica vaginalis 959.14
 tympanum, tympanic membrane 959.09
 ultraviolet rays NEC 990
 ureter - *see* Injury, internal, ureter
 urethra (sphincter) - *see* Injury, internal, urethra
 uterus - *see* Injury, internal, uterus
 uvula 959.09
 vagina 959.14
 vascular - *see* Injury, blood vessel
 vas deferens - *see* Injury, internal, vas deferens
 vein (*see also* Injury, blood vessel, by site) 904.9
 vena cava
  inferior 902.10
  superior 901.2
 vesical (sphincter) - *see* Injury, internal, vesical
 viscera (abdominal) - *see* Injury, internal, viscera
  with fracture, pelvis - *see* Fracture, pelvis
 visual 950.9
  cortex 950.3
 vitreous (humor) 871.2
 vulva 959.14
 whiplash (cervical spine) 847.0
 wringer - *see* Crush, by site
 wrist (and elbow) (and forearm) 959.3
 x-ray NEC 990
Inoculation - *see also* Vaccination
 complication or reaction - *see* Complication, vaccination
INPH (idiopathic normal pressure hydrocephalus) 331.5

Insanity, insane (*see also* Psychosis) 298.9
 adolescent (*see also* Schizophrenia) 295.9●
 alternating (*see also* Psychosis, affective, circular) 296.7
 confusional 298.9
  acute 293.0
  subacute 293.1
 delusional 298.9
 paralysis, general 094.1
  progressive 094.1
 paresis, general 094.1
 senile 290.20
Insect
 bite - *see* Injury, superficial, by site
 venomous, poisoning by 989.5
Insemination, artificial V26.1
Insensitivity
 adrenocorticotropin hormone (ACTH) 255.41
 androgen 259.50
  complete 259.51
  partial 259.52
Insertion
 cord (umbilical) lateral or velamentous 663.8●
  affecting fetus or newborn 762.6
 intrauterine contraceptive device V25.1
 placenta, vicious - *see* Placenta, previa
 subdermal implantable contraceptive V25.5
 velamentous, umbilical cord 663.8●
  affecting fetus or newborn 762.6
Insolation 992.0
 meaning sunstroke 992.0
Insomnia, unspecified 780.52
 with sleep apnea, unspecified 780.51
 adjustment 307.41
 alcohol induced 291.82
 behavioral, of childhood V69.5
 drug induced 292.85
 due to
  medical condition classified elsewhere 327.01
  mental disorder 327.02
 fatal familial (FFI) 046.72
 idiopathic 307.42
 nonorganic origin 307.41
  persistent (primary) 307.42
  transient 307.41
 organic 327.00
  other 327.09
 paradoxical 307.42
 primary 307.42
 psychophysiological 307.42
 subjective complaint 307.49
Inspiration
 food or foreign body (*see also* Asphyxia, food or foreign body) 933.1
 mucus (*see also* Asphyxia, mucus) 933.1
Inspissated bile syndrome, newborn 774.4
Instability
 detrusor 596.59
 emotional (excessive) 301.3
 joint (posttraumatic) 718.80
  ankle 718.87
  elbow 718.82
  foot 718.87
  hand 718.84
  hip 718.85
  knee 718.86
  lumbosacral 724.6
  multiple sites 718.89
  pelvic region 718.85

Instability *(Continued)*
 joint *(Continued)*
  sacroiliac 724.6
  shoulder (region) 718.81
  specified site NEC 718.88
  wrist 718.83
 lumbosacral 724.6
 nervous 301.89
 personality (emotional) 301.59
 thyroid, paroxysmal 242.9●
 urethral 599.83
 vasomotor 780.2
Insufficiency, insufficient
 accommodation 367.4
 adrenal (gland) (acute) (chronic) 255.41
  medulla 255.5
  primary 255.41
  specified site NEC 255.5
 adrenocortical 255.41
 anterior (occlusal) guidance 524.54
 anus 569.49
 aortic (valve) 424.1
  with
   mitral (valve) disease 396.1
    insufficiency, incompetence, or regurgitation 396.3
    stenosis or obstruction 396.1
   stenosis or obstruction 424.1
    with mitral (valve) disease 396.8
  congenital 746.4
  rheumatic 395.1
   with
    mitral (valve) disease 396.1
     insufficiency, incompetence, or regurgitation 396.3
     stenosis or obstruction 396.1
    stenosis or obstruction 395.2
     with mitral (valve) disease 396.8
  specified cause NEC 424.1
  syphilitic 093.22
 arterial 447.1
  basilar artery 435.0
  carotid artery 435.8
  cerebral 437.1
  coronary (acute or subacute) 411.89
  mesenteric 557.1
  peripheral 443.9
  precerebral 435.9
  vertebral artery 435.1
  vertebrobasilar 435.3
 arteriovenous 459.9
 basilar artery 435.0
 biliary 575.8
 cardiac (*see also* Insufficiency, myocardial) 428.0
  complicating surgery 997.1
  due to presence of (cardiac) prosthesis 429.4
  postoperative 997.1
   long-term effect of cardiac surgery 429.4
  specified during or due to a procedure 997.1
   long-term effect of cardiac surgery 429.4
 cardiorenal (*see also* Hypertension, cardiorenal) 404.90
 cardiovascular (*see also* Disease, cardiovascular) 429.2
  renal (*see also* Hypertension, cardiorenal) 404.90
 carotid artery 435.8

◀ New   ◀▥ Revised   ~~deleted~~ Deleted   ● Use Additional Digit(s)   ▨ Omit code

Insufficiency, insufficient (Continued)
cerebral (vascular) 437.9
cerebrovascular 437.9
with transient focal neurological
signs and symptoms 435.9
acute 437.1
with transient focal neurological
signs and symptoms 435.9
circulatory NEC 459.9
fetus or newborn 779.89
convergence 378.83
coronary (acute or subacute) 411.89
chronic or with a stated duration of
over 8 weeks 414.8
corticoadrenal 255.41
dietary 269.9
divergence 378.85
food 994.2
gastroesophageal 530.89
gonadal
ovary 256.39
testis 257.2
gonadotropic hormone secretion 253.4
heart - see also Insufficiency, myocardial
fetus or newborn 779.89
valve (see also Endocarditis) 424.90
congenital NEC 746.89
hepatic 573.8
idiopathic autonomic 333.0
interocclusal distance of teeth (ridge)
524.36
kidney
acute 593.9
chronic 585.9
labyrinth, labyrinthine (function)
386.53
bilateral 386.54
unilateral 386.53
lacrimal 375.15
liver 573.8
lung (acute) (see also Insufficiency,
pulmonary) 518.82
following trauma, surgery, or shock
518.5
newborn 770.89
mental (congenital) (see also
Retardation, mental) 319
mesenteric 557.1
mitral (valve) 424.0
with
aortic (valve) disease 396.3
insufficiency, incompetence, or
regurgitation 396.3
stenosis or obstruction 396.2
obstruction or stenosis 394.2
with aortic valve disease 396.8
congenital 746.6
rheumatic 394.1
with
aortic (valve) disease 396.3
insufficiency, incompetence,
or regurgitation 396.3
stenosis or obstruction 396.2
obstruction or stenosis 394.2
with aortic valve disease
396.8
active or acute 391.1
with chorea, rheumatic
(Sydenham's) 392.0
specified cause, except rheumatic
424.0
muscle
heart - see Insufficiency, myocardial
ocular (see also Strabismus) 378.9

Insufficiency, insufficient (Continued)
myocardial, myocardium (with
arteriosclerosis) 428.0
with rheumatic fever (conditions
classifiable to 390)
active, acute, or subacute 391.2
with chorea 392.0
inactive or quiescent (with
chorea) 398.0
congenital 746.89
due to presence of (cardiac)
prosthesis 429.4
fetus or newborn 779.89
following cardiac surgery 429.4
hypertensive (see also Hypertension,
heart) 402.91
benign 402.11
malignant 402.01
postoperative 997.1
long-term effect of cardiac
surgery 429.4
rheumatic 398.0
active, acute, or subacute 391.2
with chorea (Sydenham's)
392.0
syphilitic 093.82
nourishment 994.2
organic 799.89
ovary 256.39
postablative 256.2
pancreatic 577.8
parathyroid (gland) 252.1
peripheral vascular (arterial) 443.9
pituitary (anterior) 253.2
posterior 253.5
placental - see Placenta, insufficiency
platelets 287.5
prenatal care in current pregnancy
V23.7
progressive pluriglandular 258.9
pseudocholinesterase 289.89
pulmonary (acute) 518.82
following
shock 518.5
surgery 518.5
trauma 518.5
newborn 770.89
valve (see also Endocarditis,
pulmonary) 424.3
congenital 746.09
pyloric 537.0
renal 593.9
acute 593.9
chronic 585.9
due to a procedure 997.5
respiratory 786.09
acute 518.82
following shock, surgery, or
trauma 518.5
newborn 770.89
rotation - see Malrotation
suprarenal 255.41
medulla 255.5
tarso-orbital fascia, congenital 743.66
tear film 375.15
testis 257.2
thyroid (gland) (acquired) - see also
Hypothyroidism
congenital 243
tricuspid (see also Endocarditis,
tricuspid) 397.0
congenital 746.89
syphilitic 093.23
urethral sphincter 599.84

Insufficiency, insufficient (Continued)
valve, valvular (heart) (see also
Endocarditis) 424.90
vascular 459.9
intestine NEC 557.9
mesenteric 557.1
peripheral 443.9
renal (see also Hypertension, kidney)
403.90
velopharyngeal
acquired 528.9
congenital 750.29
venous (peripheral) 459.81
ventricular - see Insufficiency,
myocardial
vertebral artery 435.1
vertebrobasilar artery 435.3
weight gain during pregnancy
646.8●
zinc 269.3
Insufflation
fallopian
fertility testing V26.21
following sterilization reversal
V26.22
meconium 770.11
with respiratory symptoms 770.12
Insular - see condition
Insulinoma (M8151/0)
malignant (M8151/3)
pancreas 157.4
specified site - see Neoplasm, by site,
malignant
unspecified site 157.4
pancreas 211.7
specified site - see Neoplasm, by site,
benign
unspecified site 211.7
Insuloma - see Insulinoma
Insult
brain 437.9
acute 436
cerebral 437.9
acute 436
cerebrovascular 437.9
acute 436
vascular NEC 437.9
acute 436
Insurance examination (certification)
V70.3
Intemperance (see also Alcoholism)
303.9●
Interception of pregnancy (menstrual
extraction) V25.3
Interference
balancing side 524.56
non-working side 524.56
Intermenstrual
bleeding 626.6
irregular 626.6
regular 626.5
hemorrhage 626.6
irregular 626.6
regular 626.5
pain(s) 625.2
Intermittent - see condition
Internal - see condition
Interproximal wear 521.10
Interruption
aortic arch 747.11
bundle of His 426.50
fallopian tube (for sterilization) V25.2
phase-shift, sleep cycle 307.45
repeated REM-sleep 307.48

Interruption *(Continued)*
  sleep
    due to perceived environmental
      disturbances 307.48
    phase-shift, of 24-hour sleep-wake
      cycle 307.45
    repeated REM-sleep type 307.48
  vas deferens (for sterilization) V25.2
Intersexuality 752.7
Interstitial - *see* condition
Intertrigo 695.89
  labialis 528.5
Intervertebral disc - *see* condition
Intestine, intestinal - *see also* condition
  flu 487.8
Intolerance
  carbohydrate NEC 579.8
  cardiovascular exercise, with pain (at
    rest) (with less than ordinary
    activity) (with ordinary activity)
    V47.2
  cold 780.99
  dissacharide (hereditary) 271.3
  drug
    correct substance properly
      administered 995.27
    wrong substance given or taken in
      error 977.9
    specified drug - *see* Table of
      Drugs and Chemicals
  effort 306.2
  fat NEC 579.8
  foods NEC 579.8
  fructose (hereditary) 271.2
  glucose (-galactose) (congenital) 271.3
  gluten 579.0
  lactose (hereditary) (infantile) 271.3
  lysine (congenital) 270.7
  milk NEC 579.8
  protein (familial) 270.7
  starch NEC 579.8
  sucrose (-isomaltose) (congenital) 271.3
Intoxicated NEC *(see also* Alcoholism)
  305.0●
Intoxication
  acid 276.2
  acute
    alcoholic 305.0●
      with alcoholism 303.0●
      hangover effects 305.0●
    caffeine 305.9●
    hallucinogenic *(see also* Abuse,
      drugs, nondependent) 305.3●
  alcohol (acute) 305.0●
    with alcoholism 303.0●
    hangover effects 305.0●
    idiosyncratic 291.4
    pathological 291.4
  alimentary canal 558.2
  ammonia (hepatic) 572.2
  caffeine 305.9●
  chemical - *see also* Table of Drugs and
    Chemicals
    via placenta or breast milk 760.70
      alcohol 760.71
      anticonvulsants 760.77
      antifungals 760.74
      anti-infective agents 760.74
      antimetabolics 760.78
      cocaine 760.75
      "crack" 760.75
      hallucinogenic agents NEC 760.73
      medicinal agents NEC 760.79
      narcotics 760.72

Intoxication *(Continued)*
  chemical *(Continued)*
    via placenta or breast milk
      (Continued)
      obstetric anesthetic or analgesic
        drug 763.5
      specified agent NEC 760.79
      suspected, affecting
        management of
          pregnancy 655.5●
    cocaine, through placenta or breast
      milk 760.75
  delirium
    alcohol 291.0
    drug 292.81
  drug 292.89
    with delirium 292.81
    correct substance properly
      administered *(see also* Allergy,
        drug) 995.27
    newborn 779.4
    obstetric anesthetic or sedation
      668.9●
      affecting fetus or newborn 763.5
    overdose or wrong substance given
      or taken - *see* Table of Drugs
      and Chemicals
    pathologic 292.2
    specific to newborn 779.4
    via placenta or breast milk 760.70
      alcohol 760.71
      anticonvulsants 760.77
      antifungals 760.74
      anti-infective agents 760.74
      antimetabolics 760.78
      cocaine 760.75
      "crack" 760.75
      hallucinogenic agents 760.73
      medicinal agents NEC 760.79
      narcotics 760.72
      obstetric anesthetic or analgesic
        drug 763.5
      specified agent NEC 760.79
      suspected, affecting
        management of
          pregnancy 655.5●
  enteric - *see* Intoxication, intestinal
  fetus or newborn, via placenta or breast
    milk 760.70
    alcohol 760.71
    anticonvulsants 760.77
    antifungals 760.74
    anti-infective agents 760.74
    antimetabolics 760.78
    cocaine 760.75
    "crack" 760.75
    hallucinogenic agents 760.73
    medicinal agents NEC 760.79
    narcotics 760.72
    obstetric anesthetic or analgesic
      drug 763.5
    specified agent NEC 760.79
    suspected, affecting management of
      pregnancy 655.5●
  food - *see* Poisoning, food
  gastrointestinal 558.2
  hallucinogenic (acute) 305.3●
  hepatocerebral 572.2
  idiosyncratic alcohol 291.4
  intestinal 569.89
    due to putrefaction of food 005.9
  methyl alcohol *(see also* Alcoholism)
    305.0●
    with alcoholism 303.0●

Intoxication *(Continued)*
  non-foodborne due to toxins of
    Clostridium botulinum [C.
    botulinum] - *see* Botulism
  pathologic 291.4
    drug 292.2
  potassium (K) 276.7
  septic
    with
      abortion - *see* Abortion, by type,
        with sepsis
      ectopic pregnancy *(see also*
        categories 633.0–633.9) 639.0
      molar pregnancy *(see also*
        categories 630–632) 639.0
    during labor 659.3●
    following
      abortion 639.0
      ectopic or molar pregnancy 639.0
    generalized - *see* Septicemia
    puerperal, postpartum,
      childbirth 670.2   ◀▥
  serum (prophylactic) (therapeutic)
    999.5
  uremic - *see* Uremia
  water 276.6
Intracranial - *see* condition
Intrahepatic gallbladder 751.69
Intraligamentous - *see also* condition
  pregnancy - *see* Pregnancy, cornual
Intraocular - *see also* condition
  sepsis 360.00
Intrathoracic - *see also* condition
  kidney 753.3
  stomach - *see* Hernia, diaphragm
Intrauterine contraceptive device
  checking V25.42
  insertion V25.1
  in situ V45.51
  management V25.42
  prescription V25.02
    repeat V25.42
  reinsertion V25.42
  removal V25.42
Intraventricular - *see* condition
Intrinsic deformity - *see* Deformity
Intruded tooth 524.34
Intrusion, repetitive, of sleep (due to
    environmental disturbances) (with
    atypical polysomnographic features)
    307.48
Intumescent, lens (eye) NEC 366.9
  senile 366.12
Intussusception (colon) (enteric)
    (intestine) (rectum) 560.0
  appendix 543.9
  congenital 751.5
  fallopian tube 620.8
  ileocecal 560.0
  ileocolic 560.0
  ureter (obstruction) 593.4
Invagination
  basilar 756.0
  colon or intestine 560.0
Invalid (since birth) 799.89
Invalidism (chronic) 799.89
Inversion
  albumin-globulin (A-G) ratio 273.8
  bladder 596.8
  cecum *(see also* Intussusception) 560.0
  cervix 622.8
  nipple 611.79
    congenital 757.6
    puerperal, postpartum 676.3●

◀ New   ◀▥ Revised   ~~deleted~~ Deleted   ● Use Additional Digit(s)   ▨ Omit code

Inversion *(Continued)*
　　optic papilla 743.57
　　organ or site, congenital NEC - *see*
　　　　Anomaly, specified type NEC
　　sleep rhythm 327.39
　　　　nonorganic origin 307.45
　　testis (congenital) 752.51
　　uterus (postinfectional) (postpartal,
　　　　old) 621.7
　　　　chronic 621.7
　　　　complicating delivery 665.2●
　　　　　　affecting fetus or newborn 763.89
　　vagina - *see* Prolapse, vagina
Investigation
　　allergens V72.7
　　clinical research (control) (normal
　　　　comparison) (participant) V70.7
Inviability - *see* Immaturity
Involuntary movement, abnormal 781.0
Involution, involutional - *see also*
　　　　condition
　　breast, cystic or fibrocystic 610.1
　　depression *(see also* Psychosis, affective)
　　　　296.2●
　　　　recurrent episode 296.3●
　　　　single episode 296.2●
　　melancholia *(see also* Psychosis,
　　　　affective) 296.2●
　　　　recurrent episode 296.3●
　　　　single episode 296.2●
　　ovary, senile 620.3
　　paranoid state (reaction) 297.2
　　paraphrenia (climacteric) (menopause)
　　　　297.2
　　psychosis 298.8
　　thymus failure 254.8
IQ
　　under 20 318.2
　　20–34 318.1
　　35–49 318.0
　　50–70 317
IRDS 769
Irideremia 743.45
Iridis rubeosis 364.42
　　diabetic 250.5● *[364.42]*
　　　　due to secondary diabetes 249.5●
　　　　　　[364.42]
Iridochoroiditis (panuveitis) 360.12
Iridocyclitis NEC 364.3
　　acute 364.00
　　　　primary 364.01
　　　　recurrent 364.02
　　chronic 364.10
　　　　in
　　　　　　lepromatous leprosy 030.0
　　　　　　　　[364.11]
　　　　　　sarcoidosis 135 *[364.11]*
　　　　　　tuberculosis *(see also* Tuberculosis)
　　　　　　　　017.3● *[364.11]*
　　due to allergy 364.04
　　endogenous 364.01
　　gonococcal 098.41
　　granulomatous 364.10
　　herpetic (simplex) 054.44
　　　　zoster 053.22
　　hypopyon 364.05
　　lens induced 364.23
　　nongranulomatous 364.00
　　primary 364.01
　　recurrent 364.02
　　rheumatic 364.10
　　secondary 364.04
　　　　infectious 364.03
　　　　noninfectious 364.04

Iridocyclitis NEC *(Continued)*
　　subacute 364.00
　　　　primary 364.01
　　　　recurrent 364.02
　　sympathetic 360.11
　　syphilitic (secondary) 091.52
　　tuberculous (chronic) *(see also*
　　　　Tuberculosis) 017.3● *[364.11]*
Iridocyclochoroiditis (panuveitis)
　　360.12
Iridodialysis 364.76
Iridodonesis 364.89
Iridoplegia (complete) (partial) (reflex)
　　379.49
Iridoschisis 364.52
Iris - *see* condition
Iritis 364.3
　　acute 364.00
　　　　primary 364.01
　　　　recurrent 364.02
　　chronic 364.10
　　　　in
　　　　　　sarcoidosis 135 *[364.11]*
　　　　　　tuberculosis *(see also*
　　　　　　　　Tuberculosis) 017.3●
　　　　　　　　[364.11]
　　diabetic 250.5● *[364.42]*
　　　　due to secondary diabetes 249.5●
　　　　　　[364.42]
　　due to
　　　　allergy 364.04
　　　　herpes simplex 054.44
　　　　leprosy 030.0 *[364.11]*
　　endogenous 364.01
　　gonococcal 098.41
　　gouty 274.89 *[364.11]*
　　granulomatous 364.10
　　hypopyon 364.05
　　lens induced 364.23
　　nongranulomatous 364.00
　　papulosa 095.8 *[364.11]*
　　primary 364.01
　　recurrent 364.02
　　rheumatic 364.10
　　secondary 364.04
　　　　infectious 364.03
　　　　noninfectious 364.04
　　subacute 364.00
　　　　primary 364.01
　　　　recurrent 364.02
　　sympathetic 360.11
　　syphilitic (secondary) 091.52
　　　　congenital 090.0 *[364.11]*
　　　　late 095.8 *[364.11]*
　　tuberculous *(see also* Tuberculosis)
　　　　017.3● *[364.11]*
　　uratic 274.89 *[364.11]*
Iron
　　deficiency anemia 280.9
　　metabolism disease 275.0
　　storage disease 275.0
Iron-miners' lung 503
Irradiated enamel (tooth, teeth) 521.89
Irradiation
　　burn - *see* Burn, by site
　　effects, adverse 990
Irreducible, irreducibility - *see*
　　　　condition
Irregular, irregularity
　　action, heart 427.9
　　alveolar process 525.8
　　bleeding NEC 626.4
　　breathing 786.09
　　colon 569.89

Irregular, irregularity *(Continued)*
　　contour
　　　　of cornea 743.41
　　　　　　acquired 371.70
　　　　reconstructed breast 612.0
　　dentin in pulp 522.3
　　eye movements NEC 379.59
　　menstruation (cause unknown) 626.4
　　periods 626.4
　　prostate 602.9
　　pupil 364.75
　　respiratory 786.09
　　septum (nasal) 470
　　shape, organ or site, congenital NEC -
　　　　see Distortion
　　sleep-wake rhythm (non-24-hour)
　　　　327.39
　　　　nonorganic origin 307.45
　　vertebra 733.99
Irritability ~~(nervous)~~ 799.22　　　◄▥
　　bladder 596.8
　　　　neurogenic 596.54
　　　　　　with cauda equina syndrome
　　　　　　　　344.61
　　bowel (syndrome) 564.1
　　bronchial *(see also* Bronchitis) 490
　　cerebral, newborn 779.1
　　colon 564.1
　　　　psychogenic 306.4
　　duodenum 564.89
　　heart (psychogenic) 306.2
　　ileum 564.89
　　jejunum 564.89
　　myocardium 306.2
　　nervousness 799.21　　　　　　◄
　　rectum 564.89
　　stomach 536.9
　　　　psychogenic 306.4
　　sympathetic (nervous system) *(see also*
　　　　Neuropathy, peripheral,
　　　　autonomic) 337.9
　　urethra 599.84
　　ventricular (heart) (psychogenic) 306.2
Irritable *(see also* Irritability) 799.22　◄▥
Irritation
　　anus 569.49
　　axillary nerve 353.0
　　bladder 596.8
　　brachial plexus 353.0
　　brain (traumatic) *(see also* Injury,
　　　　intracranial) 854.0●
　　　　nontraumatic - *see* Encephalitis
　　bronchial *(see also* Bronchitis) 490
　　cerebral (traumatic) *(see also* Injury,
　　　　intracranial) 854.0●
　　　　nontraumatic - *see* Encephalitis
　　cervical plexus 353.2
　　cervix *(see also* Cervicitis) 616.0
　　choroid, sympathetic 360.11
　　cranial nerve - *see* Disorder, nerve,
　　　　cranial
　　digestive tract 536.9
　　　　psychogenic 306.4
　　gastric 536.9
　　　　psychogenic 306.4
　　gastrointestinal (tract) 536.9
　　　　functional 536.9
　　　　psychogenic 306.4
　　globe, sympathetic 360.11
　　intestinal (bowel) 564.9
　　labyrinth 386.50
　　lumbosacral plexus 353.1
　　meninges (traumatic) *(see also* Injury,
　　　　intracranial) 854.0●
　　　　nontraumatic - *see* Meningitis

Irritation *(Continued)*
  myocardium 306.2
  nerve - *see* Disorder, nerve
  nervous 799.21 ◄▥
  nose 478.19
  penis 607.89
  perineum 709.9
  peripheral
    autonomic nervous system *(see also* Neuropathy, peripheral, autonomic)* 337.9
    nerve - *see* Disorder, nerve
  peritoneum *(see also* Peritonitis)* 567.9
  pharynx 478.29
  plantar nerve 355.6
  spinal (cord) (traumatic) - *see also* Injury, spinal, by site
    nerve - *see also* Disorder, nerve
    root NEC 724.9
      traumatic - *see* Injury, nerve, spinal
    nontraumatic - *see* Myelitis
  stomach 536.9
    psychogenic 306.4
  sympathetic nerve NEC *(see also* Neuropathy, peripheral, autonomic)* 337.9
  ulnar nerve 354.2
  vagina 623.9
Isambert's disease 012.3●
Ischemia, ischemic 459.9
  basilar artery (with transient neurologic deficit) 435.0
  bone NEC 733.40
  bowel (transient) 557.9
    acute 557.0
    chronic 557.1
    due to mesenteric artery insufficiency 557.1
  brain - *see also* Ischemia, cerebral
    recurrent focal 435.9
  cardiac *(see also* Ischemia, heart)* 414.9
  cardiomyopathy 414.8
  carotid artery (with transient neurologic deficit) 435.8
  cerebral (chronic) (generalized) 437.1
    arteriosclerotic 437.0
    intermittent (with transient neurologic deficit) 435.9
    newborn 779.2
    puerperal, postpartum, childbirth 674.0●
    recurrent focal (with transient neurologic deficit) 435.9
    transient (with transient neurologic deficit) 435.9
  colon 557.9
    acute 557.0
    chronic 557.1
    due to mesenteric artery insufficiency 557.1
  coronary (chronic) *(see also* Ischemia, heart)* 414.9

Ischemia, ischemic *(Continued)*
  heart (chronic or with a stated duration of over 8 weeks) 414.9
    acute or with a stated duration of 8 weeks or less *(see also* Infarct, myocardium)* 410.9●
      without myocardial infarction 411.89
        with coronary (artery) occlusion 411.81
    subacute 411.89
  intestine (transient) 557.9
    acute 557.0
    chronic 557.1
    due to mesenteric artery insufficiency 557.1
  kidney 593.81
  labyrinth 386.50
  muscles, leg 728.89
  myocardium, myocardial (chronic or with a stated duration of over 8 weeks) 414.8
    acute *(see also* Infarct, myocardium)* 410.9●
      without myocardial infarction 411.89
        with coronary (artery) occlusion 411.81
  renal 593.81
  retina, retinal 362.84
  small bowel 557.9
    acute 557.0
    chronic 557.1
    due to mesenteric artery insufficiency 557.1
  spinal cord 336.1
  subendocardial *(see also* Insufficiency, coronary)* 411.89
  vertebral artery (with transient neurologic deficit) 435.1
Ischialgia *(see also* Sciatica)* 724.3
Ischiopagus 759.4
Ischium, ischial - *see* condition
Ischomenia 626.8
Ischuria 788.5
Iselin's disease or osteochondrosis 732.5
Islands of
  parotid tissue in
    lymph nodes 750.26
    neck structures 750.26
  submaxillary glands in
    fascia 750.26
    lymph nodes 750.26
    neck muscles 750.26
Islet cell tumor, pancreas (M8150/0) 211.7
Isoimmunization NEC *(see also* Incompatibility)* 656.2●
  anti-E 656.2●
  fetus or newborn 773.2
    ABO blood groups 773.1
    Rhesus (Rh) factor 773.0

Isolation V07.0
  social V62.4
Isosporosis 007.2
Issue
  medical certificate NEC V68.09
    cause of death V68.09
    disability examination V68.01
    fitness V68.09
    incapacity V68.09
  repeat prescription NEC V68.1
    appliance V68.1
    contraceptive V25.40
      device NEC V25.49
        intrauterine V25.42
        specified type NEC V25.49
      pill V25.41
    glasses V68.1
    medicinal substance V68.1
Itch *(see also* Pruritus)* 698.9
  bakers' 692.89
  barbers' 110.0
  bricklayers' 692.89
  cheese 133.8
  clam diggers' 120.3
  coolie 126.9
  copra 133.8
  Cuban 050.1
  dew 126.9
  dhobie 110.3
  eye 379.99
  filarial *(see also* Infestation, filarial)* 125.9
  grain 133.8
  grocers' 133.8
  ground 126.9
  harvest 133.8
  jock 110.3
  Malabar 110.9
    beard 110.0
    foot 110.4
    scalp 110.0
  meaning scabies 133.0
  Norwegian 133.0
  perianal 698.0
  poultrymen's 133.8
  sarcoptic 133.0
  scrub 134..1
  seven year V61.10
    meaning scabies 133.0
  straw 133.8
  swimmers' 120.3
  washerwoman's 692.4
  water 120.3
  winter 698.8
Itsenko-Cushing syndrome (pituitary basophilism) 255.0
Ivemark's syndrome (asplenia with congenital heart disease) 759.0
Ivory bones 756.52
Ixodes 134.8
Ixodiasis 134.8

◄ New   ◄▥ Revised   ~~deleted~~ Deleted   ● Use Additional Digit(s)   ▨ Omit code

J

Jaccoud's nodular fibrositis, chronic (Jaccoud's syndrome) 714.4
Jackson's
  membrane 751.4
  paralysis or syndrome 344.89
  veil 751.4
Jacksonian
  epilepsy (*see also* Epilepsy) 345.5●
  seizures (focal) (*see also* Epilepsy) 345.5●
Jacob's ulcer (M8090/3) - *see* Neoplasm, skin, malignant, by site
Jacquet's dermatitis (diaper dermatitis) 691.0
Jadassohn's
  blue nevus (M8780/0) - *see* Neoplasm, skin, benign
  disease (maculopapular erythroderma) 696.2
  intraepidermal epithelioma (M8096/0) - *see* Neoplasm, skin, benign
Jadassohn-Lewandowski syndrome (pachyonychia congenita) 757.5
Jadassohn-Pellizari's disease (anetoderma) 701.3
Jadassohn-Tièche nevus (M8780/0) - *see* Neoplasm, skin, benign
Jaffe-Lichtenstein (-Uehlinger) syndrome 252.01
Jahnke's syndrome (encephalocutaneous angiomatosis) 759.6
Jakob-Creutzfeldt disease (CJD) (syndrome) 046.19
  with dementia
    with behavioral disturba nce 046.19 [294.11]
    without behavioral disturbance 046.19 [294.10]
  familial 046.19
  iatrogenic 046.19
  specified NEC 046.19
  sporadic 046.19
  variant (vCJD) 046.11
    with dementia
      with behavioral disturbance 046.11 [294.11]
      without behavioral disturbance 046.11 [294.10]
Jaksch (-Luzet) disease or syndrome (pseudoleukemia infantum) 285.8
Jamaican
  neuropathy 349.82
  paraplegic tropical ataxic-spastic syndrome 349.82
Janet's disease (psychasthenia) 300.89
Janiceps 759.4
Jansky-Bielschowsky amaurotic familial idiocy 330.1
Japanese
  B-type encephalitis 062.0
  river fever 081.2
  seven-day fever 100.89
Jaundice (yellow) 782.4
  acholuric (familial) (splenomegalic) (*see also* Spherocytosis) 282.0
    acquired 283.9
  breast milk 774.39
  catarrhal (acute) 070.1
    with hepatic coma 070.0
    chronic 571.9
    epidemic - *see* Jaundice, epidemic
  cholestatic (benign) 782.4
  chronic idiopathic 277.4

Jaundice (*Continued*)
  epidemic (catarrhal) 070.1
    with hepatic coma 070.0
    leptospiral 100.0
    spirochetal 100.0
  febrile (acute) 070.1
    with hepatic coma 070.0
    leptospiral 100.0
    spirochetal 100.0
  fetus or newborn 774.6
    due to or associated with
      ABO
        antibodies 773.1
        incompatibility, maternal/fetal 773.1
        isoimmunization 773.1
      absence or deficiency of enzyme system for bilirubin conjugation (congenital) 774.39
      blood group incompatibility NEC 773.2
      breast milk inhibitors to conjugation 774.39
      associated with preterm delivery 774.2
      bruising 774.1
      Crigler-Najjar syndrome 277.4 [774.31]
      delayed conjugation 774.30
      associated with preterm delivery 774.2
      development 774.39
      drugs or toxins transmitted from mother 774.1
      G-6-PD deficiency 282.2 [774.0]
      galactosemia 271.1 [774.5]
      Gilbert's syndrome 277.4 [774.31]
      hepatocellular damage 774.4
      hereditary hemolytic anemia (*see also* Anemia, hemolytic) 282.9 [774.0]
      hypothyroidism, congenital 243 [774.31]
      incompatibility, maternal/fetal NEC 773.2
      infection 774.1
      inspissated bile syndrome 774.4
      isoimmunization NEC 773.2
      mucoviscidosis 277.01 [774.5]
      obliteration of bile duct, congenital 751.61 [774.5]
      polycythemia 774.1
      preterm delivery 774.2
      red cell defect 282.9 [774.0]
      Rh
        antibodies 773.0
        incompatibility, maternal/fetal 773.0
        isoimmunization 773.0
      spherocytosis (congenital) 282.0 [774.0]
      swallowed maternal blood 774.1
    physiological NEC 774.6
  from injection, inoculation, infusion, or transfusion (blood) (plasma) (serum) (other substance) (onset within 8 months after administration) - *see* Hepatitis, viral
  Gilbert's (familial nonhemolytic) 277.4
  hematogenous 283.9
  hemolytic (acquired) 283.9
    congenital (*see also* Spherocytosis) 282.0

Jaundice (*Continued*)
  hemorrhagic (acute) 100.0
    leptospiral 100.0
    newborn 776.0
    spirochetal 100.0
  hepatocellular 573.8
  homologous (serum) - *see* Hepatitis, viral
  idiopathic, chronic 277.4
  infectious (acute) (subacute) 070.1
    with hepatic coma 070.0
    leptospiral 100.0
    spirochetal 100.0
  leptospiral 100.0
  malignant (*see also* Necrosis, liver) 570
  newborn (physiological) (*see also* Jaundice, fetus or newborn) 774.6
  nonhemolytic, congenital familial (Gilbert's) 277.4
  nuclear, newborn (*see also* Kernicterus of newborn) 774.7
  obstructive NEC (*see also* Obstruction, biliary) 576.8
  postimmunization - *see* Hepatitis, viral
  posttransfusion - *see* Hepatitis, viral
  regurgitation (*see also* Obstruction, biliary) 576.8
  serum (homologous) (prophylactic) (therapeutic) - *see* Hepatitis, viral
  spirochetal (hemorrhagic) 100.0
  symptomatic 782.4
    newborn 774.6
Jaw - *see* condition
Jaw-blinking 374.43
  congenital 742.8
Jaw-winking phenomenon or syndrome 742.8
Jealousy
  alcoholic 291.5
  childhood 313.3
  sibling 313.3
Jejunitis (*see also* Enteritis) 558.9
Jejunostomy status V44.4
Jejunum, jejunal - *see* condition
Jensen's disease 363.05
Jericho boil 085.1
Jerks, myoclonic 333.2
Jervell-Lange-Nielsen syndrome 426.82
Jeune's disease or syndrome (asphyxiating thoracic dystrophy) 756.4
Jigger disease 134.1
Job's syndrome (chronic granulomatous disease) 288.1
Jod-Basedow phenomenon 242.8●
Johnson-Stevens disease (erythema multiforme exudativum) 695.13
Joint - *see also* condition
  Charcôt's 094.0 [713.5]
  false 733.82
  flail - *see* Flail, joint
  mice - *see* Loose, body, joint, by site
  sinus to bone 730.9●
  von Gies' 095.8
Jordan's anomaly or syndrome 288.2
Josephs-Diamond-Blackfan anemia (congenital hypoplastic) 284.01
Joubert syndrome 759.89
Jumpers' knee 727.2
Jungle yellow fever 060.0
Jungling's disease (sarcoidosis) 135
Junin virus hemorrhagic fever 078.7
Juvenile - *see also* condition
  delinquent 312.9
    group (*see also* Disturbance, conduct) 312.2●
  neurotic 312.4

K

Kabuki syndrome 759.89
Kahler (-Bozzolo) disease (multiple
   myeloma) (M9730/3) 203.0●
Kakergasia 300.9
Kakke 265.0
Kala-azar (Indian) (infantile)
   (Mediterranean) (Sudanese) 085.0
Kalischer's syndrome
   (encephalocutaneous angiomatosis)
   759.6
Kallmann's syndrome (hypogonadotropic
   hypogonadism with anosmia)
   253.4
Kanner's syndrome (autism) (see also
   Psychosis, childhood) 299.0●
Kaolinosis 502
Kaposi's
   disease 757.33
      lichen ruber 696.4
         acuminatus 696.4
         moniliformis 697.8
      xeroderma pigmentosum 757.33
   sarcoma (M9140/3) 176.9
      adipose tissue 176.1
      aponeurosis 176.1
      artery 176.1
      associated herpesvirus infection
         058.89
      blood vessel 176.1
      bursa 176.1
      connective tissue 176.1
      external genitalia 176.8
      fascia 176.1
      fatty tissue 176.1
      fibrous tissue 176.1
      gastrointestinal tract NEC 176.3
      ligament 176.1
      lung 176.4
      lymph
         gland(s) 176.5
         node(s) 176.5
      lymphatic(s) NEC 176.1
      muscle (skeletal) 176.1
      oral cavity NEC 176.8
      palate 176.2
      scrotum 176.8
      skin 176.0
      soft tissue 176.1
      specified site NEC 176.8
      subcutaneous tissue 176.1
      synovia 176.1
      tendon (sheath) 176.1
      vein 176.1
      vessel 176.1
      viscera NEC 176.9
      vulva 176.8
   varicelliform eruption 054.0
      vaccinia 999.0
Kartagener's syndrome or triad (sinusitis,
   bronchiectasis, situs inversus) 759.3
Kasabach-Merritt syndrome (capillary
   hemangioma associated with
   thrombocytopenic purpura) 287.39
Kaschin-Beck disease (endemic
   polyarthritis) - see Disease, Kaschin-
   Beck
Kast's syndrome (dyschondroplasia with
   hemangiomas) 756.4
Katatonia- see Catatonia
Katayama disease or fever 120.2
Kathisophobia 781.0
Kawasaki disease 446.1

Kayser-Fleischer ring (cornea)
   (pseudosclerosis) 275.1 [371.14]
Kaznelson's syndrome (congenital
   hypoplastic anemia) 284.01
Kearns-Sayre syndrome 277.87
Kedani fever 081.2
Kelis 701.4
Kelly (-Patterson) syndrome (sideropenic
   dysphagia) 280.8
Keloid, cheloid 701.4
   Addison's (morphea) 701.0
   cornea 371.00
   Hawkins' 701.4
   scar 701.4
Keloma 701.4
Kenya fever 082.1
Keratectasia 371.71
   congenital 743.41
Keratinization NEC
   alveolar ridge mucosa
      excessive 528.72
      minimal 528.71
Keratitis (nodular) (nonulcerative)
   (simple) (zonular) NEC 370.9
   with ulceration (see also Ulcer, cornea)
      370.00
   actinic 370.24
   arborescens 054.42
   areolar 370.22
   bullosa 370.8
   deep - see Keratitis, interstitial
   dendritic(a) 054.42
   desiccation 370.34
   diffuse interstitial 370.52
   disciform(is) 054.43
      varicella 052.7 [370.44]
   epithelialis vernalis 372.13 [370.32]
   exposure 370.34
   filamentary 370.23
   gonococcal (congenital) (prenatal)
      098.43
   herpes, herpetic (simplex) NEC 054.43
      zoster 053.21
   hypopyon 370.04
   in
      chickenpox 052.7 [370.44]
      exanthema (see also Exanthem) 057.9
         [370.44]
      paravaccinia (see also Paravaccinia)
         051.9 [370.44]
      smallpox (see also Smallpox) 050.9
         [370.44]
      vernal conjunctivitis 372.13 [370.32]
   interstitial (nonsyphilitic) 370.50
      with ulcer (see also Ulcer, cornea)
         370.00
      diffuse 370.52
      herpes, herpetic (simplex) 054.43
         zoster 053.21
      syphilitic (congenital) (hereditary)
         090.3
      tuberculous (see also Tuberculosis)
         017.3● [370.59]
   lagophthalmic 370.34
   macular 370.22
   neuroparalytic 370.35
   neurotrophic 370.35
   nummular 370.22
   oyster-shuckers' 370.8
   parenchymatous - see Keratitis,
      interstitial
   petrificans 370.8
   phlyctenular 370.31
   postmeasles 055.71

Keratitis (Continued)
   punctata, punctate 370.21
      leprosa 030.0 [370.21]
      profunda 090.3
      superficial (Thygeson's) 370.21
   purulent 370.8
   pustuliformis profunda 090.3
   rosacea 695.3 [370.49]
   sclerosing 370.54
   specified type NEC 370.8
   stellate 370.22
   striate 370.22
   superficial 370.20
      with conjunctivitis (see also
         Keratoconjunctivitis) 370.40
      punctate (Thygeson's) 370.21
   suppurative 370.8
   syphilitic (congenital) (prenatal)
      090.3
   trachomatous 076.1
      late effect 139.1
   tuberculous (phlyctenular) (see also
      Tuberculosis) 017.3● [370.31]
   ulcerated (see also Ulcer, cornea)
      370.00
   vesicular 370.8
   welders' 370.24
   xerotic (see also Keratomalacia)
      371.45
      vitamin A deficiency 264.4
Keratoacanthoma 238.2
Keratocele 371.72
Keratoconjunctivitis (see also Keratitis)
   370.40
   adenovirus type 8 077.1
   epidemic 077.1
   exposure 370.34
   gonococcal 098.43
   herpetic (simplex) 054.43
      zoster 053.21
   in
      chickenpox 052.7 [370.44]
      exanthema (see also Exanthem)
         057.9 [370.44]
      paravaccinia (see also Paravaccinia)
         051.9 [370.44]
      smallpox (see also Smallpox) 050.9
         [370.44]
   infectious 077.1
   neurotrophic 370.35
   phlyctenular 370.31
   postmeasles 055.71
   shipyard 077.1
   sicca (Sjögren's syndrome) 710.2
      not in Sjögren's syndrome 370.33
   specified type NEC 370.49
   tuberculous (phlyctenular) (see also
      Tuberculosis) 017.3● [370.31]
Keratoconus 371.60
   acute hydrops 371.62
   congenital 743.41
   stable 371.61
Keratocyst (dental) 526.0
Keratoderma, keratodermia (congenital)
   (palmaris et plantaris) (symmetrical)
   757.39
   acquired 701.1
   blennorrhagica 701.1
      gonococcal 098.81
   climacterium 701.1
   eccentrica 757.39
   gonorrheal 098.81
   punctata 701.1
   tylodes, progressive 701.1

◀ New   ◀⫿⫿ Revised   ~~deleted~~ Deleted   ● Use Additional Digit(s)   ▨ Omit code

Keratodermatocele 371.72
Keratoglobus 371.70
  congenital 743.41
    associated with buphthalmos 743.22
Keratohemia 371.12
Keratoiritis (see also Iridocyclitis) 364.3
  syphilitic 090.3
  tuberculous (see also Tuberculosis) 017.3● [364.11]
Keratolysis exfoliativa (congenital) 757.39
  acquired 695.89
  neonatorum 757.39
Keratoma 701.1
  congenital 757.39
  malignum congenitale 757.1
  palmaris et plantaris hereditarium 757.39
  senile 702.0
Keratomalacia 371.45
  vitamin A deficiency 264.4
Keratomegaly 743.41
Keratomycosis 111.1
  nigricans (palmaris) 111.1
Keratopathy 371.40
  band (see also Keratitis) 371.43
  bullous (see also Keratitis) 371.23
  degenerative (see also Degeneration, cornea) 371.40
    hereditary (see also Dystrophy, cornea) 371.50
  discrete colliquative 371.49
Keratoscleritis, tuberculous (see also Tuberculosis) 017.3● [370.31]
Keratosis 701.1
  actinic 702.0
  arsenical 692.4
  blennorrhagica 701.1
    gonococcal 098.81
  congenital (any type) 757.39
  ear (middle) (see also Cholesteatoma) 385.30
  female genital (external) 629.89
  follicular, vitamin A deficiency 264.8
  follicularis 757.39
    acquired 701.1
    congenital (acneiformis) (Siemens') 757.39
    spinulosa (decalvans) 757.39
    vitamin A deficiency 264.8
  gonococcal 098.81
  larynx, laryngeal 478.79
  male genital (external) 608.89
  middle ear (see also Cholesteatoma) 385.30
  nigricans 701.2
    congenital 757.39
  obturans 380.21
  oral epithelium
    residual ridge mucosa
      excessive 528.72
      minimal 528.71
  palmaris et plantaris (symmetrical) 757.39
  penile 607.89
  pharyngeus 478.29
  pilaris 757.39
    acquired 701.1
  punctata (palmaris et plantaris) 701.1
  scrotal 608.89
  seborrheic 702.19
    inflamed 702.11
  senilis 702.0
  solar 702.0

Keratosis (Continued)
  suprafollicularis 757.39
  tonsillaris 478.29
  vagina 623.1
  vegetans 757.39
  vitamin A deficiency 264.8
Kerato-uveitis (see also Iridocyclitis) 364.3
Keraunoparalysis 994.0
Kerion (celsi) 110.0
Kernicterus of newborn (not due to isoimmunization) 774.7
  due to isoimmunization (conditions classifiable to 773.0–773.2) 773.4
Ketoacidosis 276.2
  diabetic 250.1●
    due to secondary diabetes 249.1●
Ketonuria 791.6
  branched-chain, intermittent 270.3
Ketosis 276.2
  diabetic 250.1●
    due to secondary diabetes 249.1●
Kidney - see condition
Kienböck's
  disease 732.3
    adult 732.8
  osteochondrosis 732.3
Kimmelstiel (-Wilson) disease or syndrome (intercapillary glomerulosclerosis) 250.4● [581.81]
  due to secondary diabetes 249.4● [581.81]
Kink, kinking
  appendix 543.9
  artery 447.1
  cystic duct, congenital 751.61
  hair (acquired) 704.2
  ileum or intestine (see also Obstruction, intestine) 560.9
  Lane's (see also Obstruction, intestine) 560.9
  organ or site, congenital NEC - see Anomaly, specified type NEC, by site
  ureter (pelvic junction) 593.3
    congenital 753.20
  vein(s) 459.2
    caval 459.2
    peripheral 459.2
Kinnier Wilson's disease (hepatolenticular degeneration) 275.1
Kissing
  osteophytes 721.5
  spine 721.5
  vertebra 721.5
Klauder's syndrome (erythema multiforme exudativum) 695.19
Klebs' disease (see also Nephritis) 583.9
Klein-Waardenburg syndrome (ptosis-epicanthus) 270.2
Kleine-Levin syndrome 327.13
Kleptomania 312.32
Klinefelter's syndrome 758.7
Klinger's disease 446.4
Klippel's disease 723.8
Klippel-Feil disease or syndrome (brevicollis) 756.16
Klippel-Trenaunay syndrome 759.89
Klumpke (-Déjérine) palsy, paralysis (birth) (newborn) 767.6
Klüver-Bucy (-Terzian) syndrome 310.0
Knee - see condition

Knifegrinders' rot (see also Tuberculosis) 011.4●
Knock-knee (acquired) 736.41
  congenital 755.64
Knot
  intestinal, syndrome (volvulus) 560.2
  umbilical cord (true) 663.2●
    affecting fetus or newborn 762.5
Knots, surfer 919.8
  infected 919.9
Knotting (of)
  hair 704.2
  intestine 560.2
Knuckle pads (Garrod's) 728.79
Köbner's disease (epidermolysis bullosa) 757.39
Koch's
  infection (see also Tuberculosis, pulmonary) 011.9●
  relapsing fever 087.9
Koch-Weeks conjunctivitis 372.03
Koenig-Wichman disease (pemphigus) 694.4
Köhler's disease (osteochondrosis) 732.5
  first (osteochondrosis juvenilis) 732.5
  second (Freiburg's infarction, metatarsal head) 732.5
  patellar 732.4
  tarsal navicular (bone) (osteoarthrosis juvenilis) 732.5
Köhler-Mouchet disease (osteoarthrosis juvenilis) 732.5
Köhler-Pellegrini-Stieda disease or syndrome (calcification, knee joint) 726.62
Koilonychia 703.8
  congenital 757.5
Kojevnikov's, Kojewnikoff's epilepsy (see also Epilepsy) 345.7●
König's
  disease (osteochondritis dissecans) 732.7
  syndrome 564.89
Koniophthisis (see also Tuberculosis) 011.4●
Koplik's spots 055.9
Kopp's asthma 254.8
Korean hemorrhagic fever 078.6
Korsakoff (-Wernicke) disease, psychosis, or syndrome (nonalcoholic) 294.0
  alcoholic 291.1
Korsakov's disease - see Korsakoff's disease
Korsakow's disease - see Korsakoff's disease
Kostmann's disease or syndrome (infantile genetic agranulocytosis) 288.01
Krabbe's
  disease (leukodystrophy) 330.0
  syndrome
    congenital muscle hypoplasia 756.89
    cutaneocerebral angioma 759.6
Kraepelin-Morel disease (see also Schizophrenia) 295.9●
Kraft-Weber-Dimitri disease 759.6
Kraurosis
  ani 569.49
  penis 607.0
  vagina 623.8
  vulva 624.09
Kreotoxism 005.9

Krukenberg's
  spindle 371.13
  tumor (M8490/6) 198.6
Kufs' disease 330.1
Kugelberg-Welander disease 335.11
Kuhnt-Junius degeneration or disease
    362.52
Kulchitsky's cell carcinoma (carcinoid
    tumor of intestine) 259.2
Kümmell's disease or spondylitis 721.7
Kundrat's disease (lymphosarcoma)
    200.1●
Kunekune - see Dermatophytosis
Kunkel syndrome (lupoid hepatitis)
    571.49
Kupffer cell sarcoma (M9124/3) 155.0
Kuru 046.0
Kussmaul's
  coma (diabetic) 250.3●
    due to secondary diabetes
        249.3●
  disease (polyarteritis nodosa) 446.0
  respiration (air hunger) 786.09
Kwashiorkor (marasmus type) 260
Kyasanur Forest disease 065.2

Kyphoscoliosis, kyphoscoliotic
    (acquired) (see also Scoliosis)
    737.30
  congenital 756.19
  due to radiation 737.33
  heart (disease) 416.1
  idiopathic 737.30
    infantile
        progressive 737.32
        resolving 737.31
  late effect of rickets 268.1 [737.43]
  specified NEC 737.39
  thoracogenic 737.34
  tuberculous (see also Tuberculosis)
      015.0● [737.43]
Kyphosis, kyphotic (acquired) (postural)
    737.10
  adolescent postural 737.0
  congenital 756.19
  dorsalis juvenilis 732.0
  due to or associated with
      Charcôt-Marie-Tooth disease 356.1
          [737.41]
      mucopolysaccharidosis 277.5
          [737.41]

Kyphosis, kyphotic (Continued)
  due to or associated with (Continued)
      neurofibromatosis 237.71 [737.41]
      osteitis
          deformans 731.0 [737.41]
          fibrosa cystica 252.01 [737.41]
      osteoporosis (see also Osteoporosis)
          733.0 [737.41]
      poliomyelitis (see also Poliomyelitis)
          138 [737.41]
      radiation 737.11
      tuberculosis (see also Tuberculosis)
          015.0● [737.41]
  Kümmell's 721.7
  late effect of rickets 268.1 [737.41]
  Morquio-Brailsford type (spinal) 277.5
      [737.41]
  pelvis 738.6
  postlaminectomy 737.12
  specified cause NEC 737.19
  syphilitic, congenital 090.5 [737.41]
  tuberculous (see also Tuberculosis)
      015.0● [737.41]
Kyrle's disease (hyperkeratosis
    follicularis in cutem penetrans) 701.1

◄ New   ◄▥ Revised   ~~deleted~~ Deleted   ● Use Additional Digit(s)   ▨ Omit code

L

Labia, labium - see condition
Labiated hymen 752.49
Labile
  blood pressure 796.2
  emotions, emotionality 301.3
  vasomotor system 443.9
Lability, emotional 799.24
Labioglossal paralysis 335.22
Labium leporinum (see also Cleft, lip) 749.10
Labor (see also Delivery)
  with complications - see Delivery, complicated
  abnormal NEC 661.9●
    affecting fetus or newborn 763.7
  arrested active phase 661.1●
    affecting fetus or newborn 763.7
  desultory 661.2●
    affecting fetus or newborn 763.7
  dyscoordinate 661.4●
    affecting fetus or newborn 763.7
  early onset (22–36 weeks gestation) 644.2●
  failed
    induction 659.1●
      mechanical 659.0●
      medical 659.1●
      surgical 659.0●
    trial (vaginal delivery) 660.6●
  false 644.1●
  forced or induced, affecting fetus or newborn 763.89
  hypertonic 661.4●
    affecting fetus or newborn 763.7
  hypotonic 661.2●
    affecting fetus or newborn 763.7
    primary 661.0●
      affecting fetus or newborn 763.7
    secondary 661.1●
      affecting fetus or newborn 763.7
  incoordinate 661.4●
    affecting fetus or newborn 763.7
  irregular 661.2●
    affecting fetus or newborn 763.7
  long - see Labor, prolonged
  missed (at or near term) 656.4●
  obstructed NEC 660.9●
    affecting fetus or newborn 763.1
    due to female genital mutilation 660.8●
    specified cause NEC 660.8●
      affecting fetus or newborn 763.1
  pains, spurious 644.1●
  precipitate 661.3●
    affecting fetus or newborn 763.6
  premature 644.2●
    threatened 644.0●
  prolonged or protracted 662.1●
    affecting fetus or newborn 763.89
    first stage 662.0●
      affecting fetus or newborn 763.89
    second stage 662.2●
      affecting fetus or newborn 763.89
  threatened NEC 644.1●
  undelivered 644.1●
Labored breathing (see also Hyperventilation) 786.09
Labyrinthitis (inner ear) (destructive) (latent) 386.30
  circumscribed 386.32
  diffuse 386.31
  focal 386.32
  purulent 386.33

Labyrinthitis (Continued)
  serous 386.31
  suppurative 386.33
  syphilitic 095.8
  toxic 386.34
  viral 386.35
Laceration - see also Wound, open, by site
  accidental, complicating surgery 998.2
  Achilles tendon 845.09
    with open wound 892.2
  anus (sphincter) 879.6
    with
      abortion - see Abortion, by type, with damage to pelvic organs
      ectopic pregnancy (see also categories 633.0–633.9) 639.2
      molar pregnancy (see also categories 630–632) 639.2
    complicated 879.7
    complicating delivery (healed) (old) 654.8●
      with laceration of anal or rectal mucosa 664.3●
      not associated with third-degree perineal laceration 664.6●
    following
      abortion 639.2
      ectopic or molar pregnancy 639.2
    nontraumatic, nonpuerperal (healed) (old) 569.43
  bladder (urinary)
    with
      abortion - see Abortion, by type, with damage to pelvic organs
      ectopic pregnancy (see also categories 633.0–633.9) 639.2
      molar pregnancy (see also categories 630–632) 639.2
    following
      abortion 639.2
      ectopic or molar pregnancy 639.2
    obstetrical trauma 665.5●
  blood vessel - see Injury, blood vessel, by site
  bowel
    with
      abortion - see Abortion, by type, with damage to pelvic organs
      ectopic pregnancy (see also categories 633.0–633.9) 639.2
      molar pregnancy (see also categories 630–632) 639.2
    following
      abortion 639.2
      ectopic or molar pregnancy 639.2
    obstetrical trauma 665.5●
  brain (cerebral) (membrane) (with hemorrhage) 851.8●

> Note 50 Use the following fifth-digit subclassification with categories 851–854:
>
> 0 unspecified state of consciousness
> 1 with no loss of consciousness
> 2 with brief [less than one hour] loss of consciousness
> 3 with moderate [1–24 hours] loss of consciousness

Laceration (Continued)
  brain (Continued)

> 4 with prolonged [more than 24 hours] loss of consciousness and return to pre-existing conscious level
> 5 with prolonged [more than 24 hours] loss of consciousness, without return to pre-existing conscious level
>
> Use fifth-digit 5 to designate when a patient is unconscious and dies before regaining consciousness, regardless of the duration of the loss of consciousness
>
> 6 with loss of consciousness of unspecified duration
> 9 with concussion, unspecified

    with
      open intracranial wound 851.9●
      skull fracture - see Fracture, skull, by site
    cerebellum 851.6●
      with open intracranial wound 851.7●
    cortex 851.2●
      with open intracranial wound 851.3●
    during birth 767.0
    stem 851.6●
      with open intracranial wound 851.7●
  broad ligament
    with
      abortion - see Abortion, by type, with damage to pelvic organs
      ectopic pregnancy (see also categories 633.0–633.9) 639.2
      molar pregnancy (see also categories 630–632) 639.2
    following
      abortion 639.2
      ectopic or molar pregnancy 639.2
    nontraumatic 620.6
    obstetrical trauma 665.6●
    syndrome (nontraumatic) 620.6
  capsule, joint - see Sprain, by site
  cardiac - see Laceration, heart
  causing eversion of cervix uteri (old) 622.0
  central, complicating delivery 664.4●
  cerebellum - see Laceration, brain, cerebellum
  cerebral - see also Laceration, brain
    during birth 767.0
  cervix (uteri)
    with
      abortion - see Abortion, by type, with damage to pelvic organs
      ectopic pregnancy (see also categories 633.0–633.9) 639.2
      molar pregnancy (see also categories 630–632) 639.2
    following
      abortion 639.2
      ectopic or molar pregnancy 639.2

Laceration (Continued)
  cervix (Continued)
    nonpuerperal, nontraumatic 622.3
    obstetrical trauma (current) 665.3●
    old (postpartal) 622.3
    traumatic - see Injury, internal, cervix
  chordae heart 429.5
  complicated 879.9
  cornea - see Laceration, eyeball
    superficial 918.1
  cortex (cerebral) - see Laceration, brain,
    cortex
  esophagus 530.89
  eye(s) - see Laceration, ocular
  eyeball NEC 871.4
    with prolapse or exposure of
      intraocular tissue 871.1
    penetrating - see Penetrating wound,
      eyeball
    specified as without prolapse of
      intraocular tissue 871.0
  eyelid NEC 870.8
    full thickness 870.1
      involving lacrimal passages 870.2
    skin (and periocular area) 870.0
    penetrating - see Penetrating
      wound, orbit
  fourchette
    with
      abortion - see Abortion, by type,
        with damage to pelvic
        organs
      ectopic pregnancy (see also
        categories 633.0–633.9) 639.2
      molar pregnancy (see also
        categories 630–632) 639.2
    complicating delivery 664.0●
    following
      abortion 639.2
      ectopic or molar pregnancy 639.2
  heart (without penetration of heart
    chambers) 861.02
    with
      open wound into thorax 861.12
      penetration of heart chambers
        861.03
        with open wound into thorax
          861.13
  hernial sac - see Hernia, by site
  internal organ (abdomen) (chest)
    (pelvis) NEC - see Injury, internal,
    by site
  kidney (parenchyma) 866.02
    with
      complete disruption of
        parenchyma (rupture)
        866.03
        with open wound into cavity
          866.13
      open wound into cavity 866.12
  labia
    complicating delivery 664.0●
  ligament - see also Sprain, by site
    with open wound - see Wound,
      open, by site
  liver 864.05
    with open wound into cavity 864.15
    major (disruption of hepatic
      parenchyma) 864.04
      with open wound into cavity
        864.14
    minor (capsule only) 864.02
      with open wound into cavity
        864.12

Laceration (Continued)
  liver (Continued)
    moderate (involving parenchyma
      without major disruption)
      864.03
      with open wound into cavity
        864.13
    multiple 864.04
      with open wound into cavity
        864.14
    stellate 864.04
      with open wound into cavity
        864.14
  lung 861.22
    with open wound into thorax
      861.32
  meninges - see Laceration, brain
  meniscus (knee) (see also Tear,
    meniscus) 836.2
    old 717.5
    site other than knee - see also Sprain,
      by site
      old NEC (see also Disorder,
        cartilage, articular) 718.0●
  muscle - see also Sprain, by site
    with open wound - see Wound,
      open, by site
  myocardium - see Laceration, heart
  nerve - see Injury, nerve, by site
  ocular NEC (see also Laceration,
    eyeball) 871.4
    adnexa NEC 870.8
      penetrating 870.3
        with foreign body 870.4
  orbit (eye) 870.8
    penetrating 870.3
      with foreign body 870.4
  pelvic
    floor (muscles)
      with
        abortion - see Abortion, by type,
          with damage to pelvic
          organs
        ectopic pregnancy (see also
          categories 633.0–633.9)
          639.2
        molar pregnancy (see also
          categories 630–632)
          639.2
      complicating delivery 664.1●
      following
        abortion 639.2
        ectopic or molar pregnancy
          639.2
      nonpuerperal 618.7
      old (postpartal) 618.7
    organ NEC
      with
        abortion - see Abortion, by type,
          with damage to pelvic
          organs
        ectopic pregnancy (see also
          categories 633.0–633.9)
          639.2
        molar pregnancy (see also
          categories 630–632) 639.2
      complicating delivery 665.5●
        affecting fetus or newborn
          763.89
      following
        abortion 639.2
        ectopic or molar pregnancy
          639.2
      obstetrical trauma 665.5●

Laceration (Continued)
  perineum, perineal (old) (postpartal)
    618.7
    with
      abortion - see Abortion, by type,
        with damage to pelvic floor
      ectopic pregnancy (see also
        categories 633.0–633.9) 639.2
      molar pregnancy (see also
        categories 630–632) 639.2
    complicating delivery 664.4●
      first degree 664.0●
      second degree 664.1●
      third degree 664.2●
      fourth degree 664.3●
      central 664.4●
      involving
        anal sphincter (healed) (old)
          654.8●
        fourchette 664.0●
        hymen 664.0●
        labia 664.0●
        not associated with third-
          degree perineal
          laceration 664.6●
        pelvic floor 664.1●
        perineal muscles 664.1●
        rectovaginal with septum
          664.2●
          with anal mucosa 664.3●
        skin 664.0●
        sphincter (anal) (healed) (old)
          654.8●
          with anal mucosa 664.3●
          not associated with third-
            degree perineal
            laceration 664.6●
        vagina 664.0●
        vaginal muscles 664.1●
        vulva 664.0●
      secondary 674.2●
    following
      abortion 639.2
      ectopic or molar pregnancy 639.2
    male 879.6
      complicated 879.7
    muscles, complicating delivery
      664.1●
    nonpuerperal, current injury 879.6
      complicated 879.7
    secondary (postpartal) 674.2●
  peritoneum
    with
      abortion - see Abortion, by type,
        with damage to pelvic
        organs
      ectopic pregnancy (see also
        categories 633.0–633.9)
        639.2
      molar pregnancy (see also
        categories 630–632) 639.2
    following
      abortion 639.2
      ectopic or molar pregnancy 639.2
    obstetrical trauma 665.5●
  periurethral tissue
    with
      abortion - see Abortion, by type,
        with damage to pelvic
        organs
      ectopic pregnancy (see also
        categories 633.0–633.9) 639.2
      molar pregnancy (see also
        categories 630–632) 639.2

◄ New   ◄║║ Revised   ~~deleted~~ Deleted   ● Use Additional Digit(s)   ▨ Omit code

Laceration *(Continued)*
  periurethral tissue *(Continued)*
    following
      abortion 639.2
      ectopic or molar pregnancy 639.2
    obstetrical trauma 665.5●
  rectovaginal (septum)
    with
      abortion - *see* Abortion, by type,
        with damage to pelvic
        organs
      ectopic pregnancy *(see also*
        categories 633.0–633.9) 639.2
      molar pregnancy *(see also*
        categories 630–632) 639.2
    complicating delivery 665.4●
      with perineum 664.2●
        involving anal or rectal
          mucosa 664.3●
    following
      abortion 639.2
      ectopic or molar pregnancy
        639.2
    nonpuerperal 623.4
    old (postpartal) 623.4
  spinal cord (meninges) - *see also* Injury,
    spinal, by site
    due to injury at birth 767.4
    fetus or newborn 767.4
  spleen 865.09
    with
      disruption of parenchyma
        (massive) 865.04
        with open wound into cavity
          865.14
      open wound into cavity 865.19
    capsule (without disruption of
      parenchyma) 865.02
      with open wound into cavity
        865.12
    parenchyma 865.03
      with open wound into cavity
        865.13
      massive disruption (rupture)
        865.04
        with open wound into cavity
          865.14
  tendon 848.9
    with open wound - *see* Wound,
      open, by site
    Achilles 845.09
      with open wound 892.2
    lower limb NEC 844.9
      with open wound NEC 894.2
    upper limb NEC 840.9
      with open wound NEC 884.2
  tentorium cerebelli - *see* Laceration,
    brain, cerebellum
  tongue 873.64
    complicated 873.74
  urethra
    with
      abortion - *see* Abortion, by type,
        with damage to pelvic
        organs
      ectopic pregnancy *(see also*
        categories 633.0–633.9) 639.2
      molar pregnancy *(see also*
        categories 630–632) 639.2
    following
      abortion 639.2
      ectopic or molar pregnancy 639.2
    nonpuerperal, nontraumatic 599.84
    obstetrical trauma 665.5●

Laceration *(Continued)*
  uterus
    with
      abortion - *see* Abortion, by type,
        with damage to pelvic
        organs
      ectopic pregnancy *(see also*
        categories 633.0–633.9) 639.2
      molar pregnancy *(see also*
        categories 630–632) 639.2
    following
      abortion 639.2
      ectopic or molar pregnancy 639.2
    nonpuerperal, nontraumatic 621.8
    obstetrical trauma NEC 665.5●
    old (postpartal) 621.8
  vagina
    with
      abortion - *see* Abortion, by type,
        with damage to pelvic
        organs
      ectopic pregnancy *(see also*
        categories 633.0–633.9) 639.2
      molar pregnancy *(see also*
        categories 630–632) 639.2
      perineal involvement,
        complicating delivery
        664.0●
    complicating delivery 665.4●
      first degree 664.0●
      second degree 664.1●
      third degree 664.2●
      fourth degree 664.3●
      high 665.4●
      muscles 664.1●
      sulcus 665.4●
      wall 665.4●
    following
      abortion 639.2
      ectopic or molar pregnancy 639.2
    nonpuerperal, nontraumatic 623.4
    old (postpartal) 623.4
  valve, heart - *see* Endocarditis
  vulva
    with
      abortion - *see* Abortion, by type,
        with damage to pelvic
        organs
      ectopic pregnancy *(see also*
        categories 633.0–633.9) 639.2
      molar pregnancy *(see also*
        categories 630–632) 639.2
    complicating delivery 664.0●
    following
      abortion 639.2
      ectopic or molar pregnancy 639.2
    nonpuerperal, nontraumatic 624.4
    old (postpartal) 624.4
Lachrymal - *see* condition
Lachrymonasal duct - *see* condition
Lack of
  adequate intermaxillary vertical
    dimension 524.36
  appetite *(see also* Anorexia) 783.0
  care
    in home V60.4
    of adult 995.84
    of infant (at or after birth) 995.52
  coordination 781.3
  development - *see also* Hypoplasia
    physiological in childhood 783.40
  education V62.3
  energy 780.79
  financial resources V60.2

Lack of *(Continued)*
  food 994.2
    in environment V60.89 ◀▥
  growth in childhood 783.43
  heating V60.1
  housing (permanent) (temporary)
    V60.0
    adequate V60.1
  material resources V60.2
  medical attention 799.89
  memory *(see also* Amnesia) 780.93
    mild, following organic brain
      damage 310.8 ◀▥
  ovulation 628.0
  person able to render necessary care
    V60.4
  physical exercise V69.0
  physiologic development in childhood
    783.40
  posterior occlusal support 524.57
  prenatal care in current pregnancy
    V23.7
  shelter V60.0
  sleep V69.4
  water 994.3
Lacrimal - *see* condition
Lacrimation, abnormal *(see also* Epiphora)
  375.20
Lacrimonasal duct - *see* condition
Lactation, lactating (breast) (puerperal)
  (postpartum)
  defective 676.4●
  disorder 676.9●
    specified type NEC 676.8●
  excessive 676.6●
  failed 676.4●
  mastitis NEC 675.2●
  mother (care and/or examination)
    V24.1
  nonpuerperal 611.6
  suppressed 676.5●
Lacticemia 271.3
  excessive 276.2
Lactosuria 271.3
Lacunar skull 756.0
Laennec's cirrhosis (alcoholic) 571.2
  nonalcoholic 571.5
Lafora's disease 333.2
Lag, lid (nervous) 374.41
Lagleyze-von Hippel disease
  (retinocerebral angiomatosis) 759.6
Lagophthalmos (eyelid) (nervous)
  374.20
  cicatricial 374.23
  keratitis *(see also* Keratitis) 370.34
  mechanical 374.22
  paralytic 374.21
La grippe - *see* Influenza
Lahore sore 085.1
Lakes, venous (cerebral) 437.8
Laki-Lorand factor deficiency *(see also*
  Defect, coagulation) 286.3
Lalling 307.9
Lambliasis 007.1
Lame back 724.5
Lancereaux's diabetes (diabetes mellitus
  with marked emaciation) 250.8●
  [261]
  due to secondary diabetes 249.8●
  [261]
Landau-Kleffner syndrome 345.8●
Landouzy-Déjérine dystrophy
  (fascioscapulohumeral atrophy)
  359.1

Landry's disease or paralysis 357.0
Landry-Guillain-Barré syndrome 357.0
Lane's
    band 751.4
    disease 569.89
    kink (*see also* Obstruction, intestine)
        560.9
Langdon Down's syndrome (mongolism)
    758.0
Language abolition 784.69
Lanugo (persistent) 757.4
Laparoscopic surgical procedure
    converted to open procedure V64.41
Lardaceous
    degeneration (any site) 277.39
    disease 277.39
    kidney 277.39 [583.81]
    liver 277.39
Large
    baby (regardless of gestational age)
        766.1
        exceptionally (weight of 4500 grams
            or more) 766.0
        of diabetic mother 775.0
    ear 744.22
    fetus - *see also* Oversize, fetus
        causing disproportion 653.5●
            with obstructed labor 660.1●
    for dates
        fetus or newborn (regardless of
            gestational age) 766.1
        affecting management of
            pregnancy 656.6●
        exceptionally (weight of 4500
            grams or more) 766.0
    physiological cup 743.57
    stature 783.9
    waxy liver 277.39
    white kidney - *see* Nephrosis
Larsen's syndrome (flattened facies and
    multiple congenital dislocations)
    755.8
Larsen-Johansson disease (juvenile
    osteopathia patellae) 732.4
Larva migrans
    cutaneous NEC 126.9
        ancylostoma 126.9
    of Diptera in vitreous 128.0
    visceral NEC 128.0
Laryngeal - *see also* condition
    syncope 786.2
Laryngismus (acute) (infectious)
    (stridulous) 478.75
    congenital 748.3
    diphtheritic 032.3
Laryngitis (acute) (edematous) (fibrinous)
    (gangrenous) (infective) (infiltrative)
    (malignant) (membranous)
    (phlegmonous) (pneumococcal)
    (pseudomembranous) (septic)
    (subglottic) (suppurative) (ulcerative)
    (viral) 464.00
    with
        influenza, flu, or grippe 487.1
        obstruction 464.01
        tracheitis (*see also* Laryngotracheitis)
            464.20
            with obstruction 464.21
            acute 464.20
                with obstruction 464.21
            chronic 476.1
    atrophic 476.0
    Borrelia vincentii 101
    catarrhal 476.0

Laryngitis (*Continued*)
    chronic 476.0
        with tracheitis (chronic) 476.1
        due to external agent - *see*
            Condition, respiratory, chronic,
            due to
    diphtheritic (membranous) 032.3
    due to external agent - *see*
        Inflammation, respiratory, upper,
        due to
    H. influenzae 464.00
        with obstruction 464.01
    Hemophilus influenzae 464.00
        with obstruction 464.01
    hypertrophic 476.0
    influenzal 487.1
    pachydermic 478.79
    sicca 476.0
    spasmodic 478.75
        acute 464.00
            with obstruction 464.01
    streptococcal 034.0
    stridulous 478.75
    syphilitic 095.8
        congenital 090.5
    tuberculous (*see also* Tuberculosis,
        larynx) 012.3●
    Vincent's 101
Laryngocele (congenital) (ventricular)
    748.3
Laryngofissure 478.79
    congenital 748.3
Laryngomalacia (congenital) 748.3
Laryngopharyngitis (acute) 465.0
    chronic 478.9
        due to external agent - *see*
            Condition, respiratory, chronic,
            due to
    due to external agent - *see*
        Inflammation, respiratory, upper,
        due to
    septic 034.0
Laryngoplegia (*see also* Paralysis, vocal
    cord) 478.30
Laryngoptosis 478.79
Laryngospasm 478.75
    due to external agent - *see* Condition,
        respiratory, acute, due to
Laryngostenosis 478.74
    congenital 748.3
Laryngotracheitis (acute) (infectional)
    (viral) (*see also* Laryngitis) 464.20
    with obstruction 464.21
    atrophic 476.1
    Borrelia vincentii 101
    catarrhal 476.1
    chronic 476.1
        due to external agent - *see*
            Condition, respiratory, chronic,
            due to
    diphtheritic (membranous) 032.3
    due to external agent - *see*
        Inflammation, respiratory, upper,
        due to
    H. influenzae 464.20
        with obstruction 464.21
    hypertrophic 476.1
    influenzal 487.1
    pachydermic 478.75
    sicca 476.1
    spasmodic 478.75
        acute 464.20
            with obstruction 464.21
    streptococcal 034.0

Laryngotracheitis (*Continued*)
    stridulous 478.75
    syphilitic 095.8
        congenital 090.5
    tuberculous (*see also* Tuberculosis,
        larynx) 012.3●
    Vincent's 101
Laryngotracheobronchitis (*see also*
    Bronchitis) 490
    acute 466.0
    chronic 491.8
    viral 466.0
Laryngotracheobronchopneumonitis - *see*
    Pneumonia, broncho-
Larynx, laryngeal - *see* condition
Lasègue's disease (persecution mania)
    297.9
Lassa fever 078.89
Lassitude (*see also* Weakness) 780.79
Late - *see also* condition
    effect(s) (of) - *see also* condition
        abscess
            intracranial or intraspinal
                (conditions classifiable to
                324) - *see* category 326
        adverse effect of drug, medicinal or
            biological substance 909.5
        allergic reaction 909.9
        amputation
            postoperative (late) 997.60
            traumatic (injury classifiable to
                885–887 and 895–897)
                905.9
        burn (injury classifiable to 948–949)
            906.9
            extremities NEC (injury
                classifiable to 943 or 945)
                906.7
            hand or wrist (injury
                classifiable to 944) 906.6
            eye (injury classifiable to 940)
                906.5
            face, head, and neck (injury
                classifiable to 941) 906.5
            specified site NEC (injury
                classifiable to 942 and
                946–947) 906.8
        cerebrovascular disease (conditions
            classifiable to 430–437) 438.9
            with
                alterations of sensations
                    438.6
                aphasia 438.11
                apraxia 438.81
                ataxia 438.84
                cognitive deficits 438.0
                disturbances of vision 438.7
                dysarthria 438.13 ◀
                dysphagia 438.82
                dysphasia 438.12
                facial droop 438.83
                facial weakness 438.83
                fluency disorder 438.14 ◀
                hemiplegia/hemiparesis
                    affecting
                        dominant side 438.21
                        nondominant side 438.22
                        unspecified side 438.20
                monoplegia of lower limb
                    affecting
                        dominant side 438.41
                        nondominant side
                            438.42
                        unspecified side 438.40

◀ New   ◀▥ Revised   ~~deleted~~ Deleted   ● Use Additional Digit(s)   ▨ Omit code

Late *(Continued)*
  effect(s) (of) *(Continued)*
    cerebrovascular disease *(Continued)*
      with *(Continued)*
        monoplegia of upper limb
          affecting
            dominant side 438.31
            nondominant side 438.32
            unspecified side 438.30
        paralytic syndrome NEC
          affecting
            bilateral 438.53
            dominant side 438.51
            nondominant side
              438.52
            unspecified side 438.50
        speech and language deficit
          438.10
        specified type NEC
          438.19
        stuttering 438.14 ◄
        vertigo 438.85
      specified type NEC 438.89
    childbirth complication(s) 677
    complication(s) of
      childbirth 677
      delivery 677
      pregnancy 677
      puerperium 677
      surgical and medical care
        (conditions classifiable to
        996–999) 909.3
      trauma (conditions classifiable to
        958) 908.6
    contusion (injury classifiable to
      920–924) 906.3
    crushing (injury classifiable to
      925–929) 906.4
    delivery complication(s) 677
    dislocation (injury classifiable to
      830–839) 905.6
    encephalitis or encephalomyelitis
      (conditions classifiable to
      323) - *see* category 326
      in infectious diseases 139.8
        viral (conditions classifiable to
          049.8, 049.9, 062–064)
          139.0
    external cause NEC (conditions
      classifiable to 995) 909.9
      certain conditions classifiable to
        categories 991–994 909.4
    foreign body in orifice (injury
      classifiable to 930–939) 908.5
    fracture (multiple) (injury
      classifiable to 828–829) 905.5
      extremity
        lower (injury classifiable to
          821–827) 905.4
          neck of femur (injury
            classifiable to 820)
            905.3
        upper (injury classifiable to
          810–819) 905.2
      face and skull (injury classifiable
        to 800–804) 905.0
      skull and face (injury classifiable
        to 800–804) 905.0
      spine and trunk (injury
        classifiable to 805 and
        807–809) 905.1
        with spinal cord lesion (injury
          classifiable to 806)
          907.2

Late *(Continued)*
  effect(s) (of) *(Continued)*
    infection
      pyogenic, intracranial - *see*
        category 326
    infectious diseases (conditions
      classifiable to 001–136) NEC
      139.8
    injury (injury classifiable to 959)
      908.9
      blood vessel 908.3
        abdomen and pelvis (injury
          classifiable to 902) 908.4
        extremity (injury classifiable to
          903–904) 908.3
        head and neck (injury
          classifiable to 900) 908.3
        intracranial (injury
          classifiable to 850–854)
          907.0
          with skull fracture 905.0
        thorax (injury classifiable to
          901) 908.4
      internal organ NEC (injury
        classifiable to 867 and 869)
        908.2
        abdomen (injury classifiable to
          863–866 and 868) 908.1
        thorax (injury classifiable to
          860–862) 908.0
      intracranial (injury classifiable to
        850–854) 907.0
        with skull fracture (injury
          classifiable to 800–801
          and 803–804) 905.0
      nerve NEC (injury classifiable to
        957) 907.9
        cranial (injury classifiable to
          950–951) 907.1
        peripheral NEC (injury
          classifiable to 957)
          907.9
          lower limb and pelvic
            girdle (injury
            classifiable to 956)
            907.5
          upper limb and shoulder
            girdle (injury
            classifiable to 955)
            907.4
        roots and plexus(es), spinal
          (injury classifiable to 953)
          907.3
        trunk (injury classifiable to
          954) 907.3
      spinal
        cord (injury classifiable to 806
          and 952) 907.2
        nerve root(s) and plexus(es)
          (injury classifiable to 953)
          907.3
      superficial (injury classifiable to
        910–919) 906.2
      tendon (tendon injury classifiable
        to 840–848, 880–884 with .2,
        and 890–894 with .2) 905.8
    meningitis
      bacterial (conditions classifiable
        to 320) - *see* category 326
      unspecified cause (conditions
        classifiable to 322) - *see*
        category 326
    myelitis (*see also* Late, effect(s) (of),
      encephalitis) - *see* category 326

Late *(Continued)*
  effect(s) (of) *(Continued)*
    parasitic diseases (conditions
      classifiable to 001–136 NEC)
      139.8
    phlebitis or thrombophlebitis of
      intracranial venous sinuses
      (conditions classifiable to
      325) - *see* category 326
    poisoning due to drug, medicinal or
      biological substance
      (conditions classifiable to
      960–979) 909.0
    poliomyelitis, acute (conditions
      classifiable to 045) 138
    pregnancy complication(s) 677
    puerperal complication(s) 677
    radiation (conditions classifiable to
      990) 909.2
    rickets 268.1
    sprain and strain without mention
      of tendon injury (injury
      classifiable to 840–848, except
      tendon injury) 905.7
      tendon involvement 905.8
    toxic effect of
      drug, medicinal or biological
        substance (conditions
        classifiable to 960–979)
        909.0
      nonmedical substance
        (conditions classifiable
        to 980–989) 909.1
    trachoma (conditions classifiable
      to 076) 139.1
    tuberculosis 137.0
      bones and joints (conditions
        classifiable to 015) 137.3
      central nervous system
        (conditions classifiable to
        013) 137.1
      genitourinary (conditions
        classifiable to 016) 137.2
      pulmonary (conditions
        classifiable to 010–012)
        137.0
      specified organs NEC (conditions
        classifiable to 014, 017–018)
        137.4
    viral encephalitis (conditions
      classifiable to 049.8, 049.9,
      062–064) 139.0
    wound, open
      extremity (injury classifiable to
        880–884 and 890–894,
        except .2) 906.1
      tendon (injury classifiable to
        880–884 with .2 and
        890–894 with .2) 905.8
      head, neck, and trunk (injury
        classifiable to 870–879)
        906.0
  infant
    post-term (gestation period
      over 40 completed weeks
      to 42 completed weeks)
      766.21
    prolonged gestation (period
      over 42 completed weeks)
      766.22
Latent - *see* condition
Lateral - *see* condition
Laterocession - *see* Lateroversion
Lateroflexion - *see* Lateroversion

Lateroversion
  cervix - *see* Lateroversion, uterus
  uterus, uterine (cervix) (postinfectional)
    (postpartal, old) 621.6
    congenital 752.3
    in pregnancy or childbirth 654.4●
      affecting fetus or newborn 763.89
Lathyrism 988.2
Launois' syndrome (pituitary gigantism)
  253.0
Launois-Bensaude's lipomatosis 272.8
Launois-Cleret syndrome (adiposogenital
  dystrophy) 253.8
Laurence-Moon-Biedl syndrome (obesity,
  polydactyly, and mental retardation)
  759.89
LAV (disease) (illness) (infection) - *see*
  Human immunodeficiency virus
  (disease) (illness) (infection)
LAV/HTLV-III (disease) (illness)
  (infection) - *see* Human
  immunodeficiency virus (disease)
  (illness) (infection)
Lawford's syndrome
  (encephalocutaneous angiomatosis)
  759.6
Lax, laxity - *see also* Relaxation
  ligament 728.4
  skin (acquired) 701.8
    congenital 756.83
Laxative habit (*see also* Abuse, drugs,
  nondependent) 305.9●
Lazy leukocyte syndrome 288.09
LCAD (long chain/very long chain acyl
  CoA dehydrogenase deficiency,
  VLCAD) 277.85
LCHAD (long chain 3-hydroxyacyl CoA
  dehydrogenase deficiency) 277.85
Lead - *see also* condition
  exposure (suspected) to V15.86 ◀▥
  incrustation of cornea 371.15
  poisoning 984.9
    specified type of lead - *see* Table of
      Drugs and Chemicals
Lead miners' lung 503
Leakage
  amniotic fluid 658.1●
    with delayed delivery 658.2●
    affecting fetus or newborn 761.1
  bile from drainage tube (T tube) 997.4
  blood (microscopic), fetal, into
    maternal circulation 656.0●
    affecting management of pregnancy
      or puerperium 656.0●
  device, implant, or graft - *see*
    Complications, mechanical
  spinal fluid at lumbar puncture site
    997.09
  urine, continuous 788.37
Leaky heart - *see* Endocarditis
Learning defect, specific NEC
  (strephosymbolia) 315.2
Leather bottle stomach (M8142/3) 151.9
Leber's
  congenital amaurosis 362.76
  optic atrophy (hereditary) 377.16
Lederer's anemia or disease (acquired
  infectious hemolytic anemia) 283.19
Lederer-Brill syndrome (acquired
  infectious hemolytic anemia) 283.19
Leeches (aquatic) (land) 134.2
Left-sided neglect 781.8
Leg - *see* condition
Legal investigation V62.5

Legg (-Calvé)-Perthes disease or
  syndrome (osteochondrosis, femoral
  capital) 732.1
Legionnaires' disease 482.84
Leigh's disease 330.8
Leiner's disease (exfoliative dermatitis)
  695.89
Leiofibromyoma (M8890/0) - *see also*
  Leiomyoma
  uterus (cervix) (corpus) (*see also*
    Leiomyoma, uterus) 218.9
Leiomyoblastoma (M8891/1) - *see*
  Neoplasm, connective tissue,
  uncertain behavior
Leiomyofibroma (M8890/0) - *see also*
  Neoplasm, connective tissue, benign
  uterus (cervix) (corpus) (*see also*
    Leiomyoma, uterus) 218.9
Leiomyoma (M8890/0) - *see also*
  Neoplasm, connective tissue, benign
  bizarre (M8893/0) - *see* Neoplasm,
    connective tissue, benign
  cellular (M8892/1) - *see* Neoplasm,
    connective tissue, uncertain
    behavior
  epithelioid (M8891/1) - *see* Neoplasm,
    connective tissue, uncertain
    behavior
  prostate (polypoid) 600.20
    with
      other lower urinary tract
        symptoms (LUTS) 600.21
      urinary
        obstruction 600.21
        retention 600.21
  uterus (cervix) (corpus) 218.9
    interstitial 218.1
    intramural 218.1
    submucous 218.0
    subperitoneal 218.2
    subserous 218.2
  vascular (M8894/0) - *see* Neoplasm,
    connective tissue, benign
Leiomyomatosis (intravascular)
  (M8890/1) - *see* Neoplasm,
  connective tissue, uncertain
  behavior
Leiomyosarcoma (M8890/3) - *see also*
  Neoplasm, connective tissue,
  malignant
  epithelioid (M8891/3) - *see* Neoplasm,
    connective tissue, malignant
Leishmaniasis 085.9
  American 085.5
    cutaneous 085.4
    mucocutaneous 085.5
  Asian desert 085.2
  Brazilian 085.5
  cutaneous 085.9
    acute necrotizing 085.2
    American 085.4
    Asian desert 085.2
    diffuse 085.3
    dry form 085.1
    Ethiopian 085.3
    eyelid 085.5 [373.6]
    late 085.1
    lepromatous 085.3
    recurrent 085.1
    rural 085.2
    ulcerating 085.1
    urban 085.1
    wet form 085.2
    zoonotic form 085.2

Leishmaniasis (*Continued*)
  dermal - *see also* Leishmaniasis,
    cutaneous
    post kala-azar 085.0
  eyelid 085.5 [373.6]
  infantile 085.0
  Mediterranean 085.0
  mucocutaneous (American) 085.5
  naso-oral 085.5
  nasopharyngeal 085.5
  Old World 085.1
  tegumentaria diffusa 085.4
  vaccination, prophylactic (against)
    V05.2
  visceral (Indian) 085.0
Leishmanoid, dermal - *see also*
  Leishmaniasis, cutaneous
  post kala-azar 085.0
Leloir's disease 695.4
Lemiere syndrome 451.89
Lenegre's disease 426.0
Lengthening, leg 736.81
Lennox-Gastaut syndrome 345.0●
  with tonic seizures 345.1●
Lennox's syndrome (*see also* Epilepsy)
  345.0●
Lens - *see* condition
Lenticonus (anterior) (posterior)
  (congenital) 743.36
Lenticular degeneration, progressive
  275.1
Lentiglobus (posterior) (congenital) 743.36
Lentigo (congenital) 709.09
  juvenile 709.09
  Maligna (M8742/2) - *see also* Neoplasm,
    skin, in situ
    melanoma (M8742/3) - *see*
      Melanoma
  senile 709.09
Leonine leprosy 030.0
Leontiasis
  ossium 733.3
  syphilitic 095.8
    congenital 090.5
Léopold-Lévi's syndrome (paroxysmal
  thyroid instability) 242.9●
Lepore hemoglobin syndrome 282.49
Lepothrix 039.0
Lepra 030.9
  Willan's 696.1
Leprechaunism 259.8
Lepromatous leprosy 030.0
Leprosy 030.9
  anesthetic 030.1
  beriberi 030.1
  borderline (group B) (infiltrated)
    (neuritic) 030.3
  cornea (*see also* Leprosy, by type) 030.9
    [371.89]
  dimorphous (group B) (infiltrated)
    (lepromatous) (neuritic)
    (tuberculoid) 030.3
  eyelid 030.0 [373.4]
  indeterminate (group I) (macular)
    (neuritic) (uncharacteristic) 030.2
  leonine 030.0
  lepromatous (diffuse) (infiltrated)
    (macular) (neuritic) (nodular)
    (type L) 030.0
  macular (early) (neuritic) (simple) 030.2
  maculoanesthetic 030.1
  mixed 030.0
  neuro 030.1
  nodular 030.0

◀ New   ◀▥ Revised   ~~deleted~~ Deleted   ● Use Additional Digit(s)   ▨ Omit code

Leprosy *(Continued)*
  primary neuritic 030.3
  specified type or group NEC 030.8
  tubercular 030.1
  tuberculoid (macular)
      (maculoanesthetic) (major)
      (minor) (neuritic) (type T)
      030.1
Leptocytosis, hereditary 282.49
Leptomeningitis (chronic)
      (circumscribed) (hemorrhagic)
      (nonsuppurative) *(see also*
      Meningitis) 322.9
  aseptic 047.9
      adenovirus 049.1
      Coxsackie virus 047.0
      ECHO virus 047.1
      enterovirus 047.9
      lymphocytic choriomeningitis
          049.0
  epidemic 036.0
  late effect - *see* category 326
  meningococcal 036.0
  pneumococcal 320.1
  syphilitic 094.2
  tuberculous *(see also* Tuberculosis,
      meninges) 013.0●
Leptomeningopathy *(see also* Meningitis)
      322.9
Leptospiral - *see* condition
Leptospirochetal - *see* condition
Leptospirosis 100.9
  autumnalis 100.89
  canicula 100.89
  grippotyphosa 100.89
  hebdomadis 100.89
  icterohemorrhagica 100.0
  nanukayami 100.89
  pomona 100.89
  Weil's disease 100.0
Leptothricosis - *see* Actinomycosis
Leptothrix infestation - *see*
      Actinomycosis
Leptotricosis - *see* Actinomycosis
Leptus dermatitis 133.8
Léris pleonosteosis 756.89
Léri-Weill syndrome 756.59
Leriche's syndrome (aortic bifurcation
      occlusion) 444.0
Lermoyez's syndrome *(see also* Disease,
      Ménière's) 386.00
Lesbianism - *omit code*
  ego-dystonic 302.0
  problems with 302.0
Lesch-Nyhan syndrome (hypoxanthine-
      guanine-phosphoribosyltransferase
      deficiency) 277.2
Lesion(s)
  abducens nerve 378.54
  alveolar process 525.8
  anorectal 569.49
  aortic (valve) - *see* Endocarditis, aortic
  auditory nerve 388.5
  basal ganglion 333.90
  bile duct *(see also* Disease, biliary)
      576.8
  bladder 596.9
  bone 733.90
  brachial plexus 353.0
  brain 348.89 ◀▦
      congenital 742.9
      vascular *(see also* Lesion,
          cerebrovascular) 437.9
          degenerative 437.1

Lesion(s) *(Continued)*
  brain *(Continued)*
      vascular *(Continued)*
          healed or old without residuals
              V12.54
          hypertensive 437.2
          late effect - *see* Late effect(s) (of)
              cerebrovascular disease
  buccal 528.9
  calcified - *see* Calcification
  canthus 373.9
  carate - *see* Pinta, lesions
  cardia 537.89
  cardiac - *see also* Disease, heart
      congenital 746.9
      valvular - *see* Endocarditis
  cauda equina 344.60
      with neurogenic bladder 344.61
  cecum 569.89
  cerebral - *see* Lesion, brain
  cerebrovascular *(see also* Disease,
      cerebrovascular NEC) 437.9
      degenerative 437.1
      healed or old without residuals
          V12.54
      hypertensive 437.2
      specified type NEC 437.8
  cervical root (nerve) NEC 353.2
  chiasmal 377.54
      associated with
          inflammatory disorders
              377.54
          neoplasm NEC 377.52
              pituitary 377.51
          pituitary disorders 377.51
          vascular disorders 377.53
  chorda tympani 351.8
  coin, lung 793.1
  colon 569.89
  congenital - *see* Anomaly
  conjunctiva 372.9
  coronary artery *(see also* Ischemia,
      heart) 414.9
  cranial nerve 352.9
      first 352.0
      second 377.49
      third
          partial 378.51
          total 378.52
      fourth 378.53
      fifth 350.9
      sixth 378.54
      seventh 351.9
      eighth 388.5
      ninth 352.2
      tenth 352.3
      eleventh 352.4
      twelfth 352.5
  cystic - *see* Cyst
  degenerative - *see* Degeneration
  dermal (skin) 709.9
  Dieulafoy (hemorrhagic)
      of
          duodenum 537.84
          intestine 569.86
          stomach 537.84
  duodenum 537.89
      with obstruction 537.3
  eyelid 373.9
  gasserian ganglion 350.8
  gastric 537.89
  gastroduodenal 537.89
  gastrointestinal 569.89
  glossopharyngeal nerve 352.2

Lesion(s) *(Continued)*
  heart (organic) - *see also* Disease, heart
      vascular - *see* Disease,
          cardiovascular
  helix (ear) 709.9
  high grade myelodysplastic syndrome
      238.73
  hyperchromic, due to pinta (carate)
      103.1
  hyperkeratotic *(see also* Hyperkeratosis)
      701.1
  hypoglossal nerve 352.5
  hypopharynx 478.29
  hypothalamic 253.9
  ileocecal coil 569.89
  ileum 569.89
  iliohypogastric nerve 355.79
  ilioinguinal nerve 355.79
  in continuity - *see* Injury, nerve, by site
  inflammatory - *see* Inflammation
  intestine 569.89
  intracerebral - *see* Lesion, brain
  intrachiasmal (optic) *(see also* Lesion,
      chiasmal) 377.54
  intracranial, space-occupying NEC 784.2
  joint 719.90
      ankle 719.97
      elbow 719.92
      foot 719.97
      hand 719.94
      hip 719.95
      knee 719.96
      multiple sites 719.99
      pelvic region 719.95
      sacroiliac (old) 724.6
      shoulder (region) 719.91
      specified site NEC 719.98
      wrist 719.93
  keratotic *(see also* Keratosis) 701.1
  kidney *(see also* Disease, renal) 593.9
  laryngeal nerve (recurrent) 352.3
  leonine 030.0
  lip 528.5
  liver 573.8
  low grade myelodysplastic syndrome
      238.72
  lumbosacral
      plexus 353.1
      root (nerve) NEC 353.4
  lung 518.89
      coin 793.1
  maxillary sinus 473.0
  mitral - *see* Endocarditis, mitral
  Morel Lavallée - *see* Hematoma,
      by site ◀
  motor cortex 348.89 ◀▦
  nerve *(see also* Disorder, nerve) 355.9
  nervous system 349.9
      congenital 742.9
  nonallopathic NEC 739.9
      in region (of)
          abdomen 739.9
          acromioclavicular 739.7
          cervical, cervicothoracic 739.1
          costochondral 739.8
          costovertebral 739.8
          extremity
              lower 739.6
              upper 739.7
          head 739.0
          hip 739.5
          lower extremity 739.6
          lumbar, lumbosacral 739.3
          occipitocervical 739.0

Lesion(s) *(Continued)*
  nonallopathic NEC *(Continued)*
    in region (of) *(Continued)*
      pelvic 739.5
      pubic 739.5
      rib cage 739.8
      sacral, sacrococcygeal, sacroiliac 739.4
      sternochondral 739.8
      sternoclavicular 739.7
      thoracic, thoracolumbar 739.2
      upper extremity 739.7
  nose (internal) 478.19
  obstructive - *see* Obstruction
  obturator nerve 355.79
  occlusive
    artery - *see* Embolism, artery
  organ or site NEC - *see* Disease, by site
  osteolytic 733.90
  paramacular, of retina 363.32
  peptic 537.89
  periodontal, due to traumatic occlusion 523.8
  perirectal 569.49
  peritoneum (granulomatous) 568.89
  pigmented (skin) 709.00
  pinta - *see* Pinta, lesions
  polypoid - *see* Polyp
  prechiasmal (optic) *(see also* Lesion, chiasmal) 377.54
  primary - *see also* Syphilis, primary
    carate 103.0
    pinta 103.0
    yaws 102.0
  pulmonary 518.89
    valve *(see also* Endocarditis, pulmonary) 424.3
  pylorus 537.89
  radiation NEC 990
  radium NEC 990
  rectosigmoid 569.89
  retina, retinal - *see also* Retinopathy
    vascular 362.17
  retroperitoneal 568.89
  romanus 720.1
  sacroiliac (joint) 724.6
  salivary gland 527.8
    benign lymphoepithelial 527.8
  saphenous nerve 355.79
  secondary - *see* Syphilis, secondary
  sigmoid 569.89
  sinus (accessory) (nasal) *(see also* Sinusitis) 473.9
  skin 709.9
    suppurative 686.00
  SLAP (superior glenoid labrum) 840.7
  space-occupying, intracranial NEC 784.2
  spinal cord 336.9
    congenital 742.9
    traumatic (complete) (incomplete) (transverse) - *see also* Injury, spinal, by site
      with
        broken
          back - *see* Fracture, vertebra, by site, with spinal cord injury
          neck - *see* Fracture, vertebra, cervical, with spinal cord injury

Lesion(s) *(Continued)*
  spinal cord *(Continued)*
    traumatic *(Continued)*
      with *(Continued)*
        fracture, vertebra - *see* Fracture, vertebra, by site, with spinal cord injury
  spleen 289.50
  stomach 537.89
  superior glenoid labrum (SLAP) 840.7
  syphilitic - *see* Syphilis
  tertiary - *see* Syphilis, tertiary
  thoracic root (nerve) 353.3
  tonsillar fossa 474.9
  tooth, teeth 525.8
    white spot 521.01
  traumatic NEC *(see also* nature and site of injury) 959.9
  tricuspid (valve) - *see* Endocarditis, tricuspid
  trigeminal nerve 350.9
  ulcerated or ulcerative - *see* Ulcer
  uterus NEC 621.9
  vagina 623.8
  vagus nerve 352.3
  valvular - *see* Endocarditis
  vascular 459.9
    affecting central nervous system *(see also* Lesion, cerebrovascular) 437.9
    following trauma *(see also* Injury, blood vessel, by site) 904.9
    retina 362.17
    traumatic - *see* Injury, blood vessel, by site
    umbilical cord 663.6 ●
      affecting fetus or newborn 762.6
  visual
    cortex NEC *(see also* Disorder, visual, cortex) 377.73
    pathway NEC *(see also* Disorder, visual, pathway) 377.63
  warty - *see* Verruca
  white spot, on teeth 521.01
  x-ray NEC 990
Lethargic - *see* condition
Lethargy 780.79
Letterer-Siwe disease (acute histiocytosis X) (M9722/3) 202.5 ●
Leucinosis 270.3
Leucocoria 360.44
Leucosarcoma (M9850/3) 207.8 ●
Leukasmus 270.2
Leukemia, leukemic (congenital) (M9800/3) 208.9 ●

> Note 51 Use the following fifth-digit subclassification for categories 203–208:
>
> 0 without mention of having achieved remission
>   failed remission
> 1 with remission
> 2 in relapse

  acute NEC (M9801/3) 208.0 ●
  aleukemic NEC (M9804/3) 208.8 ●
    granulocytic (M9864/3) 205.8 ●
  basophilic (M9870/3) 205.1 ●
  blast (cell) (M9801/3) 208.0 ●
  blastic (M9801/3) 208.0 ●
    granulocytic (M9861/3) 205.0 ●

Leukemia, leukemic *(Continued)*
  chronic NEC (M9803/3) 208.1 ●
  compound (M9810/3) 207.8 ●
  eosinophilic (M9880/3) 205.1 ●
  giant cell (M9910/3) 207.2 ●
  granulocytic (M9860/3) 205.9 ●
    acute (M9861/3) 205.0 ●
    aleukemic (M9864/3) 205.8 ●
    blastic (M9861/3) 205.0 ●
    chronic (M9863/3) 205.1 ●
    subacute (M9862/3) 205.2 ●
    subleukemic (M9864/3) 205.8 ●
  hairy cell (M9940/3) 202.4 ●
  hemoblastic (M9801/3) 208.0 ●
  histiocytic (M9890/3) 206.9 ●
  lymphatic (M9820/3) 204.9 ●
    acute (M9821/3) 204.0 ●
    aleukemic (M9824/3) 204.8 ●
    chronic (M9823/3) 204.1 ●
    subacute (M9822/3) 204.2 ●
    subleukemic (M9824/3) 204.8 ●
  lymphoblastic (M9821/3) 204.0 ●
  lymphocytic (M9820/3) 204.9 ●
    acute (M9821/3) 204.0 ●
    aleukemic (M9824/3) 204.8 ●
    chronic (M9823/3) 204.1 ●
    granular
      large T-cell 204.8 ●
    subacute (M9822/3) 204.2 ●
    subleukemic (M9824/3) 204.8 ●
  lymphogenous (M9820/3) - *see* Leukemia, lymphoid
  lymphoid (M9820/3) 204.9 ●
    acute (M9821/3) 204.0 ●
    aleukemic (M9824/3) 204.8 ●
    blastic (M9821/3) 204.0 ●
    chronic (M9823/3) 204.1 ●
    subacute (M9822/3) 204.2 ●
    subleukemic (M9824/3) 204.8 ●
  lymphosarcoma cell (M9850/3) 207.8 ●
  mast cell (M9900/3) 207.8 ●
  megakaryocytic (M9910/3) 207.2 ●
  megakaryocytoid (M9910/3) 207.2 ●
  mixed (cell) (M9810/3) 207.8 ●
  monoblastic (M9891/3) 206.0 ●
  monocytic (Schilling-type) (M9890/3) 206.9 ●
    acute (M9891/3) 206.0 ●
    aleukemic (M9894/3) 206.8 ●
    chronic (M9893/3) 206.1 ●
    Naegeli-type (M9863/3) 205.1 ●
    subacute (M9892/3) 206.2 ●
    subleukemic (M9894/3) 206.8 ●
  monocytoid (M9890/3) 206.9 ●
    acute (M9891/3) 206.0 ●
    aleukemic (M9894/3) 206.8 ●
    chronic (M9893/3) 206.1 ●
    myelogenous (M9863/3) 205.1 ●
    subacute (M9892/3) 206.2 ●
    subleukemic (M9894/3) 206.8 ●
  monomyelocytic (M9860/3) - *see* Leukemia, myelomonocytic
  myeloblastic (M9861/3) 205.0 ●
  myelocytic (M9863/3) 205.1 ●
    acute (M9861/3) 205.0 ●
  myelogenous (M9860/3) 205.9 ●
    acute (M9861/3) 205.0 ●
    aleukemic (M9864/3) 205.8 ●
    chronic (M9863/3) 205.1 ●
    monocytoid (M9863/3) 205.1 ●
    subacute (M9862/3) 205.2 ●
    subleukemic (M9864) 205.8 ●
  myeloid (M9860/3) 205.9 ●
    acute (M9861/3) 205.0 ●

◀ New   ◀▦ Revised   ~~deleted~~ Deleted   ● Use Additional Digit(s)   ▦ Omit code

Lichen *(Continued)*
  spinulosus 757.39
    mycotic 117.9
  striata 697.8
  urticatus 698.2
Lichenification 698.3
  nodular 698.3
Lichenoides tuberculosis (primary) *(see also* Tuberculosis) 017.0
Lichtheim's disease or syndrome (subacute combined sclerosis with pernicious anemia) 281.0 *[336.2]*
Lien migrans 289.59
Lientery *(see also* Diarrhea) 787.91
  infectious 009.2
Life circumstance problem NEC V62.89
Li-Fraumeni cancer syndrome V84.01
Ligament - *see* condition
Light-for-dates (infant) 764.0●
  with signs of fetal malnutrition 764.1●
  affecting management of pregnancy 656.5●
Light-headedness 780.4
Lightning (effects) (shock) (stroke) (struck by) 994.0
  burn - *see* Burn, by site
  foot 266.2
Lightwood's disease or syndrome (renal tubular acidosis) 588.89
Lignac's disease (cystinosis) 270.0
Lignac (-de Toni) (-Fanconi) (-Debré) syndrome (cystinosis) 270.0
Lignac (-Fanconi) syndrome (cystinosis) 270.0
Ligneous thyroiditis 245.3
Likoff's syndrome (angina in menopausal women) 413.9
Limb - *see* condition
Limitation of joint motion *(see also* Stiffness, joint) 719.5●
  sacroiliac 724.6
Limit dextrinosis 271.0
Limited
  cardiac reserve - *see* Disease, heart
  duction, eye NEC 378.63
  mandibular range of motion 524.52
Lindau's disease (retinocerebral angiomatosis) 759.6
Lindau (-von Hippel) disease (angiomatosis retinocerebellosa) 759.6
Linea corneae senilis 371.41
Lines
  Beau's (transverse furrows on fingernails) 703.8
  Harris' 733.91
  Hudson-Stähli 371.11
  Stähli's 371.11
Lingua
  geographical 529.1
  nigra (villosa) 529.3
  plicata 529.5
    congenital 750.13
  tylosis 528.6
Lingual (tongue) - *see also* condition
  thyroid 759.2
Linitis (gastric) 535.4●
  plastica (M8142/3) 151.9
Lioderma essentialis (cum melanosis et telangiectasia) 757.33
Lip - *see also* condition
  biting 528.9
Lipalgia 272.8
Lipedema - *see* Edema

Lipemia *(see also* Hyperlipidemia) 272.4
  retina, retinalis 272.3
Lipidosis 272.7
  cephalin 272.7
  cerebral (infantile) (juvenile) (late) 330.1
  cerebroretinal 330.1 *[362.71]*
  cerebroside 272.7
  cerebrospinal 272.7
  chemically-induced 272.7
  cholesterol 272.7
  diabetic 250.8● *[272.7]*
    due to secondary diabetes 249.8● *[272.7]*
  dystopic (hereditary) 272.7
  glycolipid 272.7
  hepatosplenomegalic 272.3
  hereditary, dystopic 272.7
  sulfatide 330.0
Lipoadenoma (M8324/0 - *see* Neoplasm, by site, benign
Lipoblastoma (M8881/0) - *see* Lipoma, by site
Lipoblastomatosis (M8881/0) - *see* Lipoma, by site
Lipochondrodystrophy 277.5
Lipochrome histiocytosis (familial) 288.1
Lipodystrophia progressiva 272.6
Lipodystrophy (progressive) 272.6
  insulin 272.6
  intestinal 040.2
  mesenteric 567.82
Lipofibroma (M8851/0) - *see* Lipoma, by site
Lipoglycoproteinosis 272.8
Lipogranuloma, sclerosing 709.8
Lipogranulomatosis (disseminated) 272.8
  kidney 272.8
Lipoid - *see also* condition
  histiocytosis 272.7
    essential 272.7
  nephrosis *(see also* Nephrosis) 581.3
  proteinosis of Urbach 272.8
Lipoidemia *(see also* Hyperlipidemia) 272.4
Lipoidosis *(see also* Lipidosis) 272.7
Lipoma (M8850/0) 214.9
  breast (skin) 214.1
  face 214.0
  fetal (M8881/0) - *see also* Lipoma, by site
    fat cell (M8880/0) - *see* Lipoma, by site
  infiltrating (M8856/0) - *see* Lipoma, by site
  intra-abdominal 214.3
  intramuscular (M8856/0) - *see* Lipoma, by site
  intrathoracic 214.2
  kidney 214.3
  mediastinum 214.2
  muscle 214.8
  peritoneum 214.3
  retroperitoneum 214.3
  skin 214.1
    face 214.0
  spermatic cord 214.4
  spindle cell (M8857/0) - *see* Lipoma, by site
  stomach 214.3
  subcutaneous tissue 214.1
    face 214.0
  thymus 214.2
  thyroid gland 214.2

Lipomatosis (dolorosa) 272.8
  epidural 214.8
  fetal (M8881/0) - *see* Lipoma, by site
  Launois-Bensaude's 272.8
Lipomyohemangioma (M8860/0)
  specified site - *see* Neoplasm, connective tissue, benign
  unspecified site 223.0
Lipomyoma (M8860/0)
  specified site - *see* Neoplasm, connective tissue, benign
  unspecified site 223.0
Lipomyxoma (M8852/0) - *see* Lipoma, by site
Lipomyxosarcoma (M8852/3) - *see* Neoplasm, connective tissue, malignant
Lipophagocytosis 289.89
Lipoproteinemia (alpha) 272.4
  broad-beta 272.2
  floating-beta 272.2
  hyper-pre-beta 272.1
Lipoproteinosis (Rossle-Urbach-Wiethe) 272.8
Liposarcoma (M8850/3) - *see also* Neoplasm, connective tissue, malignant
  differentiated type (M8851/3) - *see* Neoplasm, connective tissue, malignant
  embryonal (M8852/3) - *see* Neoplasm, connective tissue, malignant
  mixed type (M8855/3) - *see* Neoplasm, connective tissue, malignant
  myxoid (M8852/3) - *see* Neoplasm, connective tissue, malignant
  pleomorphic (M8854/3) - *see* Neoplasm, connective tissue, malignant
  round cell (M8853/3) - *see* Neoplasm, connective tissue, malignant
  well differentiated type (M8851/3) - *see* Neoplasm, connective tissue, malignant
Liposynovitis prepatellaris 272.8
Lipping
  cervix 622.0
  spine *(see also* Spondylosis) 721.90
  vertebra *(see also* Spondylosis) 721.90
Lip pits (mucus), congenital 750.25
Lipschütz disease or ulcer 616.50
Lipuria 791.1
  bilharziasis 120.0
Liquefaction, vitreous humor 379.21
Lisping 307.9
Lissauer's paralysis 094.1
Lissencephalia, lissencephaly 742.2
Listerellose 027.0
Listeriose 027.0
Listeriosis 027.0
  congenital 771.2
  fetal 771.2
  suspected fetal damage affecting management of pregnancy 655.4●
Listlessness 780.79
Lithemia 790.6
Lithiasis - *see also* Calculus
  hepatic (duct) - *see* Choledocholithiasis
  urinary 592.9
Lithopedion 779.9
  affecting management of pregnancy 656.8●

◀ New   ◀▥ Revised   ~~deleted~~ Deleted   ● Use Additional Digit(s)   ▨ Omit code

Lithosis (occupational) 502
   with tuberculosis - see Tuberculosis,
      pulmonary
Lithuria 791.9
Litigation V62.5
Little
   league elbow 718.82
   stroke syndrome 435.9
Little's disease - see Palsy, cerebral
Littre's
   gland - see condition
   hernia - see Hernia, Littre's
Littritis (see also Urethritis) 597.89
Livedo 782.61
   annularis 782.61
   racemose 782.61
   reticularis 782.61
Live flesh 781.0
Liver - see also condition
   donor V59.6
Livida, asphyxia
   newborn 768.6
Living
   alone V60.3
      with handicapped person V60.4
Lloyd's syndrome 258.1
Loa loa 125.2
Loasis 125.2
Lobe, lobar - see condition
Lobo's disease or blastomycosis
      116.2
Lobomycosis 116.2
Lobotomy syndrome 310.0
Lobstein's disease (brittle bones and
      blue sclera) 756.51
Lobster-claw hand 755.58
Lobulation (congenital) - see also
      Anomaly, specified type NEC, by
      site
   kidney, fetal 753.3
   liver, abnormal 751.69
   spleen 759.0
Lobule, lobular - see condition
Local, localized - see condition
Locked bowel or intestine (see also
      Obstruction, intestine) 560.9
Locked-in state 344.81
Locked twins 660.5●
   affecting fetus or newborn 763.1
Locking
   joint (see also Derangement, joint)
      718.90
   knee 717.9
Lockjaw (see also Tetanus) 037
Locomotor ataxia (progressive) 094.0
Löffler's
   endocarditis 421.0
   eosinophilia or syndrome 518.3
   pneumonia 518.3
   syndrome (eosinophilic
      pneumonitis) 518.3
Löfgren's syndrome (sarcoidosis)
      135
Loiasis 125.2
   eyelid 125.2 [373.6]
Loneliness V62.89
Lone Star fever 082.8
Long labor 662.1●
   affecting fetus or newborn 763.89
   first stage 662.0●
   second stage 662.2●
Longitudinal stripes or grooves, nails
      703.8
   congenital 757.5

Long-term (current) drug use V58.69
   antibiotics V58.62
   anticoagulants V58.61
   anti-inflammatories, non-steroidal
      (NSAID) V58.64
   antiplatelets/antithrombotics
      V58.63
   aspirin V58.66
   high-risk medications NEC V58.69
   insulin V58.67
   methadone V58.69
   opiate analgesic V58.69
   pain killers V58.69
      anti-inflammatories, non-steroidal
         (NSAID) V58.64
      aspirin V58.66
   steroids V58.65
   tamoxifen V07.51   ◀▥
Loop
   intestine (see also Volvulus) 560.2
   intrascleral nerve 379.29
   vascular on papilla (optic) 743.57
Loose - see also condition
   body
      in tendon sheath 727.82
      joint 718.10
         ankle 718.17
         elbow 718.12
         foot 718.17
         hand 718.14
         hip 718.15
         knee 717.6
         multiple sites 718.19
         pelvic region 718.15
         prosthetic implant - see
            Complications, mechanical
         shoulder (region) 718.11
         specified site NEC 718.18
         wrist 718.13
      cartilage (joint) (see also Loose, body,
            joint) 718.1●
         knee 717.6
      facet (vertebral) 724.9
      prosthetic implant - see Complications,
         mechanical
      sesamoid, joint (see also Loose, body,
            joint) 718.1●
      tooth, teeth 525.8
Loosening epiphysis 732.9
Looser (-Debray)-Milkman syndrome
      (osteomalacia with
      pseudofractures) 268.2
Lop ear (deformity) 744.29
Lorain's disease or syndrome (pituitary
      dwarfism) 253.3
Lorain-Levi syndrome (pituitary
      dwarfism) 253.3
Lordosis (acquired) (postural) 737.20
   congenital 754.2
   due to or associated with
      Charcôt-Marie-Tooth disease 356.1
         [737.42]
      mucopolysaccharidosis 277.5
         [737.42]
      neurofibromatosis 237.71 [737.42]
      osteitis
         deformans 731.0 [737.42]
         fibrosa cystica 252.01 [737.42]
      osteoporosis (see also Osteoporosis)
         733.00 [737.42]
      poliomyelitis (see also Poliomyelitis)
         138 [737.42]
      tuberculosis (see also Tuberculosis)
         015.0● [737.42]

Lordosis (Continued)
   late effect of rickets 268.1 [737.42]
   postlaminectomy 737.21
   postsurgical NEC 737.22
   rachitic 268.1 [737.42]
   specified NEC 737.29
   tuberculous (see also Tuberculosis)
      015.0● [737.42]
Loss
   appetite 783.0
      hysterical 300.11
      nonorganic origin 307.59
      psychogenic 307.59
   blood - see Hemorrhage
   central vision 368.41
   consciousness 780.09
      transient 780.2
   control, sphincter, rectum 787.6
      nonorganic origin 307.7
   ear ossicle, partial 385.24
   elasticity, skin 782.8
   extremity or member, traumatic,
      current - see Amputation,
      traumatic
   fluid (acute) 276.50
      with
         hypernatremia 276.0
         hyponatremia 276.1
      fetus or newborn 775.5
   hair 704.00
   hearing - see also Deafness
      central 389.14
      conductive (air) 389.00
         with sensorineural hearing loss
            389.20
            bilateral 389.22
            unilateral 389.21
         bilateral 389.06
         combined types 389.08
         external ear 389.01
         inner ear 389.04
         middle ear 389.03
         multiple types 389.08
         tympanic membrane 389.02
         unilateral 389.05
      mixed conductive and sensorineural
            389.20
         bilateral 389.22
         unilateral 389.21
      mixed type 389.20
         bilateral 389.22
         unilateral 389.21
      nerve
         bilateral 389.12
         unilateral 389.13
      neural
         bilateral 389.12
         unilateral 389.13
      noise-induced 388.12
      perceptive NEC (see also Loss,
         hearing, sensorineural)
         389.10
      sensorineural 389.10
         with conductive hearing loss
            389.20
            bilateral 389.22
            unilateral 389.21
         asymmetrical 389.16
         bilateral 389.18
         central 389.14
         neural
            bilateral 389.12
            unilateral 389.13

Loss *(Continued)*
  hearing *(Continued)*
    sensorineural *(Continued)*
      sensory
        bilateral 389.11
          unilateral 389.17
        unilateral 389.15
      sensory
        bilateral 389.11
        unilateral 389.17
      specified type NEC 389.8
      sudden NEC 388.2
  height 781.91
  labyrinthine reactivity (unilateral) 386.55
    bilateral 386.56
  memory *(see also* Amnesia) 780.93
    mild, following organic brain damage 310.8 ◀▥
  mind *(see also* Psychosis) 298.9
  occusal vertical dimension 524.37
  organ or part - *see* Absence, by site, acquired
  sensation 782.0
  sense of
    smell *(see also* Disturbance, sensation) 781.1
    taste *(see also* Disturbance, sensation) 781.1
    touch *(see also* Disturbance, sensation) 781.1
  sight (acquired) (complete) (congenital) - *see* Blindness
  spinal fluid
    headache 349.0
  substance of
    bone *(see also* Osteoporosis) 733.00
    cartilage 733.99
      ear 380.32
    vitreous (humor) 379.26
  tooth, teeth
    acquired 525.10
      due to
        caries 525.13
        extraction 525.10
        periodontal disease 525.12
        specified NEC 525.19
        trauma 525.11
  vision, visual *(see also* Blindness) 369.9
    both eyes *(see also* Blindness, both eyes) 369.3
    complete *(see also* Blindness, both eyes) 369.00
    one eye 369.8
    sudden 368.11
    transient 368.12
  vitreous 379.26
  voice *(see also* Aphonia) 784.41
  weight (cause unknown) 783.21
Lou Gehrig's disease 335.20
Louis-Bar syndrome (ataxia-telangiectasia) 334.8
Louping ill 063.1
Lousiness - *see* Lice
Low
  back syndrome 724.2
  basal metabolic rate (BMR) 794.7
  birthweight 765.1●
    extreme (less than 1000 grams) 765.0●
    for gestational age 764.0●
    status *(see also* Status, low birth weight) V21.30
  bladder compliance 596.52

Low *(Continued)*
  blood pressure *(see also* Hypotension) 458.9
    reading (incidental) (isolated) (nonspecific) 796.3
  cardiac reserve - *see* Disease, heart
  compliance bladder 596.52
  frequency deafness - *see* Disorder, hearing
  function - *see also* Hypofunction
    kidney *(see also* Disease, renal) 593.9
    liver 573.9
  hemoglobin 285.9
  implantation, placenta - *see* Placenta, previa
  insertion, placenta - *see* Placenta, previa
  lying
    kidney 593.0
    organ or site, congenital - *see* Malposition, congenital
    placenta - *see* Placenta, previa
  output syndrome (cardiac) *(see also* Failure, heart) 428.9
  platelets (blood) *(see also* Thrombocytopenia) 287.5
  reserve, kidney *(see also* Disease, renal) 593.9
  risk
    human papillomavirus (HPV) DNA test positive
      anal 796.79
      cervical 795.09
      vaginal 795.19
  salt syndrome 593.9
  tension glaucoma 365.12
  vision 369.9
    both eyes 369.20
    one eye 369.70
Lowe (-Terrey-MacLachlan) syndrome (oculocerebrorenal dystrophy) 270.8
Lower extremity - *see* condition
Lown (-Ganong)-Levine syndrome (short P-R interval, normal QRS complex, and paroxysmal supraventricular tachycardia) 426.81
LSD reaction *(see also* Abuse, drugs, nondependent) 305.3●
L-shaped kidney 753.3
Lucas-Championnière disease (fibrinous bronchitis) 466.0
Lucey-Driscoll syndrome (jaundice due to delayed conjugation) 774.30
Ludwig's
  angina 528.3
  disease (submaxillary cellulitis) 528.3
Lues (venerea), luetic - *see* Syphilis
Luetscher's syndrome (dehydration) 276.51
Lumbago 724.2
  due to displacement, intervertebral disc 722.10
Lumbalgia 724.2
  due to displacement, intervertebral disc 722.10
Lumbar - *see* condition
Lumbarization, vertebra 756.15
Lumbermen's itch 133.8
Lump - *see also* Mass
  abdominal 789.3●
  breast 611.72
  chest 786.6
  epigastric 789.3●

Lump *(Continued)*
  head 784.2
  kidney 753.3
  liver 789.1
  lung 786.6
  mediastinal 786.6
  neck 784.2
  nose or sinus 784.2
  pelvic 789.3●
  skin 782.2
  substernal 786.6
  throat 784.2
  umbilicus 789.3●
Lunacy *(see also* Psychosis) 298.9
Lunatomalacia 732.3
Lung - *see also* condition
  donor V59.8
  drug addict's 417.8
  mainliners' 417.8
  vanishing 492.0
Lupoid (miliary) of Boeck 135
Lupus 710.0
  anticoagulant 289.81
  Cazenave's (erythematosus) 695.4
  discoid (local) 695.4
  disseminated 710.0
  erythematodes (discoid) (local) 695.4
  erythematosus (discoid) (local) 695.4
    disseminated 710.0
    eyelid 373.34
    systemic 710.0
      with
        encephalitis 710.0 *[323.81]*
        lung involvement 710.0 *[517.8]*
      inhibitor (presence of) 286.5
  exedens 017.0●
  eyelid *(see also* Tuberculosis) 017.0● *[373.4]*
  Hilliard's 017.0●
  hydralazine
    correct substance properly administered 695.4
    overdose or wrong substance given or taken 972.6
  miliaris disseminatus faciei 017.0●
  nephritis 710.0 *[583.81]*
    acute 710.0 *[580.81]*
    chronic 710.0 *[582.81]*
  nontuberculous, not disseminated 695.4
  pernio (Besnier) 135
  tuberculous *(see also* Tuberculosis) 017.0●
    eyelid *(see also* Tuberculosis) 017.0● *[373.4]*
  vulgaris 017.0●
Luschka's joint disease 721.90
Luteinoma (M8610/0) 220
Lutembacher's disease or syndrome (atrial septal defect with mitral stenosis) 745.5
Luteoma (M8610/0) 220
Lutz-Miescher disease (elastosis perforans serpiginosa) 701.1
Lutz-Splendore-de Almeida disease (Brazilian blastomycosis) 116.1
Luxatio
  bulbi due to birth injury 767.8
  coxae congenita *(see also* Dislocation, hip, congenital) 754.30
  erecta - *see* Dislocation, shoulder
  imperfecta - *see* Sprain, by site
  perinealis - *see* Dislocation, hip

◀ New   ◀▥ Revised   ~~deleted~~ Deleted   ● Use Additional Digit(s)   ▨ Omit code

Luxation - *see also* Dislocation, by site
  eyeball 360.81
    due to birth injury 767.8
    lateral 376.36
  genital organs (external) NEC - *see*
      Wound, open, genital organs
  globe (eye) 360.81
    lateral 376.36
  lacrimal gland (postinfectional) 375.16
  lens (old) (partial) 379.32
    congenital 743.37
      syphilitic 090.49 [379.32]
    Marfan's disease 090.49
    spontaneous 379.32
  penis - *see* Wound, open, penis
  scrotum - *see* Wound, open, scrotum
  testis - *see* Wound, open, testis
L-xyloketosuria 271.8
Lycanthropy (*see also* Psychosis) 298.9
Lyell's disease or syndrome (toxic
    epidermal necrolysis) 695.15
  due to drug
    correct substance properly
      administered 695.15
    overdose or wrong substance given
      or taken 977.9
      specified drug - *see* Table of
        Drugs and Chemicals
Lyme disease 088.81
Lymph
  gland or node - *see* condition
  scrotum (*see also* Infestation, filarial)
    125.9
Lymphadenitis 289.3
  with
    abortion - *see* Abortion, by type,
      with sepsis
    ectopic pregnancy (*see also*
      categories 633.0–633.9)
      639.0
    molar pregnancy (*see also* categories
      630–632) 639.0
  acute 683
    mesenteric 289.2
  any site, except mesenteric 289.3
    acute 683
    chronic 289.1
    mesenteric (acute) (chronic)
      (nonspecific) (subacute)
      289.2
    subacute 289.1
      mesenteric 289.2
  breast, puerperal, postpartum
    675.2●
  chancroidal (congenital) 099.0
  chronic 289.1
    mesenteric 289.2
  dermatopathic 695.89
  due to
    anthracosis (occupational) 500
    Brugia (Wuchereria) malayi
      125.1
    diphtheria (toxin) 032.89
    lymphogranuloma venereum
      099.1
    Wuchereria bancrofti 125.0
  following
    abortion 639.0
    ectopic or molar pregnancy
      639.0
  generalized 289.3
  gonorrheal 098.89
  granulomatous 289.1
  infectional 683

Lymphadenitis (*Continued*)
  mesenteric (acute) (chronic)
    (nonspecific) (subacute) 289.2
    due to Bacillus typhi 002.0
    tuberculous (*see also* Tuberculosis)
      014.8●
  mycobacterial 031.8
  purulent 683
  pyogenic 683
  regional 078.3
  septic 683
  streptococcal 683
  subacute, unspecified site 289.1
  suppurative 683
  syphilitic (early) (secondary) 091.4
    late 095.8
  tuberculous - *see* Tuberculosis, lymph
    gland
  venereal 099.1
Lymphadenoid goiter 245.2
Lymphadenopathy (general) 785.6
  due to toxoplasmosis (acquired)
    130.7
    congenital (active) 771.2
Lymphadenopathy-associated virus
  (disease) (illness) (infection) - *see*
    Human immunodeficiency virus
    (disease) (illness) (infection)
Lymphadenosis 785.6
  acute 075
Lymphangiectasis 457.1
  conjunctiva 372.89
  postinfectional 457.1
  scrotum 457.1
Lymphangiectatic elephantiasis,
    nonfilarial 457.1
Lymphangioendothelioma (M9170/0)
    228.1
  malignant (M9170/3) - *see* Neoplasm,
    connective tissue, malignant
Lymphangioma (M9170/0) 228.1
  capillary (M9171/0) 228.1
  cavernous (M9172/0) 228.1
  cystic (M9173/0) 228.1
  malignant (M9170/3) - *see* Neoplasm,
    connective tissue, malignant
Lymphangiomyoma (M9174/0) 228.1
Lymphangiomyomatosis (M9174/1) - *see*
    Neoplasm, connective tissue,
    uncertain behavior
Lymphangiosarcoma (M9170/3) - *see*
    Neoplasm, connective tissue,
    malig-nant
Lymphangitis 457.2
  with
    abortion - *see* Abortion, by type,
      with sepsis
    abscess - *see* Abscess, by site
    cellulitis - *see* Abscess, by site
    ectopic pregnancy (*see also*
      categories 633.0–633.9)
      639.0
    molar pregnancy (*see also* categories
      630–632) 639.0
  acute (with abscess or cellulitis)
    682.9
    specified site - *see* Abscess, by site
  breast, puerperal, postpartum
    675.2●
  chancroidal 099.0
  chronic (any site) 457.2
  due to
    Brugia (Wuchereria) malayi 125.1
    Wuchereria bancrofti 125.0

Lymphangitis (*Continued*)
  following
    abortion 639.0
    ectopic or molar pregnancy
      639.0
  gangrenous 457.2
  penis
    acute 607.2
    gonococcal (acute) 098.0
      chronic or duration of 2 months
        or more 098.2
  puerperal, postpartum,
    childbirth 670.8   ◀▥
  strumous, tuberculous (*see also*
    Tuberculosis) 017.2●
  subacute (any site) 457.2
  tuberculous - *see* Tuberculosis, lymph
    gland
Lymphatic (vessel) - *see* condition
Lymphatism 254.8
  scrofulous (*see also* Tuberculosis)
    017.2●
Lymphectasia 457.1
Lymphedema (*see also* Elephantiasis)
    457.1
  acquired (chronic) 457.1
  chronic hereditary 757.0
  congenital 757.0
  idiopathic hereditary 757.0
  praecox 457.1
  secondary 457.1
  surgical NEC 997.99
    postmastectomy (syndrome) 457.0
Lymph-hemangioma (M9120/0) - *see*
    Hemangioma, by site
Lymphoblastic - *see* condition
Lymphoblastoma (diffuse) (M9630/3)
    200.1●
  giant follicular (M9690/3) 202.0●
  macrofollicular (M9690/3) 202.0●
Lymphoblastosis, acute benign 075
Lymphocele 457.8
Lymphocythemia 288.51
Lymphocytic - *see also* condition
  chorioencephalitis (acute) (serous)
    049.0
  choriomeningitis (acute) (serous)
    049.0
Lymphocytoma (diffuse) (malignant)
    (M9620/3) 200.1●
Lymphocytomatosis (M9620/3) 200.1●
Lymphocytopenia 288.51
Lymphocytosis (symptomatic) 288.61
  infectious (acute) 078.89
Lymphoepithelioma (M8082/3) - *see*
    Neoplasm, by site, malignant
Lymphogranuloma (malignant)
    (M9650/3) 201.9●
  inguinale 099.1
  venereal (any site) 099.1
    with stricture of rectum 099.1
  venereum 099.1
Lymphogranulomatosis (malignant)
    (M9650/3) 201.9●
  benign (Boeck's sarcoid) (Schaumann's)
    135
  Hodgkin's (M9650/3) 201.9●
Lymphohistiocytosis, familial
    hemophagocytic 288.4
Lymphoid - *see* condition
Lympholeukoblastoma (M9850/3)
    207.8●
Lympholeukosarcoma (M9850/3)
    207.8●

Lymphoma (malignant) (M9590/3) 202.8●

Note 52   Use the following fifth-digit subclassification with categories 200–202:

0   unspecified site, extranodal and solid organ sites
1   lymph nodes of head, face, and neck
2   intrathoracic lymph nodes
3   intra-abdominal lymph nodes
4   lymph nodes of axilla and upper limb
5   lymph nodes of inguinal region and lower limb
6   intrapelvic lymph nodes
7   spleen
8   lymph nodes of multiple sites

benign (M9590/0) - see Neoplasm, by site, benign
Burkitt's type (lymphoblastic) (undifferentiated) (M9750/3) 200.2●
Castleman's (mediastinal lymph node hyperplasia) 785.6
centroblastic-centrocytic
    diffuse (M9614/3) 202.8●
    follicular (M9692/3) 202.0●
centroblastic type (diffuse) (M9632/3) 202.8●
    follicular (M9697/3) 202.0●
centrocytic (M9622/3) 202.8●
compound (M9613/3) 200.8●
convoluted cell type (lymphoblastic) (M9602/3) 202.8●
diffuse NEC (M9590/3) 202.8●
    large B cell 202.8●
follicular (giant) (M9690/3) 202.0●
    center cell (diffuse) (M9615/3) 202.8●
        cleaved (diffuse) (M9623/3) 202.8●
            follicular (M9695/3) 202.0●
        non-cleaved (diffuse) (M9633/3) 202.8●
            follicular (M9698/3) 202.0●
    centroblastic-centrocytic (M9692/3) 202.0●
    centroblastic type (M9697/3) 202.0●
    large cell 202.0● ◄
    lymphocytic
        intermediate differentiation (M9694/3) 202.0●
        poorly differentiated (M9696/3) 202.0●
    mixed (cell type) (lymphocytic-histiocytic) (small cell and large cell) (M9691/3) 202.0●
germinocytic (M9622/3) 202.8●
giant, follicular or follicle (M9690/3) 202.0●

Lymphoma (Continued)
histiocytic (diffuse) (M9640/3) 200.0●
    nodular (M9642/3) 200.0●
    pleomorphic cell type (M9641/3) 200.0●
Hodgkin's (M9650/3) (see also Disease, Hodgkin's) 201.9●
immunoblastic (type) (M9612/3) 200.8●
large cell (M9640/3) 200.7●
    anaplastic 200.6●
    nodular (M9642/3) 202.0●   ◄▥
    pleomorphic cell type (M9641/3) 200.0●
lymphoblastic (diffuse) (M9630/3) 200.1●
    Burkitt's type (M9750/3) 200.2●
    convoluted cell type (M9602/3) 202.8●
lymphocytic (cell type) (diffuse) (M9620/3) 200.1●
    with plasmacytoid differentiation, diffuse (M9611/3) 200.8●
    intermediate differentiation (diffuse) (M9621/3) 200.1●
        follicular (M9694/3) 202.0●
        nodular (M9694/3) 202.0●
    nodular (M9690/3) 202.0●
    poorly differentiated (diffuse) (M9630/3) 200.1●
        follicular (M9696/3) 202.0●
        nodular (M9696/3) 202.0●
    well differentiated (diffuse) (M9620/3) 200.1●
        follicular (M9693/3) 202.0●
        nodular (M9693/3) 202.0●
lymphocytic-histiocytic, mixed (diffuse) (M9613/3) 200.8●
    follicular (M9691/3) 202.0●
    nodular (M9691/3) 202.0●
lymphoplasmacytoid type (M9611/3) 200.8●
lymphosarcoma type (M9610/3) 200.1●
macrofollicular (M9690/3) 202.0●
mantle cell 200.4●
marginal zone 200.3●
    extranodal B-cell 200.3●
    nodal B-cell 200.3●
    splenic B-cell 200.3●
mixed cell type (diffuse) (M9613/3) 200.8●
    follicular (M9691/3) 202.0●
    nodular (M9691/3) 202.0●
nodular (M9690/3) 202.0●
    histiocytic (M9642/3) 200.0●
    lymphocytic (M9690/3) 202.0●
        intermediate differentiation (M9694/3) 202.0●
        poorly differentiated (M9696/3) 202.0●
    mixed (cell type) (lymphocytic-histiocytic) (small cell and large cell) (M9691/3) 202.0●
non-Hodgkin's type NEC (M9591/3) 202.8●

Lymphoma (Continued)
peripheral T-cell 202.7●
primary central nervous system 200.5●
reticulum cell (type) (M9640/3) 200.0●
small cell and large cell, mixed (diffuse) (M9613/3) 200.8●
    follicular (M9691/3) 202.0●
    nodular (9691/3) 202.0●
stem cell (type) (M9601/3) 202.8●
T-cell 202.1●
    peripheral 202.7●
undifferentiated (cell type) (non-Burkitt's) (M9600/3) 202.8●
    Burkitt's type (M9750/3) 200.2●
Lymphomatosis (M9590/3) - see also Lymphoma
    granulomatous 099.1
Lymphopathia
    venereum 099.1
    veneris 099.1
Lymphopenia 288.51
    familial 279.2
Lymphoreticulosis, benign (of inoculation) 078.3
Lymphorrhea 457.8
Lymphosarcoma (M9610/3) 200.1●
    diffuse (M9610/3) 200.1●
        with plasmacytoid differentiation (M9611/3) 200.8●
        lymphoplasmacytic (M9611/3) 200.8●
    follicular (giant) (M9690/3) 202.0●
        lymphoblastic (M9696/3) 202.0●
        lymphocytic, intermediate differentiation (M9694/3) 202.0●
    mixed cell type (M9691/3) 202.0●
    giant follicular (M9690/3) 202.0●
    Hodgkin's (M9650/3) 201.9●
    immunoblastic (M9612/3) 200.8●
    lymphoblastic (diffuse) (M9630/3) 200.1●
        follicular (M9696/3) 202.0●
        nodular (M9696/3) 202.0●
    lymphocytic (diffuse) (M9620/3) 200.1
        intermediate differentiation (diffuse) (M9621/3) 200.1●
            follicular (M9694/3) 202.0●
            nodular (M9694/3) 202.0●
    mixed cell type (diffuse) (M9613/3) 200.8●
        follicular (M9691/3) 202.0●
        nodular (M9691/3) 202.0●
    nodular (M9690/3) 202.0●
        lymphoblastic (M9696/3) 202.0●
        lymphocytic, intermediate differentiation (M9694/3) 202.0●
    mixed cell type (M9691/3) 202.0●
    prolymphocytic (M9631/3) 200.1●
    reticulum cell (M9640/3) 200.0●
Lymphostasis 457.8
Lypemania (see also Melancholia) 296.2●
Lyssa 071

◄ New   ◄▥ Revised   ~~deleted~~ Deleted   ● Use Additional Digit(s)   ▨ Omit code

M

Macacus ear 744.29
Maceration
  fetus (cause not stated) 779.9
  wet feet, tropical (syndrome) 991.4
Machado-Joseph disease 334.8
Machupo virus hemorrhagic fever 078.7
Macleod's syndrome (abnormal
    transradiancy, one lung) 492.8
Macrocephalia, macrocephaly 756.0
Macrocheilia (congenital) 744.81
Macrochilia (congenital) 744.81
Macrocolon (congenital) 751.3
Macrocornea 743.41
  associated with buphthalmos 743.22
Macrocytic - see condition
Macrocytosis 289.89
Macrodactylia, macrodactylism (fingers)
    (thumbs) 755.57
  toes 755.65
Macrodontia 520.2
Macroencephaly 742.4
Macrogenia 524.05
Macrogenitosomia (female) (male)
    (praecox) 255.2
Macrogingivae 523.8
Macroglobulinemia (essential)
    (idiopathic) (monoclonal) (primary)
    (syndrome) (Waldenström's) 273.3
Macroglossia (congenital) 750.15
  acquired 529.8
Macrognathia, macrognathism
    (congenital) 524.00
  mandibular 524.02
    alveolar 524.72
  maxillary 524.01
    alveolar 524.71
Macrogyria (congenital) 742.4
Macrohydrocephalus (see also
    Hydrocephalus) 331.4
Macromastia (see also Hypertrophy,
    breast) 611.1
Macrophage activation syndrome 288.4
Macropsia 368.14
Macrosigmoid 564.7
  congenital 751.3
Macrospondylitis, acromegalic 253.0
Macrostomia (congenital) 744.83
Macrotia (external ear) (congenital)
    744.22
Macula
  cornea, corneal
    congenital 743.43
      interfering with vision 743.42
      interfering with central vision 371.03
      not interfering with central vision 371.02
  degeneration (see also Degeneration,
    macula) 362.50
  hereditary (see also Dystrophy,
    retina) 362.70
  edema, cystoid 362.53
Maculae ceruleae 132.1
Macules and papules 709.8
Maculopathy, toxic 362.55
Madarosis 374.55
Madelung's
  deformity (radius) 755.54
  disease (lipomatosis) 272.8
  lipomatosis 272.8
Madness (see also Psychosis) 298.9
  myxedema (acute) 293.0
    subacute 293.1

Madura
  disease (actinomycotic) 039.9
    mycotic 117.4
  foot (actinomycotic) 039.4
    mycotic 117.4
Maduromycosis (actinomycotic) 039.9
  mycotic 117.4
Maffucci's syndrome (dyschondroplasia
    with hemangiomas) 756.4
Magenblase syndrome 306.4
Main en griffe (acquired) 736.06
  congenital 755.59
Maintenance
  chemotherapy regimen or treatment
    V58.11
  dialysis regimen or treatment
    extracorporeal (renal) V56.0
    peritoneal V56.8
    renal V56.0
  drug therapy or regimen
    chemotherapy, antineoplastic
      V58.11
    immunotherapy, antineoplastic
      V58.12
  external fixation NEC V54.89
  radiotherapy V58.0
  traction NEC V54.89
Majocchi's
  disease (purpura annularis
    telangiectodes) 709.1
  granuloma 110.6
Major - see condition
Mal
  cerebral (idiopathic) (see also Epilepsy)
    345.9●
  comital (see also Epilepsy) 345.9●
  de los pintos (see also Pinta) 103.9
  de Meleda 757.39
  de mer 994.6
  lie - see Presentation, fetal
  perforant (see also Ulcer, lower
    extremity) 707.15
Malabar itch 110.9
  beard 110.0
  foot 110.4
  scalp 110.0
Malabsorption 579.9
  calcium 579.8
  carbohydrate 579.8
  disaccharide 271.3
  drug-induced 579.8
  due to bacterial overgrowth 579.8
  fat 579.8
  folate, congenital 281.2
  galactose 271.1
  glucose-galactose (congenital) 271.3
  intestinal 579.9
  isomaltose 271.3
  lactose (hereditary) 271.3
  methionine 270.4
  monosaccharide 271.8
  postgastrectomy 579.3
  postsurgical 579.3
  protein 579.8
  sucrose (-isomaltose) (congenital)
    271.3
  syndrome 579.9
    postgastrectomy 579.3
    postsurgical 579.3
Malacia, bone 268.2
  juvenile (see also Rickets) 268.0
  Kienböck's (juvenile) (lunate) (wrist)
    732.3
    adult 732.8

Malacoplakia
  bladder 596.8
  colon 569.89
  pelvis (kidney) 593.89
  ureter 593.89
  urethra 599.84
Malacosteon 268.2
  juvenile (see also Rickets) 268.0
Maladaptation - see Maladjustment
Maladie de Roger 745.4
Maladjustment
  conjugal V61.10
    involving
      divorce V61.03
      estrangement V61.09
  educational V62.3
  family V61.9
    specified circumstance NEC
      V61.8
  marital V61.10
    involving
      divorce V61.03
      estrangement V61.09
  occupational V62.29
    current military deployment status
      V62.21
  simple, adult (see also Reaction,
    adjustment) 309.9
  situational acute (see also Reaction,
    adjustment) 309.9
  social V62.4
Malaise 780.79
Malakoplakia - see Malacoplakia
Malaria, malarial (fever) 084.6
  algid 084.9
  any type, with
    algid malaria 084.9
    blackwater fever 084.8
    fever
      blackwater 084.8
      hemoglobinuric (bilious)
        084.8
    hemoglobinuria, malarial 084.8
    hepatitis 084.9 [573.2]
    nephrosis 084.9 [581.81]
    pernicious complication NEC
      084.9
      cardiac 084.9
      cerebral 084.9
  cardiac 084.9
  carrier (suspected) of V02.9
  cerebral 084.9
  complicating pregnancy, childbirth,
    or puerperium 647.4●
  congenital 771.2
  congestion, congestive 084.6
    brain 084.9
  continued 084.0
  estivo-autumnal 084.0
  falciparum (malignant tertian)
    084.0
  hematinuria 084.8
  hematuria 084.8
  hemoglobinuria 084.8
  hemorrhagic 084.6
  induced (therapeutically) 084.7
    accidental - see Malaria, by type
  liver 084.9 [573.2]
  malariae (quartan) 084.2
  malignant (tertian) 084.0
  mixed infections 084.5
  monkey 084.4
  ovale 084.3
  pernicious, acute 084.0

Malaria, malarial (Continued)
  Plasmodium, P.
    falciparum 084.0
    malariae 084.2
    ovale 084.3
    vivax 084.1
  quartan 084.2
  quotidian 084.0
  recurrent 084.6
    induced (therapeutically) 084.7
      accidental - see Malaria, by type
  remittent 084.6
  specified types NEC 084.4
  spleen 084.6
  subtertian 084.0
  tertian (benign) 084.1
    malignant 084.0
  tropical 084.0
  typhoid 084.6
  vivax (benign tertian) 084.1
Malassez's disease (testicular cyst)
    608.89
Malassimilation 579.9
Maldescent, testis 752.51
Maldevelopment - see also Anomaly, by
    site
  brain 742.9
  colon 751.5
  hip (joint) 755.63
    congenital dislocation (see also
        Dislocation, hip, congenital)
        754.30
  mastoid process 756.0
  middle ear, except ossicles 744.03
    ossicles 744.04
  newborn (not malformation) 764.9●
  ossicles, ear 744.04
  spine 756.10
  toe 755.66
Male type pelvis 755.69
  with disproportion (fetopelvic) 653.2●
    affecting fetus or newborn 763.1
    causing obstructed labor 660.1●
      affecting fetus or newborn
          763.1
Malformation (congenital) - see also
    Anomaly
  bone 756.9
  bursa 756.9
  Chiari
    type I 348.4
    type II (see also Spina bifida)
        741.0●
    type III 742.0
    type IV 742.2
  circulatory system NEC 747.9
    specified type NEC 747.89
  cochlea 744.05
  digestive system NEC 751.9
    lower 751.5
    specified type NEC 751.8
    upper 750.9
  eye 743.9
  gum 750.9
  heart NEC 746.9
    specified type NEC 746.89
    valve 746.9
  internal ear 744.05
  joint NEC 755.9
    specified type NEC 755.8
  Mondini's (congenital) (malformation,
      cochlea) 744.05
  muscle 756.9
  nervous system (central) 742.9

Malformation (Continued)
  pelvic organs or tissues
    in pregnancy or childbirth 654.9●
      affecting fetus or newborn
          763.89
      causing obstructed labor 660.2●
        affecting fetus or newborn
            763.1
  placenta (see also Placenta, abnormal)
      656.7●
  respiratory organs 748.9
    specified type NEC 748.8
  Rieger's 743.44
  sense organs NEC 742.9
    specified type NEC 742.8
  skin 757.9
    specified type NEC 757.8
  spinal cord 742.9
  teeth, tooth NEC 520.9
  tendon 756.9
  throat 750.9
  umbilical cord (complicating delivery)
      663.9●
    affecting fetus or newborn 762.6
  umbilicus 759.9
  urinary system NEC 753.9
    specified type NEC 753.8
  venous - see Anomaly, vein
Malfunction - see also Dysfunction
  arterial graft 996.1
  cardiac pacemaker 996.01
  catheter device - see Complications,
      mechanical, catheter
  colostomy 569.62
    valve 569.62
  cystostomy 997.5
  device, implant, or graft NEC - see
      Complications, mechanical
  enteric stoma 569.62
  enterostomy 569.62
  esophagostomy 530.87
  gastroenteric 536.8
  gastrostomy 536.42
  ileostomy
    valve 569.62
  nephrostomy 997.5
  pacemaker - see Complications,
      mechanical, pacemaker
  prosthetic device, internal - see
      Complications, mechanical
  tracheostomy 519.02
  valve
    colostomy 569.62
    ileostomy 569.62
  vascular graft or shunt 996.1
Malgaigne's fracture (closed) 808.43
  open 808.53
Malherbe's
  calcifying epithelioma (M8110/0) - see
      Neoplasm, skin, benign
  tumor (M8110/0) - see Neoplasm, skin,
      benign
Malibu disease 919.8
  infected 919.9
Malignancy (M8000/3) - see Neoplasm,
    by site, malignant
Malignant - see condition
Malingerer, malingering V65.2
Mallet, finger (acquired) 736.1
  congenital 755.59
  late effect of rickets 268.1
Malleus 024
Mallory's bodies 034.1
Mallory-Weiss syndrome 530.7

Malnutrition (calorie) 263.9
  complicating pregnancy 648.9●
  degree
    first 263.1
    second 263.0
    third 262
    mild 263.1
    moderate 263.0
    severe 261
      protein-calorie 262
  fetus 764.2●
  "light-for-dates" 764.1●
  following gastrointestinal surgery 579.3
  intrauterine or fetal 764.2●
    fetus or infant "light-for-dates"
        764.1●
  lack of care, or neglect (child) (infant)
      995.52
    adult 995.84
  malignant 260
  mild 263.1
  moderate 263.0
  protein 260
  protein-calorie 263.9
    severe 262
    specified type NEC 263.8
  severe 261
    protein-calorie NEC 262
Malocclusion (teeth) 524.4
  angle's class I 524.21
  angle's class II 524.22
  angle's class III 524.23
  due to
    abnormal swallowing 524.59
    accessory teeth (causing crowding)
        524.31
    dentofacial abnormality NEC 524.89
    impacted teeth (causing crowding)
        520.6
    missing teeth 524.30
    mouth breathing 524.59
    sleep postures 524.59
    supernumerary teeth (causing
        crowding) 524.31
    thumb sucking 524.59
    tongue, lip, or finger habits 524.59
  temporomandibular (joint) 524.69
Malposition
  cardiac apex (congenital) 746.87
  cervix - see Malposition, uterus
  congenital
    adrenal (gland) 759.1
    alimentary tract 751.8
      lower 751.5
      upper 750.8
    aorta 747.21
    appendix 751.5
    arterial trunk 747.29
    artery (peripheral) NEC (see also
        Malposition, congenital,
        peripheral vascular system)
        747.60
      coronary 746.85
      pulmonary 747.3
    auditory canal 744.29
      causing impairment of hearing
          744.02
    auricle (ear) 744.29
      causing impairment of hearing
          744.02
      cervical 744.43
    biliary duct or passage 751.69
    bladder (mucosa) 753.8
      exteriorized or extroverted 753.5

Malposition (Continued)
  congenital (Continued)
    brachial plexus 742.8
    brain tissue 742.4
    breast 757.6
    bronchus 748.3
    cardiac apex 746.87
    cecum 751.5
    clavicle 755.51
    colon 751.5
    digestive organ or tract NEC 751.8
      lower 751.5
      upper 750.8
    ear (auricle) (external) 744.29
      ossicles 744.04
    endocrine (gland) NEC 759.2
    epiglottis 748.3
    Eustachian tube 744.24
    eye 743.8
    facial features 744.89
    fallopian tube 752.19
    finger(s) 755.59
      supernumerary 755.01
    foot 755.67
    gallbladder 751.69
    gastrointestinal tract 751.8
    genitalia, genital organ(s) or tract
      female 752.89
        external 752.49
        internal NEC 752.89
      male 752.89
        penis 752.69
        scrotal transposition 752.81
    glottis 748.3
    hand 755.59
    heart 746.87
      dextrocardia 746.87
        with complete transposition of
          viscera 759.3
    hepatic duct 751.69
    hip (joint) (see also Dislocation, hip,
      congenital) 754.30
    intestine (large) (small) 751.5
      with anomalous adhesions,
        fixation, or malrotation
        751.4
    joint NEC 755.8
    kidney 753.3
    larynx 748.3
    limb 755.8
      lower 755.69
      upper 755.59
    liver 751.69
    lung (lobe) 748.69
    nail(s) 757.5
    nerve 742.8
    nervous system NEC 742.8
    nose, nasal (septum) 748.1
    organ or site NEC - see Anomaly,
      specified type NEC, by site
    ovary 752.0
    pancreas 751.7
    parathyroid (gland) 759.2
    patella 755.64
    peripheral vascular system 747.60
      gastrointestinal 747.61
      lower limb 747.64
      renal 747.62
      specified NEC 747.69
      spinal 747.82
      upper limb 747.63
    pituitary (gland) 759.2
    respiratory organ or system NEC
      748.9

Malposition (Continued)
  congenital (Continued)
    rib (cage) 756.3
      supernumerary in cervical region
        756.2
    scapula 755.59
    shoulder 755.59
    spinal cord 742.59
    spine 756.19
    spleen 759.0
    sternum 756.3
    stomach 750.7
    symphysis pubis 755.69
    testis (undescended) 752.51
    thymus (gland) 759.2
    thyroid (gland) (tissue) 759.2
      cartilage 748.3
    toe(s) 755.66
      supernumerary 755.02
    tongue 750.19
    trachea 748.3
    uterus 752.3
    vein(s) (peripheral) NEC (see also
      Malposition, congenital,
      peripheral vascular system)
      747.60
      great 747.49
      portal 747.49
      pulmonary 747.49
    vena cava (inferior) (superior)
      747.49
  device, implant, or graft - see
    Complications, mechanical
  fetus NEC (see also Presentation, fetal)
    652.9●
    with successful version 652.1●
    affecting fetus or newborn 763.1
    before labor, affecting fetus or
      newborn 761.7
    causing obstructed labor 660.0●
    in multiple gestation (one fetus or
      more) 652.6●
      with locking 660.5●
      causing obstructed labor 660.0●
  gallbladder (see also Disease,
    gallbladder) 575.8
  gastrointestinal tract 569.89
    congenital 751.8
  heart (see also Malposition, congenital,
    heart) 746.87
  intestine 569.89
    congenital 751.5
  pelvic organs or tissues
    in pregnancy or childbirth 654.4●
      affecting fetus or newborn
        763.89
      causing obstructed labor 660.2●
        affecting fetus or newborn
          763.1
  placenta - see Placenta, previa
  stomach 537.89
    congenital 750.7
  tooth, teeth 524.30
    with impaction 520.6
  uterus (acquired) (acute) (adherent)
    (any degree) (asymptomatic)
    (postinfectional) (postpartal, old)
    621.6
    anteflexion or anteversion (see also
      Anteversion, uterus) 621.6
    congenital 752.3
    flexion 621.6
      lateral (see also Lateroversion,
        uterus) 621.6

Malposition (Continued)
  uterus (Continued)
    in pregnancy or childbirth 654.4●
      affecting fetus or newborn
        763.89
      causing obstructed labor 660.2●
        affecting fetus or newborn
          763.1
    inversion 621.6
    lateral (flexion) (version) (see also
      Lateroversion, uterus) 621.6
    lateroflexion (see also Lateroversion,
      uterus) 621.6
    lateroversion (see also Lateroversion,
      uterus) 621.6
    retroflexion or retroversion (see also
      Retroversion, uterus) 621.6
Malposture 729.90
Malpresentation, fetus (see also
  Presentation, fetal) 652.9●
Malrotation
  cecum 751.4
  colon 751.4
  intestine 751.4
  kidney 753.3
MALT (mucosa associated lymphoid
  tissue) 200.3●
Malt workers' lung 495.4
Malta fever (see also Brucellosis) 023.9
Maltosuria 271.3
Maltreatment (of)
  adult 995.80
    emotional 995.82
    multiple forms 995.85
    neglect (nutritional) 995.84
    physical 995.81
    psychological 995.82
    sexual 995.83
  child 995.50
    emotional 995.51
    multiple forms 995.59
    neglect (nutritional) 995.52
    physical 995.54
    shaken infant syndrome 995.55
    psychological 995.51
    sexual 995.53
  spouse (see also Maltreatment, adult)
    995.80
Malum coxae senilis 715.25
Malunion, fracture 733.81
Mammillitis (see also Mastitis) 611.0
  puerperal, postpartum 675.2●
Mammitis (see also Mastitis) 611.0
  puerperal, postpartum 675.2●
Mammographic
  calcification 793.89
  calculus 793.89
  microcalcification 793.81
Mammoplasia 611.1
Management
  contraceptive V25.9
    specified type NEC V25.8
  procreative V26.9
    specified type NEC V26.89
Mangled NEC (see also nature and site of
  injury) 959.9
Mania (monopolar) (see also Psychosis,
  affective) 296.0●
  alcoholic (acute) (chronic) 291.9
  Bell's - see Mania, chronic
  chronic 296.0●
    recurrent episode 296.1●
    single episode 296.0●
  compulsive 300.3

Mania *(Continued)*
   delirious (acute) 296.0●
      recurrent episode 296.1●
      single episode 296.0●
   epileptic *(see also* Epilepsy) 345.4●
   hysterical 300.10
   inhibited 296.89
   puerperal (after delivery) 296.0●
      recurrent episode 296.1●
      single episode 296.0●
   recurrent episode 296.1●
   senile 290.8
   single episode 296.0●
   stupor 296.89
   stuporous 296.89
   unproductive 296.89
Manic-depressive insanity, psychosis,
      reaction, or syndrome *(see also*
      Psychosis, affective) 296.80
   circular (alternating) 296.7
      currently
         depressed 296.5●
         episode unspecified 296.7
         hypomanic, previously depressed
            296.4●
         manic 296.4●
         mixed 296.6●
   depressed (type), depressive 296.2●
      atypical 296.82
      recurrent episode 296.3●
      single episode 296.2●
   hypomanic 296.0●
      recurrent episode 296.1●
      single episode 296.0●
   manic 296.0●
      atypical 296.81
      recurrent episode 296.1●
      single episode 296.0●
   mixed NEC 296.89
   perplexed 296.89
   stuporous 296.89
Manifestations, rheumatoid
   lungs 714.81
   pannus - *see* Arthritis, rheumatoid
   subcutaneous nodules - *see* Arthritis,
      rheumatoid
Mankowsky's syndrome (familial
      dysplastic osteopathy) 731.2
Mannoheptulosuria 271.8
Mannosidosis 271.8
Manson's
   disease (schistosomiasis) 120.1
   pyosis (pemphigus contagiosus) 684
   schistosomiasis 120.1
Mansonellosis 125.5
Manual - *see* condition
Maple bark disease 495.6
Maple bark-strippers' lung 495.6
Maple syrup (urine) disease or syndrome
   270.3
Marable's syndrome (celiac artery
      compression) 447.4
Marasmus 261
   brain 331.9
   due to malnutrition 261
   intestinal 569.89
   nutritional 261
   senile 797
   tuberculous NEC *(see also* Tuberculosis)
      011.9●
Marble
   bones 756.52
   skin 782.61
Marburg disease (virus) 078.89

March
   foot 733.94
   hemoglobinuria 283.2
Marchand multiple nodular hyperplasia
   (liver) 571.5
Marchesani (-Weill) syndrome
      (brachymorphism and ectopia
      lentis) 759.89
Marchiafava (-Bignami) disease or
      syndrome 341.8
Marchiafava-Micheli syndrome
      (paroxysmal nocturnal
      hemoglobinuria) 283.2
Marcus Gunn's syndrome (jaw-winking
      syndrome) 742.8
Marfan's
   congenital syphilis 090.49
   disease 090.49
   syndrome (arachnodactyly) 759.82
      meaning congenital syphilis
         090.49
      with luxation of lens 090.49
         [379.32]
Marginal
   implantation, placenta - *see* Placenta,
      previa
   placenta - *see* Placenta, previa
   sinus (hemorrhage) (rupture) 641.2●
      affecting fetus or newborn 762.1
Marie's
   cerebellar ataxia 334.2
   syndrome (acromegaly) 253.0
Marie-Bamberger disease or syndrome
      (hypertrophic) (pulmonary)
      (secondary) 731.2
   idiopathic (acropachyderma) 757.39
   primary (acropachyderma) 757.39
Marie-Charcôt-Tooth neuropathic
      atrophy, muscle 356.1
Marie-Strümpell arthritis or disease
      (ankylosing spondylitis) 720.0
Marihuana, marijuana
   abuse *(see also* Abuse, drugs,
      nondependent) 305.2●
   dependence *(see also* Dependence)
      304.3●
Marion's disease (bladder neck
      obstruction) 596.0
Marital conflict V61.10
Mark
   port wine 757.32
   raspberry 757.32
   strawberry 757.32
   stretch 701.3
   tattoo 709.09
Maroteaux-Lamy syndrome
      (mucopolysaccharidosis VI) 277.5
Marriage license examination V70.3
Marrow (bone)
   arrest 284.9
   megakaryocytic 287.30
   poor function 289.9
Marseilles fever 082.1
Marsh's disease (exophthalmic goiter)
   242.0●
Marshall's (hidrotic) ectodermal
      dysplasia 757.31
Marsh fever *(see also* Malaria) 084.6
Martin's disease 715.27
Martin-Albright syndrome
      (pseudohypoparathyroidism)
      275.49
Martorell-Fabre syndrome (pulseless
      disease) 446.7

Masculinization, female, with adrenal
      hyperplasia 255.2
Masculinovoblastoma (M8670/0)
   220
Masochism 302.83
Masons' lung 502
Mass
   abdominal 789.3●
   anus 787.99
   bone 733.90
   breast 611.72
   cheek 784.2
   chest 786.6
   cystic - *see* Cyst
   ear 388.8
   epigastric 789.3●
   eye 379.92
   female genital organ 625.8
   gum 784.2
   head 784.2
   intracranial 784.2
   joint 719.60
      ankle 719.67
      elbow 719.62
      foot 719.67
      hand 719.64
      hip 719.65
      knee 719.66
      multiple sites 719.69
      pelvic region 719.65
      shoulder (region) 719.61
      specified site NEC 719.68
      wrist 719.63
   kidney *(see also* Disease, kidney)
      593.9
   lung 786.6
   lymph node 785.6
   malignant (M8000/3) - *see* Neoplasm,
      by site, malignant
   mediastinal 786.6
   mouth 784.2
   muscle (limb) 729.89
   neck 784.2
   nose or sinus 784.2
   palate 784.2
   pelvis, pelvic 789.3●
   penis 607.89
   perineum 625.8
   rectum 787.99
   scrotum 608.89
   skin 782.2
   specified organ NEC - *see* Disease of
      specified organ or site
   splenic 789.2
   substernal 786.6
      thyroid *(see also* Goiter) 240.9
   superficial (localized) 782.2
   testes 608.89
   throat 784.2
   tongue 784.2
   umbilicus 789.3●
   uterus 625.8
   vagina 625.8
   vulva 625.8
Massive - *see* condition
Mastalgia 611.71
   psychogenic 307.89
Mast cell
   disease 757.33
      systemic (M9741/3) 202.6●
   leukemia (M9900/3) 207.8●
   sarcoma (M9742/3) 202.6●
   tumor (M9740/1) 238.5
      malignant (M9740/3) 202.6●

◀ New   ◀▥ Revised   ~~deleted~~ Deleted   ● Use Additional Digit(s)   ▨ Omit code

Masters-Allen syndrome 620.6
Mastitis (acute) (adolescent)
(diffuse) (interstitial) (lobular)
(nonpuerperal) (nonsuppurative)
(parenchymatous) (phlegmonous)
(simple) (subacute) (suppurative)
611.0
chronic (cystic) (fibrocystic) 610.1
cystic 610.1
Schimmelbusch's type 610.1
fibrocystic 610.1
infective 611.0
lactational 675.2●
lymphangitis 611.0
neonatal (noninfective) 778.7
infective 771.5
periductal 610.4
plasma cell 610.4
puerperal, postpartum, (interstitial)
(nonpurulent) (parenchymatous)
675.2●
purulent 675.1●
stagnation 676.2●
puerperalis 675.2●
retromammary 611.0
puerperal, postpartum 675.1●
submammary 611.0
puerperal, postpartum 675.1●
Mastocytoma (M9740/1) 238.5
malignant (M9740/3) 202.6●
Mastocytosis 757.33
malignant (M9741/3) 202.6●
systemic (M9741/3) 202.6●
Mastodynia 611.71
psychogenic 307.89
Mastoid - *see* condition
Mastoidalgia (*see also* Otalgia) 388.70
Mastoiditis (coalescent) (hemorrhagic)
(pneumococcal) (streptococcal)
(suppurative) 383.9
acute or subacute 383.00
with
Gradenigo's syndrome 383.02
petrositis 383.02
specified complication NEC
383.02
subperiosteal abscess 383.01
chronic (necrotic) (recurrent) 383.1
tuberculous (*see also* Tuberculosis)
015.6●
Mastopathy, mastopathia 611.9
chronica cystica 610.1
diffuse cystic 610.1
estrogenic 611.89
ovarian origin 611.89
Mastoplasia 611.1
Masturbation 307.9
Maternal condition, affecting fetus or
newborn
acute yellow atrophy of liver 760.8
albuminuria 760.1
anesthesia or analgesia 763.5
blood loss 762.1
chorioamnionitis 762.7
circulatory disease, chronic
(conditions classifiable
to 390–459, 745–747) 760.3
congenital heart disease (conditions
classifiable to 745–746) 760.3
cortical necrosis of kidney 760.1
death 761.6
diabetes mellitus 775.0
manifest diabetes in the infant
775.1

Maternal condition, affecting fetus or
newborn (*Continued*)
disease NEC 760.9
circulatory system, chronic
(conditions classifiable to
390–459, 745–747) 760.3
genitourinary system (conditions
classifiable to 580–599)
760.1
respiratory (conditions classifiable
to 490–519, 748) 760.3
eclampsia 760.0
hemorrhage NEC 762.1
hepatitis acute, malignant, or subacute
760.8
hyperemesis (gravidarum) 761.8
hypertension (arising during
pregnancy) (conditions
classifiable to 642) 760.0
infection
disease classifiable to 001–136
760.2
genital tract NEC 760.8
urinary tract 760.1
influenza 760.2
manifest influenza in the infant
771.2
injury (conditions classifiable to
800–996) 760.5
malaria 760.2
manifest malaria in infant or fetus
771.2
malnutrition 760.4
necrosis of liver 760.8
nephritis (conditions classifiable to
580–583) 760.1
nephrosis (conditions classifiable to
581) 760.1
noxious substance transmitted via
breast milk or placenta 760.70
alcohol 760.71
anticonvulsants 760.77
antifungals 760.74
anti-infective agents 760.74
antimetabolics 760.78
cocaine 760.75
"crack" 760.75
diethylstilbestrol [DES] 760.76
hallucinogenic agents 760.73
medicinal agents NEC 760.79
narcotics 760.72
obstetric anesthetic or analgesic
drug 760.72
specified agent NEC 760.79
nutritional disorder (conditions
classifiable to 260–269) 760.4
operation unrelated to current delivery
(*see also* Newborn, affected by)
760.64
pre-eclampsia 760.0
pyelitis or pyelonephritis, arising
during pregnancy (conditions
classifiable to 590) 760.1
renal disease or failure 760.1
respiratory disease, chronic
(conditions classifiable to
490–519, 748) 760.3
rheumatic heart disease (chronic)
(conditions classifiable to 393–
398) 760.3
rubella (conditions classifiable to 056)
760.2
manifest rubella in the infant or
fetus 771.0

Maternal condition, affecting fetus or
newborn (*Continued*)
surgery unrelated to current delivery
(*see also* Newborn, affected by)
760.64
to uterus or pelvic organs 760.64
syphilis (conditions classifiable to 090–
097) 760.2
manifest syphilis in the infant or
fetus 090.0
thrombophlebitis 760.3
toxemia (of pregnancy) 760.0
pre-eclamptic 760.0
toxoplasmosis (conditions classifiable
to 130) 760.2
manifest toxoplasmosis in the infant
or fetus 771.2
transmission of chemical substance
through the placenta 760.70
alcohol 760.71
anticonvulsants 760.77
antifungals 760.74
anti-infective 760.74
antimetabolics 760.78
cocaine 760.75
"crack" 760.75
diethylstilbestrol [DES] 760.76
hallucinogenic agents 760.73
narcotics 760.72
specified substance NEC 760.79
uremia 760.1
urinary tract conditions (conditions
classifiable to 580–599) 760.1
vomiting (pernicious) (persistent)
(vicious) 761.8
Maternity - *see* Delivery
Matheiu's disease (leptospiral jaundice)
100.0
Mauclaire's disease or osteochondrosis
732.3
Maxcy's disease 081.0
Maxilla, maxillary - *see* condition
May (-Hegglin) anomaly or syndrome 288.2
Mayaro fever 066.3
Mazoplasia 610.8
MBD (minimal brain dysfunction), child
(*see also* Hyperkinesia) 314.9
MCAD (medium chain acyl CoA
dehydrogenase deficiency) 277.85
McArdle (-Schmid-Pearson) disease or
syndrome (glycogenosis V) 271.0
McCune-Albright syndrome (osteitis
fibrosa disseminata) 756.59
MCLS (mucocutaneous lymph node
syndrome) 446.1
McQuarrie's syndrome (idiopathic
familial hypoglycemia) 251.2
Measles (black) (hemorrhagic)
(suppressed) 055.9
with
encephalitis 055.0
keratitis 055.71
keratoconjunctivitis 055.71
otitis media 055.2
pneumonia 055.1
complication 055.8
specified type NEC 055.79
encephalitis 055.0
French 056.9
German 056.9
keratitis 055.71
keratoconjunctivitis 055.71
liberty 056.9
otitis media 055.2

Ɯ

Measles (Continued)
  pneumonia 055.1
  specified complications NEC 055.79
  vaccination, prophylactic (against)
    V04.2
Meatitis, urethral (see also Urethritis)
  597.89
Meat poisoning - see Poisoning, food
Meatus, meatal - see condition
Meat-wrappers' asthma 506.9
Meckel's
  diverticulitis 751.0
  diverticulum (displaced)
    (hypertrophic) 751.0
Meconium
  aspiration 770.11
    with
      pneumonia 770.12
      pneumonitis 770.12
      respiratory symptoms 770.12
    below vocal cords 770.11
      with respiratory symptoms
        770.12
    syndrome 770.12
  delayed passage in newborn 777.1
  ileus 777.1
    due to cystic fibrosis 277.01
  in liquor 792.3
    noted during delivery - 656.8●
  insufflation 770.11
    with respiratory symptoms 770.12
  obstruction
    fetus or newborn 777.1
      in mucoviscidosis 277.01
  passage of 792.3
    noted during delivery 763.84
  peritonitis 777.6
  plug syndrome (newborn) NEC
    777.1
  staining 779.84
Median - see also condition
  arcuate ligament syndrome 447.4
  bar (prostate) 600.90
    with
      other lower urinary tract
        symptoms (LUTS)
        600.91
      urinary
        obstruction 600.91
        retention 600.91
  rhomboid glossitis 529.2
  vesical orifice 600.90
    with
      other lower urinary tract
        symptoms (LUTS)
        600.91
      urinary
        obstruction 600.91
        retention 600.91
Mediastinal shift 793.2
Mediastinitis (acute) (chronic) 519.2
  actinomycotic 039.8
  syphilitic 095.8
  tuberculous (see also Tuberculosis)
    012.8●
Mediastinopericarditis (see also
    Pericarditis) 423.9
  acute 420.90
  chronic 423.8
    rheumatic 393
  rheumatic, chronic 393
Mediastinum, mediastinal - see condition
Medical services provided for - see Health,
    services provided because (of)

Medicine poisoning (by overdose)
    (wrong substance given or taken in
    error) 977.9
  specified drug or substance - see Table
    of Drugs and Chemicals
Medin's disease (poliomyelitis) 045.9●
Mediterranean
  anemia (with other hemoglobinopathy)
    282.49
  disease or syndrome (hemipathic)
    282.49
  fever (see also Brucellosis) 023.9
    familial 277.31
  kala-azar 085.0
  leishmaniasis 085.0
  tick fever 082.1
Medulla - see condition
Medullary
  cystic kidney 753.16
  sponge kidney 753.17
Medullated fibers
  optic (nerve) 743.57
  retina 362.85
Medulloblastoma (M9470/3)
  desmoplastic (M9471/3) 191.6
  specified site - see Neoplasm, by site,
    malignant
  unspecified site 191.6
Medulloepithelioma (M9501/3) - see also
    Neoplasm, by site, malignant
  teratoid (M9502/3) - see Neoplasm, by
    site, malignant
Medullomyoblastoma (M9472/3)
  specified site - see Neoplasm, by site,
    malignant
  unspecified site 191.6
Meekeren-Ehlers-Danlos syndrome
  756.83
Megacaryocytic - see condition
Megacolon (acquired) (functional) (not
    Hirschsprung's disease) 564.7
  aganglionic 751.3
  congenital, congenitum 751.3
  Hirschsprung's (disease) 751.3
  psychogenic 306.4
  toxic (see also Colitis, ulcerative) 556.9
Megaduodenum 537.3
Megaesophagus (functional) 530.0
  congenital 750.4
Megakaryocytic - see condition
Megalencephaly 742.4
Megalerythema (epidermicum)
    (infectiosum) 057.0
Megalia, cutis et ossium 757.39
Megaloappendix 751.5
Megalocephalus, megalocephaly NEC
  756.0
Megalocornea 743.41
  associated with buphthalmos 743.22
Megalocytic anemia 281.9
Megalodactylia (fingers) (thumbs) 755.57
  toes 755.65
Megaloduodenum 751.5
Megaloesophagus (functional) 530.0
  congenital 750.4
Megalogastria (congenital) 750.7
Megalomania 307.9
Megalophthalmos 743.8
Megalopsia 368.14
Megalosplenia (see also Splenomegaly)
  789.2
Megaloureter 593.89
  congenital 753.22
Megarectum 569.49

Megasigmoid 564.7
  congenital 751.3
Megaureter 593.89
  congenital 753.22
Megrim 346.9●
Meibomian
  cyst 373.2
    infected 373.12
  gland - see condition
  infarct (eyelid) 374.85
  stye 373.11
Meibomitis 373.12
Meige
  -Milroy disease (chronic hereditary
    edema) 757.0
  syndrome (blepharospasm-
    oromandibular dystonia) 333.82
Melalgia, nutritional 266.2
Melancholia (see also Psychosis, affective)
  296.90
  climacteric 296.2●
    recurrent episode 296.3●
    single episode 296.2●
  hypochondriac 300.7
  intermittent 296.2●
    recurrent episode 296.3●
    single episode 296.2●
  involutional 296.2●
    recurrent episode 296.3●
    single episode 296.2●
  menopausal 296.2●
    recurrent episode 296.3●
    single episode 296.2●
  puerperal 296.2●
  reactive (from emotional stress,
    psychological trauma) 298.0
  recurrent 296.3●
  senile 290.21
  stuporous 296.2●
    recurrent episode 296.3●
    single episode 296.2●
Melanemia 275.0
Melanoameloblastoma (M9363/0) - see
    Neoplasm, bone, benign
Melanoblastoma (M8720/3) - see
    Melanoma
Melanoblastosis
  Block-Sulzberger 757.33
  cutis linearis sive systematisata 757.33
Melanocarcinoma (M8720/3) - see
    Melanoma
Melanocytoma, eyeball (M8726/0) 224.0
Melanoderma, melanodermia 709.09
  Addison's (primary adrenal
    insufficiency) 255.41
Melanodontia, infantile 521.05
Melanodontoclasia 521.05
Melanoepithelioma (M8720/3) - see
    Melanoma
Melanoma (malignant) (M8720/3) 172.9

Note 53   Except where otherwise
indicated, the morphological varieties
of melanoma in the list below should
be coded by site as for "Melanoma
(malignant)." Internal sites should be
coded to malignant neoplasm of those
sites.

  abdominal wall 172.5
  ala nasi 172.3
  amelanotic (M8730/3) - see Melanoma,
    by site

◄ New   ◄▓▓ Revised   ~~deleted~~ Deleted   ● Use Additional Digit(s)   ▓▓ Omit code

Melanoma *(Continued)*
ankle 172.7
anus, anal 154.3
canal 154.2
arm 172.6
auditory canal (external) 172.2
auricle (ear) 172.2
auricular canal (external) 172.2
axilla 172.5
axillary fold 172.5
back 172.5
balloon cell (M8722/3) - *see* Melanoma, by site
benign (M8720/0) - *see* Neoplasm, skin, benign
breast (female) (male) 172.5
brow 172.3
buttock 172.5
canthus (eye) 172.1
cheek (external) 172.3
chest wall 172.5
chin 172.3
choroid 190.6
conjunctiva 190.3
ear (external) 172.2
epithelioid cell (M8771/3) - *see also* Melanoma, by site
and spindle cell, mixed (M8775/3) - *see* Melanoma, by site
external meatus (ear) 172.2
eye 190.9
eyebrow 172.3
eyelid (lower) (upper) 172.1
face NEC 172.3
female genital organ (external) NEC 184.4
finger 172.6
flank 172.5
foot 172.7
forearm 172.6
forehead 172.3
foreskin 187.1
gluteal region 172.5
groin 172.5
hand 172.6
heel 172.7
helix 172.2
hip 172.7
in
giant pigmented nevus (M8761/3) - *see* Melanoma, by site
Hutchinson's melanotic freckle (M8742/3) - *see* Melanoma, by site
junctional nevus (M8740/3) - *see* Melanoma, by site
precancerous melanosis (M8741/3) - *see* Melanoma, by site
in situ - *see* Melanoma, by site
skin 172.9
interscapular region 172.5
iris 190.0
jaw 172.3
juvenile (M8770/0) - *see* Neoplasm, skin, benign
knee 172.7
labium
majus 184.1
minus 184.2
lacrimal gland 190.2
leg 172.7
lip (lower) (upper) 172.0
liver 197.7
lower limb NEC 172.7

Melanoma *(Continued)*
male genital organ (external) NEC 187.9
meatus, acoustic (external) 172.2
meibomian gland 172.1
metastatic
of or from specified site - *see* Melanoma, by site
site not of skin - *see* Neoplasm, by site, malignant, secondary
to specified site - *see* Neoplasm, by site, malignant, secondary
unspecified site 172.9
nail 172.9
finger 172.6
toe 172.7
neck 172.4
nodular (M8721/3) - *see* Melanoma, by site
nose, external 172.3
orbit 190.1
penis 187.4
perianal skin 172.5
perineum 172.5
pinna 172.2
popliteal (fossa) (space) 172.7
prepuce 187.1
pubes 172.5
pudendum 184.4
retina 190.5
scalp 172.4
scrotum 187.7
septum nasal (skin) 172.3
shoulder 172.6
skin NEC 172.8
in situ 172.9
spindle cell (M8772/3) - *see also* Melanoma, by site
type A (M8773/3) 190.0
type B (M8774/3) 190.0
submammary fold 172.5
superficial spreading (M8743/3) - *see* Melanoma, by site
temple 172.3
thigh 172.7
toe 172.7
trunk NEC 172.5
umbilicus 172.5
upper limb NEC 172.6
vagina vault 184.0
vulva 184.4
Melanoplakia 528.9
Melanosarcoma (M8720/3) - *see also* Melanoma
epithelioid cell (M8771/3) - *see* Melanoma
Melanosis 709.09
addisonian (primary adrenal insufficiency) 255.41
tuberculous (*see also* Tuberculosis) 017.6●
adrenal 255.41
colon 569.89
conjunctiva 372.55
congenital 743.49
corii degenerativa 757.33
cornea (presenile) (senile) 371.12
congenital 743.43
interfering with vision 743.42
prenatal 743.43
interfering with vision 743.42
eye 372.55
congenital 743.49
jute spinners' 709.09

Melanosis *(Continued)*
lenticularis progressiva 757.33
liver 573.8
precancerous (M8741/2) - *see also* Neoplasm, skin, in situ
malignant melanoma in (M8741/3) - *see* Melanoma
Riehl's 709.09
sclera 379.19
congenital 743.47
suprarenal 255.41
tar 709.09
toxic 709.09
Melanuria 791.9
MELAS syndrome (mitochondrial encephalopathy, lactic acidosis and stroke-like episodes) 277.87
Melasma 709.09
adrenal (gland) 255.41
suprarenal (gland) 255.41
Melena 578.1
due to
swallowed maternal blood 777.3
ulcer - *see* Ulcer, by site, with hemorrhage
newborn 772.4
due to swallowed maternal blood 777.3
Meleney's
gangrene (cutaneous) 686.09
ulcer (chronic undermining) 686.09
Melioidosis 025
Melitensis, febris 023.0
Melitococcosis 023.0
Melkersson (-Rosenthal) syndrome 351.8
Mellitus, diabetes - *see* Diabetes
Melorheostosis (bone) (leri) 733.99
Meloschisis 744.83
Melotia 744.29
Membrana
capsularis lentis posterior 743.39
epipapillaris 743.57
Membranacea placenta - *see* Placenta, abnormal
Membranaceous uterus 621.8
Membrane, membranous - *see also* condition
folds, congenital - *see* Web
Jackson's 751.4
over face (causing asphyxia), fetus or newborn 768.9
premature rupture - *see* Rupture, membranes, premature
pupillary 364.74
persistent 743.46
retained (complicating delivery) (with hemorrhage) 666.2●
without hemorrhage 667.1●
secondary (eye) 366.50
unruptured (causing asphyxia) 768.9
vitreous humor 379.25
Membranitis, fetal 658.4
affecting fetus or newborn 762.7
Memory disturbance, loss or lack (*see also* Amnesia) 780.93
mild, following organic brain damage 310.8 ◀▥
MEN (multiple endocrine neoplasia) syndromes
type I 258.01
type IIA 258.02
type IIB 258.03

Menadione (vitamin K) deficiency 269.0
Menarche, precocious 259.1
Mendacity, pathologic 301.7
Mende's syndrome (ptosis-epicanthus) 270.2
Mendelson's syndrome (resulting from a procedure) 997.39
  obstetric 668.0●
Ménétrier's disease or syndrome (hypertrophic gastritis) 535.2●
Ménière's disease, syndrome, or vertigo 386.00
  cochlear 386.02
  cochleovestibular 386.01
  inactive 386.04
  in remission 386.04
  vestibular 386.03
Meninges, meningeal - see condition
Meningioma (M9530/0) - see also Neoplasm, meninges, benign
  angioblastic (M9535/0) - see Neoplasm, meninges, benign
  angiomatous (M9534/0) - see Neoplasm, meninges, benign
  endotheliomatous (M9531/0) - see Neoplasm, meninges, benign
  fibroblastic (M9532/0) - see Neoplasm, meninges, benign
  fibrous (M9532/0) - see Neoplasm, meninges, benign
  hemangioblastic (M9535/0) - see Neoplasm, meninges, benign
  hemangiopericytic (M9536/0) - see Neoplasm, meninges, benign
  malignant (M9530/3) - see Neoplasm, meninges, malignant
  meningiothelial (M9531/0) - see Neoplasm, meninges, benign
  meningotheliomatous (M9531/0) - see Neoplasm, meninges, benign
  mixed (M9537/0) - see Neoplasm, meninges, benign
  multiple (M9530/1) 237.6
  papillary (M9538/1) 237.6
  psammomatous (M9533/0) - see Neoplasm, meninges, benign
  syncytial (M9531/0) - see Neoplasm, meninges, benign
  transitional (M9537/0) - see Neoplasm, meninges, benign
Meningiomatosis (diffuse) (M9530/1) 237.6
Meningism (see also Meningismus) 781.6
Meningismus (infectional) (pneumococcal) 781.6
  due to serum or vaccine 997.09 [321.8]
  influenzal NEC 487.8
Meningitis (basal) (basic) (basilar) (brain) (cerebral) (cervical) (congestive) (diffuse) (hemorrhagic) (infantile) (membranous) (metastatic) (nonspecific) (pontine) (progressive) (simple) (spinal) (subacute) (sympathetica) (toxic) 322.9
  abacterial NEC (see also Meningitis, aseptic) 047.9
  actinomycotic 039.8 [320.7]
  adenoviral 049.1
  aerobacter aerogenes 320.82
  anaerobes (cocci) (gram-negative) (gram-positive) (mixed) (NEC) 320.81
  arbovirus NEC 066.9 [321.2]
    specified type NEC 066.8 [321.2]

Meningitis (Continued)
  aseptic (acute) NEC 047.9
    adenovirus 049.1
    Coxsackie virus 047.0
    due to
      adenovirus 049.1
      Coxsackie virus 047.0
      ECHO virus 047.1
      enterovirus 047.9
      mumps 072.1
      poliovirus (see also Poliomyelitis) 045.2● [321.2]
    ECHO virus 047.1
    herpes (simplex) virus 054.72
    zoster 053.0
    leptospiral 100.81
    lymphocytic choriomeningitis 049.0
    noninfective 322.0
  Bacillus pyocyaneus 320.89
  bacterial NEC 320.9
    anaerobic 320.81
    gram-negative 320.82
      anaerobic 320.81
  Bacteroides (fragilis) (oralis) (melaninogenicus) 320.81
  cancerous (M8000/6) 198.4
  candidal 112.83
  carcinomatous (M8010/6) 198.4
  caseous (see also Tuberculosis, meninges) 013.0●
  cerebrospinal (acute) (chronic) (diplococcal) (endemic) (epidemic) (fulminant) (infectious) (malignant) (meningococcal) (sporadic) 036.0
    carrier (suspected) of V02.59
  chronic NEC 322.2
  clear cerebrospinal fluid NEC 322.0
  Clostridium (haemolyticum) (novyi) NEC 320.81
  coccidioidomycosis 114.2
  Coxsackie virus 047.0
  cryptococcal 117.5 [321.0]
  diplococcal 036.0
    gram-negative 036.0
    gram-positive 320.1
  Diplococcus pneumoniae 320.1
  due to
    actinomycosis 039.8 [320.7]
    adenovirus 049.1
    coccidiomycosis 114.2
    enterovirus 047.9
      specified NEC 047.8
    histoplasmosis (see also Histoplasmosis) 115.91
    Listerosis 027.0 [320.7]
    Lyme disease 088.81 [320.7]
    moniliasis 112.83
    mumps 072.1
    neurosyphilis 094.2
    nonbacterial organisms NEC 321.8
    oidiomycosis 112.83
    poliovirus (see also Poliomyelitis) 045.2● [321.2]
    preventive immunization, inoculation, or vaccination 997.09 [321.8]
    sarcoidosis 135 [321.4]
    sporotrichosis 117.1 [321.1]
    syphilis 094.2
      acute 091.81
      congenital 090.42
      secondary 091.81

Meningitis (Continued)
  due to (Continued)
    trypanosomiasis (see also Trypanosomiasis) 086.9 [321.3]
    whooping cough 033.9 [320.7]
  E. coli 320.82
  ECHO virus 047.1
  endothelial-leukocytic, benign, recurrent 047.9
  Enterobacter aerogenes 320.82
  enteroviral 047.9
    specified type NEC 047.8
  enterovirus 047.9
    specified NEC 047.8
  eosinophilic 322.1
  epidemic NEC 036.0
  Escherichia coli (E. coli) 320.82
  Eubacterium 320.81
  fibrinopurulent NEC 320.9
    specified type NEC 320.89
  Friedländer (bacillus) 320.82
  fungal NEC 117.9 [321.1]
  Fusobacterium 320.81
  gonococcal 098.82
  gram-negative bacteria NEC 320.82
    anaerobic 320.81
    cocci 036.0
      specified NEC 320.82
  gram-negative cocci NEC 036.0
    specified NEC 320.82
  gram-positive cocci NEC 320.9
  H. influenzae 320.0
  herpes (simplex) virus 054.72
    zoster 053.0
  infectious NEC 320.9
  influenzal 320.0
  Klebsiella pneumoniae 320.82
  late effect - see Late, effect, meningitis
  leptospiral (aseptic) 100.81
  Listerella (monocytogenes) 027.0 [320.7]
  Listeria monocytogenes 027.0 [320.7]
  lymphocytic (acute) (benign) (serous) 049.0
    choriomeningitis virus 049.0
  meningococcal (chronic) 036.0
  Mima polymorpha 320.82
  Mollaret's 047.9
  monilial 112.83
  mumps (virus) 072.1
  mycotic NEC 117.9 [321.1]
  Neisseria 036.0
  neurosyphilis 094.2
  nonbacterial NEC (see also Meningitis, aseptic) 047.9
  nonpyogenic NEC 322.0
  oidiomycosis 112.83
  ossificans 349.2
  Peptococcus 320.81
  PeptoStreptococcus 320.81
  pneumococcal 320.1
  poliovirus (see also Poliomyelitis) 045.2● [321.2]
  Proprionibacterium 320.81
  Proteus morganii 320.82
  Pseudomonas (aeruginosa) (pyocyaneus) 320.82
  purulent NEC 320.9
    specified organism NEC 320.89
  pyogenic NEC 320.9
    specified organism NEC 320.89
  Salmonella 003.21
  septic NEC 320.9
    specified organism NEC 320.89

◄ New   ◄▥ Revised   ~~deleted~~ Deleted   ● Use Additional Digit(s)   ▒ Omit code

Meningitis (Continued)
  serosa circumscripta NEC 322.0
  serous NEC (see also Meningitis,
      aseptic) 047.9
    lymphocytic 049.0
    syndrome 348.2
  Serratia (marcescens) 320.82
  specified organism NEC 320.89
  sporadic cerebrospinal 036.0
  sporotrichosis 117.1 [321.1]
  staphylococcal 320.3
  sterile 997.09
  streptococcal (acute) 320.2
  suppurative 320.9
    specified organism NEC 320.89
  syphilitic 094.2
    acute 091.81
    congenital 090.42
    secondary 091.81
  torula 117.5 [321.0]
  traumatic (complication of injury)
      958.8
  Treponema (denticola)
      (macrodenticum) 320.81
  trypanosomiasis 086.1 [321.3]
  tuberculous (see also Tuberculosis,
      meninges) 013.0●
  typhoid 002.0 [320.7]
  Veillonella 320.81
  Vibrio vulnificus 320.82
  viral, virus NEC (see also Meningitis,
      aseptic) 047.9
  Wallgren's (see also Meningitis, aseptic)
      047.9
Meningocele (congenital) (spinal) (see also
    Spina bifida) 741.9●
  acquired (traumatic) 349.2
  cerebral 742.0
  cranial 742.0
Meningocerebritis - see
    Meningoencephalitis
Meningococcemia (acute) (chronic)
    036.2
Meningococcus, meningococcal (see also
    condition) 036.9
  adrenalitis, hemorrhagic 036.3
  carditis 036.40
  carrier (suspected) of V02.59
  cerebrospinal fever 036.0
  encephalitis 036.1
  endocarditis 036.42
  exposure to V01.84
  infection NEC 036.9
  meningitis (cerebrospinal) 036.0
  myocarditis 036.43
  optic neuritis 036.81
  pericarditis 036.41
  septicemia (chronic) 036.2
Meningoencephalitis (see also
    Encephalitis) 323.9
  acute NEC 048
  bacterial, purulent, pyogenic, or
      septic - see Meningitis
  chronic NEC 094.1
  diffuse NEC 094.1
  diphasic 063.2
  due to
    actinomycosis 039.8 [320.7]
    blastomycosis NEC (see also
        Blastomycosis) 116.0 [323.41]
    free-living amebae 136.29
    Listeria monocytogenes 027.0 [320.7]
    Lyme disease 088.81 [320.7]
    mumps 072.2

Meningoencephalitis (Continued)
  due to (Continued)
    Naegleria (amebae) (gruberi)
        (organisms) 136.29
    rubella 056.01
    sporotrichosis 117.1 [321.1]
    toxoplasmosis (acquired) 130.0
      congenital (active) 771.2
        [323.41]
    Trypanosoma 086.1 [323.2]
  epidemic 036.0
  herpes 054.3
  herpetic 054.3
  H. influenzae 320.0
  infectious (acute) 048
  influenzal 320.0
  late effect - see category 326
  Listeria monocytogenes 027.0 [320.7]
  lymphocytic (serous) 049.0
  mumps 072.2
  parasitic NEC 123.9 [323.41]
  pneumococcal 320.1
  primary amebic 136.29
  rubella 056.01
  serous 048
    lymphocytic 049.0
  specific 094.2
  staphylococcal 320.3
  streptococcal 320.2
  syphilitic 094.2
  toxic NEC 989.9 [323.71]
    due to
      carbon tetrachloride (vapor)
          987.8 [323.71]
      hydroxyquinoline derivatives
          poisoning 961.3 [323.71]
      lead 984.9 [323.71]
      mercury 985.0 [323.71]
      thallium 985.8 [323.71]
  toxoplasmosis (acquired) 130.0
  trypanosomic 086.1 [323.2]
  tuberculous (see also Tuberculosis,
      meninges) 013.0●
  virus NEC 048
Meningoencephalocele 742.0
  syphilitic 094.89
    congenital 090.49
Meningoencephalomyelitis (see also
    Meningoencephalitis) 323.9
  acute NEC 048
    disseminated (postinfectious) 136.9
        [323.61]
      postimmunization or
          postvaccination 323.51
  due to
    actinomycosis 039.8 [320.7]
    torula 117.5 [323.41]
    toxoplasma or toxoplasmosis
        (acquired) 130.0
      congenital (active) 771.2
          [323.41]
  late effect - see category 326
Meningoencephalomyelopathy (see also
    Meningoencephalomyelitis) 349.9
Meningoencephalopathy (see also
    Meningoencephalitis) 348.39
Meningoencephalopoliomyelitis (see also
    Poliomyelitis, bulbar) 045.0●
  late effect 138
Meningomyelitis (see also
    Meningoencephalitis) 323.9
  blastomycotic NEC (see also
      Blastomycosis) 116.0
      [323.41]

Meningomyelitis (Continued)
  due to
    actinomycosis 039.8 [320.7]
    blastomycosis (see also
        Blastomycosis) 116.0 [323.41]
    Meningococcus 036.0
    sporotrichosis 117.1 [323.41]
    torula 117.5 [323.41]
  late effect - see category 326
  lethargic 049.8
  meningococcal 036.0
  syphilitic 094.2
  tuberculous (see also Tuberculosis,
      meninges) 013.0●
Meningomyelocele (see also Spina bifida)
    741.9●
  syphilitic 094.89
Meningomyeloneuritis - see
    Meningoencephalitis
Meningoradiculitis - see Meningitis
Meningovascular - see condition
Meniscocytosis 282.60
Menkes' syndrome - see Syndrome,
    Menkes'
Menolipsis 626.0
Menometrorrhagia 626.2
Menopause, menopausal (symptoms)
    (syndrome) 627.2
  arthritis (any site) NEC 716.3●
  artificial 627.4
  bleeding 627.0
  crisis 627.2
  depression (see also Psychosis, affective)
      296.2●
    agitated 296.2●
      recurrent episode 296.3●
      single episode 296.2●
    psychotic 296.2●
      recurrent episode 296.3●
      single episode 296.2●
    recurrent episode 296.3●
    single episode 296.2●
  melancholia (see also Psychosis,
      affective) 296.2●
    recurrent episode 296.3●
    single episode 296.2●
  paranoid state 297.2
  paraphrenia 297.2
  postsurgical 627.4
  premature 256.31
    postirradiation 256.2
    postsurgical 256.2
  psychoneurosis 627.2
  psychosis NEC 298.8
  surgical 627.4
  toxic polyarthritis NEC 716.39
Menorrhagia (primary) 626.2
  climacteric 627.0
  menopausal 627.0
  postclimacteric 627.1
  postmenopausal 627.1
  preclimacteric 627.0
  premenopausal 627.0
  puberty (menses retained) 626.3
Menorrhalgia 625.3
Menoschesis 626.8
Menostaxis 626.2
Menses, retention 626.8
Menstrual - see also Menstruation
  cycle, irregular 626.4
  disorders NEC 626.9
  extraction V25.3
  fluid, retained 626.8
  molimen 625.4

M

Menstrual *(Continued)*
  period, normal V65.5
  regulation V25.3
Menstruation
  absent 626.0
  anovulatory 628.0
  delayed 626.8
  difficult 625.3
  disorder 626.9
    psychogenic 306.52
    specified NEC 626.8
  during pregnancy 640.8●
  excessive 626.2
  frequent 626.2
  infrequent 626.1
  irregular 626.4
  latent 626.8
  membranous 626.8
  painful (primary) (secondary) 625.3
    psychogenic 306.52
  passage of clots 626.2
  precocious 626.8
  protracted 626.8
  retained 626.8
  retrograde 626.8
  scanty 626.1
  suppression 626.8
  vicarious (nasal) 625.8
Mentagra *(see also* Sycosis) 704.8
Mental - *see also* condition
  deficiency *(see also* Retardation, mental) 319
  deterioration *(see also* Psychosis) 298.9
  disorder *(see also* Disorder, mental) 300.9
  exhaustion 300.5
  insufficiency (congenital) *(see also* Retardation, mental) 319
  observation without need for further medical care NEC V71.09
  retardation *(see also* Retardation, mental) 319
  subnormality *(see also* Retardation, mental) 319
    mild 317
    moderate 318.0
    profound 318.2
    severe 318.1
  upset *(see also* Disorder, mental) 300.9
Meralgia paresthetica 355.1
Mercurial - *see* condition
Mercurialism NEC 985.0
Merergasia 300.9
Merkel cell tumor - see ~~Neoplasm, by site, malignant~~ Carcinoma, Merkel cell ◀▥
Merocele *(see also* Hernia, femoral) 553.00
Meromelia 755.4
  lower limb 755.30
    intercalary 755.32
      femur 755.34
        tibiofibular (complete) (incomplete) 755.33
      fibula 755.37
      metatarsal(s) 755.38
      tarsal(s) 755.38
      tibia 755.36
      tibiofibular 755.35
    terminal (complete) (partial) (transverse) 755.31
    longitudinal 755.32
      metatarsal(s) 755.38
      phalange(s) 755.39
      tarsal(s) 755.38
    transverse 755.31

Meromelia *(Continued)*
  upper limb 755.20
    intercalary 755.22
      carpal(s) 755.28
      humeral 755.24
        radioulnar (complete) (incomplete) 755.23
      metacarpal(s) 755.28
      phalange(s) 755.29
      radial 755.26
      radioulnar 755.25
      ulnar 755.27
    terminal (complete) (partial) (transverse) 755.21
    longitudinal 755.22
      carpal(s) 755.28
      metacarpal(s) 755.28
      phalange(s) 755.29
    transverse 755.21
Merosmia 781.1
MERRF syndrome (myoclonus with epilepsy and with ragged red fibers) 277.87
Merycism - *see also* Vomiting
  psychogenic 307.53
Merzbacher-Pelizaeus disease 330.0
Mesaortitis - *see* Aortitis
Mesarteritis - *see* Arteritis
Mesencephalitis *(see also* Encephalitis) 323.9
  late effect - *see* category 326
Mesenchymoma (M8990/1) - *see also* Neoplasm, connective tissue, uncertain behavior
  benign (M8990/0) - *see* Neoplasm, connective tissue, benign
  malignant (M8990/3) - *see* Neoplasm, connective tissue, malignant
Mesenteritis
  retractile 567.82
  sclerosing 567.82
Mesentery, mesenteric - *see* condition
Mesiodens, mesiodentes 520.1
  causing crowding 524.31
Mesio-occlusion 524.23
Mesocardia (with asplenia) 746.87
Mesocolon - *see* condition
Mesonephroma (malignant) (M9110/3) - *see also* Neoplasm, by site, malignant
  benign (M9110/0) - *see* Neoplasm, by site, benign
Mesophlebitis - *see* Phlebitis
Mesostromal dysgenesis 743.51
Mesothelioma (malignant) (M9050/3) - *see also* Neoplasm, by site, malignant
  benign (M9050/0) - *see* Neoplasm, by site, benign
  biphasic type (M9053/3) - *see also* Neoplasm, by site, malignant
    benign (M9053/0) - *see* Neoplasm, by site, benign
  epithelioid (M9052/3) - *see also* Neoplasm, by site, malignant
    benign (M9052/0) - *see* Neoplasm, by site, benign
  fibrous (M9051/3) - *see also* Neoplasm, by site, malignant
    benign (M9051/0) - *see* Neoplasm, by site, benign
Metabolic syndrome 277.7
Metabolism disorder 277.9
  specified type NEC 277.89
Metagonimiasis 121.5

Metagonimus infestation (small intestine) 121.5
Metal
  pigmentation (skin) 709.00
    polishers' disease 502
Metalliferous miners' lung 503
Metamorphopsia 368.14
Metaplasia
  bone, in skin 709.3
  breast 611.89
  cervix - *omit code*
  endometrium (squamous) 621.8
  esophagus 530.85
  intestinal, of gastric mucosa 537.89
  kidney (pelvis) (squamous) *(see also* Disease, renal) 593.89
  myelogenous 289.89
  myeloid 289.89
    agnogenic 238.76
    megakaryocytic 238.76
  spleen 289.59
  squamous cell
    amnion 658.8●
    bladder 596.8
    cervix - *see* condition
    trachea 519.19
    tracheobronchial tree 519.19
    uterus 621.8
      cervix - *see* condition
Metastasis, metastatic
  abscess - *see* Abscess
  calcification 275.40
  cancer, neoplasm, or disease
    from specified site (M8000/3) - *see* Neoplasm, by site, malignant
    to specified site (M8000/6) - *see* Neoplasm, by site, secondary
  deposits (in) (M8000/6) - *see* Neoplasm, by site, secondary
  mesentery, of neuroendocrine tumor 209.71 ◀
  pneumonia 038.8 *[484.8]*
  spread (to) (M8000/6) - *see* Neoplasm, by site, secondary
Metatarsalgia 726.70
  anterior 355.6
  due to Freiberg's disease 732.5
  Morton's 355.6
Metatarsus, metatarsal - *see also* condition
  abductus valgus (congenital) 754.60
  adductus varus (congenital) 754.53
  primus varus 754.52
  valgus (adductus) (congenital) 754.60
  varus (abductus) (congenital) 754.53
    primus 754.52
Methadone use 304.00
Methemoglobinemia 289.7
  acquired (with sulfhemoglobinemia) 289.7
  congenital 289.7
  enzymatic 289.7
  Hb-M disease 289.7
  hereditary 289.7
  toxic 289.7
Methemoglobinuria *(see also* Hemoglobinuria) 791.2
Methicillin
  resistant staphylococcus aureus (MRSA) 041.12
    colonization V02.54
    personal history of V12.04
  susceptible staphylococcus aureus (MSSA) 041.11
    colonization V02.53

Methioninemia 270.4
Metritis (catarrhal) (septic) (suppurative)
   (*see also* Endometritis) 615.9
  blennorrhagic 098.16
    chronic or duration of 2 months or
      over 098.36
  cervical (*see also* Cervicitis) 616.0
  gonococcal 098.16
    chronic or duration of 2 months or
      over 098.36
  hemorrhagic 626.8
  puerperal, postpartum, childbirth
    670.1 ◀▥
  septic 670.2 ◀
  tuberculous (*see also* Tuberculosis)
    016.7 ●
Metropathia hemorrhagica 626.8
Metroperitonitis (*see also* Peritonitis,
  pelvic, female) 614.5
Metrorrhagia 626.6
  arising during pregnancy - *see*
    Hemorrhage, pregnancy
  postpartum NEC 666.2 ●
  primary 626.6
  psychogenic 306.59
  puerperal 666.2 ●
Metrorrhexis - *see* Rupture, uterus
Metrosalpingitis (*see also* Salpingo-
  oophoritis) 614.2
Metrostaxis 626.6
Metrovaginitis (*see also* Endometritis) 615.9
  gonococcal (acute) 098.16
    chronic or duration of 2 months or
      over 098.36
Mexican fever - *see* Typhus, Mexican
Meyenburg-Altherr-Uehlinger syndrome
  733.99
Meyer-Schwickerath and Weyers
  syndrome (dysplasia
  oculodentodigitalis) 759.89
Meynert's amentia (nonalcoholic) 294.0
  alcoholic 291.1
Mibelli's disease 757.39
Mice, joint (*see also* Loose, body, joint)
  718.1 ●
  knee 717.6
Micheli-Rietti syndrome (thalassemia
  minor) 282.49
Michotte's syndrome 721.5
Micrencephalon, micrencephaly 742.1
Microalbuminuria 791.0
Microaneurysm, retina 362.14
  diabetic 250.5 ● [362.01]
    due to secondary diabetes 249.5 ●
      [362.01]
Microangiopathy 443.9
  diabetic (peripheral) 250.7 ●
    [443.81]
    due to secondary diabetes 249.7 ●
      [443.81]
    retinal 250.5 ● [362.01]
      due to secondary diabetes 249.5 ●
        [362.01]
  peripheral 443.9
    diabetic 250.7 ● [443.81]
      due to secondary diabetes 249.7 ●
        [443.81]
  retinal 362.18
    diabetic 250.5 ● [362.01]
      due to secondary diabetes 249.5 ●
        [362.01]
  thrombotic 446.6
    Moschcowitz's (thrombotic
      thrombocytopenic purpura)
      446.6

Microcalcification, mammographic
  793.81
Microcephalus, microcephalic,
  microcephaly 742.1
  due to toxoplasmosis (congenital)
    771.2
Microcheilia 744.82
Microcolon (congenital) 751.5
Microcornea (congenital) 743.41
Microcytic - *see* condition
Microdeletions NEC 758.33
Microdontia 520.2
Microdrepanocytosis (thalassemia-Hb-S
  disease) 282.49
Microembolism
  atherothrombotic - *see*
    Atheroembolism
  retina 362.33
Microencephalon 742.1
Microfilaria streptocerca infestation
  125.3
Microgastria (congenital) 750.7
Microgenia 524.06
Microgenitalia (congenital) 752.89
  penis 752.64
Microglioma (M9710/3)
  specified site - *see* Neoplasm, by site,
    malignant
  unspecified site 191.9
Microglossia (congenital) 750.16
Micrognathia, micrognathism
  (congenital) 524.00
  mandibular 524.04
    alveolar 524.74
  maxillary 524.03
    alveolar 524.73
Microgyria (congenital) 742.2
Microinfarct, heart (*see also* Insufficiency,
  coronary) 411.89
Microlithiasis, alveolar, pulmonary
  516.2
Micromastia 611.82
Micromyelia (congenital) 742.59
Micropenis 752.64
Microphakia (congenital) 743.36
Microphthalmia (congenital) (*see also*
  Microphthalmos) 743.10
Microphthalmos (congenital) 743.10
  associated with eye and adnexal
    anomalies NEC 743.12
  due to toxoplasmosis (congenital)
    771.2
  isolated 743.11
  simple 743.11
  syndrome 759.89
Micropsia 368.14
Microsporidiosis 136.8
Microsporosis (*see also* Dermatophytosis)
  110.9
  nigra 111.1
Microsporum furfur infestation 111.0
Microstomia (congenital) 744.84
Microthelia 757.6
Microthromboembolism - *see* Embolism
Microtia (congenital) (external ear)
  744.23
Microtropia 378.34
Micturition
  disorder NEC 788.69
    psychogenic 306.53
  frequency 788.41
    psychogenic 306.53
  nocturnal 788.43
  painful 788.1
    psychogenic 306.53

Middle
  ear - *see* condition
  lobe (right) syndrome 518.0
Midplane - *see* condition
Miescher's disease 709.3
  cheilitis 351.8
  granulomatosis disciformis 709.3
Miescher-Leder syndrome or
  granulomatosis 709.3
Mieten's syndrome 759.89
Migraine (idiopathic) 346.9 ●

> Note The following fifth digit
> subclassification is for use with
> category 346:
>
> 0 without mention of intractable
>   migraine without mention
>   of status migrainosus
> 1 with intractable migraine, so
>   stated, without mention of
>   status migrainosus
> 2 without mention of intractable
>   migraine with status
>   migrainosus
> 3 with intractable migraine, so
>   stated, with status
>   migrainosus

  with aura (acute-onset) (without
    headache) (prolonged) (typical)
    346.0 ●
  without aura 346.1 ●
    chronic 346.7 ●
    transformed 346.7 ●
  abdominal (syndrome) 346.2 ●
  allergic (histamine) 346.2 ●
  atypical 346.8 ●
  basilar 346.0 ●
  chronic without aura 346.7 ●
  classic(al) 346.0 ●
  common 346.1 ●
  hemiplegic 346.3 ●
    familial 346.3 ●
    sporadic 346.3 ●
  lower-half 339.00
  menstrual 346.4 ●
  menstrually related 346.4 ●
  ophthalmic 346.8 ●
  ophthalmoplegic 346.2 ●
  premenstrual 346.4 ●
  pure menstrual 346.4 ●
  retinal 346.0 ●
  specified form NEC 346.8 ●
  transformed without aura 346.7 ●
  variant 346.2 ●
Migrant, social V60.0
Migratory, migrating - *see also* condition
  person V60.0
  testis, congenital 752.52
Mikulicz's disease or syndrome (dryness
  of mouth, absent or decreased
  lacrimation) 527.1
Milian atrophia blanche 701.3
Miliaria (crystallina) (rubra) (tropicalis)
  705.1
  apocrine 705.82
Miliary - *see* condition
Milium (*see also* Cyst, sebaceous)
  706.2
  colloid 709.3
  eyelid 374.84
Milk
  crust 690.11
  excess secretion 676.6 ●

Milk (Continued)
  fever, female 672●
  poisoning 988.8
  retention 676.2●
  sickness 988.8
  spots 423.1
Milkers' nodes 051.1
Milk-leg (deep vessels) 671.4●
  complicating pregnancy 671.3●
  nonpuerperal 451.19
  puerperal, postpartum, childbirth
      671.4●
Milkman (-Looser) disease or syndrome
    (osteomalacia with pseudofractures)
    268.2
Milky urine (see also Chyluria) 791.1
Millar's asthma (laryngismus stridulus)
    478.75
Millard-Gubler paralysis or syndrome
    344.89
Millard-Gubler-Foville paralysis 344.89
Miller-Dieker syndrome 758.33
Miller's disease (osteomalacia) 268.2
Miller Fisher's syndrome 357.0
Milles' syndrome (encephalocutaneous
    angiomatosis) 759.6
Mills' disease 335.29
Millstone makers' asthma or lung 502
Milroy's disease (chronic hereditary
    edema) 757.0
Miners' - see also condition
  asthma 500
  elbow 727.2
  knee 727.2
  lung 500
  nystagmus 300.89
  phthisis (see also Tuberculosis) 011.4●
  tuberculosis (see also Tuberculosis)
      011.4●
Minkowski-Chauffard syndrome (see also
    Spherocytosis) 282.0
Minor - see condition
Minor's disease 336.1
Minot's disease (hemorrhagic disease,
    newborn) 776.0
Minot-von Willebrand (-Jürgens) disease
    or syndrome (angiohemophilia)
    286.4
Minus (and plus) hand (intrinsic) 736.09
Miosis (persistent) (pupil) 379.42
Mirizzi's syndrome (hepatic duct
    stenosis) (see also Obstruction,
    biliary) 576.2
  with calculus, cholelithiasis, or stones -
      see Choledocholithiasis
Mirror writing 315.09
  secondary to organic lesion 784.69
Misadventure (prophylactic) (therapeutic)
    (see also Complications) 999.9
  administration of insulin 962.3
  infusion - see Complications, infusion
  local applications (of fomentations,
      plasters, etc.) 999.9
    burn or scald - see Burn, by site
  medical care (early) (late) NEC 999.9
    adverse effect of drugs or
        chemicals - see Table of Drugs
        and Chemicals
    burn or scald - see Burn, by site
  radiation NEC 990
  radiotherapy NEC 990
  surgical procedure (early) (late) - see
      Complications, surgical
      procedure

Misadventure (Continued)
  transfusion - see Complications,
      transfusion
  vaccination or other immunological
      procedure - see Complications,
      vaccination
Misanthropy 301.7
Miscarriage - see Abortion, spontaneous
Mischief, malicious, child (see also
    Disturbance, conduct) 312.0●
Misdirection
  aqueous 365.83
Mismanagement, feeding 783.3
Misplaced, misplacement
  kidney (see also Disease, renal)
      593.0
    congenital 753.3
  organ or site, congenital NEC - see
      Malposition, congenital
Missed
  abortion 632
  delivery (at or near term) 656.4●
  labor (at or near term) 656.4●
Misshapen reconstructed breast 612.0
Missing - see also Absence
  teeth (acquired) 525.10
    congenital (see also Anodontia)
        520.0
    due to
      caries 525.13
      extraction 525.10
      periodontal disease 525.12
      specified NEC 525.19
      trauma 525.11
  vertebrae (congenital) 756.13
Misuse of drugs NEC (see also Abuse,
    drug, nondependent) 305.9●
Mitchell's disease (erythromelalgia)
    443.82
Mite(s)
  diarrhea 133.8
  grain (itch) 133.8
  hair follicle (itch) 133.8
  in sputum 133.8
Mitochondrial encephalopathy, lactic
    acidosis and stroke-like episodes
    (MELAS syndrome) 277.87
Mitochondrial neurogastrointestinal
    encephalopathy syndrome
    (MNGIE) 277.87
Mitral - see condition
Mittelschmerz 625.2
Mixed - see condition
Mljet disease (mal de Meleda) 757.39
Mobile, mobility
  cecum 751.4
  coccyx 733.99
  excessive - see Hypermobility
  gallbladder 751.69
  kidney 593.0
    congenital 753.3
  organ or site, congenital NEC - see
      Malposition, congenital
  spleen 289.59
Mobitz heart block (atrioventricular)
    426.10
  type I (Wenckebach's) 426.13
  type II 426.12
Möbius'
  disease 346.2●
  syndrome
    congenital oculofacial paralysis
        352.6
    ophthalmoplegic migraine 346.2●

Moeller (-Barlow) disease (infantile
    scurvy) 267
  glossitis 529.4
Mohr's syndrome (types I and II) 759.89
Mola destruens (M9100/1) 236.1
Molarization, premolars 520.2
Molar pregnancy 631
  hydatidiform (delivered) (undelivered)
      630
Mold(s) in vitreous 117.9
Molding, head (during birth) - omit code
Mole (pigmented) (M8720/0) - see also
    Neoplasm, skin, benign
  blood 631
  Breus' 631
  cancerous (M8720/3) - see Melanoma
  carneous 631
  destructive (M9100/1) 236.1
  ectopic - see Pregnancy, ectopic
  fleshy 631
  hemorrhagic 631
  hydatid, hydatidiform (benign)
      (complicating pregnancy)
      (delivered) (undelivered) (see also
      Hydatidiform mole) 630
    invasive (M9100/1) 236.1
    malignant (M9100/1) 236.1
    previous, affecting management of
        pregnancy V23.1
  invasive (hydatidiform) (M9100/1)
      236.1
  malignant
    meaning
      malignant hydatidiform mole
          (9100/1) 236.1
      melanoma (M8720/3) - see
          Melanoma
  nonpigmented (M8730/0) - see
      Neoplasm, skin, benign
  pregnancy NEC 631
  skin (M8720/0) - see Neoplasm, skin,
      benign
  tubal - see Pregnancy, tubal
  vesicular (see also Hydatidiform mole)
      630
Molimen, molimina (menstrual) 625.4
Mollaret's meningitis 047.9
Mollities (cerebellar) (cerebral) 437.8
  ossium 268.2
Molluscum
  contagiosum 078.0
  epitheliale 078.0
  fibrosum (M8851/0) - see Lipoma, by
      site
  pendulum (M8851/0) - see Lipoma, by
      site
Mönckeberg's arteriosclerosis,
    degeneration, disease, or sclerosis
    (see also Arteriosclerosis, extremities)
    440.20
Monday fever 504
Monday morning dyspnea or asthma
    504
Mondini's malformation (cochlea) 744.05
Mondor's disease (thrombophlebitis of
    breast) 451.89
Mongolian, mongolianism, mongolism,
    mongoloid 758.0
  spot 757.33
Monilethrix (congenital) 757.4
Monilia infestation - see Candidiasis
Moniliasis - see also Candidiasis
  neonatal 771.7
  vulvovaginitis 112.1

◀ New   ◀▥ Revised   ~~deleted~~ Deleted   ● Use Additional Digit(s)   ▥ Omit code

Monkeypox 059.01
Monoarthritis 716.60
    ankle 716.67
    arm 716.62
        lower (and wrist) 716.63
        upper (and elbow) 716.62
    foot (and ankle) 716.67
    forearm (and wrist) 716.63
    hand 716.64
    leg 716.66
        lower 716.66
        upper 716.65
    pelvic region (hip) (thigh) 716.65
    shoulder (region) 716.61
    specified site NEC 716.68
Monoblastic - *see* condition
Monochromatism (cone) (rod)
    368.54
Monocytic - *see* condition
Monocytopenia 288.59
Monocytosis (symptomatic) 288.63
Monofixation syndrome 378.34
Monomania (*see also* Psychosis) 298.9
Mononeuritis 355.9
    cranial nerve - *see* Disorder, nerve,
        cranial
    femoral nerve 355.2
    lateral
        cutaneous nerve of thigh 355.1
        popliteal nerve 355.3
    lower limb 355.8
        specified nerve NEC 355.79
    medial popliteal nerve 355.4
    median nerve 354.1
    multiplex 354.5
    plantar nerve 355.6
    posterior tibial nerve 355.5
    radial nerve 354.3
    sciatic nerve 355.0
    ulnar nerve 354.2
    upper limb 354.9
        specified nerve NEC 354.8
    vestibular 388.5
Mononeuropathy (*see also* Mononeuritis)
    355.9
    diabetic NEC 250.6● [355.9]
        due to secondary diabetes 249.6●
            [355.9]
    lower limb 250.6● [355.8]
        due to secondary diabetes 249.6●
            [355.8]
    upper limb 250.6● [354.9]
        due to secondary diabetes 249.6●
            [354.9]
    iliohypogastric nerve 355.79
    ilioinguinal nerve 355.79
    obturator nerve 355.79
    saphenous nerve 355.79
Mononucleosis, infectious 075
    with hepatitis 075 [573.1]
Monoplegia 344.5
    brain (current episode) (*see also*
        Paralysis, brain) 437.8
        fetus or newborn 767.8
    cerebral (current episode) (*see also*
        Paralysis, brain) 437.8
    congenital or infantile (cerebral)
        (spastic) (spinal) 343.3
    embolic (current) (*see also* Embolism,
        brain) 434.1●
        late effect - *see* Late effect(s) (of)
            cerebrovascular disease
    infantile (cerebral) (spastic) (spinal)
        343.3

Monoplegia (*Continued*)
    lower limb 344.30
        affecting
            dominant side 344.31
            nondominant side 344.32
        due to late effect of cerebrovascular
            accident - *see* Late effect(s) (of)
            cerebrovascular accident
    newborn 767.8
    psychogenic 306.0
        specified as conversion reaction
            300.11
    thrombotic (current) (*see also*
        Thrombosis, brain) 434.0●
        late effect - *see* Late effect(s) (of)
            cerebrovascular disease
    transient 781.4
    upper limb 344.40
        affecting
            dominant side 344.41
            nondominant side 344.42
        due to late effect of cerebrovascular
            accident - *see* Late effect(s) (of)
            cerebrovascular accident
Monorchism, monorchidism 752.89
Monteggia's fracture (closed) 813.03
    open 813.13
Mood swings
    brief compensatory 296.99
    rebound 296.99
Moore's syndrome (*see also* Epilepsy)
    345.5●
Mooren's ulcer (cornea) 370.07
Mooser-Neill reaction 081.0
Mooser bodies 081.0
Moral
    deficiency 301.7
    imbecility 301.7
Morax-Axenfeld conjunctivitis 372.03
Morbilli (*see also* Measles) 055.9
Morbus
    anglicus, anglorum 268.0
    Beigel 111.2
    caducus (*see also* Epilepsy) 345.9●
    caeruleus 746.89
    celiacus 579.0
    comitialis (*see also* Epilepsy) 345.9●
    cordis - *see also* Disease, heart
        valvulorum - *see* Endocarditis
    coxae 719.95
        tuberculous (*see also* Tuberculosis)
            015.1●
    hemorrhagicus neonatorum 776.0
    maculosus neonatorum 772.6
    renum 593.0
    senilis (*see also* Osteoarthrosis) 715.9●
Morel-Kraepelin disease (*see also*
    Schizophrenia) 295.9●
Morel-Moore syndrome (hyperostosis
    frontalis interna) 733.3
Morel-Morgagni syndrome (hyperostosis
    frontalis interna) 733.3
Morgagni
    cyst, organ, hydatid, or appendage
        752.89
        fallopian tube 752.11
    disease or syndrome (hyperostosis
        frontalis interna) 733.3
Morgagni-Adams-Stokes syndrome
    (syncope with heart block) 426.9
Morgagni-Stewart-Morel syndrome
    (hyperostosis frontalis interna) 733.3
Moria (*see also* Psychosis) 298.9
Morning sickness 643.0●

Moron 317
Morphea (guttate) (linear) 701.0
Morphine dependence (*see also*
    Dependence) 304.0●
Morphinism (*see also* Dependence)
    304.0●
Morphinomania (*see also* Dependence)
    304.0●
Morphoea 701.0
Morquio (-Brailsford) (-Ullrich) disease or
    syndrome (mucopolysaccharidosis
    IV) 277.5
    kyphosis 277.5
Morris syndrome (testicular feminization)
    259.51
Morsus humanus (open wound) - *see also*
    Wound, open, by site
    skin surface intact - *see* Contusion
Mortification (dry) (moist) (*see also*
    Gangrene) 785.4
Morton's
    disease 355.6
    foot 355.6
    metatarsalgia (syndrome) 355.6
    neuralgia 355.6
    neuroma 355.6
    syndrome (metatarsalgia) (neuralgia)
        355.6
    toe 355.6
Morvan's disease 336.0
Mosaicism, mosaic (chromosomal) 758.9
    autosomal 758.5
    sex 758.81
Moschcowitz's syndrome (thrombotic
    thrombocytopenic purpura) 446.6
Mother yaw 102.0
Motion sickness (from travel, any
    vehicle) (from roundabouts or
    swings) 994.6
Mottled teeth (enamel) (endemic)
    (nonendemic) 520.3
Mottling enamel (endemic) (nonendemic)
    (teeth) 520.3
Mouchet's disease 732.5
Mould(s) (in vitreous) 117.9
Moulders'
    bronchitis 502
    tuberculosis (*see also* Tuberculosis)
        011.4●
Mounier-Kuhn syndrome 748.3
    with
        acute exacerbation 494.1
        bronchiectasis 494.0
            with (acute) exacerbation 494.1
    acquired 519.19
        with bronchiectasis 494.0
            with (acute) exacerbation 494.1
Mountain
    fever - *see* Fever, mountain
    sickness 993.2
        with polycythemia, acquired 289.0
        acute 289.0
    tick fever 066.1
Mouse, joint (*see also* Loose, body, joint)
    718.1●
    knee 717.6
Mouth - *see* condition
Movable
    coccyx 724.71
    kidney (*see also* Disease, renal) 593.0
        congenital 753.3
    organ or site, congenital NEC - *see*
        Malposition, congenital
    spleen 289.59

Movement
abnormal (dystonic) (involuntary) 781.0
decreased fetal 655.7●
paradoxical facial 374.43
Moya Moya disease 437.5
Mozart's ear 744.29
MRSA (methicillin resistant staphylococcus aureus) 041.12
colonization V02.54
personal history of V12.04
MSSA (methicillin susceptible staphylococcus aureus) 041.11
colonization V02.53
Mucha's disease (acute parapsoriasis varioliformis) 696.2
Mucha-Haberman syndrome (acute parapsoriasis varioliformis) 696.2
Mu-chain disease 273.2
Mucinosis (cutaneous) (papular) 701.8
Mucocele
appendix 543.9
buccal cavity 528.9
gallbladder (see also Disease, gallbladder) 575.3
lacrimal sac 375.43
orbit (eye) 376.81
salivary gland (any) 527.6
sinus (accessory) (nasal) 478.19
turbinate (bone) (middle) (nasal) 478.19
uterus 621.8
Mucocutaneous lymph node syndrome (acute) (febrile) (infantile) 446.1
Mucoenteritis 564.9
Mucolipidosis I, II, III 272.7
Mucopolysaccharidosis (types 1–6) 277.5
cardiopathy 277.5 [425.7]
Mucormycosis (lung) 117.7
Mucosa associated lymphoid tissue (MALT) 200.3●
Mucositis - see also Inflammation, by site 528.00
cervix (ulcerative) 616.81
due to
antineoplastic therapy (ulcerative) 528.01
other drugs (ulcerative) 528.02
specified NEC 528.09
gastrointestinal (ulcerative) 538
nasal (ulcerative) 478.11
necroticans agranulocytica (see also Agranulocytosis) 288.09
ulcerative 528.00
vagina (ulcerative) 616.81
vulva (ulcerative) 616.81
Mucous - see also condition
patches (syphilitic) 091.3
congenital 090.0
Mucoviscidosis 277.00
with meconium obstruction 277.01
Mucus
asphyxia or suffocation (see also Asphyxia, mucus) 933.1
newborn 770.18
in stool 792.1
plug (see also Asphyxia, mucus) 933.1
aspiration, of newborn 770.17
tracheobronchial 519.19
newborn 770.18
Muguet 112.0
Mulberry molars 090.5
Müllerian mixed tumor (M8950/3) - see Neoplasm, by site, malignant

Multicystic kidney 753.19
Multilobed placenta - see Placenta, abnormal
Multinodular prostate 600.10
with
urinary
obstruction 600.11
retention 600.11
Multiparity V61.5
affecting
fetus or newborn 763.89
management of
labor and delivery 659.4●
pregnancy V23.3
requiring contraceptive management (see also Contraception) V25.9
Multipartita placenta - see Placenta, abnormal
Multiple, multiplex - see also condition
birth
affecting fetus or newborn 761.5
healthy liveborn - see Newborn, multiple
digits (congenital) 755.00
fingers 755.01
toes 755.02
organ or site NEC - see Accessory
personality 300.14
renal arteries 747.62
Mumps 072.9
with complication 072.8
specified type NEC 072.79
encephalitis 072.2
hepatitis 072.71
meningitis (aseptic) 072.1
meningoencephalitis 072.2
oophoritis 072.79
orchitis 072.0
pancreatitis 072.3
polyneuropathy 072.72
vaccination, prophylactic (against) V04.6
Mumu (see also Infestation, filarial) 125.9
Münchausen syndrome 301.51
Münchmeyer's disease or syndrome (exostosis luxurians) 728.11
Mural - see condition
Murmur (cardiac) (heart) (nonorganic) (organic) 785.2
abdominal 787.5
aortic (valve) (see also Endocarditis, aortic) 424.1
benign - omit code
cardiorespiratory 785.2
diastolic - see condition
Flint (see also Endocarditis, aortic) 424.1
functional - omit code
Graham Steell (pulmonic regurgitation) (see also Endocarditis, pulmonary) 424.3
innocent - omit code
insignificant - omit code
midsystolic 785.2
mitral (valve) - see Stenosis
physiologic - see condition
presystolic, mitral - see Insufficiency, mitral
pulmonic (valve) (see also Endocarditis, pulmonary) 424.3
Still's (vibratory) - omit code
systolic (valvular) - see condition
tricuspid (valve) - see Endocarditis, tricuspid

Murmur (Continued)
undiagnosed 785.2
valvular - see condition
vibratory - omit code
Murri's disease (intermittent hemoglobinuria) 283.2
Muscae volitantes 379.24
Muscle, muscular - see condition
Musculoneuralgia 729.1
Mushrooming hip 718.95
Mushroom workers' (pickers') lung 495.5
Mutation
factor V leiden 289.81
prothrombin gene 289.81
Mutism (see also Aphasia) 784.3
akinetic 784.3
deaf (acquired) (congenital) 389.7
hysterical 300.11
selective (elective) 313.23
adjustment reaction 309.83
Myà's disease (congenital dilation, colon) 751.3
Myalgia (intercostal) 729.1
eosinophilia syndrome 710.5
epidemic 074.1
cervical 078.89
psychogenic 307.89
traumatic NEC 959.9
Myasthenia 358.00
cordis - see Failure, heart
gravis 358.00
with exacerbation (acute) 358.01
in crisis 358.01
neonatal 775.2
pseudoparalytica 358.00
stomach 536.8
psychogenic 306.4
syndrome
in
botulism 005.1 [358.1]
diabetes mellitus 250.6● [358.1]
due to secondary diabetes 249.6● [358.1]
hypothyroidism (see also Hypothyroidism) 244.9 [358.1]
malignant neoplasm NEC 199.1 [358.1]
pernicious anemia 281.0 [358.1]
thyrotoxicosis (see also Thyrotoxicosis) 242.9● [358.1]
Myasthenic 728.87
Mycelium infection NEC 117.9
Mycetismus 988.1
Mycetoma (actinomycotic) 039.9
bone 039.8
mycotic 117.4
foot 039.4
mycotic 117.4
madurae 039.9
mycotic 117.4
maduromycotic 039.9
mycotic 117.4
mycotic 117.4
nocardial 039.9
Mycobacteriosis - see Mycobacterium
Mycobacterium, mycobacterial (infection) 031.9
acid-fast (bacilli) 031.9
anonymous (see also Mycobacterium, atypical) 031.9

◄ New ◄ Revised ~~deleted~~ Deleted ● Use Additional Digit(s) ▒ Omit code

Mycobacterium, mycobacterial
   (Continued)
   atypical (acid-fast bacilli) 031.9
      cutaneous 031.1
      pulmonary 031.0
         tuberculous (see also Tuberculosis,
            pulmonary) 011.9●
      specified site NEC 031.8
   avium 031.0
      intracellulare complex bacteremia
         (MAC) 031.2
   balnei 031.1
   Battey 031.0
   cutaneous 031.1
   disseminated 031.2
      avium-intracellulare complex
         (DMAC) 031.2
   fortuitum 031.0
   intracellulare (battey bacillus) 031.0
   kakerifu 031.8
   kansasii 031.0
   kasongo 031.8
   leprae - see Leprosy
   luciflavum 031.0
   marinum 031.1
   pulmonary 031.0
      tuberculous (see also Tuberculosis,
         pulmonary) 011.9●
   scrofulaceum 031.1
   tuberculosis (human, bovine) - see also
      Tuberculosis
      avian type 031.0
   ulcerans 031.1
   xenopi 031.0
Mycosis, mycotic 117.9
   cutaneous NEC 111.9
   ear 111.8 [380.15]
   fungoides (M9700/3) 202.1●
   mouth 112.0
   pharynx 117.9
   skin NEC 111.9
   stomatitis 112.0
   systemic NEC 117.9
   tonsil 117.9
   vagina, vaginitis 112.1
Mydriasis (persistent) (pupil)
   379.43
Myelatelia 742.59
Myelinoclasis, perivascular, acute
   (postinfectious) NEC 136.9
   [323.61]
   postimmunization or postvaccinal
      323.51
Myelinosis, central pontine 341.8
Myelitis (ascending) (cerebellar)
   (childhood) (chronic) (descending)
   (diffuse) (disseminated) (pressure)
   (progressive) (spinal cord)
   (subacute) (see also Encephalitis)
   323.9
   acute (transverse) 341.20
      idiopathic 341.22
      in conditions classified elsewhere
         341.21
   due to
      infection classified elsewhere 136.9
         [323.42]
      specified cause NEC 323.82
      vaccination (any) 323.52
      viral diseases classified elsewhere
         323.02
   herpes simplex 054.74
   herpes zoster 053.14
   late effect - see category 326

Myelitis (Continued)
   optic neuritis in 341.0
   postchickenpox 052.2
   postimmunization 323.52
   postinfectious 136.9 [323.63]
   postvaccinal 323.52
   postvaricella 052.2
   syphilitic (transverse) 094.89
   toxic 989.9 [323.72]
   transverse 323.82
      acute 341.20
         idiopathic 341.22
         in conditions classified elsewhere
            341.21
      idiopathic 341.22
      tuberculous (see also Tuberculosis)
         013.6●
   virus 049.9
Myeloblastic - see condition
Myelocele (see also Spina bifida) 741.9●
   with hydrocephalus 741.0●
Myelocystocele (see also Spina bifida)
   741.9●
Myelocytic - see condition
Myelocytoma 205.1●
Myelodysplasia (spinal cord) 742.59
   meaning myelodysplastic syndrome -
      see Syndrome, myelodysplastic
Myeloencephalitis - see Encephalitis
Myelofibrosis 289.83
   with myeloid metaplasia 238.76
   idiopathic (chronic) 238.76
   megakaryocytic 238.79
   primary 238.76
   secondary 289.83
Myelogenous - see condition
Myeloid - see condition
Myelokathexis 288.09
Myeloleukodystrophy 330.0
Myelolipoma (M8870/0) - see Neoplasm,
   by site, benign
Myeloma (multiple) (plasma cell)
   (plasmacytic) (M9730/3) 203.0●
   monostotic (M9731/1) 238.6
   solitary (M9731/1) 238.6
Myelomalacia 336.8
Myelomata, multiple (M9730/3) 203.0●
Myelomatosis (M9730/3) 203.0●
Myelomeningitis - see
   Meningoencephalitis
Myelomeningocele (spinal cord) (see also
   Spina bifida) 741.9●
   fetal, causing fetopelvic disproportion
      653.7●
Myelo-osteo-musculodysplasia
   hereditaria 756.89
Myelopathic - see condition
Myelopathy (spinal cord) 336.9
   cervical 721.1
   diabetic 250.6● [336.3]
      due to secondary diabetes 249.6●
         [336.3]
   drug-induced 336.8
   due to or with
      carbon tetrachloride 987.8
         [323.72]
      degeneration or displacement,
         intervertebral disc 722.70
         cervical, cervicothoracic 722.71
         lumbar, lumbosacral 722.73
         thoracic, thoracolumbar 722.72
      hydroxyquinoline derivatives 961.3
         [323.72]
      infection - see Encephalitis

Myelopathy (Continued)
   due to or with (Continued)
      intervertebral disc disorder
         722.70
         cervical, cervicothoracic
            722.71
         lumbar, lumbosacral 722.73
         thoracic, thoracolumbar
            722.72
      lead 984.9 [323.72]
      mercury 985.0 [323.72]
      neoplastic disease (see also
         Neoplasm, by site) 239.9
         [336.3]
      pernicious anemia 281.0 [336.3]
      spondylosis 721.91
         cervical 721.1
         lumbar, lumbosacral 721.42
         thoracic 721.41
      thallium 985.8 [323.72]
   lumbar, lumbosacral 721.42
   necrotic (subacute) 336.1
   radiation-induced 336.8
   spondylogenic NEC 721.91
      cervical 721.1
      lumbar, lumbosacral 721.42
      thoracic 721.41
   thoracic 721.41
   toxic NEC 989.9 [323.72]
   transverse (see also Myelitis) 323.82
   vascular 336.1
Myelophthisis 284.2
Myeloproliferative disease (M9960/1)
   238.79
Myeloradiculitis (see also
   Polyneuropathy) 357.0
Myeloradiculodysplasia (spinal)
   742.59
Myelosarcoma (M9930/3) 205.3●
Myelosclerosis 289.89
   with myeloid metaplasia (M9961/1)
      238.76
   disseminated, of nervous system
      340
   megakaryocytic (M9961/1) 238.79
Myelosis (M9860/3) (see also Leukemia,
   myeloid) 205.9●
   acute (M9861/3) 205.0●
   aleukemic (M9864/3) 205.8●
   chronic (M9863/3) 205.1●
   erythremic (M9840/3) 207.0●
      acute (M9841/3) 207.0●
   megakaryocytic (M9920/3) 207.2●
   nonleukemic (chronic) 288.8
   subacute (M9862/3) 205.2●
Myesthenia - see Myasthenia
Myiasis (cavernous) 134.0
   orbit 134.0 [376.13]
Myoadenoma, prostate 600.20
   with
      other lower urinary tract symptoms
         (LUTS) 600.21
      urinary
         obstruction 600.21
         retention 600.21
Myoblastoma
   granular cell (M9580/0) - see also
      Neoplasm, connective tissue,
      benign
      malignant (M9580/3) - see
         Neoplasm, connective tissue,
         malignant
   tongue (M9580/0) 210.1
Myocardial - see condition

M

Myocardiopathy (congestive)
  (constrictive) (familial)
  (hypertrophic nonobstructive)
  (idiopathic) (infiltrative)
  (obstructive) (primary) (restrictive)
  (sporadic) 425.4
  alcoholic 425.5
  amyloid 277.39 [425.7]
  beriberi 265.0 [425.7]
  cobalt-beer 425.5
  due to
    amyloidosis 277.39 [425.7]
    beriberi 265.0 [425.7]
    cardiac glycogenosis 271.0 [425.7]
    Chagas' disease 086.0
    Friedreich's ataxia 334.0 [425.8]
    influenza 487.8 [425.8]
    mucopolysaccharidosis 277.5 [425.7]
    myotonia atrophica 359.21 [425.8]
    progressive muscular dystrophy
      359.1 [425.8]
    sarcoidosis 135 [425.8]
  glycogen storage 271.0 [425.7]
  hypertrophic obstructive 425.1
  metabolic NEC 277.9 [425.7]
  nutritional 269.9 [425.7]
  obscure (African) 425.2
  peripartum 674.5●
  postpartum 674.5●
  secondary 425.9
  thyrotoxic (see also Thyrotoxicosis)
    242.9 ● [425.7]
  toxic NEC 425.9
Myocarditis (fibroid) (interstitial) (old)
  (progressive) (senile) (with
  arteriosclerosis) 429.0
  with
    rheumatic fever (conditions
      classifiable to 390) 398.0
      active (see also Myocarditis, acute,
        rheumatic) 391.2
      inactive or quiescent (with
        chorea) 398.0
  active (nonrheumatic) 422.90
    rheumatic 391.2
      with chorea (acute) (rheumatic)
        (Sydenham's) 392.0
  acute or subacute (interstitial) 422.90
    due to Streptococcus (beta-
      hemolytic) 391.2
    idiopathic 422.91
    rheumatic 391.2
      with chorea (acute) (rheumatic)
        (Sydenham's) 392.0
    specified type NEC 422.99
  aseptic of newborn 074.23
  bacterial (acute) 422.92
  chagasic 086.0
  chronic (interstitial) 429.0
  congenital 746.89
  constrictive 425.4
  Coxsackie (virus) 074.23
  diphtheritic 032.82
  due to or in
    Coxsackie (virus) 074.23
    diphtheria 032.82
    epidemic louse-borne typhus 080
      [422.0]
    influenza 487.8 [422.0]
    Lyme disease 088.81 [422.0]
    scarlet fever 034.1 [422.0]
    toxoplasmosis (acquired) 130.3
    tuberculosis (see also Tuberculosis)
      017.9● [422.0]

Myocarditis (Continued)
  due to or in (Continued)
    typhoid 002.0 [422.0]
    typhus NEC 081.9 [422.0]
  eosinophilic 422.91
  epidemic of newborn 074.23
  Fiedler's (acute) (isolated) (subacute)
    422.91
  giant cell (acute) (subacute) 422.91
  gonococcal 098.85
  granulomatous (idiopathic) (isolated)
    (nonspecific) 422.91
  hypertensive (see also Hypertension,
    heart) 402.90
  idiopathic 422.91
    granulomatous 422.91
  infective 422.92
  influenzal 487.8 [422.0]
  isolated (diffuse) (granulomatous)
    422.91
  malignant 422.99
  meningococcal 036.43
  nonrheumatic, active 422.90
  parenchymatous 422.90
  pneumococcal (acute) (subacute) 422.92
  rheumatic (chronic) (inactive) (with
    chorea) 398.0
    active or acute 391.2
      with chorea (acute) (rheumatic)
        (Sydenham's) 392.0
  septic 422.92
  specific (giant cell) (productive)
    422.91
  staphylococcal (acute) (subacute)
    422.92
  suppurative 422.92
  syphilitic (chronic) 093.82
  toxic 422.93
    rheumatic (see also Myocarditis,
      acute rheumatic) 391.2
  tuberculous (see also Tuberculosis)
    017.9● [422.0]
  typhoid 002.0 [422.0]
  valvular - see Endocarditis
  viral, except Coxsackie 422.91
    Coxsackie 074.23
    of newborn (Coxsackie) 074.23
Myocardium, myocardial - see condition
Myocardosis (see also Cardiomyopathy)
  425.4
Myoclonia (essential) 333.2
  epileptica 345.1 ◄▥
  Friedrich's 333.2
  massive 333.2
Myoclonic
  epilepsy, familial (progressive) 345.1 ◄▥
  jerks 333.2
Myoclonus (familial essential)
  (multifocal) (simplex) 333.2
  with epilepsy and with ragged red
    fibers (MERRF syndrome)
    277.87
  facial 351.8
  massive (infantile) 333.2
  palatal 333.2 ◄
  pharyngeal 333.2 ◄▥
Myocytolysis 429.1 ◄
Myodiastasis 728.84
Myoendocarditis - see also Endocarditis
  acute or subacute 421.9
Myoepithelioma (M8982/0) - see
  Neoplasm, by site, benign
Myofascitis (acute) 729.1
  low back 724.2

Myofibroma (M8890/0) - see also
  Neoplasm, connective tissue, benign
  uterus (cervix) (corpus) (see also
    Leiomyoma) 218.9
Myofibromatosis
  infantile 759.89
Myofibrosis 728.2
  heart (see also Myocarditis) 429.0
  humeroscapular region 726.2
  scapulohumeral 726.2
Myofibrositis (see also Myositis) 729.1
  scapulohumeral 726.2
Myogelosis (occupational) 728.89
Myoglobinuria 791.3
Myoglobulinuria, primary 791.3
Myokymia - see also Myoclonus
  facial 351.8
Myolipoma (M8860/0)
  specified site - see Neoplasm,
    connective tissue, benign
  unspecified site 223.0
Myoma (M8895/0) - see also Neoplasm,
  connective tissue, benign
  cervix (stump) (uterus) (see also
    Leiomyoma) 218.9
  malignant (M8895/3) - see Neoplasm,
    connective tissue, malignant
  prostate 600.20
    with
      other lower urinary tract
        symptoms (LUTS) 600.21
      urinary
        obstruction 600.21
        retention 600.21
  uterus (cervix) (corpus) (see also
    Leiomyoma) 218.9
    in pregnancy or childbirth 654.1●
      affecting fetus or newborn 763.89
      causing obstructed labor 660.2●
        affecting fetus or newborn
          763.1
Myomalacia 728.9
  cordis, heart (see also Degeneration,
    myocardial) 429.1
Myometritis (see also Endometritis)
  615.9
Myometrium - see condition
Myonecrosis, clostridial 040.0
Myopathy 359.9
  alcoholic 359.4
  amyloid 277.39 [359.6]
  benign, congenital 359.0
  central core 359.0
  centronuclear 359.0
  congenital (benign) 359.0
  critical illness 359.81
  distal 359.1
  due to drugs 359.4
  endocrine 259.9 [359.5]
    specified type NEC 259.8 [359.5]
  extraocular muscles 376.82
  facioscapulohumeral 359.1
  in
    Addison's disease 255.41 [359.5]
    amyloidosis 277.39 [359.6]
    cretinism 243 [359.5]
    Cushing's syndrome 255.0 [359.5]
    disseminated lupus erythematosus
      710.0 [359.6]
    giant cell arteritis 446.5 [359.6]
    hyperadrenocorticism NEC 255.3
      [359.5]
    hyperparathyroidism 252.01 [359.5]
    hypopituitarism 253.2 [359.5]

◄ New   ◄▥ Revised   ~~deleted~~ Deleted   ● Use Additional Digit(s)   ▨ Omit code

Myopathy *(Continued)*
  in *(Continued)*
    hypothyroidism *(see also*
      Hypothyroidism) 244.9 *[359.5]*
    malignant neoplasm NEC
      (M8000/3) 199.1 *[359.6]*
    myxedema *(see also* Myxedema)
      244.9 *[359.5]*
    polyarteritis nodosa 446.0 *[359.6]*
    rheumatoid arthritis 714.0 *[359.6]*
    sarcoidosis 135 *[359.6]*
    scleroderma 710.1 *[359.6]*
    Sjögren's disease 710.2 *[359.6]*
    thyrotoxicosis *(see also*
      Thyrotoxicosis) 242.9● *[359.5]*
  inflammatory 359.79
    immune NEC 359.79
    specified NEC 359.79
  intensive care (ICU) 359.81
  limb-girdle 359.1
  myotubular 359.0
  necrotizing, acute 359.81
  nemaline 359.0
  ocular 359.1
  oculopharyngeal 359.1
  of critical illness 359.81
  primary 359.89
  progressive NEC 359.89
  proximal myotonic (PROMM) 359.21
  quadriplegic, acute 359.81
  rod body 359.0
  scapulohumeral 359.1
  specified type NEC 359.89
  toxic 359.4
Myopericarditis *(see also* Pericarditis)
  423.9
Myopia (axial) (congenital) (increased
  curvature or refraction, nucleus of
  lens) 367.1
  degenerative, malignant 360.21
  malignant 360.21
  progressive high (degenerative) 360.21
Myosarcoma (M8895/3) - *see* Neoplasm,
  connective tissue, malignant

Myosis (persistent) 379.42
  stromal (endolymphatic) (M8931/1)
    236.0
Myositis 729.1
  clostridial 040.0
  due to posture 729.1
  epidemic 074.1
  fibrosa or fibrous (chronic) 728.2
    Volkmann's (complicating trauma)
      958.6
  inclusion body (IBM) 359.71 ◄
  infective 728.0
  interstitial 728.81
  multiple - *see* Polymyositis
  occupational 729.1
  orbital, chronic 376.12
  ossificans 728.12
    circumscribed 728.12
    progressive 728.11
    traumatic 728.12
  progressive fibrosing 728.11
  purulent 728.0
  rheumatic 729.1
  rheumatoid 729.1
  suppurative 728.0
  syphilitic 095.6
  traumatic (old) 729.1
Myospasia impulsiva 307.23
Myotonia (acquisita) (intermittens) 728.85
  atrophica 359.21
  congenita 359.22
    acetazolamide responsive 359.22
    dominant form 359.22
    recessive form 359.22
  drug-induced 359.24
  dystrophica 359.21
  fluctuans 359.29
  levior 359.22 ◄▥
  permanens 359.29
Myotonic pupil 379.46
Myriapodiasis 134.1
Myringitis
  with otitis media - *see* Otitis media
  acute 384.00
    specified type NEC 384.09

Myringitis *(Continued)*
  bullosa hemorrhagica 384.01
  bullous 384.01
  chronic 384.1
Mysophobia 300.29
Mytilotoxism 988.0
Myxadenitis labialis 528.5
Myxedema (adult) (idiocy) (infantile)
  (juvenile) (thyroid gland) *(see also*
  Hypothyroidism) 244.9
  circumscribed 242.9●
  congenital 243
  cutis 701.8
  localized (pretibial) 242.9●
  madness (acute) 293.0
    subacute 293.1
  papular 701.8
  pituitary 244.8
  postpartum 674.8●
  pretibial 242.9●
  primary 244.9
Myxochondrosarcoma (M9220/3) -
  see Neoplasm, cartilage,
  malignant
Myxofibroma (M8811/0) - *see also*
  Neoplasm, connective tissue,
  benign
  odontogenic (M9320/0) 213.1
    upper jaw (bone) 213.0
Myxofibrosarcoma (M8811/3) - *see*
  Neoplasm, connective tissue,
  malignant
Myxolipoma (M8852/0) *(see also* Lipoma,
  by site) 214.9
Myxoliposarcoma (M8852/3) - *see*
  Neoplasm, connective tissue,
  malignant
Myxoma (M8840/0) - *see also* Neoplasm,
  connective tissue, benign
  odontogenic (M9320/0) 213.1
    upper jaw (bone) 213.0
Myxosarcoma (M8840/3) - *see* Neoplasm,
  connective tissue, malignant

N

Naegeli's
  disease (hereditary hemorrhagic
      thrombasthenia) 287.1
  leukemia, monocytic (M9863/3)
      205.1 ●
  syndrome (incontinentia pigmenti)
      757.33
Naffziger's syndrome 353.0
Naga sore (*see also* Ulcer, skin) 707.9
Nägele's pelvis 738.6
  with disproportion (fetopelvic)
      653.0 ●
      affecting fetus or newborn 763.1
      causing obstructed labor 660.1 ●
          affecting fetus or newborn 763.1
Nager-de Reynier syndrome (dysostosis
      mandibularis) 756.0
Nail - *see also* condition
  biting 307.9
  patella syndrome (hereditary
      osteoonychodysplasia) 756.89
Nanism, nanosomia (*see also* Dwarfism)
      259.4
  hypophyseal 253.3
  pituitary 253.3
  renis, renalis 588.0
Nanukayami 100.89
Napkin rash 691.0
Narcissism 301.81
Narcolepsy 347.00
  with cataplexy 347.01
  in conditions classified elsewhere
      347.10
      with cataplexy 347.11
Narcosis
  carbon dioxide (respiratory) 786.09
  due to drug
      correct substance properly
          administered 780.09
      overdose or wrong substance given
          or taken 977.9
      specified drug - *see* Table of
          Drugs and Chemicals
Narcotism (chronic) (*see also* Dependence)
      304.9 ●
  acute
      correct substance properly
          administered 349.82
      overdose or wrong substance given
          or taken 967.8
      specified drug - *see* Table of
          Drugs and Chemicals
NARP (ataxia and retinitis pigmentosa
      syndrome) 277.87
Narrow
  anterior chamber angle 365.02
  pelvis (inlet) (outlet) - *see* Contraction,
      pelvis
Narrowing
  artery NEC 447.1
      auditory, internal 433.8 ●
      basilar 433.0 ●
          with other precerebral artery
              433.3 ●
          bilateral 433.3 ●
      carotid 433.1 ●
          with other precerebral artery
              433.3 ●
          bilateral 433.3 ●
      cerebellar 433.8 ●
      choroidal 433.8 ●
      communicating posterior 433.8 ●

Narrowing (*Continued*)
  artery NEC (*Continued*)
      coronary - *see also* Arteriosclerosis,
          coronary
          congenital 746.85
              due to syphilis 090.5
      hypophyseal 433.8 ●
      pontine 433.8 ●
      precerebral NEC 433.9 ●
          multiple or bilateral 433.3 ●
          specified NEC 433.8 ●
      vertebral 433.2 ●
          with other precerebral artery
              433.3 ●
          bilateral 433.3 ●
  auditory canal (external) (*see also*
      Stricture, ear canal, acquired)
      380.50
  cerebral arteries 437.0
  cicatricial - *see* Cicatrix
  congenital - *see* Anomaly, congenital
  coronary artery - *see* Narrowing, artery,
      coronary
  ear, middle 385.22
  Eustachian tube (*see also* Obstruction,
      Eustachian tube) 381.60
  eyelid 374.46
      congenital 743.62
  intervertebral disc or space NEC - *see*
      Degeneration, intervertebral disc
  joint space, hip 719.85
  larynx 478.74
  lids 374.46
      congenital 743.62
  mesenteric artery (with gangrene) 557.0
  palate 524.89
  palpebral fissure 374.46
  retinal artery 362.13
  ureter 593.3
  urethra (*see also* Stricture, urethra) 598.9
Narrowness, abnormal, eyelid 743.62
Nasal - *see* condition
Nasolacrimal - *see* condition
Nasopharyngeal - *see also* condition
  bursa 478.29
  pituitary gland 759.2
  torticollis 723.5
Nasopharyngitis (acute) (infective)
      (subacute) 460
  chronic 472.2
      due to external agent - *see*
          Condition, respiratory, chronic,
          due to
  due to external agent - *see* Condition,
      respiratory, due to
  septic 034.0
  streptococcal 034.0
  suppurative (chronic) 472.2
  ulcerative (chronic) 472.2
Nasopharynx, nasopharyngeal - *see*
      condition
Natal tooth, teeth 520.6
Nausea (*see also* Vomiting) 787.02
  with vomiting 787.01
  epidemic 078.82
  gravidarum - *see* Hyperemesis,
      gravidarum
  marina 994.6
Naval - *see* condition
Neapolitan fever (*see also* Brucellosis)
      023.9
Near drowning 994.1
Nearsightedness 367.1
Near-syncope 780.2

Nebécourt's syndrome 253.3
Nebula, cornea (eye) 371.01
  congenital 743.43
      interfering with vision 743.42
Necator americanus infestation 126.1
Necatoriasis 126.1
Neck - *see* condition
Necrencephalus (*see also* Softening, brain)
      437.8
Necrobacillosis 040.3
Necrobiosis 799.89
  brain or cerebral (*see also* Softening,
      brain) 437.8
  lipoidica 709.3
      diabeticorum 250.8 ● [709.3]
          due to secondary diabetes 249.8 ●
              [709.3]
Necrodermolysis 695.15
Necrolysis, toxic epidermal 695.15
  due to drug
      correct substance properly
          administered 695.15
      overdose or wrong substance given
          or taken 977.9
      specified drug - *see* Table of
          Drugs and Chemicals
  Stevens-Johnson syndrome overlap
      (SJS-TEN overlap syndrome)
      695.14
Necrophilia 302.89
Necrosis, necrotic
  adrenal (capsule) (gland) 255.8
  antrum, nasal sinus 478.19
  aorta (hyaline) (*see also* Aneurysm,
      aorta) 441.9
      cystic medial 441.00
          abdominal 441.02
          thoracic 441.01
          thoracoabdominal 441.03
      ruptured 441.5
  arteritis 446.0
  artery 447.5
  aseptic, bone 733.40
      femur (head) (neck) 733.42
          medial condyle 733.43
      humoral head 733.41
      jaw 733.45
      medial femoral condyle 733.43
      specific site NEC 733.49
      talus 733.44
  avascular, bone NEC (*see also* Necrosis,
      aseptic, bone) 733.40
  bladder (aseptic) (sphincter) 596.8
  bone (*see also* Osteomyelitis) 730.1 ●
      acute 730.0 ●
      aseptic or avascular 733.40
          femur (head) (neck) 733.42
              medial condyle 733.43
          humoral head 733.41
          jaw 733.45
          medial femoral condyle 733.43
          specified site NEC 733.49
          talus 733.44
      ethmoid 478.19
      ischemic 733.40
      jaw 526.4
          aseptic 733.45
      marrow 289.89
      Paget's (osteitis deformans) 731.0
      tuberculous - *see* Tuberculosis, bone
  brain (softening) (*see also* Softening,
      brain) 437.8
  breast (aseptic) (fat) (segmental)
      611.3

◀ New   ◀▥ Revised   ~~deleted~~ Deleted   ● Use Additional Digit(s)   ▨ Omit code

Necrosis, necrotic (Continued)
bronchus, bronchi 519.19
central nervous system NEC (see also
Softening, brain) 437.8
cerebellar (see also Softening, brain) 437.8
cerebral (softening) (see also Softening,
brain) 437.8
cerebrospinal (softening) (see also
Softening, brain) 437.8
colon 557.0
cornea (see also Keratitis) 371.40
cortical, kidney 583.6
cystic medial (aorta) 441.00
abdominal 441.02
thoracic 441.01
thoracoabdominal 441.03
dental 521.09
pulp 522.1
due to swallowing corrosive
substance - see Burn, by site
ear (ossicle) 385.24
esophagus 530.89
ethmoid (bone) 478.19
eyelid 374.50
fat, fatty (generalized) (see also
Degeneration, fatty) 272.8
abdominal wall 567.82
breast (aseptic) (segmental) 611.3
intestine 569.89
localized - see Degeneration, by site,
fatty
mesentery 567.82
omentum 567.82
pancreas 577.8
peritoneum 567.82
skin (subcutaneous) 709.3
newborn 778.1
femur (aseptic) (avascular) 733.42
head 733.42
medial condyle 733.43
neck 733.42
gallbladder (see also Cholecystitis,
acute) 575.0
gangrenous 785.4
gastric 537.89
glottis 478.79
heart (myocardium) - see Infarct,
myocardium
hepatic (see also Necrosis, liver) 570
hip (aseptic) (avascular) 733.42
intestine (acute) (hemorrhagic)
(massive) 557.0
ischemic 785.4
jaw 526.4
aseptic 733.45
kidney (bilateral) 583.9
acute 584.9
cortical 583.6
acute 584.6
with
abortion - see Abortion, by
type, with renal
failure
ectopic pregnancy (see also
categories 633.0–633.9)
639.3
molar pregnancy (see also
categories 630–632)
639.3
complicating pregnancy 646.2●
affecting fetus or newborn
760.1
following labor and delivery
669.3●

Necrosis, necrotic (Continued)
kidney (Continued)
medullary (papillary) (see also
Pyelitis) 590.80
in
acute renal failure 584.7
nephritis, nephropathy 583.7
papillary (see also Pyelitis) 590.80
in
acute renal failure 584.7
nephritis, nephropathy 583.7
tubular 584.5
with
abortion - see Abortion, by
type, with renal failure
ectopic pregnancy (see also
categories 633.0–633.9)
639.3
molar pregnancy (see also
categories 630–632)
639.3
complicating
abortion 639.3
ectopic or molar pregnancy
639.3
pregnancy 646.2●
affecting fetus or newborn
760.1
following labor and delivery
669.3●
traumatic 958.5
larynx 478.79
liver (acute) (congenital) (diffuse)
(massive) (subacute) 570
with
abortion - see Abortion, by type,
with specified complication
NEC
ectopic pregnancy (see also
categories 633.0–633.9)
639.8
molar pregnancy (see also
categories 630–632) 639.8
complicating pregnancy 646.7●
affecting fetus or newborn
760.8
following
abortion 639.8
ectopic or molar pregnancy
639.8
obstetrical 646.7●
postabortal 639.8
puerperal, postpartum 674.8●
toxic 573.3
lung 513.0
lymphatic gland 683
mammary gland 611.3
mastoid (chronic) 383.1
mesentery 557.0
fat 567.82
mitral valve - see Insufficiency, mitral
myocardium, myocardial - see Infarct,
myocardium
nose (septum) 478.19
omentum 557.0
with mesenteric infarction 557.0
fat 567.82
orbit, orbital 376.10
ossicles, ear (aseptic) 385.24
ovary (see also Salpingo-oophoritis)
614.2
pancreas (aseptic) (duct) (fat) 577.8
acute 577.0
infective 577.0

Necrosis, necrotic (Continued)
papillary, kidney (see also Pyelitis)
590.80
perineum 624.8
peritoneum 557.0
with mesenteric infarction 557.0
fat 567.82
pharynx 462
in granulocytopenia 288.09
phosphorus 983.9
pituitary (gland) (postpartum)
(Sheehan) 253.2
placenta (see also Placenta, abnormal)
656.7●
pneumonia 513.0
pulmonary 513.0
pulp (dental) 522.1
pylorus 537.89
radiation - see Necrosis, by site
radium - see Necrosis, by site
renal - see Necrosis, kidney
sclera 379.19
scrotum 608.89
skin or subcutaneous tissue 709.8
due to burn - see Burn, by site
gangrenous 785.4
spine, spinal (column) 730.18
acute 730.18
cord 336.1
spleen 289.59
stomach 537.89
stomatitis 528.1
subcutaneous fat 709.3
fetus or newborn 778.1
subendocardial - see Infarct, myocardium
suprarenal (capsule) (gland) 255.8
teeth, tooth 521.09
testis 608.89
thymus (gland) 254.8
tonsil 474.8
trachea 519.19
tuberculous NEC - see Tuberculosis
tubular (acute) (anoxic) (toxic) 584.5
due to a procedure 997.5
umbilical cord, affecting fetus or
newborn 762.6
vagina 623.8
vertebra (lumbar) 730.18
acute 730.18
tuberculous (see also Tuberculosis)
015.0● [730.8]
vesical (aseptic) (bladder) 596.8
vulva 624.8
x-ray - see Necrosis, by site
Necrospermia 606.0
Necrotizing angiitis 446.0
Negativism 301.7
Neglect (child) (newborn) NEC 995.52
adult 995.84
after or at birth 995.52
hemispatial 781.8
left-sided 781.8
sensory 781.8
visuospatial 781.8
Negri bodies 071
Neill-Dingwall syndrome
(microcephaly and dwarfism)
759.89
Neisserian infection NEC - see
Gonococcus
Nematodiasis NEC (see also Infestation,
Nematode) 127.9
ancylostoma (see also Ancylostomiasis)
126.9

Neoformans cryptococcus infection
117.5
Neonatal - *see also* condition
abstinence syndrome 779.5 ◀
adrenoleukodystrophy
277.86
teeth, tooth 520.6
Neonatorum - *see* condition
Neoplasia
anal intraepithelial I [AIN I]
(histologically confirmed)
569.44

Neoplasia (*Continued*)
anal intraepithelial II [AIN II]
(histologically confirmed)
569.44
anal intraepithelial III [AIN III] 230.6
anal canal 230.5
endometrial intraepithelial
[EIN] 621.35 ◀
multiple endocrine [MEN]
type I 258.01
type IIA 258.02
type IIB 258.03

Neoplasia (*Continued*)
vaginal intraepithelial I [VAIN I]
623.0
vaginal intraepithelial II [VAIN II]
623.0
vaginal intraepithelial III [VAIN III]
233.31
vulvar intraepithelial I [VIN I] 624.01
vulvar intraepithelial II [VIN II] 624.02
vulvar intraepithelial III [VIN III]
233.32
Neoplasm, neoplastic see page 423–467

◀ New   ◀ⁿ Revised   ~~deleted~~ Deleted   ● Use Additional Digit(s)   ▨ Omit code

	Malignant					
	Primary	Secondary	Ca in situ	Benign	Uncertain Behavior	Unspecified
Neoplasm, neoplastic	199.1	199.1	234.9	229.9	238.9	239.9

Notes — 1. The list below gives the code numbers for neoplasms by anatomical site. For each site there are six possible code numbers according to whether the neoplasm in question is malignant, benign, in situ, of uncertain behavior, or of unspecified nature. The description of the neoplasm will often indicate which of the six columns is appropriate; e.g., malignant melanoma of skin, benign fibroadenoma of breast, carcinoma in situ of cervix uteri.

Where such descriptors are not present, the remainder of the Index should be consulted where guidance is given to the appropriate column for each morphological (histological) variety listed; e.g., Mesonephroma—see Neoplasm, malignant; Embryoma—see also Neoplasm, uncertain behavior; Disease, Bowen's—see Neoplasm, skin, in situ. However, the guidance in the Index can be overridden if one of the descriptors mentioned above is present; e.g., malignant adenoma of colon is coded to 153.9 and not to 211.3 as the adjective "malignant" overrides the Index entry "Adenoma - see also Neoplasm, benign."

*2. Sites marked with the sign * (e.g., face NEC*) should be classified to malignant neoplasm of skin of these sites if the variety of neoplasm is a squamous cell carcinoma or an epidermoid carcinoma and to benign neoplasm of skin of these sites if the variety of neoplasm is a papilloma (any type).*

	Primary	Secondary	Ca in situ	Benign	Uncertain Behavior	Unspecified
abdomen, abdominal	195.2	198.89	234.8	229.8	238.8	239.89◄
cavity	195.2	198.89	234.8	229.8	238.8	239.89◄
organ	195.2	198.89	234.8	229.8	238.8	239.89◄
viscera	195.2	198.89	234.8	229.8	238.8	239.89◄
wall	173.5	198.2	232.5	216.5	238.2	239.2
connective tissue	171.5	198.89	—	215.5	238.1	239.2
abdominopelvic	195.8	198.89	234.8	229.8	238.8	239.89◄
accessory sinus - *see* Neoplasm, sinus						
acoustic nerve	192.0	198.4	—	225.1	237.9	239.7
acromion (process)	170.4	198.5	—	213.4	238.0	239.2
adenoid (pharynx) (tissue)	147.1	198.89	230.0	210.7	235.1	239.0
adipose tissue (*see also* Neoplasm, connective tissue)	171.9	198.89	—	215.9	238.1	239.2
adnexa (uterine)	183.9	198.82	233.39	221.8	236.3	239.5
adrenal (cortex) (gland) (medulla)	194.0	198.7	234.8	227.0	237.2	239.7
ala nasi (external)	173.3	198.2	232.3	216.3	238.2	239.2
alimentary canal or tract NEC	159.9	197.8	230.9	211.9	235.5	239.0
alveolar	143.9	198.89	230.0	210.4	235.1	239.0
mucosa	143.9	198.89	230.0	210.4	235.1	239.0
lower	143.1	198.89	230.0	210.4	235.1	239.0
upper	143.0	198.89	230.0	210.4	235.1	239.0
ridge or process	170.1	198.5	—	213.1	238.0	239.2
carcinoma	143.9	—	—	—	—	—
lower	143.1	—	—	—	—	—
upper	143.0	—	—	—	—	—
lower	170.1	198.5	—	213.1	238.0	239.2
mucosa	143.9	198.89	230.0	210.4	235.1	239.0
lower	143.1	198.89	230.0	210.4	235.1	239.0
upper	143.0	198.89	230.0	210.4	235.1	239.0
upper	170.0	198.5	—	213.0	238.0	239.2
sulcus	145.1	198.89	230.0	210.4	235.1	239.0

	Malignant					
	Primary	Secondary	Ca in situ	Benign	Uncertain Behavior	Unspecified
Neoplasm *(Continued)*						
alveolus	143.9	198.89	230.0	210.4	235.1	239.0
lower	143.1	198.89	230.0	210.4	235.1	239.0
upper	143.0	198.89	230.0	210.4	235.1	239.0
ampulla of Vater	156.2	197.8	230.8	211.5	235.3	239.0
ankle NEC*	195.5	198.89	232.7	229.8	238.8	239.89◄
anorectum, anorectal (junction)	154.8	197.5	230.7	211.4	235.2	239.0
antecubital fossa or space*	195.4	198.89	232.6	229.8	238.8	239.89◄
antrum (Highmore) (maxillary)	160.2	197.3	231.8	212.0	235.9	239.1
pyloric	151.2	197.8	230.2	211.1	235.2	239.0
tympanicum	160.1	197.3	231.8	212.0	235.9	239.1
anus, anal	154.3	197.5	230.6	211.4	235.5	239.0
canal	154.2	197.5	230.5	211.4	235.5	239.0
contiguous sites with rectosigmoid junction or rectum	154.8	—	—	—	—	—
margin	173.5	198.2	232.5	216.5	238.2	239.2
skin	173.5	198.2	232.5	216.5	238.2	239.2
sphincter	154.2	197.5	230.5	211.4	235.5	239.0
aorta (thoracic)	171.4	198.89	—	215.4	238.1	239.2
abdominal	171.5	198.89	—	215.5	238.1	239.2
aortic body	194.6	198.89	—	227.6	237.3	239.7
aponeurosis	171.9	198.89	—	215.9	238.1	239.2
palmar	171.2	198.89	—	215.2	238.1	239.2
plantar	171.3	198.89	—	215.3	238.1	239.2
appendix	153.5	197.5	230.3	211.3	235.2	239.0
arachnoid (cerebral)	192.1	198.4	—	225.2	237.6	239.7
spinal	192.3	198.4	—	225.4	237.6	239.7
areola (female)	174.0	198.81	233.0	217	238.3	239.3
male	175.0	198.81	233.0	217	238.3	239.3
arm NEC*	195.4	198.89	232.6	229.8	238.8	239.89◄
artery - *see* Neoplasm, connective tissue						
aryepiglottic fold	148.2	198.89	230.0	210.8	235.1	239.0
hypopharyngeal aspect	148.2	198.89	230.0	210.8	235.1	239.0
laryngeal aspect	161.1	197.3	231.0	212.1	235.6	239.1
marginal zone	148.2	198.89	230.0	210.8	235.1	239.0
arytenoid (cartilage)	161.3	197.3	231.0	212.1	235.6	239.1
fold - *see* Neoplasm, aryepiglottic						
associated with transplanted organ	199.2	—	—	—	—	—
atlas	170.2	198.5	—	213.2	238.0	239.2
atrium, cardiac	164.1	198.89	—	212.7	238.8	239.89◄
auditory						
canal (external) (skin)	173.2	198.2	232.2	216.2	238.2	239.2
internal	160.1	197.3	231.8	212.0	235.9	239.1

◄ New   ◄▥ Revised   ~~deleted~~ Deleted   ● Use Additional Digit(s)   ▨ Omit code

	Malignant			Benign	Uncertain Behavior	Unspecified
	Primary	Secondary	Ca in situ	Benign	Uncertain Behavior	Unspecified
Neoplasm *(Continued)*						
auditory *(Continued)*						
nerve	192.0	198.4	—	225.1	237.9	239.7
tube	160.1	197.3	231.8	212.0	235.9	239.1
opening	147.2	198.89	230.0	210.7	235.1	239.0
auricle, ear	173.2	198.2	232.2	216.2	238.2	239.2
cartilage	171.0	198.89	—	215.0	238.1	239.2
auricular canal (external)	173.2	198.2	232.2	216.2	238.2	239.2
internal	160.1	197.3	231.8	212.0	235.9	239.1
autonomic nerve or nervous system NEC	171.9	198.89	—	215.9	238.1	239.2
axilla, axillary	195.1	198.89	234.8	229.8	238.8	239.89◄▦
fold	173.5	198.2	232.5	216.5	238.2	239.2
back NEC*	195.8	198.89	232.5	229.8	238.8	239.89◄▦
Bartholin's gland	184.1	198.82	233.39	221.2	236.3	239.5
basal ganglia	191.0	198.3	—	225.0	237.5	239.6
basis pedunculi	191.7	198.3	—	225.0	237.5	239.6
bile or biliary (tract)	156.9	197.8	230.8	211.5	235.3	239.0
canaliculi (biliferi) (intrahepatic)	155.1	197.8	230.8	211.5	235.3	239.0
canals, interlobular	155.1	197.8	230.8	211.5	235.3	239.0
contiguous sites	156.8	—	—	—	—	—
duct or passage (common) (cystic) (extrahepatic)	156.1	197.8	230.8	211.5	235.3	239.0
contiguous sites						
with gallbladder	156.8	—	—	—	—	—
interlobular	155.1	197.8	230.8	211.5	235.3	239.0
intrahepatic	155.1	197.8	230.8	211.5	235.3	239.0
and extrahepatic	156.9	197.8	230.8	211.5	235.3	239.0
bladder (urinary)	188.9	198.1	233.7	223.3	236.7	239.4
contiguous sites	188.8	—	—	—	—	—
dome	188.1	198.1	233.7	223.3	236.7	239.4
neck	188.5	198.1	233.7	223.3	236.7	239.4
orifice	188.9	198.1	233.7	223.3	236.7	239.4
ureteric	188.6	198.1	233.7	223.3	236.7	239.4
urethral	188.5	198.1	233.7	223.3	236.7	239.4
sphincter	188.8	198.1	233.7	223.3	236.7	239.4
trigone	188.0	198.1	233.7	223.3	236.7	239.4
urachus	188.7	—	233.7	223.3	236.7	239.4
wall	188.9	198.1	233.7	223.3	236.7	239.4
anterior	188.3	198.1	233.7	223.3	236.7	239.4
lateral	188.2	198.1	233.7	223.3	236.7	239.4
posterior	188.4	198.1	233.7	223.3	236.7	239.4
blood vessel - *see* Neoplasm, connective tissue						

◄ New   ◄▦ Revised   ~~deleted~~ Deleted   ● Use Additional Digit(s)   ▦ Omit code

	Malignant					
	Primary	Secondary	Ca in situ	Benign	Uncertain Behavior	Unspecified
Neoplasm *(Continued)*						
bone (periosteum)	170.9	198.5	—	213.9	238.0	239.2
Note — Carcinomas and adenocarcinomas, of any type other than intraosseous or odontogenic, of the sites listed under "Neoplasm, bone" should be considered as constituting metastatic spread from an unspecified primary site and coded to 198.5 for morbidity coding.						
acetabulum	170.6	198.5	—	213.6	238.0	239.2
acromion (process)	170.4	198.5	—	213.4	238.0	239.2
ankle	170.8	198.5	—	213.8	238.0	239.2
arm NEC	170.4	198.5	—	213.4	238.0	239.2
astragalus	170.8	198.5	—	213.8	238.0	239.2
atlas	170.2	198.5	—	213.2	238.0	239.2
axis	170.2	198.5	—	213.2	238.0	239.2
back NEC	170.2	198.5	—	213.2	238.0	239.2
calcaneus	170.8	198.5	—	213.8	238.0	239.2
calvarium	170.0	198.5	—	213.0	238.0	239.2
carpus (any)	170.5	198.5	—	213.5	238.0	239.2
cartilage NEC	170.9	198.5	—	213.9	238.0	239.2
clavicle	170.3	198.5	—	213.3	238.0	239.2
clivus	170.0	198.5	—	213.0	238.0	239.2
coccygeal vertebra	170.6	198.5	—	213.6	238.0	239.2
coccyx	170.6	198.5	—	213.6	238.0	239.2
costal cartilage	170.3	198.5	—	213.3	238.0	239.2
costovertebral joint	170.3	198.5	—	213.3	238.0	239.2
cranial	170.0	198.5	—	213.0	238.0	239.2
cuboid	170.8	198.5	—	213.8	238.0	239.2
cuneiform	170.9	198.5	—	213.9	238.0	239.2
ankle	170.8	198.5	—	213.8	238.0	239.2
wrist	170.5	198.5	—	213.5	238.0	239.2
digital	170.9	198.5	—	213.9	238.0	239.2
finger	170.5	198.5	—	213.5	238.0	239.2
toe	170.8	198.5	—	213.8	238.0	239.2
elbow	170.4	198.5	—	213.4	238.0	239.2
ethmoid (labyrinth)	170.0	198.5	—	213.0	238.0	239.2
face	170.0	198.5	—	213.0	238.0	239.2
lower jaw	170.1	198.5	—	213.1	238.0	239.2
femur (any part)	170.7	198.5	—	213.7	238.0	239.2
fibula (any part)	170.7	198.5	—	213.7	238.0	239.2
finger (any)	170.5	198.5	—	213.5	238.0	239.2
foot	170.8	198.5	—	213.8	238.0	239.2
forearm	170.4	198.5	—	213.4	238.0	239.2
frontal	170.0	198.5	—	213.0	238.0	239.2
hand	170.5	198.5	—	213.5	238.0	239.2

◀ New   ◀▥ Revised   ~~deleted~~ Deleted   ● Use Additional Digit(s)   ▨ Omit code

	Malignant			Benign	Uncertain Behavior	Unspecified
	Primary	Secondary	Ca in situ			
Neoplasm *(Continued)*						
bone *(Continued)*						
heel	170.8	198.5	—	213.8	238.0	239.2
hip	170.6	198.5	—	213.6	238.0	239.2
humerus (any part)	170.4	198.5	—	213.4	238.0	239.2
hyoid	170.0	198.5	—	213.0	238.0	239.2
ilium	170.6	198.5	—	213.6	238.0	239.2
innominate	170.6	198.5	—	213.6	238.0	239.2
intervertebral cartilage or disc	170.2	198.5	—	213.2	238.0	239.2
ischium	170.6	198.5	—	213.6	238.0	239.2
jaw (lower)	170.1	198.5	—	213.1	238.0	239.2
upper	170.0	198.5	—	213.0	238.0	239.2
knee	170.7	198.5	—	213.7	238.0	239.2
leg NEC	170.7	198.5	—	213.7	238.0	239.2
limb NEC	170.9	198.5	—	213.9	238.0	239.2
lower (long bones)	170.7	198.5	—	213.7	238.0	239.2
short bones	170.8	198.5	—	213.8	238.0	239.2
upper (long bones)	170.4	198.5	—	213.4	238.0	239.2
short bones	170.5	198.5	—	213.5	238.0	239.2
long	170.9	198.5	—	213.9	238.0	239.2
lower limbs NEC	170.7	198.5	—	213.7	238.0	239.2
upper limbs NEC	170.4	198.5	—	213.4	238.0	239.2
malar	170.0	198.5	—	213.0	238.0	239.2
mandible	170.1	198.5	—	213.1	238.0	239.2
marrow NEC	202.9●	198.5	—	—	—	238.79
mastoid	170.0	198.5	—	213.0	238.0	239.2
maxilla, maxillary (superior)	170.0	198.5	—	213.0	238.0	239.2
inferior	170.1	198.5	—	213.1	238.0	239.2
metacarpus (any)	170.5	198.5	—	213.5	238.0	239.2
metatarsus (any)	170.8	198.5	—	213.8	238.0	239.2
navicular (ankle)	170.8	198.5	—	213.8	238.0	239.2
hand	170.5	198.5	—	213.5	238.0	239.2
nose, nasal	170.0	198.5	—	213.0	238.0	239.2
occipital	170.0	198.5	—	213.0	238.0	239.2
orbit	170.0	198.5	—	213.0	238.0	239.2
parietal	170.0	198.5	—	213.0	238.0	239.2
patella	170.8	198.5	—	213.8	238.0	239.2
pelvic	170.6	198.5	—	213.6	238.0	239.2
phalanges	170.9	198.5	—	213.9	238.0	239.2
foot	170.8	198.5	—	213.8	238.0	239.2
hand	170.5	198.5	—	213.5	238.0	239.2

	Malignant					
	Primary	Secondary	Ca in situ	Benign	Uncertain Behavior	Unspecified
Neoplasm *(Continued)*						
bone *(Continued)*						
pubic	170.6	198.5	—	213.6	238.0	239.2
radius (any part)	170.4	198.5	—	213.4	238.0	239.2
rib	170.3	198.5	—	213.3	238.0	239.2
sacral vertebra	170.6	198.5	—	213.6	238.0	239.2
sacrum	170.6	198.5	—	213.6	238.0	239.2
scaphoid (of hand)	170.5	198.5	—	213.5	238.0	239.2
of ankle	170.8	198.5	—	213.8	238.0	239.2
scapula (any part)	170.4	198.5	—	213.4	238.0	239.2
sella turcica	170.0	198.5	—	213.0	238.0	239.2
short	170.9	198.5	—	213.9	238.0	239.2
lower limb	170.8	198.5	—	213.8	238.0	239.2
upper limb	170.5	198.5	—	213.5	238.0	239.2
shoulder	170.4	198.5	—	213.4	238.0	239.2
skeleton, skeletal NEC	170.9	198.5	—	213.9	238.0	239.2
skull	170.0	198.5	—	213.0	238.0	239.2
sphenoid	170.0	198.5	—	213.0	238.0	239.2
spine, spinal (column)	170.2	198.5	—	213.2	238.0	239.2
coccyx	170.6	198.5	—	213.6	238.0	239.2
sacrum	170.6	198.5	—	213.6	238.0	239.2
sternum	170.3	198.5	—	213.3	238.0	239.2
tarsus (any)	170.8	198.5	—	213.8	238.0	239.2
temporal	170.0	198.5	—	213.0	238.0	239.2
thumb	170.5	198.5	—	213.5	238.0	239.2
tibia (any part)	170.7	198.5	—	213.7	238.0	239.2
toe (any)	170.8	198.5	—	213.8	238.0	239.2
trapezium	170.5	198.5	—	213.5	238.0	239.2
trapezoid	170.5	198.5	—	213.5	238.0	239.2
turbinate	170.0	198.5	—	213.0	238.0	239.2
ulna (any part)	170.4	198.5	—	213.4	238.0	239.2
unciform	170.5	198.5	—	213.5	238.0	239.2
vertebra (column)	170.2	198.5	—	213.2	238.0	239.2
coccyx	170.6	198.5	—	213.6	238.0	239.2
sacrum	170.6	198.5	—	213.6	238.0	239.2
vomer	170.0	198.5	—	213.0	238.0	239.2
wrist	170.5	198.5	—	213.5	238.0	239.2
xiphoid process	170.3	198.5	—	213.3	238.0	239.2
zygomatic	170.0	198.5	—	213.0	238.0	239.2
book-leaf (mouth)	145.8	198.89	230.0	210.4	235.1	239.0
bowel - *see* Neoplasm, intestine						

◀ New   ◀▬ Revised   ~~deleted~~ Deleted   ● Use Additional Digit(s)   ▨ Omit code

	Malignant					
	Primary	**Secondary**	**Ca in situ**	**Benign**	**Uncertain Behavior**	**Unspecified**
Neoplasm *(Continued)*						
brachial plexus	171.2	198.89	—	215.2	238.1	239.2
brain NEC	191.9	198.3	—	225.0	237.5	239.6
basal ganglia	191.0	198.3	—	225.0	237.5	239.6
cerebellopontine angle	191.6	198.3	—	225.0	237.5	239.6
cerebellum NOS	191.6	198.3	—	225.0	237.5	239.6
cerebrum	191.0	198.3	—	225.0	237.5	239.6
choroid plexus	191.5	198.3	—	225.0	237.5	239.6
contiguous sites	191.8	—	—	—	—	—
corpus callosum	191.8	198.3	—	225.0	237.5	239.6
corpus striatum	191.0	198.3	—	225.0	237.5	239.6
cortex (cerebral)	191.0	198.3	—	225.0	237.5	239.6
frontal lobe	191.1	198.3	—	225.0	237.5	239.6
globus pallidus	191.0	198.3	—	225.0	237.5	239.6
hippocampus	191.2	198.3	—	225.0	237.5	239.6
hypothalamus	191.0	198.3	—	225.0	237.5	239.6
internal capsule	191.0	198.3	—	225.0	237.5	239.6
medulla oblongata	191.7	198.3	—	225.0	237.5	239.6
meninges	192.1	198.4	—	225.2	237.6	239.7
midbrain	191.7	198.3	—	225.0	237.5	239.6
occipital lobe	191.4	198.3	—	225.0	237.5	239.6
parietal lobe	191.3	198.3	—	225.0	237.5	239.6
peduncle	191.7	198.3	—	225.0	237.5	239.6
pons	191.7	198.3	—	225.0	237.5	239.6
stem	191.7	198.3	—	225.0	237.5	239.6
tapetum	191.8	198.3	—	225.0	237.5	239.6
temporal lobe	191.2	198.3	—	225.0	237.5	239.6
thalamus	191.0	198.3	—	225.0	237.5	239.6
uncus	191.2	198.3	—	225.0	237.5	239.6
ventricle (floor)	191.5	198.3	—	225.0	237.5	239.6
branchial (cleft) (vestiges)	146.8	198.89	230.0	210.6	235.1	239.0
breast (connective tissue) (female) (glandular tissue) (soft parts)	174.9	198.81	233.0	217	238.3	239.3
areola	174.0	198.81	233.0	217	238.3	239.3
male	175.0	198.81	233.0	217	238.3	239.3
axillary tail	174.6	198.81	233.0	217	238.3	239.3
central portion	174.1	198.81	233.0	217	238.3	239.3
contiguous sites	174.8	—	—	—	—	—
ectopic sites	174.8	198.81	233.0	217	238.3	239.3
inner	174.8	198.81	233.0	217	238.3	239.3
lower	174.8	198.81	233.0	217	238.3	239.3
lower-inner quadrant	174.3	198.81	233.0	217	238.3	239.3

◀ New   ◀▥ Revised   ~~deleted~~ Deleted   ● Use Additional Digit(s)   ▨ Omit code

	Malignant					
	Primary	Secondary	Ca in situ	Benign	Uncertain Behavior	Unspecified
Neoplasm *(Continued)*						
breast *(Continued)*						
lower-outer quadrant	174.5	198.81	233.0	217	238.3	239.3
male	175.9	198.81	233.0	217	238.3	239.3
areola	175.0	198.81	233.0	217	238.3	239.3
ectopic tissue	175.9	198.81	233.0	217	238.3	239.3
nipple	175.0	198.81	233.0	217	238.3	239.3
mastectomy site (skin)	173.5	198.2	—	—	—	—
specified as breast tissue	174.8	198.81	—	—	—	—
midline	174.8	198.81	233.0	217	238.3	239.3
nipple	174.0	198.81	233.0	217	238.3	239.3
male	175.0	198.81	233.0	217	238.3	239.3
outer	174.8	198.81	233.0	217	238.3	239.3
skin	173.5	198.2	232.5	216.5	238.2	239.2
tail (axillary)	174.6	198.81	233.0	217	238.3	239.3
upper	174.8	198.81	233.0	217	238.3	239.3
upper-inner quadrant	174.2	198.81	233.0	217	238.3	239.3
upper-outer quadrant	174.4	198.81	233.0	217	238.3	239.3
broad ligament	183.3	198.82	233.39	221.0	236.3	239.5
bronchiogenic, bronchogenic (lung)	162.9	197.0	231.2	212.3	235.7	239.1
bronchiole	162.9	197.0	231.2	212.3	235.7	239.1
bronchus	162.9	197.0	231.2	212.3	235.7	239.1
carina	162.2	197.0	231.2	212.3	235.7	239.1
contiguous sites with lung or trachea	162.8	—	—	—	—	—
lower lobe of lung	162.5	197.0	231.2	212.3	235.7	239.1
main	162.2	197.0	231.2	212.3	235.7	239.1
middle lobe of lung	162.4	197.0	231.2	212.3	235.7	239.1
upper lobe of lung	162.3	197.0	231.2	212.3	235.7	239.1
brow	173.3	198.2	232.3	216.3	238.2	239.2
buccal (cavity)	145.9	198.89	230.0	210.4	235.1	239.0
commissure	145.0	198.89	230.0	210.4	235.1	239.0
groove (lower) (upper)	145.1	198.89	230.0	210.4	235.1	239.0
mucosa	145.0	198.89	230.0	210.4	235.1	239.0
sulcus (lower) (upper)	145.1	198.89	230.0	210.4	235.1	239.0
bulbourethral gland	189.3	198.1	233.9	223.81	236.99	239.5
bursa - *see* Neoplasm, connective tissue						
buttock NEC*	195.3	198.89	232.5	229.8	238.8	239.89◀▥
calf*	195.5	198.89	232.7	229.8	238.8	239.89◀▥
calvarium	170.0	198.5	—	213.0	238.0	239.2
calyx, renal	189.1	198.0	233.9	223.1	236.91	239.5

◀ New   ◀▥ Revised   ~~deleted~~ Deleted   ● Use Additional Digit(s)   ▨ Omit code

	Malignant					
	Primary	Secondary	Ca in situ	Benign	Uncertain Behavior	Unspecified
Neoplasm *(Continued)*						
canal						
anal	154.2	197.5	230.5	211.4	235.5	239.0
auditory (external)	173.2	198.2	232.2	216.2	238.2	239.2
auricular (external)	173.2	198.2	232.2	216.2	238.2	239.2
canaliculi, biliary (biliferi) (intrahepatic)	155.1	197.8	230.8	211.5	235.3	239.0
canthus (eye) (inner) (outer)	173.1	198.2	232.1	216.1	238.2	239.2
capillary - *see* Neoplasm, connective tissue						
caput coli	153.4	197.5	230.3	211.3	235.2	239.0
cardia (gastric)	151.0	197.8	230.2	211.1	235.2	239.0
cardiac orifice (stomach)	151.0	197.8	230.2	211.1	235.2	239.0
cardio-esophageal junction	151.0	197.8	230.2	211.1	235.2	239.0
cardio-esophagus	151.0	197.8	230.2	211.1	235.2	239.0
carina (bronchus) (trachea)	162.2	197.0	231.2	212.3	235.7	239.1
carotid (artery)	171.0	198.89	—	215.0	238.1	239.2
body	194.5	198.89	—	227.5	237.3	239.7
carpus (any bone)	170.5	198.5	—	213.5	238.0	239.2
cartilage (articular) (joint) NEC - *see also* Neoplasm, bone	170.9	198.5	—	213.9	238.0	239.2
arytenoid	161.3	197.3	231.0	212.1	235.6	239.1
auricular	171.0	198.89	—	215.0	238.1	239.2
bronchi	162.2	197.3	—	212.3	235.7	239.1
connective tissue - *see* Neoplasm, connective tissue						
costal	170.3	198.5	—	213.3	238.0	239.2
cricoid	161.3	197.3	231.0	212.1	235.6	239.1
cuneiform	161.3	197.3	231.0	212.1	235.6	239.1
ear (external)	171.0	198.89	—	215.0	238.1	239.2
ensiform	170.3	198.5	—	213.3	238.0	239.2
epiglottis	161.1	197.3	231.0	212.1	235.6	239.1
anterior surface	146.4	198.89	230.0	210.6	235.1	239.0
eyelid	171.0	198.89	—	215.0	238.1	239.2
intervertebral	170.2	198.5	—	213.2	238.0	239.2
larynx, laryngeal	161.3	197.3	231.0	212.1	235.6	239.1
nose, nasal	160.0	197.3	231.8	212.0	235.9	239.1
pinna	171.0	198.89	—	215.0	238.1	239.2
rib	170.3	198.5	—	213.3	238.0	239.2
semilunar (knee)	170.7	198.5	—	213.7	238.0	239.2
thyroid	161.3	197.3	231.0	212.1	235.6	239.1
trachea	162.0	197.3	231.1	212.2	235.7	239.1
cauda equina	192.2	198.3	—	225.3	237.5	239.7

	Malignant					
	Primary	Secondary	Ca in situ	Benign	Uncertain Behavior	Unspecified
Neoplasm *(Continued)*						
cavity						
buccal	145.9	198.89	230.0	210.4	235.1	239.0
nasal	160.0	197.3	231.8	212.0	235.9	239.1
oral	145.9	198.89	230.0	210.4	235.1	239.0
peritoneal	158.9	197.6	—	211.8	235.4	239.0
tympanic	160.1	197.3	231.8	212.0	235.9	239.1
cecum	153.4	197.5	230.3	211.3	235.2	239.0
central						
nervous system - *see* Neoplasm, nervous system						
white matter	191.0	198.3	—	225.0	237.5	239.6
cerebellopontine (angle)	191.6	198.3	—	225.0	237.5	239.6
cerebellum, cerebellar	191.6	198.3	—	225.0	237.5	239.6
cerebrum, cerebral (cortex) (hemisphere) (white matter)	191.0	198.3	—	225.0	237.5	239.6
meninges	192.1	198.4	—	225.2	237.6	239.7
peduncle	191.7	198.3	—	225.0	237.5	239.6
ventricle (any)	191.5	198.3	—	225.0	237.5	239.6
cervical region	195.0	198.89	234.8	229.8	238.8	239.89◄
cervix (cervical) (uteri) (uterus)	180.9	198.82	233.1	219.0	236.0	239.5
canal	180.0	198.82	233.1	219.0	236.0	239.5
contiguous sites	180.8	—	—	—	—	—
endocervix (canal) (gland)	180.0	198.82	233.1	219.0	236.0	239.5
exocervix	180.1	198.82	233.1	219.0	236.0	239.5
external os	180.1	198.82	233.1	219.0	236.0	239.5
nabothian gland	180.0	198.82	233.1	219.0	236.0	239.5
squamocolumnar junction	180.8	198.82	233.1	219.0	236.0	239.5
stump	180.8	198.82	233.1	219.0	236.0	239.5
cheek	195.0	198.89	234.8	229.8	238.8	239.89◄
external	173.3	198.2	232.3	216.3	238.2	239.2
inner aspect	145.0	198.89	230.0	210.4	235.1	239.0
internal	145.0	198.89	230.0	210.4	235.1	239.0
mucosa	145.0	198.89	230.0	210.4	235.1	239.0
chest (wall) NEC	195.1	198.89	234.8	229.8	238.8	239.89◄
chiasma opticum	192.0	198.4	—	225.1	237.9	239.7
chin	173.3	198.2	232.3	216.3	238.2	239.2
choana	147.3	198.89	230.0	210.7	235.1	239.0
cholangiole	155.1	197.8	230.8	211.5	235.3	239.0
choledochal duct	156.1	197.8	230.8	211.5	235.3	239.0
choroid	190.6	198.4	234.0	224.6	238.8	239.81◄
plexus	191.5	198.3	—	225.0	237.5	239.6
ciliary body	190.0	198.4	234.0	224.0	238.8	239.89◄

◄ New   ◄▥ Revised   ~~deleted~~ Deleted   ● Use Additional Digit(s)   Omit code

	Malignant			Benign	Uncertain Behavior	Unspecified
	Primary	Secondary	Ca in situ			
Neoplasm *(Continued)*						
clavicle	170.3	198.5	—	213.3	238.0	239.2
clitoris	184.3	198.82	233.32	221.2	236.3	239.5
clivus	170.0	198.5	—	213.0	238.0	239.2
cloacogenic zone	154.8	197.5	230.7	211.4	235.5	239.0
coccygeal						
body or glomus	194.6	198.89	—	227.6	237.3	239.7
vertebra	170.6	198.5	—	213.6	238.0	239.2
coccyx	170.6	198.5	—	213.6	238.0	239.2
colon - *see also* Neoplasm, intestine, large and rectum	154.0	197.5	230.4	211.4	235.2	239.0
column, spinal - *see* Neoplasm, spine						
columnella	173.3	198.2	232.3	216.3	238.2	239.2
commissure						
labial, lip	140.6	198.89	230.0	210.4	235.1	239.0
laryngeal	161.0	197.3	231.0	212.1	235.6	239.1
common (bile) duct	156.1	197.8	230.8	211.5	235.3	239.0
concha	173.2	198.2	232.2	216.2	238.2	239.2
nose	160.0	197.3	231.8	212.0	235.9	239.1
conjunctiva	190.3	198.4	234.0	224.3	238.8	239.89◀
connective tissue NEC	171.9	198.89	—	215.9	238.1	239.2

Note — For neoplasms of connective tissue (blood vessel, bursa, fascia, ligament, muscle, peripheral nerves, sympathetic and parasympathetic nerves and ganglia, synovia, tendon, etc.) or of morphological types that indicate connective tissue, code according to the list under "Neoplasm, connective tissue;" for sites that do not appear in this list, code to neoplasm of that site; e.g.,

> *liposarcoma, shoulder 171.2*
> *leiomyosarcoma, stomach 151.9*
> *neurofibroma, chest wall 215.4*

Morphological types that indicate connective tissue appear in their proper place in the alphabetic index with the instruction "see Neoplasm, connective tissue ...."

	Primary	Secondary	Ca in situ	Benign	Uncertain Behavior	Unspecified
abdomen	171.5	198.89	—	215.5	238.1	239.2
abdominal wall	171.5	198.89	—	215.5	238.1	239.2
ankle	171.3	198.89	—	215.3	238.1	239.2
antecubital fossa or space	171.2	198.89	—	215.2	238.1	239.2
arm	171.2	198.89	—	215.2	238.1	239.2
auricle (ear)	171.0	198.89	—	215.0	238.1	239.2
axilla	171.4	198.89	—	215.4	238.1	239.2
back	171.7	198.89	—	215.7	238.1	239.2
breast (female) *(see also* Neoplasm, breast)	174.9	198.81	233.0	217	238.3	239.3
male	175.9	198.81	233.0	217	238.3	239.3
buttock	171.6	198.89	—	215.6	238.1	239.2
calf	171.3	198.89	—	215.3	238.1	239.2
cervical region	171.0	198.89	—	215.0	238.1	239.2
cheek	171.0	198.89	—	215.0	238.1	239.2

	Malignant					
	Primary	Secondary	Ca in situ	Benign	Uncertain Behavior	Unspecified
Neoplasm *(Continued)*						
connective tissue NEC *(Continued)*						
chest (wall)	171.4	198.89	—	215.4	238.1	239.2
chin	171.0	198.89	—	215.0	238.1	239.2
contiguous sites	171.8	—	—	—	—	—
diaphragm	171.4	198.89	—	215.4	238.1	239.2
ear (external)	171.0	198.89	—	215.0	238.1	239.2
elbow	171.2	198.89	—	215.2	238.1	239.2
extrarectal	171.6	198.89	—	215.6	238.1	239.2
extremity	171.8	198.89	—	215.8	238.1	239.2
lower	171.3	198.89	—	215.3	238.1	239.2
upper	171.2	198.89	—	215.2	238.1	239.2
eyelid	171.0	198.89	—	215.0	238.1	239.2
face	171.0	198.89	—	215.0	238.1	239.2
finger	171.2	198.89	—	215.2	238.1	239.2
flank	171.7	198.89	—	215.7	238.1	239.2
foot	171.3	198.89	—	215.3	238.1	239.2
forearm	171.2	198.89	—	215.2	238.1	239.2
forehead	171.0	198.89	—	215.0	238.1	239.2
gastric	171.5	198.89	—	215.5	238.1	—
gastrointestinal	171.5	198.89	—	215.5	238.1	—
gluteal region	171.6	198.89	—	215.6	238.1	239.2
great vessels NEC	171.4	198.89	—	215.4	238.1	239.2
groin	171.6	198.89	—	215.6	238.1	239.2
hand	171.2	198.89	—	215.2	238.1	239.2
head	171.0	198.89	—	215.0	238.1	239.2
heel	171.3	198.89	—	215.3	238.1	239.2
hip	171.3	198.89	—	215.3	238.1	239.2
hypochondrium	171.5	198.89	—	215.5	238.1	239.2
iliopsoas muscle	171.6	198.89	—	215.5	238.1	239.2
infraclavicular region	171.4	198.89	—	215.4	238.1	239.2
inguinal (canal) (region)	171.6	198.89	—	215.6	238.1	239.2
intestine	171.5	198.89	—	215.5	238.1	—
intrathoracic	171.4	198.89	—	215.4	238.1	239.2
ischorectal fossa	171.6	198.89	—	215.6	238.1	239.2
jaw	143.9	198.89	230.0	210.4	235.1	239.0
knee	171.3	198.89	—	215.3	238.1	239.2
leg	171.3	198.89	—	215.3	238.1	239.2
limb NEC	171.9	198.89	—	215.8	238.1	239.2
lower	171.3	198.89	—	215.3	238.1	239.2
upper	171.2	198.89	—	215.2	238.1	239.2

◄ New   ◄▪▪ Revised   ~~deleted~~ Deleted   ● Use Additional Digit(s)   ▨ Omit code

	Malignant					
	Primary	Secondary	Ca in situ	Benign	Uncertain Behavior	Unspecified
Neoplasm *(Continued)*						
connective tissue NEC *(Continued)*						
nates	171.6	198.89	—	215.6	238.1	239.2
neck	171.0	198.89	—	215.0	238.1	239.2
orbit	190.1	198.4	234.0	224.1	238.8	239.89◀
pararectal	171.6	198.89	—	215.6	238.1	239.2
para-urethral	171.6	198.89	—	215.6	238.1	239.2
paravaginal	171.6	198.89	—	215.6	238.1	239.2
pelvis (floor)	171.6	198.89	—	215.6	238.1	239.2
pelvo-abdominal	171.8	198.89	—	215.8	238.1	239.2
perineum	171.6	198.89	—	215.6	238.1	239.2
perirectal (tissue)	171.6	198.89	—	215.6	238.1	239.2
periurethral (tissue)	171.6	198.89	—	215.6	238.1	239.2
popliteal fossa or space	171.3	198.89	—	215.3	238.1	239.2
presacral	171.6	198.89	—	215.6	238.1	239.2
psoas muscle	171.5	198.89	—	215.5	238.1	239.2
pterygoid fossa	171.0	198.89	—	215.0	238.1	239.2
rectovaginal septum or wall	171.6	198.89	—	215.6	238.1	239.2
rectovesical	171.6	198.89	—	215.6	238.1	239.2
retroperitoneum	158.0	197.6	—	211.8	235.4	239.0
sacrococcygeal region	171.6	198.89	—	215.6	238.1	239.2
scalp	171.0	198.89	—	215.0	238.1	239.2
scapular region	171.4	198.89	—	215.4	238.1	239.2
shoulder	171.2	198.89	—	215.2	238.1	239.2
skin (dermis) NEC	173.9	198.2	232.9	216.9	238.2	239.2
stomach	171.5	198.89	—	215.5	238.1	—
submental	171.0	198.89	—	215.0	238.1	239.2
supraclavicular region	171.0	198.89	—	215.0	238.1	239.2
temple	171.0	198.89	—	215.0	238.1	239.2
temporal region	171.0	198.89	—	215.0	238.1	239.2
thigh	171.3	198.89	—	215.3	238.1	239.2
thoracic (duct) (wall)	171.4	198.89	—	215.4	238.1	239.2
thorax	171.4	198.89	—	215.4	238.1	239.2
thumb	171.2	198.89	—	215.2	238.1	239.2
toe	171.3	198.89	—	215.3	238.1	239.2
trunk	171.7	198.89	—	215.7	238.1	239.2
umbilicus	171.5	198.89	—	215.5	238.1	239.2
vesicorectal	171.6	198.89	—	215.6	238.1	239.2
wrist	171.2	198.89	—	215.2	238.1	239.2
conus medullaris	192.2	198.3	—	225.3	237.5	239.7

	Malignant					
	Primary	Secondary	Ca in situ	Benign	Uncertain Behavior	Unspecified
Neoplasm *(Continued)*						
cord (true) (vocal)	161.0	197.3	231.0	212.1	235.6	239.1
false	161.1	197.3	231.0	212.1	235.6	239.1
spermatic	187.6	198.82	233.6	222.8	236.6	239.5
spinal (cervical) (lumbar) (thoracic)	192.2	198.3	—	225.3	237.5	239.7
cornea (limbus)	190.4	198.4	234.0	224.4	238.8	239.89◀
corpus						
albicans	183.0	198.6	233.39	220	236.2	239.5
callosum, brain	191.8	198.3	—	225.0	237.5	239.6
cavernosum	187.3	198.82	233.5	222.1	236.6	239.5
gastric	151.4	197.8	230.2	211.1	235.2	239.0
penis	187.3	198.82	233.5	222.1	236.6	239.5
striatum, cerebrum	191.0	198.3	—	225.0	237.5	239.6
uteri	182.0	198.82	233.2	219.1	236.0	239.5
isthmus	182.1	198.82	233.2	219.1	236.0	239.5
cortex						
adrenal	194.0	198.7	234.8	227.0	237.2	239.7
cerebral	191.0	198.3	—	225.0	237.5	239.6
costal cartilage	170.3	198.5	—	213.3	238.0	239.2
costovertebral joint	170.3	198.5	—	213.3	238.0	239.2
Cowper's gland	189.3	198.1	233.9	223.81	236.99	239.5
cranial (fossa, any)	191.9	198.3	—	225.0	237.5	239.6
meninges	192.1	198.4	—	225.2	237.6	239.7
nerve (any)	192.0	198.4	—	225.1	237.9	239.7
craniobuccal pouch	194.3	198.89	234.8	227.3	237.0	239.7
craniopharyngeal (duct) (pouch)	194.3	198.89	234.8	227.3	237.0	239.7
cricoid	148.0	198.89	230.0	210.8	235.1	239.0
cartilage	161.3	197.3	231.0	212.1	235.6	239.1
cricopharynx	148.0	198.89	230.0	210.8	235.1	239.0
crypt of Morgagni	154.8	197.5	230.7	211.4	235.2	239.0
crystalline lens	190.0	198.4	234.0	224.0	238.8	239.89◀
cul-de-sac (Douglas')	158.8	197.6	—	211.8	235.4	239.0
cuneiform cartilage	161.3	197.3	231.0	212.1	235.6	239.1
cutaneous - *see* Neoplasm, skin						
cutis - *see* Neoplasm, skin						
cystic (bile) duct (common)	156.1	197.8	230.8	211.5	235.3	239.0
dermis - *see* Neoplasm, skin						
diaphragm	171.4	198.89	—	215.4	238.1	239.2
digestive organs, system, tube, or tract NEC	159.9	197.8	230.9	211.9	235.5	239.0
contiguous sites with peritoneum	159.8	—	—	—	—	—
disc, intervertebral	170.2	198.5	—	213.2	238.0	239.2

◀ New   ◀▥ Revised   ~~deleted~~ Deleted   ● Use Additional Digit(s)   ▭ Omit code

	Malignant					
	Primary	Secondary	Ca in situ	Benign	Uncertain Behavior	Unspecified
Neoplasm *(Continued)*						
disease, generalized	199.0	199.0	234.9	229.9	238.9	199.0
disseminated	199.0	199.0	234.9	229.9	238.9	199.0
Douglas' cul-de-sac or pouch	158.8	197.6	—	211.8	235.4	239.0
duodenojejunal junction	152.8	197.4	230.7	211.2	235.2	239.0
duodenum	152.0	197.4	230.7	211.2	235.2	239.0
dura (cranial) (mater)	192.1	198.4	—	225.2	237.6	239.7
cerebral	192.1	198.4	—	225.2	237.6	239.7
spinal	192.3	198.4	—	225.4	237.6	239.7
ear (external)	173.2	198.2	232.2	216.2	238.2	239.2
auricle or auris	173.2	198.2	232.2	216.2	238.2	239.2
canal, external	173.2	198.2	232.2	216.2	238.2	239.2
cartilage	171.0	198.89	—	215.0	238.1	239.2
external meatus	173.2	198.2	232.2	216.2	238.2	239.2
inner	160.1	197.3	231.8	212.0	235.9	239.89◄
lobule	173.2	198.2	232.2	216.2	238.2	239.2
middle	160.1	197.3	231.8	212.0	235.9	239.89◄
contiguous sites with accessory sinuses or nasal cavities	160.8	—	—	—	—	—
skin	173.2	198.2	232.2	216.2	238.2	239.2
earlobe	173.2	198.2	232.2	216.2	238.2	239.2
ejaculatory duct	187.8	198.82	233.6	222.8	236.6	239.5
elbow NEC*	195.4	198.89	232.6	229.8	238.8	239.89◄
endocardium	164.1	198.89	—	212.7	238.8	239.89◄
endocervix (canal) (gland)	180.0	198.82	233.1	219.0	236.0	239.5
endocrine gland NEC	194.9	198.89	—	227.9	237.4	239.7
pluriglandular NEC	194.8	198.89	234.8	227.8	237.4	239.7
endometrium (gland) (stroma)	182.0	198.82	233.2	219.1	236.0	239.5
ensiform cartilage	170.3	198.5	—	213.3	238.0	239.2
enteric - *see* Neoplasm, intestine						
ependyma (brain)	191.5	198.3	—	225.0	237.5	239.6
epicardium	164.1	198.89	—	212.7	238.8	239.89◄
epididymis	187.5	198.82	233.6	222.3	236.6	239.5
epidural	192.9	198.4	—	225.9	237.9	239.7
epiglottis	161.1	197.3	231.0	212.1	235.6	239.1
anterior aspect or surface	146.4	198.89	230.0	210.6	235.1	239.0
cartilage	161.3	197.3	231.0	212.1	235.6	239.1
free border (margin)	146.4	198.89	230.0	210.6	235.1	239.0
junctional region	146.5	198.89	230.0	210.6	235.1	239.0
posterior (laryngeal) surface	161.1	197.3	231.0	212.1	235.6	239.1
suprahyoid portion	161.1	197.3	231.0	212.1	235.6	239.1
esophagogastric junction	151.0	197.8	230.2	211.1	235.2	239.0

◄ New ◄▥ Revised ~~deleted~~ Deleted ● Use Additional Digit(s) ▨ Omit code

	Malignant					
	Primary	Secondary	Ca in situ	Benign	Uncertain Behavior	Unspecified
Neoplasm *(Continued)*						
esophagus	150.9	197.8	230.1	211.0	235.5	239.0
abdominal	150.2	197.8	230.1	211.0	235.5	239.0
cervical	150.0	197.8	230.1	211.0	235.5	239.0
contiguous sites	150.8	—	—	—	—	—
distal (third)	150.5	197.8	230.1	211.0	235.5	239.0
lower (third)	150.5	197.8	230.1	211.0	235.5	239.0
middle (third)	150.4	197.8	230.1	211.0	235.5	239.0
proximal (third)	150.3	197.8	230.1	211.0	235.5	239.0
specified part NEC	150.8	197.8	230.1	211.0	235.5	239.0
thoracic	150.1	197.8	230.1	211.0	235.5	239.0
upper (third)	150.3	197.8	230.1	211.0	235.5	239.0
ethmoid (sinus)	160.3	197.3	231.8	212.0	235.9	239.1
bone or labyrinth	170.0	198.5	—	213.0	238.0	239.2
Eustachian tube	160.1	197.3	231.8	212.0	235.9	239.1
exocervix	180.1	198.82	233.1	219.0	236.0	239.5
external						
meatus (ear)	173.2	198.2	232.2	216.2	238.2	239.2
os, cervix uteri	180.1	198.82	233.1	219.0	236.0	239.5
extradural	192.9	198.4	—	225.9	237.9	239.7
extrahepatic (bile) duct	156.1	197.8	230.8	211.5	235.3	239.0
contiguous sites with gallbladder	156.8	—	—	—	—	—
extraocular muscle	190.1	198.4	234.0	224.1	238.8	239.89◀▥
extrarectal	195.3	198.89	234.8	229.8	238.8	239.89◀▥
extremity*	195.8	198.89	232.8	229.8	238.8	239.89◀▥
lower*	195.5	198.89	232.7	229.8	238.8	239.89◀▥
upper*	195.4	198.89	232.6	229.8	238.8	239.89◀▥
eye NEC	190.9	198.4	234.0	224.9	238.8	239.89◀▥
contiguous sites	190.8	—	—	—	—	—
specified sites NEC	190.8	198.4	234.0	224.8	238.8	239.89◀▥
eyeball	190.0	198.4	234.0	224.0	238.8	239.89◀▥
eyebrow	173.3	198.2	232.3	216.3	238.2	239.2
eyelid (lower) (skin) (upper)	173.1	198.2	232.1	216.1	238.2	239.2
cartilage	171.0	198.89	—	215.0	238.1	239.2
face NEC*	195.0	198.89	232.3	229.8	238.8	239.89◀▥
Fallopian tube (accessory)	183.2	198.82	233.39	221.0	236.3	239.5
falx (cerebella) (cerebri)	192.1	198.4	—	225.2	237.6	239.7
fascia - *see also* Neoplasm, connective tissue						
palmar	171.2	198.89	—	215.2	238.1	239.2
plantar	171.3	198.89	—	215.3	238.1	239.2
fatty tissue - *see* Neoplasm, connective tissue						

◀ New ◀▥ Revised ~~deleted~~ Deleted ● Use Additional Digit(s) ▨ Omit code

| | Malignant | | | | | |
	Primary	Secondary	Ca in situ	Benign	Uncertain Behavior	Unspecified
Neoplasm *(Continued)*						
fauces, faucial NEC	146.9	198.89	230.0	210.6	235.1	239.0
pillars	146.2	198.89	230.0	210.6	235.1	239.0
tonsil	146.0	198.89	230.0	210.5	235.1	239.0
femur (any part)	170.7	198.5	—	213.7	238.0	239.2
fetal membrane	181	198.82	233.2	219.8	236.1	239.5
fibrous tissue - *see* Neoplasm, connective tissue						
fibula (any part)	170.7	198.5	—	213.7	238.0	239.2
filum terminale	192.2	198.3	—	225.3	237.5	239.7
finger NEC*	195.4	198.89	232.6	229.8	238.8	239.89◀
flank NEC*	195.8	198.89	232.5	229.8	238.8	239.89◀
follicle, nabothian	180.0	198.82	233.1	219.0	236.0	239.5
foot NEC*	195.5	198.89	232.7	229.8	238.8	239.89◀
forearm NEC*	195.4	198.89	232.6	229.8	238.8	239.89◀
forehead (skin)	173.3	198.2	232.3	216.3	238.2	239.2
foreskin	187.1	198.82	233.5	222.1	236.6	239.5
fornix						
pharyngeal	147.3	198.89	230.0	210.7	235.1	239.0
vagina	184.0	198.82	233.31	221.1	236.3	239.5
fossa (of)						
anterior (cranial)	191.9	198.3	—	225.0	237.5	239.6
cranial	191.9	198.3	—	225.0	237.5	239.6
ischiorectal	195.3	198.89	234.8	229.8	238.8	239.89◀
middle (cranial)	191.9	198.3	—	225.0	237.5	239.6
pituitary	194.3	198.89	234.8	227.3	237.0	239.7
posterior (cranial)	191.9	198.3	—	225.0	237.5	239.6
pterygoid	171.0	198.89	—	215.0	238.1	239.2
pyriform	148.1	198.89	230.0	210.8	235.1	239.0
Rosenmüller	147.2	198.89	230.0	210.7	235.1	239.0
tonsillar	146.1	198.89	230.0	210.6	235.1	239.0
fourchette	184.4	198.82	233.32	221.2	236.3	239.5
frenulum						
labii - *see* Neoplasm, lip, internal						
linguae	141.3	198.89	230.0	210.1	235.1	239.0
frontal						
bone	170.0	198.5	—	213.0	238.0	239.2
lobe, brain	191.1	198.3	—	225.0	237.5	239.6
meninges	192.1	198.4	—	225.2	237.6	239.7
pole	191.1	198.3	—	225.0	237.5	239.6
sinus	160.4	197.3	231.8	212.0	235.9	239.1

	Malignant					
	Primary	Secondary	Ca in situ	Benign	Uncertain Behavior	Unspecified
Neoplasm (Continued)						
fundus						
stomach	151.3	197.8	230.2	211.1	235.2	239.0
uterus	182.0	198.82	233.2	219.1	236.0	239.5
gall duct (extrahepatic)	156.1	197.8	230.8	211.5	235.3	239.0
intrahepatic	155.1	197.8	230.8	211.5	235.3	239.0
gallbladder	156.0	197.8	230.8	211.5	235.3	239.0
contiguous sites with extrahepatic bile ducts	156.8	—	—	—	—	—
ganglia (see also Neoplasm, connective tissue)	171.9	198.89	—	215.9	238.1	239.2
basal	191.0	198.3	—	225.0	237.5	239.6
ganglion (see also Neoplasm, connective tissue)	171.9	198.89	—	215.9	238.1	239.2
cranial nerve	192.0	198.4	—	225.1	237.9	239.7
Gartner's duct	184.0	198.82	233.31	221.1	236.3	239.5
gastric - see Neoplasm, stomach						
gastrocolic	159.8	197.8	230.9	211.9	235.5	239.0
gastroesophageal junction	151.0	197.8	230.2	211.1	235.2	239.0
gastrointestinal (tract) NEC	159.9	197.8	230.9	211.9	235.5	239.0
generalized	199.0	199.0	234.9	229.9	238.9	199.0
genital organ or tract						
female NEC	184.9	198.82	233.39	221.9	236.3	239.5
contiguous sites	184.8					
specified site NEC	184.8	198.82	233.39	221.8	236.3	239.5
male NEC	187.9	198.82	233.6	222.9	236.6	239.5
contiguous sites	187.8	—	—	—	—	—
specified site NEC	187.8	198.82	233.6	222.8	236.6	239.5
genitourinary tract						
female	184.9	198.82	233.39	221.9	236.3	239.5
male	187.9	198.82	233.6	222.9	236.6	239.5
gingiva (alveolar) (marginal)	143.9	198.89	230.0	210.4	235.1	239.0
lower	143.1	198.89	230.0	210.4	235.1	239.0
mandibular	143.1	198.89	230.0	210.4	235.1	239.0
maxillary	143.0	198.89	230.0	210.4	235.1	239.0
upper	143.0	198.89	230.0	210.4	235.1	239.0
gland, glandular (lymphatic) (system) - see also Neoplasm, lymph gland						
endocrine NEC	194.9	198.89	—	227.9	237.4	239.7
salivary - see Neoplasm, salivary, gland						
glans penis	187.2	198.82	233.5	222.1	236.6	239.5
globus pallidus	191.0	198.3	—	225.0	237.5	239.6
glomus						
coccygeal	194.6	198.89	—	227.6	237.3	239.7
jugularis	194.6	198.89	—	227.6	237.3	239.7

◀ New   ◀▥ Revised   ~~deleted~~ Deleted   ● Use Additional Digit(s)   ▨ Omit code

	Malignant					
	Primary	Secondary	Ca in situ	Benign	Uncertain Behavior	Unspecified
Neoplasm *(Continued)*						
glosso-epiglottic fold(s)	146.4	198.89	230.0	210.6	235.1	239.0
glossopalatine fold	146.2	198.89	230.0	210.6	235.1	239.0
glossopharyngeal sulcus	146.1	198.89	230.0	210.6	235.1	239.0
glottis	161.0	197.3	231.0	212.1	235.6	239.1
gluteal region*	195.3	198.89	232.5	229.8	238.8	239.89◀
great vessels NEC	171.4	198.89	—	215.4	238.1	239.2
groin NEC	195.3	198.89	232.5	229.8	238.8	239.89◀
gum	143.9	198.89	230.0	210.4	235.1	239.0
contiguous sites	143.8	—	—	—	—	—
lower	143.1	198.89	230.0	210.4	235.1	239.0
upper	143.0	198.89	230.0	210.4	235.1	239.0
hand NEC*	195.4	198.89	232.6	229.8	238.8	239.89◀
head NEC*	195.0	198.89	232.4	229.8	238.8	239.89◀
heart	164.1	198.89	—	212.7	238.8	239.89◀
contiguous sites with mediastinum or thymus	164.8	—	—	—	—	—
heel NEC*	195.5	198.89	232.7	229.8	238.8	239.89◀
helix	173.2	198.2	232.2	216.2	238.2	239.2
hematopoietic, hemopoietic tissue NEC	202.8●	198.89	—	—	—	238.79
hemisphere, cerebral	191.0	198.3	—	225.0	237.5	239.6
hemorrhoidal zone	154.2	197.5	230.5	211.4	235.5	239.0
hepatic	155.2	197.7	230.8	211.5	235.3	239.0
duct (bile)	156.1	197.8	230.8	211.5	235.3	239.0
flexure (colon)	153.0	197.5	230.3	211.3	235.2	239.0
primary	155.0	—	—	—	—	—
hilus of lung	162.2	197.0	231.2	212.3	235.7	239.1
hip NEC*	195.5	198.89	232.7	229.8	238.8	239.89◀
hippocampus, brain	191.2	198.3	—	225.0	237.5	239.6
humerus (any part)	170.4	198.5	—	213.4	238.0	239.2
hymen	184.0	198.82	233.31	221.1	236.3	239.5
hypopharynx, hypopharyngeal NEC	148.9	198.89	230.0	210.8	235.1	239.0
contiguous sites	148.8	—	—	—	—	—
postcricoid region	148.0	198.89	230.0	210.8	235.1	239.0
posterior wall	148.3	198.89	230.0	210.8	235.1	239.0
pyriform fossa (sinus)	148.1	198.89	230.0	210.8	235.1	239.0
specified site NEC	148.8	198.89	230.0	210.8	235.1	239.0
wall	148.9	198.89	230.0	210.8	235.1	239.0
posterior	148.3	198.89	230.0	210.8	235.1	239.0
hypophysis	194.3	198.89	234.8	227.3	237.0	239.7
hypothalamus	191.0	198.3	—	225.0	237.5	239.6
ileocecum, ileocecal (coil) (junction) (valve)	153.4	197.5	230.3	211.3	235.2	239.0

	Malignant					
	Primary	Secondary	Ca in situ	Benign	Uncertain Behavior	Unspecified
Neoplasm *(Continued)*						
ileum	152.2	197.4	230.7	211.2	235.2	239.0
ilium	170.6	198.5	—	213.6	238.0	239.2
immunoproliferative NEC	203.8●	—	—	—	—	—
infraclavicular (region)*	195.1	198.89	232.5	229.8	238.8	239.89◄
inguinal (region)*	195.3	198.89	232.5	229.8	238.8	239.89◄
insula	191.0	198.3	—	225.0	237.5	239.6
insular tissue (pancreas)	157.4	197.8	230.9	211.7	235.5	239.0
brain	191.0	198.3	—	225.0	237.5	239.6
interarytenoid fold	148.2	198.89	230.0	210.8	235.1	239.0
hypopharyngeal aspect	148.2	198.89	230.0	210.8	235.1	239.0
laryngeal aspect	161.1	197.3	231.0	212.1	235.6	239.1
marginal zone	148.2	198.89	230.0	210.8	235.1	239.0
interdental papillae	143.9	198.89	230.0	210.4	235.1	239.0
lower	143.1	198.89	230.0	210.4	235.1	239.0
upper	143.0	198.89	230.0	210.4	235.1	239.0
internal						
capsule	191.0	198.3	—	225.0	237.5	239.6
os (cervix)	180.0	198.82	233.1	219.0	236.0	239.5
intervertebral cartilage or disc	170.2	198.5	—	213.2	238.0	239.2
intestine, intestinal	159.0	197.8	230.7	211.9	235.2	239.0
large	153.9	197.5	230.3	211.3	235.2	239.0
appendix	153.5	197.5	230.3	211.3	235.2	239.0
caput coli	153.4	197.5	230.3	211.3	235.2	239.0
cecum	153.4	197.5	230.3	211.3	235.2	239.0
colon	153.9	197.5	230.3	211.3	235.2	239.0
and rectum	154.0	197.5	230.4	211.4	235.2	239.0
ascending	153.6	197.5	230.3	211.3	235.2	239.0
caput	153.4	197.5	230.3	211.3	235.2	239.0
contiguous sites	153.8	—	—	—	—	—
descending	153.2	197.5	230.3	211.3	235.2	239.0
distal	153.2	197.5	230.3	211.3	235.2	239.0
left	153.2	197.5	230.3	211.3	235.2	239.0
pelvic	153.3	197.5	230.3	211.3	235.2	239.0
right	153.6	197.5	230.3	211.3	235.2	239.0
sigmoid (flexure)	153.3	197.5	230.3	211.3	235.2	239.0
transverse	153.1	197.5	230.3	211.3	235.2	239.0
contiguous sites	153.8	—	—	—	—	—
hepatic flexure	153.0	197.5	230.3	211.3	235.2	239.0
ileocecum, ileocecal (coil) (valve)	153.4	197.5	230.3	211.3	235.2	239.0
sigmoid flexure (lower) (upper)	153.3	197.5	230.3	211.3	235.2	239.0
splenic flexure	153.7	197.5	230.3	211.3	235.2	239.0

◄ New   ◄▥ Revised   deleted Deleted   ● Use Additional Digit(s)   ▨ Omit code

| | Malignant | | | | | |
	Primary	Secondary	Ca in situ	Benign	Uncertain Behavior	Unspecified
Neoplasm *(Continued)*						
intestine, intestinal *(Continued)*						
small	152.9	197.4	230.7	211.2	235.2	239.0
contiguous sites	152.8	—	—	—	—	—
duodenum	152.0	197.4	230.7	211.2	235.2	239.0
ileum	152.2	197.4	230.7	211.2	235.2	239.0
jejunum	152.1	197.4	230.7	211.2	235.2	239.0
tract NEC	159.0	197.8	230.7	211.9	235.2	239.0
intra-abdominal	195.2	198.89	234.8	229.8	238.8	239.89◄
intracranial NEC	191.9	198.3	—	225.0	237.5	239.6
intrahepatic (bile) duct	155.1	197.8	230.8	211.5	235.3	239.0
intraocular	190.0	198.4	234.0	224.0	238.8	239.89◄
intraorbital	190.1	198.4	234.0	224.1	238.8	239.89◄
intrasellar	194.3	198.89	234.8	227.3	237.0	239.7
intrathoracic (cavity) (organs NEC)	195.1	198.89	234.8	229.8	238.8	239.89◄
contiguous sites with respiratory organs	165.8	—	—	—	—	—
iris	190.0	198.4	234.0	224.0	238.8	239.89◄
ischiorectal (fossa)	195.3	198.89	234.8	229.8	238.8	239.89◄
ischium	170.6	198.5	—	213.6	238.0	239.2
island of Reil	191.0	198.3	—	225.0	237.5	239.6
islands or islets of Langerhans	157.4	197.8	230.9	211.7	235.5	239.0
isthmus uteri	182.1	198.82	233.2	219.1	236.0	239.5
jaw	195.0	198.89	234.8	229.8	238.8	239.89◄
bone	170.1	198.5	—	213.1	238.0	239.2
carcinoma	143.9	—	—	—	—	—
lower	143.1	—	—	—	—	—
upper	143.0	—	—	—	—	—
lower	170.1	198.5	—	213.1	238.0	239.2
upper	170.0	198.5	—	213.0	238.0	239.2
carcinoma (any type) (lower) (upper)	195.0	—	—	—	—	—
skin	173.3	198.2	232.3	216.3	238.2	239.2
soft tissues	143.9	198.89	230.0	210.4	235.1	239.0
lower	143.1	198.89	230.0	210.4	235.1	239.0
upper	143.0	198.89	230.0	210.4	235.1	239.0
jejunum	152.1	197.4	230.7	211.2	235.2	239.0
joint NEC *(see also* Neoplasm, bone)	170.9	198.5	—	213.9	238.0	239.2
acromioclavicular	170.4	198.5	—	213.4	238.0	239.2
bursa or synovial membrane - *see* Neoplasm, connective tissue						
costovertebral	170.3	198.5	—	213.3	238.0	239.2
sternocostal	170.3	198.5	—	213.3	238.0	239.2
temporomandibular	170.1	198.5	—	213.1	238.0	239.2

| | Malignant | | | | | |
	Primary	Secondary	Ca in situ	Benign	Uncertain Behavior	Unspecified
Neoplasm *(Continued)*						
junction						
anorectal	154.8	197.5	230.7	211.4	235.5	239.0
cardioesophageal	151.0	197.8	230.2	211.1	235.2	239.0
esophagogastric	151.0	197.8	230.2	211.1	235.2	239.0
gastroesophageal	151.0	197.8	230.2	211.1	235.2	239.0
hard and soft palate	145.5	198.89	230.0	210.4	235.1	239.0
ileocecal	153.4	197.5	230.3	211.3	235.2	239.0
pelvirectal	154.0	197.5	230.4	211.4	235.2	239.0
pelviureteric	189.1	198.0	233.9	223.1	236.91	239.5
rectosigmoid	154.0	197.5	230.4	211.4	235.2	239.0
squamocolumnar, of cervix	180.8	198.82	233.1	219.0	236.0	239.5
kidney (parenchymal)	189.0	198.0	233.9	223.0	236.91	239.5
calyx	189.1	198.0	233.9	223.1	236.91	239.5
hilus	189.1	198.0	233.9	223.1	236.91	239.5
pelvis	189.1	198.0	233.9	223.1	236.91	239.5
knee NEC*	195.5	198.89	232.7	229.8	238.8	239.89◀
labia (skin)	184.4	198.82	233.32	221.2	236.3	239.5
majora	184.1	198.82	233.32	221.2	236.3	239.5
minora	184.2	198.82	233.32	221.2	236.3	239.5
labial - *see also* Neoplasm, lip sulcus (lower) (upper)	145.1	198.89	230.0	210.4	235.1	239.0
labium (skin)	184.4	198.82	233.32	221.2	236.3	239.5
majus	184.1	198.82	233.32	221.2	236.3	239.5
minus	184.2	198.82	233.32	221.2	236.3	239.5
lacrimal						
canaliculi	190.7	198.4	234.0	224.7	238.8	239.89◀
duct (nasal)	190.7	198.4	234.0	224.7	238.8	239.89◀
gland	190.2	198.4	234.0	224.2	238.8	239.89◀
punctum	190.7	198.4	234.0	224.7	238.8	239.89◀
sac	190.7	198.4	234.0	224.7	238.8	239.89◀
Langerhans, islands or islets	157.4	197.8	230.9	211.7	235.5	239.0
laryngopharynx	148.9	198.89	230.0	210.8	235.1	239.0
larynx, laryngeal NEC	161.9	197.3	231.0	212.1	235.6	239.1
aryepiglottic fold	161.1	197.3	231.0	212.1	235.6	239.1
cartilage (arytenoid) (cricoid) (cuneiform) (thyroid)	161.3	197.3	231.0	212.1	235.6	239.1
commissure (anterior) (posterior)	161.0	197.3	231.0	212.1	235.6	239.1
contiguous sites	161.8	—	—	—	—	—
extrinsic NEC	161.1	197.3	231.0	212.1	235.6	239.1
meaning hypopharynx	148.9	198.89	230.0	210.8	235.1	239.0
interarytenoid fold	161.1	197.3	231.0	212.1	235.6	239.1
intrinsic	161.0	197.3	231.0	212.1	235.6	239.1

◀ New　◀▥ Revised　~~deleted~~ Deleted　● Use Additional Digit(s)　▨ Omit code

| | Malignant | | | | | |
	Primary	Secondary	Ca in situ	Benign	Uncertain Behavior	Unspecified
Neoplasm *(Continued)*						
larynx, laryngeal NEC *(Continued)*						
ventricular band	161.1	197.3	231.0	212.1	235.6	239.1
leg NEC*	195.5	198.89	232.7	229.8	238.8	239.89◀
lens, crystalline	190.0	198.4	234.0	224.0	238.8	239.89◀
lid (lower) (upper)	173.1	198.2	232.1	216.1	238.2	239.2
ligament - *see also* Neoplasm, connective tissue						
broad	183.3	198.82	233.39	221.0	236.3	239.5
Mackenrodt's	183.8	198.82	233.39	221.8	236.3	239.5
non-uterine - *see* Neoplasm, connective tissue						
round	183.5	198.82	—	221.0	236.3	239.5
sacro-uterine	183.4	198.82	—	221.0	236.3	239.5
uterine	183.4	198.82	—	221.0	236.3	239.5
utero-ovarian	183.8	198.82	233.39	221.8	236.3	239.5
uterosacral	183.4	198.82	—	221.0	236.3	239.5
limb*	195.8	198.89	232.8	229.8	238.8	239.89◀
lower*	195.5	198.89	232.7	229.8	238.8	239.89◀
upper*	195.4	198.89	232.6	229.8	238.8	239.89◀
limbus of cornea	190.4	198.4	234.0	224.4	238.8	239.89◀
lingual NEC (*see also* Neoplasm, tongue)	141.9	198.89	230.0	210.1	235.1	239.0
lingula, lung	162.3	197.0	231.2	212.3	235.7	239.1
lip (external) (lipstick area) (vermillion border)	140.9	198.89	230.0	210.0	235.1	239.0
buccal aspect - *see* Neoplasm, lip, internal						
commissure	140.6	198.89	230.0	210.4	235.1	239.0
contiguous sites	140.8	—	—	—	—	—
with oral cavity or pharynx	149.8	—	—	—	—	—
frenulum - *see* Neoplasm, lip, internal						
inner aspect - *see* Neoplasm, lip, internal						
internal (buccal) (frenulum) (mucosa) (oral)	140.5	198.89	230.0	210.0	235.1	239.0
lower	140.4	198.89	230.0	210.0	235.1	239.0
upper	140.3	198.89	230.0	210.0	235.1	239.0
lower	140.1	198.89	230.0	210.0	235.1	239.0
internal (buccal) (frenulum) (mucosa) (oral)	140.4	198.89	230.0	210.0	235.1	239.0
mucosa - *see* Neoplasm, lip, internal						
oral aspect - *see* Neoplasm, lip, internal						
skin (commissure) (lower) (upper)	173.0	198.2	232.0	216.0	238.2	239.2
upper	140.0	198.89	230.0	210.0	235.1	239.0
internal (buccal) (frenulum) (mucosa) (oral)	140.3	198.89	230.0	210.0	235.1	239.0
liver	155.2	197.7	230.8	211.5	235.3	239.0
primary	155.0	—	—	—	—	—

	Malignant					
	Primary	Secondary	Ca in situ	Benign	Uncertain Behavior	Unspecified
Neoplasm *(Continued)*						
lobe						
azygos	162.3	197.0	231.2	212.3	235.7	239.1
frontal	191.1	198.3	—	225.0	237.5	239.6
lower	162.5	197.0	231.2	212.3	235.7	239.1
middle	162.4	197.0	231.2	212.3	235.7	239.1
occipital	191.4	198.3	—	225.0	237.5	239.6
parietal	191.3	198.3	—	225.0	237.5	239.6
temporal	191.2	198.3	—	225.0	237.5	239.6
upper	162.3	197.0	231.2	212.3	235.7	239.1
lumbosacral plexus	171.6	198.4	—	215.6	238.1	239.2
lung	162.9	197.0	231.2	212.3	235.7	239.1
azygos lobe	162.3	197.0	231.2	212.3	235.7	239.1
carina	162.2	197.0	231.2	212.3	235.7	239.1
contiguous sites with bronchus or trachea	162.8	—	—	—	—	—
hilus	162.2	197.0	231.2	212.3	235.7	239.1
lingula	162.3	197.0	231.2	212.3	235.7	239.1
lobe NEC	162.9	197.0	231.2	212.3	235.7	239.1
lower lobe	162.5	197.0	231.2	212.3	235.7	239.1
main bronchus	162.2	197.0	231.2	212.3	235.7	239.1
middle lobe	162.4	197.0	231.2	212.3	235.7	239.1
upper lobe	162.3	197.0	231.2	212.3	235.7	239.1
lymph, lymphatic						
channel NEC (*see also* Neoplasm, connective tissue)	171.9	198.89	—	215.9	238.1	239.2
gland (secondary)	—	196.9	—	229.0	238.8	239.89◀
abdominal	—	196.2	—	229.0	238.8	239.89◀
aortic	—	196.2	—	229.0	238.8	239.89◀
arm	—	196.3	—	229.0	238.8	239.89◀
auricular (anterior) (posterior)	—	196.0	—	229.0	238.8	239.89◀
axilla, axillary	—	196.3	—	229.0	238.8	239.89◀
brachial	—	196.3	—	229.0	238.8	239.89◀
bronchial	—	196.1	—	229.0	238.8	239.89◀
bronchopulmonary	—	196.1	—	229.0	238.8	239.89◀
celiac	—	196.2	—	229.0	238.8	239.89◀
cervical	—	196.0	—	229.0	238.8	239.89◀
cervicofacial	—	196.0	—	229.0	238.8	239.89◀
Cloquet	—	196.5	—	229.0	238.8	239.89◀
colic	—	196.2	—	229.0	238.8	239.89◀
common duct	—	196.2	—	229.0	238.8	239.89◀
cubital	—	196.3	—	229.0	238.8	239.89◀
diaphragmatic	—	196.1	—	229.0	238.8	239.89◀

◀ New   ◀IIII Revised   ~~deleted~~ Deleted   ● Use Additional Digit(s)   ▨ Omit code

	Malignant					
	Primary	Secondary	Ca in situ	Benign	Uncertain Behavior	Unspecified
Neoplasm *(Continued)*						
lymph, lymphatic *(Continued)*						
gland *(Continued)*						
epigastric, inferior	—	196.6	—	229.0	238.8	239.89◀
epitrochlear	—	196.3	—	229.0	238.8	239.89◀
esophageal	—	196.1	—	229.0	238.8	239.89◀
face	—	196.0	—	229.0	238.8	239.89◀
femoral	—	196.5	—	229.0	238.8	239.89◀
gastric	—	196.2	—	229.0	238.8	239.89◀
groin	—	196.5	—	229.0	238.8	239.89◀
head	—	196.0	—	229.0	238.8	239.89◀
hepatic	—	196.2	—	229.0	238.8	239.89◀
hilar (pulmonary)	—	196.1	—	229.0	238.8	239.89◀
splenic	—	196.2	—	229.0	238.8	239.89◀
hypogastric	—	196.6	—	229.0	238.8	239.89◀
ileocolic	—	196.2	—	229.0	238.8	239.89◀
iliac	—	196.6	—	229.0	238.8	239.89◀
infraclavicular	—	196.3	—	229.0	238.8	239.89◀
inguina, inguinal	—	196.5	—	229.0	238.8	239.89◀
innominate	—	196.1	—	229.0	238.8	239.89◀
intercostal	—	196.1	—	229.0	238.8	239.89◀
intestinal	—	196.2	—	229.0	238.8	239.89◀
intrabdominal	—	196.2	—	229.0	238.8	239.89◀
intrapelvic	—	196.6	—	229.0	238.8	239.89◀
intrathoracic	—	196.1	—	229.0	238.8	239.9
jugular	—	196.0	—	229.0	238.8	239.89◀
leg	—	196.5	—	229.0	238.8	239.89◀
limb						
lower	—	196.5	—	229.0	238.8	239.89◀
upper	—	196.3	—	229.0	238.8	239.89◀
lower limb	—	196.5	—	229.0	238.8	238.9
lumbar	—	196.2	—	229.0	238.8	239.89◀
mandibular	—	196.0	—	229.0	238.8	239.89◀
mediastinal	—	196.1	—	229.0	238.8	239.89◀
mesenteric (inferior) (superior)	—	196.2	—	229.0	238.8	239.89◀
midcolic	—	196.2	—	229.0	238.8	239.89◀
multiple sites in categories 196.0–196.6	—	196.8	—	229.0	238.8	239.89◀
neck	—	196.0	—	229.0	238.8	239.89◀
obturator	—	196.6	—	229.0	238.8	239.89◀
occipital	—	196.0	—	229.0	238.8	239.89◀
pancreatic	—	196.2	—	229.0	238.8	239.89◀

	Malignant					
	Primary	**Secondary**	**Ca in situ**	**Benign**	**Uncertain Behavior**	**Unspecified**
Neoplasm *(Continued)*						
lymph, lymphatic *(Continued)*						
gland *(Continued)*						
para-aortic	—	196.2	—	229.0	238.8	239.89
paracervical	—	196.6	—	229.0	238.8	239.89
parametrial	—	196.6	—	229.0	238.8	239.89
parasternal	—	196.1	—	229.0	238.8	239.89
parotid	—	196.0	—	229.0	238.8	239.89
pectoral	—	196.3	—	229.0	238.8	239.89
pelvic	—	196.6	—	229.0	238.8	239.89
peri-aortic	—	196.2	—	229.0	238.8	239.89
peripancreatic	—	196.2	—	229.0	238.8	239.89
popliteal	—	196.5	—	229.0	238.8	239.89
porta hepatis	—	196.2	—	229.0	238.8	239.89
portal	—	196.2	—	229.0	238.8	239.89
preauricular	—	196.0	—	229.0	238.8	239.89
prelaryngeal	—	196.0	—	229.0	238.8	239.89
presymphysial	—	196.6	—	229.0	238.8	239.89
pretracheal	—	196.0	—	229.0	238.8	239.89
primary (any site) NEC	202.9●	—	—	—	—	—
pulmonary (hiler)	—	196.1	—	229.0	238.8	239.89
pyloric	—	196.2	—	229.0	238.8	239.89
retroperitoneal	—	196.2	—	229.0	238.8	239.89
retropharyngeal	—	196.0	—	229.0	238.8	239.89
Rosenmüller's	—	196.5	—	229.0	238.8	239.89
sacral	—	196.6	—	229.0	238.8	239.89
scalene	—	196.0	—	229.0	238.8	239.89
site NEC	—	196.9	—	229.0	238.8	239.89
splenic (hilar)	—	196.2	—	229.0	238.8	239.89
subclavicular	—	196.3	—	229.0	238.8	239.89
subinguinal	—	196.5	—	229.0	238.8	239.89
sublingual	—	196.0	—	229.0	238.8	239.89
submandibular	—	196.0	—	229.0	238.8	239.89
submaxillary	—	196.0	—	229.0	238.8	239.89
submental	—	196.0	—	229.0	238.8	239.89
subscapular	—	196.3	—	229.0	238.8	239.89
supraclavicular	—	196.0	—	229.0	238.8	239.89
thoracic	—	196.1	—	229.0	238.8	239.89
tibial	—	196.5	—	229.0	238.8	239.89
tracheal		196.1	—	229.0	238.8	239.89
tracheobronchial	—	196.1	—	229.0	238.8	239.89

◀ New   ◀ Revised   ~~deleted~~ Deleted   ● Use Additional Digit(s)   Omit code

| | Malignant | | | | | |
	Primary	Secondary	Ca in situ	Benign	Uncertain Behavior	Unspecified
Neoplasm *(Continued)*						
lymph, lymphatic *(Continued)*						
gland *(Continued)*						
upper limb	—	196.3	—	229.0	238.8	239.89◀
Virchow's	—	196.0	—	229.0	238.8	239.89◀
node - *see also* Neoplasm, lymph gland	202.9●	—	—	—	—	—
primary NEC						
vessel *(see also* Neoplasm, connective tissue)	171.9	198.89	—	215.9	238.1	239.2
Mackenrodt's ligament	183.8	198.82	233.39	221.8	236.3	239.5
malar region - *see* Neoplasm, cheek	170.0	198.5	—	213.0	238.0	239.2
mammary gland - *see* Neoplasm, breast						
mandible	170.1	198.5	—	213.1	238.0	239.2
alveolar						
mucosa	143.1	198.89	230.0	210.4	235.1	239.0
ridge or process	170.1	198.5	—	213.1	238.0	239.2
carcinoma	143.1	—	—	—	—	—
carcinoma	143.1	—	—	—	—	—
marrow (bone) NEC	202.9●	198.5	—	—	—	238.79
mastectomy site (skin)	173.5	198.2	—	—	—	—
specified as breast tissue	174.8	198.81	—	—	—	—
mastoid (air cells) (antrum) (cavity)	160.1	197.3	231.8	212.0	235.9	239.1
bone or process	170.0	198.5	—	213.0	238.0	239.2
maxilla, maxillary (superior)	170.0	198.5	—	213.0	238.0	239.2
alveolar						
mucosa	143.0	198.89	230.0	210.4	235.1	239.0
ridge or process	170.0	198.5	—	213.0	238.0	239.2
carcinoma	143.0	—	—	—	—	—
antrum	160.2	197.3	231.8	212.0	235.9	239.1
carcinoma	143.0	—	—	—	—	—
inferior - *see* Neoplasm, mandible						
sinus	160.2	197.3	231.8	212.0	235.9	239.1
meatus						
external (ear)	173.2	198.2	232.2	216.2	238.2	239.2
Meckel's diverticulum	152.3	197.4	230.7	211.2	235.2	239.0
mediastinum, mediastinal	164.9	197.1	—	212.5	235.8	239.89◀
anterior	164.2	197.1	—	212.5	235.8	239.89◀
contiguous sites with heart and thymus	164.8	—	—	—	—	—
posterior	164.3	197.1	—	212.5	235.8	239.89◀
medulla						
adrenal	194.0	198.7	234.8	227.0	237.2	239.7
oblongata	191.7	198.3	—	225.0	237.5	239.6

◀ New   ◀▥ Revised   ~~deleted~~ Deleted   ● Use Additional Digit(s)   ▨ Omit code

	Malignant					
	Primary	Secondary	Ca in situ	Benign	Uncertain Behavior	Unspecified
Neoplasm *(Continued)*						
meibomian gland	173.1	198.2	232.1	216.1	238.2	239.2
melanoma - *see* Melanoma						
meninges (brain) (cerebral) (cranial) (intracranial)	192.1	198.4	—	225.2	237.6	239.7
spinal (cord)	192.3	198.4	—	225.4	237.6	239.7
meniscus, knee joint (lateral) (medial)	170.7	198.5	—	213.7	238.0	239.2
mesentery, mesenteric	158.8	197.6	—	211.8	235.4	239.0
mesoappendix	158.8	197.6	—	211.8	235.4	239.0
mesocolon	158.8	197.6	—	211.8	235.4	239.0
mesopharynx - *see* Neoplasm, oropharynx						
mesosalpinx	183.3	198.82	233.39	221.0	236.3	239.5
mesovarium	183.3	198.82	233.39	221.0	236.3	239.5
metacarpus (any bone)	170.5	198.5	—	213.5	238.0	239.2
metastatic NEC - *see also* Neoplasm, by site, secondary	—	199.1	—	—	—	—
metatarsus (any bone)	170.8	198.5	—	213.8	238.0	239.2
midbrain	191.7	198.3	—	225.0	237.5	239.6
milk duct - *see* Neoplasm, breast						
mons						
pubis	184.4	198.82	233.32	221.2	236.3	239.5
veneris	184.4	198.82	233.32	221.2	236.3	239.5
motor tract	192.9	198.4	—	225.9	237.9	239.7
brain	191.9	198.3	—	225.0	237.5	239.6
spinal	192.2	198.3	—	225.3	237.5	239.7
mouth	145.9	198.89	230.0	210.4	235.1	239.0
contiguous sites	145.8	—	—	—	—	—
floor	144.9	198.89	230.0	210.3	235.1	239.0
anterior portion	144.0	198.89	230.0	210.3	235.1	239.0
contiguous sites	144.8	—	—	—	—	—
lateral portion	144.1	198.89	230.0	210.3	235.1	239.0
roof	145.5	198.89	230.0	210.4	235.1	239.0
specified part NEC	145.8	198.89	230.0	210.4	235.1	239.0
vestibule	145.1	198.89	230.0	210.4	235.1	239.0
mucosa						
alveolar (ridge or process)	143.9	198.89	230.0	210.4	235.1	239.0
lower	143.1	198.89	230.0	210.4	235.1	239.0
upper	143.0	198.89	230.0	210.4	235.1	239.0
buccal	145.0	198.89	230.0	210.4	235.1	239.0
cheek	145.0	198.89	230.0	210.4	235.1	239.0
lip - *see* Neoplasm, lip, internal						
nasal	160.0	197.3	231.8	212.0	235.9	239.1
oral	145.0	198.89	230.0	210.4	235.1	239.0

◀ New   ◀▥ Revised   ~~deleted~~ Deleted   ● Use Additional Digit(s)   ▨ Omit code

	Malignant					
	Primary	Secondary	Ca in situ	Benign	Uncertain Behavior	Unspecified
Neoplasm *(Continued)*						
Müllerian duct						
female	184.8	198.82	233.39	221.8	236.3	239.5
male	187.8	198.82	233.6	222.8	236.6	239.5
multiple sites NEC	199.0	199.0	234.9	229.9	238.9	199.0
muscle - *see also* Neoplasm, connective tissue extraocular	190.1	198.4	234.0	224.1	238.8	239.89◀
myocardium	164.1	198.89	—	212.7	238.8	239.89◀
myometrium	182.0	198.82	233.2	219.1	236.0	239.5
myopericardium	164.1	198.89	—	212.7	238.8	239.89◀
nabothian gland (follicle)	180.0	198.82	233.1	219.0	236.0	239.5
nail	173.9	198.2	232.9	216.9	238.2	239.2
finger	173.6	198.2	232.6	216.6	238.2	239.2
toe	173.7	198.2	232.7	216.7	238.2	239.2
nares, naris (anterior) (posterior)	160.0	197.3	231.8	212.0	235.9	239.1
nasal - *see* Neoplasm, nose						
nasolabial groove	173.3	198.2	232.3	216.3	238.2	239.2
nasolacrimal duct	190.7	198.4	234.0	224.7	238.8	239.89◀
nasopharynx, nasopharyngeal	147.9	198.89	230.0	210.7	235.1	239.0
contiguous sites	147.8	—	—	—	—	—
floor	147.3	198.89	230.0	210.7	235.1	239.0
roof	147.0	198.89	230.0	210.7	235.1	239.0
specified site NEC	147.8	198.89	230.0	210.7	235.1	239.0
wall	147.9	198.89	230.0	210.7	235.1	239.0
anterior	147.3	198.89	230.0	210.7	235.1	239.0
lateral	147.2	198.89	230.0	210.7	235.1	239.0
posterior	147.1	198.89	230.0	210.7	235.1	239.0
superior	147.0	198.89	230.0	210.7	235.1	239.0
nates	173.5	198.2	232.5	216.5	238.2	239.2
neck NEC*	195.0	198.89	234.8	229.8	238.8	239.89◀
nerve (autonomic) (ganglion) (parasympathetic) (peripheral) (sympathetic) - *see also* Neoplasm, connective tissue						
abducens	192.0	198.4	—	225.1	237.9	239.7
accessory (spinal)	192.0	198.4	—	225.1	237.9	239.7
acoustic	192.0	198.4	—	225.1	237.9	239.7
auditory	192.0	198.4	—	225.1	237.9	239.7
brachial	171.2	198.89	—	215.2	238.1	239.2
cranial (any)	192.0	198.4	—	225.1	237.9	239.7
facial	192.0	198.4	—	225.1	237.9	239.7
femoral	171.3	198.89	—	215.3	238.1	239.2
glossopharyngeal	192.0	198.4	—	225.1	237.9	239.7
hypoglossal	192.0	198.4	—	225.1	237.9	239.7

	Malignant			Benign	Uncertain Behavior	Unspecified
	Primary	Secondary	Ca in situ			
Neoplasm *(Continued)*						
nerve *(Continued)*						
intercostal	171.4	198.89	—	215.4	238.1	239.2
lumbar	171.7	198.89	—	215.7	238.1	239.2
median	171.2	198.89	—	215.2	238.1	239.2
obturator	171.3	198.89	—	215.3	238.1	239.2
oculomotor	192.0	198.4	—	225.1	237.9	239.7
olfactory	192.0	198.4	—	225.1	237.9	239.7
optic	192.0	198.4	—	225.1	237.9	239.7
peripheral NEC	171.9	198.89	—	215.9	238.1	239.2
radial	171.2	198.89	—	215.2	238.1	239.2
sacral	171.6	198.89	—	215.6	238.1	239.2
sciatic	171.3	198.89	—	215.3	238.1	239.2
spinal NEC	171.9	198.89	—	215.9	238.1	239.2
trigeminal	192.0	198.4	—	225.1	237.9	239.7
trochlear	192.0	198.4	—	225.1	237.9	239.7
ulnar	171.2	198.89	—	215.2	238.1	239.2
vagus	192.0	198.4	—	225.1	237.9	239.7
nervous system (central) NEC	192.9	198.4	—	225.9	237.9	239.7
autonomic NEC	171.9	198.89	—	215.9	238.1	239.2
brain - *see also* Neoplasm, brain membrane or meninges	192.1	198.4	—	225.2	237.6	239.7
contiguous sites	192.8	—	—	—	—	—
parasympathetic NEC	171.9	198.89	—	215.9	238.1	239.2
sympathetic NEC	171.9	198.89	—	215.9	238.1	239.2
nipple (female)	174.0	198.81	233.0	217	238.3	239.3
male	175.0	198.81	233.0	217	238.3	239.3
nose, nasal	195.0	198.89	234.8	229.8	238.8	239.89◄◖◖
ala (external)	173.3	198.2	232.3	216.3	238.2	239.2
bone	170.0	198.5	—	213.0	238.0	239.2
cartilage	160.0	197.3	231.8	212.0	235.9	239.1
cavity	160.0	197.3	231.8	212.0	235.9	239.1
contiguous sites with accessory sinuses or middle ear	160.8	—	—	—	—	—
choana	147.3	198.89	230.0	210.7	235.1	239.0
external (skin)	173.3	198.2	232.3	216.3	238.2	239.2
fossa	160.0	197.3	231.8	212.0	235.9	239.1
internal	160.0	197.3	231.8	212.0	235.9	239.1
mucosa	160.0	197.3	231.8	212.0	235.9	239.1
septum	160.0	197.3	231.8	212.0	235.9	239.1
posterior margin	147.3	198.89	230.0	210.7	235.1	239.0
sinus - *see* Neoplasm, sinus						
skin	173.3	198.2	232.3	216.3	238.2	239.2

◄ New   ◖◖◖ Revised   ~~deleted~~ Deleted   ● Use Additional Digit(s)   ▨ Omit code

	Malignant					
	Primary	**Secondary**	**Ca in situ**	**Benign**	**Uncertain Behavior**	**Unspecified**
Neoplasm *(Continued)*						
nose, nasal *(Continued)*						
turbinate (mucosa)	160.0	197.3	231.8	212.0	235.9	239.1
bone	170.0	198.5	—	213.0	238.0	239.2
vestibule	160.0	197.3	231.8	212.0	235.9	239.1
nostril	160.0	197.3	231.8	212.0	235.9	239.1
nucleus pulposus	170.2	198.5	—	213.2	238.0	230.2
occipital						
bone	170.0	198.5	—	213.0	238.0	239.2
lobe or pole, brain	191.4	198.3	—	225.0	237.5	239.6
odontogenic - *see* Neoplasm, jaw bone						
oesophagus - *see* Neoplasm, esophagus						
olfactory nerve or bulb	192.0	198.4	—	225.1	237.9	239.7
olive (brain)	191.7	198.3	—	225.0	237.5	239.6
omentum	158.8	197.6	—	211.8	235.4	239.0
operculum (brain)	191.0	198.3	—	225.0	237.5	239.6
optic nerve, chiasm, or tract	192.0	198.4	—	225.1	237.9	239.7
oral (cavity)	145.9	198.89	230.0	210.4	235.1	239.0
contiguous sites with lip or pharynx	149.8	—	—	—	—	—
ill-defined	149.9	198.89	230.0	210.4	235.1	239.0
mucosa	145.9	198.89	230.0	210.4	235.1	239.0
orbit	190.1	198.4	234.0	224.1	238.8	239.89◄
bone	170.0	198.5	—	213.0	238.0	239.2
eye	190.1	198.4	234.0	224.1	238.8	239.89◄
soft parts	190.1	198.4	234.0	224.1	238.8	239.89◄
organ of Zuckerkandl	194.6	198.89	—	227.6	237.3	239.7
oropharynx	146.9	198.89	230.0	210.6	235.1	239.0
branchial cleft (vestige)	146.8	198.89	230.0	210.6	235.1	239.0
contiguous sites	146.8	—	—	—	—	—
junctional region	146.5	198.89	230.0	210.6	235.1	239.0
lateral wall	146.6	198.89	230.0	210.6	235.1	239.0
pillars of fauces	146.2	198.89	230.0	210.6	235.1	239.0
posterior wall	146.7	198.89	230.0	210.6	235.1	239.0
specified part NEC	146.8	198.89	230.0	210.6	235.1	239.0
vallecula	146.3	198.89	230.0	210.6	235.1	239.0
os						
external	180.1	198.82	233.1	219.0	236.0	239.5
internal	180.0	198.82	233.1	219.0	236.0	239.5
ovary	183.0	198.6	233.39	220	236.2	239.5
oviduct	183.2	198.82	233.39	221.0	236.3	239.5

	Malignant					
	Primary	Secondary	Ca in situ	Benign	Uncertain Behavior	Unspecified
Neoplasm (Continued)						
palate	145.5	198.89	230.0	210.4	235.1	239.0
hard	145.2	198.89	230.0	210.4	235.1	239.0
junction of hard and soft palate	145.5	198.89	230.0	210.4	235.1	239.0
soft	145.3	198.89	230.0	210.4	235.1	239.0
nasopharyngeal surface	147.3	198.89	230.0	210.7	235.1	239.0
posterior surface	147.3	198.89	230.0	210.7	235.1	239.0
superior surface	147.3	198.89	230.0	210.7	235.1	239.0
palatoglossal arch	146.2	198.89	230.0	210.6	235.1	239.0
palatopharyngeal arch	146.2	198.89	230.0	210.6	235.1	239.0
pallium	191.0	198.3	—	225.0	237.5	239.6
palpebra	173.1	198.2	232.1	216.1	238.2	239.2
pancreas	157.9	197.8	230.9	211.6	235.5	239.0
body	157.1	197.8	230.9	211.6	235.5	239.0
contiguous sites	157.8	—	—	—	—	—
duct (of Santorini) (of Wirsung)	157.3	197.8	230.9	211.6	235.5	239.0
ectopic tissue	157.8	197.8				
head	157.0	197.8	230.9	211.6	235.5	239.0
islet cells	157.4	197.8	230.9	211.7	235.5	239.0
neck	157.8	197.8	230.9	211.6	235.5	239.0
tail	157.2	197.8	230.9	211.6	235.5	239.0
para-aortic body	194.6	198.89	—	227.6	237.3	239.7
paraganglion NEC	194.6	198.89	—	227.6	237.3	239.7
parametrium	183.4	198.82	—	221.0	236.3	239.5
paranephric	158.0	197.6	—	211.8	235.4	239.0
pararectal	195.3	198.89	—	229.8	238.8	239.89◀▪▪
parasagittal (region)	195.0	198.89	234.8	229.8	238.8	239.89◀▪▪
parasellar	192.9	198.4	—	225.9	237.9	239.7
parathyroid (gland)	194.1	198.89	234.8	227.1	237.4	239.7
paraurethral	195.3	198.89	—	229.8	238.8	239.89◀▪▪
gland	189.4	198.1	233.9	223.89	236.99	239.5
paravaginal	195.3	198.89	—	229.8	238.8	239.89◀▪▪
parenchyma, kidney	189.0	198.0	233.9	223.0	236.91	239.5
parietal						
bone	170.0	198.5	—	213.0	238.0	239.2
lobe, brain	191.3	198.3	—	225.0	237.5	239.6
paroophoron	183.3	198.82	233.39	221.0	236.3	239.5
parotid (duct) (gland)	142.0	198.89	230.0	210.2	235.0	239.0
parovarium	183.3	198.82	233.39	221.0	236.3	239.5
patella	170.8	198.5	—	213.8	238.0	239.2
peduncle, cerebral	191.7	198.3	—	225.0	237.5	239.6

◀ New ◀▪▪ Revised deleted Deleted ● Use Additional Digit(s) ▨ Omit code

	Malignant					
	Primary	Secondary	Ca in situ	Benign	Uncertain Behavior	Unspecified
Neoplasm *(Continued)*						
pelvirectal junction	154.0	197.5	230.4	211.4	235.2	239.0
pelvis, pelvic	195.3	198.89	234.8	229.8	238.8	239.89◄
bone	170.6	198.5	—	213.6	238.0	239.2
floor	195.3	198.89	234.8	229.8	238.8	239.89◄
renal	189.1	198.0	233.9	223.1	236.91	239.5
viscera	195.3	198.89	234.8	229.8	238.8	239.89◄
wall	195.3	198.89	234.8	229.8	238.8	239.89◄
pelvo-abdominal	195.8	198.89	234.8	229.8	238.8	239.89◄
penis	187.4	198.82	233.5	222.1	236.6	239.5
body	187.3	198.82	233.5	222.1	236.6	239.5
corpus (cavernosum)	187.3	198.82	233.5	222.1	236.6	239.5
glans	187.2	198.82	233.5	222.1	236.6	239.5
skin NEC	187.4	198.82	233.5	222.1	236.6	239.5
periadrenal (tissue)	158.0	197.6	—	211.8	235.4	239.0
perianal (skin)	173.5	198.2	232.5	216.5	238.2	239.2
pericardium	164.1	198.89	—	212.7	238.8	239.89◄
perinephric	158.0	197.6	—	211.8	235.4	239.0
perineum	195.3	198.89	234.8	229.8	238.8	239.89◄
periodontal tissue NEC	143.9	198.89	230.0	210.4	235.1	239.0
periosteum - *see* Neoplasm, bone						
peripancreatic	158.0	197.6	—	211.8	235.4	239.0
peripheral nerve NEC	171.9	198.89	—	215.9	238.1	239.2
perirectal (tissue)	195.3	198.89	—	229.8	238.8	239.89◄
perirenal (tissue)	158.0	197.6	—	211.8	235.4	239.0
peritoneum, peritoneal (cavity)	158.9	197.6	—	211.8	235.4	239.0
contiguous sites	158.8	—	—	—	—	—
with digestive organs	159.8	—	—	—	—	—
parietal	158.8	197.6	—	211.8	235.4	239.0
pelvic	158.8	197.6	—	211.8	235.4	239.0
specified part NEC	158.8	197.6	—	211.8	235.4	239.0
peritonsillar (tissue)	195.0	198.89	234.8	229.8	238.8	239.89◄
periurethral tissue	195.3	198.89	—	229.8	238.8	239.89◄
phalanges	170.9	198.5	—	213.9	238.0	239.2
foot	170.8	198.5	—	213.8	238.0	239.2
hand	170.5	198.5	—	213.5	238.0	239.2
pharynx, pharyngeal	149.0	198.89	230.0	210.9	235.1	239.0
bursa	147.1	198.89	230.0	210.7	235.1	239.0
fornix	147.3	198.89	230.0	210.7	235.1	239.0
recess	147.2	198.89	230.0	210.7	235.1	239.0
region	149.0	198.89	230.0	210.9	235.1	239.0

◄ New ◄▥ Revised deleted Deleted ● Use Additional Digit(s) ▨ Omit code

	Malignant			Benign	Uncertain Behavior	Unspecified
	Primary	Secondary	Ca in situ			
Neoplasm *(Continued)*						
pharynx, pharyngeal *(Continued)*						
tonsil	147.1	198.89	230.0	210.7	235.1	239.0
wall (lateral) (posterior)	149.0	198.89	230.0	210.9	235.1	239.0
pia mater (cerebral) (cranial)	192.1	198.4	—	225.2	237.6	239.7
spinal	192.3	198.4	—	225.4	237.6	239.7
pillars of fauces	146.2	198.89	230.0	210.6	235.1	239.0
pineal (body) (gland)	194.4	198.89	234.8	227.4	237.1	239.7
pinna (ear) NEC	173.2	198.2	232.2	216.2	238.2	239.2
cartilage	171.0	198.89	—	215.0	238.1	239.2
piriform fossa or sinus	148.1	198.89	230.0	210.8	235.1	239.0
pituitary (body) (fossa) (gland) (lobe)	194.3	198.89	234.8	227.3	237.0	239.7
placenta	181	198.82	233.2	219.8	236.1	239.5
pleura, pleural (cavity)	163.9	197.2	—	212.4	235.8	239.1
contiguous sites	163.8	—	—	—	—	—
parietal	163.0	197.2	—	212.4	235.8	239.1
visceral	163.1	197.2	—	212.4	235.8	239.1
plexus						
brachial	171.2	198.89	—	215.2	238.1	239.2
cervical	171.0	198.89	—	215.0	238.1	239.2
choroid	191.5	198.3	—	225.0	237.5	239.6
lumbosacral	171.6	198.89	—	215.6	238.1	239.2
sacral	171.6	198.89	—	215.6	238.1	239.2
pluri-endocrine	194.8	198.89	234.8	227.8	237.4	239.7
pole						
frontal	191.1	198.3	—	225.0	237.5	239.6
occipital	191.4	198.3	—	225.0	237.5	239.6
pons (varolii)	191.7	198.3	—	225.0	237.5	239.6
popliteal fossa or space*	195.5	198.89	234.8	229.8	238.8	239.89◄
postcricoid (region)	148.0	198.89	230.0	210.8	235.1	239.0
posterior fossa (cranial)	191.9	198.3	—	225.0	237.5	239.6
postnasal space	147.9	198.89	230.0	210.7	235.1	239.0
prepuce	187.1	198.82	233.5	222.1	236.6	239.5
prepylorus	151.1	197.8	230.2	211.1	235.2	239.0
presacral (region)	195.3	198.89	—	229.8	238.8	239.89◄
prostate (gland)	185	198.82	233.4	222.2	236.5	239.5
utricle	189.3	198.1	233.9	223.81	236.99	239.5
pterygoid fossa	171.0	198.89	—	215.0	238.1	239.2
pubic bone	170.6	198.5	—	213.6	238.0	239.2
pudenda, pudendum (female)	184.4	198.82	233.32	221.2	236.3	239.5
pulmonary	162.9	197.0	231.2	212.3	235.7	239.1

◄ New   ◄▦ Revised   ~~deleted~~ Deleted   ● Use Additional Digit(s)   ▦ Omit code

Neoplasm (Continued)	Malignant			Benign	Uncertain Behavior	Unspecified
	Primary	Secondary	Ca in situ			
putamen	191.0	198.3	—	225.0	237.5	239.6
pyloric						
antrum	151.2	197.8	230.2	211.1	235.2	239.0
canal	151.1	197.8	230.2	211.1	235.2	239.0
pylorus	151.1	197.8	230.2	211.1	235.2	239.0
pyramid (brain)	191.7	198.3	—	225.0	237.5	239.6
pyriform fossa or sinus	148.1	198.89	230.0	210.8	235.1	239.0
radius (any part)	170.4	198.5	—	213.4	238.0	239.2
Rathke's pouch	194.3	198.89	234.8	227.3	237.0	239.7
rectosigmoid (colon) (junction)	154.0	197.5	230.4	211.4	235.2	239.0
contiguous sites with anus or rectum	154.8	—	—	—	—	—
rectouterine pouch	158.8	197.6	—	211.8	235.4	239.0
rectovaginal septum or wall	195.3	198.89	234.8	229.8	238.8	239.89◄
rectovesical septum	195.3	198.89	234.8	229.8	238.8	239.89◄
rectum (ampulla)	154.1	197.5	230.4	211.4	235.2	239.0
and colon	154.0	197.5	230.4	211.4	235.2	239.0
contiguous sites with anus or rectosigmoid junction	154.8	—	—	—	—	—
renal	189.0	198.0	233.9	223.0	236.91	239.5
calyx	189.1	198.0	233.9	223.1	236.91	239.5
hilus	189.1	198.0	233.9	223.1	236.91	239.5
parenchyma	189.0	198.0	233.9	223.0	236.91	239.5
pelvis	189.1	198.0	233.9	223.1	236.91	239.5
respiratory						
organs or system NEC	165.9	197.3	231.9	212.9	235.9	239.1
contiguous sites with intrathoracic organs	165.8	—	—	—	—	—
specified sites NEC	165.8	197.3	231.8	212.8	235.9	239.1
tract NEC	165.9	197.3	231.9	212.9	235.9	239.1
upper	165.0	197.3	231.9	212.9	235.9	239.1
retina	190.5	198.4	234.0	224.5	238.8	239.81◄
retrobulbar	190.1	198.4	—	224.1	238.8	239.89◄
retrocecal	158.0	197.6	—	211.8	235.4	239.0
retromolar (area) (triangle) (trigone)	145.6	198.89	230.0	210.4	235.1	239.0
retro-orbital	195.0	198.89	234.8	229.8	238.8	239.89◄
retroperitoneal (space) (tissue)	158.0	197.6	—	211.8	235.4	239.0
contiguous sites	158.8	—	—	—	—	—
retroperitoneum	158.0	197.6	—	211.8	235.4	239.0
contiguous sites	158.8	—	—	—	—	—
retropharyngeal	149.0	198.89	230.0	210.9	235.1	239.0
retrovesical (septum)	195.3	198.89	234.8	229.8	238.8	239.89◄
rhinencephalon	191.0	198.3	—	225.0	237.5	239.6

◄ New   ◄▥ Revised   deleted Deleted   ● Use Additional Digit(s)   ▨ Omit code

| | Malignant | | | | | |
	Primary	Secondary	Ca in situ	Benign	Uncertain Behavior	Unspecified
Neoplasm *(Continued)*						
rib	170.3	198.5	—	213.3	238.0	239.2
Rosenmüller's fossa	147.2	198.89	230.0	210.7	235.1	239.0
round ligament	183.5	198.82	—	221.0	236.3	239.5
sacrococcyx, sacrococcygeal	170.6	198.5	—	213.6	238.0	239.2
region	195.3	198.89	234.8	229.8	238.8	239.89◄
sacrouterine ligament	183.4	198.82	—	221.0	236.3	239.5
sacrum, sacral (vertebra)	170.6	198.5	—	213.6	238.0	239.2
salivary gland or duct (major)	142.9	198.89	230.0	210.2	235.0	239.0
contiguous sites	142.8	—	—	—	—	—
minor NEC	145.9	198.89	230.0	210.4	235.1	239.0
parotid	142.0	198.89	230.0	210.2	235.0	239.0
pluriglandular	142.8	198.89	230.0	210.2	235.0	239.0
sublingual	142.2	198.89	230.0	210.2	235.0	239.0
submandibular	142.1	198.89	230.0	210.2	235.0	239.0
submaxillary	142.1	198.89	230.0	210.2	235.0	239.0
salpinx (uterine)	183.2	198.82	233.39	221.0	236.3	239.5
Santorini's duct	157.3	197.8	230.9	211.6	235.5	239.0
scalp	173.4	198.2	232.4	216.4	238.2	239.2
scapula (any part)	170.4	198.5	—	213.4	238.0	239.2
scapular region	195.1	198.89	234.8	229.8	238.8	239.89◄
scar NEC (*see also* Neoplasm, skin)	173.9	198.2	232.9	216.9	238.2	239.2
sciatic nerve	171.3	198.89	—	215.3	238.1	239.2
sclera	190.0	198.4	234.0	224.0	238.8	239.89◄
scrotum (skin)	187.7	198.82	233.6	222.4	236.6	239.5
sebaceous gland - *see* Neoplasm, skin						
sella turcica	194.3	198.89	234.8	227.3	237.0	239.7
bone	170.0	198.5	—	213.0	238.0	239.2
semilunar cartilage (knee)	170.7	198.5	—	213.7	238.0	239.2
seminal vesicle	187.8	198.82	233.6	222.8	236.6	239.5
septum						
nasal	160.0	197.3	231.8	212.0	235.9	239.1
posterior margin	147.3	198.89	230.0	210.7	235.1	239.0
rectovaginal	195.3	198.89	234.8	229.8	238.8	239.89◄
rectovesical	195.3	198.89	234.8	229.8	238.8	239.89◄
urethrovaginal	184.9	198.82	233.39	221.9	236.3	239.5
vesicovaginal	184.9	198.82	233.39	221.9	236.3	239.5
shoulder NEC*	195.4	198.89	232.6	229.8	238.8	239.89◄
sigmoid flexure (lower) (upper)	153.3	197.5	230.3	211.3	235.2	239.0
sinus (accessory)	160.9	197.3	231.8	212.0	235.9	239.1
bone (any)	170.0	198.5	—	213.0	238.0	239.2

◄ New   ◄▦ Revised   ~~deleted~~ Deleted   ● Use Additional Digit(s)   ▦ Omit code

	Malignant					
	Primary	Secondary	Ca in situ	Benign	Uncertain Behavior	Unspecified
Neoplasm *(Continued)*						
sinus *(Continued)*						
contiguous sites with middle ear or nasal cavities	160.8	—	—	—	—	—
ethmoidal	160.3	197.3	231.8	212.0	235.9	239.1
frontal	160.4	197.3	231.8	212.0	235.9	239.1
maxillary	160.2	197.3	231.8	212.0	235.9	239.1
nasal, paranasal NEC	160.9	197.3	231.8	212.0	235.9	239.1
pyriform	148.1	198.89	230.0	210.8	235.1	239.0
sphenoidal	160.5	197.3	231.8	212.0	235.9	239.1
skeleton, skeletal NEC	170.9	198.5	—	213.9	238.0	239.2
Skene's gland	189.4	198.1	233.9	223.89	236.99	239.5
skin NEC	173.9	198.2	232.9	216.9	238.2	239.2
abdominal wall	173.5	198.2	232.5	216.5	238.2	239.2
ala nasi	173.3	198.2	232.3	216.3	238.2	239.2
ankle	173.7	198.2	232.7	216.7	238.2	239.2
antecubital space	173.6	198.2	232.6	216.6	238.2	239.2
anus	173.5	198.2	232.5	216.5	238.2	239.2
arm	173.6	198.2	232.6	216.6	238.2	239.2
auditory canal (external)	173.2	198.2	232.2	216.2	238.2	239.2
auricle (ear)	173.2	198.2	232.2	216.2	238.2	239.2
auricular canal (external)	173.2	198.2	232.2	216.2	238.2	239.2
axilla, axillary fold	173.5	198.2	232.5	216.5	238.2	239.2
back	173.5	198.2	232.5	216.5	238.2	239.2
breast	173.5	198.2	232.5	216.5	238.2	239.2
brow	173.3	198.2	232.3	216.3	238.2	239.2
buttock	173.5	198.2	232.5	216.5	238.2	239.2
calf	173.7	198.2	232.7	216.7	238.2	239.2
canthus (eye) (inner) (outer)	173.1	198.2	232.1	216.1	238.2	239.2
cervical region	173.4	198.2	232.4	216.4	238.2	239.2
cheek (external)	173.3	198.2	232.3	216.3	238.2	239.2
chest (wall)	173.5	198.2	232.5	216.5	238.2	239.2
chin	173.3	198.2	232.3	216.3	238.2	239.2
clavicular area	173.5	198.2	232.5	216.5	238.2	239.2
clitoris	184.3	198.82	233.32	221.2	236.3	239.5
columnella	173.3	198.2	232.3	216.3	238.2	239.2
concha	173.2	198.2	232.2	216.2	238.2	239.2
contiguous sites	173.8	—	—	—	—	—
ear (external)	173.2	198.2	232.2	216.2	238.2	239.2
elbow	173.6	198.2	232.6	216.6	238.2	239.2
eyebrow	173.3	198.2	232.3	216.3	238.2	239.2
eyelid	173.1	198.2	232.1	216.1	238.2	239.2

	Malignant					
	Primary	Secondary	Ca in situ	Benign	Uncertain Behavior	Unspecified
Neoplasm (Continued)						
skin NEC (Continued)						
face NEC	173.3	198.2	232.3	216.3	238.2	239.2
female genital organs (external)	184.4	198.82	233.30	221.2	236.3	239.5
clitoris	184.3	198.82	233.32	221.2	236.3	239.5
labium NEC	184.4	198.82	233.32	221.2	236.3	239.5
majus	184.1	198.82	233.32	221.2	236.3	239.5
minus	184.2	198.82	233.32	221.2	236.3	239.5
pudendum	184.4	198.82	233.32	221.2	236.3	239.5
vulva	184.4	198.82	233.32	221.2	236.3	239.5
finger	173.6	198.2	232.6	216.6	238.2	239.2
flank	173.5	198.2	232.5	216.5	238.2	239.2
foot	173.7	198.2	232.7	216.7	238.2	239.2
forearm	173.6	198.2	232.6	216.6	238.2	239.2
forehead	173.3	198.2	232.3	216.3	238.2	239.2
glabella	173.3	198.2	232.3	216.3	238.2	239.2
gluteal region	173.5	198.2	232.5	216.5	238.2	239.2
groin	173.5	198.2	232.5	216.5	238.2	239.2
hand	173.6	198.2	232.6	216.6	238.2	239.2
head NEC	173.4	198.2	232.4	216.4	238.2	239.2
heel	173.7	198.2	232.7	216.7	238.2	239.2
helix	173.2	198.2	232.2	216.2	238.2	239.2
hip	173.7	198.2	232.7	216.7	238.2	239.2
infraclavicular region	173.5	198.2	232.5	216.5	238.2	239.2
inguinal region	173.5	198.2	232.5	216.5	238.2	239.2
jaw	173.3	198.2	232.3	216.3	238.2	239.2
knee	173.7	198.2	232.7	216.7	238.2	239.2
labia						
majora	184.1	198.82	233.32	221.2	236.3	239.5
minora	184.2	198.82	233.32	221.2	236.3	239.5
leg	173.7	198.2	232.7	216.7	238.2	239.2
lid (lower) (upper)	173.1	198.2	232.1	216.1	238.2	239.2
limb NEC	173.9	198.2	232.9	216.9	238.2	239.5
lower	173.7	198.2	232.7	216.7	238.2	239.2
upper	173.6	198.2	232.6	216.6	238.2	239.2
lip (lower) (upper)	173.0	198.2	232.0	216.0	238.2	239.2
male genital organs	187.9	198.82	233.6	222.9	236.6	239.5
penis	187.4	198.82	233.5	222.1	236.6	239.5
prepuce	187.1	198.82	233.5	222.1	236.6	239.5
scrotum	187.7	198.82	233.6	222.4	236.6	239.5

◀ New   ◀━━ Revised   ~~deleted~~ Deleted   ● Use Additional Digit(s)   ▓ Omit code

	Malignant			Benign	Uncertain Behavior	Unspecified
	Primary	Secondary	Ca in situ			
Neoplasm *(Continued)*						
skin NEC *(Continued)*						
mastectomy site	173.5	198.2	—	—	—	—
specified as breast tissue	174.8	198.81	—	—	—	—
meatus, acoustic (external)	173.2	198.2	232.2	216.2	238.2	239.2
nates	173.5	198.2	232.5	216.5	238.2	239.2
neck	173.4	198.2	232.4	216.4	238.2	239.2
nose (external)	173.3	198.2	232.3	216.3	238.2	239.2
palm	173.6	198.2	232.6	216.6	238.2	239.2
palpebra	173.1	198.2	232.1	216.1	238.2	239.2
penis NEC	187.4	198.82	233.5	222.1	236.6	239.5
perianal	173.5	198.2	232.5	216.5	238.2	239.2
perineum	173.5	198.2	232.5	216.5	238.2	239.2
pinna	173.2	198.2	232.2	216.2	238.2	239.2
plantar	173.7	198.2	232.7	216.7	238.2	239.2
popliteal fossa or space	173.7	198.2	232.7	216.7	238.2	239.2
prepuce	187.1	198.82	233.5	222.1	236.6	239.5
pubes	173.5	198.2	232.5	216.5	238.2	239.2
sacrococcygeal region	173.5	198.2	232.5	216.5	238.2	239.2
scalp	173.4	198.2	232.4	216.4	238.2	239.2
scapular region	173.5	198.2	232.5	216.5	238.2	239.2
scrotum	187.7	198.82	233.6	222.4	236.6	239.5
shoulder	173.6	198.2	232.6	216.6	238.2	239.2
sole (foot)	173.7	198.2	232.7	216.7	238.2	239.2
specified sites NEC	173.8	198.2	232.8	216.8	232.8	239.2
submammary fold	173.5	198.2	232.5	216.5	238.2	239.2
supraclavicular region	173.4	198.2	232.4	216.4	238.2	239.2
temple	173.3	198.2	232.3	216.3	238.2	239.2
thigh	173.7	198.2	232.7	216.7	238.2	239.2
thoracic wall	173.5	198.2	232.5	216.5	238.2	239.2
thumb	173.6	198.2	232.6	216.6	238.2	239.2
toe	173.7	198.2	232.7	216.7	238.2	239.2
tragus	173.2	198.2	232.2	216.2	238.2	239.2
trunk	173.5	198.2	232.5	216.5	238.2	239.2
umbilicus	173.5	198.2	232.5	216.5	238.2	239.2
vulva	184.4	198.82	233.32	221.2	236.3	239.5
wrist	173.6	198.2	232.6	216.6	238.2	239.2
skull	170.0	198.5	—	213.0	238.0	239.2
soft parts or tissues - *see* Neoplasm, connective tissue						
specified site NEC	195.8	198.89	234.8	229.8	238.8	239.89◀

	Malignant					
	Primary	Secondary	Ca in situ	Benign	Uncertain Behavior	Unspecified
Neoplasm *(Continued)*						
spermatic cord	187.6	198.82	233.6	222.8	236.6	239.5
sphenoid	160.5	197.3	231.8	212.0	235.9	239.1
bone	170.0	198.5	—	213.0	238.0	239.2
sinus	160.5	197.3	231.8	212.0	235.9	239.1
sphincter						
anal	154.2	197.5	230.5	211.4	235.5	239.0
of Oddi	156.1	197.8	230.8	211.5	235.3	239.0
spine, spinal (column)	170.2	198.5	—	213.2	238.0	239.2
bulb	191.7	198.3	—	225.0	237.5	239.6
coccyx	170.6	198.5	—	213.6	238.0	239.2
cord (cervical) (lumbar) (sacral) (thoracic)	192.2	198.3	—	225.3	237.5	239.7
dura mater	192.3	198.4	—	225.4	237.6	239.7
lumbosacral	170.2	198.5	—	213.2	238.0	239.2
membrane	192.3	198.4	—	225.4	237.6	239.7
meninges	192.3	198.4	—	225.4	237.6	239.7
nerve (root)	171.9	198.89	—	215.9	238.1	239.2
pia mater	192.3	198.4	—	225.4	237.6	239.7
root	171.9	198.89	—	215.9	238.1	239.2
sacrum	170.6	198.5	—	213.6	238.0	239.2
spleen, splenic NEC	159.1	197.8	230.9	211.9	235.5	239.0
flexure (colon)	153.7	197.5	230.3	211.3	235.2	239.0
stem, brain	191.7	198.3	—	225.0	237.5	239.6
Stensen's duct	142.0	198.89	230.0	210.2	235.0	239.0
sternum	170.3	198.5	—	213.3	238.0	239.2
stomach	151.9	197.8	230.2	211.1	235.2	239.0
antrum (pyloric)	151.2	197.8	230.2	211.1	235.2	239.0
body	151.4	197.8	230.2	211.1	235.2	239.0
cardia	151.0	197.8	230.2	211.1	235.2	239.0
cardiac orifice	151.0	197.8	230.2	211.1	235.2	239.0
contiguous sites	151.8	—	—	—	—	—
corpus	151.4	197.8	230.2	211.1	235.2	239.0
fundus	151.3	197.8	230.2	211.1	235.2	239.0
greater curvature NEC	151.6	197.8	230.2	211.1	235.2	239.0
lesser curvature NEC	151.5	197.8	230.2	211.1	235.2	239.0
prepylorus	151.1	197.8	230.2	211.1	235.2	239.0
pylorus	151.1	197.8	230.2	211.1	235.2	239.0
wall NEC	151.9	197.8	230.2	211.1	235.2	239.0
anterior NEC	151.8	197.8	230.2	211.1	235.2	239.0
posterior NEC	151.8	197.8	230.2	211.1	235.2	239.0
stroma, endometrial	182.0	198.82	233.2	219.1	236.0	239.5

◀ New   ◀▥ Revised   deleted Deleted   ● Use Additional Digit(s)   ▨ Omit code

	Malignant					
	Primary	Secondary	Ca in situ	Benign	Uncertain Behavior	Unspecified
Neoplasm *(Continued)*						
stump, cervical	180.8	198.82	233.1	219.0	236.0	239.5
subcutaneous (nodule) (tissue) NEC - *see* Neoplasm, connective tissue						
subdural	192.1	198.4	—	225.2	237.6	239.7
subglottis, subglottic	161.2	197.3	231.0	212.1	235.6	239.1
sublingual	144.9	198.89	230.0	210.3	235.1	239.0
gland or duct	142.2	198.89	230.0	210.2	235.0	239.0
submandibular gland	142.1	198.89	230.0	210.2	235.0	239.0
submaxillary gland or duct	142.1	198.89	230.0	210.2	235.0	239.0
submental	195.0	198.89	234.8	229.8	238.8	239.89◄
subpleural	162.9	197.0	—	212.3	235.7	239.1
substernal	164.2	197.1	—	212.5	235.8	239.89◄
sudoriferous, sudoriparous gland, site unspecified	173.9	198.2	232.9	216.9	238.2	239.2
specified site - *see* Neoplasm, skin						
supraclavicular region	195.0	198.89	234.8	229.8	238.8	239.89◄
supraglottis	161.1	197.3	231.0	212.1	235.6	239.1
suprarenal (capsule) (cortex) (gland) (medulla)	194.0	198.7	234.8	227.0	237.2	239.7
suprasellar (region)	191.9	198.3	—	225.0	237.5	239.6
sweat gland (apocrine) (eccrine), site unspecified	173.9	198.2	232.9	216.9	238.2	239.2
specified site - *see* Neoplasm, skin						
sympathetic nerve or nervous system NEC	171.9	198.89	—	215.9	238.1	239.2
symphysis pubis	170.6	198.5	—	213.6	238.0	239.2
synovial membrane - *see* Neoplasm, connective tissue						
tapetum, brain	191.8	198.3	—	225.0	237.5	239.6
tarsus (any bone)	170.8	198.5	—	213.8	238.0	239.2
temple (skin)	173.3	198.2	232.3	216.3	238.2	239.2
temporal						
bone	170.0	198.5	—	213.0	238.0	239.2
lobe or pole	191.2	198.3	—	225.0	237.5	239.6
region	195.0	198.89	234.8	229.8	238.8	239.89◄
skin	173.3	198.2	232.3	216.3	238.2	239.2
tendon (sheath) - *see* Neoplasm, connective tissue						
tentorium (cerebelli)	192.1	198.4	—	225.2	237.6	239.7
testis, testes (descended) (scrotal)	186.9	198.82	233.6	222.0	236.4	239.5
ectopic	186.0	198.82	233.6	222.0	236.4	239.5
retained	186.0	198.82	233.6	222.0	236.4	239.5
undescended	186.0	198.82	233.6	222.0	236.4	239.5
thalamus	191.0	198.3	—	225.0	237.5	239.6
thigh NEC*	195.5	198.89	234.8	229.8	238.8	239.89◄
thorax, thoracic (cavity) (organs NEC)	195.1	198.89	234.8	229.8	238.8	239.89◄
duct	171.4	198.89	—	215.4	238.1	239.2
wall NEC	195.1	198.89	234.8	229.8	238.8	239.89◄

◄ New   ◄ Revised   ~~deleted~~ Deleted   ● Use Additional Digit(s)   ▓ Omit code

Neoplasm *(Continued)*	Malignant			Benign	Uncertain Behavior	Unspecified
	Primary	Secondary	Ca in situ			
throat	149.0	198.89	230.0	210.9	235.1	239.0
thumb NEC*	195.4	198.89	232.6	229.8	238.8	239.89◀
thymus (gland)	164.0	198.89	—	212.6	235.8	239.89◀
contiguous sites with heart and mediastinum	164.8	—	—	—	—	—
thyroglossal duct	193	198.89	234.8	226	237.4	239.7
thyroid (gland)	193	198.89	234.8	226	237.4	239.7
cartilage	161.3	197.3	231.0	212.1	235.6	239.1
tibia (any part)	170.7	198.5	—	213.7	238.0	239.2
toe NEC*	195.5	198.89	232.7	229.8	238.8	239.89◀
tongue	141.9	198.89	230.0	210.1	235.1	239.0
anterior (two-thirds) NEC	141.4	198.89	230.0	210.1	235.1	239.0
dorsal surface	141.1	198.89	230.0	210.1	235.1	239.0
ventral surface	141.3	198.89	230.0	210.1	235.1	239.0
base (dorsal surface)	141.0	198.89	230.0	210.1	235.1	239.0
border (lateral)	141.2	198.89	230.0	210.1	235.1	239.0
contiguous sites	141.8	—	—	—	—	—
dorsal surface NEC	141.1	198.89	230.0	210.1	235.1	239.0
fixed part NEC	141.0	198.89	230.0	210.1	235.1	239.0
foramen cecum	141.1	198.89	230.0	210.1	235.1	239.0
frenulum linguae	141.3	198.89	230.0	210.1	235.1	239.0
junctional zone	141.5	198.89	230.0	210.1	235.1	239.0
margin (lateral)	141.2	198.89	230.0	210.1	235.1	239.0
midline NEC	141.1	198.89	230.0	210.1	235.1	239.0
mobile part NEC	141.4	198.89	230.0	210.1	235.1	239.0
posterior (third)	141.0	198.89	230.0	210.1	235.1	239.0
root	141.0	198.89	230.0	210.1	235.1	239.0
surface (dorsal)	141.1	198.89	230.0	210.1	235.1	239.0
base	141.0	198.89	230.0	210.1	235.1	239.0
ventral	141.3	198.89	230.0	210.1	235.1	239.0
tip	141.2	198.89	230.0	210.1	235.1	239.0
tonsil	141.6	198.89	230.0	210.1	235.1	239.0
tonsil	146.0	198.89	230.0	210.5	235.1	239.0
fauces, faucial	146.0	198.89	230.0	210.5	235.1	239.0
lingual	141.6	198.89	230.0	210.1	235.1	239.0
palatine	146.0	198.89	230.0	210.5	235.1	239.0
pharyngeal	147.1	198.89	230.0	210.7	235.1	239.0
pillar (anterior) (posterior)	146.2	198.89	230.0	210.6	235.1	239.0
tonsillar fossa	146.1	198.89	230.0	210.6	235.1	239.0
tooth socket NEC	143.9	198.89	230.0	210.4	235.1	239.0

◀ New   ◀▥ Revised   ~~deleted~~ Deleted   ● Use Additional Digit(s)   ▨ Omit code

	Malignant					
	Primary	Secondary	Ca in situ	Benign	Uncertain Behavior	Unspecified
Neoplasm *(Continued)*						
trachea (cartilage) (mucosa)	162.0	197.3	231.1	212.2	235.7	239.1
contiguous sites with bronchus or lung	162.8	—	—	—	—	—
tracheobronchial	162.8	197.3	231.1	212.2	235.7	239.1
contiguous sites with lung	162.8	—	—	—	—	—
tragus	173.2	198.2	232.2	216.2	238.2	239.2
trunk NEC*	195.8	198.89	232.5	229.8	238.8	239.89◀
tubo-ovarian	183.8	198.82	233.39	221.8	236.3	239.5
tunica vaginalis	187.8	198.82	233.6	222.8	236.6	239.5
turbinate (bone)	170.0	198.5	—	213.0	238.0	239.2
nasal	160.0	197.3	231.8	212.0	235.9	239.1
tympanic cavity	160.1	197.3	231.8	212.0	235.9	239.1
ulna (any part)	170.4	198.5	—	213.4	238.0	239.2
umbilicus, umbilical	173.5	198.2	232.5	216.5	238.2	239.2
uncus, brain	191.2	198.3	—	225.0	237.5	239.6
unknown site or unspecified	199.1	199.1	234.9	229.9	238.9	239.9
urachus	188.7	198.1	233.7	223.3	236.7	239.4
ureter, ureteral	189.2	198.1	233.9	223.2	236.91	239.5
orifice (bladder)	188.6	198.1	233.7	223.3	236.7	239.4
ureter-bladder (junction)	188.6	198.1	233.7	223.3	236.7	239.4
urethra, urethral (gland)	189.3	198.1	233.9	223.81	236.99	239.5
orifice, internal	188.5	198.1	233.7	223.3	236.7	239.4
urethrovaginal (septum)	184.9	198.82	233.39	221.9	236.3	239.5
urinary organ or system NEC	189.9	198.1	233.9	223.9	236.99	239.5
bladder - *see* Neoplasm, bladder						
contiguous sites	189.8	—	—	—	—	—
specified sites NEC	189.8	198.1	233.9	223.89	236.99	239.5
utero-ovarian	183.8	198.82	233.39	221.8	236.3	239.5
ligament	183.3	198.82	—	221.0	236.3	239.5
uterosacral ligament	183.4	198.82	—	221.0	236.3	239.5
uterus, uteri, uterine	179	198.82	233.2	219.9	236.0	239.5
adnexa NEC	183.9	198.82	233.39	221.8	236.3	239.5
contiguous sites	183.8	—	—	—	—	—
body	182.0	198.82	233.2	219.1	236.0	239.5
contiguous sites	182.8	—	—	—	—	—
cervix	180.9	198.82	233.1	219.0	236.0	239.5
cornu	182.0	198.82	233.2	219.1	236.0	239.5
corpus	182.0	198.82	233.2	219.1	236.0	239.5
endocervix (canal) (gland)	180.0	198.82	233.1	219.0	236.0	239.5
endometrium	182.0	198.82	233.2	219.1	236.0	239.5

◀ New   ◀⁍ Revised   ~~deleted~~ Deleted   ● Use Additional Digit(s)   ▓ Omit code

	Malignant					
	Primary	Secondary	Ca in situ	Benign	Uncertain Behavior	Unspecified
Neoplasm *(Continued)*						
uterus, uteri, uterine *(Continued)*						
exocervix	180.1	198.82	233.1	219.0	236.0	239.5
external os	180.1	198.82	233.1	219.0	236.0	239.5
fundus	182.0	198.82	233.2	219.1	236.0	239.5
internal os	180.0	198.82	233.1	219.0	236.0	239.5
isthmus	182.1	198.82	233.2	219.1	236.0	239.5
ligament	183.4	198.82	—	221.0	236.3	239.5
broad	183.3	198.82	233.39	221.0	236.3	239.5
round	183.5	198.82	—	221.0	236.3	239.5
lower segment	182.1	198.82	233.2	219.1	236.0	239.5
myometrium	182.0	198.82	233.2	219.1	236.0	239.5
squamocolumnar junction	180.8	198.82	233.1	219.0	236.0	239.5
tube	183.2	198.82	233.39	221.0	236.3	239.5
utricle, prostatic	189.3	198.1	233.9	223.81	236.99	239.5
uveal tract	190.0	198.4	234.0	224.0	238.8	239.89◀
uvula	145.4	198.89	230.0	210.4	235.1	239.0
vagina, vaginal (fornix) (vault) (wall)	184.0	198.82	233.31	221.1	236.3	239.5
vaginovesical	184.9	198.82	233.39	221.9	236.3	239.5
septum	184.9	198.82	233.39	221.9	236.3	239.5
vallecula (epiglottis)	146.3	198.89	230.0	210.6	235.1	239.0
vascular - *see* Neoplasm, connective tissue						
vas deferens	187.6	198.82	233.6	222.8	236.6	239.5
Vater's ampulla	156.2	197.8	230.8	211.5	235.3	239.0
vein, venous - *see* Neoplasm, connective tissue						
vena cava (abdominal) (inferior)	171.5	198.89	—	215.5	238.1	239.2
superior	171.4	198.89	—	215.4	238.1	239.2
ventricle (cerebral) (floor) (fourth) (lateral) (third)	191.5	198.3	—	225.0	237.5	239.6
cardiac (left) (right)	164.1	198.89	—	212.7	238.8	239.89◀
ventricular band of larynx	161.1	197.3	231.0	212.1	235.6	239.1
ventriculus - *see* Neoplasm, stomach						
vermillion border - *see* Neoplasm, lip						
vermis, cerebellum	191.6	198.3	—	225.0	237.5	239.6
vertebra (column)	170.2	198.5	—	213.2	238.0	239.2
coccyx	170.6	198.5	—	213.6	238.0	239.2
sacrum	170.6	198.5	—	213.6	238.0	239.2
vesical - *see* Neoplasm, bladder						
vesicle, seminal	187.8	198.82	233.6	222.8	236.6	239.5
vesicocervical tissue	184.9	198.82	233.39	221.9	236.3	239.5
vesicorectal	195.3	198.89	234.8	229.8	238.8	239.89◀
vesicovaginal	184.9	198.82	233.39	221.9	236.3	239.5
septum	184.9	198.82	233.39	221.9	236.3	239.5

◀ New ◀▥ Revised ~~deleted~~ Deleted ● Use Additional Digit(s) ▦ Omit code

	Malignant			Benign	Uncertain Behavior	Unspecified
	Primary	Secondary	Ca in situ			
Neoplasm *(Continued)*						
vessel (blood) - *see* Neoplasm, connective tissue						
vestibular gland, greater	184.1	198.82	233.32	221.2	236.3	239.5
vestibule						
mouth	145.1	198.89	230.0	210.4	235.1	239.0
nose	160.0	197.3	231.8	212.0	235.9	239.1
Virchow's gland	—	196.0	—	229.0	238.8	239.89◀
viscera NEC	195.8	198.89	234.8	229.8	238.8	239.89◀
vocal cords (true)	161.0	197.3	231.0	212.1	235.6	239.1
false	161.1	197.3	231.0	212.1	235.6	239.1
vomer	170.0	198.5	—	213.0	238.0	239.2
vulva	184.4	198.82	233.32	221.2	236.3	239.5
vulvovaginal gland	184.4	198.82	233.32	221.2	236.3	239.5
Waldeyer's ring	149.1	198.89	230.0	210.9	235.1	239.0
Wharton's duct	142.1	198.89	230.0	210.2	235.0	239.0
white matter (central) (cerebral)	191.0	198.3	—	225.0	237.5	239.6
windpipe	162.0	197.3	231.1	212.2	235.7	239.1
Wirsung's duct	157.3	197.8	230.9	211.6	235.5	239.0
wolffian (body) (duct)						
female	184.8	198.82	233.39	221.8	236.3	239.5
male	187.8	198.82	233.6	222.8	236.6	239.5
womb - *see* Neoplasm, uterus						
wrist NEC*	195.4	198.89	232.6	229.8	238.8	239.89◀
xiphoid process	170.3	198.5	—	213.3	238.0	239.2
Zuckerkandl's organ	194.6	198.89	—	227.6	237.3	239.7

◀ New   ◀▥ Revised   ~~deleted~~ Deleted   ● Use Additional Digit(s)   ▨ Omit code   467

Neovascularization
 choroid 362.16
 ciliary body 364.42
 cornea 370.60
  deep 370.63
  localized 370.61
 iris 364.42
 retina 362.16
 subretinal 362.16
Nephralgia 788.0
Nephritis, nephritic (albuminuric)
 (azotemic) (congenital)
 (degenerative) (diffuse)
 (disseminated) (epithelial) (familial)
 (focal) (granulomatous)
 (hemorrhagic) (infantile)
 (nonsuppurative, excretory)
 (uremic) 583.9
 with
  edema - *see* Nephrosis
  lesion of
   glomerulonephritis
    hypocomplementemic
     persistent 583.2
     with nephrotic syndrome
      581.2
     chronic 582.2
    lobular 583.2
     with nephrotic syndrome
      581.2
     chronic 582.2
    membranoproliferative
     583.2
     with nephrotic syndrome
      581.2
     chronic 582.2
    membranous 583.1
     with nephrotic syndrome
      581.1
     chronic 582.1
    mesangiocapillary 583.2
     with nephrotic syndrome
      581.2
     chronic 582.2
    mixed membranous and
     proliferative 583.2
     with nephrotic syndrome
      581.2
     chronic 582.2
    proliferative (diffuse) 583.0
     with nephrotic syndrome
      581.0
     acute 580.0
     chronic 582.0
    rapidly progressive 583.4
     acute 580.4
     chronic 582.4
   interstitial nephritis (diffuse)
    (focal) 583.89
    with nephrotic syndrome
     581.89
    acute 580.89
    chronic 582.89
   necrotizing glomerulitis 583.4
    acute 580.4
    chronic 582.4
   renal necrosis 583.9
    cortical 583.6
    medullary 583.7
   specified pathology NEC 583.89
    with nephrotic syndrome
     581.89
    acute 580.89
    chronic 582.89

Nephritis, nephritic *(Continued)*
 with *(Continued)*
  necrosis, renal 583.9
   cortical 583.6
   medullary (papillary) 583.7
  nephrotic syndrome (*see also*
   Nephrosis) 581.9
  papillary necrosis 583.7
  specified pathology NEC 583.89
 acute 580.9
  extracapillary with epithelial
   crescents 580.4
  hypertensive (*see also* Hypertension,
   kidney) 403.90
  necrotizing 580.4
  poststreptococcal 580.0
  proliferative (diffuse) 580.0
  rapidly progressive 580.4
  specified pathology NEC 580.89
 amyloid 277.39 *[583.81]*
  chronic 277.39 *[582.81]*
 arteriolar (*see also* Hypertension,
  kidney) 403.90
 arteriosclerotic (*see also* Hypertension,
  kidney) 403.90
 ascending (*see also* Pyelitis) 590.80
 atrophic 582.9
 basement membrane NEC 583.89
  with pulmonary hemorrhage
   (Goodpasture's syndrome)
   446.21 *[583.81]*
 calculous, calculus 592.0
 cardiac (*see also* Hypertension, kidney)
  403.90
 cardiovascular (*see also* Hypertension,
  kidney) 403.90
 chronic 582.9
  arteriosclerotic (*see also*
   Hypertension, kidney) 403.90
  hypertensive (*see also* Hypertension,
   kidney) 403.90
 cirrhotic (*see also* Sclerosis, renal) 587
 complicating pregnancy, childbirth, or
  puerperium 646.2●
  with hypertension 642.1●
   affecting fetus or newborn 760.0
  affecting fetus or newborn 760.1
 croupous 580.9
 desquamative - *see* Nephrosis
 due to
  amyloidosis 277.39 *[583.81]*
   chronic 277.39 *[582.81]*
  arteriosclerosis (*see also*
   Hypertension, kidney) 403.90
  diabetes mellitus 250.4● *[583.81]*
   due to secondary diabetes 249.4●
    [583.81] ◀▥
   with nephrotic syndrome 250.4●
    [581.81]
    due to secondary diabetes
     249.4● *[581.81]*
  diphtheria 032.89 *[580.81]*
  gonococcal infection (acute) 098.19
   [583.81]
   chronic or duration of 2 months
    or over 098.39 *[583.81]*
  gout 274.10
  infectious hepatitis 070.9 *[580.81]*
  mumps 072.79 *[580.81]*
  specified kidney pathology NEC
   583.89
   acute 580.89
   chronic 582.89
  streptotrichosis 039.8 *[583.81]*

Nephritis, nephritic *(Continued)*
 due to *(Continued)*
  subacute bacterial endocarditis 421.0
   [580.81]
  systemic lupus erythematosus 710.0
   [583.81]
   chronic 710.0 *[582.81]*
  typhoid fever 002.0 *[580.81]*
 endothelial 582.2
 end state (chronic) (terminal) NEC
  585.6
 epimembranous 581.1
 exudative 583.89
  with nephrotic syndrome 581.89
  acute 580.89
  chronic 582.89
 gonococcal (acute) 098.19 *[583.81]*
  chronic or duration of 2 months or
   over 098.39 *[583.81]*
 gouty 274.10
 hereditary (Alport's syndrome)
  759.89
 hydremic - *see* Nephrosis
 hypertensive (*see also* Hypertension,
  kidney) 403.90
 hypocomplementemic persistent
  583.2
  with nephrotic syndrome 581.2
  chronic 582.2
 immune complex NEC 583.89
 infective (*see also* Pyelitis) 590.80
 interstitial (diffuse) (focal) 583.89
  with nephrotic syndrome 581.89
  acute 580.89
  chronic 582.89
 latent or quiescent - *see* Nephritis,
  chronic
 lead 984.9
  specified type of lead - *see* Table of
   Drugs and Chemicals
 lobular 583.2
  with nephrotic syndrome
   581.2
  chronic 582.2
 lupus 710.0 *[583.81]*
  acute 710.0 *[580.81]*
  chronic 710.0 *[582.81]*
 membranoproliferative 583.2
  with nephrotic syndrome 581.2
  chronic 582.2
 membranous 583.1
  with nephrotic syndrome 581.1
  chronic 582.1
 mesangiocapillary 583.2
  with nephrotic syndrome 581.2
  chronic 582.2
 minimal change 581.3
 mixed membranous and proliferative
  583.2
  with nephrotic syndrome 581.2
  chronic 582.2
 necrotic, necrotizing 583.4
  acute 580.4
  chronic 582.4
 nephrotic - *see* Nephrosis
 old - *see* Nephritis, chronic
 parenchymatous 581.89
 polycystic 753.12
  adult type (APKD) 753.13
  autosomal dominant 753.13
  autosomal recessive 753.14
  childhood type (CPKD) 753.14
  infantile type 753.14
 poststreptococcal 580.0

◀ New ◀▥ Revised ~~deleted~~ Deleted ● Use Additional Digit(s) ▥ Omit code

Nephritis, nephritic *(Continued)*
  pregnancy - *see* Nephritis, complicating
        pregnancy
  proliferative 583.0
    with nephrotic syndrome 581.0
    acute 580.0
    chronic 582.0
  purulent *(see also* Pyelitis) 590.80
  rapidly progressive 583.4
    acute 580.4
    chronic 582.4
  salt-losing or salt-wasting *(see also*
        Disease, renal) 593.9
  saturnine 584.9
    specified type of lead - *see* Table of
        Drugs and Chemicals
  septic *(see also* Pyelitis) 590.80
  specified pathology NEC 583.89
    acute 580.89
    chronic 582.89
  staphylococcal *(see also* Pyelitis) 590.80
  streptotrichosis 039.8 *[583.81]*
  subacute *(see also* Nephrosis) 581.9
  suppurative *(see also* Pyelitis) 590.80
  syphilitic (late) 095.4
    congenital 090.5 *[583.81]*
    early 091.69 *[583.81]*
  terminal (chronic) (end-stage) NEC
        585.6
  toxic - *see* Nephritis, acute
  tubal, tubular - *see* Nephrosis, tubular
  tuberculous *(see also* Tuberculosis)
        016.0● *[583.81]*
  type II (Ellis) - *see* Nephrosis
  vascular - *see also* Hypertension, kidney
  war 580.9
Nephroblastoma (M8960/3) 189.0
  epithelial (M8961/3) 189.0
  mesenchymal (M8962/3) 189.0
Nephrocalcinosis 275.49
Nephrocystitis, pustular *(see also* Pyelitis)
        590.80
Nephrolithiasis (congenital) (pelvis)
        (recurrent) 592.0
  uric acid 274.11
Nephroma (M8960/3) 189.0
  mesoblastic (M8960/1) 236.9
Nephronephritis *(see also* Nephrosis)
        581.9
Nephronopthisis 753.16
Nephropathy *(see also* Nephritis) 583.9
  with
    exudative nephritis 583.89
    interstitial nephritis (diffuse) (focal)
        583.89
    medullary necrosis 583.7
    necrosis 583.9
        cortical 583.6
        medullary or papillary 583.7
    papillary necrosis 583.7
    specified lesion or cause NEC 583.89
  analgesic 583.89
    with medullary necrosis, acute 584.7
  arteriolar *(see also* Hypertension,
        kidney) 403.90
  arteriosclerotic *(see also* Hypertension,
        kidney) 403.90
  complicating pregnancy 646.2●
  diabetic 250.4● *[583.81]*
    due to secondary diabetes 249.4●
        [583.81] ◀▥
  gouty 274.10
    specified type NEC 274.19
  hereditary amyloid 277.31

Nephropathy *(Continued)*
  hypercalcemic 588.89
  hypertensive *(see also* Hypertension,
        kidney) 403.90
  hypokalemic (vacuolar) 588.89
  IgA 583.9
  obstructive 593.89
    congenital 753.20
  phenacetin 584.7
  phosphate-losing 588.0
  potassium depletion 588.89
  proliferative *(see also* Nephritis,
        proliferative) 583.0
  protein-losing 588.89
  salt-losing or salt-wasting *(see also*
        Disease, renal) 593.9
  sickle-cell *(see also* Disease, sickle-cell)
        282.60 *[583.81]*
  toxic 584.5
  vasomotor 584.5
  water-losing 588.89
Nephroptosis *(see also* Disease, renal)
        593.0
  congenital (displaced) 753.3
Nephropyosis *(see also* Abscess, kidney)
        590.2
Nephrorrhagia 593.81
Nephrosclerosis (arteriolar)
        (arteriosclerotic) (chronic) (hyaline)
        (see also Hypertension, kidney)
        403.90
  gouty 274.10
  hyperplastic (arteriolar) *(see also*
        Hypertension, kidney) 403.90
  senile *(see also* Sclerosis, renal) 587
Nephrosis, nephrotic (Epstein's)
        (syndrome) 581.9
  with
    lesion of
        focal glomerulosclerosis 581.1
        glomerulonephritis
            endothelial 581.2
            hypocomplementemic
                persistent 581.2
            lobular 581.2
            membranoproliferative 581.2
            membranous 581.1
            mesangiocapillary 581.2
            minimal change 581.3
            mixed membranous and
                proliferative 581.2
            proliferative 581.0
        segmental hyalinosis 581.1
        specified pathology NEC 581.89
  acute - *see* Nephrosis, tubular
  anoxic - *see* Nephrosis, tubular
  arteriosclerotic *(see also* Hypertension,
        kidney) 403.90
  chemical - *see* Nephrosis, tubular
  cholemic 572.4
  complicating pregnancy, childbirth, or
        puerperium - *see* Nephritis,
        complicating pregnancy
  diabetic 250.4● *[581.81]*
    due to secondary diabetes 249.4●
        [581.81]
  Finnish type (congenital) 759.89
  hemoglobinuric - *see* Nephrosis,
        tubular
  in
    amyloidosis 277.39 *[581.81]*
    diabetes mellitus 250.4● *[581.81]*
        due to secondary diabetes 249.4●
            [581.81]

Nephrosis, nephrotic *(Continued)*
  in *(Continued)*
    epidemic hemorrhagic fever
        078.6
    malaria 084.9 *[581.81]*
    polyarteritis 446.0 *[581.81]*
    systemic lupus erythematosus
        710.0 *[581.81]*
  ischemic - *see* Nephrosis, tubular
  lipoid 581.3
  lower nephron - *see* Nephrosis,
        tubular
  lupoid 710.0 *[581.81]*
  lupus 710.0 *[581.81]*
  malarial 084.9 *[581.81]*
  minimal change 581.3
  necrotizing - *see* Nephrosis, tubular
  osmotic (sucrose) 588.89
  polyarteritic 446.0 *[581.81]*
  radiation 581.9
  specified lesion or cause NEC
        581.89
  syphilitic 095.4
  toxic - *see* Nephrosis, tubular
  tubular (acute) 584.5
    due to a procedure 997.5
    radiation 581.9
Nephrosonephritis hemorrhagic
        (endemic) 078.6
Nephrostomy status V44.6
  with complication 997.5
Nerve - *see* condition
Nerves 799.21   ◀▥
Nervous *(see also* condition) 799.21   ◀▥
  breakdown 300.9
  heart 306.2
  stomach 306.4
  tension 799.21   ◀▥
Nervousness 799.21   ◀▥
Nesidioblastoma (M8150/0)
  pancreas 211.7
  specified site NEC - *see* Neoplasm, by
        site, benign
  unspecified site 211.7
Netherton's syndrome (ichthyosiform
        erythroderma) 757.1
Nettle rash 708.8
Nettleship's disease (urticaria
        pigmentosa) 757.33
Neumann's disease (pemphigus
        vegetans) 694.4
Neuralgia, neuralgic (acute) *(see also*
        Neuritis) 729.2
  accessory (nerve) 352.4
  acoustic (nerve) 388.5
  ankle 355.8
  anterior crural 355.8
  anus 787.99
  arm 723.4
  auditory (nerve) 388.5
  axilla 353.0
  bladder 788.1
  brachial 723.4
  brain - *see* Disorder, nerve, cranial
  broad ligament 625.9
  cerebral - *see* Disorder, nerve, cranial
  ciliary 339.00
  cranial nerve - *see also* Disorder, nerve,
        cranial
    fifth or trigeminal *(see also*
        Neuralgia, trigeminal)
        350.1
  ear 388.71
    middle 352.1

Neuralgia, neuralgic (*Continued*)
  facial 351.8
  finger 354.9
  flank 355.8
  foot 355.8
  forearm 354.9
  Fothergill's (*see also* Neuralgia,
      trigeminal) 350.1
    postherpetic 053.12
  glossopharyngeal (nerve) 352.1
  groin 355.8
  hand 354.9
  heel 355.8
  Horton's 339.00
  Hunt's 053.11
  hypoglossal (nerve) 352.5
  iliac region 355.8
  infraorbital (*see also* Neuralgia,
      trigeminal) 350.1
  inguinal 355.8
  intercostal (nerve) 353.8
    postherpetic 053.19
  jaw 352.1
  kidney 788.0
  knee 355.8
  loin 355.8
  malarial (*see also* Malaria) 084.6
  mastoid 385.89
  maxilla 352.1
  median thenar 354.1
  metatarsal 355.6
  middle ear 352.1
  migrainous 339.00
  Morton's 355.6
  nerve, cranial - *see* Disorder, nerve,
      cranial
  nose 352.0
  occipital 723.8
  olfactory (nerve) 352.0
  ophthalmic 377.30
    postherpetic 053.19
  optic (nerve) 377.30
  penis 607.9
  perineum 355.8
  pleura 511.0
  postherpetic NEC 053.19
    geniculate ganglion 053.11
    ophthalmic 053.19
    trifacial 053.12
    trigeminal 053.12
  pubic region 355.8
  radial (nerve) 723.4
  rectum 787.99
  sacroiliac joint 724.3
  sciatic (nerve) 724.3
  scrotum 608.9
  seminal vesicle 608.9
  shoulder 354.9
  sluder's 337.09
  specified nerve NEC - *see* Disorder,
      nerve
  spermatic cord 608.9
  sphenopalatine (ganglion)
      337.09
  subscapular (nerve) 723.4
  suprascapular (nerve) 723.4
  testis 608.89
  thenar (median) 354.1
  thigh 355.8
  tongue 352.5
  trifacial (nerve) (*see also* Neuralgia,
      trigeminal) 350.1
  trigeminal (nerve) 350.1
    postherpetic 053.12
  tympanic plexus 388.71

Neuralgia, neuralgic (*Continued*)
  ulnar (nerve) 723.4
  vagus (nerve) 352.3
  wrist 354.9
  writers' 300.89
    organic 333.84
Neurapraxia - *see* Injury, nerve, by site
Neurasthenia 300.5
  cardiac 306.2
  gastric 306.4
  heart 306.2
  postfebrile 780.79
  postviral 780.79
Neurilemmoma (M9560/0) - *see also*
      Neoplasm, connective tissue,
      benign
  acoustic (nerve) 225.1
  malignant (M9560/3) - *see also*
      Neoplasm, connective tissue,
      malignant
    acoustic (nerve) 192.0
Neurilemmosarcoma (M9560/3) - *see*
      Neoplasm, connective tissue,
      malignant
Neurilemoma - *see* Neurilemmoma
Neurinoma (M9560/0) - *see*
      Neurilemmoma
Neurinomatosis (M9560/1) - *see also*
      Neoplasm, connective tissue,
      uncertain behavior
  centralis 759.5
Neuritis (*see also* Neuralgia) 729.2
  abducens (nerve) 378.54
  accessory (nerve) 352.4
  acoustic (nerve) 388.5
    syphilitic 094.86
  alcoholic 357.5
    with psychosis 291.1
  amyloid, any site 277.39 [357.4]
  anterior crural 355.8
  arising during pregnancy 646.4●
  arm 723.4
  ascending 355.2
  auditory (nerve) 388.5
  brachial (nerve) NEC 723.4
    due to displacement, intervertebral
        disc 722.0
  cervical 723.4
  chest (wall) 353.8
  costal region 353.8
  cranial nerve - *see also* Disorder, nerve,
      cranial
    first or olfactory 352.0
    second or optic 377.30
    third or oculomotor 378.52
    fourth or trochlear 378.53
    fifth or trigeminal (*see also*
        Neuralgia, trigeminal)
        350.1
    sixth or abducens 378.54
    seventh or facial 351.8
      newborn 767.5
    eighth or acoustic 388.5
    ninth or glossopharyngeal
        352.1
    tenth or vagus 352.3
    eleventh or accessory 352.4
    twelfth or hypoglossal 352.5
  Déjérine-Sottas 356.0
  diabetic 250.6● [357.2]
    due to secondary diabetes
        249.6● [357.2]
  diphtheritic 032.89 [357.4]

Neuritis (*Continued*)
  due to
    beriberi 265.0 [357.4]
    displacement, prolapse, protrusion,
        or rupture of intervertebral
        disc 722.2
      cervical 722.0
      lumbar, lumbosacral 722.10
      thoracic, thoracolumbar 722.11
    herniation, nucleus pulposus 722.2
      cervical 722.0
      lumbar, lumbosacral 722.10
      thoracic, thoracolumbar 722.11
  endemic 265.0 [357.4]
  facial (nerve) 351.8
    newborn 767.5
  general - *see* Polyneuropathy
  geniculate ganglion 351.1
    due to herpes 053.11
  glossopharyngeal (nerve) 352.1
  gouty 274.89 [357.4]
  hypoglossal (nerve) 352.5
  ilioinguinal (nerve) 355.8
  in diseases classified elsewhere - *see*
      Polyneuropathy,
  infectious (multiple) 357.0
  intercostal (nerve) 353.8
  interstitial hypertrophic progressive
      NEC 356.9
  leg 355.8
  lumbosacral NEC 724.4
  median (nerve) 354.1
    thenar 354.1
  multiple (acute) (infective) 356.9
    endemic 265.0 [357.4]
  multiplex endemica 265.0 [357.4]
  nerve root (*see also* Radiculitis) 729.2
  oculomotor (nerve) 378.52
  olfactory (nerve) 352.0
  optic (nerve) 377.30
    in myelitis 341.0
    meningococcal 036.81
  pelvic 355.8
  peripheral (nerve) - *see also*
      Neuropathy, peripheral
    complicating pregnancy or
        puerperium 646.4●
    specified nerve NEC - *see*
        Mononeuritis
  pneumogastric (nerve) 352.3
  postchickenpox 052.7
  postherpetic 053.19
  progressive hypertrophic interstitial
      NEC 356.9
  puerperal, postpartum 646.4●
  radial (nerve) 723.4
  retrobulbar 377.32
    syphilitic 094.85
  rheumatic (chronic) 729.2
  sacral region 355.8
  sciatic (nerve) 724.3
    due to displacement of
        intervertebral disc 722.10
  serum 999.5
  specified nerve NEC - *see* Disorder,
      nerve
  spinal (nerve) 355.9
    root (*see also* Radiculitis) 729.2
  subscapular (nerve) 723.4
  suprascapular (nerve) 723.4
  syphilitic 095.8
  thenar (median) 354.1
  thoracic NEC 724.4
  toxic NEC 357.7
  trochlear (nerve) 378.53

◀ New   ◀▥ Revised   ~~deleted~~ Deleted   ● Use Additional Digit(s)   ▨ Omit code

Neuritis (Continued)
  ulnar (nerve) 723.4
  vagus (nerve) 352.3
Neuroangiomatosis, encephalofacial
    759.6
Neuroastrocytoma (M9505/1) - see
    Neoplasm, by site, uncertain
    behavior
Neuro-avitaminosis 269.2
Neuroblastoma (M9500/3)
  olfactory (M9522/3) 160.0
  specified site - see Neoplasm, by site,
    malignant
  unspecified site 194.0
Neurochorioretinitis (see also
    Chorioretinitis) 363.20
Neurocirculatory asthenia 306.2
Neurocytoma (M9506/0) - see Neoplasm,
    by site, benign
Neurodermatitis (circumscribed)
    (circumscripta) (local) 698.3
  atopic 691.8
  diffuse (Brocq) 691.8
  disseminated 691.8
  nodulosa 698.3
Neuroencephalomyelopathy, optic 341.0
Neuroendocrine tumor - see Tumor,
    neuroendocrine
Neuroepithelioma (M9503/3) - see also
    Neoplasm, by site, malignant
  olfactory (M9521/3) 160.0
Neurofibroma (M9540/0) - see also
    Neoplasm, connective tissue, benign
  melanotic (M9541/0) - see Neoplasm,
    connective tissue, benign
  multiple (M9540/1) 237.70
    type 1 237.71
    type 2 237.72
  plexiform (M9550/0) - see Neoplasm,
    connective tissue, benign
Neurofibromatosis (multiple) (M9540/1)
    237.70
  acoustic 237.72
  malignant (M9540/3) - see Neoplasm,
    connective tissue, malignant
  type 1 237.71
  type 2 237.72
  von Recklinghausen's 237.71
Neurofibrosarcoma (M9540/3) - see
    Neoplasm, connective tissue,
    malignant
Neurogenic - see also condition
  bladder (atonic) (automatic)
    (autonomic) (flaccid) (hypertonic)
    (hypotonic) (inertia)
    (infranuclear) (irritable) (motor)
    (nonreflex) (nuclear) (paralysis)
    (reflex) (sensory) (spastic)
    (supranuclear) (uninhibited)
    596.54
    with cauda equina syndrome 344.61
  bowel 564.81
  heart 306.2
Neuroglioma (M9505/1) - see Neoplasm,
    by site, uncertain behavior
Neurolabyrinthitis (of Dix and Hallpike)
    386.12
Neurolathyrism 988.2
Neuroleprosy 030.1
Neuroleptic malignant syndrome 333.92
Neurolipomatosis 272.8
Neuroma (M9570/0) - see also Neoplasm,
    connective tissue, benign
  acoustic (nerve) (M9560/0) 225.1
  amputation (traumatic) - see also Injury,
    nerve, by site
    surgical complication (late) 997.61

Neuroma (Continued)
  appendix 211.3
  auditory nerve 225.1
  digital 355.6
    toe 355.6
  interdigital (toe) 355.6
  intermetatarsal 355.6
  Morton's 355.6
  multiple 237.70
    type 1 237.71
    type 2 237.72
  nonneoplastic 355.9
    arm NEC 354.9
    leg NEC 355.8
    lower extremity NEC 355.8
    specified site NEC - see
      Mononeuritis, by site
    upper extremity NEC 354.9
  optic (nerve) 225.1
  plantar 355.6
  plexiform (M9550/0) - see Neoplasm,
    connective tissue, benign
  surgical (nonneoplastic) 355.9
    arm NEC 354.9
    leg NEC 355.8
    lower extremity NEC 355.8
    upper extremity NEC 354.9
  traumatic - see also Injury, nerve,
    by site old - see Neuroma,
    nonneoplastic
Neuromyalgia 729.1
Neuromyasthenia (epidemic) 049.8
Neuromyelitis 341.8
  ascending 357.0
  optica 341.0
Neuromyopathy NEC 358.9
Neuromyositis 729.1
Neuronevus (M8725/0) - see Neoplasm,
    skin, benign
Neuronitis 357.0
  ascending (acute) 355.2
  vestibular 386.12
Neuroparalytic - see condition
Neuropathy, neuropathic (see also
    Disorder, nerve) 355.9
  acute motor 357.82
  alcoholic 357.5
    with psychosis 291.1
  arm NEC 354.9
  ataxia and retinitis pigmentosa (NARP
    syndrome) 277.87
  autonomic (peripheral) - see
    Neuropathy, peripheral,
    autonomic
  axillary nerve 353.0
  brachial plexus 353.0
  cervical plexus 353.2
  chronic
    progressive segmentally
      demyelinating 357.89
    relapsing demyelinating 357.89
  congenital sensory 356.2
  Déjérine-Sottas 356.0
  diabetic 250.6● [357.2]
    autonomic (peripheral) 250.6
      [337.1]   ◄
    due to secondary diabetes 249.6●
      [357.2]
      autonomic (peripheral) 249.6
        [337.1]   ◄
  entrapment 355.9
    iliohypogastric nerve
      355.79
    ilioinguinal nerve 355.79

Neuropathy, neuropathic (Continued)
  entrapment (Continued)
    lateral cutaneous nerve of thigh 355.1
    median nerve 354.0
    obturator nerve 355.79
    peroneal nerve 355.3
    posterior tibial nerve 355.5
    saphenous nerve 355.79
    ulnar nerve 354.2
  facial nerve 351.9
  hereditary 356.9
    peripheral 356.0
    sensory (radicular) 356.2
  hypertrophic
    Charcôt-Marie-Tooth 356.1
    Déjérine-Sottas 356.0
    interstitial 356.9
    Refsum 356.3
  intercostal nerve 354.8
  ischemic - see Disorder, nerve
  Jamaican (ginger) 357.7
  leg NEC 355.8
  lower extremity NEC 355.8
  lumbar plexus 353.1
  median nerve 354.1
  motor
    acute 357.82
  multiple (acute) (chronic) (see also
    Polyneuropathy) 356.9
  optic 377.39
    ischemic 377.41
    nutritional 377.33
    toxic 377.34
  peripheral (nerve) (see also
    Polyneuropathy) 356.9
    arm NEC 354.9
    autonomic 337.9
      amyloid 277.39 [337.1]
      idiopathic 337.00
      in
        amyloidosis 277.39 [337.1]
        diabetes (mellitus) 250.6●
          [337.1]
          due to secondary diabetes
            249.6● [337.1]
        diseases classified elsewhere
          337.1
        gout 274.89 [337.1]
        hyperthyroidism 242.9●
          [337.1]
      due to
        antitetanus serum 357.6
        arsenic 357.7
        drugs 357.6
        lead 357.7
        organophosphate compounds
          357.7
        toxic agent NEC 357.7
    hereditary 356.0
    idiopathic 356.9
      progressive 356.4
      specified type NEC 356.8
    in diseases classified elsewhere - see
      Polyneuropathy, in
    leg NEC 355.8
    lower extremity NEC 355.8
    upper extremity NEC 354.9
  plantar nerves 355.6
  progressive hypertrophic interstitial
    356.9   ◄▦
    hypertrophic interstitial 356.9   ◄
    inflammatory 357.89   ◄
  radicular NEC 729.2
    brachial 723.4
    cervical NEC 723.4

Neuropathy, neuropathic *(Continued)*
  radicular NEC *(Continued)*
    hereditary sensory 356.2
      lumbar 724.4
      lumbosacral 724.4
      thoracic NEC 724.4
    sacral plexus 353.1
    sciatic 355.0
    spinal nerve NEC 355.9
      root *(see also* Radiculitis) 729.2
    toxic 357.7
    trigeminal sensory 350.8
    ulnar nerve 354.2
    upper extremity NEC 354.9
    uremic 585.9 *[357.4]*
    vitamin B_{12} 266.2 *[357.4]*
      with anemia (pernicious) 281.0
        [357.4]
        due to dietary deficiency 281.1
          [357.4]
Neurophthisis - *see also* Disorder, nerve
  peripheral 356.9
  diabetic 250.6● *[357.2]*
    due to secondary diabetes 249.6●
      [357.2]
Neuropraxia - *see* Injury, nerve
Neuroretinitis 363.05
  syphilitic 094.85
Neurosarcoma (M9540/3) - *see* Neoplasm,
  connective tissue, malignant
Neurosclerosis - *see* Disorder, nerve
Neurosis, neurotic 300.9
  accident 300.16
  anancastic, anankastic 300.3
  anxiety (state) 300.00
    generalized 300.02
    panic type 300.01
  asthenic 300.5
  bladder 306.53
  cardiac (reflex) 306.2
  cardiovascular 306.2
  climacteric, unspecified type 627.2
  colon 306.4
  compensation 300.16
  compulsive, compulsion 300.3
  conversion 300.11
  craft 300.89
  cutaneous 306.3
  depersonalization 300.6
  depressive (reaction) (type) 300.4
  endocrine 306.6
  environmental 300.89
  fatigue 300.5
  functional *(see also* Disorder,
    psychosomatic) 306.9
  gastric 306.4
  gastrointestinal 306.4
  genitourinary 306.50
  heart 306.2
  hypochondriacal 300.7
  hysterical 300.10
    conversion type 300.11
    dissociative type 300.15
  impulsive 300.3
  incoordination 306.0
    larynx 306.1
    vocal cord 306.1
  intestine 306.4
  larynx 306.1
    hysterical 300.11
    sensory 306.1
  menopause, unspecified type
    627.2
  mixed NEC 300.89

Neurosis, neurotic *(Continued)*
  musculoskeletal 306.0
  obsessional 300.3
    phobia 300.3
  obsessive-compulsive 300.3
  occupational 300.89
  ocular 306.7
  oral 307.0
  organ *(see also* Disorder,
    psychosomatic) 306.9
  pharynx 306.1
  phobic 300.20
  posttraumatic (acute) (situational)
    309.81
    chronic 309.81
  psychasthenic (type) 300.89
  railroad 300.16
  rectum 306.4
  respiratory 306.1
  rumination 306.4
  senile 300.89
  sexual 302.70
  situational 300.89
  specified type NEC 300.89
  state 300.9
    with depersonalization episode
      300.6
  stomach 306.4
  vasomotor 306.2
  visceral 306.4
  war 300.16
Neurospongioblastosis diffusa 759.5
Neurosyphilis (arrested) (early)
  (inactive) (late) (latent) (recurrent)
  094.9
  with ataxia (cerebellar) (locomotor)
    (spastic) (spinal) 094.0
  acute meningitis 094.2
  aneurysm 094.89
  arachnoid (adhesive) 094.2
  arteritis (any artery) 094.89
  asymptomatic 094.3
  congenital 090.40
  dura (mater) 094.89
  general paresis 094.1
  gumma 094.9
  hemorrhagic 094.9
  juvenile (asymptomatic) (meningeal)
    090.40
  leptomeninges (aseptic) 094.2
  meningeal 094.2
  meninges (adhesive) 094.2
  meningovascular (diffuse) 094.2
  optic atrophy 094.84
  parenchymatous (degenerative) 094.1
  paresis *(see also* Paresis, general) 094.1
  paretic *(see also* Paresis, general) 094.1
  relapse 094.9
  remission in (sustained) 094.9
  serological 094.3
  specified nature or site NEC
    094.89
  tabes (dorsalis) 094.0
    juvenile 090.40
  tabetic 094.0
    juvenile 090.40
  taboparesis 094.1
    juvenile 090.40
  thrombosis 094.89
  vascular 094.89
Neurotic *(see also* Neurosis) 300.9
  excoriation 698.4
    psychogenic 306.3
Neurotmesis - *see* Injury, nerve, by site

Neurotoxemia - *see* Toxemia
Neutro-occlusion 524.21
Neutropenia, neutropenic (idiopathic)
  (pernicious) (primary) 288.00
  chronic 288.09
    hypoplastic 288.09
  congenital (nontransient) 288.01
  cyclic 288.02
  drug induced 288.03
  due to infection 288.04
  fever 288.00
  genetic 288.01
  immune 288.09
  infantile 288.01
  malignant 288.09
  neonatal, transitory (isoimmune)
    (maternal transfer) 776.7
  periodic 288.02
  splenic 289.53
  splenomegaly 289.53
  toxic 288.09
Neutrophilia, hereditary giant
  288.2
Nevocarcinoma (M8720/3) - *see*
  Melanoma
Nevus (M8720/0) - *see also* Neoplasm,
  skin, benign

> **Note 55**   Except where otherwise indicated, varieties of nevus in the list below that are followed by a morphology code number (M----/0) should be coded by site as for "Neoplasm, skin, benign."

  acanthotic 702.8
  achromic (M8730/0)
  amelanotic (M8730/0)
  anemic, anemicus 709.09
  angiomatous (M9120/0) *(see also*
    Hemangioma) 228.00
  araneus 448.1
  avasculosus 709.09
  balloon cell (M8722/0)
  bathing trunk (M8761/1) 238.2
  blue (M8780/0)
    cellular (M8790/0)
    giant (M8790/0)
    Jadassohn's (M8780/0)
    malignant (M8780/3) - *see*
      Melanoma
  capillary (M9131/0) *(see also*
    Hemangioma) 228.00
  cavernous (M9121/0) *(see also*
    Hemangioma) 228.00
  cellular (M8720/0)
    blue (M8790/0)
  comedonicus 757.33
  compound (M8760/0)
  conjunctiva (M8720/0) 224.3
  dermal (8750/0)
    and epidermal (M8760/0)
  epithelioid cell (and spindle cell)
    (M8770/0)
  flammeus 757.32
    osteohypertrophic 759.89
  hairy (M8720/0)
  halo (M8723/0)
  hemangiomatous (M9120/0) *(see also*
    Hemangioma) 228.00
  intradermal (M8750/0)
  intraepidermal (M8740/0)
  involuting (M8724/0)
  Jadassohn's (blue) (M8780/0)

◀ New   ◀▬ Revised   ~~deleted~~ Deleted   ● Use Additional Digit(s)   ▨ Omit code

Nevus *(Continued)*
   junction, junctional (M8740/0)
      malignant melanoma in (M8740/3) -
        see Melanoma
   juvenile (M8770/0)
   lymphatic (M9170/0) 228.1
   magnocellular (M8726/0)
      specified site - *see* Neoplasm, by site,
        benign
      unspecified site 224.0
   malignant (M8720/3) - *see* Melanoma
   meaning hemangioma (M9120/0) (*see
      also* Hemangioma) 228.00
   melanotic (pigmented) (M8720/0)
   multiplex 759.5
   nonneoplastic 448.1
   nonpigmented (M8730/0)
   nonvascular (M8720/0)
   oral mucosa, white sponge 750.26
   osteohypertrophic, flammeus
      759.89
   papillaris (M8720/0)
   papillomatosus (M8720/0)
   pigmented (M8720/0)
      giant (M8761/1) - *see also* Neoplasm,
        skin, uncertain behavior
        malignant melanoma in
          (M8761/3) - *see* Melanoma
      systematicus 757.33
   pilosus (M8720/0)
   port wine 757.32
   sanguineous 757.32
   sebaceous (senile) 702.8
   senile 448.1
   spider 448.1
   spindle cell (and epithelioid cell)
      (M8770/0)
   stellar 448.1
   strawberry 757.32
   syringocystadenomatous papilliferous
      (M8406/0)
   unius lateris 757.33
   Unna's 757.32
   vascular 757.32
   verrucous 757.33
   white sponge (oral mucosa) 750.26
Newborn (infant) (liveborn) ◄
   abstinence syndrome 779.5
   affected by
      amniocentesis 760.61
      maternal abuse of drugs
         (gestational) (via placenta) (via
         breast milk) (*see also* Noxious,
         substances transmitted
         through placenta
         or breast milk (affecting fetus
         or newborn)) 760.70
         methamphetamine(s) 760.72
      procedure
         amniocentesis 760.61
         in utero NEC 760.62
         surgical on mother
          during pregnancy NEC
           760.63
          previous not associated with
           pregnancy 760.64
   apnea 770.81
      obstructive 770.82
      specified NEC 770.82
   breast buds 779.89
   cardiomyopathy 425.4
      congenital 425.3
   convulsion 779.0
   electrolyte imbalance NEC (transitory)
      775.5

Newborn *(Continued)*
   fever (environmentally-induced)
      778.4
   gestation
      24 completed weeks 765.22
      25–26 completed weeks 765.23
      27–28 completed weeks 765.24
      29–30 completed weeks 765.25
      31–32 completed weeks 765.26
      33–34 completed weeks 765.27
      35–36 completed weeks 765.28
      37 or more completed weeks 765.29
      less than 24 completed weeks
        765.21
      unspecified completed weeks
        765.20
   infection 771.89
      candida 771.7
      mastitis 771.5
      specified NEC 771.89
      urinary tract 771.82
   mastitis 771.5
   multiple NEC
      born in hospital (without mention of
        cesarean delivery or section)
        V37.00
        with cesarean delivery or section
          V37.01
      born outside hospital
        hospitalized V37.1●
        not hospitalized V37.2●
      mates all liveborn
        born in hospital (without
          mention of cesarean
          delivery or section)
          V34.00
          with cesarean delivery or
           section V34.01
        born outside hospital
          hospitalized V34.1●
          not hospitalized V34.2●
      mates all stillborn
        born in hospital (without
          mention of cesarean
          delivery or section)
          V35.00
          with cesarean delivery or
           section V35.01
        born outside hospital
          hospitalized V35.1●
          not hospitalized V35.2●
      mates liveborn and stillborn
        born in hospital (without
          mention of cesarean
          delivery or section)
          V36.00
          with cesarean delivery or
           section V36.01
        born outside hospital
          hospitalized V36.1●
          not hospitalized V36.2●
   omphalitis 771.4
   seizure 779.0
   sepsis 771.81
   single
      born in hospital (without mention of
        cesarean delivery or section)
        V30.00
        with cesarean delivery or section
          V30.01
      born outside hospital
        hospitalized V30.1●
        not hospitalized V30.2●
   specified condition NEC 779.89

Newborn *(Continued)*
   twin NEC
      born in hospital (without mention of
        cesarean delivery or section)
        V33.00
        with cesarean delivery or section
          V33.01
      born outside hospital
        hospitalized V33.1●
        not hospitalized V33.2●
      mate liveborn
        born in hospital V31.0●
        born outside hospital
          hospitalized V31.1●
          not hospitalized V31.2●
      mate stillborn
        born in hospital V32.0●
        born outside hospital
          hospitalized V32.1●
          not hospitalized V32.2●
   unspecified as to single or multiple
      birth
      born in hospital (without mention of
        cesarean delivery or section)
        V39.00
        with cesarean delivery or section
          V39.01
      born outside hospital
        hospitalized V39.1●
        not hospitalized V39.2●
   weight check V20.32 ◄
Newcastle's conjunctivitis or disease
   077.8
Nezelof's syndrome (pure
   alymphocytosis) 279.13
Niacin (amide) deficiency 265.2
Nicolas-Durand-Favre disease (climatic
   bubo) 099.1
Nicolas-Favre disease (climatic bubo)
   099.1
Nicotinic acid (amide) deficiency
   265.2
Niemann-Pick disease (lipid
   histiocytosis) (splenomegaly)
   272.7
Night
   blindness (*see also* Blindness, night)
      368.60
      congenital 368.61
      vitamin A deficiency 264.5
   cramps 729.82
   sweats 780.8
   terrors, child 307.46
Nightmare 307.47
   REM-sleep type 307.47
Nipple - *see* condition
Nisbet's chancre 099.0
Nishimoto (-Takeuchi) disease 437.5
Nitritoid crisis or reaction - *see* Crisis,
   nitritoid
Nitrogen retention, extrarenal 788.99
Nitrosohemoglobinemia 289.89
Njovera 104.0
No
   diagnosis 799.9
   disease (found) V71.9
   room at the inn V65.0
Nocardiasis - *see* Nocardiosis
Nocardiosis 039.9
   with pneumonia 039.1
   lung 039.1
   specified type NEC 039.8
Nocturia 788.43
   psychogenic 306.53

Nocturnal - *see also* condition
  dyspnea (paroxysmal) 786.09
  emissions 608.89
  enuresis 788.36
    psychogenic 307.6
  frequency (micturition) 788.43
    psychogenic 306.53
Nodal rhythm disorder 427.89
Nodding of head 781.0
Node(s) - *see also* Nodules
  Heberden's 715.04
  larynx 478.79
  lymph - *see* condition
  milkers' 051.1
  Osler's 421.0
  rheumatic 729.89
  Schmorl's 722.30
    lumbar, lumbosacral 722.32
    specified region NEC 722.39
    thoracic, thoracolumbar 722.31
  singers' 478.5
  skin NEC 782.2
  tuberculous - *see* Tuberculosis, lymph
    gland
  vocal cords 478.5
Nodosities, Haygarth's 715.04
Nodule(s), nodular
  actinomycotic (*see also* Actinomycosis)
    039.9
  arthritic - *see* Arthritis, nodosa
  breast 793.89
  cutaneous 782.2
  Haygarth's 715.04
  inflammatory - *see* Inflammation
  juxta-articular 102.7
    syphilitic 095.7
    yaws 102.7
  larynx 478.79
  lung, solitary 518.89
    emphysematous 492.8
  milkers' 051.1
  prostate 600.10
    with
      urinary
        obstruction 600.11
        retention 600.11
  retrocardiac 785.9
  rheumatic 729.89
  rheumatoid - *see* Arthritis rheumatoid
  scrotum (inflammatory) 608.4
  singers' 478.5
  skin NEC 782.2
  solitary, lung 518.89
    emphysematous 492.8
  subcutaneous 782.2
  thyroid (gland) (nontoxic) (uninodular)
    241.0
    with
      hyperthyroidism 242.1●
      thyrotoxicosis 242.1●
    toxic or with hyperthyroidism
      242.1●
  vocal cords 478.5
Noma (gangrenous) (hospital) (infective)
  528.1
  auricle (*see also* Gangrene) 785.4
  mouth 528.1
  pudendi (*see also* Vulvitis) 616.10
  vulvae (*see also* Vulvitis) 616.10
Nomadism V60.0
Non-adherence
  artificial skin graft 996.55
  decellularized allodermis graft
    996.55

Non-autoimmune hemolytic anemia
  NEC 283.10
Nonclosure - *see also* Imperfect, closure
  ductus
    arteriosus 747.0
    Botalli 747.0
  Eustachian valve 746.89
  foramen
    Botalli 745.5
    ovale 745.5
Noncompliance with medical treatment
  V15.81
  renal dialysis V45.12
Nondescent (congenital) - *see also*
  Malposition, congenital
  cecum 751.4
  colon 751.4
  testis 752.51
Nondevelopment
  brain 742.1
    specified part 742.2
  heart 746.89
  organ or site, congenital NEC - *see*
    Hypoplasia
Nonengagement
  head NEC 652.5●
    in labor 660.1●
      affecting fetus or newborn 763.1
Nonexanthematous tick fever 066.1
Nonexpansion, lung (newborn) NEC 770.4
Nonfunctioning
  cystic duct (*see also* Disease,
    gallbladder) 575.8
  gallbladder (*see also* Disease,
    gallbladder) 575.8
  kidney (*see also* Disease, renal) 593.9
  labyrinth 386.58
Nonhealing
  stump (surgical) 997.69
  wound, surgical 998.83
Nonimplantation of ovum, causing
  infertility 628.3
Noninsufflation, fallopian tube 628.2
Nonne-Milroy-Meige syndrome (chronic
  hereditary edema) 757.0
Nonovulation 628.0
Nonpatent fallopian tube 628.2
Nonpneumatization, lung NEC 770.4
Nonreflex bladder 596.54
  with cauda equina 344.61
Nonretention of food - *see* Vomiting
Nonrotation - *see* Malrotation
Nonsecretion, urine (*see also* Anuria)
  788.5
  newborn 753.3
Nonunion
  fracture 733.82
  organ or site, congenital NEC - *see*
    Imperfect, closure
  symphysis pubis, congenital 755.69
  top sacrum, congenital 756.19
Nonviability 765.0●
Nonvisualization, gallbladder 793.3
Nonvitalized tooth 522.9
Non-working side interference 524.56
Normal
  delivery - *see* category 650
  menses V65.5
  state (feared complaint unfounded)
    V65.5
Normoblastosis 289.89
Normocytic anemia (infectional) 285.9
  due to blood loss (chronic) 280.0
    acute 285.1

Norrie's disease (congenital) (progressive
  oculoacousticocerebral
  degeneration) 743.8
North American blastomycosis
  116.0
Norwegian itch 133.0
Nose, nasal - *see* condition
Nosebleed 784.7
Nosomania 298.9
Nosophobia 300.29
Nostalgia 309.89
Notch of iris 743.46
Notched lip, congenital (*see also* Cleft,
  lip) 749.10
Notching nose, congenital (tip) 748.1
Nothnagel's
  syndrome 378.52
  vasomotor acroparesthesia 443.89
Novy's relapsing fever (American)
  087.1
Noxious
  foodstuffs, poisoning by
    fish 988.0
    fungi 988.1
    mushrooms 988.1
    plants (food) 988.2
    shellfish 988.0
    specified type NEC 988.8
    toadstool 988.1
  substances transmitted through
    placenta or breast milk
    (affecting fetus or newborn)
    760.70
    acetretin 760.78
    alcohol 760.71
    aminopterin 760.78
    antiandrogens 760.79
    anticonvulsant 760.77
    antifungal 760.74
    anti-infective agents 760.74
    antimetabolic 760.78
    atorvastatin 760.78
    carbamazepine 760.77
    cocaine 760.75
    "crack" 760.75
    diethylstilbestrol (DES) 760.76
    divalproex sodium 760.77
    endocrine disrupting chemicals
      760.79
    estrogens 760.79
    etretinate 760.78
    fluconazole 760.74
    fluvastatin 760.78
    hallucinogenic agents NEC 760.73
    hormones 760.79
    lithium 760.79
    lovastatin 760.78
    medicinal agents NEC 760.79
    methotrexate 760.78
    misoprostil 760.79
    narcotics 760.72
    obstetric anesthetic or analgesic
      763.5
    phenobarbital 760.77
    phenytoin 760.77
    pravastatin 760.78
    progestins 760.79
    retinoic acid 760.78
    simvastatin 760.78
    solvents 760.79
    specified agent NEC 760.79
    statins 760.78
    suspected, affecting management of
      pregnancy 655.5●

Noxious *(Continued)*
  substances transmitted through placenta
    or breast milk *(Continued)*
    tetracycline 760.74
    thalidomide 760.79
    trimethadione 760.77
    valproate 760.77
    valproic acid 760.77
    vitamin A 760.78
NPDH (new persistent daily headache)
  339.42
Nuchal hitch (arm) 652.8●
Nucleus pulposus - *see* condition
Numbness 782.0
Nuns' knee 727.2
Nursemaid's
  elbow 832.2●   ◀▥
  shoulder 831.0●

Nutmeg liver 573.8
Nutrition, deficient or insufficient
  (particular kind of food)
  269.9
  due to
    insufficient food 994.2
    lack of
      care (child) (infant) 995.52
        adult 995.84
      food 994.2
Nyctalopia (*see also* Blindness, night)
  368.60
  vitamin A deficiency 264.5
Nycturia 788.43
  psychogenic 306.53
Nymphomania 302.89

Nystagmus 379.50
  associated with vestibular system
    disorders 379.54
  benign paroxysmal positional 386.11
  central positional 386.2
  congenital 379.51
  deprivation 379.53
  dissociated 379.55
  latent 379.52
  miners' 300.89
  positional
    benign paroxysmal 386.11
    central 386.2
  specified NEC 379.56
  vestibular 379.54
  visual deprivation 379.53

O

Oasthouse urine disease 270.2
Obermeyer's relapsing fever (European) 087.0
Obesity (constitutional) (exogenous) (familial) (nutritional) (simple) 278.00
  adrenal 255.8
  complicating pregnancy, childbirth, or puerperium 649.1●
  due to hyperalimentation 278.00
  endocrine NEC 259.9
  endogenous 259.9
  Fröhlich's (adiposogenital dystrophy) 253.8
  glandular NEC 259.9
  hypothyroid (see also Hypothyroidism) 244.9
  morbid 278.01
  of pregnancy 649.1●
  pituitary 253.8
  severe 278.01
  thyroid (see also Hypothyroidism) 244.9
Oblique - see also condition
  lie before labor, affecting fetus or newborn 761.7
Obliquity, pelvis 738.6
Obliteration
  abdominal aorta 446.7
  appendix (lumen) 543.9
  artery 447.1
  ascending aorta 446.7
  bile ducts 576.8
    with calculus, choledocholithiasis, or stones - see Choledocholithiasis
    congenital 751.61
      jaundice from 751.61 [774.5]
  common duct 576.8
    with calculus, choledocholithiasis, or stones - see Choledocholithiasis
    congenital 751.61
  cystic duct 575.8
    with calculus, choledocholithiasis, or stones - see Choledocholithiasis
  disease, arteriolar 447.1
  endometrium 621.8
  eye, anterior chamber 360.34
  fallopian tube 628.2
  lymphatic vessel 457.1
    postmastectomy 457.0
  organ or site, congenital NEC - see Atresia
  placental blood vessels - see Placenta, abnormal
  supra-aortic branches 446.7
  ureter 593.89
  urethra 599.84
  vein 459.9
  vestibule (oral) 525.8
Observation (for) V71.9
  without need for further medical care V71.9
  accident NEC V71.4
    at work V71.3
  criminal assault V71.6
  deleterious agent ingestion V71.89
  disease V71.9
    cardiovascular V71.7
    heart V71.7

Observation (Continued)
  disease (Continued)
    mental V71.09
    specified condition NEC V71.89
  foreign body ingestion V71.89
  growth and development variations V21.8
  injuries (accidental) V71.4
    inflicted NEC V71.6
      during alleged rape or seduction V71.5
  malignant neoplasm, suspected V71.1
  postpartum
    immediately after delivery V24.0
    routine follow-up V24.2
  pregnancy
    high-risk V23.9
      specified problem NEC V23.89
    normal (without complication) V22.1
      with nonobstetric complication V22.2
    first V22.0
  rape or seduction, alleged V71.5
    injury during V71.5
  suicide attempt, alleged V71.89
  suspected (undiagnosed) (unproven)
    abuse V71.81
    cardiovascular disease V71.7
    child or wife battering victim V71.6
    concussion (cerebral) V71.6
    condition NEC V71.89
      infant - see Observation, suspected, condition, newborn
    maternal and fetal
      amniotic cavity and membrane problem V89.01
      cervical shortening V89.05
      fetal anomaly V89.03
      fetal growth problem V89.04
      oligohydramnios V89.01
      other specified problem NEC V89.09
      placental problem V89.02
      polyhydramnios V89.01
    newborn V29.9
      cardiovascular disease V29.8
      congenital anomaly V29.8
      genetic V29.3
      infectious V29.0
      ingestion foreign object V29.8
      injury V29.8
      metabolic V29.3
      neoplasm V29.8
      neurological V29.1
      poison, poisoning V29.8
      respiratory V29.2
      specified NEC V29.8
    exposure
      anthrax V71.82
      biologic agent NEC V71.83
      SARS V71.83
    infectious disease not requiring isolation V71.89
    malignant neoplasm V71.1
    mental disorder V71.09
    neglect V71.81
    neoplasm
      benign V71.89
      malignant V71.1
    specified condition NEC V71.89
    tuberculosis V71.2
  tuberculosis, suspected V71.2

Obsession, obsessional 300.3
  ideas and mental images 300.3
  impulses 300.3
  neurosis 300.3
  phobia 300.3
  psychasthenia 300.3
  ruminations 300.3
  state 300.3
  syndrome 300.3
Obsessive-compulsive 300.3
  neurosis 300.3
  personality 301.4
  reaction 300.3
Obstetrical trauma NEC (complicating delivery) 665.9●
  with
    abortion - see Abortion, by type, with damage to pelvic organs
    ectopic pregnancy (see also categories 633.0-633.9) 639.2
    molar pregnancy (see also categories 630-632) 639.2
  affecting fetus or newborn 763.89
  following
    abortion 639.2
    ectopic or molar pregnancy 639.2
Obstipation (see also Constipation) 564.00
  psychogenic 306.4
Obstruction, obstructed, obstructive
  airway NEC 519.8
    with
      allergic alveolitis NEC 495.9
      asthma NEC (see also Asthma) 493.9●
      bronchiectasis 494.0
        with acute exacerbation 494.1
      bronchitis (see also Bronchitis, with, obstruction) 491.20
      emphysema NEC 492.8
    chronic 496
      with
        allergic alveolitis NEC 495.5
        asthma NEC (see also Asthma) 493.2●
        bronchiectasis 494.0
          with acute exacerbation 494.1
        bronchitis (chronic) (see also Bronchitis, chronic, obstructive) 491.20
        emphysema NEC 492.8
    due to
      bronchospasm 519.11
      foreign body 934.9
      inhalation of fumes or vapors 506.9
      laryngospasm 478.75
  alimentary canal (see also Obstruction, intestine) 560.9
  ampulla of Vater 576.2
    with calculus, cholelithiasis, or stones - see Choledocholithiasis
  aortic (heart) (valve) (see also Stenosis, aortic) 424.1
    rheumatic (see also Stenosis, aortic, rheumatic) 395.0
  aortoiliac 444.0
  aqueduct of Sylvius 331.4
    congenital 742.3
      with spina bifida (see also Spina bifida) 741.0●
  Arnold-Chiari (see also Spina bifida) 741.0●

◀ New   ◀▥ Revised   ~~deleted~~ Deleted   ● Use Additional Digit(s)   ▭ Omit code

Obstruction, obstructed, obstructive
(Continued)
artery (see also Embolism, artery) 444.9
  basilar (complete) (partial) (see also
      Occlusion, artery, basilar)
      433.0●
  carotid (complete) (partial) (see also
      Occlusion, artery, carotid)
      433.1●
  precerebral - see Occlusion, artery,
      precerebral NEC
  retinal (central) (see also Occlusion,
      retina) 362.30
  vertebral (complete) (partial) (see
      also Occlusion, artery,
      vertebral) 433.2●
asthma (chronic) (with obstructive
    pulmonary disease) 493.2●
band (intestinal) 560.81
bile duct or passage (see also
    Obstruction, biliary) 576.2
  congenital 751.61
    jaundice from 751.61 [774.5]
biliary (duct) (tract) 576.2
  with calculus 574.51
    with cholecystitis (chronic) 574.41
      acute 574.31
  congenital 751.61
    jaundice from 751.61 [774.5]
  gallbladder 575.2
    with calculus 574.21
      with cholecystitis (chronic)
          574.11
        acute 574.01
bladder neck (acquired) 596.0
  congenital 753.6
bowel (see also Obstruction, intestine)
    560.9
bronchus 519.19
canal, ear (see also Stricture, ear canal,
    acquired) 380.50
cardia 537.89
caval veins (inferior) (superior) 459.2
cecum (see also Obstruction, intestine)
    560.9
circulatory 459.9
colon (see also Obstruction, intestine)
    560.9
  sympathicotonic 560.89
common duct (see also Obstruction,
    biliary) 576.2
  congenital 751.61
coronary (artery) (heart) - (see also
    Arteriosclerosis, coronary)
  acute (see also Infarct, myocardium)
      410.9●
    without myocardial infarction
        411.81
cystic duct (see also Obstruction,
    gallbladder) 575.2
  congenital 751.61
device, implant, or graft - see
    Complications, due to (presence
    of) any device, implant, or graft
    classified to 996.0–996.5 NEC
due to foreign body accidentally left in
    operation wound 998.4
duodenum 537.3
  congenital 751.1
  due to
    compression NEC 537.3
    cyst 537.3
    intrinsic lesion or disease NEC
        537.3

Obstruction, obstructed, obstructive
(Continued)
duodenum (Continued)
  due to (Continued)
    scarring 537.3
    torsion 537.3
    ulcer 532.91
    volvulus 537.3
ejaculatory duct 608.89
endocardium 424.90
  arteriosclerotic 424.99
  specified cause, except rheumatic
      424.99
esophagus 530.3
Eustachian tube (complete) (partial)
    381.60
  cartilaginous
    extrinsic 381.63
    intrinsic 381.62
  due to
    cholesteatoma 381.61
    osseous lesion NEC 381.61
    polyp 381.61
  osseous 381.61
fallopian tube (bilateral) 628.2
fecal 560.39
  with hernia - see also Hernia, by site,
      with obstruction
    gangrenous - see Hernia, by site,
        with gangrene
foramen of Monro (congenital)
    742.3
  with spina bifida (see also Spina
      bifida) 741.0●
foreign body - see Foreign body
gallbladder 575.2
  with calculus, cholelithiasis, or
      stones 574.21
    with cholecystitis (chronic)
        574.11
      acute 574.01
  congenital 751.69
    jaundice from 751.69 [774.5]
gastric outlet 537.0
gastrointestinal (see also Obstruction,
    intestine) 560.9
glottis 478.79
hepatic 573.8
  duct (see also Obstruction, biliary)
      576.2
    congenital 751.61
  icterus (see also Obstruction, biliary)
      576.8
    congenital 751.61
ileocecal coil (see also Obstruction,
    intestine) 560.9
ileum (see also Obstruction, intestine)
    560.9
iliofemoral (artery) 444.81
internal anastomosis - see
    Complications, mechanical, graft
intestine (mechanical) (neurogenic)
    (paroxysmal) (postinfectional)
    (reflex) 560.9
  with
    adhesions (intestinal) (peritoneal)
        560.81
    hernia - see also Hernia, by site,
        with obstruction
      gangrenous - see Hernia, by
          site, with gangrene
  adynamic (see also Ileus)
      560.1
  by gallstone 560.31

Obstruction, obstructed, obstructive
(Continued)
intestine (Continued)
  congenital or infantile (small)
      751.1
    large 751.2
  due to
    Ascaris lumbricoides 127.0
    mural thickening 560.89
    procedure 997.4
      involving urinary tract
          997.5
  impaction 560.39
  infantile - see Obstruction, intestine,
      congenital
  newborn
    due to
      fecaliths 777.1
      inspissated milk 777.2
      meconium (plug) 777.1
        in mucoviscidosis
            277.01
      transitory 777.4
    specified cause NEC 560.89
    transitory, newborn 777.4
  volvulus 560.2
intracardiac ball valve prosthesis
    996.02
jaundice (see also Obstruction, biliary)
    576.8
  congenital 751.61
jejunum (see also Obstruction, intestine)
    560.9
kidney 593.89
labor 660.9●
  affecting fetus or newborn
      763.1
  by
    bony pelvis (conditions
        classifiable to 653.0–653.9)
        660.1●
    deep transverse arrest 660.3●
    impacted shoulder 660.4●
    locked twins 660.5●
    malposition (fetus) (conditions
        classifiable to 652.0–652.9)
        660.0●
    head during labor 660.3●
    persistent occipitoposterior
        position 660.3●
    soft tissue, pelvic (conditions
        classifiable to 654.0–654.9)
        660.2●
lacrimal
  canaliculi 375.53
  congenital 743.65
  punctum 375.52
  sac 375.54
lacrimonasal duct 375.56
  congenital 743.65
  neonatal 375.55
lacteal, with steatorrhea 579.2
laryngitis (see also Laryngitis) 464.01
larynx 478.79
  congenital 748.3
liver 573.8
  cirrhotic (see also Cirrhosis, liver)
      571.5
lung 518.89
  with
    asthma - see Asthma
    bronchitis (chronic) 491.20
    emphysema NEC 492.8
  airway, chronic 496

Obstruction, obstructed, obstructive
(Continued)
  lung *(Continued)*
    chronic NEC 496
      with
        asthma (chronic) (obstructive)
          493.2●
    disease, chronic 496
      with
        asthma (chronic) (obstructive)
          493.2●
    emphysematous 492.8
  lymphatic 457.1
  meconium
    fetus or newborn 777.1
      in mucoviscidosis 277.01
    newborn due to fecaliths 777.1
  mediastinum 519.3
  mitral (rheumatic) - *see* Stenosis,
    mitral
  nasal 478.19
    duct 375.56
      neonatal 375.55
    sinus - *see* Sinusitis
  nasolacrimal duct 375.56
    congenital 743.65
    neonatal 375.55
  nasopharynx 478.29
  nose 478.19
  organ or site, congenital NEC - *see*
    Atresia
  pancreatic duct 577.8
  parotid gland 527.8
  pelviureteral junction *(see also*
    Obstruction, ureter) 593.4
  pharynx 478.29
  portal (circulation) (vein) 452
  prostate 600.90
    with
      other lower urinary tract
        symptoms (LUTS) 600.91
      urinary
        obstruction 600.91
        retention 600.91
    valve (urinary) 596.0
  pulmonary
    valve (heart) *(see also* Endocarditis,
      pulmonary) 424.3
    vein, isolated 747.49
  pyemic - *see* Septicemia
  pylorus (acquired) 537.0
    congenital 750.5
    infantile 750.5
  rectosigmoid *(see also* Obstruction,
    intestine) 560.9
  rectum 569.49
  renal 593.89
  respiratory 519.8
    chronic 496
  retinal (artery) (vein) (central) *(see also*
    Occlusion, retina) 362.30
  salivary duct (any) 527.8
    with calculus 527.5
  sigmoid *(see also* Obstruction, intestine)
    560.9
  sinus (accessory) (nasal) *(see also*
    Sinusitis) 473.9
  Stensen's duct 527.8
  stomach 537.89
    acute 536.1
    congenital 750.7
  submaxillary gland 527.8
    with calculus 527.5
  thoracic duct 457.1
  thrombotic - *see* Thrombosis
  tooth eruption 520.6

Obstruction, obstructed, obstructive
(Continued)
  trachea 519.19
  tracheostomy airway 519.09
  tricuspid - *see* Endocarditis, tricuspid
  upper respiratory, congenital 748.8
  ureter (functional) 593.4
    congenital 753.20
    due to calculus 592.1
  ureteropelvic junction, congenital
    753.21
  ureterovesical junction, congenital
    753.22
  urethra 599.60
    congenital 753.6
  urinary (moderate) 599.60
    organ or tract (lower) 599.60
      due to
        benign prostatic hypertrophy
          (BPH) - *see* category
          600
      specified NEC 599.69
        due to
          benign prostatic
            hypertrophy (BPH) -
            see category 600
    prostatic valve 596.0
    specified NEC 599.69
      due to
        benign prostatic hypertrophy
          (BPH) - *see* category
          600
  uropathy 599.60
  uterus 621.8
  vagina 623.2
  valvular - *see* Endocarditis
  vascular graft or shunt 996.1
    atherosclerosis - *see* Arteriosclerosis,
      coronary
    embolism 996.74
    occlusion NEC 996.74
    thrombus 996.74
  vein, venous 459.2
    caval (inferior) (superior) 459.2
    thrombotic - *see* Thrombosis
  vena cava (inferior) (superior)
    459.2
  ventricular shunt 996.2
  vesical 596.0
  vesicourethral orifice 596.0
  vessel NEC 459.9
Obturator - *see* condition
Occlusal
  plane deviation 524.76
  wear, teeth 521.10
Occlusion
  anus 569.49
    congenital 751.2
    infantile 751.2
  aortoiliac (chronic) 444.0
  aqueduct of Sylvius 331.4
    congenital 742.3
      with spina bifida *(see also* Spina
        bifida) 741.0●
  arteries of extremities, lower 444.22
    without thrombus or embolus *(see*
      also Arteriosclerosis,
      extremities) 440.20
    due to stricture or stenosis 447.1
    upper 444.21
      without thrombus or embolus
        (see also Arteriosclerosis,
        extremities) 440.20
      due to stricture or stenosis
        447.1

Occlusion *(Continued)*
  artery NEC *(see also* Embolism, artery)
    444.9
    auditory, internal 433.8●
    basilar 433.0●
      with other precerebral artery
        433.3●
      bilateral 433.3●
    brain or cerebral *(see also* Infarct,
      brain) 434.9●
    carotid 433.1●
      with other precerebral artery
        433.3●
      bilateral 433.3●
    cerebellar (anterior inferior)
      (posterior inferior) (superior)
      433.8●
    cerebral *(see also* Infarct, brain)
      434.9●
    choroidal (anterior) 433.8●
    chronic total
      coronary 414.2
      extremity(ies) 440.4
    communicating posterior 433.8●
    complete
      coronary 414.2
      extremity(ies) 440.4
    coronary (thrombotic) *(see also*
      Infarct, myocardium)
      410.9●
      acute 410.9●
        without myocardial infarction
          411.81
      chronic total 414.2
      complete 414.2
      healed or old 412
      total 414.2
    extremity(ies)
      chronic total 440.4
      complete 440.4
      total 440.4
    hypophyseal 433.8●
    iliac 444.81
    mesenteric (embolic) (thrombotic)
      (with gangrene) 557.0
    pontine 433.8●
    precerebral NEC 433.9●
      late effect - *see* Late effect(s) (of)
        cerebrovascular disease
      multiple or bilateral 433.3●
      puerperal, postpartum, childbirth
        674.0●
      specified NEC 433.8●
    renal 593.81
    retinal - *see* Occlusion, retina, artery
    spinal 433.8●
    vertebral 433.2●
      with other precerebral artery
        433.3●
      bilateral 433.3●
  basilar (artery) - *see* Occlusion, artery,
    basilar
  bile duct (any) *(see also* Obstruction,
    biliary) 576.2
  bowel *(see also* Obstruction, intestine)
    560.9
  brain (artery) (vascular) *(see also* Infarct,
    brain) 434.9●
  breast (duct) 611.89
  carotid (artery) (common) (internal) -
    see Occlusion, artery, carotid
  cerebellar (anterior inferior) (artery)
    (posterior inferior) (superior)
    433.8●
  cerebral (artery) *(see also* Infarct, brain)
    434.9●

◄ New   ◄||| Revised   ~~deleted~~ Deleted   ● Use Additional Digit(s)   � Omit code

Occlusion (*Continued*)
  cerebrovascular (*see also* Infarct, brain) 434.9●
    diffuse 437.0
  cervical canal (*see also* Stricture, cervix) 622.4
    by falciparum malaria 084.0
  cervix (uteri) (*see also* Stricture, cervix) 622.4
  choanal 748.0
  choroidal (artery) 433.8●
  colon (*see also* Obstruction, intestine) 560.9
  communicating posterior artery 433.8●
  coronary (artery) (thrombotic) (*see also* Infarct, myocardium) 410.9●
    acute 410.9●
      without myocardial infarction 411.81
    healed or old 412
  cystic duct (*see also* Obstruction, gallbladder) 575.2
    congenital 751.69
  disto
    division I 524.22
    division II 524.22
  embolic - *see* Embolism
  fallopian tube 628.2
    congenital 752.19
  gallbladder (*see also* Obstruction, gallbladder) 575.2
    congenital 751.69
      jaundice from 751.69 [744.5]
  gingiva, traumatic 523.8
  hymen 623.3
    congenital 752.42
  hypophyseal (artery) 433.8●
  iliac (artery) 444.81
  intestine (*see also* Obstruction, intestine) 560.9
  kidney 593.89
  lacrimal apparatus - *see* Stenosis, lacrimal
  lung 518.89
  lymph or lymphatic channel 457.1
  mammary duct 611.89
  mesenteric artery (embolic) (thrombotic) (with gangrene) 557.0
  nose 478.19
    congenital 748.0
  organ or site, congenital NEC - *see* Atresia
  oviduct 628.2
    congenital 752.19
  periodontal, traumatic 523.8
  peripheral arteries (lower extremity) 444.22
    without thrombus or embolus (*see also* Arteriosclerosis, extremities) 440.20
    due to stricture or stenosis 447.1
    upper extremity 444.21
      without thrombus or embolus (*see also* Arteriosclerosis, extremities) 440.20
      due to stricture or stenosis 447.1
  pontine (artery) 433.8●
  posterior lingual, of mandibular teeth 524.29
  precerebral artery - *see* Occlusion, artery, precerebral NEC
  puncta lacrimalia 375.52
  pupil 364.74
  pylorus (*see also* Stricture, pylorus) 537.0

Occlusion (*Continued*)
  renal artery 593.81
  retina, retinal (vascular) 362.30
    artery, arterial 362.30
      branch 362.32
      central (total) 362.31
      partial 362.33
      transient 362.34
      tributary 362.32
    vein 362.30
      branch 362.36
      central (total) 362.35
      incipient 362.37
      partial 362.37
      tributary 362.36
  spinal artery 433.8●
  stent
    coronary 996.72
  teeth (mandibular) (posterior lingual) 524.29
  thoracic duct 457.1
  tubal 628.2
  ureter (complete) (partial) 593.4
    congenital 753.29
  urethra (*see also* Stricture, urethra) 598.9
    congenital 753.6
  uterus 621.8
  vagina 623.2
  vascular NEC 459.9
  vein - *see* Thrombosis
  vena cava ~~(inferior) (superior)~~ ◀‖‖
    ~~453.2~~
    inferior 453.2 ◀
    superior 453.2 ◀
      acute 453.87 ◀
      chronic 453.77 ◀
  ventricle (brain) NEC 331.4
  vertebral (artery) - *see* Occlusion, artery, vertebral
  vessel (blood) NEC 459.9
  vulva 624.8
Occlusio pupillae 364.74
Occupational
  problems NEC V62.29
  therapy V57.21
Ochlophobia 300.29
Ochronosis (alkaptonuric) (congenital) (endogenous) 270.2
  with chloasma of eyelid 270.2
Ocular muscle - *see also* condition
  myopathy 359.1
  torticollis 781.93
Oculoauriculovertebral dysplasia 756.0
Oculogyric
  crisis or disturbance 378.87
    psychogenic 306.7
Oculomotor syndrome 378.81
Oddi's sphincter spasm 576.5
Odelberg's disease (juvenile osteochondrosis) 732.1
Odontalgia 525.9
Odontoameloblastoma (M9311/0) 213.1
  upper jaw (bone) 213.0
Odontoclasia 521.05
Odontoclasis 873.63
  complicated 873.73
Odontodysplasia, regional 520.4
Odontogenesis imperfecta 520.5
Odontoma (M9280/0) 213.1
  ameloblastic (M9311/0) 213.1
    upper jaw (bone) 213.0
  calcified (M9280/0) 213.1
    upper jaw (bone) 213.0
  complex (M9282/0) 213.1
    upper jaw (bone) 213.0

Odontoma (*Continued*)
  compound (M9281/0) 213.1
    upper jaw (bone) 213.0
  fibroameloblastic (M9290/0) 213.1
    upper jaw (bone) 213.0
  follicular 526.0
    upper jaw (bone) 213.0
Odontomyelitis (closed) (open) 522.0
Odontonecrosis 521.09
Odontorrhagia 525.8
Odontosarcoma, ameloblastic (M9290/3) 170.1
  upper jaw (bone) 170.0
Odynophagia 787.20
Oesophagostomiasis 127.7
Oesophagostomum infestation 127.7
Oestriasis 134.0
Ogilvie's syndrome (sympathicotonic colon obstruction) 560.89
Oguchi's disease (retina) 368.61
Ohara's disease (*see also* Tularemia) 021.9
Oidiomycosis (*see also* Candidiasis) 112.9
Oidiomycotic meningitis 112.83
Oidium albicans infection (*see also* Candidiasis) 112.9
Old age 797
  dementia (of) 290.0
Olfactory - *see* condition
Oligemia 285.9
Oligergasia (*see also* Retardation, mental) 319
Oligoamnios 658.0●
  affecting fetus or newborn 761.2
Oligoastrocytoma, mixed (M9382/3)
  specified site - *see* Neoplasm, by site, malignant
  unspecified site 191.9
Oligocythemia 285.9
Oligodendroblastoma (M9460/3)
  specified site - *see* Neoplasm, by site, malignant
  unspecified site 191.9
Oligodendroglioma (M9450/3)
  anaplastic type (M9451/3)
    specified site - *see* Neoplasm, by site, malignant
    unspecified site 191.9
  specified site - *see* Neoplasm, by site, malignant
  unspecified site 191.9
Oligodendroma - *see* Oligodendroglioma
Oligodontia (*see also* Anodontia) 520.0
Oligoencephalon 742.1
Oligohydramnios 658.0●
  affecting fetus or newborn 761.2
  due to premature rupture of membranes 658.1●
    affecting fetus or newborn 761.2
Oligohydrosis 705.0
Oligomenorrhea 626.1
Oligophrenia (*see also* Retardation, mental) 319
  phenylpyruvic 270.1
Oligospermia 606.1
Oligotrichia 704.09
  congenita 757.4
Oliguria 788.5
  with
    abortion - *see* Abortion, by type, with renal failure
    ectopic pregnancy (*see also* categories 633.0–633.9) 639.3
    molar pregnancy (*see also* categories 630–632) 639.3

Oliguria *(Continued)*
  complicating
    abortion 639.3
    ectopic or molar pregnancy 639.3
    pregnancy 646.2●
      with hypertension - *see* Toxemia,
        of pregnancy
  due to a procedure 997.5
  following labor and delivery 669.3●
  heart or cardiac - *see* Failure, heart
  puerperal, postpartum 669.3●
  specified due to a procedure 997.5
Ollier's disease (chondrodysplasia)
    756.4
Omentitis *(see also* Peritonitis) 567.9
Omentocele *(see also* Hernia, omental)
    553.8
Omentum, omental - *see* condition
Omphalitis (congenital) (newborn)
    771.4
  not of newborn 686.9
  tetanus 771.3
Omphalocele 756.72   ◀▥
Omphalomesenteric duct, persistent
    751.0
Omphalorrhagia, newborn 772.3
Omsk hemorrhagic fever 065.1
Onanism 307.9
Onchocerciasis 125.3
  eye 125.3 *[360.13]*
Onchocercosis 125.3
Oncocytoma (M8290/0) - *see* Neoplasm,
    by site, benign
Ondine's curse 348.89   ◀▥
Oneirophrenia *(see also* Schizophrenia)
    295.4●
Onychauxis 703.8
  congenital 757.5
Onychia (with lymphangitis) 681.9
  dermatophytic 110.1
  finger 681.02
  toe 681.11
Onychitis (with lymphangitis) 681.9
  finger 681.02
  toe 681.11
Onychocryptosis 703.0
Onychodystrophy 703.8
  congenital 757.5
Onychogryphosis 703.8
Onychogryposis 703.8
Onycholysis 703.8
Onychomadesis 703.8
Onychomalacia 703.8
Onychomycosis 110.1
  finger 110.1
  toe 110.1
Onycho-osteodysplasia 756.89
Onychophagy 307.9
Onychoptosis 703.8
Onychorrhexis 703.8
  congenital 757.5
Onychoschizia 703.8
Onychotrophia *(see also* Atrophy, nail)
    703.8
O'Nyong Nyong fever 066.3
Onyxis (finger) (toe) 703.0
Onyxitis (with lymphangitis) 681.9
  finger 681.02
  toe 681.11
Oocyte (egg) (ovum)
  donor V59.70
    over age 35 V59.73
      anonymous recipient V59.73
      designated recipient V59.74

Oocyte *(Continued)*
  donor *(Continued)*
    under age 35 V59.71
      anonymous recipient V59.71
      designated recipient V59.72
Oophoritis (cystic) (infectional)
    (interstitial) *(see also* Salpingo-
    oophoritis) 614.2
  complicating pregnancy 646.6●
  fetal (acute) 752.0
  gonococcal (acute) 098.19
    chronic or duration of 2 months or
      over 098.39
  tuberculous *(see also* Tuberculosis)
    016.6●
Opacity, opacities
  cornea 371.00
    central 371.03
    congenital 743.43
      interfering with vision 743.42
    degenerative *(see also* Degeneration,
      cornea) 371.40
    hereditary *(see also* Dystrophy,
      cornea) 371.50
    inflammatory *(see also* Keratitis)
      370.9
    late effect of trachoma (healed) 139.1
    minor 371.01
    peripheral 371.02
  enamel (fluoride) (nonfluoride) (teeth)
    520.3
  lens *(see also* Cataract) 366.9
  snowball 379.22
  vitreous (humor) 379.24
    congenital 743.51
Opalescent dentin (hereditary) 520.5
Open, opening
  abnormal, organ or site, congenital - *see*
    Imperfect, closure
  angle with
    borderline intraocular pressure
      365.01
    cupping of discs 365.01
  bite
    anterior 524.24
    posterior 524.25
  false - *see* Imperfect, closure
  margin on tooth restoration 525.61
  restoration margins 525.61
  wound - *see* Wound, open, by site
Operation
  causing mutilation of fetus 763.89
  destructive, on live fetus, to facilitate
    birth 763.89
  for delivery, fetus or newborn 763.89
  maternal, unrelated to current
    delivery, affecting fetus or
    newborn *(see also* Newborn,
    affected by) 760.64
Operational fatigue 300.89
Operative - *see* condition
Operculitis (chronic) 523.40
  acute 523.30
Operculum, retina 361.32
  with detachment 361.01
Ophiasis 704.01
Ophthalmia *(see also* Conjunctivitis)
    372.30
  actinic rays 370.24
  allergic (acute) 372.05
    chronic 372.14
  blennorrhagic (neonatorum) 098.40
  catarrhal 372.03
  diphtheritic 032.81

Ophthalmia *(Continued)*
  Egyptian 076.1
  electric, electrica 370.24
  gonococcal (neonatorum) 098.40
  metastatic 360.11
  migraine 346.8●
  neonatorum, newborn 771.6
    gonococcal 098.40
  nodosa 360.14
  phlyctenular 370.31
    with ulcer *(see also* Ulcer, cornea)
      370.00
  sympathetic 360.11
Ophthalmitis - *see* Ophthalmia
Ophthalmocele (congenital) 743.66
Ophthalmoneuromyelitis 341.0
Ophthalmopathy, infiltrative with
    thyrotoxicosis 242.0●
Ophthalmoplegia *(see also* Strabismus)
    378.9
  anterior internuclear 378.86
  ataxia-areflexia syndrome 357.0
  bilateral 378.9
  diabetic 250.5● *[378.86]*
    due to secondary diabetes 249.5●
      [378.86]
  exophthalmic 242.0● *[376.22]*
  external 378.55
    progressive 378.72
    total 378.56
  internal (complete) (total) 367.52
  internuclear 378.86
  migraine 346.2●
  painful 378.55
  Parinaud's 378.81
  progressive external 378.72
  supranuclear, progressive 333.0
  total (external) 378.56
    internal 367.52
  unilateral 378.9
Opisthognathism 524.00
Opisthorchiasis (felineus) (tenuicollis)
    (viverrini) 121.0
Opisthotonos, opisthotonus 781.0
Opitz's disease (congestive
    splenomegaly) 289.51
Opiumism *(see also* Dependence) 304.0●
Oppenheim's disease 358.8
Oppenheim-Urbach disease or syndrome
    (necrobiosis lipoidica diabeticorum)
    250.8● *[709.3]*
  due to secondary diabetes 249.8● *[709.3]*
Opsoclonia 379.59
Optic nerve - *see* condition
Orbit - *see* condition
Orchioblastoma (M9071/3) 186.9
Orchitis (nonspecific) (septic) 604.90
  with abscess 604.0
  blennorrhagic (acute) 098.13
    chronic or duration of 2 months or
      over 098.33
  diphtheritic 032.89 *[604.91]*
  filarial 125.9 *[604.91]*
  gangrenous 604.99
  gonococcal (acute) 098.13
    chronic or duration of 2 months or
      over 098.33
  mumps 072.0
  parotidea 072.0
  suppurative 604.99
  syphilitic 095.8 *[604.91]*
  tuberculous *(see also* Tuberculosis)
    016.5● *[608.81]*
Orf 051.2

◀ New   ◀▥ Revised   ~~deleted~~ Deleted   ● Use Additional Digit(s)   ▨ Omit code

Organic - *see also* condition
heart - *see* Disease, heart
insufficiency 799.89
Oriental
bilharziasis 120.2
schistosomiasis 120.2
sore 085.1
Orientation
ego-dystonic sexual 302.0
Orifice - *see* condition
Origin, both great vessels from right
ventricle 745.11
Ormond's disease or syndrome 593.4
Ornithosis 073.9
with
complication 073.8
specified NEC 073.7
pneumonia 073.0
pneumonitis (lobular) 073.0
Orodigitofacial dysostosis 759.89
Oropouche fever 066.3
Orotaciduria, oroticaciduria (congenital)
(hereditary) (pyrimidine deficiency)
281.4
Oroya fever 088.0
Orthodontics V58.5
adjustment V53.4
aftercare V58.5
fitting V53.4
Orthopnea 786.02
Os, uterus - *see* condition
Osgood-Schlatter
disease 732.4
osteochondrosis 732.4
Osler's
disease (M9950/1) (polycythemia vera)
238.4
nodes 421.0
Osler-Rendu disease (familial
hemorrhagic telangiectasia) 448.0
Osler-Vaquez disease (M9950/1)
(polycythemia vera) 238.4
Osler-Weber-Rendu syndrome (familial
hemorrhagic telangiectasia) 448.0
Osmidrosis 705.89
Osseous - *see* condition
Ossification
artery - *see* Arteriosclerosis
auricle (ear) 380.39
bronchus 519.19
cardiac (*see also* Degeneration,
myocardial) 429.1
cartilage (senile) 733.99
coronary - *see* Arteriosclerosis, coronary
diaphragm 728.10
ear 380.39
middle (*see also* Otosclerosis) 387.9
falx cerebri 349.2
fascia 728.10
fontanel
defective or delayed 756.0
premature 756.0
heart (*see also* Degeneration,
myocardial) 429.1
valve - *see* Endocarditis
larynx 478.79
ligament
posterior longitudinal 724.8
cervical 723.7
meninges (cerebral) 349.2
spinal 336.8
multiple, eccentric centers 733.99
muscle 728.10
heterotopic, postoperative 728.13

Ossification *(Continued)*
myocardium, myocardial (*see also*
Degeneration, myocardial) 429.1
penis 607.81
periarticular 728.89
sclera 379.16
tendon 727.82
trachea 519.19
tympanic membrane (*see also*
Tympanosclerosis) 385.00
vitreous (humor) 360.44
Osteitis (*see also* Osteomyelitis) 730.2●
acute 730.0●
alveolar 526.5
chronic 730.1●
condensans (ilii) 733.5
deformans (Paget's) 731.0
due to or associated with malignant
neoplasm (*see also* Neoplasm,
bone, malignant) 170.9 [731.1]
due to yaws 102.6
fibrosa NEC 733.29
cystica (generalisata) 252.01
disseminata 756.59
osteoplastica 252.01
fragilitans 756.51
Garré's (sclerosing) 730.1●
infectious (acute) (subacute) 730.0●
chronic or old 730.1●
jaw (acute) (chronic) (lower) (neonatal)
(suppurative) (upper) 526.4
parathyroid 252.01
petrous bone (*see also* Petrositis) 383.20
pubis 733.5
sclerotic, nonsuppurative 730.1●
syphilitic 095.5
tuberculosa
cystica (of Jüngling) 135
multiplex cystoides 135
Osteoarthritica spondylitis (spine) (*see
also* Spondylosis) 721.90
Osteoarthritis (*see also* Osteoarthrosis)
715.9●
distal interphalangeal 715.9●
hyperplastic 731.2
interspinalis (*see also* Spondylosis)
721.90
spine, spinal NEC (*see also* Spondylosis)
721.90
Osteoarthropathy (*see also* Osteoarthrosis)
715.9●
chronic idiopathic hypertrophic 757.39
familial idiopathic 757.39
hypertrophic pulmonary 731.2
secondary 731.2
idiopathic hypertrophic 757.39
primary hypertrophic 731.2
pulmonary hypertrophic 731.2
secondary hypertrophic 731.2
Osteoarthrosis (degenerative)
(hypertrophic) (rheumatoid) 715.9●

Note 56   Use the following fifth-digit
subclassification with category 715:

0   site unspecified
1   shoulder region
2   upper arm
3   forearm
4   hand
5   pelvic region and thigh
6   lower leg
7   ankle and foot
8   other specified sites except spine
9   multiple sites

Osteoarthrosis *(Continued)*
Deformans alkaptonurica 270.2
generalized 715.09
juvenilis (Köhler's) 732.5
localized 715.3●
idiopathic 715.1●
primary 715.1●
secondary 715.2●
multiple sites, not specified as
generalized 715.89
polyarticular 715.09
spine (*see also* Spondylosis) 721.90
temporomandibular joint 524.69
Osteoblastoma (M9200/0) - *see*
Neoplasm, bone, benign
Osteochondritis (*see also*
Osteochondrosis) 732.9
dissecans 732.7
hip 732.7
ischiopubica 732.1
multiple 756.59
syphilitic (congenital) 090.0
Osteochondrodermodysplasia 756.59
Osteochondrodystrophy 277.5
deformans 277.5
familial 277.5
fetalis 756.4
Osteochondrolysis 732.7
Osteochondroma (M9210/0) - *see also*
Neoplasm, bone, benign
multiple, congenital 756.4
Osteochondromatosis (M9210/1) 238.0
synovial 727.82
Osteochondromyxosarcoma (M9180/3) -
see Neoplasm, bone, malignant
Osteochondropathy NEC 732.9
Osteochondrosarcoma (M9180/3) - *see*
Neoplasm, bone, malignant
Osteochondrosis 732.9
acetabulum 732.1
adult spine 732.8
astragalus 732.5
Blount's 732.4
Buchanan's (juvenile osteochondrosis
of iliac crest) 732.1
Buchman's (juvenile osteochondrosis)
732.1
Burns' 732.3
calcaneus 732.5
capitular epiphysis (femur) 732.1
carpal
lunate (wrist) 732.3
scaphoid 732.3
coxae juvenilis 732.1
deformans juvenilis (coxae) (hip)
732.1
Scheuermann's 732.0
spine 732.0
tibia 732.4
vertebra 732.0
Diaz's (astragalus) 732.5
dissecans (knee) (shoulder) 732.7
femoral capital epiphysis 732.1
femur (head) (juvenile) 732.1
foot (juvenile) 732.5
Freiberg's (disease) (second metatarsal)
732.5
Haas' 732.3
Haglund's (os tibiale externum)
732.5
hand (juvenile) 732.3
head of
femur 732.1
humerus (juvenile) 732.3

Osteochondrosis (*Continued*)
hip (juvenile) 732.1
humerus (juvenile) 732.3
iliac crest (juvenile) 732.1
ilium (juvenile) 732.1
ischiopubic synchondrosis 732.1
Iselin's (osteochondrosis fifth
　metatarsal) 732.5
juvenile, juvenilis 732.6
　arm 732.3
　capital femoral epiphysis 732.1
　capitellum humeri 732.3
　capitular epiphysis 732.1
　carpal scaphoid 732.3
　clavicle, sternal epiphysis 732.6
　coxae 732.1
　deformans 732.1
　foot 732.5
　hand 732.3
　hip and pelvis 732.1
　lower extremity, except foot 732.4
　lunate, wrist 732.3
　medial cuneiform bone 732.5
　metatarsal (head) 732.5
　metatarsophalangeal 732.5
　navicular, ankle 732.5
　patella 732.4
　primary patellar center (of Köhler)
　　732.4
　specified site NEC 732.6
　spine 732.0
　tarsal scaphoid 732.5
　tibia (epiphysis) (tuberosity) 732.4
　upper extremity 732.3
　vertebra (body) (Calvé) 732.0
　　epiphyseal plates (of
　　　Scheuermann) 732.0
Kienböck's (disease) 732.3
Köhler's (disease) (navicular, ankle)
　732.5
　patellar 732.4
　tarsal navicular 732.5
Legg-Calvé-Perthes (disease) 732.1
lower extremity (juvenile) 732.4
lunate bone 732.3
Mauclaire's 732.3
metacarpal heads (of Mauclaire) 732.3
metatarsal (fifth) (head) (second) 732.5
navicular, ankle 732.5
os calcis 732.5
Osgood-Schlatter 732.4
os tibiale externum 732.5
Panner's 732.3
patella (juvenile) 732.4
patellar center
　primary (of Köhler) 732.4
　secondary (of Sinding-Larsen) 732.4
pelvis (juvenile) 732.1
Pierson's 732.1
radial head (juvenile) 732.3
Scheuermann's 732.0
Sever's (calcaneum) 732.5
Sinding-Larsen (secondary patellar
　center) 732.4
spine (juvenile) 732.0
　adult 732.8
symphysis pubis (of Pierson) (juvenile)
　732.1
syphilitic (congenital) 090.0
tarsal (navicular) (scaphoid) 732.5
tibia (proximal) (tubercle) 732.4
tuberculous - *see* Tuberculosis, bone
ulna 732.3
upper extremity (juvenile) 732.3

Osteochondrosis (*Continued*)
van Neck's (juvenile osteochondrosis)
　732.1
vertebral (juvenile) 732.0
　adult 732.8
Osteoclastoma (M9250/1) 238.0
malignant (M9250/3) - *see* Neoplasm,
　bone, malignant
Osteocopic pain 733.90
Osteodynia 733.90
Osteodystrophy
azotemic 588.0
chronica deformans hypertrophica
　731.1
congenital 756.50
　specified type NEC 756.59
deformans 731.0
fibrosa localisata 731.0
parathyroid 252.01
renal 588.0
Osteofibroma (M9262/0) - *see* Neoplasm,
　bone, benign
Osteofibrosarcoma (M9182/3) - *see*
　Neoplasm, bone, malignant
Osteogenesis imperfecta 756.51
Osteogenic - *see* condition
Osteoma (M9180/0) - *see also* Neoplasm,
　bone, benign
osteoid (M9191/0) - *see also* Neoplasm,
　bone, benign
　giant (M9200/0) - *see* Neoplasm,
　　bone, benign
Osteomalacia 268.2
chronica deformans hypertrophica
　731.0
due to vitamin D deficiency 268.2
infantile (*see also* Rickets) 268.0
juvenile (*see also* Rickets) 268.0
pelvis 268.2
vitamin D-resistant 275.3
Osteomalacic bone 268.2
Osteomalacosis 268.2
Osteomyelitis (general) (infective)
　(localized) (neonatal) (purulent)
　(pyogenic) (septic) (staphylococcal)
　(streptococcal) (suppurative) (with
　periostitis) 730.2●

Note 57　Use the following fifth-digit
subclassification with category 730:

0　site unspecified
1　shoulder region
2　upper arm
3　forearm
4　hand
5　pelvic region and thigh
6　lower leg
7　ankle and foot
8　other specified sites
9　multiple sites

acute or subacute 730.0●
chronic or old 730.1●
due to or associated with
　diabetes mellitus 250.8● [731.8]
　　due to secondary diabetes 249.8●
　　　[731.8]
　tuberculosis (*see also* Tuberculosis,
　　bone) 015.9● [730.8]●
　　limb bones 015.5● [730.8]●
　　specified bones NEC 015.7●
　　　[730.8]●
　　spine 015.0● [730.8]●
　typhoid 002.0 [730.8]●

Osteomyelitis (*Continued*)
Garré's 730.1●
jaw (acute) (chronic) (lower) (neonatal)
　(suppurative) (upper) 526.4
nonsuppurating 730.1●
orbital 376.03
petrous bone (*see also* Petrositis)
　383.20
Salmonella 003.24
sclerosing, nonsuppurative 730.1●
sicca 730.1●
syphilitic 095.5
　congenital 090.0 [730.8]●
tuberculous - *see* Tuberculosis, bone
typhoid 002.0 [730.8]●
Osteomyelofibrosis 289.89
Osteomyelosclerosis 289.89
Osteonecrosis 733.40
meaning osteomyelitis 730.1●
Osteo-onycho-arthro dysplasia 756.89
Osteo-onychodysplasia, hereditary
　756.89
Osteopathia
condensans disseminata 756.53
hyperostotica multiplex infantilis
　756.59
hypertrophica toxica 731.2
striata 756.4
Osteopathy resulting from poliomyelitis
　(*see also* Poliomyelitis) 045.9●
　[730.7]
familial dysplastic 731.2
Osteopecilia 756.53
Osteopenia 733.90
borderline 733.90
Osteoperiostitis (*see also* Osteomyelitis)
　730.2●
ossificans toxica 731.2
toxica ossificans 731.2
Osteopetrosis (familial) 756.52
Osteophyte - *see* Exostosis
Osteophytosis - *see* Exostosis
Osteopoikilosis 756.53
Osteoporosis (generalized) 733.00
circumscripta 731.0
disuse 733.03
drug-induced 733.09
idiopathic 733.02
postmenopausal 733.01
posttraumatic 733.7
screening V82.81
senile 733.01
specified type NEC 733.09
Osteoporosis-osteomalacia syndrome
　268.2
Osteopsathyrosis 756.51
Osteoradionecrosis, jaw 526.89
Osteosarcoma (M9180/3) - *see also*
　Neoplasm, bone, malignant
chondroblastic (M9181/3) - *see*
　Neoplasm, bone, malignant
fibroblastic (M9182/3) - *see* Neoplasm,
　bone, malignant
in Paget's disease of bone (M9184/3) -
　see Neoplasm, bone, malignant
juxtacortical (M9190/3) - *see* Neoplasm,
　bone malignant
parosteal (M9190/3) - *see* Neoplasm,
　bone, malignant
telangiectatic (M9183/3) - *see*
　Neoplasm, bone, malignant
Osteosclerosis 756.52
fragilis (generalisata) 756.52
Osteosclerotic anemia 289.89

Osteosis
acromegaloid 757.39
cutis 709.3
parathyroid 252.01
renal fibrocystic 588.0
Österreicher-Turner syndrome 756.89
Ostium
atrioventriculare commune 745.69
primum (arteriosum) (defect)
(persistent) 745.61
secundum (arteriosum) (defect)
(patent) (persistent) 745.5
Ostrum-Furst syndrome 756.59
Otalgia 388.70
otogenic 388.71
referred 388.72
Othematoma 380.31
Otitic hydrocephalus 348.2
Otitis 382.9
with effusion 381.4
purulent 382.4
secretory 381.4
serous 381.4
suppurative 382.4
acute 382.9
adhesive (see also Adhesions, middle
ear) 385.10
chronic 382.9
with effusion 381.3
mucoid, mucous (simple) 381.20
purulent 382.3
secretory 381.3
serous 381.10
suppurative 382.3
diffuse parasitic 136.8
externa (acute) (diffuse) (hemorrhagica)
380.10
actinic 380.22
candidal 112.82
chemical 380.22
chronic 380.23
mycotic - see Otitis, externa,
mycotic
specified type NEC 380.23
circumscribed 380.10
contact 380.22
due to
erysipelas 035 [380.13]
impetigo 684 [380.13]
seborrheic dermatitis 690.10
[380.13]
eczematoid 380.22
furuncular 680.0 [380.13]
infective 380.10
chronic 380.16
malignant 380.14
mycotic (chronic) 380.15
due to
aspergillosis 117.3 [380.15]
moniliasis 112.82
otomycosis 111.8 [380.15]
reactive 380.22
specified type NEC 380.22
tropical 111.8 [380.15]
insidiosa (see also Otosclerosis) 387.9
interna (see also Labyrinthitis) 386.30
media (hemorrhagic) (staphylococcal)
(streptococcal) 382.9
acute 382.9
with effusion 381.00
allergic 381.04
mucoid 381.05
sanguineous 381.06
serous 381.04

Otitis (Continued)
media (Continued)
acute (Continued)
catarrhal 381.00
exudative 381.00
mucoid 381.02
allergic 381.05
necrotizing 382.00
with spontaneous rupture of
ear drum 382.01
in
influenza 487.8 [382.02]
measles 055.2
scarlet fever 034.1 [382.02]
nonsuppurative 381.00
purulent 382.00
with spontaneous rupture of
ear drum 382.01
sanguineous 381.03
allergic 381.06
secretory 381.01
seromucinous 381.02
serous 381.01
allergic 381.04
suppurative 382.00
with spontaneous rupture of
ear drum 382.01
due to
influenza 487.8 [382.02]
scarlet fever 034.1 [382.02]
transudative 381.00
adhesive (see also Adhesions, middle
ear) 385.10
allergic 381.4
acute 381.04
mucoid 381.05
sanguineous 381.06
serous 381.04
chronic 381.3
catarrhal 381.4
acute 381.00
chronic (simple) 381.10
chronic 382.9
with effusion 381.3
adhesive (see also Adhesions,
middle ear) 385.10
allergic 381.3
atticoantral, suppurative (with
posterior or superior
marginal perforation of ear
drum) 382.2
benign suppurative (with
anterior perforation of ear
drum) 382.1
catarrhal 381.10
exudative 381.3
mucinous 381.20
mucoid, mucous (simple)
381.20
mucosanguineous 381.29
nonsuppurative 381.3
purulent 382.3
secretory 381.3
seromucinous 381.3
serosanguineous 381.19
serous (simple) 381.10
suppurative 382.3
atticoantral (with posterior or
superior marginal
perforation of ear drum)
382.2
benign (with anterior
perforation of ear drum)
382.1

Otitis (Continued)
media (Continued)
chronic (Continued)
suppurative (Continued)
tuberculous (see also
Tuberculosis) 017.4●
tubotympanic 382.1
transudative 381.3
exudative 381.4
acute 381.00
chronic 381.3
fibrotic (see also Adhesions, middle
ear) 385.10
mucoid, mucous 381.4
acute 381.02
chronic (simple) 381.20
mucosanguineous, chronic 381.29
nonsuppurative 381.4
acute 381.00
chronic 381.3
postmeasles 055.2
purulent 382.4
acute 382.00
with spontaneous rupture of
ear drum 382.01
chronic 382.3
sanguineous, acute 381.03
allergic 381.06
secretory 381.4
acute or subacute 381.01
chronic 381.3
seromucinous 381.4
acute or subacute 381.02
chronic 381.3
serosanguineous, chronic 381.19
serous 381.4
acute or subacute 381.01
chronic (simple) 381.10
subacute - see Otitis, media, acute
suppurative 382.4
acute 382.00
with spontaneous rupture of
ear drum 382.01
chronic 382.3
atticoantral 382.2
benign 382.1
tuberculous (see also
Tuberculosis)
017.4●
tubotympanic 382.1
transudative 381.4
acute 381.00
chronic 381.3
tuberculous (see also Tuberculosis)
017.4●
postmeasles 055.2
Otoconia 386.8
Otolith syndrome 386.19
Otomycosis 111.8 [380.15]
in
aspergillosis 117.3 [380.15]
moniliasis 112.82
Otopathy 388.9
Otoporosis (see also Otosclerosis)
387.9
Otorrhagia 388.69
traumatic - see nature of injury
Otorrhea 388.60
blood 388.69
cerebrospinal (fluid) 388.61
Otosclerosis (general) 387.9
cochlear (endosteal) 387.2
involving
otic capsule 387.2

Otosclerosis (Continued)
  involving (Continued)
    oval window
      nonobliterative 387.0
      obliterative 387.1
    round window 387.2
  nonobliterative 387.0
  obliterative 387.1
  specified type NEC 387.8
Otospongiosis (see also Otosclerosis) 387.9
Otto's disease or pelvis 715.35
Outburst, aggressive (see also
    Disturbance, conduct) 312.0●
  in children or adolescents 313.9
Outcome of delivery
  multiple birth NEC V27.9
    all liveborn V27.5
    all stillborn V27.7
    some liveborn V27.6
    unspecified V27.9
  single V27.9
    liveborn V27.0
    stillborn V27.1
  twins V27.9
    both liveborn V27.2
    both stillborn V27.4
    one liveborn, one stillborn V27.3
Outlet - see also condition
  syndrome (thoracic) 353.0
Outstanding ears (bilateral) 744.29
Ovalocytosis (congenital) (hereditary) (see
    also Elliptocytosis) 282.1
Ovarian - see also condition
  pregnancy - see Pregnancy, ovarian
  remnant syndrome 620.8
  vein syndrome 593.4
Ovaritis (cystic) (see also Salpingo-
    oophoritis) 614.2
Ovary, ovarian - see condition
Overactive - see also Hyperfunction
  bladder 596.51
  eye muscle (see also Strabismus) 378.9
  hypothalamus 253.8
  thyroid (see also Thyrotoxicosis) 242.9●
Overactivity, child 314.01
Overbite (deep) (excessive) (horizontal)
    (vertical) 524.29

Overbreathing (see also Hyperventilation)
    786.01
Overconscientious personality 301.4
Overdevelopment - see also Hypertrophy
  breast (female) (male) 611.1
  nasal bones 738.0
  prostate, congenital 752.89
Overdistention - see Distention
Overdose overdosage (drug) 977.9
  specified drug or substance - see Table
    of Drugs and Chemicals
Overeating 783.6
  nonorganic origin 307.51
Overexertion (effects) (exhaustion)
    994.5
Overexposure (effects) 994.9
  exhaustion 994.4
Overfeeding (see also Overeating)
    783.6
Overfill, endodontic 526.62
Overgrowth, bone NEC 733.99
Overhanging
  tooth restoration 525.62
  unrepairable, dental restorative
    materials 525.62
Overheated (effects) (places) - see Heat
Overinhibited child 313.0
Overjet 524.29
  excessive horizontal 524.26
Overlaid, overlying (suffocation)
    994.7
Overlap
  excessive horizontal 524.26
Overlapping toe (acquired) 735.8
  congenital (fifth toe) 755.66
Overload
  fluid 276.6
  potassium (K) 276.7
  sodium (Na) 276.0
Overnutrition (see also
    Hyperalimentation) 783.6
Overproduction - see also Hypersecretion
  ACTH 255.3
  cortisol 255.0
  growth hormone 253.0
  thyroid-stimulating hormone (TSH)
    242.8●

Overriding
  aorta 747.21
  finger (acquired) 736.29
    congenital 755.59
  toe (acquired) 735.8
    congenital 755.66
Oversize
  fetus (weight of 4500 grams or more)
    766.0
    affecting management of pregnancy
      656.6●
    causing disproportion 653.5●
      with obstructed labor 660.1●
    affecting fetus or newborn 763.1
Overstimulation, ovarian 256.1
Overstrained 780.79
  heart - see Hypertrophy, cardiac
Overweight (see also Obesity) 278.02
Overwork 780.79
Oviduct - see condition
Ovotestis 752.7
Ovulation (cycle)
  failure or lack of 628.0
  pain 625.2
Ovum
  blighted 631
  donor V59.70
    over age 35 V59.73
      anonymous recipient V59.73
      designated recipient V59.74
    under age 35 V59.71
      anonymous recipient V59.71
      designated recipient V59.72
  dropsical 631
  pathologic 631
Owren's disease or syndrome
    (parahemophilia) (see also Defect,
    coagulation) 286.3
Oxalosis 271.8
Oxaluria 271.8
Ox heart - see Hypertrophy, cardiac
OX syndrome 758.6
Oxycephaly, oxycephalic 756.0
  syphilitic, congenital 090.0
Oxyuriasis 127.4
Oxyuris vermicularis (infestation) 127.4
Ozena 472.0

◀ New   ◀▪▪ Revised   ~~deleted~~ Deleted   ● Use Additional Digit(s)   ▨ Omit code

P

Pacemaker syndrome 429.4
Pachyderma, pachydermia 701.8
  laryngis 478.5
  laryngitis 478.79
  larynx (verrucosa) 478.79
Pachydermatitis 701.8
Pachydermatocele (congenital) 757.39
  acquired 701.8
Pachydermatosis 701.8
Pachydermoperiostitis
  secondary 731.2
Pachydermoperiostosis
  primary idiopathic 757.39
  secondary 731.2
Pachymeningitis (adhesive) (basal)
    (brain) (cerebral) (cervical) (chronic)
    (circumscribed) (external) (fibrous)
    (hemorrhagic) (hypertrophic)
    (internal) (purulent) (spinal)
    (suppurative) (see also Meningitis)
    322.9
  gonococcal 098.82
Pachyonychia (congenital) 757.5
  acquired 703.8
Pachyperiosteodermia
  primary or idiopathic 757.39
  secondary 731.2
Pachyperiostosis
  primary or idiopathic 757.39
  secondary 731.2
Pacinian tumor (M9507/0) - see
    Neoplasm, skin, benign
Pads, knuckle or Garrod's 728.79
Paget's disease (osteitis deformans)
    731.0
  with infiltrating duct carcinoma of the
    breast (M8541/3) - see Neoplasm,
    breast, malignant
  bone 731.0
    osteosarcoma in (M9184/3) - see
      Neoplasm, bone, malignant
  breast (M8540/3) 174.0
  extramammary (M8542/3) - see also
    Neoplasm, skin, malignant
    anus 154.3
      skin 173.5
  malignant (M8540/3)
    breast 174.0
    specified site NEC (M8542/3) - see
      Neoplasm, skin, malignant
    unspecified site 174.0
  mammary (M8540/3) 174.0
  necrosis of bone 731.0
  nipple (M8540/3) 174.0
  osteitis deformans 731.0
Paget-Schroetter syndrome (intermittent
    venous claudication) 453.89 ◀▥
Pain(s) (see also Painful) 780.96
  abdominal 789.0●
  acute 338.19
    due to trauma 338.11
    postoperative 338.18
      post-thoracotomy 338.12
  adnexa (uteri) 625.9
  alimentary, due to vascular
    insufficiency 557.9
  anginoid (see also Pain, precordial)
    786.51
  anus 569.42
  arch 729.5
  arm 729.5
  axillary 729.5

Pain(s) (Continued)
  back (postural) 724.5
    low 724.2
    psychogenic 307.89
  bile duct 576.9
  bladder 788.99
  bone 733.90
  breast 611.71
    psychogenic 307.89
  broad ligament 625.9
  cancer associated 338.3
  cartilage NEC 733.90
  cecum 789.0●
  cervicobrachial 723.3
  chest (central) 786.50
    atypical 786.59
    midsternal 786.51
    musculoskeletal 786.59
    noncardiac 786.59
    substernal 786.51
    wall (anterior) 786.52
  chronic 338.29
    associated with significant
      psychosocial dysfunction
      338.4
    due to trauma 338.21
    postoperative 338.28
      post-thoracotomy 338.22
    syndrome 338.4
  coccyx 724.79
  colon 789.0●
  common duct 576.9
  coronary - see Angina
  costochondral 786.52
  diaphragm 786.52
  due to (presence of) any device,
    implant, or graft classifiable to
    996.0–996.5 - see Complications,
    due to (presence of) any device,
    implant, or graft classified to
    996.0–996.5 NEC
  malignancy (primary) (secondary)
    338.3
  ear (see also Otalgia) 388.70
  epigastric, epigastrium 789.06
  extremity (lower) (upper) 729.5
  eye 379.91
  face, facial 784.0
    atypical 350.2
    nerve 351.8
  false (labor) 644.1●
  female genital organ NEC 625.9
    psychogenic 307.89
  finger 729.5
  flank 789.0●
  foot 729.5
  gallbladder 575.9
  gas (intestinal) 787.3
  gastric 536.8
  generalized 780.96
  genital organ
    female 625.9
    male 608.9
    psychogenic 307.89
  groin 789.0●
  growing 781.99
  hand 729.5
  head (see also Headache) 784.0
  heart (see also Pain, precordial)
    786.51
  infraorbital (see also Neuralgia,
    trigeminal) 350.1
  intermenstrual 625.2
  jaw 526.9

Pain(s) (Continued)
  joint 719.40
    ankle 719.47
    elbow 719.42
    foot 719.47
    hand 719.44
    hip 719.45
    knee 719.46
    multiple sites 719.49
    pelvic region 719.45
    psychogenic 307.89
    shoulder (region) 719.41
    specified site NEC 719.48
    wrist 719.43
  kidney 788.0
  labor, false or spurious 644.1●
  laryngeal 784.1
  leg 729.5
  limb 729.5
  low back 724.2
  lumbar region 724.2
  mastoid (see also Otalgia) 388.70
  maxilla 526.9
  menstrual 625.3
  metacarpophalangeal (joint)
    719.44
  metatarsophalangeal (joint)
    719.47
  mouth 528.9
  muscle 729.1
    intercostal 786.59
  musculoskeletal (see also Pain, by site)
    729.1
  nasal 478.19
  nasopharynx 478.29
  neck NEC 723.1
    psychogenic 307.89
  neoplasm related (acute) (chronic)
    338.3
  nerve NEC 729.2
  neuromuscular 729.1
  nose 478.19
  ocular 379.91
  ophthalmic 379.91
  orbital region 379.91
  osteocopic 733.90
  ovary 625.9
    psychogenic 307.89
  over heart (see also Pain, precordial)
    786.51
  ovulation 625.2
  pelvic (female) 625.9
    male NEC 789.0●
      psychogenic 307.89
    psychogenic 307.89
  penis 607.9
    psychogenic 307.89
  pericardial (see also Pain, precordial)
    786.51
  perineum
    female 625.9
    male 608.9
  pharynx 478.29
  pleura, pleural, pleuritic 786.52
  postoperative 338.18
    acute 338.18
    chronic 338.28
  post-thoracotomy 338.12
    acute 338.12
    chronic 338.22
  preauricular 388.70
  precordial (region) 786.51
    psychogenic 307.89
  premenstrual 625.4

Pain(s) *(Continued)*
  psychogenic 307.80
    cardiovascular system 307.89
    gastrointestinal system 307.89
    genitourinary system 307.89
    heart 307.89
    musculoskeletal system 307.89
    respiratory system 307.89
    skin 306.3
  radicular (spinal) *(see also* Radiculitis)
    729.2
  rectum 569.42
  respiration 786.52
  retrosternal 786.51
  rheumatic NEC 729.0
    muscular 729.1
  rib 786.50
  root (spinal) *(see also* Radiculitis)
    729.2
  round ligament (stretch) 625.9
  sacroiliac 724.6
  sciatic 724.3
  scrotum 608.9
    psychogenic 307.89
  seminal vesicle 608.9
  sinus 478.19
  skin 782.0
  spermatic cord 608.9
  spinal root *(see also* Radiculitis)
    729.2
  stomach 536.8
    psychogenic 307.89
  substernal 786.51
  temporomandibular (joint) 524.62
  temporomaxillary joint 524.62
  testis 608.9
    psychogenic 307.89
  thoracic spine 724.1
    with radicular and visceral pain
     724.4
  throat 784.1
  tibia 733.90
  toe 729.5
  tongue 529.6
  tooth 525.9
  trigeminal *(see also* Neuralgia,
    trigeminal) 350.1
  tumor associated 338.3
  umbilicus 789.05
  ureter 788.0
  urinary (organ) (system) 788.0
  uterus 625.9
    psychogenic 307.89
  vagina 625.9
  vertebrogenic (syndrome) 724.5
  vesical 788.99
  vulva 625.9
  xiphoid 733.90
Painful - *see also* Pain
  arc syndrome 726.19
  coitus
    female 625.0
    male 608.89
    psychogenic 302.76
  ejaculation (semen) 608.89
    psychogenic 302.79
  erection 607.3
  feet syndrome 266.2
  menstruation 625.3
    psychogenic 306.52
  micturition 788.1
  ophthalmoplegia 378.55
  respiration 786.52
  scar NEC 709.2

Painful *(Continued)*
  total hip replacement 996.77
  total knee replacement 996.77
  urination 788.1
  wire sutures 998.89
Painters' colic 984.9
  specified type of lead - *see* Table of
    Drugs and Chemicals
Palate - *see* condition
Palatoplegia 528.9
Palatoschisis *(see also* Cleft, palate) 749.00
Palilalia 784.69
Palindromic arthritis *(see also*
    Rheumatism, palindromic) 719.3●
Palliative care V66.7
Pallor 782.61
  temporal, optic disc 377.15
Palmar - *see also* condition
  fascia - *see* condition
Palpable
  cecum 569.89
  kidney 593.89
  liver 573.9
  lymph nodes 785.6
  ovary 620.8
  prostate 602.9
  spleen *(see also* Splenomegaly) 789.2
  uterus 625.8
Palpitation (heart) 785.1
  psychogenic 306.2
Palsy *(see also* Paralysis) 344.9
  atrophic diffuse 335.20
  Bell's 351.0
    newborn 767.5
  birth 767.7
  brachial plexus 353.0
    fetus or newborn 767.6
  brain - *see also* Palsy, cerebral
    noncongenital or noninfantile 344.89
     late effect - *see* Late effect(s) (of)
      cerebrovascular disease
    syphilitic 094.89
     congenital 090.49
  bulbar (chronic) (progressive) 335.22
    pseudo NEC 335.23
    supranuclear NEC 344.89
  cerebral (congenital) (infantile)
    (spastic) 343.9
    athetoid 333.71
    diplegic 343.0
     late effect - *see* Late effect(s) (of)
      cerebrovascular disease
    hemiplegic 343.1
    monoplegic 343.3
    noncongenital or noninfantile 437.8
     late effect - *see* Late effect(s) (of)
      cerebrovascular disease
    paraplegic 343.0
    quadriplegic 343.2
    spastic, not congenital or infantile
     344.89
    syphilitic 094.89
     congenital 090.49
    tetraplegic 343.2
  cranial nerve - *see also* Disorder, nerve,
    cranial
    multiple 352.6
  creeping 335.21
  divers' 993.3
  Erb's (birth injury) 767.6
  facial 351.0
    newborn 767.5
  glossopharyngeal 352.2
  Klumpke (-Déjérine) 767.6

Palsy *(Continued)*
  lead 984.9
    specified type of lead - *see* Table of
     Drugs and Chemicals
  median nerve (tardy) 354.0
  peroneal nerve (acute) (tardy) 355.3
  progressive supranuclear 333.0
  pseudobulbar NEC 335.23
  radial nerve (acute) 354.3
  seventh nerve 351.0
    newborn 767.5
  shaking *(see also* Parkinsonism)
    332.0
  spastic (cerebral) (spinal) 343.9
    hemiplegic 343.1
  specified nerve NEC - *see* Disorder,
    nerve
  supranuclear NEC 356.8
    progressive 333.0
  ulnar nerve (tardy) 354.2
  wasting 335.21
Paltauf-Sternberg disease 201.9●
Paludism - *see* Malaria
Panama fever 084.0
Panaris (with lymphangitis) 681.9
  finger 681.02
  toe 681.11
Panaritium (with lymphangitis) 681.9
  finger 681.02
  toe 681.11
Panarteritis (nodosa) 446.0
  brain or cerebral 437.4
Pancake heart 793.2
  with cor pulmonale (chronic) 416.9
Pancarditis (acute) (chronic) 429.89
  with
    rheumatic
     fever (active) (acute) (chronic)
      (subacute) 391.8
      inactive or quiescent 398.99
  rheumatic, acute 391.8
    chronic or inactive 398.99
Pancoast's syndrome or tumor
  (carcinoma, pulmonary apex)
  (M8010/3) 162.3
Pancoast-Tobias syndrome (M8010/3)
  (carcinoma, pulmonary apex)
  162.3
Pancolitis 556.6
Pancreas, pancreatic - *see* condition
Pancreatitis 577.0
  acute (edematous) (hemorrhagic)
    (recurrent) 577.0
  annular 577.0
  apoplectic 577.0
  calcereous 577.0
  chronic (infectious) 577.1
    recurrent 577.1
  cystic 577.2
  fibrous 577.8
  gangrenous 577.0
  hemorrhagic (acute) 577.0
  interstitial (chronic) 577.1
    acute 577.0
  malignant 577.0
  mumps 072.3
  painless 577.1
  recurrent 577.1
  relapsing 577.1
  subacute 577.0
  suppurative 577.0
  syphilitic 095.8
Pancreatolithiasis 577.8
Pancytolysis 289.9

◀ New   ◀▥ Revised   ~~deleted~~ Deleted   ● Use Additional Digit(s)   ▨ Omit code

Pancytopenia (acquired) 284.1
  with malformations 284.09
  congenital 284.09
Panencephalitis - *see also* Encephalitis
  subacute, sclerosing 046.2
Panhematopenia 284.81
  congenital 284.09
  constitutional 284.09
  splenic, primary 289.4
Panhemocytopenia 284.81
  congenital 284.09
  constitutional 284.09
Panhypogonadism 257.2
Panhypopituitarism 253.2
  prepubertal 253.3
Panic (attack) (state) 300.01
  reaction to exceptional stress (transient) 308.0
Panmyelopathy, familial constitutional 284.09
Panmyelophthisis 284.2
  acquired (secondary) 284.81
  congenital 284.2
  idiopathic 284.9
Panmyelosis (acute) (M9951/1) 238.79
Panner's disease 732.3
  capitellum humeri 732.3
  head of humerus 732.3
  tarsal navicular (bone) (osteochondrosis) 732.5
Panneuritis endemica 265.0 [357.4]
Panniculitis 729.30
  back 724.8
  knee 729.31
  mesenteric 567.82
  neck 723.6
  nodular, nonsuppurative 729.30
  sacral 724.8
  specified site NEC 729.39
Panniculus adiposus (abdominal) 278.1
Pannus (corneal) 370.62
  abdominal (symptomatic) 278.1
  allergic eczematous 370.62
  degenerativus 370.62
  keratic 370.62
  rheumatoid - *see* Arthritis, rheumatoid
  trachomatosus, trachomatous (active) 076.1 [370.62]
    late effect 139.1
Panophthalmitis 360.02
Panotitis - *see* Otitis media
Pansinusitis (chronic) (hyperplastic) (nonpurulent) (purulent) 473.8
  acute 461.8
  due to fungus NEC 117.9
  tuberculous (*see also* Tuberculosis) 012.8●
Panuveitis 360.12
  sympathetic 360.11
Panvalvular disease - *see* Endocarditis, mitral
Papageienkrankheit 073.9
Papanicolaou smear
  anus 796.70
    with
      atypical squamous cells
        cannot exclude high grade squamous intraepithelial lesion (ASC-H) 796.72
        of undetermined significance (ASC-US) 796.71
      cytologic evidence of malignancy 796.76

Papanicolaou smear *(Continued)*
  anus *(Continued)*
    with *(Continued)*
      high grade squamous intraepithelial lesion (HGSIL) 796.74
      low grade squamous intraepithelial lesion (LGSIL) 796.73
    glandular 796.70
    specified finding NEC 796.79
    unsatisfactory cytology 796.78
  cervix (screening test) V76.2
    as part of gynecological examination V72.31
    for suspected malignant neoplasm V76.2
    no disease found V71.1
    inadequate cytology sample 795.08
    nonspecific abnormal finding 795.00
    with
      atypical squamous cells
        cannot exclude high grade squamous intraepithelial lesion (ASC-H) 795.02
        of undetermined significance (ASC-US) 795.01
      cytologic evidence of malignancy 795.06
      high grade squamous intraepithelial lesion (HGSIL) 795.04
      low grade squamous intraepithelial lesion (LGSIL) 795.03
      nonspecific finding NEC 795.09
      to confirm findings of recent normal smear following initial abnormal smear V72.32
    satisfactory smear but lacking transformation zone 795.07
    unsatisfactory cervical cytology 795.08
  other specified site - *see also* Screening, malignant neoplasm
    for suspected malignant neoplasm - *see also* Screening, malignant neoplasm
    no disease found V71.1
    nonspecific abnormal finding 796.9
    vagina V76.47
      with
        atypical squamous cells
          cannot exclude high grade squamous intraepithelial lesion (ASC-H) 795.12
          of undetermined significance (ASC-US) 795.11
        cytologic evidence of malignancy 795.16
        high grade squamous intraepithelial lesion (HGSIL) 795.14
        low grade squamous intraepithelial lesion (LGSIL) 795.13

Papanicolaou smear *(Continued)*
  other specified site *(Continued)*
    vagina *(Continued)*
      abnormal NEC 795.19
      following hysterectomy for malignant condition V67.01
      inadequate cytology sample 795.18
      unsatisfactory cytology 795.18
Papilledema 377.00
  associated with
    decreased ocular pressure 377.02
    increased intracranial pressure 377.01
    retinal disorder 377.03
  choked disc 377.00
  infectional 377.00
Papillitis 377.31
  anus 569.49
  chronic lingual 529.4
  necrotizing, kidney 584.7
  optic 377.31
  rectum 569.49
  renal, necrotizing 584.7
  tongue 529.0
Papilloma (M8050/0) - *see also* Neoplasm, by site, benign

> Note 58 Except where otherwise indicated, the morphological varieties of papilloma in the list below should be coded by site as for "Neoplasm, benign".

  acuminatum (female) (male) 078.11
  bladder (urinary) (transitional cell) (M8120/1) 236.7
    benign (M8120/0) 223.3
  choroid plexus (M9390/0) 225.0
    anaplastic type (M9390/3) 191.5
    malignant (M9390/3) 191.5
  ductal (M8503/0)
  dyskeratotic (M8052/0)
  epidermoid (M8052/0)
  hyperkeratotic (M8052/0)
  intracystic (M8504/0)
  intraductal (M8503/0)
  inverted (M8053/0)
  keratotic (M8052/0)
  parakeratotic (M8052/0)
  pinta (primary) 103.0
  renal pelvis (transitional cell) (M8120/1) 236.99
    benign (M8120/0) 223.1
  Schneiderian (M8121/0)
    specified site - *see* Neoplasm, by site, benign
    unspecified site 212.0
  serous surface (M8461/0)
    borderline malignancy (M8461/1)
      specified site - *see* Neoplasm, by site, uncertain behavior
      unspecified site 236.2
    specified site - *see* Neoplasm, by site, benign
    unspecified site 220
  squamous (cell) (M8052/0)
  transitional (cell) (M8120/0)
    bladder (urinary) (M8120/1) 236.7
    inverted type (M8121/1) - *see* Neoplasm, by site, uncertain behavior
    renal pelvis (M8120/1) 236.91
    ureter (M8120/1) 236.91

Papilloma *(Continued)*
  ureter (transitional cell) (M8120/1)
    236.91
    benign (M8120/0) 223.2
  urothelial (M8120/1) - *see* Neoplasm,
    by site, uncertain behavior
  verrucous (M8051/0)
  villous (M8261/1) - *see* Neoplasm, by
    site, uncertain behavior
  yaws, plantar or palmar 102.1
Papillomata, multiple, of yaws 102.1
Papillomatosis (M8060/0) - *see also*
    Neoplasm, by site, benign
  confluent and reticulate 701.8
  cutaneous 701.8
  ductal, breast 610.1
  Gougerot-Carteaud (confluent
    reticulate) 701.8
  intraductal (diffuse) (M8505/0) - *see*
    Neoplasm, by site, benign
  subareolar duct (M8506/0) 217
Papillon-Léage and Psaume syndrome
    (orodigitofacial dysostosis)
    759.89
Papule 709.8
  carate (primary) 103.0
  fibrous, of nose (M8724/0) 216.3
  pinta (primary) 103.0
Papulosis, malignant 447.8
Papyraceous fetus 779.89
  complicating pregnancy 646.0●
Paracephalus 759.7
Parachute mitral valve 746.5
Paracoccidioidomycosis 116.1
  mucocutaneous-lymphangitic 116.1
  pulmonary 116.1
  visceral 116.1
Paracoccidiomycosis - *see*
    Paracoccidioidomycosis
Paracusis 388.40
Paradentosis 523.5
Paradoxical facial movements 374.43
Paraffinoma 999.9
Paraganglioma (M8680/1)
  adrenal (M8700/0) 227.0
    malignant (M8700/3) 194.0
  aortic body (M8691/1) 237.3
    malignant (M8691/3) 194.6
  carotid body (M8692/1) 237.3
    malignant (M8692/3) 194.5
  chromaffin (M8700/0) - *see also*
    Neoplasm, by site, benign
    malignant (M8700/3) - *see*
      Neoplasm, by site, malignant
  extra-adrenal (M8693/1)
    malignant (M8693/3)
      specified site - *see* Neoplasm, by
        site, malignant
      unspecified site 194.6
    specified site - *see* Neoplasm, by site,
      uncertain behavior
    unspecified site 237.3
  glomus jugulare (M8690/1) 237.3
    malignant (M8690/3) 194.6
  jugular (M8690/1) 237.3
  malignant (M8680/3)
    specified site - *see* Neoplasm, by site,
      malignant
    unspecified site 194.6
  nonchromaffin (M8693/1)
    malignant (M8693/3)
      specified site - *see* Neoplasm, by
        site, malignant
      unspecified site 194.6

Paraganglioma *(Continued)*
  nonchromaffin *(Continued)*
    specified site - *see* Neoplasm, by site,
      uncertain behavior
    unspecified site 237.3
  parasympathetic (M8682/1)
    specified site - *see* Neoplasm, by site,
      uncertain behavior
    unspecified site 237.3
  specified site - *see* Neoplasm, by site,
    uncertain behavior
  sympathetic (M8681/1)
    specified site - *see* Neoplasm, by site,
      uncertain behavior
    unspecified site 237.3
  unspecified site 237.3
Parageusia 781.1
  psychogenic 306.7
Paragonimiasis 121.2
Paragranuloma, Hodgkin's (M9660/3)
    201.0●
Parahemophilia (*see also* Defect,
    coagulation) 286.3
Parakeratosis 690.8
  psoriasiformis 696.2
  variegata 696.2
Paralysis, paralytic (complete)
    (incomplete) 344.9
  with
    broken
      back - *see* Fracture, vertebra, by
        site, with spinal cord injury
      neck - *see* Fracture, vertebra,
        cervical, with spinal cord
        injury
    fracture, vertebra - *see* Fracture,
      vertebra, by site, with spinal
      cord injury
    syphilis 094.89
  abdomen and back muscles 355.9
  abdominal muscles 355.9
  abducens (nerve) 378.54
  abductor 355.9
    lower extremity 355.8
    upper extremity 354.9
  accessory nerve 352.4
  accommodation 367.51
    hysterical 300.11
  acoustic nerve 388.5
  agitans 332.0
    arteriosclerotic 332.0
  alternating 344.89
    oculomotor 344.89
  amyotrophic 335.20
  ankle 355.8
  anterior serratus 355.9
  anus (sphincter) 569.49
  apoplectic (current episode) (*see also*
    Disease, cerebrovascular, acute)
    436
    late effect - *see* Late effect(s) (of)
      cerebrovascular disease
  arm 344.40
    affecting
      dominant side 344.41
      nondominant side 344.42
    both 344.2
    hysterical 300.11
    late effect - *see* Late effect(s) (of)
      cerebrovascular disease
    psychogenic 306.0
    transient 781.4
      traumatic NEC (*see also* Injury,
        nerve, upper limb) 955.9

Paralysis, paralytic *(Continued)*
  arteriosclerotic (current episode) 437.0
    late effect - *see* Late effect(s) (of)
      cerebrovascular disease
  ascending (spinal), acute 357.0
  associated, nuclear 344.89
  asthenic bulbar 358.00
  ataxic NEC 334.9
    general 094.1
  athetoid 333.71
  atrophic 356.9
    infantile, acute (*see also*
      Poliomyelitis, with paralysis)
      045.1●
    muscle NEC 355.9
    progressive 335.21
    spinal (acute) (*see also* Poliomyelitis,
      with paralysis) 045.1●
  attack (*see also* Disease, cerebrovascular,
    acute) 436
  axillary 353.0
  Babinski-Nageotte's 344.89
  Bell's 351.0
    newborn 767.5
  Benedikt's 344.89
  birth (injury) 767.7
    brain 767.0
    intracranial 767.0
    spinal cord 767.4
  bladder (sphincter) 596.53
    neurogenic 596.54
      with cauda equina syndrome
        344.61
    puerperal, postpartum, childbirth
      665.5●
    sensory 596.54
      with cauda equina 344.61
    spastic 596.54
      with cauda equina 344.61
  bowel, colon, or intestine (*see also* Ileus)
    560.1
  brachial plexus 353.0
    due to birth injury 767.6
    newborn 767.6
  brain
    congenital - *see* Palsy, cerebral
    current episode 437.8
    diplegia 344.2
      late effect - *see* Late effect(s) (of)
        cerebrovascular disease
    hemiplegia 342.9●
      late effect - *see* Late effect(s) (of)
        cerebrovascular disease
    infantile - *see* Palsy, cerebral
    monoplegia - *see also* Monoplegia
      late effect - *see* Late effect(s) (of)
        cerebrovascular disease
    paraplegia 344.1
    quadriplegia - *see* Quadriplegia
    syphilitic, congenital 090.49
    triplegia 344.89
  bronchi 519.19
  Brown-Séquard's 344.89
  bulbar (chronic) (progressive)
    335.22
    infantile (*see also* Poliomyelitis,
      bulbar) 045.0●
    poliomyelitic (*see also* Poliomyelitis,
      bulbar) 045.0●
    pseudo 335.23
    supranuclear 344.89
  bulbospinal 358.00
  cardiac (*see also* Failure, heart)
    428.9

◀ New   ◀▥ Revised   ~~deleted~~ Deleted   ● Use Additional Digit(s)   ▨ Omit code

Paralysis, paralytic (Continued)
cerebral
current episode 437.8
spastic, infantile - see Palsy, cerebral
cerebrocerebellar 437.8
diplegic infantile 343.0
cervical
plexus 353.2
sympathetic NEC 337.09
Céstan-Chenais 344.89
Charcôt-Marie-Tooth type 356.1
childhood - see Palsy, cerebral
Clark's 343.9
colon (see also Ileus) 560.1
compressed air 993.3
compression
arm NEC 354.9
cerebral - see Paralysis, brain
leg NEC 355.8
lower extremity NEC 355.8
upper extremity NEC 354.9
congenital (cerebral) (spastic) (spinal) -
see Palsy, cerebral
conjugate movement (of eye) 378.81
cortical (nuclear) (supranuclear)
378.81
convergence 378.83
cordis (see also Failure, heart) 428.9
cortical (see also Paralysis, brain)
437.8
cranial or cerebral nerve (see also
Disorder, nerve, cranial) 352.9
creeping 335.21
crossed leg 344.89
crutch 953.4
deglutition 784.99
hysterical 300.11
dementia 094.1
descending (spinal) NEC 335.9
diaphragm (flaccid) 519.4
due to accidental section of phrenic
nerve during procedure 998.2
digestive organs NEC 564.89
diplegic - see Diplegia
divergence (nuclear) 378.85
divers' 993.3
Duchenne's 335.22
due to intracranial or spinal birth
injury - see Palsy, cerebral
embolic (current episode) (see also
Embolism, brain) 434.1●
late effect - see Late effect(s) (of)
cerebrovascular disease
enteric (see also Ileus) 560.1
with hernia - see Hernia, by site,
with obstruction
Erb's syphilitic spastic spinal 094.89
Erb (-Duchenne) (birth) (newborn)
767.6
esophagus 530.89
essential, infancy (see also Poliomyelitis)
045.9●
extremity
lower - see Paralysis, leg
spastic (hereditary) 343.3
noncongenital or noninfantile
344.1
transient (cause unknown) 781.4
upper - see Paralysis, arm
eye muscle (extrinsic) 378.55
intrinsic 367.51
facial (nerve) 351.0
birth injury 767.5
congenital 767.5

Paralysis, paralytic (Continued)
facial (Continued)
following operation NEC 998.2
newborn 767.5
familial 359.3
periodic 359.3
spastic 334.1
fauces 478.29
finger NEC 354.9
foot NEC 355.8
gait 781.2
gastric nerve 352.3
gaze 378.81
general 094.1
ataxic 094.1
insane 094.1
juvenile 090.40
progressive 094.1
tabetic 094.1
glossopharyngeal (nerve) 352.2
glottis (see also Paralysis, vocal cord)
478.30
gluteal 353.4
Gubler (-Millard) 344.89
hand 354.9
hysterical 300.11
psychogenic 306.0
heart (see also Failure, heart) 428.9
hemifacial, progressive 349.89
hemiplegic - see Hemiplegia
hyperkalemic periodic (familial) 359.3
hypertensive (current episode) 437.8
hypoglossal (nerve) 352.5
hypokalemic periodic 359.3
Hyrtl's sphincter (rectum) 569.49
hysterical 300.11
ileus (see also Ileus) 560.1
infantile (see also Poliomyelitis) 045.9●
atrophic acute 045.1●
bulbar 045.0●
cerebral - see Palsy, cerebral
paralytic 045.1●
progressive acute 045.9●
spastic - see Palsy, cerebral
spinal 045.9●
infective (see also Poliomyelitis) 045.9●
inferior nuclear 344.9
insane, general or progressive 094.1
internuclear 378.86
interosseous 355.9
intestine (see also Ileus) 560.1
intracranial (current episode) (see also
Paralysis, brain) 437.8
due to birth injury 767.0
iris 379.49
due to diphtheria (toxin) 032.81
[379.49]
ischemic, Volkmann's (complicating
trauma) 958.6
isolated sleep, recurrent 327.43
Jackson's 344.89
jake 357.7
Jamaica ginger (jake) 357.7
juvenile general 090.40
Klumpke (-Déjérine) (birth) (newborn)
767.6
labioglossal (laryngeal) (pharyngeal)
335.22
Landry's 357.0
laryngeal nerve (recurrent) (superior)
(see also Paralysis, vocal cord)
478.30
larynx (see also Paralysis, vocal cord)
478.30
due to diphtheria (toxin) 032.3

Paralysis, paralytic (Continued)
late effect
due to
birth injury, brain or spinal
(cord) - see Palsy, cerebral
edema, brain or cerebral - see
Paralysis, brain
lesion
late effect - see Late effect(s)
(of) cerebrovascular
disease
spinal (cord) - see Paralysis,
spinal
lateral 335.24
lead 984.9
specified type of lead - see Table of
Drugs and Chemicals
left side - see Hemiplegia
leg 344.30
affecting
dominant side 344.31
nondominant side 344.32
both (see also Paraplegia) 344.1
crossed 344.89
hysterical 300.11
psychogenic 306.0
transient or transitory 781.4
traumatic NEC (see also
Injury, nerve, lower limb)
956.9
levator palpebrae superioris 374.31
limb NEC 344.5
all four - see Quadriplegia
quadriplegia - see Quadriplegia
lip 528.5
Lissauer's 094.1
local 355.9
lower limb - see also Paralysis,
leg
both (see also Paraplegia) 344.1
lung 518.89
newborn 770.89
median nerve 354.1
medullary (tegmental) 344.89
mesencephalic NEC 344.89
tegmental 344.89
middle alternating 344.89
Millard-Gubler-Foville 344.89
monoplegic - see Monoplegia
motor NEC 344.9
cerebral - see Paralysis, brain
spinal - see Paralysis, spinal
multiple
cerebral - see Paralysis, brain
spinal - see Paralysis, spinal
muscle (flaccid) 359.9
due to nerve lesion NEC 355.9
eye (extrinsic) 378.55
intrinsic 367.51
oblique 378.51
iris sphincter 364.89
ischemic (complicating trauma)
(Volkmann's) 958.6
pseudohypertrophic 359.1
muscular (atrophic) 359.9
progressive 335.21
musculocutaneous nerve 354.9
musculospiral 354.9
nerve - see also Disorder, nerve
third or oculomotor (partial)
378.51
total 378.52
fourth or trochlear 378.53
sixth or abducens 378.54

Paralysis, paralytic (Continued)
  nerve (Continued)
    seventh or facial 351.0
      birth injury 767.5
      due to
        injection NEC 999.9
        operation NEC 997.09
      newborn 767.5
    accessory 352.4
    auditory 388.5
    birth injury 767.7
    cranial or cerebral (see also Disorder, nerve, cranial) 352.9
    facial 351.0
      birth injury 767.5
      newborn 767.5
    laryngeal (see also Paralysis, vocal cord) 478.30
    newborn 767.7
    phrenic 354.8
      newborn 767.7
    radial 354.3
      birth injury 767.6
      newborn 767.6
    syphilitic 094.89
    traumatic NEC (see also Injury, nerve, by site) 957.9
    trigeminal 350.9
    ulnar 354.2
  newborn NEC 767.0
  normokalemic periodic 359.3
  obstetrical, newborn 767.7
  ocular 378.9
  oculofacial, congenital 352.6
  oculomotor (nerve) (partial) 378.51
    alternating 344.89
    external bilateral 378.55
    total 378.52
  olfactory nerve 352.0
  palate 528.9
  palatopharyngolaryngeal 352.6
  paratrigeminal 350.9
  periodic (familial) (hyperkalemic) (hypokalemic) (normokalemic) (potassium sensitive) (secondary) 359.3
  peripheral
    autonomic nervous system - see Neuropathy, peripheral, autonomic
    nerve NEC 355.9
  peroneal (nerve) 355.3
  pharynx 478.29
  phrenic nerve 354.8
  plantar nerves 355.6
  pneumogastric nerve 352.3
  poliomyelitis (current) (see also Poliomyelitis, with paralysis) 045.1●
    bulbar 045.0●
  popliteal nerve 355.3
  pressure (see also Neuropathy, entrapment) 355.9
  progressive 335.21
    atrophic 335.21
    bulbar 335.22
    general 094.1
    hemifacial 349.89
    infantile, acute (see also Poliomyelitis) 045.9●
    multiple 335.20
  pseudobulbar 335.23
  pseudohypertrophic 359.1
    muscle 359.1

Paralysis, paralytic (Continued)
  psychogenic 306.0
  pupil, pupillary 379.49
  quadriceps 355.8
  quadriplegic (see also Quadriplegia) 344.0
  radial nerve 354.3
    birth injury 767.6
  rectum (sphincter) 569.49
  rectus muscle (eye) 378.55
  recurrent
    isolated sleep 327.43
    laryngeal nerve (see also Paralysis, vocal cord) 478.30
  respiratory (muscle) (system) (tract) 786.09
    center NEC 344.89
      fetus or newborn 770.87
    congenital 768.9
    newborn 768.9
  right side - see Hemiplegia
  Saturday night 354.3
  saturnine 984.9
    specified type of lead - see Table of Drugs and Chemicals
  sciatic nerve 355.0
  secondary - see Paralysis, late effect
  seizure (cerebral) (current episode) (see also Disease, cerebrovascular, acute) 436
    late effect - see Late effect(s) (of) cerebrovascular disease
  senile NEC 344.9
  serratus magnus 355.9
  shaking (see also Parkinsonism) 332.0
  shock (see also Disease, cerebrovascular, acute) 436
    late effect - see Late effect(s) (of) cerebrovascular disease
  shoulder 354.9
  soft palate 528.9
  spasmodic - see Paralysis, spastic
  spastic 344.9
    cerebral infantile - see Palsy, cerebral
    congenital (cerebral) - see Palsy, cerebral
    familial 334.1
    hereditary 334.1
    infantile 343.9
    noncongenital or noninfantile, cerebral 344.9
    syphilitic 094.0
      spinal 094.89
  sphincter, bladder (see also Paralysis, bladder) 596.53
  spinal (cord) NEC 344.1
    accessory nerve 352.4
    acute (see also Poliomyelitis) 045.9●
    ascending acute 357.0
    atrophic (acute) (see also Poliomyelitis, with paralysis) 045.1●
      spastic, syphilitic 094.89
    congenital NEC 343.9
    hemiplegic - see Hemiplegia
    hereditary 336.8
    infantile (see also Poliomyelitis) 045.9●
    late effect NEC 344.89
    monoplegic - see Monoplegia
    nerve 355.9
    progressive 335.10
    quadriplegic - see Quadriplegia

Paralysis, paralytic (Continued)
  spinal (cord) NEC (Continued)
    spastic NEC 343.9
    traumatic - see Injury, spinal, by site
  sternomastoid 352.4
  stomach 536.3
    diabetic 250.6● [536.3]
      due to secondary diabetes 249.6● [536.3]
    nerve (nondiabetic) 352.3
  stroke (current episode) - see Infarct, brain
    late effect - see Late effect(s) (of) cerebrovascular disease
  subscapularis 354.8
  superior nuclear NEC 334.9
  supranuclear 356.8
  sympathetic
    cervical NEC 337.09
    nerve NEC (see also Neuropathy, peripheral, autonomic) 337.9
    nervous system - see Neuropathy, peripheral, autonomic
  syndrome 344.9
    specified NEC 344.89
  syphilitic spastic spinal (Erb's) 094.89
  tabetic general 094.1
  thigh 355.8
  throat 478.29
    diphtheritic 032.0
    muscle 478.29
  thrombotic (current episode) (see also Thrombosis, brain) 434.0●
    late effect - see Late effect(s) (of) cerebrovascular disease
  thumb NEC 354.9
  tick (-bite) 989.5
  Todd's (postepileptic transitory paralysis) 344.89
  toe 355.6
  tongue 529.8
  transient
    arm or leg NEC 781.4
    traumatic NEC (see also Injury, nerve, by site) 957.9
  trapezius 352.4
  traumatic, transient NEC (see also Injury, nerve, by site) 957.9
  trembling (see also Parkinsonism) 332.0
  triceps brachii 354.9
  trigeminal nerve 350.9
  trochlear nerve 378.53
  ulnar nerve 354.2
  upper limb - see also Paralysis, arm
    both (see also Diplegia) 344.2
  uremic - see Uremia
  uveoparotitic 135
  uvula 528.9
    hysterical 300.11
    postdiphtheritic 032.0
  vagus nerve 352.3
  vasomotor NEC 337.9
  velum palati 528.9
  vesical (see also Paralysis, bladder) 596.53
  vestibular nerve 388.5
  visual field, psychic 368.16
  vocal cord 478.30
    bilateral (partial) 478.33
      complete 478.34
    complete (bilateral) 478.34
    unilateral (partial) 478.31
      complete 478.32

◀ New   ◀▥ Revised   deleted Deleted   ● Use Additional Digit(s)   ▨ Omit code

Paralysis, paralytic (Continued)
Volkmann's (complicating trauma) 958.6
wasting 335.21
Weber's 344.89
wrist NEC 354.9
Paramedial orifice, urethrovesical 753.8
Paramenia 626.9
Parametritis (chronic) (see also Disease, pelvis, inflammatory) 614.4
acute 614.3
puerperal, postpartum, childbirth 670.8 ◀▥
Parametrium, parametric - see condition
Paramnesia (see also Amnesia) 780.93
Paramolar 520.1
causing crowding 524.31
Paramyloidosis 277.30
Paramyoclonus multiplex 333.2
Paramyotonia 359.29
congenita (of von Eulenburg) 359.29
Paraneoplastic syndrome - see condition
Parangi (see also Yaws) 102.9
Paranoia 297.1
alcoholic 291.5
querulans 297.8
senile 290.20
Paranoid
dementia (see also Schizophrenia) 295.3●
praecox (acute) 295.3●
senile 290.20
personality 301.0
psychosis 297.9
alcoholic 291.5
climacteric 297.2
drug-induced 292.11
involutional 297.2
menopausal 297.2
protracted reactive 298.4
psychogenic 298.4
acute 298.3
senile 290.20
reaction (chronic) 297.9
acute 298.3
schizophrenia (acute) (see also Schizophrenia) 295.3●
state 297.9
alcohol-induced 291.5
climacteric 297.2
drug-induced 292.11
due to or associated with arteriosclerosis (cerebrovascular) 290.42
presenile brain disease 290.12
senile brain disease 290.20
involutional 297.2
menopausal 297.2
senile 290.20
simple 297.0
specified type NEC 297.8
tendencies 301.0
traits 301.0
trends 301.0
type, psychopathic personality 301.0
Paraparesis (see also Paraplegia) 344.1
Paraphasia 784.3
Paraphilia (see also Deviation, sexual) 302.9
Paraphimosis (congenital) 605
chancroidal 099.0
Paraphrenia, paraphrenic (late) 297.2
climacteric 297.2
dementia (see also Schizophrenia) 295.3●

Paraphrenia, paraphrenic (Continued)
involutional 297.2
menopausal 297.2
schizophrenia (acute) (see also Schizophrenia) 295.3●
Paraplegia 344.1
with
broken back - see Fracture, vertebra, by site, with spinal cord injury
fracture, vertebra - see Fracture, vertebra, by site, with spinal cord injury
ataxic - see Degeneration, combined, spinal cord
brain (current episode) (see also Paralysis, brain) 437.8
cerebral (current episode) (see also Paralysis, brain) 437.8
congenital or infantile (cerebral) (spastic) (spinal) 343.0
cortical - see Paralysis, brain
familial spastic 334.1
functional (hysterical) 300.11
hysterical 300.11
infantile 343.0
late effect 344.1
Pott's (see also Tuberculosis) 015.0● [730.88]
psychogenic 306.0
spastic
Erb's spinal 094.89
hereditary 334.1
not infantile or congenital 344.1
spinal (cord)
traumatic NEC - see Injury, spinal, by site
syphilitic (spastic) 094.89
traumatic NEC - see Injury, spinal, by site
Paraproteinemia 273.2
benign (familial) 273.1
monoclonal 273.1
secondary to malignant or inflammatory disease 273.1
Parapsoriasis 696.2
en plaques 696.2
guttata 696.2
lichenoides chronica 696.2
retiformis 696.2
varioliformis (acuta) 696.2
Parascarlatina 057.8
Parasitic - see also condition
disease NEC (see also Infestation, parasitic) 136.9
contact V01.89
exposure to V01.89
intestinal NEC 129
skin NEC 134.9
stomatitis 112.0
sycosis 110.0
beard 110.0
scalp 110.0
twin 759.4
Parasitism NEC 136.9
intestinal NEC 129
skin NEC 134.9
specified - see Infestation
Parasitophobia 300.29
Parasomnia 307.47
alcohol induced 291.82
drug induced 292.85
nonorganic origin 307.47

Parasomnia (Continued)
organic 327.40
in conditions classified elsewhere 327.44
other 327.49
Paraspadias 752.69
Paraspasm facialis 351.8
Parathyroid gland - see condition
Parathyroiditis (autoimmune) 252.1
Parathyroprival tetany 252.1
Paratrachoma 077.0
Paratyphilitis (see also Appendicitis) 541
Paratyphoid (fever) - see Fever, paratyphoid
Paratyphus - see Fever, paratyphoid
Paraurethral duct 753.8
Para-urethritis 597.89
gonococcal (acute) 098.0
chronic or duration of 2 months or over 098.2
Paravaccinia NEC 051.9
milkers' node 051.1
Paravaginitis (see also Vaginitis) 616.10
Parencephalitis (see also Encephalitis) 323.9
late effect - see category 326
Parergasia 298.9
Paresis (see also Paralysis) 344.9
accommodation 367.51
bladder (spastic) (sphincter) (see also Paralysis, bladder) 596.53
tabetic 094.0
bowel, colon, or intestine (see also Ileus) 560.1
brain or cerebral - see Paralysis, brain
extrinsic muscle, eye 378.55
general 094.1
arrested 094.1
brain 094.1
cerebral 094.1
insane 094.1
juvenile 090.40
remission 090.49
progressive 094.1
remission (sustained) 094.1
tabetic 094.1
heart (see also Failure, heart) 428.9
infantile (see also Poliomyelitis) 045.9●
insane 094.1
juvenile 090.40
late effect - see Paralysis, late effect
luetic (general) 094.1
peripheral progressive 356.9
pseudohypertrophic 359.1
senile NEC 344.9
stomach 536.3
diabetic 250.6● [536.3]
due to secondary diabetes 249.6● [536.3]
syphilitic (general) 094.1
congenital 090.40
transient, limb 781.4
vesical (sphincter) NEC 596.53
Paresthesia (see also Disturbance, sensation) 782.0
Berger's (paresthesia of lower limb) 782.0
Bernhardt 355.1
Magnan's 782.0
Paretic - see condition
Parinaud's
conjunctivitis 372.02
oculoglandular syndrome 372.02
ophthalmoplegia 378.81

Parinaud's (Continued)
  syndrome (paralysis of conjugate
      upward gaze) 378.81
Parkes Weber and Dimitri syndrome
      (encephalocutaneous angiomatosis)
      759.6
Parkinson's disease, syndrome, or
      tremor - see Parkinsonism
Parkinsonism (arteriosclerotic)
      (idiopathic) (primary) 332.0
  associated with orthostatic hypotension
      (idiopathic) (symptomatic) 333.0
  due to drugs 332.1
  neuroleptic-induced 332.1
  secondary 332.1
  syphilitic 094.82
Parodontitis 523.40
Parodontosis 523.5
Paronychia (with lymphangitis) 681.9
  candidal (chronic) 112.3
  chronic 681.9
      candidal 112.3
      finger 681.02
      toe 681.11
  finger 681.02
  toe 681.11
  tuberculous (primary) (see also
      Tuberculosis) 017.0●
Parorexia NEC 307.52
  hysterical 300.11
Parosmia 781.1
  psychogenic 306.7
Parotid gland - see condition
Parotiditis (see also Parotitis) 527.2
  epidemic 072.9
  infectious 072.9
Parotitis 527.2
  allergic 527.2
  chronic 527.2
  epidemic (see also Mumps) 072.9
  infectious (see also Mumps) 072.9
  noninfectious 527.2
  nonspecific toxic 527.2
  not mumps 527.2
  postoperative 527.2
  purulent 527.2
  septic 527.2
  suppurative (acute) 527.2
  surgical 527.2
  toxic 527.2
Paroxysmal - see also condition
  dyspnea (nocturnal) 786.09
Parrot's disease (syphilitic
      osteochondritis) 090.0
Parrot fever 073.9
Parry's disease or syndrome
      (exophthalmic goiter) 242.0●
Parry-Romberg syndrome 349.89
Parson's disease (exophthalmic goiter)
      242.0●
Parsonage-Aldren-Turner syndrome 353.5
Parsonage-Turner syndrome 353.5
Pars planitis 363.21
Particolored infant 757.39
Parturition - see Delivery
Parvovirus 079.83
  B19 079.83
  human 079.83
Passage
  false, urethra 599.4
  meconium noted during delivery
      763.84
  of sounds or bougies (see also Attention
      to artificial opening) V55.9

Passive - see condition
Pasteurella septica 027.2
Pasteurellosis (see also Infection,
      Pasteurella) 027.2
PAT (paroxysmal atrial tachycardia)
      427.0
Patau's syndrome (trisomy D1) 758.1
Patch
  herald 696.3
Patches
  mucous (syphilitic) 091.3
      congenital 090.0
  smokers' (mouth) 528.6
Patellar - see condition
Patellofemoral syndrome 719.46
Patent - see also Imperfect closure
  atrioventricular ostium 745.69
  canal of Nuck 752.41
  cervix 622.5
      complicating pregnancy 654.5●
          affecting fetus or newborn 761.0
  ductus arteriosus or Botalli 747.0
  Eustachian
      tube 381.7
      valve 746.89
  foramen
      Botalli 745.5
      ovale 745.5
  interauricular septum 745.5
  interventricular septum 745.4
  omphalomesenteric duct 751.0
  os (uteri) - see Patent, cervix
  ostium secundum 745.5
  urachus 753.7
  vitelline duct 751.0
Paternity testing V70.4
Paterson's syndrome (sideropenic
      dysphagia) 280.8
Paterson (-Brown) (-Kelly) syndrome
      (sideropenic dysphagia) 280.8
Paterson-Kelly syndrome or web
      (sideropenic dysphagia) 280.8
Pathologic, pathological - see also
      condition
  asphyxia 799.01
  drunkenness 291.4
  emotionality 301.3
  fracture - see Fracture, pathologic
  liar 301.7
  personality 301.9
  resorption, tooth 521.40
      external 521.42
      internal 521.41
      specified NEC 521.49
  sexuality (see also Deviation, sexual)
      302.9
Pathology (of) - see also Disease
  periradicular, associated with previous
      endodontic treatment 526.69
Patterned motor discharge, idiopathic
      (see also Epilepsy) 345.5●
Patulous - see also Patent
  anus 569.49
  Eustachian tube 381.7
Pause, sinoatrial 427.81
Pavor nocturnus 307.46
Pavy's disease 593.6
Paxton's disease (white piedra) 111.2
Payr's disease or syndrome (splenic
      flexure syndrome) 569.89
PBA (pseudobulbar affect) 310.8
Pearls
  Elschnig 366.51
  enamel 520.2

Pearl-workers' disease (chronic
      osteomyelitis) (see also
      Osteomyelitis) 730.1●
Pectenitis 569.49
Pectenosis 569.49
Pectoral - see condition
Pectus
  carinatum (congenital) 754.82
      acquired 738.3
      rachitic (see also Rickets) 268.0
  excavatum (congenital) 754.81
      acquired 738.3
      rachitic (see also Rickets) 268.0
  recurvatum (congenital) 754.81
      acquired 738.3
Pedatrophia 261
Pederosis 302.2
Pediculosis (infestation) 132.9
  capitis (head louse) (any site) 132.0
  corporis (body louse) (any site) 132.1
  eyelid 132.0 [373.6]
  mixed (classifiable to more than one
      category in 132.0–132.2) 132.3
  pubis (pubic louse) (any site) 132.2
  vestimenti 132.1
  vulvae 132.2
Pediculus (infestation) - see Pediculosis
Pedophilia 302.2
Peg-shaped teeth 520.2
Pel's crisis 094.0
Pel-Ebstein disease - see Disease,
      Hodgkin's
Pelade 704.01
Pelger-Huët anomaly or syndrome
      (hereditary hyposegmentation) 288.2
Peliosis (rheumatica) 287.0
Pelizaeus-Merzbacher
  disease 330.0
  sclerosis, diffuse cerebral 330.0
Pellagra (alcoholic or with alcoholism)
      265.2
  with polyneuropathy 265.2 [357.4]
Pellagra-cerebellar-ataxia-renal
      aminoaciduria syndrome 270.0
Pellegrini's disease (calcification, knee
      joint) 726.62
Pellegrini (-Stieda) disease or syndrome
      (calcification, knee joint) 726.62
Pellizzi's syndrome (pineal) 259.8
Pelvic - see also condition
  congestion-fibrosis syndrome 625.5
  kidney 753.3
Pelvioectasis 591
Pelviolithiasis 592.0
Pelviperitonitis
  female (see also Peritonitis, pelvic,
      female) 614.5
  male (see also Peritonitis) 567.21
Pelvis, pelvic - see also condition or type
  infantile 738.6
  Nägele's 738.6
  obliquity 738.6
  Robert's 755.69
Pemphigoid 694.5
  benign, mucous membrane 694.60
      with ocular involvement 694.61
  bullous 694.5
  cicatricial 694.60
      with ocular involvement 694.61
  juvenile 694.2
Pemphigus 694.4
  benign 694.5
      chronic familial 757.39
  Brazilian 694.4

◄ New   ◄▌▌▌ Revised   ~~deleted~~ Deleted   ● Use Additional Digit(s)   ▨ Omit code

Pemphigus (Continued)
    circinatus 694.0
    congenital, traumatic 757.39
    conjunctiva 694.61
    contagiosus 684
    erythematodes 694.4
    erythematosus 694.4
    foliaceus 694.4
    frambesiodes 694.4
    gangrenous (see also Gangrene) 785.4
    malignant 694.4
    neonatorum, newborn 684
    ocular 694.61
    papillaris 694.4
    seborrheic 694.4
    South American 694.4
    syphilitic (congenital) 090.0
    vegetans 694.4
    vulgaris 694.4
    wildfire 694.4
Pendred's syndrome (familial goiter with
    deaf-mutism) 243
Pendulous
    abdomen 701.9
        in pregnancy or childbirth 654.4●
            affecting fetus or newborn
                763.89
    breast 611.89
Penetrating wound - see also Wound,
    open, by site
    with internal injury - see Injury,
        internal, by site, with open
        wound
    eyeball 871.7
        with foreign body (nonmagnetic)
            871.6
            magnetic 871.5
    ocular (see also Penetrating wound,
        eyeball) 871.7
        adnexa 870.3
            with foreign body 870.4
    orbit 870.3
        with foreign body 870.4
Penetration, pregnant uterus by
    instrument
    with
        abortion - see Abortion, by type,
            with damage to pelvic organs
        ectopic pregnancy (see also
            categories 633.0–633.9) 639.2
        molar pregnancy (see also categories
            630–632) 639.2
    complication of delivery 665.1●
        affecting fetus or newborn 763.89
    following
        abortion 639.2
        ectopic or molar pregnancy 639.2
Penfield's syndrome (see also Epilepsy)
    345.5●
Penicilliosis of lung 117.3
Penis - see condition
Penitis 607.2
Penta X syndrome 758.81
Pentalogy (of Fallot) 745.2
Pentosuria (benign) (essential) 271.8
Peptic acid disease 536.8
Peregrinating patient V65.2
Perforated - see Perforation
Perforation, perforative (nontraumatic)
    antrum (see also Sinusitis, maxillary)
        473.0
    appendix 540.0
        with peritoneal abscess 540.1
    atrial septum, multiple 745.5

Perforation, perforative (Continued)
    attic, ear 384.22
        healed 384.81
    bile duct, except cystic (see also Disease,
        biliary) 576.3
        cystic 575.4
    bladder (urinary) 596.6
        with
            abortion - see Abortion, by type,
                with damage to pelvic
                organs
            ectopic pregnancy (see also
                categories 633.0–633.9) 639.2
            molar pregnancy (see also
                categories 630–632) 639.2
        following
            abortion 639.2
            ectopic or molar pregnancy 639.2
        obstetrical trauma 665.5●
    bowel 569.83
        with
            abortion - see Abortion, by type,
                with damage to pelvic
                organs
            ectopic pregnancy (see also
                categories 633.0–633.9) 639.2
            molar pregnancy (see also
                categories 630–632) 639.2
        fetus or newborn 777.6
        following
            abortion 639.2
            ectopic or molar pregnancy 639.2
        obstetrical trauma 665.5●
    broad ligament
        with
            abortion - see Abortion, by type,
                with damage to pelvic
                organs
            ectopic pregnancy (see also
                categories 633.0–633.9) 639.2
            molar pregnancy (see also
                categories 630–632) 639.2
        following
            abortion 639.2
            ectopic or molar pregnancy 639.2
        obstetrical trauma 665.6●
    by
        device, implant, or graft - see
            Complications, mechanical
        foreign body left accidentally in
            operation wound 998.4
        instrument (any) during a
            procedure, accidental 998.2
    cecum 540.0
        with peritoneal abscess 540.1
    cervix (uteri) - see also Injury, internal,
        cervix
        with
            abortion - see Abortion, by type,
                with damage to pelvic
                organs
            ectopic pregnancy (see also
                categories 633.0–633.9) 639.2
            molar pregnancy (see also
                categories 630–632) 639.2
        following
            abortion 639.2
            ectopic or molar pregnancy 639.2
        obstetrical trauma 665.3●
    colon 569.83
    common duct (bile) 576.3
    cornea (see also Ulcer, cornea) 370.00
        due to ulceration 370.06
    cystic duct 575.4

Perforation, perforative (Continued)
    diverticulum (see also Diverticula)
        562.10
        small intestine 562.00
    duodenum, duodenal (ulcer) - see
        Ulcer, duodenum, with
        perforation
    ear drum - see Perforation, tympanum
    enteritis - see Enteritis
    esophagus 530.4
    ethmoidal sinus (see also Sinusitis,
        ethmoidal) 473.2
    foreign body (external site) - see also
        Wound, open, by site,
        complicated
        internal site, by ingested object - see
            Foreign body
    frontal sinus (see also Sinusitis, frontal)
        473.1
    gallbladder or duct (see also Disease,
        gallbladder) 575.4
    gastric (ulcer) - see Ulcer, stomach, with
        perforation
    heart valve - see Endocarditis
    ileum (see also Perforation, intestine)
        569.83
    instrumental
        external - see Wound, open, by site
        pregnant uterus, complicating
            delivery 665.9●
        surgical (accidental) (blood vessel)
            (nerve) (organ) 998.2
    intestine 569.83
        with
            abortion - see Abortion, by type,
                with damage to pelvic
                organs
            ectopic pregnancy (see also
                categories 633.0–633.9) 639.2
            molar pregnancy (see also
                categories 630–632) 639.2
        fetus or newborn 777.6
        obstetrical trauma 665.5●
        ulcerative NEC 569.83
    jejunum, jejunal 569.83
        ulcer - see Ulcer, gastrojejunal, with
            perforation
    mastoid (antrum) (cell) 383.89
    maxillary sinus (see also Sinusitis,
        maxillary) 473.0
    membrana tympani - see Perforation,
        tympanum
    nasal
        septum 478.19
            congenital 748.1
            syphilitic 095.8
        sinus (see also Sinusitis) 473.9
            congenital 748.1
    palate (hard) 526.89
        soft 528.9
            syphilitic 095.8
        syphilitic 095.8
    palatine vault 526.89
        syphilitic 095.8
            congenital 090.5
    pelvic
        floor
            with
                abortion - see Abortion, by
                    type, with damage to
                    pelvic organs
                ectopic pregnancy (see also
                    categories 633.0–633.9)
                    639.2

Perforation, perforative *(Continued)*
  pelvic *(Continued)*
    floor *(Continued)*
      with *(Continued)*
        molar pregnancy (*see also*
            categories 630–632)
            639.2
        obstetrical trauma 664.1●
    organ
      with
        abortion - *see* Abortion, by
            type, with damage to
            pelvic organs
        ectopic pregnancy (*see also*
            categories 633.0–633.9)
            639.2
        molar pregnancy (*see also*
            categories 630–632)
            639.2
      following
        abortion 639.2
        ectopic or molar pregnancy
            639.2
      obstetrical trauma 665.5●
  perineum - *see* Laceration, perineum
  periurethral tissue
    with
      abortion - *see* Abortion, by type,
          with damage to pelvic
          organs
      ectopic pregnancy (*see also*
          categories 630–632) 639.2
      molar pregnancy (*see also*
          categories 630–632) 639.2
  pharynx 478.29
  pylorus, pyloric (ulcer) - *see* Ulcer,
      stomach, with perforation
  rectum 569.49
  root canal space 526.61
  sigmoid 569.83
  sinus (accessory) (chronic) (nasal) (*see*
      also Sinusitis) 473.9
  sphenoidal sinus (*see also* Sinusitis,
      sphenoidal) 473.3
  stomach (due to ulcer) - *see* Ulcer,
      stomach, with perforation
  surgical (accidental) (by instrument)
      (blood vessel) (nerve) (organ)
      998.2
  traumatic
    external - *see* Wound, open, by
        site
    eye (*see also* Penetrating wound,
        ocular) 871.7
    internal organ - *see* Injury, internal,
        by site
  tympanum (membrane) (persistent
      posttraumatic)
      (postinflammatory) 384.20
    with
      otitis media - *see* Otitis media
    attic 384.22
    central 384.21
    healed 384.81
    marginal NEC 384.23
    multiple 384.24
    pars flaccida 384.22
    total 384.25
    traumatic - *see* Wound, open, ear,
        drum
  typhoid, gastrointestinal 002.0
  ulcer - *see* Ulcer, by site, with
      perforation
  ureter 593.89

Perforation, perforative *(Continued)*
  urethra
    with
      abortion - *see* Abortion, by type,
          with damage to pelvic
          organs
      ectopic pregnancy (*see also*
          categories 633.0–633.9) 639.2
      molar pregnancy (*see also*
          categories 630–632) 639.2
    following
      abortion 639.2
      ectopic or molar pregnancy 639.2
    obstetrical trauma 665.5●
  uterus - *see also* Injury, internal, uterus
    with
      abortion - *see* Abortion, by type,
          with damage to pelvic
          organs
      ectopic pregnancy (*see also*
          categories 633.0–633.9) 639.2
      molar pregnancy (*see also*
          categories 630–632) 639.2
    by intrauterine contraceptive device
        996.32
    following
      abortion 639.2
      ectopic or molar pregnancy 639.2
    obstetrical trauma - *see* Injury,
        internal, uterus, obstetrical
        trauma
  uvula 528.9
    syphilitic 095.8
  vagina - *see* Laceration, vagina
  viscus NEC 799.89
    traumatic 868.00
      with open wound into cavity
          868.10

Periadenitis mucosa necrotica recurrens
    528.2
Periangiitis 446.0
Periantritis 535.4●
Periappendicitis (acute) (*see also*
    Appendicitis) 541
Periarteritis (disseminated) (infectious)
    (necrotizing) (nodosa) 446.0
Periarthritis (joint) 726.90
  Duplay's 726.2
  gonococcal 098.50
  humeroscapularis 726.2
  scapulohumeral 726.2
  shoulder 726.2
  wrist 726.4
Periarthrosis (angioneural) - *see*
    Periarthritis
Peribronchitis 491.9
  tuberculous (*see also* Tuberculosis)
      011.3●
Pericapsulitis, adhesive (shoulder) 726.0
Pericarditis (granular) (with
    decompensation) (with effusion)
    423.9
  with
    rheumatic fever (conditions
        classifiable to 390)
      active (*see also* Pericarditis,
          rheumatic) 391.0
      inactive or quiescent 393
  actinomycotic 039.8 *[420.0]*
  acute (nonrheumatic) 420.90
    with chorea (acute) (rheumatic)
        (Sydenham's) 392.0
    bacterial 420.99
    benign 420.91

Pericarditis *(Continued)*
  acute *(Continued)*
    hemorrhagic 420.90
    idiopathic 420.91
    infective 420.90
    nonspecific 420.91
    rheumatic 391.0
      with chorea (acute) (rheumatic)
          (Sydenham's) 392.0
    sicca 420.90
    viral 420.91
  adhesive or adherent (external)
      (internal) 423.1
    acute - *see* Pericarditis, acute
    rheumatic (external) (internal) 393
  amebic 006.8 *[420.0]*
  bacterial (acute) (subacute) (with
      serous or seropurulent effusion)
      420.99
  calcareous 423.2
  cholesterol (chronic) 423.8
    acute 420.90
  chronic (nonrheumatic) 423.8
    rheumatic 393
  constrictive 423.2
  Coxsackie 074.21
  due to
    actinomycosis 039.8 *[420.0]*
    amebiasis 006.8 *[420.0]*
    Coxsackie (virus) 074.21
    histoplasmosis (*see also*
        Histoplasmosis) 115.93
    nocardiosis 039.8 *[420.0]*
    tuberculosis (*see also* Tuberculosis)
        017.9● *[420.0]*
  fibrinocaseous (*see also* Tuberculosis)
      017.9● *[420.0]*
  fibrinopurulent 420.99
  fibrinous - *see* Pericarditis, rheumatic
  fibropurulent 420.99
  fibrous 423.1
  gonococcal 098.83
  hemorrhagic 423.0
  idiopathic (acute) 420.91
  infective (acute) 420.90
  meningococcal 036.41
  neoplastic (chronic) 423.8
    acute 420.90
  nonspecific 420.91
  obliterans, obliterating 423.1
  plastic 423.1
  pneumococcal (acute) 420.99
  postinfarction 411.0
  purulent (acute) 420.99
  rheumatic (active) (acute) (with
      effusion) (with pneumonia)
      391.0
    with chorea (acute) (rheumatic)
        (Sydenham's) 392.0
    chronic or inactive (with chorea)
        393
  septic (acute) 420.99
  serofibrinous - *see* Pericarditis,
      rheumatic
  staphylococcal (acute) 420.99
  streptococcal (acute) 420.99
  suppurative (acute) 420.99
  syphilitic 093.81
  tuberculous (acute) (chronic) (*see also*
      Tuberculosis) 017.9● *[420.0]*
  uremic 585.9 *[420.0]*
  viral (acute) 420.91
Pericardium, pericardial - *see* condition
Pericellulitis (*see also* Cellulitis) 682.9

◀ New   ◀ⅢⅢ Revised   ~~deleted~~ Deleted   ● Use Additional Digit(s)   ▨ Omit code

Pericementitis 523.40
  acute 523.30
  chronic (suppurative) 523.40
Pericholecystitis (see also Cholecystitis)
    575.10
Perichondritis
  auricle 380.00
    acute 380.01
    chronic 380.02
  bronchus 491.9
  ear (external) 380.00
    acute 380.01
    chronic 380.02
  larynx 478.71
    syphilitic 095.8
    typhoid 002.0 [478.71]
  nose 478.19
  pinna 380.00
    acute 380.01
    chronic 380.02
  trachea 478.9
Periclasia 523.5
Pericolitis 569.89
Pericoronitis (chronic) 523.40
  acute 523.33
Pericystitis (see also Cystitis) 595.9
Pericytoma (M9150/1) - see also
    Neoplasm, connective tissue,
    uncertain behavior
  benign (M9150/0) - see Neoplasm,
    connective tissue, benign
  malignant (M9150/3) - see Neoplasm,
    connective tissue, malignant
Peridacryocystitis, acute 375.32
Peridiverticulitis (see also Diverticulitis)
    562.11
Periduodenitis 535.6●
Periendocarditis (see also Endocarditis)
    424.90
  acute or subacute 421.9
Periepididymitis (see also Epididymitis)
    604.90
Perifolliculitis (abscedens) 704.8
  capitis, abscedens et suffodiens 704.8
  dissecting, scalp 704.8
  scalp 704.8
  superficial pustular 704.8
Perigastritis (acute) 535.0●
Perigastrojejunitis (acute) 535.0●
Perihepatitis (acute) 573.3
  chlamydial 099.56
  gonococcal 098.86
Peri-ileitis (subacute) 569.89
Perilabyrinthitis (acute) - see Labyrinthitis
Perimeningitis - see Meningitis
Perimetritis (see also Endometritis) 615.9
Perimetrosalpingitis (see also Salpingo-
    oophoritis) 614.2
Perineocele 618.05
Perinephric - see condition
Perinephritic - see condition
Perinephritis (see also Infection, kidney)
    590.9
  purulent (see also Abscess, kidney)
    590.2
Perineum, perineal - see condition
Perineuritis NEC 729.2
Periodic - see also condition
  disease (familial) 277.31
  edema 995.1
    hereditary 277.6
  fever 277.31
  headache syndromes in child or
    adolescent 346.2●

Periodic (Continued)
  limb movement disorder 327.51
  paralysis (familial) 359.3
  peritonitis 277.31
  polyserositis 277.31
  somnolence (see also Narcolepsy) 347.00
Periodontal
  cyst 522.8
  pocket 523.8
Periodontitis (chronic) (complex)
    (compound) (simplex) 523.40
  acute 523.33
  aggressive 523.30
    generalized 523.32
    localized 523.31
  apical 522.6
    acute (pulpal origin) 522.4
  generalized 523.42
  localized 523.41
Periodontoclasia 523.5
Periodontosis 523.5
Periods - see also Menstruation
  heavy 626.2
  irregular 626.4
Perionychia (with lymphangitis) 681.9
  finger 681.02
  toe 681.11
Periophoritis (see also Salpingo-
    oophoritis) 614.2
Periorchitis (see also Orchitis) 604.90
Periosteum, periosteal - see condition
Periostitis (circumscribed) (diffuse)
    (infective) 730.3●

┌───┐
│ Note 59   Use the following fifth-digit │
│ subclassification with category 730:   │
│   │
│   0   site unspecified   │
│   1   shoulder region   │
│   2   upper arm   │
│   3   forearm   │
│   4   hand   │
│   5   pelvic region and thigh   │
│   6   lower leg   │
│   7   ankle and foot   │
│   8   other specified sites   │
│   9   multiple sites   │
└───┘

  with osteomyelitis (see also
    Osteomyelitis) 730.2●
    acute or subacute 730.0●
    chronic or old 730.1●
  albuminosa, albuminosus 730.3●
  alveolar 526.5
  alveolodental 526.5
  dental 526.5
  gonorrheal 098.89
  hyperplastica, generalized 731.2
  jaw (lower) (upper) 526.4
  monomelic 733.99
  orbital 376.02
  syphilitic 095.5
    congenital 090.0 [730.8]●
    secondary 091.61
  tuberculous (see also Tuberculosis,
    bone) 015.9● [730.8]●
  yaws (early) (hypertrophic) (late)
    102.6
Periostosis (see also Periostitis) 730.3●
  with osteomyelitis (see also
    Osteomyelitis) 730.2●
    acute or subacute 730.0●
    chronic or old 730.1●
  hyperplastic 756.59
Peripartum cardiomyopathy 674.5●

Periphlebitis (see also Phlebitis) 451.9
  lower extremity 451.2
    deep (vessels) 451.19
    superficial (vessels) 451.0
  portal 572.1
  retina 362.18
  superficial (vessels) 451.0
  tuberculous (see also Tuberculosis)
    017.9●
    retina 017.3● [362.18]
Peripneumonia - see Pneumonia
Periproctitis 569.49
Periprostatitis (see also Prostatitis) 601.9
Perirectal - see condition
Perirenal - see condition
Perisalpingitis (see also Salpingo-
    oophoritis) 614.2
Perisigmoiditis 569.89
Perisplenitis (infectional) 289.59
Perispondylitis - see Spondylitis
Peristalsis reversed or visible 787.4
Peritendinitis (see also Tenosynovitis)
    726.90
  adhesive (shoulder) 726.0
Perithelioma (M9150/1) - see Pericytoma
Peritoneum, peritoneal - see also condition
  equilibration test V56.32
Peritonitis (acute) (adhesive) (fibrinous)
    (hemorrhagic) (idiopathic)
    (localized) (perforative) (primary)
    (with adhesions) (with effusion)
    567.9
  with or following
    abortion - see Abortion, by type,
      with sepsis
    abscess 567.21
    appendicitis 540.0
      with peritoneal abscess 540.1
    ectopic pregnancy (see also
      categories 633.0–633.9) 639.0
    molar pregnancy (see also categories
      630–632) 639.0
  aseptic 998.7
  bacterial 567.29
    spontaneous 567.23
  bile, biliary 567.81
  chemical 998.7
  chlamydial 099.56
  chronic proliferative 567.89
  congenital NEC 777.6
  diaphragmatic 567.22
  diffuse NEC 567.29
  diphtheritic 032.83
  disseminated NEC 567.29
  due to
    bile 567.81
    foreign
      body or object accidentally left
        during a procedure
        (instrument) (sponge)
        (swab) 998.4
      substance accidentally left during
        a procedure (chemical)
        (powder) (talc) 998.7
    talc 998.7
    urine 567.89
  fibrinopurulent 567.29
  fibrinous 567.29
  fibrocaseous (see also Tuberculosis)
    014.0●
  fibropurulent 567.29
  general, generalized (acute) 567.21
  gonococcal 098.86
  in infective disease NEC 136.9 [567.0]

Peritonitis *(Continued)*
  meconium (newborn) 777.6
  pancreatic 577.8
  paroxysmal, benign 277.31
  pelvic
    female (acute) 614.5
      chronic NEC 614.7
        with adhesions 614.6
        puerperal, postpartum, childbirth
          670.8 ◀▥
    male (acute) 567.21
  periodic (familial) 277.31
  phlegmonous 567.29
  pneumococcal 567.1
  postabortal 639.0
  proliferative, chronic 567.89
  puerperal, postpartum, childbirth
    670.8 ◀▥
  purulent 567.29
  septic 567.29
  spontaneous bacterial 567.23
  staphylococcal 567.29
  streptococcal 567.29
  subdiaphragmatic 567.29
  subphrenic 567.29
  suppurative 567.29
  syphilitic 095.2
    congenital 090.0 *[567.0]*
  talc 998.7
  tuberculous *(see also* Tuberculosis)
    014.0●
  urine 567.89
Peritonsillar - *see* condition
Peritonsillitis 475
Perityphlitis *(see also* Appendicitis) 541
Periureteritis 593.89
Periurethral - *see* condition
Periurethritis (gangrenous) 597.89
Periuterine - *see* condition
Perivaginitis *(see also* Vaginitis) 616.10
Perivasculitis, retinal 362.18
Perivasitis (chronic) 608.4
Periventricular leukomalacia 779.7
Perivesiculitis (seminal) *(see also*
  Vesiculitis) 608.0
Perlèche 686.8
  due to
    moniliasis 112.0
    riboflavin deficiency 266.0
Pernicious - *see* condition
Pernio, perniosis 991.5
Persecution
  delusion 297.9
  social V62.4
Perseveration (tonic) 784.69
Persistence, persistent (congenital)
  759.89
  anal membrane 751.2
  arteria stapedia 744.04
  atrioventricular canal 745.69
  bloody ejaculate 792.2
  branchial cleft 744.41
  bulbus cordis in left ventricle 745.8
  canal of Cloquet 743.51
  capsule (opaque) 743.51
  cilioretinal artery or vein 743.51
  cloaca 751.5
  communication - *see* Fistula, congenital
  convolutions
    aortic arch 747.21
    fallopian tube 752.19
    oviduct 752.19
    uterine tube 752.19
  double aortic arch 747.21

Persistence, persistent *(Continued)*
  ductus
    arteriosus 747.0
    Botalli 747.0
  fetal
    circulation 747.83
    form of cervix (uteri) 752.49
    hemoglobin (hereditary) ("Swiss
      variety") 282.7
    pulmonary hypertension 747.83
  foramen
    Botalli 745.5
    ovale 745.5
  Gartner's duct 752.41
  hemoglobin, fetal (hereditary) (HPFH)
    282.7
  hyaloid
    artery (generally incomplete) 743.51
    system 743.51
  hymen (tag)
    in pregnancy or childbirth
      654.8●
      causing obstructed labor
        660.2●
  lanugo 757.4
  left
    posterior cardinal vein 747.49
    root with right arch of aorta 747.21
    superior vena cava 747.49
  Meckel's diverticulum 751.0
  mesonephric duct 752.89
    fallopian tube 752.11
  mucosal disease (middle ear) (with
    posterior or superior marginal
    perforation of ear drum) 382.2
  nail(s), anomalous 757.5
  occiput, anterior or posterior
    660.3●
    fetus or newborn 763.1
  omphalomesenteric duct 751.0
  organ or site NEC - *see* Anomaly,
    specified type NEC
  ostium
    atrioventriculare commune 745.69
    primum 745.61
    secundum 745.5
  ovarian rests in fallopian tube 752.19
  pancreatic tissue in intestinal tract
    751.5
  primary (deciduous)
    teeth 520.6
    vitreous hyperplasia 743.51
  pulmonary hypertension 747.83
  pupillary membrane 743.46
    iris 743.46
    Rhesus (Rh) titer 999.7
  right aortic arch 747.21
  sinus
    urogenitalis 752.89
    venosus with imperfect
      incorporation in right auricle
      747.49
  thymus (gland) 254.8
    hyperplasia 254.0
  thyroglossal duct 759.2
  thyrolingual duct 759.2
  truncus arteriosus or communis
    745.0
  tunica vasculosa lentis 743.39
  umbilical sinus 753.7
  urachus 753.7
  vegetative state 780.03
  vitelline duct 751.0
  wolffian duct 752.89

Person (with)
  admitted for clinical research, as
    participant or control subject
    V70.7
  affected by
    family member
      currently on deployment
        (military) V61.01
      returned from deployment
        (military) (current or past
        conflict) V61.02
  awaiting admission to adequate facility
    elsewhere V63.2
    undergoing social agency
      investigation V63.8
  concern (normal) about sick person in
    family V61.49
  consulting on behalf of another V65.19
    pediatric ~~pre-birth visit for~~
      ~~expectant mother V65.11~~ ◀▥
    pre-adoption visit for adoptive
      parents V65.11 ◀
    pre-birth visit for expectant
      parents V65.11 ◀
  currently deployed in theater or in
    support of military war,
    peacekeeping and humanitarian
    operations V62.21
  feared
    complaint in whom no diagnosis
      was made V65.5
    condition not demonstrated V65.5
  feigning illness V65.2
  healthy, accompanying sick person
    V65.0
  history of military war, peacekeeping
    and humanitarian deployment
    (current or past conflict) V62.22
  living (in)
    alone V60.3
    boarding school V60.6
    residence remote from hospital or
      medical care facility V63.0
    residential institution V60.6
    without
      adequate
        financial resources V60.2
        housing (heating) (space)
          V60.1
      housing (permanent) (temporary)
        V60.0
      material resources V60.2
      person able to render necessary
        care V60.4
      shelter V60.0
  medical services in home not available
    V63.1
  on waiting list V63.2
    undergoing social agency
      investigation V63.8
  sick or handicapped in family V61.49
  "worried well" V65.5
Personality
  affective 301.10
  aggressive 301.3
  amoral 301.7
  anancastic, anankastic 301.4
  antisocial 301.7
  asocial 301.7
  asthenic 301.6
  avoidant 301.82
  borderline 301.83
  change 310.1
  compulsive 301.4

◀ New ◀▥ Revised ~~deleted~~ Deleted ● Use Additional Digit(s) ▥ Omit code

Personality *(Continued)*
    cycloid 301.13
    cyclothymic 301.13
    dependent 301.6
    depressive (chronic) 301.12
    disorder, disturbance NEC 301.9
        with
            antisocial disturbance 301.7
            pattern disturbance NEC 301.9
            sociopathic disturbance 301.7
            trait disturbance 301.9
    dual 300.14
    dyssocial 301.7
    eccentric 301.89
        "haltlose" type 301.89
    emotionally unstable 301.59
    epileptoid 301.3
    explosive 301.3
    fanatic 301.0
    histrionic 301.50
    hyperthymic 301.11
    hypomanic 301.11
    hypothymic 301.12
    hysterical 301.50
    immature 301.89
    inadequate 301.6
    labile 301.59
    masochistic 301.89
    morally defective 301.7
    multiple 300.14
    narcissistic 301.81
    obsessional 301.4
    obsessive-compulsive 301.4
    overconscientious 301.4
    paranoid 301.0
    passive (-dependent) 301.6
    passive-aggressive 301.84
    pathologic NEC 301.9
    pattern defect or disturbance 301.9
    pseudosocial 301.7
    psychoinfantile 301.59
    psychoneurotic NEC 301.89
    psychopathic 301.9
        with
            amoral trend 301.7
            antisocial trend 301.7
            asocial trend 301.7
            pathologic sexuality (*see also*
                Deviation, sexual) 302.9
        mixed types 301.9
    schizoid 301.20
        introverted 301.21
        schizotypal 301.22
    type A 301.4
    unstable (emotional) 301.59
Perthes' disease (capital femoral
    osteochondrosis) 732.1
Pertussis (*see also* Whooping cough) 033.9
    vaccination, prophylactic (against)
        V03.6
Peruvian wart 088.0
Perversion, perverted
    appetite 307.52
        hysterical 300.11
    function
        pineal gland 259.8
        pituitary gland 253.9
            anterior lobe
                deficient 253.2
                excessive 253.1
            posterior lobe 253.6
        placenta - *see* Placenta, abnormal
    sense of smell or taste 781.1
        psychogenic 306.7
    sexual (*see also* Deviation, sexual) 302.9

Pervious, congenital - *see also* Imperfect,
    closure
    ductus arteriosus 747.0
Pes (congenital) (*see also* Talipes) 754.70
    abductus (congenital) 754.60
        acquired 736.79
    acquired NEC 736.79
        planus 734
    adductus (congenital) 754.79
        acquired 736.79
    cavus 754.71
        acquired 736.73
    planovalgus (congenital) 754.69
        acquired 736.79
    planus (acquired) (any degree) 734
        congenital 754.61
        rachitic 268.1
    valgus (congenital) 754.61
        acquired 736.79
    varus (congenital) 754.50
        acquired 736.79
Pest (*see also* Plague) 020.9
Pestis (*see also* Plague) 020.9
    bubonica 020.0
    fulminans 020.0
    minor 020.8
    pneumonica - *see* Plague, pneumonic
Petechia, petechiae 782.7
    fetus or newborn 772.6
Petechial
    fever 036.0
    typhus 081.9
Petges-Cléjat or Petges-Clégat syndrome
    (poikilodermatomyositis) 710.3
Petit's
    disease (*see also* Hernia, lumbar) 553.8
Petit mal (idiopathic) (*see also* Epilepsy)
    345.0●
    status 345.2
Petrellidosis 117.6
Petrositis 383.20
    acute 383.21
    chronic 383.22
Peutz-Jeghers disease or syndrome 759.6
Peyronie's disease 607.85
Pfeiffer's disease 075
Phacentocele 379.32
    traumatic 921.3
Phacoanaphylaxis 360.19
Phacocele (old) 379.32
    traumatic 921.3
Phaehyphomycosis 117.8
Phagedena (dry) (moist) (*see also*
    Gangrene) 785.4
    arteriosclerotic 440.24
    geometric 686.09
    penis 607.89
    senile 440.24
    sloughing 785.4
    tropical (*see also* Ulcer, skin) 707.9
    vulva 616.50
Phagedenic - *see also* condition
    abscess - *see also* Abscess
        chancroid 099.0
    bubo NEC 099.8
    chancre 099.0
    ulcer (tropical) (*see also* Ulcer, skin)
        707.9
Phagomania 307.52
Phakoma 362.89
Phantom limb (syndrome) 353.6
Pharyngeal - *see also* condition
    arch remnant 744.41
    pouch syndrome 279.11

Pharyngitis (acute) (catarrhal)
    (gangrenous) (infective)
    (malignant) (membranous)
    (phlegmonous) (pneumococcal)
    (pseudomembranous) (simple)
    (staphylococcal) (subacute)
    (suppurative) (ulcerative) (viral)
    462
    with influenza, flu, or grippe 487.1
    aphthous 074.0
    atrophic 472.1
    chlamydial 099.51
    chronic 472.1
    Coxsackie virus 074.0
    diphtheritic (membranous) 032.0
    follicular 472.1
    fusospirochetal 101
    gonococcal 098.6
    granular (chronic) 472.1
    herpetic 054.79
    hypertrophic 472.1
    infectional, chronic 472.1
    influenzal 487.1
    lymphonodular, acute 074.8
    septic 034.0
    streptococcal 034.0
    tuberculous (*see also* Tuberculosis)
        012.8●
    vesicular 074.0
Pharyngoconjunctival fever 077.2
Pharyngoconjunctivitis, viral 077.2
Pharyngolaryngitis (acute) 465.0
    chronic 478.9
    septic 034.0
Pharyngoplegia 478.29
Pharyngotonsillitis 465.8
    tuberculous 012.8●
Pharyngotracheitis (acute) 465.8
    chronic 478.9
Pharynx, pharyngeal - *see* condition
Phase of life problem NEC V62.89
Phenomenon
    Arthus 995.21
    flashback (drug) 292.89
    jaw-winking 742.8
    Jod-Basedow 242.8●
    L. E. cell 710.0
    lupus erythematosus cell 710.0
    Pelger-Huët (hereditary
        hyposegmentation) 288.2
    Raynaud's (paroxysmal digital
        cyanosis) (secondary) 443.0
    Reilly's (*see also* Neuropathy,
        peripheral, autonomic)
        337.9
    vasomotor 780.2
    vasospastic 443.9
    vasovagal 780.2
    Wenckebach's, heart block (second
        degree) 426.13
Phenylketonuria (PKU) 270.1
Phenylpyruvicaciduria 270.1
Pheochromoblastoma (M8700/3)
    specified site - *see* Neoplasm, by site,
        malignant
    unspecified site 194.0
Pheochromocytoma (M8700/0)
    malignant (M8700/3)
        specified site - *see* Neoplasm, by site,
            malignant
        unspecified site 194.0
    specified site - *see* Neoplasm, by site,
        benign
    unspecified site 227.0

Phimosis (congenital) 605
  chancroidal 099.0
  due to infection 605
Phlebectasia (see also Varicose, vein)
  454.9
  congenital NEC 747.60
  esophagus (see also Varix, esophagus)
    456.1
    with hemorrhage (see also Varix,
      esophagus, bleeding) 456.0
Phlebitis (infective) (pyemic) (septic)
  (suppurative) 451.9
  antecubital vein 451.82
  arm NEC 451.84
    axillary vein 451.89
    basilic vein 451.82
    deep 451.83
    superficial 451.82
  axillary vein 451.89
  basilic vein 451.82
  blue 451.9
  brachial vein 451.83
  breast, superficial 451.89
  cavernous (venous) sinus - see
    Phlebitis, intracranial sinus
  cephalic vein 451.82
  cerebral (venous) sinus - see Phlebitis,
    intracranial sinus
  chest wall, superficial 451.89
  complicating pregnancy or puerperium
    671.2● ◀▥
    affecting fetus or newborn 760.3
  cranial (venous) sinus - see Phlebitis,
    intracranial sinus
  deep (vessels) 451.19
    femoral vein 451.11
    specified vessel NEC 451.19
  due to implanted device - see
    Complications, due to (presence
    of) any device, implant, or graft
    classified to 996.0–996.5 NEC
  during or resulting from a procedure
    997.2
  femoral vein (deep) (superficial)
    451.11
  femoropopliteal 451.19
  following infusion, perfusion, or
    transfusion 999.2
  gouty 274.89 [451.9]
  hepatic veins 451.89
  iliac vein 451.81
  iliofemoral 451.11
  intracranial sinus (any) (venous) 325
    late effect - see category 326
    nonpyogenic 437.6
      in pregnancy or puerperium
        671.5●
  jugular vein 451.89
  lateral (venous) sinus - see Phlebitis,
    intracranial sinus
  leg 451.2
    deep (vessels) 451.19
      specified vessel NEC 451.19
    superficial (vessels) 451.0
      femoral vein 451.11
  longitudinal sinus - see Phlebitis,
    intracranial sinus
  lower extremity 451.2
    deep (vessels) 451.19
      specified vessel NEC 451.19
    superficial (vessels) 451.0
      femoral vein 451.11
  migrans, migrating (superficial)
    453.1

Phlebitis (Continued)
  pelvic
    with
      abortion - see Abortion, by type,
        with sepsis
      ectopic pregnancy (see also
        categories 633.0–633.9)
        639.0
      molar pregnancy (see also
        categories 630–632)
        639.0
    following
      abortion 639.0
      ectopic or molar pregnancy
        639.0
    puerperal, postpartum 671.4●
  popliteal vein 451.19
  portal (vein) 572.1
  postoperative 997.2
  pregnancy 671.2● ◀▥
    deep 671.3●
    specified type NEC 671.5●
  superficial 671.2●
  puerperal, postpartum, childbirth
    671.2● ◀▥
    deep 671.4●
    lower extremities 671.2●
    pelvis 671.4●
    specified site NEC 671.5●
    superficial 671.2●
  radial vein 451.83
  retina 362.18
  saphenous (great) (long) 451.0
    accessory or small 451.0
  sinus (meninges) - see Phlebitis,
    intracranial sinus
  specified site NEC 451.89
  subclavian vein 451.89
  syphilitic 093.89
  tibial vein 451.19
  ulcer, ulcerative 451.9
    leg 451.2
      deep (vessels) 451.19
        specified vessel NEC 451.19
      superficial (vessels) 451.0
        femoral vein 451.11
    lower extremity 451.2
      deep (vessels) 451.19
        femoral vein 451.11
        specified vessel NEC
          451.19
      superficial (vessels) 451.0
  ulnar vein 451.83
  umbilicus 451.89
  upper extremity - see Phlebitis, arm
    deep (veins) 451.83
      brachial vein 451.83
      radial vein 451.83
      ulnar vein 451.83
    superficial (veins) 451.82
      antecubital vein 451.82
      basilic vein 451.82
      cephalic vein 451.82
  uterus (septic) (see also Endometritis)
    615.9
  varicose (leg) (lower extremity)
    (see also Varicose, vein)
    454.1
Phlebofibrosis 459.89
Phleboliths 459.89
Phlebosclerosis 459.89
Phlebothrombosis - see Thrombosis
Phlebotomus fever 066.0
Phlegm, choked on 933.1

Phlegmasia
  alba dolens (deep vessels) 451.19
    complicating pregnancy 671.3●
    nonpuerperal 451.19
    puerperal, postpartum, childbirth
      671.4●
  cerulea dolens 451.19
Phlegmon (see also Abscess) 682.9
  erysipelatous (see also Erysipelas) 035
  iliac 682.2
    fossa 540.1
  throat 478.29
Phlegmonous - see condition
Phlyctenulosis (allergic)
  (keratoconjunctivitis)
  (nontuberculous) 370.31
  cornea 370.31
    with ulcer (see also Ulcer, cornea)
      370.00
  tuberculous (see also Tuberculosis)
    017.3● [370.31]
Phobia, phobic (reaction) 300.20
  animal 300.29
  isolated NEC 300.29
  obsessional 300.3
  simple NEC 300.29
  social 300.23
  specified NEC 300.29
  state 300.20
Phocas' disease 610.1
Phocomelia 755.4
  lower limb 755.32
    complete 755.33
    distal 755.35
    proximal 755.34
  upper limb 755.22
    complete 755.23
    distal 755.25
    proximal 755.24
Phoria (see also Heterophoria) 378.40
Phosphate-losing tubular disorder 588.0
Phosphatemia 275.3
Phosphaturia 275.3
Photoallergic response 692.72
Photocoproporphyria 277.1
Photodermatitis (sun) 692.72
  light other than sun 692.82
Photokeratitis 370.24
Photo-ophthalmia 370.24
Photophobia 368.13
Photopsia 368.15
Photoretinitis 363.31
Photoretinopathy 363.31
Photosensitiveness (sun) 692.72
  light other than sun 692.82
Photosensitization skin (sun) 692.72
  light other than sun 692.82
Phototoxic response 692.72
Phrenitis 323.9
Phrynoderma 264.8
Phthiriasis (pubis) (any site) 132.2
  with any infestation classifiable to 132.0
    and 132.1 132.3
Phthirus infestation - see Phthiriasis
Phthisis (see also Tuberculosis) 011.9●
  bulbi (infectional) 360.41
  colliers' 011.4●
  cornea 371.05
  eyeball (due to infection) 360.41
  millstone makers' 011.4●
  miners' 011.4●
  potters' 011.4●
  sandblasters' 011.4●
  stonemasons' 011.4●

◀ New　◀▥ Revised　~~deleted~~ Deleted　● Use Additional Digit(s)　▨ Omit code

Phycomycosis 117.7
Physalopteriasis 127.7
Physical therapy NEC V57.1
  breathing exercises V57.0
Physiological cup, optic papilla
  borderline, glaucoma suspect 365.00
  enlarged 377.14
  glaucomatous 377.14
Phytobezoar 938
  intestine 936
  stomach 935.2
Pian (see also Yaws) 102.9
Pianoma 102.1
Piarhemia, piarrhemia (see also
      Hyperlipemia) 272.4
  bilharziasis 120.9
Pica 307.52
  hysterical 300.11
Pick's
  cerebral atrophy 331.11
    with dementia
      with behavioral disturbance
        331.11 [294.11]
      without behavioral disturbance
        331.11 [294.10]
  disease
    brain 331.11
      dementia in
        with behavioral disturbance
          331.11 [294.11]
        without behavioral
          disturbance 331.11
          [294.10]
    lipid histiocytosis 272.7
    liver (pericardial pseudocirrhosis of
      liver) 423.2
    pericardium (pericardial
      pseudocirrhosis of liver)
      423.2
    polyserositis (pericardial
      pseudocirrhosis of liver) 423.2
  syndrome
    heart (pericardial pseudocirrhosis of
      liver) 423.2
    liver (pericardial pseudocirrhosis of
      liver) 423.2
  tubular adenoma (M8640/0)
    specified site - see Neoplasm, by site,
      benign
    unspecified site
      female 220
      male 222.0
Pick-Herxheimer syndrome (diffuse
      idiopathic cutaneous atrophy) 701.8
Pick-Niemann disease (lipid
      histiocytosis) 272.7
Pickwickian syndrome (cardiopulmonary
      obesity) 278.8
Piebaldism, classic 709.09
Piedra 111.2
  beard 111.2
    black 111.3
    white 111.2
  black 111.3
  scalp 111.3
    black 111.3
    white 111.2
  white 111.2
Pierre Marie's syndrome (pulmonary
      hypertrophic osteoarthropathy)
      731.2
Pierre Marie-Bamberger syndrome
      (hypertrophic pulmonary
      osteoarthropathy) 731.2

Pierre Mauriac's syndrome (diabetes-
      dwarfism-obesity) 258.1
Pierre Robin deformity or syndrome
      (congenital) 756.0
Pierson's disease or osteochondrosis 732.1
Pigeon
  breast or chest (acquired) 738.3
    congenital 754.82
    rachitic (see also Rickets) 268.0
  breeders' disease or lung 495.2
  fanciers' disease or lung 495.2
  toe 735.8
Pigmentation (abnormal) 709.00
  anomalies NEC 709.00
    congenital 757.33
    specified NEC 709.09
  conjunctiva 372.55
  cornea 371.10
    anterior 371.11
    posterior 371.13
    stromal 371.12
  lids (congenital) 757.33
    acquired 374.52
  limbus corneae 371.10
  metals 709.00
  optic papilla, congenital 743.57
  retina (congenital) (grouped) (nevoid)
    743.53
    acquired 362.74
  scrotum, congenital 757.33
Piles - see Hemorrhoids
Pili
  annulati or torti (congenital) 757.4
  incarnati 704.8
Pill roller hand (intrinsic) 736.09
Pilomatrixoma (M8110/0) - see Neoplasm,
    skin, benign
Pilonidal - see condition
Pimple 709.8
PIN I (prostatic intraepithelial
    neoplasia I) 602.3
PIN II (prostatic intraepithelial
    neoplasia II) 602.3
PIN III (prostatic intraepithelial
    neoplasia III) 233.4
Pinched nerve - see Neuropathy,
    entrapment
Pineal body or gland - see condition
Pinealoblastoma (M9362/3) 194.4
Pinealoma (M9360/1) 237.1
  malignant (M9360/3) 194.4
Pineoblastoma (M9362/3) 194.4
Pineocytoma (M9361/1) 237.1
Pinguecula 372.51
Pingueculitis 372.34
Pinhole meatus (see also Stricture, urethra)
    598.9
Pink
  disease 985.0
  eye 372.03
  puffer 492.8
Pinkus' disease (lichen nitidus) 697.1
Pinpoint
  meatus (see also Stricture, urethra)
    598.9
  os (uteri) (see also Stricture, cervix)
    622.4
Pinselhaare (congenital) 757.4
Pinta 103.9
  cardiovascular lesions 103.2
  chancre (primary) 103.0
  erythematous plaques 103.1
  hyperchromic lesions 103.1
  hyperkeratosis 103.1

Pinta (Continued)
  lesions 103.9
    cardiovascular 103.2
    hyperchromic 103.1
    intermediate 103.1
    late 103.2
    mixed 103.3
    primary 103.0
    skin (achromic) (cicatricial)
      (dyschromic) 103.2
      hyperchromic 103.1
      mixed (achromic and
        hyperchromic) 103.3
  papule (primary) 103.0
  skin lesions (achromic) (cicatricial)
    (dyschromic) 103.2
    hyperchromic 103.1
    mixed (achromic and hyperchromic)
      103.3
  vitiligo 103.2
Pintid 103.0
Pinworms (disease) (infection)
    (infestation) 127.4
Piry fever 066.8
Pistol wound - see Gunshot wound
Pit, lip (mucus), congenital 750.25
Pitchers' elbow 718.82
Pithecoid pelvis 755.69
  with disproportion (fetopelvic)
    653.2●
    affecting fetus or newborn 763.1
    causing obstructed labor 660.1●
Pithiatism 300.11
Pitted - see also Pitting
  teeth 520.4
Pitting (edema) (see also Edema) 782.3
  lip 782.3
  nail 703.8
    congenital 757.5
Pituitary gland - see condition
Pituitary snuff-takers' disease 495.8
Pityriasis 696.5
  alba 696.5
  capitis 690.11
  circinata (et maculata) 696.3
  Hebra's (exfoliative dermatitis) 695.89
  lichenoides et varioliformis 696.2
  maculata (et circinata) 696.3
  nigra 111.1
  pilaris 757.39
    acquired 701.1
    Hebra's 696.4
  rosea 696.3
  rotunda 696.3
  rubra (I Iebra) 695.89
    pilaris 696.4
  sicca 690.18
  simplex 690.18
  specified type NEC 696.5
  streptogenes 696.5
  versicolor 111.0
    scrotal 111.0
Placenta, placental
  ablatio 641.2●
    affecting fetus or newborn 762.1
  abnormal, abnormality 656.7●
    with hemorrhage 641.8●
      affecting fetus or newborn 762.1
    affecting fetus or newborn 762.2
  abruptio 641.2●
    affecting fetus or newborn 762.1
  accessory lobe - see Placenta, abnormal
  accreta (without hemorrhage) 667.0●
    with hemorrhage 666.0●

Placenta, placental (Continued)
adherent (without hemorrhage) 667.0 ●
with hemorrhage 666.0 ●
apoplexy - see Placenta, separation
battledore - see Placenta, abnormal
bilobate - see Placenta, abnormal
bipartita - see Placenta, abnormal
carneous mole 631
centralis - see Placenta, previa
circumvallata - see Placenta, abnormal
cyst (amniotic) - see Placenta, abnormal
deficiency - see Placenta, insufficiency
degeneration - see Placenta,
insufficiency
detachment (partial) (premature) (with
hemorrhage) 641.2 ●
affecting fetus or newborn 762.1
dimidiata - see Placenta, abnormal
disease 656.7 ●
affecting fetus or newborn 762.2
duplex - see Placenta, abnormal
dysfunction - see Placenta,
insufficiency
fenestrata - see Placenta, abnormal
fibrosis - see Placenta, abnormal
fleshy mole 631
hematoma - see Placenta, abnormal
hemorrhage NEC - see Placenta,
separation
hormone disturbance or malfunction -
see Placenta, abnormal
hyperplasia - see Placenta, abnormal
increta (without hemorrhage) 667.0 ●
with hemorrhage 666.0 ●
infarction 656.7 ●
affecting fetus or newborn 762.2
insertion, vicious - see Placenta, previa
insufficiency
affecting
fetus or newborn 762.2
management of pregnancy
656.5 ●
lateral - see Placenta, previa
low implantation or insertion - see
Placenta, previa
low-lying - see Placenta, previa
malformation - see Placenta, abnormal
malposition - see Placenta, previa
marginalis, marginata - see Placenta,
previa
marginal sinus (hemorrhage) (rupture)
641.2 ●
affecting fetus or newborn 762.1
membranacea - see Placenta, abnormal
multilobed - see Placenta, abnormal
multipartita - see Placenta, abnormal
necrosis - see Placenta, abnormal
percreta (without hemorrhage) 667.0 ●
with hemorrhage 666.0 ●
polyp 674.4 ●
previa (central) (centralis) (complete)
(lateral) (marginal) (marginalis)
(partial) (partialis) (total) (with
hemorrhage) 641.1 ●
affecting fetus or newborn 762.0
noted
before labor, without hemorrhage
(with cesarean delivery)
641.0 ●
during pregnancy (without
hemorrhage) 641.0 ●
without hemorrhage (before labor
and delivery) (during
pregnancy) 641.0 ●

Placenta, placental (Continued)
retention (with hemorrhage) 666.0
fragments, complicating
puerperium (delayed
hemorrhage) 666.2 ●
without hemorrhage 667.1 ●
postpartum, puerperal 666.2 ●
without hemorrhage 667.0 ●
separation (normally implanted)
(partial) (premature) (with
hemorrhage) 641.2 ●
affecting fetus or newborn 762.1
septuplex - see Placenta, abnormal
small - see Placenta, insufficiency
softening (premature) - see Placenta,
abnormal
spuria - see Placenta, abnormal
succenturiata - see Placenta, abnormal
syphilitic 095.8
transfusion syndromes 762.3
transmission of chemical substance -
see Absorption, chemical, through
placenta
trapped (with hemorrhage) 666.0 ●
without hemorrhage 667.0 ●
trilobate - see Placenta, abnormal
tripartita - see Placenta, abnormal
triplex - see Placenta, abnormal
varicose vessel - see Placenta, abnormal
vicious insertion - see Placenta, previa
Placentitis
affecting fetus or newborn 762.7
complicating pregnancy 658.4 ●
Plagiocephaly (skull) 754.0
Plague 020.9
abortive 020.8
ambulatory 020.8
bubonic 020.0
cellulocutaneous 020.1
lymphatic gland 020.0
pneumonic 020.5
primary 020.3
secondary 020.4
pulmonary - see Plague, pneumonic
pulmonic - see Plague, pneumonic
septicemic 020.2
tonsillar 020.9
septicemic 020.2
vaccination, prophylactic (against)
V03.3
Planning, family V25.09
contraception V25.9
natural
procreative V26.41
to avoid pregnancy V25.04
procreation V26.49
natural V26.41
Plaque
artery, arterial - see Arteriosclerosis
calcareous - see Calcification
Hollenhorst's (retinal) 362.33
tongue 528.6
Plasma cell myeloma 203.0 ●
Plasmacytoma, plasmocytoma (solitary)
(M9731/1) 238.6
benign (M9731/0) - see Neoplasm, by
site, benign
malignant (M9731/3) 203.8 ●
Plasmacytopenia 288.59
Plasmacytosis 288.64
Plaster ulcer (see also Ulcer, pressure)
707.00
Plateau iris syndrome 364.82
Platybasia 756.0

Platyonychia (congenital) 757.5
acquired 703.8
Platypelloid pelvis 738.6
with disproportion (fetopelvic) 653.2 ●
affecting fetus or newborn 763.1
causing obstructed labor 660.1 ●
affecting fetus or newborn 763.1
congenital 755.69
Platyspondylia 756.19
Plethora 782.62
newborn 776.4
Pleura, pleural - see condition
Pleuralgia 786.52
Pleurisy (acute) (adhesive) (chronic)
(costal) (diaphragmatic) (double)
(dry) (fetid) (fibrinous) (fibrous)
(interlobar) (latent) (lung) (old)
(plastic) (primary) (residual) (sicca)
(sterile) (subacute) (unresolved)
(with adherent pleura) 511.0
with
effusion (without mention of cause)
511.9
bacterial, nontuberculous 511.1
nontuberculous NEC 511.9
bacterial 511.1
pneumococcal 511.1
specified type NEC 511.89
staphylococcal 511.1
streptococcal 511.1
tuberculous (see also Tuberculosis,
pleura) 012.0 ●
primary, progressive 010.1 ●
influenza, flu, or grippe 487.1
tuberculosis - see Pleurisy,
tuberculous
encysted 511.89
exudative (see also Pleurisy, with
effusion) 511.9
bacterial, nontuberculous 511.1
fibrinopurulent 510.9
with fistula 510.0
fibropurulent 510.9
with fistula 510.0
hemorrhagic 511.89
influenzal 487.1
pneumococcal 511.0
with effusion 511.1
purulent 510.9
with fistula 510.0
septic 510.9
with fistula 510.0
serofibrinous (see also Pleurisy, with
effusion) 511.9
bacterial, nontuberculous 511.1
seropurulent 510.9
with fistula 510.0
serous (see also Pleurisy, with effusion)
511.9
bacterial, nontuberculous 511.1
staphylococcal 511.0
with effusion 511.1
streptococcal 511.0
with effusion 511.1
suppurative 510.9
with fistula 510.0
traumatic (post) (current) 862.29
with open wound into cavity 862.39
tuberculous (with effusion) (see also
Tuberculosis, pleura) 012.0 ●
primary, progressive 010.1 ●
Pleuritis sicca - see Pleurisy
Pleurobronchopneumonia (see also
Pneumonia, broncho-) 485

◀ New   ◀▥ Revised   ~~deleted~~ Deleted   ● Use Additional Digit(s)   ▦ Omit code

Pleurodynia 786.52
  epidemic 074.1
  viral 074.1
Pleurohepatitis 573.8
Pleuropericarditis (see also Pericarditis)
    423.9
  acute 420.90
Pleuropneumonia (acute) (bilateral)
    (double) (septic) (see also
    Pneumonia) 486
  chronic (see also Fibrosis, lung) 515
Pleurorrhea (see also Hydrothorax) 511.89

Plexitis, brachial 353.0
Plica
  knee 727.83
  polonica 132.0
  tonsil 474.8
Plicae dysphonia ventricularis 784.49
Plicated tongue 529.5
  congenital 750.13
Plug
  bronchus NEC 519.19
  meconium (newborn) NEC 777.1
  mucus - see Mucus, plug
Plumbism 984.9
  specified type of lead - see Table of
    Drugs and Chemicals
Plummer's disease (toxic nodular goiter)
    242.3 ●
Plummer-Vinson syndrome (sideropenic
    dysphagia) 280.8
Pluricarential syndrome of infancy 260
Plurideficiency syndrome of infancy 260
Plus (and minus) hand (intrinsic) 736.09
PMDD (premenstrual dysphoric
    disorder) 625.4
PMS 625.4
Pneumathemia - see Air, embolism, by type
Pneumatic drill or hammer disease 994.9
Pneumatocele (lung) 518.89
  intracranial 348.89   ◀▥
  tension 492.0
Pneumatosis
  cystoides intestinalis 569.89
  peritonei 568.89
  pulmonum 492.8
Pneumaturia 599.84
Pneumoblastoma (M8981/3) - see
    Neoplasm, lung, malignant
Pneumocephalus 348.89   ◀▥
Pneumococcemia 038.2
Pneumococcus, pneumococcal - see
    condition
Pneumoconiosis (due to) (inhalation of)
    505
  aluminum 503
  asbestos 501
  bagasse 495.1
  bauxite 503
  beryllium 503
  carbon electrode makers' 503
  coal
    miners' (simple) 500
    workers' (simple) 500
  cotton dust 504
  diatomite fibrosis 502
  dust NEC 504
    inorganic 503
    lime 502
    marble 502
    organic NEC 504
  fumes or vapors (from silo) 506.9
  graphite 503

Pneumoconiosis (Continued)
  hard metal 503
  mica 502
  moldy hay 495.0
  rheumatoid 714.81
  silica NEC 502
    and carbon 500
  silicate NEC 502
  talc 502
Pneumocystis carinii pneumonia
    136.3
Pneumocystis jiroveci pneumonia
    136.3
Pneumocystosis 136.3
  with pneumonia 136.3
Pneumoenteritis 025
Pneumohemopericardium (see also
    Pericarditis) 423.9
Pneumohemothorax (see also
    Hemothorax) 511.89
  traumatic 860.4
    with open wound into thorax
      860.5
Pneumohydropericardium (see also
    Pericarditis) 423.9
Pneumohydrothorax (see also
    Hydrothorax) 511.89
Pneumomediastinum 518.1
  congenital 770.2
  fetus or newborn 770.2
Pneumomycosis 117.9
Pneumonia (acute) (Alpenstich) (benign)
    (bilateral) (brain) (cerebral)
    (circumscribed) (congestive)
    (creeping) (delayed resolution)
    (double) (epidemic) (fever) (flash)
    (fulminant) (fungoid)
    (granulomatous) (hemorrhagic)
    (incipient) (infantile) (infectious)
    (infiltration) (insular) (intermittent)
    (latent) (lobe) (migratory) (newborn)
    (organized) (overwhelming)
    (primary) (progressive)
    (pseudolobar) (purulent) (resolved)
    (secondary) (senile) (septic)
    (suppurative) (terminal) (true)
    (unresolved) (vesicular) 486
  with influenza, flu, or grippe 487.0
  adenoviral 480.0
  adynamic 514
  alba 090.0
  allergic 518.3
  alveolar - see Pneumonia, lobar
  anaerobes 482.81
  anthrax 022.1 [484.5]
  apex, apical - see Pneumonia, lobar
  ascaris 127.0 [484.8]
  aspiration 507.0
    due to
      aspiration of microorganisms
        bacterial 482.9
          specified type NEC
            482.89
        specified organism NEC
          483.8
          bacterial NEC 482.89
        viral 480.9
          specified type NEC 480.8
      food (regurgitated) 507.0
      gastric secretions 507.0
      milk 507.0
      oils, essences 507.1
      solids, liquids NEC 507.8
      vomitus 507.0

Pneumonia (Continued)
  aspiration (Continued)
    fetal 770.18
      due to
        blood 770.16
        clear amniotic fluid
          770.14
        meconium 770.12
        postnatal stomach contents
          770.86
    newborn 770.18
      due to
        blood 770.16
        clear amniotic fluid
          770.14
        meconium 770.12
        postnatal stomach contents
          770.86
  asthenic 514
  atypical (disseminated) (focal)
    (primary) 486
    with influenza 487.0
  bacillus 482.9
    specified type NEC 482.89
  bacterial 482.9
    specified type NEC 482.89
  Bacteroides (fragilis) (oralis)
    (melaninogenicus) 482.81
  basal, basic, basilar - see Pneumonia,
    lobar
  bronchiolitis obliterans organized
    (BOOP) 516.8
  broncho-, bronchial (confluent)
    (croupous) (diffuse)
    (disseminated) (hemorrhagic)
    (involving lobes) (lobar)
    (terminal) 485
    with influenza 487.0
    allergic 518.3
    aspiration (see also Pneumonia,
      aspiration) 507.0
    bacterial 482.9
      specified type NEC 482.89
    capillary 466.19
      with bronchospasm or
        obstruction 466.19
    chronic (see also Fibrosis, lung)
      515
  congenital (infective) 770.0
  diplococcal 481
  Eaton's agent 483.0
  Escherichia coli (E. coli) 482.82
  Friedländer's bacillus 482.0
  Hemophilus influenzae 482.2
  hiberno-vernal 083.0 [484.8]
  hypostatic 514
  influenzal 487.0
  inhalation (see also Pneumonia,
    aspiration) 507.0
    due to fumes or vapors
      (chemical) 506.0
  Klebsiella 482.0
  lipid 507.1
    endogenous 516.8
  Mycoplasma (pneumoniae)
    483.0
  ornithosis 073.0
  pleuropneumonia-like organisms
    (PPLO) 483.0
  pneumococcal 481
  Proteus 482.83
  Pseudomonas 482.1
  specified organism NEC 483.8
    bacterial NEC 482.89

Pneumonia (Continued)
  broncho-, bronchial (Continued)
    staphylococcal 482.40
      aureus 482.41
        methicillin
          resistant (MRSA) 482.42
          susceptible (MSSA) 482.41
        specified type NEC 482.49
    streptococcal - see Pneumonia,
      streptococcal
    typhoid 002.0 [484.8]
    viral, virus (see also Pneumonia,
      viral) 480.9
  Butyrivibrio (fibriosolvens) 482.81
  Candida 112.4
  capillary 466.19
    with bronchospasm or obstruction
      466.19
  caseous (see also Tuberculosis) 011.6●
  catarrhal - see Pneumonia, broncho-
  central - see Pneumonia, lobar
  Chlamydia, chlamydial 483.1
    pneumoniae 483.1
    psittaci 073.0
    specified type NEC 483.1
    trachomatis 483.1
  cholesterol 516.8
  chronic (see also Fibrosis, lung) 515
  cirrhotic (chronic) (see also Fibrosis,
    lung) 515
  Clostridium (haemolyticum) (novyi)
    NEC 482.81
  confluent - see Pneumonia, broncho-
  congenital (infective) 770.0
    aspiration 770.18
  croupous - see Pneumonia, lobar
  cytomegalic inclusion 078.5 [484.1]
  deglutition (see also Pneumonia,
    aspiration) 507.0
  desquamative interstitial 516.8
  diffuse - see Pneumonia, broncho-
  diplococcal, diplococcus (broncho-)
    (lobar) 481
  disseminated (focal) - see Pneumonia,
    broncho-
  due to
    adenovirus 480.0
    anaerobes 482.81
    Bacterium anitratum 482.83
    Chlamydia, chlamydial 483.1
      pneumoniae 483.1
      psittaci 073.0
      specified type NEC 483.1
      trachomatis 483.1
    coccidioidomycosis 114.0
    Diplococcus (pneumoniae) 481
    Eaton's agent 483.0
    Escherichia coli (E. coli) 482.82
    Friedländer's bacillus 482.0
    fumes or vapors (chemical)
      (inhalation) 506.0
    fungus NEC 117.9 [484.7]
      coccidioidomycosis 114.0
    Hemophilus influenzae (H.
      influenzae) 482.2
    Herellea 482.83
    influenza 487.0
    Klebsiella pneumoniae 482.0
    Mycoplasma (pneumoniae) 483.0
    parainfluenza virus 480.2
    pleuropneumonia-like organism
      (PPLO) 483.0
    Pneumococcus 481
    Pneumocystis carinii 136.3

Pneumonia (Continued)
  due to (Continued)
    Pneumocystis jiroveci 136.3
    Proteus 482.83
    Pseudomonas 482.1
    respiratory syncytial virus 480.1
    rickettsia 083.9 [484.8]
    SARS-associated coronavirus 480.3
    specified
      bacteria NEC 482.89
      organism NEC 483.8
      virus NEC 480.8
    Staphylococcus 482.40
      aureus 482.41
        methicillin
          resistant (MRSA) 482.42
          susceptible (MSSA) 482.41
        specified type NEC 482.49
    Streptococcus - see also Pneumonia,
      streptococcal
      pneumoniae 481
    virus (see also Pneumonia, viral)
      480.9
      SARS-associated coronavirus
        480.3
  Eaton's agent 483.0
  embolic, embolism (see Embolism,
    pulmonary) 415.1●
  eosinophilic 518.3
  Escherichia coli (E. coli) 482.82
  Eubacterium 482.81
  fibrinous - see Pneumonia, lobar
  fibroid (chronic) (see also Fibrosis, lung)
    515
  fibrous (see also Fibrosis, lung) 515
  Friedländer's bacillus 482.0
  fusobacterium (nucleatum) 482.81
  gangrenous 513.0
  giant cell (see also Pneumonia, viral)
    480.9
  gram-negative bacteria NEC 482.83
    anaerobic 482.81
  grippal 487.0
  Hemophilus influenzae (bronchial)
    (lobar) 482.2
  hypostatic (broncho-) (lobar) 514
  in
    actinomycosis 039.1
    anthrax 022.1 [484.5]
    aspergillosis 117.3 [484.6]
    candidiasis 112.4
    coccidioidomycosis 114.0
    cytomegalic inclusion disease 078.5
      [484.1]
    histoplasmosis (see also
      Histoplasmosis) 115.95
    infectious disease NEC 136.9 [484.8]
    measles 055.1
    mycosis, systemic NEC 117.9 [484.7]
    nocardiasis, nocardiosis 039.1
    ornithosis 073.0
    pneumocystosis 136.3
    psittacosis 073.0
    Q fever 083.0 [484.8]
    salmonellosis 003.22
    toxoplasmosis 130.4
    tularemia 021.2
    typhoid (fever) 002.0 [484.8]
    varicella 052.1
    whooping cough (see also Whooping
      cough) 033.9 [484.3]
  infective, acquired prenatally 770.0
  influenzal (broncho) (lobar) (virus)
    487.0

Pneumonia (Continued)
  inhalation (see also Pneumonia,
    aspiration) 507.0
    fumes or vapors (chemical) 506.0
  interstitial 516.8
    with influenzal 487.0
    acute 136.3
    chronic (see also Fibrosis, lung) 515
    desquamative 516.8
    hypostatic 514
    lipoid 507.1
    lymphoid 516.8
    plasma cell 136.3
    Pseudomonas 482.1
  intrauterine (infective) 770.0
    aspiration 770.18
    blood 770.16
    clear amniotic fluid 770.14
    meconium 770.12
    postnatal stomach contents 770.86
  Klebsiella pneumoniae 482.0
  Legionnaires' 482.84
  lipid, lipoid (exogenous) (interstitial)
    507.1
    endogenous 516.8
  lobar (diplococcal) (disseminated)
    (double) (interstitial)
    (pneumococcal, any type) 481
    with influenza 487.0
    bacterial 482.9
      specified type NEC 482.89
    chronic (see also Fibrosis, lung) 515
    Escherichia coli (E. coli) 482.82
    Friedländer's bacillus 482.0
    Hemophilus influenzae (H.
      influenzae) 482.2
    hypostatic 514
    influenzal 487.0
    Klebsiella 482.0
    ornithosis 073.0
    Proteus 482.83
    Pseudomonas 482.1
    psittacosis 073.0
    specified organism NEC 483.8
      bacterial NEC 482.89
    staphylococcal 482.40
      aureus 482.41
        methicillin
          resistant (MRSA) 482.42
          susceptible (MSSA) 482.41
        specified type NEC 482.49
    streptococcal - see Pneumonia,
      streptococcal
    viral, virus (see also Pneumonia,
      viral) 480.9
  lobular (confluent) - see Pneumonia,
    broncho-
  Löffler's 518.3
  massive - see Pneumonia, lobar
  meconium aspiration 770.12
  metastatic NEC 038.8 [484.8]
  methicillin resistant Staphylococcus
    aureus (MRSA) 482.42
  methicillin susceptible Staphylococcus
    aureus (MSSA) 482.41
  MRSA (methicillin resistant
    Staphylococcus aureus) 482.42
  MSSA (methicillin susceptible
    Staphylococcus aureus) 482.41
  Mycoplasma (pneumoniae) 483.0
  necrotic 513.0
  nitrogen dioxide 506.9
  orthostatic 514
  parainfluenza virus 480.2

◀ New   ◀III Revised   ~~deleted~~ Deleted   ● Use Additional Digit(s)   ▨ Omit code

Pneumonia *(Continued)*
   parenchymatous *(see also* Fibrosis, lung) 515
   passive 514
   patchy - *see* Pneumonia, broncho
   Peptococcus 482.81
   Peptostreptococcus 482.81
   plasma cell 136.3
   pleurolobar - *see* Pneumonia, lobar
   pleuropneumonia-like organism (PPLO) 483.0
   pneumococcal (broncho) (lobar) 481
   Pneumocystis (carinii) (jiroveci) 136.3
   postinfectional NEC 136.9 *[484.8]*
   postmeasles 055.1
   postoperative 997.39
   primary atypical 486
   Proprionibacterium 482.81
   Proteus 482.83
   Pseudomonas 482.1
   psittacosis 073.0
   radiation 508.0
   respiratory syncytial virus 480.1
   resulting from a procedure 997.39
   rheumatic 390 *[517.1]*
   Salmonella 003.22
   SARS-associated coronavirus 480.3
   segmented, segmental - *see* Pneumonia, broncho-
   Serratia (marcascens) 482.83
   specified
      bacteria NEC 482.89
      organism NEC 483.8
      virus NEC 480.8
   spirochetal 104.8 *[484]*
   staphylococcal (broncho) (lobar) 482.40
      aureus 482.41
         methicillin
            resistant (MRSA) 482.42
            susceptible (MSSA) 482.41
      specified type NEC 482.49
   static, stasis 514
   streptococcal (broncho) (lobar) NEC 482.30
      Group
         A 482.31
         B 482.32
         specified NEC 482.39
      pneumoniae 481
      specified type NEC 482.39
   Streptococcus pneumoniae 481
   traumatic (complication) (early) (secondary) 958.8
   tuberculous (any) *(see also* Tuberculosis) 011.6●
   tularemic 021.2
   TWAR agent 483.1
   varicella 052.1
   Veillonella 482.81
   ventilator associated 997.31
   viral, virus (broncho) (interstitial) (lobar) 480.9
      with influenza, flu, or grippe 487.0
      adenoviral 480.0
      parainfluenza 480.2
      respiratory syncytial 480.1
      SARS-associated coronavirus 480.3
      specified type NEC 480.8
   white (congenital) 090.0
Pneumonic - *see* condition

Pneumonitis (acute) (primary) *(see also* Pneumonia) 486
   allergic 495.9
      specified type NEC 495.8
   aspiration 507.0
      due to fumes or gases 506.0
      fetal 770.18
         due to
            blood 770.16
            clear amniotic fluid 770.14
            meconium 770.12
            postnatal stomach contents 770.86
      newborn 770.18
         due to
            blood 770.16
            clear amniotic fluid 770.14
            meconium 770.12
            postnatal stomach contents 770.86
      obstetric 668.0●
   chemical 506.0
      due to fumes or gases 506.0
   cholesterol 516.8
   chronic *(see also* Fibrosis, lung) 515
   congenital rubella 771.0
   crack 506.0
   due to
      crack (cocaine) 506.0
      fumes or vapors 506.0
      inhalation
         food (regurgitated), milk, vomitus 507.0
         oils, essences 507.1
         saliva 507.0
         solids, liquids NEC 507.8
      toxoplasmosis (acquired) 130.4
         congenital (active) 771.2 *[484.8]*
   eosinophilic 518.3
   fetal aspiration 770.18
      due to
         blood 770.16
         clear amniotic fluid 770.14
         meconium 770.12
         postnatal stomach contents 770.86
   hypersensitivity 495.9
   interstitial (chronic) *(see also* Fibrosis, lung) 515
      lymphoid 516.8
   lymphoid, interstitial 516.8
   meconium aspiration 770.12
   postanesthetic
      correct substance properly administered 507.0
      obstetric 668.0●
      overdose or wrong substance given 968.4
      specified anesthetic - *see* Table of Drugs and Chemicals
   postoperative 997.39
      obstetric 668.0●
   radiation 508.0
   rubella, congenital 771.0
   "ventilation" 495.7
   ventilator associated 997.31 ◄▬
   wood-dust 495.8
Pneumonoconiosis - *see* Pneumoconiosis
Pneumoparotid 527.8
Pneumopathy NEC 518.89
   alveolar 516.9
      specified NEC 516.8
      due to dust NEC 504
   parietoalveolar 516.9
      specified condition NEC 516.8

Pneumopericarditis *(see also* Pericarditis) 423.9
   acute 420.90
Pneumopericardium - *see also* Pericarditis
   congenital 770.2
   fetus or newborn 770.2
   traumatic (post) *(see also* Pneumothorax, traumatic) 860.0
      with open wound into thorax 860.1
Pneumoperitoneum 568.89
   fetus or newborn 770.2
Pneumophagia (psychogenic) 306.4
Pneumopleurisy, pneumopleuritis *(see also* Pneumonia) 486
Pneumopyopericardium 420.99
Pneumopyothorax *(see also* Pyopneumothorax) 510.9
   with fistula 510.0
Pneumorrhagia 786.3
   newborn 770.3
   tuberculous *(see also* Tuberculosis, pulmonary) 011.9●
Pneumosiderosis (occupational) 503
Pneumothorax (acute) (chronic) 512.8
   congenital 770.2
   due to operative injury of chest wall or lung 512.1
      accidental puncture or laceration 512.1
   fetus or newborn 770.2
   iatrogenic 512.1
   postoperative 512.1
   spontaneous 512.8
      fetus or newborn 770.2
      tension 512.0
   sucking 512.8
      iatrogenic 512.1
      postoperative 512.1
   tense valvular, infectional 512.0
   tension 512.0
      iatrogenic 512.1
      postoperative 512.1
      spontaneous 512.0
   traumatic 860.0
      with
         hemothorax 860.4
            with open wound into thorax 860.5
         open wound into thorax 860.1
   tuberculous *(see also* Tuberculosis) 011.7●
Pocket(s)
   endocardial *(see also* Endocarditis) 424.90
   periodontal 523.8
Podagra 274.01 ◄▬
Podencephalus 759.89
Poikilocytosis 790.09
Poikiloderma 709.09
   Civatte's 709.09
   congenital 757.33
   vasculare atrophicans 696.2
Poikilodermatomyositis 710.3
Pointed ear 744.29
Poise imperfect 729.90
Poisoned - *see* Poisoning
Poisoning (acute) - *see also* Table of Drugs and Chemicals
   Bacillus, B.
      aertrycke *(see also* Infection, Salmonella) 003.9
      botulinus 005.1
      cholerae (suis) *(see also* Infection, Salmonella) 003.9

Poisoning *(Continued)*
  Bacillus, B. *(Continued)*
    paratyphosus *(see also* Infection, Salmonella) 003.9
    suipestifer *(see also* Infection, Salmonella) 003.9
  bacterial toxins NEC 005.9
  berries, noxious 988.2
  blood (general) - *see* Septicemia
  botulism 005.1
  bread, moldy, mouldy - *see* Poisoning, food
  Ciguatera 988.0
  damaged meat - *see* Poisoning, food
  death-cap (Amanita phalloides) (Amanita verna) 988.1
  decomposed food - *see* Poisoning, food
  diseased food - *see* Poisoning, food
  drug - *see* Table of Drugs and Chemicals
  epidemic, fish, meat, or other food - *see* Poisoning, food
  fava bean 282.2
  fish (bacterial) - *see also* Poisoning, food
    noxious 988.0
  food (acute) (bacterial) (diseased) (infected) NEC 005.9
    due to
      bacillus
        aertrycke *(see also* Poisoning, food, due to Salmonella) 003.9
        botulinus 005.1
        cereus 005.89
        choleraesuis *(see also* Poisoning, food, due to Salmonella) 003.9
        paratyphosus *(see also* Poisoning, food, due to Salmonella) 003.9
        suipestifer *(see also* Poisoning, food, due to Salmonella) 003.9
      Clostridium 005.3
        botulinum 005.1
        perfringens 005.2
        welchii 005.2
      Salmonella (aertrycke) (callinarum) (choleraesuis) (enteritidis) (paratyphi) (suipestifer) 003.9
        with
          gastroenteritis 003.0
          localized infection(s) *(see also* Infection, Salmonella) 003.20
          septicemia 003.1
          specified manifestation NEC 003.8
      specified bacterium NEC 005.89
      Staphylococcus 005.0
      Streptococcus 005.89
      Vibrio parahaemolyticus 005.4
      Vibrio vulnificus 005.81
    noxious or naturally toxic 988.0
      berries 988.2
      fish 988.0
      mushroom 988.1
      plants NEC 988.2
  ice cream - *see* Poisoning, food
  ichthyotoxism (bacterial) 005.9
  kreotoxism, food 005.9
  malarial - *see* Malaria
  meat - *see* Poisoning, food

Poisoning *(Continued)*
  mushroom (noxious) 988.1
  mussel - *see also* Poisoning, food
    noxious 988.0
  noxious foodstuffs *(see also* Poisoning, food, noxious) 988.9
    specified type NEC 988.8
  plants, noxious 988.2
  pork - *see also* Poisoning, food
    specified NEC 988.8
    Trichinosis 124
  ptomaine - *see* Poisoning, food
  putrefaction, food - *see* Poisoning, food
  radiation 508.0
  Salmonella *(see also* Infection, Salmonella) 003.9
  sausage - *see also* Poisoning, food
    Trichinosis 124
  saxitoxin 988.0
  shellfish - *see also* Poisoning, food
    noxious (amnesic) (azaspiracid) (diarrheic) (neurotoxic) (paralytic) 988.0
  Staphylococcus, food 005.0
  toxic, from disease NEC 799.89
  truffles - *see* Poisoning, food
  uremic - *see* Uremia
  uric acid 274.9
  water 276.6

Poison ivy, oak, sumac or other plant dermatitis 692.6
Poker spine 720.0
Policeman's disease 729.2
Polioencephalitis (acute) (bulbar) *(see also* Poliomyelitis, bulbar) 045.0●
  inferior 335.22
  influenzal 487.8
  superior hemorrhagic (acute) (Wernicke's) 265.1
  Wernicke's (superior hemorrhagic) 265.1
Polioencephalomyelitis (acute) (anterior) (bulbar) *(see also* Polioencephalitis) 045.0●
Polioencephalopathy, superior hemorrhagic 265.1
  with
    beriberi 265.0
    pellagra 265.2
Poliomeningoencephalitis - *see* Meningoencephalitis
Poliomyelitis (acute) (anterior) (epidemic) 045.9●

> Note 60　Use the following fifth-digit subclassification with category 045:
>
> 0　poliovirus, unspecified type
> 1　poliovirus, type I
> 2　poliovirus, type II
> 3　poliovirus, type III

  with
    paralysis 045.1●
      bulbar 045.0●
  abortive 045.2●
  ascending 045.9●
    progressive 045.9●
  bulbar 045.0●
  cerebral 045.0●
  chronic 335.21
  congenital 771.2
  contact V01.2
  deformities 138
  exposure to V01.2

Poliomyelitis *(Continued)*
  late effect 138
  nonepidemic 045.9●
  nonparalytic 045.2●
  old with deformity 138
  posterior, acute 053.19
  residual 138
  sequelae 138
  spinal, acute 045.9●
  syphilitic (chronic) 094.89
  vaccination, prophylactic (against) V04.0
Poliosis (eyebrow) (eyelashes) 704.3
  circumscripta (congenital) 757.4
    acquired 704.3
  congenital 757.4
Pollakiuria 788.41
  psychogenic 306.53
Pollinosis 477.0
Pollitzer's disease (hidradenitis suppurativa) 705.83
Polyadenitis *(see also* Adenitis) 289.3
  malignant 020.0
Polyalgia 729.99
Polyangiitis (essential) 446.0
Polyarteritis (nodosa) (renal) 446.0
Polyarthralgia 719.49
  psychogenic 306.0
Polyarthritis, polyarthropathy NEC 716.59
  due to or associated with other specified conditions - *see* Arthritis, due to or associated with
  endemic *(see also* Disease, Kaschin-Beck) 716.0●
  inflammatory 714.9
    specified type NEC 714.89
  juvenile (chronic) 714.30
    acute 714.31
  migratory - *see* Fever, rheumatic
  rheumatic 714.0
    fever (acute) - *see* Fever, rheumatic
Polycarential syndrome of infancy 260
Polychondritis (atrophic) (chronic) (relapsing) 733.99
Polycoria 743.46
Polycystic (congenital) (disease) 759.89
  degeneration, kidney - *see* Polycystic, kidney
  kidney (congenital) 753.12
    adult type (APKD) 753.13
    autosomal dominant 753.13
    autosomal recessive 753.14
    childhood type (CPKD) 753.14
    infantile type 753.14
  liver 751.62
  lung 518.89
    congenital 748.4
  ovary, ovaries 256.4
  spleen 759.0
Polycythemia (primary) (rubra) (vera) (M9950/1) 238.4
  acquired 289.0
  benign 289.0
    familial 289.6
  due to
    donor twin 776.4
    fall in plasma volume 289.0
    high altitude 289.0
    maternal-fetal transfusion 776.4
    stress 289.0

Polycythemia (Continued)
  emotional 289.0
  erythropoietin 289.0
  familial (benign) 289.6
  Gaisböck's (hypertonica) 289.0
  high altitude 289.0
  hypertonica 289.0
  hypoxemic 289.0
  neonatorum 776.4
  nephrogenous 289.0
  relative 289.0
  secondary 289.0
  spurious 289.0
  stress 289.0
Polycytosis cryptogenica 289.0
Polydactylism, polydactyly 755.00
  fingers 755.01
  toes 755.02
Polydipsia 783.5
Polydystrophic oligophrenia 277.5
Polyembryoma (M9072/3) - see
  Neoplasm, by site, malignant
Polygalactia 676.6●
Polyglandular
  deficiency 258.9
  dyscrasia 258.9
  dysfunction 258.9
  syndrome 258.8
Polyhydramnios (see also Hydramnios)
  657●
Polymastia 757.6
Polymenorrhea 626.2
Polymicrogyria 742.2
Polymyalgia 725
  arteritica 446.5
  rheumatica 725
Polymyositis (acute) (chronic)
  (hemorrhagic) 710.4
  with involvement of
    lung 710.4 [517.8]
    skin 710.3
  ossificans (generalisata) (progressiva)
    728.19
  Wagner's (dermatomyositis) 710.3
Polyneuritis, polyneuritic (see also
  Polyneuropathy) 356.9
  alcoholic 357.5
    with psychosis 291.1
  cranialis 352.6
  demyelinating, chronic inflammatory
    (CIDP) 357.81
  diabetic 250.6● [357.2]
    due to secondary diabetes 249.6●
      [357.2]
  due to lack of vitamin NEC 269.2
    [357.4]
  endemic 265.0 [357.4]
  erythredema 985.0
  febrile 357.0
  hereditary ataxic 356.3
  idiopathic, acute 357.0
  infective (acute) 357.0
  nutritional 269.9 [357.4]
  postinfectious 357.0
Polyneuropathy (peripheral) 356.9
  alcoholic 357.5
  amyloid 277.39 [357.4]
  arsenical 357.7
  critical illness 357.82
  demyelinating, chronic inflammatory
    (CIDP) 357.81
  diabetic 250.6● [357.2]
    due to secondary diabetes 249.6●
      [357.2]

Polyneuropathy (Continued)
  due to
    antitetanus serum 357.6
    arsenic 357.7
    drug or medicinal substance 357.6
      correct substance properly
        administered 357.6
      overdose or wrong substance
        given or taken 977.9
      specified drug - see Table of
        Drugs and Chemicals
    lack of vitamin NEC 269.2 [357.4]
    lead 357.7
    organophosphate compounds 357.7
    pellagra 265.2 [357.4]
    porphyria 277.1 [357.4]
    serum 357.6
    toxic agent NEC 357.7
  hereditary 356.0
  idiopathic 356.9
    progressive 356.4
  in
    amyloidosis 277.39 [357.4]
    avitaminosis 269.2 [357.4]
      specified NEC 269.1 [357.4]
    beriberi 265.0 [357.4]
    collagen vascular disease NEC 710.9
      [357.1]
    deficiency
      B-complex NEC 266.2 [357.4]
      vitamin B 266.9 [357.4]
      vitamin B_6 266.1 [357.4]
    diabetes 250.6● [357.2]
      due to secondary diabetes 249.6●
        [357.2]
    diphtheria (see also Diphtheria)
      032.89 [357.4]
    disseminated lupus erythematosus
      710.0 [357.1]
    herpes zoster 053.13
    hypoglycemia 251.2 [357.4]
    malignant neoplasm (M8000/3)
      NEC 199.1 [357.3]
    mumps 072.72
    pellagra 265.2 [357.4]
    polyarteritis nodosa 446.0 [357.1]
    porphyria 277.1 [357.4]
    rheumatoid arthritis 714.0 [357.1]
    sarcoidosis 135 [357.4]
    uremia 585.9 [357.4]
  lead 357.7
  nutritional 269.9 [357.4]
    specified NEC 269.8 [357.4]
  postherpetic 053.13
  progressive 356.4
  sensory (hereditary) 356.2
  specified NEC 356.8
Polyonychia 757.5
Polyopia 368.2
  refractive 368.15
Polyorchism, polyorchidism (three testes)
  752.89
Polyorrhymenitis (peritoneal) (see also
  Polyserositis) 568.82
  pericardial 423.2
Polyostotic fibrous dysplasia 756.54
Polyotia 744.1
Polyp, polypus

Note 61   Polyps of organs or sites that
do not appear in the list below should
be coded to the residual category for
diseases of the organ or site concerned.

Polyp, polypus (Continued)
  accessory sinus 471.8
  adenoid tissue 471.0
  adenomatous (M8210/0) - see also
    Neoplasm, by site, benign
    adenocarcinoma in (M8210/3) - see
      Neoplasm, by site, malignant
    carcinoma in (M8210/3) - see
      Neoplasm, by site, malignant
    multiple (M8221/0) - see Neoplasm,
      by site, benign
  antrum 471.8
  anus, anal (canal) (nonadenomatous)
    569.0
    adenomatous 211.4
  Bartholin's gland 624.6
  bladder (M8120/1) 236.7
  broad ligament 620.8
  cervix (uteri) 622.7
    adenomatous 219.0
    in pregnancy or childbirth 654.6●
      affecting fetus or newborn
        763.89
      causing obstructed labor 660.2●
    mucous 622.7
    nonneoplastic 622.7
  choanal 471.0
  cholesterol 575.6
  clitoris 624.6
  colon (M8210/0) (see also Polyp,
    adenomatous) 211.3
  corpus uteri 621.0
  dental 522.0
  ear (middle) 385.30
  endometrium 621.0
  ethmoidal (sinus) 471.8
  fallopian tube 620.8
  female genital organs NEC 624.8
  frontal (sinus) 471.8
  gallbladder 575.6
  gingiva 523.8
  gum 523.8
  labia 624.6
  larynx (mucous) 478.4
  malignant (M8000/3) - see Neoplasm,
    by site, malignant
  maxillary (sinus) 471.8
  middle ear 385.30
  myometrium 621.0
  nares
    anterior 471.9
    posterior 471.0
  nasal (mucous) 471.9
    cavity 471.0
    septum 471.9
  nasopharyngeal 471.0
  neoplastic (M8210/0) - see Neoplasm,
    by site, benign
  nose (mucous) 471.9
  oviduct 620.8
  paratubal 620.8
  pharynx 478.29
    congenital 750.29
  placenta, placental 674.4●
  prostate 600.20
    with
      other lower urinary tract
        symptoms (LUTS) 600.21
      urinary
        obstruction 600.21
        retention 600.21
  pudenda 624.6
  pulp (dental) 522.0
  rectosigmoid 211.4

Polyp, polypus *(Continued)*
  rectum (nonadenomatous) 569.0
    adenomatous 211.4
  septum (nasal) 471.9
  sinus (accessory) (ethmoidal) (frontal)
      (maxillary) (sphenoidal) 471.8
  sphenoidal (sinus) 471.8
  stomach (M8210/0) 211.1
  tube, fallopian 620.8
  turbinate, mucous membrane 471.8
  ureter 593.89
  urethra 599.3
  uterine
    ligament 620.8
    tube 620.8
  uterus (body) (corpus) (mucous) 621.0
    in pregnancy or childbirth 654.1●
      affecting fetus or newborn 763.89
      causing obstructed labor 660.2●
  vagina 623.7
  vocal cord (mucous) 478.4
  vulva 624.6
Polyphagia 783.6
Polypoid - *see* condition
Polyposis - *see also* Polyp
  coli (adenomatous) (M8220/0) 211.3
    adenocarcinoma in (M8220/3) 153.9
    carcinoma in (M8220/3) 153.9
  familial (M8220/0) 211.3
  intestinal (adenomatous) (M8220/0)
      211.3
  multiple (M8221/0) - *see* Neoplasm, by
      site, benign
Polyradiculitis (acute) 357.0
Polyradiculoneuropathy (acute)
    (segmentally demyelinating) 357.0
Polysarcia 278.00
Polyserositis (peritoneal) 568.82
  due to pericarditis 423.2
  paroxysmal (familial) 277.31
  pericardial 423.2
  periodic (familial) 277.31
  pleural - *see* Pleurisy
  recurrent 277.31
  tuberculous (*see also* Tuberculosis,
      polyserositis) 018.9●
Polysialia 527.7
Polysplenia syndrome 759.0
Polythelia 757.6
Polytrichia (*see also* Hypertrichosis)
    704.1
Polyunguia (congenital) 757.5
  acquired 703.8
Polyuria 788.42
Pompe's disease (glycogenosis II) 271.0
Pompholyx 705.81
Poncet's disease (tuberculous
    rheumatism) (*see also* Tuberculosis)
    015.9●
Pond fracture - *see* Fracture, skull, vault
Ponos 085.0
Pons, pontine - *see* condition
Poor
  aesthetics of existing restoration of
      tooth 525.67
  contractions, labor 661.2●
    affecting fetus or newborn 763.7
  fetal growth NEC 764.9●
    affecting management of pregnancy
        656.5●
  incorporation
    artificial skin graft 996.55
    decellularized allodermis graft
        996.55

Poor *(Continued)*
  obstetrical history V13.29
    affecting management of current
        pregnancy V23.49
      pre-term labor V23.41
    pre-term labor V13.21
  sucking reflex (newborn) 796.1
  vision NEC 369.9
Poradenitis, nostras 099.1
Porencephaly (congenital)
    (developmental) (true) 742.4
  acquired 348.0
  nondevelopmental 348.0
  traumatic (post) 310.2
Porocephaliasis 134.1
Porokeratosis 757.39
  disseminated superficial actinic (DSAP)
      692.75
Poroma, eccrine (M8402/0) - *see*
    Neoplasm, skin, benign
Porphyria (acute) (congenital)
    (constitutional) (erythropoietic)
    (familial) (hepatica) (idiopathic)
    (idiosyncratic) (intermittent) (latent)
    (mixed hepatic) (photosensitive)
    (South African genetic) (Swedish)
    277.1
  acquired 277.1
  cutaneatarda
    hereditaria 277.1
    symptomatica 277.1
  due to drugs
    correct substance properly
        administered 277.1
    overdose or wrong substance given
        or taken 977.9
      specified drug - *see* Table of
          Drugs and Chemicals
  secondary 277.1
  toxic NEC 277.1
  variegata 277.1
Porphyrinuria (acquired) (congenital)
    (secondary) 277.1
Porphyruria (acquired) (congenital) 277.1
Portal - *see* condition
Port wine nevus or mark 757.32
Posadas-Wernicke disease 114.9
Position
  fetus, abnormal (*see also* Presentation,
      fetal) 652.9●
  teeth, faulty (*see also* Anomaly, position
      tooth) 524.30
Positive
  culture (nonspecific) 795.39
    AIDS virus V08
    blood 790.7
    HIV V08
    human immunodeficiency virus V08
    nose 795.39
      Staphylococcus - *see* Carrier
          (suspected) of,
          Staphylococcus
    skin lesion NEC 795.39
    spinal fluid 792.0
    sputum 795.39
    stool 792.1
    throat 795.39
    urine 791.9
    wound 795.39
  findings, anthrax 795.31
  HIV V08
  human immunodeficiency virus (HIV)
      V08
  PPD 795.5

Positive *(Continued)*
  serology
    AIDS virus V08
      inconclusive 795.71
    HIV V08
      inconclusive 795.71
    human immunodeficiency virus V08
      inconclusive 795.71
    syphilis 097.1
      with signs or symptoms - *see*
          Syphilis, by site and stage
      false 795.6
    skin test 795.7
      tuberculin (without active
          tuberculosis) 795.5
    VDRL 097.1
      with signs or symptoms - *see*
          Syphilis, by site and stage
      false 795.6
    Wassermann reaction 097.1
      false 795.6
Postcardiotomy syndrome 429.4
Postcaval ureter 753.4
Postcholecystectomy syndrome
    576.0
Postclimacteric bleeding 627.1
Postcommissurotomy syndrome
    429.4
Postconcussional syndrome 310.2
Postcontusional syndrome 310.2
Postcricoid region - *see* condition
Post-dates (pregnancy) - *see* Pregnancy
Postencephalitic - *see also* condition
  syndrome 310.8
Posterior - *see* condition
Posterolateral sclerosis (spinal cord) - *see*
    Degeneration, combined
Postexanthematous - *see* condition
Postfebrile - *see* condition
Postgastrectomy dumping syndrome
    564.2
Posthemiplegic chorea 344.89
Posthemorrhagic anemia (chronic) 280.0
  acute 285.1
  newborn 776.5
Posthepatitis syndrome 780.79
Postherpetic neuralgia (intercostal)
    (syndrome) (zoster) 053.19
  geniculate ganglion 053.11
  ophthalmica 053.19
  trigeminal 053.12
Posthitis 607.1
Postimmunization complication or
    reaction - *see* Complications,
    vaccination
Postinfectious - *see* condition
Postinfluenzal syndrome 780.79
Postlaminectomy syndrome 722.80
  cervical, cervicothoracic 722.81
  kyphosis 737.12
  lumbar, lumbosacral 722.83
  thoracic, thoracolumbar 722.82
Postleukotomy syndrome 310.0
Postlobectomy syndrome 310.0
Postmastectomy lymphedema
    (syndrome) 457.0
Postmaturity, postmature (fetus or
    newborn) (gestation period
    over 42 completed weeks)
    766.22
  affecting management of pregnancy
    post-term pregnancy 645.1●
    prolonged pregnancy 645.2●
  syndrome 766.22

◀ New   ◀|||| Revised   ~~deleted~~ Deleted   ● Use Additional Digit(s)   ▓ Omit code

Postmeasles - *see also* condition
  complication 055.8
    specified NEC 055.79
Postmenopausal
  endometrium (atrophic) 627.8
    suppurative (*see also* Endometritis)
      615.9
  hormone replacement therapy
    V07.4
  status (age related) (natural)
    V49.81
Postnasal drip 784.91
Postnatal - *see* condition
Postoperative - *see also* condition
  confusion state 293.9
  psychosis 293.9
  status NEC (*see also* Status (post))
    V45.89
Postpancreatectomy hyperglycemia
  251.3
Postpartum - *see also* condition
  anemia 648.2●
    cardiomyopathy 674.5●
  observation
    immediately after delivery
      V24.0
    routine follow-up V24.2
Postperfusion syndrome NEC
  999.89
  bone marrow 996.85
Postpoliomyelitic - *see* condition
Postsurgery status NEC (*see also* Status
  (post)) V45.89
Post-term (pregnancy) 645.1●
  infant (gestation period over 40
    completed weeks to 42
    completed weeks) 766.21
Post-transplant lymphoproliferative
  disorder (PTLD) 238.77
Posttraumatic - *see* condition
Posttraumatic brain syndrome,
  nonpsychotic 310.2
Post-Traumatic Stress Disorder (PTSD)
  309.81
Post-typhoid abscess 002.0
Postures, hysterical 300.11
Postvaccinal reaction or complication -
  see Complications, vaccination
Postvagotomy syndrome 564.2
Postvalvulotomy syndrome 429.4
Postvasectomy sperm count V25.8
Potain's disease (pulmonary edema)
  514
Potain's syndrome (gastrectasis with
  dyspepsia) 536.1
Pott's
  curvature (spinal) (*see also*
    Tuberculosis) 015.0● [737.43]
  disease or paraplegia (*see also*
    Tuberculosis) 015.0● [730.88]
  fracture (closed) 824.4
    open 824.5
  gangrene 440.24
  osteomyelitis (*see also* Tuberculosis)
    015.0● [730.88]
  spinal curvature (*see also* Tuberculosis)
    015.0● [737.43]
  tumor, puffy (*see also* Osteomyelitis)
    730.2●
Potter's
  asthma 502
  disease 753.0
  facies 754.0
  lung 502

Potter's (*Continued*)
  syndrome (with renal agenesis)
    753.0
Pouch
  bronchus 748.3
  Douglas' - *see* condition
  esophagus, esophageal (congenital)
    750.4
    acquired 530.6
  gastric 537.1
  Hartmann's (abnormal sacculation of
    gallbladder neck) 575.8
    of intestine V44.3
      attention to V55.3
  pharynx, pharyngeal (congenital)
    750.27
Pouchitis 569.71 ◄
Poulet's disease 714.2
Poultrymen's itch 133.8
Poverty V60.2
PPE (palmar plantar erythrodysesthesia)
  693.0
Prader-Labhart-Willi-Fanconi syndrome
  (hypogenital dystrophy with
  diabetic tendency) 759.81
Prader-Willi syndrome (hypogenital
  dystrophy with diabetic tendency)
  759.81
Preachers' voice 784.49
Pre-AIDS - *see* Human
  immunodeficiency virus
  (disease) (illness) (infection)
Preauricular appendage 744.1
Prebetalipoproteinemia (acquired)
  (essential) (familial) (hereditary)
  (primary) (secondary) 272.1
  with chylomicronemia 272.3
Precipitate labor 661.3●
  affecting fetus or newborn 763.6
Preclimacteric bleeding 627.0
  menorrhagia 627.0
Precocious
  adrenarche 259.1
  menarche 259.1
  menstruation 626.8
  pubarche 259.1
  puberty NEC 259.1
  sexual development NEC 259.1
  thelarche 259.1
Precocity, sexual (constitutional)
  (cryptogenic) (female) (idiopathic)
  (male) NEC 259.1
  with adrenal hyperplasia 255.2
Precordial pain 786.51
  psychogenic 307.89
Predeciduous teeth 520.2
Prediabetes, prediabetic 790.29
  complicating pregnancy, childbirth, or
    puerperium 648.8●
  fetus or newborn 775.89
Predislocation status of hip, at birth (*see
  also* Subluxation, congenital, hip)
  754.32
Pre-eclampsia (mild) 642.4●
  with pre-existing hypertension642.7●
  affecting fetus or newborn 760.0
  severe 642.5●
  superimposed on pre-existing
    hypertensive disease 642.7●
Preeruptive color change, teeth, tooth
  520.8
Preexcitation 426.7
  atrioventricular conduction 426.7
  ventricular 426.7

Preglaucoma 365.00
Pregnancy (single) (uterine) (without
  sickness) V22.2

```
┌─────────────────────────────────────┐
│ Note 62   Use the following fifth-digit
│ subclassification with categories
│ 640-649, 651-679:              ◄━━━
│
│   0   unspecified as to episode of care
│   1   delivered, with or without
│         mention of antepartum
│         condition
│   2   delivered, with mention of
│         postpartum complication
│   3   antepartum condition or
│         complication
│   4   postpartum condition or
│         complication
└─────────────────────────────────────┘
```

  abdominal (ectopic) 633.00
    with intrauterine pregnancy 633.01
    affecting fetus or newborn 761.4
  abnormal NEC 646.9●
  ampullar - *see* Pregnancy, tubal
  broad ligament - *see* Pregnancy, cornual
  cervical - *see* Pregnancy, cornual
  chemical 631 ◄
  combined (extrauterine and
    intrauterine) - *see* Pregnancy,
    cornual
  complicated (by) 646.9●
    abnormal, abnormality NEC 646.9●
      cervix 654.6●
      cord (umbilical) 663.9●
      glucose tolerance (conditions
        classifiable to 790.21-790.29)
        648.8●
      pelvic organs or tissues NEC
        654.9●
      pelvis (bony) 653.0●
      perineum or vulva 654.8●
      placenta, placental (vessel)
        656.7●
      position
        cervix 654.4●
        placenta 641.1●
          without hemorrhage 641.0●
        uterus 654.4●
      size, fetus 653.5●
      uterus (congenital) 654.0●
    abscess or cellulitis
      bladder 646.6●
      genitourinary tract (conditions
        classifiable to 590, 595,
        597, 599.0, 614.0-614.5,
        614.7-614.9, 615) 646.6●
      kidney 646.6●
      urinary tract NEC 646.6●
    adhesion, pelvic peritoneal 648.9●
    air embolism 673.0●
    albuminuria 646.2●
      with hypertension - *see* Toxemia,
        of pregnancy
    amnionitis 658.4●
    amniotic fluid embolism 673.1●
    anemia (conditions classifiable to
      280-285) 648.2●
    appendicitis 648.9●
    atrophy, yellow (acute) (liver)
      (subacute) 646.7●
    bacilluria, asymptomatic 646.5●
    bacteriuria, asymptomatic 646.5●
    bariatric surgery status 649.2●
    bicornis or bicornuate uterus
      654.0●
    biliary problems 646.8●

Pregnancy (*Continued*)
  complicated (*Continued*)
    bone and joint disorders
      (conditions classifiable to
      720–724 or conditions
      affecting lower limbs
      classifiable to 711–719,
      725–738) 648.7●
    breech presentation (buttocks)
      (complete) (frank) 652.2●
      with successful version 652.1
    cardiovascular disease (conditions
      classifiable to 390–398, 410–
      429) 648.6●
      congenital (conditions classifiable
        to 745–747) 648.5●
    cerebrovascular disorders
      (conditions classifiable to
      430–434, 436–437) 674.0●
    cervicitis (conditions classifiable to
      616.0) 646.6●
    chloasma (gravidarum) 646.8●
    cholelithiasis 646.8●
    chorea (gravidarum) - *see* Eclampsia,
      pregnancy
    coagulation defect 649.3●
    conjoined twins 678.1●
    contraction, pelvis (general)
      653.1●
      inlet 653.2●
      outlet 653.3●
    convulsions (eclamptic) (uremic)
      642.6●
      with pre-existing hypertension
        642.7●
    current disease or condition
      (nonobstetric)
      abnormal glucose tolerance
        648.8●
      anemia 648.2●
      bone and joint (lower limb)
        648.7●
      cardiovascular 648.6●
        congenital 648.5●
      cerebrovascular 674.0●
      diabetes (conditions
        classifiable to 249 and
        250) 648.0●
      drug dependence 648.3●
      female genital mutilation
        648.9●
      genital organ or tract 646.6●
      gonorrheal 647.1●
      hypertensive 642.2●
        chronic kidney 642.2●
        renal 642.1●
      infectious 647.9
        specified type NEC 647.8●
      liver 646.7●
      malarial 647.4●
      nutritional deficiency 648.9●
      parasitic NEC 647.8●
      periodontal disease 648.9●
      renal 646.2●
        hypertensive 642.1●
      rubella 647.5●
      specified condition NEC
        648.9●
      syphilitic 647.0●
      thyroid 648.1●
      tuberculous 647.3●
      urinary 646.6●
      venereal 647.2●
      viral NEC 647.6●
    cystitis 646.6●
    cystocele 654.4●

Pregnancy (*Continued*)
  complicated (*Continued*)
    death of fetus (near term) 656.4●
      early pregnancy (before 22
        completed weeks'
        gestation) 632
    deciduitis 646.6●
    decreased fetal movements 655.7●
    diabetes (mellitus) (conditions
      classifiable to 249 and 250)
      648.0●
    disorders of liver 646.7●
    displacement, uterus NEC 654.4●
    disproportion - *see* Disproportion
    double uterus 654.0●
    drug dependence (conditions
      classifiable to 304) 648.3●
    dysplasia, cervix 654.6●
    early onset of delivery
      (spontaneous) 644.2●
    eclampsia, eclamptic (coma)
      (convulsions) (delirium)
      (nephritis) (uremia) 642.6●
      with pre-existing hypertension
        642.7●
    edema 646.1●
      with hypertension - *see* Toxemia,
        of pregnancy
    effusion, amniotic fluid 658.1●
      delayed delivery following
        658.2●
    embolism
      air 673.0●
      amniotic fluid 673.1●
      blood-clot 673.2●
      cerebral 674.0●
      pulmonary NEC 673.2●
      pyemic 673.3●
      septic 673.3●
    emesis (gravidarum) - *see* Pregnancy,
      complicated, vomiting
    endometritis (conditions classifiable
      to 615.0–615.9) 670.1●   ◀▥
    decidual 646.6●
    epilepsy 649.4●
    excessive weight gain NEC 646.1●
    face presentation 652.4●
    failure, fetal head to enter pelvic
      brim 652.5●
    false labor (pains) 644.1●
    fatigue 646.8●
    fatty metamorphosis of liver
      646.7●
    female genital mutilation 648.9●
    fetal
      anemia 678.0●   ◀
      complications from in utero
        procedure 679.1●   ◀
      conjoined twins 678.1●
      death (near term) 656.4●
        early (before 22 completed
          weeks' gestation) 632
      deformity 653.7●
      distress 656.8●
      hematologic conditions
        678.0●   ◀
      reduction of multiple fetuses
        reduced to single fetus
        651.7●
      thrombocytopenia 678.0● ◀
      twin to twin transfusion
        678.0●   ◀
    fibroid (tumor) (uterus) 654.1●
    footling presentation 652.8●
      with successful version 652.1●
    gallbladder disease 646.8●

Pregnancy (*Continued*)
  complicated (*Continued*)
    gastric banding status 649.2●
    gastric bypass status for obesity
      649.2●
    goiter 648.1●
    gonococcal infection (conditions
      classifiable to 098) 647.1●
    gonorrhea (conditions classifiable to
      098) 647.1●
    hemorrhage 641.9●
      accidental 641.2●
      before 22 completed weeks'
        gestation NEC 640.9●
      cerebrovascular 674.0●
      due to
        afibrinogenemia or other
          coagulation defect
          (conditions classifiable t
          o 286.0–286.9) 641.3●
        leiomyoma, uterine 641.8●
        marginal sinus (rupture)
          641.2●
        premature separation, placenta
          641.2●
        trauma 641.8●
      early (before 22 completed weeks'
        gestation) 640.9●
      threatened abortion 640.0●
      unavoidable 641.1●
    hepatitis (acute) (malignant)
      (subacute) 646.7●
      viral 647.6●
    herniation of uterus 654.4●
    high head at term 652.5●
    hydatidiform mole (delivered)
      (undelivered) 630
    hydramnios 657●
    hydrocephalic fetus 653.6●
    hydrops amnii 657●
    hydrorrhea 658.1●
    hyperemesis (gravidarum) - *see*
      Hyperemesis, gravidarum
    hypertension - *see* Hypertension,
      complicating pregnancy
    hypertensive
      chronic kidney disease
        642.2●
      heart and chronic kidney
        disease 642.2●
      heart and renal disease 642.2●
      heart disease 642.2●
      renal disease 642.2●
    hypertensive heart and chronic
      kidney disease 642.2●
    hyperthyroidism 648.1●
    hypothyroidism 648.1●
    hysteralgia 646.8●
    icterus gravis 646.7●
    incarceration, uterus 654.3●
    incompetent cervix (os)
      654.5●
    infection 647.9●
      amniotic fluid 658.4●
      bladder 646.6●
      genital organ (conditions
        classifiable to 614.0–
        614.5, 614.7–614.9, 615)
        646.6●
      kidney (conditions classifiable to
        590.0–590.9) 646.6●
      urinary (tract) 646.6●
        asymptomatic 646.5●
    infective and parasitic diseases NEC
      647.8●

◀ New   ◀▥ Revised   ~~deleted~~ Deleted   ● Use Additional Digit(s)   ▥ Omit code

P

Pregnancy *(Continued)*
  complicated *(Continued)*
    inflammation●
      bladder 646.6●
      genital organ (conditions
          classifiable to 614.0–614.5,
          614.7–614.9, 615) 646.6●
      urinary tract NEC 646.6
    injury 648.9●
      obstetrical NEC 665.9●
    insufficient weight gain 646.8●
    intrauterine fetal death (near term)
        NEC 656.4●
      early (before 22 completed weeks'
          gestation) 632
    malaria (conditions classifiable to
        084) 647.4●
    malformation, uterus (congenital)
        654.0●
    malnutrition (conditions classifiable
        to 260–269) 648.9●
    malposition
      fetus - *see* Pregnancy,
          complicated,
          malpresentation
      uterus or cervix 654.4●
    malpresentation 652.9●
      with successful version 652.1●
      in multiple gestation 652.6●
      specified type NEC 652.8●
    marginal sinus hemorrhage or
        rupture 641.2●
    maternal complications from in
        utero procedure 679.0● ◄
    maternal drug abuse 648.4●
    maternal obesity syndrome 646.1●
    menstruation 640.8●
    mental disorders (conditions
        classifiable to 290–303, 305.0,
        305.2–305.9, 306–316, 317–319)
        648.4●
    mentum presentation 652.4●
    missed
      abortion 632
      delivery (at or near term) 656.4●
      labor (at or near term) 656.4●
    necrosis
      genital organ or tract (conditions
          classifiable to 614.0–614.5,
          614.7–614.9, 615) 646.6●
      liver (conditions classifiable to
          570) 646.7●
      renal, cortical 646.2●
    nephritis or nephrosis (conditions
        classifiable to 580–589)
        646.2●
      with hypertension 642.1●
    nephropathy NEC 646.2●
    neuritis (peripheral) 646.4●
    nutritional deficiency (conditions
        classifiable to 260–269) 648.9●
    obesity 649.1●
      surgery status 649.2●
    oblique lie or presentation 652.3●
      with successful version 652.1●
    obstetrical trauma NEC 665.9●
    oligohydramnios NEC 658.0●
    onset of contractions before 37
        weeks 644.0●
    oversize fetus 653.5●
    papyraceous fetus 646.0●
    patent cervix 654.5●
    pelvic inflammatory disease
        (conditions classifiable to
        614.0–614.5, 614.7–614.9, 615)
        646.6●

Pregnancy *(Continued)*
  complicated *(Continued)*
    pelvic peritoneal adhesion 648.9●
    placenta, placental
      abnormality 656.7●
      abruptio or ablatio 641.2●
      detachment 641.2●
      disease 656.7●
      infarct 656.7●
      low implantation 641.1●
        without hemorrhage 641.0●
      malformation 656.7●
      malposition 641.1●
        without hemorrhage 641.0●
      marginal sinus hemorrhage
          641.2●
      previa 641.1●
        without hemorrhage 641.0●
      separation (premature)
          (undelivered) 641.2●
    placentitis 658.4●
    polyhydramnios 657●
    postmaturity
      post-term 645.1●
      prolonged 645.2●
    prediabetes 648.8●
    pre-eclampsia (mild) 642.4●
      severe 642.5●
      superimposed on pre-existing
          hypertensive disease 642.7●
    premature rupture of membranes
        658.1●
      with delayed delivery 658.2●
    previous
      infertility V23.0
      in utero procedure during
          previous pregnancy
          V23.86
      nonobstetric condition V23.89
      poor obstetrical history V23.49
      premature delivery V23.41
      trophoblastic disease (conditions
          classifiable to 630) V23.1
    prolapse, uterus 654.4●
    proteinuria (gestational) 646.2●
      with hypertension - *see* Toxemia,
          of pregnancy
    pruritus (neurogenic) 646.8●
    psychosis or psychoneurosis 648.4●
    ptyalism 646.8●
    pyelitis (conditions classifiable to
        590.0–590.9) 646.6●
    renal disease or failure NEC 646.2●
      with secondary hypertension
          642.1●
      hypertensive 642.2●
    retention, retained dead
        ovum 631●
    retroversion, uterus 654.3●
    Rh immunization, incompatibility,
        or sensitization 656.1●
    rubella (conditions classifiable to
        056) 647.5●
    rupture
      amnion (premature) 658.1●
        with delayed delivery 658.2●
      marginal sinus (hemorrhage)
          641.2●
      membranes (premature) 658.1●
        with delayed delivery 658.2●
      uterus (before onset of labor)
          665.0●
    salivation (excessive) 646.8●
    salpingo-oophoritis (conditions
        classifiable to 614.0–614.2)
        646.6●

Pregnancy *(Continued)*
  complicated *(Continued)*
    septicemia (conditions classifiable to
        038.0–038.9) 647.8●
      postpartum 670.2●   ◄▥
      puerperal 670.2●   ◄▥
      smoking 649.0●
    spasms, uterus (abnormal) 646.8●
    specified condition NEC 646.8●
    spotting 649.5●
    spurious labor pains 644.1●
    status post
      bariatric surgery 649.2●
      gastric banding 649.2●
      gastric bypass for obesity
          649.2●
      obesity surgery 649.2●
    superfecundation 651.9●
    superfetation 651.9●
    syphilis (conditions classifiable to
        090–097) 647.0●
    threatened
      abortion 640.0●
      premature delivery 644.2●
      premature labor 644.0●
    thrombophlebitis (superficial)
        671.2●
      deep 671.3●
      septic 670.3●   ◄
    thrombosis 671.2●   ◄▥
      venous (superficial) 671.2●
        deep 671.3●
    thyroid dysfunction (conditions
        classifiable to 240–246) 648.1●
    thyroiditis 648.1●
    thyrotoxicosis 648.1●
    tobacco use disorder 649.0●
    torsion of uterus 654.4●
    toxemia - *see* Toxemia, of pregnancy
    transverse lie or presentation 652.3●
      with successful version 652.1●
    trauma 648.9●
      obstetrical 665.9●
    tuberculosis (conditions classifiable
        to 010–018) 647.3●
    tumor
      cervix 654.6●
      ovary 654.4●
      pelvic organs or tissue NEC
          654.4●
      uterus (body) 654.1●
        cervix 654.6●
      vagina 654.7●
      vulva 654.8●
    unstable lie 652.0●
    uremia - *see* Pregnancy, complicated,
        renal disease
    urethritis 646.6●
    vaginitis or vulvitis (conditions
        classifiable to 616.1) 646.6●
    varicose
      placental vessels 656.7●
      veins (legs) 671.0●
        perineum 671.1●
        vulva 671.1●
    varicosity, labia or vulva 671.1●
    venereal disease NEC (conditions
        classifiable to 099) 647.2●
    venous complication 671.9●   ◄
    viral disease NEC (conditions
        classifiable to 042, 050–055,
        057–079, 795.05, 795.15, 796.75)
        647.6●
    vomiting (incoercible) (pernicious)
        (persistent) (uncontrollable)
        (vicious) 643.9●

Pregnancy (Continued)
  complicated (Continued)
    vomiting (Continued)
      due to organic disease or other
        cause 643.8●
      early - see Hyperemesis,
        gravidarum
      late (after 22 completed weeks
        gestation) 643.2●
      young maternal age 659.8●
  complications NEC 646.9●
  cornual 633.80
    with intrauterine pregnancy 633.81
    affecting fetus or newborn 761.4
  death, maternal NEC 646.9●
  delivered - see Delivery
  ectopic (ruptured) NEC 633.90
    with intrauterine pregnancy 633.91
    abdominal - see Pregnancy,
      abdominal
    affecting fetus or newborn 761.4
    combined (extrauterine and
      intrauterine) - see Pregnancy,
      cornual
    ovarian - see Pregnancy, ovarian
    specified type NEC 633.80
      with intrauterine pregnancy
        633.81
      affecting fetus or newborn 761.4
    tubal - see Pregnancy, tubal
  examination, pregnancy
    negative result V72.41
    not confirmed V72.40
    positive result V72.42
  extrauterine - see Pregnancy, ectopic
  fallopian - see Pregnancy, tubal
  false 300.11
    labor (pains) 644.1●
  fatigue 646.8●
  illegitimate V61.6
  incidental finding V22.2
  in double uterus 654.0●
  interstitial - see Pregnancy, cornual
  intraligamentous - see Pregnancy,
    cornual
  intramural - see Pregnancy, cornual
  intraperitoneal - see Pregnancy,
    abdominal
  isthmian - see Pregnancy, tubal
  management affected by
    abnormal, abnormality
      fetus (suspected) 655.9●
        specified NEC 655.8●
      placenta 656.7●
    advanced maternal age NEC 659.6●
      multigravida 659.6●
      primigravida 659.5●
    antibodies (maternal)
      anti-c 656.1●
      anti-d 656.1●
      anti-e 656.1●
      blood group (ABO) 656.2●
        Rh(esus) 656.1●
    appendicitis 648.9●
    bariatric surgery status 649.2●
    coagulation defect 649.3●
    elderly multigravida 659.6●
    elderly primigravida 659.5●
    epilepsy 649.4●
    fetal (suspected)●
      abnormality 655.9●
        abdominal 655.8●
        acid-base balance 656.8●
        cardiovascular 655.8●
        facial 655.8●
        gastrointestinal 655.8●

Pregnancy (Continued)
  management affected by (Continued)
    fetal (Continued)
      abnormality (Continued)
        genitourinary 655.8●
        heart rate or rhythm 659.7●
        limb 655.8●
        specified NEC 655.8●
      acidemia 656.3●
      anencephaly 655.0●
      aneuploidy 655.1●
      bradycardia 659.7●
      central nervous system
        malformation 655.0●
      chromosomal abnormalities
        (conditions classifiable to
        758.0–758.9) 655.1●
      damage from
        drugs 655.5●
          obstetric, anesthetic, or
            sedative 655.5●
        environmental toxins 655.8
        intrauterine contraceptive
          device 655.8●
        maternal
          alcohol addiction 655.4●
          disease NEC 655.4●
          drug use 655.5●
          listeriosis 655.4●
          rubella 655.3●
          toxoplasmosis 655.4●
          viral infection 655.3●
        radiation 655.6●
      death (near term) 656.4●
        early (before 22 completed
          weeks' gestation) 632
      distress 656.8●
      excessive growth 656.6●
      growth retardation 656.5●
      hereditary disease 655.2●
      hydrocephalus 655.0●
      intrauterine death 656.4●
      poor growth 656.5●
      spina bifida (with
        myelomeningocele)
        655.0●
    fetal-maternal hemorrhage 656.0●
    gastric banding status 649.2●
    gastric bypass status for obesity
      649.2●
    hereditary disease in family
      (possibly) affecting fetus
      655.2●
    incompatibility, blood groups (ABO)
      656.2●
      Rh(esus) 656.1●
    insufficient prenatal care V23.7
    intrauterine death 656.4●
    isoimmunization (ABO) 656.2●
      Rh(esus) 656.1●
    large-for-dates fetus 656.6●
    light-for-dates fetus 656.5●
    meconium in liquor 656.8●
    mental disorder (conditions
      classifiable to 290–303, 305.0,
      305.2–305.9, 306–316, 317–319)
      648.4●
    multiparity (grand) 659.4●
    obesity 649.1●
      surgery status 649.2●
    poor obstetric history V23.49
      pre-term labor V23.41
    postmaturity
      post-term 645.1●
      prolonged 645.2●
    post-term pregnancy 645.1●

Pregnancy (Continued)
  management affected by (Continued)
    previous
      abortion V23.2
        habitual 646.3●
      cesarean delivery 654.2●
      difficult delivery V23.49
      forceps delivery V23.49
      habitual abortions 646.3●
      hemorrhage, antepartum or
        postpartum V23.49
      hydatidiform mole V23.1
      infertility V23.0
      in utero procedure during
        previous pregnancy V23.86
      malignancy NEC V23.89
      nonobstetrical conditions V23.89
      premature delivery V23.41
      trophoblastic disease (conditions
        in 630) V23.1
      vesicular mole V23.1
    prolonged pregnancy 645.2●
    small-for-dates fetus 656.5●
    smoking 649.0●
    spotting 649.5●
    suspected conditions not found
      amniotic cavity and membrane
        problem V89.01
      cervical shortening V89.05
      fetal anomaly V89.03
      fetal growth problem V89.04
      oligohydramnios V89.01
      other specified problem NEC
        V89.09
      placental problem V89.02
      polyhydramnios V89.01
    tobacco use disorder 649.0●
    venous complication 671.9● ◀
    young maternal age 659.8●
  maternal death NEC 646.9●
  mesometric (mural) - see Pregnancy,
    cornual
  molar 631
    hydatidiform (see also Hydatidiform
      mole) 630
      previous, affecting management
        of pregnancy V23.1
    previous, affecting management of
      pregnancy V23.49
  multiple NEC 651.9●
    with fetal loss and retention of one
      or more fetus(es) 651.6●
    affecting fetus or newborn 761.5
    following (elective) fetal reduction
      651.7●
    specified type NEC 651.8●
      with fetal loss and retention of one
        or more fetus(es) 651.6●
      following (elective) fetal
        reduction 651.7●
  mural - see Pregnancy, cornual
  observation NEC V22.1
    first pregnancy V22.0
    high-risk V23.9
      specified problem NEC V23.89
  ovarian 633.20
    with intrauterine pregnancy 633.21
    affecting fetus or newborn 761.4
  possible, not (yet) confirmed V72.40
  postmature
    post-term 645.1●
    prolonged 645.2●
  post-term 645.1●
  prenatal care only V22.1
    first pregnancy V22.0
    high-risk V23.9
      specified problem NEC V23.89

◀ New   ◀▥ Revised   ~~deleted~~ Deleted   ● Use Additional Digit(s)   ▨ Omit code

Pregnancy *(Continued)*
  prolonged 645.2●
  quadruplet NEC 651.2●
    with fetal loss and retention of one
      or more fetus(es) 651.5●
    affecting fetus or newborn 761.5
    following (elective) fetal reduction
      651.7●
  quintuplet NEC 651.8●
    with fetal loss and retention of one
      or more fetus(es) 651.6●
    affecting fetus or newborn 761.5
    following (elective) fetal reduction
      651.7●
  resulting from
    assisted reproductive technology
      V23.85
    in vitro fertilization V23.85
  sextuplet NEC 651.8●
    with fetal loss and retention of one
      or more fetus(es) 651.6●
    affecting fetus or newborn 761.5
    following (elective) fetal reduction
      651.7●
  spurious 300.11
  superfecundation NEC 651.9●
    with fetal loss and retention of one
      or more fetus(es) 651.6●
    following (elective) fetal reduction
      651.7●
  superfetation NEC 651.9●
    with fetal loss and retention of one
      or more fetus(es) 651.6●
    following (elective) fetal reduction
      651.7●
  supervision (of) (for) - *see also*
    Pregnancy, management
    affected by
    elderly
      multigravida V23.82
      primigravida V23.81
    high-risk V23.9
      insufficient prenatal care V23.7
      specified problem NEC
        V23.89
    multiparity V23.3
    normal NEC V22.1
      first V22.0
    poor
      obstetric history V23.49
        pre-term labor V23.41
      reproductive history V23.5
    previous
      abortion V23.2
      hydatidiform mole V23.1
      infertility V23.0
      neonatal death V23.5
      stillbirth V23.5
      trophoblastic disease V23.1
      vesicular mole V23.1
    specified problem NEC V23.89
    young
      multigravida V23.84
      primigravida V23.83
  triplet NEC 651.1●
    with fetal loss and retention of one
      or more fetus(es) 651.4●
    affecting fetus or newborn 761.5
    following (elective) fetal reduction
      651.7●
  tubal (with rupture) 633.10
    with intrauterine pregnancy
      633.11
    affecting fetus or newborn
      761.4

Pregnancy *(Continued)*
  twin NEC 651.0●
    with fetal loss and retention of one
      fetus 651.3●
    affecting fetus or newborn 761.5
    conjoined 678.1●
    following (elective) fetal reduction
      651.7●
  unconfirmed V72.40
  undelivered (no other diagnosis) V22.2
    with false labor 644.1●
    high-risk V23.9
      specified problem NEC V23.89
  unwanted NEC V61.7
Pregnant uterus - *see* condition
Preiser's disease (osteoporosis) 733.09
Prekwashiorkor 260
Preleukemia 238.75
Preluxation of hip, congenital *(see also*
  Subluxation, congenital, hip) 754.32
Premature - *see also* condition
  beats (nodal) 427.60
    atrial 427.61
    auricular 427.61
    postoperative 997.1
    specified type NEC 427.69
    supraventricular 427.61
    ventricular 427.69
  birth NEC 765.1●
  closure
    cranial suture 756.0
    fontanel 756.0
    foramen ovale 745.8
  contractions 427.60
    atrial 427.61
    auricular 427.61
    auriculoventricular 427.61
    heart (extrasystole) 427.60
    junctional 427.60
    nodal 427.60
    postoperative 997.1
    ventricular 427.69
  ejaculation 302.75
  infant NEC 765.1●
    excessive 765.0●
    light-for-dates - *see* Light-for-dates
  labor 644.2●
    threatened 644.0●
  lungs 770.4
  menopause 256.31
  puberty 259.1
  rupture of membranes or amnion
    658.1●
    affecting fetus or newborn 761.1
    delayed delivery following 658.2●
  senility (syndrome) 259.8
  separation, placenta (partial) - *see*
    Placenta, separation
  ventricular systole 427.69
Prematurity NEC 765.1●
  extreme 765.0●
Premenstrual syndrome 625.4
Premenstrual tension 625.4
Premolarization, cuspids 520.2
Premyeloma 273.1
Prenatal
  care, normal pregnancy V22.1
    first V22.0
  death, cause unknown - *see* Death,
    fetus
  screening - *see* Antenatal, screening
  teeth 520.6
Prepartum - *see* condition
Preponderance, left or right ventricular
  429.3

Prepuce - *see* condition
PRES (posterior reversible
  encephalopathy syndrome) 348.39
Presbycardia 797
  hypertensive *(see also* Hypertension,
    heart) 402.90
Presbycusis 388.01
Presbyesophagus 530.89
Presbyophrenia 310.1
Presbyopia 367.4
Prescription of contraceptives NEC
  V25.02
  diaphragm V25.02
  oral (pill) V25.01
    emergency V25.03
    postcoital V25.03
    repeat V25.41
  repeat V25.40
    oral (pill) V25.41
Presenile - *see also* condition
  aging 259.8
  dementia *(see also* Dementia, presenile)
    290.10
Presenility 259.8
Presentation, fetal
  abnormal 652.9●
    with successful version 652.1●
    before labor, affecting fetus or
      newborn 761.7
    causing obstructed labor 660.0●
      affecting fetus or newborn, any,
        except breech 763.1
    in multiple gestation (one or more)
      652.6●
    specified NEC 652.8●
  arm 652.7●
    causing obstructed labor 660.0●
  breech (buttocks) (complete) (frank)
    652.2●
    with successful version 652.1●
    before labor, affecting fetus or
      newborn 761.7
    before labor, affecting fetus or
      newborn 761.7
  brow 652.4●
    causing obstructed labor 660.0●
  buttocks 652.2●
  chin 652.4●
  complete 652.2●
  compound 652.8●
  cord 663.0●
  extended head 652.4●
  face 652.4●
    to pubes 652.8●
  footling 652.8●
  frank 652.2●
  hand, leg, or foot NEC 652.8●
  incomplete 652.8●
  mentum 652.4●
  multiple gestation (one fetus or more)
    652.6●
  oblique 652.3●
    with successful version 652.1●
  shoulder 652.8●
    affecting fetus or newborn 763.1
  transverse 652.3●
    with successful version 652.1●
  umbilical cord 663.0●
  unstable 652.0●
Prespondylolisthesis (congenital)
  (lumbosacral) 756.11
Pressure
  area, skin ulcer *(see also* Ulcer, pressure)
    707.00
  atrophy, spine 733.99

Pressure (*Continued*)
  birth, fetus or newborn NEC 767.9
  brachial plexus 353.0
  brain 348.4
    injury at birth 767.0
  cerebral - *see* Pressure, brain
  chest 786.59
  cone, tentorial 348.4
    injury at birth 767.0
  funis - *see* Compression, umbilical cord
  hyposystolic (*see also* Hypotension)
      458.9
  increased
    intracranial 781.99
      due to
        benign intracranial
              hypertension 348.2
        hydrocephalus - *see*
              hydrocephalus
        injury at birth 767.8
    intraocular 365.00
  lumbosacral plexus 353.1
  mediastinum 519.3
  necrosis (chronic) (skin) (*see also*
      Decubitus) 707.00
  nerve - *see* Compression, nerve
  paralysis (*see also* Neuropathy,
      entrapment) 355.9
  pre-ulcer skin changes limited to
      persistent focal erythema (*see also*
      Ulcer, pressure) 707.21
  sore (chronic) (*see also* Ulcer, pressure)
      707.00
  spinal cord 336.9
  ulcer (chronic) (*see also* Ulcer, pressure)
      707.00
  umbilical cord - *see* Compression,
      umbilical cord
  venous, increased 459.89
Pre-syncope 780.2
Preterm infant NEC 765.1●
  extreme 765.0●
Priapism (penis) 607.3
Prickling sensation (*see also* Disturbance,
    sensation) 782.0
Prickly heat 705.1
Primary - *see* condition
Primigravida, elderly
  affecting
    fetus or newborn 763.89
    management of pregnancy, labor,
        and delivery 659.5●
Primipara, old
  affecting
    fetus or newborn 763.89
    management of pregnancy, labor,
        and delivery 659.5●
Primula dermatitis 692.6
Primus varus (bilateral) (metatarsus) 754.52
PRIND (prolonged reversible ischemic
    neurologic deficit) 434.91
  history of (personal) V12.54
Pringle's disease (tuberous sclerosis) 759.5
Prinzmetal's angina 413.1
Prinzmetal-Massumi syndrome (anterior
    chest wall) 786.52
Prizefighter ear 738.7
Problem (with) V49.9
  academic V62.3
  acculturation V62.4
  adopted child V61.24 ◀▥
  aged
    in-law V61.3
    parent V61.3
    person NEC V61.8

Problem (*Continued*)
  alcoholism in family V61.41
  anger reaction (*see also* Disturbance,
      conduct) 312.0●
  behavior, child 312.9
  behavioral V40.9
    specified NEC V40.3
  betting V69.3
  biological child V61.23 ◀
  cardiorespiratory NEC V47.2
  care of sick or handicapped person in
      family or household V61.49
  career choice V62.29
  communication V40.1
  conscience regarding medical care
      V62.6
  delinquency (juvenile) 312.9
  diet, inappropriate V69.1
  digestive NEC V47.3
  ear NEC V41.3
  eating habits, inappropriate V69.1
  economic V60.2
    affecting care V60.9
      specified type NEC V60.89 ◀▥
  educational V62.3
  enuresis, child 307.6
  exercise, lack of V69.0
  eye NEC V41.1
  family V61.9
    specified circumstance NEC V61.8
  fear reaction, child 313.0
  feeding (elderly) (infant) 783.3
    newborn 779.31 ◀▥
    nonorganic 307.59
  fetal, affecting management of
      pregnancy 656.9●
    specified type NEC 656.8●
  financial V60.2
  foster child V61.25 ◀▥
  ~~specified NEC V41.8~~
  functional V41.9
    specified type NEC V41.8
  gambling V69.3
  genital NEC V47.5
  head V48.9
    deficiency V48.0
    disfigurement V48.6
    mechanical V48.2
    motor V48.2
    movement of V48.2
    sensory V48.4
    specified condition NEC V48.8
  hearing V41.2
  high-risk sexual behavior V69.2
  identity 313.82
  influencing health status
      NEC V49.89
  internal organ NEC V47.9
    deficiency V47.0
    mechanical or motor V47.1
  interpersonal NEC V62.81
  jealousy, child 313.3
  learning V40.0
  legal V62.5
  life circumstance NEC V62.89
  lifestyle V69.9
    specified NEC V69.8
  limb V49.9
    deficiency V49.0
    disfigurement V49.4
    mechanical V49.1
    motor V49.2
    movement, involving
        musculoskeletal system V49.1
        nervous system V49.2

Problem (*Continued*)
  limb, (*Continued*)
      sensory V49.3
      specified condition NEC V49.5
  litigation V62.5
  living alone V60.3
  loneliness NEC V62.89
  marital V61.10
    involving
        divorce V61.03
        estrangement V61.09
        psychosexual disorder 302.9
        sexual function V41.7
    relationship V61.10
  mastication V41.6
  medical care, within family V61.49
  mental V40.9
    specified NEC V40.2
  mental hygiene, adult V40.9
  multiparity V61.5
  nail biting, child 307.9
  neck V48.9
    deficiency V48.1
    disfigurement V48.7
    mechanical V48.3
    motor V48.3
    movement V48.3
    sensory V48.5
    specified condition NEC V48.8
  neurological NEC 781.99
  none (feared complaint unfounded)
      V65.5
  occupational V62.29
  parent-child V61.20
    adopted child V61.24 ◀
    biological child V61.23 ◀
    foster child V61.25 ◀
    relationship V61.20
  partner V61.10
    relationship V61.10
  personal NEC V62.89
    interpersonal conflict NEC
        V62.81
  personality (*see also* Disorder,
      personality) 301.9
  phase of life V62.89
  placenta, affecting management of
      pregnancy 656.9●
    specified type NEC 656.8●
  poverty V60.2
  presence of sick or handicapped
      person in family or household
      V61.49
  psychiatric 300.9
  psychosocial V62.9
    specified type NEC V62.89
  relational NEC V62.81
  relationship, childhood 313.3
  religious or spiritual belief
    other than medical care V62.89
    regarding medical care V62.6
  self-damaging behavior V69.8
  sexual
    behavior, high-risk V69.2
    function NEC V41.7
  sibling
    relational V61.8
    relationship V61.8
  sight V41.0
  sleep, lack of V69.4
  sleep disorder, child 307.40
  smell V41.5
  speech V40.1
  spite reaction, child (*see also*
      Disturbance, conduct) 312.0●

◀ New   ◀▥ Revised   ~~deleted~~ Deleted   ● Use Additional Digit(s)   ▥ Omit code

Problem (*Continued*)
  spoiled child reaction (*see also* Disturbance, conduct) 312.1 ●
  substance abuse in family V61.42 ◄
  swallowing V41.6
  tantrum, child (*see also* Disturbance, conduct) 312.1 ●
  taste V41.5
  thumb sucking, child 307.9
  tic (child) 307.21
  trunk V48.9
    deficiency V48.1
    disfigurement V48.7
    mechanical V48.3
    motor V48.3
    movement V48.3
    sensory V48.5
    specified condition NEC V48.8
  unemployment V62.0
  urinary NEC V47.4
  voice production V41.4
Procedure (surgical) not done NEC V64.3
  because of
    contraindication V64.1
    patient's decision V64.2
      for reasons of conscience or religion V62.6
    specified reason NEC V64.3
Procidentia
  anus (sphincter) 569.1
  rectum (sphincter) 569.1
  stomach 537.89
  uteri 618.1
Proctalgia 569.42
  fugax 564.6
  spasmodic 564.6
    psychogenic 307.89
Proctitis 569.49
  amebic 006.8
  chlamydial 099.52
  gonococcal 098.7
  granulomatous 555.1
  idiopathic 556.2
    with ulcerative sigmoiditis 556.3
  tuberculous (*see also* Tuberculosis) 014.8 ●
  ulcerative (chronic) (nonspecific) 556.2
    with ulcerative sigmoiditis 556.3
Proctocele
  female (without uterine prolapse) 618.04
    with uterine prolapse 618.4
      complete 618.3
      incomplete 618.2
  male 569.49
Proctocolitis, idiopathic 556.2
  with ulcerative sigmoiditis 556.3
Proctoptosis 569.1
Proctosigmoiditis 569.89
  ulcerative (chronic) 556.3
Proctospasm 564.6
  psychogenic 306.4
Prodromal-AIDS - *see* Human immunodeficiency virus (disease) (illness) (infection)
Profichet's disease or syndrome 729.90
Progeria (adultorum) (syndrome) 259.8
Prognathism (mandibular) (maxillary) 524.00
Progonoma (melanotic) (M9363/0) - *see* Neoplasm, by site, benign

Progressive - *see* condition
Prolapse, prolapsed
  anus, anal (canal) (sphincter) 569.1
  arm or hand, complicating delivery 652.7 ●
    causing obstructed labor 660.0 ●
      affecting fetus or newborn 763.1
    fetus or newborn 763.1
  bladder (acquired) (mucosa) (sphincter)
    congenital (female) (male) 756.71
    female (*see also* Cystocele, female) 618.01
    male 596.8
  breast implant (prosthetic) 996.54
  cecostomy 569.69
  cecum 569.89
  cervix, cervical (hypertrophied) 618.1
    anterior lip, obstructing labor 660.2 ●
      affecting fetus or newborn 763.1
    congenital 752.49
    postpartal (old) 618.1
    stump 618.84
  ciliary body 871.1
  colon (pedunculated) 569.89
  colostomy 569.69
  conjunctiva 372.73
  cord - *see* Prolapse, umbilical cord
  disc (intervertebral) - *see* Displacement, intervertebral disc
  duodenum 537.89
  eye implant (orbital) 996.59
    lens (ocular) 996.53
  fallopian tube 620.4
  fetal extremity, complicating delivery 652.8 ●
    causing obstructed labor 660.0 ●
    fetus or newborn 763.1
  funis - *see* Prolapse, umbilical cord
  gastric (mucosa) 537.89
  genital, female 618.9
    specified NEC 618.89
  globe 360.81
  ileostomy bud 569.69
  intervertebral disc - *see* Displacement, intervertebral disc
  intestine (small) 569.89
  iris 364.89
    traumatic 871.1
  kidney (*see also* Disease, renal) 593.0
    congenital 753.3
  laryngeal muscles or ventricle 478.79
  leg, complicating delivery 652.8 ●
    causing obstructed labor 660.0 ●
    fetus or newborn 763.1
  liver 573.8
  meatus urinarius 599.5
  mitral valve 424.0
  ocular lens implant 996.53
  organ or site, congenital NEC - *see* Malposition, congenital
  ovary 620.4
  pelvic (floor), female 618.89
  perineum, female 618.89
  pregnant uterus 654.4 ●
  rectum (mucosa) (sphincter) 569.1
    due to Trichuris trichiuria 127.3
  spleen 289.59
  stomach 537.89
  umbilical cord
    affecting fetus or newborn 762.4
    complicating delivery 663.0 ●

Prolapse, prolapsed (*Continued*)
  ureter 593.89
    with obstruction 593.4
  ureterovesical orifice 593.89
  urethra (acquired) (infected) (mucosa) 599.5
    congenital 753.8
  uterovaginal 618.4
    complete 618.3
    incomplete 618.2
    specified NEC 618.89
  uterus (first degree) (second degree) (third degree) (complete) (without vaginal wall prolapse) 618.1
    with mention of vaginal wall prolapse - *see* Prolapse, uterovaginal
    congenital 752.3
    in pregnancy or childbirth 654.4 ●
      affecting fetus or newborn 763.1
      causing obstructed labor 660.2 ●
        affecting fetus or newborn 763.1
    postpartal (old) 618.1
  uveal 871.1
  vagina (anterior) (posterior) (vault) (wall) (without uterine prolapse) 618.00
    with uterine prolapse 618.4
      complete 618.3
      incomplete 618.2
    paravaginal 618.02
    posthysterectomy 618.5
    specified NEC 618.09
  vitreous (humor) 379.26
    traumatic 871.1
  womb - *see* Prolapse, uterus
Prolapsus, female 618.9
Proliferative - *see* condition
Prolinemia 270.8
Prolinuria 270.8
Prolonged, prolongation
  bleeding time (*see also* Defect, coagulation) 790.92
  "idiopathic" (in von Willebrand's disease) 286.4
  coagulation time (*see also* Defect, coagulation) 790.92
  gestation syndrome 766.22
  labor 662.1 ●
    affecting fetus or newborn 763.89
    first stage 662.0 ●
    second stage 662.2 ●
  PR interval 426.11
  pregnancy 645.2 ●
  prothrombin time (*see also* Defect, coagulation) 790.92
  QT interval 794.31
    syndrome 426.82
  rupture of membranes (24 hours or more prior to onset of labor) 658.2 ●
  uterine contractions in labor 661.4 ●
    affecting fetus or newborn 763.7
Prominauris 744.29
Prominence
  auricle (ear) (congenital) 744.29
    acquired 380.32

◄ New   ◄▥ Revised   ~~deleted~~ Deleted   ● Use Additional Digit(s)   ▨ Omit code   **513**

Prominence (Continued)
  ischial spine or sacral promontory
      with disproportion (fetopelvic)
      653.3●
      affecting fetus or newborn
          763.1
      causing obstructed labor
          660.1●
          affecting fetus or newborn
              763.1
  nose (congenital) 748.1
      acquired 738.0
PROMM (proximal myotonic myotonia)
    359.21
Pronation
  ankle 736.79
  foot 736.79
      congenital 755.67
Prophylactic
  administration of
      agents affecting estrogen receptors
          and estrogen levels NEC
          V07.59
      anastrozole (Arimidex) V07.52
      antibiotics V07.39
      antitoxin, any V07.2
      antivenin V07.2
      aromatase inhibitors V07.52
      chemotherapeutic agent NEC V07.39
          fluoride V07.31
      diphtheria antitoxin V07.2
      drug V07.39
      estrogen receptor downregulators
          V07.59
      exemestane (Aromasin) V07.52 ◄▥
      fulvestrant (Faslodex) V07.59
      gamma globulin V07.2
      gonadotropin-releasing hormone
          (GnRH) agonist V07.59
      goserelin acetate (Zoladex) V07.59
      immune sera (gamma globulin)
          V07.2
      letrozole (Femara) V07.52
      leuprolide acetate (leuprorelin)
          (Lupron) V07.59
      megestrol acetate (Megace)
          V07.59
      raloxifene (Evista) V07.51
      RhoGAM V07.2
      selective estrogen receptor
          modulators (SERMs)
          V07.51
      tamoxifen (Nolvadex) V07.51
      tetanus antitoxin V07.2
      toremifene (Fareston) V07.51
  chemotherapy NEC V07.39
      fluoride V07.31
  hormone replacement
      (postmenopausal) V07.4
  immunotherapy V07.2
  measure V07.9
      specified type NEC V07.8
  medication V07.39
  postmenopausal hormone replacement
      V07.4
  sterilization V25.2
Proptosis (ocular) (see also Exophthalmos)
    376.30
  thyroid 242.0●
Propulsion
  eyeball 360.81
Prosecution, anxiety concerning V62.5
Prosopagnosia 368.16
Prostate, prostatic - see condition

Prostatism 600.90
  with
      other lower urinary tract symptoms
          (LUTS) 600.91
      urinary
          obstruction 600.91
          retention 600.91
Prostatitis (congestive) (suppurative)
    601.9
  acute 601.0
  cavitary 601.8
  chlamydial 099.54
  chronic 601.1
  diverticular 601.8
  due to Trichomonas (vaginalis) 131.03
  fibrous 600.90
      with
          other lower urinary tract
              symptoms (LUTS) 600.91
          urinary
              obstruction 600.91
              retention 600.91
      gonococcal (acute) 098.12
      chronic or duration of 2 months or
          over 098.32
  granulomatous 601.8
  hypertrophic 600.00
      with
          other lower urinary tract
              symptoms (LUTS) 600.01
          urinary
              obstruction 600.01
              retention 600.01
  specified type NEC 601.8
  subacute 601.1
  trichomonal 131.03
  tuberculous (see also Tuberculosis)
      016.5● [601.4]
Prostatocystitis 601.3
Prostatorrhea 602.8
Prostatoseminovesiculitis, trichomonal
    131.03
Prostration 780.79
  heat 992.5
      anhydrotic 992.3
      due to
          salt (and water) depletion
              992.4
          water depletion 992.3
  nervous 300.5
  newborn 779.89
  senile 797
Protanomaly 368.51
Protanopia (anomalous trichromat)
    (complete) (incomplete) 368.51
Protection (against) (from) - see
    Prophylactic
Protein
  deficiency 260
  malnutrition 260
  sickness (prophylactic) (therapeutic)
      999.5
Proteinemia 790.99
Proteinosis
  alveolar, lung or pulmonary 516.0
  lipid 272.8
  lipoid (of Urbach) 272.8
Proteinuria (see also Albuminuria) 791.0
  Bence-Jones NEC 791.0
  gestational 646.2●
      with hypertension - see Toxemia, of
          pregnancy
  orthostatic 593.6
  postural 593.6

Proteolysis, pathologic 286.6
Protocoproporphyria 277.1
Protoporphyria (erythrohepatic)
    (erythropoietic) 277.1
Protrusio acetabuli 718.65
Protrusion
  acetabulum (into pelvis) 718.65
  device, implant, or graft - see
      Complications, mechanical
  ear, congenital 744.29
  intervertebral disc - see Displacement,
      intervertebral disc
  nucleus pulposus - see Displacement,
      intervertebral disc
Proud flesh 701.5
Prune belly (syndrome) 756.71
Prurigo (ferox) (gravis) (Hebra's) (hebrae)
    (mitis) (simplex) 698.2
  agria 698.3
  asthma syndrome 691.8
  Besnier's (atopic dermatitis) (infantile
      eczema) 691.8
  eczematodes allergicum 691.8
  estivalis (Hutchinson's) 692.72
  Hutchinson's 692.72
  nodularis 698.3
  psychogenic 306.3
Pruritus, pruritic 698.9
  ani 698.0
      psychogenic 306.3
  conditions NEC 698.9
      psychogenic 306.3
  due to Onchocerca volvulus 125.3
  ear 698.9
  essential 698.9
  genital organ(s) 698.1
      psychogenic 306.3
  gravidarum 646.8●
  hiemalis 698.8
  neurogenic (any site) 306.3
  perianal 698.0
  psychogenic (any site) 306.3
  scrotum 698.1
      psychogenic 306.3
  senile, senilis 698.8
  Trichomonas 131.9
  vulva, vulvae 698.1
      psychogenic 306.3
Psammocarcinoma (M8140/3) - see
    Neoplasm, by site, malignant
Pseudarthrosis, pseudoarthrosis (bone)
    733.82
  joint following fusion V45.4
Pseudoacanthosis
  nigricans 701.8
Pseudoaneurysm - see Aneurysm
Pseudoangina (pectoris) - see Angina
Pseudoangioma 452
Pseudo-Argyll-Robertson pupil
    379.45
Pseudoarteriosus 747.89
Pseudoarthrosis - see Pseudarthrosis
Pseudoataxia 799.89
Pseudobulbar affect (PBA) 310.8
Pseudobursa 727.89
Pseudocholera 025
Pseudochromidrosis 705.89
Pseudocirrhosis, liver, pericardial
    423.2
Pseudocoarctation 747.21
Pseudocowpox 051.1
Pseudocoxalgia 732.1
Pseudocroup 478.75
Pseudocyesis 300.11

◄ New   ◄▥ Revised   ~~deleted~~ Deleted   ● Use Additional Digit(s)   ▨ Omit code

Pseudocyst
   lung 518.89
   pancreas 577.2
   retina 361.19
Pseudodementia 300.16
Pseudoelephantiasis neuroarthritica
   757.0
Pseudoemphysema 518.89
Pseudoencephalitis
   superior (acute) hemorrhagic 265.1
Pseudoerosion cervix, congenital 752.49
Pseudoexfoliation, lens capsule 366.11
Pseudofracture (idiopathic) (multiple)
   (spontaneous) (symmetrical) 268.2
Pseudoglanders 025
Pseudoglioma 360.44
Pseudogout - see Chondrocalcinosis
Pseudohallucination 780.1
Pseudohemianesthesia 782.0
Pseudohemophilia (Bernuth's)
   (hereditary) (type B) 286.4
   type A 287.8
   vascular 287.8
Pseudohermaphroditism 752.7
   with chromosomal anomaly - see
      Anomaly, chromosomal
   adrenal 255.2
   female (without adrenocortical
      disorder) 752.7
      with adrenocortical disorder
         255.2
      adrenal 255.2
   male (without gonadal disorder)
      752.7
      with
         adrenocortical disorder 255.2
         cleft scrotum 752.7
         feminizing testis 259.51
         gonadal disorder 257.9
      adrenal 255.2
Pseudohole, macula 362.54
Pseudo-Hurler's disease (mucolipidosis
   III) 272.7
Pseudohydrocephalus 348.2
Pseudohypertrophic muscular dystrophy
   (Erb's) 359.1
Pseudohypertrophy, muscle 359.1
Pseudohypoparathyroidism 275.49
Pseudoinfluenza 487.1
Pseudoinsomnia 307.49
Pseudoleukemia 288.8
   infantile 285.8
Pseudomembranous - see condition
Pseudomeningocele (cerebral) (infective)
   349.2
   postprocedural 997.01
   spinal 349.2
Pseudomenstruation 626.8
Pseudomucinous
   cyst (ovary) (M8470/0) 220
   peritoneum 568.89
Pseudomyeloma 273.1
Pseudomyxoma peritonei (M8480/6)
   197.6
Pseudoneuritis optic (nerve) 377.24
   papilla 377.24
      congenital 743.57
Pseudoneuroma - see Injury, nerve, by site
Pseudo-obstruction
   intestine (chronic) (idiopathic)
      (intermittent secondary)
      (primary) 564.89
      acute 560.89
Pseudopapilledema 377.24

Pseudoparalysis
   arm or leg 781.4
   atonic, congenital 358.8
Pseudopelade 704.09
Pseudophakia V43.1
Pseudopolycythemia 289.0
Pseudopolyposis, colon 556.4
Pseudoporencephaly 348.0
Pseudopseudohypoparathyroidism 275.49
Pseudopsychosis 300.16
Pseudopterygium 372.52
Pseudoptosis (eyelid) 374.34
Pseudorabies 078.89
Pseudoretinitis, pigmentosa 362.65
Pseudorickets 588.0
   senile (Pozzi's) 731.0
Pseudorubella 057.8
Pseudoscarlatina 057.8
Pseudosclerema 778.1
Pseudosclerosis (brain)
   Jakob's 046.19
   of Westphal (-Strümpell)
      (hepatolenticular degeneration)
      275.1
   spastic 046.19
      with dementia
         with behavioral disturbance
            046.19 [294.11]
         without behavioral disturbance
            046.19 [294.10]
Pseudoseizure 780.39
   non-psychiatric 780.39
   psychiatric 300.11
Pseudotabes 799.89
   diabetic 250.6 ● [337.1]
      due to secondary diabetes 249.6 ●
         [337.1]
Pseudotetanus (see also Convulsions)
   780.39
Pseudotetany 781.7
   hysterical 300.11
Pseudothalassemia 285.0
Pseudotrichinosis 710.3
Pseudotruncus arteriosus 747.29
Pseudotuberculosis, pasteurella
   (infection) 027.2
Pseudotumor
   cerebri 348.2
   orbit (inflammatory) 376.11
Pseudo-Turner's syndrome 759.89
Pseudoxanthoma elasticum 757.39
Psilosis (sprue) (tropical) 579.1
   Monilia 112.89
   nontropical 579.0
   not sprue 704.00
Psittacosis 073.9
Psoitis 728.89
Psora NEC 696.1
Psoriasis 696.1
   any type, except arthropathic 696.1
   arthritic, arthropathic 696.0
   buccal 528.6
   flexural 696.1
   follicularis 696.1
   guttate 696.1
   inverse 696.1
   mouth 528.6
   nummularis 696.1
   psychogenic 316 [696.1]
   punctata 696.1
   pustular 696.1
   rupioides 696.1
   vulgaris 696.1
Psorospermiasis 136.4

Psorospermosis 136.4
   follicularis (vegetans) 757.39
Psychalgia 307.80
Psychasthenia 300.89
   compulsive 300.3
   mixed compulsive states 300.3
   obsession 300.3
Psychiatric disorder or problem NEC
   300.9
Psychogenic - see also condition
   factors associated with physical
      conditions 316
Psychoneurosis, psychoneurotic (see also
   Neurosis) 300.9
   anxiety (state) 300.00
   climacteric 627.2
   compensation 300.16
   compulsion 300.3
   conversion hysteria 300.11
   depersonalization 300.6
   depressive type 300.4
   dissociative hysteria 300.15
   hypochondriacal 300.7
   hysteria 300.10
      conversion type 300.11
      dissociative type 300.15
   mixed NEC 300.89
   neurasthenic 300.5
   obsessional 300.3
   obsessive-compulsive 300.3
   occupational 300.89
   personality NEC 301.89
   phobia 300.20
   senile NEC 300.89
Psychopathic - see also condition
   constitution, posttraumatic 310.2
      with psychosis 293.9
   personality 301.9
      amoral trends 301.7
      antisocial trends 301.7
      asocial trends 301.7
      mixed types 301.7
   state 301.9
Psychopathy, sexual (see also Deviation,
   sexual) 302.9
Psychophysiologic, psychophysiological
   condition - see Reaction,
   psychophysiologic
Psychose passionelle 297.8
Psychosexual identity disorder 302.6
   adult-life 302.85
   childhood 302.6
Psychosis 298.9
   acute hysterical 298.1
   affecting management of pregnancy,
      childbirth, or puerperium 648.4 ●
   affective (see also Disorder, mood) 296.90

> **Note 63**   Use the following fifth-digit subclassification with categories 296.0–296.6:
>
> 0   unspecified
> 1   mild
> 2   moderate
> 3   severe, without mention of
>   psychotic behavior
> 4   severe, specified as with
>   psychotic behavior
> 5   in partial or unspecified remission
> 6   in full remission

   drug-induced 292.84
   due to or associated with physical
      condition 293.9

Psychosis (Continued)
  affective (Continued)
    involutional 293.83
      recurrent episode 296.3●
      single episode 296.2●
    manic-depressive 296.80
      circular (alternating) 296.7
        currently depressed 296.5●
        currently manic 296.4●
      depressed type 296.2●
        atypical 296.82
        recurrent episode 296.3●
        single episode 296.2●
      manic 296.0●
        atypical 296.81
        recurrent episode 296.1●
        single episode 296.0●
      mixed type NEC 296.89
      specified type NEC 296.89
    senile 290.21
    specified type NEC 296.99
  alcoholic 291.9
    with
      anxiety 291.89
      delirium tremens 291.0
      delusions 291.5
      dementia 291.2
      hallucinosis 291.3
      jealousy 291.5
      mood disturbance 291.89
      paranoia 291.5
      persisting amnesia 291.1
      sexual dysfunction 291.89
      sleep disturbance 291.89
    amnestic confabulatory 291.1
    delirium tremens 291.0
    hallucinosis 291.3
    Korsakoff's, Korsakov's, Korsakow's 291.1
    paranoid type 291.5
    pathological intoxication 291.4
    polyneuritic 291.1
    specified type NEC 291.89
  alternating (see also Psychosis, manic-depressive, circular) 296.7
  anergastic (see also Psychosis, organic) 294.9
  arteriosclerotic 290.40
    with
      acute confusional state 290.41
      delirium 290.41
      delusions 290.42
      depressed mood 290.43
    depressed type 290.43
    paranoid type 290.42
    simple type 290.40
    uncomplicated 290.40
  atypical 298.9
    depressive 296.82
    manic 296.81
  borderline (schizophrenia) (see also Schizophrenia) 295.5●
    of childhood (see also Psychosis, childhood) 299.8●
    prepubertal 299.8●
  brief reactive 298.8
  childhood, with origin specific to 299.9●

Note 64 Use the following fifth-digit subclassification with category 299:

  0 current or active state
  1 residual state

Psychosis (Continued)
  childhood, with origin specific to (Continued)
    atypical 299.8●
    specified type NEC 299.8●
  circular (see also Psychosis, manic-depressive, circular) 296.7
  climacteric (see also Psychosis, involutional) 298.8
  confusional 298.9
    acute 293.0
    reactive 298.2
    subacute 293.1
  depressive (see also Psychosis, affective) 296.2●
    atypical 296.82
    involutional 296.2●
      with hypomania (bipolar II) 296.89
      recurrent episode 296.3●
      single episode 296.2●
    psychogenic 298.0
    reactive (emotional stress) (psychological trauma) 298.0
    recurrent episode 296.3●
      with hypomania (bipolar II) 296.89
    single episode 296.2●
  disintegrative, childhood (see also Psychosis, childhood) 299.1●
  drug 292.9
    with
      affective syndrome 292.84
      amnestic syndrome 292.83
      anxiety 292.89
      delirium 292.81
        withdrawal 292.0
      delusions 292.11
      dementia 292.82
      depressive state 292.84
      hallucinations 292.12
      hallucinosis 292.12
      mood disorder 292.84
      mood disturbance 292.84
      organic personality syndrome NEC 292.89
      sexual dysfunction 292.89
      sleep disturbance 292.89
      withdrawal syndrome (and delirium) 292.0
    affective syndrome 292.84
    delusions 292.11
    hallucinatory state 292.12
    hallucinosis 292.12
    paranoid state 292.11
    specified type NEC 292.89
    withdrawal syndrome (and delirium) 292.0
  due to or associated with physical condition (see also Psychosis, organic) 294.9
  epileptic NEC 293.9
  excitation (psychogenic) (reactive) 298.1
  exhaustive (see also Reaction, stress, acute) 308.9
  hypomanic (see also Psychosis, affective) 296.0●
    recurrent episode 296.1●
    single episode 296.0●
  hysterical 298.8
    acute 298.1
  incipient 298.8
    schizophrenic (see also Schizophrenia) 295.5●

Psychosis (Continued)
  induced 297.3
  infantile (see also Psychosis, childhood) 299.0●
  infective 293.9
    acute 293.0
    subacute 293.1
  in
    conditions classified elsewhere
      with
        delusions 293.81
        hallucinations 293.82
    pregnancy, childbirth, or puerperium 648.4●
  interactional (childhood) (see also Psychosis, childhood) 299.1●
  involutional 298.8
    depressive (see also Psychosis, affective) 296.2●
      recurrent episode 296.3●
      single episode 296.2●
    melancholic 296.2●
      recurrent episode 296.3●
      single episode 296.2●
    paranoid state 297.2
    paraphrenia 297.2
  Korsakoff's, Korakov's, Korsakow's (nonalcoholic) 294.0
    alcoholic 291.1
  mania (phase) (see also Psychosis, affective) 296.0●
    recurrent episode 296.1●
    single episode 296.0●
  manic (see also Psychosis, affective) 296.0●
    atypical 296.81
    recurrent episode 296.1●
    single episode 296.0●
  manic-depressive 296.80
    circular 296.7
      currently
        depressed 296.5●
        manic 296.4●
      mixed 296.6●
    depressive 296.2●
      recurrent episode 296.3●
        with hypomania (bipolar II) 296.89
      single episode 296.2●
    hypomanic 296.0●
      recurrent episode 296.1●
      single episode 296.0●
    manic 296.0●
      atypical 296.81
      recurrent episode 296.1●
      single episode 296.0●
    mixed NEC 296.89
    perplexed 296.89
    stuporous 296.89
  menopausal (see also Psychosis, involutional) 298.8
  mixed schizophrenic and affective (see also Schizophrenia) 295.7●
  multi-infarct (cerebrovascular) (see also Psychosis, arteriosclerotic) 290.40
  organic NEC 294.9
    due to or associated with
      addiction
        alcohol (see also Psychosis, alcoholic) 291.9
        drug (see also Psychosis, drug) 292.9

◀ New   ◀▥ Revised   ~~deleted~~ Deleted   ● Use Additional Digit(s)   ▨ Omit code

Psychosis *(Continued)*
  organic NEC *(Continued)*
    due to or associated with *(Continued)*
      alcohol intoxication, acute *(see also* Psychosis, alcoholic) 291.9
      alcoholism *(see also* Psychosis, alcoholic) 291.9
      arteriosclerosis (cerebral) *(see also* Psychosis, arteriosclerotic) 290.40
      cerebrovascular disease
        acute (psychosis) 293.0
        arteriosclerotic *(see also* Psychosis, arteriosclerotic) 290.40
      childbirth - *see* Psychosis, puerperal
      dependence
        alcohol *(see also* Psychosis, alcoholic) 291.9
        drug 292.9
      disease
        alcoholic liver *(see also* Psychosis, alcoholic) 291.9
        brain
          arteriosclerotic *(see also* Psychosis, arteriosclerotic) 290.40
          cerebrovascular
            acute (psychosis) 293.0
            arteriosclerotic *(see also* Psychosis, arteriosclerotic) 290.40
          endocrine or metabolic 293.9
            acute (psychosis) 293.0
            subacute (psychosis) 293.1
          Jakob-Creutzfeldt 046.19
            with behavioral disturbance 046.19 *[294.11]*
            without behavioral disturbance 046.19 *[294.10]*
            familial 046.19
            iatrogenic 046.19
            specified NEC 046.19
            sporadic 046.19
            variant 046.11
              with dementia
                with behavioral disturbance 046.11 *[294.11]*
                without behavioral disturbance 046.11 *[294.10]*
          liver, alcoholic *(see also* Psychosis, alcoholic) 291.9
      disorder
        cerebrovascular
          acute (psychosis) 293.0
        endocrine or metabolic 293.9
          acute (psychosis) 293.0
          subacute (psychosis) 293.1
        epilepsy
          with behavioral disturbance 345.9 *[294.11]*●
          without behavioral disturbance 345.9 *[294.10]*●
          transient (acute) 293.0

Psychosis *(Continued)*
  organic NEC *(Continued)*
    due to or associated with *(Continued)*
      Huntington's chorea
        with behavioral disturbance 333.4 *[294.11]*
        without behavioral disturbance 333.4 *[294.10]*
      infection
        brain 293.9
          acute (psychosis) 293.0
          chronic 294.8
          subacute (psychosis) 293.1
        intracranial NEC 293.9
          acute (psychosis) 293.0
          chronic 294.8
          subacute (psychosis) 293.1
      intoxication
        alcoholic (acute) *(see also* Psychosis, alcoholic) 291.9
          pathological 291.4
        drug *(see also* Psychosis, drug) 292.9
      ischemia
        cerebrovascular (generalized) *(see also* Psychosis, arteriosclerotic) 290.40
      Jakob-Creutzfeldt disease (syndrome) 046.19
        with behavioral disturbance 046.19 *[294.11]*
        without behavioral disturbance 046.19 *[294.10]*
        variant 046.11
          with dementia
            with behavioral disturbance 046.11 *[294.11]*
            without behavioral disturbance 046.11 *[294.10]*
      multiple sclerosis
        with behavioral disturbance 340 *[294.11]*
        without behavioral disturbance 340 *[294.10]*
      physical condition NEC 293.9
        with
          delusions 293.81
          hallucinations 293.82
      presenility 290.10
      puerperium - *see* Psychosis, puerperal
      sclerosis, multiple
        with behavioral disturbance 340 *[294.11]*
        without behavioral disturbance 340 *[294.10]*
      senility 290.20
      status epilepticus
        with behavioral disturbance 345.3 *[294.11]*
        without behavioral disturbance 345.3 *[294.10]*
      trauma
        brain (birth) (from electrical current) (surgical) 293.9
          acute (psychosis) 293.0
          chronic 294.8
          subacute (psychosis) 293.1

Psychosis *(Continued)*
  organic NEC *(Continued)*
    due to or associated with *(Continued)*
      unspecified physical condition 293.9
        with
          delusions 293.81
          hallucinations 293.82
      infective 293.9
        acute (psychosis) 293.0
        subacute 293.1
      posttraumatic 293.9
        acute 293.0
        subacute 293.1
      specified type NEC 294.8
      transient 293.9
        with
          anxiety 293.84
          delusions 293.81
          depression 293.83
          hallucinations 293.82
        depressive type 293.83
        hallucinatory type 293.82
        paranoid type 293.81
        specified type NEC 293.89
  paranoic 297.1
  paranoid (chronic) 297.9
    alcoholic 291.5
    chronic 297.1
    climacteric 297.2
    involutional 297.2
    menopausal 297.2
    protracted reactive 298.4
    psychogenic 298.4
      acute 298.3
    schizophrenic *(see also* Schizophrenia) 295.3●
    senile 290.20
  paroxysmal 298.9
    senile 290.20
  polyneuritic, alcoholic 291.1
  postoperative 293.9
  postpartum - *see* Psychosis, puerperal
  prepsychotic *(see also* Schizophrenia) 295.5●
  presbyophrenic (type) 290.8
  presenile *(see also* Dementia, presenile) 290.10
  prison 300.16
  psychogenic 298.8
    depressive 298.0
    paranoid 298.4
      acute 298.3
  puerperal
    specified type - *see* categories 295–298
    unspecified type 293.89
      acute 293.0
      chronic 293.89
      subacute 293.1
  reactive (emotional stress) (psychological trauma) 298.8
    brief 298.8
    confusion 298.2
    depressive 298.0
    excitation 298.1
  schizo-affective (depressed) (excited) *(see also* Schizophrenia) 295.7●
  schizophrenia, schizophrenic *(see also* Schizophrenia) 295.9●
    borderline type 295.5●
      of childhood *(see also* Psychosis, childhood) 299.8●

Psychosis (Continued)
  schizophrenia, schizophrenic
    (Continued)
    catatonic (excited) (withdrawn)
      295.2●
    childhood type (see also Psychosis,
      childhood) 299.9●
    hebephrenic 295.1●
    incipient 295.5●
    latent 295.5●
    paranoid 295.3●
    prepsychotic 295.5●
    prodromal 295.5●
    pseudoneurotic 295.5●
    pseudopsychopathic 295.5●
    schizophreniform 295.4●
    simple 295.0●
    undifferentiated type 295.9●
  schizophreniform 295.4●
  senile NEC 290.20
    with
      delusional features 290.20
      depressive features 290.21
    depressed type 290.21
    paranoid type 290.20
    simple deterioration 290.20
    specified type - see categories 295–298
  shared 297.3
  situational (reactive) 298.8
  symbiotic (childhood) (see also
    Psychosis, childhood) 299.1●
  toxic (acute) 293.9
Psychotic (see also condition) 298.9
  episode 298.9
    due to or associated with physical
      conditions (see also Psychosis,
      organic) 293.9
Pterygium (eye) 372.40
  central 372.43
  colli 744.5
  double 372.44
  peripheral (stationary) 372.41
    progressive 372.42
  recurrent 372.45
Ptilosis 374.55
PTLD (post-transplant
  lymphoproliferative disorder)
  238.77
Ptomaine (poisoning) (see also Poisoning,
  food) 005.9
Ptosis (adiposa) 374.30
  breast 611.81
  cecum 569.89
  colon 569.89
  congenital (eyelid) 743.61
    specified site NEC - see Anomaly,
      specified type NEC
  epicanthus syndrome 270.2
  eyelid 374.30
    congenital 743.61
    mechanical 374.33
    myogenic 374.32
    paralytic 374.31
  gastric 537.5
  intestine 569.89
  kidney (see also Disease, renal) 593.0
    congenital 753.3
  liver 573.8
  renal (see also Disease, renal) 593.0
    congenital 753.3
  splanchnic 569.89
  spleen 289.59
  stomach 537.5
  viscera 569.89

PTSD (Post-Traumatic Stress Disorder)
  309.81
Ptyalism 527.7
  hysterical 300.11
  periodic 527.2
  pregnancy 646.8●
  psychogenic 306.4
Ptyalolithiasis 527.5
Pubalgia 848.8
Pubarche, precocious 259.1
Pubertas praecox 259.1
Puberty V21.1
  abnormal 259.9
  bleeding 626.3
  delayed 259.0
  precocious (constitutional)
    (cryptogenic) (idiopathic) NEC
    259.1
    due to
      adrenal
        cortical hyperfunction 255.2
        hyperplasia 255.2
      cortical hyperfunction 255.2
      ovarian hyperfunction 256.1
        estrogen 256.0
      pineal tumor 259.8
      testicular hyperfunction 257.0
  premature 259.1
    due to
      adrenal cortical hyperfunction
        255.2
      pineal tumor 259.8
      pituitary (anterior) hyperfunction
        253.1
Puckering, macula 362.56
Pudenda, pudendum - see condition
Puente's disease (simple glandular
  cheilitis) 528.5
Puerperal
  abscess
    areola 675.1●
    Bartholin's gland 646.6●
    breast 675.1●
    cervix (uteri) 670.8 ◀▥
    fallopian tube 670.8 ◀▥
    genital organ 670.8 ◀▥
    kidney 646.6●
    mammary 675.1●
    mesosalpinx 670.8 ◀▥
    nabothian 646.6●
    nipple 675.0●
    ovary, ovarian 670.8 ◀▥
    oviduct 670.8 ◀▥
    parametric 670.8 ◀▥
    para-uterine 670.8 ◀▥
    pelvic 670.8 ◀▥
    perimetric 670.8 ◀▥
    periuterine 670.8 ◀▥
    retro-uterine 670.8 ◀▥
    subareolar 675.1●
    suprapelvic 670.8 ◀▥
    tubal (ruptured) 670.8 ◀▥
    tubo-ovarian 670.8 ◀▥
    urinary tract NEC 646.6●
    uterine, uterus 670.8 ◀▥
    vagina (wall) 646.6●
    vaginorectal 646.6●
    vulvovaginal gland 646.6●
  accident 674.9●
  adnexitis 670.8 ◀▥
  afibrinogenemia, or other coagulation
    defect 666.3●
  albuminuria (acute) (subacute) 646.2●
    pre-eclamptic 642.4●

Puerperal (Continued)
  anemia (conditions classifiable to
    280–285) 648.2●
  anuria 669.3●
  apoplexy 674.0●
  asymptomatic bacteriuria 646.5●
  atrophy, breast 676.3●
  blood dyscrasia 666.3●
  caked breast 676.2●
  cardiomyopathy 674.5●
  cellulitis - see Puerperal, abscess
  cerebrovascular disorder (conditions
    classifiable to 430–434, 436–437)
    674.0●
  cervicitis (conditions classifiable to
    616.0) 646.6●
  coagulopathy (any) 666.3●
  complications 674.9●
    specified type NEC 674.8●
  convulsions (eclamptic) (uremic)
    642.6●
    with pre-existing hypertension
      642.7●
  cracked nipple 676.1●
  cystitis 646.6●
  cystopyelitis 646.6●
  deciduitis (acute) 670.8 ◀▥
  delirium NEC 293.9
  diabetes (mellitus) (conditions
    classifiable to 249 and 250)
    648.0●
  disease 674.9●
    breast NEC 676.3●
    cerebrovascular (acute) 674.0●
    nonobstetric NEC (see also
      Pregnancy, complicated,
      current disease or condition)
      648.9●
    pelvis inflammatory 670.8 ◀▥
    renal NEC 646.2●
    tubo-ovarian 670.8 ◀▥
    Valsuani's (progressive pernicious
      anemia) 648.2●
  disorder
    lactation 676.9●
      specified type NEC 676.8●
    nonobstetric NEC (see also
      Pregnancy, complicated,
      current disease or condition)
      648.9●
  disruption
    cesarean wound 674.1●
    episiotomy wound 674.2●
    perineal laceration wound 674.2●
  drug dependence (conditions
    classifiable to 304) 648.3●
  eclampsia 642.6●
    with pre-existing hypertension
      642.7●
  embolism (pulmonary) 673.2●
    air 673.0●
    amniotic fluid 673.1●
    blood clot 673.2●
    brain or cerebral 674.0●
    cardiac 674.8●
    fat 673.8●
    intracranial sinus (venous) 671.5●
    pyemic 673.3●
    septic 673.3●
    spinal cord 671.5●
  endometritis (conditions classifiable to
    615.0–615.9) 670.1 ◀▥
  endophlebitis - see Puerperal, phlebitis
  endotrachelitis 646.6●

◀ New   ◀▥ Revised   ~~deleted~~ Deleted   ● Use Additional Digit(s)   ▨ Omit code

Puerperal *(Continued)*
  engorgement, breasts 676.2●
  erysipelas 670.8 ◀━
  failure
    lactation 676.4●
    renal, acute 669.3●
  fever 670.8 ◀━
    meaning pyrexia (of unknown
      origin) 672●
    meaning sepsis 670.2 ◀━
    fissure, nipple 676.1●
  fistula
    breast 675.1●
    mammary gland 675.1●
    nipple 675.0●
  galactophoritis 675.2●
  galactorrhea 676.6●
  gangrene
    gas 670.8 ◀━
      with sepsis 670.2 ◀
    uterus 670.8 ◀━
  gonorrhea (conditions classifiable to
    098) 647.1●
  hematoma, subdural 674.0●
  hematosalpinx, infectional 670.8 ◀━
  hemiplegia, cerebral 674.0●
  hemorrhage 666.1●
    brain 674.0●
    bulbar 674.0●
    cerebellar 674.0●
    cerebral 674.0●
    cortical 674.0●
    delayed (after 24 hours) (uterine)
      666.2●
    extradural 674.0●
    internal capsule 674.0●
    intracranial 674.0●
    intrapontine 674.0●
    meningeal 674.0●
    pontine 674.0●
    subarachnoid 674.0●
    subcortical 674.0●
    subdural 674.0●
    uterine, delayed 666.2●
    ventricular 674.0●
  hemorrhoids 671.8●
  hepatorenal syndrome 674.8●
  hypertrophy
    breast 676.3●
    mammary gland 676.3●
  induration breast (fibrous) 676.3●
  infarction
    lung - *see* Puerperal, embolism
    pulmonary - *see* Puerperal,
      embolism
  infection
    Bartholin's gland 646.6●
    breast 675.2●
      with nipple 675.9●
        specified type NEC 675.8●
    cervix 646.6●
    endocervix 646.6●
    fallopian tube 670.8 ◀━
    generalized 670.0 ◀━
    genital tract (major) 670.0 ◀━
      minor or localized 646.6●
    kidney (bacillus coli) 646.6●
    mammary gland 675.2●
      with nipple 675.9●
        specified type NEC 675.8●
    nipple 675.0●
      with breast 675.9●
        specified type NEC 675.8●
    ovary 670.8 ◀━

Puerperal *(Continued)*
  infection *(Continued)*
    pelvic 670.8 ◀━
    peritoneum 670.8 ◀━
    renal 646.6●
    tubo-ovarian 670.8 ◀━
    urinary (tract) NEC 646.6●
      asymptomatic 646.5●
    uterus, uterine 670.8 ◀━
    vagina 646.6●
  inflammation - *see also* Puerperal,
    infection
    areola 675.1●
    Bartholin's gland 646.6●
    breast 675.2●
    broad ligament 670.8 ◀━
    cervix (uteri) 646.6●
    fallopian tube 670.8 ◀━
    genital organs 670.8 ◀━
      localized 646.6●
    mammary gland 675.2●
    nipple 675.0●
    ovary 670.8 ◀━
    oviduct 670.8 ◀━
    pelvis 670.8 ◀━
    periuterine 670.8 ◀━
    tubal 670.8 ◀━
    vagina 646.6●
    vein - *see* Puerperal, phlebitis●
  inversion, nipple 676.3●
  ischemia, cerebral 674.0●
  lymphangitis 670.8 ◀━
    breast 675.2●
  malaria (conditions classifiable to 084)
    647.4●
  malnutrition 648.9●
  mammillitis 675.0●
  mammitis 675.2●
  mania 296.0●
    recurrent episode 296.1●
    single episode 296.0●
  mastitis 675.2●
    purulent 675.1●
    retromammary 675.1●
    submammary 675.1●
  melancholia 296.2●
    recurrent episode 296.3●
    single episode 296.2●
  mental disorder (conditions
    classifiable to 290–303, 305.0,
    305.2–305.9, 306–316, 317–319)
    648.4●
  metritis (septic) (suppurative) 670.1 ◀━
    septic 670.2 ◀
  metroperitonitis 670.8 ◀━
  metrorrhagia 666.2●
  metrosalpingitis 670.8 ◀━
  metrovaginitis 670.8 ◀━
  milk leg 671.4●
  monoplegia, cerebral 674.0●
  necrosis
    kidney, tubular 669.3●
    liver (acute) (subacute) (conditions
      classifiable to 570) 674.8●
    ovary 670.8 ◀━
    renal cortex 669.3●
  nephritis or nephrosis (conditions
    classifiable to 580–589) 646.2●
    with hypertension 642.1●
  nutritional deficiency (conditions
    classifiable to 260–269) 648.9●
  occlusion, precerebral artery 674.0●
  oliguria 669.3●
  oophoritis 670.8 ◀━
  ovaritis 670.8 ◀━

Puerperal *(Continued)*
  paralysis●
    bladder (sphincter) 665.5●
    cerebral 674.0●
  paralytic stroke 674.0●
  parametritis 670.8 ◀━
  paravaginitis 646.6●
  pelviperitonitis 670.8 ◀━
  perimetritis 670.8 ◀━
  perimetrosalpingitis 670.8 ◀━
  perinephritis 646.6●
  perioophoritis 670.8 ◀━
  periphlebitis - *see* Puerperal, phlebitis
  perisalpingitis 670.8 ◀━
  peritoneal infection 670.8 ◀━
  peritonitis (pelvic) 670.8 ◀━
  perivaginitis 646.6●
  phlebitis 671.2 ◀━
    deep 671.4●
    intracranial sinus (venous) 671.5●
    pelvic 671.4●
    specified site NEC 671.5●
    superficial 671.2●
  phlegmasia alba dolens 671.4●
  placental polyp 674.4●
  pneumonia, embolic - *see* Puerperal,
    embolism
  prediabetes 648.8●
  pre-eclampsia (mild) 642.4●
    with pre-existing hypertension
      642.7●
    severe 642.5●
  psychosis, unspecified (*see also*
    Psychosis, puerperal) 293.89●
  pyelitis 646.6●
  pyelocystitis 646.6●
  pyelohydronephrosis 646.6●
  pyelonephritis 646.6●
  pyelonephrosis 646.6●
  pyemia 670.2 ◀━
  pyocystitis 646.6●
  pyohemia 670.2 ◀━
  pyometra 670.8 ◀━
  pyonephritis 646.6●
  pyonephrosis 646.6●
  pyo-oophoritis 670.8 ◀━
  pyosalpingitis 670.8 ◀━
  pyosalpinx 670.8 ◀━
  pyrexia (of unknown origin) 672●
  renal
    disease NEC 646.2●
    failure, acute 669.3●
  retention
    decidua (fragments) (with delayed
      hemorrhage) 666.2●
      without hemorrhage 667.1●
    placenta (fragments) (with delayed
      hemorrhage) 666.2●
      without hemorrhage 667.1●
    secundines (fragments) (with
      delayed hemorrhage) 666.2●
      without hemorrhage 667.1●
  retracted nipple 676.0●
  rubella (conditions classifiable to 056)
    647.5●
  salpingitis 670.8 ◀━
  salpingo-oophoritis 670.8 ◀━
  salpingo-ovaritis 670.8 ◀━
  salpingoperitonitis 670.8 ◀━
  sapremia 670.2 ◀━
  secondary perineal tear 674.2●
  sepsis (pelvic) 670.2 ◀━
  septicemia 670.2 ◀━
  subinvolution (uterus) 674.8●

Puerperal *(Continued)*
 sudden death (cause unknown)
  674.9●
 suppuration - *see* Puerperal, abscess
 syphilis (conditions classifiable to 090–
  097) 647.0●
 tetanus 670.8 ◀‖‖
 thelitis 675.0●
 thrombocytopenia 666.3●
 thrombophlebitis (superficial) 671.2●
  deep 671.4●
  pelvic 671.4●
  septic 670.3 ◀
  specified site NEC 671.5●
 thrombosis (venous) - *see* Thrombosis,
  puerperal
 thyroid dysfunction (conditions
  classifiable to 240–246) 648.1●
 toxemia (*see also* Toxemia, of
  pregnancy) 642.4●
  eclamptic 642.6●
   with pre-existing hypertension
    642.7●
  pre-eclamptic (mild) 642.4●
   with
    convulsions 642.6●
    pre-existing hypertension
     642.7●
   severe 642.5●
 tuberculosis (conditions classifiable to
  010–018) 647.3●
 uremia 669.3●
 vaginitis (conditions classifiable to
  616.1) 646.6●
 varicose veins (legs) 671.0●
  vulva or perineum 671.1●
 venous complication 671.9 ◀
 vulvitis (conditions classifiable to
  616.1) 646.6●
 vulvovaginitis (conditions classifiable
  to 616.1) 646.6●
 white leg 671.4●
Pulled muscle - *see* Sprain, by site
Pulmolithiasis 518.89
Pulmonary - *see* condition
Pulmonitis (unknown etiology) 486
Pulpitis (acute) (anachoretic) (chronic)
  (hyperplastic) (putrescent)
  (suppurative) (ulcerative) 522.0
Pulpless tooth 522.9
Pulse
 alternating 427.89
  psychogenic 306.2
 bigeminal 427.89
 fast 785.0
 feeble, rapid, due to shock following
  injury 958.4
 rapid 785.0
 slow 427.89
 strong 785.9
 trigeminal 427.89
 water-hammer (*see also* Insufficiency,
  aortic) 424.1
 weak 785.9
Pulseless disease 446.7
Pulsus
 alternans or trigeminy 427.89
  psychogenic 306.2
Punch drunk 310.2
Puncta lacrimalia occlusion 375.52
Punctiform hymen 752.49
Puncture (traumatic) - *see also* Wound,
  open, by site
 accidental, complicating surgery 998.2
 bladder, nontraumatic 596.6

Puncture *(Continued)*
 by
  device, implant, or graft - *see*
   Complications, mechanical
  foreign body
   internal organs - *see also* Injury,
    internal, by site
    by ingested object - *see* Foreign
     body
   left accidentally in operation
    wound 998.4
  instrument (any) during a
   procedure, accidental 998.2
 internal organs, abdomen, chest, or
  pelvis - *see* Injury, internal, by site
 kidney, nontraumatic 593.89
Pupil - *see* condition
Pupillary membrane 364.74
 persistent 743.46
Pupillotonia 379.46
 pseudotabetic 379.46
Purpura 287.2
 abdominal 287.0
 allergic 287.0
 anaphylactoid 287.0
 annularis telangiectodes 709.1
 arthritic 287.0
 autoerythrocyte sensitization 287.2
 autoimmune 287.0
 bacterial 287.0
 Bateman's (senile) 287.2
 capillary fragility (hereditary)
  (idiopathic) 287.8
 cryoglobulinemic 273.2
 devil's pinches 287.2
 fibrinolytic (*see also* Fibrinolysis)
  286.6
 fulminans, fulminous 286.6
 gangrenous 287.0
 hemorrhagic (*see also* Purpura,
  thrombocytopenic) 287.39
  nodular 272.7
  nonthrombocytopenic 287.0
  thrombocytopenic 287.39
 Henoch's (purpura nervosa) 287.0
 Henoch-Schönlein (allergic) 287.0
 hypergammaglobulinemic (benign
  primary) (Waldenström's) 273.0
 idiopathic 287.31
  nonthrombocytopenic 287.0
  thrombocytopenic 287.31
 immune thrombocytopenic 287.31
 infectious 287.0
 malignant 287.0
 neonatorum 772.6
 nervosa 287.0
 newborn NEC 772.6
 nonthrombocytopenic 287.2
  hemorrhagic 287.0
  idiopathic 287.0
 nonthrombopenic 287.2
 peliosis rheumatica 287.0
 pigmentaria, progressiva 709.09
 posttransfusion 287.4
 primary 287.0
 primitive 287.0
 red cell membrane sensitivity 287.2
 rheumatica 287.0
 Schönlein (-Henoch) (allergic) 287.0
 scorbutic 267
 senile 287.2
 simplex 287.2
 symptomatica 287.0
 telangiectasia annularis 709.1

Purpura *(Continued)*
 thrombocytopenic (*see also*
  Thrombocytopenia) 287.30
  congenital 287.33
  essential 287.30
  hereditary 287.31
  idiopathic 287.31
  immune 287.31
  neonatal, transitory (*see also*
   Thrombocytopenia, neonatal
   transitory) 776.1
  primary 287.30
  puerperal, postpartum 666.3●
  thrombotic 446.6
 thrombohemolytic (*see also* Fibrinolysis)
  286.6
 thrombopenic (*see also*
  Thrombocytopenia) 287.30
  congenital 287.33
  essential 287.30
 thrombotic 446.6
  thrombocytic 446.6
  thrombocytopenic 446.6
 toxic 287.0
 variolosa 050.0
 vascular 287.0
 visceral symptoms 287.0
 Werlhof's (*see also* Purpura,
  thrombocytopenic) 287.39
Purpuric spots 782.7
Purulent - *see* condition
Pus
 absorption, general - *see* Septicemia
 in
  stool 792.1
  urine 791.9
  tube (rupture) (*see also* Salpingo-
   oophoritis) 614.2
Pustular rash 782.1
Pustule 686.9
 malignant 022.0
 nonmalignant 686.9
Putnam's disease (subacute combined
  sclerosis with pernicious anemia)
  281.0 [336.2]
Putnam-Dana syndrome (subacute
  combined sclerosis with pernicious
  anemia) 281.0 [336.2]
Putrefaction, intestinal 569.89
Putrescent pulp (dental) 522.1
Pyarthritis - *see* Pyarthrosis
Pyarthrosis (*see also* Arthritis, pyogenic)
  711.0●
 tuberculous - *see* Tuberculosis, joint
Pycnoepilepsy, pycnolepsy (idiopathic)
  (*see also* Epilepsy) 345.0●
Pyelectasia 593.89
Pyelectasis 593.89
Pyelitis (congenital) (uremic) 590.80
 with
  abortion - *see* Abortion, by type,
   with specified complication
   NEC
  contracted kidney 590.00
  ectopic pregnancy (*see also*
   categories 633.0–633.9) 639.8
  molar pregnancy (*see also* categories
   630–632) 639.8
 acute 590.10
  with renal medullary necrosis
   590.11
 chronic 590.00
  with
   renal medullary necrosis 590.01

◀ New ◀‖‖ Revised ~~deleted~~ Deleted ● Use Additional Digit(s) ▮ Omit code

Pyelitis (Continued)
  complicating pregnancy, childbirth, or
      puerperium 646.6●
    affecting fetus or newborn 760.1
  cystica 590.3
  following
    abortion 639.8
    ectopic or molar pregnancy 639.8
  gonococcal 098.19
    chronic or duration of 2 months or
      over 098.39
  tuberculous (see also Tuberculosis)
    016.0● [590.81]
Pyelocaliectasis 593.89
Pyelocystitis (see also Pyelitis) 590.80
Pyelohydronephrosis 591
Pyelonephritis (see also Pyelitis) 590.80
  acute 590.10
    with renal medullary necrosis 590.11
  chronic 590.00
  syphilitic (late) 095.4
  tuberculous (see also Tuberculosis)
    016.0● [590.81]
Pyelonephrosis (see also Pyelitis) 590.80
  chronic 590.00
Pyelophlebitis 451.89
Pyelo-ureteritis cystica 590.3
Pyemia, pyemic (purulent) (see also
    Septicemia) 038.9
  abscess - see Abscess
  arthritis (see also Arthritis, pyogenic)
    711.0●
  Bacillus coli 038.42
  embolism (see also Septicemia) 415.12
  fever 038.9
  infection 038.9
  joint (see also Arthritis, pyogenic)
    711.0●
  liver 572.1
  meningococcal 036.2
  newborn 771.81
  phlebitis - see Phlebitis
  pneumococcal 038.2
  portal 572.1
  postvaccinal 999.39
  puerperal 670.2
  specified organism NEC 038.8
  staphylococcal 038.10
    aureus 038.11
      methicillin
        resistant 038.12
        susceptible 038.11
    specified organism NEC 038.19

Pyemia, pyemic (Continued)
  streptococcal 038.0
  tuberculous - see Tuberculosis,
    miliary
Pygopagus 759.4
Pykno-epilepsy, pyknolepsy
    (idiopathic) (see also Epilepsy)
    345.0●
Pyle (-Cohn) disease (craniometaphyseal
    dysplasia) 756.89
Pylephlebitis (suppurative) 572.1
Pylethrombophlebitis 572.1
Pylethrombosis 572.1
Pyloritis (see also Gastritis) 535.5●
Pylorospasm (reflex) 537.81
  congenital or infantile 750.5
  neurotic 306.4
  newborn 750.5
  psychogenic 306.4
Pylorus, pyloric - see condition
Pyoarthrosis - see Pyarthrosis
Pyocele
  mastoid 383.00
  sinus (accessory) (nasal) (see also
    Sinusitis) 473.9
  turbinate (bone) 473.9
  urethra (see also Urethritis) 597.0
Pyococcal dermatitis 686.00
Pyococcide, skin 686.00
Pyocolpos (see also Vaginitis)
    616.10
Pyocyaneus dermatitis 686.09
Pyocystitis (see also Cystitis) 595.9
Pyoderma, pyodermia 686.00
  gangrenosum 686.01
  specified type NEC 686.09
  vegetans 686.8
Pyodermatitis 686.00
  vegetans 686.8
Pyogenic - see condition
Pyohemia - see Septicemia
Pyohydronephrosis (see also Pyelitis)
    590.80
Pyometra 615.9
Pyometritis (see also Endometritis)
    615.9
Pyometrium (see also Endometritis)
    615.9
Pyomyositis 728.0
  ossificans 728.19
  tropical (bungpagga) 040.81
Pyonephritis (see also Pyelitis) 590.80
  chronic 590.00

Pyonephrosis (congenital) (see also
    Pyelitis) 590.80
  acute 590.10
Pyo-oophoritis (see also Salpingo-
    oophoritis) 614.2
Pyo-ovarium (see also Salpingo-
    oophoritis) 614.2
Pyopericarditis 420.99
Pyopericardium 420.99
Pyophlebitis - see Phlebitis
Pyopneumopericardium 420.99
Pyopneumothorax (infectional) 510.9
  with fistula 510.0
  subdiaphragmatic (see also Peritonitis)
    567.29
  subphrenic (see also Peritonitis)
    567.29
  tuberculous (see also Tuberculosis,
    pleura) 012.0●
Pyorrhea (alveolar) (alveolaris) 523.40
  degenerative 523.5
Pyosalpingitis (see also Salpingo-
    oophoritis) 614.2
Pyosalpinx (see also Salpingo-oophoritis)
    614.2
Pyosepticemia - see Septicemia
Pyosis
  Corlett's (impetigo) 684
  Manson's (pemphigus contagiosus)
    684
Pyothorax 510.9
  with fistula 510.0
  tuberculous (see also Tuberculosis,
    pleura) 012.0●
Pyoureter 593.89
  tuberculous (see also Tuberculosis)
    016.2●
Pyramidopallidonigral syndrome 332.0
Pyrexia (of unknown origin) (P.U.O.)
    780.60
  atmospheric 992.0
  during labor 659.2●
  environmentally-induced newborn
    778.4
  heat 992.0
  newborn, environmentally-induced
    778.4
  puerperal 672●
Pyroglobulinemia 273.8
Pyromania 312.33
Pyrosis 787.1
Pyrroloporphyria 277.1
Pyuria (bacterial) 791.9

Q

Q fever 083.0
  with pneumonia 083.0 [484.8]
Quadricuspid aortic valve 746.89
Quadrilateral fever 083.0
Quadriparesis - *see* Quadriplegia
  meaning muscle weakness 728.87
Quadriplegia 344.00
  with fracture, vertebra (process) - *see*
      Fracture, vertebra, cervical, with
      spinal cord injury
  brain (current episode) 437.8
  C$_1$–C$_4$
    complete 344.01
    incomplete 344.02
  C$_5$–C$_7$
    complete 344.03
    incomplete 344.04
  cerebral (current episode) 437.8
  congenital or infantile (cerebral)
      (spastic) (spinal) 343.2
  cortical 437.8
  embolic (current episode) (*see also*
      Embolism, brain) 434.1●
  functional 780.72

Quadriplegia (*Continued*)
  infantile (cerebral) (spastic) (spinal)
      343.2
  newborn NEC 767.0
  specified NEC 344.09
  thrombotic (current episode) (*see also*
      Thrombosis, brain) 434.0●
  traumatic - *see* Injury, spinal, cervical
Quadruplet
  affected by maternal complications of
      pregnancy 761.5
  healthy liveborn - *see* Newborn,
      multiple
  pregnancy (complicating delivery)
      NEC 651.8●
    with fetal loss and retention
        of one or more fetus(es)
        651.5●
    following (elective) fetal reduction
        651.7●
Quarrelsomeness 301.3
Quartan
  fever 084.2
  malaria (fever) 084.2
Queensland fever 083.0
  coastal 083.0
  seven-day 100.89

Quervain's disease 727.04
  thyroid (subacute granulomatous
      thyroiditis) 245.1
Queyrat's erythroplasia (M8080/2)
  specified site - *see* Neoplasm, skin, in
      situ
  unspecified site 233.5
Quincke's disease or edema - *see* Edema,
      angioneurotic
Quinquaud's disease (acne decalvans)
      704.09
Quinsy (gangrenous) 475
Quintan fever 083.1
Quintuplet
  affected by maternal complications of
      pregnancy 761.5
  healthy liveborn - *see* Newborn,
      multiple
  pregnancy (complicating delivery)
      NEC 651.2●
    with fetal loss and retention of one
        or more fetus(es) 651.6●
    following (elective) fetal reduction
        651.7●
Quotidian
  fever 084.0
  malaria (fever) 084.0

◀ New   ◀▥ Revised   ~~deleted~~ Deleted   ● Use Additional Digit(s)   ▨ Omit code

R

Rabbia 071
Rabbit fever (*see also* Tularemia) 021.9
Rabies 071
    contact V01.5
    exposure to V01.5
    inoculation V04.5
        reaction - *see* Complications,
            vaccination
    vaccination, prophylactic (against)
        V04.5
Rachischisis (*see also* Spina bifida) 741.9●
Rachitic - *see also* condition
    deformities of spine 268.1
    pelvis 268.1
        with disproportion (fetopelvic)
            653.2●
            affecting fetus or newborn 763.1
            causing obstructed labor 660.1●
                affecting fetus or newborn
                    763.1
Rachitis, rachitism - *see also* Rickets
    acute 268.0
    fetalis 756.4
    renalis 588.0
    tarda 268.0
Racket nail 757.5
Radial nerve - *see* condition
Radiation effects or sickness - *see also*
    Effect, adverse, radiation
    cataract 366.46
    dermatitis 692.82
        sunburn (*see also* Sunburn) 692.71
Radiculitis (pressure) (vertebrogenic)
    729.2
    accessory nerve 723.4
    anterior crural 724.4
    arm 723.4
    brachial 723.4
    cervical NEC 723.4
    due to displacement of intervertebral
        disc - *see* Neuritis, due to,
        displacement intervertebral disc
    leg 724.4
    lumbar NEC 724.4
    lumbosacral 724.4
    rheumatic 729.2
    syphilitic 094.89
    thoracic (with visceral pain) 724.4
Radiculomyelitis 357.0
    toxic, due to
        Clostridium tetani 037
        corynebacterium diphtheriae 032.89
Radiculopathy (*see also* Radiculitis) 729.2
Radioactive substances, adverse effect -
    see Effect, adverse, radioactive
    substance
Radiodermal burns (acute) (chronic)
    (occupational) - *see* Burn, by site
Radiodermatitis 692.82
Radionecrosis - *see* Effect, adverse,
    radiation
Radiotherapy session V58.0
Radium, adverse effect - *see* Effect,
    adverse, radioactive substance
Raeder-Harbitz syndrome (pulseless
    disease) 446.7
Rage (*see also* Disturbance, conduct)
    312.0●
    meaning rabies 071
Rag sorters' disease 022.1
Raillietiniasis 123.8
Railroad neurosis 300.16

Railway spine 300.16
Raised - *see* Elevation
Raiva 071
Rake teeth, tooth 524.39
Rales 786.7
Ramifying renal pelvis 753.3
Ramsay Hunt syndrome (herpetic
    geniculate ganglionitis) 053.11
    meaning dyssynergia cerebellaris
        myoclonica 334.2
Ranke's primary infiltration (*see also*
    Tuberculosis) 010.0●
Ranula 527.6
    congenital 750.26
Rape
    adult 995.83
    alleged, observation or examination
        V71.5
    child 995.53
Rapid
    feeble pulse, due to shock, following
        injury 958.4
    heart (beat) 785.0
        psychogenic 306.2
    respiration 786.06
        psychogenic 306.1
    second stage (delivery) 661.3●
        affecting fetus or newborn 763.6
    time-zone change syndrome 327.35
Rarefaction, bone 733.99
Rash 782.1
    canker 034.1
    diaper 691.0
    drug (internal use) 693.0
        contact 692.3
    ECHO 9 virus 078.89
    enema 692.89
    food (*see also* Allergy, food) 693.1
    heat 705.1
    napkin 691.0
    nettle 708.8
    pustular 782.1
    rose 782.1
        epidemic 056.9
        of infants 057.8
    scarlet 034.1
    serum (prophylactic) (therapeutic)
        999.5
    toxic 782.1
    wandering tongue 529.1
Rasmussen's aneurysm (*see also*
    Tuberculosis) 011.2●
Rat-bite fever 026.9
    due to Streptobacillus moniliformis
        026.1
    spirochetal (morsus muris) 026.0
Rathke's pouch tumor (M9350/1) 237.0
Raymond (-Céstan) syndrome 433.8●
Raynaud's
    disease or syndrome (paroxysmal
        digital cyanosis) 443.0
    gangrene (symmetric) 443.0 [785.4]
    phenomenon (paroxysmal digital
        cyanosis) (secondary) 443.0
RDS 769
Reaction
    acute situational maladjustment (*see*
        also Reaction, adjustment) 309.9
    adaptation (*see also* Reaction,
        adjustment) 309.9
    adjustment 309.9
        with
            anxious mood 309.24
                with depressed mood 309.28

Reaction (*Continued*)
    adjustment (*Continued*)
        with (*Continued*)
            conduct disturbance 309.3
                combined with disturbance of
                    emotions 309.4
            depressed mood 309.0
                brief 309.0
                    with anxious mood
                      309.28
                prolonged 309.1
            elective mutism 309.83
            mixed emotions and conduct
                309.4
            mutism, elective 309.83
            physical symptoms 309.82
            predominant disturbance (of)
                conduct 309.3
                emotions NEC 309.29
                    mixed 309.28
                mixed, emotions and conduct
                    309.4
            specified type NEC 309.89
            specific academic or work
                inhibition 309.23
            withdrawal 309.83
        depressive 309.0
            with conduct disturbance
                309.4
            brief 309.0
            prolonged 309.1
        specified type NEC 309.89
    adverse food NEC 995.7
    affective (*see also* Psychosis, affective)
        296.90
        specified type NEC 296.99
    aggressive 301.3
        unsocialized (*see also* Disturbance,
            conduct) 312.0●
    allergic (*see also* Allergy) 995.3
        drug, medicinal substance, and
            biological - *see* Allergy, drug
        food - *see* Allergy, food
        serum 999.5
    anaphylactic - *see* Shock, anaphylactic
    anesthesia - *see* Anesthesia,
        complication
    anger 312.0●
    antisocial 301.7
    antitoxin (prophylactic) (therapeutic) -
        see Complications, vaccination
    anxiety 300.00
    Arthus 995.21
    asthenic 300.5
    compulsive 300.3
    conversion (anesthetic) (autonomic)
        (hyperkinetic) (mixed paralytic)
        (paresthetic) 300.11
    deoxyribonuclease (DNA)
        (DNase) hypersensitivity
        NEC 287.2
    depressive 300.4
        acute 309.0
        affective (*see also* Psychosis,
            affective) 296.2●
            recurrent episode 296.3●
            single episode 296.2●
        brief 309.0
        manic (*see also* Psychosis, affective)
            296.80
        neurotic 300.4
        psychoneurotic 300.4
        psychotic 298.0
    dissociative 300.15

Reaction (*Continued*)
 drug NEC (*see also* Table of Drugs and
  Chemicals) 995.20
  allergic - *see also* Allergy, drug
   995.27
  correct substance properly
   administered 995.20
  obstetric anesthetic or analgesic
   NEC 668.9●
   affecting fetus or newborn 763.5
   specified drug - *see* Table of
    Drugs and Chemicals
  overdose or poisoning 977.9
   specified drug - *see* Table of
    Drugs and Chemicals
  specific to newborn 779.4
  transmitted via placenta or breast
   milk - *see* Absorption, drug,
   through placenta
  withdrawal NEC 292.0
   infant of dependent mother
    779.5
  wrong substance given or taken in
   error 977.9
   specified drug - *see* Table of
    Drugs and Chemicals
 dyssocial 301.7
 dystonic, acute, due to drugs 333.72
 erysipeloid 027.1
 fear 300.20
  child 313.0
 fluid loss, cerebrospinal 349.0
 food - *see also* Allergy, food
  adverse NEC 995.7
  anaphylactic shock - *see*
   Anaphylactic shock, due to,
   food
 foreign
  body NEC 728.82
   in operative wound
    (inadvertently left) 998.4
    due to surgical material
     intentionally left - *see*
     Complications, due to
     (presence of) any device,
     implant, or graft
     classified to 996.0–996.5
     NEC
  substance accidentally left during a
   procedure (chemical) (powder)
   (talc) 998.7
   body or object (instrument)
    (sponge) (swab) 998.4
 graft-versus-host (GVH) 279.50
 grief (acute) (brief) 309.0
  prolonged 309.1
 gross stress (*see also* Reaction, stress,
  acute) 308.9
 group delinquent (*see also* Disturbance,
  conduct) 312.2●
 Herxheimer's 995.0
 hyperkinetic (*see also* Hyperkinesia)
  314.9
 hypochondriacal 300.7
 hypoglycemic, due to insulin 251.0
  therapeutic misadventure 962.3
 hypomanic (*see also* Psychosis,
  affective) 296.0●
  recurrent episode 296.1●
  single episode 296.0●
 hysterical 300.10
  conversion type 300.11
  dissociative 300.15
 id (bacterial cause) 692.89

Reaction (*Continued*)
 immaturity NEC 301.89
  aggressive 301.3
  emotional instability 301.59
 immunization - *see* Complications,
  vaccination
 incompatibility
  blood group (ABO) (infusion)
   (transfusion) 999.6 ◀▥
   ABO 999.6 ◀
   minor blood group 999.89 ◀
   Rh (factor) (infusion) (transfusion)
    999.7
 inflammatory - *see* Infection
 infusion - *see* Complications, infusion
 inoculation (immune serum) - *see*
  Complications, vaccination
 insulin 995.23
 involutional
  paranoid 297.2
  psychotic (*see also* Psychosis,
   affective, depressive) 296.2●
 leukemoid (basophilic) (lymphocytic)
  (monocytic) (myelocytic)
  (neutrophilic) 288.62
 LSD (*see also* Abuse, drugs,
  nondependent) 305.3●
 lumbar puncture 349.0
 manic-depressive (*see also* Psychosis,
  affective) 296.80
  depressed 296.2●
   recurrent episode 296.3●
   single episode 296.2●
  hypomanic 296.0●
 neurasthenic 300.5
 neurogenic (*see also* Neurosis) 300.9
 neurotic NEC 300.9
 neurotic-depressive 300.4
 nitritoid - *see* Crisis, nitritoid
 obsessive-compulsive 300.3
 organic 293.9
  acute 293.0
  subacute 293.1
 overanxious, child or adolescent 313.0
 paranoid (chronic) 297.9
  acute 298.3
  climacteric 297.2
  involutional 297.2
  menopausal 297.2
  senile 290.20
  simple 297.0
 passive
  aggressive 301.84
  dependency 301.6
 personality (*see also* Disorder,
  personality) 301.9
 phobic 300.20
 postradiation - *see* Effect, adverse,
  radiation
 psychogenic NEC 300.9
 psychoneurotic (*see also* Neurosis) 300.9
  anxiety 300.00
  compulsive 300.3
  conversion 300.11
  depersonalization 300.6
  depressive 300.4
  dissociative 300.15
  hypochondriacal 300.7
  hysterical 300.10
   conversion type 300.11
   dissociative type 300.15
  neurasthenic 300.5
  obsessive 300.3
  obsessive-compulsive 300.3
  phobic 300.20
  tension state 300.9

Reaction (*Continued*)
 psychophysiologic NEC (*see also*
  Disorder, psychosomatic) 306.9
  cardiovascular 306.2
  digestive 306.4
  endocrine 306.6
  gastrointestinal 306.4
  genitourinary 306.50
  heart 306.2
  hemic 306.8
  intestinal (large) (small) 306.4
  laryngeal 306.1
  lymphatic 306.8
  musculoskeletal 306.0
  pharyngeal 306.1
  respiratory 306.1
  skin 306.3
  special sense organs 306.7
 psychosomatic (*see also* Disorder,
  psychosomatic) 306.9
 psychotic (*see also* Psychosis) 298.9
  depressive 298.0
  due to or associated with physical
   condition (*see also* Psychosis,
   organic) 293.9
  involutional (*see also* Psychosis,
   affective) 296.2●
   recurrent episode 296.3●
   single episode 296.2●
 pupillary (myotonic) (tonic) 379.46
 radiation - *see* Effect, adverse,
  radiation
 runaway - *see also* Disturbance,
  conduct
  socialized 312.2●
  undersocialized, unsocialized
   312.1●
 scarlet fever toxin - *see* Complications,
  vaccination
 schizophrenic (*see also* Schizophrenia)
  295.9●
  latent 295.5●
 serological for syphilis - *see* Serology
  for syphilis
 serum (prophylactic) (therapeutic)
  999.5
  immediate 999.4
 situational (*see also* Reaction,
  adjustment) 309.9
  acute, to stress 308.3
  adjustment (*see also* Reaction,
   adjustment) 309.9
 somatization (*see also* Disorder,
  psychosomatic) 306.9
 spinal puncture 349.0
 spite, child (*see also* Disturbance,
  conduct) 312.0●
 stress, acute 308.9
  with predominant disturbance (of)
   consciousness 308.1
   emotions 308.0
   mixed 308.4
   psychomotor 308.2
   specified type NEC 308.3
  bone or cartilage - *see* Fracture, stress
 surgical procedure - *see* Complications,
  surgical procedure
 tetanus antitoxin - *see* Complications,
  vaccination
 toxin-antitoxin - *see* Complications,
  vaccination
 transfusion (blood) (bone marrow)
  (lymphocytes) (allergic) - *see*
  Complications, transfusion

Reaction (*Continued*)
  tuberculin skin test, nonspecific
      (without active tuberculosis)
      795.5
    positive (without active
        tuberculosis) 795.5
  ultraviolet - *see* Effect, adverse,
      ultraviolet
  undersocialized, unsocialized - *see also*
      Disturbance, conduct
    aggressive (type) 312.0●
    unaggressive (type) 312.1●
  vaccination (any) - *see* Complications,
      vaccination
  white graft (skin) 996.52
  withdrawing, child or adolescent
      313.22
  x-ray - *see* Effect, adverse, x-rays
Reactive depression (*see also* Reaction,
    depressive) 300.4
  neurotic 300.4
  psychoneurotic 300.4
  psychotic 298.0
Rebound tenderness 789.6●
Recalcitrant patient V15.81
Recanalization, thrombus - *see*
    Thrombosis
Recession, receding
  chamber angle (eye) 364.77
  chin 524.06
  gingival (postinfective) (postoperative)
      523.20
    generalized 523.25
    localized 523.24
    minimal 523.21
    moderate 523.22
    severe 523.23
Recklinghausen's disease (M9540/1)
    237.71
  bones (osteitis fibrosa cystica) 252.01
Recklinghausen-Applebaum disease
    (hemochromatosis) 275.0
Reclus' disease (cystic) 610.1
Recrudescent typhus (fever) 081.1
Recruitment, auditory 388.44
Rectalgia 569.42
Rectitis 569.49
Rectocele
  female (without uterine prolapse)
      618.04
    with uterine prolapse 618.4
        complete 618.3
        incomplete 618.2
  in pregnancy or childbirth 654.4●
    causing obstructed labor 660.2●
        affecting fetus or newborn 763.1
  male 569.49
  vagina, vaginal (outlet) 618.04
Rectosigmoiditis 569.89
  ulcerative (chronic) 556.3
Rectosigmoid junction - *see* condition
Rectourethral - *see* condition
Rectovaginal - *see* condition
Rectovesical - *see* condition
Rectum, rectal - *see* condition
Recurrent - *see* condition
Red bugs 133.8
Red cedar asthma 495.8
Redness
  conjunctiva 379.93
  eye 379.93
  nose 478.19
Reduced ventilatory or vital capacity
    794.2

Reduction
  function
    kidney (*see also* Disease, renal)
        593.9
    liver 573.8
    ventilatory capacity 794.2
    vital capacity 794.2
Redundant, redundancy
  abdomen 701.9
  anus 751.5
  cardia 537.89
  clitoris 624.2
  colon (congenital) 751.5
  foreskin (congenital) 605
  intestine 751.5
  labia 624.3
  organ or site, congenital NEC - *see*
      Accessory
  panniculus (abdominal) 278.1
  prepuce (congenital) 605
  pylorus 537.89
  rectum 751.5
  scrotum 608.89
  sigmoid 751.5
  skin (of face) 701.9
    eyelids 374.30
  stomach 537.89
  uvula 528.9
  vagina 623.8
Reduplication - *see* Duplication
Referral
  adoption (agency) V68.89
  nursing care V63.8
  patient without examination or
      treatment V68.81
  social services V63.8
Reflex - *see also* condition
  blink, deficient 374.45
  hyperactive gag 478.29
  neurogenic bladder NEC 596.54
    atonic 596.54
      with cauda equina syndrome
          344.61
  vasoconstriction 443.9
  vasovagal 780.2
Reflux 530.81
  acid 530.81
  esophageal 530.81
    with esophagitis 530.11
  esophagitis 530.11
  gastroesophageal 530.81
  mitral - *see* Insufficiency, mitral
  ureteral - *see* Reflux, vesicoureteral
  vesicoureteral 593.70
    with
      reflux nephropathy 593.73
        bilateral 593.72
        unilateral 593.71
Reformed gallbladder 576.0
Reforming, artificial openings (*see also*
    Attention to, artificial, opening)
    V55.9
Refractive error (*see also* Error, refractive)
    367.9
Refsum's disease or syndrome
    (heredopathia atactica
    polyneuritiformis) 356.3
Refusal of
  food 307.59
    hysterical 300.11
  treatment because of, due to
    patient's decision NEC V64.2
    reason of conscience or religion
        V62.6

Regaud
  tumor (M8082/3) - *see* Neoplasm,
      nasopharynx, malignant
  type carcinoma (M8082/3) - *see*
      Neoplasm, nasopharynx,
      malignant
Regional - *see* condition
Regulation feeding (elderly)
    (infant) 783.3
  newborn 779.31 ◄▮▮▮
Regurgitated
  food, choked on 933.1
  stomach contents, choked on 933.1
Regurgitation 787.03
  aortic (valve) (*see also* Insufficiency,
      aortic) 424.1
    congenital 746.4
    syphilitic 093.22
  food - *see also* Vomiting
    with reswallowing - *see* Rumination
    newborn 779.33 ◄▮▮▮
  gastric contents - *see* Vomiting
  heart - *see* Endocarditis
  mitral (valve) - *see also* Insufficiency,
      mitral
    congenital 746.6
  myocardial - *see* Endocarditis
  pulmonary (heart) (valve) (*see also*
      Endocarditis, pulmonary) 424.3
  stomach - *see* Vomiting
  tricuspid - *see* Endocarditis, tricuspid
  valve, valvular - *see* Endocarditis
  vesicoureteral - *see* Reflux,
      vesicoureteral
Rehabilitation V57.9
  multiple types V57.89
  occupational V57.21
  specified type NEC V57.89
  speech (-language) V57.3 ◄▮▮▮
  vocational V57.22
Reichmann's disease or syndrome
    (gastrosuccorrhea) 536.8
Reifenstein's syndrome (hereditary
    familial hypogonadism, male)
    259.52
Reilly's syndrome or phenomenon (*see
    also* Neuropathy, peripheral,
    autonomic) 337.9
Reimann's periodic disease 277.31
Reinsertion, contraceptive device V25.42
Reiter's disease, syndrome, or urethritis
    099.3 [711.1]●
Rejection
  food, hysterical 300.11
  transplant 996.80
    bone marrow 996.85
    corneal 996.51
    organ (immune or nonimmune
        cause) 996.80
      bone marrow 996.85
      heart 996.83
      intestines 996.87
      kidney 996.81
      liver 996.82
      lung 996.84
      pancreas 996.86
      specified NEC 996.89
    skin 996.52
      artificial 996.55
      decellularized allodermis 996.55
Relapsing fever 087.9
  Carter's (Asiatic) 087.0
  Dutton's (West African) 087.1
  Koch's 087.9

Relapsing fever *(Continued)*
  louse-borne (epidemic) 087.0
  Novy's (American) 087.1
  Obermeyer's (European) 087.0
  Spirillum 087.9
  tick-borne (endemic) 087.1
Relaxation
  anus (sphincter) 569.49
    due to hysteria 300.11
  arch (foot) 734
    congenital 754.61
  back ligaments 728.4
  bladder (sphincter) 596.59
  cardio-esophageal 530.89
  cervix *(see also* Incompetency, cervix)
      622.5
  diaphragm 519.4
  inguinal rings - *see* Hernia, inguinal
  joint (capsule) (ligament) (paralytic)
      (see also Derangement, joint)
      718.90
    congenital 755.8
  lumbosacral joint 724.6
  pelvic floor 618.89
  pelvis 618.89
  perineum 618.89
  posture 729.90
  rectum (sphincter) 569.49
  sacroiliac (joint) 724.6
  scrotum 608.89
  urethra (sphincter) 599.84
  uterus (outlet) 618.89
  vagina (outlet) 618.89
  vesical 596.59
Remains
  canal of Cloquet 743.51
  capsule (opaque) 743.51
Remittent fever (malarial) 084.6
Remnant
  canal of Cloquet 743.51
  capsule (opaque) 743.51
  cervix, cervical stump (acquired)
      (postoperative) 622.8
  cystic duct, postcholecystectomy 576.0
  fingernail 703.8
    congenital 757.5
  meniscus, knee 717.5
  thyroglossal duct 759.2
  tonsil 474.8
    infected 474.00
  urachus 753.7
Remote effect of cancer - *see* condition
Removal (of)
  catheter (urinary) (indwelling) V53.6
    from artificial opening - *see*
        Attention to, artificial, opening
    non-vascular V58.82
    vascular V58.81
  cerebral ventricle (communicating)
      shunt V53.01
  device - *see also* Fitting (of)
    contraceptive V25.42
    fixation
      external V54.89
      internal V54.01
    traction V54.89
  drains V58.49
  dressing
    wound V58.30
      nonsurgical V58.30
      surgical V58.31
  ileostomy V55.2
  Kirschner wire V54.89
  non-vascular catheter V58.82

Removal (of) *(Continued)*
  pin V54.01
  plaster cast V54.89
  plate (fracture) V54.01
  rod V54.01
  screw V54.01
  splint, external V54.89
  staples V58.32
  subdermal implantable contraceptive
      V25.43
  sutures V58.32
  traction device, external V54.89
  vascular catheter V58.81
  wound packing V58.30
    nonsurgical V58.30
    surgical V58.31
Ren
  arcuatus 753.3
  mobile, mobilis *(see also* Disease, renal)
      593.0
    congenital 753.3
  unguliformis 753.3
Renal - *see also* condition
  glomerulohyalinosis-diabetic
      syndrome 250.4● *[581.81]*
    due to secondary diabetes 249.4●
        [581.81]
Rendu-Osler-Weber disease or syndrome
    (familial hemorrhagic telangiectasia)
    448.0
Reninoma (M8361/1) 236.91
Rénon-Delille syndrome 253.8
Repair
  pelvic floor, previous, in pregnancy or
      childbirth 654.4●
    affecting fetus or newborn 763.89
  scarred tissue V51.8
Replacement by artificial or mechanical
    device or prosthesis of *(see also*
    Fitting (of))
  artificial skin V43.83
  bladder V43.5
  blood vessel V43.4
  breast V43.82
  eye globe V43.0
  heart
    with
      assist device V43.21
      fully implantable artificial heart
          V43.22
    valve V43.3
  intestine V43.89
  joint V43.60
    ankle V43.66
    elbow V43.62
    finger V43.69
    hip (partial) (total) V43.64
    knee V43.65
    shoulder V43.61
    specified NEC V43.69
    wrist V43.63
  kidney V43.89
  larynx V43.81
  lens V43.1
  limb(s) V43.7
  liver V43.89
  lung V43.89
  organ NEC V43.89
  pancreas V43.89
  skin (artificial) V43.83
  tissue NEC V43.89
Reprogramming
  cardiac pacemaker V53.31
Request for expert evidence V68.2

Reserve, decreased or low
  cardiac - *see* Disease, heart
  kidney *(see also* Disease, renal) 593.9
Residual - *see also* condition
  bladder 596.8
  foreign body - *see* Retention, foreign
      body
  state, schizophrenic *(see also*
      Schizophrenia) 295.6●
  urine 788.69
Resistance, resistant (to)
  activated protein C 289.81

Note 65   Use the following
subclassification for categories V09.5,
V09.7, V09.8, V09.9

  0   without mention of resistance to
       multiple drugs
  1   with resistance to multiple drugs
     V09.5   quinolones and
              fluoro-quinolones
     V09.7   antimycobacterial agents
     V09.8   specified drugs NEC
     V09.9   unspecified drugs

---

  drugs by microorganisms V09.90
    amikacin V09.4
    aminoglycosides V09.4
    amodiaquine V09.5●
    amoxicillin V09.0
    ampicillin V09.0
    antimycobacterial agents V09.7●
    azithromycin V09.2
    azlocillin V09.0
    aztreonam V09.1
    B-lactam antibiotics V09.1
    bacampicillin V09.0
    bacitracin V09.8●
    benznidazole V09.8●
    capreomycin V09.7●
    carbenicillin V09.0
    cefaclor V09.1
    cefadroxil V09.1
    cefamandole V09.1
    cefatetan V09.1
    cefazolin V09.1
    cefixime V09.1
    cefonicid V09.1
    cefoperazone V09.1
    ceforanide V09.1
    cefotaxime V09.1
    cefoxitin V09.1
    ceftazidine V09.1
    ceftizoxime V09.1
    ceftriaxone V09.1
    cefuroxime V09.1
    cephalexin V09.1
    cephaloglycin V09.1
    cephaloridine V09.1
    cephalosporins V09.1
    cephalothin V09.1
    cephapirin V09.1
    cephradine V09.1
    chloramphenicol V09.8●
    chloraquine V09.5●
    chlorguanide V09.8●
    chlorproguanil V09.8●
    chlortetracycline V09.3
    cinoxacin V09.5●
    ciprofloxacin V09.5●
    clarithromycin V09.2
    clindamycin V09.8●
    clioquinol V09.5●
    clofazimine V09.7●

◀ New   ◀▥ Revised   ~~deleted~~ Deleted   ● Use Additional Digit(s)   ▨ Omit code

Resistance, resistant *(Continued)*
    drugs by microorganisms *(Continued)*
        cloxacillin V09.0
        cyclacillin V09.0
        cycloserine V09.7●
        dapsone [Dz] V09.7●
        demeclocycline V09.3
        dicloxacillin V09.0
        doxycycline V09.3
        enoxacin V09.5●
        erythromycin V09.2
        ethambutol [EMB] V09.7●
        ethionamide [ETA] V09.7●
        fluoroquinolones NEC V09.5●
        gentamicin V09.4
        halofantrine V09.8●
        imipenem V09.1
        iodoquinol V09.5●
        isoniazid [INH] V09.7●
        kanamycin V09.4
        macrolides V09.2
        mafenide V09.6
        MDRO (multiple drug resistant
            organisms) NOS V09.91
        mefloquine V09.8●
        melarsoprol V09.8●
        methicillin - *see* Infection,
            Methicillin
        methacycline V09.3
        methenamine V09.8●
        metronidazole V09.8●
        mezlocillin V09.0
        minocycline V09.3
        multiple drug resistant organisms
            NOS V09.91
        nafcillin V09.0
        nalidixic acid V09.5●
        natamycin V09.2
        neomycin V09.4
        netilmicin V09.4
        nimorazole V09.8●
        nitrofurantoin V09.8●
        norfloxacin V09.5●
        nystatin V09.2
        ofloxacin V09.5●
        oleandomycin V09.2
        oxacillin V09.0
        oxytetracycline V09.3
        para-amino salicyclic acid [PAS]
            V09.7●
        paromomycin V09.4
        penicillin (G) (V) (Vk) V09.0
        penicillins V09.0
        pentamidine V09.8●
        piperacillin V09.0
        primaquine V09.5●
        proguanil V09.8●
        pyrazinamide [PZA] V09.7●
        pyrimethamine/sulfalene V09.8●
        pyrimethamine/sulfodoxine V09.8●
        quinacrine V09.5●
        quinidine V09.8●
        quinine V09.8●
        quinolones V09.5●
        rifabutin V09.7●
        rifampin [Rif] V09.7●
        rifamycin V09.7●
        rolitetracycline V09.3
        specified drugs NEC V09.8●
        spectinomycin V09.8●
        spiramycin V09.2
        streptomycin [Sm] V09.4
        sulfacetamide V09.6
        sulfacytine V09.6

Resistance, resistant *(Continued)*
    drugs by microorganisms *(Continued)*
        sulfadiazine V09.6
        sulfadoxine V09.6
        sulfamethoxazole V09.6
        sulfapyridine V09.6
        sulfasalizine V09.6
        sulfasoxazone V09.6
        sulfonamides V09.6
        sulfoxone V09.7●
        tetracycline V09.3
        tetracyclines V09.3
        thiamphenicol V09.8●
        ticarcillin V09.0
        tinidazole V09.8●
        tobramycin V09.4
        triamphenicol V09.8●
        trimethoprim V09.8●
        vancomycin V09.8●
    insulin 277.7
    thyroid hormone 246.8
Resorption
    biliary 576.8
        purulent or putrid *(see also*
            Cholecystitis) 576.8
    dental (roots) 521.40
        alveoli 525.8
        pathological
            external 521.42
            internal 521.41
            specified NEC 521.49
    septic - *see* Septicemia
    teeth (roots) 521.40
        pathological
            external 521.42
            internal 521.41
            specified NEC 521.49
Respiration
    asymmetrical 786.09
    bronchial 786.09
    Cheyne-Stokes (periodic respiration)
        786.04
    decreased, due to shock following
        injury 958.4
    disorder of 786.00
        psychogenic 306.1
        specified NEC 786.09
    failure 518.81
        acute 518.81
        acute and chronic 518.84
        chronic 518.83
        newborn 770.84
    insufficiency 786.09
        acute 518.82
        newborn NEC 770.89
    Kussmaul (air hunger) 786.09
    painful 786.52
    periodic 786.09
    high altitude 327.22
    poor 786.09
        newborn NEC 770.89
    sighing 786.7
        psychogenic 306.1
    wheezing 786.07
Respiratory - *see also* condition
    distress 786.09
        acute 518.82
        fetus or newborn NEC 770.89
        syndrome (newborn) 769
            adult (following shock,
                surgery, or trauma)
                518.5
            specified NEC 518.82

Respiratory *(Continued)*
    failure 518.81
        acute 518.81
        acute and chronic 518.84
        chronic 518.83
Respiratory syncytial virus (RSV) 079.6
    bronchiolitis 466.11
    pneumonia 480.1
    vaccination, prophylactic (against)
        V04.82
Response
    photoallergic 692.72
    phototoxic 692.72
Rest, rests
    mesonephric duct 752.89
        fallopian tube 752.11
    ovarian, in fallopian tubes 752.19
    wolffian duct 752.89
Restless legs syndrome (RLS) 333.94
Restlessness 799.29   ◀▮▮▮
Restoration of organ continuity from
        previous sterilization (tuboplasty)
        (vasoplasty) V26.0
Restriction of housing space V60.1
Restzustand, schizophrenic *(see also*
        Schizophrenia) 295.6●
Retained - *see* Retention
Retardation
    development, developmental, specific
        (see also Disorder, development,
        specific) 315.9
        learning, specific 315.2
            arithmetical 315.1
            language (skills) 315.31
                expressive 315.31
                mixed receptive-expressive
                    315.32
            mathematics 315.1
            reading 315.00
                phonological 315.39
            written expression 315.2
        motor 315.4
    endochondral bone growth 733.91
    growth (physical) in childhood 783.43
        due to malnutrition 263.2
        fetal (intrauterine) 764.9●
            affecting management of
                pregnancy 656.5●
    intrauterine growth 764.9●
        affecting management of pregnancy
            656.5●
    mental 319
        borderline V62.89
        mild, IQ 50–70 317
        moderate, IQ 35–49 318.0
        profound, IQ under 20 318.2
        severe, IQ 20–34 318.1
    motor, specific 315.4
    physical 783.43
        child 783.43
        due to malnutrition 263.2
        fetus (intrauterine) 764.9●
            affecting management of
                pregnancy 656.5●
    psychomotor NEC 307.9
    reading 315.00
Retching - *see* Vomiting
Retention, retained
    bladder *(see also* Retention, urine)
        788.20
        psychogenic 306.53
    carbon dioxide 276.2
    cholelithisis 997.4
    cyst - *see* Cyst

Retention, retained (Continued)
   dead
      fetus (after 22 completed weeks'
         gestation) 656.4●
      early fetal death (before 22
         completed weeks'
         gestation) 632
      ovum 631
   decidua (following delivery)
      (fragments) (with hemorrhage)
      666.2●
      without hemorrhage 667.1●
   deciduous tooth 520.6
   dental root 525.3
   fecal (see also Constipation) 564.00
   fluid 276.6
   foreign body - see also Foreign body,
      retained
      bone 733.99
      current trauma - see Foreign body,
         by site or type
      middle ear 385.83
      muscle 729.6
      soft tissue NEC 729.6
   gallstones 997.4
   gastric 536.8
   membranes (following delivery) (with
      hemorrhage) 666.2●
      with abortion - see Abortion, by type
      without hemorrhage 667.1●
   menses 626.8
   milk (puerperal) 676.2●
   nitrogen, extrarenal 788.99
   placenta (total) (with hemorrhage)
      666.0●
      with abortion - see Abortion, by type
      portions or fragments 666.2●
         without hemorrhage 667.1●
      without hemorrhage 667.0●
   products of conception
      early pregnancy (fetal death before
         22 completed weeks'
         gestation) 632
      following
         abortion - see Abortion, by type
         delivery 666.2●
            with hemorrhage 666.2●
            without hemorrhage 667.1●
   secundines (following delivery) (with
      hemorrhage) 666.2●
      with abortion - see Abortion, by type
      complicating puerperium (delayed
         hemorrhage) 666.2●
      without hemorrhage 667.1●
   smegma, clitoris 624.8
   urine NEC 788.20
      bladder, incomplete emptying
         788.21
         due to
            benign prostatic hypertrophy
               (BPH) - see category 600
      due to
         benign prostatic hypertrophy
            (BPH) - see category 600
      psychogenic 306.53
      specified NEC 788.29
   water (in tissue) (see also Edema) 782.3
Reticulation, dust (occupational) 504
Reticulocytosis NEC 790.99
Reticuloendotheliosis
   acute infantile (M9722/3) 202.5●
   leukemic (M9940/3) 202.4●
   malignant (M9720/3) 202.3●
   nonlipid (M9722/3) 202.5●

Reticulohistiocytoma (giant cell) 277.89
Reticulohistiocytosis, multicentric
   272.8
Reticulolymphosarcoma (diffuse)
   (M9613/3) 200.8●
   follicular (M9691/3) 202.0●
   nodular (M9691/3) 202.0●
Reticulosarcoma (M9640/3) 200.0●
   nodular (M9642/3) 200.0●
   pleomorphic cell type (M9641/3)
      200.0●
Reticulosis (skin)
   acute of infancy (M9722/3) 202.5●
   familial hemophagocytic 288.4
   histiocytic medullary (M9721/3)
      202.3●
   lipomelanotic 695.89
   malignant (M9720/3) 202.3●
   Sezary's (M9701/3) 202.2●
Retina, retinal - see condition
Retinitis (see also Chorioretinitis) 363.20
   albuminurica 585.9 [363.10]
   arteriosclerotic 440.8 [362.13]
   central angiospastic 362.41
   Coat's 362.12
   diabetic 250.5● [362.01]
      due to secondary diabetes 249.5●
         [362.01]
   disciformis 362.52
   disseminated 363.10
      metastatic 363.14
      neurosyphilitic 094.83
      pigment epitheliopathy 363.15
   exudative 362.12
   focal 363.00
      in histoplasmosis 115.92
         capsulatum 115.02
         duboisii 115.12
      juxtapapillary 363.05
      macular 363.06
      paramacular 363.06
      peripheral 363.08
      posterior pole NEC 363.07
   gravidarum 646.8●
   hemorrhagica externa 362.12
   juxtapapillary (Jensen's) 363.05
   luetic - see Retinitis, syphilitic
   metastatic 363.14
   pigmentosa 362.74
   proliferans 362.29
   proliferating 362.29
   punctata albescens 362.76
   renal 585.9 [363.13]
   syphilitic (secondary) 091.51
      congenital 090.0 [363.13]
      early 091.51
      late 095.8 [363.13]
   syphilitica, central, recurrent 095.8
      [363.13]
   tuberculous (see also Tuberculous)
      017.3● [363.13]
Retinoblastoma (M9510/3) 190.5
   differentiated type (M9511/3) 190.5
   undifferentiated type (M9512/3) 190.5
Retinochoroiditis (see also Chorioretinitis)
   363.20
   central angiospastic 362.41
   disseminated 363.10
      metastatic 363.14
      neurosyphilitic 094.83
      pigment epitheliopathy 363.15
      syphilitic 094.83
   due to toxoplasmosis (acquired) (focal)
      130.2

Retinochoroiditis (Continued)
   focal 363.00
      in histoplasmosis 115.92
         capsulatum 115.02
         duboisii 115.12
      juxtapapillary (Jensen's) 363.05
      macular 363.06
      paramacular 363.06
      peripheral 363.08
      posterior pole NEC 363.07
   juxtapapillaris 363.05
   syphilitic (disseminated) 094.83
Retinopathy (background) 362.10
   arteriosclerotic 440.8 [362.13]
   atherosclerotic 440.8 [362.13]
   central serous 362.41
   circinate 362.10
   Coat's 362.12
   diabetic 250.5● [362.01]
      due to secondary diabetes 249.5●
         [362.01]
      nonproliferative 250.5● [362.03]
         due to secondary diabetes
            249.5● [362.03]
         mild 250.5● [362.04]
            due to secondary diabetes
               249.5● [362.04]
         moderate 250.5● [362.05]
            due to secondary diabetes
               249.5● [362.05]
         severe 250.5● [362.06]
            due to secondary diabetes
               249.5● [362.06]
      proliferative 250.5● [362.02]
         due to secondary diabetes 249.5●
            [362.02]
   exudative 362.12
   hypertensive 362.11
   nonproliferative
      diabetic 250.5● [362.03]
         due to secondary diabetes 249.5●
            [362.03]
         mild 250.5● [362.04]
            due to secondary diabetes
               249.5● [362.04]
         moderate 250.5● [362.05]
            due to secondary diabetes
               249.5● [362.05]
         severe 250.5● [362.06]
            due to secondary diabetes
               249.5● [362.06]
   of prematurity 362.20
      cicatricial 362.21
      stage
         0 362.22
         1 362.23
         2 362.24
         3 362.25
         4 362.26
         5 362.27
   pigmentary, congenital 362.74
   proliferative 362.29
      diabetic 250.5● [362.02]
         due to secondary diabetes
            249.5● [362.02]
      sickle-cell 282.60 [362.29]
   solar 363.31
Retinoschisis 361.10
   bullous 361.12
   congenital 743.56
   flat 361.11
   juvenile 362.73
Retractile testis 752.52

◀ New   ◀║ Revised   deleted Deleted   ● Use Additional Digit(s)   ▨ Omit code

Retraction
cervix *see* Retraction, uterus
drum (membrane) 384.82
eyelid 374.41
finger 736.29
head 781.0
lid 374.41
lung 518.89
mediastinum 519.3
nipple 611.79
   congenital 757.6
   puerperal, postpartum 676.0●
palmar fascia 728.6
pleura (*see also* Pleurisy) 511.0
ring, uterus (Bandl's) (pathological)
   661.4●
   affecting fetus or newborn 763.7
sternum (congenital) 756.3
   acquired 738.3
   during respiration 786.9
substernal 738.3
supraclavicular 738.8
syndrome (Duane's) 378.71
uterus 621.6
valve (heart) - *see* Endocarditis
Retrobulbar - *see* condition
Retrocaval ureter 753.4
Retrocecal - *see also* condition
appendix (congenital) 751.5
Retrocession - *see* Retroversion
Retrodisplacement - *see* Retroversion
Retroflection, retroflexion - *see*
Retroversion
Retrognathia, retrognathism
(mandibular) (maxillary) 524.10
Retrograde
ejaculation 608.87
menstruation 626.8
Retroiliac ureter 753.4
Retroperineal - *see* condition
Retroperitoneal - *see* condition
Retroperitonitis 567.39
Retropharyngeal - *see* condition
Retroplacental - *see* condition
Retroposition - *see* Retroversion
Retrosternal thyroid (congenital) 759.2
Retroversion, retroverted
cervix - *see* Retroversion, uterus
female NEC (*see also* Retroversion,
   uterus) 621.6
iris 364.70
testis (congenital) 752.51
uterus, uterine (acquired) (acute)
   (adherent) (any degree)
   (asymptomatic) (cervix)
   (postinfectional) (postpartal, old)
   621.6
   congenital 752.3
   in pregnancy or childbirth
      654.3●
      affecting fetus or newborn
         763.89
      causing obstructed labor
         660.2●
         affecting fetus or newborn
            763.1
Retrusion, premaxilla (developmental)
524.04
Rett's syndrome 330.8
Reverse, reversed
peristalsis 787.4
Reye's syndrome 331.81
Reye-Sheehan syndrome (postpartum
pituitary necrosis) 253.2

Rh (factor)
hemolytic disease 773.0
incompatibility, immunization, or
   sensitization
   affecting management of pregnancy
      656.1●
   fetus or newborn 773.0
   transfusion reaction 999.7
negative mother, affecting fetus or
   newborn 773.0
titer elevated 999.7
transfusion reaction 999.7
Rhabdomyolysis (idiopathic) 728.88
Rhabdomyoma (M8900/0) - *see also*
Neoplasm, connective tissue,
benign
adult (M8904/0) - *see* Neoplasm,
   connective tissue, benign
fetal (M8903/0) - *see* Neoplasm,
   connective tissue, benign
glycogenic (M8904/0) - *see* Neoplasm,
   connective tissue, benign
Rhabdomyosarcoma (M8900/3) - *see also*
Neoplasm, connective tissue,
malignant
alveolar (M8920/3) - *see* Neoplasm,
   connective tissue, malignant
embryonal (M8910/3) - *see* Neoplasm,
   connective tissue, malignant
mixed type (M8902/3) - *see* Neoplasm,
   connective tissue, malignant
pleomorphic (M8901/3) - *see*
   Neoplasm, connective tissue,
   malignant
Rhabdosarcoma (M8900/3) - *see*
Rhabdomyosarcoma
Rhesus (factor) (Rh) incompatibility - *see*
Rh, incompatibility
Rheumaticosis - *see* Rheumatism
Rheumatism, rheumatic (acute NEC)
729.0
adherent pericardium 393
arthritis
   acute or subacute - *see* Fever,
      rheumatic
   chronic 714.0
      spine 720.0
articular (chronic) NEC (*see also*
   Arthritis) 716.9●
   acute or subacute - *see* Fever,
      rheumatic
back 724.9
blennorrhagic 098.59
carditis - *see* Disease, heart, rheumatic
cerebral - *see* Fever, rheumatic
chorea (acute) - *see* Chorea, rheumatic
chronic NEC 729.0
coronary arteritis 391.9
   chronic 398.99
degeneration, myocardium (*see also*
   Degeneration, myocardium, with
   rheumatic fever) 398.0
desert 114.0
febrile - *see* Fever, rheumatic
fever - *see* Fever, rheumatic
gonococcal 098.59
gout 274.00   ◀▥
heart
   disease (*see also* Disease, heart,
      rheumatic) 398.90
   failure (chronic) (congestive)
      (inactive) 398.91
   hemopericardium - *see* Rheumatic,
      pericarditis

Rheumatism, rheumatic *(Continued)*
hydropericardium - *see* Rheumatic,
   pericarditis
inflammatory (acute) (chronic)
   (subacute) - *see* Fever, rheumatic
intercostal 729.0
   meaning Tietze's disease 733.6
joint (chronic) NEC (*see also* Arthritis)
   716.9●
   acute - *see* Fever, rheumatic
mediastinopericarditis - *see* Rheumatic,
   pericarditis
muscular 729.0
myocardial degeneration (*see also*
   Degeneration, myocardium, with
   rheumatic fever) 398.0
myocarditis (chronic) (inactive) (with
   chorea) 398.0
   active or acute 391.2
      with chorea (acute) (rheumatic)
         (Sydenham's) 392.0
myositis 729.1
neck 724.9
neuralgic 729.0
neuritis (acute) (chronic) 729.2
neuromuscular 729.0
nodose - *see* Arthritis, nodosa
nonarticular 729.0
palindromic 719.30
   ankle 719.37
   elbow 719.32
   foot 719.37
   hand 719.34
   hip 719.35
   knee 719.36
   multiple sites 719.39
   pelvic region 719.35
   shoulder (region) 719.31
   specified site NEC 719.38
   wrist 719.33
pancarditis, acute 391.8
   with chorea (acute) (rheumatic)
      (Sydenham's) 392.0
   chronic or inactive 398.99
pericarditis (active) (acute) (with
   effusion) (with pneumonia)
   391.0
   with chorea (acute) (rheumatic)
      (Sydenham's) 392.0
   chronic or inactive 393
pericardium - *see* Rheumatic,
   pericarditis
pleuropericarditis - *see* Rheumatic,
   pericarditis
pneumonia 390 [517.1]
pneumonitis 390 [517.1]
pneumopericarditis - *see* Rheumatic,
   pericarditis
polyarthritis
   acute or subacute - *see* Fever,
      rheumatic
   chronic 714.0
polyarticular NEC (*see also* Arthritis)
   716.9●
psychogenic 306.0
radiculitis 729.2
sciatic 724.3
septic - *see* Fever, rheumatic
spine 724.9
subacute NEC 729.0
torticollis 723.5
tuberculous NEC (*see also* Tuberculosis)
   015.9●
typhoid fever 002.0

Rheumatoid - *see also* condition
  lungs 714.81
Rhinitis (atrophic) (catarrhal) (chronic)
      (croupous) (fibrinous) (hyperplastic)
      (hypertrophic) (membranous)
      (purulent) (suppurative) (ulcerative)
      472.0
  with
      hay fever (*see also* Fever, hay) 477.9
          with asthma (bronchial) 493.0●
      sore throat - *see* Nasopharyngitis
  acute 460
  allergic (nonseasonal) (seasonal) (*see
      also* Fever, hay) 477.9
      with asthma (*see also* Asthma)
          493.0●
      due to food 477.1
  granulomatous 472.0
  infective 460
  obstructive 472.0
  pneumococcal 460
  syphilitic 095.8
      congenital 090.0
  tuberculous (*see also* Tuberculosis)
      012.8●
  vasomotor (*see also* Fever, hay) 477.9
Rhinoantritis (chronic) 473.0
  acute 461.0
Rhinodacryolith 375.57
Rhinolalia (aperta) (clausa) (open)
      784.43   ◀▥
Rhinolith 478.19
  nasal sinus (*see also* Sinusitis) 473.9
Rhinomegaly 478.19
Rhinopharyngitis (acute) (subacute) (*see
      also* Nasopharyngitis) 460
  chronic 472.2
  destructive ulcerating 102.5
  mutilans 102.5
Rhinophyma 695.3
Rhinorrhea 478.19
  cerebrospinal (fluid) 349.81
  paroxysmal (*see also* Fever, hay) 477.9
  spasmodic (*see also* Fever, hay) 477.9
Rhinosalpingitis 381.50
  acute 381.51
  chronic 381.52
Rhinoscleroma 040.1
Rhinosporidiosis 117.0
Rhinovirus infection 079.3
Rhizomelic chrondrodysplasia punctata
      277.86
Rhizomelique, pseudopolyarthritic 446.5
Rhoads and Bomford anemia (refractory)
      238.72
Rhus
  diversiloba dermatitis 692.6
  radicans dermatitis 692.6
  toxicodendron dermatitis 692.6
  venenata dermatitis 692.6
  verniciflua dermatitis 692.6
Rhythm
  atrioventricular nodal 427.89
  disorder 427.9
      coronary sinus 427.89
      ectopic 427.89
      nodal 427.89
  escape 427.89
  heart, abnormal 427.9
      fetus or newborn - *see* Abnormal,
          heart rate
  idioventricular 426.89
      accelerated 427.89
  nodal 427.89

Rhythm (*Continued*)
  sleep, inversion 327.39
      nonorganic origin 307.45
Rhytidosis facialis 701.8
Rib - *see also* condition
  cervical 756.2
Riboflavin deficiency 266.0
Rice bodies (*see also* Loose, body, joint)
      718.1●
  knee 717.6
Richter's hernia - *see* Hernia, Richter's
Ricinism 988.2
Rickets (active) (acute) (adolescent)
      (adult) (chest wall) (congenital)
      (current) (infantile) (intestinal) 268.0
  celiac 579.0
  fetal 756.4
  hemorrhagic 267
  hypophosphatemic with nephrotic-
      glycosuric dwarfism 270.0
  kidney 588.0
  late effect 268.1
  renal 588.0
  scurvy 267
  vitamin D-resistant 275.3
Rickettsial disease 083.9
  specified type NEC 083.8
Rickettsialpox 083.2
Rickettsiosis NEC 083.9
  specified type NEC 083.8
  tick-borne 082.9
      specified type NEC 082.8
  vesicular 083.2
Ricord's chancre 091.0
Riddoch's syndrome (visual
      disorientation) 368.16
Rider's
  bone 733.99
  chancre 091.0
Ridge, alveolus - *see also* condition
  edentulous
      atrophy 525.20
          mandible 525.20
              minimal 525.21
              moderate 525.22
              severe 525.23
          maxilla 525.20
              minimal 525.24
              moderate 525.25
              severe 525.26
      flabby 525.20
Ridged ear 744.29
Riedel's
  disease (ligneous thyroiditis) 245.3
  lobe, liver 751.69
  struma (ligneous thyroiditis) 245.3
  thyroiditis (ligneous) 245.3
Rieger's anomaly or syndrome
      (mesodermal dysgenesis, anterior
      ocular segment) 743.44
Riehl's melanosis 709.09
Rietti-Greppi-Micheli anemia or
      syndrome 282.49
Rieux's hernia - *see* Hernia, Rieux's
Rift Valley fever 066.3
Riga's disease (cachectic aphthae) 529.0
Riga-Fede disease (cachectic aphthae)
      529.0
Riggs' disease (compound periodontitis)
      523.40
Right middle lobe syndrome 518.0
Rigid, rigidity - *see also* condition
  abdominal 789.4●
  articular, multiple congenital 754.89

Rigid, rigidity (*Continued*)
  back 724.8
  cervix uteri
      in pregnancy or childbirth 654.6●
          affecting fetus or newborn 763.89
          causing obstructed labor 660.2●
              affecting fetus or newborn
                  763.1
  hymen (acquired) (congenital) 623.3
  nuchal 781.6
  pelvic floor
      in pregnancy or childbirth 654.4●
          affecting fetus or newborn 763.89
          causing obstructed labor 660.2●
              affecting fetus or newborn
                  763.1
  perineum or vulva
      in pregnancy or childbirth 654.8●
          affecting fetus or newborn 763.89
          causing obstructed labor 660.2●
              affecting fetus or newborn
                  763.1
  spine 724.8
  vagina
      in pregnancy or childbirth 654.7●
          affecting fetus or newborn 763.89
          causing obstructed labor 660.2●
              affecting fetus or newborn 763.1
Rigors 780.99
Riley-Day syndrome (familial
      dysautonomia) 742.8
RIND (reversible ischemic neurological
      deficit) 434.91
  history of (personal) V12.54
Ring(s)
  aorta 747.21
  Bandl's, complicating delivery 661.4●
      affecting fetus or newborn 763.7
  contraction, complicating delivery
      661.4●
      affecting fetus or newborn 763.7
  esophageal (congenital) 750.3
  Fleischer (-Kayser) (cornea) 275.1
      [371.14]
  hymenal, tight (acquired) (congenital)
      623.3
  Kayser-Fleischer (cornea) 275.1 *[371.14]*
  retraction, uterus, pathological 661.4●
      affecting fetus or newborn 763.7
  Schatzki's (esophagus) (congenital)
      (lower) 750.3
      acquired 530.3
  Soemmering's 366.51
  trachea, abnormal 748.3
  vascular (congenital) 747.21
  Vossius' 921.3
      late effect 366.21
Ringed hair (congenital) 757.4
Ringing in the ear (*see also* Tinnitus)
      388.30
Ringworm 110.9
  beard 110.0
  body 110.5
  Burmese 110.9
  corporeal 110.5
  foot 110.4
  groin 110.3
  hand 110.2
  honeycomb 110.0
  nails 110.1
  perianal (area) 110.3
  scalp 110.0
  specified site NEC 110.8
  Tokelau 110.5

◀ New   ◀▥ Revised   ~~deleted~~ Deleted   ● Use Additional Digit(s)   ▨ Omit code

Rise, venous pressure 459.89
Risk
  factor - see Problem
  falling V15.88
  suicidal 300.9
Ritter's disease (dermatitis exfoliativa
  neonatorum) 695.81
Rivalry, sibling 313.3
Rivalta's disease (cervicofacial
  actinomycosis) 039.3
River blindness 125.3 [360.13]
Robert's pelvis 755.69
  with disproportion (fetopelvic)
    653.0●
    affecting fetus or newborn 763.1
    causing obstructed labor 660.1●
      affecting fetus or newborn
      763.1
Robin's syndrome 756.0
Robinson's (hidrotic) ectodermal
  dysplasia 757.31
Robles' disease (onchocerciasis) 125.3
  [360.13]
Rochalimea - see Rickettsial disease
Rocky Mountain fever (spotted) 082.0
Rodent ulcer (M8090/3) - see also
  Neoplasm, skin, malignant
  cornea 370.07
Roentgen ray, adverse effect - see Effect,
  adverse, x-ray
Roetheln 056.9
Roger's disease (congenital
  interventricular septal defect) 745.4
Rokitansky's
  disease (see also Necrosis, liver) 570
  tumor 620.2
Rokitansky-Aschoff sinuses (mucosal
  outpouching of gallbladder) (see also
  Disease, gallbladder) 575.8
Rokitansky-Kuster-Hauser syndrome
  (congenital absence vagina)
  752.49
Rollet's chancre (syphilitic) 091.0
Rolling of head 781.0
Romano-Ward syndrome (prolonged QT
  interval syndrome) 426.82
Romanus lesion 720.1
Romberg's disease or syndrome
  349.89
Roof, mouth - see condition
Rosacea 695.3
  acne 695.3
  keratitis 695.3 [370.49]
Rosary, rachitic 268.0
Rose
  cold 477.0
  fever 477.0
  rash 782.1
    epidemic 056.9
    of infants 057.8
Rosen-Castleman-Liebow syndrome
  (pulmonary proteinosis) 516.0
Rosenbach's erysipelatoid or erysipeloid
  027.1
Rosenthal's disease (factor XI deficiency)
  286.2
Roseola 057.8
  infantum, infantilis (see also Exanthem
    subitum) 058.10
Rossbach's disease (hyperchlorhydria)
  536.8
  psychogenic 306.4
Rossle-Urbach-Wiethe lipoproteinosis
  272.8

Ross river fever 066.3
Rostan's asthma (cardiac) (see also Failure,
  ventricular, left) 428.1
Rot
  Barcoo (see also Ulcer, skin) 707.9
  knife-grinders' (see also Tuberculosis)
    011.4●
Rot-Bernhardt disease 355.1
Rotation
  anomalous, incomplete or insufficient -
    see Malrotation
  cecum (congenital) 751.4
  colon (congenital) 751.4
  manual, affecting fetus or newborn
    763.89
  spine, incomplete or insufficient
    737.8
  tooth, teeth 524.35
  vertebra, incomplete or insufficient
    737.8
Röteln 056.9
Roth's disease or meralgia 355.1
Roth-Bernhardt disease or syndrome
  355.1
Rothmund (-Thomson) syndrome 757.33
Rotor's disease or syndrome (idiopathic
  hyperbilirubinemia) 277.4
Rotundum ulcus - see Ulcer, stomach
Round
  back (with wedging of vertebrae)
    737.10
    late effect of rickets 268.1
  hole, retina 361.31
    with detachment 361.01
  ulcer (stomach) - see Ulcer, stomach
  worms (infestation) (large) NEC
    127.0
Roussy-Lévy syndrome 334.3
Routine postpartum follow-up V24.2
Roy (-Jutras) syndrome (acropachyderma)
  757.39
Rubella (German measles) 056.9
  complicating pregnancy, childbirth, or
    puerperium 647.5●
  complication 056.8
    neurological 056.00
      encephalomyelitis 056.01
      specified type NEC 056.09
    specified type NEC 056.79
  congenital 771.0
  contact V01.4
  exposure to V01.4
  maternal
    with suspected fetal damage
      affecting management of
      pregnancy 655.3●
    affecting fetus or newborn 760.2
      manifest rubella in infant 771.0
  specified complications NEC 056.79
  vaccination, prophylactic (against)
    V04.3
Rubeola (measles) (see also Measles) 055.9
  complicated 055.8
  meaning rubella (see also Rubella) 056.9
  scarlatinosis 057.8
Rubeosis iridis 364.42
  diabetica 250.5● [364.42]
    due to secondary diabetes 249.5●
    [364.42]
Rubinstein-Taybi's syndrome
  (brachydactylia, short stature and
  mental retardation) 759.89
Rud's syndrome (mental deficiency,
  epilepsy, and infantilism) 759.89

Rudimentary (congenital) - see also
  Agenesis
  arm 755.22
  bone 756.9
  cervix uteri 752.49
  eye (see also Microphthalmos) 743.10
  fallopian tube 752.19
  leg 755.32
  lobule of ear 744.21
  patella 755.64
  respiratory organs in thoracopagus
    759.4
  tracheal bronchus 748.3
  uterine horn 752.3
  uterus 752.3
    in male 752.7
    solid or with cavity 752.3
  vagina 752.49
Ruiter-Pompen (-Wyers) syndrome
  (angiokeratoma corporis diffusum)
  272.7
Ruled out condition (see also Observation,
  suspected) V71.9
Rumination - see also Vomiting
  disorder 307.53
  neurotic 300.3
  obsessional 300.3
  psychogenic 307.53
Runaway reaction - see also Disturbance,
  conduct
  socialized 312.2●
  undersocialized, unsocialized 312.1●
Runeberg's disease (progressive
  pernicious anemia) 281.0
Runge's syndrome (postmaturity)
  766.22
Runny nose 784.99
Rupia 091.3
  congenital 090.0
  tertiary 095.9
Rupture, ruptured 553.9
  abdominal viscera NEC 799.89
    obstetrical trauma 665.5●
  abscess (spontaneous) - see Abscess, by
    site
  amnion - see Rupture, membranes
  aneurysm - see Aneurysm
  anus (sphincter) - see Laceration, anus
  aorta, aortic 441.5
    abdominal 441.3
    arch 441.1
    ascending 441.1
    descending 441.5
      abdominal 441.3
      thoracic 441.1
    syphilitic 093.0
    thoracoabdominal 441.6
    thorax, thoracic 441.1
    transverse 441.1
    traumatic (thoracic) 901.0
      abdominal 902.0
    valve or cusp (see also Endocarditis,
      aortic) 424.1
  appendix (with peritonitis) 540.0
    with peritoneal abscess 540.1
    traumatic - see Injury, internal,
      gastrointestinal tract
  arteriovenous fistula, brain (congenital)
    430
  artery 447.2
    brain (see also Hemorrhage, brain)
      431
    coronary (see also Infarct,
      myocardium) 410.9●

Rupture, ruptured (Continued)
 artery (Continued)
  heart (see also Infarct, myocardium)
    410.9●
  pulmonary 417.8
  traumatic (complication) (see also
    Injury, blood vessel, by site)
    904.9
 bile duct, except cystic (see also Disease,
    biliary) 576.3
  cystic 575.4
  traumatic - see Injury, internal, intra-
    abdominal
 bladder (sphincter) 596.6
  with
   abortion - see Abortion, by type,
    with damage to pelvic
    organs
   ectopic pregnancy (see also
    categories 633.0–633.9)
    639.2
   molar pregnancy (see also
    categories 630–632) 639.2
  following
   abortion 639.2
   ectopic or molar pregnancy
    639.2
  nontraumatic 596.6
  obstetrical trauma 665.5●
  spontaneous 596.6
  traumatic - see Injury, internal,
    bladder
 blood vessel (see also Hemorrhage)
    459.0
  brain (see also Hemorrhage, brain)
    431
  heart (see also Infarct, myocardium)
    410.9●
  traumatic (complication) (see also
    Injury, blood vessel, by site)
    904.9
 bone - see Fracture, by site
 bowel 569.89
  traumatic - see Injury, internal,
    intestine
 Bowman's membrane 371.31
 brain
  aneurysm (congenital) (see also
    Hemorrhage, subarachnoid)
    430
   late effect - see Late effect(s) (of)
    cerebrovascular disease
  syphilitic 094.87
  hemorrhagic (see also Hemorrhage,
    brain) 431
  injury at birth 767.0
  syphilitic 094.89
 capillaries 448.9
 cardiac (see also Infarct, myocardium)
    410.9●
 cartilage (articular) (current) - see also
    Sprain, by site
  knee - see Tear, meniscus
  semilunar - see Tear, meniscus
 cecum (with peritonitis) 540.0
  with peritoneal abscess 540.1
  traumatic 863.89
   with open wound into cavity
    863.99
 cerebral aneurysm (congenital) (see
    also Hemorrhage, subarachnoid)
    430
   late effect - see Late effect(s) (of)
    cerebrovascular disease

Rupture, ruptured (Continued)
 cervix (uteri)
  with
   abortion - see Abortion, by type,
    with damage to pelvic
    organs
   ectopic pregnancy (see also
    categories 633.0–633.9) 639.2
   molar pregnancy (see also
    categories 630–632) 639.2
  following
   abortion 639.2
   ectopic or molar pregnancy 639.2
  obstetrical trauma 665.3●
  traumatic - see Injury, internal, cervix
 chordae tendineae 429.5
 choroid (direct) (indirect) (traumatic)
    363.63
 circle of Willis (see also Hemorrhage,
    subarachnoid) 430
  late effect - see Late effect(s) (of)
    cerebrovascular disease
 colon 569.89
  traumatic - see Injury, internal, colon
 cornea (traumatic) - see also Rupture,
    eye
  due to ulcer 370.00
 coronary (artery) (thrombotic) (see also
    Infarct, myocardium) 410.9●
 corpus luteum (infected) (ovary) 620.1
 cyst - see Cyst
 cystic duct (see also Disease,
    gallbladder) 575.4
 Descemet's membrane 371.33
  traumatic - see Rupture, eye
 diaphragm - see also Hernia, diaphragm
  traumatic - see Injury, internal,
    diaphragm
 diverticulum
  bladder 596.3
  intestine (large) (see also Diverticula)
    562.10
   small 562.00
 duodenal stump 537.89
 duodenum (ulcer) - see Ulcer,
    duodenum, with perforation
 ear drum (see also Perforation,
    tympanum) 384.20
  with otitis media - see Otitis media
  traumatic - see Wound, open, ear
 esophagus 530.4
  traumatic 862.22
   with open wound into cavity
    862.32
   cervical region - see Wound, open,
    esophagus
 eye (without prolapse of intraocular
    tissue) 871.0
  with
   exposure of intraocular tissue
    871.1
   partial loss of intraocular tissue
    871.2
   prolapse of intraocular tissue
    871.1
  due to burn 940.5
 fallopian tube 620.8
  due to pregnancy - see Pregnancy,
    tubal
  traumatic - see Injury, internal,
    fallopian tube
 fontanel 767.3
 free wall (ventricle) (see also Infarct,
    myocardium) 410.9●

Rupture, ruptured (Continued)
 gallbladder or duct (see also Disease,
    gallbladder) 575.4
  traumatic - see Injury, internal,
    gallbladder
 gastric (see also Rupture, stomach)
    537.89
  vessel 459.0
 globe (eye) (traumatic) - see Rupture,
    eye
 graafian follicle (hematoma) 620.0
 heart (auricle) (ventricle) (see also
    Infarct, myocardium) 410.9●
  infectional 422.90
  traumatic - see Rupture,
    myocardium, traumatic
 hymen 623.8
 internal
  organ, traumatic - see also Injury,
    internal, by site
   heart - see Rupture, myocardium,
    traumatic
   kidney - see Rupture, kidney
   liver - see Rupture, liver
   spleen - see Rupture, spleen,
    traumatic
  semilunar cartilage - see Tear,
    meniscus
 intervertebral disc - see Displacement,
    intervertebral disc
  traumatic (current) - see Dislocation,
    vertebra
 intestine 569.89
  traumatic - see Injury, internal,
    intestine
 intracranial, birth injury 767.0
 iris 364.76
  traumatic - see Rupture, eye
 joint capsule - see Sprain, by site
 kidney (traumatic) 866.03
  with open wound into cavity
    866.13
  due to birth injury 767.8
  nontraumatic 593.89
 lacrimal apparatus (traumatic) 870.2
 lens (traumatic) 366.20
 ligament - see also Sprain, by site
  with open wound - see Wound,
    open, by site
  old (see also Disorder, cartilage,
    articular) 718.0●
 liver (traumatic) 864.04
  with open wound into cavity
    864.14
  due to birth injury 767.8
  nontraumatic 573.8
 lymphatic (node) (vessel) 457.8
 marginal sinus (placental) (with
    hemorrhage) 641.2●
  affecting fetus or newborn 762.1
 meaning hernia - see Hernia
 membrana tympani (see also
    Perforation, tympanum) 384.20
  with otitis media - see Otitis media
  traumatic - see Wound, open, ear
 membranes (spontaneous)
  artificial
   delayed delivery following
    658.3●
    affecting fetus or newborn
    761.1
   fetus or newborn 761.1
  delayed delivery following 658.2●
   affecting fetus or newborn 761.1

◄ New   ◄▥ Revised   ~~deleted~~ Deleted   ● Use Additional Digit(s)   ▨ Omit code

Rupture, ruptured *(Continued)*
  membranes *(Continued)*
    premature (less than 24 hours prior
        to onset of labor) 658.1●
      affecting fetus or newborn 761.1
      delayed delivery following
          658.2●
        affecting fetus or newborn
            761.1
    meningeal artery *(see also* Hemorrhage,
        subarachnoid) 430
      late effect - *see* Late effect(s) (of)
          cerebrovascular disease
    meniscus (knee) - *see also* Tear,
        meniscus
      old *(see also* Derangement, meniscus)
          717.5
      site other than knee - *see* Disorder,
          cartilage, articular
      site other than knee - *see* Sprain, by
          site
    mesentery 568.89
      traumatic - *see* Injury, internal,
          mesentery
    mitral - *see* Insufficiency, mitral
    muscle (traumatic) NEC - *see also*
        Sprain, by site
      with open wound - *see* Wound,
          open, by site
      nontraumatic 728.83
    musculotendinous cuff (nontraumatic)
        (shoulder) 840.4
    mycotic aneurysm, causing cerebral
        hemorrhage *(see also*
        Hemorrhage, subarachnoid) 430
      late effect - *see* Late effect(s) (of)
          cerebrovascular disease
    myocardium, myocardial *(see also*
        Infarct, myocardium) 410.9●
      traumatic 861.03
        with open wound into thorax
            861.13
    nontraumatic (meaning hernia) *(see also*
        Hernia, by site) 553.9
      obstructed *(see also* Hernia, by site, with
          obstruction) 552.9
      gangrenous *(see also* Hernia, by site,
          with gangrene) 551.9
    operation wound *(see also* Dehiscence)
        998.32
      internal 998.31
    ovary, ovarian 620.8
      corpus luteum 620.1
      follicle (graafian) 620.0
    oviduct 620.8
      due to pregnancy - *see* Pregnancy,
          tubal
    pancreas 577.8
      traumatic - *see* Injury, internal,
          pancreas
    papillary muscle (ventricular) 429.6
    pelvic
      floor, complicating delivery
          664.1●
      organ NEC - *see* Injury, pelvic,
          organs
    penis (traumatic) - *see* Wound, open,
        penis
    perineum 624.8
      during delivery *(see also* Laceration,
          perineum, complicating
          delivery) 664.4●
    pharynx (nontraumatic) (spontaneous)
        478.29

Rupture, ruptured *(Continued)*
  pregnant uterus (before onset of labor)
      665.0●
  prostate (traumatic) - *see* Injury,
      internal, prostate
  pulmonary
    artery 417.8
    valve (heart) *(see also* Endocarditis,
        pulmonary) 424.3
    vein 417.8
    vessel 417.8
  pupil, sphincter 364.75
  pus tube *(see also* Salpingo-oophoritis)
      614.2
  pyosalpinx *(see also* Salpingo-
      oophoritis) 614.2
  rectum 569.49
    traumatic - *see* Injury, internal,
        rectum
  retina, retinal (traumatic) (without
      detachment) 361.30
    with detachment *(see also*
        Detachment, retina, with
        retinal defect) 361.00
  rotator cuff (capsule) (traumatic) 840.4
    nontraumatic, complete 727.61
  sclera 871.0
  semilunar cartilage, knee *(see also* Tear,
      meniscus) 836.2
    old *(see also* Derangement, meniscus)
        717.5
  septum (cardiac) 410.8●
  sigmoid 569.89
    traumatic - *see* Injury, internal, colon,
        sigmoid
  sinus of Valsalva 747.29
  spinal cord - *see also* Injury, spinal, by
      site
    due to injury at birth 767.4
    fetus or newborn 767.4
    syphilitic 094.89
    traumatic - *see also* Injury, spinal, by
        site
      with fracture - *see* Fracture,
          vertebra, by site, with
          spinal cord injury
  spleen 289.59
    congenital 767.8
    due to injury at birth 767.8
    malarial 084.9
    nontraumatic 289.59
    spontaneous 289.59
    traumatic 865.04
      with open wound into cavity
          865.14
  splenic vein 459.0
  stomach 537.89
    due to injury at birth 767.8
    traumatic - *see* Injury, internal,
        stomach
    ulcer - *see* Ulcer, stomach, with
        perforation
  synovium 727.50
    specified site NEC 727.59
  tendon (traumatic) - *see also* Sprain, by
      site
    with open wound - *see* Wound,
        open, by site
    Achilles 845.09
      nontraumatic 727.67
    ankle 845.09
      nontraumatic 727.68
    biceps (long bead) 840.8
      nontraumatic 727.62

Rupture, ruptured *(Continued)*
  tendon *(Continued)*
    foot 845.10
      interphalangeal (joint) 845.13
      metatarsophalangeal (joint)
          845.12
      nontraumatic 727.68
      specified site NEC 845.19
      tarsometatarsal (joint) 845.11
    hand 842.10
      carpometacarpal (joint) 842.11
      interphalangeal (joint) 842.13
      metacarpophalangeal (joint)
          842.12
      nontraumatic 727.63
        extensors 727.63
        flexors 727.64
      specified site NEC 842.19
    nontraumatic 727.60
      specified site NEC 727.69
    patellar 844.8
      nontraumatic 727.66
    quadriceps 844.8
      nontraumatic 727.65
    rotator cuff (capsule) 840.4
      nontraumatic, complete
          727.61
    wrist 842.00
      carpal (joint) 842.01
      nontraumatic 727.63
        extensors 727.63
        flexors 727.64
      radiocarpal (joint) (ligament)
          842.02
      radioulnar (joint), distal
          842.09
      specified site NEC 842.09
  testis (traumatic) 878.2
    complicated 878.3
    due to syphilis 095.8
  thoracic duct 457.8
  tonsil 474.8
  traumatic
    with open wound - *see* Wound,
        open, by site
    aorta - *see* Rupture, aorta, traumatic
    ear drum - *see* Wound, open, ear,
        drum
    external site - *see* Wound, open, by
        site
    eye 871.2
    globe (eye) - *see* Wound, open,
        eyeball
    internal organ (abdomen, chest, or
        pelvis) - *see also* Injury,
        internal, by site
      heart - *see* Rupture, myocardium,
          traumatic
      kidney - *see* Rupture, kidney
      liver - *see* Rupture, liver
      spleen - *see* Rupture, spleen,
          traumatic
    ligament, muscle, or tendon - *see also*
        Sprain, by site
      with open wound - *see* Wound,
          open, by site
    meaning hernia - *see* Hernia
  tricuspid (heart) (valve) - *see*
      Endocarditis, tricuspid
  tube, tubal 620.8
    abscess *(see also* Salpingo-oophoritis)
        614.2
    due to pregnancy - *see* Pregnancy,
        tubal

◀ New   ◀▥ Revised   ~~deleted~~ Deleted   ● Use Additional Digit(s)   ▨ Omit code   **533**

Rupture, ruptured (Continued)
 tympanum, tympanic (membrane) (see
  also Perforation, tympanum)
  384.20
  with otitis media - see Otitis media
  traumatic - see Wound, open, ear,
   drum
 umbilical cord 663.8●
  fetus or newborn 772.0
 ureter (traumatic) (see also Injury,
  internal, ureter) 867.2
  nontraumatic 593.89
 urethra 599.84
  with
   abortion - see Abortion, by type,
    with damage to pelvic
    organs
   ectopic pregnancy (see also
    categories 633.0–633.9)
    639.2
   molar pregnancy (see also
    categories 630–632)
    639.2
  following
   abortion 639.2
   ectopic or molar pregnancy
    639.2

Rupture, ruptured (Continued)
 urethra (Continued)
  obstetrical trauma 665.5●
  traumatic - see Injury, internal
   urethra
 uterosacral ligament 620.8
 uterus (traumatic) - see also Injury,
  internal uterus
  affecting fetus or newborn 763.89
  during labor 665.1●
  nonpuerperal, nontraumatic 621.8
  nontraumatic 621.8
  pregnant (during labor) 665.1●
   before labor 665.0●
 vagina 878.6
  complicated 878.7
  complicating delivery - see
   Laceration, vagina,
   complicating delivery
 valve, valvular (heart) - see
  Endocarditis
 varicose vein - see Varicose, vein
 varix - see Varix
 vena cava 459.0
 ventricle (free wall) (left) (see also
  Infarct, myocardium)
  410.9●

Rupture, ruptured (Continued)
 vesical (urinary) 596.6
  traumatic - see Injury, internal,
   bladder
 vessel (blood) 459.0
  pulmonary 417.8
 viscus 799.89
 vulva 878.4
  complicated 878.5
  complicating delivery 664.0●
Russell's dwarf (uterine dwarfism and
 craniofacial dysostosis) 759.89
Russell's dysentery 004.8
Russell (-Silver) syndrome (congenital
 hemihypertrophy and short stature)
 759.89
Russian spring-summer type
 encephalitis 063.0
Rust's disease (tuberculous spondylitis)
 015.0● [720.81]
Rustitskii's disease (multiple myeloma)
 (M9730/3) 203.0●
Ruysch's disease (Hirschsprung's
 disease) 751.3
Rytand-Lipsitch syndrome (complete
 atrioventricular block) 426.0

◄ New ◄▥ Revised ~~deleted~~ Deleted ● Use Additional Digit(s) ▨ Omit code

S

Saber
  shin 090.5
  tibia 090.5
Sac, lacrimal - *see* condition
Saccharomyces infection (*see also*
    Candidiasis) 112.9
Saccharopinuria 270.7
Saccular - *see* condition
Sacculation
  aorta (nonsyphilitic) (*see also*
      Aneurysm, aorta) 441.9
    ruptured 441.5
    syphilitic 093.0
  bladder 596.3
  colon 569.89
  intralaryngeal (congenital)
      (ventricular) 748.3
  larynx (congenital) (ventricular)
      748.3
  organ or site, congenital - *see*
      Distortion
  pregnant uterus, complicating delivery
      654.4●
    affecting fetus or newborn 763.1
    causing obstructed labor
        660.2●
      affecting fetus or newborn
          763.1
  rectosigmoid 569.89
  sigmoid 569.89
  ureter 593.89
  urethra 599.2
  vesical 596.3
Sachs (-Tay) disease (amaurotic familial
    idiocy) 330.1
Sacks-Libman disease 710.0 *[424.91]*
Sacralgia 724.6
Sacralization
  fifth lumbar vertebra 756.15
  incomplete (vertebra) 756.15
Sacrodynia 724.6
Sacroiliac joint - *see* condition
Sacroiliitis NEC 720.2
Sacrum - *see* condition
Saddle
  back 737.8
  embolus, aorta 444.0
  nose 738.0
    congenital 754.0
    due to syphilis 090.5
Sadism (sexual) 302.84
Saemisch's ulcer 370.04
Saenger's syndrome 379.46
Sago spleen 277.39
Sailors' skin 692.74
Saint
  Anthony's fire (*see also* Erysipelas)
      035
  Guy's dance - *see* Chorea
  Louis-type encephalitis 062.3
  triad (*see also* Hernia, diaphragm)
      553.3
  Vitus' dance - *see* Chorea
Salicylism
  correct substance properly
      administered 535.4●
  overdose or wrong substance given or
      taken 965.1
Salivary duct or gland - *see also* condition
  virus disease 078.5
Salivation (excessive) (*see also* Ptyalism)
    527.7

Salmonella (aertrycke) (choleraesuis)
    (enteritidis) (gallinarum)
    (suipestifer) (typhimurium) (*see also*
    Infection, Salmonella) 003.9
  arthritis 003.23
  carrier (suspected) of V02.3
  meningitis 003.21
  osteomyelitis 003.24
  pneumonia 003.22
  septicemia 003.1
  typhosa 002.0
    carrier (suspected) of V02.1
Salmonellosis 003.0
  with pneumonia 003.22
Salpingitis (catarrhal) (fallopian tube)
    (nodular) (pseudofollicular)
    (purulent) (septic) (*see also* Salpingo-
    oophoritis) 614.2
  ear 381.50
    acute 381.51
    chronic 381.52
  Eustachian (tube) 381.50
    acute 381.51
    chronic 381.52
  follicularis 614.1
  gonococcal (chronic) 098.37
    acute 098.17
  interstitial, chronic 614.1
  isthmica nodosa 614.1
  old - *see* Salpingo-oophoritis, chronic
  puerperal, postpartum, childbirth
      670.8 ◀▥
  specific (chronic) 098.37
    acute 098.17
  tuberculous (acute) (chronic) (*see also*
      Tuberculosis) 016.6●
  venereal (chronic) 098.37
    acute 098.17
Salpingocele 620.4
Salpingo-oophoritis (catarrhal) (purulent)
    (ruptured) (septic) (suppurative)
    614.2
  acute 614.0
    with
        abortion - *see* Abortion, by type,
            with sepsis
        ectopic pregnancy (*see also*
            categories 633.0–633.9)
            639.0
        molar pregnancy (*see also*
            categories 630–632) 639.0
    following
        abortion 639.0
        ectopic or molar pregnancy
            639.0
    gonococcal 098.17
    puerperal, postpartum, childbirth
        670.8 ◀▥
    tuberculous (*see also* Tuberculosis)
        016.6●
  chronic 614.1
    gonococcal 098.37
    tuberculous (*see also* Tuberculosis)
        016.6●
  complicating pregnancy 646.6●
    affecting fetus or newborn 760.8
  gonococcal (chronic) 098.37
    acute 098.17
  old - *see* Salpingo-oophoritis, chronic
  puerperal 670.8 ◀▥
  specific - *see* Salpingo-oophoritis,
      gonococcal
  subacute (*see also* Salpingo-oophoritis,
      acute) 614.0

Salpingo-oophoritis (*Continued*)
  tuberculous (acute) (chronic) (*see also*
      Tuberculosis) 016.6●
  venereal - *see* Salpingo-oophoritis,
      gonococcal
Salpingo-ovaritis (*see also* Salpingo-
    oophoritis) 614.2
Salpingoperitonitis (*see also* Salpingo-
    oophoritis) 614.2
Salt-losing
  nephritis (*see also* Disease, renal)
      593.9
  syndrome (*see also* Disease, renal)
      593.9
Salt-rheum (*see also* Eczema) 692.9
Salzmann's nodular dystrophy 371.46
Sampling
  chorionic villus V28.89
Sampson's cyst or tumor 617.1
Sandblasters'
  asthma 502
  lung 502
Sander's disease (paranoia) 297.1
Sandfly fever 066.0
Sandhoff's disease 330.1
Sanfilippo's syndrome
    (mucopolysaccharidosis III) 277.5
Sanger-Brown's ataxia 334.2
San Joaquin Valley fever 114.0
Sao Paulo fever or typhus 082.0
Saponification, mesenteric 567.89
Sapremia - *see* Septicemia
Sarcocele (benign)
  syphilitic 095.8
    congenital 090.5
Sarcoepiplocele (*see also* Hernia) 553.9
Sarcoepiplomphalocele (*see also* Hernia,
    umbilicus) 553.1
Sarcoid (any site) 135
  with lung involvement 135 *[517.8]*
  Boeck's 135
  Darier-Roussy 135
  Spiegler-Fendt 686.8
Sarcoidosis 135
  cardiac 135 *[425.8]*
  lung 135 *[517.8]*
Sarcoma (M8800/3) - *see also* Neoplasm,
    connective tissue, malignant
  alveolar soft part (M9581/3) - *see*
      Neoplasm, connective tissue,
      malignant
  ameloblastic (M9330/3) 170.1
    upper jaw (bone) 170.0
  botryoid (M8910/3) - *see* Neoplasm,
      connective tissue, malignant
  botryoides (M8910/3) - *see* Neoplasm,
      connective tissue, malignant
  cerebellar (M9480/3) 191.6
    circumscribed (arachnoidal)
        (M9471/3) 191.6
  circumscribed (arachnoidal) cerebellar
      (M9471/3) 191.6
  clear cell, of tendons and aponeuroses
      (M9044/3) - *see* Neoplasm,
      connective tissue, malignant
  embryonal (M8991/3) - *see* Neoplasm,
      connective tissue, malignant
  endometrial (stromal) (M8930/3) 182.0
    isthmus 182.1
  endothelial (M9130/3) - *see also*
      Neoplasm, connective tissue,
      malignant
    bone (M9260/3) - *see* Neoplasm,
        bone, malignant

Sarcoma (Continued)
  epithelioid cell (M8804/3) - see
      Neoplasm, connective tissue,
      malignant
  Ewing's (M9260/3) - see Neoplasm,
      bone, malignant
  follicular dendritic cell 202.9●
  germinoblastic (diffuse) (M9632/3)
      202.8●
      follicular (M9697/3) 202.0●
  giant cell (M8802/3) - see also
      Neoplasm, connective tissue,
      malignant
      bone (M9250/3) - see Neoplasm,
          bone, malignant
  glomoid (M8710/3) - see Neoplasm,
      connective tissue, malignant
  granulocytic (M9930/3) 205.3●
  hemangioendothelial (M9130/3) - see
      Neoplasm, connective tissue,
      malignant
  hemorrhagic, multiple (M9140/3) - see
      Kaposi's, sarcoma
  Hodgkin's (M9662/3) 201.2●
  immunoblastic (M9612/3) 200.8●
  interdigitating dendritic cell 202.9●
  Kaposi's (M9140/3) - see Kaposi's,
      sarcoma
  Kupffer cell (M9124/3) 155.0
  Langerhans cell 202.9●
  leptomeningeal (M9530/3) - see
      Neoplasm, meninges,
      malignant
  lymphangioendothelial (M9170/3) - see
      Neoplasm, connective tissue,
      malignant
  lymphoblastic (M9630/3) 200.1●
  lymphocytic (M9620/3) 200.1●
  mast cell (M9740/3) 202.6●
  melanotic (M8720/3) - see Melanoma
  meningeal (M9530/3) - see Neoplasm,
      meninges, malignant
  meningothelial (M9530/3) - see
      Neoplasm, meninges,
      malignant
  mesenchymal (M8800/3) - see also
      Neoplasm, connective tissue,
      malignant
      mixed (M8990/3) - see Neoplasm,
          connective tissue, malignant
  mesothelial (M9050/3) - see Neoplasm,
      by site, malignant
  monstrocellular (M9481/3)
      specified site - see Neoplasm, by site,
          malignant
      unspecified site 191.9
  myeloid (M9930/3) 205.3●
  neurogenic (M9540/3) - see Neoplasm,
      connective tissue, malignant
  odontogenic (M9270/3) 170.1
      upper jaw (bone) 170.0
  osteoblastic (M9180/3) - see Neoplasm,
      bone, malignant
  osteogenic (M9180/3) - see also
      Neoplasm, bone, malignant
      juxtacortical (M9190/3) - see
          Neoplasm, bone, malignant
      periosteal (M9190/3) - see
          Neoplasm, bone, malignant
  periosteal (M8812/3) - see also
      Neoplasm, bone, malignant
      osteogenic (M9190/3) - see
          Neoplasm, bone, malignant
  plasma cell (M9731/3) 203.8●

Sarcoma (Continued)
  pleomorphic cell (M8802/3) - see
      Neoplasm, connective tissue,
      malignant
  reticuloendothelial (M9720/3)
      202.3●
  reticulum cell (M9640/3) 200.0●
      nodular (M9642/3) 200.0●
      pleomorphic cell type (M9641/3)
          200.0●
  round cell (M8803/3) - see
      Neoplasm, connective
      tissue, malignant
  small cell (M8803/3) - see
      Neoplasm, connective
      tissue, malignant
  spindle cell (M8801/3) - see
      Neoplasm, connective
      tissue, malignant
  stromal (endometrial) (M8930/3)
      182.0
      isthmus 182.1
  synovial (M9040/3) - see also
      Neoplasm, connective tissue,
      malignant
      biphasic type (M9043/3) - see
          Neoplasm, connective tissue,
          malignant
      epithelioid cell type (M9042/3) - see
          Neoplasm, connective tissue,
          malignant
      spindle cell type (M9041/3) - see
          Neoplasm, connective tissue,
          malignant
Sarcomatosis
  meningeal (M9539/3) - see Neoplasm,
      meninges, malignant
  specified site NEC (M8800/3) - see
      Neoplasm, connective tissue,
      malignant
  unspecified site (M8800/6) 171.9
Sarcosinemia 270.8
Sarcosporidiosis 136.5
Satiety, early 780.94
Satisfactory smear but lacking
      transformation zone
  anal 796.77
  cervical 795.07
Saturnine - see condition
Saturnism 984.9
  specified type of lead - see Table of
      Drugs and Chemicals
Satyriasis 302.89
Sauriasis - see Ichthyosis
Sauriderma 757.39
Sauriosis - see Ichthyosis
Savill's disease (epidemic exfoliative
      dermatitis) 695.89
SBE (subacute bacterial endocarditis)
      421.0
Scabies (any site) 133.0
Scabs 782.8
Scaglietti-Dagnini syndrome
      (acromegalic macrospondylitis)
      253.0
Scald, scalded - see also Burn, by site
  skin syndrome 695.81
Scalenus anticus (anterior) syndrome
      353.0
Scales 782.8
Scalp - see condition
Scaphocephaly 756.0
Scaphoiditis, tarsal 732.5
Scapulalgia 733.90

Scapulohumeral myopathy 359.1
Scar, scarring (see also Cicatrix) 709.2
  adherent 709.2
  atrophic 709.2
  cervix
      in pregnancy or childbirth 654.6●
          affecting fetus or newborn
              763.89
          causing obstructed labor 660.2●
              affecting fetus or newborn
                  763.1
  cheloid 701.4
  chorioretinal 363.30
      disseminated 363.35
      macular 363.32
      peripheral 363.34
      posterior pole NEC 363.33
  choroid (see also Scar, chorioretinal)
      363.30
  compression, pericardial 423.9
  congenital 757.39
  conjunctiva 372.64
  cornea 371.00
      xerophthalmic 264.6
  due to previous cesarean delivery,
      complicating pregnancy or
      childbirth 654.2●
      affecting fetus or newborn 763.89
  duodenal (bulb) (cap) 537.3
  hypertrophic 701.4
  keloid 701.4
  labia 624.4
  lung (base) 518.89
  macula 363.32
      disseminated 363.35
      peripheral 363.34
  muscle 728.89
  myocardium, myocardial 412
  painful 709.2
  papillary muscle 429.81
  posterior pole NEC 363.33
      macular - see Scar, macula
  postnecrotic (hepatic) (liver) 571.9
  psychic V15.49
  retina (see also Scar, chorioretinal)
      363.30
  trachea 478.9
  uterus 621.8
      in pregnancy or childbirth NEC
          654.9●
          affecting fetus or newborn
              763.89
          from previous cesarean delivery
              654.2●
  vulva 624.4
Scarabiasis 134.1
Scarlatina 034.1
  anginosa 034.1
  maligna 034.1
  myocarditis, acute 034.1 [422.0]
      old (see also Myocarditis) 429.0
  otitis media 034.1 [382.02]
  ulcerosa 034.1
Scarlatinella 057.8
Scarlet fever (albuminuria) (angina)
      (convulsions) (lesions of lid) (rash)
      034.1
Schamberg's disease, dermatitis, or
      dermatosis (progressive pigmentary
      dermatosis) 709.09
Schatzki's ring (esophagus) (lower)
      (congenital) 750.3
  acquired 530.3
Schaufenster krankheit 413.9

◀ New   ◀‖‖ Revised   ~~deleted~~ Deleted   ● Use Additional Digit(s)   ▨ Omit code

Schaumann's
　　benign lymphogranulomatosis 135
　　disease (sarcoidosis) 135
　　syndrome (sarcoidosis) 135
Scheie's syndrome
　　　(mucopolysaccharidosis IS) 277.5
Schenck's disease (sporotrichosis) 117.1
Scheuermann's disease or
　　osteochondrosis 732.0
Scheuthauer-Marie-Sainton syndrome
　　　(cleidocranialis dysostosis) 755.59
Schilder (-Flatau) disease 341.1
Schilling-type monocytic leukemia
　　　(M9890/3) 206.9●
Schimmelbusch's disease, cystic mastitis,
　　or hyperplasia 610.1
Schirmer's syndrome
　　　(encephalocutaneous angiomatosis)
　　　759.6
Schistocelia 756.79
Schistoglossia 750.13
Schistosoma infestation - *see* Infestation,
　　Schistosoma
Schistosomiasis 120.9
　　Asiatic 120.2
　　bladder 120.0
　　chestermani 120.8
　　colon 120.1
　　cutaneous 120.3
　　due to
　　　S. hematobium 120.0
　　　S. japonicum 120.2
　　　S. mansoni 120.1
　　　S. mattheii 120.8
　　eastern 120.2
　　genitourinary tract 120.0
　　intestinal 120.1
　　lung 120.2
　　Manson's (intestinal) 120.1
　　Oriental 120.2
　　pulmonary 120.2
　　specified type NEC 120.8
　　vesical 120.0
Schizencephaly 742.4
Schizo-affective psychosis (*see also*
　　Schizophrenia) 295.7●
Schizodontia 520.2
Schizoid personality 301.20
　　introverted 301.21
　　schizotypal 301.22
Schizophrenia, schizophrenic (reaction)
　　295.9●

Note 66　Use the following fifth-digit
subclassification with category 295:

　0　unspecified
　1　subchronic
　2　chronic
　3　subchronic with acute
　　　exacerbation
　4　chronic with acute exacerbation
　5　in remission

acute (attack) NEC 295.8●
　　episode 295.4●
atypical form 295.8●
borderline 295.5●
catalepsy 295.2●
catatonic (type) (acute) (excited)
　　(withdrawn) 295.2●
childhood (type) (*see also* Psychosis,
　　childhood) 299.9●
chronic NEC 295.6●
coenesthesiopathic 295.8●

Schizophrenia, schizophrenic (*Continued*)
　　cyclic (type) 295.7●
　　disorganized (type) 295.1●
　　flexibilitas cerea 295.2●
　　hebephrenic (type) (acute) 295.1●
　　incipient 295.5●
　　latent 295.5●
　　paranoid (type) (acute) 295.3●
　　paraphrenic (acute) 295.3●
　　prepsychotic 295.5●
　　primary (acute) 295.0●
　　prodromal 295.5●
　　pseudoneurotic 295.5●
　　pseudopsychopathic 295.5●
　　reaction 295.9●
　　residual type (state) 295.6●
　　restzustand 295.6●
　　schizo-affective (type) (depressed)
　　　(excited) 295.7●
　　schizophreniform type 295.4●
　　simple (type) (acute) 295.0●
　　simplex (acute) 295.0●
　　specified type NEC 295.8●
　　syndrome of childhood NEC (*see also*
　　　Psychosis, childhood) 299.9●
　　undifferentiated type 295.9●
　　　acute 295.8●
　　　chronic 295.6●
Schizothymia 301.20
　　introverted 301.21
　　schizotypal 301.22
Schlafkrankheit 086.5
Schlatter's tibia (osteochondrosis) 732.4
Schlatter-Osgood disease
　　　(osteochondrosis, tibial tubercle)
　　　732.4
Schloffer's tumor (*see also* Peritonitis) 567.29
Schmidt's syndrome
　　sphallo-pharyngo-laryngeal
　　　hemiplegia 352.6
　　thyroid-adrenocortical insufficiency
　　　258.1
　　vagoaccessory 352.6
Schmincke
　　carcinoma (M8082/3) - *see* Neoplasm,
　　　nasopharynx, malignant
　　tumor (M8082/3) - *see* Neoplasm,
　　　nasopharynx, malignant
Schmitz (-Stutzer) dysentery 004.0
Schmorl's disease or nodes 722.30
　　lumbar, lumbosacral 722.32
　　specified region NEC 722.39
　　thoracic, thoracolumbar 722.31
Schneider's syndrome 047.9
Schnciderian
　　carcinoma (M8121/3)
　　　specified site - *see* Neoplasm, by site,
　　　　malignant
　　　unspecified site 160.0
　　papilloma (M8121/0)
　　　specified site - *see* Neoplasm, by site,
　　　　benign
　　　unspecified site 212.0
Schnitzler syndrome 273.1
Schoffer's tumor (*see also* Peritonitis) 567.29
Scholte's syndrome (malignant carcinoid)
　　259.2
Scholz's disease 330.0
Scholz (-Bielschowsky-Henneberg)
　　syndrome 330.0
Schönlein (-Henoch) disease (primary)
　　(purpura) (rheumatic) 287.0
School examination V70.3
　　following surgery V67.09　　◄

Schottmüller's disease (*see also* Fever,
　　paratyphoid) 002.9
Schroeder's syndrome (endocrine-
　　hypertensive) 255.3
Schüller-Christian disease or syndrome
　　　(chronic histiocytosis X) 277.89
Schultz's disease or syndrome
　　　(agranulocytosis) 288.09
Schultze's acroparesthesia, simple 443.89
Schwalbe-Ziehen-Oppenheimer disease
　　333.6
Schwannoma (M9560/0) - *see also*
　　Neoplasm, connective tissues,
　　benign
　　malignant (M9560/3) - *see* Neoplasm,
　　　connective tissue, malignant
Schwartz (-Jampel) syndrome 359.23
Schwartz-Bartter syndrome
　　　(inappropriate secretion of
　　　antidiuretic hormone) 253.6
Schweninger-Buzzi disease (macular
　　atrophy) 701.3
Sciatic - *see* condition
Sciatica (infectional) 724.3
　　due to
　　　displacement of intervertebral disc
　　　722.10
　　　herniation, nucleus pulposus 722.10
　　wallet 724.3
Scimitar syndrome (anomalous venous
　　drainage, right lung to inferior vena
　　cava) 747.49
Sclera - *see* condition
Sclerectasia 379.11
Scleredema
　　adultorum 710.1
　　Buschke's 710.1
　　newborn 778.1
Sclerema
　　adiposum (newborn) 778.1
　　adultorum 710.1
　　edematosum (newborn) 778.1
　　neonatorum 778.1
　　newborn 778.1
Scleriasis - *see* Scleroderma
Scleritis 379.00
　　with corneal involvement 379.05
　　anterior (annular) (localized) 379.03
　　brawny 379.06
　　granulomatous 379.09
　　posterior 379.07
　　specified NEC 379.09
　　suppurative 379.09
　　syphilitic 095.0
　　tuberculous (nodular) (*see also*
　　　Tuberculosis) 017.3● [*379.09*]
Sclerochoroiditis (*see also* Scleritis)
　　379.00
Scleroconjunctivitis (*see also* Scleritis)
　　379.00
Sclerocystic ovary (syndrome) 256.4
Sclerodactylia 701.0
Scleroderma, sclerodermia (acrosclerotic)
　　　(diffuse) (generalized) (progressive)
　　　(pulmonary) 710.1
　　circumscribed 701.0
　　linear 701.0
　　localized (linear) 701.0
　　newborn 778.1
Sclerokeratitis 379.05
　　meaning sclerosing keratitis 370.54
　　tuberculous (*see also* Tuberculosis)
　　　017.3● [*379.09*]
Scleroma, trachea 040.1

Scleromalacia
 multiple 731.0
 perforans 379.04
Scleromyxedema 701.8
Scleroperikeratitis 379.05
Sclerose en plaques 340
Sclerosis, sclerotic
 adrenal (gland) 255.8
 Alzheimer's 331.0
  with dementia - see Alzheimer's,
   dementia
 amyotrophic (lateral) 335.20
 annularis fibrosi
  aortic 424.1
  mitral 424.0
 aorta, aortic 440.0
  valve (see also Endocarditis, aortic)
   424.1
 artery, arterial, arteriolar,
   arteriovascular - see
   Arteriosclerosis
 ascending multiple 340
 Baló's (concentric) 341.1
 basilar - see Sclerosis, brain
 bone (localized) NEC 733.99
 brain (general) (lobular) 348.89   ◀▥
  Alzheimer's - see Alzheimer's,
   dementia
  artery, arterial 437.0
  atrophic lobar 331.0
   with dementia
    with behavioral disturbance
     331.0 [294.11]
    without behavioral
     disturbance 331.0
     [294.10]
  diffuse 341.1
   familial (chronic) (infantile) 330.0
   infantile (chronic) (familial) 330.0
   Pelizaeus-Merzbacher type 330.0
  disseminated 340
  hereditary 334.2
  hippocampal 348.81   ◀
  infantile (degenerative) (diffuse) 330.0
  insular 340
  Krabbe's 330.0
  mesial temporal 348.81   ◀
  miliary 340
  multiple 340
  Pelizaeus-Merzbacher 330.0
  progressive familial 330.0
  senile 437.0
  temporal 348.81   ◀
   mesial 348.81   ◀
  tuberous 759.5
 bulbar, progressive 340
 bundle of His 426.50
  left 426.3
  right 426.4
 cardiac - see Arteriosclerosis, coronary
 cardiorenal (see also Hypertension,
   cardiorenal) 404.90
 cardiovascular (see also Disease,
   cardiovascular) 429.2
  renal (see also Hypertension,
   cardiorenal) 404.90
 centrolobar, familial 330.0
 cerebellar - see Sclerosis, brain
 cerebral - see Sclerosis, brain
 cerebrospinal 340
  disseminated 340
  multiple 340
 cerebrovascular 437.0
 choroid 363.40
  diffuse 363.56

Sclerosis, sclerotic (Continued)
 combined (spinal cord) - see also
   Degeneration, combined
  multiple 340
 concentric, Baló's 341.1
 cornea 370.54
 coronary (artery) - see Arteriosclerosis,
   coronary
 corpus cavernosum
  female 624.8
  male 607.89
 Dewitzky's
  aortic 424.1
  mitral 424.0
 diffuse NEC 341.1
 disease, heart - see Arteriosclerosis,
   coronary
 disseminated 340
 dorsal 340
 dorsolateral (spinal cord) - see
   Degeneration, combined
 endometrium 621.8
 extrapyramidal 333.90
 eye, nuclear (senile) 366.16
 Friedreich's (spinal cord) 334.0
 funicular (spermatic cord) 608.89
 gastritis 535.4●
 general (vascular) - see Arteriosclerosis
 gland (lymphatic) 457.8
 hepatic 571.9
 hereditary
  cerebellar 334.2
  spinal 334.0
 hippocampal 348.81   ◀
 idiopathic cortical (Garre's) (see also
   Osteomyelitis) 730.1●
 ilium, piriform 733.5
 insular 340
  pancreas 251.8
 Islands of Langerhans 251.8
 kidney - see Sclerosis, renal
 larynx 478.79
 lateral 335.24
  amyotrophic 335.20
  descending 335.24
  primary 335.24
  spinal 335.24
 liver 571.9
 lobar, atrophic (of brain) 331.0
  with dementia
   with behavioral disturbance 331.0
    [294.11]
   without behavioral disturbance
    331.0 [294.10]
 lung (see also Fibrosis, lung) 515
 mastoid 383.1
 mesial temporal 348.81   ◀
 mitral - see Endocarditis, mitral
 Mönckeberg's (medial) (see also
   Arteriosclerosis, extremities)
   440.20
 multiple (brain stem) (cerebral)
   (generalized) (spinal cord) 340
 myocardium, myocardial - see
   Arteriosclerosis, coronary
 nuclear (senile), eye 366.16
 ovary 620.8
 pancreas 577.8
 penis 607.89
 peripheral arteries (see also
   Arteriosclerosis, extremities)
   440.20
 plaques 340
 pluriglandular 258.8
 polyglandular 258.8

Sclerosis, sclerotic (Continued)
 posterior (spinal cord) (syphilitic) 094.0
 posterolateral (spinal cord) - see
   Degeneration, combined
 prepuce 607.89
 primary lateral 335.24
 progressive systemic 710.1
 pulmonary (see also Fibrosis, lung) 515
  artery 416.0
  valve (heart) (see also Endocarditis,
   pulmonary) 424.3
 renal 587
  with
   cystine storage disease 270.0
   hypertension (see also
    Hypertension, kidney)
    403.90
   hypertensive heart disease
    (conditions classifiable to
    402) (see also Hypertension,
    cardiorenal) 404.90
   arteriolar (hyaline) (see also
    Hypertension, kidney) 403.90
   hyperplastic (see also
    Hypertension, kidney)
    403.90
 retina (senile) (vascular) 362.17
 rheumatic
  aortic valve 395.9
  mitral valve 394.9
 Schilder's 341.1
 senile - see Arteriosclerosis
 spinal (cord) (general) (progressive)
   (transverse) 336.8
  ascending 357.0
  combined - see also Degeneration,
   combined
   multiple 340
   syphilitic 094.89
  disseminated 340
  dorsolateral - see Degeneration,
   combined
  hereditary (Friedreich's) (mixed
   form) 334.0
  lateral (amyotrophic) 335.24
  multiple 340
  posterior (syphilitic) 094.0
 stomach 537.89
 subendocardial, congenital 425.3
 systemic (progressive) 710.1
  with lung involvement 710.1 [517.2]   ◀
 temporal 348.81   ◀
  mesial 348.81   ◀
 tricuspid (heart) (valve) - see
   Endocarditis, tricuspid
 tuberous (brain) 759.5
 tympanic membrane (see also
   Tympanosclerosis) 385.00
 valve, valvular (heart) - see
   Endocarditis
 vascular - see Arteriosclerosis
 vein 459.89
Sclerotenonitis 379.07
Sclerotitis (see also Scleritis) 379.00
 syphilitic 095.0
 tuberculous (see also Tuberculosis) 017.3
   ●[379.09]
Scoliosis (acquired) (postural) 737.30
 congenital 754.2
 due to or associated with
  Charcôt-Marie-Tooth disease 356.1
   [737.43]
  mucopolysaccharidosis 277.5
   [737.43]
  neurofibromatosis 237.71 [737.43]

◀ New   ◀▥ Revised   ~~deleted~~ Deleted   ● Use Additional Digit(s)   ▨ Omit code

Scoliosis *(Continued)*
  due to or associated with *(Continued)*
    osteitis
      deformans 731.0 *[737.43]*
      fibrosa cystica 252.01 *[737.43]*
    osteoporosis *(see also* Osteoporosis)
      733.00 *[737.43]*
    poliomyelitis 138 *[737.43]*
    radiation 737.33
    tuberculosis *(see also* Tuberculosis)
      015.0● *[737.43]*
  idiopathic 737.30
    infantile
      progressive 737.32
      resolving 737.31
  paralytic 737.39
  rachitic 268.1
  sciatic 724.3
  specified NEC 737.39
  thoracogenic 737.34
  tuberculous *(see also* Tuberculosis)
    015.0● *[737.43]*
Scoliotic pelvis 738.6
  with disproportion (fetopelvic) 653.0●
    affecting fetus or newborn 763.1
    causing obstructed labor 660.1●
      affecting fetus or newborn 763.1
Scorbutus, scorbutic 267
  anemia 281.8
Scotoma (ring) 368.44
  arcuate 368.43
  Bjerrum 368.43
  blind spot area 368.42
  central 368.41
  centrocecal 368.41
  paracecal 368.42
  paracentral 368.41
  scintillating 368.12
  Seidel 368.43
Scratch - *see* Injury, superficial, by site
Scratchy throat 784.99
Screening (for) V82.9
  alcoholism V79.1
  anemia, deficiency NEC V78.1
    iron V78.0
  anomaly, congenital V82.89
  antenatal, of mother V28.9
    alphafetoprotein levels, raised V28.1
    based on amniocentesis V28.2
      chromosomal anomalies V28.0
      raised alphafetoprotein levels
        V28.1
    fetal growth retardation using
      ultrasonics V28.4
    genomic V28.89
    isoimmunization V28.5
    malformations using ultrasonics
      V28.3
    proteomic V28.89
    raised alphafetoprotein levels V28.1
    risk
      pre-term labor V28.82
    specified condition NEC V28.89
    Streptococcus B V28.6
  arterial hypertension V81.1
  arthropod-borne viral disease NEC
    V73.5
  asymptomatic bacteriuria V81.5
  bacterial
    and spirochetal sexually transmitted
      diseases V74.5
    conjunctivitis V74.4
    disease V74.9
      sexually transmitted V74.5
      specified condition NEC V74.8

Screening *(Continued)*
  bacteriuria, asymptomatic V81.5
  blood disorder NEC V78.9
    specified type NEC V78.8
  bronchitis, chronic V81.3
  brucellosis V74.8
  cancer - *see* Screening, malignant
    neoplasm
  cardiovascular disease NEC V81.2
  cataract V80.2
  Chagas' disease V75.3
  chemical poisoning V82.5
  cholera V74.0
  cholesterol level V77.91
  chromosomal
    anomalies
      by amniocentesis, antenatal V28.0
      maternal postnatal V82.4
    athletes V70.3
  condition
    cardiovascular NEC V81.2
    eye NEC V80.2
    genitourinary NEC V81.6
    neurological NEC V80.09 ◀▥
    respiratory NEC V81.4
    skin V82.0
    specified NEC V82.89
  congenital
    anomaly V82.89
      eye V80.2
    dislocation of hip V82.3
    eye condition or disease V80.2
  conjunctivitis, bacterial V74.4
  contamination NEC *(see also* Poisoning)
    V82.5
  coronary artery disease V81.0
  cystic fibrosis V77.6
  deficiency anemia NEC V78.1
    iron V78.0
  dengue fever V73.5
  depression V79.0
  developmental handicap V79.9
    in early childhood V79.3
    specified type NEC V79.8
  diabetes mellitus V77.1
  diphtheria V74.3
  disease or disorder V82.9
    bacterial V74.9
      specified NEC V74.8
    blood V78.9
      specified type NEC V78.8
    blood-forming organ V78.9
      specified type NEC V78.8
    cardiovascular NEC V81.2
      hypertensive V81.1
      ischemic V81.0
    Chagas' V75.3
    chlamydial V73.98
      specified NEC V73.88
    ear NEC V80.3
    endocrine NEC V77.99
    eye NEC V80.2
    genitourinary NEC V81.6
    heart NEC V81.2
      hypertensive V81.1
      ischemic V81.0
    HPV (human papillomavirus)
      V73.81
    human papillomavirus (HPV)
      V73.81
    immunity NEC V77.99
    infectious NEC V75.9
    lipoid NEC V77.91
    mental V79.9
      specified type NEC V79.8

Screening *(Continued)*
  disease or disorder *(Continued)*
    metabolic NEC V77.99
      inborn NEC V77.7
    neurological NEC V80.09 ◀▥
    nutritional NEC V77.99
    rheumatic NEC V82.2
    rickettsial V75.0
    sexually transmitted V74.5
      bacterial V74.5
      spirochetal V74.5
    sickle-cell V78.2
      trait V78.2
    specified type NEC V82.89
    thyroid V77.0
    vascular NEC V81.2
      ischemic V81.0
    venereal V74.5
    viral V73.99
      arthropod-borne NEC V73.5
      specified type NEC V73.89
  dislocation of hip, congenital V82.3
  drugs in athletes V70.3
  elevated titer V82.9
  emphysema (chronic) V81.3
  encephalitis, viral (mosquito or tick
    borne) V73.5
  endocrine disorder NEC V77.99
  eye disorder NEC V80.2
    congenital V80.2
  fever
    dengue V73.5
    hemorrhagic V73.5
    yellow V73.4
  filariasis V75.6
  galactosemia V77.4
  genetic V82.79
    disease carrier status V82.71
  genitourinary condition NEC V81.6
  glaucoma V80.1
  gonorrhea V74.5
  gout V77.5
  Hansen's disease V74.2
  heart disease NEC V81.2
    hypertensive V81.1
    ischemic V81.0
  heavy metal poisoning V82.5
  helminthiasis, intestinal V75.7
  hematopoietic malignancy V76.89
  hemoglobinopathies NEC V78.3
  hemorrhagic fever V73.5
  Hodgkin's disease V76.89
  hormones in athletes V70.3
  HPV (human papillomavirus) V73.81
  human papillomavirus (HPV) V73.81
  hypercholesterolemia V77.91
  hyperlipidemia V77.91
  hypertension V81.1
  immunity disorder NEC V77.99
  inborn errors of metabolism NEC
    V77.7
  infection
    bacterial V74.9
      specified type NEC V74.8
    mycotic V75.4
    parasitic NEC V75.8
  infectious disease V75.9
    specified type NEC V75.8
  ingestion of radioactive substance
    V82.5
  intestinal helminthiasis V75.7
  iron deficiency anemia V78.0
  ischemic heart disease V81.0
  lead poisoning V82.5
  leishmaniasis V75.2

Screening *(Continued)*
  leprosy V74.2
  leptospirosis V74.8
  leukemia V76.89
  lipoid disorder NEC V77.91
  lymphoma V76.89
  malaria V75.1
  malignant neoplasm (of) V76.9
    bladder V76.3
    blood V76.89
    breast V76.10
      mammogram NEC V76.12
        for high-risk patient V76.11
      specified type NEC V76.19
    cervix V76.2
    colon V76.51
    colorectal V76.51
    hematopoietic system V76.89
    intestine V76.50
      colon V76.51
      small V76.52
    lung V76.0
    lymph (glands) V76.89
    nervous system V76.81
    oral cavity V76.42
    other specified neoplasm NEC
        V76.89
    ovary V76.46
    prostate V76.44
    rectum V76.41
    respiratory organs V76.0
    skin V76.43
    specified sites NEC V76.49
    testis V76.45
    vagina V76.47
      following hysterectomy for
          malignant condition
          V67.01
  malnutrition V77.2
  mammogram NEC V76.12
    for high-risk patient V76.11
  maternal postnatal chromosomal
      anomalies V82.4
  measles V73.2
  mental
    disorder V79.9
      specified type NEC V79.8
    retardation V79.2
  metabolic disorder NEC V77.99
  metabolic errors, inborn V77.7
  mucoviscidosis V77.6
  multiphasic V82.6
  mycosis V75.4
  mycotic infection V75.4
  nephropathy V81.5
  neurological condition NEC V80.09 ◄▥
  nutritional disorder NEC V77.99
  obesity V77.8
  osteoporosis V82.81
  parasitic infection NEC V75.8
  phenylketonuria V77.3
  plague V74.8
  poisoning
    chemical NEC V82.5
    contaminated water supply V82.5
    heavy metal V82.5
  poliomyelitis V73.0
  postnatal chromosomal anomalies,
      maternal V82.4
  prenatal - *see* Screening, antenatal
  pulmonary tuberculosis V74.1
  radiation exposure V82.5
  renal disease V81.5
  respiratory condition NEC V81.4

Screening *(Continued)*
  rheumatic disorder NEC V82.2
  rheumatoid arthritis V82.1
  rickettsial disease V75.0
  rubella V73.3
  schistosomiasis V75.5
  senile macular lesions of eye V80.2
  sexually transmitted diseases V74.5
    bacterial V74.5
    spirochetal V74.5
  sickle-cell anemia, disease, or trait
      V78.2
  skin condition V82.0
  sleeping sickness V75.3
  smallpox V73.1
  special V82.9
    specified condition NEC V82.89
  specified type NEC V82.89
  spirochetal disease V74.9
    sexually transmitted V74.5
    specified type NEC V74.8
  stimulants in athletes V70.3
  syphilis V74.5
  tetanus V74.8
  thyroid disorder V77.0
  trachoma V73.6
  traumatic brain injury V80.01 ◄
  trypanosomiasis V75.3
  tuberculosis, pulmonary V74.1
  venereal disease V74.5
  viral encephalitis
    mosquito-borne V73.5
    tick-borne V73.5
  whooping cough V74.8
  worms, intestinal V75.7
  yaws V74.6
  yellow fever V73.4
Scrofula *(see also* Tuberculosis) 017.2 ●
Scrofulide (primary) *(see also*
    Tuberculosis) 017.0 ●
Scrofuloderma, scrofulodermia
    (any site) (primary) *(see also*
    Tuberculosis) 017.0 ●
Scrofulosis (universal) *(see also*
    Tuberculosis) 017.2 ●
Scrofulosis lichen (primary) *(see also*
    Tuberculosis) 017.0 ●
Scrofulous - *see* condition
Scrotal tongue 529.5
  congenital 750.13
Scrotum - *see* condition
Scurvy (gum) (infantile) (rickets)
    (scorbutic) 267
Sea-blue histiocyte syndrome 272.7
Seabright-Bantam syndrome
    (pseudohypoparathyroidism) 275.49
Sealpox 059.12
Seasickness 994.6
Seatworm 127.4
Sebaceous
  cyst *(see also* Cyst, sebaceous)
      706.2
  gland disease NEC 706.9
Sebocystomatosis 706.2
Seborrhea, seborrheic 706.3
  adiposa 706.3
  capitis 690.11
  congestiva 695.4
  corporis 706.3
  dermatitis 690.10
    infantile 690.12
  diathesis in infants 695.89
  eczema 690.18
    infantile 690.12

Seborrhea, seborrheic *(Continued)*
  keratosis 702.19
    inflamed 702.11
  nigricans 759.89
  sicca 690.18
  wart 702.19
    inflamed 702.11
Seckel's syndrome 759.89
Seclusion pupil 364.74
Seclusiveness, child 313.22
Secondary - *see also* condition
  neoplasm - *see* Neoplasm, by site,
      malignant, secondary
Secretan's disease or syndrome
    (posttraumatic edema) 782.3
Secretion
  antidiuretic hormone, inappropriate
      (syndrome) 253.6
  catecholamine, by pheochromocytoma
      255.6
  hormone
    antidiuretic, inappropriate
        (syndrome) 253.6
    by
      carcinoid tumor 259.2
      pheochromocytoma 255.6
    ectopic NEC 259.3
  urinary
    excessive 788.42
    suppression 788.5
Section
  cesarean
    affecting fetus or newborn 763.4
    post mortem, affecting fetus or
        newborn 761.6
    previous, in pregnancy or childbirth
        654.2 ●
      affecting fetus or newborn 763.89
  nerve, traumatic - *see* Injury, nerve, by
      site
Seeligmann's syndrome (ichthyosis
    congenita) 757.1
Segmentation, incomplete (congenital) -
    see also Fusion
  bone NEC 756.9
  lumbosacral (joint) 756.15
  vertebra 756.15
    lumbosacral 756.15
Seizure(s) 780.39
  akinetic (idiopathic) *(see also* Epilepsy)
      345.0 ●
    psychomotor 345.4 ●
  apoplexy, apoplectic *(see also* Disease,
      cerebrovascular, acute) 436
  atonic *(see also* Epilepsy) 345.0 ●
  autonomic 300.11
  brain or cerebral *(see also* Disease,
      cerebrovascular, acute) 436
  convulsive *(see also* Convulsions)
      780.39
  cortical (focal) (motor) *(see also*
      Epilepsy) 345.5 ●
  disorder *(see also* Epilepsy) 345.9 ◄
  due to stroke 438.89
  epilepsy, epileptic (cryptogenic) *(see*
      also Epilepsy) 345.9 ●
  epileptiform, epileptoid 780.39
    focal *(see also* Epilepsy) 345.5 ●
  febrile (simple) 780.31
    with status epilepticus 345.3
    atypical 780.32
    complex 780.32
    complicated 780.32
  heart - *see* Disease, heart
  hysterical 300.11

Seizure(s) (Continued)
  Jacksonian (focal) (see also Epilepsy)
      345.5●
    motor type 345.5●
    sensory type 345.5●
  migraine triggered 346.0●
  newborn 779.0
  paralysis (see also Disease,
      cerebrovascular, acute) 436
  recurrent 345.9●
    epileptic - see Epilepsy
  repetitive 780.39
    epileptic - see Epilepsy
  salaam (see also Epilepsy) 345.6●
  uncinate (see also Epilepsy) 345.4●
Self-mutilation 300.9
Semicoma 780.09
Semiconsciousness 780.09
Seminal
  vesicle - see condition
  vesiculitis (see also Vesiculitis) 608.0
Seminoma (M9061/3)
  anaplastic type (M9062/3)
    specified site - see Neoplasm, by site,
        malignant
    unspecified site 186.9
  specified site - see Neoplasm, by site,
      malignant
  spermatocytic (M9063/3)
    specified site - see Neoplasm, by site,
        malignant
    unspecified site 186.9
  unspecified site 186.9
Semliki Forest encephalitis 062.8
Senear-Usher disease or syndrome
    (pemphigus erythematosus)
    694.4
Senecio jacobae dermatitis 692.6
Senectus 797
Senescence 797
Senile (see also condition) 797
  cervix (atrophic) 622.8
  degenerative atrophy, skin 701.3
  endometrium (atrophic) 621.8
  fallopian tube (atrophic) 620.3
  heart (failure) 797
  lung 492.8
  ovary (atrophic) 620.3
  syndrome 259.8
  vagina, vaginitis (atrophic) 627.3
  wart 702.0
Senility 797
  with
    acute confusional state 290.3
    delirium 290.3
    mental changes 290.9
    psychosis NEC (see also Psychosis,
        senile) 290.20
  premature (syndrome) 259.8
Sensation
  burning (see also Disturbance,
      sensation) 782.0
    tongue 529.6
  choking 784.99
  loss of (see also Disturbance, sensation)
      782.0
  prickling (see also Disturbance,
      sensation) 782.0
  tingling (see also Disturbance,
      sensation) 782.0
Sense loss (touch) (see also Disturbance,
      sensation) 782.0
  smell 781.1
  taste 781.1

Sensibility disturbance NEC (cortical)
    (deep) (vibratory) (see also
    Disturbance, sensation) 782.0
Sensitive dentine 521.89
Sensitiver Beziehungswahn 297.8
Sensitivity, sensitization - see also
    Allergy
  autoerythrocyte 287.2
  carotid sinus 337.01
  child (excessive) 313.21
  cold, autoimmune 283.0
  methemoglobin 289.7
  suxamethonium 289.89
  tuberculin, without clinical or
      radiological symptoms 795.5
Sensory
  extinction 781.8
  neglect 781.8
Separation
  acromioclavicular - see Dislocation,
      acromioclavicular
  anxiety, abnormal 309.21
  apophysis, traumatic - see Fracture, by
      site
  choroid 363.70
    hemorrhagic 363.72
    serous 363.71
  costochondral (simple) (traumatic) - see
      Dislocation, costochondral
  delayed
    umbilical cord 779.83
  epiphysis, epiphyseal
    nontraumatic 732.9
      upper femoral 732.2
    traumatic - see Fracture, by site
  fracture - see Fracture, by site
  infundibulum cardiac from right
      ventricle by a partition 746.83
  joint (current) (traumatic) - see
      Dislocation, by site
  placenta (normally implanted) - see
      Placenta, separation
  pubic bone, obstetrical trauma
      665.6●
  retina, retinal (see also Detachment,
      retina) 361.9
    layers 362.40
      sensory (see also Retinoschisis)
          361.10
      pigment epithelium (exudative)
          362.42
        hemorrhagic 362.43
  sternoclavicular (traumatic) - see
      Dislocation, sternoclavicular
  symphysis pubis, obstetrical trauma
      665.6●
  tracheal ring, incomplete (congenital)
      748.3
Sepsis (generalized) 995.91
  with
    abortion - see Abortion, by type,
        with sepsis
    acute organ dysfunction 995.92
    ectopic pregnancy (see also
        categories 633.0–633.9) 639.0
    molar pregnancy (see also categories
        630–632) 639.0
    multiple organ dysfunction (MOD)
        995.92
  buccal 528.3
  complicating labor 659.3●
  dental (pulpal origin) 522.4
  female genital organ NEC 614.9
  fetus (intrauterine) 771.81

Sepsis (Continued)
  following
    abortion 639.0
    ectopic or molar pregnancy 639.0
    infusion, perfusion, or transfusion
        999.39
  Friedländer's 038.49
  intraocular 360.00
  localized
    in operation wound 998.59
    skin (see also Abscess) 682.9
  malleus 024
  nadir 038.9
  newborn (organism unspecified) NEC
      771.81
  oral 528.3
  puerperal, postpartum, childbirth
      (pelvic) 670.2   ◀▥
  resulting from infusion, injection,
      transfusion, or vaccination
      999.39
  severe 995.92
  skin, localized (see also Abscess) 682.9
  umbilical (newborn) (organism
      unspecified) 771.89
    tetanus 771.3
  urinary 599.0
    meaning sepsis 995.91
    meaning urinary tract infection
        599.0
Septate - see also Septum
Septic - see also condition
  adenoids 474.01
    and tonsils 474.02
  arm (with lymphangitis) 682.3
  embolus - see Embolism
  finger (with lymphangitis) 681.00
  foot (with lymphangitis) 682.7
  gallbladder (see also Cholecystitis)
      575.8
  hand (with lymphangitis) 682.4
  joint (see also Arthritis, septic) 711.0●
  kidney (see also Infection, kidney)
      590.9
  leg (with lymphangitis) 682.6
  mouth 528.3
  nail 681.9
    finger 681.02
    toe 681.11
  shock (endotoxic) 785.52
  sore (see also Abscess) 682.9
    throat 034.0
      milk-borne 034.0
      streptococcal 034.0
  spleen (acute) 289.59
  teeth (pulpal origin) 522.4
  throat 034.0
  thrombus - see Thrombosis
  toe (with lymphangitis) 681.10
  tonsils 474.00
    and adenoids 474.02
  umbilical cord (newborn) (organism
      unspecified) 771.89
  uterus (see also Endometritis) 615.9
Septicemia, septicemic (generalized)
    (suppurative) 038.9
  with
    abortion - see Abortion, by type,
        with sepsis
    ectopic pregnancy (see also
        categories 633.0–633.9) 639.0
    molar pregnancy (see also categories
        630–632) 639.0
  Aerobacter aerogenes 038.49

Septicemia, septicemic (Continued)
 anaerobic 038.3
 anthrax 022.3
 Bacillus coli 038.42
 Bacteroides 038.3
 Clostridium 038.3
 complicating labor 659.3●
 cryptogenic 038.9
 enteric gram-negative bacilli
  038.40
 Enterobacter aerogenes 038.49
 Erysipelothrix (insidiosa)
  (rhusiopathiae) 027.1
 Escherichia coli 038.42
 following
  abortion 639.0
  ectopic or molar pregnancy
   639.0
  infusion, injection, transfusion, or
   vaccination 999.39
 Friedländer's (bacillus) 038.49
 gangrenous 038.9
 gonococcal 098.89
 gram-negative (organism)
  038.40
  anaerobic 038.3
 Hemophilus influenzae 038.41
 herpes (simplex) 054.5
 herpetic 054.5
 Listeria monocytogenes 027.0
 meningeal - see Meningitis
 meningococcal (chronic) (fulminating)
  036.2
 methicillin
  resistant Staphylococcus aureus
   (MRSA) 038.12
  susceptible Staphylococcus aureus
   (MSSA) 038.11
 MRSA (methicillin resistant
  Staphylococcus aureus)
  038.12
 MSSA (methicillin susceptible
  Staphylococcus aureus) 038.11
 navel, newborn (organism unspecified)
  771.89
 newborn (organism unspecified)
  771.81
 plague 020.2
 pneumococcal 038.2
 postabortal 639.0
 postoperative 998.59
 Proteus vulgaris 038.49
 Pseudomonas (aeruginosa) 038.43
 puerperal, postpartum 670.2 ◀▥
 Salmonella (aertrycke) (callinarum)
  (choleraesuis) (enteritidis)
  (suipestifer) 003.1
 Serratia 038.44
 Shigella (see also Dysentery, bacillary)
  004.9
 specified organism NEC 038.8
 staphylococcal 038.10
  aureus 038.11
   methicillin
    resistant (MRSA) 038.12
    susceptible (MSSA) 038.11
  specified organism NEC 038.19
 streptococcal (anaerobic) 038.0
 Streptococcus pneumoniae 038.2
 suipestifer 003.1
 umbilicus, newborn (organism
  unspecified) 771.89
 viral 079.99
 Yersinia enterocolitica 038.49

Septum, septate (congenital) - see also
  Anomaly, specified type NEC
 anal 751.2
 aqueduct of Sylvius 742.3
  with spina bifida (see also Spina
   bifida) 741.0●
 hymen 752.49
 uterus (see also Double, uterus)
  752.2
 vagina 752.49
  in pregnancy or childbirth
   654.7●
   affecting fetus or newborn 763.89
   causing obstructed labor
    660.2●
     affecting fetus or newborn
      763.1
Sequestration
 lung (congenital) (extralobar)
  (intralobar) 748.5
 orbit 376.10
 pulmonary artery (congenital)
  747.3
 splenic 289.52
Sequestrum
 bone (see also Osteomyelitis)
  730.1●
 jaw 526.4
 dental 525.8
 jaw bone 526.4
 sinus (accessory) (nasal) (see also
  Sinusitis) 473.9
  maxillary 473.0
Sequoiosis asthma 495.8
Serology for syphilis
 doubtful
  with signs or symptoms - see
   Syphilis, by site and stage
  follow-up of latent syphilis - see
   Syphilis, latent
 false positive 795.6
 negative, with signs or symptoms - see
   Syphilis, by site and stage
 positive 097.1
  with signs or symptoms - see
   Syphilis, by site and stage
  false 795.6
  follow-up of latent syphilis - see
   Syphilis, latent
  only finding - see Syphilis, latent
 reactivated 097.1
Seroma - (postoperative) (non-infected)
  998.13
 infected 998.51
 post-traumatic 729.91
Seropurulent - see condition
Serositis, multiple 569.89
 pericardial 423.2
 peritoneal 568.82
 pleural - see Pleurisy
Serotonin syndrome 333.99
Serous - see condition
Sertoli cell
 adenoma (M8640/0)
  specified site - see Neoplasm, by site,
   benign
  unspecified site
   female 220
   male 222.0
 carcinoma (M8640/3)
  specified site - see Neoplasm, by site,
   malignant
  unspecified site 186.9
 syndrome (germinal aplasia) 606.0

Sertoli cell (Continued)
 tumor (M8640/0)
  with lipid storage (M8641/0)
   specified site - see Neoplasm, by
    site, benign
   unspecified site
    female 220
    male 222.0
  specified site - see Neoplasm, by site,
   benign
  unspecified site
   female 220
   male 222.0
Sertoli-Leydig cell tumor (M8631/0)
 specified site - see Neoplasm, by site,
  benign
 unspecified site
  female 220
  male 222.0
Serum
 allergy, allergic reaction 999.5
  shock 999.4
 arthritis 999.5 [713.6]
 complication or reaction NEC 999.5
 disease NEC 999.5
 hepatitis 070.3●
 intoxication 999.5
 jaundice (homologous) - see Hepatitis,
  viral, type B
 neuritis 999.5
 poisoning NEC 999.5
 rash NEC 999.5
 reaction NEC 999.5
 sickness NEC 999.5
Sesamoiditis 733.99
Seven-day fever 061
 of
  Japan 100.89
  Queensland 100.89
Sever's disease or osteochondrosis
  (calcaneum) 732.5
Sex chromosome mosaics 758.81
Sex reassignment surgery status (see also
  Trans-sexualism) 302.50   ◀▥
Sextuplet
 affected by maternal complication of
  pregnancy 761.5
 healthy liveborn - see Newborn,
  multiple
 pregnancy (complicating delivery)
  NEC 651.8●
  with fetal loss and retention of one
   or more fetus(es) 651.6●
  following (elective) fetal reduction
   651.7●
Sexual
 anesthesia 302.72
 deviation (see also Deviation, sexual)
  302.9
 disorder (see also Deviation, sexual)
  302.9
 frigidity (female) 302.72
 function, disorder of (psychogenic)
  302.70
  specified type NEC 302.79
 immaturity (female) (male) 259.0
 impotence 607.84
  organic origin NEC 607.84
  psychogenic 302.72
 precocity (constitutional) (cryptogenic)
  (female) (idiopathic) (male) NEC
  259.1
  with adrenal hyperplasia 255.2
 sadism 302.84

◀ New   ◀▥ Revised   d̶e̶l̶e̶t̶e̶d̶ Deleted   ● Use Additional Digit(s)   ▨ Omit code

Sexuality, pathological (*see also* Deviation, sexual) 302.9
Sézary's disease, reticulosis, or syndrome (M9701/3) 202.2●
Shadow, lung 793.1
Shaken infant syndrome 995.55
Shaking
    head (tremor) 781.0
    palsy or paralysis (*see also* Parkinsonism) 332.0
Shallowness, acetabulum 736.39
Shaver's disease or syndrome (bauxite pneumoconiosis) 503
Shearing
    artificial skin graft 996.55
    decellularized allodermis graft 996.55
Sheath (tendon) - *see* condition
Shedding
    nail 703.8
    teeth, premature, primary (deciduous) 520.6
Sheehan's disease or syndrome (postpartum pituitary necrosis) 253.2
Shelf, rectal 569.49
Shell
    shock (current) (*see also* Reaction, stress, acute) 308.9
        lasting state 300.16
    teeth 520.5
Shield kidney 753.3
Shift, mediastinal 793.2
Shifting
    pacemaker 427.89
    sleep-work schedule (affecting sleep) 327.36
Shiga's
    bacillus 004.0
    dysentery 004.0
Shigella (dysentery) (*see also* Dysentery, bacillary) 004.9
    carrier (suspected) of V02.3
Shigellosis (*see also* Dysentery, bacillary) 004.9
Shingles (*see also* Herpes, zoster) 053.9
    eye NEC 053.29
Shin splints 844.9
Shipyard eye or disease 077.1
Shirodkar suture, in pregnancy 654.5●
Shock 785.50
    with
        abortion - *see* Abortion, by type, with shock
        ectopic pregnancy (*see also* categories 633.0–633.9) 639.5
        molar pregnancy (*see also* categories 630–632) 639.5
    allergic - *see* Shock, anaphylactic
    anaclitic 309.21
    anaphylactic 995.0
        chemical - *see* Table of Drugs and Chemicals
        correct medicinal substance properly administered 995.0
        drug or medicinal substance
            correct substance properly administered 995.0
            overdose or wrong substance given or taken 977.9
            specified drug - *see* Table of Drugs and Chemicals
        following sting(s) 989.5

Shock (*Continued*)
    anaphylactic (*Continued*)
        food - *see* Anaphylactic shock, due to, food
        immunization 999.4
        serum 999.4
    anaphylactoid - *see* Shock, anaphylactic
    anesthetic
        correct substance properly administered 995.4
        overdose or wrong substance given 968.4
            specified anesthetic - *see* Table of Drugs and Chemicals
    birth, fetus or newborn NEC 779.89
    cardiogenic 785.51
    chemical substance - *see* Table of Drugs and Chemicals
    circulatory 785.59
    complicating
        abortion - *see* Abortion, by type, with shock
        ectopic pregnancy - (*see also* categories 633.0–633.9) 639.5
        labor and delivery 669.1●
        molar pregnancy (*see also* categories 630–632) 639.5
    culture 309.29
    due to
        drug 995.0
            correct substance properly administered 995.0
            overdose or wrong substance given or taken 977.9
            specified drug - *see* Table of Drugs and Chemicals
        food - *see* Anaphylactic shock, due to, food
    during labor and delivery 669.1●
    electric 994.8
        from electroshock gun (taser) 994.8
    endotoxic 785.52
        due to surgical procedure 998.0
    following
        abortion 639.5
        ectopic or molar pregnancy 639.5
        injury (immediate) (delayed) 958.4
        labor and delivery 669.1●
    gram-negative 785.52
    hematogenic 785.59
    hemorrhagic
        due to
            disease 785.59
            surgery (intraoperative) (postoperative) 998.0
            trauma 958.4
    hypovolemic NEC 785.59
        surgical 998.0
        traumatic 958.4
    insulin 251.0
        therapeutic misadventure 962.3
    kidney 584.5
        traumatic (following crushing) 958.5
    lightning 994.0
    lung 518.5
    nervous (*see also* Reaction, stress, acute) 308.9

Shock (*Continued*)
    obstetric 669.1●
        with
            abortion - *see* Abortion, by type, with shock
            ectopic pregnancy (*see also* categories 633.0–633.9) 639.5
            molar pregnancy (*see also* categories 630–632) 639.5
        following
            abortion 639.5
            ectopic or molar pregnancy 639.5
    paralysis, paralytic (*see also* Disease, cerebrovascular, acute) 436
        late effect - *see* Late effect(s) (of) cerebrovascular disease
    pleural (surgical) 998.0
        due to trauma 958.4
    postoperative 998.0
        with
            abortion - *see* Abortion, by type, with shock
            ectopic pregnancy (*see also* categories 633.0–633.9) 639.5
            molar pregnancy (*see also* categories 630–632) 639.5
        following
            abortion 639.5
            ectopic or molar pregnancy 639.5
    psychic (*see also* Reaction, stress, acute) 308.9
        past history (of) V15.49
    psychogenic (*see also* Reaction, stress, acute) 308.9
    septic 785.52
        with
            abortion - *see* Abortion, by type, with shock
            ectopic pregnancy (*see also* categories 633.0–633.9) 639.5
            molar pregnancy (*see also* categories 630–632) 639.5
        due to
            surgical procedure 998.0
            transfusion NEC 999.89 ◀▥
                bone marrow 996.85
        following
            abortion 639.5
            ectopic or molar pregnancy 639.5
            surgical procedure 998.0
            transfusion NEC 999.89 ◀▥
                bone marrow 996.85
    spinal - *see also* Injury, spinal, by site
        with spinal bone injury - *see* Fracture, vertebra, by site, with spinal cord injury
    surgical 998.0
    therapeutic misadventure NEC (*see also* Complications) 998.89
    thyroxin 962.7
    toxic 040.82
    transfusion - *see* Complications, transfusion
    traumatic (immediate) (delayed) 958.4
Shoemakers' chest 738.3
Short, shortening, shortness
    Achilles tendon (acquired) 727.81
    arm 736.89
        congenital 755.20
    back 737.9
    bowel syndrome 579.3
    breath 786.05

Short, shortening, shortness (Continued)
  cervical, cervix 649.7●
    gravid uterus 649.7●
    non-gravid uterus 622.5
      acquired 622.5
      congenital 752.49
  chain acyl CoA dehydrogenase
      deficiency (SCAD) 277.85
  common bile duct, congenital 751.69
  cord (umbilical) 663.4●
    affecting fetus or newborn 762.6
  cystic duct, congenital 751.69
  esophagus (congenital) 750.4
  femur (acquired) 736.81
    congenital 755.34
  frenulum linguae 750.0
  frenum, lingual 750.0
  hamstrings 727.81
  hip (acquired) 736.39
    congenital 755.63
  leg (acquired) 736.81
    congenital 755.30
  metatarsus (congenital) 754.79
    acquired 736.79
  organ or site, congenital NEC - see
      Distortion
  palate (congenital) 750.26
  P-R interval syndrome 426.81
  radius (acquired) 736.09
    congenital 755.26
  round ligament 629.89
  sleeper 307.49
  stature, constitutional (hereditary)
      (idiopathic) 783.43
  tendon 727.81
    Achilles (acquired) 727.81
      congenital 754.79
    congenital 756.89
  thigh (acquired) 736.81
    congenital 755.34
  tibialis anticus 727.81
  umbilical cord 663.4●
    affecting fetus or newborn 762.6
  urethra 599.84
  uvula (congenital) 750.26
  vagina 623.8
Shortsightedness 367.1
Shoshin (acute fulminating beriberi) 265.0
Shoulder - see condition
Shovel-shaped incisors 520.2
Shower, thromboembolic - see Embolism
Shunt (status)
  aortocoronary bypass V45.81
  arterial-venous (dialysis) V45.11
  arteriovenous, pulmonary (acquired)
      417.0
    congenital 747.3
    traumatic (complication) 901.40
  cerebral ventricle (communicating) in
      situ V45.2
  coronary artery bypass V45.81
  surgical, prosthetic, with
      complications - see
      Complications, shunt
  vascular NEC V45.89
Shutdown
  renal 586
    with
      abortion - see Abortion, by type,
          with renal failure
      ectopic pregnancy (see also
          categories 633.0–633.9) 639.3
      molar pregnancy (see also
          categories 630–632) 639.3

Shutdown (Continued)
  complicating
    abortion 639.3
    ectopic or molar pregnancy 639.3
    following labor and delivery 669.3●
Shwachman's syndrome 288.02
Shy-Drager syndrome (orthostatic
    hypotension with multisystem
    degeneration) 333.0
Sialadenitis (any gland) (chronic)
    (supportive) 527.2
  epidemic - see Mumps
Sialadenosis, periodic 527.2
Sialaporia 527.7
Sialectasia 527.8
Sialitis 527.2
Sialoadenitis (see also Sialadenitis) 527.2
Sialoangitis 527.2
Sialodochitis (fibrinosa) 527.2
Sialodocholithiasis 527.5
Sialolithiasis 527.5
Sialorrhea (see also Ptyalism) 527.7
  periodic 527.2
Sialosis 527.8
  rheumatic 710.2
Siamese twin 759.4
  complicating pregnancy 678.1●
Sicard's syndrome 352.6
Sicca syndrome (keratoconjunctivitis)
    710.2
Sick 799.9
  cilia syndrome 759.89
  or handicapped person in family
      V61.49
Sickle-cell
  anemia (see also Disease, sickle-cell)
      282.60
  disease (see also Disease, sickle-cell)
      282.60
  hemoglobin
    C disease (without crisis) 282.63
      with
        crisis 282.64
        vaso-occlusive pain 282.64
    D disease (without crisis) 282.68
      with crisis 282.69
    E disease (without crisis) 282.68
      with crisis 282.69
  thalassemia (without crisis) 282.41
    with
      crisis 282.42
      vaso-occlusive pain 282.42
  trait 282.5
Sicklemia (see also Disease, sickle-cell)
    282.60
  trait 282.5
Sickness
  air (travel) 994.6
  airplane 994.6
  alpine 993.2
  altitude 993.2
  Andes 993.2
  aviators' 993.2
  balloon 993.2
  car 994.6
  compressed air 993.3
  decompression 993.3
  green 280.9
  harvest 100.89
  milk 988.8
  morning 643.0●
  motion 994.6
  mountain 993.2
    acute 289.0

Sickness (Continued)
  protein (see also Complications,
      vaccination) 999.5
  radiation NEC 990
  roundabout (motion) 994.6
  sea 994.6
  serum NEC 999.5
  sleeping (African) 086.5
    by Trypanosoma 086.5
      gambiense 086.3
      rhodesiense 086.4
    Gambian 086.3
    late effect 139.8
    Rhodesian 086.4
  sweating 078.2
  swing (motion) 994.6
  train (railway) (travel) 994.6
  travel (any vehicle) 994.6
Sick sinus syndrome 427.81
Sideropenia (see also Anemia, iron
    deficiency) 280.9
Siderosis (lung) (occupational) 503
  cornea 371.15
  eye (bulbi) (vitreous) 360.23
  lens 360.23
Siegal-Cattan-Mamou disease (periodic)
    277.31
Siemens' syndrome
  ectodermal dysplasia 757.31
  keratosis follicularis spinulosa
      (decalvans) 757.39
Sighing respiration 786.7
Sigmoid
  flexure - see condition
  kidney 753.3
Sigmoiditis - see Enteritis
Silfverskiöld's syndrome 756.50
Silicosis, silicotic (complicated)
    (occupational) (simple) 502
  fibrosis, lung (confluent) (massive)
      (occupational) 502
  non-nodular 503
  pulmonum 502
Silicotuberculosis (see also Tuberculosis)
    011.4●
Silo fillers' disease 506.9
Silver's syndrome (congenital
    hemihypertrophy and short
    stature) 759.89
Silver wire arteries, retina 362.13
Silvestroni-Bianco syndrome
    (thalassemia minima) 282.49
Simian crease 757.2
Simmonds' cachexia or disease
    (pituitary cachexia) 253.2
Simons' disease or syndrome
    (progressive lipodystrophy)
    272.6
Simple, simplex - see condition
Sinding-Larsen disease (juvenile
    osteopathia patellae) 732.4
Singapore hemorrhagic fever 065.4
Singers' node or nodule 478.5
Single
  atrium 745.69
  coronary artery 746.85
  umbilical artery 747.5
  ventricle 745.3
Singultus 786.8
  epidemicus 078.89
Sinus - see also Fistula
  abdominal 569.81
  arrest 426.6
  arrhythmia 427.89

◀ New   ◀|||| Revised   ~~deleted~~ Deleted   ● Use Additional Digit(s)   ▨ Omit code

Sinus (Continued)
  bradycardia 427.89
    chronic 427.81
  branchial cleft (external) (internal)
    744.41
  coccygeal (infected) 685.1
    with abscess 685.0
  dental 522.7
  dermal (congenital) 685.1
    with abscess 685.0
  draining - see Fistula
  infected, skin NEC 686.9
  marginal, rupture or bleeding
    641.2●
    affecting fetus or newborn
      762.1
  pause 426.6
  pericranii 742.0
  pilonidal (infected) (rectum) 685.1
    with abscess 685.0
  preauricular 744.46
  rectovaginal 619.1
  sacrococcygeal (dermoid) (infected)
    685.1
    with abscess 685.0
  skin
    infected NEC 686.9
    noninfected- see Ulcer, skin
  tachycardia 427.89
  tarsi syndrome 726.79
  testis 608.89
  tract (postinfectional) - see Fistula
  urachus 753.7
Sinuses, Rokitansky-Aschoff (see also
    Disease, gallbladder) 575.8
Sinusitis (accessory) (chronic)
    (hyperplastic) (nasal)
    (nonpurulent) (purulent)
    473.9
  with influenza, flu, or grippe
    487.1
  acute 461.9
    ethmoidal 461.2
    frontal 461.1
    maxillary 461.0
    specified type NEC 461.8
    sphenoidal 461.3
  allergic (see also Fever, hay)
    477.9
  antrum - see Sinusitis, maxillary
  due to
    fungus, any sinus 117.9
    high altitude 993.1
  ethmoidal 473.2
    acute 461.2
  frontal 473.1
    acute 461.1
  influenzal 487.1
  maxillary 473.0
    acute 461.0
  specified site NEC 473.8
  sphenoidal 473.3
    acute 461.3
  syphilitic, any sinus 095.8
  tuberculous, any sinus (see also
    Tuberculosis) 012.8●
Sinusitis-bronchiectasis-situs inversus
    (syndrome) (triad) 759.3
Sipple's syndrome (medullary thyroid
    carcinoma-pheochromocytoma)
    258.02
Sirenomelia 759.89
Siriasis 992.0
Sirkari's disease 085.0

SIRS (systemic inflammatory response
    syndrome) 995.90
  due to
    infectious process 995.91
      with acute organ dysfunction
        995.92
    non-infectious process 995.93
      with acute organ dysfunction
        995.94
Siti 104.0
Sitophobia 300.29
Situation, psychiatric 300.9
Situational
  disturbance (transient) (see also
    Reaction, adjustment) 309.9
    acute 308.3
  maladjustment, acute (see also Reaction,
    adjustment) 309.9
  reaction (see also Reaction, adjustment)
    309.9
    acute 308.3
Situs inversus or transversus 759.3
  abdominalis 759.3
  thoracis 759.3
Sixth disease
  due to
    human herpesvirus 6 058.11
    human herpesvirus 7 058.12
Sjögren (-Gougerot) syndrome or disease
    (keratoconjunctivitis sicca) 710.2
  with lung involvement 710.2 [517.8]
Sjögren-Larsson syndrome (ichthyosis
    congenita) 757.1
SJS-TEN (Stevens-Johnson syndrome-
    toxic epidermal necrolysis overlap
    syndrome) 695.14
Skeletal - see condition
Skene's gland - see condition
Skenitis (see also Urethritis) 597.89
  gonorrheal (acute) 098.0
    chronic or duration of 2 months or
      over 098.2
Skerljevo 104.0
Skevas-Zerfus disease 989.5
Skin - see also condition
  donor V59.1
  hidebound 710.9
SLAP lesion (superior glenoid labrum)
    840.7
Slate-dressers' lung 502
Slate-miners' lung 502
Sleep
  deprivation V69.4
  disorder 780.50
    with apnea - see Apnea, sleep
    child 307.40
    movement, unspecified 780.58
    nonorganic origin 307.40
      specified type NEC 307.49
  disturbance 780.50
    with apnea - see Apnea, sleep
    nonorganic origin 307.40
      specified type NEC 307.49
  drunkenness 307.47
  movement disorder, unspecified
    780.58
  paroxysmal (see also Narcolepsy)
    347.00
  related movement disorder,
    unspecified 780.58
  rhythm inversion 327.39
    nonorganic origin 307.45
  walking 307.46
    hysterical 300.13

Sleeping sickness 086.5
  late effect 139.8
Sleeplessness (see also Insomnia) 780.52
  menopausal 627.2
  nonorganic origin 307.41
Slipped, slipping
  epiphysis (postinfectional) 732.9
    traumatic (old) 732.9
      current - see Fracture, by site
      upper femoral (nontraumatic)
        732.2
  intervertebral disc - see Displacement,
    intervertebral disc
  ligature, umbilical 772.3
  patella 717.89
  rib 733.99
  sacroiliac joint 724.6
  tendon 727.9
  ulnar nerve, nontraumatic 354.2
  vertebra NEC (see also
    Spondylolisthesis) 756.12
Slocumb's syndrome 255.3
Sloughing (multiple) (skin) 686.9
  abscess - see Abscess, by site
  appendix 543.9
  bladder 596.8
  fascia 728.9
  graft - see Complications, graft
  phagedena (see also Gangrene) 785.4
  reattached extremity (see also
    Complications, reattached
    extremity) 996.90
  rectum 569.49
  scrotum 608.89
  tendon 727.9
  transplanted organ (see also Rejection,
    transplant, organ, by site)
    996.80
  ulcer (see also Ulcer, skin) 707.9
Slow
  feeding newborn 779.31   ◀▥
  fetal, growth NEC 764.9●
    affecting management of pregnancy
      656.5●
Slowing
  heart 427.89
  urinary stream 788.62
Sluder's neuralgia or syndrome 337.09
Slurred, slurring, speech 784.59   ◀▥
Small, smallness
  cardia reserve - see Disease, heart
  for dates
    fetus or newborn 764.0●
      with malnutrition 764.1●
      affecting management of
        pregnancy 656.5●
  infant, term 764.0●
    with malnutrition 764.1●
    affecting management of pregnancy
      656.5●
  introitus, vagina 623.3
  kidney, unknown cause 589.9
    bilateral 589.1
    unilateral 589.0
  ovary 620.8
  pelvis
    with disproportion (fetopelvic)
      653.1●
      affecting fetus or newborn 763.1
    causing obstructed labor 660.1●
      affecting fetus or newborn 763.1
  placenta - see Placenta, insufficiency
  uterus 621.8
  white kidney 582.9

Small-for-dates (see also Light-for-dates)
764.0●
  affecting management of pregnancy
    656.5●
Smallpox 050.9
  contact V01.3
  exposure to V01.3
  hemorrhagic (pustular) 050.0
  malignant 050.0
  modified 050.2
  vaccination
    complications - see Complications,
      vaccination
    prophylactic (against) V04.1
Smith's fracture (separation) (closed)
    813.41
  open 813.51
Smith-Lemli-Opitz syndrome
    (cerebrohepatorenal syndrome)
    759.89
Smith-Magenis syndrome 758.33
Smith-Strang disease (oasthouse urine)
    270.2
Smokers'
  bronchitis 491.0
  cough 491.0
  syndrome (see also Abuse, drugs,
    nondependent) 305.1
  throat 472.1
  tongue 528.6
Smoking complicating pregnancy,
    childbirth, or the puerperium
    649.0●
Smothering spells 786.09
Snaggle teeth, tooth 524.39
Snapping
  finger 727.05
  hip 719.65
  jaw 524.69
    temporomandibular joint sounds on
      opening or closing 524.64
  knee 717.9
  thumb 727.05
Sneddon-Wilkinson disease or
    syndrome (subcorneal pustular
    dermatosis) 694.1
Sneezing 784.99
  intractable 478.19
Sniffing
  cocaine (see also Dependence) 304.2●
  either (see also Dependence) 304.6●
  glue (airplane) (see also Dependence)
    304.6●
Snoring 786.09
Snow blindness 370.24
Snuffles (nonsyphilitic) 460
  syphilitic (infant) 090.0
Social migrant V60.0
Sodoku 026.0
Soemmering's ring 366.51
Soft - see also condition
  enlarged prostate 600.00
    with
      other lower urinary tract
        symptoms (LUTS) 600.01
      urinary
        obstruction 600.01
        retention 600.01
  nails 703.8
Softening
  bone 268.2
  brain (necrotic) (progressive) 434.9●
    arteriosclerotic 437.0
    congenital 742.4

Softening (Continued)
  brain (Continued)
    embolic (see also Embolism, brain)
      434.1●
    hemorrhagic (see also Hemorrhage,
      brain) 431
    occlusive 434.9●
    thrombotic (see also Thrombosis,
      brain) 434.0●
  cartilage 733.92
  cerebellar - see Softening, brain
  cerebral - see Softening, brain
  cerebrospinal - see Softening, brain
  myocardial, heart (see also
    Degeneration, myocardial) 429.1
  nails 703.8
  spinal cord 336.8
  stomach 537.89
Solar fever 061
Soldier's
  heart 306.2
  patches 423.1
Solitary
  cyst
    bone 733.21
    kidney 593.2
  kidney (congenital) 753.0
  tubercle, brain (see also Tuberculosis,
    brain) 013.2●
  ulcer, bladder 596.8
Somatization reaction, somatic reaction
    (see also Disorder, psychosomatic)
    306.9
  disorder 300.81
Somatoform disorder 300.82
  atypical 300.82
  severe 300.81
  undifferentiated 300.82
Somnambulism 307.46
  hysterical 300.13
Somnolence 780.09
  nonorganic origin 307.43
  periodic 349.89
Sonne dysentery 004.3
Soor 112.0
Sore
  Delhi 085.1
  desert (see also Ulcer, skin) 707.9
  eye 379.99
  Lahore 085.1
  mouth 528.9
    canker 528.2
    due to dentures 528.9
  muscle 729.1
  naga (see also Ulcer, skin) 707.9
  oriental 085.1
  pressure (see also Ulcer, pressure)
    707.00
    with gangrene (see also Ulcer,
      pressure) 707.00 [785.4]
  skin NEC 709.9
  soft 099.0
  throat 462
    with influenza, flu, or grippe 487.1
    acute 462
    chronic 472.1
    clergyman's 784.49
    Coxsackie (virus) 074.0
    diphtheritic 032.0
    epidemic 034.0
    gangrenous 462
    herpetic 054.79
    influenzal 487.1
    malignant 462

Sore (Continued)
  throat (Continued)
    purulent 462
    putrid 462
    septic 034.0
    streptococcal (ulcerative) 034.0
    ulcerated 462
    viral NEC 462
      Coxsackie 074.0
  tropical (see also Ulcer, skin) 707.9
  veldt (see also Ulcer, skin) 707.9
Sotos' syndrome (cerebral gigantism)
    253.0
Sounds
  friction, pleural 786.7
  succussion, chest 786.7
  temporomandibular joint
    on opening or closing 524.64
South African cardiomyopathy
    syndrome 425.2
South American
  blastomycosis 116.1
  trypanosomiasis - see Trypanosomiasis
Southeast Asian hemorrhagic fever 065.4
Spacing, teeth, abnormal 524.30
  excessive 524.32
Spade-like hand (congenital) 754.89
Spading nail 703.8
  congenital 757.5
Spanemia 285.9
Spanish collar 605
Sparganosis 123.5
Spasm, spastic, spasticity (see also
    condition) 781.0
  accommodation 367.53
  ampulla of Vater (see also Disease,
    gallbladder) 576.8
  anus, ani (sphincter) (reflex) 564.6
    psychogenic 306.4
  artery NEC 443.9
    basilar 435.0
    carotid 435.8
    cerebral 435.9
      specified artery NEC 435.8
    retinal (see also Occlusion, retinal,
      artery) 362.30
    vertebral 435.1
    vertebrobasilar 435.3
  Bell's 351.0
  bladder (sphincter, external or internal)
    596.8
  bowel 564.9
    psychogenic 306.4
  bronchus, bronchiole 519.11
  cardia 530.0
  cardiac - see Angina
  carpopedal (see also Tetany) 781.7
  cecum 564.9
    psychogenic 306.4
  cerebral (arteries) (vascular) 435.9
    specified artery NEC 435.8
  cerebrovascular 435.9
  cervix, complicating delivery 661.4●
    affecting fetus or newborn 763.7
  ciliary body (of accommodation)
    367.53
  colon 564.1
    psychogenic 306.4
  common duct (see also Disease, biliary)
    576.8
  compulsive 307.22
  conjugate 378.82
  convergence 378.84
  coronary (artery) - see Angina

◄ New   ◄▮▮ Revised   ~~deleted~~ Deleted   ● Use Additional Digit(s)   ▒ Omit code

Spasm, spastic, spasticity (Continued)
  diaphragm (reflex) 786.8
    psychogenic 306.1
  duodenum, duodenal (bulb) 564.89
  esophagus (diffuse) 530.5
    psychogenic 306.4
  facial 351.8
  fallopian tube 620.8
  gait 781.2
  gastrointestinal (tract) 536.8
    psychogenic 306.4
  glottis 478.75
    hysterical 300.11
    psychogenic 306.1
      specified as conversion reaction
        300.11
    reflex through recurrent laryngeal
      nerve 478.75
  habit 307.20
    chronic 307.22
    transient (of childhood) 307.21
  heart - see Angina
  hourglass - see Contraction, hourglass
  hysterical 300.11
  infantile (see also Epilepsy) 345.6●
  internal oblique, eye 378.51
  intestinal 564.9
    psychogenic 306.4
  larynx, laryngeal 478.75
    hysterical 300.11
    psychogenic 306.1
      specified as conversion reaction
        300.11
  levator palpebrae superioris 333.81
  lightning (see also Epilepsy) 345.6●
  mobile 781.0
  muscle 728.85
    back 724.8
    psychogenic 306.0
  nerve, trigeminal 350.1
  nervous 306.0
  nodding 307.3
    infantile (see also Epilepsy) 345.6●
  occupational 300.89
  oculogyric 378.87
  ophthalmic artery 362.30
  orbicularis 781.0
  perineal 625.8
  peroneo-extensor (see also Flat, foot)
    734
  pharynx (reflex) 478.29
    hysterical 300.11
    psychogenic 306.1
      specified as conversion reaction
        300.11
  pregnant uterus, complicating delivery
    661.4●
  psychogenic 306.0
  pylorus 537.81
    adult hypertrophic 537.0
    congenital or infantile 750.5
    psychogenic 306.4
  rectum (sphincter) 564.6
    psychogenic 306.4
  retinal artery NEC (see also Occlusion,
    retina, artery) 362.30
  sacroiliac 724.6
  salaam (infantile) (see also Epilepsy)
    345.6●
  saltatory 781.0
  sigmoid 564.9
    psychogenic 306.4
  sphincter of Oddi (see also Disease,
    gallbladder) 576.5

Spasm, spastic, spasticity (Continued)
  stomach 536.8
    neurotic 306.4
  throat 478.29
    hysterical 300.11
    psychogenic 306.1
      specified as conversion reaction
        300.11
  tic 307.20
    chronic 307.22
    transient (of childhood) 307.21
  tongue 529.8
  torsion 333.6
  trigeminal nerve 350.1
    postherpetic 053.12
  ureter 593.89
  urethra (sphincter) 599.84
  uterus 625.8
    complicating labor 661.4●
      affecting fetus or newborn
        763.7
  vagina 625.1
    psychogenic 306.51
  vascular NEC 443.9
  vasomotor NEC 443.9
  vein NEC 459.89
  vesical (sphincter, external or internal)
    596.8
  viscera 789.0●
Spasmodic - see condition
Spasmophilia (see also Tetany) 781.7
Spasmus nutans 307.3
Spastic - see also Spasm
  child 343.9
Spasticity - see also Spasm
  cerebral, child 343.9
Speakers' throat 784.49
Specific, specified - see condition
Speech
  defect, disorder, disturbance,
    impediment NEC 784.59 ◀▦
    psychogenic 307.9
  (language) therapy V57.3 ◀▦
Spells 780.39
  breath-holding 786.9
Spencer's disease (epidemic vomiting)
  078.82
Spens' syndrome (syncope with heart
  block) 426.9
Spermatic cord - see condition
Spermatocele 608.1
  congenital 752.89
Spermatocystitis 608.4
Spermatocytoma (M9063/3)
  specified site - see Neoplasm, by site,
    malignant
  unspecified site 186.9
Spermatorrhea 608.89
Sperm counts
  fertility testing V26.21
  following sterilization reversal V26.22
  postvasectomy V25.8
Sphacelus (see also Gangrene) 785.4
Sphenoidal - see condition
Sphenoiditis (chronic) (see also Sinusitis,
  sphenoidal) 473.3
Sphenopalatine ganglion neuralgia
  337.09
Sphericity, increased, lens 743.36
Spherocytosis (congenital) (familial)
  (hereditary) 282.0
  hemoglobin disease 282.7
  sickle-cell (disease) 282.60
Spherophakia 743.36

Sphincter - see condition
Sphincteritis, sphincter of Oddi (see also
  Cholecystitis) 576.8
Sphingolipidosis 272.7
Sphingolipodystrophy 272.7
Sphingomyelinosis 272.7
Spicule tooth 520.2
Spider
  finger 755.59
  nevus 448.1
  vascular 448.1
Spiegler-Fendt sarcoid 686.8
Spielmeyer-Stock disease 330.1
Spielmeyer-Vogt disease 330.1
Spina bifida (aperta) 741.9●

Note 67   Use the following fifth-digit
subclassification with category 741:

  0   unspecified region
  1   cervical region
  2   dorsal [thoracic] region
  3   lumbar region

---

  with hydrocephalus 741.0●
    fetal (suspected), affecting
      management of pregnancy
      655.0●
  occulta 756.17
Spindle, Krukenberg's 371.13
Spine, spinal - see condition
Spiradenoma (eccrine) (M8403/0) - see
  Neoplasm, skin, benign
Spirillosis NEC (see also Fever, relapsing)
  087.9
Spirillum minus 026.0
Spirillum obermeieri infection 087.0
Spirochetal - see condition
Spirochetosis 104.9
  arthritic, arthritica 104.9 [711.8]●
  bronchopulmonary 104.8
  icterohemorrhagica 100.0
  lung 104.8
Spitting blood (see also Hemoptysis) 786.3
Splanchnomegaly 569.89
Splanchnoptosis 569.89
Spleen, splenic - see also condition
  agenesis 759.0
  flexure syndrome 569.89
  neutropenia syndrome 289.53
  sequestration syndrome 289.52
Splenectasis (see also Splenomegaly)
  789.2
Splenitis (interstitial) (malignant)
  (nonspecific) 289.59
  malarial (see also Malaria) 084.6
  tuberculous (see also Tuberculosis)
    017.7●
Splenocele 289.59
Splenomegalia - see Splenomegaly
Splenomegalic - see condition
Splenomegaly 789.2
  Bengal 789.2
  cirrhotic 289.51
  congenital 759.0
  congestive, chronic 289.51
  cryptogenic 789.2
  Egyptian 120.1
  Gaucher's (cerebroside lipidosis) 272.7
  idiopathic 789.2
  malarial (see also Malaria) 084.6
  neutropenic 289.53
  Niemann-Pick (lipid histiocytosis)
    272.7
  siderotic 289.51

Splenomegaly *(Continued)*
  syphilitic 095.8
    congenital 090.0
  tropical (Bengal) (idiopathic) 789.2
Splenopathy 289.50
Splenopneumonia - *see* Pneumonia
Splenoptosis 289.59
Splinter - *see* Injury, superficial, by site
Split, splitting
  heart sounds 427.89
  lip, congenital *(see also* Cleft, lip)
    749.10
  nails 703.8
  urinary stream 788.61
Spoiled child reaction *(see also*
    Disturbance, conduct) 312.1●
Spondylarthritis *(see also* Spondylosis)
    721.90
Spondylarthrosis *(see also* Spondylosis)
    721.90
Spondylitis 720.9
  ankylopoietica 720.0
  ankylosing (chronic) 720.0
  atrophic 720.9
    ligamentous 720.9
  chronic (traumatic) *(see also*
    Spondylosis) 721.90
  deformans (chronic) *(see also*
    Spondylosis) 721.90
  gonococcal 098.53
  gouty 274.00   ◀▥
  hypertrophic *(see also* Spondylosis)
    721.90
  infectious NEC 720.9
  juvenile (adolescent) 720.0
  Kummell's 721.7
  Marie-Strümpell (ankylosing) 720.0
  muscularis 720.9
  ossificans ligamentosa 721.6
  osteoarthritica *(see also* Spondylosis)
    721.90
  posttraumatic 721.7
  proliferative 720.0
  rheumatoid 720.0
  rhizomelica 720.0
  sacroiliac NEC 720.2
  senescent *(see also* Spondylosis)
    721.90
  senile *(see also* Spondylosis) 721.90
  static *(see also* Spondylosis) 721.90
  traumatic (chronic) *(see also*
    Spondylosis) 721.90
  tuberculous *(see also* Tuberculosis)
    015.0● [720.81]
  typhosa 002.0 [720.81]
Spondyloarthrosis *(see also* Spondylosis)
    721.90
Spondylolisthesis (congenital)
    (lumbosacral) 756.12
  with disproportion (fetopelvic)
    653.3●
    affecting fetus or newborn
      763.1
    causing obstructed labor
      660.1●
      affecting fetus or newborn
        763.1
  acquired 738.4
  degenerative 738.4
  traumatic 738.4
    acute (lumbar) - *see* Fracture,
      vertebra, lumbar
    site other than lumbosacral - *see*
      Fracture, vertebra, by site

Spondylolysis (congenital) 756.11
  acquired 738.4
  cervical 756.19
  lumbosacral region 756.11
    with disproportion (fetopelvic)
      653.3●
      affecting fetus or newborn
        763.1
      causing obstructed labor 660.1●
        affecting fetus or newborn
          763.1
Spondylopathy
  inflammatory 720.9
    specified type NEC 720.89
  traumatic 721.7
Spondylose rhizomelique 720.0
Spondylosis 721.90
  with
    disproportion 653.3●
      affecting fetus or newborn
        763.1
      causing obstructed labor 660.1●
        affecting fetus or newborn
          763.1
    myelopathy NEC 721.91
  cervical, cervicodorsal 721.0
    with myelopathy 721.1
  inflammatory 720.9
  lumbar, lumbosacral 721.3
    with myelopathy 721.42
  sacral 721.3
    with myelopathy 721.42
  thoracic 721.2
    with myelopathy 721.41
  traumatic 721.7
Sponge
  divers' disease 989.5
  inadvertently left in operation wound
    998.4
  kidney (medullary) 753.17
Spongioblastoma (M9422/3)
  multiforme (M9440/3)
    specified site - *see* Neoplasm, by site,
      malignant
    unspecified site 191.9
  polare (M9423/3)
    specified site - *see* Neoplasm, by site,
      malignant
    unspecified site 191.9
  primitive polar (M9443/3)
    specified site - *see* Neoplasm, by site,
      malignant
    unspecified site 191.9
  specified site - *see* Neoplasm, by site,
    malignant
  unspecified site 191.9
Spongiocytoma (M9400/3)
  specified site - *see* Neoplasm, by site,
    malignant
  unspecified site 191.9
Spongioneuroblastoma (M9504/3) - *see*
    Neoplasm, by site, malignant
Spontaneous - *see also* condition
  fracture - *see* Fracture, pathologic
Spoon nail 703.8
  congenital 757.5
Sporadic - *see* condition
Sporotrichosis (bones) (cutaneous)
    (disseminated) (epidermal)
    (lymphatic) (lymphocutaneous)
    (mucous membranes) (pulmonary)
    (skeletal) (visceral) 117.1
Sporotrichum schenckii infection
    117.1

Spots, spotting
  atrophic (skin) 701.3
  Bitôt's (in the young child) 264.1
  café au lait 709.09
  cayenne pepper 448.1
  complicating pregnancy 649.5●
  cotton wool (retina) 362.83
  de Morgan's (senile angiomas) 448.1
  Fúchs' black (myopic) 360.21
  intermenstrual
    irregular 626.6
    regular 626.5
  interpalpebral 372.53
  Koplik's 055.9
  liver 709.09
  Mongolian (pigmented) 757.33
  of pregnancy 649.5●
  purpuric 782.7
  ruby 448.1
Spotted fever - *see* Fever, spotted
Sprain, strain (joint) (ligament) (muscle)
    (tendon) 848.9
  abdominal wall (muscle) 848.8
  Achilles tendon 845.09
  acromioclavicular 840.0
  ankle 845.00
    and foot 845.00
  anterior longitudinal, cervical 847.0
  arm 840.9
    upper 840.9
      and shoulder 840.9
  astragalus 845.00
  atlanto-axial 847.0
  atlanto-occipital 847.0
  atlas 847.0
  axis 847.0
  back *(see also* Sprain, spine) 847.9
  breast bone 848.40
  broad ligaments - *see* Injury, internal,
    broad ligament
  calcaneofibular 845.02
  carpal 842.01
  carpometacarpal 842.11
  cartilage
    costal, without mention of injury to
      sternum 848.3
      involving sternum 848.42
    ear 848.8
    knee 844.9
      with current tear *(see also* Tear,
        meniscus) 836.2
    semilunar (knee) 844.8
      with current tear *(see also* Tear,
        meniscus) 836.2
    septal, nose 848.0
    thyroid region 848.2
    xiphoid 848.49
  cervical, cervicodorsal, cervicothoracic
    847.0
  chondrocostal, without mention of
    injury to sternum 848.3
    involving sternum 848.42
  chondrosternal 848.42
  chronic (joint) - *see* Derangement,
    joint
  clavicle 840.9
  coccyx 847.4
  collar bone 840.9
  collateral, knee (medial) (tibial)
    844.1
    lateral (fibular) 844.0
    recurrent or old 717.89
      lateral 717.81
      medial 717.82

Sprain, strain *(Continued)*
  coracoacromial 840.8
  coracoclavicular 840.1
  coracohumeral 840.2
  coracoid (process) 840.9
  coronary, knee 844.8
  costal cartilage, without mention of
      injury to sternum 848.3
    involving sternum 848.42
  cricoarytenoid articulation 848.2
  cricothyroid articulation 848.2
  cruciate
    knee 844.2
    old 717.89
      anterior 717.83
      posterior 717.84
  deltoid
    ankle 845.01
    shoulder 840.8
  dorsal (spine) 847.1
  ear cartilage 848.8
  elbow 841.9
    and forearm 841.9
    specified site NEC 841.8
  femur (proximal end) 843.9
    distal end 844.9
  fibula (proximal end) 844.9
    distal end 845.00
  fibulocalcaneal 845.02
  finger(s) 842.10
  foot 845.10
    and ankle 845.00
  forearm 841.9
    and elbow 841.9
    specified site NEC 841.8
  glenoid (shoulder) - *(see also* SLAP
      lesion) 840.8
  hand 842.10
  hip 843.9
    and thigh 843.9
  humerus (proximal end) 840.9
    distal end 841.9
  iliofemoral 843.0
  infraspinatus 840.3
  innominate
    acetabulum 843.9
    pubic junction 848.5
    sacral junction 846.1
  internal
    collateral, ankle 845.01
    semilunar cartilage 844.8
      with current tear *(see also* Tear,
          meniscus) 836.2
      old 717.5
  interphalangeal
    finger 842.13
    toe 845.13
  ischiocapsular 843.1
  jaw (cartilage) (meniscus) 848.1
    old 524.69
  knee 844.9
    and leg 844.9
    old 717.5
      collateral
        lateral 717.81
        medial 717.82
      cruciate
        anterior 717.83
        posterior 717.84
  late effect - *see* Late, effects (of), sprain
  lateral collateral, knee 844.0
    old 717.81
  leg 844.9
    and knee 844.9

Sprain, strain *(Continued)*
  ligamentum teres femoris 843.8
  low back 846.9
  lumbar (spine) 847.2
  lumbosacral 846.0
    chronic or old 724.6
  mandible 848.1
    old 524.69
  maxilla 848.1
  medial collateral, knee 844.1
    old 717.82
  meniscus
    jaw 848.1
      old 524.69
    knee 844.8
      with current tear *(see also* Tear,
          meniscus) 836.2
      old 717.5
    mandible 848.1
      old 524.69
    specified site NEC 848.8
  metacarpal 842.10
    distal 842.12
    proximal 842.11
  metacarpophalangeal 842.12
  metatarsal 845.10
  metatarsophalangeal 845.12
  midcarpal 842.19
  midtarsal 845.19
  multiple sites, except fingers alone or
      toes alone 848.8
  neck 847.0
  nose (septal cartilage) 848.0
  occiput from atlas 847.0
  old - *see* Derangement, joint
  orbicular, hip 843.8
  patella(r) 844.8
    old 717.89
  pelvis 848.5
  phalanx
    finger 842.10
    toe 845.10
  radiocarpal 842.02
  radiohumeral 841.2
  radioulnar 841.9
    distal 842.09
  radius, radial (proximal end) 841.9
    and ulna 841.9
      distal 842.09
    collateral 841.0
    distal end 842.00
  recurrent - *see* Sprain, by site
  rib (cage), without mention of injury to
      sternum 848.3
    involving sternum 848.42
  rotator cuff (capsule) 840.4
  round ligament - *see also* Injury,
      internal, round ligament
    femur 843.8
  sacral (spine) 847.3
  sacrococcygeal 847.3
  sacroiliac (region) 846.9
    chronic or old 724.6
    ligament 846.1
    specified site NEC 846.8
  sacrospinatus 846.2
  sacrospinous 846.2
  sacrotuberous 846.3
  scaphoid bone, ankle 845.00
  scapula(r) 840.9
  semilunar cartilage (knee) 844.8
    with current tear *(see also* Tear,
        meniscus) 836.2
    old 717.5

Sprain, strain *(Continued)*
  septal cartilage (nose) 848.0
  shoulder 840.9
    and arm, upper 840.9
    blade 840.9
  specified site NEC 848.8
  spine 847.9
    cervical 847.0
    coccyx 847.4
    dorsal 847.1
    lumbar 847.2
    lumbosacral 846.0
      chronic or old 724.6
    sacral 847.3
    sacroiliac *(see also* Sprain, sacroiliac)
        846.9
      chronic or old 724.6
    thoracic 847.1
  sternoclavicular 848.41
  sternum 848.40
  subglenoid - *(see also* SLAP lesion)
      840.8
  subscapularis 840.5
  supraspinatus 840.6
  symphysis
    jaw 848.1
      old 524.69
    mandibular 848.1
      old 524.69
    pubis 848.5
  talofibular 845.09
  tarsal 845.10
  tarsometatarsal 845.11
  temporomandibular 848.1
    old 524.69
  teres
    ligamentum femoris 843.8
    major or minor 840.8
  thigh (proximal end) 843.9
    and hip 843.9
    distal end 844.9
  thoracic (spine) 847.1
  thorax 848.8
  thumb 842.10
  thyroid cartilage or region 848.2
  tibia (proximal end) 844.9
    distal end 845.00
  tibiofibular
    distal 845.03
    superior 844.3
  toe(s) 845.10
  trachea 848.8
  trapezoid 840.8
  ulna, ulnar (proximal end) 841.9
    collateral 841.1
    distal end 842.00
  ulnohumeral 841.3
  vertebrae *(see also* Sprain, spine)
      847.9
    cervical, cervicodorsal,
        cervicothoracic 847.0
  wrist (cuneiform) (scaphoid)
      (semilunar) 842.00
  xiphoid cartilage 848.49
Sprengel's deformity (congenital)
    755.52
Spring fever 309.23
Sprue 579.1
  celiac 579.0
  idiopathic 579.0
  meaning thrush 112.0
  nontropical 579.0
  tropical 579.1

Spur - *see also* Exostosis
  bone 726.91
    calcaneal 726.73
  calcaneal 726.73
  iliac crest 726.5
  nose (septum) 478.19
    bone 726.91
  septal 478.19
Spuria placenta - *see* Placenta, abnormal
Spurway's syndrome (brittle bones and
    blue sclera) 756.51
Sputum, abnormal (amount) (color)
    (excessive) (odor) (purulent) 786.4
  bloody 786.3
Squamous - *see also* condition
  cell metaplasia
    bladder 596.8
    cervix - *see* condition
  epithelium in
    cervical canal (congenital) 752.49
    uterine mucosa (congenital) 752.3
  metaplasia
    bladder 596.8
    cervix - *see* condition
Squashed nose 738.0
  congenital 754.0
Squeeze, divers' 993.3
Squint (*see also* Strabismus) 378.9
  accommodative (*see also* Esotropia)
    378.00
  concomitant (*see also* Heterotropia)
    378.30
Stab - *see also* Wound, open, by site
  internal organs - *see* Injury, internal, by
    site, with open wound
Staggering gait 781.2
  hysterical 300.11
Staghorn calculus 592.0
Stähl's
  ear 744.29
  pigment line (cornea) 371.11
Stähli's pigment lines (cornea) 371.11
Stain, staining
  meconium 779.84
  port wine 757.32
  tooth, teeth (hard tissues) 521.7
    due to
      accretions 523.6
      deposits (betel) (black) (green)
        (materia alba) (orange)
        (tobacco) 523.6
      metals (copper) (silver) 521.7
      nicotine 523.6
      pulpal bleeding 521.7
      tobacco 523.6
Stammering 307.0
Standstill
  atrial 426.6
  auricular 426.6
  cardiac (*see also* Arrest, cardiac) 427.5
  sinoatrial 426.6
  sinus 426.6
  ventricular (*see also* Arrest, cardiac)
    427.5
Stannosis 503
Stanton's disease (melioidosis) 025
Staphylitis (acute) (catarrhal) (chronic)
    (gangrenous) (membranous)
    (suppurative) (ulcerative) 528.3
Staphylococcemia 038.10
  aureus 038.11
  specified organism NEC 038.19
Staphylococcus, staphylococcal - *see*
  condition

Staphyloderma (skin) 686.00
Staphyloma 379.11
  anterior, localized 379.14
  ciliary 379.11
  cornea 371.73
  equatorial 379.13
  posterior 379.12
  posticum 379.12
  ring 379.15
  sclera NEC 379.11
Starch eating 307.52
Stargardt's disease 362.75
Starvation (inanition) (due to lack of
    food) 994.2
  edema 262
  voluntary NEC 307.1
Stasis
  bile (duct) (*see also* Disease, biliary)
    576.8
  bronchus (*see also* Bronchitis) 490
  cardiac (*see also* Failure, heart)
    428.0
  cecum 564.89
  colon 564.89
  dermatitis (*see also* Varix, with stasis
    dermatitis) 454.1
  duodenal 536.8
  eczema (*see also* Varix, with stasis
    dermatitis) 454.1
  edema (*see also* Hypertension, venous)
    459.30
  foot 991.4
  gastric 536.3
  ileocecal coil 564.89
  ileum 564.89
  intestinal 564.89
  jejunum 564.89
  kidney 586
  liver 571.9
    cirrhotic - *see* Cirrhosis, liver
  lymphatic 457.8
  pneumonia 514
  portal 571.9
  pulmonary 514
  rectal 564.89
  renal 586
    tubular 584.5
  stomach 536.3
  ulcer
    with varicose veins 454.0
    without varicose veins 459.81
  urine NEC (*see also* Retention, urine)
    788.20
  venous 459.81
State
  affective and paranoid, mixed, organic
    psychotic 294.8
  agitated 307.9
    acute reaction to stress 308.2
  anxiety (neurotic) (*see also* Anxiety)
    300.00
    specified type NEC 300.09
  apprehension (*see also* Anxiety) 300.00
    specified type NEC 300.09
  climacteric, female 627.2
    following induced menopause
      627.4
  clouded
    epileptic (*see also* Epilepsy)
      345.9●
    paroxysmal (idiopathic) (*see also*
      Epilepsy) 345.9●
  compulsive (mixed) (with obsession)
    300.3

State (*Continued*)
  confusional 298.9
    acute 293.0
      with
        arteriosclerotic dementia
          290.41
        presenile brain disease 290.11
        senility 290.3
    alcoholic 291.0
    drug-induced 292.81
    epileptic 293.0
    postoperative 293.9
    reactive (emotional stress)
      (psychological trauma) 298.2
    subacute 293.1
  constitutional psychopathic 301.9
  convulsive (*see also* Convulsions) 780.39
  depressive NEC 311
    induced by drug 292.84
    neurotic 300.4
  dissociative 300.15
  hallucinatory 780.1
    induced by drug 292.12
  hypercoagulable (primary) 289.81
    secondary 289.82
  hyperdynamic beta-adrenergic
    circulatory 429.82
  locked-in 344.81
  menopausal 627.2
    artificial 627.4
    following induced menopause
      627.4
  neurotic NEC 300.9
    with depersonalization episode
      300.6
  obsessional 300.3
  oneiroid (*see also* Schizophrenia)
    295.4●
  panic 300.01
  paranoid 297.9
    alcohol-induced 291.5
    arteriosclerotic 290.42
    climacteric 297.2
    drug-induced 292.11
    in
      presenile brain disease 290.12
      senile brain disease 290.20
    involutional 297.2
    menopausal 297.2
    senile 290.20
    simple 297.0
  postleukotomy 310.0
  pregnant (*see also* Pregnancy) V22.2
  psychogenic, twilight 298.2
  psychotic, organic (*see also* Psychosis,
    organic) 294.9
    mixed paranoid and affective
      294.8
    senile or presenile NEC 290.9
    transient NEC 293.9
      with
        anxiety 293.84
        delusions 293.81
        depression 293.83
        hallucinations 293.82
  residual schizophrenic (*see also*
    Schizophrenia) 295.6●
  tension (*see also* Anxiety) 300.9
  transient organic psychotic 293.9
    anxiety type 293.84
    depressive type 293.83
    hallucinatory type 293.83
    paranoid type 293.81
    specified type NEC 293.89

◀ New   ◀▥ Revised   ~~deleted~~ Deleted   ● Use Additional Digit(s)   ▨ Omit code

State *(Continued)*
  twilight
    epileptic 293.0
    psychogenic 298.2
  vegetative (persistent) 780.03
Status (post)
  absence
    epileptic *(see also* Epilepsy) 345.2
    of organ, acquired (postsurgical) -
      see Absence, by site, acquired
  administration of tPA (rtPA) in a
    different institution within the
    last 24 hours prior to admission
    to facility V45.88
  anastomosis of intestine (for bypass)
    V45.3
  anginosus 413.9
  angioplasty, percutaneous
    transluminal coronary
    V45.82
  ankle prosthesis V43.66
  aortocoronary bypass or shunt
    V45.81
  arthrodesis V45.4
  artificially induced condition NEC
    V45.89
  artificial opening (of) V44.9
    gastrointestinal tract NEC
      V44.4
    specified site NEC V44.8
    urinary tract NEC V44.6
    vagina V44.7
  aspirator V46.0
  asthmaticus *(see also* Asthma)
    493.9●
  awaiting organ transplant V49.83
  bariatric surgery V45.86
    complicating pregnancy,
      childbirth, or the
      puerperium 649.2●
  bed confinement V49.84
  breast
    correction V43.82
    implant removal V45.83
    reconstruction V43.82
  cardiac
    device (in situ) V45.00
      carotid sinus V45.09
        fitting or adjustment V53.39
      defibrillator, automatic
        implantable V45.02
      pacemaker V45.01
        fitting or adjustment V53.31
  carotid sinus stimulator V45.09
  cataract extraction V45.61
  chemotherapy V66.2
    current V58.69
  circumcision, female 629.20
  clitorectomy (female genital mutilation
    type I) 629.21
    with excision of labia minora
      (female genital mutilation
      type II) 629.22
  colonization - *see* Carrier (suspected) of
  colostomy V44.3
  contraceptive device V45.59
    intrauterine V45.51
    subdermal V45.52
  convulsivus idiopathicus *(see also*
    Epilepsy) 345.3
  coronary artery bypass or shunt
    V45.81
  ~~current military deployment status~~
    ~~V62.21~~

Status *(Continued)*
  cutting
    female genital 629.20
      specified NEC 629.29
      type I 629.21
      type II 629.22
      type III 629.23
      type IV 629.29
  cystostomy V44.50
    appendico-vesicostomy V44.52
    cutaneous-vesicostomy V44.51
    specifed type NEC V44.59
  defibrillator, automatic implantable
    cardiac V45.02
  delinquent immunization V15.83 ◄
  dental crowns V45.84
  dental fillings V45.84
  dental restoration V45.84
  dental sealant V49.82
  dialysis (hemo) (peritoneal) V45.11
  donor V59.9
  drug therapy or regimen V67.59
    high-risk medication NEC V67.51
  elbow prosthesis V43.62
  enterostomy V44.4
  epileptic, epilepticus (absence) (grand
    mal) *(see also* Epilepsy) 345.3
    focal motor 345.7●
    partial 345.7●
    petit mal 345.2
    psychomotor 345.7●
    temporal lobe 345.7●
  estrogen receptor
    negative [ER-] V86.1
    positive [ER+] V86.0
  eye (adnexa) surgery V45.69
  female genital
    cutting 629.20
      specified NEC 629.29
      type I 629.21
      type II 629.22
      type III 629.23
      type IV 629.29
    mutilation 629.20
      type I 629.21
      type II 629.22
      type III 629.23
      type IV 629.29
  filtering bleb (eye) (postglaucoma)
    V45.69
    with rupture or complication
      997.99
    postcataract extraction
      (complication) 997.99
  finger joint prosthesis V43.69
  foster care V60.81 ◄
  gastric
    banding V45.86
      complicating pregnancy,
      childbirth, or the
      puerperium 649.2●
    bypass for obesity V45.86
      complicating pregnancy,
      childbirth, or the
      puerperium 649.2●
  gastrostomy V44.1
  grand mal 345.3
  heart valve prosthesis V43.3
  hemodialysis V45.11
  hip prosthesis (joint) (partial) (total)
    V43.64
  hysterectomy V88.01
    partial with remaining cervical
      stump V88.02
    total V88.01
  ileostomy V44.2

Status *(Continued)*
  infibulation (female genital mutilation
    type III) 629.23
  insulin pump V45.85
  intestinal bypass V45.3
  intrauterine contraceptive device
    V45.51
  jejunostomy V44.4
  knee joint prosthesis V43.65
  lacunaris 437.8
  lacunosis 437.8
  lapsed immunization schedule
    V15.83 ◄
  low birth weight V21.30
    less than 500 grams V21.31
    500–999 grams V21.32
    1000–1499 grams V21.33
    1500–1999 grams V21.34
    2000–2500 grams V21.35
  lymphaticus 254.8
  malignant neoplasm, ablated or
    excised - *see* History, malignant
    neoplasm
  marmoratus 333.79
  military deployment V62.22 ◄
  mutilation, female 629.20
    type I 629.21
    type II 629.22
    type III 629.23
    type IV 629.29
  nephrostomy V44.6
  neuropacemaker NEC V45.89
    brain V45.89
    carotid sinus V45.09
    neurologic NEC V45.89
  obesity surgery V45.86
    complicating pregnancy, childbirth,
      or the puerperium 649.2●
  organ replacement
    by artificial or mechanical device or
      prosthesis of
      artery V43.4
      artificial skin V43.83
      bladder V43.5
      blood vessel V43.4
      breast V43.82
      eye globe V43.0
      heart
        assist device V43.21
        fully implantable artificial
          heart V43.22
        valve V43.3
      intestine V43.89
      joint V43.60
        ankle V43.66
        elbow V43.62
        finger V43.69
        hip (partial) (total) V43.64
        knee V43.65
        shoulder V43.61
        specified NEC V43.69
        wrist V43.63
      kidney V43.89
      larynx V43.81
      lens V43.1
      limb(s) V43.7
      liver V43.89
      lung V43.89
      organ NEC V43.89
      pancreas V43.89
      skin (artificial) V43.83
      tissue NEC V43.89
      vein V43.4
    by organ transplant (heterologous)
      (homologous) - *see* Status,
      transplant

Status *(Continued)*
    pacemaker
        brain V45.89
        cardiac V45.01
        carotid sinus V45.09
        neurologic NEC V45.89
        specified site NEC V45.89
    percutaneous transluminal coronary
        angioplasty V45.82
    peritoneal dialysis V45.11
    petit mal 345.2
    postcommotio cerebri 310.2
    postmenopausal (age related) (natural)
        V49.81
    postoperative NEC V45.89
    postpartum NEC V24.2
        care immediately following delivery
            V24.0
        routine follow-up V24.2
    postsurgical NEC V45.89
    renal dialysis V45.11
        noncompliance V45.12
    respirator [ventilator] V46.11
        encounter
            during
                mechanical failure V46.14
                power failure V46.12
            for weaning V46.13
    reversed jejunal transposition (for
        bypass) V45.3
    sex reassignment surgery *(see also*
        Trans-sexualism) 302.50   ◀▥
    shoulder prosthesis V43.61
    shunt
        aortocoronary bypass V45.81
        arteriovenous (for dialysis) V45.11
        cerebrospinal fluid V45.2
        vascular NEC V45.89
            aortocoronary (bypass) V45.81
        ventricular (communicating) (for
            drainage) V45.2
    sterilization
        tubal ligation V26.51
        vasectomy V26.52
    subdermal contraceptive device
        V45.52
    thymicolymphaticus 254.8
    thymicus 254.8
    thymolymphaticus 254.8
    tooth extraction 525.10
    tracheostomy V44.0
    transplant
        blood vessel V42.89
        bone V42.4
            marrow V42.81
        cornea V42.5
        heart V42.1
            valve V42.2
        intestine V42.84
        kidney V42.0
        liver V42.7
        lung V42.6
        organ V42.9
            removal (due to complication,
                failure, rejection or
                infection) V45.87
            specified site NEC V42.89
        pancreas V42.83
        peripheral stem cells V42.82
        skin V42.3
        stem cells, peripheral V42.82
        tissue V42.9
            specified type NEC V42.89
        vessel, blood V42.89

Status *(Continued)*
    tubal ligation V26.51
    underimmunization V15.83   ◀
    ureterostomy V44.6
    urethrostomy V44.6
    vagina, artificial V44.7
    vascular shunt NEC V45.89
        aortocoronary (bypass) V45.81
    vasectomy V26.52
    ventilator [respirator] V46.11
        encounter
            during
                mechanical failure V46.14
                power failure V46.12
            for weaning V46.13
    wheelchair confinement V46.3
    wrist prosthesis V43.63
Stave fracture - *see* Fracture, metacarpus,
    metacarpal bone(s)
Steal
    subclavian artery 435.2
    vertebral artery 435.1
Stealing, solitary, child problem *(see also*
    Disturbance, conduct) 312.1●
Steam burn - *see* Burn, by site
Steatocystoma multiplex 706.2
Steatoma (infected) 706.2
    eyelid (cystic) 374.84
        infected 373.13
Steatorrhea (chronic) 579.8
    with lacteal obstruction 579.2
    idiopathic 579.0
        adult 579.0
        infantile 579.0
    pancreatic 579.4
    primary 579.0
    secondary 579.8
    specified cause NEC 579.8
    tropical 579.1
Steatosis 272.8
    heart *(see also* Degeneration,
        myocardial) 429.1
    kidney 593.89
    liver 571.8
Steele-Richardson (-Olszewski)
    syndrome 333.0
Stein's syndrome (polycystic ovary) 256.4
Stein-Leventhal syndrome (polycystic
    ovary) 256.4
Steinbrocker's syndrome *(see also*
    Neuropathy, peripheral, autonomic)
    337.9
Steinert's disease 359.21
STEMI (ST elevation myocardial
    infarction) *(see also* - Infarct,
    myocardium, ST elevation) 410.9●
Stenocardia *(see also* Angina) 413.9
Stenocephaly 756.0
Stenosis (cicatricial) - *see also* Stricture
    ampulla of Vater 576.2
        with calculus, cholelithiasis, or
            stones - *see* Choledocholithiasis
    anus, anal (canal) (sphincter) 569.2
        congenital 751.2
    aorta (ascending) 747.22
        arch 747.10
        arteriosclerotic 440.0
        calcified 440.0
    aortic (valve) 424.1
        with
            mitral (valve)
                insufficiency or incompetence
                    396.2
                stenosis or obstruction 396.0

Stenosis *(Continued)*
    aortic *(Continued)*
        atypical 396.0
        congenital 746.3
        rheumatic 395.0
            with
                insufficiency, incompetency or
                    regurgitation 395.2
                    with mitral (valve) disease
                        396.8
                mitral (valve)
                    disease (stenosis) 396.0
                    insufficiency or
                        incompetence 396.2
                    stenosis or obstruction 396.0
        specified cause, except rheumatic
            424.1
        syphilitic 093.22
    aqueduct of Sylvius (congenital) 742.3
        with spina bifida *(see also* Spina
            bifida) 741.0●
        acquired 331.4
    artery NEC *(see also* Arteriosclerosis)
        447.1
        basilar - *see* Narrowing, artery,
            basilar
        carotid (common) (internal) - *see*
            Narrowing, artery, carotid
        celiac 447.4
        cerebral 437.0
            due to
                embolism *(see also* Embolism,
                    brain) 434.1●
                thrombus *(see also* Thrombosis,
                    brain) 434.0●
        extremities 440.20
        precerebral - *see* Narrowing, artery,
            precerebral
        pulmonary (congenital) 747.3
            acquired 417.8
        renal 440.1
        vertebral - *see* Narrowing, artery,
            vertebral
    bile duct or biliary passage *(see also*
        Obstruction, biliary) 576.2
        congenital 751.61
    bladder neck (acquired) 596.0
        congenital 753.6
    brain 348.89   ◀▥
    bronchus 519.19
        syphilitic 095.8
    cardia (stomach) 537.89
        congenital 750.7
    cardiovascular *(see also* Disease,
        cardiovascular) 429.2
    carotid artery - *see* Narrowing, artery,
        carotid
    cervix, cervical (canal) 622.4
        congenital 752.49
        in pregnancy or childbirth 654.6●
            affecting fetus or newborn
                763.89
            causing obstructed labor 660.2●
                affecting fetus or newborn
                    763.1
    colon *(see also* Obstruction, intestine)
        560.9
        congenital 751.2
    colostomy 569.62
    common bile duct *(see also* Obstruction,
        biliary) 576.2
        congenital 751.61
    coronary (artery) - *see* Arteriosclerosis,
        coronary

Stenosis (Continued)
  cystic duct (see also Obstruction,
    gallbladder) 575.2
    congenital 751.61
  due to (presence of) any device, implant,
    or graft classifiable to 996.0–996.5 -
    see Complications, due to
    (presence of) any device, implant,
    or graft classified to 996.0–996.5
    NEC
  duodenum 537.3
    congenital 751.1
  ejaculatory duct NEC 608.89
  endocervical os - see Stenosis, cervix
  enterostomy 569.62
  esophagostomy 530.87
  esophagus 530.3
    congenital 750.3
    syphilitic 095.8
      congenital 090.5
  external ear canal 380.50
    secondary to
      inflammation 380.53
      surgery 380.52
      trauma 380.51
  gallbladder (see also Obstruction,
    gallbladder) 575.2
  glottis 478.74
  heart valve (acquired) - see also
    Endocarditis
    congenital NEC 746.89
      aortic 746.3
      mitral 746.5
      pulmonary 746.02
      tricuspid 746.1
  hepatic duct (see also Obstruction,
    biliary) 576.2
  hymen 623.3
  hypertrophic subaortic (idiopathic)
    425.1
  infundibulum cardiac 746.83
  intestine (see also Obstruction, intestine)
    560.9
    congenital (small) 751.1
      large 751.2
  lacrimal
    canaliculi 375.53
    duct 375.56
      congenital 743.65
    punctum 375.52
      congenital 743.65
    sac 375.54
      congenital 743.65
  lacrimonasal duct 375.56
    congenital 743.65
    neonatal 375.55
  larynx 478.74
    congenital 748.3
    syphilitic 095.8
      congenital 090.5
  mitral (valve) (chronic) (inactive) 394.0
    with
      aortic (valve)
        disease (insufficiency) 396.1
        insufficiency or incompetence
          396.1
        stenosis or obstruction 396.0
      incompetency, insufficiency or
        regurgitation 394.2
        with aortic valve disease
          396.8
    active or acute 391.1
      with chorea (acute) (rheumatic)
        (Sydenham's) 392.0

Stenosis (Continued)
  mitral (Continued)
    congenital 746.5
    specified cause, except rheumatic
      424.0
    syphilitic 093.21
  myocardium, myocardial (see also
    Degeneration, myocardial)
    429.1
    hypertrophic subaortic (idiopathic)
      425.1
  nares (anterior) (posterior) 478.19
    congenital 748.0
  nasal duct 375.56
    congenital 743.65
  nasolacrimal duct 375.56
    congenital 743.65
    neonatal 375.55
  organ or site, congenital NEC - see
    Atresia
  papilla of Vater 576.2
    with calculus, cholelithiasis, or
      stones - see Choledocholithiasis
  pulmonary (artery) (congenital) 747.3
    with ventricular septal defect,
      dextraposition of aorta and
      hypertrophy of right ventricle
      745.2
    acquired 417.8
    infundibular 746.83
    in tetralogy of Fallot 745.2
    subvalvular 746.83
    valve (see also Endocarditis,
      pulmonary) 424.3
      congenital 746.02
    vein 747.49
      acquired 417.8
    vessel NEC 417.8
  pulmonic (congenital) 746.02
    infundibular 746.83
    subvalvular 746.83
  pylorus (hypertrophic) 537.0
    adult 537.0
    congenital 750.5
    infantile 750.5
  rectum (sphincter) (see also Stricture,
    rectum) 569.2
  renal artery 440.1
  salivary duct (any) 527.8
  sphincter of Oddi (see also Obstruction,
    biliary) 576.2
  spinal 724.00
    cervical 723.0
    lumbar, lumbosacral 724.02
    nerve (root) NEC 724.9
    specified region NEC 724.09
    thoracic, thoracolumbar 724.01
  stomach, hourglass 537.6
  subaortic 746.81
    hypertrophic (idiopathic) 425.1
  supra (valvular)-aortic 747.22
  trachea 519.19
    congenital 748.3
    syphilitic 095.8
    tuberculous (see also Tuberculosis)
      012.8●
  tracheostomy 519.02
  tricuspid (valve) (see also Endocarditis,
    tricuspid) 397.0
    congenital 746.1
    nonrheumatic 424.2
  tubal 628.2
  ureter (see also Stricture, ureter) 593.3
    congenital 753.29

Stenosis (Continued)
  urethra (see also Stricture, urethra)
    598.9
  vagina 623.2
    congenital 752.49
    in pregnancy or childbirth 654.7●
      affecting fetus or newborn
        763.89
      causing obstructed labor
        660.2●
        affecting fetus or newborn
          763.1
  valve (cardiac) (heart) (see also
    Endocarditis) 424.90
    congenital NEC 746.89
      aortic 746.3
      mitral 746.5
      pulmonary 746.02
      tricuspid 746.1
      urethra 753.6
  valvular (see also Endocarditis) 424.90
    congenital NEC 746.89
      urethra 753.6
  vascular graft or shunt 996.1
    atherosclerosis - see Arteriosclerosis,
      extremities
    embolism 996.74
    occlusion NEC 996.74
    thrombus 996.74
  vena cava (inferior) (superior) 459.2
    congenital 747.49
  ventricular shunt 996.2
  vulva 624.8
Stercolith (see also Fecalith) 560.39
  appendix 543.9
Stercoraceous, stercoral ulcer 569.82
  anus or rectum 569.41
Stereopsis, defective
  with fusion 368.33
  without fusion 368.32
Stereotypies NEC 307.3
Sterility
  female - see Infertility, female
  male (see also Infertility, male) 606.9
Sterilization, admission for V25.2
  status
    tubal ligation V26.51
    vasectomy V26.52
Sternalgia (see also Angina) 413.9
Sternopagus 759.4
Sternum bifidum 756.3
Sternutation 784.99
Steroid
  effects (adverse) (iatrogenic)
    cushingoid
      correct substance properly
        administered 255.0
      overdose or wrong substance
        given or taken 962.0
    diabetes - see Diabetes, secondary
      correct substance properly
        administered 251.8
      overdose or wrong substance
        given or taken 962.0
    due to
      correct substance properly
        administered 255.8
      overdose or wrong substance
        given or taken 962.0
    fever
      correct substance properly
        administered 780.60
      overdose or wrong substance
        given or taken 962.0

Steroid (*Continued*)
　effects (*Continued*)
　　withdrawal
　　　correct substance properly
　　　　administered 255.41
　　　overdose or wrong substance
　　　　given or taken 962.0
　　responder 365.03
Stevens-Johnson disease or syndrome
　(erythema multiforme exudativum)
　695.13
　toxic epidermal necrolysis overlap
　　(SJS-TEN overlap syndrome)
　　695.14
Stewart-Morel syndrome (hyperostosis
　frontalis interna) 733.3
Sticker's disease (erythema infectiosum)
　057.0
Stickler syndrome 759.89
Sticky eye 372.03
Stieda's disease (calcification, knee joint)
　726.62
Stiff
　back 724.8
　neck (*see also* Torticollis) 723.5
Stiff-baby 759.89
Stiff-man syndrome 333.91
Stiffness, joint NEC 719.50
　ankle 719.57
　back 724.8
　elbow 719.52
　finger 719.54
　hip 719.55
　knee 719.56
　multiple sites 719.59
　sacroiliac 724.6
　shoulder 719.51
　specified site NEC 719.58
　spine 724.9
　surgical fusion V45.4
　wrist 719.53
Stigmata, congenital syphilis 090.5
Still's disease or syndrome 714.30
　adult onset 714.2
Still-Felty syndrome (rheumatoid
　arthritis with splenomegaly and
　leukopenia) 714.1
Stillbirth, stillborn NEC 779.9
Stiller's disease (asthenia) 780.79
Stilling-Türk-Duane syndrome (ocular
　retraction syndrome) 378.71
Stimulation, ovary 256.1
Sting (animal) (bee) (fish) (insect)
　(jellyfish) (Portuguese man-o-war)
　(wasp) (venomous) 989.5
　anaphylactic shock or reaction
　　989.5
　plant 692.6
Stippled epiphyses 756.59
Stitch
　abscess 998.59
　burst (in external operation
　　wound) (*see also* Dehiscence)
　　998.32
　　internal 998.31
　in back 724.5
Stojano's (subcostal) syndrome 098.86
Stokes' disease (exophthalmic goiter)
　242.0●
Stokes-Adams syndrome (syncope with
　heart block) 426.9
Stokvis' (-Talma) disease (enterogenous
　cyanosis) 289.7
Stomach - *see* condition

Stoma malfunction
　colostomy 569.62
　cystostomy 997.5
　enterostomy 569.62
　esophagostomy 530.87
　gastrostomy 536.42
　ileostomy 569.62
　nephrostomy 997.5
　tracheostomy 519.02
　ureterostomy 997.5
Stomatitis 528.00
　angular 528.5
　　due to dietary or vitamin deficiency
　　　266.0
　aphthous 528.2
　bovine 059.11
　candidal 112.0
　catarrhal 528.00
　denture 528.9
　diphtheritic (membranous) 032.0
　due to
　　dietary deficiency 266.0
　　thrush 112.0
　　vitamin deficiency 266.0
　epidemic 078.4
　epizootic 078.4
　follicular 528.00
　gangrenous 528.1
　herpetic 054.2
　herpetiformis 528.2
　malignant 528.00
　membranous acute 528.00
　monilial 112.0
　mycotic 112.0
　necrotic 528.1
　　ulcerative 101
　necrotizing ulcerative 101
　parasitic 112.0
　septic 528.00
　specified NEC 528.09
　spirochetal 101
　suppurative (acute) 528.00
　ulcerative 528.00
　　necrotizing 101
　ulceromembranous 101
　vesicular 528.00
　　with exanthem 074.3
　Vincent's 101
Stomatocytosis 282.8
Stomatomycosis 112.0
Stomatorrhagia 528.9
Stone(s) - *see also* Calculus
　bladder 594.1
　　diverticulum 594.0
　cystine 270.0
　heart syndrome (*see also* Failure,
　　ventricular, left) 428.1
　kidney 592.0
　prostate 602.0
　pulp (dental) 522.2
　renal 592.0
　salivary duct or gland (any) 527.5
　ureter 592.1
　urethra (impacted) 594.2
　urinary (duct) (impacted) (passage)
　　592.9
　　bladder 594.1
　　　diverticulum 594.0
　　lower tract NEC 594.9
　　specified site 594.8
　xanthine 277.2
Stonecutters' lung 502
　tuberculous (*see also* Tuberculosis)
　　011.4●

Stonemasons'
　asthma, disease, or lung 502
　　tuberculous (*see also* Tuberculosis)
　　　011.4●
　phthisis (*see also* Tuberculosis) 011.4●
Stoppage
　bowel (*see also* Obstruction, intestine)
　　560.9
　heart (*see also* Arrest, cardiac) 427.5
　intestine (*see also* Obstruction, intestine)
　　560.9
　urine NEC (*see also* Retention, urine)
　　788.20
Storm, thyroid (apathetic) (*see also*
　Thyrotoxicosis) 242.9●
Strabismus (alternating) (congenital)
　(nonparalytic) 378.9
　concomitant (*see also* Heterotropia)
　　378.30
　　convergent (*see also* Esotropia)
　　　378.00
　　divergent (*see also* Exotropia)
　　　378.10
　convergent (*see also* Esotropia) 378.00
　divergent (*see also* Exotropia) 378.10
　due to adhesions, scars - *see*
　　Strabismus, mechanical
　in neuromuscular disorder NEC
　　378.73
　intermittent 378.20
　　vertical 378.31
　latent 378.40
　　convergent (esophoria) 378.41
　　divergent (exophoria) 378.42
　　vertical 378.43
　mechanical 378.60
　　due to
　　　Brown's tendon sheath syndrome
　　　　378.61
　　　specified musculofascial disorder
　　　　NEC 378.62
　paralytic 378.50
　　third or oculomotor nerve (partial)
　　　378.51
　　　total 378.52
　　fourth or trochlear nerve 378.53
　　sixth or abducens nerve 378.54
　specified type NEC 378.73
　vertical (hypertropia) 378.31
Strain - *see also* Sprain, by site
　eye NEC 368.13
　heart - *see* Disease, heart
　meaning gonorrhea - *see* Gonorrhea
　on urination 788.65
　physical NEC V62.89
　postural 729.90
　psychological NEC V62.89
Strands
　conjunctiva 372.62
　vitreous humor 379.25
Strangulation, strangulated 994.7
　appendix 543.9
　asphyxiation or suffocation by 994.7
　bladder neck 596.0
　bowel - *see* Strangulation, intestine
　colon - *see* Strangulation, intestine
　cord (umbilical) - *see* Compression,
　　umbilical cord
　due to birth injury 767.8
　food or foreign body (*see also* Asphyxia,
　　food) 933.1
　hemorrhoids 455.8
　　external 455.5
　　internal 455.2

◀ New　　◀▥ Revised　　~~deleted~~ Deleted　　● Use Additional Digit(s)　　▨ Omit code

Strangulation, strangulated (*Continued*)
hernia - *see also* Hernia, by site, with
  obstruction
  gangrenous - *see* Hernia, by site,
    with gangrene
  intestine (large) (small) 560.2
    with hernia - *see also* Hernia, by site,
      with obstruction
      gangrenous - *see* Hernia, by site,
        with gangrene
    congenital (small) 751.1
      large 751.2
  mesentery 560.2
  mucus (*see also* Asphyxia, mucus)
    933.1
    newborn 770.18
  omentum 560.2
  organ or site, congenital NEC - *see*
    Atresia
  ovary 620.8
    due to hernia 620.4
  penis 607.89
    foreign body 939.3
  rupture (*see also* Hernia, by site, with
    obstruction) 552.9
    gangrenous (*see also* Hernia, by site,
      with gangrene) 551.9
  stomach, due to hernia (*see also*
    Hernia, by site, with obstruction)
    552.9
    with gangrene (*see also* Hernia, by
      site, with gangrene) 551.9
  umbilical cord - *see* Compression,
    umbilical cord
  vesicourethral orifice 596.0
Stranguary 788.1
Strawberry
  gallbladder (*see also* Disease,
    gallbladder) 575.6
  mark 757.32
  tongue (red) (white) 529.3
Straw itch 133.8
Streak, ovarian 752.0
Strephosymbolia 315.01
  secondary to organic lesion 784.69
Streptobacillary fever 026.1
Streptobacillus moniliformis 026.1
Streptococcemia 038.0
Streptococcicosis - *see* Infection,
  streptococcal
Streptococcus, streptococcal - *see*
  condition
Streptoderma 686.00
Streptomycosis - *see* Actinomycosis
Streptothricosis - *see* Actinomycosis
Streptothrix - *see* Actinomycosis
Streptotrichosis - *see* Actinomycosis
Stress 308.9
  fracture - *see* Fracture, stress
  polycythemia 289.0
  reaction (gross) (*see also* Reaction,
    stress, acute) 308.9
Stretching, nerve - *see* Injury, nerve, by
  site
Striae (albicantes) (atrophicae) (cutis
  distensae) (distensae) 701.3
Striations of nails 703.8
Stricture (*see also* Stenosis) 799.89
  ampulla of Vater 576.2
    with calculus, cholelithiasis, or
      stones - *see* Choledocholithiasis
  anus (sphincter) 569.2
    congenital 751.2
    infantile 751.2

Stricture (*Continued*)
aorta (ascending) 747.22
  arch 747.10
  arteriosclerotic 440.0
  calcified 440.0
aortic (valve) (*see also* Stenosis, aortic)
  424.1
  congenital 746.3
aqueduct of Sylvius (congenital)
  742.3
  with spina bifida (*see also* Spina
    bifida) 741.0●
  acquired 331.4
artery 447.1
  basilar - *see* Narrowing, artery,
    basilar
  carotid (common) (internal) - *see*
    Narrowing, artery, carotid
  celiac 447.4
  cerebral 437.0
    congenital 747.81
    due to
      embolism (*see also* Embolism,
        brain) 434.1●
      thrombus (*see also* Thrombosis,
        brain) 434.0●
  congenital (peripheral) 747.60
    cerebral 747.81
    coronary 746.85
    gastrointestinal 747.61
    lower limb 747.64
    renal 747.62
    retinal 743.58
    specified NEC 747.69
    spinal 747.82
    umbilical 747.5
    upper limb 747.63
  coronary - *see* Arteriosclerosis,
    coronary
    congenital 746.85
  precerebral - *see* Narrowing, artery,
    precerebral NEC
  pulmonary (congenital) 747.3
    acquired 417.8
  renal 440.1
  vertebral - *see* Narrowing, artery,
    vertebral
auditory canal (congenital) (external)
  744.02
  acquired (*see also* Stricture, ear canal,
    acquired) 380.50
bile duct or passage (any)
  (postoperative) (*see also*
    Obstruction, biliary) 576.2
  congenital 751.61
bladder 596.8
  congenital 753.6
  neck 596.0
    congenital 753.6
bowel (*see also* Obstruction, intestine)
  560.9
brain 348.89   ◄▥
bronchus 519.19
  syphilitic 095.8
cardia (stomach) 537.89
  congenital 750.7
cardiac - *see also* Disease, heart orifice
  (stomach) 537.89
cardiovascular (*see also* Disease,
  cardiovascular) 429.2
carotid artery - *see* Narrowing, artery,
  carotid
cecum (*see also* Obstruction, intestine)
  560.9

Stricture (*Continued*)
cervix, cervical (canal) 622.4
  congenital 752.49
  in pregnancy or childbirth
    654.6●
    affecting fetus or newborn
      763.89
    causing obstructed labor
      660.2●
      affecting fetus or newborn
        763.1
colon (*see also* Obstruction, intestine)
  560.9
  congenital 751.2
colostomy 569.62
common bile duct (*see also* Obstruction,
  biliary) 576.2
  congenital 751.61
coronary (artery) - *see* Arteriosclerosis,
  coronary
  congenital 746.85
cystic duct (*see also* Obstruction,
  gallbladder) 575.2
  congenital 751.61
cystostomy 997.5
digestive organs NEC, congenital
  751.8
duodenum 537.3
  congenital 751.1
ear canal (external) (congenital)
  744.02
  acquired 380.50
    secondary to
      inflammation 380.53
      surgery 380.52
      trauma 380.51
ejaculatory duct 608.85
enterostomy 569.62
esophagostomy 530.87
esophagus (corrosive) (peptic)
  530.3
  congenital 750.3
  syphilitic 095.8
    congenital 090.5
Eustachian tube (*see also* Obstruction,
  Eustachian tube) 381.60
  congenital 744.24
fallopian tube 628.2
  gonococcal (chronic) 098.37
    acute 098.17
  tuberculous (*see also* Tuberculosis)
    016.6●
gallbladder (*see also* Obstruction,
  gallbladder) 575.2
  congenital 751.69
glottis 478.74
heart - *see also* Disease, heart
  congenital NEC 746.89
  valve - *see also* Endocarditis
    congenital NEC 746.89
      aortic 746.3
      mitral 746.5
      pulmonary 746.02
      tricuspid 746.1
hepatic duct (*see also* Obstruction,
  biliary) 576.2
hourglass, of stomach 537.6
hymen 623.3
hypopharynx 478.29
intestine (*see also* Obstruction, intestine)
  560.9
  congenital (small) 751.1
    large 751.2
  ischemic 557.1

Stricture (Continued)
  lacrimal
    canaliculi 375.53
      congenital 743.65
    punctum 375.52
      congenital 743.65
    sac 375.54
      congenital 743.65
  lacrimonasal duct 375.56
    congenital 743.65
    neonatal 375.55
  larynx 478.79
    congenital 748.3
    syphilitic 095.8
      congenital 090.5
  lung 518.89
  meatus
    ear (congenital) 744.02
      acquired (see also Stricture, ear
        canal, acquired) 380.50
    osseous (congenital) (ear) 744.03
      acquired (see also Stricture, ear
        canal, acquired) 380.50
    urinarius (see also Stricture, urethra)
      598.9
      congenital 753.6
  mitral (valve) (see also Stenosis, mitral)
    394.0
    congenital 746.5
    specified cause, except rheumatic
      424.0
  myocardium, myocardial (see also
    Degeneration, myocardial)
    429.1
    hypertrophic subaortic (idiopathic)
      425.1
  nares (anterior) (posterior) 478.19
    congenital 748.0
  nasal duct 375.56
    congenital 743.65
    neonatal 375.55
  nasolacrimal duct 375.56
    congenital 743.65
    neonatal 375.55
  nasopharynx 478.29
    syphilitic 095.8
  nephrostomy 997.5
  nose 478.19
    congenital 748.0
  nostril (anterior) (posterior) 478.19
    congenital 748.0
  organ or site, congenital NEC - see
    Atresia
  osseous meatus (congenital) (ear)
    744.03
    acquired (see also Stricture, ear canal,
      acquired) 380.50
  os uteri (see also Stricture, cervix)
    622.4
  oviduct - see Stricture, fallopian tube
  pelviureteric junction 593.3
  pharynx (dilation) 478.29
  prostate 602.8
  pulmonary, pulmonic
    artery (congenital) 747.3
      acquired 417.8
      noncongenital 417.8
    infundibulum (congenital) 746.83
    valve (see also Endocarditis,
      pulmonary) 424.3
      congenital 746.02
    vein (congenital) 747.49
      acquired 417.8
    vessel NEC 417.8

Stricture (Continued)
  punctum lacrimale 375.52
    congenital 743.65
  pylorus (hypertrophic) 537.0
    adult 537.0
    congenital 750.5
    infantile 750.5
  rectosigmoid 569.89
  rectum (sphincter) 569.2
    congenital 751.2
    due to
      chemical burn 947.3
      irradiation 569.2
      lymphogranuloma venereum
        099.1
    gonococcal 098.7
    inflammatory 099.1
    syphilitic 095.8
    tuberculous (see also Tuberculosis)
      014.8●
  renal artery 440.1
  salivary duct or gland (any) 527.8
  sigmoid (flexure) (see also Obstruction,
    intestine) 560.9
  spermatic cord 608.85
  stoma (following) (of)
    colostomy 569.62
    cystostomy 997.5
    enterostomy 569.62
    esophagostomy 530.87
    gastrostomy 536.42
    ileostomy 569.62
    nephrostomy 997.5
    tracheostomy 519.02
    ureterostomy 997.5
  stomach 537.89
    congenital 750.7
    hourglass 537.6
  subaortic 746.81
    hypertrophic (acquired) (idiopathic)
      425.1
  subglottic 478.74
  syphilitic NEC 095.8
  tendon (sheath) 727.81
  trachea 519.19
    congenital 748.3
    syphilitic 095.8
    tuberculous (see also Tuberculosis)
      012.8●
  tracheostomy 519.02
  tricuspid (valve) (see also Endocarditis,
    tricuspid) 397.0
    congenital 746.1
    nonrheumatic 424.2
  tunica vaginalis 608.85
  ureter (postoperative) 593.3
    congenital 753.29
    tuberculous (see also Tuberculosis)
      016.2●
  ureteropelvic junction 593.3
    congenital 753.21
  ureterovesical orifice 593.3
    congenital 753.22
  urethra (anterior) (meatal) (organic)
    (posterior) (spasmodic) 598.9
    associated with schistosomiasis (see
      also Schistosomiasis) 120.9
      [598.01]
    congenital (valvular) 753.6
    due to
      infection 598.00
        syphilis 095.8 [598.01]
      trauma 598.1
    gonococcal 098.2 [598.01]

Stricture (Continued)
  urethra (Continued)
    gonorrheal 098.2 [598.01]
    infective 598.00
    late effect of injury 598.1
    postcatheterization 598.2
    postobstetric 598.1
    postoperative 598.2
    specified cause NEC 598.8
    syphilitic 095.8 [598.01]
    traumatic 598.1
    valvular, congenital 753.6
  urinary meatus (see also Stricture,
    urethra) 598.9
    congenital 753.6
  uterus, uterine 621.5
    os (external) (internal) - see Stricture,
      cervix
  vagina (outlet) 623.2
    congenital 752.49
  valve (cardiac) (heart) (see also
    Endocarditis) 424.90
    congenital (cardiac) (heart) NEC
      746.89
      aortic 746.3
      mitral 746.5
      pulmonary 746.02
      tricuspid 746.1
      urethra 753.6
  valvular (see also Endocarditis)
    424.90
  vascular graft or shunt 996.1
    atherosclerosis - see Arteriosclerosis,
      extremities
    embolism 996.74
    occlusion NEC 996.74
    thrombus 996.74
  vas deferens 608.85
    congenital 752.89
  vein 459.2
  vena cava (inferior) (superior) NEC
    459.2
    congenital 747.49
  ventricular shunt 996.2
  vesicourethral orifice 596.0
    congenital 753.6
  vulva (acquired) 624.8
Stridor 786.1
  congenital (larynx) 748.3
Stridulous - see condition
Strippling of nails 703.8
Stroke 434.91
  apoplectic (see also Disease,
    cerebrovascular, acute) 436
  brain - see Infarct, brain
  embolic 434.11
  epileptic - see Epilepsy
  healed or old V12.54
  heart - see Disease, heart
  heat 992.0
  hemorrhagic - see Hemorrhage, brain
  iatrogenic 997.02
  in evolution 434.91
  ischemic 434.91
  late effect - see Late effect(s) (of)
    cerebrovascular disease
  lightning 994.0
  paralytic - see Infarct, brain
  postoperative 997.02
  progressive 435.9
  thrombotic 434.01
Stromatosis, endometrial (M8931/1)
  236.0
Strong pulse 785.9

◀ New   ◀▥ Revised   ~~deleted~~ Deleted   ● Use Additional Digit(s)   ▨ Omit code

Strongyloides stercoralis infestation 127.2
Strongyloidiasis 127.2
Strongyloidosis 127.2
Strongylus (gibsoni) infestation 127.7
Strophulus (newborn) 779.89
　　pruriginosus 698.2
Struck by lighting 994.0
Struma (see also Goiter) 240.9
　　fibrosa 245.3
　　Hashimoto (struma lymphomatosa)
　　　　245.2
　　lymphomatosa 245.2
　　nodosa (simplex) 241.9
　　　　endemic 241.9
　　　　multinodular 241.1
　　　　sporadic 241.9
　　　　toxic or with hyperthyroidism
　　　　　　242.3●
　　　　　　multinodular 242.2●
　　　　　　uninodular 242.1●
　　　　toxicosa 242.3●
　　　　　　multinodular 242.2●
　　　　　　uninodular 242.1●
　　　　uninodular 241.0
　　ovarii (M9090/0) 220
　　　　and carcinoid (M9091/1) 236.2
　　　　malignant (M9090/3) 183.0
　　Riedel's (ligneous thyroiditis) 245.3
　　scrofulous (see also Tuberculosis) 017.2●
　　tuberculous (see also Tuberculosis)
　　　　017.2●
　　　　abscess 017.2●
　　　　adenitis 017.2●
　　　　lymphangitis 017.2●
　　　　ulcer 017.2●
Strumipriva cachexia (see also
　　Hypothyroidism) 244.9
Strümpell-Marie disease or spine
　　(ankylosing spondylitis) 720.0
Strümpell-Westphal pseudosclerosis
　　(hepatolenticular degeneration) 275.1
Stuart's disease (congenital factor X
　　deficiency) (see also Defect,
　　coagulation) 286.3
Stuart-Prower factor deficiency
　　(congenital factor X deficiency) (see
　　also Defect, coagulation) 286.3
Students' elbow 727.2
Stuffy nose 478.19
Stump - see also Amputation
　　cervix, cervical (healed) 622.8
Stupor 780.09
　　catatonic (see also Schizophrenia)
　　　　295.2●
　　circular (see also Psychosis, manic-
　　　　depressive, circular) 296.7
　　manic 296.89
　　manic-depressive (see also Psychosis,
　　　　affective) 296.89
　　mental (anergic) (delusional) 298.9
　　psychogenic 298.8
　　reaction to exceptional stress (transient)
　　　　308.2
　　traumatic NEC - see also Injury,
　　　　intracranial
　　　　with spinal (cord)
　　　　　　lesion - see Injury, spinal, by site
　　　　　　shock - see Injury, spinal, by site
Sturge (-Weber) (-Dimitri) disease or
　　syndrome (encephalocutaneous
　　angiomatosis) 759.6
Sturge-Kalischer-Weber syndrome
　　(encephalocutaneous angiomatosis)
　　759.6

Stuttering 307.0
　　due to late effect of cerebrovascular
　　　　disease (see also Late effect(s) (of)
　　　　cerebrovascular disease) 438.14 ◄
Sty, stye 373.11
　　external 373.11
　　internal 373.12
　　meibomian 373.12
Subacidity, gastric 536.8
　　psychogenic 306.4
Subacute - see condition
Subarachnoid - see condition
Subclavian steal syndrome 435.2
Subcortical - see condition
Subcostal syndrome 098.86
　　nerve compression 354.8
Subcutaneous, subcuticular - see
　　condition
Subdelirium 293.1
Subdural - see condition
Subendocardium - see condition
Subependymoma (M9383/1) 237.5
Suberosis 495.3
Subglossitis - see Glossitis
Subhemophilia 286.0
Subinvolution (uterus) 621.1
　　breast (postlactational) (postpartum)
　　　　611.89
　　chronic 621.1
　　puerperal, postpartum 674.8●
Sublingual - see condition
Sublinguitis 527.2
Subluxation - see also Dislocation, by site
　　congenital NEC - see also Malposition,
　　　　congenital
　　　　hip (unilateral) 754.32
　　　　　　with dislocation of other hip
　　　　　　　　754.35
　　　　　　bilateral 754.33
　　　　joint
　　　　　　lower limb 755.69
　　　　　　shoulder 755.59
　　　　　　upper limb 755.59
　　　　lower limb (joint) 755.69
　　　　shoulder (joint) 755.59
　　　　upper limb (joint) 755.59
　　lens 379.32
　　　　anterior 379.33
　　　　posterior 379.34
　　radial head 832.2　　　　　　　　　◄
　　rotary, cervical region of spine - see
　　　　Fracture, vertebra, cervical
Submaxillary - see condition
Submersion (fatal) (nonfatal) 994.1
Submissiveness (undue), in child
　　313.0
Submucous - see condition
Subnormal, subnormality
　　accommodation (see also Disorder,
　　　　accommodation) 367.9
　　mental (see also Retardation, mental)
　　　　319
　　　　mild 317
　　　　moderate 318.0
　　　　profound 318.2
　　　　severe 318.1
　　temperature (accidental) 991.6
　　　　not associated with low
　　　　　　environmental temperature
　　　　　　780.99
Subphrenic - see condition
Subscapular nerve - see condition
Subseptus uterus 752.3
Subsiding appendicitis 542

Substance abuse in family V61.42　　◄
Substernal thyroid (see also Goiter) 240.9
　　congenital 759.2
Substitution disorder 300.11
Subtentorial - see condition
Subtertian
　　fever 084.0
　　malaria (fever) 084.0
Subthyroidism (acquired) (see also
　　Hypothyroidism) 244.9
　　congenital 243
Succenturiata placenta - see Placenta,
　　abnormal
Succussion sounds, chest 786.7
Sucking thumb, child 307.9
Sudamen 705.1
Sudamina 705.1
Sudanese kala-azar 085.0
Sudden
　　death, cause unknown (less than 24
　　　　hours) 798.1
　　　　cardiac (SCD)
　　　　　　family history of V17.41
　　　　　　personal history of, successfully
　　　　　　　　resuscitated V12.53
　　　　during childbirth 669.9●
　　　　infant 798.0
　　　　puerperal, postpartum 674.9●
　　hearing loss NEC 388.2
　　heart failure (see also Failure, heart)
　　　　428.9
　　infant death syndrome 798.0
Sudeck's atrophy, disease, or syndrome
　　733.7
SUDS (Sudden unexplained death) 798.2
Suffocation (see also Asphyxia) 799.01
　　by
　　　　bed clothes 994.7
　　　　bunny bag 994.7
　　　　cave-in 994.7
　　　　constriction 994.7
　　　　drowning 994.1
　　　　inhalation
　　　　　　food or foreign body (see also
　　　　　　　　Asphyxia, food or foreign
　　　　　　　　body) 933.1
　　　　　　oil or gasoline (see also Asphyxia,
　　　　　　　　food or foreign body)
　　　　　　　　933.1
　　　　overlying 994.7
　　　　plastic bag 994.7
　　　　pressure 994.7
　　　　strangulation 994.7
　　during birth 768.1
　　mechanical 994.7
Sugar
　　blood
　　　　high 790.29
　　　　low 251.2
　　in urine 791.5
Suicide, suicidal (attempted)
　　by poisoning - see Table of Drugs and
　　　　Chemicals
　　ideation V62.84
　　risk 300.9
　　tendencies 300.9
　　trauma NEC (see also nature and site of
　　　　injury) 959.9
Suipestifer infection (see also Infection,
　　Salmonella) 003.9
Sulfatidosis 330.0
Sulfhemoglobinemia,
　　sulphemoglobinemia (acquired)
　　(congenital) 289.7

Sumatran mite fever 081.2
Summer - see condition
Sunburn 692.71
  dermatitis 692.71
  due to
    other ultraviolet radiation
      692.82
    tanning bed 692.82
  first degree 692.71
  second degree 692.76
  third degree 692.77
SUNCT (short lasting unilateral
  neuralgiform headache with
  conjunctival injection and tearing)
  339.05
Sunken
  acetabulum 718.85
  fontanels 756.0
Sunstroke 992.0
Superfecundation 651.9●
  with fetal loss and retention of one or
    more fetus(es) 651.6●
  following (elective) fetal reduction
    651.7●
Superfetation 651.9●
  with fetal loss and retention of one or
    more fetus(es) 651.6●
  following (elective) fetal reduction
    651.7●
Superinvolution uterus 621.8
Supernumerary (congenital)
  aortic cusps 746.89
  auditory ossicles 744.04
  bone 756.9
  breast 757.6
  carpal bones 755.56
  cusps, heart valve NEC 746.89
    mitral 746.5
    pulmonary 746.09
  digit(s) 755.00
    finger 755.01
    toe 755.02
  ear (lobule) 744.1
  fallopian tube 752.19
  finger 755.01
  hymen 752.49
  kidney 753.3
  lacrimal glands 743.64
  lacrimonasal duct 743.65
  lobule (ear) 744.1
  mitral cusps 746.5
  muscle 756.82
  nipples 757.6
  organ or site NEC - see Accessory
  ossicles, auditory 744.04
  ovary 752.0
  oviduct 752.19
  pulmonic cusps 746.09
  rib 756.3
    cervical or first 756.2
      syndrome 756.2
  roots (of teeth) 520.2
  spinal vertebra 756.19
  spleen 759.0
  tarsal bones 755.67
  teeth 520.1
    causing crowding 524.31
  testis 752.89
  thumb 755.01
  toe 755.02
  uterus 752.2
  vagina 752.49
  vertebra 756.19

Supervision (of)
  contraceptive method previously
    prescribed V25.40
    intrauterine device V25.42
    oral contraceptive (pill) V25.41
    specified type NEC V25.49
    subdermal implantable
      contraceptive V25.43
  dietary (for) V65.3
    allergy (food) V65.3
    colitis V65.3
    diabetes mellitus V65.3
    food allergy intolerance V65.3
    gastritis V65.3
    hypercholesterolemia V65.3
    hypoglycemia V65.3
    intolerance (food) V65.3
    obesity V65.3
    specified NEC V65.3
  lactation V24.1
  newborn health ◄
    8 to 28 days old V20.32 ◄
    under 8 days old V20.31 ◄
  pregnancy - see Pregnancy,
    supervision of
Supplemental teeth 520.1
  causing crowding 524.31
Suppression
  binocular vision 368.31
  lactation 676.5●
  menstruation 626.8
  ovarian secretion 256.39
  renal 586
  urinary secretion 788.5
  urine 788.5
Suppuration, suppurative - see also
    condition
  accessory sinus (chronic) (see also
    Sinusitis) 473.9
  adrenal gland 255.8
  antrum (chronic) (see also Sinusitis,
    maxillary) 473.0
  bladder (see also Cystitis) 595.89
  bowel 569.89
  brain 324.0
    late effect 326
  breast 611.0
    puerperal, postpartum 675.1●
  dental periosteum 526.5
  diffuse (skin) 686.00
  ear (middle) (see also Otitis media)
    382.4
    external (see also Otitis, externa)
      380.10
    internal 386.33
  ethmoidal (sinus) (chronic) (see also
    Sinusitis, ethmoidal) 473.2
  fallopian tube (see also Salpingo-
    oophoritis) 614.2
  frontal (sinus) (chronic) (see also
    Sinusitis, frontal) 473.1
  gallbladder (see also Cholecystitis,
    acute) 575.0
  gum 523.30
  hernial sac - see Hernia, by site
  intestine 569.89
  joint (see also Arthritis, suppurative)
    711.0●
  labyrinthine 386.33
  lung 513.0
  mammary gland 611.0
    puerperal, postpartum 675.1●
  maxilla, maxillary 526.4
    sinus (chronic) (see also Sinusitis,
      maxillary) 473.0
  muscle 728.0

Suppuration, suppurative (Continued)
  nasal sinus (chronic) (see also Sinusitis)
    473.9
  pancreas 577.0
  parotid gland 527.2
  pelvis, pelvic
    female (see also Disease, pelvis,
      inflammatory) 614.4
    acute 614.3
    male (see also Peritonitis) 567.21
  pericranial (see also Osteomyelitis)
    730.2●
  salivary duct or gland (any) 527.2
  sinus (nasal) (see also Sinusitis) 473.9
  sphenoidal (sinus) (chronic) (see also
    Sinusitis, sphenoidal) 473.3
  thymus (gland) 254.1
  thyroid (gland) 245.0
  tonsil 474.8
  uterus (see also Endometritis) 615.9
  vagina 616.10
  wound - see also Wound, open, by site,
    complicated
    dislocation - see Dislocation, by site,
      compound
    fracture - see Fracture, by site, open
    scratch or other superficial injury -
      see Injury, superficial, by site
Supraeruption, teeth 524.34
Supraglottitis 464.50
  with obstruction 464.51
Suprapubic drainage 596.8
Suprarenal (gland) - see condition
Suprascapular nerve - see condition
Suprasellar - see condition
Supraspinatus syndrome 726.10
Surfer knots 919.8
  infected 919.9
Surgery
  cosmetic NEC V50.1
    breast reconstruction following
      mastectomy V51.0
    following healed injury or operation
      V51.8
    hair transplant V50.0
  elective V50.9
    breast
      augmentation or reduction
        V50.1
      reconstruction following
        mastectomy V51.0
    circumcision, ritual or routine (in
      absence of medical indication)
      V50.2
    cosmetic NEC V50.1
    ear piercing V50.3
    face-lift V50.1
    following healed injury or operation
      V51.8
    hair transplant V50.0
  not done because of
    contraindication V64.1
    patient's decision V64.2
    specified reason NEC V64.3
  plastic
    breast
      augmentation or reduction
        V50.1
      reconstruction following
        mastectomy V51.0
    cosmetic V50.1
    face-lift V50.1
    following healed injury or operation
      V51.8

◄ New   ◄▮▮▮ Revised   ~~deleted~~ Deleted   ● Use Additional Digit(s)   ▒ Omit code

Surgery (Continued)
  plastic (Continued)
    repair of scarred tissue (following
        healed injury or operation)
        V51.8
    specified type NEC V50.8
  previous, in pregnancy or childbirth
    cervix 654.6●
      affecting fetus or newborn (see
          also Newborn, affected by)
          760.63
      causing obstructed labor 660.2●
        affecting fetus or newborn
            763.1
    pelvic soft tissues NEC 654.9●
      affecting fetus or newborn (see
          also Newborn, affected by)
          760.63
      causing obstructed labor
          660.2●
        affecting fetus or newborn
            763.1
    perineum or vulva 654.8●
    uterus NEC 654.9●
      affecting fetus or newborn (see
          also Newborn, affected by)
          760.63
      causing obstructed labor
          660.2●
        affecting fetus or newborn
            763.1
      from previous cesarean delivery
          654.2●
    vagina 654.7●
Surgical
  abortion - see Abortion, legal
  emphysema 998.81
  kidney (see also Pyelitis) 590.80
  operation NEC 799.9
  procedures, complication or
      misadventure - see Complications,
      surgical procedure
  shock 998.0
Survey
  fetal anatomic V28.81
Susceptibility
  genetic
    to
      MEN (multiple endocrine
          neoplasia) V84.81
      neoplasia
        multiple endocrine [MEN]
            V84.81
      neoplasm
        malignant, of
          breast V84.01
          endometrium V84.04
          other V84.09
          ovary V84.02
          prostate V84.03
          specified disease NEC
              V84.89
Suspected condition, ruled out (see also
    Observation, suspected) V71.9
  specified condition NEC V71.89
Suspended uterus, in pregnancy or
    childbirth 654.4●
  affecting fetus or newborn 763.89
  causing obstructed labor 660.2●
    affecting fetus or newborn 763.1
Sutton's disease 709.09
Sutton and Gull's disease (arteriolar
    nephrosclerosis) (see also
    Hypertension, kidney) 403.90

Suture
  burst (in external operation wound)
      (see also Dehiscence) 998.32
    internal 998.31
  inadvertently left in operation wound
      998.4
  removal V58.32
  Shirodkar, in pregnancy (with or
      without cervical incompetence)
      654.5●
Swab inadvertently left in operation
    wound 998.4
Swallowed, swallowing
  difficulty (see also Dysphagia) 787.20
  foreign body NEC (see also Foreign
      body) 938
Swamp fever 100.89
Swan neck hand (intrinsic) 736.09
Sweat(s), sweating
  disease or sickness 078.2
  excessive (see also Hyperhidrosis)
      780.8
  fetid 705.89
  fever 078.2
  gland disease 705.9
    specified type NEC 705.89
  miliary 078.2
  night 780.8
Sweeley-Klionsky disease
    (angiokeratoma corporis diffusum)
    272.7
Sweet's syndrome (acute febrile
    neutrophilic dermatosis) 695.89
Swelling 782.3
  abdominal (not referable to specific
      organ) 789.3●
  adrenal gland, cloudy 255.8
  ankle 719.07
  anus 787.99
  arm 729.81
  breast 611.72
  Calabar 125.2
  cervical gland 785.6
  cheek 784.2
  chest 786.6
  ear 388.8
  epigastric 789.3●
  extremity (lower) (upper) 729.81
  eye 379.92
  female genital organ 625.8
  finger 729.81
  foot 729.81
  glands 785.6
  gum 784.2
  hand 729.81
  head 784.2
  inflammatory - see Inflammation
  joint (see also Effusion, joint) 719.0●
    tuberculous - see Tuberculosis, joint
  kidney, cloudy 593.89
  leg 729.81
  limb 729.81
  liver 573.8
  lung 786.6
  lymph nodes 785.6
  mediastinal 786.6
  mouth 784.2
  muscle (limb) 729.81
  neck 784.2
  nose or sinus 784.2
  palate 784.2
  pelvis 789.3●
  penis 607.83
  perineum 625.8

Swelling (Continued)
  rectum 787.99
  scrotum 608.86
  skin 782.2
  splenic (see also Splenomegaly) 789.2
  substernal 786.6
  superficial, localized (skin) 782.2
  testicle 608.86
  throat 784.2
  toe 729.81
  tongue 784.2
  tubular (see also Disease, renal) 593.9
  umbilicus 789.3●
  uterus 625.8
  vagina 625.8
  vulva 625.8
  wandering, due to Gnathostoma
      (spinigerum) 128.1
  white - see Tuberculosis, arthritis
Swift's disease 985.0
Swimmers'
  ear (acute) 380.12
  itch 120.3
Swimming in the head 780.4
Swollen - see also Swelling
  glands 785.6
Swyer-James syndrome (unilateral
    hyperlucent lung) 492.8
Swyer's syndrome (XY pure gonadal
    dysgenesis) 752.7
Sycosis 704.8
  barbae (not parasitic) 704.8
  contagiosa 110.0
  lupoid 704.8
  mycotic 110.0
  parasitic 110.0
  vulgaris 704.8
Sydenham's chorea - see Chorea,
    Sydenham's
Sylvatic yellow fever 060.0
Sylvest's disease (epidemic pleurodynia)
    074.1
Symblepharon 372.63
  congenital 743.62
Symonds' syndrome 348.2
Sympathetic - see condition
Sympatheticotonia (see also Neuropathy,
    peripheral, autonomic) 337.9
Sympathicoblastoma (M9500/3)
  specified site - see Neoplasm, by site,
      malignant
  unspecified site 194.0
Sympathicogonioma (M9500/3) - see
    Sympathicoblastoma
Sympathoblastoma (M9500/3) - see
    Sympathicoblastoma
Sympathogonioma (M9500/3) - see
    Sympathicoblastoma
Symphalangy (see also Syndactylism) 755.10
Symptoms, specified (general) NEC
    780.99
  abdomen NEC 789.9
  bone NEC 733.90
  breast NEC 611.79
  cardiac NEC 785.9
  cardiovascular NEC 785.9
  chest NEC 786.9
  development NEC 783.9
  digestive system NEC 787.99
  emotional state NEC 799.29
  eye NEC 379.99
  gastrointestinal tract NEC 787.99
  genital organs NEC
    female 625.9
    male 608.9

Symptoms, specified *(Continued)*
  head and neck NEC 784.99
  heart NEC 785.9
  joint NEC 719.60
    ankle 719.67
    elbow 719.62
    foot 719.67
    hand 719.64
    hip 719.65
    knee 719.66
    multiple sites 719.69
    pelvic region 719.65
    shoulder (region) 719.61
    specified site NEC 719.68
    wrist 719.63
  larynx NEC 784.99
  limbs NEC 729.89
  lymphatic system NEC 785.9
  menopausal 627.2
  metabolism NEC 783.9
  mouth NEC 528.9
  muscle NEC 728.9
  musculoskeletal NEC 781.99
    limbs NEC 729.89
  nervous system NEC 781.99
  neurotic NEC 300.9
  nutrition, metabolism, and
    development NEC 783.9
  pelvis NEC 789.9
    female 625.9
  peritoneum NEC 789.9
  respiratory system NEC 786.9
  skin and integument NEC 782.9
  subcutaneous tissue NEC 782.9
  throat NEC 784.99
  tonsil NEC 784.99
  urinary system NEC 788.99
  vascular NEC 785.9
Sympus 759.89
Synarthrosis 719.80
  ankle 719.87
  elbow 719.82
  foot 719.87
  hand 719.84
  hip 719.85
  knee 719.86
  multiple sites 719.89
  pelvic region 719.85
  shoulder (region) 719.81
  specified site NEC 719.88
  wrist 719.83
Syncephalus 759.4
Synchondrosis 756.9
  abnormal (congenital) 756.9
  ischiopubic (van Neck's) 732.1
Synchysis (senile) (vitreous humor)
  379.21
  scintillans 379.22
Syncope (near) (pre-) 780.2
  anginosa 413.9
  bradycardia 427.89
  cardiac 780.2
  carotid sinus 337.01
  complicating delivery 669.2●
  due to lumbar puncture 349.0
  fatal 798.1
  heart 780.2
  heat 992.1
  laryngeal 786.2
  tussive 786.2
  vasoconstriction 780.2
  vasodepressor 780.2
  vasomotor 780.2
  vasovagal 780.2

Syncytial infarct - *see* Placenta, abnormal
Syndactylism, syndactyly (multiple sites)
  755.10
  fingers (without fusion of bone) 755.11
    with fusion of bone 755.12
  toes (without fusion of bone) 755.13
    with fusion of bone 755.14
Syndrome - *see also* Disease
  5q minus 238.74
  abdominal
    acute 789.0●
    migraine 346.2●
    muscle deficiency 756.79
  Abercrombie's (amyloid degeneration)
    277.39
  abnormal innervation 374.43
  abstinence
    alcohol 291.81
    drug 292.0
    neonatal 779.5　　　　　　　◀
  Abt-Letterer-Siwe (acute histiocytosis
    X) (M9722/3) 202.5●
  Achard-Thiers (adrenogenital) 255.2
  acid pulmonary aspiration 997.39
    obstetric (Mendelson's) 668.0●
  acquired immune deficiency 042
  acquired immunodeficiency 042
  acrocephalosyndactylism 755.55
  acute abdominal 789.0●
  acute chest 517.3
  acute coronary 411.1
  Adair-Dighton (brittle bones and blue
    sclera, deafness) 756.51
  Adams-Stokes (-Morgagni) (syncope
    with heart block) 426.9
  Addisonian 255.41
  Adie (-Holmes) (pupil) 379.46
  adiposogenital 253.8
  adrenal
    hemorrhage 036.3
    meningococcic 036.3
  adrenocortical 255.3
  adrenogenital (acquired) (congenital)
    255.2
    feminizing 255.2
    iatrogenic 760.79
    virilism (acquired) (congenital) 255.2
  affective organic NEC 293.89
    drug-induced 292.84
  afferent loop NEC 537.89
  African macroglobulinemia 273.3
  Ahumada-Del Castillo (nonpuerperal
    galactorrhea and amenorrhea)
    253.1
  air blast concussion - *see* Injury,
    internal, by site
  Alagille 759.89
  Albright (-Martin)
    (pseudohypoparathyroidism)
    275.49
  Albright-McCune-Sternberg (osteitis
    fibrosa disseminata) 756.59
  alcohol withdrawal 291.81
  Alder's (leukocyte granulation
    anomaly) 288.2
  Aldrich (-Wiskott) (eczema-
    thrombocytopenia) 279.12
  Alibert-Bazin (mycosis fungoides)
    (M9700/3) 202.1●
  Alice in Wonderland 293.89
  alien hand 781.8
  Allen-Masters 620.6
  Alligator baby (ichthyosis congenita)
    757.1

Syndrome *(Continued)*
  Alport's (hereditary hematuria-
    nephropathy-deafness) 759.89
  Alvarez (transient cerebral ischemia)
    435.9
  alveolar capillary block 516.3
  Alzheimer's 331.0
    with dementia - *see* Alzheimer's,
      dementia
  amnestic (confabulatory) 294.0
    alcohol-induced persisting 291.1
    drug-induced 292.83
    posttraumatic 294.0
  amotivational 292.89
  amyostatic 275.1
  amyotrophic lateral sclerosis 335.20
  androgen insensitivity 259.51
    partial 259.52
  Angelman 759.89
  angina (*see also* Angina) 413.9
  ankyloglossia superior 750.0
  anterior
    chest wall 786.52
    compartment (tibial) 958.8
    spinal artery 433.8●
      compression 721.1
    tibial (compartment) 958.8
  antibody deficiency 279.00
    agammaglobulinemic 279.00
    congenital 279.04
    hypogammaglobulinemic 279.00
  anticardiolipin antibody 289.81
  antimongolism 758.39
  antiphospholipid antibody 289.81
  Anton (-Babinski)
    (hemiasomatognosia) 307.9
  anxiety (*see also* Anxiety) 300.00
    organic 293.84
  aortic
    arch 446.7
    bifurcation (occlusion) 444.0
    ring 747.21
  Apert's (acrocephalosyndactyly)
    755.55
  Apert-Gallais (adrenogenital) 255.2
  aphasia-apraxia-alexia 784.69
  apical ballooning 429.83
  "approximate answers" 300.16
  arcuate ligament (-celiac axis) 447.4
  arcus aortae 446.7
  arc welders' 370.24
  argentaffin, argentaffinoma 259.2
  Argonz-Del Castillo (nonpuerperal
    galactorrhea and amenorrhea)
    253.1
  Argyll Robertson's (syphilitic) 094.89
    nonsyphilitic 379.45
  Armenian 277.31
  arm-shoulder (*see also* Neuropathy,
    peripheral, autonomic) 337.9
  Arnold-Chiari (*see also* Spina bifida)
    741.0●
    type I 348.4
    type II 741.0●
    type III 742.0
    type IV 742.2
  Arrillaga-Ayerza (pulmonary artery
    sclerosis with pulmonary
    hypertension) 416.0
  arteriomesenteric duodenum occlusion
    537.89
  arteriovenous steal 996.73
  arteritis, young female (obliterative
    brachiocephalic) 446.7

◀ New　　◀▥ Revised　　~~deleted~~ Deleted　　● Use Additional Digit(s)　　▨ Omit code

Syndrome (Continued)
aseptic meningitis - see Meningitis,
   aseptic
Asherman's 621.5
Asperger's 299.8●
asphyctic (see also Anxiety) 300.00
aspiration, of newborn (massive
   770.18)
   meconium 770.12
ataxia-telangiectasia 334.8
Audry's (acropachyderma) 757.39
auriculotemporal 350.8
autoimmune lymphoproliferative
   (ALPS) 279.41   ◄
autosomal - see also Abnormal,
   autosomes NEC
   deletion 758.39
      5p 758.31
      22q11.2 758.32
Avellis' 344.89
Axenfeld's 743.44
Ayerza (-Arrillaga) (pulmonary artery
   sclerosis with pulmonary
   hypertension) 416.0
Baader's (erythema multiforme
   exudativum) 695.19
Baastrup's 721.5
Babinski (-Vaquez) (cardiovascular
   syphilis) 093.89
Babinski-Fröhlich (adiposogenital
   dystrophy) 253.8
Babinski-Nageotte 344.89
Bagratuni's (temporal arteritis) 446.5
Bakwin-Krida (craniometaphyseal
   dysplasia) 756.89
Balint's (psychic paralysis of visual
   disorientation) 368.16
Ballantyne (-Runge) (postmaturity)
   766.22
ballooning posterior leaflet 424.0
Banti's - see Cirrhosis, liver
Bard-Pic's (carcinoma, head of
   pancreas) 157.0
Bardet-Biedl (obesity, polydactyly, and
   mental retardation) 759.89
Barlow's (mitral valve prolapse) 424.0
Barlow (-Möller) (infantile scurvy) 267
Baron Munchausen's 301.51
Barré-Guillain 357.0
Barré-Liéou (posterior cervical
   sympathetic) 723.2
Barrett's (chronic peptic ulcer of
   esophagus) 530.85
Bársony-Pólgar (corkscrew esophagus)
   530.5
Bársony-Teschendorf (corkscrew
   esophagus) 530.5
Barth 759.89
Bartter's (secondary
   hyperaldosteronism with
   juxtaglomerular hyperplasia)
   255.13
basal cell nevus 759.89   ◄
Basedow's (exophthalmic goiter)
   242.0●
basilar artery 435.0
basofrontal 377.04
Bassen-Kornzweig
   (abetalipoproteinemia) 272.5
Batten-Steinert 359.21
battered
   adult 995.81
   baby or child 995.54
   spouse 995.81
Baumgarten-Cruveilhier (cirrhosis of
   liver) 571.5

Syndrome (Continued)
Beals 759.82
Bearn-Kunkel (-Slater) (lupoid
   hepatitis) 571.49
Beau's (see also Degeneration,
   myocardial) 429.1
Bechterew-Strümpell-Marie
   (ankylosing spondylitis) 720.0
Beck's (anterior spinal artery occlusion)
   433.8●
Beckwith (-Wiedemann) 759.89
Behçet's 136.1
Bekhterev-Strümpell-Marie
   (ankylosing spondylitis) 720.0
Benedikt's 344.89
Béquez César (-Steinbrinck-Chédiak-
   Higashi) (congenital gigantism of
   peroxidase granules) 288.2
Bernard-Horner (see also Neuropathy,
   peripheral, autonomic) 337.9
Bernard-Sergent (acute adrenocortical
   insufficiency) 255.41
Bernhardt-Roth 355.1
Bernheim's (see also Failure, heart) 428.0
Bertolotti's (sacralization of fifth
   lumbar vertebra) 756.15
Besnier-Boeck-Schaumann (sarcoidosis)
   135
Bianchi's (aphasia-apraxia-alexia
   syndrome) 784.69
Biedl-Bardet (obesity, polydactyly, and
   mental retardation) 759.89
Biemond's (obesity, polydactyly, and
   mental retardation) 759.89
big spleen 289.4
bilateral polycystic ovarian 256.4
Bing-Horton's 339.00
Biörck (-Thorson) (malignant carcinoid)
   259.2
Birt-Hogg-Dube 759.89
Blackfan-Diamond (congenital
   hypoplastic anemia) 284.01
black lung 500
black widow spider bite 989.5
bladder neck (see also Incontinence,
   urine) 788.30
blast (concussion) - see Blast, injury
blind loop (postoperative) 579.2
Block-Siemens (incontinentia pigmenti)
   757.33
Bloch-Sulzberger (incontinentia
   pigmenti) 757.33
Bloom (-Machacek) (-Torre) 757.39
Blount-Barber (tibia vara) 732.4
blue
   bloater 491.20
      with
         acute bronchitis 491.22
         exacerbation (acute) 491.21
   diaper 270.0
   drum 381.02
   sclera 756.51
   toe 445.02
Boder-Sedgwick (ataxia-telangiectasia)
   334.8
Boerhaave's (spontaneous esophageal
   rupture) 530.4
Bonnevie-Ullrich 758.6
Bonnier's 386.19
Borjeson-Forssman-Lehmann 759.89
Bouillaud's (rheumatic heart disease)
   391.9
Bourneville (-Pringle) (tuberous
   sclerosis) 759.5

Syndrome (Continued)
Bouveret (-Hoffmann) (paroxysmal
   tachycardia) 427.2
brachial plexus 353.0
Brachman-de Lange (Amsterdam
   dwarf, mental retardation, and
   brachycephaly) 759.89
bradycardia-tachycardia 427.81
Brailsford-Morquio (dystrophy)
   (mucopolysaccharidosis IV) 277.5
brain (acute) (chronic) (nonpsychotic)
   (organic) (with behavioral
   reaction) (with neurotic reaction)
   310.9
   with
      presenile brain disease (see also
         Dementia, presenile) 290.10
      psychosis, psychotic reaction (see
         also Psychosis, organic)
         294.9
   chronic alcoholic 291.2
   congenital (see also Retardation,
      mental) 319
   postcontusional 310.2
   posttraumatic
      nonpsychotic 310.2
      psychotic 293.9
         acute 293.0
         chronic (see also Psychosis,
            organic) 294.8
         subacute 293.1
   psycho-organic (see also Syndrome,
      psycho-organic) 310.9
   psychotic (see also Psychosis,
      organic) 294.9
   senile (see also Dementia, senile)
      290.0
branchial arch 744.41
Brandt's (acrodermatitis enteropathica)
   686.8
Brennemann's 289.2
Briquet's 300.81
Brissaud-Meige (infantile myxedema)
   244.9
broad ligament laceration 620.6
Brock's (atelectasis due to enlarged
   lymph nodes) 518.0
broken heart 429.83
Brown's tendon sheath 378.61
Brown-Séquard 344.89
brown spot 756.59
Brugada 746.89
Brugsch's (acropachyderma) 757.39
bubbly lung 770.7
Buchem's (hyperostosis corticalis)
   733.3
Budd-Chiari (hepatic vein thrombosis)
   453.0
Büdinger-Ludloff-Läwen 717.89
bulbar 335.22
   lateral (see also Disease,
      cerebrovascular, acute) 436
Bullis fever 082.8
bundle of Kent (anomalous
   atrioventricular excitation) 426.7
Bürger-Grutz (essential familial
   hyperlipemia) 272.3
Burke's (pancreatic insufficiency and
   chronic neutropenia) 577.8
Burnett's (milk-alkali) 275.42
Burnier's (hypophyseal dwarfism)
   253.3
burning feet 266.2
Bywaters' 958.5

Syndrome (Continued)

Caffey's (infantile cortical hyperostosis) 756.59
Calvé-Legg-Perthes (osteochrondrosis, femoral capital) 732.1
Caplan (-Colinet) syndrome 714.81
capsular thrombosis (see also Thrombosis, brain) 434.0●
carbohydrate-deficient glycoprotein (CDGS) 271.8
carcinogenic thrombophlebitis 453.1
carcinoid 259.2
cardiac asthma (see also Failure, ventricular, left) 428.1
cardiacos negros 416.0
cardiofaciocutaneous 759.89 ◀
cardiopulmonary obesity 278.8
cardiorenal (see also Hypertension, cardiorenal) 404.90
cardiorespiratory distress (idiopathic), newborn 769
cardiovascular renal (see also Hypertension, cardiorenal) 404.90
cardiovasorenal 272.7
Carini's (ichthyosis congenita) 757.1
carotid
    artery (internal) 435.8
    body or sinus 337.01
carpal tunnel 354.0
Carpenter's 759.89
Cassidy (-Scholte) (malignant carcinoid) 259.2
cat-cry 758.31
cauda equina 344.60
causalgia 355.9
    lower limb 355.71
    upper limb 354.4
cavernous sinus 437.6
celiac 579.0
    artery compression 447.4
    axis 447.4
central pain 338.0
cerebellomedullary malformation (see also Spina bifida) 741.0●
cerebral gigantism 253.0
cerebrohepatorenal 759.89
cervical (root) (spine) NEC 723.8
    disc 722.71
    posterior, sympathetic 723.2
    rib 353.0
    sympathetic paralysis 337.09
    traumatic (acute) NEC 847.0
cervicobrachial (diffuse) 723.3
cervicocranial 723.2
cervicodorsal outlet 353.2
Céstan's 344.89
Céstan (-Raymond) 433.8●
Céstan-Chenais 344.89
chancriform 114.1
Charcôt's (intermittent claudication) 443.9
    angina cruris 443.9
    due to atherosclerosis 440.21
Charcôt-Marie-Tooth 356.1
Charcôt-Weiss-Baker 337.01
CHARGE association 759.89
Cheadle (-Möller) (-Barlow) (infantile scurvy) 267
Chédiak-Higashi (-Steinbrinck) (congenital gigantism of peroxidase granules) 288.2
chest wall 786.52
Chiari's (hepatic vein thrombosis) 453.0
Chiari-Frommel 676.6●

Syndrome (Continued)

chiasmatic 368.41
Chilaiditi's (subphrenic displacement, colon) 751.4
chondroectodermal dysplasia 756.55
chorea-athetosis-agitans 275.1
Christian's (chronic histiocytosis X) 277.89
chromosome 4 short arm deletion 758.39
chronic pain 338.4
Churg-Strauss 446.4
Clarke-Hadfield (pancreatic infantilism) 577.8
Claude's 352.6
Claude Bernard-Horner (see also Neuropathy, peripheral, autonomic) 337.9
Clérambault's
    automatism 348.89 ◀▮▮▮
    erotomania 297.8
Clifford's (postmaturity) 766.22
climacteric 627.2
Clouston's (hidrotic ectodermal dysplasia) 757.31
clumsiness 315.4
Cockayne's (microencephaly and dwarfism) 759.89
Cockayne-Weber (epidermolysis bullosa) 757.39
Coffin-Lowry 759.89
Cogan's (nonsyphilitic interstitial keratitis) 370.52
cold injury (newborn) 778.2
Collet (-Sicard) 352.6
combined immunity deficiency 279.2
compartment(al) (anterior) (deep) (posterior) 958.8
    nontraumatic
        abdomen 729.73
        arm 729.71
        buttock 729.72
        fingers 729.71
        foot 729.72
        forearm 729.71
        hand 729.71
        hip 729.72
        leg 729.72
        lower extremity 729.72
        shoulder 729.71
        specified site NEC 729.79
        thigh 729.72
        toes 729.72
        upper extremity 729.71
        wrist 729.71
    post-surgical (see also Syndrome, compartment, non-traumatic) 998.89
    traumatic 958.90
        abdomen 958.93
        arm 958.91
        buttock 958.92
        fingers 958.91
        foot 958.92
        forearm 958.91
        hand 958.91
        hip 958.92
        leg 958.92
        lower extremity 958.92
        shoulder 958.91
        specified site NEC 958.99
        thigh 958.92
        tibial 958.92

Syndrome (Continued)

compartment(al) (Continued)
    traumatic (Continued)
        toes 958.92
        upper extremity 958.91
        wrist 958.91
complex regional pain - see also Dystrophy, sympathetic
    type I - see Dystrophy, sympathetic (posttraumatic) (reflex)
    type II - see Causalgia
compression 958.5
    cauda equina 344.60
        with neurogenic bladder 344.61
concussion 310.2
congenital
    affecting more than one system 759.7
        specified type NEC 759.89
    congenital central alveolar hypoventilation 327.25
    facial diplegia 352.6
    muscular hypertrophy-cerebral 759.89
congestion-fibrosis (pelvic) 625.5
conjunctivourethrosynovial 099.3
Conn (-Louis) (primary aldosteronism) 255.12
Conradi (-Hünermann) (chondrodysplasia calcificans congenita) 756.59
conus medullaris 336.8
Cooke-Apert-Gallais (adrenogenital) 255.2
Cornelia de Lange's (Amsterdam dwarf, mental retardation, and brachycephaly) 759.8
coronary insufficiency or intermediate 411.1
cor pulmonale 416.9
corticosexual 255.2
Costen's (complex) 524.60
costochondral junction 733.6
costoclavicular 353.0
costovertebral 253.0
Cotard's (paranoia) 297.1
Cowden 759.6
craniovertebral 723.2
Creutzfeldt-Jakob 046.19
    with dementia
        with behavioral disturbance 046.19 [294.11]
        without behavioral disturbance 046.19 [294.10]
    variant 046.11
        with dementia
            with behavioral disturbance 046.11 [294.11]
            without behavioral disturbance 046.11 [294.10]
crib death 798.0
cricopharyngeal 787.20
cri-du-chat 758.31
Crigler-Najjar (congenital hyperbilirubinemia) 277.4
crocodile tears 351.8
Cronkhite-Canada 211.3
croup 464.4
CRST (cutaneous systemic sclerosis) 710.1
crush 958.5
crushed lung (see also Injury, internal, lung) 861.20

Syndrome (Continued)

Cruveilhier-Baumgarten (cirrhosis of liver) 571.5
cubital tunnel 354.2
Cuiffini-Pancoast (M8010/3) (carcinoma, pulmonary apex) 162.3
Curschmann (-Batten) (-Steinert) 359.21
Cushing's (iatrogenic) (idiopathic) (pituitary basophilism) (pituitary-dependent) 255.0
   overdose or wrong substance given or taken 962.0
Cyriax's (slipping rib) 733.99
cystic duct stump 576.0
Da Costa's (neurocirculatory asthenia) 306.2
Dameshek's (erythroblastic anemia) 282.49
Dana-Putnam (subacute combined sclerosis with pernicious anemia) 281.0 [336.2]
Danbolt (-Closs) (acrodermatitis enteropathica) 686.8
Dandy-Walker (atresia, foramen of Magendie) 742.3
   with spina bifida (see also Spina bifida) 741.0●
Danlos' 756.83
Davies-Colley (slipping rib) 733.99
dead fetus 641.3●
defeminization 255.2
defibrination (see also Fibrinolysis) 286.6
Degos' 447.8
Deiters' nucleus 386.19
Déjérine-Roussy 338.0
Déjérine-Thomas 333.0
de Lange's (Amsterdam dwarf, mental retardation, and brachycephaly) (Cornelia) 759.89
Del Castillo's (germinal aplasia) 606.0
deletion chromosomes 758.39
delusional
   induced by drug 292.11
dementia-aphonia, of childhood (see also Psychosis, childhood) 299.1●
demyelinating NEC 341.9
denial visual hallucination 307.9
depersonalization 300.6
de Quervain's 259.51
Dercum's (adiposis dolorosa) 272.8
de Toni-Fanconi (-Debre) (cystinosis) 270.0
diabetes-dwarfism-obesity (juvenile) 258.1
diabetes mellitus-hypertension-nephrosis 250.4● [581.81]
   due to secondary diabetes 249.4● [581.81]
diabetes mellitus in newborn infant 775.1
diabetes-nephrosis 250.4● [581.81]
   due to secondary diabetes 249.4● [581.81]
diabetic amyotrophy 250.6● [353.5]
   due to secondary diabetes 249.6● [353.5]
Diamond-Blackfan (congenital hypoplastic anemia) 284.01
Diamond-Gardner (autoerythrocyte sensitization) 287.2

Syndrome (Continued)

DIC (diffuse or disseminated intravascular coagulopathy) (see also Fibrinolysis) 286.6
diencephalohypophyseal NEC 253.8
diffuse cervicobrachial 723.3
diffuse obstructive pulmonary 496
DiGeorge's (thymic hypoplasia) 279.11
Dighton's 756.51
Di Guglielmo's (erythremic myelosis) (M9841/3) 207.0●
disequilibrium 276.9
disseminated platelet thrombosis 446.6
Ditthomska 307.81
Doan-Wiseman (primary splenic neutropenia) 289.53
Döhle body-panmyelopathic 288.2
Donohue's (leprechaunism) 259.8
dorsolateral medullary (see also Disease, cerebrovascular, acute) 436
double athetosis 333.71
double whammy 360.81
Down's (mongolism) 758.0
Dresbach's (elliptocytosis) 282.1
Dressler's (postmyocardial infarction) 411.0
   hemoglobinuria 283.2
   postcardiotomy 429.4
drug withdrawal, infant, of dependent mother 779.5
dry skin 701.1
   eye 375.15
DSAP (disseminated superficial actinic porokeratosis) 692.75
Duane's (retraction) 378.71
Duane-Stilling-Türk (ocular retraction syndrome) 378.71
Dubin-Johnson (constitutional hyperbilirubinemia) 277.4
Dubin-Sprinz (constitutional hyperbilirubinemia) 277.4
Duchenne's 335.22
due to abnormality
   autosomal NEC (see also Abnormal, autosomes NEC) 758.5
      13 758.1
      18 758.2
      21 or 22 758.0
      D₁ 758.1
      E₃ 758.2
      G 758.0
   chromosomal 758.89
      sex 758.81
dumping 564.2
   nonsurgical 536.8
Duplay's 726.2
Dupré's (meningism) 781.6
Dyke-Young (acquired macrocytic hemolytic anemia) 283.9
dyspraxia 315.4
dystocia, dystrophia 654.9●
Eagle-Barret 756.71
Eales' 362.18
Eaton-Lambert (see also Neoplasm, by site, malignant) 199.1 [358.1]
Ebstein's (downward displacement, tricuspid valve into right ventricle) 746.2
ectopic ACTH secretion 255.0
eczema-thrombocytopenia 279.12
Eddowes' (brittle bones and blue sclera) 756.51

Syndrome (Continued)

Edwards' 758.2
efferent loop 537.89
effort (aviators') (psychogenic) 306.2
Ehlers-Danlos 756.83
Eisenmenger's (ventricular septal defect) 745.4
Ekbom's (restless legs) 333.94
Ekman's (brittle bones and blue sclera) 756.51
electric feet 266.2
Elephant man 237.71
Ellison-Zollinger (gastric hypersecretion with pancreatic islet cell tumor) 251.5
Ellis-van Creveld (chondroectodermal dysplasia) 756.55
embryonic fixation 270.2
empty sella (turcica) 253.8
endocrine-hypertensive 255.3
Engel-von Recklinghausen (osteitis fibrosa cystica) 252.01
enteroarticular 099.3
entrapment - see Neuropathy, entrapment
eosinophilia myalgia 710.5
epidemic vomiting 078.82
Epstein's - see Nephrosis
Erb (-Oppenheim)-Goldflam 358.00
Erdheim-Chester 277.89 ◄
Erdheim's (acromegalic macrospondylitis) 253.0
Erlacher-Blount (tibia vara) 732.4
erythrocyte fragmentation 283.19
euthyroid sick 790.94
Evans' (thrombocytopenic purpura) 287.32
excess cortisol, iatrogenic 255.0
exhaustion 300.5
extrapyramidal 333.90
eyelid-malar-mandible 756.0
eye retraction 378.71
Faber's (achlorhydric anemia) 280.9
Fabry (-Anderson) (angiokeratoma corporis diffusum) 272.7
facet 724.8
Fallot's 745.2
falx (see also Hemorrhage, brain) 431
familial eczema-thrombocytopenia 279.12
Fanconi's (anemia) (congenital pancytopenia) 284.09
Fanconi (-de Toni) (-Debré) (cystinosis) 270.0
Farber (-Uzman) (disseminated lipogranulomatosis) 272.8
fatigue NEC 300.5
   chronic 780.71
faulty bowel habit (idiopathic megacolon) 564.7
FDH (focal dermal hypoplasia) 757.39
fecal reservoir 560.39
Feil-Klippel (brevicollis) 756.16
Felty's (rheumatoid arthritis with splenomegaly and leukopenia) 714.1
fertile eunuch 257.2
fetal alcohol 760.71
   late effect 760.71
fibrillation-flutter 427.32
fibrositis (periarticular) 729.0
Fiedler's (acute isolated myocarditis) 422.91
Fiessinger-Leroy (-Reiter) 099.3

Syndrome *(Continued)*
Fiessinger-Rendu (erythema
multiforme exudativum)
695.19
first arch 756.0
Fisher's 357.0
fish odor 270.8
Fitz's (acute hemorrhagic pancreatitis)
577.0
Fitz-Hugh and Curtis 098.86
due to
Chlamydia trachomatis 099.56
Neisseria gonorrhoeae
(gonococcal peritonitis)
098.86
Flajani (-Basedow) (exophthalmic
goiter) 242.0●
flat back
acquired 737.29
postprocedural 738.5
floppy
infant 781.99
iris 364.81
valve (mitral) 424.0
flush 259.2
Foix-Alajouanine 336.1
Fong's (hereditary osteo-
onychodysplasia) 756.89
foramen magnum 348.4
Forbes-Albright (nonpuerperal
amenorrhea and lactation
associated with pituitary tumor)
253.1
Foster-Kennedy 377.04
Foville's (peduncular) 344.89
fragile X 759.83
Franceschetti's (mandibulofacial
dysostosis) 756.0
Fraser's 759.89
Freeman-Sheldon 759.89
Frey's (auriculotemporal) 705.22
Friderichsen-Waterhouse 036.3
Friedrich-Erb-Arnold
(acropachyderma) 757.39
Fröhlich's (adiposogenital dystrophy)
253.8
Froin's 336.8
Frommel-Chiari 676.6●
frontal lobe 310.0
Fukuhara 277.87
Fuller Albright's (osteitis fibrosa
disseminata) 756.59
functional
bowel 564.9
prepubertal castrate 752.89
Gaisböck's (polycythemia hypertonica)
289.0
ganglion (basal, brain) 333.90
geniculi 351.1
Ganser's, hysterical 300.16
Gardner-Diamond (autoerythrocyte
sensitization) 287.2
gastroesophageal junction 530.0
gastroesophageal laceration-
hemorrhage 530.7
gastrojejunal loop obstruction 537.89
Gayet-Wernicke's (superior
hemorrhagic polioencephalitis)
265.1
Gee-Herter-Heubner (nontropical
sprue) 579.0
Gélineau's (*see also* Narcolepsy)
347.00
genito-anorectal 099.1

Syndrome *(Continued)*
Gerhardt's (vocal cord paralysis)
478.30
Gerstmann's (finger agnosia) 784.69
Gerstmann-Sträussler-Scheinker (GSS)
046.71
Gianotti Crosti 057.8
due to known virus - *see* Infection,
virus
due to unknown virus 057.8
Gilbert's 277.4
Gilford (-Hutchinson) (progeria) 259.8
Gilles de la Tourette's 307.23
Gillespie's (dysplasia
oculodentodigitalis) 759.89
Glénard's (enteroptosis) 569.89
Glinski-Simmonds (pituitary cachexia)
253.2
glucuronyl transferase 277.4
glue ear 381.20
Goldberg (-Maxwell) (-Morris)
(testicular feminization) 259.51
Goldenhar's (oculoauriculovertebral
dysplasia) 756.0
Goldflam-Erb 358.00
Goltz-Gorlin (dermal hypoplasia)
757.39
Goodpasture's (pneumorenal) 446.21
Good's 279.06
Gopalan's (burning feet) 266.2
Gorlin-Chaudhry-Moss 759.89
Gorlin's 759.89 ◀
Gougerot (-Houwer)-Sjögren
(keratoconjunctivitis sicca) 710.2
Gougerot-Blum (pigmented purpuric
lichenoid dermatitis) 709.1
Gougerot-Carteaud (confluent
reticulate papillomatosis) 701.8
Gouley's (constrictive pericarditis)
423.2
Gowers' (vasovagal attack) 780.2
Gowers-Paton-Kennedy 377.04
Gradenigo's 383.02
Gray or grey (chloramphenicol)
(newborn) 779.4
Greig's (hypertelorism) 756.0
GSS (Gerstmann-Sträussler-Scheinker)
046.71
Gubler-Millard 344.89
Guérin-Stern (arthrogryposis multiplex
congenita) 754.89
Guillain-Barré (-Strohl) 357.0
Gunn's (jaw-winking syndrome)
742.8
Günther's (congenital erythropoietic
porphyria) 277.1
gustatory sweating 350.8
H_2O 759.81
Hadfield-Clarke (pancreatic
infantilism) 577.8
Haglund-Läwen-Fründ 717.89
hair tourniquet - *see also* Injury,
superficial, by site
finger 915.8
infected 915.9
penis 911.8
infected 911.9
toe 917.8
infected 917.9
hairless women 257.8
Hallermann-Strieff 756.0
Hallervorden-Spatz 333.0
Hamman's (spontaneous mediastinal
emphysema) 518.1

Syndrome *(Continued)*
Hamman-Rich (diffuse interstitial
pulmonary fibrosis) 516.3
Hand-Schüller-Christian (chronic
histiocytosis X) 277.89
hand-foot 693.0
Hanot-Chauffard (-Troisier) (bronze
diabetes) 275.0
Harada's 363.22
Hare's (M8010/3) (carcinoma,
pulmonary apex) 162.3
Harkavy's 446.0
harlequin color change 779.89
Harris' (organic hyperinsulinism)
251.1
Hart's (pellagra-cerebellar ataxia-renal
aminoaciduria) 270.0
Hayem-Faber (achlorhydric anemia)
280.9
Hayem-Widal (acquired hemolytic
jaundice) 283.9
headache - *see* Headache, syndrome
Heberden's (angina pectoris) 413.9
Hedinger's (malignant carcinoid)
259.2
Hegglin's 288.2
Heller's (infantile psychosis) (*see also*
Psychosis, childhood) 299.1●
H.E.L.L.P. 642.5●
hemolytic-uremic (adult) (child) 283.11
hemophagocytic 288.4
infection-associated 288.4
Hench-Rosenberg (palindromic
arthritis) (*see also* Rheumatism,
palindromic) 719.3●
Henoch-Schönlein (allergic purpura)
287.0
hepatic flexure 569.89
hepatorenal 572.4
due to a procedure 997.4
following delivery 674.8●
hepatourologic 572.4
Herrick's (hemoglobin S disease)
282.61
Herter (-Gee) (nontropical sprue) 579.0
Heubner-Herter (nontropical sprue)
579.0
Heyd's (hepatorenal) 572.4
HHHO 759.81
high grade myelodysplastic 238.73
with 5q deletion 238.73
Hilger's 337.09
histiocytic 288.4
Hoffa (-Kastert) (liposynovitis
prepatellaris) 272.8
Hoffmann's 244.9 [359.5]
Hoffmann-Bouveret (paroxysmal
tachycardia) 427.2
Hoffmann-Werdnig 335.0
Holländer-Simons (progressive
lipodystrophy) 272.6
Holmes' (visual disorientation) 368.16
Holmes-Adie 379.46
Hoppe-Goldflam 358.00
Horner's (*see also* Neuropathy,
peripheral, autonomic) 337.9
traumatic - *see* Injury, nerve, cervical
sympathetic
hospital addiction 301.51
hungry bone 275.5
Hunt's (herpetic geniculate
ganglionitis) 053.11
dyssynergia cerebellaris myoclonica
334.2

◀ New   ◀ Revised   ~~deleted~~ Deleted   ● Use Additional Digit(s)   ▓ Omit code

Syndrome *(Continued)*
  Hunter (-Hurler)
    (mucopolysaccharidosis II) 277.5
  hunterian glossitis 529.4
  Hurler (-Hunter)
    (mucopolysaccharidosis II)
    277.5
  Hutchinson's incisors or teeth 090.5
  Hutchinson-Boeck (sarcoidosis) 135
  Hutchinson-Gilford (progeria) 259.8
  hydralazine
    correct substance properly
      administered 695.4
    overdose or wrong substance given
      or taken 972.6
  hydraulic concussion (abdomen) *(see also* Injury, internal, abdomen) 868.00
  hyperabduction 447.8
  hyperactive bowel 564.9
  hyperaldosteronism with hypokalemic alkalosis (Bartter's) 255.13
  hypercalcemic 275.42
  hypercoagulation NEC 289.89
  hypereosinophilic (idiopathic) 288.3
  hyperkalemic 276.7
  hyperkinetic - *see also* Hyperkinesia, heart 429.82
  hyperlipemia-hemolytic anemia-icterus 571.1
  hypermobility 728.5
  hypernatremia 276.0
  hyperosmolarity 276.0
  hyperperfusion 997.01
  hypersomnia-bulimia 349.89
  hypersplenic 289.4
  hypersympathetic *(see also* Neuropathy, peripheral, autonomic) 337.9
  hypertransfusion, newborn 776.4
  hyperventilation, psychogenic 306.1
  hyperviscosity (of serum) NEC 273.3
    polycythemic 289.0
    sclerothymic 282.8
  hypoglycemic (familial) (neonatal) 251.2
    functional 251.1
  hypokalemic 276.8
  hypophyseal 253.8
  hypophyseothalamic 253.8
  hypopituitarism 253.2
  hypoplastic left heart 746.7
  hypopotassemia 276.8
  hyposmolality 276.1
  hypotension, maternal 669.2●
  hypothenar hammer 443.89
  hypotonia-hypomentia-hypogonadism-obesity 759.81
  ICF (intravascular coagulation-fibrinolysis) *(see also* Fibrinolysis) 286.6
  idiopathic cardiorespiratory distress, newborn 769
  idiopathic nephrotic (infantile) 581.9
  iliotibial band 728.89
  Imerslund (-Gräsbeck) (anemia due to familial selective vitamin B$_{12}$ malabsorption) 281.1
  immobility (paraplegic) 728.3
  immunity deficiency, combined 279.2
  impending coronary 411.1
  impingement
    shoulder 726.2
    vertebral bodies 724.4

Syndrome *(Continued)*
  inappropriate secretion of antidiuretic hormone (ADH) 253.6
  incomplete
    mandibulofacial 756.0
  infant
    death, sudden (SIDS) 798.0
    Hercules 255.2
    of diabetic mother 775.0
    shaken 995.55
  infantilism 253.3
  inferior vena cava 459.2
  influenza-like 487.1
  inspissated bile, newborn 774.4
  insufficient sleep 307.44
  intermediate coronary (artery) 411.1
  internal carotid artery *(see also* Occlusion, artery, carotid) 433.1●
  interspinous ligament 724.8
  intestinal
    carcinoid 259.2
    gas 787.3
    knot 560.2
  intraoperative floppy iris (IFIS) 364.81
  intravascular
    coagulation-fibrinolysis (ICF) *(see also* Fibrinolysis) 286.6
    coagulopathy *(see also* Fibrinolysis) 286.6
  inverted Marfan's 759.89
  IRDS (idiopathic respiratory distress, newborn) 769
  irritable
    bowel 564.1
    heart 306.2
    weakness 300.5
  ischemic bowel (transient) 557.9
    chronic 557.1
    due to mesenteric artery insufficiency 557.1
  Itsenko-Cushing (pituitary basophilism) 255.0
  IVC (intravascular coagulopathy) *(see also* Fibrinolysis) 286.6
  Ivemark's (asplenia with congenital heart disease) 759.0
  Jaccoud's 714.4
  Jackson's 344.89
  Jadassohn-Lewandowski (pachyonchia congenita) 757.5
  Jaffe-Lichtenstein (-Uehlinger) 252.01
  Jahnke's (encephalocutaneous angiomatosis) 759.6
  Jakob-Creutzfeldt 046.19
    with dementia
      with behavioral disturbance 046.19 *[294.11]*
      without behavioral disturbance 046.19 *[294.10]*
    variant 046.11
      with dementia
        with behavioral disturbance 046.11 *[294.11]*
        without behavioral disturbance 046.11 *[294.10]*
  Jaksch's (pseudoleukemia infantum) 285.8
  Jaksch-Hayem (-Luzet) (pseudoleukemia infantum) 285.8
  jaw-winking 742.8
  jejunal 564.2

Syndrome *(Continued)*
  Jervell-Lange-Nielsen 426.82
  jet lag 327.35
  Jeune's (asphyxiating thoracic dystrophy of newborn) 756.4
  Job's (chronic granulomatous disease) 288.1
  Jordan's 288.2
  Joseph-Diamond-Blackfan (congenital hypoplastic anemia) 284.01
  Joubert 759.89
  jugular foramen 352.6
  Kabuki 759.89
  Kahler's (multiple myeloma) (M9730/3) 203.0●
  Kalischer's (encephalocutaneous angiomatosis) 759.6
  Kallmann's (hypogonadotropic hypogonadism with anosmia) 253.4
  Kanner's (autism) *(see also* Psychosis, childhood) 299.0●
  Kartagener's (sinusitis, bronchiectasis, situs inversus) 759.3
  Kasabach-Merritt (capillary hemangioma associated with thrombocytopenic purpura) 287.39
  Kast's (dyschondroplasia with hemangiomas) 756.4
  Kaznelson's (congenital hypoplastic anemia) 284.01
  Kearns-Sayre 277.87
  Kelly's (sideropenic dysphagia) 280.8
  Kimmelstiel-Wilson (intercapillary glomerulosclerosis) 250.4● *[581.81]*
    due to secondary diabetes 249.4● *[581.81]*
  Klauder's (erythema multiforme exudativum) 695.19
  Klein-Waardenburg (ptosis-epicanthus) 270.2
  Kleine-Levin 327.13
  Klinefelter's 758.7
  Klippel-Feil (brevicollis) 756.16
  Klippel-Trenaunay 759.89
  Klumpke (-Déjérine) (injury to brachial plexus at birth) 767.6
  Klüver-Bucy (-Terzian) 310.0
  Köhler-Pelligrini-Stieda (calcification, knee joint) 726.62
  König's 564.89
  Korsakoff's (nonalcoholic) 294.0
    alcoholic 291.1
  Korsakoff (-Wernicke) (nonalcoholic) 294.0
    alcoholic 291.1
  Kostmann's (infantile genetic agranulocytosis) 288.01
  Krabbe's
    congenital muscle hypoplasia 756.89
    cutaneocerebral angioma 759.6
  Kunkel (lupoid hepatitis) 571.49
  labyrinthine 386.50
  laceration, broad ligament 620.6
  Landau-Kleffner 345.8●
  Langdon Down (mongolism) 758.0
  Larsen's (flattened facies and multiple congenital dislocations) 755.8
  lateral
    cutaneous nerve of thigh 355.1
    medullary *(see also* Disease, cerebrovascular, acute) 436

Syndrome *(Continued)*

Launois' (pituitary gigantism) 253.0
Launois-Cléret (adiposogenital
    dystrophy) 253.8
Laurence-Moon (-Bardet)-Biedl
    (obesity, polydactyly, and mental
    retardation) 759.89
Lawford's (encephalocutaneous
    angiomatosis) 759.6
lazy
    leukocyte 288.09
    posture 728.3
Lederer-Brill (acquired infectious
    hemolytic anemia) 283.19
Legg-Calvé-Perthes (osteochondrosis
    capital femoral) 732.1
Lemiere 451.89
Lennox-Gastaut syndrome 345.0●
    with tonic seizures 345.1●
Lennox's (*see also* Epilepsy) 345.0●
lenticular 275.1
Léopold-Lévi's (paroxysmal thyroid
    instability) 242.9●
Lepore hemoglobin 282.49
Léri-Weill 756.59
Leriche's (aortic bifurcation occlusion)
    444.0
Lermoyez's (*see also* Disease, Ménière's)
    386.00
Lesch-Nyhan (hypoxanthine-guanine-
    phosphoribosyltransferase
    deficiency) 277.2
leukoencephalopathy, reversible,
    posterior 348.5
Lev's (acquired complete heart block)
    426.0
Levi's (pituitary dwarfism) 253.3
Lévy-Roussy 334.3
Lichtheim's (subacute combined
    sclerosis with pernicious anemia)
    281.0 *[336.2]*
Li-Fraumeni V84.01
Lightwood's (renal tubular acidosis)
    588.89
Lignac (-de Toni) (-Fanconi) (-Debré)
    (cystinosis) 270.0
Likoff's (angina in menopausal
    women) 413.9
liver-kidney 572.4
Lloyd's 258.1
lobotomy 310.0
Löffler's (eosinophilic pneumonitis)
    518.3
Löfgren's (sarcoidosis) 135
long arm 18 or 21 deletion 758.39
Looser (-Debray)-Milkman
    (osteomalacia with
    pseudofractures) 268.2
Lorain-Levi (pituitary dwarfism)
    253.3
Louis-Bar (ataxia-telangiectasia)
    334.8
low
    atmospheric pressure 993.2
    back 724.2
        psychogenic 306.0
    output (cardiac) (*see also* Failure,
        heart) 428.9
Lowe's (oculocerebrorenal dystrophy)
    270.8
Lowe-Terrey-MacLachlan
    (oculocerebrorenal
    dystrophy) 270.8
lower radicular, newborn 767.4

Syndrome *(Continued)*

Lown (-Ganong)-Levine (short P-R
    internal, normal QRS complex,
    and supraventricular tachycardia)
    426.81
Lucey-Driscoll (jaundice due to
    delayed conjugation) 774.30
Luetscher's (dehydration) 276.51
lumbar vertebral 724.4
Lutembacher's (atrial septal defect
    with mitral stenosis) 745.5
Lyell's (toxic epidermal necrolysis)
    695.15
    due to drug
        correct substance properly
            administered 695.15
        overdose or wrong substance
            given or taken 977.9
        specified drug - *see* Table of
            Drugs and Chemicals
MacLeod's 492.8
macrogenitosomia praecox 259.8
macroglobulinemia 273.3
macrophage activation 288.4
Maffucci's (dyschondroplasia with
    hemangiomas) 756.4
Magenblase 306.4
magnesium-deficiency 781.7
malabsorption 579.9
    postsurgical 579.3
    spinal fluid 331.3
Mal de Debarquement 780.4
malignant carcinoid 259.2
Mallory-Weiss 530.7
mandibulofacial dysostosis 756.0
manic-depressive (*see also* Psychosis,
    affective) 296.80
Mankowsky's (familial dysplastic
    osteopathy) 731.2
maple syrup (urine) 270.3
Marable's (celiac artery compression)
    447.4
Marchesani (-Weill) (brachymorphism
    and ectopia lentis) 759.89
Marchiafava-Bignami 341.8
Marchiafava-Micheli (paroxysmal
    nocturnal hemoglobinuria)
    283.2
Marcus Gunn's (jaw-winking
    syndrome) 742.8
Marfan's (arachnodactyly) 759.82
    meaning congenital syphilis 090.49
        with luxation of lens 090.49
        [379.32]
Marie's (acromegaly) 253.0
    primary or idiopathic
        (acropachyderma) 757.39
    secondary (hypertrophic pulmonary
        osteoarthropathy) 731.2
Markus-Adie 379.46
Maroteaux-Lamy
    (mucopolysaccharidosis VI)
    277.5
Martin's 715.27
Martin-Albright
    (pseudohypoparathyroidism)
    275.49
Martorell-Fabré (pulseless disease)
    446.7
massive aspiration of newborn 770.18
Masters-Allen 620.6
mastocytosis 757.33
maternal hypotension 669.2●
maternal obesity 646.1●

Syndrome *(Continued)*

May (-Hegglin) 288.2
McArdle (-Schmid) (-Pearson)
    (glycogenosis V) 271.0
McCune-Albright (osteitis fibrosa
    disseminata) 756.59
McQuarrie's (idiopathic familial
    hypoglycemia) 251.2
meconium
    aspiration 770.12
    plug (newborn) NEC 777.1
median arcuate ligament 447.4
mediastinal fibrosis 519.3
Meekeren-Ehlers-Danlos 756.83
Meige (blepharospasm-oromandibular
    dystonia) 333.82
    -Milroy (chronic hereditary edema)
        757.0
MELAS (mitochondrial
    encephalopathy, lactic acidosis
    and stroke-like episodes)
    277.87
Melkersson (-Rosenthal) 351.8
MEN (multiple endocrine neoplasia)
    type I 258.01
    type IIA 258.02
    type IIB 258.03
Mende's (ptosis-epicanthus) 270.2
Mendelson's (resulting from a
    procedure) 997.39
    during labor 668.0●
    obstetric 668.0●
Ménétrier's (hypertrophic gastritis)
    535.2●
Ménière's (*see also* Disease, Ménière's)
    386.00
meningo-eruptive 047.1
Menkes' 759.89
    glutamic acid 759.89
    maple syrup (urine) disease 270.3
menopause 627.2
    postartificial 627.4
menstruation 625.4
MERRF (myoclonus with epilepsy and
    with ragged red fibers) 277.87
mesenteric
    artery, superior 557.1
    vascular insufficiency (with
        gangrene) 557.1
metabolic 277.7
metastatic carcinoid 259.2
Meyenburg-Altherr-Uehlinger 733.99
Meyer-Schwickerath and Weyers
    (dysplasia oculodentodigitalis)
    759.89
Micheli-Rietti (thalassemia minor)
    282.49
Michotte's 721.5
micrognathia-glossoptosis 756.0
microphthalmos (congenital) 759.89
midbrain 348.89 ◀▥
middle
    lobe (lung) (right) 518.0
    radicular 353.0
Miescher's
    familial acanthosis nigricans 701.2
    granulomatosis disciformis 709.3
Mieten's 759.89
migraine 346.0●
Mikity-Wilson (pulmonary
    dysmaturity) 770.7
Mikulicz's (dryness of mouth, absent
    or decreased lacrimation) 527.1
milk alkali (milk drinkers') 275.42

◀ New   ◀▥ Revised   ~~deleted~~ Deleted   ● Use Additional Digit(s)   ▨ Omit code

Syndrome *(Continued)*
  Milkman (-Looser) (osteomalacia with pseudofractures) 268.2
  Millard-Gubler 344.89
  Miller-Dieker 758.33
  Miller Fisher's 357.0
  Milles' (encephalocutaneous angiomatosis) 759.6
  Minkowski-Chauffard *(see also* Spherocytosis) 282.0
  Mirizzi's (hepatic duct stenosis) 576.2
    with calculus, cholelithiasis, or stones - *see* Choledocholithiasis
  mitochondrial neurogastrointestinal encephalopathy (MNGIE) 277.87
  mitral
    click (-murmur) 785.2
    valve prolapse 424.0
  MNGIE (mitochondrial neurogastrointestinal encephalopathy) 277.87
  Möbius'
    congenital oculofacial paralysis 352.6
    ophthalmoplegic migraine 346.2●
  Mohr's (types I and II) 759.89
  monofixation 378.34
  Moore's *(see also* Epilepsy) 345.5●
  Morel-Moore (hyperostosis frontalis interna) 733.3
  Morel-Morgagni (hyperostosis frontalis interna) 733.3
  Morgagni (-Stewart-Morel) (hyperostosis frontalis interna) 733.3
  Morgagni-Adams-Stokes (syncope with heart block) 426.9
  Morquio (-Brailsford) (-Ullrich) (mucopolysaccharidosis IV) 277.5
  Morris (testicular feminization) 259.51
  Morton's (foot) (metatarsalgia) (metatarsal neuralgia) (neuralgia) (neuroma) (toe) 355.6
  Moschcowitz (-Singer-Symmers) (thrombotic thrombocytopenic purpura) 446.6
  Mounier-Kuhn 748.3
    with
      acute exacerbation 494.1
      bronchiectasis 494.0
        with (acute) exacerbation 494.1
    acquired 519.19
      with bronchiectasis 494.0
        with (acute) exacerbation 494.1
  Mucha-Haberman (acute parapsoriasis varioliformis) 696.2
  mucocutaneous lymph node (acute) (febrile) (infantile) (MCLS) 446.1
  multiple
    deficiency 260
    endocrine neoplasia (MEN)
      type I 258.01
      type IIA 258.02
      type IIB 258.03
    operations 301.51
  Munchausen's 301.51
  Munchmeyer's (exostosis luxurians) 728.11
  Murchison-Sanderson - *see* Disease, Hodgkin's
  myasthenic - *see* Myasthenia, syndrome

Syndrome *(Continued)*
  myelodysplastic 238.75
    with 5q deletion 238.74
    high grade with 5q deletion 238.73
    therapy-related 289.83
  myeloproliferative (chronic) (M9960/1) 238.79
  myofascial pain NEC 729.1
  Naffziger's 353.0
  Nager-de Reynier (dysostosis mandibularis) 756.0
  nail-patella (hereditary osteo-onychodysplasia) 756.89
  NARP (neuropathy, ataxia and retinitis pigmentosa) 277.87
  Nebécourt's 253.3
  Neill Dingwall (microencephaly and dwarfism) 759.89
  nephrotic *(see also* Nephrosis) 581.9
    diabetic 250.4● *[581.81]*
      due to secondary diabetes 249.4● *[581.81]*
  Netherton's (ichthyosiform erythroderma) 757.1
  neurocutaneous 759.6
  neuroleptic malignant 333.92
  Nezelof's (pure alymphocytosis) 279.13
  Niemann-Pick (lipid histiocytosis) 272.7
  Nonne-Milroy-Meige (chronic hereditary edema) 757.0
  nonsense 300.16
  Noonan's 759.89
  Nothnagel's
    ophthalmoplegia-cerebellar ataxia 378.52
    vasomotor acroparesthesia 443.89
  nucleus ambiguous-hypoglossal 352.6
  OAV (oculoauriculovertebral dysplasia) 756.0
  obsessional 300.3
  oculocutaneous 364.24
  oculomotor 378.81
  oculourethroarticular 099.3
  Ogilvie's (sympathicotonic colon obstruction) 560.89
  ophthalmoplegia-cerebellar ataxia 378.52
  Oppenheim-Urbach (necrobiosis lipoidica diabeticorum) 250.8● *[709.3]*
    due to secondary diabetes 249.8● *[709.3]*
  oral-facial-digital 759.89
  organic
    affective NEC 293.83
      drug-induced 292.84
    anxiety 293.84
    delusional 293.81
      alcohol-induced 291.5
      drug-induced 292.11
      due to or associated with
        arteriosclerosis 290.42
          presenile brain disease 290.12
          senility 290.20
    depressive 293.83
      drug-induced 292.84
      due to or associated with
        arteriosclerosis 290.43
          presenile brain disease 290.13
          senile brain disease 290.21
    hallucinosis 293.82
      drug-induced 292.84

Syndrome *(Continued)*
  organic affective 293.83
    induced by drug 292.84
  organic personality 310.1
    induced by drug 292.89
  Ormond's 593.4
  orodigitofacial 759.89
  orthostatic hypotensive-dysautonomic-dyskinetic 333.0
  Osler-Weber-Rendu (familial hemmorrhagic telangiectasia) 448.0
  osteodermopathic hyperostosis 757.39
  osteoporosis-osteomalacia 268.2
  Österreicher-Turner (hereditary osteo-onychodysplasia) 756.89
  os trigonum 755.69
  Ostrum-Furst 756.59
  otolith 386.19
  otopalatodigital 759.89
  outlet (thoracic) 353.0
  ovarian remnant 620.8
  Owren's *(see also* Defect, coagulation) 286.3
  OX 758.6
  pacemaker 429.4
  Paget-Schroetter (intermittent venous claudication) 453.89 ◀▥
  pain - *see also* Pain
    central 338.0
    chronic 338.4
    complex regional 355.9
      type I 337.20
        lower limb 337.22
        specified site NEC 337.29
        upper limb 337.21
      type II
        lower limb 355.71
        upper limb 354.4
    myelopathic 338.0
    thalamic (hyperesthetic) 338.0
  painful
    apicocostal vertebral (M8010/3) 162.3
    arc 726.19
    bruising 287.2
    feet 266.2
  Pancoast's (carcinoma, pulmonary apex) (M8010/3) 162.3
  panhypopituitary (postpartum) 253.2
  papillary muscle 429.81
    with myocardial infarction 410.8●
  Papillon-Léage and Psaume (orodigitofacial dysostosis) 759.89
  parabiotic (transfusion)
    donor (twin) 772.0
    recipient (twin) 776.4
  paralysis agitans 332.0
  paralytic 344.9
    specified type NEC 344.89
  paraneoplastic - *see* Condition
  Parinaud's (paralysis of conjugate upward gaze) 378.81
    oculoglandular 372.02
  Parkes Weber and Dimitri (encephalocutaneous angiomatosis) 759.6
  Parkinson's *(see also* Parkinsonism) 332.0
  parkinsonian *(see also* Parkinsonism) 332.0
  Parry's (exophthalmic goiter) 242.0●
  Parry-Romberg 349.89

Syndrome *(Continued)*

Parsonage-Aldren-Turner 353.5
Parsonage-Turner 353.5
Patau's (trisomy D₁) 758.1
patella clunk 719.66
patellofemoral 719.46
Paterson (-Brown) (-Kelly) (sideropenic dysphagia) 280.8
Payr's (splenic flexure syndrome) 569.89
pectoral girdle 447.8
pectoralis minor 447.8
Pelger-Huët (hereditary hyposegmentation) 288.2
pellagra-cerebellar ataxia-renal aminoaciduria 270.0
Pellegrini-Stieda 726.62
pellagroid 265.2
Pellizzi's (pineal) 259.8
pelvic congestion (-fibrosis) 625.5
Pendred's (familial goiter with deaf-mutism) 243
Penfield's *(see also* Epilepsy) 345.5●
Penta X 758.81
peptic ulcer - *see* Ulcer, peptic 533.9
perabduction 447.8
periodic 277.31
periurethral fibrosis 593.4
persistent fetal circulation 747.83
Petges-Cléjat (poikilodermatomyositis) 710.3
Peutz-Jeghers 759.6
Pfeiffer (acrocephalosyndactyly) 755.55
phantom limb 353.6
pharyngeal pouch 279.11
Pick's (pericardial pseudocirrhosis of liver) 423.2
  heart 423.2
  liver 423.2
Pick-Herxheimer (diffuse idiopathic cutaneous atrophy) 701.8
Pickwickian (cardiopulmonary obesity) 278.8
PIE (pulmonary infiltration with eosinophilia) 518.3
Pierre Marie-Bamberger (hypertrophic pulmonary osteoarthropathy) 731.2
Pierre Mauriac's (diabetes-dwarfism-obesity) 258.1
Pierre Robin 756.0
pigment dispersion, iris 364.53
pineal 259.8
pink puffer 492.8
pituitary 253.0
placental
  dysfunction 762.2
  insufficiency 762.2
  transfusion 762.3
plantar fascia 728.71
plateau iris 364.82
plica knee 727.83
Plummer-Vinson (sideropenic dysphagia) 280.8
pluricarential of infancy 260
plurideficiency of infancy 260
pluriglandular (compensatory) 258.8
polycarential of infancy 260
polyglandular 258.8
polysplenia 759.0
pontine 433.8●
popliteal
  artery entrapment 447.8
  web 756.89

Syndrome *(Continued)*

postartificial menopause 627.4
postcardiac injury
  postcardiotomy 429.4
  postmyocardial infarction 411.0
postcardiotomy 429.4
postcholecystectomy 576.0
postcommissurotomy 429.4
postconcussional 310.2
postcontusional 310.2
postencephalitic 310.8
posterior
  cervical sympathetic 723.2
  fossa compression 348.4
  inferior cerebellar artery *(see also* Disease, cerebrovascular, acute)* 436
  reversible encephalopathy (PRES) 348.39
postgastrectomy (dumping) 564.2
post-gastric surgery 564.2
posthepatitis 780.79
posttherpetic (neuralgia) (zoster) 053.19
  geniculate ganglion 053.11
  ophthalmica 053.19
postimmunization - *see* Complications, vaccination
postinfarction 411.0
postinfluenza (asthenia) 780.79
postirradiation 990
postlaminectomy 722.80
  cervical, cervicothoracic 722.81
  lumbar, lumbosacral 722.83
  thoracic, thoracolumbar 722.82
postleukotomy 310.0
postlobotomy 310.0
postmastectomy lymphedema 457.0
postmature (of newborn) 766.22
postmyocardial infarction 411.0
postoperative NEC 998.9
  blind loop 579.2
postpartum panhypopituitary 253.2
postperfusion NEC 999.89
  bone marrow 996.85
postpericardiotomy 429.4
postphlebitic (asymptomatic) 459.10
  with
    complications NEC 459.19
    inflammation 459.12
      and ulcer 459.13
    stasis dermatitis 459.12
      with ulcer 459.13
    ulcer 459.11
      with inflammation 459.13
postpolio (myelitis) 138
postvagotomy 564.2
postvalvulotomy 429.4
postviral (asthenia) NEC 780.79
Potain's (gastrectasis with dyspepsia) 536.1
potassium intoxication 276.7
Potter's 753.0
Prader (-Labhart)-Willi (-Fanconi) 759.81
preinfarction 411.1
preleukemic 238.75
premature senility 259.8
premenstrual 625.4
premenstrual tension 625.4
pre ulcer 536.9

Syndrome *(Continued)*

Prinzmetal-Massumi (anterior chest wall syndrome) 786.52
Profichet's 729.90
progeria 259.8
progressive pallidal degeneration 333.0
prolonged gestation 766.22
Proteus (dermal hypoplasia) 757.39
prune belly 756.71
prurigo-asthma 691.8
pseudocarpal tunnel (sublimis) 354.0
pseudohermaphroditism-virilismhirsutism 255.2
pseudoparalytica 358.00
pseudo-Turner's 759.89
psycho-organic 293.9
  acute 293.0
  anxiety type 293.84
  depressive type 293.83
  hallucinatory type 293.82
  nonpsychotic severity 310.1
    specified focal (partial) NEC 310.8
  paranoid type 293.81
  specified type NEC 293.89
  subacute 293.1
pterygolymphangiectasia 758.6
ptosis-epicanthus 270.2
pulmonary
  arteriosclerosis 416.0
  hypoperfusion (idiopathic) 769
  renal (hemorrhagic) 446.21
pulseless 446.7
Putnam-Dana (subacute combined sclerosis with pernicious anemia) 281.0 *[336.2]*
pyloroduodenal 537.89
pyramidopallidonigral 332.0
pyriformis 355.0
QT interval prolongation 426.82
radicular NEC 729.2
  lower limbs 724.4
  upper limbs 723.4
  newborn 767.4
Raeder-Harbitz (pulseless disease) 446.7
Ramsay Hunt's
  dyssynergia cerebellaris myoclonica 334.2
  herpetic geniculate ganglionitis 053.11
rapid time-zone change 327.35
Raymond (-Céstan) 433.8●
Raynaud's (paroxysmal digital cyanosis) 443.0
RDS (respiratory distress syndrome, newborn) 769
Refsum's (heredopathia atactica polyneuritiformis) 356.3
Reichmann's (gastrosuccorrhea) 536.8
Reifenstein's (hereditary familial hypogonadism, male) 259.52
Reilly's *(see also* Neuropathy, peripheral, autonomic)* 337.9
Reiter's 099.3
renal glomerulohyalinosis-diabetic 250.4● *[581.81]*
  due to secondary diabetes 249.4● *[581.81]*
Rendu-Osler-Weber (familial hemorrhagic telangiectasia) 448.0
renofacial (congenital biliary fibroangiomatosis) 753.0
Rénon-Delille 253.8

◀ New   ◀▥ Revised   ~~deleted~~ Deleted   ● Use Additional Digit(s)   ▨ Omit code

Syndrome *(Continued)*
    respiratory distress (idiopathic)
            (newborn) 769
        adult (following shock, surgery, or
                trauma) 518.5
            specified NEC 518.82
        type II 770.6
    restless legs (RLS) 333.94
    retinoblastoma (familial) 190.5
    retraction (Duane's) 378.71
    retroperitoneal fibrosis 593.4
    retroviral seroconversion (acute) V08
    Rett's 330.8
    Reye's 331.81
    Reye-Sheehan (postpartum pituitary
            necrosis) 253.2
    Riddoch's (visual disorientation) 368.16
    Ridley's (*see also* Failure, ventricular,
            left) 428.1
    Rieger's (mesodermal dysgenesis,
            anterior ocular segment) 743.44
    Rietti-Greppi-Micheli (thalassemia
            minor) 282.49
    right ventricular obstruction - *see*
            Failure, heart
    Riley-Day (familial dysautonomia)
            742.8
    Robin's 756.0
    Rokitansky-Kuster-Hauser (congenital
            absence, vagina) 752.49
    Romano-Ward (prolonged QT interval
            syndrome) 426.82
    Romberg's 349.89
    Rosen-Castleman-Liebow (pulmonary
            proteinosis) 516.0
    rotator cuff, shoulder 726.10
    Roth's 355.1
    Rothmund's (congenital poikiloderma)
            757.33
    Rotor's (idiopathic hyperbilirubinemia)
            277.4
    Roussy-Lévy 334.3
    Roy (-Jutras) (acropachyderma)
            757.39
    rubella (congenital) 771.0
    Rubinstein-Taybi's (brachydactylia,
            short stature, and mental
            retardation) 759.89
    Rud's (mental deficiency, epilepsy, and
            infantilism) 759.89
    Ruiter-Pompen (-Wyers)
            (angiokeratoma corporis
            diffusum) 272.7
    Runge's (postmaturity) 766.22
    Russell (-Silver) (congenital
            hemihypertrophy and short
            stature) 759.89
    Rytand-Lipsitch (complete
            atrioventricular block) 426.0
    sacralization-scoliosis-sciatica 756.15
    sacroiliac 724.6
    Saenger's 379.46
    salt
        depletion (*see also* Disease, renal)
                593.9
            due to heat NEC 992.8
                causing heat exhaustion or
                        prostration 992.4
        low (*see also* Disease, renal) 593.9
    salt-losing (*see also* Disease, renal) 593.9
    Sanfilippo's (mucopolysaccharidosis
            III) 277.5
    Scaglietti-Dagnini (acromegalic
            macrospondylitis) 253.0

Syndrome *(Continued)*
    scalded skin 695.81
    scalenus anticus (anterior) 353.0
    scapulocostal 354.8
    scapuloperoneal 359.1
    scapulovertebral 723.4
    Schaumann's (sarcoidosis) 135
    Scheie's (mucopolysaccharidosis IS)
            277.5
    Scheuthauer-Marie-Sainton
            (cleidocranialis dysostosis) 755.59
    Schirmer's (encephalocutaneous
            angiomatosis) 759.6
    schizophrenic, of childhood NEC (*see
            also* Psychosis, childhood) 299.9 ●
    Schmidt's
        sphallo-pharyngo-laryngeal
                hemiplegia 352.6
        thyroid-adrenocortical insufficiency
                258.1
        vagoaccessory 352.6
    Schneider's 047.9
    Schnitzler 273.1
    Scholte's (malignant carcinoid) 259.2
    Scholz (-Bielschowsky-Henneberg)
            330.0
    Schroeder's (endocrine-hypertensive)
            255.3
    Schüller-Christian (chronic
            histiocytosis X) 277.89
    Schultz's (agranulocytosis) 288.09
    Schwachman's - *see* Syndrome,
            Shwachman's
    Schwartz (-Jampel) 359.23
    Schwartz-Bartter (inappropriate
            secretion of antidiuretic hormone)
            253.6
    Scimitar (anomalous venous drainage,
            right lung to inferior vena cava)
            747.49
    sclerocystic ovary 256.4
    sea-blue histiocyte 272.7
    Seabright-Bantam
            (pseudohypoparathyroidism)
            275.49
    Seckel's 759.89
    Secretan's (posttraumatic edema) 782.3
    secretoinhibitor (keratoconjunctivitis
            sicca) 710.2
    Seeligmann's (ichthyosis congenita)
            757.1
    Senear-Usher (pemphigus
            erythematosus) 694.4
    senilism 259.8
    seroconversion, retroviral (acute) V08
    serotonin 333.99
    serous meningitis 348.2
    Sertoli cell (germinal aplasia) 606.0
    sex chromosome mosaic 758.81
    Sézary's (reticulosis) (M9701/3) 202.2 ●
    shaken infant 995.55
    Shaver's (bauxite pneumoconiosis) 503
    Sheehan's (postpartum pituitary
            necrosis) 253.2
    shock (traumatic) 958.4
        kidney 584.5
            following crush injury 958.5
        lung 518.5
        neurogenic 308.9
        psychic 308.9
    Shone's 746.84
    short
        bowel 579.3
        P-R interval 426.81

Syndrome *(Continued)*
    shoulder-arm (*see also* Neuropathy,
            peripheral, autonomic) 337.9
    shoulder-girdle 723.4
    shoulder-hand (*see also* Neuropathy,
            peripheral, autonomic) 337.9
    Shwachman's 288.02
    Shy-Drager (orthostatic hypotension
            with multisystem degeneration)
            333.0
    Sicard's 352.6
    sicca (keratoconjunctivitis) 710.2
    sick
        cell 276.1
        cilia 759.89
        sinus 427.81
    sideropenic 280.8
    Siemens'
        ectodermal dysplasia 757.31
        keratosis follicularis spinulosa
                (decalvans) 757.39
    Silfverskiöld's (osteochondrodystrophy,
            extremities) 756.50
    Silver's (congenital hemihypertrophy
            and short stature) 759.89
    Silvestroni-Bianco (thalassemia
            minima) 282.49
    Simons' (progressive lipodystrophy)
            272.6
    sinus tarsi 726.79
    sinusitis-bronchiectasis-situs inversus
            759.3
    Sipple's (medullary thyroid carcinoma-
            pheochromocytoma) 258.02
    Sjögren (-Gougerot)
            (keratoconjunctivitis sicca) 710.2
        with lung involvement 710.2 [*517.8*]
    Sjögren-Larsson (ichthyosis congenita)
            757.1
    SJS-TEN (Stevens-Johnson syndrome-
            toxic epidermal necrolysis
            overlap) 695.14
    Slocumb's 255.3
    Sluder's 337.09
    Smith-Lemli-Opitz (cerebrohepatorenal
            syndrome) 759.89
    Smith-Magenis 758.33
    smokers' 305.1
    Sneddon-Wilkinson (subcorneal
            pustular dermatosis) 694.1
    Sotos' (cerebral gigantism) 253.0
    South African cardiomyopathy 425.2
    spasmodic
        upward movement, eye(s) 378.82
        winking 307.20
    Spens' (syncope with heart block) 426.9
    spherophakia-brachymorphia 759.89
    spinal cord injury - *see also* Injury,
            spinal, by site
        with fracture, vertebra - *see* Fracture,
                vertebra, by site, with spinal
                cord injury
        cervical - *see* Injury, spinal, cervical
        fluid malabsorption (acquired)
                331.3
    splenic
        agenesis 759.0
        flexure 569.89
        neutropenia 289.53
        sequestration 289.52
    Spurway's (brittle bones and blue
            sclera) 756.51
    staphylococcal scalded skin 695.81
    Stein's (polycystic ovary) 256.4

Syndrome *(Continued)*
Stein-Leventhal (polycystic ovary) 256.4
Steinbrocker's *(see also* Neuropathy, peripheral, autonomic) 337.9
Stevens-Johnson (erythema multiforme exudativum) 695.13
    toxic epidermal necrolysis overlap (SJS-TEN overlap syndrome) 695.14
Stewart-Morel (hyperostosis frontalis interna) 733.3
Stickler 759.89
stiff-baby 759.89
stiff-man 333.91
Still's (juvenile rheumatoid arthritis) 714.30
Still-Felty (rheumatoid arthritis with splenomegaly and leukopenia) 714.1
Stilling-Türk-Duane (ocular retraction syndrome) 378.71
Stojano's (subcostal) 098.86
Stokes (-Adams) (syncope with heart block) 426.9
Stokvis-Talma (enterogenous cyanosis) 289.7
stone heart *(see also* Failure, ventricular, left) 428.1
straight-back 756.19
stroke *(see also* Disease, cerebrovascular, acute) 436
    little 435.9
Sturge-Kalischer-Weber (encephalotrigeminal angiomatosis) 759.6
Sturge-Weber (-Dimitri) (encephalocutaneous angiomatosis) 759.6
subclavian-carotid obstruction (chronic) 446.7
subclavian steal 435.2
subcoracoid-pectoralis minor 447.8
subcostal 098.86
    nerve compression 354.8
subperiosteal hematoma 267
subphrenic interposition 751.4
sudden infant death (SIDS) 798.0
Sudeck's 733.7
Sudeck-Leriche 733.7
superior
    cerebellar artery *(see also* Disease, cerebrovascular, acute) 436
    mesenteric artery 557.1
    pulmonary sulcus (tumor) (M8010/3) 162.3
    vena cava 459.2
suprarenal cortical 255.3
supraspinatus 726.10
Susac 348.39
swallowed blood 777.3
sweat retention 705.1
Sweet's (acute febrile neutrophilic dermatosis) 695.89
Swyer-James (unilateral hyperlucent lung) 492.8
Swyer's (XY pure gonadal dysgenesis) 752.7
Symonds' 348.2
sympathetic
    cervical paralysis 337.09
    pelvic 625.5
syndactylic oxycephaly 755.55
syphilitic-cardiovascular 093.89

Syndrome *(Continued)*
systemic
    fibrosclerosing 710.8
    inflammatory response (SIRS) 995.90
    due to
        infectious process 995.91
            with acute organ dysfunction 995.92
        non-infectious process 995.93
            with acute organ dysfunction 995.94
systolic click (-murmur) 785.2
Tabagism 305.1
tachycardia-bradycardia 427.81
Takayasu (-Onishi) (pulseless disease) 446.7
Takotsubo 429.83
Tapia's 352.6
tarsal tunnel 355.5
Taussig-Bing (transposition, aorta and overriding pulmonary artery) 745.11
Taybi's (otopalatodigital) 759.89
Taylor's 625.5
teething 520.7
tegmental 344.89
telangiectasis-pigmentation-cataract 757.33
temporal 383.02
    lobectomy behavior 310.0
temporomandibular joint-pain-dysfunction [TMJ] NEC 524.60
    specified NEC 524.69
Terry's *(see also* Retinopathy of prematurity) 362.21
testicular feminization 259.51
testis, nonvirilizing 257.8
tethered (spinal) cord 742.59
thalamic 338.0
Thibierge-Weissenbach (cutaneous systemic sclerosis) 710.1
Thiele 724.6
thoracic outlet (compression) 353.0
thoracogenous rheumatic (hypertrophic pulmonary osteoarthropathy) 731.2
Thorn's *(see also* Disease, renal) 593.9
Thorson-Biörck (malignant carcinoid) 259.2
thrombopenia-hemangioma 287.39
thyroid-adrenocortical insufficiency 258.1
Tietze's 733.6
time-zone (rapid) 327.35
Tobias' (carcinoma, pulmonary apex) (M8010/3) 162.3
toilet seat 926.0
Tolosa-Hunt 378.55
Toni-Fanconi (cystinosis) 270.0
Touraine's (hereditary osteo-onychodysplasia) 756.89
Touraine-Solente-Golé (acropachyderma) 757.39
toxic
    oil 710.5
    shock 040.82
transfusion
    fetal-maternal 772.0
    twin
        donor (infant) 772.0
        recipient (infant) 776.4
transient left ventricular apical ballooning 429.83

Syndrome *(Continued)*
Treacher Collins' (incomplete mandibulofacial dysostosis) 756.0
trigeminal plate 259.8
triplex X female 758.81
trisomy NEC 758.5
    13 or D$_1$ 758.1
    16–18 or E 758.2
    18 or E$_3$ 758.2
    20 758.5
    21 or G (mongolism) 758.0
    22 or G (mongolism) 758.0
    G 758.0
Troisier-Hanot-Chauffard (bronze diabetes) 275.0
tropical wet feet 991.4
Trousseau's (thrombophlebitis migrans visceral cancer) 453.1
tumor lysis (following antineoplastic drug therapy) (spontaneous) 277.88 ◀
Türk's (ocular retraction syndrome) 378.71
Turner's 758.6
Turner-Varny 758.6
Twiddler's (due to)
    automatic implantable defibrillator 996.04
    pacemaker 996.01
twin-to-twin transfusion 762.3
    recipient twin 776.4
Uehlinger's (acropachyderma) 757.39
Ullrich (-Bonnevie) (-Turner) 758.6
Ullrich-Feichtiger 759.89
underwater blast injury (abdominal) *(see also* Injury, internal, abdomen) 868.00
universal joint, cervix 620.6
Unverricht (-Lundborg) 345.1 ◀═
Unverricht-Wagner (dermatomyositis) 710.3
upward gaze 378.81
Urbach-Oppenheim (necrobiosis lipoidica diabeticorum) 250.8● *[709.3]*
    due to secondary diabetes 249.8● *[709.3]*
Urbach-Wiethe (lipoid proteinosis) 272.8
uremia, chronic 585.9
urethral 597.81
urethro-oculoarticular 099.3
urethro-oculosynovial 099.3
urohepatic 572.4
uveocutaneous 364.24
uveomeningeal, uveomeningitis 363.22
vagohypoglossal 352.6
vagovagal 780.2
van Buchem's (hyperostosis corticalis) 733.3
van der Hoeve's (brittle bones and blue sclera, deafness) 756.51
van der Hoeve-Halbertsma-Waardenburg (ptosis-epicanthus) 270.2
van der Hoeve-Waarderburg-Gualdi (ptosis-epicanthus) 270.2
vanishing twin 651.33
van Neck-Odelberg (juvenile osteochondrosis) 732.1
vascular splanchnic 557.0
vasomotor 443.9
vasovagal 780.2

◀ New   ◀═ Revised   ~~deleted~~ Deleted   ● Use Additional Digit(s)   ▨ Omit code

Syndrome (Continued)
  VATER 759.89
  Velo-cardio-facial 758.32
  vena cava (inferior) (superior)
      (obstruction) 459.2
  Verbiest's (claudicatio intermittens
      spinalis) 435.1
  Vernet's 352.6
  vertebral
      artery 435.1
          compression 721.1
          lumbar 724.4
          steal 435.1
  vertebrogenic (pain) 724.5
  vertiginous NEC 386.9
  video display tube 723.8
  Villaret's 352.6
  Vinson-Plummer (sideropenic
      dysphagia) 280.8
  virilizing adrenocortical hyperplasia,
      congenital 255.2
  virus, viral 079.99
  visceral larval migrans 128.0
  visual disorientation 368.16
  vitamin B_6 deficiency 266.1
  vitreous touch 997.99
  Vogt's (corpus striatum) 333.71
  Vogt-Koyanagi 364.24
  Volkmann's 958.6
  von Bechterew-Stumpell (ankylosing
      spondylitis) 720.0
  von Graefe's 378.72
  von Hippel-Lindau (angiomatosis
      retinocerebellosa) 759.6
  von Schroetter's (intermittent venous
      claudication) 453.89
  von Willebrand (-Jürgens)
      (angiohemophilia) 286.4
  Waardenburg-Klein (ptosis epicanthus)
      270.2
  Wagner (-Unverricht)
      (dermatomyositis) 710.3
  Waldenström's (macroglobulinemia)
      273.3
  Waldenström-Kjellberg (sideropenic
      dysphagia) 280.8
  Wallenberg's (posterior inferior
      cerebellar artery) (see also Disease,
      cerebrovascular, acute) 436
  Waterhouse (-Friderichsen) 036.3
  water retention 276.6
  Weber's 344.89
  Weber-Christian (nodular
      nonsuppurative panniculitis)
      729.30
  Weber-Cockayne (epidermolysis
      bullosa) 757.39
  Weber-Dimitri (encephalocutaneous
      angiomatosis) 759.6
  Weber-Gubler 344.89
  Weber-Leyden 344.89
  Weber-Osler (familial hemorrhagic
      telangiectasia) 448.0
  Wegener's (necrotizing respiratory
      granulomatosis) 446.4
  Weill-Marchesani (brachymorphism
      and ectopia lentis) 759.89
  Weingarten's (tropical eosinophilia)
      518.3
  Weiss-Baker (carotid sinus syncope)
      337.01
  Weissenbach-Thibierge (cutaneous
      systemic sclerosis) 710.1
  Werdnig-Hoffmann 335.0

Syndrome (Continued)
  Werlhof-Wichmann (see also Purpura,
      thrombocytopenic) 287.39
  Wermer's (polyendocrine
      adenomatosis) 258.01
  Werner's (progeria adultorum) 259.8
  Wernicke's (nonalcoholic) (superior
      hemorrhagic polioencephalitis)
      265.1
  Wernicke-Korsakoff (nonalcoholic) 294.0
      alcoholic 291.1
  Westphal-Strümpell (hepatolenticular
      degeneration) 275.1
  wet
      brain (alcoholic) 303.9●
      feet (maceration) (tropical) 991.4
      lung
          adult 518.5
          newborn 770.6
  whiplash 847.0
  Whipple's (intestinal lipodystrophy)
      040.2
  "whistling face" (craniocarpotarsal
      dystrophy) 759.89
  Widal (-Abrami) (acquired hemolytic
      jaundice) 283.9
  Wilkie's 557.1
  Wilkinson-Sneddon (subcorneal
      pustular dermatosis) 694.1
  Willan-Plumbe (psoriasis) 696.1
  Willebrand (-Jürgens)
      (angiohemophilia) 286.4
  Willi-Prader (hypogenital dystrophy
      with diabetic tendency) 759.81
  Wilson's (hepatolenticular
      degeneration) 275.1
  Wilson-Mikity 770.7
  Wiskott-Aldrich (eczema-
      thrombocytopenia) 279.12
  withdrawal
      alcohol 291.81
      drug 292.0
          infant of dependent mother
              779.5
  Woakes' (ethmoiditis) 471.1
  Wolff-Parkinson-White (anomalous
      atrioventricular excitation)
      426.7
  Wright's (hyperabduction) 447.8
  X
      cardiac 413.9
      dysmetabolic 277.7
  xiphoidalgia 733.99
  XO 758.6
  XXX 758.81
  XXXXY 758.81
  XXY 758.7
  yellow vernix (placental dysfunction)
      762.2
  Zahorsky's 074.0
  Zellweger 277.86
  Zieve's (jaundice, hyperlipemia and
      hemolytic anemia) 571.1
  Zollinger-Ellison (gastric
      hypersecretion with pancreatic
      islet cell tumor) 251.5
  Zuelzer-Ogden (nutritional
      megaloblastic anemia) 281.2
Synechia (iris) (pupil) 364.70
  anterior 364.72
      peripheral 364.73
  intrauterine (traumatic) 621.5
  posterior 364.71
  vulvae, congenital 752.49

Synesthesia (see also Disturbance,
      sensation) 782.0
Synodontia 520.2
Synophthalmus 759.89
Synorchidism 752.89
Synorchism 752.89
Synostosis (congenital) 756.59
  astragaloscaphoid 755.67
  radioulnar 755.53
  talonavicular (bar) 755.67
  tarsal 755.67
Synovial - see condition
Synovioma (M9040/3) - see also
      Neoplasm, connective tissue,
      malignant
  benign (M9040/0) - see Neoplasm,
      connective tissue, benign
Synoviosarcoma (M9040/3) - see
      Neoplasm, connective tissue,
      malignant
Synovitis (see also Tenosynovitis)
      727.00
  chronic crepitant, wrist 727.2
  due to crystals - see Arthritis, due to
      crystals
  gonococcal 098.51
  gouty 274.00
  specified NEC 727.09
  syphilitic 095.7
      congenital 090.0
  traumatic, current - see Sprain, by site
  tuberculous - see Tuberculosis,
      synovitis
  villonodular 719.20
      ankle 719.27
      elbow 719.22
      foot 719.27
      hand 719.24
      hip 719.25
      knee 719.26
      multiple sites 719.29
      pelvic region 719.25
      shoulder (region) 719.21
      specified site NEC 719.28
      wrist 719.23
Syphilide 091.3
  congenital 090.0
  newborn 090.0
  tubercular 095.8
      congenital 090.0
Syphilis, syphilitic (acquired) 097.9
  with lung involvement 095.1
  abdomen (late) 095.2
  acoustic nerve 094.86
  adenopathy (secondary) 091.4
  adrenal (gland) 095.8
      with cortical hypofunction 095.8
  age under 2 years NEC (see also
      Syphilis, congenital) 090.9
      acquired 097.9
  alopecia (secondary) 091.82
  anemia 095.8
  aneurysm (artery) (ruptured) 093.89
      aorta 093.0
      central nervous system 094.89
      congenital 090.5
  anus 095.8
      primary 091.1
      secondary 091.3
  aorta, aortic (arch) (abdominal)
      (insufficiency) (pulmonary)
      (regurgitation) (stenosis)
      (thoracic) 093.89
      aneurysm 093.0

Syphilis, syphilitic (Continued)
  arachnoid (adhesive) 094.2
  artery 093.89
    cerebral 094.89
    spinal 094.89
  arthropathy (neurogenic) (tabetic) 094.0
    [713.5]
  asymptomatic - see Syphilis, latent
  ataxia, locomotor (progressive) 094.0
  atrophoderma maculatum 091.3
  auricular fibrillation 093.89
  Bell's palsy 094.89
  bladder 095.8
  bone 095.5
    secondary 091.61
  brain 094.89
  breast 095.8
  bronchus 095.8
  bubo 091.0
  bulbar palsy 094.89
  bursa (late) 095.7
  cardiac decompensation 093.89
  cardiovascular (early) (late) (primary)
    (secondary) (tertiary) 093.9
    specified type and site NEC 093.89
  causing death under 2 years of age (see
    also Syphilis, congenital) 090.9
    stated to be acquired NEC 097.9
  central nervous system (any site) (early)
    (late) (latent) (primary) (recurrent)
    (relapse) (secondary) (tertiary)
    094.9
    with
      ataxia 094.0
      paralysis, general 094.1
        juvenile 090.40
      paresis (general) 094.1
        juvenile 090.40
      tabes (dorsalis) 094.0
        juvenile 090.40
      taboparesis 094.1
        juvenile 090.40
    aneurysm (ruptured) 094.87
    congenital 090.40
    juvenile 090.40
    remission in (sustained) 094.9
    serology doubtful, negative, or
      positive 094.9
    specified nature or site NEC 094.89
    vascular 094.89
  cerebral 094.89
    meningovascular 094.2
    nerves 094.89
    sclerosis 094.89
    thrombosis 094.89
  cerebrospinal 094.89
    tabetic 094.0
  cerebrovascular 094.89
  cervix 095.8
  chancre (multiple) 091.0
    extragenital 091.2
    Rollet's 091.2
  Charcôt's joint 094.0 [713.5]
  choked disc 094.89 [377.00]
  chorioretinitis 091.51
    congenital 090.0 [363.13]
    late 094.83
  choroiditis 091.51
    congenital 090.0 [363.13]
    late 094.83
    prenatal 090.0 [363.13]
  choroidoretinitis (secondary) 091.51
    congenital 090.0 [363.13]
    late 094.83

Syphilis, syphilitic (Continued)
  ciliary body (secondary) 091.52
    late 095.8 [364.11]
  colon (late) 095.8
  combined sclerosis 094.89
  complicating pregnancy, childbirth, or
    puerperium 647.0●
    affecting fetus or newborn 760.2
  condyloma (latum) 091.3
  congenital 090.9
    with
      encephalitis 090.41
      paresis (general) 090.40
      tabes (dorsalis) 090.40
      taborparesis 090.40
    chorioretinitis, choroiditis 090.0
      [363.13]
    early or less than 2 years after birth
      NEC 090.2
      with manifestations 090.0
      latent (without manifestations)
        090.1
        negative spinal fluid test
          090.1
        serology, positive 090.1
      symptomatic 090.0
    interstitial keratitis 090.3
    juvenile neurosyphilis 090.40
    late or 2 years or more after birth
      NEC 090.7
      chorioretinitis, choroiditis 090.5
        [363.13]
      interstitial keratitis 090.3
      juvenile neurosyphilis NEC
        090.40
      latent (without manifestations)
        090.6
        negative spinal fluid test
          090.6
        serology, positive 090.6
      symptomatic or with
        manifestations NEC 090.5
      interstitial keratitis 090.3
  conjugal 097.9
    tabes 094.0
  conjunctiva 095.8 [372.10]
  contact V01.6
  cord, bladder 094.0
  cornea, late 095.8 [370.59]
  coronary (artery) 093.89
    sclerosis 093.89
  coryza 095.8
    congenital 090.0
  cranial nerve 094.89
  cutaneous - see Syphilis, skin
  dacryocystitis 095.8
  degeneration, spinal cord 094.89
  d'emblée 095.8
  dementia 094.1
    paralytica 094.1
      juvenilis 090.40
  destruction of bone 095.5
  dilatation, aorta 093.0
  due to blood transfusion 097.9
  dura mater 094.89
  ear 095.8
    inner 095.8
      nerve (eighth) 094.86
      neurorecurrence 094.86
  early NEC 091.0
    cardiovascular 093.9
    central nervous system 094.9
      paresis 094.1
      tabes 094.0

Syphilis, syphilitic (Continued)
  early NEC (Continued)
    latent (without manifestations) (less
      than 2 years after infection)
      092.9
      negative spinal fluid test 092.9
      serological relapse following
        treatment 092.0
      serology positive 092.9
    paresis 094.1
    relapse (treated, untreated) 091.7
    skin 091.3
    symptomatic NEC 091.89
      extragenital chancre 091.2
      primary, except extragenital
        chancre 091.0
      secondary (see also Syphilis,
        secondary) 091.3
      relapse (treated, untreated)
        091.7
    tabes 094.0
    ulcer 091.3
  eighth nerve 094.86
  endemic, nonveneral 104.0
  endocarditis 093.20
    aortic 093.22
    mitral 093.21
    pulmonary 093.24
    tricuspid 093.23
  epididymis (late) 095.8
  epiglottis 095.8
  epiphysitis (congenital) 090.0
  esophagus 095.8
  Eustachian tube 095.8
  exposure to V01.6
  eye 095.8 [363.13]
    neuromuscular mechanism
      094.85
  eyelid 095.8 [373.5]
    with gumma 095.8 [373.5]
    ptosis 094.89
  fallopian tube 095.8
  fracture 095.5
  gallbladder (late) 095.8
  gastric 095.8
    crisis 094.0
    polyposis 095.8
  general 097.9
    paralysis 094.1
      juvenile 090.40
  genital (primary) 091.0
  glaucoma 095.8
  gumma (late) NEC 095.9
    cardiovascular system 093.9
    central nervous system 094.9
    congenital 090.5
    heart or artery 093.89
  heart 093.89
    block 093.89
    decompensation 093.89
    disease 093.89
    failure 093.89
    valve (see also Syphilis, endocarditis)
      093.20
  hemianesthesia 094.89
  hemianopsia 095.8
  hemiparesis 094.89
  hemiplegia 094.89
  hepatic artery 093.89
  hepatitis 095.3
  hepatomegaly 095.3
    congenital 090.0
  hereditaria tarda (see also Syphilis,
    congenital, late) 090.7

◀ New   ◀||| Revised   ~~deleted~~ Deleted   ● Use Additional Digit(s)   ▨ Omit code

Syphilis, syphilitic (Continued)
  hereditary (see also Syphilis, congenital)
      090.9
    interstitial keratitis 090.3
  Hutchinson's teeth 090.5
  hyalitis 095.8
  inactive - see Syphilis, latent
  infantum NEC (see also Syphilis,
      congenital) 090.9
  inherited - see Syphilis, congenital
  internal ear 095.8
  intestine (late) 095.8
  iris, iritis (secondary) 091.52
    late 095.8 [364.11]
  joint (late) 095.8
  keratitis (congenital) (early)
      (interstitial) (late)
      (parenchymatous) (punctata
      profunda) 090.3
  kidney 095.4
  lacrimal apparatus 095.8
  laryngeal paralysis 095.8
  larynx 095.8
  late 097.0
    cardiovascular 093.9
    central nervous system 094.9
    latent or 2 years or more after
        infection (without
        manifestation) 096
      negative spinal fluid test 096
      serology positive 096
    paresis 094.1
    specified site NEC 095.8
    symptomatic or with symptoms
        095.9
    tabes 094.0
  latent 097.1
    central nervous system 094.9
    date of infection unspecified
        097.1
    early or less than 2 years after
        infection 092.9
    late or 2 years or more after infection
        096
    serology
      doubtful
        follow-up of latent syphilis
            097.1
          central nervous system
              094.9
          date of infection unspecified
              097.1
          early or less than 2 years
              after infection 092.9
          late or 2 years or more after
              infection 096
      positive, only finding 097.1
        date of infection unspecified
            097.1
        early or less than 2 years after
            infection 097.1
        late or 2 years or more after
            infection 097.1
  lens 095.8
  leukoderma 091.3
    late 095.8
  lienis 095.8
  lip 091.3
    chancre 091.2
    late 095.8
    primary 091.2
  Lissauer's paralysis 094.1
  liver 095.3
    secondary 091.62

Syphilis, syphilitic (Continued)
  locomotor ataxia 094.0
  lung 095.1
  lymphadenitis (secondary) 091.4
  lymph gland (early) (secondary) 091.4
    late 095.8
  macular atrophy of skin 091.3
    striated 095.8
  maternal, affecting fetus or newborn
      760.2
    manifest syphilis in newborn - see
        Syphilis, congenital
  mediastinum (late) 095.8
  meninges (adhesive) (basilar) (brain)
      (spinal cord) 094.2
  meningitis 094.2
    acute 091.81
    congenital 090.42
  meningoencephalitis 094.2
  meningovascular 094.2
    congenital 090.49
  mesarteritis 093.89
    brain 094.89
    spine 094.89
  middle ear 095.8
  mitral stenosis 093.21
  monoplegia 094.89
  mouth (secondary) 091.3
    late 095.8
  mucocutaneous 091.3
    late 095.8
  mucous
    membrane 091.3
      late 095.8
    patches 091.3
      congenital 090.0
  mulberry molars 090.5
  muscle 095.6
  myocardium 093.82
  myositis 095.6
  nasal sinus 095.8
  neonatorum NEC (see also Syphilis,
      congenital) 090.9
  nerve palsy (any cranial nerve)
      094.89
  nervous system, central 094.9
  neuritis 095.8
    acoustic nerve 094.86
  neurorecidive of retina 094.83
  neuroretinitis 094.85
  newborn (see also Syphilis, congenital)
      090.9
  nodular superficial 095.8
  nonvenereal, endemic 104.0
  nose 095.8
    saddle back deformity 090.5
    septum 095.8
      perforated 095.8
  occlusive arterial disease 093.89
  ophthalmic 095.8 [363.13]
  ophthalmoplegia 094.89
  optic nerve (atrophy) (neuritis)
      (papilla) 094.84
  orbit (late) 095.8
  orchitis 095.8
  organic 097.9
  osseous (late) 095.5
  osteochondritis (congenital) 090.0
  osteoporosis 095.5
  ovary 095.8
  oviduct 095.8
  palate 095.8
    gumma 095.8
    perforated 090.5

Syphilis, syphilitic (Continued)
  pancreas (late) 095.8
  pancreatitis 095.8
  paralysis 094.89
    general 094.1
    juvenile 090.40
  paraplegia 094.89
  paresis (general) 094.1
    juvenile 090.40
  paresthesia 094.89
  Parkinson's disease or syndrome
      094.82
  paroxysmal tachycardia 093.89
  pemphigus (congenital) 090.0
  penis 091.0
    chancre 091.0
    late 095.8
  pericardium 093.81
  perichondritis, larynx 095.8
  periosteum 095.5
    congenital 090.0
    early 091.61
    secondary 091.61
  peripheral nerve 095.8
  petrous bone (late) 095.5
  pharynx 095.8
    secondary 091.3
  pituitary (gland) 095.8
  placenta 095.8
  pleura (late) 095.8
  pneumonia, white 090.0
  pontine (lesion) 094.89
  portal vein 093.89
  primary NEC 091.2
    anal 091.1
    and secondary (see also Syphilis,
        secondary) 091.9
    cardiovascular 093.9
    central nervous system 094.9
    extragenital chancre NEC 091.2
    fingers 091.2
    genital 091.0
    lip 091.2
    specified site NEC 091.2
    tonsils 091.2
  prostate 095.8
  psychosis (intracranial gumma) 094.89
  ptosis (eyelid) 094.89
  pulmonary (late) 095.1
    artery 093.89
  pulmonum 095.1
  pyelonephritis 095.4
  recently acquired, symptomatic NEC
      091.89
  rectum 095.8
  respiratory tract 095.8
  retina
    late 094.83
    neurorecidive 094.83
  retrobulbar neuritis 094.85
  salpingitis 095.8
  sclera (late) 095.0
  sclerosis
    cerebral 094.89
    coronary 093.89
    multiple 094.89
    subacute 094.89
  scotoma (central) 095.8
  scrotum 095.8
  secondary (and primary) 091.9
    adenopathy 091.4
    anus 091.3
    bone 091.61
    cardiovascular 093.9

Syphilis, syphilitic *(Continued)*
  secondary *(Continued)*
    central nervous system 094.9
    chorioretinitis, choroiditis 091.51
    hepatitis 091.62
    liver 091.62
    lymphadenitis 091.4
    meningitis, acute 091.81
    mouth 091.3
    mucous membranes 091.3
    periosteum 091.61
    periostitis 091.61
    pharynx 091.3
    relapse (treated) (untreated) 091.7
    skin 091.3
    specified form NEC 091.89
    tonsil 091.3
    ulcer 091.3
    viscera 091.69
    vulva 091.3
  seminal vesicle (late) 095.8
  seronegative
    with signs or symptoms - *see*
      Syphilis, by site and stage
  seropositive
    with signs or symptoms - *see*
      Syphilis, by site or stage
    follow-up of latent syphilis - *see*
      Syphilis, latent
    only finding - *see* Syphilis, latent
  seventh nerve (paralysis) 094.89
  sinus 095.8
  sinusitis 095.8
  skeletal system 095.5
  skin (early) (secondary) (with
    ulceration) 091.3
    late or tertiary 095.8
  small intestine 095.8
  spastic spinal paralysis 094.0
  spermatic cord (late) 095.8
  spinal (cord) 094.89
    with
      paresis 094.1
      tabes 094.0
  spleen 095.8
  splenomegaly 095.8
  spondylitis 095.5
  staphyloma 095.8
  stigmata (congenital) 090.5
  stomach 095.8
  synovium (late) 095.7

Syphilis, syphilitic *(Continued)*
  tabes dorsalis (early) (late) 094.0
    juvenile 090.40
  tabetic type 094.0
    juvenile 090.40
  taboparesis 094.1
    juvenile 090.40
  tachycardia 093.89
  tendon (late) 095.7
  tertiary 097.0
    with symptoms 095.8
    cardiovascular 093.9
    central nervous system 094.9
    multiple NEC 095.8
    specified site NEC 095.8
  testis 095.8
  thorax 095.8
  throat 095.8
  thymus (gland) 095.8
  thyroid (late) 095.8
  tongue 095.8
  tonsil (lingual) 095.8
    primary 091.2
    secondary 091.3
  trachea 095.8
  tricuspid valve 093.23
  tumor, brain 094.89
  tunica vaginalis (late) 095.8
  ulcer (any site) (early) (secondary)
    091.3
    late 095.9
    perforating 095.9
      foot 094.0
  urethra (stricture) 095.8
  urogenital 095.8
  uterus 095.8
  uveal tract (secondary) 091.50
    late 095.8 *[363.13]*
  uveitis (secondary) 091.50
    late 095.8 *[363.13]*
  uvula (late) 095.8
    perforated 095.8
  vagina 091.0
    late 095.8
  valvulitis NEC 093.20
  vascular 093.89
    brain or cerebral 094.89
  vein 093.89
    cerebral 094.89
  ventriculi 095.8
  vesicae urinariae 095.8

Syphilis, syphilitic *(Continued)*
  viscera (abdominal) 095.2
    secondary 091.69
  vitreous (hemorrhage) (opacities) 095.8
  vulva 091.0
    late 095.8
    secondary 091.3
Syphiloma 095.9
  cardiovascular system 093.9
  central nervous system 094.9
  circulatory system 093.9
  congenital 090.5
Syphilophobia 300.29
Syringadenoma (M8400/0) - *see also*
  Neoplasm, skin, benign
  papillary (M8406/0) - *see* Neoplasm,
    skin, benign
Syringobulbia 336.0
Syringocarcinoma (M8400/3) - *see*
  Neoplasm, skin, malignant
Syringocystadenoma (M8400/0) - *see also*
  Neoplasm, skin, benign
  papillary (M8406/0) - *see* Neoplasm,
    skin, benign
Syringocystoma (M8407/0) - *see*
  Neoplasm, skin, benign
Syringoma (M8407/0) - *see also*
  Neoplasm, skin, benign
  chondroid (M8940/0) - *see* Neoplasm,
    by site, benign
Syringomyelia 336.0
Syringomyelitis 323.9
  late effect - *see* category 326
Syringomyelocele (*see also* Spina bifida)
  741.9●
Syringopontia 336.0
System, systemic - *see also* condition
  disease, combined - *see* Degeneration,
    combined
  fibrosclerosing syndrome 710.8
  inflammatory response syndrome
    (SIRS) 995.90
    due to
      infectious process 995.91
        with acute organ dysfunction
          995.92
      non-infectious process 995.93
        with acute organ dysfunction
          995.94
  lupus erythematosus 710.0
    inhibitor 286.5

T

Tab - *see* Tag
Tabacism 989.84
Tabacosis 989.84
Tabardillo 080
  flea-borne 081.0
  louse-borne 080
Tabes, tabetic
  with
    central nervous system syphilis
      094.0
    Charcôt's joint 094.0 [713.5]
    cord bladder 094.0
    crisis, viscera (any) 094.0
    paralysis, general 094.1
    paresis (general) 094.1
    perforating ulcer 094.0
  arthropathy 094.0 [713.5]
  bladder 094.0
  bone 094.0
  cerebrospinal 094.0
  congenital 090.40
  conjugal 094.0
  dorsalis 094.0
    neurosyphilis 094.0
  early 094.0
  juvenile 090.40
  latent 094.0
  mesenterica (*see also* Tuberculosis)
    014.8●
  paralysis insane, general 094.1
  peripheral (nonsyphilitic) 799.89
  spasmodic 094.0
    not dorsal or dorsalis 343.9
  syphilis (cerebrospinal) 094.0
Taboparalysis 094.1
Taboparesis (remission) 094.1
  with
    Charcôt's joint 094.1 [713.5]
    cord bladder 094.1
    perforating ulcer 094.1
  juvenile 090.40
Tache noir 923.20
Tachyalimentation 579.3
Tachyarrhythmia, tachyrhythmia - *see also*
  Tachycardia
  paroxysmal with sinus bradycardia
    427.81
Tachycardia 785.0
  atrial 427.89
  auricular 427.89
  AV nodal re-entry (re-entrant)
    427.89
  junctional ectopic 427.0
  newborn 779.82
  nodal 427.89
    nonparoxysmal atrioventricular
      426.89
    nonparoxysmal atrioventricular (nodal)
      426.89
  nonsustained 427.2
  paroxysmal 427.2
    with sinus bradycardia 427.81
    atrial (PAT) 427.0
      psychogenic 316 [427.0]
    atrioventricular (AV) 427.0
      psychogenic 316 [427.0]
    essential 427.2
    junctional 427.0
    nodal 427.0
    psychogenic 316 [427.2]
      atrial 316 [427.0]
      supraventricular 316 [427.0]
      ventricular 316 [427.1]

Tachycardia (*Continued*)
  paroxysmal (*Continued*)
    supraventricular 427.0
      psychogenic 316 [427.0]
    ventricular 427.1
      psychogenic 316 [427.1]
  postoperative 997.1
  psychogenic 306.2
  sick sinus 427.81
  sinoauricular 427.89
  sinus 427.89
  supraventricular 427.89
  sustained 427.2
    supraventricular 427.0
    ventricular 427.1
  ventricular (paroxysmal) 427.1
    psychogenic 316 [427.1]
Tachygastria 536.8
Tachypnea 786.06
  hysterical 300.11
  newborn (idiopathic) (transitory) 770.6
  psychogenic 306.1
  transitory, of newborn 770.6
Taenia (infection) (infestation) (*see also*
  Infestation, taenia) 123.3
  diminuta 123.6
  echinococcal infestation (*see also*
    Echinococcus) 122.9
  nana 123.6
  saginata infestation 123.2
  solium (intestinal form) 123.0
    larval form 123.1
Taeniasis (intestine) (*see also* Infestation,
  taenia) 123.3
  saginata 123.2
  solium 123.0
Taenzer's disease 757.4
Tag (hypertrophied skin) (infected) 701.9
  adenoid 474.8
  anus 455.9
  endocardial (*see also* Endocarditis)
    424.90
  hemorrhoidal 455.9
  hymen 623.8
  perineal 624.8
  preauricular 744.1
  rectum 455.9
  sentinel 455.9
  skin 701.9
    accessory 757.39
    anus 455.9
    congenital 757.39
    preauricular 744.1
    rectum 455.9
  tonsil 474.8
  urethra, urethral 599.84
  vulva 624.8
Tahyna fever 062.5
Takayasu (-Onishi) disease or syndrome
  (pulseless disease) 446.7
Takotsubo syndrome 429.83
Talc granuloma 728.82
  in operation wound 998.7
Talcosis 502
Talipes (congenital) 754.70
  acquired NEC 736.79
    planus 734
  asymmetric 754.79
    acquired 736.79
  calcaneovalgus 754.62
    acquired 736.76
  calcaneovarus 754.59
    acquired 736.76
  calcaneus 754.79
    acquired 736.76

Talipes (*Continued*)
  cavovarus 754.59
    acquired 736.75
  cavus 754.71
    acquired 736.73
  equinovalgus 754.69
    acquired 736.72
  equinovarus 754.51
    acquired 736.71
  equinus 754.79
    acquired, NEC 736.72
  percavus 754.71
    acquired 736.73
  planovalgus 754.69
    acquired 736.79
  planus (acquired) (any degree) 734
    congenital 754.61
    due to rickets 268.1
  valgus 754.60
    acquired 736.79
  varus 754.50
    acquired 736.79
Talma's disease 728.85
Talon noir 924.20
  hand 923.20
  heel 924.20
  toe 924.3
Tamponade heart (Rose's) (*see also*
  Pericarditis) 423.3
Tanapox 059.21
Tangier disease (familial high-density
  lipoprotein deficiency) 272.5
Tank ear 380.12
Tantrum (childhood) (*see also* Disturbance,
  conduct) 312.1●
Tapeworm (infection) (infestation) (*see
  also* Infestation, tapeworm) 123.9
Tapia's syndrome 352.6
Tarantism 297.8
Target-oval cell anemia 282.49
Tarlov's cyst 355.9
Tarral-Besnier disease (pityriasis rubra
  pilaris) 696.4
Tarsalgia 729.2
Tarsal tunnel syndrome 355.5
Tarsitis (eyelid) 373.00
  syphilitic 095.8 [373.00]
  tuberculous (*see also* Tuberculosis)
    017.0● [373.4]
Tartar (teeth) 523.6
Tattoo (mark) 709.09
Taurodontism 520.2
Taussig-Bing defect, heart, or syndrome
  (transposition, aorta and overriding
  pulmonary artery) 745.11
Tay's choroiditis 363.41
Tay-Sachs
  amaurotic familial idiocy 330.1
  disease 330.1
Taybi's syndrome (otopalatodigital)
  759.89
Taylor's
  disease (diffuse idiopathic cutaneous
    atrophy) 701.8
  syndrome 625.5
TBI (traumatic brain injury) (*see also*
  Injury, intracranial) 854.0 ◀
  with skull fracture - *see* Fracture,
    skull, by site ◀
Tear, torn (traumatic) - *see also* Wound,
  open, by site
  anus, anal (sphincter) 863.89
    with open wound in cavity 863.99
    complicating delivery (healed) (old)
      654.8●
      with mucosa 664.3●

Tear, torn *(Continued)*
  anus, anal *(Continued)*
    complicating delivery *(Continued)*
      not associated with third-degree
        perineal laceration 664.6●
    nontraumatic, nonpuerperal
        (healed) (old) 569.43
  articular cartilage, old *(see also*
      Disorder, cartilage, articular)
      718.0●
  bladder
    with
      abortion - *see* Abortion, by type,
        with damage to pelvic
        organs
      ectopic pregnancy *(see also*
        categories 633.0–633.9)
        639.2
      molar pregnancy *(see also*
        categories 630–632) 639.2
    following
      abortion 639.2
      ectopic or molar pregnancy 639.2
    obstetrical trauma 665.5●
  bowel
    with
      abortion - *see* Abortion, by type,
        with damage to pelvic
        organs
      ectopic pregnancy *(see also*
        categories 633.0–633.9) 639.2
      molar pregnancy *(see also*
        categories 630–632) 639.2
    following
      abortion 639.2
      ectopic or molar pregnancy
        639.2
    obstetrical trauma 665.5●
  broad ligament
    with
      abortion - *see* Abortion, by type,
        with damage to pelvic
        organs
      ectopic pregnancy *(see also*
        categories 633.0–633.9)
        639.2
      molar pregnancy *(see also*
        categories 630–632) 639.2
    following
      abortion 639.2
      ectopic or molar pregnancy
        639.2
    obstetrical trauma 665.6●
  bucket handle (knee) (meniscus) - *see*
      Tear, meniscus
  capsule
    joint - *see* Sprain, by site
    spleen - *see* Laceration, spleen,
        capsule
  cartilage - *see also* Sprain, by site
    articular, old *(see also* Disorder,
        cartilage, articular) 718.0●
    knee - *see* Tear, meniscus
    semilunar (knee) (current injury) -
        see Tear, meniscus
  cervix
    with
      abortion - *see* Abortion, by type,
        with damage to pelvic
        organs
      ectopic pregnancy *(see also*
        categories 633.0–633.9)
        639.2
      molar pregnancy *(see also*
        categories 630–632) 639.2

Tear, torn *(Continued)*
  cervix *(Continued)*
    following
      abortion 639.2
      ectopic or molar pregnancy 639.2
    obstetrical trauma (current) 665.3●
    old 622.3
  dural 349.31
    accidental puncture or laceration
        during a procedure 349.31
    incidental (inadvertent) 349.31
    nontraumatic NEC 349.39
  internal organ (abdomen, chest, or
      pelvis) - *see* Injury, internal, by
      site
  ligament - *see also* Sprain, by site
    with open wound - *see* Wound,
        open, by site
  meniscus (knee) (current injury) 836.2
    bucket handle 836.0
      old 717.0
    lateral 836.1
      anterior horn 836.1
        old 717.42
      bucket handle 836.1
        old 717.41
      old 717.40
      posterior horn 836.1
        old 717.43
      specified site NEC 836.1
        old 717.49
    medial 836.0
      anterior horn 836.0
        old 717.1
      bucket handle 836.0
        old 717.0
      old 717.3
      posterior horn 836.0
        old 717.2
    old NEC 717.5
    site other than knee - *see* Sprain, by
        site
  muscle - *see also* Sprain, by site
    with open wound - *see* Wound,
        open, by site
  pelvic
    floor, complicating delivery 664.1●
    organ NEC
      with
        abortion - *see* Abortion, by
          type, with damage to
          pelvic organs
        ectopic pregnancy *(see also*
          categories 633.0–633.9)
          639.2
        molar pregnancy *(see also*
          categories 630–632) 639.2
      following
        abortion 639.2
        ectopic or molar pregnancy
          639.2
      obstetrical trauma 665.5●
  perineum - *see also* Laceration,
      perineum
    obstetrical trauma 665.5●
  periurethral tissue
    with
      abortion - *see* Abortion, by type,
        with damage to pelvic
        organs
      ectopic pregnancy *(see also*
        categories 633.0–633.9) 639.2
      molar pregnancy *(see also*
        categories 630–632) 639.2
    following
      abortion 639.2
      ectopic or molar pregnancy 639.2

Tear, torn *(Continued)*
  periurethral tissue *(Continued)*
    obstetrical trauma 665.5●
  rectovaginal septum - *see* Laceration,
      rectovaginal septum
  retina, retinal (recent) (with
      detachment) 361.00
    without detachment 361.30
    dialysis (juvenile) (with detachment)
        361.04
    giant (with detachment) 361.03
    horseshoe (without detachment)
        361.32
    multiple (with detachment) 361.02
      without detachment 361.33
    old
      delimited (partial) 361.06
      partial 361.06
      total or subtotal 361.07
    partial (without detachment)
      giant 361.03
      multiple defects 361.02
      old (delimited) 361.06
      single defect 361.01
    round hole (without detachment)
        361.31
    single defect (with detachment)
        361.01
    total or subtotal (recent) 361.05
      old 361.07
  rotator cuff (traumatic) 840.4
    current injury 840.4
    degenerative 726.10
    nontraumatic 727.61
  semilunar cartilage, knee (*see also* Tear,
      meniscus) 836.2
    old 717.5
  tendon - *see also* Sprain, by site
    with open wound - *see* Wound,
        open, by site
  tentorial, at birth 767.0
  umbilical cord
    affecting fetus or newborn 772.0
    complicating delivery 663.8●
  urethra
    with
      abortion - *see* Abortion, by type,
        with damage to pelvic
        organs
      ectopic pregnancy *(see also*
        categories 633.0–633.9) 639.2
      molar pregnancy *(see also*
        categories 630–632) 639.2
    following
      abortion 639.2
      ectopic or molar pregnancy
        639.2
    obstetrical trauma 665.5●
  uterus - *see* Injury, internal, uterus
  vagina - *see* Laceration, vagina
  vessel, from catheter 998.2
  vulva, complicating delivery
      664.0●
Tear stone 375.57
Teeth, tooth - *see also* condition
  grinding 306.8
  prenatal 520.6
Teething 520.7
  syndrome 520.7
Tegmental syndrome 344.89
Telangiectasia, telangiectasis (verrucous)
    448.9
  ataxic (cerebellar) 334.8
  familial 448.0
  hemorrhagic, hereditary (congenital)
      (senile) 448.0

◄ New   ◄▥ Revised   ~~deleted~~ Deleted   ● Use Additional Digit(s)   ▨ Omit code

Telangiectasia, telangiectasis *(Continued)*
  hereditary hemorrhagic 448.0
  retina 362.15
  spider 448.1
Telecanthus (congenital) 743.63
Telescoped bowel or intestine *(see also*
    Intussusception) 560.0
Teletherapy, adverse effect NEC 990
Telogen effluvium 704.02
Temperature
  body, high (of unknown origin) *(see also*
      Pyrexia) 780.60
  cold, trauma from 991.9
    newborn 778.2
    specified effect NEC 991.8
  high
    body (of unknown origin) *(see also*
        Pyrexia) 780.60
    trauma from - *see* Heat
Temper tantrum (childhood) *(see also*
    Disturbance, conduct) 312.1 ●
Temple - *see* condition
Temporal - *see also* condition
  lobe syndrome 310.0
Temporomandibular joint-pain-
    dysfunction syndrome 524.60
Temporosphenoidal - *see* condition
Tendency
  bleeding *(see also* Defect, coagulation)
      286.9
  homosexual, ego-dystonic
      302.0
  paranoid 301.0
  suicide 300.9
Tenderness
  abdominal (generalized) (localized)
      789.6 ●
  rebound 789.6 ●
  skin 782.0
Tendinitis, tendonitis *(see also*
    Tenosynovitis) 726.90
  Achilles 726.71
  adhesive 726.90
    shoulder 726.0
  calcific 727.82
    shoulder 726.11
  gluteal 726.5
  patellar 726.64
  peroneal 726.79
  pes anserinus 726.61
  psoas 726.5
  tibialis (anterior) (posterior) 726.72
  trochanteric 726.5
Tendon - *see* condition
Tendosynovitis - *see* Tenosynovitis
Tendovaginitis - *see* Tenosynovitis
Tenesmus 787.99
  rectal 787.99
  vesical 788.99
Tenia - *see* Taenia
Teniasis - *see* Taeniasis
Tennis elbow 726.32
Tenonitis - *see also* Tenosynovitis
  eye (capsule) 376.04
Tenontosynovitis - *see* Tenosynovitis
Tenontothecitis - *see* Tenosynovitis
Tenophyte 727.9
Tenosynovitis *(see also* Synovitis) 727.00
  adhesive 726.90
    shoulder 726.0
  ankle 727.06
  bicipital (calcifying) 726.12
  buttock 727.09
  due to crystals - *see* Arthritis, due to
      crystals
  elbow 727.09

Tenosynovitis *(Continued)*
  finger 727.05
  foot 727.06
  gonococcal 098.51
  hand 727.05
  hip 727.09
  knee 727.09
  radial styloid 727.04
  shoulder 726.10
    adhesive 726.0
  specified NEC 727.09
  spine 720.1
  supraspinatus 726.10
  toe 727.06
  tuberculous - *see* Tuberculosis,
      tenosynovitis
  wrist 727.05
Tenovaginitis - *see* Tenosynovitis
Tension
  arterial, high *(see also* Hypertension)
      401.9
    without diagnosis of hypertension
        796.2
  headache 307.81
  intraocular (elevated) 365.00
  nervous 799.21   ◀▥
  ocular (elevated) 365.00
  pneumothorax 512.0
    iatrogenic 512.1
    postoperative 512.1
    spontaneous 512.0
  premenstrual 625.4
  state 300.9
Tentorium - *see* condition
Teratencephalus 759.89
Teratism 759.7
Teratoblastoma (malignant)
    (M9080/3) - *see* Neoplasm,
    by site, malignant
Teratocarcinoma (M9081/3) - *see also*
    Neoplasm, by site, malignant
  liver 155.0
Teratoma (solid) (M9080/1) - *see also*
    Neoplasm, by site, uncertain
    behavior
  adult (cystic) (M9080/0) - *see*
      Neoplasm, by site, benign
  and embryonal carcinoma, mixed
      (M9081/3) - *see* Neoplasm, by
      site, malignant
  benign (M9080/0) - *see* Neoplasm, by
      site, benign
  combined with choriocarcinoma
      (M9101/3) - *see* Neoplasm, by
      site, malignant
  cystic (adult) (M9080/0) - *see*
      Neoplasm, by site, benign
  differentiated type (M9080/0) - *see*
      Neoplasm, by site, benign
  embryonal (M9080/3) - *see also*
      Neoplasm, by site, malignant
    liver 155.0
  fetal
    sacral, causing fetopelvic
        disproportion 653.7 ●
  immature (M9080/3) - *see* Neoplasm,
      by site, malignant
  liver (M9080/3) 155.0
    adult, benign, cystic, differentiated
        type, or mature (M9080/0)
        211.5
  malignant (M9080/3) - *see also*
      Neoplasm, by site, malignant
    anaplastic type (M9082/3) - *see*
        Neoplasm, by site, malignant

Teratoma *(Continued)*
  malignant *(Continued)*
    intermediate type (M9083/3) - *see*
        Neoplasm, by site, malignant
    liver (M9080/3) 155.0
    trophoblastic (M9102/3)
      specified site - *see* Neoplasm, by
          site, malignant
      unspecified site 186.9
    undifferentiated type (M9082/3) -
        see Neoplasm, by site,
        malignant
  mature (M9080/0) - *see* Neoplasm, by
      site, benign
    malignant (M9080/3) - *see*
        Neoplasm, by site,
        malignant
  ovary (M9080/0) 220
    embryonal, immature, or malignant
        (M9080/3) 183.0
  suprasellar (M9080/3) - *see* Neoplasm,
      by site, malignant
  testis (M9080/3) 186.9
    adult, benign, cystic, differentiated
        type or mature (M9080/0)
        222.0
    undescended 186.0
Terminal care V66.7
Termination
  anomalous - *see also* Malposition,
      congenital
    portal vein 747.49
    right pulmonary vein 747.42
  pregnancy (legal) (therapeutic) *(see*
      Abortion, legal) 635.9 ●
    fetus NEC 779.6
    illegal *(see also* Abortion, illegal)
        636.9 ●
Ternidens diminutus infestation 127.7
Terrors, night (child) 307.46
Terry's syndrome *(see also* Retinopathy
    of prematurity) 362.21
Tertiary - *see* condition
Tessellated fundus, retina (tigroid)
    362.89
Test(s)
  adequacy
    hemodialysis V56.31
    peritoneal dialysis V56.32
  AIDS virus V72.69   ◀▥
  allergen V72.7
  bacterial disease NEC *(see also*
      Screening, by name of disease)
      V74.9
  basal metabolic rate V72.69   ◀▥
  blood ~~alcohol V70.4~~   ◀▥
    alcohol V70.4   ◀
    drug V70.4   ◀
      for therapeutic drug monitoring
          V58.83   ◀
    for routine general physical
        examination V72.62   ◀
    prior to treatment or procedure
        V72.63   ◀
    typing V72.86   ◀
      Rh typing V72.86   ◀
  ~~blood-drug V70.4~~
      ~~for therapeutic drug monitoring~~
          ~~V58.83~~
  ~~blood typing V72.86~~
      ~~Rh typing V72.86~~
  developmental, infant or child
      V20.2
  Dick V74.8
  fertility V26.21

Test(s) (Continued)
genetic
  female V26.32
  for genetic disease carrier status
    female V26.31
    male V26.34
  male V26.39
hearing V72.19
  following failed hearing screening
    V72.11
  routine, for infant and child V20.2 ◄
HIV V72.69 ◄▥
human immunodeficiency virus
  V72.69 ◄▥
immunity status V72.61 ◄
Kveim V82.89
laboratory V72.60 ◄▥
  for medicolegal reason V70.4
  ordered as part of a routine
    general medical
    examination V72.62 ◄
  pre-operative V72.63 ◄
  pre-procedural V72.63 ◄
  specified NEC V72.69 ◄
male partner of habitual aborter V26.35
Mantoux (for tuberculosis) V74.1
mycotic organism V75.4
nuchal translucency V28.89
parasitic agent NEC V75.8
paternity V70.4
peritoneal equilibration V56.32
pregnancy
  negative result V72.41
  positive result V72.42
    first pregnancy V72.42
  unconfirmed V72.40
preoperative V72.84
  cardiovascular V72.81
  respiratory V72.82
  specified NEC V72.83
procreative management NEC V26.29
  genetic disease carrier status
    female V26.31
    male V26.34
Rh typing V72.86
sarcoidosis V82.89
Schick V74.3
Schultz-Charlton V74.8
skin, diagnostic
  allergy V72.7
  bacterial agent NEC (see also
    Screening, by name of
    disease) V74.9
  Dick V74.8
  hypersensitivity V72.7
  Kveim V82.89
  Mantoux V74.1
  mycotic organism V75.4
  parasitic agent NEC V75.8
  sarcoidosis V82.89
  Schick V74.3
  Schultz-Charlton V74.8
  tuberculin V74.1
specified type NEC V72.85
tuberculin V74.1
vision V72.0
  routine, for infant and child
    V20.2 ◄
Wassermann
  positive (see also Serology for
    syphilis, positive) 097.1
  false 795.6
Testicle, testicular, testis - see also
  condition
  feminization (syndrome) 259.51
Tetanus, tetanic (cephalic) (convulsions)
  037

Tetanus, tetanic (Continued)
with
  abortion - see Abortion, by type,
    with sepsis
  ectopic pregnancy (see also
    categories 633.0–633.9) 639.0
  molar pregnancy (see categories
    630–632) 639.0
following
  abortion 639.0
  ectopic or molar pregnancy 639.0
inoculation V03.7
  reaction (due to serum) - see
    Complications, vaccination
neonatorum 771.3
puerperal, postpartum, childbirth
  670.8 ◄▥
Tetany, tetanic 781.7
alkalosis 276.3
associated with rickets 268.0
convulsions 781.7
  hysterical 300.11
functional (hysterical) 300.11
hyperkinetic 781.7
  hysterical 300.11
hyperpnea 786.01
  hysterical 300.11
  psychogenic 306.1
hyperventilation 786.01
  hysterical 300.11
  psychogenic 306.1
hypocalcemic, neonatal 775.4
hysterical 300.11
neonatal 775.4
parathyroid (gland) 252.1
parathyroprival 252.1
postoperative 252.1
postthyroidectomy 252.1
pseudotetany 781.7
  hysterical 300.11
psychogenic 306.1
  specified as conversion reaction
    300.11
Tetralogy of Fallot 745.2
Tetraplegia - see Quadriplegia
Thailand hemorrhagic fever 065.4
Thalassanemia 282.49
Thalassemia (alpha) (beta) (disease)
  (Hb-C) (Hb-D) (Hb-E) (Hb-H)
  (Hb-I) (high fetal gene) (high fetal
  hemoglobin) (intermedia) (major)
  (minima) (minor) (mixed) (trait)
  (with other hemoglobinopathy)
  282.49
Hb-S (without crisis) 282.41
  with
    crisis 282.42
    vaso-occlusive pain 282.42
sickle-cell (without crisis) 282.41
  with
    crisis 282.42
    vaso-occlusive pain 282.42
Thalassemic variants 282.49
Thaysen-Gee disease (nontropical
  sprue) 579.0
Thecoma (M8600/0) 220
  malignant (M8600/3) 183.0
Thelarche, precocious 259.1
Thelitis 611.0
  puerperal, postpartum 675.0●
Therapeutic - see condition
Therapy V57.9
  blood transfusion, without reported
    diagnosis V58.2
  breathing V57.0
  chemotherapy, antineoplastic
    V58.11

Therapy (Continued)
chemotherapy, (Continued)
  fluoride V07.31
  prophylactic NEC V07.39
dialysis (intermittent) (treatment)
  extracorporeal V56.0
  peritoneal V56.8
  renal V56.0
  specified type NEC V56.8
exercise NEC V57.1
  breathing V57.0
extracorporeal dialysis (renal) V56.0
fluoride prophylaxis V07.31
hemodialysis V56.0
hormone replacement
  (postmenopausal) V07.4
immunotherapy antineoplastic V58.12
long term oxygen therapy V46.2
occupational V57.21
orthoptic V57.4
orthotic V57.81
peritoneal dialysis V56.8
physical NEC V57.1
postmenopausal hormone replacement
  V07.4
radiation V58.0
speech (-language) V57.3 ◄▥
vocational V57.22
Thermalgesia 782.0
Thermalgia 782.0
Thermanalgesia 782.0
Thermanesthesia 782.0
Thermic - see condition
Thermography (abnormal) 793.99
  breast 793.89
Thermoplegia 992.0
Thesaurismosis
  amyloid 277.39
  bilirubin 277.4
  calcium 275.40
  cystine 270.0
  glycogen (see also Disease, glycogen
    storage) 271.0
  kerasin 272.7
  lipoid 272.7
  melanin 255.41
  phosphatide 272.7
  urate 274.9
Thiaminic deficiency 265.1
  with beriberi 265.0
Thibierge-Weissenbach syndrome
  (cutaneous systemic sclerosis)
  710.1
Thickened endometrium 793.5
Thickening
  bone 733.99
    extremity 733.99
  breast 611.79
  hymen 623.3
  larynx 478.79
  nail 703.8
    congenital 757.5
  periosteal 733.99
  pleura (see also Pleurisy) 511.0
  skin 782.8
  subepiglottic 478.79
  tongue 529.8
  valve, heart - see Endocarditis
Thiele syndrome 724.6
Thigh - see condition
Thinning vertebra (see also Osteoporosis)
  733.00
Thirst, excessive 783.5
  due to deprivation of water 994.3
Thomsen's disease 359.22
Thomson's disease (congenital
  poikiloderma) 757.33

◄ New   ◄▥ Revised   ~~deleted~~ Deleted   ● Use Additional Digit(s)   ▨ Omit code

Thoracic - *see also* condition
kidney 753.3
outlet syndrome 353.0
stomach - *see* Hernia, diaphragm
Thoracogastroschisis (congenital) 759.89
Thoracopagus 759.4
Thoracoschisis 756.3
Thoracoscopic surgical procedure
converted to open procedure V64.42
Thorax - *see* condition
Thorn's syndrome (*see also* Disease, renal)
593.9
Thornwaldt's, Tornwaldt's
bursitis (pharyngeal) 478.29
cyst 478.26
disease (pharyngeal bursitis) 478.29
Thorson-Biörck syndrome (malignant
carcinoid) 259.2
Threadworm (infection) (infestation) 127.4
Threatened
abortion or miscarriage 640.0●
with subsequent abortion (*see also*
Abortion, spontaneous) 634.9●
affecting fetus 762.1
labor 644.1●
affecting fetus or newborn 761.8
premature 644.0●
miscarriage 640.0●
affecting fetus 762.1
premature
delivery 644.2●
affecting fetus or newborn 761.8
labor 644.0●
before 22 completed weeks
gestation 640.0●
Three-day fever 066.0
Threshers' lung 495.0
Thrix annulata (congenital) 757.4
Throat - *see* condition
Thrombasthenia (Glanzmann's)
(hemorrhagic) (hereditary) 287.1
Thromboangiitis 443.1
obliterans (general) 443.1
cerebral 437.1
vessels
brain 437.1
spinal cord 437.1
Thromboarteritis - *see* Arteritis
Thromboasthenia (Glanzmann's)
(hemorrhagic) (hereditary) 287.1
Thrombocytasthenia (Glanzmann's) 287.1
Thrombocythemia (primary) (M9962/1)
238.71
essential 238.71
hemorrhagic 238.71
idiopathic (hemorrhagic) (M9962/1)
238.71
Thrombocytopathy (dystrophic)
(granulopenic) 287.1
Thrombocytopenia, thrombocytopenic
287.5
with
absent radii (TAR) syndrome 287.33
giant hemangioma 287.39
amegakaryocytic, congenital 287.33
congenital 287.33
cyclic 287.39
dilutional 287.4
due to
drugs 287.4
extracorporeal circulation of blood
287.4
massive blood transfusion 287.4
platelet alloimmunization 287.4
essential 287.30
fetal 678.0●
heparin-induced (HIT) 289.84

Thrombocytopenia,
thrombocytopenic (*Continued*)
hereditary 287.33
Kasabach-Merritt 287.39
neonatal, transitory 776.1
due to
exchange transfusion 776.1
idiopathic maternal
thrombocytopenia 776.1
isoimmunization 776.1
primary 287.30
puerperal, postpartum 666.3●
purpura (*see also* Purpura,
thrombocytopenic) 287.30
thrombotic 446.6
secondary 287.4
sex-linked 287.39
Thrombocytosis 238.71
essential 238.71
primary 238.71
Thromboembolism - *see* Embolism
Thrombopathy (Bernard-Soulier)
287.1
constitutional 286.4
Willebrand-Jürgens (angiohemophilia)
286.4
Thrombopenia (*see also*
Thrombocytopenia) 287.5
Thrombophlebitis 451.9
antecubital vein 451.82
antepartum (superficial) 671.2●
affecting fetus or newborn 760.3
deep 671.3●
arm 451.89
deep 451.83
superficial 451.82
breast, superficial 451.89
cavernous (venous) sinus - *see*
Thrombophlebitis, intracranial
venous sinus
cephalic vein 451.82
cerebral (sinus) (vein) 325
late effect - *see* category 326
nonpyogenic 437.6
in pregnancy or puerperium
671.5●
late effect - *see* Late effect(s) (of)
cerebrovascular disease
due to implanted device - *see*
Complications, due to (presence
of) any device, implant, or graft
classified to 996.0–996.5 NEC
during or resulting from a procedure
NEC 997.2
femoral 451.11
femoropopliteal 451.19
following infusion, perfusion, or
transfusion 999.2
hepatic (vein) 451.89
idiopathic, recurrent 453.1
iliac vein 451.81
iliofemoral 451.11
intracranial venous sinus (any) 325
late effect - *see* category 326
nonpyogenic 437.6
in pregnancy or puerperium
671.5
late effect - *see* Late effect(s) (of)
cerebrovascular disease
jugular vein 451.89
lateral (venous) sinus - *see*
Thrombophlebitis, intracranial
venous sinus
leg 451.2
deep (vessels) 451.19
femoral vein 451.11
specified vessel NEC 451.19

Thrombophlebitis (*Continued*)
leg (*Continued*)
superficial (vessels) 451.0
femoral vein 451.11
longitudinal (venous) sinus - *see*
Thrombophlebitis, intracranial
venous sinus
lower extremity 451.2
deep (vessels) 451.19
femoral vein 451.11
specified vessel NEC 451.19
superficial (vessels) 451.0
migrans, migrating 453.1
pelvic
with
abortion - *see* Abortion, by type,
with sepsis
ectopic pregnancy (*see also*
categories 633.0–633.9) 639.0
molar pregnancy (*see also*
categories 630–632) 639.0
following
abortion 639.0
ectopic or molar pregnancy 639.0
puerperal 671.4●
popliteal vein 451.19
portal (vein) 572.1
postoperative 997.2
pregnancy (superficial) 671.2●
affecting fetus or newborn 760.3
deep 671.3●
puerperal, postpartum, childbirth
(extremities) (superficial)
671.2●
deep 671.4●
pelvic 671.4●
septic 670.3 ◀
specified site NEC 671.5●
radial vein 451.82
saphenous (greater) (lesser) 451.0
sinus (intracranial) - *see*
Thrombophlebitis, intracranial
venous sinus
specified site NEC 451.89
tibial vein 451.19
Thrombosis, thrombotic (marantic)
(multiple) (progressive) (vein)
(vessel) 453.9
with childbirth or during the
puerperium - *see* Thrombosis,
puerperal, postpartum
antepartum - *see* Thrombosis,
pregnancy
aorta, aortic 444.1
abdominal 444.0
bifurcation 444.0
saddle 444.0
terminal 444.0
thoracic 444.1
valve - *see* Endocarditis, aortic
apoplexy (*see also* Thrombosis, brain)
434.0●
late effect - *see* Late effect(s) (of)
cerebrovascular disease
appendix, septic - *see* Appendicitis,
acute
arteriolar-capillary platelet,
disseminated 446.6
artery, arteries (postinfectional) 444.9
auditory, internal 433.8●
basilar (*see also* Occlusion, artery,
basilar) 433.0●
carotid (common) (internal) (*see also*
Occlusion, artery, carotid)
433.1●
with other precerebral artery
433.3●

◄ New   ◄▥ Revised   ~~deleted~~ Deleted   ● Use Additional Digit(s)   ▥ Omit code

Thyroiditis *(Continued)*
tuberculous *(see also* Tuberculosis)
017.5●
viral 245.1
woody 245.3
Thyrolingual duct, persistent
759.2
Thyromegaly 240.9
Thyrotoxic
crisis or storm *(see also* Thyrotoxicosis)
242.9●
heart failure *(see also* Thyrotoxicosis)
242.9● *[425.7]*
Thyrotoxicosis 242.9●

Note 68   Use the following fifth-digit
subclassification with category 242:

0   without mention of thyrotoxic
crisis or storm
1   with mention of thyrotoxic crisis
or storm

---

with
goiter (diffuse) 242.0●
adenomatous 242.3●
multinodular 242.2●
uninodular 242.1●
nodular 242.3●
multinodular 242.2●
uninodular 242.1●
infiltrative●
dermopathy 242.0●
ophthalmopathy 242.0●
thyroid acropachy 242.0●
complicating pregnancy, childbirth, or
puerperium 648.1●
due to
ectopic thyroid nodule 242.4●
ingestion of (excessive) thyroid
material 242.8●
specified cause NEC 242.8●
factitia 242.8●
heart 242.9● *[425.7]*
neonatal (transient) 775.3
TIA (transient ischemic attack) 435.9
with transient neurologic deficit
435.9
late effect - *see* Late effect(s) (of)
cerebrovascular disease
Tibia vara 732.4
Tic 307.20
breathing 307.20
child problem 307.21
compulsive 307.22
convulsive 307.20
degenerative (generalized) (localized)
333.3
facial 351.8
douloureux *(see also* Neuralgia,
trigeminal) 350.1
atypical 350.2
habit 307.20
chronic (motor or vocal) 307.22
transient (of childhood) 307.21
lid 307.20
transient (of childhood) 307.21
motor-verbal 307.23
occupational 300.89
orbicularis 307.20
transient (of childhood) 307.21
organic origin 333.3
postchoreic - *see* Chorea
psychogenic 307.20
compulsive 307.22
salaam 781.0

Tic *(Continued)*
spasm 307.20
chronic (motor or vocal) 307.22
transient (of childhood) 307.21
Tick (-borne) fever NEC 066.1
American mountain 066.1
Colorado 066.1
hemorrhagic NEC 065.3
Crimean 065.0
Kyasanur Forest 065.2
Omsk 065.1
mountain 066.1
nonexanthematous 066.1
Tick-bite fever NEC 066.1
African 087.1
Colorado (virus) 066.1
Rocky Mountain 082.0
Tick paralysis 989.5
Tics and spasms, compulsive 307.22
Tietze's disease or syndrome 733.6
Tight, tightness
anus 564.89
chest 786.59
fascia (lata) 728.9
foreskin (congenital) 605
hymen 623.3
introitus (acquired) (congenital) 623.3
rectal sphincter 564.89
tendon 727.81
Achilles (heel) 727.81
urethral sphincter 598.9
Tilting vertebra 737.9
Timidity, child 313.21
Tinea (intersecta) (tarsi) 110.9
amiantacea 110.0
asbestina 110.0
barbae 110.0
beard 110.0
black dot 110.0
blanca 111.2
capitis 110.0
corporis 110.5
cruris 110.3
decalvans 704.09
flava 111.0
foot 110.4
furfuracea 111.0
imbricata (Tokelau) 110.5
lepothrix 039.0
manuum 110.2
microsporic *(see also*
Dermatophytosis) 110.9
nigra 111.1
nodosa 111.2
pedis 110.4
scalp 110.0
specified site NEC 110.8
sycosis 110.0
tonsurans 110.0
trichophytic *(see also*
Dermatophytosis) 110.9
unguium 110.1
versicolor 111.0
Tingling sensation *(see also*
Disturbance, sensation)
782.0
Tin-miners' lung 503
Tinnitus (aurium) 388.30
audible 388.32
objective 388.32
subjective 388.31
Tipped, teeth 524.33
Tipping
pelvis 738.6
with disproportion (fetopelvic)
653.0●

Tipping *(Continued)*
pelvis *(Continued)*
with disproportion *(Continued)*
affecting fetus or newborn 763.1
causing obstructed labor
660.1●
affecting fetus or newborn
763.1
teeth 524.33
Tiredness 780.79
Tissue - *see* condition
Tobacco
abuse (affecting health) NEC *(see also*
Abuse, drugs, nondependent)
305.1
heart 989.84
use disorder complicating pregnancy,
childbirth, or the puerperium
649.0●
Tobias' syndrome (carcinoma,
pulmonary apex) (M8010/3)
162.3
Tocopherol deficiency 269.1
Todd's
cirrhosis - *see* Cirrhosis, biliary
paralysis (postepileptic transitory
paralysis) 344.89
Toe - *see* condition
Toilet, artificial opening *(see also*
Attention to, artificial, opening)
V55.9
Tokelau ringworm 110.5
Tollwut 071
Tolosa-Hunt syndrome 378.55
Tommaselli's disease
correct substance properly
administered 599.70
overdose or wrong substance given or
taken 961.4
Tongue - *see also* condition
worms 134.1
Tongue tie 750.0
Toni-Fanconi syndrome (cystinosis)
270.0
Tonic pupil 379.46
Tonsil - *see* condition
Tonsillitis (acute) (catarrhal) (croupous)
(follicular) (gangrenous) (infective)
(lacunar) (lingual) (malignant)
(membranous) (phlegmonous)
(pneumococcal)
(pseudomembranous) (purulent)
(septic) (staphylococcal) (subacute)
(suppurative) (toxic) (ulcerative)
(vesicular) (viral) 463
with influenza, flu, or grippe 487.1
chronic 474.00
diphtheritic (membranous) 032.0
hypertrophic 474.00
influenzal 487.1
parenchymatous 475
streptococcal 034.0
tuberculous *(see also* Tuberculosis)
012.8●
Vincent's 101
Tonsillopharyngitis 465.8
Tooth, teeth - *see* condition
Toothache 525.9
Topagnosis 782.0
Tophi (gouty) 274.03 ◀■■
ear 274.81
heart 274.82
specified site NEC 274.82
TORCH infection - *(see also* Infection,
congenital) 760.2
Torn - *see* Tear, torn

Tornwaldt's bursitis (disease) (pharyngeal bursitis) 478.29
  cyst 478.26
Torpid liver 573.9
Torsion
  accessory tube 620.5
  adnexa (female) 620.5
  aorta (congenital) 747.29
    acquired 447.1
  appendix
    epididymis 608.24
    testis 608.23
  bile duct 576.8
    with calculus, choledocholithiasis or stones - see Choledocholithiasis
    congenital 751.69
  bowel, colon, or intestine 560.2
  cervix - see Malposition, uterus
  duodenum 537.3
  dystonia - see Dystonia, torsion
  epididymis 608.24
    appendix 608.24
  fallopian tube 620.5
  gallbladder (see also Disease, gallbladder) 575.8
    congenital 751.69
  gastric 537.89
  hydatid of Morgagni (female) 620.5
  kidney (pedicle) 593.89
  Meckel's diverticulum (congenital) 751.0
  mesentery 560.2
  omentum 560.2
  organ or site, congenital NEC - see Anomaly, specified type NEC
  ovary (pedicle) 620.5
    congenital 752.0
  oviduct 620.5
  penis 607.89
    congenital 752.69
  renal 593.89
  spasm - see Dystonia, torsion
  spermatic cord 608.22
    extravaginal 608.21
    intravaginal 608.22
  spleen 289.59
  testicle, testis 608.20
    appendix 608.23
  tibia 736.89
  umbilical cord - see Compression, umbilical cord
  uterus (see also Malposition, uterus) 621.6
Torticollis (intermittent) (spastic) 723.5
  congenital 754.1
    sternomastoid 754.1
  due to birth injury 767.8
  hysterical 300.11
  ocular 781.93
  psychogenic 306.0
    specified as conversion reaction 300.11
  rheumatic 723.5
  rheumatoid 714.0
  spasmodic 333.83
  traumatic, current NEC 847.0
Tortuous
  artery 447.1
  fallopian tube 752.19
  organ or site, congenital NEC - see Distortion
  renal vessel (congenital) 747.62
  retina vessel (congenital) 743.58
    acquired 362.17

Tortuous (Continued)
  ureter 593.4
  urethra 599.84
  vein - see Varicose, vein
Torula, torular (infection) 117.5
  histolytica 117.5
  lung 117.5
Torulosis 117.5
Torus
  fracture
    fibula 823.41
      with tibia 823.42
    humerus 812.49 ◄
    radius (alone) 813.45 ◄▥
      with ulna 813.47 ◄
    tibia 823.40
      with fibula 823.42 ◄
    ulna (alone) 813.46 ◄
      with radius 813.47 ◄
  mandibularis 526.81
  palatinus 526.81
Touch, vitreous 997.99
Touraine's syndrome (hereditary osteo-onychodysplasia) 756.89
Touraine-Solente-Golé syndrome (acropachyderma) 757.39
Tourette's disease (motor-verbal tic) 307.23
Tower skull 756.0
  with exophthalmos 756.0
Toxemia 799.89
  with
    abortion - see Abortion, by type, with toxemia
  bacterial - see Septicemia
  biliary (see also Disease, biliary) 576.8
  burn - see Burn, by site
  congenital NEC 779.89
  eclamptic 642.6●
    with pre-existing hypertension 642.7●
  erysipelatous (see also Erysipelas) 035
  fatigue 799.89
  fetus or newborn NEC 779.89
  food (see also Poisoning, food) 005.9
  gastric 537.89
  gastrointestinal 558.2
  intestinal 558.2
  kidney (see also Disease, renal) 593.9
  lung 518.89
  malarial NEC (see also Malaria) 084.6
  maternal (of pregnancy), affecting fetus or newborn 760.0
  myocardial - see Myocarditis, toxic
  of pregnancy (mild) (pre-eclamptic) 642.4●
    with
      convulsions 642.6●
      pre-existing hypertension 642.7●
    affecting fetus or newborn 760.0
    severe 642.5●
  pre-eclamptic - see Toxemia, of pregnancy
  puerperal, postpartum - see Toxemia, of pregnancy
  pulmonary 518.89
  renal (see also Disease, renal) 593.9
  septic (see also Septicemia) 038.9
  small intestine 558.2
  staphylococcal 038.10
    aureus 038.11
    due to food 005.0
    specified organism NEC 038.19
  stasis 799.89

Toxemia (Continued)
  stomach 537.89
  uremic (see also Uremia) 586
  urinary 586
Toxemica cerebropathia psychica (nonalcoholic) 294.0
  alcoholic 291.1
Toxic (poisoning) - see also condition
  from drug or poison - see Table of Drugs and Chemicals
  oil syndrome 710.5
  shock syndrome 040.82
  thyroid (gland) (see also Thyrotoxicosis) 242.9●
Toxicemia - see Toxemia
Toxicity
  dilantin
    asymptomatic 796.0
    symptomatic -see Table of Drugs and Chemicals
  drug
    asymptomatic 796.0
    symptomatic - see Table of Drugs and Chemicals
  fava bean 282.2
  from drug or poison
    asymptomatic 796.0
    symptomatic - see Table of Drugs and Chemicals
Toxicosis (see also Toxemia) 799.89
  capillary, hemorrhagic 287.0
Toxinfection 799.89
  gastrointestinal 558.2
Toxocariasis 128.0
Toxoplasma infection, generalized 130.9
Toxoplasmosis (acquired) 130.9
  with pneumonia 130.4
  congenital, active 771.2
  disseminated (multisystemic) 130.8
  maternal
    with suspected damage to fetus affecting management of pregnancy 655.4●
    affecting fetus or newborn 760.2
      manifest toxoplasmosis in fetus or newborn 771.2
  multiple sites 130.8
  multisystemic disseminated 130.8
  specified site NEC 130.7
Trabeculation, bladder 596.8
Trachea - see condition
Tracheitis (acute) (catarrhal) (infantile) (membranous) (plastic) (pneumococcal) (septic) (suppurative) (viral) 464.10
  with
    bronchitis 490
      acute or subacute 466.0
      chronic 491.8
      tuberculosis - see Tuberculosis, pulmonary
    laryngitis (acute) 464.20
      with obstruction 464.21
      chronic 476.1
      tuberculous (see also Tuberculosis, larynx) 012.3●
    obstruction 464.11
  chronic 491.8
    with
      bronchitis (chronic) 491.8
      laryngitis (chronic) 476.1
    due to external agent - see Condition, respiratory, chronic, due to

Tracheitis (*Continued*)
  diphtheritic (membranous) 032.3
    due to external agent - *see*
      Inflammation, respiratory,
      upper, due to
  edematous 464.11
  influenzal 487.1
  streptococcal 034.0
  syphilitic 095.8
  tuberculous (*see also* Tuberculosis)
    012.8●
Trachelitis (nonvenereal) (*see also*
    Cervicitis) 616.0
  trichomonal 131.09
Tracheobronchial - *see* condition
Tracheobronchitis (*see also* Bronchitis)
    490
  acute or subacute 466.0
    with bronchospasm or obstruction
      466.0
  chronic 491.8
  influenzal 487.1
  senile 491.8
Tracheobronchomegaly (congenital)
    748.3
  with bronchiectasis 494.0
    with (acute) exacerbation 494.1
  acquired 519.19
    with bronchiectasis 494.0
      with (acute) exacerbation
        494.1
Tracheobronchopneumonitis - *see*
    Pneumonia, broncho
Tracheocele (external) (internal) 519.19
  congenital 748.3
Tracheomalacia 519.19
  congenital 748.3
Tracheopharyngitis (acute) 465.8
  chronic 478.9
    due to external agent - *see*
      Condition, respiratory, chronic,
      due to
    due to external agent - *see*
      Inflammation, respiratory, upper,
      due to
Tracheostenosis 519.19
  congenital 748.3
Tracheostomy
  attention to V55.0
  complication 519.00
  granuloma 519.09
  hemorrhage 519.09
  infection 519.01
  malfunctioning 519.02
  obstruction 519.09
  sepsis 519.01
  status V44.0
  stenosis 519.02
Trachoma, trachomatous 076.9
  active (stage) 076.1
  contraction of conjunctiva 076.1
  dubium 076.0
  healed or late effect 139.1
  initial (stage) 076.0
  Türck's (chronic catarrhal laryngitis)
    476.0
Trachyphonia 784.49
Training
  insulin pump V65.46
  orthoptic V57.4
  orthotic V57.81
Train sickness 994.6
Trait
  hemoglobin
    abnormal NEC 282.7
      with thalassemia 282.49

Trait (*Continued*)
  hemoglobin (*Continued*)
    C (*see also* Disease, hemoglobin, C)
      282.7
      with elliptocytosis 282.7
    S (Hb-S) 282.5
  Lepore 282.49
    with other abnormal hemoglobin
      NEC 282.49
  paranoid 301.0
  sickle-cell 282.5
    with
      elliptocytosis 282.5
      spherocytosis 282.5
Traits, paranoid 301.0
Tramp V60.0
Trance 780.09
  hysterical 300.13
Transaminasemia 790.4
Transfusion, blood
  donor V59.01
    stem cells V59.02
  fetal twin to twin 678.0●
  incompatible 999.6
    ABO 999.6
    minor blood group 999.89
  reaction or complication - *see*
    Complications, transfusion
  related acute lung injury (TRALI) 518.7
  syndrome
    fetomaternal 772.0
    twin-to-twin
      blood loss (donor twin) 772.0
      recipient twin 776.4
  twin to twin fetal 678.0●
  without reported diagnosis V58.2
Transient - *see also* condition
  alteration of awareness 780.02
  blindness 368.12
  deafness (ischemic) 388.02
  global amnesia 437.7
  hyperglycemia (post-procedural)
    790.29 ◀
  hypoglycemia (post-procedural)
    251.2 ◀
  person (homeless) NEC V60.0
Transitional, lumbosacral joint of
    vertebra 756.19
Translocation
  autosomes NEC 758.5
    13–15 758.1
    16–18 758.2
    21 or 22 758.0
    balanced in normal individual 758.4
    D₁ 758.1
    E₃ 758.2
    G 758.0
  balanced autosomal in normal
    individual 758.4
  chromosomes NEC 758.89
  Down's syndrome 758.0
Translucency, iris 364.53
Transmission of chemical substances
    through the placenta (affecting fetus
    or newborn) 760.70
  alcohol 760.71
  anticonvulsants 760.77
  antifungals 760.74
  anti-infective agents 760.74
  antimetabolics 760.78
  cocaine 760.75
  "crack" 760.75
  diethylstilbestrol [DES] 760.76
  hallucinogenic agents 760.73
  medicinal agents NEC 760.79
  narcotics 760.72

Transmission of chemical
    substances (*Continued*)
  obstetric anesthetic or analgesic drug
    763.5
  specified agent NEC 760.79
  suspected, affecting management of
    pregnancy 655.5●
Transplant (ed)
  bone V42.4
    marrow V42.81
  complication - *see also* Complications,
    due to (presence of) any device,
    implant, or graft classified to
    996.0–996.5 NEC
    bone marrow 996.85
    corneal graft NEC 996.79
      infection or inflammation 996.69
      reaction 996.51
      rejection 996.51
    organ (failure) (immune or
      nonimmune cause) (infection)
      (rejection) 996.80
      bone marrow 996.85
      heart 996.83
      intestines 996.87
      kidney 996.81
      liver 996.82
      lung 996.84
      pancreas 996.86
      specified NEC 996.89
    previously removed due to
      complication, failure, rejection
      or infection V45.87
    removal status V45.87
    skin NEC 996.79
      infection or inflammation
        996.69
      rejection 996.52
      artificial 996.55
        decellularized allodermis
          996.55
  cornea V42.5
  hair V50.0
  heart V42.1
    valve V42.2
  intestine V42.84
  kidney V42.0
  liver V42.7
  lung V42.6
  organ V42.9
    specified NEC V42.89
  pancreas V42.83
  peripheral stem cells V42.82
  skin V42.3
  stem cells, peripheral V42.82
  tissue V42.9
    specified NEC V42.89
Transplants, ovarian, endometrial
    617.1
Transposed - *see* Transposition
Transposition (congenital) - *see also*
    Malposition, congenital
  abdominal viscera 759.3
  aorta (dextra) 745.11
  appendix 751.5
  arterial trunk 745.10
  colon 751.5
  great vessels (complete) 745.10
    both originating from right ventricle
      745.11
    corrected 745.12
    double outlet right ventricle
      745.11
    incomplete 745.11
    partial 745.11
    specified type NEC 745.19

◀ New ◀▥ Revised ~~deleted~~ Deleted ● Use Additional Digit(s) ▨ Omit code

Transposition (Continued)
  heart 746.87
    with complete transposition of
        viscera 759.3
    intestine (large) (small) 751.5
    pulmonary veins 747.49
    reversed jejunal (for bypass) (status)
        V45.3
    scrotal 752.81
    stomach 750.7
      with general transposition of viscera
          759.3
    teeth, tooth 524.30
    vessels (complete) 745.10
      partial 745.11
    viscera (abdominal) (thoracic) 759.3
Trans-sexualism 302.50
  with
    asexual history 302.51
    heterosexual history 302.53
    homosexual history 302.52
Transverse - see also condition
  arrest (deep), in labor 660.3●
    affecting fetus or newborn 763.1
  lie 652.3●
    before labor, affecting fetus or
        newborn 761.7
    causing obstructed labor 660.0●
      affecting fetus or newborn 763.1
    during labor, affecting fetus or
        newborn 763.1
Transvestism, transvestitism (transvestic
    fetishism) 302.3
Trapped placenta (with hemorrhage)
    666.0●
  without hemorrhage 667.0●
Trauma, traumatism (see also Injury, by
    site) 959.9
  birth - see Birth, injury NEC
  causing hemorrhage of pregnancy or
      delivery 641.8●
  complicating
    abortion - see Abortion, by type,
        with damage to pelvic organs
    ectopic pregnancy (see also
        categories 633.0–633.9) 639.2
    molar pregnancy (see also categories
        630–632) 639.2
  during delivery NEC 665.9●
  following
    abortion 639.2
    ectopic or molar pregnancy 639.2
  maternal, during pregnancy, affecting
      fetus or newborn 760.5
  neuroma - see Injury, nerve, by site
  previous major, affecting management
      of pregnancy, childbirth, or
      puerperium V23.89
  psychic (current) - see also Reaction,
      adjustment
    previous (history) V15.49
  psychologic, previous (affecting health)
      V15.49
  transient paralysis - see Injury, nerve,
      by site
Traumatic - see also condition   ◀▥▥
  brain injury (TBI) (see also Injury,
      intracranial) 854.0   ◀
    with skull fracture - see Fracture,
        skull, by site   ◀
Treacher Collins' syndrome (incomplete
    facial dysostosis) 756.0
Treitz's hernia - see Hernia, Treitz's
Trematode infestation NEC 121.9
Trematodiasis NEC 121.9
Trembles 988.8

Trembling paralysis (see also
    Parkinsonism) 332.0
Tremor 781.0
  essential (benign) 333.1
  familial 333.1
  flapping (liver) 572.8
  hereditary 333.1
  hysterical 300.11
  intention 333.1
  medication-induced postural 333.1
  mercurial 985.0
  muscle 728.85
  Parkinson's (see also Parkinsonism)
      332.0
  psychogenic 306.0
    specified as conversion reaction
        300.11
  senilis 797
  specified type NEC 333.1
Trench
  fever 083.1
  foot 991.4
  mouth 101
  nephritis - see Nephritis, acute
Treponema pallidum infection (see also
    Syphilis) 097.9
Treponematosis 102.9
  due to
    T. pallidum - see Syphilis
    T. pertenue (yaws) (see also Yaws)
        102.9
Triad
  Kartagener's 759.3
  Reiter's (complete) (incomplete)
      099.3
  Saint's (see also Hernia, diaphragm)
      553.3
Trichiasis 704.2
  cicatricial 704.2
  eyelid 374.05
    with entropion (see also Entropion)
        374.00
Trichinella spiralis (infection)
    (infestation) 124
Trichinelliasis 124
Trichinellosis 124
Trichiniasis 124
Trichinosis 124
Trichobezoar 938
  intestine 936
  stomach 935.2
Trichocephaliasis 127.3
Trichocephalosis 127.3
Trichocephalus infestation 127.3
Trichoclasis 704.2
Trichoepithelioma (M8100/0) - see also
    Neoplasm, skin, benign
  breast 217
  genital organ NEC - see Neoplasm, by
      site, benign
  malignant (M8100/3) - see Neoplasm,
      skin, malignant
Trichofolliculoma (M8101/0) - see
    Neoplasm, skin, benign
Tricholemmoma (M8102/0) - see
    Neoplasm, skin, benign
Trichomatosis 704.2
Trichomoniasis 131.9
  bladder 131.09
  cervix 131.09
  intestinal 007.3
  prostate 131.03
  seminal vesicle 131.09
  specified site NEC 131.8
  urethra 131.02
  urogenitalis 131.00

Trichomoniasis (Continued)
  vagina 131.01
  vulva 131.01
  vulvovaginal 131.01
Trichomycosis 039.0
  axillaris 039.0
  nodosa 111.2
  nodularis 111.2
  rubra 039.0
Trichonocardiosis (axillaris) (palmellina)
    039.0
Trichonodosis 704.2
Trichophytid, trichophyton infection (see
    also Dermatophytosis) 110.9
Trichophytide - see Dermatophytosis
Trichophytobezoar 938
  intestine 936
  stomach 935.2
Trichophytosis - see Dermatophytosis
Trichoptilosis 704.2
Trichorrhexis (nodosa) 704.2
Trichosporosis nodosa 111.2
Trichostasis spinulosa (congenital) 757.4
Trichostrongyliasis (small intestine) 127.6
Trichostrongylosis 127.6
Trichostrongylus (instabilis) infection
    127.6
Trichotillomania 312.39
Trichromat, anomalous (congenital)
    368.59
Trichromatopsia, anomalous (congenital)
    368.59
Trichuriasis 127.3
Trichuris trichiuria (any site) (infection)
    (infestation) 127.3
Tricuspid (valve) - see condition
Trifid - see also Accessory
  kidney (pelvis) 753.3
  tongue 750.13
Trigeminal neuralgia (see also Neuralgia,
    trigeminal) 350.1
Trigeminoencephaloangiomatosis 759.6
Trigeminy 427.89
  postoperative 997.1
Trigger finger (acquired) 727.03
  congenital 756.89
Trigonitis (bladder) (chronic)
    (pseudomembranous) 595.3
  tuberculous (see also Tuberculosis)
      016.1●
Trigonocephaly 756.0
Trihexosidosis 272.7
Trilobate placenta - see Placenta,
    abnormal
Trilocular heart 745.8
Trimethylaminuria 270.8
Tripartita placenta - see Placenta,
    abnormal
Triple - see also Accessory
  kidneys 753.3
  uteri 752.2
  X female 758.81
Triplegia 344.89
  congenital or infantile 343.8
Triplet
  affected by maternal complications of
      pregnancy 761.5
  healthy liveborn - see Newborn,
      multiple
  pregnancy (complicating delivery)
      NEC 651.1●
    with fetal loss and retention of one
        or more fetus(es) 651.4●
    following (elective) fetal reduction
        651.7●
Triplex placenta - see Placenta, abnormal

◀ New   ◀▥▥ Revised   ~~deleted~~ Deleted   ● Use Additional Digit(s)   ▨▨▨ Omit code   585

Triplication - *see* Accessory
Trismus 781.0
 neonatorum 771.3
 newborn 771.3
Trisomy (syndrome) NEC 758.5
 13 (partial) 758.1
 16–18 758.2
 18 (partial) 758.2
 21 (partial) 758.0
 22 758.0
 autosomes NEC 758.5
 D₁ 758.1
 E₃ 758.2
 G (group) 758.0
 group D₁ 758.1
 group E 758.2
 group G 758.0
Tritanomaly 368.53
Tritanopia 368.53
Troisier-Hanot-Chauffard syndrome
  (bronze diabetes) 275.0
Trombidiosis 133.8
Trophedema (hereditary) 757.0
 congenital 757.0
Trophoblastic disease (*see also*
  Hydatidiform mole) 630
 previous, affecting management of
  pregnancy V23.1
Tropholymphedema 757.0
Trophoneurosis NEC 356.9
 arm NEC 354.9
 disseminated 710.1
 facial 349.89
 leg NEC 355.8
 lower extremity NEC 355.8
 upper extremity NEC 354.9
Tropical - *see also* condition
 maceration feet (syndrome) 991.4
 wet foot (syndrome) 991.4
Trouble - *see also* Disease
 bowel 569.9
 heart - *see* Disease, heart
 intestine 569.9
 kidney (*see also* Disease, renal)
  593.9
 nervous 799.21   ◀▥
 sinus (*see also* Sinusitis) 473.9
Trousseau's syndrome (thrombophlebitis
  migrans) 453.1
Truancy, childhood - *see also* Disturbance,
  conduct
 socialized 312.2●
 undersocialized, unsocialized 312.1●
Truncus
 arteriosus (persistent) 745.0
 common 745.0
 communis 745.0
Trunk - *see* condition
Trychophytide - *see* Dermatophytosis
Trypanosoma infestation - *see*
  Trypanosomiasis
Trypanosomiasis 086.9
 with meningoencephalitis 086.9
  [323.2]
 African 086.5
  due to Trypanosoma 086.5
   gambiense 086.3
   rhodesiense 086.4
 American 086.2
  with
   heart involvement 086.0
   other organ involvement 086.1
  without mention of organ
   involvement 086.2
 Brazilian - *see* Trypanosomiasis,
  American

Trypanosomiasis (Continued)
 Chagas' - *see* Trypanosomiasis,
  American
 due to Trypanosoma
  cruzi - *see* Trypanosomiasis,
   American
  gambiense 086.3
  rhodesiense 086.4
 gambiensis, Gambian 086.3
 North American - *see* Trypanosomiasis,
  American
 rhodesiensis, Rhodesian 086.4
 South American - *see* Trypanosomiasis,
  American
T-shaped incisors 520.2
Tsutsugamushi fever 081.2
Tube, tubal, tubular - *see also* condition
 ligation, admission for V25.2
Tubercle - *see also* Tuberculosis
 brain, solitary 013.2●
 Darwin's 744.29
 epithelioid noncaseating 135
 Ghon, primary infection 010.0●
Tuberculid, tuberculide (indurating)
  (lichenoid) (miliary)
  (papulonecrotic) (primary) (skin)
  (subcutaneous) (*see also*
  Tuberculosis) 017.0●
Tuberculoma - *see also* Tuberculosis
 brain (any part) 013.2●
 meninges (cerebral) (spinal) 013.1●
 spinal cord 013.4●
Tuberculosis, tubercular, tuberculous
  (calcification) (calcified) (caseous)
  (chromogenic acid-fast bacilli)
  (congenital) (degeneration) (disease)
  (fibrocaseous) (fistula) (gangrene)
  (interstitial) (isolated circumscribed
  lesions) (necrosis) (parenchymatous)
  (ulcerative) 011.9●

Note 69 Use the following fifth-digit
subclassification with categories
010–018:

 0 unspecified
 1 bacteriological or histological
   examination not done
 2 bacteriological or histological
   examination unknown (at
   present)
 3 tubercle bacilli found (in sputum)
   by microscopy
 4 tubercle bacilli not found (in
   sputum) by microscopy, but
   found by bacterial culture
 5 tubercle bacilli not found by
   bacteriological examination,
   but tuberculosis confirmed
   histologically
 6 tubercle bacilli not found by
   bacteriological or
   histological examination,
   but tuberculosis confirmed
   by other methods
   [inoculation of animals]

For tuberculous conditions specified as
late effects or sequelae, *see* category
137.

---

 abdomen 014.8●
  lymph gland 014.8●
 abscess 011.9●
  arm 017.9
  bone (*see also* Osteomyelitis, due to,
   tuberculosis) 015.9● [730.8]●
   hip 015.1● [730.85]

Tuberculosis, tubercular, tuberculous
  (Continued)
 abscess (Continued)
  bone (Continued)
   knee 015.2● [730.86]
   sacrum 015.0● [730.88]
   specified site NEC 015.7●
    [730.88]
   spinal 015.0● [730.88]
   vertebra 015.0● [730.88]
  brain 013.3●
  breast 017.9●
  Cowper's gland 016.5●
  dura (mater) 013.8●
   brain 013.3●
   spinal cord 013.5●
  epidural 013.8●
   brain 013.3●
   spinal cord 013.5●
  frontal sinus - *see* Tuberculosis, sinus
  genital organs NEC 016.9●
   female 016.7●
   male 016.5●
  genitourinary NEC 016.9●
  gland (lymphatic) - *see* Tuberculosis,
   lymph gland
  hip 015.1●
  iliopsoas 015.0● [730.88]
  intestine 014.8●
  ischiorectal 014.8●
  joint 015.9●
   hip 015.1●
   knee 015.2●
   specified joint NEC 015.8●
   vertebral 015.0● [730.88]
  kidney 016.0● [590.81]
  knee 015.2●
  lumbar 015.0● [730.88]
  lung 011.2●
   primary, progressive 010.8●
  meninges (cerebral) (spinal) 013.0●
  pelvic 016.9●
   female 016.7●
   male 016.5●
  perianal 014.8●
   fistula 014.8●
  perinephritic 016.0● [590.81]
  perineum 017.9●
  perirectal 014.8●
  psoas 015.0● [730.88]
  rectum 014.8●
  retropharyngeal 012.8●
  sacrum 015.0● [730.88]
  scrofulous 017.2●
  scrotum 016.5●
  skin 017.0●
   primary 017.0●
  spinal cord 013.5●
  spine or vertebra (column) 015.0●
   [730.88]
  strumous 017.2●
  subdiaphragmatic 014.8●
  testis 016.5●
  thigh 017.9●
  urinary 016.3●
   kidney 016.0● [590.81]
  uterus 016.7●
 accessory sinus - *see* Tuberculosis, sinus
 Addison's disease 017.6●
 adenitis (*see also* Tuberculosis, lymph
  gland) 017.2●
 adenoids 012.8●
 adenopathy (*see also* Tuberculosis,
  lymph gland) 017.2●
  tracheobronchial 012.1●
   primary progressive 010.8●

◀ New   ◀▥ Revised   ~~deleted~~ Deleted   ● Use Additional Digit(s)   ▨ Omit code

Tuberculosis, tubercular, tuberculous
   (Continued)
   adherent pericardium 017.9● *[420.0]*
   adnexa (uteri) 016.7●
   adrenal (capsule) (gland) 017.6●
   air passage NEC 012.8●
   alimentary canal 014.8●
   anemia 017.9●
   ankle (joint) 015.8●
      bone 015.5● *[730.87]*
   anus 014.8●
   apex (*see also* Tuberculosis, pulmonary)
      011.9●
   apical (*see also* Tuberculosis,
      pulmonary) 011.9●
   appendicitis 014.8●
   appendix 014.8●
   arachnoid 013.0●
   artery 017.9●
   arthritis (chronic) (synovial) 015.9●
      [711.40]
      ankle 015.8● *[730.87]*
      hip 015.1● *[711.45]*
      knee 015.2 *[711.46]*
      specified site NEC 015.8 ● *[711.48]*
      spine or vertebra (column) 015.0●
         [720.81]
      wrist 015.8● *[730.83]*
   articular - *see* Tuberculosis, joint
   ascites 014.0●
   asthma (*see also* Tuberculosis,
      pulmonary) 011.9●
   axilla, axillary 017.2●
      gland 017.2●
   bilateral (*see also* Tuberculosis,
      pulmonary) 011.9●
   bladder 016.1●
   bone (*see also* Osteomyelitis, due to,
      tuberculosis) 015.9● *[730.8]*
      hip 015.1● *[730.85]*
      knee 015.2● *[730.86]*
      limb NEC 015.5● *[730.88]*
      sacrum 015.0● *[730.88]*
      specified site NEC 015.7● *[730.88]*
      spinal or vertebral column 015.0●
         [730.88]
   bowel 014.8●
      miliary 018.9●
   brain 013.2●
   breast 017.9●
   broad ligament 016.7●
   bronchi, bronchial, bronchus 011.3●
      ectasia, ectasis 011.5●
      fistula 011.3●
         primary, progressive 010.8●
      gland 012.1●
         primary, progressive 010.8●
         isolated 012.2●
      lymph gland or node 012.1●
         primary, progressive 010.8●
   bronchiectasis 011.5●
   bronchitis 011.3●
   bronchopleural 012.0●
   bronchopneumonia,
      bronchopneumonic 011.6●
   bronchorrhagia 011.3●
   bronchotracheal 011.3●
      isolated 012.2●
   bronchus - *see* Tuberculosis, bronchi
   bronze disease (Addison's) 017.6●
   buccal cavity 017.9●
   bulbourethral gland 016.5●
   bursa (*see also* Tuberculosis, joint)
      015.9●
   cachexia NEC (*see also* Tuberculosis,
      pulmonary) 011.9●

Tuberculosis, tubercular, tuberculous
   (Continued)
   cardiomyopathy 017.9● *[425.8]*
   caries (*see also* Tuberculosis, bone)
      015.9● *[730.8]*
   cartilage (*see also* Tuberculosis, bone)
      015.9● *[730.8]*
      intervertebral 015.0● *[730.88]*
   catarrhal (*see also* Tuberculosis,
      pulmonary) 011.9●
   cecum 014.8●
   cellular tissue (primary) 017.0●
   cellulitis (primary) 017.0●
   central nervous system 013.9●
      specified site NEC 013.8●
   cerebellum (current) 013.2●
   cerebral (current) 013.2●
      meninges 013.0●
   cerebrospinal 013.6●
      meninges 013.0●
   cerebrum (current) 013.2●
   cervical 017.2●
      gland 017.2●
      lymph nodes 017.2●
   cervicitis (uteri) 016.7●
   cervix 016.7●
   chest (*see also* Tuberculosis, pulmonary)
      011.9●
   childhood type or first infection
      010.0●
   choroid 017.3● *[363.13]*
   choroiditis 017.3● *[363.13]*
   ciliary body 017.3● *[364.11]*
   colitis 014.8●
   colliers' 011.4●
   colliquativa (primary) 017.0●
   colon 014.8●
      ulceration 014.8●
   complex, primary 010.0●
   complicating pregnancy, childbirth, or
      puerperium 647.3●
      affecting fetus or newborn 760.2
   congenital 771.2
   conjunctiva 017.3● *[370.31]*
   connective tissue 017.9●
      bone - *see* Tuberculosis, bone
   contact V01.1
   converter (tuberculin skin test)
      (without disease) 795.5
   cornea (ulcer) 017.3● *[370.31]*
   Cowper's gland 016.5●
   coxae 015.1● *[730.85]*
   coxalgia 015.1● *[730.85]*
   cul-de-sac of Douglas 014.8●
   curvature, spine 015.0● *[737.40]*
   cutis (colliquativa) (primary) 017.0●
   cyst, ovary 016.6●
   cystitis 016.1●
   dacryocystitis 017.3● *[375.32]*
   dactylitis 015.5●
   diarrhea 014.8●
   diffuse (*see also* Tuberculosis, miliary)
      018.9●
      lung - *see* Tuberculosis, pulmonary
      meninges 013.0●
   digestive tract 014.8●
   disseminated (*see also* Tuberculosis,
      miliary) 018.9●
      meninges 013.0●
   duodenum 014.8●
   dura (mater) 013.9●
      abscess 013.8●
         cerebral 013.3●
         spinal 013.5●
   dysentery 014.8●

Tuberculosis, tubercular, tuberculous
   (Continued)
   ear (inner) (middle) 017.4●
      bone 015.6●
      external (primary) 017.0●
      skin (primary) 017.0●
   elbow 015.8●
   emphysema - *see* Tuberculosis,
      pulmonary
   empyema 012.0●
   encephalitis 013.6●
   endarteritis 017.9●
   endocarditis (any valve) 017.9●
      [424.91]
   endocardium (any valve) 017.9●
      [424.91]
   endocrine glands NEC 017.9●
   endometrium 016.7●
   enteric, enterica 014.8●
   enteritis 014.8●
   enterocolitis 014.8●
   epididymis 016.4●
   epididymitis 016.4●
   epidural abscess 013.8●
      brain 013.3●
      spinal cord 013.5●
   epiglottis 012.3●
   episcleritis 017.3● *[379.00]*
   erythema (induratum) (nodosum)
      (primary) 017.1●
   esophagus 017.8●
   Eustachian tube 017.4●
   exposure to V01.1
   exudative 012.0●
      primary, progressive 010.1●
   eye 017.3●
   eyelid (primary) 017.0●
      lupus 017.0● *[373.4]*
   fallopian tube 016.6●
   fascia 017.9●
   fauces 012.8●
   finger 017.9●
   first infection 010.0●
   fistula, perirectal 014.8●
   Florida 011.6●
   foot 017.9●
   funnel pelvis 137.3
   gallbladder 017.9●
   galloping (*see also* Tuberculosis,
      pulmonary) 011.9●
   ganglionic 015.9●
   gastritis 017.9●
   gastrocolic fistula 014.8●
   gastroenteritis 014.8●
   gastrointestinal tract 014.8●
   general, generalized 018.9●
      acute 018.0●
      chronic 018.8●
   genital organs NEC 016.9●
      female 016.7●
      male 016.5●
   genitourinary NEC 016.9●
   genu 015.2●
   glandulae suprarenalis 017.6●
   glandular, general 017.2●
   glottis 012.3●
   grinders' 011.4●
   groin 017.2●
   gum 017.9●
   hand 017.9●
   heart 017.9 ● *[425.8]*●
   hematogenous - *see* Tuberculosis,
      miliary

Tuberculosis, tubercular, tuberculous
    (Continued)
    hemoptysis (see also Tuberculosis,
        pulmonary) 011.9●
    hemorrhage NEC (see also Tuberculosis,
        pulmonary) 011.9●
    hemothorax 012.0●
    hepatitis 017.9●
    hilar lymph nodes 012.1●
        primary, progressive 010.8●
    hip (disease) (joint) 015.1●
        bone 015.1● [730.85]
    hydrocephalus 013.8●
    hydropneumothorax 012.0●
    hydrothorax 012.0●
    hypoadrenalism 017.6●
    hypopharynx 012.8●
    ileocecal (hyperplastic) 014.8●
    ileocolitis 014.8●
    ileum 014.8●
    iliac spine (superior) 015.0● [730.88]
    incipient NEC (see also Tuberculosis,
        pulmonary) 011.9●
    indurativa (primary) 017.1●
    infantile 010.0●
    infection NEC 011.9●
        without clinical manifestation
            010.0●
    infraclavicular gland 017.2●
    inguinal gland 017.2●
    inguinalis 017.2●
    intestine (any part) 014.8●
    iris 017.3● [364.11]
    iritis 017.3● [364.11]
    ischiorectal 014.8●
    jaw 015.7● [730.88]
    jejunum 014.8●
    joint 015.9●
        hip 015.1●
        knee 015.2●
        specified site NEC 015.8●
        vertebral 015.0● [730.88]
    keratitis 017.3● [370.31]
        interstitial 017.3● [370.59]
    keratoconjunctivitis 017.3● [370.31]
    kidney 016.0●
    knee (joint) 015.2●
    kyphoscoliosis 015.0● [737.43]
    kyphosis 015.0● [737.41]
    lacrimal apparatus, gland 017.3●
    laryngitis 012.3●
    larynx 012.3●
    leptomeninges, leptomeningitis
        (cerebral) (spinal) 013.0●
    lichenoides (primary) 017.0●
    linguae 017.9●
    lip 017.9●
    liver 017.9●
    lordosis 015.0● [737.42]
    lung - see Tuberculosis, pulmonary
    luposa 017.0●
        eyelid 017.0● [373.4]
    lymphadenitis - see Tuberculosis,
        lymph gland
    lymphangitis - see Tuberculosis, lymph
        gland
    lymphatic (gland) (vessel) - see
        Tuberculosis, lymph gland
    lymph gland or node (peripheral)
        017.2●
        abdomen 014.8●
        bronchial 012.1●
            primary, progressive 010.8●
        cervical 017.2●

Tuberculosis, tubercular, tuberculous
    (Continued)
    lymph gland or node (Continued)
        hilar 012.1●
            primary, progressive 010.8●
        intrathoracic 012.1●
            primary, progressive 010.8●
        mediastinal 012.1●
            primary, progressive 010.8●
        mesenteric 014.8●
        peripheral 017.2●
        retroperitoneal 014.8●
        tracheobronchial 012.1●
            primary, progressive 010.8●
    malignant NEC (see also Tuberculosis,
        pulmonary) 011.9●
    mammary gland 017.9●
    marasmus NEC (see also Tuberculosis,
        pulmonary) 011.9●
    mastoiditis 015.6●
    maternal, affecting fetus or newborn
        760.2
    mediastinal (lymph) gland or node
        012.1●
        primary, progressive 010.8●
    mediastinitis 012.8●
        primary, progressive 010.8●
    mediastinopericarditis 017.9●
        [420.0]
    mediastinum 012.8●
        primary, progressive 010.8●
    medulla 013.9●
        brain 013.2●
        spinal cord 013.4●
    melanosis, Addisonian 017.6●
    membrane, brain 013.0●
    meninges (cerebral) (spinal) 013.0●
    meningitis (basilar) (brain) (cerebral)
        (cerebrospinal) (spinal) 013.0●
    meningoencephalitis 013.0●
    mesentery, mesenteric 014.8●
        lymph gland or node 014.8●
    miliary (any site) 018.9●
        acute 018.0●
        chronic 018.8●
        specified type NEC 018.8●
    millstone makers' 011.4●
    miners' 011.4●
    moulders' 011.4●
    mouth 017.9●
    multiple 018.9●
        acute 018.0●
        chronic 018.8●
    muscle 017.9●
    myelitis 013.6●
    myocarditis 017.9● [422.0]
    myocardium 017.9● [422.0]
    nasal (passage) (sinus) 012.8●
    nasopharynx 012.8●
    neck gland 017.2●
    nephritis 016.0● [583.81]
    nerve 017.9●
    nose (septum) 012.8●
    ocular 017.3●
    old NEC 137.0
        without residuals V12.01
    omentum 014.8●
    oophoritis (acute) (chronic) 016.6●
    optic 017.3● [377.39]
        nerve trunk 017.3● [377.39]
        papilla, papillae 017.3● [377.39]
    orbit 017.3●
    orchitis 016.5● [608.81]
    organ, specified NEC 017.9●

Tuberculosis, tubercular, tuberculous
    (Continued)
    orificialis (primary) 017.0●
    osseous (see also Tuberculosis, bone)
        015.9● [730.8]
    osteitis (see also Tuberculosis, bone)
        015.9● [730.8]
    osteomyelitis (see also Tuberculosis,
        bone) 015.9● [730.8]
    otitis (media) 017.4●
    ovaritis (acute) (chronic) 016.6●
    ovary (acute) (chronic) 016.6●
    oviducts (acute) (chronic) 016.6●
    pachymeningitis 013.0●
    palate (soft) 017.9●
    pancreas 017.9●
    papulonecrotic (primary) 017.0●
    parathyroid glands 017.9●
    paronychia (primary) 017.0●
    parotid gland or region 017.9●
    pelvic organ NEC 016.9●
        female 016.7●
        male 016.5●
    pelvis (bony) 015.7● [730.85]
    penis 016.5●
    peribronchitis 011.3●
    pericarditis 017.9● [420.0]
    pericardium 017.9● [420.0]
    perichondritis, larynx 012.3●
    perineum 017.9●
    periostitis (see also Tuberculosis, bone)
        015.9● [730.8]●
    periphlebitis 017.9●
        eye vessel 017.3● [362.18]
        retina 017.3● [362.18]
    perirectal fistula 014.8●
    peritoneal gland 014.8●
    peritoneum 014.0●
    peritonitis 014.0●
    pernicious NEC (see also Tuberculosis,
        pulmonary) 011.9●
    pharyngitis 012.8●
    pharynx 012.8●
    phlyctenulosis (conjunctiva) 017.3●
        [370.31]
    phthisis NEC (see also Tuberculosis,
        pulmonary) 011.9●
    pituitary gland 017.9●
    placenta 016.7●
    pleura, pleural, pleurisy, pleuritis
        (fibrinous) (obliterative)
        (purulent) (simple plastic) (with
        effusion) 012.0●
        primary, progressive 010.1●
    pneumonia, pneumonic 011.6●
    pneumothorax 011.7●
    polyserositis 018.9●
        acute 018.0●
        chronic 018.8●
    potters' 011.4●
    prepuce 016.5●
    primary 010.9●
        complex 010.0●
        complicated 010.8●
            with pleurisy or effusion 010.1●
        progressive 010.8●
            with pleurisy or effusion
                010.1●
        skin 017.0●
    proctitis 014.8●
    prostate 016.5● [601.4]
    prostatitis 016.5● [601.4]
    pulmonaris (see also Tuberculosis,
        pulmonary) 011.9●

◀ New   ◀▥ Revised   ~~deleted~~ Deleted   ● Use Additional Digit(s)   ▨ Omit code

Tuberculosis, tubercular, tuberculous
(Continued)
  pulmonary (artery) (incipient)
    (malignant) (multiple round foci)
    (pernicious) (reinfection stage)
    011.9●
    cavitated or with cavitation 011.2●
      primary, progressive 010.8●
    childhood type or first infection
      010.0●
    chromogenic acid-fast bacilli 795.39
    fibrosis or fibrotic 011.4●
    infiltrative 011.0●
      primary, progressive 010.9●
    nodular 011.1●
    specified NEC 011.8●
    sputum positive only 795.39
    status following surgical collapse of
      lung NEC 011.9●
  pyelitis 016.0● [590.81]
  pyelonephritis 016.0● [590.81]
  pyemia - see Tuberculosis, miliary
  pyonephrosis 016.0●
  pyopneumothorax 012.0●
  pyothorax 012.0●
  rectum (with abscess) 014.8●
    fistula 014.8●
  reinfection stage (see also Tuberculosis,
    pulmonary) 011.9●
  renal 016.0●
  renis 016.0●
  reproductive organ 016.7●
  respiratory NEC (see also Tuberculosis,
    pulmonary) 011.9●
    specified site NEC 012.8●
  retina 017.3● [363.13]
  retroperitoneal (lymph gland or node)
    014.8●
    gland 014.8●
  retropharyngeal abscess 012.8●
  rheumatism 015.9●
  rhinitis 012.8●
  sacroiliac (joint) 015.8●
  sacrum 015.0● [730.88]
  salivary gland 017.9●
  salpingitis (acute) (chronic) 016.6●
  sandblasters' 011.4●
  sclera 017.3● [379.09]
  scoliosis 015.0● [737.43]
  scrofulous 017.2●
  scrotum 016.5●
  seminal tract or vesicle 016.5●
    [608.81]
  senile NEC (see also Tuberculosis,
    pulmonary) 011.9●
  septic NEC (see also Tuberculosis,
    miliary) 018.9●
  shoulder 015.8●
    blade 015.7● [730.8] ●
  sigmoid 014.8●
  sinus (accessory) (nasal) 012.8●
    bone 015.7● [730.88]
    epididymis 016.4●
  skeletal NEC (see also Osteomyelitis,
    due to tuberculosis) 015.9●
    [730.8]●
  skin (any site) (primary) 017.0●
  small intestine 014.8●
  soft palate 017.9●
  spermatic cord 016.5●
  spinal
    column 015.0● [730.88]
    cord 013.4●
    disease 015.0● [730.88]

Tuberculosis, tubercular, tuberculous
(Continued)
  spinal (Continued)
    medulla 013.4●
    membrane 013.0●
    meninges 013.0●
  spine 015.0● [730.88]
  spleen 017.7●
  splenitis 017.7●
  spondylitis 015.0● [720.81]
  spontaneous pneumothorax - see
    Tuberculosis, pulmonary
  sternoclavicular joint 015.8●
  stomach 017.9●
  stonemasons' 011.4●
  struma 017.2●
  subcutaneous tissue (cellular)
    (primary) 017.0●
  subcutis (primary) 017.0●
  subdeltoid bursa 017.9●
  submaxillary 017.9●
    region 017.9●
  supraclavicular gland 017.2●
  suprarenal (capsule) (gland) 017.6●
  swelling, joint (see also Tuberculosis,
    joint) 015.9●
  symphysis pubis 015.7● [730.88]
  synovitis 015.9● [727.01]
    hip 015.1● [727.01]
    knee 015.2● [727.01]
    specified site NEC 015.8●
      [727.01]
    spine or vertebra 015.0● [727.01]
  systemic - see Tuberculosis, miliary
  tarsitis (eyelid) 017.0● [373.4]
    ankle (bone) 015.5● [730.87]
  tendon (sheath) - see Tuberculosis,
    tenosynovitis
  tenosynovitis 015.9● [727.01]
    hip 015.1● [727.01]
    knee 015.2● [727.01]
    specified site NEC 015.8● [727.01]
    spine or vertebra 015.0● [727.01]
  testis 016.5● [608.81]
  throat 012.8●
  thymus gland 017.9●
  thyroid gland 017.5●
  toe 017.9●
  tongue 017.9●
  tonsil (lingual) 012.8●
  tonsillitis 012.8●
  trachea, tracheal 012.8●
    gland 012.1●
      primary, progressive 010.8●
    isolated 012.2●
  tracheobronchial 011.3●
    glandular 012.1●
      primary, progressive 010.8●
    isolated 012.2●
    lymph gland or node 012.1●
      primary, progressive 010.8●
  tubal 016.6●
  tunica vaginalis 016.5●
  typhlitis 014.8●
  ulcer (primary) (skin) 017.0●
    bowel or intestine 014.8●
    specified site NEC - see Tuberculosis,
      by site
    unspecified site - see Tuberculosis,
      pulmonary
  ureter 016.2●
  urethra, urethral 016.3●
  urinary organ or tract 016.3●
    kidney 016.0●

Tuberculosis, tubercular, tuberculous
(Continued)
  uterus 016.7●
  uveal tract 017.3● [363.13]
  uvula 017.9●
  vaccination, prophylactic (against)
    V03.2
  vagina 016.7●
  vas deferens 016.5●
  vein 017.9●
  verruca (primary) 017.0●
  verrucosa (cutis) (primary) 017.0●
  vertebra (column) 015.0● [730.88]
  vesiculitis 016.5● [608.81]
  viscera NEC 014.8●
  vulva 016.7● [616.51]
  wrist (joint) 015.8●
    bone 015.5● [730.83]
Tuberculum
  auriculae 744.29
  occlusal 520.2
  paramolare 520.2
Tuberosity
  jaw, excessive 524.07
  maxillary, entire 524.07
Tuberous sclerosis (brain) 759.5
Tubo-ovarian - see condition
Tuboplasty, after previous sterilization
  V26.0
Tubotympanitis 381.10
Tularemia 021.9
  with
    conjunctivitis 021.3
    pneumonia 021.2
  bronchopneumonic 021.2
  conjunctivitis 021.3
  cryptogenic 021.1
  disseminated 021.8
  enteric 021.1
  generalized 021.8
  glandular 021.8
  intestinal 021.1
  oculoglandular 021.3
  ophthalmic 021.3
  pneumonia 021.2
  pulmonary 021.2
  specified NEC 021.8
  typhoidal 021.1
  ulceroglandular 021.0
  vaccination, prophylactic (against)
    V03.4
Tularensis conjunctivitis 021.3
Tumefaction - see also Swelling
  liver (see also Hypertrophy, liver) 789.1
Tumor (M8000/1) - see also Neoplasm,
  by site, unspecified nature
  Abrikossov's (M9580/0) - see also
    Neoplasm, connective tissue,
    benign
    malignant (M9580/3) - see
      Neoplasm, connective tissue,
      malignant
  acinar cell (M8550/1) - see
    Neoplasm, by site,
    uncertain behavior
  acinic cell (M8550/1) - see
    Neoplasm, by site,
    uncertain behavior
  adenomatoid (M9054/0) - see also
    Neoplasm, by site, benign
    odontogenic (M9300/0) 213.1
      upper jaw (bone) 213.0
  adnexal (skin) (M8390/0) - see
    Neoplasm, skin, benign

Tumor (*Continued*)
  adrenal
    cortical (benign) (M8370/0) 227.0
      malignant (M8370/3) 194.0
    rest (M8671/0) - *see* Neoplasm, by site, benign
  alpha cell (M8152/0)
    malignant (M8152/3)
      pancreas 157.4
      specified site NEC - *see* Neoplasm, by site, malignant
      unspecified site 157.4
    pancreas 211.7
    specified site NEC - *see* Neoplasm, by site, benign
    unspecified site 211.7
  aneurysmal (*see also* Aneurysm) 442.9
  aortic body (M8691/1) 237.3
    malignant (M8691/3) 194.6
  argentaffin (M8241/1) - *see* Neoplasm, by site, uncertain behavior
  basal cell (M8090/1) - *see also* Neoplasm, skin, uncertain behavior
  benign (M8000/0) - *see* Neoplasm, by site, benign
  beta cell (M8151/0)
    malignant (M8151/3)
      pancreas 157.4
      specified site - *see* Neoplasm, by site, malignant
      unspecified site 157.4
    pancreas 211.7
    specified site NEC - *see* Neoplasm, by site, benign
    unspecified site 211.7
  blood - *see* Hematoma
  brenner (M9000/0) 220
    borderline malignancy (M9000/1) 236.2
    malignant (M9000/3) 183.0
    proliferating (M9000/1) 236.2
  Brooke's (M8100/0) - *see* Neoplasm, skin, benign
  brown fat (M8880/0) - *see* Lipoma, by site
  Burkitt's (M9750/3) 200.2●
  calcifying epithelial odontogenic (M9340/0) 213.1
    upper jaw (bone) 213.0
  carcinoid (M8240/1) 209.60
    benign 209.60
      appendix 209.51
      ascending colon 209.53
      bronchus 209.61
      cecum 209.52
      colon 209.50
      descending colon 209.55
      duodenum 209.41
      foregut 209.65
      hindgut 209.67
      ileum 209.43
      jejunum 209.42
      kidney 209.64
      large intestine 209.50
      lung 209.61
      midgut 209.66
      rectum 209.57
      sigmoid colon 209.56
      small intestine 209.40
      specified NEC 209.69
      stomach 209.63

Tumor (*Continued*)
  carcinoid (*Continued*)
    benign (*Continued*)
      thymus 209.62
      transverse colon 209.54
    malignant (of) 209.20
      appendix 209.11
      ascending colon 209.13
      bronchus 209.21
      cecum 209.12
      colon 209.10
      descending colon 209.15
      duodenum 209.01
      foregut 209.25
      hindgut 209.27
      ileum 209.03
      jejunum 209.02
      kidney 209.24
      large intestine 209.10
      lung 209.21
      midgut 209.26
      rectum 209.17
      sigmoid colon 209.16
      small intestine 209.00
      specified NEC 209.29
      stomach 209.23
      thymus 209.22
      transverse colon 209.14
    secondary - *see* Tumor, neuroendocrine, secondary ◄
    ~~neuroendocrine 209.60~~
      ~~malignant poorly differentiated 209.30~~
  carotid body (M8692/1) 237.3
    malignant (M8692/3) 194.5
  Castleman's (mediastinal lymph node hyperplasia) 785.6
  cells (M8001/1) - *see also* Neoplasm, by site, unspecified nature
    benign (M8001/0) - *see* Neoplasm, by site, benign
    malignant (M8001/3) - *see* Neoplasm, by site, malignant
    uncertain whether benign or malignant (M8001/1) - *see* Neoplasm, by site, uncertain nature
  cervix
    in pregnancy or childbirth 654.6●
      affecting fetus or newborn 763.89
      causing obstructed labor 660.2●
        affecting fetus or newborn 763.1
  chondromatous giant cell (M9230/0) - *see* Neoplasm, bone, benign
  chromaffin (M8700/0) - *see also* Neoplasm, by site, benign
    malignant (M8700/3) - *see* Neoplasm, by site, malignant
  Cock's peculiar 706.2
  Codman's (benign chondroblastoma) (M9230/0) - *see* Neoplasm, bone, benign
  dentigerous, mixed (M9282/0) 213.1
    upper jaw (bone) 213.0
  dermoid (M9084/0) - *see* Neoplasm, by site, benign
    with malignant transformation (M9084/3) 183.0
  desmoid (extra-abdominal) (M8821/1) - *see also* Neoplasm, connective tissue, uncertain behavior
    abdominal (M8822/1) - *see* Neoplasm, connective tissue, uncertain behavior

Tumor (*Continued*)
  embryonal (mixed) (M9080/1) - *see also* Neoplasm, by site, uncertain behavior
    liver (M9080/3) 155.0
  endodermal sinus (M9071/3)
    specified site - *see* Neoplasm, by site, malignant
    unspecified site
      female 183.0
      male 186.9
  epithelial
    benign (M8010/0) - *see* Neoplasm, by site, benign
    malignant (M8010/3) - *see* Neoplasm, by site, malignant
  Ewing's (M9260/3) - *see* Neoplasm, bone, malignant
  fatty - *see* Lipoma
  fetal, causing disproportion 653.7●
    causing obstructed labor 660.1●
  fibroid (M8890/0) - *see* Leiomyoma
  G cell (M8153/1)
    malignant (M8153/3)
      pancreas 157.4
      specified site NEC - *see* Neoplasm, by site, malignant
      unspecified site 157.4
    specified site - *see* Neoplasm, by site, uncertain behavior
    unspecified site 235.5
  giant cell (type) (M8003/1) - *see also* Neoplasm, by site, unspecified nature
    bone (M9250/1) 238.0
      malignant (M9250/3) - *see* Neoplasm, bone, malignant
    chondromatous (M9230/0) - *see* Neoplasm, bone, benign
    malignant (M8003/3) - *see* Neoplasm, by site, malignant
    peripheral (gingiva) 523.8
    soft parts (M9251/1) - *see also* Neoplasm, connective tissue, uncertain behavior
      malignant (M9251/3) - *see* Neoplasm, connective tissue, malignant
    tendon sheath 727.02
  glomus (M8711/0) - *see also* Hemangioma, by site
    jugulare (M8690/1) 237.3
      malignant (M8690/3) 194.6
  gonadal stromal (M8590/1) - *see* Neoplasm, by site, uncertain behavior
  granular cell (M9580/0) - *see also* Neoplasm, connective tissue, benign
    malignant (M9580/3) - *see* Neoplasm, connective tissue, malignant
  granulosa cell (M8620/1) 236.2
    malignant (M8620/3) 183.0
  granulosa cell-theca cell (M8621/1) 236.2
    malignant (M8621/3) 183.0
  Grawitz's (hypernephroma) (M8312/3) 189.0
  hazard-crile (M8350/3) 193
  hemorrhoidal - *see* Hemorrhoids
  hilar cell (M8660/0) 220
  Hürthle cell (benign) (M8290/0) 226
    malignant (M8290/3) 193
  hydatid (*see also* Echinococcus) 122.9

◄ New ◄◄ Revised ~~deleted~~ Deleted ● Use Additional Digit(s) ▨ Omit code

Tumor *(Continued)*
    hypernephroid (M8311/1) - *see also*
        Neoplasm, by site, uncertain
        behavior
    interstitial cell (M8650/1) - *see also*
        Neoplasm, by site, uncertain
        behavior
        benign (M8650/0) - *see* Neoplasm,
            by site, benign
        malignant (M8650/3) - *see*
            Neoplasm, by site, malignant
    islet cell (M8150/0)
        malignant (M8150/3)
            pancreas 157.4
            specified site - *see* Neoplasm, by
                site, malignant
            unspecified site 157.4
        pancreas 211.7
        specified site NEC - *see* Neoplasm,
            by site, benign
        unspecified site 211.7
    juxtaglomerular (M8361/1) 236.91
    Krukenberg's (M8490/6) 198.6
    Leydig cell (M8650/1)
        benign (M8650/0)
            specified site - *see* Neoplasm, by
                site, benign
            unspecified site
                female 220
                male 222.0
        malignant (M8650/3)
            specified site - *see* Neoplasm, by
                site, malignant
            unspecified site
                female 183.0
                male 186.9
        specified site - *see* Neoplasm, by site,
            uncertain behavior
        unspecified site
            female 236.2
            male 236.4
    lipid cell, ovary (M8670/0) 220
    lipoid cell, ovary (M8670/0) 220
    lymphomatous, benign (M9590/0) - *see*
        also Neoplasm, by site,benign
    lysis syndrome (following
        antineoplastic drug therapy)
        (spontaneous) 277.88 ◀
    Malherbe's (M8110/0) - *see* Neoplasm,
        skin, benign
    malignant (M8000/3) - *see also*
        Neoplasm, by site, malignant
        fusiform cell (type) (M8004/3) - *see*
            Neoplasm, by site, malignant
        giant cell (type) (M8003/3) - *see*
            Neoplasm, by site, malignant
        mixed NEC (M8940/3) - *see*
            Neoplasm, by site, malignant
        small cell (type) (M8002/3) - *see*
            Neoplasm, by site, malignant
        spindle cell (type) (M8004/3) - *see*
            Neoplasm, by site, malignant
    mast cell (M9740/1) 238.5
        malignant (M9740/3) 202.6●
    melanotic, neuroectodermal
        (M9363/0) - *see* Neoplasm, by site,
        benign
    Merkel cell - *see* ~~Neoplasm, by site,~~
        ~~malignant~~ Carcinoma, Merkel
        cell ◀▥
    mesenchymal
        malignant (M8800/3) - *see*
            Neoplasm, connective tissue,
            malignant
        mixed (M8990/1) - *see* Neoplasm,
            connective tissue, uncertain
            behavior

Tumor *(Continued)*
    mesodermal, mixed (M8951/3) - *see*
        also Neoplasm, by site, malignant
        liver 155.0
    mesonephric (M9110/1) - *see also*
        Neoplasm, by site, uncertain
        behavior
        malignant (M9110/3) - *see*
            Neoplasm, by site, malignant
    metastatic
        from specified site (M8000/3) - *see*
            Neoplasm, by site, malignant
        to specified site (M8000/6) - *see*
            Neoplasm, by site, malignant,
            secondary
    mixed NEC (M8940/0) - *see also*
        Neoplasm, by site, benign
        malignant (M8940/3) - *see*
            Neoplasm, by site, malignant
    mucocarcinoid, malignant (M8243/3) -
        see Neoplasm, by site, malignant
    mucoepidermoid (M8430/1) - *see*
        Neoplasm, by site, uncertain
        behavior
    Müllerian, mixed (M8950/3) - *see*
        Neoplasm, by site, malignant
    myoepithelial (M8982/0) - *see*
        Neoplasm, by site, benign
    neuroendocrine 209.60
        malignant poorly differentiated
            209.30 ◀
        secondary 209.70 ◀
            bone 209.73 ◀
            distant lymph nodes 209.71 ◀
            liver 209.72 ◀
            peritoneum 209.74 ◀
            site specified NEC 209.79 ◀
    neurogenic olfactory (M9520/3) 160.0
    nonencapsulated sclerosing (M8350/3)
        193
    odontogenic (M9270/1) 238.0
        adenomatoid (M9300/0) 213.1
            upper jaw (bone) 213.0
        benign (M9270/0) 213.1
            upper jaw (bone) 213.0
        calcifying epithelial (M9340/0)
            213.1
            upper jaw (bone) 213.0
        malignant (M9270/3) 170.1
            upper jaw (bone) 170.0
        squamous (M9312/0) 213.1
            upper jaw (bone) 213.0
    ovarian stromal (M8590/1) 236.2
    ovary
        in pregnancy or childbirth 654.4●
            affecting fetus or newborn
                763.89
            causing obstructed labor 660.2●
                affecting fetus or newborn
                    763.1
    pacinian (M9507/0) - *see* Neoplasm,
        skin, benign
    Pancoast's (M8010/3) 162.3
    papillary - *see* Papilloma
    pelvic, in pregnancy or childbirth
        654.9●
        affecting fetus or newborn 763.89
        causing obstructed labor 660.2●
            affecting fetus or newborn 763.1
    phantom 300.11
    plasma cell (M9731/1) 238.6
        benign (M9731/0) - *see* Neoplasm,
            by site, benign
        malignant (M9731/3) 203.8●

Tumor *(Continued)*
    polyvesicular vitelline (M9071/3)
        specified site - *see* Neoplasm, by site,
            malignant
        unspecified site
            female 183.0
            male 186.9
    Pott's puffy (*see also* Osteomyelitis)
        730.2●
    Rathke's pouch (M9350/1) 237.0
    regaud's (M8082/3) - *see* Neoplasm,
        nasopharynx, malignant
    rete cell (M8140/0) 222.0
    retinal anlage (M9363/0) - *see*
        Neoplasm, by site, benign
    Rokitansky's 620.2
    salivary gland type, mixed (M8940/0) -
        see also Neoplasm, by site,
        benign
        malignant (M8940/3) - *see*
            Neoplasm, by site, malignant
    Sampson's 617.1
    Schloffer's (*see also* Peritonitis)
        567.29
    Schmincke (M8082/3) - *see* Neoplasm,
        nasopharynx, malignant
    sebaceous (*see also* Cyst, sebaceous)
        706.2
    secondary (M8000/6) - *see* Neoplasm,
        by site, secondary
        carcinoid - *see* Tumor,
            neuroendocrine, secondary ◀
        neuroendocrine - *see* Tumor,
            neuroendocrine,
            secondary ◀
    Sertoli cell (M8640/0)
        with lipid storage (M8641/0)
            specified site, - *see* Neoplasm, by
                site, benign
            unspecified site
                female 220
                male 222.0
        specified site - *see* Neoplasm, by site,
            benign
        unspecified site
            female 220
            male 222.0
    Sertoli-Leydig cell (M8631/0)
        specified site - *see* Neoplasm, by site,
            benign
        unspecified site
            female 220
            male 222.0
    sex cord (-stromal) (M8590/1) - *see*
        Neoplasm, by site, uncertain
        behavior
    skin appendage (M8390/0) - *see*
        Neoplasm, skin, benign
    soft tissue
        benign (M8800/0) - *see* Neoplasm,
            connective tissue, benign
        malignant (M8800/3) - *see*
            Neoplasm, connective tissue,
            malignant
    sternomastoid 754.1
    stromal
        abdomen
            benign 215.5
            malignant NEC 171.5
            uncertain behavior 238.1
        digestive system 238.1
            benign 215.5
            malignant NEC 171.5
            uncertain behavior 238.1

Tumor (Continued)
  stromal (Continued)
    gastric 238.1
      benign 215.5
      malignant 151.9
      uncertain behavior 238.1
    gastrointestinal 238.1
      benign 215.5
      malignant NEC 171.5
      uncertain behavior 238.1
    intestine (small) 238.1
      benign 215.5
      malignant 152.9
      uncertain behavior 238.1
    stomach 238.1
      benign 215.5
      malignant 151.9
      uncertain behavior 238.1
  superior sulcus (lung) (pulmonary)
      (syndrome) (M8010/3) 162.3
  suprasulcus (M8010/3) 162.3
  sweat gland (M8400/1) - see also
      Neoplasm, skin, uncertain
      behavior
    benign (M8400/0) - see Neoplasm,
      skin, benign
    malignant (M8400/3) - see
      Neoplasm, skin, malignant
  syphilitic brain 094.89
    congenital 090.49
  testicular stromal (M8590/1) 236.4
  theca cell (M8600/0) 220
  theca cell-granulosa cell (M8621/1)
      236.2
  theca-lutein (M8610/0) 220
  turban (M8200/0) 216.4
  uterus
    in pregnancy or childbirth 654.1●
      affecting fetus or newborn
          763.89
      causing obstructed labor
          660.2●
        affecting fetus or newborn
            763.1
  vagina
    in pregnancy or childbirth 654.7●
      affecting fetus or newborn
          763.89
      causing obstructed labor 660.2●
        affecting fetus or newborn
            763.1
  varicose (see also Varicose, vein) 454.9
  von Recklinghausen's (M9540/1)
      237.71
  vulva
    in pregnancy or childbirth 654.8●
      affecting fetus or newborn
          763.89
      causing obstructed labor
          660.2●
        affecting fetus or newborn
            763.1
  Warthin's (salivary gland) (M8561/0)
      210.2
  white - see also Tuberculosis, arthritis
  White-Darier 757.39
  Wilms' (nephroblastoma) (M8960/3)
      189.0
  yolk sac (M9071/3)
    specified site - see Neoplasm, by site,
      malignant
    unspecified site
      female 183.0
      male 186.9

Tumorlet (M8040/1) - see Neoplasm, by
    site, uncertain behavior
Tungiasis 134.1
Tunica vasculosa lentis 743.39
Tunnel vision 368.45
Turban tumor (M8200/0) 216.4
Türck's trachoma (chronic catarrhal
    laryngitis) 476.0
Türk's syndrome (ocular retraction
    syndrome) 378.71
Turner's
  hypoplasia (tooth) 520.4
  syndrome 758.6
  tooth 520.4
Turner-Kieser syndrome (hereditary
    osteo-onychodysplasia) 756.89
Turner-Varny syndrome 758.6
Turricephaly 756.0
Tussis convulsiva (see also Whooping
    cough) 033.9
Twiddler's syndrome (due to)
  automatic implantable defibrillator
      996.04
  pacemaker 996.01
Twin
  affected by maternal complications of
      pregnancy 761.5
  conjoined 759.4
    fetal 678.1●
  healthy liveborn - see Newborn, twin
  pregnancy (complicating delivery)
      NEC 651.0●
    with fetal loss and retention of one
        fetus 651.3●
    conjoined 678.1●
    following (elective) fetal reduction
        651.7●
Twinning, teeth 520.2
Twist, twisted
  bowel, colon, or intestine 560.2
  hair (congenital) 757.4
  mesentery 560.2
  omentum 560.2
  organ or site, congenital NEC - see
      Anomaly, specified type NEC
  ovarian pedicle 620.5
    congenital 752.0
  umbilical cord - see Compression,
      umbilical cord
Twitch 781.0
Tylosis 700
  buccalis 528.6
  gingiva 523.8
  linguae 528.6
  palmaris et plantaris 757.39
Tympanism 787.3
Tympanites (abdominal) (intestine)
    787.3
Tympanitis - see Myringitis
Tympanosclerosis 385.00
  involving
    combined sites NEC 385.09
      with tympanic membrane 385.03
    tympanic membrane 385.01
      with ossicles 385.02
        and middle ear 385.03
Tympanum - see condition
Tympany
  abdomen 787.3
  chest 786.7
Typhlitis (see also Appendicitis) 541
Typhoenteritis 002.0
Typhogastric fever 002.0

Typhoid (abortive) (ambulant) (any site)
    (fever) (hemorrhagic) (infection)
    (intermittent) (malignant)
    (rheumatic) 002.0
  with pneumonia 002.0 [484.8]
  abdominal 002.0
  carrier (suspected) of V02.1
  cholecystitis (current) 002.0
  clinical (Widal and blood test negative)
      002.0
  endocarditis 002.0 [421.1]
  inoculation reaction - see
      Complications, vaccination
  meningitis 002.0 [320.7]
  mesenteric lymph nodes 002.0
  myocarditis 002.0 [422.0]
  osteomyelitis (see also Osteomyelitis,
      due to, typhoid) 002.0 [730.8]●
  perichondritis, larynx 002.0 [478.71]
  pneumonia 002.0 [484.8]
  spine 002.0 [720.81]
  ulcer (perforating) 002.0
  vaccination, prophylactic (against)
      V03.1
  Widal negative 002.0
Typhomalaria (fever) (see also Malaria)
    084.6
Typhomania 002.0
Typhoperitonitis 002.0
Typhus (fever) 081.9
  abdominal, abdominalis 002.0
  African tick 082.1
  amarillic (see also Fever, Yellow)
      060.9
  brain 081.9
  cerebral 081.9
  classical 080
  endemic (flea-borne) 081.0
  epidemic (louse-borne) 080
  exanthematic NEC 080
  exanthematicus SAI 080
    brillii SAI 081.1
    Mexicanus SAI 081.0
    pediculo vestimenti causa 080
    typhus murinus 081.0
  flea-borne 081.0
  Indian tick 082.1
  Kenya tick 082.1
  louse-borne 080
  Mexican 081.0
    flea-borne 081.0
    louse-borne 080
    tabardillo 080
  mite-borne 081.2
  murine 081.0
  North Asian tick-borne 082.2
  petechial 081.9
  Queensland tick 082.3
  rat 081.0
  recrudescent 081.1
  recurrent (see also Fever, relapsing)
      087.9
  São Paulo 082.0
  scrub (China) (India) (Malaya) (New
      Guinea) 081.2
  shop (of Malaya) 081.0
  Siberian tick 082.2
  tick-borne NEC 082.9
  tropical 081.2
  vaccination, prophylactic (against)
      V05.8
Tyrosinemia 270.2
  neonatal 775.89
Tyrosinosis (Medes) (Sakai) 270.2
Tyrosinuria 270.2
Tyrosyluria 270.2

◀ New   ◀▦ Revised   ~~deleted~~ Deleted   ● Use Additional Digit(s)   ▦ Omit code

U

Uehlinger's syndrome (acropachyderma) 757.39

Uhl's anomaly or disease (hypoplasia of myocardium, right ventricle) 746.84

Ulcer, ulcerated, ulcerating, ulceration, ulcerative 707.9
- with gangrene 707.9 [785.4]
- abdomen (wall) (see also Ulcer, skin) 707.8
- ala, nose 478.19
- alveolar process 526.5
- amebic (intestine) 006.9
  - skin 006.6
- anastomotic - see Ulcer, gastrojejunal
- anorectal 569.41
- antral - see Ulcer, stomach
- anus (sphincter) (solitary) 569.41
  - varicose - see Varicose, ulcer, anus
- aorta - see Aneurysm
- aphthous (oral) (recurrent) 528.2
  - genital organ(s)
    - female 616.50
    - male 608.89
  - mouth 528.2
- arm (see also Ulcer, skin) 707.8
- arteriosclerotic plaque - see Arteriosclerosis, by site
- artery NEC 447.2
  - without rupture 447.8
- atrophic NEC - see Ulcer, skin
- Barrett's (chronic peptic ulcer of esophagus) 530.85
- bile duct 576.8
- bladder (solitary) (sphincter) 596.8
  - bilharzial (see also Schistosomiasis) 120.9 [595.4]
  - submucosal (see also Cystitis) 595.1
  - tuberculous (see also Tuberculosis) 016.1●
- bleeding NEC - see Ulcer, peptic, with hemorrhage
- bone 730.9●
- bowel (see also Ulcer, intestine) 569.82
- breast 611.0
- bronchitis 491.8
- bronchus 519.19
- buccal (cavity) (traumatic) 528.9
- burn (acute) - see Ulcer, duodenum
- Buruli 031.1
- buttock (see also Ulcer, skin) 707.8
  - decubitus (see also Ulcer, pressure) 707.00
- cancerous (M8000/3) - see Neoplasm, by site, malignant
- cardia - see Ulcer, stomach
- cardio-esophageal (peptic) 530.20
  - with bleeding 530.21
- cecum (see also Ulcer, intestine) 569.82
- cervix (uteri) (trophic) 622.0
  - with mention of cervicitis 616.0
- chancroidal 099.0
- chest (wall) (see also Ulcer, skin) 707.8
- Chiclero 085.4
- chin (pyogenic) (see also Ulcer, skin) 707.8
- chronic (cause unknown) - see also Ulcer, skin
  - penis 607.89
- Cochin-China 085.1
- colitis - see Colitis, ulcerative
- colon (see also Ulcer, intestine) 569.82

Ulcer, ulcerated, ulcerating, ulceration, ulcerative (Continued)
- conjunctiva (acute) (postinfectional) 372.00
- cornea (infectional) 370.00
  - with perforation 370.06
  - annular 370.02
  - catarrhal 370.01
  - central 370.03
  - dendritic 054.42
  - marginal 370.01
  - mycotic 370.05
  - phlyctenular, tuberculous (see also Tuberculosis) 017.3● [370.31]
  - ring 370.02
  - rodent 370.07
  - serpent, serpiginous 370.04
  - superficial marginal 370.01
  - tuberculous (see also Tuberculosis) 017.3● [370.31]
- corpus cavernosum (chronic) 607.89
- crural - see Ulcer, lower extremity
- Curling's - see Ulcer, duodenum
- Cushing's - see Ulcer, peptic
- cystitis (interstitial) 595.1
- decubitus (unspecified site) (see also Ulcer, pressure) 707.00
  - with gangrene 707.00 [785.4]
  - ankle 707.06
  - back
    - lower 707.03
    - upper 707.02
  - buttock 707.05
  - coccyx 707.03
  - elbow 707.01
  - head 707.09
  - heel 707.07
  - hip 707.04
  - other site 707.09
  - sacrum 707.03
  - shoulder blades 707.02
- dendritic 054.42
- diabetes, diabetic (mellitus) 250.8● [707.9]
  - due to secondary diabetes 249.8● [707.9]
  - lower limb 250.8● [707.10]
    - due to secondary diabetes 249.8● [707.10]
    - ankle 250.8● [707.13]
      - due to secondary diabetes 249.8● [707.13]
    - calf 250.8● [707.12]
      - due to secondary diabetes 249.8● [707.12]
    - foot 250.8● [707.15]
      - due to secondary diabetes 249.8● [707.15]
    - heel 250.8● [707.14]
      - due to secondary diabetes 249.8● [707.14]
    - knee 250.8● [707.19]
      - due to secondary diabetes 249.8● [707.19]
    - specified site NEC 250.8● [707.19]
      - due to secondary diabetes 249.8● [707.19]
    - thigh 250.8● [707.11]
      - due to secondary diabetes 249.8● [707.11]
    - toes 250.8● [707.15]
      - due to secondary diabetes 249.8● [707.15]

Ulcer, ulcerated, ulcerating, ulceration, ulcerative (Continued)
- diabetes, diabetic (Continued)
  - lower limb (Continued)
    - specified site NEC 250.8● [707.8]
      - due to secondary diabetes 249.8● [707.8]
- Dieulafoy - see Lesion, Dieulafoy
  - due to
    - infection NEC - see Ulcer, skin
    - radiation, radium - see Ulcer, by site
    - trophic disturbance (any region) - see Ulcer, skin
    - x-ray - see Ulcer, by site
- duodenum, duodenal (eroded) (peptic) 532.9●

> Note 70   Use the following fifth-digit subclassification with categories 531–534:
>
> 0   without mention of obstruction
> 1   with obstruction

- with
  - hemorrhage (chronic) 532.4●
    - and perforation 532.6●
  - perforation (chronic) 532.5●
    - and hemorrhage 532.6●
- acute 532.3●
  - with
    - hemorrhage 532.0●
      - and perforation 532.2●
    - perforation 532.1●
      - and hemorrhage 532.2●
- bleeding (recurrent) - see Ulcer, duodenum, with hemorrhage
- chronic 532.7●
  - with
    - hemorrhage 532.4●
      - and perforation 532.6●
    - perforation 532.5●
      - and hemorrhage 532.6●
- penetrating - see Ulcer, duodenum, with perforation
- perforating - see Ulcer, duodenum, with perforation
- dysenteric NEC 009.0
- elusive 595.1
- endocarditis (any valve) (acute) (chronic) (subacute) 421.0
- enteritis - see Colitis, ulcerative
- enterocolitis 556.0
- epiglottis 478.79
- esophagus (peptic) 530.20
  - with bleeding 530.21
  - due to ingestion
    - aspirin 530.20
    - chemicals 530.20
    - medicinal agents 530.20
  - fungal 530.20
  - infectional 530.20
  - varicose (see also Varix, esophagus) 456.1
    - bleeding (see also Varix, esophagus, bleeding) 456.0
- eye NEC 360.00
  - dendritic 054.42
- eyelid (region) 373.01
- face (see also Ulcer, skin) 707.8
- fauces 478.29
- Fenwick (-Hunner) (solitary) (see also Cystitis) 595.1

Ulcer, ulcerated, ulcerating, ulceration,
ulcerative *(Continued)*
fistulous NEC - *see* Ulcer, skin
foot (indolent) (*see also* Ulcer, lower
extremity) 707.15
perforating 707.15
leprous 030.1
syphilitic 094.0
trophic 707.15
varicose 454.0
inflamed or infected 454.2
frambesial, initial or primary 102.0
gallbladder or duct 575.8
gall duct 576.8
gangrenous (*see also* Gangrene) 785.4
gastric - *see* Ulcer, stomach
gastrocolic - *see* Ulcer, gastrojejunal
gastroduodenal - *see* Ulcer, peptic
gastroesophageal - *see* Ulcer, stomach
gastrohepatic - *see* Ulcer, stomach
gastrointestinal - *see* Ulcer, gastrojejunal
gastrojejunal (eroded) (peptic) 534.9

Note 71   Use the following fifth-digit
subclassification with categories
531–534:

0   without mention of obstruction
1   with obstruction

---

with
hemorrhage (chronic) 534.4●
and perforation 534.6●
perforation 534.5●
and hemorrhage 534.6●
acute 534.3●
with
hemorrhage 534.0●
and perforation 534.2●
perforation 534.1●
and hemorrhage 534.2●
bleeding (recurrent) - *see* Ulcer,
gastrojejunal, with
hemorrhage
chronic 534.7●
with
hemorrhage 534.4●
and perforation 534.6●
perforation 534.5●
and hemorrhage 534.6●
penetrating - *see* Ulcer, gastrojejunal,
with perforation
perforating - *see* Ulcer, gastrojejunal,
with perforation
gastrojejunocolic - *see* Ulcer,
gastrojejunal
genital organ
female 629.89
male 608.89
gingiva 523.8
gingivitis 523.10
glottis 478.79
granuloma of pudenda 099.2
groin (*see also* Ulcer, skin) 707.8
gum 523.8
gumma, due to yaws 102.4
hand (*see also* Ulcer, skin) 707.8
hard palate 528.9
heel (*see also* Ulcer, lower extremity)
707.14
decubitus (*see also* Ulcer, pressure)
707.07
hemorrhoids 455.8
external 455.5
internal 455.2

Ulcer, ulcerated, ulcerating, ulceration,
ulcerative *(Continued)*
hip (*see also* Ulcer, skin) 707.8
decubitus (*see also* Ulcer, pressure)
707.04
Hunner's 595.1
hypopharynx 478.29
hypopyon (chronic) (subacute)
370.04
hypostaticum - *see* Ulcer, varicose
ileocolitis 556.1
ileum (*see also* Ulcer, intestine) 569.82
intestine, intestinal 569.82
with perforation 569.83
amebic 006.9
duodenal - *see* Ulcer, duodenum
granulocytopenic (with
hemorrhage) 288.09
marginal 569.82
perforating 569.83
small, primary 569.82
stercoraceous 569.82
stercoral 569.82
tuberculous (*see also* Tuberculosis)
014.8●
typhoid (fever) 002.0
varicose 456.8
ischemic 707.9
lower extremity (*see also* Ulcer, lower
extremity) 707.10
ankle 707.13
calf 707.12
foot 707.15
heel 707.14
knee 707.19
specified site NEC 707.19
thigh 707.11
toes 707.15
jejunum, jejunal - *see* Ulcer,
gastrojejunal
keratitis (*see also* Ulcer, cornea)
370.00
knee - *see* Ulcer, lower extremity
labium (majus) (minus) 616.50
laryngitis (*see also* Laryngitis) 464.00
with obstruction 464.01
larynx (aphthous) (contact) 478.79
diphtheritic 032.3
leg - *see* Ulcer, lower extremity
lip 528.5
Lipschütz's 616.50
lower extremity (atrophic) (chronic)
(neurogenic) (perforating)
(pyogenic) (trophic) (tropical)
707.10
with gangrene (*see also* Ulcer, lower
extremity) 707.10 *[785.4]*
arteriosclerotic 440.24
ankle 707.13
arteriosclerotic 440.23
with gangrene 440.24
calf 707.12
decubitus (*see also* Ulcer, pressure)
707.00
with gangrene 707.00 *[785.4]*
ankle 707.06
buttock 707.05
heel 707.07
hip 707.04
foot 707.15
heel 707.14
knee 707.19
specified site NEC 707.19
thigh 707.11

Ulcer, ulcerated, ulcerating, ulceration,
ulcerative *(Continued)*
lower extremity *(Continued)*
toes 707.15
varicose 454.0
inflamed or infected 454.2
luetic - *see* Ulcer, syphilitic
lung 518.89
tuberculous (*see also* Tuberculosis)
011.2●
malignant (M8000/3) - *see* Neoplasm,
by site, malignant
marginal NEC - *see* Ulcer, gastrojejunal
meatus (urinarius) 597.89
Meckel's diverticulum 751.0
Meleney's (chronic undermining)
686.09
Mooren's (cornea) 370.07
mouth (traumatic) 528.9
mycobacterial (skin) 031.1
nasopharynx 478.29
navel cord (newborn) 771.4
neck (*see also* Ulcer, skin) 707.8
uterus 622.0
neurogenic NEC - *see* Ulcer, skin
nose, nasal (infectional) (passage)
478.19
septum 478.19
varicose 456.8
skin - *see* Ulcer, skin
spirochetal NEC 104.8
oral mucosa (traumatic) 528.9
palate (soft) 528.9
penetrating NEC - *see* Ulcer, peptic,
with perforation
penis (chronic) 607.89
peptic (site unspecified) 533.9

Note 72   Use the following fifth-digit
subclassification with categories
531–534:

0   without mention of obstruction
1   with obstruction

---

with
hemorrhage 533.4●
and perforation 533.6●
perforation (chronic) 533.5●
and hemorrhage 533.6●
acute 533.3●
with
hemorrhage 533.0●
and perforation 533.2●
perforation 533.1●
and hemorrhage 533.2●
bleeding (recurrent) - *see* Ulcer,
peptic, with hemorrhage
chronic 533.7●
with
hemorrhage 533.4●
and perforation 533.6●
perforation 533.5●
and hemorrhage 533.6●
penetrating - *see* Ulcer, peptic, with
perforation
perforating NEC (*see also* Ulcer, peptic,
with perforation) 533.5●
skin 707.9
perineum (*see also* Ulcer, skin) 707.8
peritonsillar 474.8
phagedenic (tropical) NEC - *see* Ulcer,
skin
pharynx 478.29
phlebitis - *see* Phlebitis

◀ New   ◀||| Revised   ~~deleted~~ Deleted   ● Use Additional Digit(s)   ▨ Omit code

Ulcer, ulcerated, ulcerating, ulceration, ulcerative *(Continued)*
plaster *(see also* Ulcer, pressure) 707.00
popliteal space - *see* Ulcer, lower extremity
postpyloric - *see* Ulcer, duodenum
prepuce 607.89
prepyloric - *see* Ulcer, stomach
pressure 707.00
  with
    abrasion, blister, partial thickness skin loss involving epidermis and/or dermis 707.22
    full thickness skin loss involving damage or necrosis of subcutaneous tissue 707.23
    gangrene 707.00 *[785.4]*
    necrosis of soft tissues through to underlying muscle, tendon, or bone 707.24
  ankle 707.06
  back
    lower 707.03
    upper 707.02
  buttock 707.05
  coccyx 707.03
  elbow 707.01
  head 707.09
  healed - *omit code*
  healing - *code to* Ulcer, pressure, by stage
  heel 707.07
  hip 707.04
  other site 707.09
  sacrum 707.03
  shoulder blades 707.02
  stage
    I (healing) 707.21
    II (healing) 707.22
    III (healing) 707.23
    IV (healing) 707.24
    unspecified (healing) 707.20
  unstageable 707.25
primary of intestine 569.82
  with perforation 569.83
proctitis 556.2
  with ulcerative sigmoiditis 556.3
prostate 601.8
pseudopeptic - *see* Ulcer, peptic
pyloric - *see* Ulcer, stomach
rectosigmoid 569.82
  with perforation 569.83
rectum (sphincter) (solitary) 569.41
  stercoraceous, stercoral 569.41
  varicose - *see* Varicose, ulcer, anus
retina *(see also* Chorioretinitis) 363.20
rodent (M8090/3) - *see also* Neoplasm, skin, malignant
  cornea 370.07
round - *see* Ulcer, stomach
sacrum (region) *(see also* Ulcer, skin) 707.8
Saemisch's 370.04
scalp *(see also* Ulcer, skin) 707.8
sclera 379.09
scrofulous *(see also* Tuberculosis) 017.2●
scrotum 608.89
  tuberculous *(see also* Tuberculosis) 016.5●
  varicose 456.4
seminal vesicle 608.89

Ulcer, ulcerated, ulcerating, ulceration, ulcerative *(Continued)*
sigmoid 569.82
  with perforation 569.83
skin (atrophic) (chronic) (neurogenic) (non-healing) (perforating) (pyogenic) (trophic) 707.9
  with gangrene 707.9 *[785.4]*
  amebic 006.6
  decubitus *(see also* Ulcer, pressure) 707.00
    with gangrene 707.00 *[785.4]*
  in granulocytopenia 288.09
  lower extremity *(see also* Ulcer, lower extremity) 707.10
    with gangrene 707.10 *[785.4]*
      arteriosclerotic 440.24
    ankle 707.13
    arteriosclerotic 440.23
      with gangrene 440.24
    calf 707.12
    foot 707.15
    heel 707.14
    knee 707.19
    specified site NEC 707.19
    thigh 707.11
    toes 707.15
  mycobacterial 031.1
  syphilitic (early) (secondary) 091.3
  tuberculous (primary) *(see also* Tuberculosis) 017.0●
  varicose - *see* Ulcer, varicose
sloughing NEC - *see* Ulcer, skin
soft palate 528.9
solitary, anus or rectum (sphincter) 569.41
sore throat 462
  streptococcal 034.0
spermatic cord 608.89
spine (tuberculous) 015.0● *[730.88]*
stasis (leg) (venous) 454.0
  with varicose veins 454.0
  without varicose veins 459.81
  inflamed or infected 454.2
stercoral, stercoraceous 569.82
  with perforation 569.83
  anus or rectum 569.41
stoma, stomal - *see* Ulcer, gastrojejunal
stomach (eroded) (peptic) (round) 531.9●

> Note 73 Use the following fifth-digit subclassification with categories 531–534:
>
> 0 without mention of obstruction
> 1 with obstruction

  with
    hemorrhage 531.4●
      and perforation 531.6●
    perforation (chronic) 531.5●
      and hemorrhage 531.6●
  acute 531.3●
    with
      hemorrhage 531.0●
      and perforation 531.2●
      perforation 531.1●
      and hemorrhage 531.2●
  bleeding (recurrent) - *see* Ulcer, stomach, with hemorrhage

Ulcer, ulcerated, ulcerating, ulceration, ulcerative *(Continued)*
stomach *(Continued)*
  chronic 531.7●
    with
      hemorrhage 531.4●
        and perforation 531.6●
      perforation 531.5●
        and hemorrhage 531.6●
  penetrating - *see* Ulcer, stomach, with perforation
  perforating - *see* Ulcer, stomach, with perforation
stomatitis 528.00
stress - *see* Ulcer, peptic
strumous (tuberculous) *(see also* Tuberculosis) 017.2●
submental *(see also* Ulcer, skin) 707.8
submucosal, bladder 595.1
syphilitic (any site) (early) (secondary) 091.3
  late 095.9
  perforating 095.9
    foot 094.0
testis 608.89
thigh - *see* Ulcer, lower extremity
throat 478.29
  diphtheritic 032.0
toe - *see* Ulcer, lower extremity
tongue (traumatic) 529.0
tonsil 474.8
  diphtheritic 032.0
trachea 519.19
trophic - *see* Ulcer, skin
tropical NEC *(see also* Ulcer, skin) 707.9
tuberculous - *see* Tuberculosis, ulcer
tunica vaginalis 608.89
turbinate 730.9●
typhoid (fever) 002.0
  perforating 002.0
umbilicus (newborn) 771.4
unspecified site NEC - *see* Ulcer, skin
urethra (meatus) *(see also* Urethritis) 597.89
uterus 621.8
  cervix 622.0
    with mention of cervicitis 616.0
  neck 622.0
    with mention of cervicitis 616.0
vagina 616.89
valve, heart 421.0
varicose (lower extremity, any part) 454.0
  anus - *see* Varicose, ulcer, anus
  broad ligament 456.5
  esophagus *(see also* Varix, esophagus) 456.1
    bleeding *(see also* Varix, esophagus, bleeding) 456.0
  inflamed or infected 454.2
  nasal septum 456.8
  perineum 456.6
  rectum - *see* Varicose, ulcer, anus
  scrotum 456.4
  specified site NEC 456.8
  sublingual 456.3
  vulva 456.6
vas deferens 608.89
vesical *(see also* Ulcer, bladder) 596.8
vulva (acute) (infectional) 616.50
  Behçet's syndrome 136.1 *[616.51]*
  herpetic 054.12
  tuberculous 016.7● *[616.51]*

Ulcer, ulcerated, ulcerating, ulceration, ulcerative (Continued)
 vulvobuccal, recurring 616.50
 x-ray - see Ulcer, by site
 yaws 102.4
Ulcerosa scarlatina 034.1
Ulcus - see also Ulcer
 cutis tuberculosum (see also Tuberculosis) 017.0●
 duodeni - see Ulcer, duodenum
 durum 091.0
  extragenital 091.2
 gastrojejunale - see Ulcer, gastrojejunal
 hypostaticum - see Ulcer, varicose
 molle (cutis) (skin) 099.0
 serpens corneae (pneumococcal) 370.04
 ventriculi - see Ulcer, stomach
Ulegyria 742.4
Ulerythema
 acneiforma 701.8
 centrifugum 695.4
 ophryogenes 757.4
Ullrich (-Bonnevie) (-Turner) syndrome 758.6
Ullrich-Feichtiger syndrome 759.89
Ulnar - see condition
Ulorrhagia 523.8
Ulorrhea 523.8
Umbilicus, umbilical - see also condition
 cord necrosis, affecting fetus or newborn 762.6
Unacceptable
 existing dental restoration
  contours 525.65
  morphology 525.65
Unavailability of medical facilities (at) V63.9
 due to
  investigation by social service agency V63.8
  lack of services at home V63.1
  remoteness from facility V63.0
  waiting list V63.2
 home V63.1
 outpatient clinic V63.0
 specified reason NEC V63.8
Uncinaria americana infestation 126.1
Uncinariasis (see also Ancylostomiasis) 126.9
Unconscious, unconsciousness 780.09
Underdevelopment - see also
  Undeveloped sexual 259.0
Underfill, endodontic 526.63
Undernourishment 269.9
Undernutrition 269.9
Under observation - see Observation
Underweight 783.22
 for gestational age - see Light-for-dates
Underwood's disease (sclerema neonatorum) 778.1
Undescended - see also Malposition, congenital
 cecum 751.4
 colon 751.4
 testis 752.51
Undetermined diagnosis or cause 799.9
Undeveloped, undevelopment - see also Hypoplasia
 brain (congenital) 742.1
 cerebral (congenital) 742.1
 fetus or newborn 764.9●
 heart 746.89

Undeveloped, undevelopment (Continued)
 lung 748.5
 testis 257.2
 uterus 259.0
Undiagnosed (disease) 799.9
Undulant fever (see also Brucellosis) 023.9
Unemployment, anxiety concerning V62.0
Unequal leg (acquired) (length) 736.81
 congenital 755.30
Unerupted teeth, tooth 520.6
Unextracted dental root 525.3
Unguis incarnatus 703.0
Unicornis uterus 752.3
Unicorporeus uterus 752.3
Uniformis uterus 752.3
Unilateral - see also condition
 development, breast 611.89
 organ or site, congenital NEC - see Agenesis
 vagina 752.49
Unilateralis uterus 752.3
Unilocular heart 745.8
Uninhibited bladder 596.54
 with cauda equina syndrome 344.61
 neurogenic (see also Neurogenic, bladder) 596.54
Union, abnormal - see also Fusion
 divided tendon 727.89
 larynx and trachea 748.3
Universal
 joint, cervix 620.6
 mesentery 751.4
Unknown
 cause of death 799.9
 diagnosis 799.9
Unna's disease (seborrheic dermatitis) 690.10
Unresponsiveness, adrenocorticotropin (ACTH) 255.41
Unsatisfactory
 cytology smear
  anal 796.78
  cervical 795.08
  vaginal 795.18
 restoration, tooth (existing) 525.60
  specified NEC 525.69
Unsoundness of mind (see also Psychosis) 298.9
Unspecified cause of death 799.9
Unstable
 back NEC 724.9
 colon 569.89
 joint - see Instability, joint
 lie 652.0●
  affecting fetus or newborn (before labor) 761.7
  causing obstructed labor 660.0●
   affecting fetus or newborn 763.1
 lumbosacral joint (congenital) 756.19
  acquired 724.6
 sacroiliac 724.6
 spine NEC 724.9
Untruthfulness, child problem (see also Disturbance, conduct) 312.0●
Unverricht (-Lundborg) disease, syndrome, or epilepsy 345.1 ◀▥
Unverricht-Wagner syndrome (dermatomyositis) 710.3
Upper respiratory - see condition

Upset
 gastric 536.8
  psychogenic 306.4
 gastrointestinal 536.8
  psychogenic 306.4
  virus (see also Enteritis, viral) 008.8
 intestinal (large) (small) 564.9
  psychogenic 306.4
 menstruation 626.9
 mental 300.9
 stomach 536.8
  psychogenic 306.4
Urachus - see also condition
 patent 753.7
 persistent 753.7
Uratic arthritis 274.00 ◀▥
Urbach's lipoid proteinosis 272.8
Urbach-Oppenheim disease or syndrome (necrobiosis lipoidica diabeticorum) 250.8● [709.3]
 due to secondary diabetes 249.8● [709.3]
Urbach-Wiethe disease or syndrome (lipoid proteinosis) 272.8
Urban yellow fever 060.1
Urea, blood, high - see Uremia
Uremia, uremic (absorption) (amaurosis) (amblyopia) (aphasia) (apoplexy) (coma) (delirium) (dementia) (dropsy) (dyspnea) (fever) (intoxication) (mania) (paralysis) (poisoning) (toxemia) (vomiting) 586
 with
  abortion - see Abortion, by type, with renal failure
  ectopic pregnancy (see also categories 633.0–633.9) 639.3
  hypertension (see also Hypertension, kidney) 403.91
  molar pregnancy (see also categories 630–632) 639.3
 chronic 585.9
 complicating
  abortion 639.3
  ectopic or molar pregnancy 639.3
  hypertension (see also Hypertension, kidney) 403.91
  labor and delivery 669.3●
 congenital 779.89
 extrarenal 788.99
 hypertensive (chronic) (see also Hypertension, kidney) 403.91
 maternal NEC, affecting fetus or newborn 760.1
 neuropathy 585.9 [357.4]
 pericarditis 585.9 [420.0]
 prerenal 788.99
 pyelitic (see also Pyelitis) 590.80
Ureter, ureteral - see condition
Ureteralgia 788.0
Ureterectasis 593.89
Ureteritis 593.89
 cystica 590.3
 due to calculus 592.1
 gonococcal (acute) 098.19
  chronic or duration of 2 months or over 098.39
 nonspecific 593.89
Ureterocele (acquired) 593.89
 congenital 753.23
Ureterolith 592.1

◀ New   ◀▥ Revised   ~~deleted~~ Deleted   ● Use Additional Digit(s)   ▨ Omit code

Ureterolithiasis 592.1
Ureterostomy status V44.6
  with complication 997.5
Urethra, urethral - *see* condition
Urethralgia 788.99
Urethritis (abacterial) (acute) (allergic)
  (anterior) (chronic) (nonvenereal)
  (posterior) (recurrent) (simple)
  (subacute) (ulcerative)
  (undifferentiated) 597.80
  diplococcal (acute) 098.0
    chronic or duration of 2 months or
      over 098.2
  due to Trichomonas (vaginalis)
    131.02
  gonococcal (acute) 098.0
    chronic or duration of 2 months or
      over 098.2
  nongonococcal (sexually transmitted)
    099.40
    Chlamydia trachomatis 099.41
    Reiter's 099.3
    specified organism NEC 099.49
  nonspecific (sexually transmitted) (*see
    also* Urethritis, nongonococcal)
    099.40
  not sexually transmitted 597.80
  Reiter's 099.3
  trichomonal or due to Trichomonas
    (vaginalis) 131.02
  tuberculous (*see also* Tuberculosis)
    016.3●
  venereal NEC (*see also* Urethritis,
    nongonococcal) 099.40
Urethrocele
  female 618.03
    with uterine prolapse 618.4
      complete 618.3
      incomplete 618.2
  male 599.5
Urethrolithiasis 594.2
Urethro-oculoarticular syndrome
  099.3
Urethro-oculosynovial syndrome
  099.3
Urethrorectal - *see* condition
Urethrorrhagia 599.84
Urethrorrhea 788.7
Urethrostomy status V44.6
  with complication 997.5
Urethrotrigonitis 595.3
Urethrovaginal - *see* condition
Urhidrosis, uridrosis 705.89
Uric acid
  diathesis 274.9
  in blood 790.6
Uricacidemia 790.6
Uricemia 790.6
Uricosuria 791.9
Urination
  frequent 788.41
  painful 788.1
  urgency 788.63
Urine, urinary - *see also* condition
  abnormality NEC 788.69
  blood in (*see also* Hematuria)
    599.70
  discharge, excessive 788.42
  enuresis 788.30
    nonorganic origin 307.6
  extravasation 788.8
  frequency 788.41
  hesitancy 788.64

Urine, urinary (*Continued*)
  incontinence 788.30
    active 788.30
    female 788.30
      stress 625.6
        and urge 788.33
    male 788.30
      stress 788.32
        and urge 788.33
    mixed (stress and urge) 788.33
    neurogenic 788.39
    nonorganic origin 307.6
    overflow 788.38
    stress (female) 625.6
      male NEC 788.32
  intermittent stream 788.61
  pus in 791.9
  retention or stasis NEC 788.20
    bladder, incomplete emptying
      788.21
    psychogenic 306.53
    specified NEC 788.29
  secretion
    deficient 788.5
    excessive 788.42
    frequency 788.41
  strain 788.65
  stream
    intermittent 788.61
    slowing 788.62
    splitting 788.61
    weak 788.62
  urgency 788.63
Urinemia - *see* Uremia
Urinoma NEC 599.9
  bladder 596.8
  kidney 593.89
  renal 593.89
  ureter 593.89
  urethra 599.84
Uroarthritis, infectious 099.3
Urodialysis 788.5
Urolithiasis 592.9
Uronephrosis 593.89
Uropathy 599.9
  obstructive 599.60
Urosepsis 599.0
  meaning sepsis 995.91
  meaning urinary tract infection 599.0
Urticaria 708.9
  with angioneurotic edema 995.1
    hereditary 277.6
  allergic 708.0
  cholinergic 708.5
  chronic 708.8
  cold, familial 708.2
  dermatographic 708.3
  due to
    cold or heat 708.2
    drugs 708.0
    food 708.0
    inhalants 708.0
    plants 708.8
    serum 999.5
  factitial 708.3
  giant 995.1
    hereditary 277.6
  gigantea 995.1
    hereditary 277.6
  idiopathic 708.1
  larynx 995.1
    hereditary 277.6
  neonatorum 778.8

Urticaria (*Continued*)
  nonallergic 708.1
  papulosa (Hebra) 698.2
  perstans hemorrhagica 757.39
  pigmentosa 757.33
  recurrent periodic 708.8
  serum 999.5
  solare 692.72
  specified type NEC 708.8
  thermal (cold) (heat) 708.2
  vibratory 708.4
Urticarioides acarodermatitis 133.9
Use of
  methadone 304.00
  nonprescribed drugs (*see also* Abuse,
    drugs, nondependent) 305.9●
  patent medicines (*see also* Abuse, drugs,
    nondependent) 305.9●
Usher-Senear disease (pemphigus
  erythematosus) 694.4
Uta 085.5
Uterine size-date discrepancy 649.6●
Uteromegaly 621.2
Uterovaginal - *see* condition
Uterovesical - *see* condition
Uterus - *see* condition
Utriculitis (utriculus prostaticus) 597.89
Uveal - *see* condition
Uveitis (anterior) (*see also* Iridocyclitis)
  364.3
  acute or subacute 364.00
    due to or associated with
      gonococcal infection 098.41
      herpes (simplex) 054.44
      zoster 053.22
    primary 364.01
    recurrent 364.02
    secondary (noninfectious) 364.04
      infectious 364.03
  allergic 360.11
  chronic 364.10
    due to or associated with
      sarcoidosis 135 [*364.11*]
      tuberculosis (*see also* Tuberculosis)
        017.3● [*364.11*]
  due to
    operation 360.11
    toxoplasmosis (acquired) 130.2
      congenital (active) 771.2
  granulomatous 364.10
  heterochromic 364.21
  lens-induced 364.23
  nongranulomatous 364.00
  posterior 363.20
    disseminated - *see* Chorioretinitis,
      disseminated
    focal - *see* Chorioretinitis, focal
  recurrent 364.02
  sympathetic 360.11
  syphilitic (secondary) 091.50
    congenital 090.0 [*363.13*]
    late 095.8 [*363.13*]
  tuberculous (*see also* Tuberculosis)
    017.3● [*364.11*]
Uveoencephalitis 363.22
Uveokeratitis (*see also* Iridocyclitis) 364.3
Uveoparotid fever 135
Uveoparotitis 135
Uvula - *see* condition
Uvulitis (acute) (catarrhal) (chronic)
  (gangrenous) (membranous)
  (suppurative) (ulcerative) 528.3

V

Vaccination
complication or reaction - *see*
    Complications, vaccination
delayed V64.00
not carried out V64.00
  because of
    acute illness V64.01
    allergy to vaccine or component
      V64.04
    caregiver refusal V64.05
    chronic illness V64.02
    guardian refusal V64.05
    immune compromised state
      V64.03
    parent refusal V64.05
    patient had disease being
      vaccinated against
      V64.08
    patient refusal V64.06
    reason NEC V64.09
    religious reasons V64.07
prophylactic (against) V05.9
  arthropod-borne viral
    disease NEC V05.1
    encephalitis V05.0
  chicken pox V05.4
  cholera (alone) V03.0
    with typhoid-paratyphoid
      (cholera + TAB) V06.0
  common cold V04.7
  diphtheria (alone) V03.5
    with
      poliomyelitis (DTP + polio)
        V06.3
      tetanus V06.5
        pertussis combined [DTP]
          (DTaP) V06.1
      typhoid-paratyphoid (DTP +
        TAB) V06.2
  disease (single) NEC V05.9
    bacterial NEC V03.9
      specified type NEC V03.89
    combination NEC V06.9
      specified type NEC V06.8
    specified type NEC V05.8
  encephalitis, viral, arthropod-borne
    V05.0
  Hemophilus influenzae, type B
    [Hib] V03.81
  hepatitis, viral V05.3
  influenza V04.81
    with
      Streptococcus pneumoniae
        [pneumococcus] V06.6
  leishmaniasis V05.2
  measles (alone) V04.2
    with mumps-rubella (MMR)
      V06.4
  mumps (alone) V04.6
    with measles and rubella (MMR)
      V06.4
  pertussis alone V03.6
  plague V03.3
  poliomyelitis V04.0
    with diphtheria-tetanus-pertussis
      (DTP polio) V06.3
  rabies V04.5
  respiratory syncytial virus (RSV)
    V04.82
  rubella (alone) V04.3
    with measles and mumps (MMR)
      V06.4

Vaccination *(Continued)*
prophylactic *(Continued)*
  smallpox V04.1
  Streptococcus pneumoniae
    [pneumococcus] V03.82
    with
      influenza V06.6
  tetanus toxoid (alone) V03.7
    with diphtheria [Td] [DT] V06.5
      with
        pertussis (DTP) (DTaP)
          V06.1
          with poliomyelitis (DTP
            + polio) V06.3
  tuberculosis (BCG) V03.2
  tularemia V03.4
  typhoid-paratyphoid (TAB) (alone)
    V03.1
    with diphtheria-tetanus-pertussis
      (TAB + DTP) V06.2
  varicella V05.4
  viral
    disease NEC V04.89
    encephalitis, arthropod-borne
      V05.0
    hepatitis V05.3
  yellow fever V04.4
Vaccinia (generalized) 999.0
congenital 771.2
conjunctiva 999.39
eyelids 999.0 *[373.5]*
localized 999.39
nose 999.39
not from vaccination 051.02
  eyelid 051.02 *[373.5]*
sine vaccinatione 051.02
without vaccination 051.02
Vacuum
extraction of fetus or newborn 763.3
in sinus (accessory) (nasal) (*see also*
  Sinusitis) 473.9
Vagabond V60.0
Vagabondage V60.0
Vagabonds' disease 132.1
Vagina, vaginal - *see also* condition
high risk human papillomavirus (HPV)
  DNA test positive 795.15
low risk human papillomavirus (HPV)
  DNA test positive 795.19
Vaginalitis (tunica) 608.4
Vaginismus (reflex) 625.1
functional 306.51
hysterical 300.11
psychogenic 306.51
Vaginitis (acute) (chronic)
  (circumscribed) (diffuse)
  (emphysematous) (Hemophilus
  vaginalis) (nonspecific)
  (nonvenereal) (ulcerative) 616.10
with
  abortion - *see* Abortion, by type,
    with sepsis
  ectopic pregnancy (*see also*
    categories 633.0–633.9)
    639.0
  molar pregnancy (*see also* categories
    630–632) 639.0
adhesive, congenital 752.49
atrophic, postmenopausal 627.3
bacterial 616.10
blennorrhagic (acute) 098.0
  chronic or duration of 2 months or
    over 098.2
candidal 112.1

Vaginitis *(Continued)*
chlamydial 099.53
complicating pregnancy or puerperium
  646.6●
  affecting fetus or newborn 760.8
congenital (adhesive) 752.49
due to
  C. albicans 112.1
  Trichomonas (vaginalis) 131.01
following
  abortion 639.0
  ectopic or molar pregnancy 639.0
gonococcal (acute) 098.0
  chronic or duration of 2 months or
    over 098.2
granuloma 099.2
Monilia 112.1
mycotic 112.1
pinworm 127.4 *[616.11]*
postirradiation 616.10
postmenopausal atrophic 627.3
senile (atrophic) 627.3
syphilitic (early) 091.0
  late 095.8
trichomonal 131.01
tuberculous (*see also* Tuberculosis)
  016.7●
venereal NEC 099.8
Vaginosis - *see* Vaginitis
Vagotonia 352.3
Vagrancy V60.0
VAIN I (vaginal intraepithelial neoplasia
  I) 623.0
VAIN II (vaginal intraepithelial neoplasia
  II) 623.0
VAIN III (vaginal intraepithelial
  neoplasia III) 233.31
Vallecula - *see* condition
Valley fever 114.0
Valsuani's disease (progressive
  pernicious anemia, puerperal)
  648.2●
Valve, valvular (formation) - *see also*
  condition
cerebral ventricle (communicating) in
  situ V45.2
cervix, internal os 752.49
colon 751.5
congenital NEC - *see* Atresia
formation congenital NEC - *see* Atresia
heart defect - *see* Anomaly, heart, valve
ureter 753.29
  pelvic junction 753.21
  vesical orifice 753.22
urethra 753.6
Valvulitis (chronic) (*see also* Endocarditis)
  424.90
rheumatic (chronic) (inactive) (with
  chorea) 397.9
  active or acute (aortic) (mitral)
    (pulmonary) (tricuspid)
    391.1
syphilitic NEC 093.20
  aortic 093.22
  mitral 093.21
  pulmonary 093.24
  tricuspid 093.23
Valvulopathy - *see* Endocarditis
van Bogaert's leukoencephalitis
  (sclerosing) (subacute) 046.2
van Bogaert-Nijssen (-Peiffer) **disease**
  330.0
van Buchem's syndrome (hyperostosis
  corticalis) 733.3

◀ New   ◀▥ Revised   ~~deleted~~ Deleted   ● Use Additional Digit(s)   ▨ Omit code

Vancomycin (glycopeptide)
  intermediate staphylococcus aureus (VISA/GISA) V09.8
  resistant
    enterococcus (VRE) V09.8
    staphylococcus aureus (VRSA/GRSA) V09.8
van Creveld-von Gierke disease (glycogenosis I) 271.0
van den Bergh's disease (enterogenous cyanosis) 289.7
van der Hoeve's syndrome (brittle bones and blue sclera, deafness) 756.51
van der Hoeve-Halbertsma-Waardenburg syndrome (ptosis-epicanthus) 270.2
van der Hoeve-Waardenburg-Gualdi syndrome (ptosis-epicanthus) 270.2
Vanillism 692.89
Vanishing lung 492.0
Vanishing twin 651.33
van Neck (-Odelberg) disease or syndrome (juvenile osteochondrosis) 732.1
Vapor asphyxia or suffocation NEC 987.9
  specified agent - see Table of Drugs and Chemicals
Vaquez's disease (M9950/1) 238.4
Vaquez-Osler disease (polycythemia vera) (M9950/1) 238.4
Variance, lethal ball, prosthetic heart valve 996.02
Variants, thalassemic 282.49
Variations in hair color 704.3
Varicella 052.9
  with
    complication 052.8
      specified NEC 052.7
    pneumonia 052.1
  exposure to V01.71
  vaccination and inoculation (against) (prophylactic) V05.4
Varices - see Varix
Varicocele (scrotum) (thrombosed) 456.4
  ovary 456.5
  perineum 456.6
  spermatic cord (ulcerated) 456.4
Varicose
  aneurysm (ruptured) (see also Aneurysm) 442.9
  dermatitis (lower extremity) - see Varicose, vein, inflamed or infected
  eczema - see Varicose, vein
  phlebitis - see Varicose, vein, inflamed or infected
  placental vessel - see Placenta, abnormal
  tumor - see Varicose, vein
  ulcer (lower extremity, any part) 454.0
    anus 455.8
      external 455.5
      internal 455.2
    esophagus (see also Varix, esophagus) 456.1
      bleeding (see also Varix, esophagus, bleeding) 456.0
    inflamed or infected 454.2
    nasal septum 456.8
    perineum 456.6
    rectum - see Varicose, ulcer, anus
    scrotum 456.4
    specified site NEC 456.8

Varicose (Continued)
  vein (lower extremity) (ruptured) (see also Varix) 454.9
    with
      complications NEC 454.8
      edema 454.8
      inflammation or infection 454.1
        ulcerated 454.2
      pain 454.8
      stasis dermatitis 454.1
        with ulcer 454.2
      swelling 454.8
      ulcer 454.0
        inflamed or infected 454.2
    anus - see Hemorrhoids
    broad ligament 456.5
    congenital (peripheral) 747.60
      gastrointestinal 747.61
      lower limb 747.64
      renal 747.62
      specified NEC 747.69
      upper limb 747.63
    esophagus (ulcerated (see also Varix, esophagus) 456.1
      bleeding (see also Varix, esophagus, bleeding) 456.0
    inflamed or infected 454.1
      with ulcer 454.2
    in pregnancy or puerperium 671.0●
      vulva or perineum 671.1●
    nasal septum (with ulcer) 456.8
    pelvis 456.5
    perineum 456.6
      in pregnancy, childbirth, or puerperium 671.1●
    rectum - see Hemorrhoids
    scrotum (ulcerated) 456.4
    specified site NEC 456.8
    sublingual 456.3
    ulcerated 454.0
      inflamed or infected 454.2
    umbilical cord, affecting fetus or newborn 762.6
    urethra 456.8
    vulva 456.6
      in pregnancy, childbirth, or puerperium 671.1●
  vessel - see also Varix
    placenta - see Placenta, abnormal
Varicosis, varicosities, varicosity (see also Varix) 454.9
Variola 050.9
  hemorrhagic (pustular) 050.0
  major 050.0
  minor 050.1
  modified 050.2
Varioloid 050.2
Variolosa, purpura 050.0
Varix (lower extremity) (ruptured) 454.9
  with
    complications NEC 454.8
    edema 454.8
    inflammation or infection 454.1
      with ulcer 454.2
    pain 454.8
    stasis dermatitis 454.1
      with ulcer 454.2
    swelling 454.8
    ulcer 454.0
      with inflammation or infection 454.2

Varix (Continued)
  aneurysmal (see also Aneurysm) 442.9
  anus - see Hemorrhoids
  arteriovenous (congenital) (peripheral) NEC 747.60
    gastrointestinal 747.61
    lower limb 747.64
    renal 747.62
    specified NEC 747.69
    spinal 747.82
    upper limb 747.63
  bladder 456.5
  broad ligament 456.5
  congenital (peripheral) 747.60
  esophagus (ulcerated) 456.1
    bleeding 456.0
      in
        cirrhosis of liver 571.5 [456.20]
        portal hypertension 572.3 [456.20]
    congenital 747.69
      in
        cirrhosis of liver 571.5 [456.21]
          with bleeding 571.5 [456.20]
        portal hypertension 572.3 [456.21]
          with bleeding 572.3 [456.20]
  gastric 456.8
  inflamed or infected 454.1
    ulcerated 454.2
  in pregnancy or puerperium 671.0●
    perineum 671.1●
    vulva 671.1●
  labia (majora) 456.6
  orbit 456.8
    congenital 747.69
  ovary 456.5
  papillary 448.1
  pelvis 456.5
  perineum 456.6
    in pregnancy or puerperium 671.1●
  pharynx 456.8
  placenta - see Placenta, abnormal
  prostate 456.8
  rectum - see Hemorrhoids
  renal papilla 456.8
  retina 362.17
  scrotum (ulcerated) 456.4
  sigmoid colon 456.8
  specified site NEC 456.8
  spinal (cord) (vessels) 456.8
  spleen, splenic (vein) (with phlebolith) 456.8
  sublingual 456.3
  ulcerated 454.0
    inflamed or infected 454.2
  umbilical cord, affecting fetus or newborn 762.6
  uterine ligament 456.5
  vocal cord 456.8
  vulva 456.6
    in pregnancy, childbirth, or puerperium 671.1●
Vasa previa 663.5●
  affecting fetus or newborn 762.6
  hemorrhage from, affecting fetus or newborn 772.0
Vascular - see also condition
  loop on papilla (optic) 743.57
  sheathing, retina 362.13
  spasm 443.9
  spider 448.1

◄ New   ◄ Revised   ~~deleted~~ Deleted   ● Use Additional Digit(s)   ▨ Omit code   **599**

Vascularity, pulmonary, congenital 747.3
Vascularization
    choroid 362.16
    cornea 370.60
        deep 370.63
        localized 370.61
    retina 362.16
    subretinal 362.16
Vasculitis 447.6
    allergic 287.0
    cryoglobulinemic 273.2
    disseminated 447.6
    kidney 447.8
    leukocytoclastic 446.29
    nodular 695.2
    retinal 362.18
    rheumatic - *see* Fever, rheumatic
Vasculopathy
    cardiac allograft 996.83
Vas deferens - *see* condition
Vas deferentitis 608.4
Vasectomy, admission for V25.2
Vasitis 608.4
    nodosa 608.4
    scrotum 608.4
    spermatic cord 608.4
    testis 608.4
    tuberculous (*see also* Tuberculosis)
        016.5●
    tunica vaginalis 608.4
    vas deferens 608.4
Vasodilation 443.9
Vasomotor - *see* condition
Vasoplasty, after previous sterilization
    V26.0
Vasoplegia, splanchnic (*see also*
    Neuropathy, peripheral, autonomic)
    337.9
Vasospasm 443.9
    cerebral (artery) 435.9
        with transient neurologic deficit
            435.9
    coronary 413.1
    nerve
        arm NEC 354.9
        autonomic 337.9
        brachial plexus 353.0
        cervical plexus 353.2
        leg NEC 355.8
        lower extremity NEC 355.8
        peripheral NEC 335.9
        spinal NEC 355.9
        sympathetic 337.9
        upper extremity NEC 354.9
    peripheral NEC 443.9
    retina (artery) (*see also* Occlusion,
        retinal, artery) 362.30
Vasospastic - *see* condition
Vasovagal attack (paroxysmal) 780.2
    psychogenic 306.2
Vater's ampulla - *see* condition
VATER syndrome 759.89
vCJD (variant Creutzfeldt-Jakob disease)
    046.11
Vegetation, vegetative
    adenoid (nasal fossa) 474.2
    consciousness (persistent) 780.03
    endocarditis (acute) (any valve)
        (chronic) (subacute) 421.0
    heart (mycotic) (valve) 421.0
    state (persistent) 780.03
Veil
    Jackson's 751.4
    over face (causing asphyxia) 768.9

Vein, venous - *see* condition
Veldt sore (*see also* Ulcer, skin) 707.9
Velo-cardio-facial syndrome 758.32
Velpeau's hernia - *see* Hernia, femoral
Venereal
    balanitis NEC 099.8
    bubo 099.1
    disease 099.9
        specified nature or type NEC 099.8
    granuloma inguinale 099.2
    lymphogranuloma (Durand-Nicolas-
        Favre), any site 099.1
    salpingitis 098.37
    urethritis (*see also* Urethritis,
        nongonococcal) 099.40
    vaginitis NEC 099.8
    warts 078.11
Vengefulness, in child (*see also*
    Disturbance, conduct) 312.0●
Venofibrosis 459.89
Venom, venomous
    bite or sting (animal or insect) 989.5
    poisoning 989.5
Venous - *see* condition
Ventouse delivery NEC 669.5●
    affecting fetus or newborn 763.3
Ventral - *see* condition
Ventricle, ventricular - *see also* condition
    escape 427.69
    standstill (*see also* Arrest, cardiac)
        427.5
Ventriculitis, cerebral (*see also* Meningitis)
    322.9
Ventriculostomy status V45.2
Verbiest's syndrome (claudicatio
    intermittens spinalis) 435.1
Vernet's syndrome 352.6
Verneuil's disease (syphilitic bursitis)
    095.7
Verruca (filiformis) 078.10
    acuminata (any site) 078.11
    necrogenica (primary) (*see also*
        Tuberculosis) 017.0●
    peruana 088.0
    peruviana 088.0
    plana (juvenilis) 078.19
    plantaris 078.12
    seborrheica 702.19
        inflamed 702.11
    senilis 702.0
    tuberculosa (primary) (*see also*
        Tuberculosis) 017.0●
    venereal 078.11
    viral 078.10
        specified NEC 078.19
    vulgaris 078.10
Verrucosities (*see also* Verruca) 078.10
Verrucous endocarditis (acute) (any
    valve) (chronic) (subacute) 710.0
    [424.91]
    nonbacterial 710.0 [424.91]
Verruga
    peruana 088.0
    peruviana 088.0
Verse's disease (calcinosis
    intervertebralis) 275.49 [722.90]
Version
    before labor, affecting fetus or newborn
        761.7
    cephalic (correcting previous
        malposition) 652.1●
        affecting fetus or newborn
            763.1
    cervix - *see* Version, uterus

Version (*Continued*)
    uterus (postinfectional) (postpartal,
        old) (*see also* Malposition, uterus)
        621.6
        forward - *see* Anteversion, uterus
        lateral - *see* Lateroversion, uterus
Vertebra, vertebral - *see* condition
Vertigo 780.4
    auditory 386.19
    aural 386.19
    benign paroxysmal positional 386.11
    central origin 386.2
    cerebral 386.2
    Dix and Hallpike (epidemic) 386.12
    endemic paralytic 078.81
    epidemic 078.81
        Dix and Hallpike 386.12
        Gerlier's 078.81
        Pedersen's 386.12
        vestibular neuronitis 386.12
    epileptic - *see* Epilepsy
    Gerlier's (epidemic) 078.81
    hysterical 300.11
    labyrinthine 386.10
    laryngeal 786.2
    malignant positional 386.2
    Ménière's (*see also* Disease, Ménière's)
        386.00
    menopausal 627.2
    otogenic 386.19
    paralytic 078.81
    paroxysmal positional, benign
        386.11
    Pedersen's (epidemic) 386.12
    peripheral 386.10
        specified type NEC 386.19
    positional
        benign paroxysmal 386.11
        malignant 386.2
Verumontanitis (chronic) (*see also*
    Urethritis) 597.89
Vesania (*see also* Psychosis) 298.9
Vesical - *see* condition
Vesicle
    cutaneous 709.8
    seminal - *see* condition
    skin 709.8
Vesicocolic - *see* condition
Vesicoperineal - *see* condition
Vesicorectal - *see* condition
Vesicourethrorectal - *see* condition
Vesicovaginal - *see* condition
Vesicular - *see* condition
Vesiculitis (seminal) 608.0
    amebic 006.8
    gonorrheal (acute) 098.14
        chronic or duration of 2 months or
            over 098.34
    trichomonal 131.09
    tuberculous (*see also* Tuberculosis)
        016.5● [608.81]
Vestibulitis (ear) (*see also* Labyrinthitis)
    386.30
    nose (external) 478.19
    vulvar 625.71
Vestibulopathy, acute peripheral
    (recurrent) 386.12
Vestige, vestigial - *see also* Persistence
    branchial 744.41
    structures in vitreous 743.51
Vibriosis NEC 027.9
Vidal's disease (lichen simplex chronicus)
    698.3
Video display tube syndrome 723.8

◀ New   ◀▥ Revised   ~~deleted~~ Deleted   ● Use Additional Digit(s)   ▨ Omit code

Vulvitis *(Continued)*
  adhesive, congenital 752.49
  blennorrhagic (acute) 098.0
    chronic or duration of 2 months or
      over 098.2
  chlamydial 099.53
  complicating pregnancy or puerperium
    646.6●
  due to Ducrey's bacillus 099.0
  following
    abortion 639.0
    ectopic or molar pregnancy
      639.0

Vulvitis *(Continued)*
  gonococcal (acute) 098.0
    chronic or duration of
      2 months or over
      098.2
  herpetic 054.11
  leukoplakic 624.09
  monilial 112.1
  puerperal, postpartum, childbirth
    646.6●
  syphilitic (early) 091.0
    late 095.8
  trichomonal 131.01

Vulvodynia 625.70
  specified NEC 625.79
Vulvorectal - *see* condition
Vulvovaginitis *(see also* Vulvitis) 616.10
  amebic 006.8
  chlamydial 099.53
  gonococcal (acute) 098.0
    chronic or duration of 2 months or
      over 098.2
  herpetic 054.11
  monilial 112.1
  trichomonal (Trichomonas vaginalis)
    131.01

◀ New   ◀▥ Revised   ~~deleted~~ Deleted   ● Use Additional Digit(s)   ▨ Omit code

W

Waardenburg's syndrome 756.89
  meaning ptosis-epicanthus 270.2
Waardenburg-Klein syndrome (ptosis-epicanthus) 270.2
Wagner's disease (colloid milium) 709.3
Wagner (-Unverricht) syndrome (dermatomyositis) 710.3
Waiting list, person on V63.2
  undergoing social agency investigation V63.8
Wakefulness disorder (see also Hypersomnia) 780.54
  nonorganic origin 307.43
Waldenström's
  disease (osteochondrosis, capital femoral) 732.1
  hepatitis (lupoid hepatitis) 571.49
  hypergammaglobulinemia 273.0
  macroglobulinemia 273.3
  purpura, hypergammaglobulinemic 273.0
  syndrome (macroglobulinemia) 273.3
Waldenström-Kjellberg syndrome (sideropenic dysphagia) 280.8
Walking
  difficulty 719.7
    psychogenic 307.9
  sleep 307.46
    hysterical 300.13
Wall, abdominal - see condition
Wallenberg's syndrome (posterior inferior cerebellar artery) (see also Disease, cerebrovascular, acute) 436
Wallgren's
  disease (obstruction of splenic vein with collateral circulation) 459.89
  meningitis (see also Meningitis, aseptic) 047.9
Wandering
  acetabulum 736.39
  gallbladder 751.69
  kidney, congenital 753.3
  organ or site, congenital NEC - see Malposition, congenital
  pacemaker (atrial) (heart) 427.89
  spleen 289.59
Wardrop's disease (with lymphangitis) 681.9
  finger 681.02
  toe 681.11
War neurosis 300.16
Wart (digitate) (filiform) (infectious) (viral) 078.10
  common 078.19
  external genital organs (venereal) 078.11
  fig 078.19
  flat 078.19
  genital 078.11
  Hassall-Henle's (of cornea) 371.41
  Henle's (of cornea) 371.41
  juvenile 078.19
  moist 078.10
  Peruvian 088.0
  plantar 078.12
  prosector (see also Tuberculosis) 017.0●
  seborrheic 702.19
    inflamed 702.11
  senile 702.0

Wart (Continued)
  specified NEC 078.19
  syphilitic 091.3
  tuberculous (see also Tuberculosis) 017.0●
  venereal (female) (male) 078.11
Warthin's tumor (salivary gland) (M8561/0) 210.2
Washerwoman's itch 692.4
Wassilieff's disease (leptospiral jaundice) 100.0
Wasting
  disease 799.4
    due to malnutrition 261
  extreme (due to malnutrition) 261
  muscular NEC 728.2
  palsy, paralysis 335.21
  pelvic muscle 618.83
Water
  clefts 366.12
  deprivation of 994.3
  in joint (see also Effusion, joint) 719.0●
  intoxication 276.6
  itch 120.3
  lack of 994.3
  loading 276.6
  on
    brain - see Hydrocephalus
    chest 511.89
  poisoning 276.6
Waterbrash 787.1
Water-hammer pulse (see also Insufficiency, aortic) 424.1
Waterhouse (-Friderichsen) disease or syndrome 036.3
Water-losing nephritis 588.89
Watermelon stomach 537.82
  with hemorrhage 537.83
  without hemorrhage 537.82
Wax in ear 380.4
Waxy
  degeneration, any site 277.39
  disease 277.39
  kidney 277.39 [583.81]
  liver (large) 277.39
  spleen 277.39
Weak, weakness (generalized) 780.79
  arches (acquired) 734
    congenital 754.61
  bladder sphincter 596.59
  congenital 779.89
  eye muscle - see Strabismus
  facial 781.94
  foot (double) - see Weak, arches
  heart, cardiac (see also Failure, heart) 428.9
    congenital 746.9
  mind 317
  muscle (generalized) 728.87
  myocardium (see also Failure, heart) 428.9
  newborn 779.89
  pelvic fundus
    pubocervical tissue 618.81
    rectovaginal tissue 618.82
  pulse 785.9
  senile 797
  urinary stream 788.62
  valvular - see Endocarditis
Wear, worn, tooth, teeth (approximal) (hard tissues) (interproximal) (occlusal) - see also Attrition, teeth 521.10

Weather, weathered
  effects of
    cold NEC 991.9
      specified effect NEC 991.8
    hot (see also Heat) 992.9
  skin 692.74
Web, webbed (congenital) - see also Anomaly, specified type NEC
  canthus 743.63
  digits (see also Syndactylism) 755.10
  duodenal 751.5
  esophagus 750.3
  fingers (see also Syndactylism, fingers) 755.11
  larynx (glottic) (subglottic) 748.2
  neck (pterygium colli) 744.5
  Paterson-Kelly (sideropenic dysphagia) 280.8
  popliteal syndrome 756.89
  toes (see also Syndactylism, toes) 755.13
Weber's paralysis or syndrome 344.89
Weber-Christian disease or syndrome (nodular nonsuppurative panniculitis) 729.30
Weber-Cockayne syndrome (epidermolysis bullosa) 757.39
Weber-Dimitri syndrome 759.6
Weber-Gubler syndrome 344.89
Weber-Leyden syndrome 344.89
Weber-Osler syndrome (familial hemorrhagic telangiectasia) 448.0
Wedge-shaped or wedging vertebra (see also Osteoporosis) 733.00
Wegener's granulomatosis or syndrome 446.4
Wegner's disease (syphilitic osteochondritis) 090.0
Weight
  gain (abnormal) (excessive) 783.1
    during pregnancy 646.1●
      insufficient 646.8●
  less than 1000 grams at birth 765.0●
  loss (cause unknown) 783.21
Weightlessness 994.9
Weil's disease (leptospiral jaundice) 100.0
Weill-Marchesani syndrome (brachymorphism and ectopia lentis) 759.89
Weingarten's syndrome (tropical eosinophilia) 518.3
Weir Mitchell's disease (erythromelalgia) 443.82
Weiss-Baker syndrome (carotid sinus syncope) 337.01
Weissenbach-Thibierge syndrome (cutaneous systemic sclerosis) 710.1
Wen (see also Cyst, sebaceous) 706.2
Wenckebach's phenomenon, heart block (second degree) 426.13
Werdnig-Hoffmann syndrome (muscular atrophy) 335.0
Werlhof's disease (see also Purpura, thrombocytopenic) 287.39
Werlhof-Wichmann syndrome (see also Purpura, thrombocytopenic) 287.39
Wermer's syndrome or disease (polyendocrine adenomatosis) 258.01
Werner's disease or syndrome (progeria adultorum) 259.8
Werner-His disease (trench fever) 083.1

Werner-Schultz disease (agranulocytosis) 288.09
Wernicke's encephalopathy, disease, or syndrome (superior hemorrhagic polioencephalitis) 265.1
Wernicke-Korsakoff syndrome or psychosis (nonalcoholic) 294.0
    alcoholic 291.1
Wernicke-Posadas disease (*see also* Coccidioidomycosis) 114.9
Wesselsbron fever 066.3
West African fever 084.8
West Nile
    encephalitis 066.41
    encephalomyelitis 066.41
    fever 066.40
        with
            cranial nerve disorders 066.42
            encephalitis 066.41
            optic neuritis 066.42
            other complications 066.49
            other neurologic manifestations 066.42
            polyradiculitis 066.42
        virus 066.40
Westphal-Strümpell syndrome (hepatolenticular degeneration) 275.1
Wet
    brain (alcoholic) (*see also* Alcoholism) 303.9●
    feet, tropical (syndrome) (maceration) 991.4
    lung (syndrome)
        adult 518.5
        newborn 770.6
Wharton's duct - *see* condition
Wheal 709.8
Wheelchair confinement status V46.3
Wheezing 786.07
Whiplash injury or syndrome 847.0
Whipple's disease or syndrome (intestinal lipodystrophy) 040.2
Whipworm 127.3
"Whistling face" syndrome (craniocarpotarsal dystrophy) 759.89
White - *see also* condition
    kidney
        large - *see* Nephrosis
        small 582.9
    leg, puerperal, postpartum, childbirth 671.4●
        nonpuerperal 451.19
    mouth 112.0
    patches of mouth 528.6
    sponge nevus of oral mucosa 750.26
    spot lesions, teeth 521.01
White's disease (congenital) (keratosis follicularis) 757.39
Whitehead 706.2
Whitlow (with lymphangitis) 681.01
    herpetic 054.6
Whitmore's disease or fever (melioidosis) 025
Whooping cough 033.9
    with pneumonia 033.9 [*484.3*]
    due to
        Bordetella
            bronchoseptica 033.8
                with pneumonia 033.8 [*484.3*]
            parapertussis 033.1
                with pneumonia 033.1 [*484.3*]

Whooping cough (*Continued*)
    due to (*Continued*)
        Bordetella (*Continued*)
            pertussis 033.0
                with pneumonia 033.0 [*484.3*]
            specified organism NEC 033.8
                with pneumonia 033.8 [*484.3*]
    vaccination, prophylactic (against) V03.6
Wichmann's asthma (laryngismus stridulus) 478.75
Widal (-Abrami) syndrome (acquired hemolytic jaundice) 283.9
Widening aorta (*see also* Aneurysm, aorta) 441.9
    ruptured 441.5
Wilkie's disease or syndrome 557.1
Wilkinson-Sneddon disease or syndrome (subcorneal pustular dermatosis) 694.1
Willan's lepra 696.1
Willan-Plumbe syndrome (psoriasis) 696.1
Willebrand (-Jürgens) syndrome or thrombopathy (angiohemophilia) 286.4
Willi-Prader syndrome (hypogenital dystrophy with diabetic tendency) 759.81
Willis' disease (diabetes mellitus) (*see also* Diabetes) 250.0●
    due to secondary diabetes 249.0●
Wilms' tumor or neoplasm (nephroblastoma) (M8960/3) 189.0
Wilson's
    disease or syndrome (hepatolenticular degeneration) 275.1
    hepatolenticular degeneration 275.1
    lichen ruber 697.0
Wilson-Brocq disease (dermatitis exfoliativa) 695.89
Wilson-Mikity syndrome 770.7
Window - *see also* Imperfect, closure
    aorticopulmonary 745.0
Winged scapula 736.89
Winter - *see also* condition
    vomiting disease 078.82
Wise's disease 696.2
Wiskott-Aldrich syndrome (eczema-thrombocytopenia) 279.12
Withdrawal symptoms, syndrome
    alcohol 291.81
        delirium (acute) 291.0
            chronic 291.1
        newborn 760.71
    drug or narcotic 292.0
        newborn, infant of dependent mother 779.5
    steroid NEC
        correct substance properly administered 255.41
        overdose or wrong substance given or taken 962.0
Withdrawing reaction, child or adolescent 313.22
Witts' anemia (achlorhydric anemia) 280.9
Witzelsucht 301.9
Woakes' syndrome (ethmoiditis) 471.1
Wohlfart-Kugelberg-Welander disease 335.11
Woillez's disease (acute idiopathic pulmonary congestion) 518.5

Wolff-Parkinson-White syndrome (anomalous atrioventricular excitation) 426.7
Wolhynian fever 083.1
Wolman's disease (primary familial xanthomatosis) 272.7
Wood asthma 495.8
Woolly, wooly hair (congenital) (nevus) 757.4
Wool-sorters' disease 022.1
Word
    blindness (congenital) (developmental) 315.01
        secondary to organic lesion 784.61
    deafness (secondary to organic lesion) 784.69
    developmental 315.31
Worm(s) (colic) (fever) (infection) (infestation) (*see also* Infestation) 128.9
    guinea 125.7
    in intestine NEC 127.9
Worm-eaten soles 102.3
Worn out (*see also* Exhaustion) 780.79 ◀
    artificial heart valve 996.02 ◀
    cardiac defibrillator V53.32 ◀
    cardiac pacemaker lead or battery V53.31 ◀
    joint prosthesis (*see also* Complications, mechanical, device NEC, prosthetic NEC, joint) 996.46
"Worried well" V65.5
Wound, open (by cutting or piercing instrument) (by firearms) (cut) (dissection) (incised) (laceration) (penetration) (perforating) (puncture) (with initial hemorrhage, not internal) 879.8

Note 74   For fracture with open wound, see Fracture.

For laceration, traumatic rupture, tear, or penetrating wound of internal organs, such as heart, lung, liver, kidney, pelvic organs, etc., whether or not accompanied by open wound or fracture in the same region, see Injury, internal. For contused wound, see Contusion. For crush injury, see Crush. For abrasion, insect bite (nonvenomous), blister, or scratch, see Injury, superficial.

Complicated includes wounds with:

    delayed healing
    delayed treatment
    foreign body
    primary infection

For late effect of open wound, see Late, effect, wound, open, by site.

---

abdomen, abdominal (external) (muscle) 879.2
    complicated 879.3
    wall (anterior) 879.2
        complicated 879.3
        lateral 879.4
            complicated 879.5
alveolar (process) 873.62
    complicated 873.72
ankle 891.0
    with tendon involvement 891.2
    complicated 891.1
anterior chamber, eye (*see also* Wound, open, intraocular) 871.9

◀ New   ◀▥ Revised   ~~deleted~~ Deleted   ● Use Additional Digit(s)   ▦ Omit code

Wound, open (Continued)
anus 879.6
  complicated 879.7
arm 884.0
  with tendon involvement 884.2
  complicated 884.1
  forearm 881.00
    with tendon involvement 881.20
    complicated 881.10
  multiple sites - see Wound, open,
    multiple, upper limb
  upper 880.03
    with tendon involvement
      880.23
    complicated 880.13
    multiple sites (with axillary or
      shoulder regions) 880.09
    with tendon involvement
      880.29
    complicated 880.19
artery - see Injury, blood vessel, by site
auditory
  canal (external) (meatus) 872.02
    complicated 872.12
  ossicles (incus) (malleus) (stapes)
    872.62
    complicated 872.72
auricle, ear 872.01
  complicated 872.11
axilla 880.02
  with tendon involvement 880.22
  complicated 880.12
    with tendon involvement
      880.29
  involving other sites of upper arm
    880.09
    complicated 880.19
back 876.0
  complicated 876.1
bladder - see Injury, internal, bladder
blood vessel - see Injury, blood vessel,
    by site
brain - see Injury, intracranial, with
    open intracranial wound
breast 879.0
  complicated 879.1
brow 873.42
  complicated 873.52
buccal mucosa 873.61
  complicated 873.71
buttock 877.0
  complicated 877.1
calf 891.0
  with tendon involvement 891.2
  complicated 891.1
canaliculus lacrimalis 870.8
  with laceration of eyelid 870.2
canthus, eye 870.8
  laceration - see Laceration, eyelid
cavernous sinus - see Injury,
    intracranial
cerebellum - see Injury, intracranial
cervical esophagus 874.4
  complicated 874.5
cervix - see Injury, internal, cervix
cheek(s) (external) 873.41
  complicated 873.51
  internal 873.61
    complicated 873.71
chest (wall) (external) 875.0
  complicated 875.1
chin 873.44
  complicated 873.54
choroid 363.63
ciliary body (eye) (see also Wound,
    open, intraocular) 871.9

Wound, open (Continued)
clitoris 878.8
  complicated 878.9
cochlea 872.64
  complicated 872.74
complicated 879.9
conjunctiva - see Wound, open,
    intraocular
cornea (nonpenetrating) (see also
    Wound, open, intraocular)
    871.9
costal region 875.0
  complicated 875.1
Descemet's membrane (see also Wound,
    open, intraocular) 871.9
digit(s)
  foot 893.0
    with tendon involvement
      893.2
    complicated 893.1
  hand 883.0
    with tendon involvement
      883.2
    complicated 883.1
drumhead, ear 872.61
  complicated 872.71
ear 872.8
  canal 872.02
    complicated 872.12
  complicated 872.9
  drum 872.61
    complicated 872.71
  external 872.00
    complicated 872.10
  multiple sites 872.69
    complicated 872.79
  ossicles (incus) (malleus) (stapes)
    872.62
    complicated 872.72
  specified part NEC 872.69
    complicated 872.79
elbow 881.01
  with tendon involvement 881.21
  complicated 881.11
epididymis 878.2
  complicated 878.3
epigastric region 879.2
  complicated 879.3
epiglottis 874.01
  complicated 874.11
esophagus (cervical) 874.4
  complicated 874.5
  thoracic - see Injury, internal,
    esophagus
Eustachian tube 872.63
  complicated 872.73
extremity
  lower (multiple) NEC 894.0
    with tendon involvement 894.2
    complicated 894.1
  upper (multiple) NEC 884.0
    with tendon involvement 884.2
    complicated 884.1
eye(s) (globe) - see Wound, open,
    intraocular
eyeball NEC 871.9
  laceration (see also Laceration,
    eyeball) 871.4
  penetrating (see also Penetrating
    wound, eyeball) 871.7
eyebrow 873.42
  complicated 873.52
eyelid NEC 870.8
  laceration - see Laceration, eyelid

Wound, open (Continued)
face 873.40
  complicated 873.50
  multiple sites 873.49
    complicated 873.59
  specified part NEC 873.49
    complicated 873.59
fallopian tube - see Injury, internal,
    fallopian tube
finger(s) (nail) (subungual) 883.0
  with tendon involvement 883.2
  complicated 883.1
flank 879.4
  complicated 879.5
foot (any part, except toe(s) alone)
    892.0
  with tendon involvement 892.2
  complicated 892.1
forearm 881.00
  with tendon involvement 881.20
  complicated 881.10
forehead 873.42
  complicated 873.52
genital organs (external) NEC 878.8
  complicated 878.9
  internal - see Injury, internal, by site
globe (eye) (see also Wound, open,
    eyeball) 871.9
groin 879.4
  complicated 879.5
gum(s) 873.62
  complicated 873.72
hand (except finger(s) alone) 882.0
  with tendon involvement 882.2
  complicated 882.1
head NEC 873.8
  with intracranial injury - see Injury,
    intracranial
  due to or associated with skull
    fracture - see Fracture,
    skull
  complicated 873.9
  scalp - see Wound, open, scalp
heel 892.0
  with tendon involvement 892.2
  complicated 892.1
high-velocity (grease gun) - see
    Wound, open, complicated,
    by site
hip 890.0
  with tendon involvement 890.2
  complicated 890.1
hymen 878.6
  complicated 878.7
hypochondrium 879.4
  complicated 879.5
hypogastric region 879.2
  complicated 879.3
iliac (region) 879.4
  complicated 879.5
incidental to
  dislocation - see Dislocation, open,
    by site
  fracture - see Fracture, open, by site
  intracranial injury - see Injury,
    intracranial, with open
    intracranial wound
  nerve injury - see Injury, nerve, by
    site
inguinal region 879.4
  complicated 879.5
instep 892.0
  with tendon involvement 892.2
  complicated 892.1

Wound, open *(Continued)*
  interscapular region 876.0
    complicated 876.1
  intracranial - *see* Injury, intracranial,
    with open intracranial wound
  intraocular 871.9
    with
      partial loss (of intraocular tissue)
        871.2
      prolapse or exposure (of
        intraocular tissue) 871.1
    laceration (*see also* Laceration,
      eyeball) 871.4
    penetrating 871.7
      with foreign body (nonmagnetic)
        871.6
        magnetic 871.5
    without prolapse (of intraocular
      tissue) 871.0
  iris (*see also* Wound, open, eyeball)
    871.9
  jaw (fracture not involved) 873.44
    with fracture - *see* Fracture, jaw
    complicated 873.54
  knee 891.0
    with tendon involvement 891.2
    complicated 891.1
  labium (majus) (minus) 878.4
    complicated 878.5
  lacrimal apparatus, gland, or sac
    870.8
    with laceration of eyelid 870.2
  larynx 874.01
    with trachea 874.00
      complicated 874.10
    complicated 874.11
  leg (multiple) 891.0
    with tendon involvement 891.2
    complicated 891.1
    lower 891.0
      with tendon involvement 891.2
      complicated 891.1
    thigh 890.0
      with tendon involvement 890.2
      complicated 890.1
    upper 890.0
      with tendon involvement 890.2
      complicated 890.1
  lens (eye) (alone) (*see also* Cataract,
    traumatic) 366.20
    with involvement of other eye
      structures - *see* Wound, open,
      eyeball
  limb
    lower (multiple) NEC 894.0
      with tendon involvement 894.2
      complicated 894.1
    upper (multiple) NEC 884.0
      with tendon involvement 884.2
      complicated 884.1
  lip 873.43
    complicated 873.53
  loin 876.0
    complicated 876.1
  lumbar region 876.0
    complicated 876.1
  malar region 873.41
    complicated 873.51
  mastoid region 873.49
    complicated 873.59
  mediastinum - *see* Injury, internal,
    mediastinum
  midthoracic region 875.0
    complicated 875.1

Wound, open *(Continued)*
  mouth 873.60
    complicated 873.70
    floor 873.64
      complicated 873.74
    multiple sites 873.69
      complicated 873.79
    specified site NEC 873.69
      complicated 873.79
  multiple, unspecified site(s) 879.8

> **Note 75**   Multiple open wounds of
> sites classifiable to the same four-digit
> category should be classified to that
> category unless they are in different
> limbs.
>
> Multiple open wounds of sites
> classifiable to different four-digit
> categories, or to different limbs, should
> be coded separately.

    complicated 879.9
    lower limb(s) (one or both) (sites
      classifiable to more than one
      three-digit category in 890–
      893) 894.0
      with tendon involvement 894.2
      complicated 894.1
    upper limb(s) (one or both) (sites
      classifiable to more than one
      three-digit category in 880–
      883) 884.0
      with tendon involvement
        884.2
      complicated 884.1
  muscle - *see* Sprain, by site
  nail
    finger(s) 883.0
      complicated 883.1
    thumb 883.0
      complicated 883.1
    toe(s) 893.0
      complicated 893.1
  nape (neck) 874.8
    complicated 874.9
    specified part NEC 874.8
      complicated 874.9
  nasal - *see also* Wound, open, nose
    cavity 873.22
      complicated 873.32
    septum 873.21
      complicated 873.31
    sinuses 873.23
      complicated 873.33
  nasopharynx 873.22
    complicated 873.32
  neck 874.8
    complicated 874.9
    nape 874.8
      complicated 874.9
    specified part NEC 874.8
      complicated 874.9
  nerve - *see* Injury, nerve, by site
  non-healing surgical 998.83
  nose 873.20
    complicated 873.30
    multiple sites 873.29
      complicated 873.39
    septum 873.21
      complicated 873.31
    sinuses 873.23
      complicated 873.33
  occipital region - *see* Wound, open,
    scalp

Wound, open *(Continued)*
  ocular NEC 871.9
    adnexa 870.9
      specified region NEC 870.8
    laceration (*see also* Laceration,
      ocular) 871.4
    muscle (extraocular) 870.3
      with foreign body 870.4
      eyelid 870.1
      intraocular - *see* Wound, open,
        eyeball
    penetrating (*see also* Penetrating
      wound, ocular) 871.7
  orbit 870.8
    penetrating 870.3
      with foreign body 870.4
  orbital region 870.9
  ovary - *see* Injury, internal, pelvic
    organs
  palate 873.65
    complicated 873.75
  palm 882.0
    with tendon involvement 882.2
    complicated 882.1
  parathyroid (gland) 874.2
    complicated 874.3
  parietal region - *see* Wound, open,
    scalp
  pelvic floor or region 879.6
    complicated 879.7
  penis 878.0
    complicated 878.1
  perineum 879.6
    complicated 879.7
  periocular area 870.8
    laceration of skin 870.0
  pharynx 874.4
    complicated 874.5
  pinna 872.01
    complicated 872.11
  popliteal space 891.0
    with tendon involvement 891.2
    complicated 891.1
  prepuce 878.0
    complicated 878.1
  pubic region 879.2
    complicated 879.3
  pudenda 878.8
    complicated 878.9
  rectovaginal septum 878.8
    complicated 878.9
  sacral region 877.0
    complicated 877.1
  sacroiliac region 877.0
    complicated 877.1
  salivary (ducts) (glands) 873.69
    complicated 873.79
  scalp 873.0
    complicated 873.1
  scalpel, fetus or newborn 767.8
  scapular region 880.01
    with tendon involvement 880.21
    complicated 880.11
    involving other sites of upper arm
      880.09
      with tendon involvement
        880.29
      complicated 880.19
  sclera (*see also* Wound, open,
    intraocular) 871.9
  scrotum 878.2
    complicated 878.3
  seminal vesicle - *see* Injury, internal,
    pelvic organs

◀ New   ◀▉ Revised   ~~deleted~~ Deleted   ● Use Additional Digit(s)   ▨ Omit code

Wound, open *(Continued)*
  shin 891.0
    with tendon involvement 891.2
    complicated 891.1
  shoulder 880.00
    with tendon involvement 880.20
    complicated 880.10
    involving other sites of upper arm
      880.09
      with tendon involvement 880.29
      complicated 880.19
  skin NEC 879.8
    complicated 879.9
  skull - *see also* Injury, intracranial, with
    open intracranial wound
    with skull fracture - *see* Fracture,
      skull
  spermatic cord (scrotal) 878.2
    complicated 878.3
    pelvic region - *see* Injury, internal,
      spermatic cord
  spinal cord - *see* Injury, spinal
  sternal region 875.0
    complicated 875.1
  subconjunctival - *see* Wound, open,
    intraocular
  subcutaneous NEC 879.8
    complicated 879.9
  submaxillary region 873.44
    complicated 873.54
  submental region 873.44
    complicated 873.54
  subungual
    finger(s) (thumb) - *see* Wound, open,
      finger
    toe(s) - *see* Wound, open, toe
  supraclavicular region 874.8
    complicated 874.9
  supraorbital 873.42
    complicated 873.52

Wound, open *(Continued)*
  surgical, non-healing 998.83
  temple 873.49
    complicated 873.59
  temporal region 873.49
    complicated 873.59
  testis 878.2
    complicated 878.3
  thigh 890.0
    with tendon involvement 890.2
    complicated 890.1
  thorax, thoracic (external) 875.0
    complicated 875.1
  throat 874.8
    complicated 874.9
  thumb (nail) (subungual) 883.0
    with tendon involvement 883.2
    complicated 883.1
  thyroid (gland) 874.2
    complicated 874.3
  toe(s) (nail) (subungual) 893.0
    with tendon involvement 893.2
    complicated 893.1
  tongue 873.64
    complicated 873.74
  tonsil - *see* Wound, open, neck
  trachea (cervical region) 874.02
    with larynx 874.00
      complicated 874.10
    complicated 874.12
    intrathoracic - *see* Injury, internal,
      trachea
  trunk (multiple) NEC 879.6
    complicated 879.7
    specified site NEC 879.6
      complicated 879.7
  tunica vaginalis 878.2
    complicated 878.3
  tympanic membrane 872.61
    complicated 872.71

Wound, open *(Continued)*
  tympanum 872.61
    complicated 872.71
  umbilical region 879.2
    complicated 879.3
  ureter - *see* Injury, internal, ureter
  urethra - *see* Injury, internal, urethra
  uterus - *see* Injury, internal, uterus
  uvula 873.69
    complicated 873.79
  vagina 878.6
    complicated 878.7
  vas deferens - *see* Injury, internal, vas
    deferens
  vitreous (humor) 871.2
  vulva 878.4
    complicated 878.5
  wrist 881.02
    with tendon involvement 881.22
    complicated 881.12
Wright's syndrome (hyperabduction)
  447.8
  pneumonia 390 *[517.1]*
Wringer injury - *see* Crush injury, by site
Wrinkling of skin 701.8
Wrist - *see also* condition
  drop (acquired) 736.05
Wrong drug (given in error) NEC 977.9
  specified drug or substance - *see* Table
    of Drugs and Chemicals
Wry neck - *see also* Torticollis
  congenital 754.1
Wuchereria infestation 125.0
  bancrofti 125.0
  Brugia malayi 125.1
  malayi 125.1
Wuchereriasis 125.0
Wuchereriosis 125.0
Wuchernde struma langhans (M8332/3)
  193

X

Xanthelasma 272.2
    eyelid 272.2 *[374.51]*
    palpebrarum 272.2 *[374.51]*
Xanthelasmatosis (essential) 272.2
Xanthelasmoidea 757.33
Xanthine stones 277.2
Xanthinuria 277.2
Xanthofibroma (M8831/0) - *see*
        Neoplasm, connective tissue, benign
Xanthoma(s), xanthomatosis 272.2
    with
        hyperlipoproteinemia
            type I 272.3
            type III 272.2
            type IV 272.1
            type V 272.3
    bone 272.7
    craniohypophyseal 277.89
    cutaneotendinous 272.7
    diabeticorum 250.8● *[272.2]*
        due to secondary diabetes
            249.8● *[272.2]*   ◀▥
    disseminatum 272.7
    eruptive 272.2
    eyelid 272.2 *[374.51]*
    familial 272.7
    hereditary 272.7
    hypercholesterinemic 272.0

Xanthoma(s) *(Continued)*
    hypercholesterolemic 272.0
    hyperlipemic 272.4
    hyperlipidemic 272.4
    infantile 272.7
    joint 272.7
    juvenile 272.7
    multiple 272.7
    multiplex 272.7
    primary familial 272.7
    tendon (sheath) 272.7
    tuberosum 272.2
    tuberous 272.2
    tubo-eruptive 272.2
Xanthosis 709.09
    surgical 998.81
Xenophobia 300.29
Xeroderma (congenital) 757.39
    acquired 701.1
        eyelid 373.33
    eyelid 373.33
    pigmentosum 757.33
    vitamin A deficiency 264.8
Xerophthalmia 372.53
    vitamin A deficiency 264.7
Xerosis
    conjunctiva 372.53
        with Bitôt's spot 372.53
            vitamin A deficiency 264.1
        vitamin A deficiency 264.0

Xerosis *(Continued)*
    cornea 371.40
        with corneal ulceration
            370.00
            vitamin A deficiency
                264.3
        vitamin A deficiency
            264.2
    cutis 706.8
    skin 706.8
Xerostomia 527.7
Xiphodynia 733.90
Xiphoidalgia 733.90
Xiphoiditis 733.99
Xiphopagus 759.4
XO syndrome 758.6
X-ray
    effects, adverse, NEC 990
    of chest
        for suspected tuberculosis
            V71.2
        routine V72.5
XXX syndrome 758.81
XXXXY syndrome 758.81
XXY syndrome 758.7
Xyloketosuria 271.8
Xylosuria 271.8
Xylulosuria 271.8
XYY syndrome 758.81

◀ New   ◀▥ Revised   ~~deleted~~ Deleted   ● Use Additional Digit(s)   ▦ Omit code

Y

Yaba monkey tumor virus 059.22
Yawning 786.09
  psychogenic 306.1
Yaws 102.9
  bone or joint lesions 102.6
  butter 102.1
  chancre 102.0
  cutaneous, less than five years after
      infection 102.2
  early (cutaneous) (macular)
      (maculopapular) (micropapular)
      (papular) 102.2
    frambeside 102.2
    skin lesions NEC 102.2
  eyelid 102.9 [373.4]
  ganglion 102.6
  gangosis, gangosa 102.5
  gumma, gummata 102.4
    bone 102.6

Yaws (Continued)
  gummatous
    frambeside 102.4
    osteitis 102.6
    periostitis 102.6
  hydrarthrosis 102.6
  hyperkeratosis (early) (late) (palmar)
      (plantar) 102.3
  initial lesions 102.0
  joint lesions 102.6
  juxta-articular nodules 102.7
  late nodular (ulcerated) 102.4
  latent (without clinical
      manifestations) (with
      positive serology) 102.8
  mother 102.0
  mucosal 102.7
  multiple papillomata 102.1
  nodular, late (ulcerated) 102.4
  osteitis 102.6

Yaws (Continued)
  papilloma, papillomata (palmar)
      (plantar) 102.1
  periostitis (hypertrophic) 102.6
  ulcers 102.4
  wet crab 102.1
Yeast infection (see also Candidiasis)
    112.9
Yellow
  atrophy (liver) 570
    chronic 571.8
    resulting from administration of
        blood, plasma, serum, or other
        biological substance (within 8
        months of administration) - see
        Hepatitis, viral
  fever - see Fever, yellow
  jack (see also Fever, yellow) 060.9
  jaundice (see also Jaundice) 782.4
Yersinia septica 027.8

Z

Zagari's disease (xerostomia) 527.7
Zahorsky's disease (exanthema subitum)
  (*see also* Exanthem subitum)
  058.10
  syndrome (herpangina) 074.0
Zellweger syndrome 277.86
Zenker's diverticulum (esophagus) 530.6
Ziehen-Oppenheim disease 333.6

Zieve's syndrome (jaundice,
  hyperlipemia, and hemolytic
  anemia) 571.1
Zika fever 066.3
Zollinger-Ellison syndrome (gastric
  hypersecretion with pancreatic islet
  cell tumor) 251.5
Zona (*see also* Herpes, zoster) 053.9
Zoophilia (erotica) 302.1
Zoophobia 300.29

Zoster (herpes) (*see also* Herpes, zoster)
  053.9
Zuelzer (-Ogden) anemia or syndrome
  (nutritional megaloblastic anemia)
  281.2
Zygodactyly (*see also* Syndactylism)
  755.10
Zygomycosis 117.7
Zymotic - *see* condition

◀ New   ◀ Revised   deleted Deleted   ● Use Additional Digit(s)   Omit code

SECTION II TABLE OF DRUGS AND CHEMICALS

ALPHABETIC INDEX TO POISONING AND EXTERNAL CAUSES OF ADVERSE EFFECTS OF DRUGS AND OTHER CHEMICAL SUBSTANCES

This table contains a classification of drugs and other chemical substances to identify poisoning states and external causes of adverse effects.

Each of the listed substances in the table is assigned a code according to the poisoning classification (960–989). These codes are used when there is a statement of poisoning, overdose, wrong substance given or taken, or intoxication.

The table also contains a listing of external causes of adverse effects. An adverse effect is a pathologic manifestation due to ingestion or exposure to drugs or other chemical substances (e.g., dermatitis, hypersensitivity reaction, aspirin gastritis). The adverse effect is to be identified by the appropriate code found in Section I, Index to Diseases and Injuries. An external cause code can then be used to identify the circumstances involved. The table headings pertaining to external causes are defined below:

Accidental poisoning (E850–E869)-accidental overdose of drug, wrong substance given or taken, drug taken inadvertently, accidents in the usage of drugs and biologicals in medical and surgical procedures, and to show external causes of poisonings classifiable to 980–989.

Therapeutic use (E930–E949)-a correct substance properly administered in therapeutic or prophylactic dosage as the external cause of adverse effects.

Suicide attempt (E950–E952)-instances in which self-inflicted injuries or poisonings are involved.

Assault (E961–E962)-injury or poisoning inflicted by another person with the intent to injure or kill.

Undetermined (E980–E982)-to be used when the intent of the poisoning or injury cannot be determined whether it was intentional or accidental.

The American Hospital Formulary Service (AHFS) list numbers are included in the table to help classify new drugs not identified in the table by name. The AHFS list numbers are keyed to the continually revised AHFS (American Hospital Formulary Service, 2 vol. Washington, D.C.: American Society of Hospital Pharmacists, 1959-). These listings are found in the table under the main term **Drug.**

Excluded from the table are radium and other radioactive substances. The classification of adverse effects and complications pertaining to these substances will be found in Index to Diseases and Injuries, and Index to External Causes of Injuries.

Although certain substances are indexed with one or more subentries, the majority are listed according to one use or state. It is recognized that many substances may be used in various ways, in medicine and in industry, and may cause adverse effects whatever the state of the agent (solid, liquid, or fumes arising from a liquid). In cases in which the reported data indicate a use or state not in the table, or which is clearly different from the one listed, an attempt should be made to classify the substance in the form which most nearly expresses the reported facts.

Substance	Poisoning	External Cause (E Code)				
		Accident	Therapeutic Use	Suicide Attempt	Assault	Undetermined
1-propanol	980.3	E860.4	—	E950.9	E962.1	E980.9
2-propanol	980.2	E860.3	—	E950.9	E962.1	E980.9
2,4-D (dichlorophenoxyacetic acid)	989.4	E863.5	—	E950.6	E962.1	E980.7
2,4-toluene diisocyanate	983.0	E864.0	—	E950.7	E962.1	E980.6
2,4,5-T (trichlorophenoxyacetic acid)	989.2	E863.5	—	E950.6	E962.1	E980.7
14-hydroxydihydromorphinone	965.09	E850.2	E935.2	E950.0	E962.0	E980.0
ABOB	961.7	E857	E931.7	E950.4	E962.0	E980.4
Abrus (seed)	988.2	E865.3	—	E950.9	E962.1	E980.9
Absinthe	980.0	E860.1	—	E950.9	E962.1	E980.9
beverage	980.0	E860.0	—	E950.9	E962.1	E980.9
Acenocoumarin, acenocoumarol	964.2	E858.2	E934.2	E950.4	E962.0	E980.4
Acepromazine	969.1	E853.0	E939.1	E950.3	E962.0	E980.3
Acetal	982.8	E862.4	—	E950.9	E962.1	E980.9
Acetaldehyde (vapor)	987.8	E869.8	—	E952.8	E962.2	E982.8
liquid	989.89	E866.8	—	E950.9	E962.1	E980.9
Acetaminophen	965.4	E850.4	E935.4	E950.0	E962.0	E980.0
Acetaminosalol	965.1	E850.3	E935.3	E950.0	E962.0	E980.0
Acetanilid(e)	965.4	E850.4	E935.4	E950.0	E962.0	E980.0
Acetarsol, acetarsone	961.1	E857	E931.1	E950.4	E962.0	E980.4
Acetazolamide	974.2	E858.5	E944.2	E950.4	E962.0	E980.4
Acetic	—	—	—	—	—	—
acid	983.1	E864.1	—	E950.7	E962.1	E980.6
with sodium acetate (ointment)	976.3	E858.7	E946.3	E950.4	E962.0	E980.4
irrigating solution	974.5	E858.5	E944.5	E950.4	E962.0	E980.4
lotion	976.2	E858.7	E946.2	E950.4	E962.0	E980.4
anhydride	983.1	E864.1	—	E950.7	E962.1	E980.6
ether (vapor)	982.8	E862.4	—	E950.9	E962.1	E980.9
Acetohexamide	962.3	E858.0	E932.3	E950.4	E962.0	E980.4
Acetomenaphthone	964.3	E858.2	E934.3	E950.4	E962.0	E980.4
Acetomorphine	965.01	E850.0	E935.0	E950.0	E962.0	E980.0
Acetone (oils) (vapor)	982.8	E862.4	—	E950.9	E962.1	E980.9
Acetophenazine (maleate)	969.1	E853.0	E939.1	E950.3	E962.0	E980.3
Acetophenetidin	965.4	E850.4	E935.4	E950.0	E962.0	E980.0
Acetophenone	982.0	E862.4	—	E950.9	E962.1	E980.9
Acetorphine	965.09	E850.2	E935.2	E950.0	E962.0	E980.0
Acetosulfone (sodium)	961.8	E857	E931.8	E950.4	E962.0	E980.4
Acetrizoate (sodium)	977.8	E858.8	E947.8	E950.4	E962.0	E980.4
Acetylcarbromal	967.3	E852.2	E937.3	E950.2	E962.0	E980.2

◀ New   ◀▥ Revised   ~~deleted~~ Deleted   ⬤ Use Additional Digit(s)

Substance	Poisoning	External Cause (E Code)				
		Accident	Therapeutic Use	Suicide Attempt	Assault	Undetermined
Acetylcholine (chloride)	971.0	E855.3	E941.0	E950.4	E962.0	E980.4
Acetylcysteine	975.5	E858.6	E945.5	E950.4	E962.0	E980.4
Acetyldigitoxin	972.1	E858.3	E942.1	E950.4	E962.0	E980.4
Acetyldihydrocodeine	965.09	E850.2	E935.2	E950.0	E962.0	E980.0
Acetyldihydrocodeinone	965.09	E850.2	E935.2	E950.0	E962.0	E980.0
Acetylene (gas) (industrial)	987.1	E868.1	—	E951.8	E962.2	E981.8
incomplete combustion of - *see* Carbon monoxide, fuel, utility	—	—	—	—	—	—
tetrachloride (vapor)	982.3	E862.4	—	E950.9	E962.1	E980.9
Acetyliodosalicylic acid	965.1	E850.3	E935.3	E950.0	E962.0	E980.0
Acetylphenylhydrazine	965.8	E850.8	E935.8	E950.0	E962.0	E980.0
Acetylsalicylic acid	965.1	E850.3	E935.3	E950.0	E962.0	E980.0
Achromycin	960.4	E856	E930.4	E950.4	E962.0	E980.4
ophthalmic preparation	976.5	E858.7	E946.5	E950.4	E962.0	E980.4
topical NEC	976.0	E858.7	E946.0	E950.4	E962.0	E980.4
Acidifying agents	963.2	E858.1	E933.2	E950.4	E962.0	E980.4
Acids (corrosive) NEC	983.1	E864.1	—	E950.7	E962.1	E980.6
Aconite (wild)	988.2	E865.4	—	E950.9	E962.1	E980.9
Aconitine (liniment)	976.8	E858.7	E946.8	E950.4	E962.0	E980.4
Aconitum ferox	988.2	E865.4	—	E950.9	E962.1	E980.9
Acridine	983.0	E864.0	—	E950.7	E962.1	E980.6
vapor	987.8	E869.8	—	E952.8	E962.2	E982.8
Acriflavine	961.9	E857	E931.9	E950.4	E962.0	E980.4
Acrisorcin	976.0	E858.7	E946.0	E950.4	E962.0	E980.4
Acrolein (gas)	987.8	E869.8	—	E952.8	E962.2	E982.8
liquid	989.89	E866.8	—	E950.9	E962.1	E980.9
Actaea spicata	988.2	E865.4	—	E950.9	E962.1	E980.9
Acterol	961.5	E857	E931.5	E950.4	E962.0	E980.4
ACTH	962.4	E858.0	E932.4	E950.4	E962.0	E980.4
Acthar	962.4	E858.0	E932.4	E950.4	E962.0	E980.4
Actinomycin (C) (D)	960.7	E856	E930.7	E950.4	E962.0	E980.4
Adalin (acetyl)	967.3	E852.2	E937.3	E950.2	E962.0	E980.2
Adenosine (phosphate)	977.8	E858.8	E947.8	E950.4	E962.0	E980.4
Adhesives	989.89	E866.6	—	E950.9	E962.1	E980.9
ADH	962.5	E858.0	E932.5	E950.4	E962.0	E980.4
Adicillin	960.0	E856	E930.0	E950.4	E962.0	E980.4
Adiphenine	975.1	E855.6	E945.1	E950.4	E962.0	E980.4
Adjunct, pharmaceutical	977.4	E858.8	E947.4	E950.4	E962.0	E980.4

◀ New　◀▥ Revised　~~deleted~~ Deleted　● Use Additional Digit(s)

Substance	Poisoning	External Cause (E Code)				
		Accident	Therapeutic Use	Suicide Attempt	Assault	Undetermined
Adrenal (extract, cortex or medulla) (glucocorticoids) (hormones) (mineralocorticoids)	962.0	E858.0	E932.0	E950.4	E962.0	E980.4
ENT agent	976.6	E858.7	E946.6	E950.4	E962.0	E980.4
ophthalmic preparation	976.5	E858.7	E946.5	E950.4	E962.0	E980.4
topical NEC	976.0	E858.7	E946.0	E950.4	E962.0	E980.4
Adrenalin	971.2	E855.5	E941.2	E950.4	E962.0	E980.4
Adrenergic blocking agents	971.3	E855.6	E941.3	E950.4	E962.0	E980.4
Adrenergics	971.2	E855.5	E941.2	E950.4	E962.0	E980.4
Adrenochrome (derivatives)	972.8	E858.3	E942.8	E950.4	E962.0	E980.4
Adrenocorticotropic hormone	962.4	E858.0	E932.4	E950.4	E962.0	E980.4
Adrenocorticotropin	962.4	E858.0	E932.4	E950.4	E962.0	E980.4
Adriamycin	960.7	E856	E930.7	E950.4	E962.0	E980.4
Aerosol spray - *see* Sprays	—	—	—	—	—	—
Aerosporin	960.8	E856	E930.8	E950.4	E962.0	E980.4
ENT agent	976.6	E858.7	E946.6	E950.4	E962.0	E980.4
ophthalmic preparation	976.5	E858.7	E946.5	E950.4	E962.0	E980.4
topical NEC	976.0	E858.7	E946.0	E950.4	E962.0	E980.4
Aethusa cynapium	988.2	E865.4	—	E950.9	E962.1	E980.9
Afghanistan black	969.6	E854.1	E939.6	E950.3	E962.0	E980.3
Aflatoxin	989.7	E865.9	—	E950.9	E962.1	E980.9
African boxwood	988.2	E865.4	—	E950.9	E962.1	E980.9
Agar (-agar)	973.3	E858.4	E943.3	E950.4	E962.0	E980.4
Agricultural agent NEC	989.89	E863.9	—	E950.6	E962.1	E980.7
Agrypnal	967.0	E851	E937.0	E950.1	E962.0	E980.1
Air contaminant(s), source or type not specified	—	—	—	—	—	—
specified type - *see* specific substance	987.9	E869.9	—	E952.9	E962.2	E982.9
Akee	988.2	E865.4	—	E950.9	E962.1	E980.9
Akrinol	976.0	E858.7	E946.0	E950.4	E962.0	E980.4
Alantolactone	961.6	E857	E931.6	E950.4	E962.0	E980.4
Albamycin	960.8	E856	E930.8	E950.4	E962.0	E980.4
Albumin (normal human serum)	964.7	E858.2	E934.7	E950.4	E962.0	E980.4
Albuterol	975.7	E858.6	E945.7	E950.4	E962.0	E980.4
Alcohol	980.9	E860.9	—	E950.9	E962.1	E980.9
absolute	980.0	E860.1	—	E950.9	E962.1	E980.9
beverage	980.0	E860.0	E947.8	E950.9	E962.1	E980.9
amyl	980.3	E860.4	—	E950.9	E962.1	E980.9
antifreeze	980.1	E860.2	—	E950.9	E962.1	E980.9
butyl	980.3	E860.4	—	E950.9	E962.1	E980.9

◀ New   ◀▥ Revised   ~~deleted~~ Deleted   ● Use Additional Digit(s)

Substance	Poisoning	External Cause (E Code)				
		Accident	Therapeutic Use	Suicide Attempt	Assault	Undetermined
Alcohol *(Continued)*						
dehydrated	980.0	E860.1	—	E950.9	E862.1	E980.9
beverage	980.0	E860.0	E947.8	E950.9	E962.1	E980.9
denatured	980.0	E860.1	—	E950.9	E962.1	E980.9
deterrents	977.3	E858.8	E947.3	E950.4	E962.0	E980.4
diagnostic (gastric function)	977.8	E858.8	E947.8	E950.4	E962.0	E980.4
ethyl	980.0	E860.1	—	E950.9	E962.1	E980.9
beverage	980.0	E860.0	E947.8	E950.9	E962.1	E980.9
grain	980.0	E860.1	—	E950.9	E962.1	E980.9
beverage	980.0	E860.0	E947.8	E950.9	E962.1	E980.9
industrial	980.9	E860.9	—	E950.9	E962.1	E980.9
isopropyl	980.2	E860.3	—	E950.9	E962.1	E980.9
methyl	980.1	E860.2	—	E950.9	E962.1	E980.9
preparation for consumption	980.0	E860.0	E947.8	E950.9	E962.1	E980.9
propyl	980.3	E860.4	—	E950.9	E962.1	E980.9
secondary	980.2	E860.3	—	E950.9	E962.1	E980.9
radiator	980.1	E860.2	—	E950.9	E962.1	E980.9
rubbing	980.2	E860.3	—	E950.9	E962.1	E980.9
specified type NEC	980.8	E860.8	—	E950.9	E962.1	E980.9
surgical	980.9	E860.9	—	E950.9	E962.1	E980.9
vapor (from any type of alcohol)	987.8	E869.8	—	E952.8	E962.2	E982.8
wood	980.1	E860.2	—	E950.9	E962.1	E980.9
Alcuronium chloride	975.2	E858.6	E945.2	E950.4	E962.0	E980.4
Aldactone	974.4	E858.5	E944.4	E950.4	E962.0	E980.4
Aldicarb	989.3	E863.2	—	E950.6	E962.1	E980.7
Aldomet	972.6	E858.3	E942.6	E950.4	E962.0	E980.4
Aldosterone	962.0	E858.0	E932.0	E950.4	E962.0	E980.4
Aldrin (dust)	989.2	E863.0	—	E950.6	E962.1	E980.7
Aleve - *see* Naproxen	—	—	—	—	—	—
Algeldrate	973.0	E858.4	E943.0	E950.4	E962.0	E980.4
Alidase	963.4	E858.1	E933.4	E950.4	E962.0	E980.4
Aliphatic thiocyanates	989.0	E866.8	—	E950.9	E962.1	E980.9
Alkaline antiseptic solution (aromatic)	976.6	E858.7	E946.6	E950.4	E962.0	E980.4
Alkalinizing agents (medicinal)	963.3	E858.1	E933.3	E950.4	E962.0	E980.4
Alkalis, caustic	983.2	E864.2	—	E950.7	E962.1	E980.6
Alkalizing agents (medicinal)	963.3	E858.1	E933.3	E950.4	E962.0	E980.4
Alka-seltzer	965.1	E850.3	E935.3	E950.0	E962.0	E980.0
Alkavervir	972.6	E858.3	E942.6	E950.4	E962.0	E980.4

◀ New　◀▥ Revised　~~deleted~~ Deleted　● Use Additional Digit(s)

		External Cause (E Code)				
Substance	**Poisoning**	**Accident**	**Therapeutic Use**	**Suicide Attempt**	**Assault**	**Undetermined**
Allegron	969.05 ◀▥	E854.0	E939.0	E950.3	E962.0	E980.3
Allobarbital, allobarbitone	967.0	E851	E937.0	E950.1	E962.0	E980.1
Allopurinol	974.7	E858.5	E944.7	E950.4	E962.0	E980.4
Allylestrenol	962.2	E858.0	E932.2	E950.4	E962.0	E980.4
Allylisopropylacetylurea	967.8	E852.8	E937.8	E950.2	E962.0	E980.2
Allylisopropylmalonylurea	967.0	E851	E937.0	E950.1	E962.0	E980.1
Allyltribromide	967.3	E852.2	E937.3	E950.2	E962.0	E980.2
Aloe, aloes, aloin	973.1	E858.4	E943.1	E950.4	E962.0	E980.4
Alosetron	973.8	E858.4	E943.8	E950.4	E962.0	E980.4
Aloxidone	966.0	E855.0	E936.0	E950.4	E962.0	E980.4
Aloxiprin	965.1	E850.3	E935.3	E950.0	E962.0	E980.0
Alpha amylase	963.4	E858.1	E933.4	E950.4	E962.0	E980.4
Alpha-1 blockers	971.3	E855.6	E941.3	E950.4	E962.0	E980.4
Alphaprodine (hydrochloride)	965.09	E850.2	E935.2	E950.0	E962.0	E980.0
Alpha tocopherol	963.5	E858.1	E933.5	E950.4	E962.0	E980.4
Alseroxylon	972.6	E858.3	E942.6	E950.4	E962.0	E980.4
Alum (ammonium) (potassium)	983.2	E864.2	—	E950.7	E962.1	E980.6
medicinal (astringent) NEC	976.2	E858.7	E946.2	E950.4	E962.0	E980.4
Aluminium, aluminum (gel) (hydroxide)	973.0	E858.4	E943.0	E950.4	E962.0	E980.4
acetate solution	976.2	E858.7	E946.2	E950.4	E962.0	E980.4
aspirin	965.1	E850.3	E935.3	E950.0	E962.0	E980.0
carbonate	973.0	E858.4	E943.0	E950.4	E962.0	E980.4
glycinate	973.0	E858.4	E943.0	E950.4	E962.0	E980.4
nicotinate	972.2	E858.3	E942.2	E950.4	E962.0	E980.4
ointment (surgical) (topical)	976.3	E858.7	E946.3	E950.4	E962.0	E980.4
phosphate	973.0	E858.4	E943.0	E950.4	E962.0	E980.4
subacetate	976.2	E858.7	E946.2	E950.4	E962.0	E980.4
topical NEC	976.3	E858.7	E946.3	E950.4	E962.0	E980.4
Alurate	967.0	E851	E937.0	E950.1	E962.0	E980.1
Alverine (citrate)	975.1	E858.6	E945.1	E950.4	E962.0	E980.4
Alvodine	965.09	E850.2	E935.2	E950.0	E962.0	E980.0
Amanita phalloides	988.1	E865.5	—	E950.9	E962.1	E980.9
Amantadine (hydrochloride)	966.4	E855.0	E936.4	E950.4	E962.0	E980.4
Ambazone	961.9	E857	E931.9	E950.4	E962.0	E980.4
Ambenonium	971.0	E855.3	E941.0	E950.4	E962.0	E980.4
Ambutonium bromide	971.1	E855.4	E941.1	E950.4	E962.0	E980.4
Ametazole	977.8	E858.8	E947.8	E950.4	E962.0	E980.4
Amethocaine (infiltration) (topical)	968.5	E855.2	E938.5	E950.4	E962.0	E980.4
nerve block (peripheral) (plexus)	968.6	E855.2	E938.6	E950.4	E962.0	E980.4
spinal	968.7	E855.2	E938.7	E950.4	E962.0	E980.4

◀ New   ◀▥ Revised   ~~deleted~~ Deleted   ● Use Additional Digit(s)

Substance	Poisoning	External Cause (E Code)				
		Accident	Therapeutic Use	Suicide Attempt	Assault	Undetermined
Amethopterin	963.1	E858.1	E933.1	E950.4	E962.0	E980.4
Amfepramone	977.0	E858.8	E947.0	E950.4	E962.0	E980.4
Amidone	965.02	E850.1	E935.1	E950.0	E962.0	E980.0
Amidopyrine	965.5	E850.5	E935.5	E950.0	E962.0	E980.0
Aminacrine	976.0	E858.7	E946.0	E950.4	E962.0	E980.4
Aminitrozole	961.5	E857	E931.5	E950.4	E962.0	E980.4
Aminoacetic acid	974.5	E858.5	E944.5	E950.4	E962.0	E980.4
Amino acids	974.5	E858.5	E944.5	E950.4	E962.0	E980.4
Aminocaproic acid	964.4	E858.2	E934.4	E950.4	E962.0	E980.4
Aminoethylisothiourium	963.8	E858.1	E933.8	E950.4	E962.0	E980.4
Aminoglutethimide	966.3	E855.0	E936.3	E950.4	E962.0	E980.4
Aminometradine	974.3	E858.5	E944.3	E950.4	E962.0	E980.4
Aminopentamide	971.1	E855.4	E941.1	E950.4	E962.0	E980.4
Aminophenazone	965.5	E850.5	E935.5	E950.0	E962.0	E980.0
Aminophenol	983.0	E864.0	—	E950.7	E962.1	E980.6
Aminophenylpyridone	969.5	E853.8	E939.5	E950.3	E962.0	E980.3
Aminophylline	975.7	E858.6	E945.7	E950.4	E962.0	E980.4
Aminopterin	963.1	E858.1	E933.1	E950.4	E962.0	E980.4
Aminopyrine	965.5	E850.5	E935.5	E950.0	E962.0	E980.0
Aminosalicylic acid	961.8	E857	E931.8	E950.4	E962.0	E980.4
Amiphenazole	970.1	E854.3	E940.1	E950.4	E962.0	E980.4
Amiquinsin	972.6	E858.3	E942.6	E950.4	E962.0	E980.4
Amisometradine	974.3	E858.5	E944.3	E950.4	E962.0	E980.4
Amitriptyline	969.05 ◀	E854.0	E939.0	E950.3	E962.0	E980.3
Ammonia (fumes) (gas) (vapor)	987.8	E869.8	—	E952.8	E962.2	E982.8
liquid (household) NEC	983.2	E861.4	—	E950.7	E962.1	E980.6
spirit, aromatic	970.8	E854.3	E940.8	E950.4	E962.0	E980.4
Ammoniated mercury	976.0	E858.7	E946.0	E950.4	E962.0	E980.4
Ammonium	—	—	—	—	—	—
carbonate	983.2	E864.2	—	E950.7	E962.1	E980.6
chloride (acidifying agent)	963.2	E858.1	E933.2	E950.4	E962.0	E980.4
expectorant	975.5	E858.6	E945.5	E950.4	E962.0	E980.4
compounds (household) NEC	983.2	E861.4	—	E950.7	E962.1	E980.6
fumes (any usage)	987.8	E869.8	—	E952.8	E962.2	E982.8
industrial	983.2	E864.2	—	E950.7	E962.1	E980.6
ichthosulfonate	976.4	E858.7	E946.4	E950.4	E962.0	E980.4
mandelate	961.9	E857	E931.9	E950.4	E962.0	E980.4
Amobarbital	967.0	E851	E937.0	E950.1	E962.0	E980.1
Amodiaquin(e)	961.4	E857	E931.4	E950.4	E962.0	E980.4
Amopyroquin(e)	961.4	E857	E931.4	E950.4	E962.0	E980.4

◀ New ◀ Revised deleted Deleted ● Use Additional Digit(s)

| | External Cause (E Code) | | | | |
Substance	Poisoning	Accident	Therapeutic Use	Suicide Attempt	Assault	Undetermined
Amphenidone	969.5	E853.8	E939.5	E950.3	E962.0	E980.3
Amphetamine	969.72 ◀▥	E854.2	E939.7	E950.3	E962.0	E980.3
Amphomycin	960.8	E856	E930.8	E950.4	E962.0	E980.4
Amphotericin B	960.1	E856	E930.1	E950.4	E962.0	E980.4
topical	976.0	E858.7	E946.0	E950.4	E962.0	E980.4
Ampicillin	960.0	E856	E930.0	E950.4	E962.0	E980.4
Amprotropine	971.1	E855.4	E941.1	E950.4	E962.0	E980.4
Amygdalin	977.8	E858.8	E947.8	E950.4	E962.0	E980.4
Amyl	—	—	—	—	—	—
acetate (vapor)	982.8	E862.4	—	E950.9	E962.1	E980.9
alcohol	980.3	E860.4	—	E950.9	E962.1	E980.9
nitrite (medicinal)	972.4	E858.3	E942.4	E950.4	E962.0	E980.4
Amylase (alpha)	963.4	E858.1	E933.4	E950.4	E962.0	E980.4
Amylene hydrate	980.8	E860.8	—	E950.9	E962.1	E980.9
Amylobarbitone	967.0	E851	E937.0	E950.1	E962.0	E980.1
Amylocaine	968.9	E855.2	E938.9	E950.4	E962.0	E980.4
infiltration (subcutaneous)	968.5	E855.2	E938.5	E950.4	E962.0	E980.4
nerve block (peripheral) (plexus)	968.6	E855.2	E938.6	E950.4	E962.0	E980.4
spinal	968.7	E855.2	E938.7	E950.4	E962.0	E980.4
topical (surface)	968.5	E855.2	E938.5	E950.4	E962.0	E980.4
Amytal (sodium)	967.0	E851	E937.0	E950.1	E962.0	E980.1
Analeptics	970.0	E854.3	E940.0	E950.4	E962.0	E980.4
Analgesics	965.9	E850.9	E935.9	E950.0	E962.0	E980.0
aromatic NEC	965.4	E850.4	E935.4	E950.0	E962.0	E980.0
non-narcotic NEC	965.7	E850.7	E935.7	E950.0	E962.0	E980.0
specified NEC	965.8	E850.8	E935.8	E950.0	E962.0	E980.0
Anamirta cocculus	988.2	E865.3	—	E950.9	E962.1	E980.9
Ancillin	960.0	E856	E930.0	E950.4	E962.0	E980.4
Androgens (anabolic congeners)	962.1	E858.0	E932.1	E950.4	E962.0	E980.4
Androstalone	962.1	E858.0	E932.1	E950.4	E962.0	E980.4
Androsterone	962.1	E858.0	E932.1	E950.4	E962.0	E980.4
Anemone pulsatilia	988.2	E865.4	—	E950.9	E962.1	E980.9
Anesthesia, anesthetic (general) NEC	968.4	E855.1	E938.4	E950.4	E962.0	E980.4
block (nerve) (plexus)	968.6	E855.2	E938.6	E950.4	E962.0	E980.4
gaseous NEC	968.2	E855.1	E938.2	E950.4	E962.0	E980.4
halogenated hydrocarbon derivatives NEC	968.2	E855.1	E938.2	E950.4	E962.0	E980.4
infiltration (intradermal) (subcutaneous) (submucosal)	968.5	E855.2	E938.5	E950.4	E962.0	E980.4
intravenous	968.3	E855.1	E938.3	E950.4	E962.0	E980.4
local NEC	968.9	E855.2	E938.9	E950.4	E962.0	E980.4

◀ New   ◀▥ Revised   ~~deleted~~ Deleted   ● Use Additional Digit(s)

Substance	Poisoning	External Cause (E Code)				
		Accident	Therapeutic Use	Suicide Attempt	Assault	Undetermined
Anesthesia *(Continued)*						
nerve blocking (peripheral) (plexus)	968.6	E855.2	E938.6	E950.4	E962.0	E980.4
rectal NEC	968.3	E855.1	E938.3	E950.4	E962.0	E980.4
spinal	968.7	E855.2	E938.7	E950.4	E962.0	E980.4
surface	968.5	E855.2	E938.5	E950.4	E962.0	E980.4
topical	968.5	E855.2	E938.5	E950.4	E962.0	E980.4
Aneurine	963.5	E858.1	E933.5	E950.4	E962.0	E980.4
Anginine - *see* Glyceryl trinitrate	971.2	E855.5	E941.2	E950.4	E962.0	E980.4
Angio-Conray	977.8	E858.8	E947.8	E950.4	E962.0	E980.4
Angiotensin	971.2	E855.5	E941.2	E950.4	E962.0	E980.4
Anhydrohydroxyprogesterone	962.2	E858.0	E932.2	E950.4	E962.0	E980.4
Anhydron	974.3	E858.5	E944.3	E950.4	E962.0	E980.4
Anileridine	965.09	E850.2	E935.2	E950.0	E962.0	E980.0
Aniline (dye) (liquid)	983.0	E864.0	—	E950.7	E962.1	E980.6
analgesic	965.4	E850.4	E935.4	E950.0	E962.0	E980.0
derivatives, therapeutic NEC	965.4	E850.4	E935.4	E950.0	E962.0	E980.0
vapor	987.8	E869.8	—	E952.8	E962.2	E982.8
Aniscoropine	971.1	E855.4	E941.1	E950.4	E962.0	E980.4
Anisindione	964.2	E858.2	E934.2	E950.4	E962.0	E980.4
Anorexic agents	977.0	E858.8	E947.0	E950.4	E962.0	E980.4
Ant (bite) (sting)	989.5	E905.5	—	E950.9	E962.1	E980.9
Antabuse	977.3	E858.8	E947.3	E950.4	E962.0	E980.4
Antacids	973.0	E858.4	E943.0	E950.4	E962.0	E980.4
Antazoline	963.0	E858.1	E933.0	E950.4	E962.0	E980.4
Anthelmintics	961.6	E857	E931.6	E950.4	E962.0	E980.4
Anthralin	976.4	E858.7	E946.4	E950.4	E962.0	E980.4
Anthramycin	960.7	E856	E930.7	E950.4	E962.0	E980.4
Antiadrenergics	971.3	E855.6	E941.3	E950.4	E962.0	E980.4
Antiallergic agents	963.0	E858.1	E933.0	E950.4	E962.0	E980.4
Antianemic agents NEC	964.1	E858.2	E934.1	E950.4	E962.0	E980.4
Antiaris toxicaria	988.2	E865.4	—	E950.9	E962.1	E980.9
Antiarteriosclerotic agents	972.2	E858.3	E942.2	E950.4	E962.0	E980.4
Antiasthmatics	975.7	E858.6	E945.7	E950.4	E962.0	E980.4
Antibiotics	960.9	E856	E930.9	E950.4	E962.0	E980.4
antifungal	960.1	E856	E930.1	E950.4	E962.0	E980.4
antimycobacterial	960.6	E856	E930.6	E950.4	E962.0	E980.4
antineoplastic	960.7	E856	E930.7	E950.4	E962.0	E980.4
cephalosporin (group)	960.5	E856	E930.5	E950.4	E962.0	E980.4
chloramphenicol (group)	960.2	E856	E930.2	E950.4	E962.0	E980.4
macrolides	960.3	E856	E930.3	E950.4	E962.0	E980.4

◀ New   ◀▥ Revised   ~~deleted~~ Deleted   ● Use Additional Digit(s)

Substance	Poisoning	External Cause (E Code) Accident	Therapeutic Use	Suicide Attempt	Assault	Undetermined
Antibiotics *(Continued)*						
specified NEC	960.8	E856	E930.8	E950.4	E962.0	E980.4
tetracycline (group)	960.4	E856	E930.4	E950.4	E962.0	E980.4
Anticancer agents NEC	963.1	E858.1	E933.1	E950.4	E962.0	E980.4
antibiotics	960.7	E856	E930.7	E950.4	E962.0	E980.4
Anticholinergics	971.1	E855.4	E941.1	E950.4	E962.0	E980.4
Anticholinesterase (organophosphorus) (reversible)	971.0	E855.3	E941.0	E950.4	E962.0	E980.4
Anticoagulants	964.2	E858.2	E934.2	E950.4	E962.0	E980.4
antagonists	964.5	E858.2	E934.5	E950.4	E962.0	E980.4
Anti-common cold agents NEC	975.6	E858.6	E945.6	E950.4	E962.0	E980.4
Anticonvulsants NEC	966.3	E855.0	E936.3	E950.4	E962.0	E980.4
Antidepressants	969.00	E854.0	E939.0	E950.3	E962.0	E980.3
monoamine oxidase inhibitors (MAOI)	969.01	E854.0	E939.0	E950.3	E962.0	E980.3
specified type NEC	969.09	E854.0	E939.0	E950.3	E962.0	E980.3
SSNRI (selective serotonin and norepinephrine reuptake inhibitors)	969.02	E854.0	E939.0	E950.3	E962.0	E980.3
SSRI (selective serotonin reuptake inhibitors)	969.03	E854.0	E939.0	E950.3	E962.0	E980.3
tetracyclic	969.04	E854.0	E939.0	E950.3	E962.0	E980.3
tricyclic	969.05	E854.0	E939.0	E950.3	E962.0	E980.3
Antidiabetic agents	962.3	E858.0	E932.3	E950.4	E962.0	E980.4
Antidiarrheal agents	973.5	E858.4	E943.5	E950.4	E962.0	E980.4
Antidiuretic hormone	962.5	E858.0	E932.5	E950.4	E962.0	E980.4
Antidotes NEC	977.2	E858.8	E947.2	E950.4	E962.0	E980.4
Antiemetic agents	963.0	E858.1	E933.0	E950.4	E962.0	E980.4
Antiepilepsy agent NEC	966.3	E855.0	E936.3	E950.4	E962.0	E980.4
Antifertility pills	962.2	E858.0	E932.2	E950.4	E962.0	E980.4
Antiflatulents	973.8	E858.4	E943.8	E950.4	E962.0	E980.4
Antifreeze	989.89	E866.8	—	E950.9	E962.1	E980.9
alcohol	980.1	E860.2	—	E950.9	E962.1	E980.9
ethylene glycol	982.8	E862.4	—	E950.9	E962.1	E980.9
Antifungals (nonmedicinal) (sprays)	989.4	E863.6	—	E950.6	E962.1	E980.7
medicinal NEC	961.9	E857	E931.9	E950.4	E962.0	E980.4
antibiotic	960.1	E856	E930.1	E950.4	E962.0	E980.4
topical	976.0	E858.7	E946.0	E950.4	E962.0	E980.4
Antigastric secretion agents	973.0	E858.4	E943.0	E950.4	E962.0	E980.4
Antihelmintics	961.6	E857	E931.6	E950.4	E962.0	E980.4
Antihemophilic factor (human)	964.7	E858.2	E934.7	E950.4	E962.0	E980.4
Antihistamine	963.0	E858.1	E933.0	E950.4	E962.0	E980.4
Antihypertensive agents NEC	972.6	E858.3	E942.6	E950.4	E962.0	E980.4

◀ New   ◀▥ Revised   ~~deleted~~ Deleted   ● Use Additional Digit(s)

Substance	Poisoning	External Cause (E Code)				
		Accident	Therapeutic Use	Suicide Attempt	Assault	Undetermined
Anti-infectives NEC	961.9	E857	E931.9	E950.4	E962.0	E980.4
antibiotics	960.9	E856	E930.9	E950.4	E962.0	E980.4
specified NEC	960.8	E856	E930.8	E950.4	E962.0	E980.4
anthelmintic	961.6	E857	E931.6	E950.4	E962.0	E980.4
antimalarial	961.4	E857	E931.4	E950.4	E962.0	E980.4
antimycobacterial NEC	961.8	E857	E931.8	E950.4	E962.0	E980.4
antibiotics	960.6	E856	E930.6	E950.4	E962.0	E980.4
antiprotozoal NEC	961.5	E857	E931.5	E950.4	E962.0	E980.4
blood	961.4	E857	E931.4	E950.4	E962.0	E980.4
antiviral	961.7	E857	E931.7	E950.4	E962.0	E980.4
arsenical	961.1	E857	E931.1	E950.4	E962.0	E980.4
ENT agents	976.6	E858.7	E946.6	E950.4	E962.0	E980.4
heavy metals NEC	961.2	E857	E931.2	E950.4	E962.0	E980.4
local	976.0	E858.7	E946.0	E950.4	E962.0	E980.4
ophthalmic preparation	976.5	E858.7	E946.5	E950.4	E962.0	E980.4
topical NEC	976.0	E858.7	E946.0	E950.4	E962.0	E980.4
Anti-inflammatory agents (topical)	976.0	E858.7	E946.0	E950.4	E962.0	E980.4
Antiknock (tetraethyl lead)	984.1	E862.1	—	E950.9	E962.1	E980.9
Antilipemics	972.2	E858.3	E942.2	E950.4	E962.0	E980.4
Antimalarials	961.4	E857	E931.4	E950.4	E962.0	E980.4
Antimony (compounds) (vapor) NEC	985.4	E866.2	—	E950.9	E962.1	E980.9
anti-infectives	961.2	E857	E931.2	E950.4	E962.0	E980.4
pesticides (vapor)	985.4	E863.4	—	E950.6	E962.2	E980.7
potassium tartrate	961.2	E857	E931.2	E950.4	E962.0	E980.4
tartrated	961.2	E857	E931.2	E950.4	E962.0	E980.4
Antimuscarinic agents	971.1	E855.4	E941.1	E950.4	E962.0	E980.4
Antimycobacterials NEC	961.8	E857	E931.8	E950.4	E962.0	E980.4
antibiotics	960.6	E856	E930.6	E950.4	E962.0	E980.4
Antineoplastic agents	963.1	E858.1	E933.1	E950.4	E962.0	E980.4
antibiotics	960.7	E856	E930.7	E950.4	E962.0	E980.4
Anti-Parkinsonism agents	966.4	E855.0	E936.4	E950.4	E962.0	E980.4
Antiphlogistics	965.69	E850.6	E935.6	E950.0	E962.0	E980.0
Antiprotozoals NEC	961.5	E857	E931.5	E950.4	E962.0	E980.4
blood	961.4	E857	E931.4	E950.4	E962.0	E980.4
Antipruritics (local)	976.1	E858.7	E946.1	E950.4	E962.0	E980.4
Antipsychotic agents NEC	969.3	E853.8	E939.3	E950.3	E962.0	E980.3
Antipyretics	965.9	E850.9	E935.9	E950.0	E962.0	E980.0
specified NEC	965.8	E850.8	E935.8	E950.0	E962.0	E980.0
Antipyrine	965.5	E850.5	E935.5	E950.0	E962.0	E980.0
Antirabies serum (equine)	979.9	E858.8	E949.9	E950.4	E962.0	E980.4

◀ New   ◀▥ Revised   ~~deleted~~ Deleted   ● Use Additional Digit(s)

Substance	Poisoning	External Cause (E Code)				
		Accident	Therapeutic Use	Suicide Attempt	Assault	Undetermined
Antirheumatics	965.69	E850.6	E935.6	E950.0	E962.0	E980.0
Antiseborrheics	976.4	E858.7	E946.4	E950.4	E962.0	E980.4
Antiseptics (external) (medicinal)	976.0	E858.7	E946.0	E950.4	E962.0	E980.4
Antistine	963.0	E858.1	E933.0	E950.4	E962.0	E980.4
Antithyroid agents	962.8	E858.0	E932.8	E950.4	E962.0	E980.4
Antitoxin, any	979.9	E858.8	E949.9	E950.4	E962.0	E980.4
Antituberculars	961.8	E857	E931.8	E950.4	E962.0	E980.4
antibiotics	960.6	E856	E930.6	E950.4	E962.0	E980.4
Antitussives	975.4	E858.6	E945.4	E950.4	E962.0	E980.4
Antivaricose agents (sclerosing)	972.7	E858.3	E942.7	E950.4	E962.0	E980.4
Antivenin (crotaline) (spider-bite)	979.9	E858.8	E949.9	E950.4	E962.0	E980.4
Antivert	963.0	E858.1	E933.0	E950.4	E962.0	E980.4
Antivirals NEC	961.7	E857	E931.7	E950.4	E962.0	E980.4
Ant poisons - *see* Pesticides	—	—	—	—	—	—
Antrol	989.4	E863.4	—	E950.6	E962.1	E980.7
fungicide	989.4	E863.6	—	E950.6	E962.1	E980.7
Apomorphine hydrochloride (emetic)	973.6	E858.4	E943.6	E950.4	E962.0	E980.4
Appetite depressants, central	977.0	E858.8	E947.0	E950.4	E962.0	E980.4
Apresoline	972.6	E858.3	E942.6	E950.4	E962.0	E980.4
Aprobarbital, aprobarbitone	967.0	E851	E937.0	E950.1	E962.0	E980.1
Apronalide	967.8	E852.8	E937.8	E950.2	E962.0	E980.2
Aqua fortis	983.1	E864.1	—	E950.7	E962.1	E980.6
Arachis oil (topical)	976.3	E858.7	E946.3	E950.4	E962.0	E980.4
cathartic	973.2	E858.4	E943.2	E950.4	E962.0	E980.4
Aralen	961.4	E857	E931.4	E950.4	E962.0	E980.4
Arginine salts	974.5	E858.5	E944.5	E950.4	E962.0	E980.4
Argyrol	976.0	E858.7	E946.0	E950.4	E962.0	E980.4
ENT agent	976.6	E858.7	E946.6	E950.4	E962.0	E980.4
ophthalmic preparation	976.5	E858.7	E946.5	E950.4	E962.0	E980.4
Aristocort	962.0	E858.0	E932.0	E950.4	E962.0	E980.4
ENT agent	976.6	E858.7	E946.6	E950.4	E962.0	E980.4
ophthalmic preparation	976.5	E858.7	E946.5	E950.4	E962.0	E980.4
topical NEC	976.0	E858.7	E946.0	E950.4	E962.0	E980.4
Aromatics, corrosive	983.0	E864.0	—	E950.7	E962.1	E980.6
disinfectants	983.0	E861.4	—	E950.7	E962.1	E980.6
Arsenate of lead (insecticide)	985.1	E863.4	—	E950.8	E962.1	E980.8
herbicide	985.1	E863.5	—	E950.8	E962.1	E980.8
Arsenic, arsenicals (compounds) (dust) (fumes) (vapor) NEC	985.1	E866.3	—	E950.8	E962.1	E980.8
anti-infectives	961.1	E857	E931.1	E950.4	E962.0	E980.4
pesticide (dust) (fumes)	985.1	E863.4	—	E950.8	E962.1	E980.8

◀ New ◀║ Revised ~~deleted~~ Deleted ● Use Additional Digit(s)

Substance	Poisoning	External Cause (E Code)				
		Accident	Therapeutic Use	Suicide Attempt	Assault	Undetermined
Arsine (gas)	985.1	E866.3	—	E950.8	E962.1	E980.8
Arsphenamine (silver)	961.1	E857	E931.1	E950.4	E962.0	E980.4
Arsthinol	961.1	E857	E931.1	E950.4	E962.0	E980.4
Artane	971.1	E855.4	E941.1	E950.4	E962.0	E980.4
Arthropod (venomous) NEC	989.5	E905.5	—	E950.9	E962.1	E980.9
Asbestos	989.81	E866.8	—	E950.9	E962.1	E980.9
Ascaridole	961.6	E857	E931.6	E950.4	E962.0	E980.4
Ascorbic acid	963.5	E858.1	E933.5	E950.4	E962.0	E980.4
Asiaticoside	976.0	E858.7	E946.0	E950.4	E962.0	E980.4
Aspidium (oleoresin)	961.6	E857	E931.6	E950.4	E962.0	E980.4
Aspirin	965.1	E850.3	E935.3	E950.0	E962.0	E980.0
Astringents (local)	976.2	E858.7	E946.2	E950.4	E962.0	E980.4
Atabrine	961.3	E857	E931.3	E950.4	E962.0	E980.4
Ataractics	969.5	E853.8	E939.5	E950.3	E962.0	E980.3
Atonia drug, intestinal	973.3	E858.4	E943.3	E950.4	E962.0	E980.4
Atophan	974.7	E858.5	E944.7	E950.4	E962.0	E980.4
Atropine	971.1	E855.4	E941.1	E950.4	E962.0	E980.4
Attapulgite	973.5	E858.4	E943.5	E950.4	E962.0	E980.4
Attenuvax	979.4	E858.8	E949.4	E950.4	E962.0	E980.4
Aureomycin	960.4	E856	E930.4	E950.4	E962.0	E980.4
ophthalmic preparation	976.5	E858.7	E946.5	E950.4	E962.0	E980.4
topical NEC	976.0	E858.7	E946.0	E950.4	E962.0	E980.4
Aurothioglucose	965.69	E850.6	E935.6	E950.0	E962.0	E980.0
Aurothioglycanide	965.69	E850.6	E935.6	E950.0	E962.0	E980.0
Aurothiomalate	965.69	E850.6	E935.6	E950.0	E962.0	E980.0
Automobile fuel	981	E862.1	—	E950.9	E962.1	E980.9
Autonomic nervous system agents NEC	971.9	E855.9	E941.9	E950.4	E962.0	E980.4
Avlosulfon	961.8	E857	E931.8	E950.4	E962.0	E980.4
Avomine	967.8	E852.8	E937.8	E950.2	E962.0	E980.2
Azacyclonol	969.5	E853.8	E939.5	E950.3	E962.0	E980.3
Azapetine	971.3	E855.6	E941.3	E950.4	E962.0	E980.4
Azaribine	963.1	E858.1	E933.1	E950.4	E962.0	E980.4
Azaserine	960.7	E856	E930.7	E950.4	E962.0	E980.4
Azathioprine	963.1	E858.1	E933.1	E950.4	E962.0	E980.4
Azosulfamide	961.0	E857	E931.0	E950.4	E962.0	E980.4
Azulfidine	961.0	E857	E931.0	E950.4	E962.0	E980.4
Azuresin	977.8	E858.8	E947.8	E950.4	E962.0	E980.4
Bacimycin	976.0	E858.7	E946.0	E950.4	E962.0	E980.4
ophthalmic preparation	976.5	E858.7	E946.5	E950.4	E962.0	E980.4

◀ New   ◀▥ Revised   ~~deleted~~ Deleted   ● Use Additional Digit(s)

			External Cause (E Code)			
Substance	Poisoning	Accident	Therapeutic Use	Suicide Attempt	Assault	Undetermined
Bacitracin	960.8	E856	E930.8	E950.4	E962.0	E980.4
ENT agent	976.6	E858.7	E946.6	E950.4	E962.0	E980.4
ophthalmic preparation	976.5	E858.7	E946.5	E950.4	E962.0	E980.4
topical NEC	976.0	E858.7	E946.0	E950.4	E962.0	E980.4
Baking soda	963.3	E858.1	E933.3	E950.4	E962.0	E980.4
BAL	963.8	E858.1	E933.8	E950.4	E962.0	E980.4
Bamethan (sulfate)	972.5	E858.3	E942.5	E950.4	E962.0	E980.4
Bamipine	963.0	E858.1	E933.0	E950.4	E962.0	E980.4
Baneberry	988.2	E865.4	—	E950.9	E962.1	E980.9
Banewort	988.2	E865.4	—	E950.9	E962.1	E980.9
Barbenyl	967.0	E851	E937.0	E950.1	E962.0	E980.1
Barbital, barbitone	967.0	E851	E937.0	E950.1	E962.0	E980.1
Barbiturates, barbituric acid	967.0	E851	E937.0	E950.1	E962.0	E980.1
anesthetic (intravenous)	968.3	E855.1	E938.3	E950.4	E962.0	E980.4
Barium (carbonate) (chloride) (sulfate)	985.8	E866.4	—	E950.9	E962.1	E980.9
diagnostic agent	977.8	E858.8	E947.8	E950.4	E962.0	E980.4
pesticide	985.8	E863.4	—	E950.6	E962.1	E980.7
rodenticide	985.8	E863.7	—	E950.6	E962.1	E980.7
Barrier cream	976.3	E858.7	E946.3	E950.4	E962.0	E980.4
Battery acid or fluid	983.1	E864.1	—	E950.7	E962.1	E980.6
Bay rum	980.8	E860.8	—	E950.9	E962.1	E980.9
BCG vaccine	978.0	E858.8	E948.0	E950.4	E962.0	E980.4
Bearsfoot	988.2	E865.4	—	E950.9	E962.1	E980.9
Beclamide	966.3	E855.0	E936.3	E950.4	E962.0	E980.4
Bee (sting) (venom)	989.5	E905.3	—	E950.9	E962.1	E980.9
Belladonna (alkaloids)	971.1	E855.4	E941.1	E950.4	E962.0	E980.4
Bemegride	970.0	E854.3	E940.0	E950.4	E962.0	E980.4
Benactyzine	969.8	E855.8	E939.8	E950.3	E962.0	E980.3
Benadryl	963.0	E858.1	E933.0	E950.4	E962.0	E980.4
Bendrofluazide	974.3	E858.5	E944.3	E950.4	E962.0	E980.4
Bendroflumethiazide	974.3	E858.5	E944.3	E950.4	E962.0	E980.4
Benemid	974.7	E858.5	E944.7	E950.4	E962.0	E980.4
Benethamine penicillin G	960.0	E856	E930.0	E950.4	E962.0	E980.4
Benisone	976.0	E858.7	E946.0	E950.4	E962.0	E980.4
Benoquin	976.8	E858.7	E946.8	E950.4	E962.0	E980.4
Benoxinate	968.5	E855.2	E938.5	E950.4	E962.0	E980.4
Bentonite	976.3	E858.7	E946.3	E950.4	E962.0	E980.4
Benzalkonium (chloride)	976.0	E858.7	E946.0	E950.4	E962.0	E980.4
ophthalmic preparation	976.5	E858.7	E946.5	E950.4	E962.0	E980.4
Benzamidosalicylate (calcium)	961.8	E857	E931.8	E950.4	E962.0	E980.4

◀ New ◀▦ Revised ~~deleted~~ Deleted ● Use Additional Digit(s)

Substance	Poisoning	External Cause (E Code)				
		Accident	Therapeutic Use	Suicide Attempt	Assault	Undetermined
Benzathine penicillin	960.0	E856	E930.0	E950.4	E962.0	E980.4
Benzcarbimine	963.1	E858.1	E933.1	E950.4	E962.0	E980.4
Benzedrex	971.2	E855.5	E941.2	E950.4	E962.0	E980.4
Benzedrine (amphetamine)	969.72 ◀ⅢⅢ	E854.2	E939.7	E950.3	E962.0	E980.3
Benzene (acetyl) (dimethyl) (methyl) (solvent) (vapor)	982.0	E862.4	—	E950.9	E962.1	E980.9
hexachloride (gamma) (insecticide) (vapor)	989.2	E863.0	—	E950.6	E962.1	E980.7
Benzethonium	976.0	E858.7	E946.0	E950.4	E962.0	E980.4
Benzhexol (chloride)	966.4	E855.0	E936.4	E950.4	E962.0	E980.4
Benzilonium	971.1	E855.4	E941.1	E950.4	E962.0	E980.4
Benzin(e) - *see* Ligroin	—	—	—	—	—	—
Benziodarone	972.4	E858.3	E942.4	E950.4	E962.0	E980.4
Benzocaine	968.5	E855.2	E938.5	E950.4	E962.0	E980.4
Benzodiapin	969.4	E853.2	E939.4	E950.3	E962.0	E980.3
Benzodiazepines (tranquilizers) NEC	969.4	E853.2	E939.4	E950.3	E962.0	E980.3
Benzoic acid (with salicylic acid) (anti-infective)	976.0	E858.7	E946.0	E950.4	E962.0	E980.4
Benzoin	976.3	E858.7	E946.3	E950.4	E962.0	E980.4
Benzol (vapor)	982.0	E862.4	—	E950.9	E962.1	E980.9
Benzomorphan	965.09	E850.2	E935.2	E950.0	E962.0	E980.0
Benzonatate	975.4	E858.6	E945.4	E950.4	E962.0	E980.4
Benzothiadiazides	974.3	E858.5	E944.3	E950.4	E962.0	E980.4
Benzoylpas	961.8	E857	E931.8	E950.4	E962.0	E980.4
Benzperidol	969.5	E853.8	E939.5	E950.3	E962.0	E980.3
Benzphetamine	977.0	E858.8	E947.0	E950.4	E962.0	E980.4
Benzpyrinium	971.0	E855.3	E941.0	E950.4	E962.0	E980.4
Benzquinamide	963.0	E858.1	E933.0	E950.4	E962.0	E980.4
Benzthiazide	974.3	E858.5	E944.3	E950.4	E962.0	E980.4
Benztropine	971.1	E855.4	E941.1	E950.4	E962.0	E980.4
Benzyl	—	—	—	—	—	—
acetate	982.8	E862.4	—	E950.9	E962.1	E980.9
benzoate (anti-infective)	976.0	E858.7	E946.0	E950.4	E962.0	E980.4
morphine	965.09	E850.2	E935.2	E950.0	E962.0	E980.0
penicillin	960.0	E856	E930.0	E950.4	E962.0	E980.4
Bephenium	—	—	—	—	—	—
hydroxynapthoate	961.6	E857	E931.6	E950.4	E962.0	E980.4
Bergamot oil	989.89	E866.8	—	E950.9	E962.1	E980.9
Berries, poisonous	988.2	E865.3	—	E950.9	E962.1	E980.9
Beryllium (compounds) (fumes)	985.3	E866.4	—	E950.9	E962.1	E980.9
Beta-carotene	976.3	E858.7	E946.3	E950.4	E962.0	E980.4
Beta-Chlor	967.1	E852.0	E937.1	E950.2	E962.0	E980.2

◀ New   ◀ⅢⅢ Revised   ~~deleted~~ Deleted   ● Use Additional Digit(s)

TABLE OF DRUGS AND CHEMICALS

Substance	External Cause (E Code)					
	Poisoning	Accident	Therapeutic Use	Suicide Attempt	Assault	Undetermined
Betamethasone	962.0	E858.0	E932.0	E950.4	E962.0	E980.4
topical	976.0	E858.7	E946.0	E950.4	E962.0	E980.4
Betazole	977.8	E858.8	E947.8	E950.4	E962.0	E980.4
Bethanechol	971.0	E855.3	E941.0	E950.4	E962.0	E980.4
Bethanidine	972.6	E858.3	E942.6	E950.4	E962.0	E980.4
Betula oil	976.3	E858.7	E946.3	E950.4	E962.0	E980.4
Bhang	969.6	E854.1	E939.6	E950.3	E962.0	E980.3
Bialamicol	961.5	E857	E931.5	E950.4	E962.0	E980.4
Bichloride of mercury - see Mercury, chloride	—	—	—	—	—	—
Bichromates (calcium) (crystals) (potassium) (sodium)	983.9	E864.3	—	E950.7	E962.1	E980.6
fumes	987.8	E869.8	—	E952.8	E962.2	E982.8
Biguanide derivatives, oral	962.3	E858.0	E932.3	E950.4	E962.0	E980.4
Biligrafin	977.8	E858.8	E947.8	E950.4	E962.0	E980.4
Bilopaque	977.8	E858.8	E947.8	E950.4	E962.0	E980.4
Bioflavonoids	972.8	E858.3	E942.8	E950.4	E962.0	E980.4
Biological substance NEC	979.9	E858.8	E949.9	E950.4	E962.0	E980.4
Biperiden	966.4	E855.0	E936.4	E950.4	E962.0	E980.4
Bisacodyl	973.1	E858.4	E943.1	E950.4	E962.0	E980.4
Bishydroxycoumarin	964.2	E858.2	E934.2	E950.4	E962.0	E980.4
Bismarsen	961.1	E857	E931.1	E950.4	E962.0	E980.4
Bismuth (compounds) NEC	985.8	E866.4	—	E950.9	E962.1	E980.9
anti-infectives	961.2	E857	E931.2	E950.4	E962.0	E980.4
subcarbonate	973.5	E858.4	E943.5	E950.4	E962.0	E980.4
sulfarsphenamine	961.1	E857	E931.1	E950.4	E962.0	E980.4
Bisphosphonates	—	—	—	—	—	—
intravenous	963.1	E858.1	E933.7	E950.4	E962.0	E980.4
oral	963.1	E858.1	E933.6	E950.4	E962.0	E980.4
Bithionol	961.6	E857	E931.6	E950.4	E962.0	E980.4
Bitter almond oil	989.0	E866.8	—	E950.9	E962.1	E980.9
Bittersweet	988.2	E865.4	—	E950.9	E962.1	E930.9
Black	—	—	—	—	—	—
flag	989.4	E863.4	—	E950.6	E962.1	E980.7
henbane	988.2	E865.4	—	E950.9	E962.1	E980.9
leaf (40)	989.4	E863.4	—	E950.6	E962.1	E980.7
widow spider (bite)	989.5	E905.1	—	E950.9	E962.1	E980.9
antivenin	979.9	E858.8	E949.9	E950.4	E962.0	E980.4
Blast furnace gas (carbon monoxide from)	986	E868.8	—	E952.1	E962.2	E982.1
Bleach NEC	983.9	E864.3	—	E950.7	E962.1	E980.6
Bleaching solutions	983.9	E864.3	—	E950.7	E962.1	E980.6
Bleomycin (sulfate)	960.7	E856	E930.7	E950.4	E962.0	E980.4

◀ New   ◀▥ Revised   ~~deleted~~ Deleted   ● Use Additional Digit(s)

Substance	Poisoning	External Cause (E Code)				
		Accident	Therapeutic Use	Suicide Attempt	Assault	Undetermined
Blockain	968.9	E855.2	E938.9	E950.4	E962.0	E980.4
infiltration (subcutaneous)	968.5	E855.2	E938.5	E950.4	E962.0	E980.4
nerve block (peripheral) (plexus)	968.6	E855.2	E938.6	E950.4	E962.0	E980.4
topical (surface)	968.5	E855.2	E938.5	E950.4	E962.0	E980.4
Blood (derivatives) (natural) (plasma) (whole)	964.7	E858.2	E934.7	E950.4	E962.0	E980.4
affecting agent	964.9	E858.2	E934.9	E950.4	E962.0	E980.4
specified NEC	964.8	E858.2	E934.8	E950.4	E962.0	E980.4
substitute (macromolecular)	964.8	E858.2	E934.8	E950.4	E962.0	E980.4
Blue velvet	965.09	E850.2	E935.2	E950.0	E962.0	E980.0
Bone meal	989.89	E866.5	—	E950.9	E962.1	E980.9
Bonine	963.0	E858.1	E933.0	E950.4	E962.0	E980.4
Boracic acid	976.0	E858.7	E946.0	E950.4	E962.0	E980.4
ENT agent	976.6	E858.7	E946.6	E950.4	E962.0	E980.4
ophthalmic preparation	976.5	E858.7	E946.5	E950.4	E962.0	E980.4
Borate (cleanser) (sodium)	989.6	E861.3	—	E950.9	E962.1	E980.9
Borax (cleanser)	989.6	E861.3	—	E950.9	E962.1	E980.9
Boric acid	976.0	E858.7	E946.0	E950.4	E962.0	E980.4
ENT agent	976.6	E858.7	E946.6	E950.4	E962.0	E980.4
ophthalmic preparation	976.5	E858.7	E946.5	E950.4	E962.0	E980.4
Boron hydride NEC	989.89	E866.8	—	E950.9	E962.1	E980.9
fumes or gas	987.8	E869.8	—	E952.8	E962.2	E982.8
Botox	975.3	E858.6	E945.3	E950.4	E962.0	E980.4
Brake fluid vapor	987.8	E869.8	—	E952.8	E962.2	E982.8
Brass (compounds) (fumes)	985.8	E866.4	—	E950.9	E962.1	E980.9
Brasso	981	E861.3	—	E950.9	E962.1	E980.9
Bretylium (tosylate)	972.6	E858.3	E942.6	E950.4	E962.0	E980.4
Brevital (sodium)	968.3	E855.1	E938.3	E950.4	E962.0	E980.4
British antilewisite	963.8	E858.1	E933.8	E950.4	E962.0	E980.4
Bromal (hydrate)	967.3	E852.2	E937.3	E950.2	E962.0	E980.2
Bromelains	963.4	E858.1	E933.4	E950.4	E962.0	E980.4
Bromides NEC	967.3	E852.2	E937.3	E950.2	E962.0	E980.2
Bromine (vapor)	987.8	E869.8	—	E952.8	E962.2	E982.8
compounds (medicinal)	967.3	E852.2	E937.3	E950.2	E962.0	E980.2
Bromisovalum	967.3	E852.2	E937.3	E950.2	E962.0	E980.2
Bromobenzyl cyanide	987.5	E869.3	—	E952.8	E962.2	E982.8
Bromodiphenhydramine	963.0	E858.1	E933.0	E950.4	E962.0	E980.4
Bromoform	967.3	E852.2	E937.3	E950.2	E962.0	E980.2
Bromophenol blue reagent	977.8	E858.8	E947.8	E950.4	E962.0	E980.4
Bromosalicylhydroxamic acid	961.8	E857	E931.8	E950.4	E962.0	E980.4
Bromo-seltzer	965.4	E850.4	E935.4	E950.0	E962.0	E980.0

◄ New   ◄▮ Revised   deleted Deleted   ● Use Additional Digit(s)

Substance	Poisoning	External Cause (E Code)				
		Accident	Therapeutic Use	Suicide Attempt	Assault	Undetermined
Brompheniramine	963.0	E858.1	E933.0	E950.4	E962.0	E980.4
Bromural	967.3	E852.2	E937.3	E950.2	E962.0	E980.2
Brown spider (bite) (venom)	989.5	E905.1	—	E950.9	E962.1	E980.9
Brucia	988.2	E865.3	—	E950.9	E962.1	E980.9
Brucine	989.1	E863.7	—	E950.6	E962.1	E980.7
Brunswick green - *see* Copper	—	—	—	—	—	—
Bruten - *see* Ibuprofen	—	—	—	—	—	—
Bryonia (alba) (dioica)	988.2	E865.4	—	E950.9	E962.1	E980.9
Buclizine	969.5	E853.8	E939.5	E950.3	E962.0	E980.3
Bufferin	965.1	E850.3	E935.3	E950.0	E962.0	E980.0
Bufotenine	969.6	E854.1	E939.6	E950.3	E962.0	E980.3
Buphenine	971.2	E855.5	E941.2	E950.4	E962.0	E980.4
Bupivacaine	968.9	E855.2	E938.9	E950.4	E962.0	E980.4
infiltration (subcutaneous)	968.5	E855.2	E938.5	E950.4	E962.0	E980.4
nerve block (peripheral) (plexus)	968.6	E855.2	E938.6	E950.4	E962.0	E980.4
Busulfan	963.1	E858.1	E933.1	E950.4	E962.0	E980.4
Butabarbital (sodium)	967.0	E851	E937.0	E950.1	E962.0	E980.1
Butabarbitone	967.0	E851	E937.0	E950.1	E962.0	E980.1
Butabarpal	967.0	E851	E937.0	E950.1	E962.0	E980.1
Butacaine	968.5	E855.2	E938.5	E950.4	E962.0	E980.4
Butallylonal	967.0	E851	E937.0	E950.1	E962.0	E980.1
Butane (distributed in mobile container)	987.0	E868.0	—	E951.1	E962.2	E981.1
distributed through pipes	987.0	E867	—	E951.0	E962.2	E981.0
incomplete combustion of - *see* Carbon monoxide, butane	—	—	—	—	—	—
Butanol	980.3	E860.4	—	E950.9	E962.1	E980.9
Butanone	982.8	E862.4	—	E950.9	E962.1	E980.9
Butaperazine	969.1	E853.0	E939.1	E950.3	E962.0	E980.3
Butazolidin	965.5	E850.5	E935.5	E950.0	E962.0	E980.0
Butethal	967.0	E851	E937.0	E950.1	E962.0	E980.1
Butethamate	971.1	E855.4	E941.1	E950.4	E962.0	E980.4
Buthalitone (sodium)	968.3	E855.1	E938.3	E950.4	E962.0	E980.4
Butisol (sodium)	967.0	E851	E937.0	E950.1	E962.0	E980.1
Butobarbital, butobarbitone	967.0	E851	E937.0	E950.1	E962.0	E980.1
Butriptyline	969.05 ◄⠇⠇	E854.0	E939.0	E950.3	E962.0	E980.3
Buttercups	988.2	E865.4	—	E950.9	E962.1	E980.9
Butter of antimony - *see* Antimony	—	—	—	—	—	—
Butyl	—	—	—	—	—	—
acetate (secondary)	982.8	E862.4	—	E950.9	E962.1	E980.9
alcohol	980.3	E860.4	—	E950.9	E962.1	E980.9

◄ New   ◄⠇⠇ Revised   ~~deleted~~ Deleted   ● Use Additional Digit(s)

Substance	Poisoning	External Cause (E Code)				
		Accident	Therapeutic Use	Suicide Attempt	Assault	Undetermined
Butyl *(Continued)*						
carbinol	980.8	E860.8	—	E950.9	E962.1	E980.9
carbitol	982.8	E862.4	—	E950.9	E962.1	E980.9
cellosolve	982.8	E862.4	—	E950.9	E962.1	E980.9
chloral (hydrate)	967.1	E852.0	E937.1	E950.2	E962.0	E980.2
formate	982.8	E862.4	—	E950.9	E962.1	E980.9
scopolammonium bromide	971.1	E855.4	E941.1	E950.4	E962.0	E980.4
Butyn	968.5	E855.2	E938.5	E950.4	E962.0	E980.4
Butyrophenone (-based tranquilizers)	969.2	E853.1	E939.2	E950.3	E962.0	E980.3
Cacodyl, cacodylic acid - *see* Arsenic	—	—	—	—	—	—
Cactinomycin	960.7	E856	E930.7	E950.4	E962.0	E980.4
Cade oil	976.4	E858.7	E946.4	E950.4	E962.0	E980.4
Cadmium (chloride) (compounds) (dust) (fumes) (oxide)	985.5	E866.4	—	E950.9	E962.1	E980.9
sulfide (medicinal) NEC	976.4	E858.7	E946.4	E950.4	E962.0	E980.4
Caffeine	969.71 ◀	E854.2	E939.7	E950.3	E962.0	E980.3
Calabar bean	988.2	E865.4	—	E950.9	E962.1	E980.9
Caladium seguinium	988.2	E865.4	—	E950.9	E962.1	E980.9
Calamine (liniment) (lotion)	976.3	E858.7	E946.3	E950.4	E962.0	E980.4
Calciferol	963.5	E858.1	E933.5	E950.4	E962.0	E980.4
Calcium (salts) NEC	974.5	E858.5	E944.5	E950.4	E962.0	E980.4
acetylsalicylate	965.1	E850.3	E935.3	E950.0	E962.0	E980.0
benzamidosalicylate	961.8	E857	E931.8	E950.4	E962.0	E980.4
carbaspirin	965.1	E850.3	E935.3	E950.0	E962.0	E980.0
carbimide (citrated)	977.3	E858.8	E947.3	E950.4	E962.0	E980.4
carbonate (antacid)	973.0	E858.4	E943.0	E950.4	E962.0	E980.4
cyanide (citrated)	977.3	E858.8	E947.3	E950.4	E962.0	E980.4
dioctyl sulfosuccinate	973.2	E858.4	E943.2	E950.4	E962.0	E980.4
disodium edathamil	963.8	E858.1	E933.8	E950.4	E962.0	E980.4
disodium edetate	963.8	E858.1	E933.8	E950.4	E962.0	E980.4
EDTA	963.8	E858.1	E933.8	E950.4	E962.0	E980.4
hydrate, hydroxide	983.2	E864.2	—	E950.7	E962.1	E980.6
mandelate	961.9	E857	E931.9	E950.4	E962.0	E980.4
oxide	983.2	E864.2	—	E950.7	E962.1	E980.6
Calomel - *see* Mercury, chloride	—	—	—	—	—	—
Caloric agents NEC	974.5	E858.5	E944.5	E950.4	E962.0	E980.4
Calusterone	963.1	E858.1	E933.1	E950.4	E962.0	E980.4
Camoquin	961.4	E857	E931.4	E950.4	E962.0	E980.4
Camphor (oil)	976.1	E858.7	E946.1	E950.4	E962.0	E980.4
Candeptin	976.0	E858.7	E946.0	E950.4	E962.0	E980.4

◀ New   ◀▥ Revised   ~~deleted~~ Deleted   ● Use Additional Digit(s)

TABLE OF DRUGS AND CHEMICALS

Substance	Poisoning	External Cause (E Code)				
		Accident	Therapeutic Use	Suicide Attempt	Assault	Undetermined
Candicidin	976.0	E858.7	E946.0	E950.4	E962.0	E980.4
Cannabinols	969.6	E854.1	E939.6	E950.3	E962.0	E980.3
Cannabis (derivatives) (indica) (sativa)	969.6	E854.1	E939.6	E950.3	E962.0	E980.3
Canned heat	980.1	E860.2	—	E950.9	E962.1	E980.9
Cantharides, cantharidin, cantharis	976.8	E858.7	E946.8	E950.4	E962.0	E980.4
Capillary agents	972.8	E858.3	E942.8	E950.4	E962.0	E980.4
Capreomycin	960.6	E856	E930.6	E950.4	E962.0	E980.4
Captodiame, captodiamine	969.5	E853.8	E939.5	E950.3	E962.0	E980.3
Caramiphen (hydrochloride)	971.1	E855.4	E941.1	E950.4	E962.0	E980.4
Carbachol	971.0	E855.3	E941.0	E950.4	E962.0	E980.4
Carbacrylamine resins	974.5	E858.5	E944.5	E950.4	E962.0	E980.4
Carbamate (sedative)	967.8	E852.8	E937.8	E950.2	E962.0	E980.2
herbicide	989.3	E863.5	—	E950.6	E962.1	E980.7
insecticide	989.3	E863.2	—	E950.6	E962.1	E980.7
Carbamazepine	966.3	E855.0	E936.3	E950.4	E962.0	E980.4
Carbamic esters	967.8	E852.8	E937.8	E950.2	E962.0	E980.2
Carbamide	974.4	E858.5	E944.4	E950.4	E962.0	E980.4
topical	976.8	E858.7	E946.8	E950.4	E962.0	E980.4
Carbamylcholine chloride	971.0	E855.3	E941.0	E950.4	E962.0	E980.4
Carbarsone	961.1	E857	E931.1	E950.4	E962.0	E980.4
Carbaryl	989.3	E863.2	—	E950.6	E962.1	E980.7
Carbaspirin	965.1	E850.3	E935.3	E950.0	E962.0	E980.0
Carbazochrome	972.8	E858.3	E942.8	E950.4	E962.0	E980.4
Carbenicillin	960.0	E856	E930.0	E950.4	E962.0	E980.4
Carbenoxolone	973.8	E858.4	E943.8	E950.4	E962.0	E980.4
Carbetapentane	975.4	E858.6	E945.4	E950.4	E962.0	E980.4
Carbimazole	962.8	E858.0	E932.8	E950.4	E962.0	E980.4
Carbinol	980.1	E860.2	—	E950.9	E962.1	E980.9
Carbinoxamine	963.0	E858.1	E933.0	E950.4	E962.0	E980.4
Carbitol	982.8	E862.4	—	E950.9	E962.1	E980.9
Carbocaine	968.9	E855.2	E938.9	E950.4	E962.0	E980.4
infiltration (subcutaneous)	968.5	E855.2	E938.5	E950.4	E962.0	E980.4
nerve block (peripheral) (plexus)	968.6	E855.2	E938.6	E950.4	E962.0	E980.4
topical (surface)	968.5	E855.2	E938.5	E950.4	E962.0	E980.4
Carbol-fuchsin solution	976.0	E858.7	E946.0	E950.4	E962.0	E980.4
Carbolic acid (see also Phenol)	983.0	E864.0	—	E950.7	E962.1	E980.6
Carbomycin	960.8	E856	E930.8	E950.4	E962.0	E980.4
Carbon	—	—	—	—	—	—
bisulfide (liquid) (vapor)	982.2	E862.4	—	E950.9	E962.1	E980.9

◀ New   ⬅ Revised   ~~deleted~~ Deleted   ● Use Additional Digit(s)

Substance	Poisoning	Accident	Therapeutic Use	Suicide Attempt	Assault	Undetermined
			External Cause (E Code)			
Carbon *(Continued)*						
dioxide (gas)	987.8	E869.8	—	E952.8	E962.2	E982.8
disulfide (liquid) (vapor)	982.2	E862.4	—	E950.9	E962.1	E980.9
monoxide (from incomplete combustion of) (in) NEC	986	E868.9	—	E952.1	E962.2	E982.1
blast furnace gas	986	E868.8	—	E952.1	E962.2	E982.1
butane (distributed in mobile container)	986	E868.0	—	E951.1	E962.2	E981.1
distributed through pipes	986	E867	—	E951.0	E962.2	E981.0
charcoal fumes	986	E868.3	—	E952.1	E962.2	E982.1
coal						
gas (piped)	986	E867	—	E951.0	E962.2	E981.0
solid (in domestic stoves, fireplaces)	986	E868.3	—	E952.1	E962.2	E982.1
coke (in domestic stoves, fireplaces)	986	E868.3	—	E952.1	E962.2	E982.1
exhaust gas (motor) not in transit	986	E868.2	—	E952.0	E962.2	E982.0
combustion engine, any not in watercraft	986	E868.2	—	E952.0	E962.2	E982.0
farm tractor, not in transit	986	E868.2	—	E952.0	E962.2	E982.0
gas engine	986	E868.2	—	E952.0	E962.2	E982.0
motor pump	986	E868.2	—	E952.0	E962.2	E982.0
motor vehicle, not in transit	986	E868.2	—	E952.0	E962.2	E982.0
fuel (in domestic use)	986	E868.3	—	E952.1	E962.2	E982.1
gas (piped)	986	E867	—	E951.0	E962.2	E981.0
in mobile container	986	E868.0	—	E951.1	E962.2	E981.1
utility	986	E868.1	—	E951.8	E962.2	E981.1
in mobile container	986	E868.0	—	E951.1	E962.2	E981.1
piped (natural)	986	E867	—	E951.0	E962.2	E981.0
illuminating gas	986	E868.1	—	E951.8	E962.2	E981.8
industrial fuels or gases, any	986	E868.8	—	E952.1	E962.2	E982.1
kerosene (in domestic stoves, fireplaces)	986	E868.3	—	E952.1	E962.2	E982.1
kiln gas or vapor	986	E868.8	—	E952.1	E962.2	E982.1
motor exhaust gas, not in transit	986	E868.2	—	E952.0	E962.2	E982.0
piped gas (manufactured) (natural)	986	E867	—	E951.0	E962.2	E981.0
producer gas	986	E868.8	—	E952.1	E962.2	E982.1
propane (distributed in mobile container)	986	E868.0	—	E951.1	E962.2	E981.1
distributed through pipes	986	E867	—	E951.0	E962.2	E981.0
specified source NEC	986	E868.8	—	E952.1	E962.2	E982.1
stove gas	986	E868.1	—	E951.8	E962.2	E981.8
piped	986	E867	—	E951.0	E962.2	E981.0
utility gas	986	E868.1	—	E951.8	E962.2	E981.8
piped	986	E867	—	E951.0	E962.2	E981.0

◀ New   ◀═ Revised   ~~deleted~~ Deleted   ● Use Additional Digit(s)

Substance	Poisoning	External Cause (E Code)				
		Accident	Therapeutic Use	Suicide Attempt	Assault	Undetermined
Carbon (Continued)						
monoxide (from incomplete combustion of) (in) NEC (Continued)						
water gas	986	E868.1	—	E951.8	E962.2	E981.8
wood (in domestic stoves, fireplaces)	986	E868.3	—	E952.1	E962.2	E982.1
tetrachloride (vapor) NEC	987.8	E869.8	—	E952.8	E962.2	E982.8
liquid (cleansing agent) NEC	982.1	E861.3	—	E950.9	E962.1	E980.9
solvent	982.1	E862.4	—	E950.9	E962.1	E980.9
Carbonic acid (gas)	987.8	E869.8	—	E952.8	E962.2	E982.8
anhydrase inhibitors	974.2	E858.5	E944.2	E950.4	E962.0	E980.4
Carbowax	976.3	E858.7	E946.3	E950.4	E962.0	E980.4
Carbrital	967.0	E851	E937.0	E950.1	E962.0	E980.1
Carbromal (derivatives)	967.3	E852.2	E937.3	E950.2	E962.0	E980.2
Cardiac	—	—	—	—	—	—
depressants	972.0	E858.3	E942.0	E950.4	E962.0	E980.4
rhythm regulators	972.0	E858.3	E942.0	E950.4	E962.0	E980.4
Cardiografin	977.8	E858.8	E947.8	E950.4	E962.0	E980.4
Cardio-green	977.8	E858.8	E947.8	E950.4	E962.0	E980.4
Cardiotonic glycosides	972.1	E858.3	E942.1	E950.4	E962.0	E980.4
Cardiovascular agents NEC	972.9	E858.3	E942.9	E950.4	E962.0	E980.4
Cardrase	974.2	E858.5	E944.2	E950.4	E962.0	E980.4
Carfusin	976.0	E858.7	E946.0	E950.4	E962.0	E980.4
Carisoprodol	968.0	E855.1	E938.0	E950.4	E962.0	E980.4
Carmustine	963.1	E858.1	E933.1	E950.4	E962.0	E980.4
Carotene	963.5	E858.1	E933.5	E950.4	E962.0	E980.4
Carphenazine (maleate)	969.1	E853.0	E939.1	E950.3	E962.0	E980.3
Carter's Little Pills	973.1	E858.4	E943.1	E950.4	E962.0	E980.4
Cascara (sagrada)	973.1	E858.4	E943.1	E950.4	E962.0	E980.4
Cassava	988.2	E865.4	—	E950.9	E962.1	E980.9
Castellani's paint	976.0	E858.7	E946.0	E950.4	E962.0	E980.4
Castor	—	—	—	—	—	—
bean	988.2	E865.3	—	E950.9	E962.1	E980.9
oil	973.1	E858.4	E943.1	E950.4	E962.0	E980.4
Caterpillar (sting)	989.5	E905.5	—	E950.9	E962.1	E980.9
Catha (edulis)	970.8	E854.3	E940.8	E950.4	E962.0	E980.4
Cathartics NEC	973.3	E858.4	E943.3	E950.4	E962.0	E980.4
contact	973.1	E858.4	E943.1	E950.4	E962.0	E980.4
emollient	973.2	E858.4	E943.2	E950.4	E962.0	E980.4
intestinal irritants	973.1	E858.4	E943.1	E950.4	E962.0	E980.4
saline	973.3	E858.4	E943.3	E950.4	E962.0	E980.4
Cathomycin	960.8	E856	E930.8	E950.4	E962.0	E980.4

◀ New   ◀▥ Revised   d̶e̶l̶e̶t̶e̶d̶ Deleted   ● Use Additional Digit(s)

Substance	Poisoning	External Cause (E Code)				
		Accident	Therapeutic Use	Suicide Attempt	Assault	Undetermined
Caustic(s)	983.9	E864.4	—	E950.7	E962.1	E980.6
alkali	983.2	E864.2	—	E950.7	E962.1	E980.6
hydroxide	983.2	E864.2	—	E950.7	E962.1	E980.6
potash	983.2	E864.2	—	E950.7	E962.1	E980.6
soda	983.2	E864.2	—	E950.7	E962.1	E980.6
specified NEC	983.9	E864.3	—	E950.7	E962.1	E980.6
Ceepryn	976.0	E858.7	E946.0	E950.4	E962.0	E980.4
ENT agent	976.6	E858.7	E946.6	E950.4	E962.0	E980.4
lozenges	976.6	E858.7	E946.6	E950.4	E962.0	E980.4
Celestone	962.0	E858.0	E932.0	E950.4	E962.0	E980.4
topical	976.0	E858.7	E946.0	E950.4	E962.0	E980.4
Cellosolve	982.8	E862.4	—	E950.9	E961.1	E980.9
Cell stimulants and proliferants	976.8	E858.7	E946.8	E950.4	E962.0	E980.4
Cellulose derivatives, cathartic	973.3	E858.4	E943.3	E950.4	E962.0	E980.4
nitrates (topical)	976.3	E858.7	E946.3	E950.4	E962.0	E980.4
Centipede (bite)	989.5	E905.4	—	E950.9	E962.1	E980.9
Central nervous system	—	—	—	—	—	—
depressants	968.4	E855.1	E938.4	E950.4	E962.0	E980.4
anesthetic (general) NEC	968.4	E855.1	E938.4	E950.4	E962.0	E980.4
gases NEC	968.2	E855.1	E938.2	E950.4	E962.0	E980.4
intravenous	968.3	E855.1	E938.3	E950.4	E962.0	E980.4
barbiturates	967.0	E851	E937.0	E950.1	E962.0	E980.1
bromides	967.3	E852.2	E937.3	E950.2	E962.0	E980.2
cannabis sativa	969.6	E854.1	E939.6	E950.3	E962.0	E980.3
chloral hydrate	967.1	E852.0	E937.1	E950.2	E962.0	E980.2
hallucinogenics	969.6	E854.1	E939.6	E950.3	E962.0	E980.3
hypnotics	967.9	E852.9	E937.9	E950.2	E962.0	E980.2
specified NEC	967.8	E852.8	E937.8	E950.2	E962.0	E980.2
muscle relaxants	968.0	E855.1	E938.0	E950.4	E962.0	E980.4
paraldehyde	967.2	E852.1	E937.2	E950.2	E962.0	E980.2
sedatives	967.9	E852.9	E937.9	E950.2	E962.0	E980.2
mixed NEC	967.6	E852.5	E937.6	E950.2	E962.0	E980.2
specified NEC	967.8	E852.8	E937.8	E950.2	E962.0	E980.2
muscle-tone depressants	968.0	E855.1	E938.0	E950.4	E962.0	E980.4
stimulants	970.9	E854.3	E940.9	E950.4	E962.0	E980.4
amphetamines	969.72 ◀	E854.2	E939.7	E950.3	E962.0	E980.3
analeptics	970.0	E854.3	E940.0	E950.4	E962.0	E980.4
antidepressants	969.00 ◀	E854.0	E939.0	E950.3	E962.0	E980.3
opiate antagonists	970.1	E854.3	E940.0	E950.4	E962.0	E980.4
specified NEC	970.8	E854.3	E940.8	E950.4	E962.0	E980.4

◀ New   ◀▦ Revised   ~~deleted~~ Deleted   ● Use Additional Digit(s)

Substance	Poisoning	External Cause (E Code)				
		Accident	Therapeutic Use	Suicide Attempt	Assault	Undetermined
Cephalexin	960.5	E856	E930.5	E950.4	E962.0	E980.4
Cephaloglycin	960.5	E856	E930.5	E950.4	E962.0	E980.4
Cephaloridine	960.5	E856	E930.5	E950.4	E962.0	E980.4
Cephalosporins NEC	960.5	E856	E930.5	E950.4	E962.0	E980.4
N (adicillin)	960.0	E856	E930.0	E950.4	E962.0	E980.4
Cephalothin (sodium)	960.5	E856	E930.5	E950.4	E962.0	E980.4
Cerbera (odallam)	988.2	E865.4	—	E950.9	E962.1	E980.9
Cerberin	972.1	E858.3	E942.1	E950.4	E962.0	E980.4
Cerebral stimulants	970.9	E854.3	E940.9	E950.4	E962.0	E980.4
psychotherapeutic	969.79 ◀▥	E854.2	E939.7	E950.3	E962.0	E980.3
specified NEC	970.8	E854.3	E940.8	E950.4	E962.0	E980.4
Cetalkonium (chloride)	976.0	E858.7	E946.0	E950.4	E962.0	E980.4
Cetoxime	963.0	E858.1	E933.0	E950.4	E962.0	E980.4
Cetrimide	976.2	E858.7	E946.2	E950.4	E962.0	E980.4
Cetylpyridinium	976.0	E858.7	E946.0	E950.4	E962.0	E980.4
ENT agent	976.6	E858.7	E946.6	E950.4	E962.0	E980.4
lozenges	976.6	E858.7	E946.6	E950.4	E962.0	E980.4
Cevadilla - *see* Sabadilla	—	—	—	—	—	—
Cevitamic acid	963.5	E858.1	E933.5	E950.4	E962.0	E980.4
Chalk, precipitated	973.0	E858.4	E943.0	E950.4	E962.0	E980.4
Charcoal	—	—	—	—	—	—
fumes (carbon monoxide)	986	E868.3	—	E952.1	E962.2	E982.1
industrial	986	E868.8	—	E952.1	E962.2	E982.1
medicinal (activated)	973.0	E858.4	E943.0	E950.4	E962.0	E980.4
Chelating agents NEC	977.2	E858.8	E947.2	E950.4	E962.0	E980.4
Chelidonium majus	988.2	E865.4	—	E950.9	E962.1	E980.9
Chemical substance	989.9	E866.9	—	E950.9	E962.1	E980.9
specified NEC	989.89	E866.8	—	E950.9	E962.1	E980.9
Chemotherapy, antineoplastic	963.1	E858.1	E933.1	E950.4	E962.0	E980.4
Chenopodium (oil)	961.6	E857	E931.6	E950.4	E962.0	E980.4
Cherry laurel	988.2	E865.4	—	E950.9	E962.1	E980.9
Chiniofon	961.3	E857	E931.3	E950.4	E962.0	E980.4
Chlophedianol	975.4	E858.6	E945.4	E950.4	E962.0	E980.4
Chloral (betaine) (formamide) (hydrate)	967.1	E852.0	E937.1	E950.2	E962.0	E980.2
Chloralamide	967.1	E852.0	E937.1	E950.2	E962.0	E980.2
Chlorambucil	963.1	E858.1	E933.1	E950.4	E962.0	E980.4
Chloramphenicol	960.2	E856	E930.2	E950.4	E962.0	E980.4
ENT agent	976.6	E858.7	E946.6	E950.4	E962.0	E980.4
ophthalmic preparation	976.5	E858.7	E946.5	E950.4	E962.0	E980.4
topical NEC	976.0	E858.7	E946.0	E950.4	E962.0	E980.4

◀ New   ◀▥ Revised   ~~deleted~~ Deleted   ● Use Additional Digit(s)

| | | External Cause (E Code) | | | |
Substance	Poisoning	Accident	Therapeutic Use	Suicide Attempt	Assault	Undetermined
Chlorate(s) (potassium) (sodium) NEC	983.9	E864.3	—	E950.7	E962.1	E980.6
herbicides	989.4	E863.5	—	E950.6	E962.1	E980.7
Chlorcyclizine	963.0	E858.1	E933.0	E950.4	E962.0	E980.4
Chlordan(e) (dust)	989.2	E863.0	—	E950.6	E962.1	E980.7
Chlordantoin	976.0	E858.7	E946.0	E950.4	E962.0	E980.4
Chlordiazepoxide	969.4	E853.2	E939.4	E950.3	E962.0	E980.3
Chloresium	976.8	E858.7	E946.8	E950.4	E962.0	E980.4
Chlorethiazol	967.1	E852.0	E937.1	E950.2	E962.0	E980.2
Chlorethyl - *see* Ethyl, chloride	—	—	—	—	—	—
Chloretone	967.1	E852.0	E937.1	E950.2	E962.0	E980.2
Chlorex	982.3	E862.4	—	E950.9	E962.1	E980.9
Chlorhexadol	967.1	E852.0	E937.1	E950.2	E962.0	E980.2
Chlorhexidine (hydrochloride)	976.0	E858.7	E946.0	E950.4	E962.0	E980.4
Chlorhydroxyquinolin	976.0	E858.7	E946.0	E950.4	E962.0	E980.4
Chloride of lime (bleach)	983.9	E864.3	—	E950.7	E962.1	E980.6
Chlorinated	—	—	—	—	—	—
camphene	989.2	E863.0	—	E950.6	E962.1	E980.7
diphenyl	989.89	E866.8	—	E950.9	E962.1	E980.9
hydrocarbons NEC	989.2	E863.0	—	E950.6	E962.1	E980.7
solvent	982.3	E862.4	—	E950.9	E962.1	E980.9
lime (bleach)	983.9	E864.3	—	E950.7	E962.1	E980.6
naphthalene - *see* Naphthalene	—	—	—	—	—	—
pesticides NEC	989.2	E863.0	—	E950.6	E962.1	E980.7
soda - *see* Sodium, hypochlorite	—	—	—	—	—	—
Chlorine (fumes) (gas)	987.6	E869.8	—	E952.8	E962.2	E982.8
bleach	983.9	E864.3	—	E950.7	E962.1	E980.6
compounds NEC	983.9	E864.3	—	E950.7	E962.1	E980.6
disinfectant	983.9	E861.4	—	E950.7	E962.1	E980.6
releasing agents NEC	983.9	E864.3	—	E950.7	E962.1	E980.6
Chlorisondamine	972.3	E858.3	E942.3	E950.4	E962.0	E980.4
Chlormadinone	962.2	E858.0	E932.2	E950.4	E962.0	E980.4
Chlormerodrin	974.0	E858.5	E944.0	E950.4	E962.0	E980.4
Chlormethiazole	967.1	E852.0	E937.1	E950.2	E962.0	E980.2
Chlormethylenecycline	960.4	E856	E930.4	E950.4	E962.0	E980.4
Chlormezanone	969.5	E853.8	E939.5	E950.3	E962.0	E980.3
Chloroacetophenone	987.5	E869.3	—	E952.8	E962.2	E982.8
Chloroaniline	983.0	E864.0	—	E950.7	E962.1	E980.6
Chlorobenzene, chlorobenzol	982.0	E862.4	—	E950.9	E962.1	E980.9
Chlorobutanol	967.1	E852.0	E937.1	E950.2	E962.0	E980.2

◀ New　◀▥ Revised　~~deleted~~ Deleted　● Use Additional Digit(s)

Substance	Poisoning	External Cause (E Code)				
		Accident	Therapeutic Use	Suicide Attempt	Assault	Undetermined
Chlorodinitrobenzene	983.0	E864.0	—	E950.7	E962.1	E980.6
dust or vapor	987.8	E869.8	—	E952.8	E962.2	E982.8
Chloroethane - *see* Ethyl, chloride	—	—	—	—	—	—
Chloroform (fumes) (vapor)	987.8	E869.8	—	E952.8	E962.2	E982.8
anesthetic (gas)	968.2	E855.1	E938.2	E950.4	E962.0	E980.4
liquid NEC	968.4	E855.1	E938.4	E950.4	E962.0	E980.4
solvent	982.3	E862.4	—	E950.9	E962.1	E980.9
Chloroguanide	961.4	E857	E931.4	E950.4	E962.0	E980.4
Chloromycetin	960.2	E856	E930.2	E950.4	E962.0	E980.4
ENT agent	976.6	E858.7	E946.6	E950.4	E962.0	E980.4
ophthalmic preparation	976.5	E858.7	E946.5	E950.4	E962.0	E980.4
otic solution	976.6	E858.7	E946.6	E950.4	E962.0	E980.4
topical NEC	976.0	E858.7	E946.0	E950.4	E962.0	E980.4
Chloronitrobenzene	983.0	E864.0	—	E950.7	E962.1	E980.6
dust or vapor	987.8	E869.8	—	E952.8	E962.2	E982.8
Chlorophenol	983.0	E864.0	—	E950.7	E962.1	E980.6
Chlorophenothane	989.2	E863.0	—	E950.6	E962.1	E980.7
Chlorophyll (derivatives)	976.8	E858.7	E946.8	E950.4	E962.0	E980.4
Chloropicrin (fumes)	987.8	E869.8	—	E952.8	E962.2	E982.8
fumigant	989.4	E863.8	—	E950.6	E962.1	E980.7
fungicide	989.4	E863.6	—	E950.6	E962.1	E980.7
pesticide (fumes)	989.4	E863.4	—	E950.6	E962.1	E980.7
Chloroprocaine	968.9	E855.2	E938.9	E950.4	E962.0	E980.4
infiltration (subcutaneous)	968.5	E855.2	E938.5	E950.4	E962.0	E980.4
nerve block (peripheral) (plexus)	968.6	E855.2	E938.6	E950.4	E962.0	E980.4
Chloroptic	976.5	E858.7	E946.5	E950.4	E962.0	E980.4
Chloropurine	963.1	E858.1	E933.1	E950.4	E962.0	E980.4
Chloroquine (hydrochloride) (phosphate)	961.4	E857	E931.4	E950.4	E962.0	E980.4
Chlorothen	963.0	E858.1	E933.0	E950.4	E962.0	E980.4
Chlorothiazide	974.3	E858.5	E944.3	E950.4	E962.0	E980.4
Chlorotrianisene	962.2	E858.0	E932.2	E950.4	E962.0	E980.4
Chlorovinyldichloroarsine	985.1	E866.3	—	E950.8	E962.1	E980.8
Chloroxylenol	976.0	E858.7	E946.0	E950.4	E962.0	E980.4
Chlorphenesin (carbamate)	968.0	E855.1	E938.0	E950.4	E962.0	E980.4
topical (antifungal)	976.0	E858.7	E946.0	E950.4	E962.0	E980.4
Chlorpheniramine	963.0	E858.1	E933.0	E950.4	E962.0	E980.4
Chlorphenoxamine	966.4	E855.0	E936.4	E950.4	E962.0	E980.4
Chlorphentermine	977.0	E858.8	E947.0	E950.4	E962.0	E980.4
Chlorproguanil	961.4	E857	E931.4	E950.4	E962.0	E980.4

◀ New ◀▥ Revised ~~deleted~~ Deleted ● Use Additional Digit(s)

Substance	Poisoning	External Cause (E Code)				
		Accident	Therapeutic Use	Suicide Attempt	Assault	Undetermined
Chlorpromazine	969.1	E853.0	E939.1	E950.3	E962.0	E980.3
Chlorpropamide	962.3	E858.0	E932.3	E950.4	E962.0	E980.4
Chlorprothixene	969.3	E853.8	E939.3	E950.3	E962.0	E980.3
Chlorquinaldol	976.0	E858.7	E946.0	E950.4	E962.0	E980.4
Chlortetracycline	960.4	E856	E930.4	E950.4	E962.0	E980.4
Chlorthalidone	974.4	E858.5	E944.4	E950.4	E962.0	E980.4
Chlortrianisene	962.2	E858.0	E932.2	E950.4	E962.0	E980.4
Chlor-Trimeton	963.0	E858.1	E933.0	E950.4	E962.0	E980.4
Chlorzoxazone	968.0	E855.1	E938.0	E950.4	E962.0	E980.4
Choke damp	987.8	E869.8	—	E952.8	E962.2	E982.8
Cholebrine	977.8	E858.8	E947.8	E950.4	E962.0	E980.4
Cholera vaccine	978.2	E858.8	E948.2	E950.4	E962.0	E980.4
Cholesterol-lowering agents	972.2	E858.3	E942.2	E950.4	E962.0	E980.4
Cholestyramine (resin)	972.2	E858.3	E942.2	E950.4	E962.0	E980.4
Cholic acid	973.4	E858.4	E943.4	E950.4	E962.0	E980.4
Choline	—	—	—	—	—	—
dihydrogen citrate	977.1	E858.8	E947.1	E950.4	E962.0	E980.4
salicylate	965.1	E850.3	E935.3	E950.0	E962.0	E980.0
theophyllinate	974.1	E858.5	E944.1	E950.4	E962.0	E980.4
Cholinergics	971.0	E855.3	E941.0	E950.4	E962.0	E980.4
Cholografin	977.8	E858.8	E947.8	E950.4	E962.0	E980.4
Chorionic gonadotropin	962.4	E858.0	E932.4	E950.4	E962.0	E980.4
Chromates	983.9	E864.3	—	E950.7	E962.1	E980.6
dust or mist	987.8	E869.8	—	E952.8	E962.2	E982.8
lead	984.0	E866.0	—	E950.9	E962.1	E980.9
paint	984.0	E861.5	—	E950.9	E962.1	E980.9
Chromic acid	983.9	E864.3	—	E950.7	E962.1	E980.6
dust or mist	987.8	E869.8	—	E952.8	E962.2	E982.8
Chromium	985.6	E866.4	—	E950.9	E962.1	E980.9
compounds - *see* Chromates	—	—	—	—	—	—
Chromonar	972.4	E858.3	E942.4	E950.4	E962.0	E980.4
Chromyl chloride	983.9	E864.3	—	E950.7	E962.1	E980.6
Chrysarobin (ointment)	976.4	E858.7	E946.4	E950.4	E962.0	E980.4
Chrysazin	973.1	E858.4	E943.1	E950.4	E962.0	E980.4
Chymar	963.4	E858.1	E933.4	E950.4	E962.0	E980.4
ophthalmic preparation	976.5	E858.7	E946.5	E950.4	E962.0	E980.4
Chymotrypsin	963.4	E858.1	E933.4	E950.4	E962.0	E980.4
ophthalmic preparation	976.5	E858.7	E946.5	E950.4	E962.0	E980.4
Cicuta maculata or virosa	988.2	E865.4	—	E950.9	E962.1	E980.9

◄ New   ◄⦚ Revised   ~~deleted~~ Deleted   ● Use Additional Digit(s)   637

TABLE OF DRUGS AND CHEMICALS

		External Cause (E Code)				
Substance	**Poisoning**	**Accident**	**Therapeutic Use**	**Suicide Attempt**	**Assault**	**Undetermined**
Cigarette lighter fluid	981	E862.1	—	E950.9	E962.1	E980.9
Cinchocaine (spinal)	968.7	E855.2	E938.7	E950.4	E962.0	E980.4
topical (surface)	968.5	E855.2	E938.5	E950.4	E962.0	E980.4
Cinchona	961.4	E857	E931.4	E950.4	E962.0	E980.4
Cinchonine alkaloids	961.4	E857	E931.4	E950.4	E962.0	E980.4
Cinchophen	974.7	E858.5	E944.7	E950.4	E962.0	E980.4
Cinnarizine	963.0	E858.1	E933.0	E950.4	E962.0	E980.4
Citanest	968.9	E855.2	E938.9	E950.4	E962.0	E980.4
infiltration (subcutaneous)	968.5	E855.2	E938.5	E950.4	E962.0	E980.4
nerve block (peripheral) (plexus)	968.6	E855.2	E938.6	E950.4	E962.0	E980.4
Citric acid	989.89	E866.8	—	E950.9	E962.1	E980.9
Citrovorum factor	964.1	E858.2	E934.1	E950.4	E962.0	E980.4
Claviceps purpurea	988.2	E865.4	—	E950.9	E962.1	E980.9
Cleaner, cleansing agent NEC	989.89	E861.3	—	E950.9	E962.1	E980.9
of paint or varnish	982.8	E862.9	—	E950.9	E962.1	E980.9
Clematis vitalba	988.2	E865.4	—	E950.9	E962.1	E980.9
Clemizole	963.0	E858.1	E933.0	E950.4	E962.0	E980.4
penicillin	960.0	E856	E930.0	E950.4	E962.0	E980.4
Clidinium	971.1	E855.4	E941.1	E950.4	E962.0	E980.4
Clindamycin	960.8	E856	E930.8	E950.4	E962.0	E980.4
Cliradon	965.09	E850.2	E935.2	E950.0	E962.0	E980.0
Clocortolone	962.0	E858.0	E932.0	E950.4	E962.0	E980.4
Clofedanol	975.4	E858.6	E945.4	E950.4	E962.0	E980.4
Clofibrate	972.2	E858.3	E942.2	E950.4	E962.0	E980.4
Clomethiazole	967.1	E852.0	E937.1	E950.2	E962.0	E980.2
Clomiphene	977.8	E858.8	E947.8	E950.4	E962.0	E980.4
Clonazepam	969.4	E853.2	E939.4	E950.3	E962.0	E980.3
Clonidine	972.6	E858.3	E942.6	E950.4	E962.0	E980.4
Clopamide	974.3	E858.5	E944.3	E950.4	E962.0	E980.4
Clorazepate	969.4	E853.2	E939.4	E950.3	E962.0	E980.3
Clorexolone	974.4	E858.5	E944.4	E950.4	E962.0	E980.4
Clorox (bleach)	983.9	E864.3	—	E950.7	E962.1	E980.6
Clortermine	977.0	E858.8	E947.0	E950.4	E962.0	E980.4
Clotrimazole	976.0	E858.7	E946.0	E950.4	E962.0	E980.4
Cloxacillin	960.0	E856	E930.0	E950.4	E962.0	E980.4
Coagulants NEC	964.5	E858.2	E934.5	E950.4	E962.0	E980.4
Coal (carbon monoxide from) - *see also* Carbon, monoxide, coal	—	—	—	—	—	—
oil - *see* Kerosene	—	—	—	—	—	—

◄ New   ◄■ Revised   ~~deleted~~ Deleted   ● Use Additional Digit(s)

Substance	Poisoning	Accident	Therapeutic Use	Suicide Attempt	Assault	Undetermined
Coal (carbon monoxide from) *(Continued)*						
tar NEC	983.0	E864.0	—	E950.7	E962.1	E980.6
fumes	987.8	E869.8	—	E952.8	E962.2	E982.8
medicinal (ointment)	976.4	E858.7	E946.4	E950.4	E962.0	E980.4
analgesics NEC	965.5	E850.5	E935.5	E950.0	E962.0	E980.0
naphtha (solvent)	981	E862.0	—	E950.9	E962.1	E980.9
Cobalt (fumes) (industrial)	985.8	E866.4	—	E950.9	E962.1	E980.9
Cobra (venom)	989.5	E905.0	—	E950.9	E962.1	E980.9
Coca (leaf)	970.8	E854.3	E940.8	E950.4	E962.0	E980.4
Cocaine (hydrochloride) (salt)	970.8	E854.3	E940.8	E950.4	E962.0	E980.4
topical anesthetic	968.5	E855.2	E938.5	E950.4	E962.0	E980.4
Coccidioidin	977.8	E858.8	E947.8	E950.4	E962.0	E980.4
Cocculus indicus	988.2	E865.3	—	E950.9	E962.1	E980.9
Cochineal	989.89	E866.8	—	E950.9	E962.1	E980.9
medicinal products	977.4	E858.8	E947.4	E950.4	E962.0	E980.4
Codeine	965.09	E850.2	E935.2	E950.0	E962.0	E980.0
Coffee	989.89	E866.8	—	E950.9	E962.1	E980.9
Cogentin	971.1	E855.4	E941.1	E950.4	E962.0	E980.4
Coke fumes or gas (carbon monoxide)	986	E868.3	—	E952.1	E962.2	E982.1
industrial use	986	E868.8	—	E952.1	E962.2	E982.1
Colace	973.2	E858.4	E943.2	E950.4	E962.0	E980.4
Colchicine	974.7	E858.5	E944.7	E950.4	E962.0	E980.4
Colchicum	988.2	E865.3	—	E950.9	E962.1	E980.9
Cold cream	976.3	E858.7	E946.3	E950.4	E962.0	E980.4
Colestipol	972.2	E858.3	E942.2	E950.4	E962.0	E980.4
Colistimethate	960.8	E856	E930.8	E950.4	E962.0	E980.4
Colistin	960.8	E856	E930.8	E950.4	E962.0	E980.4
Collagen	977.8	E866.8	E947.8	E950.9	E962.1	E980.9
Collagenase	976.8	E858.7	E946.8	E950.4	E962.0	E980.4
Collodion (flexible)	976.3	E858.7	E946.3	E950.4	E962.0	E980.4
Colocynth	973.1	E858.4	E943.1	E950.4	E962.0	E980.4
Coloring matter - *see* Dye(s)	—	—	—	—	—	—
Combustion gas - *see* Carbon, monoxide	—	—	—	—	—	—
Compazine	969.1	E853.0	E939.1	E950.3	E962.0	E980.3
Compound	—	—	—	—	—	—
42 (warfarin)	989.4	E863.7	—	E950.6	E962.1	E980.7
269 (endrin)	989.2	E863.0	—	E950.6	E962.1	E980.7
497 (dieldrin)	989.2	E863.0	—	E950.6	E962.1	E980.7

		External Cause (E Code)				
Substance	**Poisoning**	**Accident**	**Therapeutic Use**	**Suicide Attempt**	**Assault**	**Undetermined**
Compound *(Continued)*						
1080 (sodium fluoroacetate)	989.4	E863.7	—	E950.6	E962.1	E980.7
3422 (parathion)	989.3	E863.1	—	E950.6	E962.1	E980.7
3911 (phorate)	989.3	E863.1	—	E950.6	E962.1	E980.7
3956 (toxaphene)	989.2	E863.0	—	E950.6	E962.1	E980.7
4049 (malathion)	989.3	E863.1	—	E950.6	E962.1	E980.7
4124 (dicapthon)	989.4	E863.4	—	E950.6	E962.1	E980.7
E (cortisone)	962.0	E858.0	E932.0	E950.4	E962.0	E980.4
F (hydrocortisone)	962.0	E858.0	E932.0	E950.4	E962.0	E980.4
Congo red	977.8	E858.8	E947.8	E950.4	E962.0	E980.4
Coniine, conine	965.7	E850.7	E935.7	E950.0	E962.0	E980.0
Conium (maculatum)	988.2	E865.4	—	E950.9	E962.1	E980.9
Conjugated estrogens (equine)	962.2	E858.0	E932.2	E950.4	E962.0	E980.4
Contac	975.6	E858.6	E945.6	E950.4	E962.0	E980.4
Contact lens solution	976.5	E858.7	E946.5	E950.4	E962.0	E980.4
Contraceptives (oral)	962.2	E858.0	E932.2	E950.4	E962.0	E980.4
vaginal	976.8	E858.7	E946.8	E950.4	E962.0	E980.4
Contrast media (roentgenographic)	977.8	E858.8	E947.8	E950.4	E962.0	E980.4
Convallaria majalis	988.2	E865.4	—	E950.9	E962.1	E980.9
Copper (dust) (fumes) (salts) NEC	985.8	E866.4	—	E950.9	E962.1	E980.9
arsenate, arsenite	985.1	E866.3	—	E950.8	E962.1	E980.8
insecticide	985.1	E863.4	—	E950.8	E962.1	E980.8
emetic	973.6	E858.4	E943.6	E950.4	E962.0	E980.4
fungicide	985.8	E863.6	—	E950.6	E962.1	E980.7
insecticide	985.8	E863.4	—	E950.6	E962.1	E980.7
oleate	976.0	E858.7	E946.0	E950.4	E962.0	E980.4
sulfate	983.9	E864.3	—	E950.7	E962.1	E980.6
fungicide	983.9	E863.6	—	E950.7	E962.1	E980.6
cupric	973.6	E858.4	E943.6	E950.4	E962.0	E980.4
cuprous	983.9	E864.3	—	E950.7	E962.1	E980.6
Copperhead snake (bite) (venom)	989.5	E905.0	—	E950.9	E962.1	E980.9
Coral (sting)	989.5	E905.6	—	E950.9	E962.1	E980.9
snake (bite) (venom)	989.5	E905.0	—	E950.9	E962.1	E980.9
Cordran	976.0	E858.7	E946.0	E950.4	E962.0	E980.4
Corn cures	976.4	E858.7	E946.4	E950.4	E962.0	E980.4
Cornhusker's lotion	976.3	E858.7	E946.3	E950.4	E962.0	E980.4
Corn starch	976.3	E858.7	E946.3	E950.4	E962.0	E980.4
Corrosive	983.9	E864.4	—	E950.7	E962.1	E980.6
acids NEC	983.1	E864.1	—	E950.7	E962.1	E980.6

◀ New   ◀▥ Revised   ~~deleted~~ Deleted   ● Use Additional Digit(s)

	External Cause (E Code)					
Substance	**Poisoning**	**Accident**	**Therapeutic Use**	**Suicide Attempt**	**Assault**	**Undetermined**
Corrosive *(Continued)*						
aromatics	983.0	E864.0	—	E950.7	E962.1	E980.6
disinfectant	983.0	E861.4	—	E950.7	E962.1	E980.6
fumes NEC	987.9	E869.9	—	E952.9	E962.2	E982.9
specified NEC	983.9	E864.3	—	E950.7	E962.1	E980.6
sublimate - *see* Mercury, chloride	—	—	—	—	—	—
Cortate	962.0	E858.0	E932.0	E950.4	E962.0	E980.4
Cort-Dome	962.0	E858.0	E932.0	E950.4	E962.0	E980.4
ENT agent	976.6	E858.7	E946.6	E950.4	E962.0	E980.4
ophthalmic preparation	976.5	E858.7	E946.5	E950.4	E962.0	E980.4
topical NEC	976.0	E858.7	E946.0	E950.4	E962.0	E980.4
Cortef	962.0	E858.0	E932.0	E950.4	E962.0	E980.4
ENT agent	976.6	E858.7	E946.6	E950.4	E962.0	E980.4
ophthalmic preparation	976.5	E858.7	E946.5	E950.4	E962.0	E980.4
topical NEC	976.0	E858.7	E946.0	E950.4	E962.0	E980.4
Corticosteroids (fluorinated)	962.0	E858.0	E932.0	E950.4	E962.0	E980.4
ENT agent	976.6	E858.7	E946.6	E950.4	E962.0	E980.4
ophthalmic preparation	976.5	E858.7	E946.5	E950.4	E962.0	E980.4
topical NEC	976.0	E858.7	E946.0	E950.4	E962.0	E980.4
Corticotropin	962.4	E858.0	E932.4	E950.4	E962.0	E980.4
Cortisol	962.0	E858.0	E932.0	E950.4	E962.0	E980.4
ENT agent	976.6	E858.7	E946.6	E950.4	E962.0	E980.4
ophthalmic preparation	976.5	E858.7	E946.5	E950.4	E962.0	E980.4
topical NEC	976.0	E858.7	E946.0	E950.4	E962.0	E980.4
Cortisone derivatives (acetate)	962.0	E858.0	E932.0	E950.4	E962.0	E980.4
ENT agent	976.6	E858.7	E946.6	E950.4	E962.0	E980.4
ophthalmic preparation	976.5	E858.7	E946.5	E950.4	E962.0	E980.4
topical NEC	976.0	E858.7	E946.0	E950.4	E962.0	E980.4
Cortogen	962.0	E858.0	E932.0	E950.4	E962.0	E980.4
ENT agent	976.6	E858.7	E946.6	E950.4	E962.0	E980.4
ophthalmic preparation	976.5	E858.7	E946.5	E950.4	E962.0	E980.4
Cortone	962.0	E858.0	E932.0	E950.4	E962.0	E980.4
ENT agent	976.6	E858.7	E946.6	E950.4	E962.0	E980.4
ophthalmic preparation	976.5	E858.7	E946.5	E950.4	E962.0	E980.4
Cortril	962.0	E858.0	E932.0	E950.4	E962.0	E980.4
ENT agent	976.6	E858.7	E946.6	E950.4	E962.0	E980.4
ophthalmic preparation	976.5	E858.7	E946.5	E950.4	E962.0	E980.4
topical NEC	976.0	E858.7	E946.0	E950.4	E962.0	E980.4
Cosmetics	989.89	E866.7	—	E950.9	E962.1	E980.9

TABLE OF DRUGS AND CHEMICALS

Substance	Poisoning	External Cause (E Code)				
		Accident	Therapeutic Use	Suicide Attempt	Assault	Undetermined
Cosyntropin	977.8	E858.8	E947.8	E950.4	E962.0	E980.4
Cotarnine	964.5	E858.2	E934.5	E950.4	E962.0	E980.4
Cottonseed oil	976.3	E858.7	E946.3	E950.4	E962.0	E980.4
Cough mixtures (antitussives)	975.4	E858.6	E945.4	E950.4	E962.0	E980.4
containing opiates	965.09	E850.2	E935.2	E950.0	E962.0	E980.0
expectorants	975.5	E858.6	E945.5	E950.4	E962.0	E980.4
Coumadin	964.2	E858.2	E934.2	E950.4	E962.0	E980.4
rodenticide	989.4	E863.7	—	E950.6	E962.1	E980.7
Coumarin	964.2	E858.2	E934.2	E950.4	E962.0	E980.4
Coumetarol	964.2	E858.2	E934.2	E950.4	E962.0	E980.4
Cowbane	988.2	E865.4	—	E950.9	E962.1	E980.9
Cozyme	963.5	E858.1	E933.5	E950.4	E962.0	E980.4
Crack	970.8	E854.3	E940.8	E950.4	E962.0	E980.4
Creolin	983.0	E864.0	—	E950.7	E962.1	E980.6
disinfectant	983.0	E861.4	—	E950.7	E962.1	E980.6
Creosol (compound)	983.0	E864.0	—	E950.7	E962.1	E980.6
Creosote (beechwood) (coal tar)	983.0	E864.0	—	E950.7	E962.1	E980.6
medicinal (expectorant)	975.5	E858.6	E945.5	E950.4	E962.0	E980.4
syrup	975.5	E858.6	E945.5	E950.4	E962.0	E980.4
Cresol	983.0	E864.0	—	E950.7	E962.1	E980.6
disinfectant	983.0	E861.4	—	E950.7	E962.1	E980.6
Cresylic acid	983.0	E864.0	—	E950.7	E962.1	E980.6
Cropropamide	965.7	E850.7	E935.7	E950.0	E962.0	E980.0
with crotethamide	970.0	E854.3	E940.0	E950.4	E962.0	E980.4
Crotamiton	976.0	E858.7	E946.0	E950.4	E962.0	E980.4
Crotethamide	965.7	E850.7	E935.7	E950.0	E962.0	E980.0
with cropropamide	970.0	E854.3	E940.0	E950.4	E962.0	E980.4
Croton (oil)	973.1	E858.4	E943.1	E950.4	E962.0	E980.4
chloral	967.1	E852.0	E937.1	E950.2	E962.0	E980.2
Crude oil	981	E862.1	—	E950.9	E962.1	E980.9
Cryogenine	965.8	E850.8	E935.8	E950.0	E962.0	E980.0
Cryolite (pesticide)	989.4	E863.4	—	E950.6	E962.1	E980.7
Cryptenamine	972.6	E858.3	E942.6	E950.4	E962.0	E980.4
Crystal violet	976.0	E858.7	E946.0	E950.4	E962.0	E980.4
Cuckoopint	988.2	E865.4	—	E950.9	E962.1	E980.9
Cumetharol	964.2	E858.2	E934.2	E950.4	E962.0	E980.4
Cupric sulfate	973.6	E858.4	E943.6	E950.4	E962.0	E980.4
Cuprous sulfate	983.9	E864.3	—	E950.7	E962.1	E980.6
Curare, curarine	975.2	E858.6	E945.2	E950.4	E962.0	E980.4

◀ New   ◀▥ Revised   ~~deleted~~ Deleted   ● Use Additional Digit(s)

Substance	Poisoning	External Cause (E Code)				
		Accident	Therapeutic Use	Suicide Attempt	Assault	Undetermined
Cyanic acid - *see* Cyanide(s)	—	—	—	—	—	—
Cyanide(s) (compounds) (hydrogen) (potassium) (sodium) NEC	989.0	E866.8	—	E950.9	E962.1	E980.9
dust or gas (inhalation) NEC	987.7	E869.8	—	E952.8	E962.2	E982.8
fumigant	989.0	E863.8	—	E950.6	E962.1	E980.7
mercuric - *see* Mercury	—	—	—	—	—	—
pesticide (dust) (fumes)	989.0	E863.4	—	E950.6	E962.1	E980.7
Cyanocobalamin	964.1	E858.2	E934.1	E950.4	E962.0	E980.4
Cyanogen (chloride) (gas)	—	—	—	—	—	—
NEC	987.8	E869.8	—	E952.8	E962.2	E982.8
Cyclaine	968.5	E855.2	E938.5	E950.4	E962.0	E980.4
Cyclamen europaeum	988.2	E865.4	—	E950.9	E962.1	E980.9
Cyclandelate	972.5	E858.3	E942.5	E950.4	E962.0	E980.4
Cyclazocine	965.09	E850.2	E935.2	E950.0	E962.0	E980.0
Cyclizine	963.0	E858.1	E933.0	E950.4	E962.0	E980.4
Cyclobarbital, cyclobarbitone	967.0	E851	E937.0	E950.1	E962.0	E980.1
Cycloguanil	961.4	E857	E931.4	E950.4	E962.0	E980.4
Cyclohexane	982.0	E862.4	—	E950.9	E962.1	E980.9
Cyclohexanol	980.8	E860.8	—	E950.9	E962.1	E980.9
Cyclohexanone	982.8	E862.4	—	E950.9	E962.1	E980.9
Cyclomethycaine	968.5	E855.2	E938.5	E950.4	E962.0	E980.4
Cyclopentamine	971.2	E855.5	E941.2	E950.4	E962.0	E980.4
Cyclopenthiazide	974.3	E858.5	E944.3	E950.4	E962.0	E980.4
Cyclopentolate	971.1	E855.4	E941.1	E950.4	E962.0	E980.4
Cyclophosphamide	963.1	E858.1	E933.1	E950.4	E962.0	E980.4
Cyclopropane	968.2	E855.1	E938.2	E950.4	E962.0	E980.4
Cycloserine	960.6	E856	E930.6	E950.4	E962.0	E980.4
Cyclothiazide	974.3	E858.5	E944.3	E950.4	E962.0	E980.4
Cycrimine	966.4	E855.0	E936.4	E950.4	E962.0	E980.4
Cymarin	972.1	E858.3	E942.1	E950.4	E962.0	E980.4
Cyproheptadine	963.0	E858.1	E933.0	E950.4	E962.0	E980.4
Cyprolidol	969.09 ◀ⅢⅢ	E854.0	E939.0	E950.3	E962.0	E980.3
Cytarabine	963.1	E858.1	E933.1	E950.4	E962.0	E980.4
Cytisus	—	—	—	—	—	—
laburnum	988.2	E865.4	—	E950.9	E962.1	E980.9
scoparius	988.2	E865.4	—	E950.9	E962.1	E980.9
Cytomel	962.7	E858.0	E932.7	E950.4	E962.0	E980.4
Cytosine (antineoplastic)	963.1	E858.1	E933.1	E950.4	E962.0	E980.4
Cytoxan	963.1	E858.1	E933.1	E950.4	E962.0	E980.4
Dacarbazine	963.1	E858.1	E933.1	E950.4	E962.0	E980.4

◀ New ◀ⅢⅢ Revised ~~deleted~~ Deleted ● Use Additional Digit(s)

Substance	Poisoning	External Cause (E Code)				
		Accident	Therapeutic Use	Suicide Attempt	Assault	Undetermined
Dactinomycin	960.7	E856	E930.7	E950.4	E962.0	E980.4
DADPS	961.8	E857	E931.8	E950.4	E962.0	E980.4
Dakin's solution (external)	976.0	E858.7	E946.0	E950.4	E962.0	E980.4
Dalmane	969.4	E853.2	E939.4	E950.3	E962.0	E980.3
DAM	977.2	E858.8	E947.2	E950.4	E962.0	E980.4
Danilone	964.2	E858.2	E934.2	E950.4	E962.0	E980.4
Danthron	973.1	E858.4	E943.1	E950.4	E962.0	E980.4
Dantrolene	975.2	E858.6	E945.2	E950.4	E962.0	E980.4
Daphne (gnidium) (mezereum)	988.2	E865.4	—	E950.9	E962.1	E980.9
berry	988.2	E865.3	—	E950.9	E962.1	E980.9
Dapsone	961.8	E857	E931.8	E950.4	E962.0	E980.4
Daraprim	961.4	E857	E931.4	E950.4	E962.0	E980.4
Darnel	988.2	E865.3	—	E950.9	E962.1	E980.9
Darvon	965.8	E850.8	E935.8	E950.0	E962.0	E980.0
Daunorubicin	960.7	E856	E930.7	E950.4	E962.0	E980.4
DBI	962.3	E858.0	E932.3	E950.4	E962.0	E980.4
D-Con (rodenticide)	989.4	E863.7	—	E950.6	E962.1	E980.7
DDS	961.8	E857	E931.8	E950.4	E962.0	E980.4
DDT	989.2	E863.0	—	E950.6	E962.1	E980.7
Deadly nightshade	988.2	E865.4	—	E950.9	E962.1	E980.9
berry	988.2	E865.3	—	E950.9	E962.1	E980.9
Deanol	969.79 ◀▥	E854.2	E939.7	E950.3	E962.0	E980.3
Debrisoquine	972.6	E858.3	E942.6	E950.4	E962.0	E980.4
Decaborane	989.89	E866.8	—	E950.9	E962.1	E980.9
fumes	987.8	E869.8	—	E952.8	E962.2	E982.8
Decadron	962.0	E858.0	E932.0	E950.4	E962.0	E980.4
ENT agent	976.6	E858.7	E946.6	E950.4	E962.0	E980.4
ophthalmic preparation	976.5	E858.7	E946.5	E950.4	E962.0	E980.4
topical NEC	976.0	E858.7	E946.0	E950.4	E962.0	E980.4
Decahydronaphthalene	982.0	E862.4	—	E950.9	E962.1	E980.9
Decalin	982.0	E862.4	—	E950.9	E962.1	E980.9
Decamethonium	975.2	E858.6	E945.2	E950.4	E962.0	E980.4
Decholin	973.4	E858.4	E943.4	E950.4	E962.0	E980.4
sodium (diagnostic)	977.8	E858.8	E947.8	E950.4	E962.0	E980.4
Declomycin	960.4	E856	E930.4	E950.4	E962.0	E980.4
Deferoxamine	963.8	E858.1	E933.8	E950.4	E962.0	E980.4
Dehydrocholic acid	973.4	E858.4	E943.4	E950.4	E962.0	E980.4
DeKalin	982.0	E862.4	—	E950.9	E962.1	E980.9
Delalutin	962.2	E858.0	E932.2	E950.4	E962.0	E980.4

◀ New   ◀▥ Revised   ~~deleted~~ Deleted   ● Use Additional Digit(s)

Substance	Poisoning	External Cause (E Code)				
		Accident	Therapeutic Use	Suicide Attempt	Assault	Undetermined
Delphinium	988.2	E865.3	—	E950.9	E962.1	E980.9
Deltasone	962.0	E858.0	E932.0	E950.4	E962.0	E980.4
Deltra	962.0	E858.0	E932.0	E950.4	E962.0	E980.4
Delvinal	967.0	E851	E937.0	E950.1	E962.0	E980.1
Demecarium (bromide)	971.0	E855.3	E941.0	E950.4	E962.0	E980.4
Demeclocycline	960.4	E856	E930.4	E950.4	E962.0	E980.4
Demecolcine	963.1	E858.1	E933.1	E950.4	E962.0	E980.4
Demelanizing agents	976.8	E858.7	E946.8	E950.4	E962.0	E980.4
Demerol	965.09	E850.2	E935.2	E950.0	E962.0	E980.0
Demethylchlortetracycline	960.4	E856	E930.4	E950.4	E962.0	E980.4
Demethyltetracycline	960.4	E856	E930.4	E950.4	E962.0	E980.4
Demeton	989.3	E863.1	—	E950.6	E962.1	E980.7
Demulcents	976.3	E858.7	E946.3	E950.4	E962.0	E980.4
Demulen	962.2	E858.0	E932.2	E950.4	E962.0	E980.4
Denatured alcohol	980.0	E860.1	—	E950.9	E962.1	E980.9
Dendrid	976.5	E858.7	E946.5	E950.4	E962.0	E980.4
Dental agents, topical	976.7	E858.7	E946.7	E950.4	E962.0	E980.4
Deodorant spray (feminine hygiene)	976.8	E858.7	E946.8	E950.4	E962.0	E980.4
Deoxyribonuclease	963.4	E858.1	E933.4	E950.4	E962.0	E980.4
Depressants	—	—	—	—	—	—
appetite, central	977.0	E858.8	E947.0	E950.4	E962.0	E980.4
cardiac	972.0	E858.3	E942.0	E950.4	E962.0	E980.4
central nervous system (anesthetic)	968.4	E855.1	E938.4	E950.4	E962.0	E980.4
psychotherapeutic	969.5	E853.9	E939.5	E950.3	E962.0	E980.3
Dequalinium	976.0	E858.7	E946.0	E950.4	E962.0	E980.4
Dermolate	976.2	E858.7	E946.2	E950.4	E962.0	E980.4
DES	962.2	E858.0	E932.2	E950.4	E962.0	E980.4
Desenex	976.0	E858.7	E946.0	E950.4	E962.0	E980.4
Deserpidine	972.6	E858.3	E942.6	E950.4	E962.0	E980.4
Desipramine	969.05 ◀▥	E854.0	E939.0	E950.3	E962.0	E980.3
Deslanoside	972.1	E858.3	E942.1	E950.4	E962.0	E980.4
Desocodeine	965.09	E850.2	E935.2	E950.0	E962.0	E980.0
Desomorphine	965.09	E850.2	E935.2	E950.0	E962.0	E980.0
Desonide	976.0	E858.7	E946.0	E950.4	E962.0	E980.4
Desoxycorticosterone derivatives	962.0	E858.0	E932.0	E950.4	E962.0	E980.4
Desoxyephedrine	969.72 ◀▥	E854.2	E939.7	E950.3	E962.0	E980.3
DET	969.6	E854.1	E939.6	E950.3	E962.0	E980.3
Detergents (ingested) (synthetic)	989.6	E861.0	—	E950.9	E962.1	E980.9
external medication	976.2	E858.7	E946.2	E950.4	E962.0	E980.4

◀ New   ◀▥ Revised   ~~deleted~~ Deleted   ● Use Additional Digit(s)

Substance	Poisoning	External Cause (E Code)				
		Accident	Therapeutic Use	Suicide Attempt	Assault	Undetermined
Deterrent, alcohol	977.3	E858.8	E947.3	E950.4	E962.0	E980.4
Detrothyronine	962.7	E858.0	E932.7	E950.4	E962.0	E980.4
Dettol (external medication)	976.0	E858.7	E946.0	E950.4	E962.0	E980.4
Dexamethasone	962.0	E858.0	E932.0	E950.4	E962.0	E980.4
ENT agent	976.6	E858.7	E946.6	E950.4	E962.0	E980.4
ophthalmic preparation	976.5	E858.7	E946.5	E950.4	E962.0	E980.4
topical NEC	976.0	E858.7	E946.0	E950.4	E962.0	E980.4
Dexamphetamine	969.72 ◀	E854.2	E939.7	E950.3	E962.0	E980.3
Dexedrine	969.72 ◀	E854.2	E939.7	E950.3	E962.0	E980.3
Dexpanthenol	963.5	E858.1	E933.5	E950.4	E962.0	E980.4
Dextran	964.8	E858.2	E934.8	E950.4	E962.0	E980.4
Dextriferron	964.0	E858.2	E934.0	E950.4	E962.0	E980.4
Dextroamphetamine	969.72 ◀	E854.2	E939.7	E950.3	E962.0	E980.3
Dextro calcium pantothenate	963.5	E858.1	E933.5	E950.4	E962.0	E980.4
Dextromethorphan	975.4	E858.6	E945.4	E950.4	E962.0	E980.4
Dextromoramide	965.09	E850.2	E935.2	E950.0	E962.0	E980.0
Dextro pantothenyl alcohol	963.5	E858.1	E933.5	E950.4	E962.0	E980.4
topical	976.8	E858.7	E946.8	E950.4	E962.0	E980.4
Dextropropoxyphene (hydrochloride)	965.8	E850.8	E935.8	E950.0	E962.0	E980.0
Dextrorphan	965.09	E850.2	E935.2	E950.0	E962.0	E980.0
Dextrose NEC	974.5	E858.5	E944.5	E950.4	E962.0	E980.4
Dextrothyroxine	962.7	E858.0	E932.7	E950.4	E962.0	E980.4
DFP	971.0	E855.3	E941.0	E950.4	E962.0	E980.4
DHE-45	972.9	E858.3	E942.9	E950.4	E962.0	E980.4
Diabinese	962.3	E858.0	E932.3	E950.4	E962.0	E980.4
Diacetyl monoxime	977.2	E858.8	E947.2	E950.4	E962.0	E980.4
Diacetylmorphine	965.01	E850.0	E935.0	E950.0	E962.0	E980.0
Diagnostic agents	977.8	E858.8	E947.8	E950.4	E962.0	E980.4
Dial (soap)	976.2	E858.7	E946.2	E950.4	E962.0	E980.4
sedative	967.0	E851	E937.0	E950.1	E962.0	E980.1
Diallylbarbituric acid	967.0	E851	E937.0	E950.1	E962.0	E980.1
Diaminodiphenyisulfone	961.8	E857	E931.8	E950.4	E962.0	E980.4
Diamorphine	965.01	E850.0	E935.0	E950.0	E962.0	E980.0
Diamox	974.2	E858.5	E944.2	E950.4	E962.0	E980.4
Diamthazole	976.0	E858.7	E946.0	E950.4	E962.0	E980.4
Diaphenyisulfone	961.8	E857	E931.8	E950.4	E962.0	E980.4
Diasone (sodium)	961.8	E857	E931.8	E950.4	E962.0	E980.4
Diazepam	969.4	E853.2	E939.4	E950.3	E962.0	E980.3
Diazinon	989.3	E863.1	—	E950.6	E962.1	E980.7

◀ New   ◀▥ Revised   ~~deleted~~ Deleted   ● Use Additional Digit(s)

Substance	Poisoning	External Cause (E Code)				
		Accident	Therapeutic Use	Suicide Attempt	Assault	Undetermined
Diazomethane (gas)	987.8	E869.8	—	E952.8	E962.2	E982.8
Diazoxide	972.5	E858.3	E942.5	E950.4	E962.0	E980.4
Dibenamine	971.3	E855.6	E941.3	E950.4	E962.0	E980.4
Dibenzheptropine	963.0	E858.1	E933.0	E950.4	E962.0	E980.4
Dibenzyline	971.3	E855.6	E941.3	E950.4	E962.0	E980.4
Diborane (gas)	987.8	E869.8	—	E952.8	E962.2	E982.8
Dibromomannitol	963.1	E858.1	E933.1	E950.4	E962.0	E980.4
Dibucaine (spinal)	968.7	E855.2	E938.7	E950.4	E962.0	E980.4
topical (surface)	968.5	E855.2	E938.5	E950.4	E962.0	E980.4
Dibunate sodium	975.4	E858.6	E945.4	E950.4	E962.0	E980.4
Dibutoline	971.1	E855.4	E941.1	E950.4	E962.0	E980.4
Dicapthon	989.4	E863.4	—	E950.6	E962.1	E980.7
Dichloralphenazone	967.1	E852.0	E937.1	E950.2	E962.0	E980.2
Dichlorodifluoromethane	987.4	E869.2	—	E952.8	E962.2	E982.8
Dichloroethane	982.3	E862.4	—	E950.9	E962.1	E980.9
Dichloroethylene	982.3	E862.4	—	E950.9	E962.1	E980.9
Dichloroethyl sulfide	987.8	E869.8	—	E952.8	E962.2	E982.8
Dichlorohydrin	982.3	E862.4	—	E950.9	E962.1	E980.9
Dichloromethane (solvent) (vapor)	982.3	E862.4	—	E950.9	E962.1	E980.9
Dichlorophen(e)	961.6	E857	E931.6	E950.4	E962.0	E980.4
Dichlorphenamide	974.2	E858.5	E944.2	E950.4	E962.0	E980.4
Dichlorvos	989.3	E863.1	—	E950.6	E962.1	E980.7
Diclofenac sodium	965.69	E850.6	E935.6	E950.0	E962.0	E980.0
Dicoumarin, dicumarol	964.2	E858.2	E934.2	E950.4	E962.0	E980.4
Dicyanogen (gas)	987.8	E869.8	—	E952.8	E962.2	E982.8
Dicyclomine	971.1	E855.4	E941.1	E950.4	E962.0	E980.4
Dieldrin (vapor)	989.2	E863.0	—	E950.6	E962.1	E980.7
Dienestrol	962.2	E858.0	E932.2	E950.4	E962.0	E980.4
Dietetics	977.0	E858.8	E947.0	E950.4	E962.0	E980.4
Diethazine	966.4	E855.0	E936.4	E950.4	E962.0	E980.4
Diethyl	—	—	—	—	—	—
barbituric acid	967.0	E851	E937.0	E950.1	E962.0	E980.1
carbamazine	961.6	E857	E931.6	E950.4	E962.0	E980.4
carbinol	980.8	E860.8	—	E950.9	E962.1	E980.9
carbonate	982.8	E862.4	—	E950.9	E962.1	E980.9
ether (vapor) - see Ether(s)	—	—	—	—	—	—
propion	977.0	E858.8	E947.0	E950.4	E962.0	E980.4
stilbestrol	962.2	E858.0	E932.2	E950.4	E962.0	E980.4

◄ New   ◄▥ Revised   ~~deleted~~ Deleted   ● Use Additional Digit(s)

Substance	Poisoning	External Cause (E Code)				
		Accident	Therapeutic Use	Suicide Attempt	Assault	Undetermined
Diethylene	—	—	—	—	—	—
dioxide	982.8	E862.4	—	E950.9	E962.1	E980.9
glycol (monoacetate) (monoethyl ether)	982.8	E862.4	—	E950.9	E962.1	E980.9
Diethylsulfone-diethylmethane	967.8	E852.8	E937.8	E950.2	E962.0	E980.2
Difencloxazine	965.09	E850.2	E935.2	E950.0	E962.0	E980.0
Diffusin	963.4	E858.1	E933.4	E950.4	E962.0	E980.4
Diflos	971.0	E855.3	E941.0	E950.4	E962.0	E980.4
Digestants	973.4	E858.4	E943.4	E950.4	E962.0	E980.4
Digitalin(e)	972.1	E858.3	E942.1	E950.4	E962.0	E980.4
Digitalis glycosides	972.1	E858.3	E942.1	E950.4	E962.0	E980.4
Digitoxin	972.1	E858.3	E942.1	E950.4	E962.0	E980.4
Digoxin	972.1	E858.3	E942.1	E950.4	E962.0	E980.4
Dihydrocodeine	965.09	E850.2	E935.2	E950.0	E962.0	E980.0
Dihydrocodeinone	965.09	E850.2	E935.2	E950.0	E962.0	E980.0
Dihydroergocristine	972.9	E858.3	E942.9	E950.4	E962.0	E980.4
Dihydroergotamine	972.9	E858.3	E942.9	E950.4	E962.0	E980.4
Dihydroergotoxine	972.9	E858.3	E942.9	E950.4	E962.0	E980.4
Dihydrohydroxycodeinone	965.09	E850.2	E935.2	E950.0	E962.0	E980.0
Dihydrohydroxymorphinone	965.09	E850.2	E935.2	E950.0	E962.0	E980.0
Dihydroisocodeine	965.09	E850.2	E935.2	E950.0	E962.0	E980.0
Dihydromorphine	965.09	E850.2	E935.2	E950.0	E962.0	E980.0
Dihydromorphinone	965.09	E850.2	E935.2	E950.0	E962.0	E980.0
Dihydrostreptomycin	960.6	E856	E930.6	E950.4	E962.0	E980.4
Dihydrotachysterol	962.6	E858.0	E932.6	E950.4	E962.0	E980.4
Dihydroxyanthraquinone	973.1	E858.4	E943.1	E950.4	E962.0	E980.4
Dihydroxycodeinone	965.09	E850.2	E935.2	E950.0	E962.0	E980.0
Diiodohydroxyquin	961.3	E857	E931.3	E950.4	E962.0	E980.4
topical	976.0	E858.7	E946.0	E950.4	E962.0	E980.4
Diiodohydroxyquinoline	961.3	E857	E931.3	E950.4	E962.0	E980.4
Dilantin	966.1	E855.0	E936.1	E950.4	E962.0	E980.4
Dilaudid	965.09	E850.2	E935.2	E950.0	E962.0	E980.0
Diloxanide	961.5	E857	E931.5	E950.4	E962.0	E980.4
Dimefline	970.0	E854.3	E940.0	E950.4	E962.0	E980.4
Dimenhydrinate	963.0	E858.1	E933.0	E950.4	E962.0	E980.4
Dimercaprol	963.8	E858.1	E933.8	E950.4	E962.0	E980.4
Dimercaptopropanol	963.8	E858.1	E933.8	E950.4	E962.0	E980.4
Dimetane	963.0	E858.1	E933.0	E950.4	E962.0	E980.4
Dimethicone	976.3	E858.7	E946.3	E950.4	E962.0	E980.4
Dimethindene	963.0	E858.1	E933.0	E950.4	E962.0	E980.4

Substance	Poisoning	External Cause (E Code)				
		Accident	Therapeutic Use	Suicide Attempt	Assault	Undetermined
Dimethisoquin	968.5	E855.2	E938.5	E950.4	E962.0	E980.4
Dimethisterone	962.2	E858.0	E932.2	E950.4	E962.0	E980.4
Dimethoxanate	975.4	E858.6	E945.4	E950.4	E962.0	E980.4
Dimethyl	—	—	—	—	—	—
arsine, arsinic acid - *see* Arsenic	—	—	—	—	—	—
carbinol	980.2	E860.3	—	E950.9	E962.1	E980.9
diguanide	962.3	E858.0	E932.3	E950.4	E962.0	E980.4
ketone	982.8	E862.4	—	E950.9	E962.1	E980.9
vapor	987.8	E869.8	—	E952.8	E962.2	E982.8
meperidine	965.09	E850.2	E935.2	E950.0	E962.0	E980.0
parathion	989.3	E863.1	—	E950.6	E962.1	E980.7
polysiloxane	973.8	E858.4	E943.8	E950.4	E962.0	E980.4
sulfate (fumes)	987.8	E869.8	—	E952.8	E962.2	E982.8
liquid	983.9	E864.3	—	E950.7	E962.1	E980.6
sulfoxide NEC	982.8	E862.4	—	E950.9	E962.1	E980.9
medicinal	976.4	E858.7	E946.4	E950.4	E962.0	E980.4
triptamine	969.6	E854.1	E939.6	E950.3	E962.0	E980.3
tubocurarine	975.2	E858.6	E945.2	E950.4	E962.0	E980.4
Dindevan	964.2	E858.2	E934.2	E950.4	E962.0	E980.4
Dinitro (-ortho-) cresol (herbicide) (spray)	989.4	E863.5	—	E950.6	E962.1	E980.7
insecticide	989.4	E863.4	—	E950.6	E962.1	E980.7
Dinitrobenzene	983.0	E864.0	—	E950.7	E962.1	E980.6
vapor	987.8	E869.8	—	E952.8	E962.2	E982.8
Dinitro-orthocresol (herbicide)	989.4	E863.5	—	E950.6	E962.1	E980.7
insecticide	989.4	E863.4	—	E950.6	E962.1	E980.7
Dinitrophenol (herbicide) (spray)	989.4	E863.5	—	E950.6	E962.1	E980.7
insecticide	989.4	E863.4	—	E950.6	E962.1	E980.7
Dinoprost	975.0	E858.6	E945.0	E950.4	E962.0	E980.4
Dioctyl sulfosuccinate (calcium) (sodium)	973.2	E858.4	E943.2	E950.4	E962.0	E980.4
Diodoquin	961.3	E857	E931.3	E950.4	E962.0	E980.4
Dione derivatives NEC	966.3	E855.0	E936.3	E950.4	E962.0	E980.4
Dionin	965.09	E850.2	E935.2	E950.0	E962.0	E980.0
Dioxane	982.8	E862.4	—	E950.9	E962.1	E980.9
Dioxin - *see* herbicide	—	—	—	—	—	—
Dioxyline	972.5	E858.3	E942.5	E950.4	E962.0	E980.4
Dipentene	982.8	E862.4	—	E950.9	E962.1	E980.9
Diphemanil	971.1	E855.4	E941.1	E950.4	E962.0	E980.4
Diphenadione	964.2	E858.2	E934.2	E950.4	E962.0	E980.4
Diphenhydramine	963.0	E858.1	E933.0	E950.4	E962.0	E980.4

◀ New　◀▥ Revised　deleted Deleted　● Use Additional Digit(s)

Substance	Poisoning	External Cause (E Code)				
		Accident	Therapeutic Use	Suicide Attempt	Assault	Undetermined
Diphenidol	963.0	E858.1	E933.0	E950.4	E962.0	E980.4
Diphenoxylate	973.5	E858.4	E943.5	E950.4	E962.0	E980.4
Diphenylchlorarsine	985.1	E866.3	—	E950.8	E962.1	E980.8
Diphenylhydantoin (sodium)	966.1	E855.0	E936.1	E950.4	E962.0	E980.4
Diphenylpyraline	963.0	E858.1	E933.0	E950.4	E962.0	E980.4
Diphtheria	—	—	—	—	—	—
antitoxin	979.9	E858.8	E949.9	E950.4	E962.0	E980.4
toxoid	978.5	E858.8	E948.5	E950.4	E962.0	E980.4
with tetanus toxoid	978.9	E858.8	E948.9	E950.4	E962.0	E980.4
with pertussis component	978.6	E858.8	E948.6	E950.4	E962.0	E980.4
vaccine	978.5	E858.8	E948.5	E950.4	E962.0	E980.4
Dipipanone	965.09	E850.2	E935.2	E950.0	E962.0	E980.0
Diplovax	979.5	E858.8	E949.5	E950.4	E962.0	E980.4
Diprophylline	975.1	E858.6	E945.1	E950.4	E962.0	E980.4
Dipyridamole	972.4	E858.3	E942.4	E950.4	E962.0	E980.4
Dipyrone	965.5	E850.5	E935.5	E950.0	E962.0	E980.0
Diquat	989.4	E863.5	—	E950.6	E962.1	E980.7
Disinfectant NEC	983.9	E861.4	—	E950.7	E962.1	E980.6
alkaline	983.2	E861.4	—	E950.7	E962.1	E980.6
aromatic	983.0	E861.4	—	E950.7	E962.1	E980.6
Disipal	966.4	E855.0	E936.4	E950.4	E962.0	E980.4
Disodium edetate	963.8	E858.1	E933.8	E950.4	E962.0	E980.4
Disulfamide	974.4	E858.5	E944.4	E950.4	E962.0	E980.4
Disulfanilamide	961.0	E857	E931.0	E950.4	E962.0	E980.4
Disulfiram	977.3	E858.8	E947.3	E950.4	E962.0	E980.4
Dithiazanine	961.6	E857	E931.6	E950.4	E962.0	E980.4
Dithioglycerol	963.8	E858.1	E933.8	E950.4	E962.0	E980.4
Dithranol	976.4	E858.7	E946.4	E950.4	E962.0	E980.4
Diucardin	974.3	E858.5	E944.3	E950.4	E962.0	E980.4
Diupres	974.3	E858.5	E944.3	E950.4	E962.0	E980.4
Diuretics NEC	974.4	E858.5	E944.4	E950.4	E962.0	E980.4
carbonic acid anhydrase inhibitors	974.2	E858.5	E944.2	E950.4	E962.0	E980.4
mercurial	974.0	E858.5	E944.0	E950.4	E962.0	E980.4
osmotic	974.4	E858.5	E944.4	E950.4	E962.0	E980.4
purine derivatives	974.1	E858.5	E944.1	E950.4	E962.0	E980.4
saluretic	974.3	E858.5	E944.3	E950.4	E962.0	E980.4
Diuril	974.3	E858.5	E944.3	E950.4	E962.0	E980.4
Divinyl ether	968.2	E855.1	E938.2	E950.4	E962.0	E980.4
D-lysergic acid diethylamide	969.6	E854.1	E939.6	E950.3	E962.0	E980.3

◀ New   ◀▥ Revised   ~~deleted~~ Deleted   ● Use Additional Digit(s)

Substance	Poisoning	External Cause (E Code)				
		Accident	Therapeutic Use	Suicide Attempt	Assault	Undetermined
DMCT	960.4	E856	E930.4	E950.4	E962.0	E980.4
DMSO	982.8	E862.4	—	E950.9	E962.1	E980.9
DMT	969.6	E854.1	E939.6	E950.3	E962.0	E980.3
DNOC	989.4	E863.5	—	E950.6	E962.1	E980.7
DOCA	962.0	E858.0	E932.0	E950.4	E962.0	E980.4
Dolophine	965.02	E850.1	E935.1	E950.0	E962.0	E980.0
Doloxene	965.8	E850.8	E935.8	E950.0	E962.0	E980.0
DOM	969.6	E854.1	E939.6	E950.3	E962.0	E980.3
Domestic gas - *see* Gas, utility	—	—	—	—	—	—
Domiphen (bromide) (lozenges)	976.6	E858.7	E946.6	E950.4	E962.0	E980.4
Dopa (levo)	966.4	E855.0	E936.4	E950.4	E962.0	E980.4
Dopamine	971.2	E855.5	E941.2	E950.4	E962.0	E980.4
Doriden	967.5	E852.4	E937.5	E950.2	E962.0	E980.2
Dormiral	967.0	E851	E937.0	E950.1	E962.0	E980.1
Dormison	967.8	E852.8	E937.8	E950.2	E962.0	E980.2
Dornase	963.4	E858.1	E933.4	E950.4	E962.0	E980.4
Dorsacaine	968.5	E855.2	E938.5	E950.4	E962.0	E980.4
Dothiepin hydrochloride	969.05 ◄▥	E854.0	E939.0	E950.3	E962.0	E980.3
Doxapram	970.0	E854.3	E940.0	E950.4	E962.0	E980.4
Doxepin	969.05 ◄▥	E854.0	E939.0	E950.3	E962.0	E980.3
Doxorubicin	960.7	E856	E930.7	E950.4	E962.0	E980.4
Doxycycline	960.4	E856	E930.4	E950.4	E962.0	E980.4
Doxylamine	963.0	E858.1	E933.0	E950.4	E962.0	E980.4
Dramamine	963.0	E858.1	E933.0	E950.4	E962.0	E980.4
Drano (drain cleaner)	983.2	E864.2	—	E950.7	E962.1	E980.6
Dromoran	965.09	E850.2	E935.2	E950.0	E962.0	E980.0
Dromostanolone	962.1	E858.0	E932.1	E950.4	E962.0	E980.4
Droperidol	969.2	E853.1	E939.2	E950.3	E962.0	E980.3
Drotrecogin alfa	964.2	E858.2	E934.2	E950.4	E962.0	E980.4
Drug	977.9	E858.9	E947.9	E950.5	E962.0	E980.5
specified NEC	977.8	E858.8	E947.8	E950.4	E962.0	E980.4
AHFS List	—	—	—	—	—	—
4:00 antihistamine drugs	963.0	E858.1	E933.0	E950.4	E962.0	E980.4
8:04 amebacides	961.5	E857	E931.5	E950.4	E962.0	E980.4
arsenical anti-infectives	961.1	E857	E931.1	E950.4	E962.0	E980.4
quinoline derivatives	961.3	E857	E931.3	E950.4	E962.0	E980.4
8:08 anthelmintics	961.6	E857	E931.6	E950.4	E962.0	E980.4
quinoline derivatives	961.3	E857	E931.3	E950.4	E962.0	E980.4
8:12.04 antifungal antibiotics	960.1	E856	E930.1	E950.4	E962.0	E980.4

Substance	Poisoning	External Cause (E Code)				
		Accident	Therapeutic Use	Suicide Attempt	Assault	Undetermined
Drug *(Continued)*						
8:12.06 cephalosporins	960.5	E856	E930.5	E950.4	E962.0	E980.4
8:12.08 chloramphenicol	960.2	E856	E930.2	E950.4	E962.0	E980.4
8:12.12 erythromycins	960.3	E856	E930.3	E950.4	E962.0	E980.4
8:12.16 penicillins	960.0	E856	E930.0	E950.4	E962.0	E980.4
8:12.20 streptomycins	960.6	E856	E930.6	E950.4	E962.0	E980.4
8:12.24 tetracyclines	960.4	E856	E930.4	E950.4	E962.0	E980.4
8:12.28 other antibiotics	960.8	E856	E930.8	E950.4	E962.0	E980.4
antimycobacterial	960.6	E856	E930.6	E950.4	E962.0	E980.4
macrolides	960.3	E856	E930.3	E950.4	E962.0	E980.4
8:16 antituberculars	961.8	E857	E931.8	E950.4	E962.0	E980.4
antibiotics	960.6	E856	E930.6	E950.4	E962.0	E980.4
8:18 antivirals	961.7	E857	E931.7	E950.4	E962.0	E980.4
8:20 plasmodicides (antimalarials)	961.4	E857	E931.4	E950.4	E962.0	E980.4
8:24 sulfonamides	961.0	E857	E931.0	E950.4	E962.0	E980.4
8:26 sulfones	961.8	E857	E931.8	E950.4	E962.0	E980.4
8:28 treponemicides	961.2	E857	E931.2	E950.4	E962.0	E980.4
8:32 trichomonacides	961.5	E857	E931.5	E950.4	E962.0	E980.4
quinoline derivatives	961.3	E857	E931.3	E950.4	E962.0	E980.4
nitrofuran derivatives	961.9	E857	E931.9	E950.4	E962.0	E980.4
8:36 urinary germicides	961.9	E857	E931.9	E950.4	E962.0	E980.4
quinoline derivatives	961.3	E857	E931.3	E950.4	E962.0	E980.4
8:40 other anti-infectives	961.9	E857	E931.9	E950.4	E962.0	E980.4
10:00 antineoplastic agents	963.1	E858.1	E933.1	E950.4	E962.0	E980.4
antibiotics	960.7	E856	E930.7	E950.4	E962.0	E980.4
progestogens	962.2	E858.0	E932.2	E950.4	E962.0	E980.4
12:04 parasympathomimetic (cholinergic) agents	971.0	E855.3	E941.0	E950.4	E962.0	E980.4
12:08 parasympatholytic (cholinergic-blocking) agents	971.1	E855.4	E941.1	E950.4	E962.0	E980.4
12:12 sympathomimetic (adrenergic) agents	971.2	E855.5	E941.2	E950.4	E962.0	E980.4
12:16 sympatholytic (adrenergic-blocking) agents	971.3	E855.6	E941.3	E950.4	E962.0	E980.4
12:20 skeletal muscle relaxants	—	—	—	—	—	—
central nervous system muscle-tone depressants	968.0	E855.1	E938.0	E950.4	E962.0	E980.4
myoneural blocking agents	975.2	E858.6	E945.2	E950.4	E962.0	E980.4
16:00 blood derivatives	964.7	E858.2	E934.7	E950.4	E962.0	E980.4
20:04 antianemia drugs	964.1	E858.2	E934.1	E950.4	E962.0	E980.4
20:04.04 iron preparations	964.0	E858.2	E934.0	E950.4	E962.0	E980.4
20:04.08 liver and stomach preparations	964.1	E858.2	E934.1	E950.4	E962.0	E980.4
20:12.04 anticoagulants	964.2	E858.2	E934.2	E950.4	E962.0	E980.4
20:12.08 antiheparin agents	964.5	E858.2	E934.5	E950.4	E962.0	E980.4

◀ New   ◀‖‖ Revised   ~~deleted~~ Deleted   ● Use Additional Digit(s)

Substance	Poisoning	External Cause (E Code)				
		Accident	Therapeutic Use	Suicide Attempt	Assault	Undetermined
Drug *(Continued)*						
20:12.12 coagulants	964.5	E858.2	E934.5	E950.4	E962.0	E980.4
20:12.16 hemostatics NEC	964.5	E858.2	E934.5	E950.4	E962.0	E980.4
capillary active drugs	972.8	E858.3	E942.8	E950.4	E962.0	E980.4
24:04 cardiac drugs	972.9	E858.3	E942.9	E950.4	E962.0	E980.4
cardiotonic agents	972.1	E858.3	E942.1	E950.4	E962.0	E980.4
rhythm regulators	972.0	E858.3	E942.0	E950.4	E962.0	E980.4
24:06 antilipemic agents	972.2	E858.3	E942.2	E950.4	E962.0	E980.4
thyroid derivatives	962.7	E858.0	E932.7	E950.4	E962.0	E980.4
24:08 hypotensive agents	972.6	E858.3	E942.6	E950.4	E962.0	E980.4
adrenergic blocking agents	971.3	E855.6	E941.3	E950.4	E962.0	E980.4
ganglion blocking agents	972.3	E858.3	E942.3	E950.4	E962.0	E980.4
vasodilators	972.5	E858.3	E942.5	E950.4	E962.0	E980.4
24:12 vasodilating agents NEC	972.5	E858.3	E942.5	E950.4	E962.0	E980.4
coronary	972.4	E858.3	E942.4	E950.4	E962.0	E980.4
nicotinic acid derivatives	972.2	E858.3	E942.2	E950.4	E962.0	E980.4
24:16 sclerosing agents	972.7	E858.3	E942.7	E950.4	E962.0	E980.4
28:04 general anesthetics	968.4	E855.1	E938.4	E950.4	E962.0	E980.4
gaseous anesthetics	968.2	E855.1	E938.2	E950.4	E962.0	E980.4
halothane	968.1	E855.1	E938.1	E950.4	E962.0	E980.4
intravenous anesthetics	968.3	E855.1	E938.3	E950.4	E962.0	E980.4
28:08 analgesics and antipyretics	965.9	E850.9	E935.9	E950.0	E962.0	E980.0
antirheumatics	965.69	E850.6	E935.6	E950.0	E962.0	E980.0
aromatic analgesics	965.4	E850.4	E935.4	E950.0	E962.0	E980.0
non-narcotic NEC	965.7	E850.7	E935.7	E950.0	E962.0	E980.0
opium alkaloids	965.00	E850.2	E935.2	E950.0	E962.0	E980.0
heroin	965.01	E850.0	E935.0	E950.0	E962.0	E980.0
methadone	965.02	E850.1	E935.1	E950.0	E962.0	E980.0
specified type NEC	965.09	E850.2	E935.2	E950.0	E962.0	E980.0
pyrazole derivatives	965.5	E850.5	E935.5	E950.0	E962.0	E980.0
salicylates	965.1	E850.3	E935.3	E950.0	E962.0	E980.0
specified NEC	965.8	E850.8	E935.8	E950.0	E962.0	E980.0
28:10 narcotic antagonists	970.1	E854.3	E940.1	E950.4	E962.0	E980.4
28:12 anticonvulsants	966.3	E855.0	E936.3	E950.4	E962.0	E980.4
barbiturates	967.0	E851	E937.0	E950.1	E962.0	E980.1
benzodiazepine-based tranquilizers	969.4	E853.2	E939.4	E950.3	E962.0	E980.3
bromides	967.3	E852.2	E937.3	E950.2	E962.0	E980.2
hydantoin derivatives	966.1	E855.0	E936.1	E950.4	E962.0	E980.4
oxazolidine (derivatives)	966.0	E855.0	E936.0	E950.4	E962.0	E980.4
succinimides	966.2	E855.0	E936.2	E950.4	E962.0	E980.4

◀ New   ◀▥ Revised   ~~deleted~~ Deleted   ● Use Additional Digit(s)

TABLE OF DRUGS AND CHEMICALS

Substance	Poisoning	External Cause (E Code)				
		Accident	Therapeutic Use	Suicide Attempt	Assault	Undetermined
Drug *(Continued)*						
28:16.04 antidepressants	969.00 ◄▦	E854.0	E939.0	E950.3	E962.0	E980.3
28:16.08 tranquilizers	969.5	E853.9	E939.5	E950.3	E962.0	E980.3
benzodiazepine-based	969.4	E853.2	E939.4	E950.3	E962.0	E980.3
butyrophenone-based	969.2	E853.1	E939.2	E950.3	E962.0	E980.3
major NEC	969.3	E853.8	E939.3	E950.3	E962.0	E980.3
phenothiazine-based	969.1	E853.0	E939.1	E950.3	E962.0	E980.3
28:16.12 other psychotherapeutic agents	969.8	E855.8	E939.8	E950.3	E962.0	E980.3
28:20 respiratory and cerebral stimulants	970.9	E854.3	E940.9	E950.4	E962.0	E980.4
analeptics	970.0	E854.3	E940.0	E950.4	E962.0	E980.4
anorexigenic agents	977.0	E858.8	E947.0	E950.4	E962.0	E980.4
psychostimulants	969.70 ◄▦	E854.2	E939.7	E950.3	E962.0	E980.3
specified NEC	970.8	E854.3	E940.8	E950.4	E962.0	E980.4
28:24 sedatives and hypnotics	967.9	E852.9	E937.9	E950.2	E962.0	E980.2
barbiturates	967.0	E851	E937.0	E950.1	E962.0	E980.1
benzodiazepine-based tranquilizers	969.4	E853.2	E939.4	E950.3	E962.0	E980.3
chloral hydrate (group)	967.1	E852.0	E937.1	E950.2	E962.0	E980.2
glutethimide group	967.5	E852.4	E937.5	E950.2	E962.0	E980.2
intravenous anesthetics	968.3	E855.1	E938.3	E950.4	E962.0	E980.4
methaqualone (compounds)	967.4	E852.3	E937.4	E950.2	E962.0	E980.2
paraldehyde	967.2	E852.1	E937.2	E950.2	E962.0	E980.2
phenothiazine-based tranquilizers	969.1	E853.0	E939.1	E950.3	E962.0	E980.3
specified NEC	967.8	E852.8	E937.8	E950.2	E962.0	E980.2
thiobarbiturates	968.3	E855.1	E938.3	E950.4	E962.0	E980.4
tranquilizer NEC	969.5	E853.9	E939.5	E950.3	E962.0	E980.3
36:04 to 36:88 diagnostic agents	977.8	E858.8	E947.8	E950.4	E962.0	E980.4
40:00 electrolyte, caloric, and water balance agents NEC	974.5	E858.5	E944.5	E950.4	E962.0	E980.4
40:04 acidifying agents	963.2	E858.1	E933.2	E950.4	E962.0	E980.4
40:08 alkalinizing agents	963.3	E858.1	E933.3	E950.4	E962.0	E980.4
40:10 ammonia detoxicants	974.5	E858.5	E944.5	E950.4	E962.0	E980.4
40:12 replacement solutions	974.5	E858.5	E944.5	E950.4	E962.0	E980.4
plasma expanders	964.8	E858.2	E934.8	E950.4	E962.0	E980.4
40:16 sodium-removing resins	974.5	E858.5	E944.5	E950.4	E962.0	E980.4
40:18 potassium-removing resins	974.5	E858.5	E944.5	E950.4	E962.0	E980.4
40:20 caloric agents	974.5	E858.5	E944.5	E950.4	E962.0	E980.4
40:24 salt and sugar substitutes	974.5	E858.5	E944.5	E950.4	E962.0	E980.4
40:28 diuretics NEC	974.4	E858.5	E944.4	E950.4	E962.0	E980.4
carbonic acid anhydrase inhibitors	974.2	E858.5	E944.2	E950.4	E962.0	E980.4

◄ New   ◄▦ Revised   ~~deleted~~ Deleted   ● Use Additional Digit(s)

Substance	Poisoning	External Cause (E Code)				
		Accident	Therapeutic Use	Suicide Attempt	Assault	Undetermined
Drug (Continued)						
40:28 diuretics NEC (Continued)						
mercurials	974.0	E858.5	E944.0	E950.4	E962.0	E980.4
purine derivatives	974.1	E858.5	E944.1	E950.4	E962.0	E980.4
saluretics	974.3	E858.5	E944.3	E950.4	E962.0	E980.4
thiazides	974.3	E858.5	E944.3	E950.4	E962.0	E980.4
40:36 irrigating solutions	974.5	E858.5	E944.5	E950.4	E962.0	E980.4
40:40 uricosuric agents	974.7	E858.5	E944.7	E950.4	E962.0	E980.4
44:00 enzymes	963.4	E858.1	E933.4	E950.4	E962.0	E980.4
fibrinolysis-affecting agents	964.4	E858.2	E934.4	E950.4	E962.0	E980.4
gastric agents	973.4	E858.4	E943.4	E950.4	E962.0	E980.4
48:00 expectorants and cough preparations	—	—	—	—	—	—
antihistamine agents	963.0	E858.1	E933.0	E950.4	E962.0	E980.4
antitussives	975.4	E858.6	E945.4	E950.4	E962.0	E980.4
codeine derivatives	965.09	E850.2	E935.2	E950.0	E962.0	E980.0
expectorants	975.5	E858.6	E945.5	E950.4	E962.0	E980.4
narcotic agents NEC	965.09	E850.2	E935.2	E950.0	E962.0	E980.0
52:04 anti-infectives (EENT)	—	—	—	—	—	—
ENT agent	976.6	E858.7	E946.6	E950.4	E962.0	E980.4
ophthalmic preparation	976.5	E858.7	E946.5	E950.4	E962.0	E980.4
52:04.04 antibiotics (EENT)	—	—	—	—	—	—
ENT agent	976.6	E858.7	E946.6	E950.4	E962.0	E980.4
ophthalmic preparation	976.5	E858.7	E946.5	E950.4	E962.0	E980.4
52:04.06 antivirals (EENT)	—	—	—	—	—	—
ENT agent	976.6	E858.7	E946.6	E950.4	E962.0	E980.4
ophthalmic preparation	976.5	E858.7	E946.5	E950.4	E962.0	E980.4
52:04.08 sulfonamides (EENT)	—	—	—	—	—	—
ENT agent	976.6	E858.7	E946.6	E950.4	E962.0	E980.4
ophthalmic preparation	976.5	E858.7	E946.5	E950.4	E962.0	E980.4
52:04.12 miscellaneous anti-infectives (EENT)	—	—	—	—	—	—
ENT agent	976.6	E858.7	E946.6	E950.4	E962.0	E980.4
ophthalmic preparation	976.5	E858.7	E946.5	E950.4	E962.0	E980.4
52:08 anti-inflammatory agents (EENT)	—	—	—	—	—	—
ENT agent	976.6	E858.7	E946.6	E950.4	E962.0	E980.4
ophthalmic preparation	976.5	E858.7	E946.5	E950.4	E962.0	E980.4
52:10 carbonic anhydrase inhibitors	974.2	E858.5	E944.2	E950.4	E962.0	E980.4
52:12 contact lens solutions	976.5	E858.7	E946.5	E950.4	E962.0	E980.4
52:16 local anesthetics (EENT)	968.5	E855.2	E938.5	E950.4	E962.0	E980.4

◀ New　◀▥ Revised　deleted Deleted　● Use Additional Digit(s)

Substance	Poisoning	External Cause (E Code)				
		Accident	Therapeutic Use	Suicide Attempt	Assault	Undetermined
Drug *(Continued)*						
52:20 miotics	971.0	E855.3	E941.0	E950.4	E962.0	E980.4
52:24 mydriatics	—	—	—	—	—	—
adrenergics	971.2	E855.5	E941.2	E950.4	E962.0	E980.4
anticholinergics	971.1	E855.4	E941.1	E950.4	E962.0	E980.4
antimuscarinics	971.1	E855.4	E941.1	E950.4	E962.0	E980.4
parasympatholytics	971.1	E855.4	E941.1	E950.4	E962.0	E980.4
spasmolytics	971.1	E855.4	E941.1	E950.4	E962.0	E980.4
sympathomimetics	971.2	E855.5	E941.2	E950.4	E962.0	E980.4
52:28 mouth washes and gargles	976.6	E858.7	E946.6	E950.4	E962.0	E980.4
52:32 vasoconstrictors (EENT)	971.2	E855.5	E941.2	E950.4	E962.0	E980.4
52:36 unclassified agents (EENT)	—	—	—	—	—	—
ENT agent	976.6	E858.7	E946.6	E950.4	E962.0	E980.4
ophthalmic preparation	976.5	E858.7	E946.5	E950.4	E962.0	E980.4
56:04 antacids and adsorbents	973.0	E858.4	E943.0	E950.4	E962.0	E980.4
56:08 antidiarrhea agents	973.5	E858.4	E943.5	E950.4	E962.0	E980.4
56:10 antiflatulents	973.8	E858.4	E943.8	E950.4	E962.0	E980.4
56:12 cathartics NEC	973.3	E858.4	E943.3	E950.4	E962.0	E980.4
emollients	973.2	E858.4	E943.2	E950.4	E962.0	E980.4
irritants	973.1	E858.4	E943.1	E950.4	E962.0	E980.4
56:16 digestants	973.4	E858.4	E943.4	E950.4	E962.0	E980.4
56:20 emetics and antiemetics	—	—	—	—	—	—
antiemetics	963.0	E858.1	E933.0	E950.4	E962.0	E980.4
emetics	973.6	E858.4	E943.6	E950.4	E962.0	E980.4
56:24 lipotropic agents	977.1	E858.8	E947.1	E950.4	E962.0	E980.4
56:40 miscellaneous G.I. drugs	973.8	E858.4	E943.8	E950.4	E962.0	E980.4
60:00 gold compounds	965.69	E850.6	E935.6	E950.0	E962.0	E980.0
64:00 heavy metal antagonists	963.8	E858.1	E933.8	E950.4	E962.0	E980.4
68:04 adrenals	962.0	E858.0	E932.0	E950.4	E962.0	E980.4
68:08 androgens	962.1	E858.0	E932.1	E950.4	E962.0	E980.4
68:12 contraceptives, oral	962.2	E858.0	E932.2	E950.4	E962.0	E980.4
68:16 estrogens	962.2	E858.0	E932.2	E950.4	E962.0	E980.4
68:18 gonadotropins	962.4	E858.0	E932.4	E950.4	E962.0	E980.4
68:20 insulins and antidiabetic agents	962.3	E858.0	E932.3	E950.4	E962.0	E980.4
68:20.08 insulins	962.3	E858.0	E932.3	E950.4	E962.0	E980.4
68:24 parathyroid	962.6	E858.0	E932.6	E950.4	E962.0	E980.4
68:28 pituitary (posterior)	962.5	E858.0	E932.5	E950.4	E962.0	E980.4
anterior	962.4	E858.0	E932.4	E950.4	E962.0	E980.4
68:32 progestogens	962.2	E858.0	E932.2	E950.4	E962.0	E980.4

◀ New　◀▥ Revised　~~deleted~~ Deleted　● Use Additional Digit(s)

Substance	Poisoning	External Cause (E Code) Accident	Therapeutic Use	Suicide Attempt	Assault	Undetermined
Drug *(Continued)*						
68:34 other corpus luteum hormones NEC	962.2	E858.0	E932.2	E950.4	E962.0	E980.4
68:36 thyroid and antithyroid	—	—	—	—	—	—
antithyroid	962.8	E858.0	E932.8	E950.4	E962.0	E980.4
thyroid (derivatives)	962.7	E858.0	E932.7	E950.4	E962.0	E980.4
72:00 local anesthetics NEC	968.9	E855.2	E938.9	E950.4	E962.0	E980.4
topical (surface)	968.5	E855.2	E938.5	E950.4	E962.0	E980.4
infiltration (intradermal) (subcutaneous) (submucosal)	968.5	E855.2	E938.5	E950.4	E962.0	E980.4
nerve blocking (peripheral) (plexus) (regional)	968.6	E855.2	E938.6	E950.4	E962.0	E980.4
spinal	968.7	E855.2	E938.7	E950.4	E962.0	E980.4
76:00 oxytocics	975.0	E858.6	E945.0	E950.4	E962.0	E980.4
78:00 radioactive agents	990	—	—	—	—	—
80:04 serums NEC	979.9	E858.8	E949.9	E950.4	E962.0	E980.4
immune gamma globulin (human)	964.6	E858.2	E934.6	E950.4	E962.0	E980.4
80:08 toxoids NEC	978.8	E858.8	E948.8	E950.4	E962.0	E980.4
diphtheria	978.5	E858.8	E948.5	E950.4	E962.0	E980.4
and tetanus	978.9	E858.8	E948.9	E950.4	E962.0	E980.4
with pertussis component	978.6	E858.8	E948.6	E950.4	E962.0	E980.4
tetanus	978.4	E858.8	E948.4	E950.4	E962.0	E980.4
and diphtheria	978.9	E858.8	E948.9	E950.4	E962.0	E980.4
with pertussis component	978.6	E858.8	E948.6	E950.4	E962.0	E980.4
80:12 vaccines	979.9	E858.8	E949.9	E950.4	E962.0	E980.4
bacterial NEC	978.8	E858.8	E948.8	E950.4	E962.0	E980.4
with	—	—	—	—	—	—
other bacterial components	978.9	E858.8	E948.9	E950.4	E962.0	E980.4
pertussis component	978.6	E858.8	E948.6	E950.4	E962.0	E980.4
viral and rickettsial components	979.7	E858.8	E949.7	E950.4	E962.0	E980.4
rickettsial NEC	979.6	E858.8	E949.6	E950.4	E962.0	E980.4
with	—	—	—	—	—	—
bacterial component	979.7	E858.8	E949.7	E950.4	E962.0	E980.4
pertussis component	978.6	E858.8	E948.6	E950.4	E962.0	E980.4
viral component	979.7	E858.8	E949.7	E950.4	E962.0	E980.4
viral NEC	979.6	E858.8	E949.6	E950.4	E962.0	E980.4
with	—	—	—	—	—	—
bacterial component	979.7	E858.8	E949.7	E950.4	E962.0	E980.4
pertussis component	978.6	E858.8	E948.6	E950.4	E962.0	E980.4
rickettsial component	979.7	E858.8	E949.7	E950.4	E962.0	E980.4
84:04.04 antibiotics (skin and mucous membrane)	976.0	E858.7	E946.0	E950.4	E962.0	E980.4
84:04.08 fungicides (skin and mucous membrane)	976.0	E858.7	E946.0	E950.4	E962.0	E980.4

Substance	Poisoning	External Cause (E Code)				
		Accident	Therapeutic Use	Suicide Attempt	Assault	Undetermined
Drug *(Continued)*						
84:04.12 scabicides and pediculicides (skin and mucous membrane)	976.0	E858.7	E946.0	E950.4	E962.0	E980.4
84:04.16 miscellaneous local anti-infectives (skin and mucous membrane)	976.0	E858.7	E946.0	E950.4	E962.0	E980.4
84:06 anti-inflammatory agents (skin and mucous membrane)	976.0	E858.7	E946.0	E950.4	E962.0	E980.4
84:08 antipruritics and local anesthetics	—	—	—	—	—	—
antipruritics	976.1	E858.7	E946.1	E950.4	E962.0	E980.4
local anesthetics	968.5	E855.2	E938.5	E950.4	E962.0	E980.4
84:12 astringents	976.2	E858.7	E946.2	E950.4	E962.0	E980.4
84:16 cell stimulants and proliferants	976.8	E858.7	E946.8	E950.4	E962.0	E980.4
84:20 detergents	976.2	E858.7	E946.2	E950.4	E962.0	E980.4
84:24 emollients, demulcents, and protectants	976.3	E858.7	E946.3	E950.4	E962.0	E980.4
84:28 keratolytic agents	976.4	E858.7	E946.4	E950.4	E962.0	E980.4
84:32 keratoplastic agents	976.4	E858.7	E946.4	E950.4	E962.0	E980.4
84:36 miscellaneous agents (skin and mucous membrane)	976.8	E858.7	E946.8	E950.4	E962.0	E980.4
86:00 spasmolytic agents	975.1	E858.6	E945.1	E950.4	E962.0	E980.4
antiasthmatics	975.7	E858.6	E945.7	E950.4	E962.0	E980.4
papaverine	972.5	E858.3	E942.5	E950.4	E962.0	E980.4
theophylline	974.1	E858.5	E944.1	E950.4	E962.0	E980.4
88:04 vitamin A	963.5	E858.1	E933.5	E950.4	E962.0	E980.4
88:08 vitamin B complex	963.5	E858.1	E933.5	E950.4	E962.0	E980.4
hematopoietic vitamin	964.1	E858.2	E934.1	E950.4	E962.0	E980.4
nicotinic acid derivatives	972.2	E858.3	E942.2	E950.4	E962.0	E980.4
88:12 vitamin C	963.5	E858.1	E933.5	E950.4	E962.0	E980.4
88:16 vitamin D	963.5	E858.1	E933.5	E950.4	E962.0	E980.4
88:20 vitamin E	963.5	E858.1	E933.5	E950.4	E962.0	E980.4
88:24 vitamin K activity	964.3	E858.2	E934.3	E950.4	E962.0	E980.4
88:28 multivitamin preparations	963.5	E858.1	E933.5	E950.4	E962.0	E980.4
92:00 unclassified therapeutic agents	977.8	E858.8	E947.8	E950.4	E962.0	E980.4
Duboisine	971.1	E855.4	E941.1	E950.4	E962.0	E980.4
Dulcolax	973.1	E858.4	E943.1	E950.4	E962.0	E980.4
Duponol (C) (EP)	976.2	E858.7	E946.2	E950.4	E962.0	E980.4
Durabolin	962.1	E858.0	E932.1	E950.4	E962.0	E980.4
Dyclone	968.5	E855.2	E938.5	E950.4	E962.0	E980.4
Dyclonine	968.5	E855.2	E938.5	E950.4	E962.0	E980.4
Dydrogesterone	962.2	E858.0	E932.2	E950.4	E962.0	E980.4
Dyes NEC	989.89	E866.8	—	E950.9	E962.1	E980.9
diagnostic agents	977.8	E858.8	E947.8	E950.4	E962.0	E980.4
pharmaceutical NEC	977.4	E858.8	E947.4	E950.4	E962.0	E980.4
Dyflos	971.0	E855.3	E941.0	E950.4	E962.0	E980.4

◄ New   ◄▥ Revised   ~~deleted~~ Deleted   ● Use Additional Digit(s)

TABLE OF DRUGS AND CHEMICALS

Substance	Poisoning	External Cause (E Code)				
		Accident	Therapeutic Use	Suicide Attempt	Assault	Undetermined
Dymelor	962.3	E858.0	E932.3	E950.4	E962.0	E980.4
Dynamite	989.89	E866.8	—	E950.9	E962.1	E980.9
fumes	987.8	E869.8	—	E952.8	E962.2	E982.8
Dyphylline	975.1	E858.6	E945.1	E950.4	E962.0	E980.4
Ear preparations	976.6	E858.7	E946.6	E950.4	E962.0	E980.4
Echothiopate, ecothiopate	971.0	E855.3	E941.0	E950.4	E962.0	E980.4
Ecstasy	969.72 ◄▥	E854.2	E939.7	E950.3	E962.0	E980.3
Ectylurea	967.8	E852.8	E937.8	E950.2	E962.0	E980.2
Edathamil disodium	963.8	E858.1	E933.8	E950.4	E962.0	E980.4
Edecrin	974.4	E858.5	E944.4	E950.4	E962.0	E980.4
Edetate, disodium (calcium)	963.8	E858.1	E933.8	E950.4	E962.0	E980.4
Edrophonium	971.0	E855.3	E941.0	E950.4	E962.0	E980.4
Elase	976.8	E858.7	E946.8	E950.4	E962.0	E980.4
Elaterium	973.1	E858.4	E943.1	E950.4	E962.0	E980.4
Elder	988.2	E865.4	—	E950.9	E962.1	E980.9
berry (unripe)	988.2	E865.3	—	E950.9	E962.1	E980.9
Electrolytes NEC	974.5	E858.5	E944.5	E950.4	E962.0	E980.4
Electrolytic agent NEC	974.5	E858.5	E944.5	E950.4	E962.0	E980.4
Embramine	963.0	E858.1	E933.0	E950.4	E962.0	E980.4
Emetics	973.6	E858.4	E943.6	E950.4	E962.0	E980.4
Emetine (hydrochloride)	961.5	E857	E931.5	E950.4	E962.0	E980.4
Emollients	976.3	E858.7	E946.3	E950.4	E962.0	E980.4
Emylcamate	969.5	E853.8	E939.5	E950.3	E962.0	E980.3
Encyprate	969.09 ◄▥	E854.0	E939.0	E950.3	E962.0	E980.3
Endocaine	968.5	E855.2	E938.5	E950.4	E962.0	E980.4
Endrin	989.2	E863.0	—	E950.6	E962.1	E980.7
Enflurane	968.2	E855.1	E938.2	E950.4	E962.0	E980.4
Enovid	962.2	E858.0	E932.2	E950.4	E962.0	E980.4
ENT preparations (anti-infectives)	976.6	E858.7	E946.6	E950.4	E962.0	E980.4
Enzodase	963.4	E858.1	E933.4	E950.4	E962.0	E980.4
Enzymes NEC	963.4	E858.1	E933.4	E950.4	E962.0	E980.4
Epanutin	966.1	E855.0	E936.1	E950.4	E962.0	E980.4
Ephedra (tincture)	971.2	E855.5	E941.2	E950.4	E962.0	E980.4
Ephedrine	971.2	E855.5	E941.2	E950.4	E962.0	E980.4
Epiestriol	962.2	E858.0	E932.2	E950.4	E962.0	E980.4
Epilim - see Sodium valproate	—	—	—	—	—	—
Epinephrine	971.2	E855.5	E941.2	E950.4	E962.0	E980.4
Epsom salt	973.3	E858.4	E943.3	E950.4	E962.0	E980.4
Equanil	969.5	E853.8	E939.5	E950.3	E962.0	E980.3

◄ New   ◄▥ Revised   ~~deleted~~ Deleted   ● Use Additional Digit(s)

Substance	Poisoning	External Cause (E Code)				
		Accident	Therapeutic Use	Suicide Attempt	Assault	Undetermined
Equisetum (diuretic)	974.4	E858.5	E944.4	E950.4	E962.0	E980.4
Ergometrine	975.0	E858.6	E945.0	E950.4	E962.0	E980.4
Ergonovine	975.0	E858.6	E945.0	E950.4	E962.0	E980.4
Ergot NEC	988.2	E865.4	—	E950.9	E962.1	E980.9
medicinal (alkaloids)	975.0	E858.6	E945.0	E950.4	E962.0	E980.4
Ergotamine (tartrate) (for migraine) NEC	972.9	E858.3	E942.9	E950.4	E962.0	E980.4
Ergotrate	975.0	E858.6	E945.0	E950.4	E962.0	E980.4
Erythrityl tetranitrate	972.4	E858.3	E942.4	E950.4	E962.0	E980.4
Erythrol tetranitrate	972.4	E858.3	E942.4	E950.4	E962.0	E980.4
Erythromycin	960.3	E856	E930.3	E950.4	E962.0	E980.4
ophthalmic preparation	976.5	E858.7	E946.5	E950.4	E962.0	E980.4
topical NEC	976.0	E858.7	E946.0	E950.4	E962.0	E980.4
Eserine	971.0	E855.3	E941.0	E950.4	E962.0	E980.4
Eskabarb	967.0	E851	E937.0	E950.1	E962.0	E980.1
Eskalith	969.8	E855.8	E939.8	E950.3	E962.0	E980.3
Estradiol (cypionate) (dipropionate) (valerate)	962.2	E858.0	E932.2	E950.4	E962.0	E980.4
Estriol	962.2	E858.0	E932.2	E950.4	E962.0	E980.4
Estrogens (with progestogens)	962.2	E858.0	E932.2	E950.4	E962.0	E980.4
Estrone	962.2	E858.0	E932.2	E950.4	E962.0	E980.4
Etafedrine	971.2	E855.5	E941.2	E950.4	E962.0	E980.4
Ethacrynate sodium	974.4	E858.5	E944.4	E950.4	E962.0	E980.4
Ethacrynic acid	974.4	E858.5	E944.4	E950.4	E962.0	E980.4
Ethambutol	961.8	E857	E931.8	E950.4	E962.0	E980.4
Ethamide	974.2	E858.5	E944.2	E950.4	E962.0	E980.4
Ethamivan	970.0	E854.3	E940.0	E950.4	E962.0	E980.4
Ethamsylate	964.5	E858.2	E934.5	E950.4	E962.0	E980.4
Ethanol	980.0	E860.1	—	E950.9	E962.1	E980.9
beverage	980.0	E860.0	—	E950.9	E962.1	E980.9
Ethchlorvynol	967.8	E852.8	E937.8	E950.2	E962.0	E980.2
Ethebenecid	974.7	E858.5	E944.7	E950.4	E962.0	E980.4
Ether(s) (diethyl) (ethyl) (vapor)	987.8	E869.8	—	E952.8	E962.2	E982.8
anesthetic	968.2	E855.1	E938.2	E950.4	E962.0	E980.4
petroleum - *see* Ligroin solvent	982.8	E862.4	—	E950.9	E962.1	E980.9
Ethidine chloride (vapor)	987.8	E869.8	—	E952.8	E962.2	E982.8
liquid (solvent)	982.3	E862.4	—	E950.9	E962.1	E980.9
Ethinamate	967.8	E852.8	E937.8	E950.2	E962.0	E980.2
Ethinylestradiol	962.2	E858.0	E932.2	E950.4	E962.0	E980.4
Ethionamide	961.8	E857	E931.8	E950.4	E962.0	E980.4
Ethisterone	962.2	E858.0	E932.2	E950.4	E962.0	E980.4

◄ New ◄▮▮ Revised ~~deleted~~ Deleted ● Use Additional Digit(s)

Substance	Poisoning	External Cause (E Code)				
		Accident	Therapeutic Use	Suicide Attempt	Assault	Undetermined
Ethobral	967.0	E851	E937.0	E950.1	E962.0	E980.1
Ethocaine (infiltration) (topical)	968.5	E855.2	E938.5	E950.4	E962.0	E980.4
nerve block (peripheral) (plexus)	968.6	E855.2	E938.6	E950.4	E962.0	E980.4
spinal	968.7	E855.2	E938.7	E950.4	E962.0	E980.4
Ethoheptazine (citrate)	965.7	E850.7	E935.7	E950.0	E962.0	E980.0
Ethopropazine	966.4	E855.0	E936.4	E950.4	E962.0	E980.4
Ethosuximide	966.2	E855.0	E936.2	E950.4	E962.0	E980.4
Ethotoin	966.1	E855.0	E936.1	E950.4	E962.0	E980.4
Ethoxazene	961.9	E857	E931.9	E950.4	E962.0	E980.4
Ethoxzolamide	974.2	E858.5	E944.2	E950.4	E962.0	E980.4
Ethyl	—	—	—	—	—	—
acetate (vapor)	982.8	E862.4	—	E950.9	E962.1	E980.9
alcohol	980.0	E860.1	—	E950.9	E962.1	E980.9
beverage	980.0	E860.0	—	E950.9	E962.1	E980.9
aldehyde (vapor)	987.8	E869.8	—	E952.8	E962.2	E982.8
liquid	989.89	E866.8	—	E950.9	E962.1	E980.9
aminobenzoate	968.5	E855.2	E938.5	E950.4	E962.0	E980.4
biscoumacetate	964.2	E858.2	E934.2	E950.4	E962.0	E980.4
bromide (anesthetic)	968.2	E855.1	E938.2	E950.4	E962.0	E980.4
carbamate (antineoplastic)	963.1	E858.1	E933.1	E950.4	E962.0	E980.4
carbinol	980.3	E860.4	—	E950.9	E962.1	E980.9
chaulmoograte	961.8	E857	E931.8	E950.4	E962.0	E980.4
chloride (vapor)	987.8	E869.8	—	E952.8	E962.2	E982.8
anesthetic (local)	968.5	E855.2	E938.5	E950.4	E962.0	E980.4
inhaled	968.2	E855.1	E938.2	E950.4	E962.0	E980.4
solvent	982.3	E862.4	—	E950.9	E962.1	E980.9
estranol	962.1	E858.0	E932.1	E950.4	E962.0	E980.4
ether - see Ether(s)	—	—	—	—	—	—
formate (solvent) NEC	982.8	E862.4	—	E950.9	E962.1	E980.9
iodoacetate	987.5	E869.3	—	E952.8	E962.2	E982.8
lactate (solvent) NEC	982.8	E862.4	—	E950.9	E962.1	E980.9
methylcarbinol	980.8	E860.8	—	E950.9	E962.1	E980.9
morphine	965.09	E850.2	E935.2	E950.0	E962.0	E980.0
Ethylene (gas)	987.1	E869.8	—	E952.8	E962.2	E982.8
anesthetic (general)	968.2	E855.1	E938.2	E950.4	E962.0	E980.4
chlorohydrin (vapor)	982.3	E862.4	—	E950.9	E962.1	E980.9
dichloride (vapor)	982.3	E862.4	—	E950.9	E962.1	E980.9
glycol(s) (any) (vapor)	982.8	E862.4	—	E950.9	E962.1	E980.9

◀ New   ◀▦ Revised   ~~deleted~~ Deleted   ● Use Additional Digit(s)

Substance	Poisoning	External Cause (E Code)				
		Accident	Therapeutic Use	Suicide Attempt	Assault	Undetermined
Ethylidene	—	—	—	—	—	—
chloride NEC	982.3	E862.4	—	E950.9	E962.1	E980.9
diethyl ether	982.8	—	E862.4	E950.9	E962.1	E980.9
Ethynodiol	962.2	E858.0	E932.2	E950.4	E962.0	E980.4
Etidocaine	968.9	E855.2	E938.9	E950.4	E962.0	E980.4
infiltration (subcutaneous)	968.5	E855.2	E938.5	E950.4	E962.0	E980.4
nerve (peripheral) (plexus)	968.6	E855.2	E938.6	E950.4	E962.0	E980.4
Etilfen	967.0	E851	E937.0	E950.1	E962.0	E980.1
Etomide	965.7	E850.7	E935.7	E950.0	E962.0	E980.0
Etorphine	965.09	E850.2	E935.2	E950.0	E962.0	E980.0
Etoval	967.0	E851	E937.0	E950.1	E962.0	E980.1
Etryptamine	969.01 ◀▥	E854.0	E939.0	E950.3	E962.0	E980.3
Eucaine	968.5	E855.2	E938.5	E950.4	E962.0	E980.4
Eucalyptus (oil) NEC	975.5	E858.6	E945.5	E950.4	E962.0	E980.4
Eucatropine	971.1	E855.4	E941.1	E950.4	E962.0	E980.4
Eucodal	965.09	E850.2	E935.2	E950.0	E962.0	E980.0
Euneryl	967.0	E851	E937.0	E950.1	E962.0	E980.1
Euphthalmine	971.1	E855.4	E941.1	E950.4	E962.0	E980.4
Eurax	976.0	E858.7	E946.0	E950.4	E962.0	E980.4
Euresol	976.4	E858.7	E946.4	E950.4	E962.0	E980.4
Euthroid	962.7	E858.0	E932.7	E950.4	E962.0	E980.4
Evans blue	977.8	E858.8	E947.8	E950.4	E962.0	E980.4
Evipal	967.0	E851	E937.0	E950.1	E962.0	E980.1
sodium	968.3	E855.1	E938.3	E950.4	E962.0	E980.4
Evipan	967.0	E851	E937.0	E950.1	E962.0	E980.1
sodium	968.3	E855.1	E938.3	E950.4	E962.0	E980.4
Exalgin	965.4	E850.4	E935.4	E950.0	E962.0	E980.0
Excipients, pharmaceutical	977.4	E858.8	E947.4	E950.4	E962.0	E980.4
Exhaust gas - *see* Carbon, monoxide	—	—	—	—	—	—
Ex-Lax (phenolphthalein)	973.1	E858.4	E943.1	E950.4	E962.0	E980.4
Expectorants	975.5	E858.6	E945.5	E950.4	E962.0	E980.4
External medications (skin) (mucous membrane)	976.9	E858.7	E946.9	E950.4	E962.0	E980.4
dental agent	976.7	E858.7	E946.7	E950.4	E962.0	E980.4
ENT agent	976.6	E858.7	E946.6	E950.4	E962.0	E980.4
ophthalmic preparation	976.5	E858.7	E946.5	E950.4	E962.0	E980.4
specified NEC	976.8	E858.7	E946.8	E950.4	E962.0	E980.4
Eye agents (anti-infective)	976.5	E858.7	E946.5	E950.4	E962.0	E980.4
Factor IX complex (human)	964.5	E858.2	E934.5	E950.4	E962.0	E980.4
Fecal softeners	973.2	E858.4	E943.2	E950.4	E962.0	E980.4

◀ New　◀▥ Revised　~~deleted~~ Deleted　● Use Additional Digit(s)

Substance	Poisoning	External Cause (E Code)				
		Accident	Therapeutic Use	Suicide Attempt	Assault	Undetermined
Fenbutrazate	977.0	E858.8	E947.0	E950.4	E962.0	E980.4
Fencamfamin	970.8	E854.3	E940.8	E950.4	E962.0	E980.4
Fenfluramine	977.0	E858.8	E947.0	E950.4	E962.0	E980.4
Fenoprofen	965.61	E850.6	E935.6	E950.0	E962.0	E980.0
Fentanyl	965.09	E850.2	E935.2	E950.0	E962.0	E980.0
Fentazin	969.1	E853.0	E939.1	E930.3	E962.0	E980.3
Fenticlor, fentichlor	976.0	E858.7	E946.0	E950.4	E962.0	E980.4
Fer de lance (bite) (venom)	989.5	E905.0	—	E950.9	E962.1	E980.9
Ferric - *see* Iron	—	—	—	—	—	—
Ferrocholinate	964.0	E858.2	E934.0	E950.4	E962.0	E980.4
Ferrous fumerate, gluconate, lactate, salt NEC, sulfate (medicinal)	964.0	E858.2	E934.0	E950.4	E962.0	E980.4
Ferrum - *see* Iron	—	—	—	—	—	—
Fertilizers NEC	989.89	E866.5	—	E950.9	E962.1	E980.4
with herbicide mixture	989.4	E863.5	—	E950.6	E962.1	E980.7
Fibrinogen (human)	964.7	E858.2	E934.7	E950.4	E962.0	E980.4
Fibrinolysin	964.4	E858.2	E934.4	E950.4	E962.0	E980.4
Fibrinolysis-affecting agents	964.4	E858.2	E934.4	E950.4	E962.0	E980.4
Filix mas	961.6	E857	E931.6	E950.4	E962.0	E980.4
Fiorinal	965.1	E850.3	E935.3	E950.0	E962.0	E980.0
Fire damp	987.1	E869.8	—	E952.8	E962.2	E982.8
Fish, nonbacterial or noxious	988.0	E865.2	—	E950.9	E962.1	E980.9
shell	988.0	E865.1	—	E950.9	E962.1	E980.9
Flagyl	961.5	E857	E931.5	E950.4	E962.0	E980.4
Flavoxate	975.1	E858.6	E945.1	E950.4	E962.0	E980.4
Flaxedil	975.2	E858.6	E945.2	E950.4	E962.0	E980.4
Flaxseed (medicinal)	976.3	E858.7	E946.3	E950.4	E962.0	E980.4
Flomax	971.3	E855.6	E941.3	E950.4	E962.0	E980.4
Florantyrone	973.4	E858.4	E943.4	E950.4	E962.0	E980.4
Floraquin	961.3	E857	E931.3	E950.4	E962.0	E980.4
Florinef	962.0	E858.0	E932.0	E950.4	E962.0	E980.4
ENT agent	976.6	E858.7	E946.6	E950.4	E962.0	E980.4
ophthalmic preparation	976.5	E858.7	E946.5	E950.4	E962.0	E980.4
topical NEC	976.0	E858.7	E946.0	E950.4	E962.0	E980.4
Flowers of sulfur	976.4	E858.7	E946.4	E950.4	E962.0	E980.4
Floxuridine	963.1	E858.1	E933.1	E950.4	E962.0	E980.4
Flucytosine	961.9	E857	E931.9	E950.4	E962.0	E980.4
Fludrocortisone	962.0	E858.0	E932.0	E950.4	E962.0	E980.4
ENT agent	976.6	E858.7	E946.6	E950.4	E962.0	E980.4
ophthalmic preparation	976.5	E858.7	E946.5	E950.4	E962.0	E980.4

◀ New   ◀▥ Revised   ~~deleted~~ Deleted   ● Use Additional Digit(s)

Substance	Poisoning	External Cause (E Code)				
		Accident	Therapeutic Use	Suicide Attempt	Assault	Undetermined
Fludrocortisone *(Continued)*						
topical NEC	976.0	E858.7	E946.0	E950.4	E962.0	E980.4
Flumethasone	976.0	E858.7	E946.0	E950.4	E962.0	E980.4
Flumethiazide	974.3	E858.5	E944.3	E950.4	E962.0	E980.4
Flumidin	961.7	E857	E931.7	E950.4	E962.0	E980.4
Flunitrazepam	969.4	E853.2	E939.4	E950.3	E962.0	E980.3
Fluocinolone	976.0	E858.7	E946.0	E950.4	E962.0	E980.4
Fluocortolone	962.0	E858.0	E932.0	E950.4	E962.0	E980.4
Fluohydrocortisone	962.0	E858.0	E932.0	E950.4	E962.0	E980.4
ENT agent	976.6	E858.7	E946.6	E950.4	E962.0	E980.4
ophthalmic preparation	976.5	E858.7	E946.5	E950.4	E962.0	E980.4
topical NEC	976.0	E858.7	E946.0	E950.4	E962.0	E980.4
Fluonid	976.0	E858.7	E946.0	E950.4	E962.0	E980.4
Fluopromazine	969.1	E853.0	E939.1	E950.3	E962.0	E980.3
Fluoracetate	989.4	E863.7	—	E950.6	E962.1	E980.7
Fluorescein (sodium)	977.8	E858.8	E947.8	E950.4	E962.0	E980.4
Fluoride(s) (pesticides) (sodium) NEC	989.4	E863.4	—	E950.6	E962.1	E980.7
hydrogen - *see* Hydrofluoric acid	—	—	—	—	—	—
medicinal	976.7	E858.7	E946.7	E950.4	E962.0	E980.4
not pesticide NEC	983.9	E864.4	—	E950.7	E962.1	E980.6
stannous	976.7	E858.7	E946.7	E950.4	E962.0	E980.4
Fluorinated corticosteroids	962.0	E858.0	E932.0	E950.4	E962.0	E980.4
Fluorine (compounds) (gas)	987.8	E869.8	—	E952.8	E962.2	E982.8
salt - *see* Fluoride(s)	—	—	—	—	—	—
Fluoristan	976.7	E858.7	E946.7	E950.4	E962.0	E980.4
Fluoroacetate	989.4	E863.7	—	E950.6	E962.1	E980.7
Fluorodeoxyuridine	963.1	E858.1	E933.1	E950.4	E962.0	E980.4
Fluorometholone (topical) NEC	976.0	E858.7	E946.0	E950.4	E962.0	E980.4
ophthalmic preparation	976.5	E858.7	E946.5	E950.4	E962.0	E980.4
Fluorouracil	963.1	E858.1	E933.1	E950.4	E962.0	E980.4
Fluothane	968.1	E855.1	E938.1	E950.4	E962.0	E980.4
Fluoxetine hydrochloride	969.03 ◀	E854.0	E939.0	E950.3	E962.0	E980.3
Fluoxymesterone	962.1	E858.0	E932.1	E950.4	E962.0	E980.4
Fluphenazine	969.1	E853.0	E939.1	E950.3	E962.0	E980.3
Fluprednisolone	962.0	E858.0	E932.0	E950.4	E962.0	E980.4
Flurandrenolide	976.0	E858.7	E946.0	E950.4	E962.0	E980.4
Flurazepam (hydrochloride)	969.4	E853.2	E939.4	E950.3	E962.0	E980.3
Flurbiprofen	965.61	E850.6	E935.6	E950.0	E962.0	E980.0

◀ New   ◀▬ Revised   ~~deleted~~ Deleted   ● Use Additional Digit(s)

Substance	Poisoning	External Cause (E Code)				
		Accident	Therapeutic Use	Suicide Attempt	Assault	Undetermined
Flurobate	976.0	E858.7	E946.0	E950.4	E962.0	E980.4
Flurothyl	969.8	E855.8	E939.8	E950.3	E962.0	E980.3
Fluroxene	968.2	E855.1	E938.2	E950.4	E962.0	E980.4
Folacin	964.1	E858.2	E934.1	E950.4	E962.0	E980.4
Folic acid	964.1	E858.2	E934.1	E950.4	E962.0	E980.4
Follicle stimulating hormone	962.4	E858.0	E932.4	E950.4	E962.0	E980.4
Food, foodstuffs, nonbacterial or noxious	988.9	E865.9	—	E950.9	E962.1	E980.9
berries, seeds	988.2	E865.3	—	E950.9	E962.1	E980.9
fish	988.0	E865.2	—	E950.9	E962.1	E980.9
mushrooms	988.1	E865.5	—	E950.9	E962.1	E980.9
plants	988.2	E865.9	—	E950.9	E962.1	E980.9
specified type NEC	988.2	E865.4	—	E950.9	E962.1	E980.9
shellfish	988.0	E865.1	—	E950.9	E962.1	E980.9
specified NEC	988.8	E865.8	—	E950.9	E962.1	E980.9
Fool's parsley	988.2	E865.4	—	E950.9	E962.1	E980.9
Formaldehyde (solution)	989.89	E861.4	—	E950.9	E962.1	E980.9
fungicide	989.4	E863.6	—	E950.6	E962.1	E980.7
gas or vapor	987.8	E869.8	—	E952.8	E962.2	E982.8
Formalin	989.89	E861.4	—	E950.9	E962.1	E980.9
fungicide	989.4	E863.6	—	E950.6	E962.1	E980.7
vapor	987.8	E869.8	—	E952.8	E962.2	E982.8
Formic acid	983.1	E864.1	—	E950.7	E962.1	E980.6
vapor	987.8	E869.8	—	E952.8	E962.2	E982.8
Fowler's solution	985.1	E866.3	—	E950.8	E962.1	E980.8
Foxglove	988.2	E865.4	—	E950.9	E962.1	E980.9
Fox green	977.8	E858.8	E947.8	E950.4	E962.0	E980.4
Framycetin	960.8	E856	E930.8	E950.4	E962.0	E980.4
Frangula (extract)	973.1	E858.4	E943.1	E950.4	E962.0	E980.4
Frei antigen	977.8	E858.8	E947.8	E950.4	E962.0	E980.4
Freons	987.4	E869.2	—	E952.8	E962.2	E982.8
Fructose	974.5	E858.5	E944.5	E950.4	E962.0	E980.4
Frusemide	974.4	E858.5	E944.4	E950.4	E962.0	E980.4
FSH	962.4	E858.0	E932.4	E950.4	E962.0	E980.4
Fuel	—	—	—	—	—	—
automobile	981	E862.1	—	E950.9	E962.1	E980.9
exhaust gas, not in transit	986	E868.2	—	E952.0	E962.2	E982.0
vapor NEC	987.1	E869.8	—	E952.8	E962.2	E982.8

◄ New ◄⁞⁞⁞ Revised deleted Deleted ● Use Additional Digit(s)

Substance	External Cause (E Code)					
	Poisoning	Accident	Therapeutic Use	Suicide Attempt	Assault	Undetermined
Fuel *(Continued)*						
gas (domestic use) - *see also* Carbon, monoxide, fuel	—	—	—	—	—	—
utility	987.1	E868.1	—	E951.8	E962.2	E981.8
incomplete combustion of - *see* Carbon, monoxide, fuel, utility	—	—	—	—	—	—
in mobile container	987.0	E868.0	—	E951.1	E962.2	E981.1
piped (natural)	987.1	E867	—	E951.0	E962.2	E981.0
industrial, incomplete combustion	986	E868.3	—	E952.1	E962.2	E982.1
Fugillin	960.8	E856	E930.8	E950.4	E962.0	E980.4
Fulminate of mercury	985.0	E866.1	—	E950.9	E962.1	E980.9
Fulvicin	960.1	E856	E930.1	E950.4	E962.0	E980.4
Fumadil	960.8	E856	E930.8	E950.4	E962.0	E980.4
Fumagillin	960.8	E856	E930.8	E950.4	E962.0	E980.4
Fumes (from)	987.9	E869.9	—	E952.9	E962.2	E982.9
carbon monoxide - *see* Carbon, monoxide	—	—	—	—	—	—
charcoal (domestic use)	986	E868.3	—	E952.1	E962.2	E982.1
chloroform - *see* Chloroform						
coke (in domestic stoves, fireplaces)	986	E868.3	—	E952.1	E962.2	E982.1
corrosive NEC	987.8	E869.8	—	E952.8	E962.2	E982.8
ether - *see* Ether(s)						
freons	987.4	E869.2	—	E952.8	E962.2	E982.8
hydrocarbons	987.1	E869.8	—	E952.8	E962.2	E982.8
petroleum (liquefied)	987.0	E868.0	—	E951.1	E962.2	E981.1
distributed through pipes (pure or mixed with air)	987.0	E867	—	E951.0	E962.2	E981.0
lead - *see* Lead	—	—	—	—	—	—
metals - *see* specified metal	—	—	—	—	—	—
nitrogen dioxide	987.2	E869.0	—	E952.8	E962.2	E982.8
pesticides - *see* Pesticides	—	—	—	—	—	—
petroleum (liquefied)	987.0	E868.0	—	E951.1	E962.2	E981.1
distributed through pipes (pure or mixed with air)	987.0	E867	—	E951.0	E962.2	E981.0
polyester	987.8	E869.8	—	E952.8	E962.2	E982.8
specified source, other (*see also* substance specified)	987.8	E869.8	—	E952.8	E962.2	E982.8
sulfur dioxide	987.3	E869.1	—	E952.8	E962.2	E982.8
Fumigants	989.4	E863.8	—	E950.6	E962.1	E980.7
Fungi, noxious, used as food	988.1	E865.5	—	E950.9	E962.1	E980.9
Fungicides (*see also* Antifungals)	989.4	E863.6	—	E950.6	E962.1	E980.7
Fungizone	960.1	E856	E930.1	E950.4	E962.0	E980.4
topical	976.0	E858.7	E946.0	E950.4	E962.0	E980.4
Furacin	976.0	E858.7	E946.0	E950.4	E962.0	E980.4

◀ New ◀▥ Revised ~~deleted~~ Deleted ● Use Additional Digit(s)

Substance	Poisoning	External Cause (E Code)				
		Accident	Therapeutic Use	Suicide Attempt	Assault	Undetermined
Furadantin	961.9	E857	E931.9	E950.4	E962.0	E980.4
Furazolidone	961.9	E857	E931.9	E950.4	E962.0	E980.4
Furnace (coal burning) (domestic), gas from	986	E868.3	—	E952.1	E962.2	E982.1
industrial	986	E868.8	—	E952.1	E962.2	E982.1
Furniture polish	989.89	E861.2	—	E950.9	E962.1	E980.9
Furosemide	974.4	E858.5	E944.4	E950.4	E962.0	E980.4
Furoxone	961.9	E857	E931.9	E950.4	E962.0	E980.4
Fusel oil (amyl) (butyl) (propyl)	980.3	E860.4	—	E950.9	E962.1	E980.9
Fusidic acid	960.8	E856	E930.8	E950.4	E962.0	E980.4
Gallamine	975.2	E858.6	E945.2	E950.4	E962.0	E980.4
Gallotannic acid	976.2	E858.7	E946.2	E950.4	E962.0	E980.4
Gamboge	973.1	E858.4	E943.1	E950.4	E962.0	E980.4
Gamimune	964.6	E858.2	E934.6	E950.4	E962.0	E980.4
Gamma-benzene hexachloride (vapor)	989.2	E863.0	—	E950.6	E962.1	E980.7
Gamma globulin	964.6	E858.2	E934.6	E950.4	E962.0	E980.4
Gamma hydroxy butyrate (GHB)	968.4	E855.1	E938.4	E950.4	E962.0	E980.4
Gamulin	964.6	E858.2	E934.6	E950.4	E962.0	E980.4
Ganglionic blocking agents	972.3	E858.3	E942.3	E950.4	E962.0	E980.4
Ganja	969.6	E854.1	E939.6	E950.3	E962.0	E980.3
Garamycin	960.8	E856	E930.8	E950.4	E962.0	E980.4
ophthalmic preparation	976.5	E858.7	E946.5	E950.4	E962.0	E980.4
topical NEC	976.0	E858.7	E946.0	E950.4	E962.0	E980.4
Gardenal	967.0	E851	E937.0	E950.1	E962.0	E980.1
Gardepanyl	967.0	E851	E937.0	E950.1	E962.0	E980.1
Gas	987.9	E869.9	—	E952.9	E962.2	E982.9
acetylene	987.1	E868.1	—	E951.8	E962.2	E981.8
incomplete combustion of - *see* Carbon, monoxide, fuel, utility	—	—	—	—	—	—
air contaminants, source or type not specified	987.9	E869.9	—	E952.9	E962.2	E982.9
anesthetic (general) NEC	968.2	E855.1	E938.2	E950.4	E962.0	E980.4
blast furnace	986	E868.8	—	E952.1	E962.2	E982.1
butane - *see* Butane	—	—	—	—	—	—
carbon monoxide - *see* Carbon, monoxide, chlorine	987.6	E869.8	—	E952.8	E962.2	E982.8
coal - *see* Carbon, monoxide, coal	—	—	—	—	—	—
cyanide	987.7	E869.8	—	E952.8	E962.2	E982.8
dicyanogen	987.8	E869.8	—	E952.8	E962.2	E982.8
domestic - *see* Gas, utility	—	—	—	—	—	—
exhaust - *see* Carbon, monoxide, exhaust gas	—	—	—	—	—	—
from wood- or coal-burning stove or fireplace	986	E868.3	—	E952.1	E962.2	E982.1

◀ New   ◀▥ Revised   ~~deleted~~ Deleted   ● Use Additional Digit(s)

Substance	External Cause (E Code)					
	Poisoning	Accident	Therapeutic Use	Suicide Attempt	Assault	Undetermined
Gas *(Continued)*						
fuel (domestic use) - *see also* Carbon, monoxide, fuel	—	—	—	—	—	—
industrial use	986	E868.8	—	E952.1	E962.2	E982.1
utility	987.1	E868.1	—	E951.8	E962.2	E981.8
incomplete combustion of - *see* Carbon, monoxide, fuel, utility	—	—	—	—	—	—
in mobile container	987.0	E868.0	—	E951.1	E962.2	E981.1
piped (natural)	987.1	E867	—	E951.0	E962.2	E981.0
garage	986	E868.2	—	E952.0	E962.2	E982.0
hydrocarbon NEC	987.1	E869.8	—	E952.8	E962.2	E982.8
incomplete combustion of - *see* Carbon, monoxide, fuel, utility	—	—	—	—	—	—
liquefied (mobile container)	987.0	E868.0	—	E951.1	E962.2	E981.1
piped	987.0	E867	—	E951.0	E962.2	E981.0
hydrocyanic acid	987.7	E869.8	—	E952.8	E962.2	E982.8
illuminating - *see* Gas, utility	—	—	—	—	—	—
incomplete combustion, any - *see* Carbon, monoxide	—	—	—	—	—	—
kiln	986	E868.8	—	E952.1	E962.2	E982.1
lacrimogenic	987.5	E869.3	—	E952.8	E962.2	E982.8
marsh	987.1	E869.8	—	E952.8	E962.2	E982.8
motor exhaust, not in transit	986	E868.8	—	E952.1	E962.2	E982.1
mustard - *see* Mustard, gas	—	—	—	—	—	—
natural	987.1	E867	—	E951.0	E962.2	E981.0
nerve (war)	987.9	E869.9	—	E952.9	E962.2	E982.9
oils	981	E862.1	—	E950.9	E962.1	E980.9
petroleum (liquefied) (distributed in mobile containers)	987.0	E868.0	—	E951.1	E962.2	E981.1
piped (pure or mixed with air)	987.0	E867	—	E951.1	E962.2	E981.1
piped (manufactured) (natural) NEC	987.1	E867	—	E951.0	E962.2	E981.0
producer	986	E868.8	—	E952.1	E962.2	E982.1
propane - *see* Propane	—	—	—	—	—	—
refrigerant (freon)	987.4	E869.2	—	E952.8	E962.2	E982.8
not freon	987.9	E869.9	—	E952.9	E962.2	E982.9
sewer	987.8	E869.8	—	E952.8	E962.2	E982.8
specified source NEC (*see also* substance specified)	987.8	E869.8	—	E952.8	E962.2	E982.8
stove - *see* Gas, utility	—	—	—	—	—	—
tear	987.5	E869.3	—	E952.8	E962.2	E982.8
utility (for cooking, heating, or lighting) (piped) NEC	987.1	E868.1	—	E951.8	E962.2	E981.8
incomplete combustion of - *see* Carbon, monoxide, fuel, utilty	—	—	—	—	—	—
in mobile container	987.0	E868.0	—	E951.1	E962.2	E981.1
piped (natural)	987.1	E867	—	E951.0	E962.2	E981.0
water	987.1	E868.1	—	E951.8	E962.2	E981.8
incomplete combustion of - *see* Carbon, monoxide, fuel, utility	—	—	—	—	—	—

◄ New   ◄▥ Revised   ~~deleted~~ Deleted   ● Use Additional Digit(s)

Substance	Poisoning	External Cause (E Code)				
		Accident	Therapeutic Use	Suicide Attempt	Assault	Undetermined
Gaseous substance - *see* Gas	—	—	—	—	—	—
Gasoline, gasolene	981	E862.1	—	E950.9	E962.1	E980.9
vapor	987.1	E869.8	—	E952.8	E962.2	E982.8
Gastric enzymes	973.4	E858.4	E943.4	E950.4	E962.0	E980.4
Gastrografin	977.8	E858.8	E947.8	E950.4	E962.0	E980.4
Gastrointestinal agents	973.9	E858.4	E943.9	E950.4	E962.0	E980.4
specified NEC	973.8	E858.4	E943.8	E950.4	E962.0	E980.4
Gaultheria procumbens	988.2	E865.4	—	E950.9	E962.1	E980.9
Gelatin (intravenous)	964.8	E858.2	E934.8	E950.4	E962.0	E980.4
absorbable (sponge)	964.5	E858.2	E934.5	E950.4	E962.0	E980.4
Gelfilm	976.8	E858.7	E946.8	E950.4	E962.0	E980.4
Gelfoam	964.5	E858.2	E934.5	E950.4	E962.0	E980.4
Gelsemine	970.8	E854.3	E940.8	E950.4	E962.0	E980.4
Gelsemium (sempervirens)	988.2	E865.4	—	E950.9	E962.1	E980.9
Gemonil	967.0	E851	E937.0	E950.1	E962.0	E980.1
Gentamicin	960.8	E856	E930.8	E950.4	E962.0	E980.4
ophthalmic preparation	976.5	E858.7	E946.5	E950.4	E962.0	E980.4
topical NEC	976.0	E858.7	E946.0	E950.4	E962.0	E980.4
Gentian violet	976.0	E858.7	E946.0	E950.4	E962.0	E980.4
Gexane	976.0	E858.7	E946.0	E950.4	E962.0	E980.4
Gila monster (venom)	989.5	E905.0	—	E950.9	E962.1	E980.9
Ginger, Jamaica	989.89	E866.8	—	E950.9	E962.1	E980.9
Gitalin	972.1	E858.3	E942.1	E950.4	E962.0	E980.4
Gitoxin	972.1	E858.3	E942.1	E950.4	E962.0	E980.4
Glandular extract (medicinal) NEC	977.9	E858.9	E947.9	E950.5	E962.0	E980.5
Glaucarubin	961.5	E857	E931.5	E950.4	E962.0	E980.4
Globin zinc insulin	962.3	E858.0	E932.3	E950.4	E962.0	E980.4
Glucagon	962.3	E858.0	E932.3	E950.4	E962.0	E980.4
Glucochloral	967.1	E852.0	E937.1	E950.2	E962.0	E980.2
Glucocorticoids	962.0	E858.0	E932.0	E950.4	E962.0	E980.4
Glucose	974.5	E858.5	E944.5	E950.4	E962.0	E980.4
oxidase reagent	977.8	E858.8	E947.8	E950.4	E962.0	E980.4
Glucosulfone sodium	961.8	E857	E931.8	E950.4	E962.0	E980.4
Glue(s)	989.89	E866.6	—	E950.9	E962.1	E980.9
Glutamic acid (hydrochloride)	973.4	E858.4	E943.4	E950.4	E962.0	E980.4
Glutaraldehyde	989.89	E861.4	—	E950.9	E962.1	E980.9
Glutathione	963.8	E858.1	E933.8	E950.4	E962.0	E980.4
Glutethimide (group)	967.5	E852.4	E937.5	E950.2	E962.0	E980.2
Glycerin (lotion)	976.3	E858.7	E946.3	E950.4	E962.0	E980.4
Glycerol (topical)	976.3	E858.7	E946.3	E950.4	E962.0	E980.4

◀ New   ◀▥ Revised   deleted Deleted   ● Use Additional Digit(s)

		External Cause (E Code)				
Substance	Poisoning	Accident	Therapeutic Use	Suicide Attempt	Assault	Undetermined
Glyceryl	—	—	—	—	—	—
guaiacolate	975.5	E858.6	E945.5	E950.4	E962.0	E980.4
triacetate (topical)	976.0	E858.7	E946.0	E950.4	E962.0	E980.4
trinitrate	972.4	E858.3	E942.4	E950.4	E962.0	E980.4
Glycine	974.5	E858.5	E944.5	E950.4	E962.0	E980.4
Glycobiarsol	961.1	E857	E931.1	E950.4	E962.0	E980.4
Glycols (ether)	982.8	E862.4	—	E950.9	E962.1	E980.9
Glycopyrrolate	971.1	E855.4	E941.1	E950.4	E962.0	E980.4
Glymidine	962.3	E858.0	E932.3	E950.4	E962.0	E980.4
Gold (compounds) (salts)	965.69	E850.6	E935.6	E950.0	E962.0	E980.0
Golden sulfide of antimony	985.4	E866.2	—	E950.9	E962.1	E980.9
Goldylocks	988.2	E865.4	—	E950.9	E962.1	E980.9
Gonadal tissue extract	962.9	E858.0	E932.9	E950.4	E962.0	E980.4
female	962.2	E858.0	E932.2	E950.4	E962.0	E980.4
male	962.1	E858.0	E932.1	E950.4	E962.0	E980.4
Gonadotropin	962.4	E858.0	E932.4	E950.4	E962.0	E980.4
Grain alcohol	980.0	E860.1	—	E950.9	E962.1	E980.9
beverage	980.0	E860.0	—	E950.9	E962.1	E980.9
Gramicidin	960.8	E856	E930.8	E950.4	E962.0	E980.4
Gratiola officinalis	988.2	E865.4	—	E950.9	E962.1	E980.9
Grease	989.89	E866.8	—	E950.9	E962.1	E980.9
Green hellebore	988.2	E865.4	—	E950.9	E962.1	E980.9
Green soap	976.2	E858.7	E946.2	E950.4	E962.0	E980.4
Grifulvin	960.1	E856	E930.1	E950.4	E962.0	E980.4
Griseofulvin	960.1	E856	E930.1	E950.4	E962.0	E980.4
Growth hormone	962.4	E858.0	E932.4	E950.4	E962.0	E980.4
Guaiacol	975.5	E858.6	E945.5	E950.4	E962.0	E980.4
Giuaiac reagent	977.8	E858.8	E947.8	E950.4	E962.0	E980.4
Guaifenesin	975.5	E858.6	E945.5	E950.4	E962.0	E980.4
Guaiphenesin	975.5	E858.6	E945.5	E950.4	E962.0	E980.4
Guanatol	961.4	E857	E931.4	E950.4	E962.0	E980.4
Guanethidine	972.6	E858.3	E942.6	E950.4	E962.0	E980.4
Guano	989.89	E866.5	—	E950.9	E962.1	E980.9
Guanochlor	972.6	E858.3	E942.6	E950.4	E962.0	E980.4
Guanoctine	972.6	E858.3	E942.6	E950.4	E962.0	E980.4
Guanoxan	972.6	E858.3	E942.6	E950.4	E962.0	E980.4
Hair treatment agent NEC	976.4	E858.7	E946.4	E950.4	E962.0	E980.4
Halcinonide	976.0	E858.7	E946.0	E950.4	E962.0	E980.4
Halethazole	976.0	E858.7	E946.0	E950.4	E962.0	E980.4

◀ New   ◀▥ Revised   ~~deleted~~ Deleted   ● Use Additional Digit(s)

Substance	Poisoning	External Cause (E Code)				
		Accident	Therapeutic Use	Suicide Attempt	Assault	Undetermined
Hallucinogens	969.6	E854.1	E939.6	E950.3	E962.0	E980.3
Haloperidol	969.2	E853.1	E939.2	E950.3	E962.0	E980.3
Haloprogin	976.0	E858.7	E946.0	E950.4	E962.0	E980.4
Halotex	976.0	E858.7	E946.0	E950.4	E962.0	E980.4
Halothane	968.1	E855.1	E938.1	E950.4	E962.0	E980.4
Halquinols	976.0	E858.7	E946.0	E950.4	E962.0	E980.4
Hand sanitizer	976.0	E858.7	E946.0	E950.4	E962.0	E980.4
Harmonyl	972.6	E858.3	E942.6	E950.4	E962.0	E980.4
Hartmann's solution	974.5	E858.5	E944.5	E950.4	E962.0	E980.4
Hashish	969.6	E854.1	E939.6	E950.3	E962.0	E980.3
Hawaiian wood rose seeds	969.6	E854.1	E939.6	E950.3	E962.0	E980.3
Headache cures, drugs, powders NEC	977.9	E858.9	E947.9	E950.5	E962.0	E980.9
Heavenly Blue (morning glory)	969.6	E854.1	E939.6	E950.3	E962.0	E980.3
Heavy metal antagonists	963.8	E858.1	E933.8	E950.4	E962.0	E980.4
anti-infectives	961.2	E857	E931.2	E950.4	E962.0	E980.4
Hedaquinium	976.0	E858.7	E946.0	E950.4	E962.0	E980.4
Hedge hyssop	988.2	E865.4	—	E950.9	E962.1	E980.9
Heet	976.8	E858.7	E946.8	E950.4	E962.0	E980.4
Helenin	961.6	E857	E931.6	E950.4	E962.0	E980.4
Hellebore (black) (green) (white)	988.2	E865.4	—	E950.9	E962.1	E980.9
Hemlock	988.2	E865.4	—	E950.9	E962.1	E980.9
Hemostatics	964.5	E858.2	E934.5	E950.4	E962.0	E980.4
capillary active drugs	972.8	E858.3	E942.8	E950.4	E962.0	E980.4
Henbane	988.2	E865.4	—	E950.9	E962.1	E980.9
Heparin (sodium)	964.2	E858.2	E934.2	E950.4	E962.0	E980.4
Heptabarbital, heptabarbitone	967.0	E851	E937.0	E950.1	E962.0	E980.1
Heptachlor	989.2	E863.0	—	E950.6	E962.1	E980.7
Heptalgin	965.09	E850.2	E935.2	E950.0	E962.0	E980.0
Herbicides	989.4	E863.5	—	E950.6	E962.1	E980.7
Heroin	965.01	E850.0	E935.0	E950.0	E962.0	E980.0
Herplex	976.5	E858.7	E946.5	E950.4	E962.0	E980.4
HES	964.8	E858.2	E934.8	E950.4	E962.0	E980.4
Hetastarch	964.8	E858.2	E934.8	E950.4	E962.0	E980.7
Hexachlorocyclohexane	989.2	E863.0	—	E950.6	E962.1	E980.7
Hexachlorophene	976.2	E858.7	E946.2	E950.4	E962.0	E980.4
Hexadimethrine (bromide)	964.5	E858.2	E934.5	E950.4	E962.0	E980.4
Hexafluorenium	975.2	E858.6	E945.2	E950.4	E962.0	E980.4
Hexa-germ	976.2	E858.7	E946.2	E950.4	E962.0	E980.4
Hexahydrophenol	980.8	E860.8	—	E950.9	E962.1	E980.9

◀ New　◀▥ Revised　~~deleted~~ Deleted　● Use Additional Digit(s)

Substance	Poisoning	External Cause (E Code)				
		Accident	Therapeutic Use	Suicide Attempt	Assault	Undetermined
Hexalen	980.8	E860.8	—	E950.9	E962.1	E980.9
Hexamethonium	972.3	E858.3	E942.3	E950.4	E962.0	E980.4
Hexamethylenamine	961.9	E857	E931.9	E950.4	E962.0	E980.4
Hexamine	961.9	E857	E931.9	E950.4	E962.0	E980.4
Hexanone	982.8	E862.4	—	E950.9	E962.1	E980.9
Hexapropymate	967.8	E852.8	E937.8	E950.2	E962.0	E980.2
Hexestrol	962.2	E858.0	E932.2	E950.4	E962.0	E980.4
Hexethal (sodium)	967.0	E851	E937.0	E950.1	E962.0	E980.1
Hexetidine	976.0	E858.7	E946.0	E950.4	E962.0	E980.4
Hexobarbital, hexobarbitone	967.0	E851	E937.0	E950.1	E962.0	E980.1
sodium (anesthetic)	968.3	E855.1	E938.3	E950.4	E962.0	E980.4
soluble	968.3	E855.1	E938.3	E950.4	E962.0	E980.4
Hexocyclium	971.1	E855.4	E941.1	E950.4	E962.0	E980.4
Hexoestrol	962.2	E858.0	E932.2	E950.4	E962.0	E980.4
Hexone	982.8	E862.4	—	E950.9	E962.1	E980.9
Hexylcaine	968.5	E855.2	E938.5	E950.4	E962.0	E980.4
Hexylresorcinol	961.6	E857	E931.6	E950.4	E962.0	E980.4
Hinkle's pills	973.1	E858.4	E943.1	E950.4	E962.0	E980.4
Histalog	977.8	E858.8	E947.8	E950.4	E962.0	E980.4
Histamine (phosphate)	972.5	E858.3	E942.5	E950.4	E962.0	E980.4
Histoplasmin	977.8	E858.8	E947.8	E950.4	E962.0	E980.4
Holly berries	988.2	E865.3	—	E950.9	E962.1	E980.9
Homatropine	971.1	E855.4	E941.1	E950.4	E962.0	E980.4
Homo-tet	964.6	E858.2	E934.6	E950.4	E962.0	E980.4
Hormones (synthetic substitute) NEC	962.9	E858.0	E932.9	E950.4	E962.0	E980.4
adrenal cortical steroids	962.0	E858.0	E932.0	E950.4	E962.0	E980.4
antidiabetic agents	962.3	E858.0	E932.3	E950.4	E962.0	E980.4
follicle stimulating	962.4	E858.0	E932.4	E950.4	E962.0	E980.4
gonadotropic	962.4	E858.0	E932.4	E950.4	E962.0	E980.4
growth	962.4	E858.0	E932.4	E950.4	E962.0	E980.4
ovarian (substitutes)	962.2	E858.0	E932.2	E950.4	E962.0	E980.4
parathyroid (derivatives)	962.6	E858.0	E932.6	E950.4	E962.0	E980.4
pituitary (posterior)	962.5	E858.0	E932.5	E950.4	E962.0	E980.4
anterior	962.4	E858.0	E932.4	E950.4	E962.0	E980.4
thyroid (derivative)	962.7	E858.0	E932.7	E950.4	E962.0	E980.4
Hornet (sting)	989.5	E905.3	—	E950.9	E962.1	E980.9
Horticulture agent NEC	989.4	E863.9	—	E950.6	E962.1	E980.7
Hyaluronidase	963.4	E858.1	E933.4	E950.4	E962.0	E980.4
Hyazyme	963.4	E858.1	E933.4	E950.4	E962.0	E980.4

◄ New   ◄▥ Revised   ~~deleted~~ Deleted   ● Use Additional Digit(s)

Substance	Poisoning	External Cause (E Code)				
		Accident	Therapeutic Use	Suicide Attempt	Assault	Undetermined
Hycodan	965.09	E850.2	E935.2	E950.0	E962.0	E980.0
Hydantoin derivatives	966.1	E855.0	E936.1	E950.4	E962.0	E980.4
Hydeltra	962.0	E858.0	E932.0	E950.4	E962.0	E980.4
Hydergine	971.3	E855.6	E941.3	E950.4	E962.0	E980.4
Hydrabamine penicillin	960.0	E856	E930.0	E950.4	E962.0	E980.4
Hydralazine, hydrallazine	972.6	E858.3	E942.6	E950.4	E962.0	E980.4
Hydrargaphen	976.0	E858.7	E946.0	E950.4	E962.0	E980.4
Hydrazine	983.9	E864.3	—	E950.7	E962.1	E980.6
Hydriodic acid	975.5	E858.6	E945.5	E950.4	E962.0	E980.4
Hydrocarbon gas	987.1	E869.8	—	E952.8	E962.2	E982.8
incomplete combustion of - *see* Carbon, monoxide, fuel, utility	—	—	—	—	—	—
liquefied (mobile container)	987.0	E868.0	—	E951.1	E962.2	E981.1
piped (natural)	987.0	E867	—	E951.0	E962.2	E981.0
Hydrochloric acid (liquid)	983.1	E864.1	—	E950.7	E962.1	E980.6
medicinal	973.4	E858.4	E943.4	E950.4	E962.0	E980.4
vapor	987.8	E869.8	—	E952.8	E962.2	E982.8
Hydrochlorothiazide	974.3	E858.5	E944.3	E950.4	E962.0	E980.4
Hydrocodone	965.09	E850.2	E935.2	E950.0	E962.0	E980.0
Hydrocortisone	962.0	E858.0	E932.0	E950.4	E962.0	E980.4
ENT agent	976.6	E858.7	E946.6	E950.4	E962.0	E980.4
ophthalmic preparation	976.5	E858.7	E946.5	E950.4	E962.0	E980.4
topical NEC	976.0	E858.7	E946.0	E950.4	E962.0	E980.4
Hydrocortone	962.0	E858.0	E932.0	E950.4	E962.0	E980.4
ENT agent	976.6	E858.7	E946.6	E950.4	E962.0	E980.4
ophthalmic preparation	976.5	E858.7	E946.5	E950.4	E962.0	E980.4
topical NEC	976.0	E858.7	E946.0	E950.4	E962.0	E980.4
Hydrocyanic acid - *see* Cyanide(s)	—	—	—	—	—	—
Hydroflumethiazide	974.3	E858.5	E944.3	E950.4	E962.0	E980.4
Hydrofluoric acid (liquid)	983.1	E864.1	—	E950.7	E962.1	E980.6
vapor	987.8	E869.8	—	E952.8	E962.2	E982.8
Hydrogen	987.8	E869.8	—	E952.8	E962.2	E982.8
arsenide	985.1	E866.3	—	E950.8	E962.1	E980.8
arseniurated	985.1	E866.3	—	E950.8	E962.1	E980.8
cyanide (salts)	989.0	E866.8	—	E950.9	E962.1	E980.9
gas	987.7	E869.8	—	E952.8	E962.2	E982.8
fluoride (liquid)	983.1	E864.1	—	E950.7	E962.1	E980.6
vapor	987.8	E869.8	—	E952.8	E962.2	E982.8
peroxide (solution)	976.6	E858.7	E946.6	E950.4	E962.0	E980.4
phosphorated	987.8	E869.8	—	E952.8	E962.2	E982.8

◀ New ◀▥ Revised ~~deleted~~ Deleted ● Use Additional Digit(s)

Substance	Poisoning	External Cause (E Code)				
		Accident	Therapeutic Use	Suicide Attempt	Assault	Undetermined
Hydrogen *(Continued)*						
sulfide (gas)	987.8	E869.8	—	E952.8	E962.2	E982.8
arseniurated	985.1	E866.3	—	E950.8	E962.1	E980.8
sulfureted	987.8	E869.8	—	E952.8	E962.2	E982.8
Hydromorphinol	965.09	E850.2	E935.2	E950.0	E962.0	E980.0
Hydromorphinone	965.09	E850.2	E935.2	E950.0	E962.0	E980.0
Hydromorphone	965.09	E850.2	E935.2	E950.0	E962.0	E980.0
Hydromox	974.3	E858.5	E944.3	E950.4	E962.0	E980.4
Hydrophilic lotion	976.3	E858.7	E946.3	E950.4	E962.0	E980.4
Hydroquinone	983.0	E864.0	—	E950.7	E962.1	E980.6
vapor	987.8	E869.8	—	E952.8	E962.2	E982.8
Hydrosulfuric acid (gas)	987.8	E869.8	—	E952.8	E962.2	E982.8
Hydrous wool fat (lotion)	976.3	E858.7	E946.3	E950.4	E962.0	E980.4
Hydroxide, caustic	983.2	E864.2	—	E950.7	E962.1	E980.6
Hydroxocobalamin	964.1	E858.2	E934.1	E950.4	E962.0	E980.4
Hydroxyamphetamine	971.2	E858.5	E941.2	E950.4	E962.0	E980.4
Hydroxychloroquine	961.4	E857	E931.4	E950.4	E962.0	E980.4
Hydroxydihydrocodeinone	965.09	E850.2	E935.2	E950.0	E962.0	E980.0
Hydroxyethyl starch	964.8	E858.2	E934.8	E950.4	E962.0	E980.4
Hydroxyphenamate	969.5	E853.8	E939.5	E950.3	E962.0	E980.3
Hydroxyphenylbutazone	965.5	E850.5	E935.5	E950.0	E962.0	E980.0
Hydroxyprogesterone	962.2	E858.0	E932.2	E950.4	E962.0	E980.4
Hydroxyquinoline derivatives	961.3	E857	E931.3	E950.4	E962.0	E980.4
Hydroxystilbamidine	961.5	E857	E931.5	E950.4	E962.0	E980.4
Hydroxyurea	963.1	E858.1	E933.1	E950.4	E962.0	E980.4
Hydroxyzine	969.5	E853.8	E939.5	E950.3	E962.0	E980.3
Hyoscine (hydrobromide)	971.1	E855.4	E941.1	E950.4	E962.0	E980.4
Hyoscyamine	971.1	E855.4	E941.1	E950.4	E962.0	E980.4
Hyoscyamus (albus) (niger)	988.2	E865.4	—	E950.9	E962.1	E980.9
Hypaque	977.8	E858.8	E947.8	E950.4	E962.0	E980.4
Hypertussis	964.6	E858.2	E934.6	E950.4	E962.0	E980.4
Hypnotics NEC	967.9	E852.9	E937.9	E950.2	E962.0	E980.2
Hypochlorites - *see* Sodium, hypochlorite	—	—	—	—	—	—
Hypotensive agents NEC	972.6	E858.3	E942.6	E950.4	E962.0	E980.4
Ibufenac	965.69	E850.6	E935.6	E950.0	E962.0	E980.0
Ibuprofen	965.61	E850.6	E935.6	E950.0	E962.0	E980.0
ICG	977.8	E858.8	E947.8	E950.4	E962.0	E980.4
Ichthammol	976.4	E858.7	E946.4	E950.4	E962.0	E980.4

◀ New   ◀▥ Revised   ~~deleted~~ Deleted   ● Use Additional Digit(s)

Substance	Poisoning	External Cause (E Code)				
		Accident	Therapeutic Use	Suicide Attempt	Assault	Undetermined
Ichthyol	976.4	E858.7	E946.4	E950.4	E962.0	E980.4
Idoxuridine	976.5	E858.7	E946.5	E950.4	E962.0	E980.4
IDU	976.5	E858.7	E946.5	E950.4	E962.0	E980.4
Iletin	962.3	E858.0	E932.3	E950.4	E962.0	E980.4
Ilex	988.2	E865.4	—	E950.9	E962.1	E980.9
Illuminating gas - *see* Gas, utility	—	—	—	—	—	—
Ilopan	963.5	E858.1	E933.5	E950.4	E962.0	E980.4
Ilotycin	960.3	E856	E930.3	E950.4	E962.0	E980.4
ophthalmic preparation	976.5	E858.7	E946.5	E950.4	E962.0	E980.4
topical NEC	976.0	E858.7	E946.0	E950.4	E962.0	E980.4
Imipramine	969.05 ◄▥	E854.0	E939.0	E950.3	E962.0	E980.3
Immu-G	964.6	E858.2	E934.6	E950.4	E962.0	E980.4
Immuglobin	964.6	E858.2	E934.6	E950.4	E962.0	E980.4
Immune serum globulin	964.6	E858.2	E934.6	E950.4	E962.0	E980.4
Immunosuppressive agents	963.1	E858.1	E933.1	E950.4	E962.0	E980.4
Immu-tetanus	964.6	E858.2	E934.6	E950.4	E962.0	E980.4
Indandione (derivatives)	964.2	E858.2	E934.2	E950.4	E962.0	E980.4
Inderal	972.0	E858.3	E942.0	E950.4	E962.0	E980.4
Indian	—	—	—	—	—	—
hemp	969.6	E854.1	E939.6	E950.3	E962.0	E980.3
tobacco	988.2	E865.4	—	E950.9	E962.1	E980.9
Indigo carmine	977.8	E858.8	E947.8	E950.4	E962.0	E980.4
Indocin	965.69	E850.6	E935.6	E950.0	E962.0	E980.0
Indocyanine green	977.8	E858.8	E947.8	E950.4	E962.0	E980.4
Indomethacin	965.69	E850.6	E935.6	E950.0	E962.0	E980.0
Industrial	—	—	—	—	—	—
alcohol	980.9	E860.9	—	E950.9	E962.1	E980.9
fumes	987.8	E869.8	—	E952.8	E962.2	E982.8
solvents (fumes) (vapors)	982.8	E862.9	—	E950.9	E962.1	E980.9
Influenza vaccine	979.6	E858.8	E949.6	E950.4	E962.0	E982.8
Ingested substances NEC	989.9	E866.9	—	E950.9	E962.1	E980.9
INH (isoniazid)	961.8	E857	E931.8	E950.4	E962.0	E980.4
Inhalation, gas (noxious) - *see* Gas	—	—	—	—	—	—
Ink	989.89	E866.8	—	E950.9	E962.1	E980.9
Innovar	967.6	E852.5	E937.6	E950.2	E962.0	E980.2
Inositol niacinate	972.2	E858.3	E942.2	E950.4	E962.0	E980.4
Inproquone	963.1	E858.1	E933.1	E950.4	E962.0	E980.4
Insect (sting), venomous	989.5	E905.5	—	E950.9	E962.1	E980.9

Substance	Poisoning	External Cause (E Code)				
		Accident	Therapeutic Use	Suicide Attempt	Assault	Undetermined
Insecticides (*see also* Pesticides)	989.4	E863.4	—	E950.6	E962.1	E980.7
chlorinated	989.2	E863.0	—	E950.6	E962.1	E980.7
mixtures	989.4	E863.3	—	E950.6	E962.1	E980.7
organochlorine (compounds)	989.2	E863.0	—	E950.6	E962.1	E980.7
organophosphorus (compounds)	989.3	E863.1	—	E950.6	E962.1	E980.7
Insular tissue extract	962.3	E858.0	E932.3	E950.4	E962.0	E980.4
Insulin (amorphous) (globin) (isophane) (Lente) (NPH) (Protamine) (Semilente) (Ultralente) (zinc)	962.3	E858.0	E932.3	E950.4	E962.0	E980.4
Intranarcon	968.3	E855.1	E938.3	E950.4	E962.0	E980.4
Inulin	977.8	E858.8	E947.8	E950.4	E962.0	E980.4
Invert sugar	974.5	E858.5	E944.5	E950.4	E962.0	E980.4
Inza - see Naproxen	—	—	—	—	—	—
Iodide NEC (*see also* Iodine)	976.0	E858.7	E946.0	E950.4	E962.0	E980.4
mercury (ointment)	976.0	E858.7	E946.0	E950.4	E962.0	E980.4
methylate	976.0	E858.7	E946.0	E950.4	E962.0	E980.4
potassium (expectorant) NEC	975.5	E858.6	E945.5	E950.4	E962.0	E980.4
Iodinated glycerol	975.5	E858.6	E945.5	E950.4	E962.0	E980.4
Iodine (antiseptic, external) (tincture) NEC	976.0	E858.7	E946.0	E950.4	E962.0	E980.4
diagnostic	977.8	E858.8	E947.8	E950.4	E962.0	E980.4
for thyroid conditions (antithyroid)	962.8	E858.0	E932.8	E950.4	E962.0	E980.4
vapor	987.8	E869.8	—	E952.8	E962.2	E982.8
Iodized oil	977.8	E858.8	E947.8	E950.4	E962.0	E980.4
Iodobismitol	961.2	E857	E931.2	E950.4	E962.0	E980.4
Iodochlorhydroxyquin	961.3	E857	E931.3	E950.4	E962.0	E980.4
topical	976.0	E858.7	E946.0	E950.4	E962.0	E980.4
Iodoform	976.0	E858.7	E946.0	E950.4	E962.0	E980.4
Iodopanoic acid	977.8	E858.8	E947.8	E950.4	E962.0	E980.4
Iodophthalein	977.8	E858.8	E947.8	E950.4	E962.0	E980.4
Ion exchange resins	974.5	E858.5	E944.5	E950.4	E962.0	E980.4
Iopanoic acid	977.8	E858.8	E947.8	E950.4	E962.0	E980.4
Iophendylate	977.8	E858.8	E947.8	E950.4	E962.0	E980.4
Iothiouracil	962.8	E858.0	E932.8	E950.4	E962.0	E980.4
Ipecac	973.6	E858.4	E943.6	E950.4	E962.0	E980.4
Ipecacuanha	973.6	E858.4	E943.6	E950.4	E962.0	E980.4
Ipodate	977.8	E858.8	E947.8	E950.4	E962.0	E980.4
Ipral	967.0	E851	E937.0	E950.1	E962.0	E980.1
Ipratropium	975.1	E858.6	E945.1	E950.4	E962.0	E980.4
Iproniazid	969.01	E854.0	E939.0	E950.3	E962.0	E980.3

◀ New   ◀▥ Revised   ~~deleted~~ Deleted   ● Use Additional Digit(s)

Substance	Poisoning	External Cause (E Code)				
		Accident	Therapeutic Use	Suicide Attempt	Assault	Undetermined
Iron (compounds) (medicinal) (preparations)	964.0	E858.2	E934.0	E950.4	E962.0	E980.4
dextran	964.0	E858.2	E934.0	E950.4	E962.0	E980.4
nonmedicinal (dust) (fumes) NEC	985.8	E866.4	—	E950.9	E962.1	E980.9
Irritant drug	977.9	E858.9	E947.9	E950.5	E962.0	E980.5
Ismelin	972.6	E858.3	E942.6	E950.4	E962.0	E980.4
Isoamyl nitrite	972.4	E858.3	E942.4	E950.4	E962.0	E980.4
Isobutyl acetate	982.8	E862.4	—	E950.9	E962.1	E980.9
Isocarboxazid	969.01 ◀▥	E854.0	E939.0	E950.3	E962.0	E980.3
Isoephedrine	971.2	E855.5	E941.2	E950.4	E962.0	E980.4
Isoetharine	971.2	E855.5	E941.2	E950.4	E962.0	E980.4
Isofluorophate	971.0	E855.3	E941.0	E950.4	E962.0	E980.4
Isoniazid (INH)	961.8	E857	E931.8	E950.4	E962.0	E980.4
Isopentaquine	961.4	E857	E931.4	E950.4	E962.0	E980.4
Isophane insulin	962.3	E858.0	E932.3	E950.4	E962.0	E980.4
Isopregnenone	962.2	E858.0	E932.2	E950.4	E962.0	E980.4
Isoprenaline	971.2	E855.5	E941.2	E950.4	E962.0	E980.4
Isopropamide	971.1	E855.4	E941.1	E950.4	E962.0	E980.4
Isopropanol	980.2	E860.3	—	E950.9	E962.1	E980.9
topical (germicide)	976.0	E858.7	E946.0	E950.4	E962.0	E980.4
Isopropyl	—	—	—	—	—	—
acetate	982.8	E862.4	—	E950.9	E962.1	E980.9
alcohol	980.2	E860.3	—	E950.9	E962.1	E980.9
topical (germicide)	976.0	E858.7	E946.0	E950.4	E962.0	E980.4
ether	982.8	E862.4	—	E950.9	E962.1	E980.9
Isoproterenol	971.2	E855.5	E941.2	E950.4	E962.0	E980.4
Isosorbide dinitrate	972.4	E858.3	E942.4	E950.4	E962.0	E980.4
Isothipendyl	963.0	E858.1	E933.0	E950.4	E962.0	E980.4
Isoxazolyl penicillin	960.0	E856	E930.0	E950.4	E962.0	E980.4
Isoxsuprine hydrochloride	972.5	E858.3	E942.5	E950.4	E962.0	E980.4
l-thyroxine sodium	962.7	E858.0	E932.7	E950.4	E962.0	E980.4
Jaborandi (pilocarpus) (extract)	971.0	E855.3	E941.0	E950.4	E962.0	E980.4
Jalap	973.1	E858.4	E943.1	E950.4	E962.0	E980.4
Jamaica	—	—	—	—	—	—
dogwood (bark)	965.7	E850.7	E935.7	E950.0	E962.0	E980.0
ginger	989.89	E866.8	—	E950.9	E962.1	E980.9
Jatropha	988.2	E865.4	—	E950.9	E962.1	E980.9
curcas	988.2	E865.3	—	E950.9	E962.1	E980.9
Jectofer	964.0	E858.2	E934.0	E950.4	E962.0	E980.4

◀ New   ◀▥ Revised   ~~deleted~~ Deleted   ● Use Additional Digit(s)

Substance	Poisoning	External Cause (E Code)				
		Accident	Therapeutic Use	Suicide Attempt	Assault	Undetermined
Jellyfish (sting)	989.5	E905.6	—	E950.9	E962.1	E980.9
Jequirity (bean)	988.2	E865.3	—	E950.9	E962.1	E980.9
Jimson weed	988.2	E865.4	—	E950.9	E962.1	E980.9
seeds	988.2	E865.3	—	E950.9	E962.1	E980.9
Juniper tar (oil) (ointment)	976.4	E858.7	E946.4	E950.4	E962.0	E980.4
Kallikrein	972.5	E858.3	E942.5	E950.4	E962.0	E980.4
Kanamycin	960.6	E856	E930.6	E950.4	E962.0	E980.4
Kantrex	960.6	E856	E930.6	E950.4	E962.0	E980.4
Kaolin	973.5	E858.4	E943.5	E950.4	E962.0	E980.4
Karaya (gum)	973.3	E858.4	E943.3	E950.4	E962.0	E980.4
Kemithal	968.3	E855.1	E938.3	E950.4	E962.0	E980.4
Kenacort	962.0	E858.0	E932.0	E950.4	E962.0	E980.4
Keratolytics	976.4	E858.7	E946.4	E950.4	E962.0	E980.4
Keratoplastics	976.4	E858.7	E946.4	E950.4	E962.0	E980.4
Kerosene, kerosine (fuel) (solvent) NEC	981	E862.1	—	E950.9	E962.1	E980.9
insecticide	981	E863.4	—	E950.6	E962.1	E980.7
vapor	987.1	E869.8	—	E952.8	E962.2	E982.8
Ketamine	968.3	E855.1	E938.3	E950.4	E962.0	E980.4
Ketobemidone	965.09	E850.2	E935.2	E950.0	E962.0	E980.0
Ketols	982.8	E862.4	—	E950.9	E962.1	E980.9
Ketone oils	982.8	E862.4	—	E950.9	E962.1	E980.9
Ketoprofen	965.61	E850.6	E935.6	E950.0	E962.0	E980.0
Kiln gas or vapor (carbon monoxide)	986	E868.8	—	E952.1	E962.2	E982.1
Konsyl	973.3	E858.4	E943.3	E950.4	E962.0	E980.4
Kosam seed	988.2	E865.3	—	E950.9	E962.1	E980.9
Krait (venom)	989.5	E905.0	—	E950.9	E962.1	E980.9
Kwell (insecticide)	989.2	E863.0	—	E950.6	E962.1	E980.7
anti-infective (topical)	976.0	E858.7	E946.0	E950.4	E962.0	E980.4
Laburnum (flowers) (seeds)	988.2	E865.3	—	E950.9	E962.1	E980.9
leaves	988.2	E865.4	—	E950.9	E962.1	E980.9
Lacquers	989.89	E861.6	—	E950.9	E962.1	E980.9
Lacrimogenic gas	987.5	E869.3	—	E952.8	E962.2	E982.8
Lactic acid	983.1	E864.1	—	E950.7	E962.1	E980.6
Lactobacillus acidophilus	973.5	E858.4	E943.5	E950.4	E962.0	E980.4
Lactoflavin	963.5	E858.1	E933.5	E950.4	E962.0	E980.4
Lactuca (virosa) (extract)	967.8	E852.8	E937.8	E950.2	E962.0	E980.2
Lactucarium	967.8	E852.8	E937.8	E950.2	E962.0	E980.2
Laevulose	974.5	E858.5	E944.5	E950.4	E962.0	E980.4
Lanatoside (C)	972.1	E858.3	E942.1	E950.4	E962.0	E980.4
Lanolin (lotion)	976.3	E858.7	E946.3	E950.4	E962.0	E980.4

◀ New ◀ Revised ~~deleted~~ Deleted ● Use Additional Digit(s)

Substance	Poisoning	External Cause (E Code)				
		Accident	Therapeutic Use	Suicide Attempt	Assault	Undetermined
Largactil	969.1	E853.0	E939.1	E950.3	E962.0	E980.3
Larkspur	988.2	E865.3	—	E950.9	E962.1	E980.9
Laroxyl	969.05 ◀▥	E854.0	E939.0	E950.3	E962.0	E980.3
Lasix	974.4	E858.5	E944.4	E950.4	E962.0	E980.4
Latex	989.82	E866.8	—	E950.9	E962.1	E980.9
Lathyrus (seed)	988.2	E865.3	—	E950.9	E962.1	E980.9
Laudanum	965.09	E850.2	E935.2	E950.0	E962.0	E980.0
Laudexium	975.2	E858.6	E945.2	E950.4	E962.0	E980.4
Laurel, black or cherry	988.2	E865.4	—	E950.9	E962.1	E980.9
Laurolinium	976.0	E858.7	E946.0	E950.4	E962.0	E980.4
Lauryl sulfoacetate	976.2	E858.7	E946.2	E950.4	E962.0	E980.4
Laxatives NEC	973.3	E858.4	E943.3	E950.4	E962.0	E980.4
emollient	973.2	E858.4	E943.2	E950.4	E962.0	E980.4
L-dopa	966.4	E855.0	E936.4	E950.4	E962.0	E980.4
L-Tryptophan - *see* amino acid	—	—	—	—	—	—
Lead (dust) (fumes) (vapor) NEC	984.9	E866.0	—	E950.9	E962.1	E980.9
acetate (dust)	984.1	E866.0	—	E950.9	E962.1	E980.9
anti-infectives	961.2	E857	E931.2	E950.4	E962.0	E980.4
antiknock compound (tetra-ethyl)	984.1	E862.1	—	E950.9	E962.1	E980.9
arsenate, arsenite (dust) (insecticide) (vapor)	985.1	E863.4	—	E950.8	E962.1	E980.8
herbicide	985.1	E863.5	—	E950.8	E962.1	E980.8
carbonate	984.0	E866.0	—	E950.9	E962.1	E980.9
paint	984.0	E861.5	—	E950.9	E962.1	E980.9
chromate	984.0	E866.0	—	E950.9	E962.1	E980.9
paint	984.0	E861.5	—	E950.9	E962.1	E980.9
dioxide	984.0	E866.0	—	E950.9	E962.1	E980.9
inorganic (compound)	984.0	E866.0	—	E950.9	E962.1	E980.9
paint	984.0	E861.5	—	E950.9	E962.1	E980.9
iodide	984.0	E866.0	—	E950.9	E962.1	E980.9
pigment (paint)	984.0	E861.5	—	E950.9	E962.1	E980.9
monoxide (dust)	984.0	E866.0	—	E950.9	E962.1	E980.9
paint	984.0	E861.5	—	E950.9	E962.1	E980.9
organic	984.1	E866.0	—	E950.9	E962.1	E980.9
oxide	984.0	E866.0	—	E950.9	E962.1	E980.9
paint	984.0	E861.5	—	E950.9	E962.1	E980.9
paint	984.0	E861.5	—	E950.9	E962.1	E980.9
salts	984.0	E866.0	—	E950.9	E962.1	E980.9
specified compound NEC	984.8	E866.0	—	E950.9	E962.1	E980.9
tetra-ethyl	984.1	E862.1	—	E950.9	E962.1	E980.9
Lebanese red	969.6	E854.1	E939.6	E950.3	E962.0	E980.3

◀ New　◀▥ Revised　~~deleted~~ Deleted　● Use Additional Digit(s)

			External Cause (E Code)			
Substance	Poisoning	Accident	Therapeutic Use	Suicide Attempt	Assault	Undetermined
Lente Iletin (insulin)	962.3	E858.0	E932.3	E950.4	E962.0	E980.4
Leptazol	970.0	E854.3	E940.0	E950.4	E962.0	E980.4
Leritine	965.09	E850.2	E935.2	E950.0	E962.0	E980.0
Letter	962.7	E858.0	E932.7	E950.4	E962.0	E980.4
Lettuce opium	967.8	E852.8	E937.8	E950.2	E962.0	E980.2
Leucovorin (factor)	964.1	E858.2	E934.1	E950.4	E962.0	E980.4
Leukeran	963.1	E858.1	E933.1	E950.4	E962.0	E980.4
Levalbuterol	975.7	E858.6	E945.7	E950.4	E962.0	E980.4
Levallorphan	970.1	E854.3	E940.1	E950.4	E962.0	E980.4
Levanil	967.8	E852.8	E937.8	E950.2	E962.0	E980.2
Levarterenol	971.2	E855.5	E941.2	E950.4	E962.0	E980.4
Levodopa	966.4	E855.0	E936.4	E950.4	E962.0	E980.4
Levo-dromoran	965.09	E850.2	E935.2	E950.0	E962.0	E980.0
Levoid	962.7	E858.0	E932.7	E950.4	E962.0	E980.4
Levo-iso-methadone	965.02	E850.1	E935.1	E950.0	E962.0	E980.0
Levomepromazine	967.8	E852.8	E937.8	E950.2	E962.0	E980.2
Levoprome	967.8	E852.8	E937.8	E950.2	E962.0	E980.2
Levopropoxyphene	975.4	E858.6	E945.4	E950.4	E962.0	E980.4
Levorphan, levophanol	965.09	E850.2	E935.2	E950.0	E962.0	E980.0
Levothyroxine (sodium)	962.7	E858.0	E932.7	E950.4	E962.0	E980.4
Levsin	971.1	E855.4	E941.1	E950.4	E962.0	E980.4
Levulose	974.5	E858.5	E944.5	E950.4	E962.0	E980.4
Lewisite (gas)	985.1	E866.3	—	E950.8	E962.1	E980.8
Librium	969.4	E853.2	E939.4	E950.3	E962.0	E980.3
Lidex	976.0	E858.7	E946.0	E950.4	E962.0	E980.4
Lidocaine (infiltration) (topical)	968.5	E855.2	E938.5	E950.4	E962.0	E980.4
nerve block (peripheral) (plexus)	968.6	E855.2	E938.6	E950.4	E962.0	E980.4
spinal	968.7	E855.2	E938.7	E950.4	E962.0	E980.4
Lighter fluid	981	E862.1	—	E950.9	E962.1	E980.9
Lignocaine (infiltration) (topical)	968.5	E855.2	E938.5	E950.4	E962.0	E980.4
nerve block (peripheral) (plexus)	968.6	E855.2	E938.6	E950.4	E962.0	E980.4
spinal	968.7	E855.2	E938.7	E950.4	E962.0	E980.4
Ligroin(e) (solvent)	981	E862.0	—	E950.9	E962.1	E980.9
vapor	987.1	E869.8	—	E952.8	E962.2	E982.8
Ligustrum vulgare	988.2	E865.3	—	E950.9	E962.1	E980.9
Lily of the valley	988.2	E865.4	—	E950.9	E962.1	E980.9
Lime (chloride)	983.2	E864.2	—	E950.7	E962.1	E980.6
solution, sulferated	976.4	E858.7	E946.4	E950.4	E962.0	E980.4
Limonene	982.8	E862.4	—	E950.9	E962.1	E980.9

◀ New   ◀▦ Revised   ~~deleted~~ Deleted   ● Use Additional Digit(s)

Substance	Poisoning	External Cause (E Code)				
		Accident	Therapeutic Use	Suicide Attempt	Assault	Undetermined
Lincomycin	960.8	E856	E930.8	E950.4	E962.0	E980.4
Lindane (insecticide) (vapor)	989.2	E863.0	—	E950.6	E962.1	E980.7
anti-infective (topical)	976.0	E858.7	E946.0	E950.4	E962.0	E980.4
Liniments NEC	976.9	E858.7	E946.9	E950.4	E962.0	E980.4
Linoleic acid	972.2	E858.3	E942.2	E950.4	E962.0	E980.4
Liothyronine	962.7	E858.0	E932.7	E950.4	E962.0	E980.4
Liotrix	962.7	E858.0	E932.7	E950.4	E962.0	E980.4
Lipancreatin	973.4	E858.4	E943.4	E950.4	E962.0	E980.4
Lipo-Lutin	962.2	E858.0	E932.2	E950.4	E962.0	E980.4
Lipotropic agents	977.1	E858.8	E947.1	E950.4	E962.0	E980.4
Liquefied petroleum gases	987.0	E868.0	—	E951.1	E962.2	E981.1
piped (pure or mixed with air)	987.0	E867	—	E951.0	E962.2	E981.0
Liquid petrolatum	973.2	E858.4	E943.2	E950.4	E962.0	E980.4
substance	989.9	E866.9	—	E950.9	E962.1	E980.9
specified NEC	989.89	E866.8	—	E950.9	E962.1	E980.9
Lirugen	979.4	E858.8	E949.4	E950.4	E962.0	E980.4
Lithane	969.8	E855.8	E939.8	E950.3	E962.0	E980.3
Lithium	985.8	E866.4	—	E950.9	E962.1	E980.9
carbonate	969.8	E855.8	E939.8	E950.3	E962.0	E980.3
Lithonate	969.8	E855.8	E939.8	E950.3	E962.0	E980.3
Liver (extract) (injection) (preparations)	964.1	E858.2	E934.1	E950.4	E962.0	E980.4
Lizard (bite) (venom)	989.5	E905.0	—	E950.9	E962.1	E980.9
LMD	964.8	E858.2	E934.8	E950.4	E962.0	E980.4
Lobelia	988.2	E865.4	—	E950.9	E962.1	E980.9
Lobeline	970.0	E854.3	E940.0	E950.4	E962.0	E980.4
Locorten	976.0	E858.7	E946.0	E950.4	E962.0	E980.4
Lolium temulentum	988.2	E865.3	—	E950.9	E962.1	E980.9
Lomotil	973.5	E858.4	E943.5	E950.4	E962.0	E980.4
Lomustine	963.1	E858.1	E933.1	E950.4	E962.0	E980.4
Lophophora williamsii	969.6	E854.1	E939.6	E950.3	E962.0	E980.3
Lorazepam	969.4	E853.2	E939.4	E950.3	E962.0	E980.3
Lotions NEC	976.9	E858.7	E946.9	E950.4	E962.0	E980.4
Lotronex	973.8	E858.4	E943.8	E950.4	E962.0	E980.4
Lotusate	967.0	E851	E937.0	E950.1	E962.0	E980.1
Lowila	976.2	E858.7	E946.2	E950.4	E962.0	E980.4
Loxapine	969.3	E853.8	E939.3	E950.3	E962.0	E980.3
Lozenges (throat)	976.6	E858.7	E946.6	E950.4	E962.0	E980.4
LSD (25)	969.6	E854.1	E939.6	E950.3	E962.0	E980.3
Lubricating oil NEC	981	E862.2	—	E950.9	E962.1	E980.9

◀ New   ◀▥ Revised   ~~deleted~~ Deleted   ● Use Additional Digit(s)

Substance	Poisoning	External Cause (E Code)				
		Accident	Therapeutic Use	Suicide Attempt	Assault	Undetermined
Lucanthone	961.6	E857	E931.6	E950.4	E962.0	E980.4
Luminal	967.0	E851	E937.0	E950.1	E962.0	E980.1
Lung irritant (gas) NEC	987.9	E869.9	—	E952.9	E962.2	E982.9
Lutocylol	962.2	E858.0	E932.2	E950.4	E962.0	E980.4
Lutromone	962.2	E858.0	E932.2	E950.4	E962.0	E980.4
Lututrin	975.0	E858.6	E945.0	E950.4	E962.0	E980.4
Lye (concentrated)	983.2	E864.2	—	E950.7	E962.1	E980.6
Lygranum (skin test)	977.8	E858.8	E947.8	E950.4	E962.0	E980.4
Lymecycline	960.4	E856	E930.4	E950.4	E962.0	E980.4
Lymphogranuloma venereum antigen	977.8	E858.8	E947.8	E950.4	E962.0	E980.4
Lynestrenol	962.2	E858.0	E932.2	E950.4	E962.0	E980.4
Lyovac Sodium Edecrin	974.4	E858.5	E944.4	E950.4	E962.0	E980.4
Lypressin	962.5	E858.0	E932.5	E950.4	E962.0	E980.4
Lysergic acid (amide) (diethylamide)	969.6	E854.1	E939.6	E950.3	E962.0	E980.3
Lysergide	969.6	E854.1	E939.6	E950.3	E962.0	E980.3
Lysine vasopressin	962.5	E858.0	E932.5	E950.4	E962.0	E980.4
Lysol	983.0	E864.0	—	E950.7	E962.1	E980.6
Lytta (vitatta)	976.8	E858.7	E946.8	E950.4	E962.0	E980.4
Mace	987.5	E869.3	—	E952.8	E962.2	E982.8
Macrolides (antibiotics)	960.3	E856	E930.3	E950.4	E962.0	E980.4
Mafenide	976.0	E858.7	E946.0	E950.4	E962.0	E980.4
Magaldrate	973.0	E858.4	E943.0	E950.4	E962.0	E980.4
Magic mushroom	969.6	E854.1	E939.6	E950.3	E962.0	E980.3
Magnamycin	960.8	E856	E930.8	E950.4	E962.0	E980.4
Magnesia magma	973.0	E858.4	E943.0	E950.4	E962.0	E980.4
Magnesium (compounds) (fumes) NEC	985.8	E866.4	—	E950.9	E962.1	E980.9
antacid	973.0	E858.4	E943.0	E950.4	E962.0	E980.4
carbonate	973.0	E858.4	E943.0	E950.4	E962.0	E980.4
cathartic	973.3	E858.4	E943.3	E950.4	E962.0	E980.4
citrate	973.3	E858.4	E943.3	E950.4	E962.0	E980.4
hydroxide	973.0	E858.4	E943.0	E950.4	E962.0	E980.4
oxide	973.0	E858.4	E943.0	E950.4	E962.0	E980.4
sulfate (oral)	973.3	E858.4	E943.3	E950.4	E962.0	E980.4
intravenous	966.3	E855.0	E936.3	E950.4	E962.0	E980.4
trisilicate	973.0	E858.4	E943.0	E950.4	E962.0	E980.4
Malathion (insecticide)	989.3	E863.1	—	E950.6	E962.1	E980.7
Male fern (oleoresin)	961.6	E857	E931.6	E950.4	E962.0	E980.4
Mandelic acid	961.9	E857	E931.9	E950.4	E962.0	E980.4
Manganese compounds (fumes) NEC	985.2	E866.4	—	E950.9	E962.1	E980.9

◀ New   ◀▦ Revised   ~~deleted~~ Deleted   ● Use Additional Digit(s)

Substance	Poisoning	External Cause (E Code)				
		Accident	Therapeutic Use	Suicide Attempt	Assault	Undetermined
Mannitol (diuretic) (medicinal) NEC	974.4	E858.5	E944.4	E950.4	E962.0	E980.4
hexanitrate	972.4	E858.3	E942.4	E950.4	E962.0	E980.4
mustard	963.1	E858.1	E933.1	E950.4	E962.0	E980.4
Mannomustine	963.1	E858.1	E933.1	E950.4	E962.0	E980.4
MAO inhibitors	969.01 ◄	E854.0	E939.0	E950.3	E962.0	E980.3
Mapharsen	961.1	E857	E931.1	E950.4	E962.0	E980.4
Marcaine	968.9	E855.2	E938.9	E950.4	E962.0	E980.4
infiltration (subcutaneous)	968.5	E855.2	E938.5	E950.4	E962.0	E980.4
nerve block (peripheral) (plexus)	968.6	E855.2	E938.6	E950.4	E962.0	E980.4
Marezine	963.0	E858.1	E933.0	E950.4	E962.0	E980.4
Marihuana, marijuana (derivatives)	969.6	E854.1	E939.6	E950.3	E962.0	E980.3
Marine animals or plants (sting)	989.5	E905.6	—	E950.9	E962.1	E980.9
Marplan	969.01 ◄	E854.0	E939.0	E950.3	E962.0	E980.3
Marsh gas	987.1	E869.8	—	E952.8	E962.2	E982.8
Marsilid	969.01 ◄	E854.0	E939.0	E950.3	E962.0	E980.3
Matulane	963.1	E858.1	E933.1	E950.4	E962.0	E980.4
Mazindol	977.0	E858.8	E947.0	E950.4	E962.0	E980.4
MDMA	969.72 ◄	E854.2	E939.7	E950.3	E962.0	E980.3
Meadow saffron	988.2	E865.3	—	E950.9	E962.1	E980.9
Measles vaccine	979.4	E858.8	E949.4	E950.4	E962.0	E980.4
Meat, noxious or nonbacterial	988.8	E865.0	—	E950.9	E962.1	E980.9
Mebanazine	969.01 ◄	E854.0	E939.0	E950.3	E962.0	E980.3
Mebaral	967.0	E851	E937.0	E950.1	E962.0	E980.1
Mebendazole	961.6	E857	E931.6	E950.4	E962.0	E980.4
Mebeverine	975.1	E858.6	E945.1	E950.4	E962.0	E980.4
Mebhydroline	963.0	E858.1	E933.0	E950.4	E962.0	E980.4
Mebrophenhydramine	963.0	E858.1	E933.0	E950.4	E962.0	E980.4
Mebutamate	969.5	E853.8	E939.5	E950.3	E962.0	E980.3
Mecamylamine (chloride)	972.3	E858.3	E942.3	E950.4	E962.0	E980.4
Mechlorethamine hydrochloride	963.1	E858.1	E933.1	E950.4	E962.0	E980.4
Meclizene (hydrochloride)	963.0	E858.1	E933.0	E950.4	E962.0	E980.4
Meclofenoxate	970.0	E854.3	E940.0	E950.4	E962.0	E980.4
Meclozine (hydrochloride)	963.0	E858.1	E933.0	E950.4	E962.0	E980.4
Medazepam	969.4	E853.2	E939.4	E950.3	E962.0	E980.3
Medicine, medicinal substance	977.9	E858.9	E947.9	E950.5	E962.0	E980.5
specified NEC	977.8	E858.8	E947.8	E950.4	E962.0	E980.4
Medinal	967.0	E851	E937.0	E950.1	E962.0	E980.1
Medomin	967.0	E851	E937.0	E950.1	E962.0	E980.1
Medroxyprogesterone	962.2	E858.0	E932.2	E950.4	E962.0	E980.4

◄ New   ◄▥ Revised   ~~deleted~~ Deleted   ● Use Additional Digit(s)

Substance	Poisoning	External Cause (E Code)				
		Accident	Therapeutic Use	Suicide Attempt	Assault	Undetermined
Medrysone	976.5	E858.7	E946.5	E950.4	E962.0	E980.4
Mefenamic acid	965.7	E850.7	E935.7	E950.0	E962.0	E980.0
Megahallucinogen	969.6	E854.1	E939.6	E950.3	E962.0	E980.3
Megestrol	962.2	E858.0	E932.2	E950.4	E962.0	E980.4
Meglumine	977.8	E858.8	E947.8	E950.4	E962.0	E980.4
Meladinin	976.3	E858.7	E946.3	E950.4	E962.0	E980.4
Melanizing agents	976.3	E858.7	E946.3	E950.4	E962.0	E980.4
Melarsoprol	961.1	E857	E931.1	E950.4	E962.0	E980.4
Melia azedarach	988.2	E865.3	—	E950.9	E962.1	E980.9
Mellaril	969.1	E853.0	E939.1	E950.3	E962.0	E980.3
Meloxine	976.3	E858.7	E946.3	E950.4	E962.0	E980.4
Melphalan	963.1	E858.1	E933.1	E950.4	E962.0	E980.4
Memantine hydrochloride	969.8	E854.8	E939.8	E950.3	E962.0	E980.3
Menadiol sodium diphosphate	964.3	E858.2	E934.3	E950.4	E962.0	E980.4
Menadione (sodium bisulfite)	964.3	E858.2	E934.3	E950.4	E962.0	E980.4
Menaphthone	964.3	E858.2	E934.3	E950.4	E962.0	E980.4
Meningococcal vaccine	978.8	E858.8	E948.8	E950.4	E962.0	E980.4
Menningovax-C	978.8	E858.8	E948.8	E950.4	E962.0	E980.4
Menotropins	962.4	E858.0	E932.4	E950.4	E962.0	E980.4
Menthol NEC	976.1	E858.7	E946.1	E950.4	E962.0	E980.4
Mepacrine	961.3	E857	E931.3	E950.4	E962.0	E980.4
Meparfynol	967.8	E852.8	E937.8	E950.2	E962.0	E980.2
Mepazine	969.1	E853.0	E939.1	E950.3	E962.0	E980.3
Mepenzolate	971.1	E855.4	E941.1	E950.4	E962.0	E980.4
Meperidine	965.09	E850.2	E935.2	E950.0	E962.0	E980.0
Mephenamin(e)	966.4	E855.0	E936.4	E950.4	E962.0	E980.4
Mephenesin (carbamate)	968.0	E855.1	E938.0	E950.4	E962.0	E980.4
Mephenoxalone	969.5	E853.8	E939.5	E950.3	E962.0	E980.3
Mephentermine	971.2	E855.5	E941.2	E950.4	E962.0	E980.4
Mephenytoin	966.1	E855.0	E936.1	E950.4	E962.0	E980.4
Mephobarbital	967.0	E851	E937.0	E950.1	E962.0	E980.1
Mepiperphenidol	971.1	E855.4	E941.1	E950.4	E962.0	E980.4
Mepivacaine	968.9	E855.2	E938.9	E950.4	E962.0	E980.4
infiltration (subcutaneous)	968.5	E855.2	E938.5	E950.4	E962.0	E980.4
nerve block (peripheral) (plexus)	968.6	E855.2	E938.6	E950.4	E962.0	E980.4
topical (surface)	968.5	E855.2	E938.5	E950.4	E962.0	E980.4
Meprednisone	962.0	E858.0	E932.0	E950.4	E962.0	E980.4
Meprobam	969.5	E853.8	E939.5	E950.3	E962.0	E980.3
Meprobamate	969.5	E853.8	E939.5	E950.3	E962.0	E980.3

◀ New   ◀▦ Revised   ~~deleted~~ Deleted   ● Use Additional Digit(s)

Substance	Poisoning	External Cause (E Code)				
		Accident	Therapeutic Use	Suicide Attempt	Assault	Undetermined
Mepyramine (maleate)	963.0	E858.1	E933.0	E950.4	E962.0	E980.4
Meralluride	974.0	E858.5	E944.0	E950.4	E962.0	E980.4
Merbaphen	974.0	E858.5	E944.0	E950.4	E962.0	E980.4
Merbromin	976.0	E858.7	E946.0	E950.4	E962.0	E980.4
Mercaptomerin	974.0	E858.5	E944.0	E950.4	E962.0	E980.4
Mercaptopurine	963.1	E858.1	E933.1	E950.4	E962.0	E980.4
Mercumatilin	974.0	E858.5	E944.0	E950.4	E962.0	E980.4
Mercuramide	974.0	E858.5	E944.0	E950.4	E962.0	E980.4
Mercuranin	976.0	E858.7	E946.0	E950.4	E962.0	E980.4
Mercurochrome	976.0	E858.7	E946.0	E950.4	E962.0	E980.4
Mercury, mercuric, mercurous (compounds) (cyanide) (fumes) (nonmedicinal) (vapor) NEC	985.0	E866.1	—	E950.9	E962.1	E980.9
ammoniated	976.0	E858.7	E946.0	E950.4	E962.0	E980.4
anti-infective	961.2	E857	E931.2	E950.4	E962.0	E980.4
topical	976.0	E858.7	E946.0	E950.4	E962.0	E980.4
chloride (antiseptic) NEC	976.0	E858.7	E946.0	E950.4	E962.0	E980.4
fungicide	985.0	E863.6	—	E950.6	E962.1	E980.7
diuretic compounds	974.0	E858.5	E944.0	E950.4	E962.0	E980.4
fungicide	985.0	E863.6	—	E950.6	E962.1	E980.7
organic (fungicide)	985.0	E863.6	—	E950.6	E962.1	E980.7
Merethoxylline	974.0	E858.5	E944.0	E950.4	E962.0	E980.4
Mersalyl	974.0	E858.5	E944.0	E950.4	E962.0	E980.4
Merthiolate (topical)	976.0	E858.7	E946.0	E950.4	E962.0	E980.4
ophthalmic preparation	976.5	E858.7	E946.5	E950.4	E962.0	E980.4
Meruvax	979.4	E858.8	E949.4	E950.4	E962.0	E980.4
Mescal buttons	969.6	E854.1	E939.6	E950.3	E962.0	E980.3
Mescaline (salts)	969.6	E854.1	E939.6	E950.3	E962.0	E980.3
Mesoridazine besylate	969.1	E853.0	E939.1	E950.3	E962.0	E980.3
Mestanolone	962.1	E858.0	E932.1	E950.4	E962.0	E980.4
Mestranol	962.2	E858.0	E932.2	E950.4	E962.0	E980.4
Metactesylacetate	976.0	E858.7	E946.0	E950.4	E962.0	E980.4
Metaldehyde (snail killer) NEC	989.4	E863.4	—	E950.6	E962.1	E980.7
Metals (heavy) (nonmedicinal) NEC	985.9	E866.4	—	E950.9	E962.1	E980.9
dust, fumes, or vapor NEC	985.9	E866.4	—	E950.9	E962.1	E980.9
light NEC	985.9	E866.4	—	E950.9	E962.1	E980.9
dust, fumes, or vapor NEC	985.9	E866.4	—	E950.9	E962.1	E980.9
pesticides (dust) (vapor)	985.9	E863.4	—	E950.6	E962.1	E980.7
Metamucil	973.3	E858.4	E943.3	E950.4	E962.0	E980.4
Metaphen	976.0	E858.7	E946.0	E950.4	E962.0	E980.4

◀ New   ◀▥ Revised   ~~deleted~~ Deleted   ● Use Additional Digit(s)

Substance	Poisoning	External Cause (E Code)				
		Accident	Therapeutic Use	Suicide Attempt	Assault	Undetermined
Metaproterenol	975.1	E858.6	E945.1	E950.4	E962.0	E980.4
Metaraminol	972.8	E858.3	E942.8	E950.4	E962.0	E980.4
Metaxalone	968.0	E855.1	E938.0	E950.4	E962.0	E980.4
Metformin	962.3	E858.0	E932.3	E950.4	E962.0	E980.4
Methacycline	960.4	E856	E930.4	E950.4	E962.0	E980.4
Methadone	965.02	E850.1	E935.1	E950.0	E962.0	E980.0
Methallenestril	962.2	E858.0	E932.2	E950.4	E962.0	E980.4
Methamphetamine	969.72 ◀▥	E854.2	E939.7	E950.3	E962.0	E980.3
Methandienone	962.1	E858.0	E932.1	E950.4	E962.0	E980.4
Methandriol	962.1	E858.0	E932.1	E950.4	E962.0	E980.4
Methandrostenolone	962.1	E858.0	E932.1	E950.4	E962.0	E980.4
Methane gas	987.1	E869.8	—	E952.8	E962.2	E982.8
Methanol	980.1	E860.2	—	E950.9	E961.1	E980.9
vapor	987.8	E869.8	—	E952.8	E962.2	E982.8
Methantheline	971.1	E855.4	E941.1	E950.4	E962.0	E980.4
Methaphenilene	963.0	E858.1	E933.0	E950.4	E962.0	E980.4
Methapyrilene	963.0	E858.1	E933.0	E950.4	E962.0	E980.4
Methaqualone (compounds)	967.4	E852.3	E937.4	E950.2	E962.0	E980.2
Metharbital, metharbitone	967.0	E851	E937.0	E950.1	E962.0	E980.1
Methazolamide	974.2	E858.5	E944.2	E950.4	E962.0	E980.4
Methdilazine	963.0	E858.1	E933.0	E950.4	E962.0	E980.4
Methedrine	969.72 ◀▥	E854.2	E939.7	E950.3	E962.0	E980.3
Methenamine (mandelate)	961.9	E857	E931.9	E950.4	E962.0	E980.4
Methenolone	962.1	E858.0	E932.1	E950.4	E962.0	E980.4
Methergine	975.0	E858.6	E945.0	E950.4	E962.0	E980.4
Methiacil	962.8	E858.0	E932.8	E950.4	E962.0	E980.4
Methicillin (sodium)	960.0	E856	E930.0	E950.4	E962.0	E980.4
Methimazole	962.8	E858.0	E932.8	E950.4	E962.0	E980.4
Methionine	977.1	E858.8	E947.1	E950.4	E962.0	E980.4
Methisazone	961.7	E857	E931.7	E950.4	E962.0	E980.4
Methitural	967.0	E851	E937.0	E950.1	E962.0	E980.1
Methixene	971.1	E855.4	E941.1	E950.4	E962.0	E980.4
Methobarbital, methobarbitone	967.0	E851	E937.0	E950.1	E962.0	E980.1
Methocarbamol	968.0	E855.1	E938.0	E950.4	E962.0	E980.4
Methohexital, methohexitone (sodium)	968.3	E855.1	E938.3	E950.4	E962.0	E980.4
Methoin	966.1	E855.0	E936.1	E950.4	E962.0	E980.4
Methopholine	965.7	E850.7	E935.7	E950.0	E962.0	E980.0
Methorate	975.4	E858.6	E945.4	E950.4	E962.0	E980.4
Methoserpidine	972.6	E858.3	E942.6	E950.4	E962.0	E980.4

◀ New   ◀▥ Revised   ~~deleted~~ Deleted   ● Use Additional Digit(s)

Substance	Poisoning	External Cause (E Code)				
		Accident	Therapeutic Use	Suicide Attempt	Assault	Undetermined
Methotrexate	963.1	E858.1	E933.1	E950.4	E962.0	E980.4
Methotrimeprazine	967.8	E852.8	E937.8	E950.2	E962.0	E980.2
Methoxa-Dome	976.3	E858.7	E946.3	E950.4	E962.0	E980.4
Methoxamine	971.2	E855.5	E941.2	E950.4	E962.0	E980.4
Methoxsalen	976.3	E858.7	E946.3	E950.4	E962.0	E980.4
Methoxybenzyl penicillin	960.0	E856	E930.0	E950.4	E962.0	E980.4
Methoxychlor	989.2	E863.0	—	E950.6	E962.1	E980.7
Methoxyflurane	968.2	E855.1	E938.2	E950.4	E962.0	E980.4
Methoxyphenamine	971.2	E855.5	E941.2	E950.4	E962.0	E980.4
Methoxypromazine	969.1	E853.0	E939.1	E950.3	E962.0	E980.3
Methoxypsoralen	976.3	E858.7	E946.3	E950.4	E962.0	E980.4
Methscopolamine (bromide)	971.1	E855.4	E941.1	E950.4	E962.0	E980.4
Methsuximide	966.2	E855.0	E936.2	E950.4	E962.0	E980.4
Methyclothiazide	974.3	E858.5	E944.3	E950.4	E962.0	E980.4
Methyl	—	—	—	—	—	—
acetate	982.8	E862.4	—	E950.9	E962.1	E980.9
acetone II	982.8	E862.4	—	E950.9	E962.1	E980.9
alcohol	980.1	E860.2	—	E950.9	E962.1	E980.9
amphetamine	969.72 ◀ⅢⅢ	E854.2	E939.7	E950.3	E962.0	E980.3
androstanolone	962.1	E858.0	E932.1	E950.4	E962.0	E980.4
atropine	971.1	E855.4	E941.1	E950.4	E962.0	E980.4
benzene	982.0	E862.4	—	E950.9	E962.1	E980.9
bromide (gas)	987.8	E869.8	—	E952.8	E962.2	E982.8
fumigant	987.8	E863.8	—	E950.6	E962.2	E980.7
butanol	980.8	E860.8	—	E950.9	E962.1	E980.9
carbinol	980.1	E860.2	—	E950.9	E962.1	E980.9
cellosolve	982.8	E862.4	—	E950.9	E962.1	E980.9
cellulose	973.3	E858.4	E943.3	E950.4	E962.0	E980.4
chloride (gas)	987.8	E869.8	—	E952.8	E962.2	E982.8
cyclohexane	982.8	E862.4	—	E950.9	E962.1	E980.9
cyclohexanone	982.8	E862.4	—	E950.9	E962.1	E980.9
dihydromorphinone	965.09	E850.2	E935.2	E950.0	E962.0	E980.0
ergometrine	975.0	E858.6	E945.0	E950.4	E962.0	E980.4
ergonovine	975.0	E858.6	E945.0	E950.4	E962.0	E980.4
ethyl ketone	982.8	E862.4	—	E950.9	E962.1	E980.9
hydrazine	983.9	E864.3	—	E950.7	E962.1	E980.6
isobutyl ketone	982.8	E862.4	—	E950.9	E962.1	E980.9
morphine NEC	965.09	E850.2	E935.2	E950.0	E962.0	E980.0
parafynol	967.8	E852.8	E937.8	E950.2	E962.0	E980.2

◀ New   ◀ⅢⅢ Revised   ~~deleted~~ Deleted   ● Use Additional Digit(s)

	External Cause (E Code)					
Substance	Poisoning	Accident	Therapeutic Use	Suicide Attempt	Assault	Undetermined
Methyl *(Continued)*						E980.7
parathion	989.3	E863.1	—	E950.6	E962.1	
pentynol NEC	967.8	E852.8	E937.8	E950.2	E962.0	E980.2
peridol	969.2	E853.1	E939.2	E950.3	E962.0	E980.3
phenidate	969.73 ◄▥	E854.2	E939.7	E950.3	E962.0	E980.3
prednisolone	962.0	E858.0	E932.0	E950.4	E962.0	E980.4
ENT agent	976.6	E858.7	E946.6	E950.4	E962.0	E980.4
ophthalmic preparation	976.5	E858.7	E946.5	E950.4	E962.0	E980.4
topical NEC	976.0	E858.7	E946.0	E950.4	E962.0	E980.4
propylcarbinol	980.8	E860.8	—	E950.9	E962.1	E980.9
rosaniline NEC	976.0	E858.7	E946.0	E950.4	E962.0	E980.4
salicylate NEC	976.3	E858.7	E946.3	E950.4	E962.0	E980.4
sulfate (fumes)	987.8	E869.8	—	E952.8	E962.2	E982.8
liquid	983.9	E864.3	—	E950.7	E962.1	E980.6
sulfonal	967.8	E852.8	E937.8	E950.2	E962.0	E980.2
testosterone	962.1	E858.0	E932.1	E950.4	E962.0	E980.4
thiouracil	962.8	E858.0	E932.8	E950.4	E962.0	E980.4
Methylated spirit	980.0	E860.1	—	E950.9	E962.1	E980.9
Methyldopa	972.6	E858.3	E942.6	E950.4	E962.0	E980.4
Methylene blue	961.9	E857	E931.9	E950.4	E962.0	E980.4
chloride or dichloride (solvent) NEC	982.3	E862.4	—	E950.9	E962.1	E980.9
Methylhexabital	967.0	E851	E937.0	E950.1	E962.0	E980.1
Methylparaben (ophthalmic)	976.5	E858.7	E946.5	E950.4	E962.0	E980.4
Methyprylon	967.5	E852.4	E937.5	E950.2	E962.0	E980.2
Methysergide	971.3	E855.6	E941.3	E950.4	E962.0	E980.4
Metoclopramide	963.0	E858.1	E933.0	E950.4	E962.0	E980.4
Metofoline	965.7	E850.7	E935.7	E950.0	E962.0	E980.0
Metopon	965.09	E850.2	E935.2	E950.0	E962.0	E980.0
Metronidazole	961.5	E857	E931.5	E950.4	E962.0	E980.4
Metycaine	968.9	E855.2	E938.9	E950.4	E962.0	E980.4
infiltration (subcutaneous)	968.5	E855.2	E938.5	E950.4	E962.0	E980.4
nerve block (peripheral) (plexus)	968.6	E855.2	E938.6	E950.4	E962.0	E980.4
topical (surface)	968.5	E855.2	E938.5	E950.4	E962.0	E980.4
Metyrapone	977.8	E858.8	E947.8	E950.4	E962.0	E980.4
Mevinphos	989.3	E863.1	—	E950.6	E962.1	E980.7
Mezereon (berries)	988.2	E865.3	—	E950.9	E962.1	E980.9
Micatin	976.0	E858.7	E946.0	E950.4	E962.0	E980.4
Miconazole	976.0	E858.7	E946.0	E950.4	E962.0	E980.4
Midol	965.1	E850.3	E935.3	E950.0	E962.0	E980.0

◄ New   ◄▥ Revised   ~~deleted~~ Deleted   ● Use Additional Digit(s)

Substance	Poisoning	External Cause (E Code)				
		Accident	Therapeutic Use	Suicide Attempt	Assault	Undetermined
Mifepristone	962.9	E858.0	E932.9	E950.4	E962.0	E980.4
Milk of magnesia	973.0	E858.4	E943.0	E950.4	E962.0	E980.4
Millipede (tropical) (venomous)	989.5	E905.4	—	E950.9	E962.1	E980.9
Miltown	969.5	E853.8	E939.5	E950.3	E962.0	E980.3
Mineral	—	—	—	—	—	—
oil (medicinal)	973.2	E858.4	E943.2	E950.4	E962.0	E980.4
nonmedicinal	981	E862.1	—	E950.9	E962.1	E980.9
topical	976.3	E858.7	E946.3	E950.4	E962.0	E980.4
salts NEC	974.6	E858.5	E944.6	E950.4	E962.0	E980.4
spirits	981	E862.0	—	E950.9	E962.1	E980.9
Minocycline	960.4	E856	E930.4	E950.4	E962.0	E980.4
Mithramycin (antineoplastic)	960.7	E856	E930.7	E950.4	E962.0	E980.4
Mitobronitol	963.1	E858.1	E933.1	E950.4	E962.0	E980.4
Mitomycin (antineoplastic)	960.7	E856	E930.7	E950.4	E962.0	E980.4
Mitotane	963.1	E858.1	E933.1	E950.4	E962.0	E980.4
Moderil	972.6	E858.3	E942.6	E950.4	E962.0	E980.4
Mogadon - *see* Nitrazepam	—	—	—	—	—	—
Molindone	969.3	E853.8	E939.3	E950.3	E962.0	E980.3
Monistat	976.0	E858.7	E946.0	E950.4	E962.0	E980.4
Monkshood	988.2	E865.4	—	E950.9	E962.1	E980.9
Monoamine oxidase inhibitors	969.01 ◂▥	E854.0	E939.0	E950.3	E962.0	E980.3
Monochlorobenzene	982.0	E862.4	—	E950.9	E962.1	E980.9
Monosodium glutamate	989.89	E866.8	—	E950.9	E962.1	E980.9
Monoxide, carbon - *see* Carbon, monoxide	—	—	—	—	—	—
Moperone	969.2	E853.1	E939.2	E950.3	E962.0	E980.3
Morning glory seeds	969.6	E854.1	E939.6	E950.3	E962.0	E980.3
Moroxydine (hydrochloride)	961.7	E857	E931.7	E950.4	E962.0	E980.4
Morphazinamide	961.8	E857	E931.8	E950.4	E962.0	E980.4
Morphinans	965.09	E850.2	E935.2	E950.0	E962.0	E980.0
Morphine NEC	965.09	E850.2	E935.2	E950.0	E962.0	E980.0
antagonists	970.1	E854.3	E940.1	E950.4	E962.0	E980.4
Morpholinylethyl morphine	965.09	E850.2	E935.2	E950.0	E962.0	E980.0
Morrhuate sodium	972.7	E858.3	E942.7	E950.4	E962.0	E980.4
Moth balls (*see also* Pesticides)	989.4	E863.4	—	E950.6	E962.1	E980.7
naphthalene	983.0	E863.4	—	E950.7	E962.1	E980.6
Motor exhaust gas - *see* Carbon, monoxide, exhaust gas	—	—	—	—	—	—
Mouth wash	976.6	E858.7	E946.6	E950.4	E962.0	E980.4
Mucolytic agent	975.5	E858.6	E945.5	E950.4	E962.0	E980.4
Mucomyst	975.5	E858.6	E945.5	E950.4	E962.0	E980.4

Substance	Poisoning	External Cause (E Code)				
		Accident	Therapeutic Use	Suicide Attempt	Assault	Undetermined
Mucous membrane agents (external)	976.9	E858.7	E946.9	E950.4	E962.0	E980.4
specified NEC	976.8	E858.7	E946.8	E950.4	E962.0	E980.4
Mumps	—	—	—	—	—	—
immune globulin (human)	964.6	E858.2	E934.6	E950.4	E962.0	E980.4
skin test antigen	977.8	E858.8	E947.8	E950.4	E962.0	E980.4
vaccine	979.6	E858.8	E949.6	E950.4	E962.0	E980.4
Mumpsvax	979.6	E858.8	E949.6	E950.4	E962.0	E980.4
Muriatic acid - see Hydrochloric acid	—	—	—	—	—	—
Muscarine	971.0	E855.3	E941.0	E950.4	E962.0	E980.4
Muscle affecting agents NEC	975.3	E858.6	E945.3	E950.4	E962.0	E980.4
oxytocic	975.0	E858.6	E945.0	E950.4	E962.0	E980.4
relaxants	975.3	E858.6	E945.3	E950.4	E962.0	E980.4
central nervous system	968.0	E855.1	E938.0	E950.4	E962.0	E980.4
skeletal	975.2	E858.6	E945.2	E950.4	E962.0	E980.4
smooth	975.1	E858.6	E945.1	E950.4	E962.0	E980.4
Mushrooms, noxious	988.1	E865.5	—	E950.9	E962.1	E980.9
Mussel, noxious	988.0	E865.1	—	E950.9	E962.1	E980.9
Mustard (emetic)	973.6	E858.4	E943.6	E950.4	E962.0	E980.4
gas	987.8	E869.8	—	E952.8	E962.2	E982.8
nitrogen	963.1	E858.1	E933.1	E950.4	E962.0	E980.4
Mustine	963.1	E858.1	E933.1	E950.4	E962.0	E980.4
M-vac	979.4	E858.8	E949.4	E950.4	E962.0	E980.4
Mycifradin	960.8	E856	E930.8	E950.4	E962.0	E980.4
topical	976.0	E858.7	E946.0	E950.4	E962.0	E980.4
Mycitracin	960.8	E856	E930.8	E950.4	E962.0	E980.4
ophthalmic preparation	976.5	E858.7	E946.5	E950.4	E962.0	E980.4
Mycostatin	960.1	E856	E930.1	E950.4	E962.0	E980.4
topical	976.0	E858.7	E946.0	E950.4	E962.0	E980.4
Mydriacyl	971.1	E855.4	E941.1	E950.4	E962.0	E980.4
Myelobromal	963.1	E858.1	E933.1	E950.4	E962.0	E980.4
Myleran	963.1	E858.1	E933.1	E950.4	E962.0	E980.4
Myochrysin(e)	965.69	E850.6	E935.6	E950.0	E962.0	E980.0
Myoneural blocking agents	975.2	E858.6	E945.2	E950.4	E962.0	E980.4
Myristica fragrans	988.2	E865.3	—	E950.9	E962.1	E980.9
Myristicin	988.2	E865.3	—	E950.9	E962.1	E980.9
Mysoline	966.3	E855.0	E936.3	E950.4	E962.0	E980.4
Nafcillin (sodium)	960.0	E856	E930.0	E950.4	E962.0	E980.4
Nail polish remover	982.8	E862.4	—	E950.9	E962.1	E980.9
Nalidixic acid	961.9	E857	E931.9	E950.4	E962.0	E980.4

◀ New   ◀▦ Revised   ~~deleted~~ Deleted   ● Use Additional Digit(s)

Substance	Poisoning	External Cause (E Code)				
		Accident	Therapeutic Use	Suicide Attempt	Assault	Undetermined
Nalorphine	970.1	E854.3	E940.1	E950.4	E962.0	E980.4
Naloxone	970.1	E854.3	E940.1	E950.4	E962.0	E980.4
Namenda	969.8	E854.8	E939.8	E950.3	E962.0	E980.3
Nandrolone (decanoate) (phenpropionate)	962.1	E858.0	E932.1	E950.4	E962.0	E980.4
Naphazoline	971.2	E855.5	E941.2	E950.4	E962.0	E980.4
Naphtha (painter's) (petroleum)	981	E862.0	—	E950.9	E962.1	E980.9
solvent	981	E862.0	—	E950.9	E962.1	E980.9
vapor	987.1	E869.8	—	E952.8	E962.2	E982.8
Naphthalene (chlorinated)	983.0	E864.0	—	E950.7	E962.1	E980.6
insecticide or moth repellent	983.0	E863.4	—	E950.7	E962.1	E980.6
vapor	987.8	E869.8	—	E952.8	E962.2	E982.8
Naphthol	983.0	E864.0	—	E950.7	E962.1	E980.6
Naphthylamine	983.0	E864.0	—	E950.7	E962.1	E980.6
Naprosyn - see Naproxen	—	—	—	—	—	—
Naproxen	965.61	E850.6	E935.6	E950.0	E962.0	E980.0
Narcotic (drug)	967.9	E852.9	E937.9	E950.2	E962.0	E980.2
analgesic NEC	965.8	E850.8	E935.8	E950.0	E962.0	E980.0
antagonist	970.1	E854.3	E940.1	E950.4	E962.0	E980.4
specified NEC	967.8	E852.8	E937.8	E950.2	E962.0	E980.2
Narcotine	975.4	E858.6	E945.4	E950.4	E962.0	E980.4
Nardil	969.01 ◀▦	E854.0	E939.0	E950.3	E962.0	E980.3
Natrium cyanide - see Cyanide(s)	—	—	—	—	—	—
Natural	—	—	—	—	—	—
blood (product)	964.7	E858.2	E934.7	E950.4	E962.0	E980.4
gas (piped)	987.1	E867	—	E951.0	E962.2	E981.0
incomplete combustion	986	E867	—	E951.0	E962.2	E981.0
Nealbarbital, nealbarbitone	967.0	E851	E937.0	E950.1	E962.0	E980.1
Nectadon	975.4	E858.6	E945.4	E950.4	E962.0	E980.4
Nematocyst (sting)	989.5	E905.6	—	E950.9	E962.1	E980.9
Nembutal	967.0	E851	E937.0	E950.1	E962.0	E980.1
Neoarsphenamine	961.1	E857	E931.1	E950.4	E962.0	E980.4
Neocinchophen	974.7	E858.5	E944.7	E950.4	E962.0	E980.4
Neomycin	960.8	E856	E930.8	E950.4	E962.0	E980.4
ENT agent	976.6	E858.7	E946.6	E950.4	E962.0	E980.4
ophthalmic preparation	976.5	E858.7	E946.5	E950.4	E962.0	E980.4
topical NEC	976.0	E858.7	E946.0	E950.4	E962.0	E980.4
Neonal	967.0	E851	E937.0	E950.1	E962.0	E980.1
Neoprontosil	961.0	E857	E931.0	E950.4	E962.0	E980.4
Neosalvarsan	961.1	E857	E931.1	E950.4	E962.0	E980.4

◀ New   ◀▦ Revised   ~~deleted~~ Deleted   ● Use Additional Digit(s)

Substance	Poisoning	External Cause (E Code)				
		Accident	Therapeutic Use	Suicide Attempt	Assault	Undetermined
Neosilversalvarsan	961.1	E857	E931.1	E950.4	E962.0	E980.4
Neosporin	960.8	E856	E930.8	E950.4	E962.0	E980.4
ENT agent	976.6	E858.7	E946.6	E950.4	E962.0	E980.4
ophthalmic preparation	976.5	E858.7	E946.5	E950.4	E962.0	E980.4
topical NEC	976.0	E858.7	E946.0	E950.4	E962.0	E980.4
Neostigmine	971.0	E855.3	E941.0	E950.4	E962.0	E980.4
Neraval	967.0	E851	E937.0	E950.1	E962.0	E980.1
Neravan	967.0	E851	E937.0	E950.1	E962.0	E980.1
Nerium oleander	988.2	E865.4	—	E950.9	E962.1	E980.9
Nerve gases (war)	987.9	E869.9	—	E952.9	E962.2	E982.9
Nesacaine	968.9	E855.2	E938.9	E950.4	E962.0	E980.4
infiltration (subcutaneous)	968.5	E855.2	E938.5	E950.4	E962.0	E980.4
nerve block (peripheral) (plexus)	968.6	E855.2	E938.6	E950.4	E962.0	E980.4
Neurobarb	967.0	E851	E937.0	E950.1	E962.0	E980.1
Neuroleptics NEC	969.3	E853.8	E939.3	E950.3	E962.0	E980.3
Neuroprotective agent	977.8	E858.8	E947.8	E950.4	E962.0	E980.4
Neutral spirits	980.0	E860.1	—	E950.9	E962.1	E980.9
beverage	980.0	E860.0	—	E950.9	E962.1	E980.9
Niacin, niacinamide	972.2	E858.3	E942.2	E950.4	E962.0	E980.4
Nialamide	969.01 ◀▥▥	E854.0	E939.0	E950.3	E962.0	E980.3
Nickle (carbonyl) (compounds) (fumes) (tetracarbonyl) (vapor)	985.8	E866.4	—	E950.9	E962.1	E980.9
Niclosamide	961.6	E857	E931.6	E950.4	E962.0	E980.4
Nicomorphine	965.09	E850.2	E935.2	E950.0	E962.0	E980.0
Nicotinamide	972.2	E858.3	E942.2	E950.4	E962.0	E980.4
Nicotine (insecticide) (spray) (sulfate) NEC	989.4	E863.4	—	E950.6	E962.1	E980.7
not insecticide	989.89	E866.8	—	E950.9	E962.1	E980.9
Nicotinic acid (derivatives)	972.2	E858.3	E942.2	E950.4	E962.0	E980.4
Nicotinyl alcohol	972.2	E858.3	E942.2	E950.4	E962.0	E980.4
Nicoumalone	964.2	E858.2	E934.2	E950.4	E962.0	E980.4
Nifenazone	965.5	E850.5	E935.5	E950.0	E962.0	E980.0
Nifuraldezone	961.9	E857	E931.9	E950.4	E962.0	E980.4
Nightshade (deadly)	988.2	E865.4	—	E950.9	E962.1	E980.9
Nikethamide	970.0	E854.3	E940.0	E950.4	E962.0	E980.4
Nilstat	960.1	E856	E930.1	E950.4	E962.0	E980.4
topical	976.0	E858.7	E946.0	E950.4	E962.0	E980.4
Nimodipine	977.8	E858.8	E947.8	E950.4	E962.0	E980.4
Niridazole	961.6	E857	E931.6	E950.4	E962.0	E980.4
Nisentil	965.09	E850.2	E935.2	E950.0	E962.0	E980.0
Nitrates	972.4	E858.3	E942.4	E950.4	E962.0	E980.4

◀ New   ◀▥▥ Revised   ~~deleted~~ Deleted   ● Use Additional Digit(s)

Substance	Poisoning	External Cause (E Code)				
		Accident	Therapeutic Use	Suicide Attempt	Assault	Undetermined
Nitrazepam	969.4	E853.2	E939.4	E950.3	E962.0	E980.3
Nitric	—	—	—	—	—	—
acid (liquid)	983.1	E864.1	—	E950.7	E962.1	E980.6
vapor	987.8	E869.8	—	E952.8	E962.2	E982.8
oxide (gas)	987.2	E869.0	—	E952.8	E962.2	E982.8
Nitrite, amyl (medicinal) (vapor)	972.4	E858.3	E942.4	E950.4	E962.0	E980.4
Nitroaniline	983.0	E864.0	—	E950.7	E962.1	E980.6
vapor	987.8	E869.8	—	E952.8	E962.2	E982.8
Nitrobenzene, nitrobenzol	983.0	E864.0	—	E950.7	E962.1	E980.6
vapor	987.8	E869.8	—	E952.8	E962.2	E982.8
Nitrocellulose	976.3	E858.7	E946.3	E950.4	E962.0	E980.4
Nitrofuran derivatives	961.9	E857	E931.9	E950.4	E962.0	E980.4
Nitrofurantoin	961.9	E857	E931.9	E950.4	E962.0	E980.4
Nitrofurazone	976.0	E858.7	E946.0	E950.4	E962.0	E980.4
Nitrogen (dioxide) (gas) (oxide)	987.2	E869.0	—	E952.8	E962.2	E982.8
mustard (antineoplastic)	963.1	E858.1	E933.1	E950.4	E962.0	E980.4
Nitroglycerin, nitroglycerol (medicinal)	972.4	E858.3	E942.4	E950.4	E962.0	E980.4
nonmedicinal	989.89	E866.8	—	E950.9	E962.1	E980.9
fumes	987.8	E869.8	—	E952.8	E962.2	E982.8
Nitrohydrochloric acid	983.1	E864.1	—	E950.7	E962.1	E980.6
Nitromersol	976.0	E858.7	E946.0	E950.4	E962.0	E980.4
Nitronaphthalene	983.0	E864.0	—	E950.7	E962.2	E980.6
Nitrophenol	983.0	E864.0	—	E950.7	E962.2	E980.6
Nitrothiazol	961.6	E857	E931.6	E950.4	E962.0	E980.4
Nitrotoluene, nitrotoluol	983.0	E864.0	—	E950.7	E962.1	E980.6
vapor	987.8	E869.8	—	E952.8	E962.2	E982.8
Nitrous	968.2	E855.1	E938.2	E950.4	E962.0	E980.4
acid (liquid)	983.1	E864.1	—	E950.7	E962.1	E980.6
fumes	987.2	E869.0	—	E952.8	E962.2	E982.8
oxide (anesthetic) NEC	968.2	E855.1	E938.2	E950.4	E962.0	E980.4
Nitrozone	976.0	E858.7	E946.0	E950.4	E962.0	E980.4
Noctec	967.1	E852.0	E937.1	E950.2	E962.0	E980.2
Noludar	967.5	E852.4	E937.5	E950.2	E962.0	E980.2
Noptil	967.0	E851	E937.0	E950.1	E962.0	E980.1
Noradrenalin	971.2	E855.5	E941.2	E950.4	E962.0	E980.4
Noramidopyrine	965.5	E850.5	E935.5	E950.0	E962.0	E980.0
Norepinephrine	971.2	E855.5	E941.2	E950.4	E962.0	E980.4
Norethandrolone	962.1	E858.0	E932.1	E950.4	E962.0	E980.4
Norethindrone	962.2	E858.0	E932.2	E950.4	E962.0	E980.4

◀ New   ◀▥ Revised   ~~deleted~~ Deleted   ● Use Additional Digit(s)

Substance	Poisoning	External Cause (E Code)				
		Accident	Therapeutic Use	Suicide Attempt	Assault	Undetermined
Norethisterone	962.2	E858.0	E932.2	E950.4	E962.0	E980.4
Norethynodrel	962.2	E858.0	E932.2	E950.4	E962.0	E980.4
Norlestrin	962.2	E858.0	E932.2	E950.4	E962.0	E980.4
Norlutin	962.2	E858.0	E932.2	E950.4	E962.0	E980.4
Normison - *see* Benzodiazepines	—	—	—	—	—	—
Normorphine	965.09	E850.2	E935.2	E950.0	E962.0	E980.0
Nortriptyline	969.05 ◀▥	E854.0	E939.0	E950.3	E962.0	E980.3
Noscapine	975.4	E858.6	E945.4	E950.4	E962.0	E980.4
Nose preparations	976.6	E858.7	E946.6	E950.4	E962.0	E980.4
Novobiocin	960.8	E856	E930.8	E950.4	E962.0	E980.4
Novocain (infiltration) (topical)	968.5	E855.2	E938.5	E950.4	E962.0	E980.4
nerve block (peripheral) (plexus)	968.6	E855.2	E938.6	E950.4	E962.0	E980.4
spinal	968.7	E855.2	E938.7	E950.4	E962.0	E980.4
Noxythiolin	961.9	E857	E931.9	E950.4	E962.0	E980.4
NPH Iletin (insulin)	962.3	E858.0	E932.3	E950.4	E962.0	E980.4
Numorphan	965.09	E850.2	E935.2	E950.0	E962.0	E980.0
Nunol	967.0	E851	E937.0	E950.1	E962.0	E980.1
Nupercaine (spinal anesthetic)	968.7	E855.2	E938.7	E950.4	E962.0	E980.4
topical (surface)	968.5	E855.2	E938.5	E950.4	E962.0	E980.4
Nutmeg oil (liniment)	976.3	E858.7	E946.3	E950.4	E962.0	E980.4
Nux vomica	989.1	E863.7	—	E950.6	E962.1	E980.7
Nydrazid	961.8	E857	E931.8	E950.4	E962.0	E980.4
Nylidrin	971.2	E855.5	E941.2	E950.4	E962.0	E980.4
Nystatin	960.1	E856	E930.1	E950.4	E962.0	E980.4
topical	976.0	E858.7	E946.0	E950.4	E962.0	E980.4
Nytol	963.0	E858.1	E933.0	E950.4	E962.0	E980.4
Oblivion	967.8	E852.8	E937.8	E950.2	E962.0	E980.2
Octyl nitrite	972.4	E858.3	E942.4	E950.4	E962.0	E980.4
Oestradiol (cypionate) (dipropionate) (valerate)	962.2	E858.0	E932.2	E950.4	E962.0	E980.4
Oestriol	962.2	E858.0	E932.2	E950.4	E962.0	E980.4
Oestrone	962.2	E858.0	E932.2	E950.4	E962.0	E980.4
Oil (of) NEC	989.89	E866.8	—	E950.9	E962.1	E980.9
bitter almond	989.0	E866.8	—	E950.9	E962.1	E980.9
camphor	976.1	E858.7	E946.1	E950.4	E962.0	E980.4
colors	989.89	E861.6	—	E950.9	E962.1	E980.9
fumes	987.8	E869.8	—	E952.8	E962.2	E982.8
lubricating	981	E862.2	—	E950.9	E962.1	E980.9
specified source, other - *see* substance specified	—	—	—	—	—	—

◀ New ◀▥ Revised ~~deleted~~ Deleted ● Use Additional Digit(s)

Substance	Poisoning	External Cause (E Code)				
		Accident	Therapeutic Use	Suicide Attempt	Assault	Undetermined
Oil (of) NEC *(Continued)*						
vitriol (liquid)	983.1	E864.1	—	E950.7	E962.1	E980.6
fumes	987.8	E869.8	—	E952.8	E962.2	E982.8
wintergreen (bitter) NEC	976.3	E858.7	E946.3	E950.4	E962.0	E980.4
Ointments NEC	976.9	E858.7	E946.9	E950.4	E962.0	E980.4
Oleander	988.2	E865.4	—	E950.9	E962.1	E980.9
Oleandomycin	960.3	E856	E930.3	E950.4	E962.0	E980.4
Oleovitamin A	963.5	E858.1	E933.5	E950.4	E962.0	E980.4
Oleum ricini	973.1	E858.4	E943.1	E950.4	E962.0	E980.4
Olive oil (medicinal) NEC	973.2	E858.4	E943.2	E950.4	E962.0	E980.4
OMPA	989.3	E863.1	—	E950.6	E962.1	E980.7
Oncovin	963.1	E858.1	E933.1	E950.4	E962.0	E980.4
Ophthaine	968.5	E855.2	E938.5	E950.4	E962.0	E980.4
Ophthetic	968.5	E855.2	E938.5	E950.4	E962.0	E980.4
Opiates, opioids, opium NEC	965.00	E850.2	E935.2	E950.0	E962.0	E980.0
antagonists	970.1	E854.3	E940.1	E950.4	E962.0	E980.4
Oracon	962.2	E858.0	E932.2	E950.4	E962.0	E980.4
Oragrafin	977.8	E858.8	E947.8	E950.4	E962.0	E980.4
Oral contraceptives	962.2	E858.0	E932.2	E950.4	E962.0	E980.4
Orciprenaline	975.1	E858.6	E945.1	E950.4	E962.0	E980.4
Organidin	975.5	E858.6	E945.5	E950.4	E962.0	E980.4
Organophosphates	989.3	E863.1	—	E950.6	E962.1	E980.7
Orimune	979.5	E858.8	E949.5	E950.4	E962.0	E980.4
Orinase	962.3	E858.0	E932.3	E950.4	E962.0	E980.4
Orphenadrine	966.4	E855.0	E936.4	E950.4	E962.0	E980.4
Ortal (sodium)	967.0	E851	E937.0	E950.1	E962.0	E980.1
Orthoboric acid	976.0	E858.7	E946.0	E950.4	E962.0	E980.4
ENT agent	976.6	E858.7	E946.6	E950.4	E962.0	E980.4
ophthalmic preparation	976.5	E858.7	E946.5	E950.4	E962.0	E980.4
Orthocaine	968.5	E855.2	E938.5	E950.4	E962.0	E980.4
Ortho-Novum	962.2	E858.0	E932.2	E950.4	E962.0	E980.4
Orthotolidine (reagent)	977.8	E858.8	E947.8	E950.4	E962.0	E980.4
Osmic acid (liquid)	983.1	E864.1	—	E950.7	E962.1	E980.6
fumes	987.8	E869.8	—	E952.8	E962.2	E982.8
Osmotic diuretics	974.4	E858.5	E944.4	E950.4	E962.0	E980.4
Ouabain	972.1	E858.3	E942.1	E950.4	E962.0	E980.4
Ovarian hormones (synthetic substitutes)	962.2	E858.0	E932.2	E950.4	E962.0	E980.4
Ovral	962.2	E858.0	E932.2	E950.4	E962.0	E980.4

◀ New   ◀▥ Revised   ~~deleted~~ Deleted   ● Use Additional Digit(s)

Substance	Poisoning	External Cause (E Code)				
		Accident	Therapeutic Use	Suicide Attempt	Assault	Undetermined
Ovulation suppressants	962.2	E858.0	E932.2	E950.4	E962.0	E980.4
Ovulen	962.2	E858.0	E932.2	E950.4	E962.0	E980.4
Oxacillin (sodium)	960.0	E856	E930.0	E950.4	E962.0	E980.4
Oxalic acid	983.1	E864.1	—	E950.7	E962.1	E980.6
Oxanamide	969.5	E853.8	E939.5	E950.3	E962.0	E980.3
Oxandrolone	962.1	E858.0	E932.1	E950.4	E962.0	E980.4
Oxaprozin	965.61	E850.6	E935.6	E950.0	E962.0	E980.0
Oxazepam	969.4	E853.2	E939.4	E950.3	E962.0	E980.3
Oxazolidine derivatives	966.0	E855.0	E936.0	E950.4	E962.0	E980.4
Ox bile extract	973.4	E858.4	E943.4	E950.4	E962.0	E980.4
Oxedrine	971.2	E855.5	E941.2	E950.4	E962.0	E980.4
Oxeladin	975.4	E858.6	E945.4	E950.4	E962.0	E980.4
Oxethazaine NEC	968.5	E855.2	E938.5	E950.4	E962.0	E980.4
Oxidizing agents NEC	983.9	E864.3	—	E950.7	E962.1	E980.6
Oxolinic acid	961.3	E857	E931.3	E950.4	E962.0	E980.4
Oxophenarsine	961.1	E857	E931.1	E950.4	E962.0	E980.4
Oxsoralen	976.3	E858.7	E946.3	E950.4	E962.0	E980.4
Oxtriphylline	976.7	E858.6	E945.7	E950.4	E962.0	E980.4
Oxybuprocaine	968.5	E855.2	E938.5	E950.4	E962.0	E980.4
Oxybutynin	975.1	E858.6	E945.1	E950.4	E962.0	E980.4
Oxycodone	965.09	E850.2	E935.2	E950.0	E962.0	E980.0
Oxygen	987.8	E869.8	—	E952.8	E962.2	E982.8
Oxylone	976.0	E858.7	E946.0	E950.4	E962.0	E980.4
ophthalmic preparation	976.5	E858.7	E946.5	E950.4	E962.0	E980.4
Oxymesterone	962.1	E858.0	E932.1	E950.4	E962.0	E980.4
Oxymetazoline	971.2	E855.5	E941.2	E950.4	E962.0	E980.4
Oxymetholone	962.1	E858.0	E932.1	E950.4	E962.0	E980.4
Oxymorphone	965.09	E850.2	E935.2	E950.0	E962.0	E980.0
Oxypertine	969.09 ◀ⅢⅢ	E854.0	E939.0	E950.3	E962.0	E980.3
Oxyphenbutazone	965.5	E850.5	E935.5	E950.0	E962.0	E980.0
Oxyphencyclimine	971.1	E855.4	E941.1	E950.4	E962.0	E980.4
Oxyphenisatin	973.1	E858.4	E943.1	E950.4	E962.0	E980.4
Oxyphenonium	971.1	E855.4	E941.1	E950.4	E962.0	E980.4
Oxyquinoline	961.3	E857	E931.3	E950.4	E962.0	E980.4
Oxytetracycline	960.4	E856	E930.4	E950.4	E962.0	E980.4
Oxytocics	975.0	E858.6	E945.0	E950.4	E962.0	E980.4
Oxytocin	975.0	E858.6	E945.0	E950.4	E962.0	E980.4
Ozone	987.8	E869.8	—	E952.8	E962.2	E982.8
PABA	976.3	E858.7	E946.3	E950.4	E962.0	E980.4

◀ New   ◀ⅢⅢ Revised   ~~deleted~~ Deleted   ● Use Additional Digit(s)

Substance	Poisoning	External Cause (E Code) Accident	Therapeutic Use	Suicide Attempt	Assault	Undetermined
Packed red cells	964.7	E858.2	E934.7	E950.4	E962.0	E980.4
Paint NEC	989.89	E861.6	—	E950.9	E962.1	E980.9
cleaner	982.8	E862.9	—	E950.9	E962.1	E980.9
fumes NEC	987.8	E869.8	—	E952.8	E962.1	E982.8
lead (fumes)	984.0	E861.5	—	E950.9	E962.1	E980.9
solvent NEC	982.8	E862.9	—	E950.9	E962.1	E980.9
stripper	982.8	E862.9	—	E950.9	E962.1	E980.9
Palfium	965.09	E850.2	E935.2	E950.0	E962.0	E980.0
Palivizumab	979.9	E858.8	E949.6	E950.4	E962.0	E980.4
Paludrine	961.4	E857	E931.4	E950.4	E962.0	E980.4
PAM	977.2	E855.8	E947.2	E950.4	E962.0	E980.4
Pamaquine (napthoate)	961.4	E857	E931.4	E950.4	E962.0	E980.4
Pamprin	965.1	E850.3	E935.3	E950.0	E962.0	E980.0
Panadol	965.4	E850.4	E935.4	E950.0	E962.0	E980.0
Pancreatic dornase (mucolytic)	963.4	E858.1	E933.4	E950.4	E962.0	E980.4
Pancreatin	973.4	E858.4	E943.4	E950.4	E962.0	E980.4
Pancrelipase	973.4	E858.4	E943.4	E950.4	E962.0	E980.4
Pangamic acid	963.5	E858.1	E933.5	E950.4	E962.0	E980.4
Panthenol	963.5	E858.1	E933.5	E950.4	E962.0	E980.4
topical	976.8	E858.7	E946.8	E950.4	E962.0	E980.4
Pantopaque	977.8	E858.8	E947.8	E950.4	E962.0	E980.4
Pantopon	965.00	E850.2	E935.2	E950.0	E962.0	E980.0
Pantothenic acid	963.5	E858.1	E933.5	E950.4	E962.0	E980.4
Panwarfin	964.2	E858.2	E934.2	E950.4	E962.0	E980.4
Papain	973.4	E858.4	E943.4	E950.4	E962.0	E980.4
Papaverine	972.5	E858.3	E942.5	E950.4	E962.0	E980.4
Para-aminobenzoic acid	976.3	E858.7	E946.3	E950.4	E962.0	E980.4
Para-aminophenol derivatives	965.4	E850.4	E935.4	E950.0	E962.0	E980.0
Para-aminosalicylic acid (derivatives)	961.8	E857	E931.8	E950.4	E962.0	E980.4
Paracetaldehyde (medicinal)	967.2	E852.1	E937.2	E950.2	E962.0	E980.2
Paracetamol	965.4	E850.4	E935.4	E950.0	E962.0	E980.0
Paracodin	965.09	E850.2	E935.2	E950.0	E962.0	E980.0
Paradione	966.0	E855.0	E936.0	E950.4	E962.0	E980.4
Paraffin(s) (wax)	981	E862.3	—	E950.9	E962.1	E980.9
liquid (medicinal)	973.2	E858.4	E943.2	E950.4	E962.0	E980.4
nonmedicinal (oil)	981	E962.1	—	E950.9	E962.1	E980.9
Paraldehyde (medicinal)	967.2	E852.1	E937.2	E950.2	E962.0	E980.2
Paramethadione	966.0	E855.0	E936.0	E950.4	E962.0	E980.4
Paramethasone	962.0	E858.0	E932.0	E950.4	E962.0	E980.4

Substance	Poisoning	External Cause (E Code)				
		Accident	Therapeutic Use	Suicide Attempt	Assault	Undetermined
Paraquat	989.4	E863.5	—	E950.6	E962.1	E980.7
Parasympatholytics	971.1	E855.4	E941.1	E950.4	E962.0	E980.4
Parasympathomimetics	971.0	E855.3	E941.0	E950.4	E962.0	E980.4
Parathion	989.3	E863.1	—	E950.6	E962.1	E980.7
Parathormone	962.6	E858.0	E932.6	E950.4	E962.0	E980.4
Parathyroid (derivatives)	962.6	E858.0	E932.6	E950.4	E962.0	E980.4
Paratyphoid vaccine	978.1	E858.8	E948.1	E950.4	E962.0	E980.4
Paredrine	971.2	E855.5	E941.2	E950.4	E962.0	E980.4
Paregoric	965.00	E850.2	E935.2	E950.0	E962.0	E980.0
Pargyline	972.3	E858.3	E942.3	E950.4	E962.0	E980.4
Paris green	985.1	E866.3	—	E950.8	E962.1	E980.8
insecticide	985.1	E863.4	—	E950.8	E962.1	E980.8
Parnate	969.01 ◀▥	E854.0	E939.0	E950.3	E962.0	E980.3
Paromomycin	960.8	E856	E930.8	E950.4	E962.0	E980.4
Paroxypropione	963.1	E858.1	E933.1	E950.4	E962.0	E980.4
Parzone	965.09	E850.2	E935.2	E950.0	E962.0	E980.0
PAS	961.8	E857	E931.8	E950.4	E962.0	E980.4
PCBs	981	E862.3	—	E950.9	E962.1	E980.9
PCP (pentachlorophenol)	989.4	E863.6	—	E950.6	E962.1	E980.7
herbicide	989.4	E863.5	—	E950.6	E962.1	E980.7
insecticide	989.4	E863.4	—	E950.6	E962.1	E980.7
phencyclidine	968.3	E855.1	E938.3	E950.4	E962.0	E980.4
Peach kernel oil (emulsion)	973.2	E858.4	E943.2	E950.4	E962.0	E980.4
Peanut oil (emulsion) NEC	973.2	E858.4	E943.2	E950.4	E962.0	E980.4
topical	976.3	E858.7	E946.3	E950.4	E962.0	E980.4
Pearly Gates (morning glory seeds)	969.6	E854.1	E939.6	E950.3	E962.0	E980.3
Pecazine	969.1	E853.0	E939.1	E950.3	E962.0	E980.3
Pecilocin	960.1	E856	E930.1	E950.4	E962.0	E980.4
Pectin (with kaolin) NEC	973.5	E858.4	E943.5	E950.4	E962.0	E980.4
Pelletierine tannate	961.6	E857	E931.6	E950.4	E962.0	E980.4
Pemoline	969.79 ◀▥	E854.2	E939.7	E950.3	E962.0	E980.3
Pempidine	972.3	E858.3	E942.3	E950.4	E962.0	E980.4
Penamecillin	960.0	E856	E930.0	E950.4	E962.0	E980.4
Penethamate hydriodide	960.0	E856	E930.0	E950.4	E962.0	E980.4
Penicillamine	963.8	E858.1	E933.8	E950.4	E962.0	E980.4
Penicillin (any type)	960.0	E856	E930.0	E950.4	E962.0	E980.4
Penicillinase	963.4	E858.1	E933.4	E950.4	E962.0	E980.4
Pentachlorophenol (fungicide)	989.4	E863.6	—	E950.6	E962.1	E980.7
herbicide	989.4	E863.5	—	E950.6	E962.1	E980.7
insecticide	989.4	E863.4	—	E950.6	E962.1	E980.7

◀ New   ◀▥ Revised   ~~deleted~~ Deleted   ● Use Additional Digit(s)

Substance	Poisoning	External Cause (E Code)				
		Accident	Therapeutic Use	Suicide Attempt	Assault	Undetermined
Pentaerythritol	972.4	E858.3	E942.4	E950.4	E962.0	E980.4
chloral	967.1	E852.0	E937.1	E950.2	E962.0	E980.2
tetranitrate NEC	972.4	E858.3	E942.4	E950.4	E962.0	E980.4
Pentagastrin	977.8	E858.8	E947.8	E950.4	E962.0	E980.4
Pentalin	982.3	E862.4	—	E950.9	E962.1	E980.9
Pentamethonium (bromide)	972.3	E858.3	E942.3	E950.4	E962.0	E980.4
Pentamidine	961.5	E857	E931.5	E950.4	E962.0	E980.4
Pentanol	980.8	E860.8	—	E950.9	E962.1	E980.9
Pentaquine	961.4	E857	E931.4	E950.4	E962.0	E980.4
Pentazocine	965.8	E850.8	E935.8	E950.0	E962.0	E980.0
Penthienate	971.1	E855.4	E941.1	E950.4	E962.0	E980.4
Pentobarbital, pentobarbitone (sodium)	967.0	E851	E937.0	E950.1	E962.0	E980.1
Pentolinium (tartrate)	972.3	E858.3	E942.3	E950.4	E962.0	E980.4
Pentothal	968.3	E855.1	E938.3	E950.4	E962.0	E980.4
Pentylenetetrazol	970.0	E854.3	E940.0	E950.4	E962.0	E980.4
Pentylsalicylamide	961.8	E857	E931.8	E950.4	E962.0	E980.4
Pepsin	973.4	E858.4	E943.4	E950.4	E962.0	E980.4
Peptavlon	977.8	E858.8	E947.8	E950.4	E962.0	E980.4
Percaine (spinal)	968.7	E855.2	E938.7	E950.4	E962.0	E980.4
topical (surface)	968.5	E855.2	E938.5	E950.4	E962.0	E980.4
Perchloroethylene (vapor)	982.3	E862.4	—	E950.9	E962.1	E980.9
medicinal	961.6	E857	E931.6	E950.4	E962.0	E980.4
Percodan	965.09	E850.2	E935.2	E950.0	E962.0	E980.0
Percogesic	965.09	E850.2	E935.2	E950.0	E962.0	E980.0
Percorten	962.0	E858.0	E932.0	E950.4	E962.0	E980.4
Pergonal	962.4	E858.0	E932.4	E950.4	E962.0	E980.4
Perhexiline	972.4	E858.3	E942.4	E950.4	E962.0	E980.4
Periactin	963.0	E858.1	E933.0	E950.4	E962.0	E980.4
Periclor	967.1	E852.0	E937.1	E950.2	E962.0	E980.2
Pericyazine	969.1	E853.0	E939.1	E950.3	E962.0	E980.3
Peritrate	972.4	E858.3	E942.4	E950.4	E962.0	E980.4
Permanganates NEC	983.9	E864.3	—	E950.7	E962.1	E980.6
potassium (topical)	976.0	E858.7	E946.0	E950.4	E962.0	E980.4
Pernocton	967.0	E851	E937.0	E950.1	E962.0	E980.1
Pernoston	967.0	E851	E937.0	E950.1	E962.0	E980.1
Peronin(e)	965.09	E850.2	E935.2	E950.0	E962.0	E980.0
Perphenazine	969.1	E853.0	E939.1	E950.3	E962.0	E980.3
Pertofrane	969.05 ◀▥	E854	E939.0	E950.3	E962.0	E980.3

◀ New   ◀▥ Revised   ~~deleted~~ Deleted   ● Use Additional Digit(s)

Substance	Poisoning	External Cause (E Code)				
		Accident	Therapeutic Use	Suicide Attempt	Assault	Undetermined
Pertussis	—	—	—	—	—	—
immune serum (human)	964.6	E858.2	E934.6	E950.4	E962.0	E980.4
vaccine (with diphtheria toxoid) (with tetanus toxoid)	978.6	E858.8	E948.6	E950.4	E962.0	E980.4
Peruvian balsam	976.8	E858.7	E946.8	E950.4	E962.0	E980.4
Pesticides (dust) (fumes) (vapor)	989.4	E863.4	—	E950.6	E962.1	E980.7
arsenic	985.1	E863.4	—	E950.8	E962.1	E980.8
chlorinated	989.2	E863.0	—	E950.6	E962.1	E980.7
cyanide	989.0	E863.4	—	E950.6	E962.1	E980.7
kerosene	981	E863.4	—	E950.6	E962.1	E980.7
mixture (of compounds)	989.4	E863.3	—	E950.6	E962.1	E980.7
naphthalene	983.0	E863.4	—	E950.7	E962.1	E980.6
organochlorine (compounds)	989.2	E863.0	—	E950.6	E962.1	E980.7
petroleum (distillate) (products) NEC	981	E863.4	—	E950.6	E962.1	E980.7
specified ingredient NEC	989.4	E863.4	—	E950.6	E962.1	E980.7
strychnine	989.1	E863.4	—	E950.6	E962.1	E980.7
thallium	985.8	E863.7	—	E950.6	E962.1	E980.7
Pethidine (hydrochloride)	965.09	E850.2	E935.2	E950.0	E962.0	E980.0
Petrichloral	967.1	E852.0	E937.1	E950.2	E962.0	E980.2
Petrol	981	E862.1	—	E950.9	E962.1	E980.9
vapor	987.1	E869.8	—	E952.8	E962.2	E982.8
Petrolatum (jelly) (ointment)	976.3	E858.7	E946.3	E950.4	E962.0	E980.4
hydrophilic	976.3	E858.7	E946.3	E950.4	E962.0	E980.4
liquid	973.2	E858.4	E943.2	E950.4	E962.0	E980.4
topical	976.3	E858.7	E946.3	E950.4	E962.0	E980.4
nonmedicinal	981	E862.1	—	E950.9	E962.1	E980.9
Petroleum (cleaners) (fuels) (products) NEC	981	E862.1	—	E950.9	E962.1	E980.9
benzin(e) - see Ligroin	—	—	—	—	—	—
ether - see Ligroin	—	—	—	—	—	—
jelly - see Petrolatum	—	—	—	—	—	—
aphtha - see Ligroin	—	—	—	—	—	—
pesticide	981	E863.4	—	E950.6	E962.1	E980.7
solids	981	E862.3	—	E950.9	E962.1	E980.9
solvents	981	E862.0	—	E950.9	E962.1	E980.9
vapor	987.1	E869.8	—	E952.8	E962.2	E982.8
Peyote	969.6	E854.1	E939.6	E950.3	E962.0	E980.3
Phanodorm, phanodorn	967.0	E851	E937.0	E950.1	E962.0	E980.1
Phanquinone, phanquone	961.5	E857	E931.5	E950.4	E962.0	E980.4
Pharmaceutical excipient or adjunct	977.4	E858.8	E947.4	E950.4	E962.0	E980.4
Phenacemide	966.3	E855.0	E936.3	E950.4	E962.0	E980.4

◀ New ◀⦙⦙ Revised ~~deleted~~ Deleted ● Use Additional Digit(s)

Substance	Poisoning	External Cause (E Code)				
		Accident	Therapeutic Use	Suicide Attempt	Assault	Undetermined
Phenacetin	965.4	E850.4	E935.4	E950.0	E962.0	E980.0
Phenadoxone	965.09	E850.2	E935.2	E950.0	E962.0	E980.0
Phenaglycodol	969.5	E853.8	E939.5	E950.3	E962.0	E980.3
Phenantoin	966.1	E855.0	E936.1	E950.4	E962.0	E980.4
Phenaphthazine reagent	977.8	E858.8	E947.8	E950.4	E962.0	E980.4
Phenazocine	965.09	E850.2	E935.2	E950.0	E962.0	E980.0
Phenazone	965.5	E850.5	E935.5	E950.0	E962.0	E980.0
Phenazopyridine	976.1	E858.7	E946.1	E950.4	E962.0	E980.4
Phenbenicillin	960.0	E856	E930.0	E950.4	E962.0	E980.4
Phenbutrazate	977.0	E858.8	E947.0	E950.4	E962.0	E980.4
Phencyclidine	968.3	E855.1	E938.3	E950.4	E962.0	E980.4
Phendimetrazine	977.0	E858.8	E947.0	E950.4	E962.0	E980.4
Phenelzine	969.01 ◄ⅢⅢ	E854.0	E939.0	E950.3	E962.0	E980.3
Phenergan	967.8	E852.8	E937.8	E950.2	E962.0	E980.2
Phenethicillin (potassium)	960.0	E856	E930.0	E950.4	E962.0	E980.4
Phenetsal	965.1	E850.3	E935.3	E950.0	E962.0	E980.0
Pheneturide	966.3	E855.0	E936.3	E950.4	E962.0	E980.4
Phenformin	962.3	E858.0	E932.3	E950.4	E962.0	E980.4
Phenglutarimide	971.1	E855.4	E941.1	E950.4	E962.0	E980.4
Phenicarbazide	965.8	E850.8	E935.8	E950.0	E962.0	E980.0
Phenindamine (tartrate)	963.0	E858.1	E933.0	E950.4	E962.0	E980.4
Phenindione	964.2	E858.2	E934.2	E950.4	E962.0	E980.4
Pheniprazine	969.01 ◄ⅢⅢ	E854.0	E939.0	E950.3	E962.0	E980.3
Pheniramine (maleate)	963.0	E858.1	E933.0	E950.4	E962.0	E980.4
Phenmetrazine	977.0	E858.8	E947.0	E950.4	E962.0	E980.4
Phenobal	967.0	E851	E937.0	E950.1	E962.0	E980.1
Phenobarbital	967.0	E851	E937.0	E950.1	E962.0	E980.1
Phenobarbitone	967.0	E851	E937.0	E950.1	E962.0	E980.1
Phenoctide	976.0	E858.7	E946.0	E950.4	E962.0	E980.4
Phenol (derivatives) NEC	983.0	E864.0	—	E950.7	E962.1	E980.6
disinfectant	983.0	E864.0	—	E950.7	E962.1	E980.6
pesticide	989.4	E863.4	—	E950.6	E962.1	E980.7
red	977.8	E858.8	E947.8	E950.4	E962.0	E980.4
Phenolphthalein	973.1	E858.4	E943.1	E950.4	E962.0	E980.4
Phenolsulfonphthalein	977.8	E858.8	E947.8	E950.4	E962.0	E980.4
Phenomorphan	965.09	E850.2	E935.2	E950.0	E962.0	E980.0
Phenonyl	967.0	E851	E937.0	E950.1	E962.0	E980.1
Phenoperidine	965.09	E850.2	E935.2	E950.0	E962.0	E980.0
Phenoquin	974.7	E858.5	E944.7	E950.4	E962.0	E980.4

◄ New   ◄ⅢⅢ Revised   ~~deleted~~ Deleted   ● Use Additional Digit(s)

Substance	Poisoning	External Cause (E Code)				
		Accident	Therapeutic Use	Suicide Attempt	Assault	Undetermined
Phenothiazines (tranquilizers) NEC	969.1	E853.0	E939.1	E950.3	E962.0	E980.3
insecticide	989.3	E863.4	—	E950.6	E962.1	E980.7
Phenoxybenzamine	971.3	E855.6	E941.3	E950.4	E962.0	E980.4
Phenoxymethyl penicillin	960.0	E856	E930.0	E950.4	E962.0	E980.4
Phenprocoumon	964.2	E858.2	E934.2	E950.4	E962.0	E980.4
Phensuximide	966.2	E855.0	E936.2	E950.4	E962.0	E980.4
Phentermine	977.0	E858.8	E947.0	E950.4	E962.0	E980.4
Phentolamine	971.3	E855.6	E941.3	E950.4	E962.0	E980.4
Phenyl	—	—	—	—	—	—
butazone	965.5	E850.5	E935.5	E950.0	E962.0	E980.0
enediamine	983.0	E864.0	—	E950.7	E962.1	E980.6
hydrazine	983.0	E864.0	—	E950.7	E962.1	E980.6
antineoplastic	963.1	E858.1	E933.1	E950.4	E962.0	E980.4
mercuric compounds - *see* Mercury	—	—	—	—	—	—
salicylate	976.3	E858.7	E946.3	E950.4	E962.0	E980.4
Phenylephrine	971.2	E855.5	E941.2	E950.4	E962.0	E980.4
Phenylethylbiguanide	962.3	E858.0	E932.3	E950.4	E962.0	E980.4
Phenylpropanolamine	971.2	E855.5	E941.2	E950.4	E962.0	E980.4
Phenylsulfthion	989.3	E863.1	—	E950.6	E962.1	E980.7
Phenyramidol, phenyramidon	965.7	E850.7	E935.7	E950.0	E962.0	E980.0
Phenytoin	966.1	E855.0	E936.1	E950.4	E962.0	E980.4
pHisoHex	976.2	E858.7	E946.2	E950.4	E962.0	E980.4
Pholcodine	965.09	E850.2	E935.2	E950.0	E962.0	E980.0
Phorate	989.3	E863.1	—	E950.6	E962.1	E980.7
Phosdrin	989.3	E863.1	—	E950.6	E962.1	E980.7
Phosgene (gas)	987.8	E869.8	—	E952.8	E962.2	E982.8
Phosphate (tricresyl)	989.89	E866.8	—	E950.9	E962.1	E980.9
organic	989.3	E863.1	—	E950.6	E962.1	E980.7
solvent	982.8	E862.4	—	E950.9	E962.1	E980.9
Phosphine	987.8	E869.8	—	E952.8	E962.2	E982.8
fumigant	987.8	E863.8	—	E950.6	E962.2	E980.7
Phospholine	971.0	E855.3	E941.0	E950.4	E962.0	E980.4
Phosphoric acid	983.1	E864.1	—	E950.7	E962.1	E980.6
Phosphorus (compounds) NEC	983.9	E864.3	—	E950.7	E962.1	E980.6
rodenticide	983.9	E863.7	—	E950.7	E962.1	E980.6
Phthalimidoglutarimide	967.8	E852.8	E937.8	E950.2	E962.0	E980.2
Phthalylsulfathiazole	961.0	E857	E931.0	E950.4	E962.0	E980.4
Phylloquinone	964.3	E858.2	E934.3	E950.4	E962.0	E980.4
Physeptone	965.02	E850.1	E935.1	E950.0	E962.0	E980.0

◀ New   ◀║ Revised   ~~deleted~~ Deleted   ● Use Additional Digit(s)

Substance	Poisoning	External Cause (E Code)				
		Accident	Therapeutic Use	Suicide Attempt	Assault	Undetermined
Physostigma venenosum	988.2	E865.4	—	E950.9	E962.1	E980.9
Physostigmine	971.0	E855.3	E941.0	E950.4	E962.0	E980.4
Phytolacca decandra	988.2	E865.4	—	E950.9	E962.1	E980.9
Phytomenadione	964.3	E858.2	E934.3	E950.4	E962.0	E980.4
Phytonadione	964.3	E858.2	E934.3	E950.4	E962.0	E980.4
Picric (acid)	983.0	E864.0	—	E950.7	E962.1	E980.6
Picrotoxin	970.0	E854.3	E940.0	E950.4	E962.0	E980.4
Pilocarpine	971.0	E855.3	E941.0	E950.4	E962.0	E980.4
Pilocarpus (jaborandi) extract	971.0	E855.3	E941.0	E950.4	E962.0	E980.4
Pimaricin	960.1	E856	E930.1	E950.4	E962.0	E980.4
Piminodine	965.09	E850.2	E935.2	E950.0	E962.0	E980.0
Pine oil, pinesol (disinfectant)	983.9	E861.4	—	E950.7	E962.1	E980.6
Pinkroot	961.6	E857	E931.6	E950.4	E962.0	E980.4
Pipadone	965.09	E850.2	E935.2	E950.0	E962.0	E980.0
Pipamazine	963.0	E858.1	E933.0	E950.4	E962.0	E980.4
Pipazethate	975.4	E858.6	E945.4	E950.4	E962.0	E980.4
Pipenzolate	971.1	E855.4	E941.1	E950.4	E962.0	E980.4
Piperacetazine	969.1	E853.0	E939.1	E950.3	E962.0	E980.3
Piperazine NEC	961.6	E857	E931.6	E950.4	E962.0	E980.4
estrone sulfate	962.2	E858.0	E932.2	E950.4	E962.0	E980.4
Piper cubeba	988.2	E865.4	—	E950.9	E962.1	E980.9
Piperidione	975.4	E858.6	E945.4	E950.4	E962.0	E980.4
Piperidolate	971.1	E855.4	E941.1	E950.4	E962.0	E980.4
Piperocaine	968.9	E855.2	E938.9	E950.4	E962.0	E980.4
infiltration (subcutaneous)	968.5	E855.2	E938.5	E950.4	E962.0	E980.4
nerve block (peripheral) (plexus)	968.6	E855.2	E938.6	E950.4	E962.0	E980.4
topical (surface)	968.5	E855.2	E938.5	E950.4	E962.0	E980.4
Pipobroman	963.1	E858.1	E933.1	E950.4	E962.0	E980.4
Pipradrol	970.8	E854.3	E940.8	E950.4	E962.0	E980.4
Piscidia (bark) (erythrina)	965.7	E850.7	E935.7	E950.0	E962.0	E980.0
Pitch	983.0	E864.0	—	E950.7	E962.1	E980.6
Pitkin's solution	968.7	E855.2	E938.7	E950.4	E962.0	E980.4
Pitocin	975.0	E858.6	E945.0	E950.4	E962.0	E980.4
Pitressin (tannate)	962.5	E858.0	E932.5	E950.4	E962.0	E980.4
Pituitary extracts (posterior)	962.5	E858.0	E932.5	E950.4	E962.0	E980.4
anterior	962.4	E858.0	E932.4	E950.4	E962.0	E980.4
Pituitrin	962.5	E858.0	E932.5	E950.4	E962.0	E980.4
Placental extract	962.9	E858.0	E932.9	E950.4	E962.0	E980.4
Placidyl	967.8	E852.8	E937.8	E950.2	E962.0	E980.2

◀ New   ◀▥ Revised   ~~deleted~~ Deleted   ● Use Additional Digit(s)

Substance	Poisoning	External Cause (E Code) Accident	External Cause (E Code) Therapeutic Use	External Cause (E Code) Suicide Attempt	External Cause (E Code) Assault	External Cause (E Code) Undetermined
Plague vaccine	978.3	E858.8	E948.3	E950.4	E962.0	E980.4
Plant foods or fertilizers NEC	989.89	E866.5	—	E950.9	E962.1	E980.9
mixed with herbicides	989.4	E863.5	—	E950.6	E962.1	E930.7
Plants, noxious, used as food	988.2	E865.9	—	E950.9	E962.1	E980.9
berries and seeds	988.2	E865.3	—	E950.9	E962.1	E980.9
specified type NEC	988.2	E865.4	—	E950.9	E962.1	E980.9
Plasma (blood)	964.7	E858.2	E934.7	E950.4	E962.0	E980.4
expanders	964.8	E858.2	E934.8	E950.4	E962.0	E980.4
Plasmanate	964.7	E858.2	E934.7	E950.4	E962.0	E980.4
Plegicil	969.1	E853.0	E939.1	E950.3	E962.0	E980.3
Podophyllin	976.4	E858.7	E946.4	E950.4	E962.0	E980.4
Podophyllum resin	976.4	E858.7	E946.4	E950.4	E962.0	E980.4
Poison NEC	989.9	E866.9	—	E950.9	E962.1	E980.9
Poisonous berries	988.2	E865.3	—	E950.9	E962.1	E980.9
Pokeweed (any part)	988.2	E865.4	—	E950.9	E962.1	E980.9
Poldine	971.1	E855.4	E941.1	E950.4	E962.0	E980.4
Poliomyelitis vaccine	979.5	E858.8	E949.5	E950.4	E962.0	E980.4
Poliovirus vaccine	979.5	E858.8	E949.5	E950.4	E962.0	E980.4
Polish (car) (floor) (furniture) (metal) (silver)	989.89	E861.2	—	E950.9	E962.1	E980.9
abrasive	989.89	E861.3	—	E950.9	E962.1	E980.9
porcelain	989.89	E861.3	—	E950.9	E962.1	E980.9
Poloxalkol	973.2	E858.4	E943.2	E950.4	E962.0	E980.4
Polyaminostyrene resins	974.5	E858.5	E944.5	E950.4	E962.0	E980.4
Polychlorinated biphenyl - see PCBs	—	—	—	—	—	—
Polycycline	960.4	E856	E930.4	E950.4	E962.0	E980.4
Polyester resin hardener	982.8	E862.4	—	E950.9	E962.1	E980.9
fumes	987.8	E869.8	—	E952.8	E962.2	E982.8
Polyestradiol (phosphate)	962.2	E858.0	E932.2	E950.4	E962.0	E980.4
Polyethanolamine alkyl sulfate	976.2	E858.7	E946.2	E950.4	E962.0	E980.4
Polyethylene glycol	976.3	E858.7	E946.3	E950.4	E962.0	E980.4
Polyferose	964.0	E858.2	E934.0	E950.4	E962.0	E980.4
Polymyxin B	960.8	E856	E930.8	E950.4	E962.0	E980.4
ENT agent	976.6	E858.7	E946.6	E950.4	E962.0	E980.4
ophthalmic preparation	976.5	E858.7	E946.5	E950.4	E962.0	E980.4
topical NEC	976.0	E858.7	E946.0	E950.4	E962.0	E980.4
Polynoxylin(e)	976.0	E858.7	E946.0	E950.4	E962.0	E980.4
Polyoxymethyleneurea	976.0	E858.7	E946.0	E950.4	E962.0	E980.4
Polytetrafluoroethylene (inhaled)	987.8	E869.8	—	E952.8	E962.2	E982.8
Polythiazide	974.3	E858.5	E944.3	E950.4	E962.0	E980.4

◀ New   ◀▦ Revised   ~~deleted~~ Deleted   ● Use Additional Digit(s)

Substance	Poisoning	External Cause (E Code)				
		Accident	Therapeutic Use	Suicide Attempt	Assault	Undetermined
Polyvinylpyrrolidone	964.8	E858.2	E934.8	E950.4	E962.0	E980.4
Pontocaine (hydrochloride) (infiltration) (topical)	968.5	E855.2	E938.5	E950.4	E962.0	E980.4
nerve block (peripheral) (plexus)	968.6	E855.2	E938.6	E950.4	E962.0	E980.4
spinal	968.7	E855.2	E938.7	E950.4	E962.0	E980.4
Pot	969.6	E854.1	E939.6	E950.3	E962.0	E980.3
Potash (caustic)	983.2	E864.2	—	E950.7	E962.1	E980.6
Potassic saline injection (lactated)	974.5	E858.5	E944.5	E950.4	E962.0	E980.4
Potassium (salts) NEC	974.5	E858.5	E944.5	E950.4	E962.0	E980.4
aminosalicylate	961.8	E857	E931.8	E950.4	E962.0	E980.4
arsenite (solution)	985.1	E866.3	—	E950.8	E962.1	E980.8
bichromate	983.9	E864.3	—	E950.7	E962.1	E980.6
bisulfate	983.9	E864.3	—	E950.7	E962.1	E980.6
bromide (medicinal) NEC	967.3	E852.2	E937.3	E950.2	E962.0	E980.2
carbonate	983.2	E864.2	—	E950.7	E962.1	E980.6
chlorate NEC	983.9	E864.3	—	E950.7	E962.1	E980.6
cyanide - see Cyanide	—	—	—	—	—	—
hydroxide	983.2	E864.2	—	E950.7	E962.1	E980.6
iodide (expectorant) NEC	975.5	E858.6	E945.5	E950.4	E962.0	E980.4
nitrate	989.89	E866.8	—	E950.9	E962.1	E980.9
oxalate	983.9	E864.3	—	E950.7	E962.1	E980.6
perchlorate NEC	977.8	E858.8	E947.8	E950.4	E962.0	E980.4
antithyroid	962.8	E858.0	E932.8	E950.4	E962.0	E980.4
permanganate	976.0	E858.7	E946.0	E950.4	E962.0	E980.4
nonmedicinal	983.9	E864.3	—	E950.7	E962.1	E980.6
Povidone-iodine (anti-infective) NEC	976.0	E858.7	E946.0	E950.4	E962.0	E980.4
Practolol	972.0	E858.3	E942.0	E950.4	E962.0	E980.4
Pralidoxime (chloride)	977.2	E858.8	E947.2	E950.4	E962.0	E980.4
Pramoxine	968.5	E855.2	E938.5	E950.4	E962.0	E980.4
Prazosin	972.6	E858.3	E942.6	E950.4	E962.0	E980.4
Prednisolone	962.0	E858.0	E932.0	E950.4	E962.0	E980.4
ENT agent	976.6	E858.7	E946.6	E950.4	E962.0	E980.4
ophthalmic preparation	976.5	E858.7	E946.5	E950.4	E962.0	E980.4
topical NEC	976.0	E858.7	E946.0	E950.4	E962.0	E980.4
Prednisone	962.0	E858.0	E932.0	E950.4	E962.0	E980.4
Pregnanediol	962.2	E858.0	E932.2	E950.4	E962.0	E980.4
Pregneninolone	962.2	E858.0	E932.2	E950.4	E962.0	E980.4
Preludin	977.0	E858.8	E947.0	E950.4	E962.0	E980.4
Premarin	962.2	E858.0	E932.2	E950.4	E962.0	E980.4
Prenylamine	972.4	E858.3	E942.4	E950.4	E962.0	E980.4

TABLE OF DRUGS AND CHEMICALS

Substance	Poisoning	External Cause (E Code)				
		Accident	Therapeutic Use	Suicide Attempt	Assault	Undetermined
Preparation H	976.8	E858.7	E946.8	E950.4	E962.0	E980.4
Preservatives	989.89	E866.8	—	E950.9	E962.1	E980.9
Pride of China	988.2	E865.3	—	E950.9	E962.1	E980.9
Prilocaine	968.9	E855.2	E938.9	E950.4	E962.0	E980.4
infiltration (subcutaneous)	968.5	E855.2	E938.5	E950.4	E962.0	E980.4
nerve block (peripheral) (plexus)	968.6	E855.2	E938.6	E950.4	E962.0	E980.4
Primaquine	961.4	E857	E931.4	E950.4	E962.0	E980.4
Primidone	966.3	E855.0	E936.3	E950.4	E962.0	E980.4
Primula (veris)	988.2	E865.4	—	E950.9	E962.1	E980.9
Prinodol	965.09	E850.2	E935.2	E950.0	E962.0	E980.0
Priscol, Priscoline	971.3	E855.6	E941.3	E950.4	E962.0	E980.4
Privet	988.2	E865.4	—	E950.9	E962.1	E980.9
Privine	971.2	E855.5	E941.2	E950.4	E962.0	E980.4
Pro-Banthine	971.1	E855.4	E941.1	E950.4	E962.0	E980.4
Probarbital	967.0	E851	E937.0	E950.1	E962.0	E980.1
Probenecid	974.7	E858.5	E944.7	E950.4	E962.0	E980.4
Procainamide (hydrochloride)	972.0	E858.3	E942.0	E950.4	E962.0	E980.4
Procaine (hydrochloride) (infiltration) (topical)	968.5	E855.2	E938.5	E950.4	E962.0	E980.4
nerve block (periphreal) (plexus)	968.6	E855.2	E938.6	E950.4	E962.0	E980.4
penicillin G	960.0	E856	E930.0	E950.4	E962.0	E980.4
spinal	968.7	E855.2	E938.7	E950.4	E962.0	E980.4
Procalmidol	969.5	E853.8	E939.5	E950.3	E962.0	E980.3
Procarbazine	963.1	E858.1	E933.1	E950.4	E962.0	E980.4
Prochlorperazine	969.1	E853.0	E939.1	E950.3	E962.0	E980.3
Procyclidine	966.4	E855.0	E936.4	E950.4	E962.0	E980.4
Producer gas	986	E868.8	—	E952.1	E962.2	E982.1
Profenamine	966.4	E855.0	E936.4	E950.4	E962.0	E980.4
Profenil	975.1	E858.6	E945.1	E950.4	E962.0	E980.4
Progesterones	962.2	E858.0	E932.2	E950.4	E962.0	E980.4
Progestin	962.2	E858.0	E932.2	E950.4	E962.0	E980.4
Progestogens (with estrogens)	962.2	E858.0	E932.2	E950.4	E962.0	E980.4
Progestone	962.2	E858.0	E932.2	E950.4	E962.0	E980.4
Proguanil	961.4	E857	E931.4	E950.4	E962.0	E980.4
Prolactin	962.4	E858.0	E932.4	E950.4	E962.0	E980.4
Proloid	962.7	E858.0	E932.7	E950.4	E962.0	E980.4
Proluton	962.2	E858.0	E932.2	E950.4	E962.0	E980.4
Promacetin	961.8	E857	E931.8	E950.4	E962.0	E980.4
Promazine	969.1	E853.0	E939.1	E950.3	E962.0	E980.3
Promedrol	965.09	E850.2	E935.2	E950.0	E962.0	E980.0

◄ New   ◀‖‖ Revised   deleted Deleted   ● Use Additional Digit(s)

Substance	Poisoning	External Cause (E Code)				
		Accident	Therapeutic Use	Suicide Attempt	Assault	Undetermined
Promethazine	967.8	E852.8	E937.8	E950.2	E962.0	E980.2
Promine	961.8	E857	E931.8	E950.4	E962.0	E980.4
Pronestyl (hydrochloride)	972.0	E858.3	E942.0	E950.4	E962.0	E980.4
Pronetalol, pronethalol	972.0	E858.3	E942.0	E950.4	E962.0	E980.4
Prontosil	961.0	E857	E931.0	E950.4	E962.0	E980.4
Propamidine isethionate	961.5	E857	E931.5	E950.4	E962.0	E980.4
Propanal (medicinal)	967.8	E852.8	E937.8	E950.2	E962.0	E980.2
Propane (gas) (distributed in mobile container)	987.0	E868.0	—	E951.1	E962.2	E981.1
distributed through pipes	987.0	E867	—	E951.0	E962.2	E981.0
incomplete combustion of - *see* Carbon monoxide, Propane	—	—	—	—	—	—
Propanidid	968.3	E855.1	E938.3	E950.4	E962.0	E980.4
Propanol	980.3	E860.4	—	E950.9	E962.1	E980.9
Propantheline	971.1	E855.4	E941.1	E950.4	E962.0	E980.4
Proparacaine	968.5	E855.2	E938.5	E950.4	E962.0	E980.4
Propatyl nitrate	972.4	E858.3	E942.4	E950.4	E962.0	E980.4
Propicillin	960.0	E856	E930.0	E950.4	E962.0	E980.4
Propiolactone (vapor)	987.8	E869.8	—	E952.8	E962.2	E982.8
Propiomazine	967.8	E852.8	E937.8	E950.2	E962.0	E980.2
Propionaldehyde (medicinal)	967.8	E852.8	E937.8	E950.2	E962.0	E980.2
Propionate compound	976.0	E858.7	E946.0	E950.4	E962.0	E980.4
Propion gel	976.0	E858.7	E946.0	E950.4	E962.0	E980.4
Propitocaine	968.9	E855.2	E938.9	E950.4	E962.0	E980.4
infiltration (subcutaneous)	968.5	E855.2	E938.5	E950.4	E962.0	E980.4
nerve block (peripheral) (plexus)	968.6	E855.2	E938.6	E950.4	E962.0	E980.4
Propoxur	989.3	E863.2	—	E950.6	E962.1	E980.7
Propoxycaine	968.9	E855.2	E938.9	E950.4	E962.0	E980.4
infiltration (subcutaneous)	968.5	E855.2	E938.5	E950.4	E962.0	E980.4
nerve block (peripheral) (plexus)	968.6	E855.2	E938.6	E950.4	E962.0	E980.4
topical (surface)	968.5	E855.2	E938.5	E950.4	E962.0	E980.4
Propoxyphene (hydrochloride)	965.8	E850.8	E935.8	E950.0	E962.0	E980.0
Propranolol	972.0	E858.3	E942.0	E950.4	E962.0	E980.4
Propyl	—	—	—	—	—	—
alcohol	980.3	E860.4	—	E950.9	E962.1	E980.9
carbinol	980.3	E860.4	—	E950.9	E962.1	E980.9
hexadrine	971.2	E855.5	E941.2	E950.4	E962.0	E980.4
iodone	977.8	E858.8	E947.8	E950.4	E962.0	E980.4
thiouracil	962.8	E858.0	E932.8	E950.4	E962.0	E980.4
Propylene	987.1	E869.8	—	E952.8	E962.2	E982.8
Propylparaben (ophthalmic)	976.5	E858.7	E946.5	E950.4	E962.0	E980.4

◀ New   ◀▥ Revised   ~~deleted~~ Deleted   ● Use Additional Digit(s)

Substance	Poisoning	External Cause (E Code)				
		Accident	Therapeutic Use	Suicide Attempt	Assault	Undetermined
Proscillaridin	972.1	E858.3	E942.1	E950.4	E962.0	E980.4
Prostaglandins	975.0	E858.6	E945.0	E950.4	E962.0	E980.4
Prostigmin	971.0	E855.3	E941.0	E950.4	E962.0	E980.4
Protamine (sulfate)	964.5	E858.2	E934.5	E950.4	E962.0	E980.4
zinc insulin	962.3	E858.0	E932.3	E950.4	E962.0	E980.4
Protectants (topical)	976.3	E858.7	E946.3	E950.4	E962.0	E980.4
Protein hydrolysate	974.5	E858.5	E944.5	E950.4	E962.0	E980.4
Prothiaden - see Dothiepin hydrochloride	—	—	—	—	—	—
Prothionamide	961.8	E857	E931.8	E950.4	E962.0	E980.4
Prothipendyl	969.5	E853.8	E939.5	E950.3	E962.0	E980.3
Protokylol	971.2	E855.5	E941.2	E950.4	E962.0	E980.4
Protopam	977.2	E858.8	E947.2	E950.4	E962.0	E980.4
Protoveratrine(s) (A) (B)	972.6	E858.3	E942.6	E950.4	E962.0	E980.4
Protriptyline	969.05 ◀▥	E854.0	E939.0	E950.3	E962.0	E980.3
Provera	962.2	E858.0	E932.2	E950.4	E962.0	E980.4
Provitamin A	963.5	E858.1	E933.5	E950.4	E962.0	E980.4
Proxymetacaine	968.5	E855.2	E938.5	E950.4	E962.0	E980.4
Proxyphylline	975.1	E858.6	E945.1	E950.4	E962.0	E980.4
Prozac - see Fluoxetine hydrochloride	—	—	—	—	—	—
Prunus	—	—	—	—	—	—
laurocerasus	988.2	E865.4	—	E950.9	E962.1	E980.9
virginiana	988.2	E865.4	—	E950.9	E962.1	E980.9
Prussic acid	989.0	E866.8	—	E950.9	E962.1	E980.9
vapor	987.7	E869.8	—	E952.8	E962.2	E982.8
Pseudoephedrine	971.2	E855.5	E941.2	E950.4	E962.0	E980.4
Psilocin	969.6	E854.1	E939.6	E950.3	E962.0	E980.3
Psilocybin	969.6	E854.1	E939.6	E950.3	E962.0	E980.3
PSP	977.8	E858.8	E947.8	E950.4	E962.0	E980.4
Psychedelic agents	969.6	E854.1	E939.6	E950.3	E962.0	E980.3
Psychodysleptics	969.6	E854.1	E939.6	E950.3	E962.0	E980.3
Psychostimulants	969.70 ◀▥	E854.2	E939.7	E950.3	E962.0	E980.3
Psychotherapeutic agents	969.9	E855.9	E939.9	E950.3	E962.0	E980.3
antidepressants	969.00 ◀▥	E854.0	E939.0	E950.3	E962.0	E980.3
specified NEC	969.8	E855.8	E939.8	E950.3	E962.0	E980.3
tranquilizers NEC	969.5	E853.9	E939.5	E950.3	E962.0	E980.3
Psychotomimetic agents	969.6	E854.1	E939.6	E950.3	E962.0	E980.3
Psychotropic agents	969.9	E854.8	E939.9	E950.3	E962.0	E980.3
specified NEC	969.8	E854.8	E939.8	E950.3	E962.0	E980.3
Psyllium	973.3	E858.4	E943.3	E950.4	E962.0	E980.4

◀ New   ◀▥ Revised   ~~deleted~~ Deleted   ● Use Additional Digit(s)

Substance	Poisoning	External Cause (E Code)				
		Accident	Therapeutic Use	Suicide Attempt	Assault	Undetermined
Pteroylglutamic acid	964.1	E858.2	E934.1	E950.4	E962.0	E980.4
Pteroyltriglutamate	963.1	E858.1	E933.1	E950.4	E962.0	E980.4
PTFE	987.8	E869.8	—	E952.8	E962.2	E982.8
Pulsatilla	988.2	E865.4	—	E950.9	E962.1	E980.9
Purex (bleach)	983.9	E864.3	—	E950.7	E962.1	E980.6
Purine diuretics	974.1	E858.5	E944.1	E950.4	E962.0	E980.4
Purinethol	963.1	E858.1	E933.1	E950.4	E962.0	E980.4
PVP	964.8	E858.2	E934.8	E950.4	E962.0	E980.4
Pyrabital	965.7	E850.7	E935.7	E950.0	E962.0	E980.0
Pyramidon	965.5	E850.5	E935.5	E950.0	E962.0	E980.0
Pyrantel (pamoate)	961.6	E857	E931.6	E950.4	E962.0	E980.4
Pyrathiazine	963.0	E858.1	E933.0	E950.4	E962.0	E980.4
Pyrazinamide	961.8	E857	E931.8	E950.4	E962.0	E980.4
Pyrazinoic acid (amide)	961.8	E857	E931.8	E950.4	E962.0	E980.4
Pyrazole (derivatives)	965.5	E850.5	E935.5	E950.0	E962.0	E980.0
Pyrazolone (analgesics)	965.5	E850.5	E935.5	E950.0	E962.0	E980.0
Pyrethrins, pyrethrum	989.4	E863.4	—	E950.6	E962.1	E980.7
Pyribenzamine	963.0	E858.1	E933.0	E950.4	E962.0	E980.4
Pyridine (liquid) (vapor)	982.0	E862.4	—	E950.9	E962.1	E980.9
aldoxime chloride	977.2	E858.8	E947.2	E950.4	E962.0	E980.4
Pyridium	976.1	E858.7	E946.1	E950.4	E962.0	E980.4
Pyridostigmine	971.0	E855.3	E941.0	E950.4	E962.0	E980.4
Pyridoxine	963.5	E858.1	E933.5	E950.4	E962.0	E980.4
Pyrilamine	963.0	E858.1	E933.0	E950.4	E962.0	E980.4
Pyrimethamine	961.4	E857	E931.4	E950.4	E962.0	E980.4
Pyrogallic acid	983.0	E864.0	—	E950.7	E962.1	E980.6
Pyroxylin	976.3	E858.7	E946.3	E950.4	E962.0	E980.4
Pyrrobutamine	963.0	E858.1	E933.0	E950.4	E962.0	E980.4
Pyrrocitine	968.5	E855.2	E938.5	E950.4	E962.0	E980.4
Pyrvinium (pamoate)	961.6	E857	E931.6	E950.4	E962.0	E980.4
PZI	962.3	E858.0	E932.3	E950.4	E962.0	E980.4
Quaalude	967.4	E852.3	E937.4	E950.2	E962.0	E980.2
Quaternary ammonium derivatives	971.1	E855.4	E941.1	E950.4	E962.0	E980.4
Quicklime	983.2	E864.2	—	E950.7	E962.1	E980.6
Quinacrine	961.3	E857	E931.3	E950.4	E962.0	E980.4
Quinaglute	972.0	E858.3	E942.0	E950.4	E962.0	E980.4
Quinalbarbitone	967.0	E851	E937.0	E950.1	E962.0	E980.1
Quinestradiol	962.2	E858.0	E932.2	E950.4	E962.0	E980.4
Quinethazone	974.3	E858.5	E944.3	E950.4	E962.0	E980.4

TABLE OF DRUGS AND CHEMICALS

Substance	Poisoning	External Cause (E Code)				
		Accident	Therapeutic Use	Suicide Attempt	Assault	Undetermined
Quinidine (gluconate) (polygalacturonate) (salts) (sulfate)	972.0	E858.3	E942.0	E950.4	E962.0	E980.4
Quinine	961.4	E857	E931.4	E950.4	E962.0	E980.4
Quiniobine	961.3	E857	E931.3	E950.4	E962.0	E980.4
Quinolines	961.3	E857	E931.3	E950.4	E962.0	E980.4
Quotane	968.5	E855.2	E938.5	E950.4	E962.0	E980.4
Rabies	—	—	—	—	—	—
immune globulin (human)	964.6	E858.2	E934.6	E950.4	E962.0	E980.4
vaccine	979.1	E858.8	E949.1	E950.4	E962.0	E980.4
Racemoramide	965.09	E850.2	E935.2	E950.0	E962.0	E980.0
Racemorphan	965.09	E850.2	E935.2	E950.0	E962.0	E980.0
Radiator alcohol	980.1	E860.2	—	E950.9	E962.1	E980.9
Radio-opaque (drugs) (materials)	977.8	E858.8	E947.8	E950.4	E962.0	E980.4
Ranunculus	988.2	E865.4	—	E950.9	E962.1	E980.9
Rat poison	989.4	E863.7	—	E950.6	E962.1	E980.7
Rattlesnake (venom)	989.5	E905.0	—	E950.9	E962.1	E980.9
Raudixin	972.6	E858.3	E942.6	E950.4	E962.0	E980.4
Rautensin	972.6	E858.3	E942.6	E950.4	E962.0	E980.4
Rautina	972.6	E858.3	E942.6	E950.4	E962.0	E980.4
Rautotal	972.6	E858.3	E942.6	E950.4	E962.0	E980.4
Rauwiloid	972.6	E858.3	E942.6	E950.4	E962.0	E980.4
Rauwoldin	972.6	E858.3	E942.6	E950.4	E962.0	E980.4
Rauwolfia (alkaloids)	972.6	E858.3	E942.6	E950.4	E962.0	E980.4
Realgar	985.1	E866.3	—	E950.8	E962.1	E980.8
Red cells, packed	964.7	E858.2	E934.7	E950.4	E962.0	E980.4
Reducing agents, industrial NEC	983.9	E864.3	—	E950.7	E962.1	E980.6
Refrigerant gas (freon)	987.4	E869.2	—	E952.8	E962.2	E982.8
not freon	987.9	E869.9	—	E952.9	E962.2	E982.9
Regroton	974.4	E858.5	E944.4	E950.4	E962.0	E980.4
Rela	968.0	E855.1	E938.0	E950.4	E962.0	E980.4
Relaxants, skeletal muscle (autonomic)	975.2	E858.6	E945.2	E950.4	E962.0	E980.4
central nervous system	968.0	E855.1	E938.0	E950.4	E962.0	E980.4
Renese	974.3	E858.5	E944.3	E950.4	E962.0	E980.4
Renografin	977.8	E858.8	E947.8	E950.4	E962.0	E980.4
Replacement solutions	974.5	E858.5	E944.5	E950.4	E962.0	E980.4
Rescinnamine	972.6	E858.3	E942.6	E950.4	E962.0	E980.4
Reserpine	972.6	E858.3	E942.6	E950.4	E962.0	E980.4
Resorcin, resorcinol	976.4	E858.7	E946.4	E950.4	E962.0	E980.4
Respaire	975.5	E858.6	E945.5	E950.4	E962.0	E980.4
Respiratory agents NEC	975.8	E858.6	E945.8	E950.4	E962.0	E980.4

◀ New   ◀▥ Revised   ~~deleted~~ Deleted   ● Use Additional Digit(s)

Substance	Poisoning	External Cause (E Code)				
		Accident	Therapeutic Use	Suicide Attempt	Assault	Undetermined
Retinoic acid	976.8	E858.7	E946.8	E950.4	E962.0	E980.4
Retinol	963.5	E858.1	E933.5	E950.4	E962.0	E980.4
Rh (D) immune globulin (human)	964.6	E858.2	E934.6	E950.4	E962.0	E980.4
Rhodine	965.1	E850.3	E935.3	E950.0	E962.0	E980.0
RhoGAM	964.6	E858.2	E934.6	E950.4	E962.0	E980.4
Riboflavin	963.5	E858.1	E933.5	E950.4	E962.0	E980.4
Ricin	989.89	E866.8	—	E950.9	E962.1	E980.9
Ricinus communis	988.2	E865.3	—	E950.9	E962.1	E980.9
Rickettsial vaccine NEC	979.6	E858.8	E949.6	E950.4	E962.0	E980.4
with viral and bacterial vaccine	979.7	E858.8	E949.7	E950.4	E962.0	E980.4
Rifampin	960.6	E856	E930.6	E950.4	E962.0	E980.4
Rimifon	961.8	E857	E931.8	E950.4	E962.0	E980.4
Ringer's injection (lactated)	974.5	E858.5	E944.5	E950.4	E962.0	E980.4
Ristocetin	960.8	E856	E930.8	E950.4	E962.0	E980.4
Ritalin	969.73 ◀▥	E854.2	E939.7	E950.3	E962.0	E980.3
Roach killers - see Pesticides	—	—	—	—	—	—
Rocky Mountain spotted fever vaccine	979.6	E858.8	E949.6	E950.4	E962.0	E980.4
Rodenticides	989.4	E863.7	—	E950.6	E962.1	E980.7
Rohypnol	969.4	E853.2	E939.4	E950.3	E962.0	E980.3
Rolaids	973.0	E858.4	E943.0	E950.4	E962.0	E980.4
Rolitetracycline	960.4	E856	E930.4	E950.4	E962.0	E980.4
Romilar	975.4	E858.6	E945.4	E950.4	E962.0	E980.4
Rose water ointment	976.3	E858.7	E946.3	E950.4	E962.0	E980.4
Rotenone	989.4	E863.7	—	E950.6	E962.1	E980.7
Rotoxamine	963.0	E858.1	E933.0	E950.4	E962.0	E980.4
Rough-on-rats	989.4	E863.7	—	E950.6	E962.1	E980.7
RU486	962.9	E858.0	E932.9	E950.4	E962.0	E980.4
Rubbing alcohol	980.2	E860.3	—	E950.9	E962.1	E980.9
Rubella virus vaccine	979.4	E858.8	E949.4	E950.4	E962.0	E980.4
Rubelogen	979.4	E858.8	E949.4	E950.4	E962.0	E980.4
Rubeovax	979.4	E858.8	E949.4	E950.4	E962.0	E980.4
Rubidomycin	960.7	E856	E930.7	E950.4	E962.0	E980.4
Rue	988.2	E865.4	—	E950.9	E962.1	E980.9
Ruta	988.2	E865.4	—	E950.9	E962.1	E980.9
Sabadilla (medicinal)	976.0	E858.7	E946.0	E950.4	E962.0	E980.4
pesticide	989.4	E863.4	—	E950.6	E962.1	E980.7
Sabin oral vaccine	979.5	E858.8	E949.5	E950.4	E962.0	E980.4
Saccharated iron oxide	964.0	E858.2	E934.0	E950.4	E962.0	E980.4
Saccharin	974.5	E858.5	E944.5	E950.4	E962.0	E980.4

Substance	Poisoning	External Cause (E Code)				
		Accident	Therapeutic Use	Suicide Attempt	Assault	Undetermined
Safflower oil	972.2	E858.3	E942.2	E950.4	E962.0	E980.4
Salbutamol sulfate	975.7	E858.6	E945.7	E950.4	E962.0	E980.4
Salicylamide	965.1	E850.3	E935.3	E950.0	E962.0	E980.0
Salicylate(s)	965.1	E850.3	E935.3	E950.0	E962.0	E980.0
methyl	976.3	E858.7	E946.3	E950.4	E962.0	E980.4
theobromine calcium	974.1	E858.5	E944.1	E950.4	E962.0	E980.4
Salicylazosulfapyridine	961.0	E857	E931.0	E950.4	E962.0	E980.4
Salicylhydroxamic acid	976.0	E858.7	E946.0	E950.4	E962.0	E980.4
Salicylic acid (keratolytic) NEC	976.4	E858.7	E946.4	E950.4	E962.0	E980.4
congeners	965.1	E850.3	E935.3	E950.0	E962.0	E980.0
salts	965.1	E850.3	E935.3	E950.0	E962.0	E980.0
Saliniazid	961.8	E857	E931.8	E950.4	E962.0	E980.4
Salol	976.3	E858.7	E946.3	E950.4	E962.0	E980.4
Salt (substitute) NEC	974.5	E858.5	E944.5	E950.4	E962.0	E980.4
Saluretics	974.3	E858.5	E944.3	E950.4	E962.0	E980.4
Saluron	974.3	E858.5	E944.3	E950.4	E962.0	E980.4
Salvarsan 606 (neosilver) (silver)	961.1	E857	E931.1	E950.4	E962.0	E980.4
Sambucus canadensis	988.2	E865.4	—	E950.9	E962.1	E980.9
berry	988.2	E865.3	—	E950.9	E962.1	E980.9
Sandril	972.6	E858.3	E942.6	E950.4	E962.0	E980.4
Sanguinaria canadensis	988.2	E865.4	—	E950.9	E962.1	E980.9
Saniflush (cleaner)	983.9	E861.3	—	E950.7	E962.1	E980.6
Santonin	961.6	E857	E931.6	E950.4	E962.0	E980.4
Santyl	976.8	E858.7	E946.8	E950.4	E962.0	E980.4
Sarkomycin	960.7	E856	E930.7	E950.4	E962.0	E980.4
Saroten	969.05 ◀	E854.0	E939.0	E950.3	E962.0	E980.3
Saturnine - *see* Lead	—	—	—	—	—	—
Savin (oil)	976.4	E858.7	E946.4	E950.4	E962.0	E980.4
Scammony	973.1	E858.4	E943.1	E950.4	E962.0	E980.4
Scarlet red	976.8	E858.7	E946.8	E950.4	E962.0	E980.4
Scheele's green	985.1	E866.3	—	E950.8	E962.1	E980.8
insecticide	985.1	E863.4	—	E950.8	E962.1	E980.8
Schradan	989.3	E863.1	—	E950.6	E962.1	E980.7
Schweinfurt(h) green	985.1	E866.3	—	E950.8	E962.1	E980.8
insecticide	985.1	E863.4	—	E950.8	E962.1	E980.8
Scilla - *see* Squill	—	—	—	—	—	—
Sclerosing agents	972.7	E858.3	E942.7	E950.4	E962.0	E980.4
Scopolamine	971.1	E855.4	E941.1	E950.4	E962.0	E980.4
Scouring powder	989.89	E861.3	—	E950.9	E962.1	E980.9

◀ New   ◀▥ Revised   ~~deleted~~ Deleted   ● Use Additional Digit(s)

Substance	Poisoning	External Cause (E Code)				
		Accident	Therapeutic Use	Suicide Attempt	Assault	Undetermined
Sea	—	—	—	—	—	—
anemone (sting)	989.5	E905.6	—	E950.9	E962.1	E980.9
cucumber (sting)	989.5	E905.6	—	E950.9	E962.1	E980.9
snake (bite) (venom)	989.5	E905.0	—	E950.9	E962.1	E980.9
urchin spine (puncture)	989.5	E905.6	—	E950.9	E962.1	E980.9
Secbutabarbital	967.0	E851	E937.0	E950.1	E962.0	E980.1
Secbutabarbitone	967.0	E851	E937.0	E950.1	E962.0	E980.1
Secobarbital	967.0	E851	E937.0	E950.1	E962.0	E980.1
Seconal	967.0	E851	E937.0	E950.1	E962.0	E980.1
Secretin	977.8	E858.8	E947.8	E950.4	E962.0	E980.4
Sedatives, nonbarbiturate	967.9	E852.9	E937.9	E950.2	E962.0	E980.2
specified NEC	967.8	E852.8	E937.8	E950.2	E962.0	E980.2
Sedormid	967.8	E852.8	E937.8	E950.2	E962.0	E980.2
Seed (plant)	988.2	E865.3	—	E950.9	E962.1	E980.9
disinfectant or dressing	989.89	E866.5	—	E950.9	E962.1	E980.9
Selective serotonin and norepinephrine reuptake inhibitors (SSNRI)	969.02	E854.0	E939.0	E950.3	E962.0	E980.3 ◄
Selective serotonin reuptake inhibitors (SSRI)	969.03	E854.0	E939.0	E950.3	E962.0	E980.3 ◄
Selenium (fumes) NEC	985.8	E866.4	—	E950.9	E962.1	E980.9
disulfide or sulfide	976.4	E858.7	E946.4	E950.4	E962.0	E980.4
Selsun	976.4	E858.7	E946.4	E950.4	E962.0	E980.4
Senna	973.1	E858.4	E943.1	E950.4	E962.0	E980.4
Septisol	976.2	E858.7	E946.2	E950.4	E962.0	E980.4
Serax	969.4	E853.2	E939.4	E950.3	E962.0	E980.3
Serenesil	967.8	E852.8	E937.8	E950.2	E962.0	E980.2
Serenium (hydrochloride)	961.9	E857	E931.9	E950.4	E962.0	E980.4
Serepax - see Oxazepam	—	—	—	—	—	—
Sernyl	968.3	E855.1	E938.3	E950.4	E962.0	E980.4
Serotonin	977.8	E858.8	E947.8	E950.4	E962.0	E980.4
Serpasil	972.6	E858.3	E942.6	E950.4	E962.0	E980.4
Sewer gas	987.8	E869.8	—	E952.8	E962.2	E982.8
Shampoo	989.6	E861.0	—	E950.9	E962.1	E980.9
Shellfish, nonbacterial or noxious	988.0	E865.1	—	E950.9	E962.1	E980.9
Silicones NEC	989.83	E866.8	E947.8	E950.9	E962.1	E980.9
Silvadene	976.0	E858.7	E946.0	E950.4	E962.0	E980.4
Silver (compound) (medicinal) NEC	976.0	E858.7	E946.0	E950.4	E962.0	E980.4
anti-infectives	976.0	E858.7	E946.0	E950.4	E962.0	E980.4
arsphenamine	961.1	E857	E931.1	E950.4	E962.0	E980.4
nitrate	976.0	E858.7	E946.0	E950.4	E962.0	E980.4
ophthalmic preparation	976.5	E858.7	E946.5	E950.4	E962.0	E980.4
toughened (keratolytic)	976.4	E858.7	E946.4	E950.4	E962.0	E980.4

◄ New   ◀▥ Revised   ~~deleted~~ Deleted   ● Use Additional Digit(s)

		External Cause (E Code)				
Substance	Poisoning	Accident	Therapeutic Use	Suicide Attempt	Assault	Undetermined
Silver (compound) (medicinal) NEC *(Continued)*						
nonmedicinal (dust)	985.8	E866.4	—	E950.9	E962.1	E980.9
protein (mild) (strong)	976.0	E858.7	E946.0	E950.4	E962.0	E980.4
salvarsan	961.1	E857	E931.1	E950.4	E962.0	E980.4
Simethicone	973.8	E858.4	E943.8	E950.4	E962.0	E980.4
Sinequan	969.05 ◀	E854.0	E939.0	E950.3	E962.0	E980.3
Singoserp	972.6	E858.3	E942.6	E950.4	E962.0	E980.4
Sintrom	964.2	E858.2	E934.2	E950.4	E962.0	E980.4
Sitosterols	972.2	E858.3	E942.2	E950.4	E962.0	E980.4
Skeletal muscle relaxants	975.2	E858.6	E945.2	E950.4	E962.0	E980.4
Skin	—	—	—	—	—	—
agents (external)	976.9	E858.7	E946.9	E950.4	E962.0	E980.4
specified NEC	976.8	E858.7	E946.8	E950.4	E962.0	E980.4
test antigen	977.8	E858.8	E947.8	E950.4	E962.0	E980.4
Sleep-eze	963.0	E858.1	E933.0	E950.4	E962.0	E980.4
Sleeping draught (drug) (pill) (tablet)	967.9	E852.9	E937.9	E950.2	E962.0	E980.2
Smallpox vaccine	979.0	E858.8	E949.0	E950.4	E962.0	E980.4
Smelter fumes NEC	985.9	E866.4	—	E950.9	E962.1	E980.9
Smog	987.3	E869.1	—	E952.8	E962.2	E982.8
Smoke NEC	987.9	E869.9	—	E952.9	E962.2	E982.9
Smooth muscle relaxant	975.1	E858.6	E945.1	E950.4	E962.0	E980.4
Snail killer	989.4	E863.4	—	E950.6	E962.1	E980.7
Snake (bite) (venom)	989.5	E905.0	—	E950.9	E962.1	E980.9
Snuff	989.89	E866.8	—	E950.9	E962.1	E980.9
Soap (powder) (product)	989.6	E861.1	—	E950.9	E962.1	E980.9
medicinal, soft	976.2	E858.7	E946.2	E950.4	E962.0	E980.4
Soda (caustic)	983.2	E864.2	—	E950.7	E962.1	E980.6
bicarb	963.3	E858.1	E933.3	E950.4	E962.0	E980.4
chlorinated - *see* Sodium, hypochlorite	—	—	—	—	—	—
Sodium	—	—	—	—	—	—
acetosulfone	961.8	E857	E931.8	E950.4	E962.0	E980.4
acetrizoate	977.8	E858.8	E947.8	E950.4	E962.0	E980.4
amytal	967.0	E851	E937.0	E950.1	E962.0	E980.1
arsenate - *see* Arsenic	—	—	—	—	—	—
bicarbonate	963.3	E858.1	E933.3	E950.4	E962.0	E980.4
bichromate	983.9	E864.3	—	E950.7	E962.1	E980.6
biphosphate	963.2	E858.1	E933.2	E950.4	E962.0	E980.4
bisulfate	983.9	E864.3	—	E950.7	E962.1	E980.6
borate (cleanser)	989.6	E861.3	—	E950.9	E962.1	E980.9
bromide NEC	967.3	E852.2	E937.3	E950.2	E962.0	E980.2

◀ New   ◀▬ Revised   ~~deleted~~ Deleted   ● Use Additional Digit(s)

Substance	Poisoning	External Cause (E Code)				
		Accident	Therapeutic Use	Suicide Attempt	Assault	Undetermined
Sodium *(Continued)*						
cacodylate (nonmedicinal) NEC	978.8	E858.8	E948.8	E950.4	E962.0	E980.4
anti-infective	961.1	E857	E931.1	E950.4	E962.0	E980.4
herbicide	989.4	E863.5	—	E950.6	E962.1	E980.7
calcium edetate	963.8	E858.1	E933.8	E950.4	E962.0	E980.4
carbonate NEC	983.2	E864.2	—	E950.7	E962.1	E980.6
chlorate NEC	983.9	E864.3	—	E950.7	E962.1	E980.6
herbicide	983.9	E863.5	—	E950.7	E962.1	E980.6
chloride NEC	974.5	E858.5	E944.5	E950.4	E962.0	E980.4
chromate	983.9	E864.3	—	E950.7	E962.1	E980.6
citrate	963.3	E858.1	E933.3	E950.4	E962.0	E980.4
cyanide - *see* Cyanide(s)	—	—	—	—	—	—
cyclamate	974.5	E858.5	E944.5	E950.4	E962.0	E980.4
diatrizoate	977.8	E858.8	E947.8	E950.4	E962.0	E980.4
dibunate	975.4	E858.6	E945.4	E950.4	E962.0	E980.4
dioctyl sulfosuccinate	973.2	E858.4	E943.2	E950.4	E962.0	E980.4
edetate	963.8	E858.1	E933.8	E950.4	E962.0	E980.4
ethacrynate	974.4	E858.5	E944.4	E950.4	E962.0	E980.4
fluoracetate (dust) (rodenticide)	989.4	E863.7	—	E950.6	E962.1	E980.7
fluoride - *see* Fluoride(s)	—	—	—	—	—	—
free salt	974.5	E858.5	E944.5	E950.4	E962.0	E980.4
glucosulfone	961.8	E857	E931.8	E950.4	E962.0	E980.4
hydroxide	983.2	E864.2	—	E950.7	E962.1	E980.6
hypochlorite (bleach) NEC	983.9	E864.3	—	E950.7	E962.1	E980.6
disinfectant	983.9	E861.4	—	E950.7	E962.1	E980.6
medicinal (anti-infective) (external)	976.0	E858.7	E946.0	E950.4	E962.0	E980.4
vapor	987.8	E869.8	—	E952.8	E962.2	E982.8
hyposulfite	976.0	E858.7	E946.0	E950.4	E962.0	E980.4
indigotindisulfonate	977.8	E858.8	E947.8	E950.4	E962.0	E980.4
iodide	977.8	E858.8	E947.8	E950.4	E962.0	E980.4
iothalamate	977.8	E858.8	E947.8	E950.4	E962.0	E980.4
iron edetate	964.0	E858.2	E934.0	E950.4	E962.0	E980.4
lactate	963.3	E858.1	E933.3	E950.4	E962.0	E980.4
lauryl sulfate	976.2	E858.7	E946.2	E950.4	E962.0	E980.4
L-triiodothyronine	962.7	E858.0	E932.7	E950.4	E962.0	E980.4
metrizoate	977.8	E858.8	E947.8	E950.4	E962.0	E980.4
monofluoracetate (dust) (rodenticide)	989.4	E863.7	—	E950.6	E962.1	E980.7
morrhuate	972.7	E858.3	E942.7	E950.4	E962.0	E980.4
nafcillin	960.0	E856	E930.0	E950.4	E962.0	E980.4

◀ New ◀▥ Revised ~~deleted~~ Deleted ⬤ Use Additional Digit(s)

Substance	Poisoning	External Cause (E Code)				
		Accident	Therapeutic Use	Suicide Attempt	Assault	Undetermined
Sodium *(Continued)*						
nitrate (oxidizing agent)	983.9	E864.3	—	E950.7	E962.1	E980.6
nitrite (medicinal)	972.4	E858.3	E942.4	E950.4	E962.0	E980.4
nitroferricyanide	972.6	E858.3	E942.6	E950.4	E962.0	E980.4
nitroprusside	972.6	E858.3	E942.6	E950.4	E962.0	E980.4
para-aminohippurate	977.8	E858.8	E947.8	E950.4	E962.0	E980.4
perborate (nonmedicinal) NEC	989.89	E866.8	—	E950.9	E962.1	E980.9
medicinal	976.6	E858.7	E946.6	E950.4	E962.0	E980.4
soap	989.6	E861.1	—	E950.9	E962.1	E980.9
percarbonate - *see* Sodium, perborate	—	—	—	—	—	—
phosphate	973.3	E858.4	E943.3	E950.4	E962.0	E980.4
polystyrene sulfonate	974.5	E858.5	E944.5	E950.4	E962.0	E980.4
propionate	976.0	E858.7	E946.0	E950.4	E962.0	E980.4
psylliate	972.7	E858.3	E942.7	E950.4	E962.0	E980.4
removing resins	974.5	E858.5	E944.5	E950.4	E962.0	E980.4
salicylate	965.1	E850.3	E935.3	E950.0	E962.0	E980.0
sulfate	973.3	E858.4	E943.3	E950.4	E962.0	E980.4
sulfoxone	961.8	E857	E931.8	E950.4	E962.0	E980.4
tetradecyl sulfate	972.7	E858.3	E942.7	E950.4	E962.0	E980.4
thiopental	968.3	E855.1	E938.3	E950.4	E962.0	E980.4
thiosalicylate	965.1	E850.3	E935.3	E950.0	E962.0	E980.0
thiosulfate	976.0	E858.7	E946.0	E950.4	E962.0	E980.4
tolbutamide	977.8	E858.8	E947.8	E950.4	E962.0	E980.4
tyropanoate	977.8	E858.8	E947.8	E950.4	E962.0	E980.4
valproate	966.3	E855.0	E936.3	E950.4	E962.0	E980.4
Solanine	977.8	E858.8	E947.8	E950.4	E962.0	E980.4
Solanum dulcamara	988.2	E865.4	—	E950.9	E962.1	E980.9
Solapsone	961.8	E857	E931.8	E950.4	E962.0	E980.4
Solasulfone	961.8	E857	E931.8	E950.4	E962.0	E980.4
Soldering fluid	983.1	E864.1	—	E950.7	E962.1	E980.6
Solid substance	989.9	E866.9	—	E950.9	E962.1	E980.9
specified NEC	989.9	E866.8	—	E950.9	E962.1	E980.9
Solvents, industrial	982.8	E862.9	—	E950.9	E962.1	E980.9
naphtha	981	E862.0	—	E950.9	E962.1	E980.9
petroleum	981	E862.0	—	E950.9	E962.1	E980.9
specified NEC	982.8	E862.4	—	E950.9	E962.1	E980.9
Soma	968.0	E855.1	E938.0	E950.4	E962.0	E980.4
Somatotropin	962.4	E858.0	E932.4	E950.4	E962.0	E980.4
Sominex	963.0	E858.1	E933.0	E950.4	E962.0	E980.4

◀ New   ◀▥ Revised   ~~deleted~~ Deleted   ● Use Additional Digit(s)

Substance	Poisoning	External Cause (E Code)				
		Accident	Therapeutic Use	Suicide Attempt	Assault	Undetermined
Somnos	967.1	E852.0	E937.1	E950.2	E962.0	E980.2
Somonal	967.0	E851	E937.0	E950.1	E962.0	E980.1
Soneryl	967.0	E851	E937.0	E950.1	E962.0	E980.1
Soothing syrup	977.9	E858.9	E947.9	E950.5	E962.0	E980.5
Sopor	967.4	E852.3	E937.4	E950.2	E962.0	E980.2
Soporific drug	967.9	E852.9	E937.9	E950.2	E962.0	E980.2
specified type NEC	967.8	E852.8	E937.8	E950.2	E962.0	E980.2
Sorbitol NEC	977.4	E858.8	E947.4	E950.4	E962.0	E980.4
Sotradecol	972.7	E858.3	E942.7	E950.4	E962.0	E980.4
Spacoline	975.1	E858.6	E945.1	E950.4	E962.0	E980.4
Spanish fly	976.8	E858.7	E946.8	E950.4	E962.0	E980.4
Sparine	969.1	E853.0	E939.1	E950.3	E962.0	E980.3
Sparteine	975.0	E858.6	E945.0	E950.4	E962.0	E980.4
Spasmolytics	975.1	E858.6	E945.1	E950.4	E962.0	E980.4
anticholinergics	971.1	E855.4	E941.1	E950.4	E962.0	E980.4
Spectinomycin	960.8	E856	E930.8	E950.4	E962.0	E980.4
Speed	969.72 ◀	E854.2	E939.7	E950.3	E962.0	E980.3
Spermicides	976.8	E858.7	E946.8	E950.4	E962.0	E980.4
Spider (bite) (venom)	989.5	E905.1	—	E950.9	E962.1	E980.9
antivenin	979.9	E858.8	E949.9	E950.4	E962.0	E980.4
Spigelia (root)	961.6	E857	E931.6	E950.4	E962.0	E980.4
Spiperone	969.2	E853.1	E939.2	E950.3	E962.0	E980.3
Spiramycin	960.3	E856	E930.3	E950.4	E962.0	E980.4
Spirilene	969.5	E853.8	E939.5	E950.3	E962.0	E980.3
Spirit(s) (neutral) NEC	980.0	E860.1	—	E950.9	E962.1	E980.9
beverage	980.0	E860.0	—	E950.9	E962.1	E980.9
industrial	980.9	E860.9	—	E950.9	E962.1	E980.9
mineral	981	E862.0	—	E950.9	E962.1	E980.9
of salt - *see* Hydrochloric acid	—	—	—	—	—	—
surgical	980.9	E860.9	—	E950.9	E962.1	E980.9
Spironolactone	974.4	E858.5	E944.4	E950.4	E962.0	E980.4
Sponge, absorbable (gelatin)	964.5	E858.2	E934.5	E950.4	E962.0	E980.4
Sporostacin	976.0	E858.7	E946.0	E950.4	E962.0	E980.4
Sprays (aerosol)	989.89	E866.8	—	E950.9	E962.1	E980.9
cosmetic	989.89	E866.7	—	E950.9	E962.1	E980.9
medicinal NEC	977.9	E858.9	E947.9	E950.5	E962.0	E980.5
pesticides - *see* Pesticides	—	—	—	—	—	—
specified content - *see* substance specified	—	—	—	—	—	—
Spurge flax	988.2	E865.4	—	E950.9	E962.1	E980.9

◀ New　◀▥ Revised　~~deleted~~ Deleted　● Use Additional Digit(s)

Substance	Poisoning	External Cause (E Code)				
		Accident	Therapeutic Use	Suicide Attempt	Assault	Undetermined
Spurges	988.2	E865.4	—	E950.9	E962.1	E980.9
Squill (expectorant) NEC	975.5	E858.6	E945.5	E950.4	E962.0	E980.4
rat poison	989.4	E863.7	—	E950.6	E962.1	E980.7
Squirting cucumber (cathartic)	973.1	E858.4	E943.1	E950.4	E962.0	E980.4
SSNRI (selective serotonin and norepinephrine reuptake inhibitors)	969.02	E854.0	E939.0	E950.3	E962.0	E980.3 ◀
SSRI (selective serotonin reuptake inhibitors)	969.03	E854.0	E939.0	E950.3	E962.0	E980.3 ◀
Stains	989.89	E866.8	—	E950.9	E962.1	E980.9
Stannous - *see also* Tin fluoride	976.7	E858.7	E946.7	E950.4	E962.0	E980.4
Stanolone	962.1	E858.0	E932.1	E950.4	E962.0	E980.4
Stanozolol	962.1	E858.0	E932.1	E950.4	E962.0	E980.4
Staphisagria or stavesacre (pediculicide)	976.0	E858.7	E946.0	E950.4	E962.0	E980.4
Stelazine	969.1	E853.0	E939.1	E950.3	E962.0	E980.3
Stemetil	969.1	E853.0	E939.1	E950.3	E962.0	E980.3
Sterculia (cathartic) (gum)	973.3	E858.4	E943.3	E950.4	E962.0	E980.4
Sternutator gas	987.8	E869.8	—	E952.8	E962.2	E982.8
Steroids NEC	962.0	E858.0	E932.0	E950.4	E962.0	E980.4
ENT agent	976.6	E858.7	E946.6	E950.4	E962.0	E980.4
ophthalmic preparation	976.5	E858.7	E946.5	E950.4	E962.0	E980.4
topical NEC	976.0	E858.7	E946.0	E950.4	E962.0	E980.4
Stibine	985.8	E866.4	—	E950.9	E962.1	E980.9
Stibophen	961.2	E857	E931.2	E950.4	E962.0	E980.4
Stilbamide, stilbamidine	961.5	E857	E931.5	E950.4	E962.0	E980.4
Stilbestrol	962.2	E858.0	E932.2	E950.4	E962.0	E980.4
Stimulants (central nervous system)	970.9	E854.3	E940.9	E950.4	E962.0	E980.4
analeptics	970.0	E854.3	E940.0	E950.4	E962.0	E980.4
opiate antagonist	970.1	E854.3	E940.1	E950.4	E962.0	E980.4
psychotherapeutic NEC	969.09 ◀	E854.0	E939.0	E950.3	E962.0	E980.3
specified NEC	970.8	E854.3	E940.8	E950.4	E962.0	E980.4
Storage batteries (acid) (cells)	983.1	E864.1	—	E950.7	E962.1	E980.6
Stovaine	968.9	E855.2	E938.9	E950.4	E962.0	E980.4
infiltration (subcutaneous)	968.5	E855.2	E938.5	E950.4	E962.0	E980.4
nerve block (peripheral) (plexus)	968.6	E855.2	E938.6	E950.4	E962.0	E980.4
spinal	968.7	E855.2	E938.7	E950.4	E962.0	E980.4
topical (surface)	968.5	E855.2	E938.5	E950.4	E962.0	E980.4
Stovarsal	961.1	E857	E931.1	E950.4	E962.0	E980.4
Stove gas - *see* Gas, utility	—	—	—	—	—	—
Stoxil	976.5	E858.7	E946.5	E950.4	E962.0	E980.4
STP	969.6	E854.1	E939.6	E950.3	E962.0	E980.3
Stramonium (medicinal) NEC	971.1	E855.4	E941.1	E950.4	E962.0	E980.4
natural state	988.2	E865.4	—	E950.9	E962.1	E980.9

◀ New ◀▦ Revised ~~deleted~~ Deleted ● Use Additional Digit(s)

Substance	Poisoning	External Cause (E Code)				
		Accident	Therapeutic Use	Suicide Attempt	Assault	Undetermined
Streptodornase	964.4	E858.2	E934.4	E950.4	E962.0	E980.4
Streptoduocin	960.6	E856	E930.6	E950.4	E962.0	E980.4
Streptokinase	964.4	E858.2	E934.4	E950.4	E962.0	E980.4
Streptomycin	960.6	E856	E930.6	E950.4	E962.0	E980.4
Streptozocin	960.7	E856	E930.7	E950.4	E962.0	E980.4
Stripper (paint) (solvent)	982.8	E862.9	—	E950.9	E962.1	E980.9
Strobane	989.2	E863.0	—	E950.6	E962.1	E980.7
Strophanthin	972.1	E858.3	E942.1	E950.4	E962.0	E980.4
Strophanthus hispidus or kombe	988.2	E865.4	—	E950.9	E962.1	E980.9
Strychnine (rodenticide) (salts)	989.1	E863.7	—	E950.6	E962.1	E980.7
medicinal NEC	970.8	E854.3	E940.8	E950.4	E962.0	E980.4
Strychnos (ignatii) - *see* Strychnine	—	—	—	—	—	—
Styramate	968.0	E855.1	E938.0	E950.4	E962.0	E980.4
Styrene	983.0	E864.0	—	E950.7	E962.1	E980.6
Succinimide (anticonvulsant)	966.2	E855.0	E936.2	E950.4	E962.0	E980.4
mercuric - *see* Mercury	—	—	—	—	—	—
Succinylcholine	975.2	E858.6	E945.2	E950.4	E962.0	E980.4
Succinylsulfathiazole	961.0	E857	E931.0	E950.4	E962.0	E980.4
Sucrose	974.5	E858.5	E944.5	E950.4	E962.0	E980.4
Sulfacetamide	961.0	E857	E931.0	E950.4	E962.0	E980.4
ophthalmic preparation	976.5	E858.7	E946.5	E950.4	E962.0	E980.4
Sulfachlorpyridazine	961.0	E857	E931.0	E950.4	E962.0	E980.4
Sulfacytine	961.0	E857	E931.0	E950.4	E962.0	E980.4
Sulfadiazine	961.0	E857	E931.0	E950.4	E962.0	E980.4
silver (topical)	976.0	E858.7	E946.0	E950.4	E962.0	E980.4
Sulfadimethoxine	961.0	E857	E931.0	E950.4	E962.0	E980.4
Sulfadimidine	961.0	E857	E931.0	E950.4	E962.0	E980.4
Sulfaethidole	961.0	E857	E931.0	E950.4	E962.0	E980.4
Sulfafurazole	961.0	E857	E931.0	E950.4	E962.0	E980.4
Sulfaguanidine	961.0	E857	E931.0	E950.4	E962.0	E980.4
Sulfamerazine	961.0	E857	E931.0	E950.4	E962.0	E980.4
Sulfameter	961.0	E857	E931.0	E950.4	E962.0	E980.4
Sulfamethizole	961.0	E857	E931.0	E950.4	E962.0	E980.4
Sulfamethoxazole	961.0	E857	E931.0	E950.4	E962.0	E980.4
Sulfamethoxydiazine	961.0	E857	E931.0	E950.4	E962.0	E980.4
Sulfamethoxypyridazine	961.0	E857	E931.0	E950.4	E962.0	E980.4
Sulfamethylthiazole	961.0	E857	E931.0	E950.4	E962.0	E980.4
Sulfamylon	976.0	E858.7	E946.0	E950.4	E962.0	E980.4
Sulfan blue (diagnostic dye)	977.8	E858.8	E947.8	E950.4	E962.0	E980.4
Sulfanilamide	961.0	E857	E931.0	E950.4	E962.0	E980.4

◀ New   ◀⃪ Revised   ~~deleted~~ Deleted   ● Use Additional Digit(s)

Substance	Poisoning	External Cause (E Code)				
		Accident	Therapeutic Use	Suicide Attempt	Assault	Undetermined
Sulfanilylguanidine	961.0	E857	E931.0	E950.4	E962.0	E980.4
Sulfaphenazole	961.0	E857	E931.0	E950.4	E962.0	E980.4
Sulfaphenylthiazole	961.0	E857	E931.0	E950.4	E962.0	E980.4
Sulfaproxyline	961.0	E857	E931.0	E950.4	E962.0	E980.4
Sulfapyridine	961.0	E857	E931.0	E950.4	E962.0	E980.4
Sulfapyrimidine	961.0	E857	E931.0	E950.4	E962.0	E980.4
Sulfarsphenamine	961.1	E857	E931.1	E950.4	E962.0	E980.4
Sulfasalazine	961.0	E857	E931.0	E950.4	E962.0	E980.4
Sulfasomizole	961.0	E857	E931.0	E950.4	E962.0	E980.4
Sulfasuxidine	961.0	E857	E931.0	E950.4	E962.0	E980.4
Sulfinpyrazone	974.7	E858.5	E944.7	E950.4	E962.0	E980.4
Sulfisoxazole	961.0	E857	E931.0	E950.4	E962.0	E980.4
ophthalmic preparation	976.5	E858.7	E946.5	E950.4	E962.0	E980.4
Sulfomyxin	960.8	E856	E930.8	E950.4	E962.0	E980.4
Sulfonal	967.8	E852.8	E937.8	E950.2	E962.0	E980.2
Sulfonamides (mixtures)	961.0	E857	E931.0	E950.4	E962.0	E980.4
Sulfones	961.8	E857	E931.8	E950.4	E962.0	E980.4
Sulfonethylmethane	967.8	E852.8	E937.8	E950.2	E962.0	E980.2
Sulfonmethane	967.8	E852.8	E937.8	E950.2	E962.0	E980.2
Sulfonphthal, sulfonphthol	977.8	E858.8	E947.8	E950.4	E962.0	E980.4
Sulfonylurea derivatives, oral	962.3	E858.0	E932.3	E950.4	E962.0	E980.4
Sulfoxone	961.8	E857	E931.8	E950.4	E962.0	E980.4
Sulfur, sulfureted, sulfuric, sulfurous, sulfuryl (compounds) NEC	989.89	E866.8	—	E950.9	E962.1	E980.9
acid	983.1	E864.1	—	E950.7	E962.1	E980.6
dioxide	987.3	E869.1	—	E952.8	E962.2	E982.8
ether - see Ether(s)	—	—	—	—	—	—
hydrogen	987.8	E869.8	—	E952.8	E962.2	E982.8
medicinal (keratolytic) (ointment) NEC	976.4	E858.7	E946.4	E950.4	E962.0	E980.4
pesticide (vapor)	989.4	E863.4	—	E950.6	E962.1	E980.7
vapor NEC	987.8	E869.8	—	E952.8	E962.2	E982.8
Sulkowitch's reagent	977.8	E858.8	E947.8	E950.4	E962.0	E980.4
Sulph - see also Sulf-	—	—	—	—	—	—
Sulphadione	961.8	E857	E931.8	E950.4	E962.0	E980.4
Sulthiame, sultiame	966.3	E855.0	E936.3	E950.4	E962.0	E980.4
Superinone	975.5	E858.6	E945.5	E950.4	E962.0	E980.4
Suramin	961.5	E857	E931.5	E950.4	E962.0	E980.4
Surfacaine	968.5	E855.2	E938.5	E950.4	E962.0	E980.4
Surital	968.3	E855.1	E938.3	E950.4	E962.0	E980.4
Sutilains	976.8	E858.7	E946.8	E950.4	E962.0	E980.4

TABLE OF DRUGS AND CHEMICALS

		External Cause (E Code)				
Substance	Poisoning	Accident	Therapeutic Use	Suicide Attempt	Assault	Undetermined
Suxamethonium (bromide) (chloride) (iodide)	975.2	E858.6	E945.2	E950.4	E962.0	E980.4
Suxethonium (bromide)	975.2	E858.6	E945.2	E950.4	E962.0	E980.4
Sweet oil (birch)	976.3	E858.7	E946.3	E950.4	E962.0	E980.4
Sym-dichloroethyl ether	982.3	E862.4	—	E950.9	E962.1	E980.9
Sympatholytics	971.3	E855.6	E941.3	E950.4	E962.0	E980.4
Sympathomimetics	971.2	E855.5	E941.2	E950.4	E962.0	E980.4
Synagis	979.6	E858.8	E949.6	E950.4	E962.0	E980.4
Synalar	976.0	E858.7	E946.0	E950.4	E962.0	E980.4
Synthroid	962.7	E858.0	E932.7	E950.4	E962.0	E980.4
Syntocinon	975.0	E858.6	E945.0	E950.4	E962.0	E950.4
Syrosingopine	972.6	E858.3	E942.6	E950.4	E962.0	E980.4
Systemic agents (primarily)	963.9	E858.1	E933.9	E950.4	E962.0	E980.4
specified NEC	963.8	E858.1	E933.8	E950.4	E962.0	E980.4
Tablets (*see also* specified substance)	977.9	E858.9	E947.9	E950.5	E962.0	E980.5
Tace	962.2	E858.0	E932.2	E950.4	E962.0	E980.4
Tacrine	971.0	E855.3	E941.0	E950.4	E962.0	E980.4
Talbutal	967.0	E851	E937.0	E950.1	E962.0	E980.1
Talc	976.3	E858.7	E946.3	E950.4	E962.0	E980.4
Talcum	976.3	E858.7	E946.3	E950.4	E962.0	E980.4
Tamsulosin	971.3	E855.6	E941.3	E950.4	E962.0	E980.4
Tandearil, tanderil	965.5	E850.5	E935.5	E950.0	E962.0	E980.0
Tannic acid	983.1	E864.1	—	E950.7	E962.1	E980.6
medicinal (astringent)	976.2	E858.7	E946.2	E950.4	E962.0	E980.4
Tannin - *see* Tannic acid	—	—	—	—	—	—
Tansy	988.2	E865.4	—	E950.9	E962.1	E980.9
TAO	960.3	E856	E930.3	E950.4	E962.0	E980.4
Tapazole	962.8	E858.0	E932.8	E950.4	E962.0	E980.4
Tar NEC	983.0	E864.0	—	E950.7	E962.1	E980.6
camphor - *see* Naphthalene	—	—	—	—	—	—
fumes	987.8	E869.8	—	E952.8	E962.2	E982.8
Taractan	969.3	E853.8	E939.3	E950.3	E962.0	E980.3
Tarantula (venomous)	989.5	E905.1	—	E950.9	E962.1	E980.9
Tartar emetic (anti-infective)	961.2	E857	E931.2	E950.4	E962.0	E980.4
Tartaric acid	983.1	E864.1	—	E950.7	E962.1	E980.6
Tartrated antimony (anti-infective)	961.2	E857	E931.2	E950.4	E962.0	E980.4
TCA - *see* Trichloroacetic acid	—	—	—	—	—	—
TDI	983.0	E864.0	—	E950.7	E962.1	E980.6
vapor	987.8	E869.8	—	E952.8	E962.2	E982.8
Tear gas	987.5	E869.3	—	E952.8	E962.2	E982.8

◄ New   ◀▥ Revised   ~~deleted~~ Deleted   ● Use Additional Digit(s)

Substance	External Cause (E Code)					
	Poisoning	Accident	Therapeutic Use	Suicide Attempt	Assault	Undetermined
Teclothiazide	974.3	E858.5	E944.3	E950.4	E962.0	E980.4
Tegretol	966.3	E855.0	E936.3	E950.4	E962.0	E980.4
Telepaque	977.8	E858.8	E947.8	E950.4	E962.0	E980.4
Tellurium	985.8	E866.4	—	E950.9	E962.1	E980.9
fumes	985.8	E866.4	—	E950.9	E962.1	E980.9
TEM	963.1	E858.1	E933.1	E950.4	E962.0	E980.4
Temazepam - see Benzodiazepines	—	—	—	—	—	—
TEPA	963.1	E858.1	E933.1	E950.4	E962.0	E980.4
TEPP	989.3	E863.1	—	E950.6	E962.1	E980.7
Terbutaline	971.2	E855.5	E941.2	E950.4	E962.0	E980.4
Teroxalene	961.6	E857	E931.6	E950.4	E962.0	E980.4
Terpin hydrate	975.5	E858.6	E945.5	E950.4	E962.0	E980.4
Terramycin	960.4	E856	E930.4	E950.4	E962.0	E980.4
Tessalon	975.4	E858.6	E945.4	E950.4	E962.0	E980.4
Testosterone	962.1	E858.0	E932.1	E950.4	E962.0	E980.4
Tetanus (vaccine)	978.4	E858.8	E948.4	E950.4	E962.0	E980.4
antitoxin	979.9	E858.8	E949.9	E950.4	E962.0	E980.4
immune globulin (human)	964.6	E858.2	E934.6	E950.4	E962.0	E980.4
toxoid	978.4	E858.8	E948.4	E950.4	E962.0	E980.4
with diphtheria toxoid	978.9	E858.8	E948.9	E950.4	E962.0	E980.4
with pertussis	978.6	E858.8	E948.6	E950.4	E962.0	E980.4
Tetrabenazine	969.5	E853.8	E939.5	E950.3	E962.0	E980.3
Tetracaine (infiltration) (topical)	968.5	E855.2	E938.5	E950.4	E962.0	E980.4
nerve block (peripheral) (plexus)	968.6	E855.2	E938.6	E950.4	E962.0	E980.4
spinal	968.7	E855.2	E938.7	E950.4	E962.0	E980.4
Tetrachlorethylene - see Tetrachloroethylene	—	—	—	—	—	—
Tetrachlormethiazide	974.3	E858.5	E944.3	E950.4	E962.0	E980.4
Tetrachloroethane (liquid) (vapor)	982.3	E862.4	—	E950.9	E962.1	E980.9
paint or varnish	982.3	E861.6	—	E950.9	E962.1	E980.9
Tetrachloroethylene (liquid) (vapor)	982.3	E862.4	—	E950.9	E962.1	E980.9
medicinal	961.6	E857	E931.6	E950.4	E962.0	E980.4
Tetrachloromethane - see Carbon, tetrachloride	—	—	—	—	—	—
Tetracycline	960.4	E856	E930.4	E950.4	E962.0	E980.4
ophthalmic preparation	976.5	E858.7	E946.5	E950.4	E962.0	E980.4
topical NEC	976.0	E858.7	E946.0	E950.4	E962.0	E980.4
Tetraethylammonium chloride	972.3	E858.3	E942.3	E950.4	E962.0	E980.4
Tetraethyl lead (antiknock compound)	984.1	E862.1	—	E950.9	E962.1	E980.9
Tetraethyl pyrophosphate	989.3	E863.1	—	E950.6	E962.1	E980.7
Tetraethylthiuram disulfide	977.3	E858.8	E947.3	E950.4	E962.0	E980.4

◀ New ◀▥ Revised ~~deleted~~ Deleted ● Use Additional Digit(s)

Substance	Poisoning	External Cause (E Code)				
		Accident	Therapeutic Use	Suicide Attempt	Assault	Undetermined
Tetrahydroaminoacridine	971.0	E855.3	E941.0	E950.4	E962.0	E980.4
Tetrahydrocannabinol	969.6	E854.1	E939.6	E950.3	E962.0	E980.3
Tetrahydronaphthalene	982.0	E862.4	—	E950.9	E962.1	E980.9
Tetrahydrozoline	971.2	E855.5	E941.2	E950.4	E962.0	E980.4
Tetralin	982.0	E862.4	—	E950.9	E962.1	E980.9
Tetramethylthiuram (disulfide) NEC	989.4	E863.6	—	E950.6	E962.1	E980.7
medicinal	976.2	E858.7	E946.2	E950.4	E962.0	E980.4
Tetronal	967.8	E852.8	E937.8	E950.2	E962.0	E980.2
Tetryl	983.0	E864.0	—	E950.7	E962.1	E980.6
Thalidomide	967.8	E852.8	E937.8	E950.2	E962.0	E980.2
Thallium (compounds) (dust) NEC	985.8	E866.4	—	E950.9	E962.1	E980.9
pesticide (rodenticide)	985.8	E863.7	—	E950.6	E962.1	E980.7
THC	969.6	E854.1	E939.6	E950.3	E962.0	E980.3
Thebacon	965.09	E850.2	E935.2	E950.0	E962.0	E980.0
Thebaine	965.09	E850.2	E935.2	E950.0	E962.0	E980.0
Theobromine (calcium salicylate)	974.1	E858.5	E944.1	E950.4	E962.0	E980.4
Theophylline (diuretic)	974.1	E858.5	E944.1	E950.4	E962.0	E980.4
ethylenediamine	975.7	E858.6	E945.7	E950.4	E962.0	E980.4
Thiabendazole	961.6	E857	E931.6	E950.4	E962.0	E980.4
Thialbarbital, thialbarbitone	968.3	E855.1	E938.3	E950.4	E962.0	E980.4
Thiamine	963.5	E858.1	E933.5	E950.4	E962.0	E980.4
Thiamylal (sodium)	968.3	E855.1	E938.3	E950.4	E962.0	E980.4
Thiazesim	969.09 ◀	E854.0	E939.0	E950.3	E962.0	E980.3
Thiazides (diuretics)	974.3	E858.5	E944.3	E950.4	E962.0	E980.4
Thiethylperazine	963.0	E858.1	E933.0	E950.4	E962.0	E980.4
Thimerosal (topical)	976.0	E858.7	E946.0	E950.4	E962.0	E980.4
ophthalmic preparation	976.5	E858.7	E946.5	E950.4	E962.0	E980.4
Thioacetazone	961.8	E857	E931.8	E950.4	E962.0	E980.4
Thiobarbiturates	968.3	E855.1	E938.3	E950.4	E962.0	E980.4
Thiobismol	961.2	E857	E931.2	E950.4	E962.0	E980.4
Thiocarbamide	962.8	E858.0	E932.8	E950.4	E962.0	E980.4
Thiocarbarsone	961.1	E857	E931.1	E950.4	E962.0	E980.4
Thiocarlide	961.8	E857	E931.8	E950.4	E962.0	E980.4
Thioguanine	963.1	E858.1	E933.1	E950.4	E962.0	E980.4
Thiomercaptomerin	974.0	E858.5	E944.0	E950.4	E962.0	E980.4
Thiomerin	974.0	E858.5	E944.0	E950.4	E962.0	E980.4
Thiopental, thiopentone (sodium)	968.3	E855.1	E938.3	E950.4	E962.0	E980.4
Thiopropazate	969.1	E853.0	E939.1	E950.3	E962.0	E980.3
Thioproperazine	969.1	E853.0	E939.1	E950.3	E962.0	E980.3

◀ New   ◀▥ Revised   ~~deleted~~ Deleted   ● Use Additional Digit(s)

Substance	Poisoning	External Cause (E Code)				
		Accident	Therapeutic Use	Suicide Attempt	Assault	Undetermined
Thioridazine	969.1	E853.0	E939.1	E950.3	E962.0	E980.3
Thio-TEPA, thiotepa	963.1	E858.1	E933.1	E950.4	E962.0	E980.4
Thiothixene	969.3	E853.8	E939.3	E950.3	E962.0	E980.3
Thiouracil	962.8	E858.0	E932.8	E950.4	E962.0	E980.4
Thiourea	962.8	E858.0	E932.8	E950.4	E962.0	E980.4
Thiphenamil	971.1	E855.4	E941.1	E950.4	E962.0	E980.4
Thiram NEC	989.4	E863.6	—	E950.6	E962.1	E980.7
medicinal	976.2	E858.7	E946.2	E950.4	E962.0	E980.4
Thonzylamine	963.0	E858.1	E933.0	E950.4	E962.0	E980.4
Thorazine	969.1	E853.0	E939.1	E950.3	E962.0	E980.3
Thornapple	988.2	E865.4	—	E950.9	E962.1	E980.9
Throat preparation (lozenges) NEC	976.6	E858.7	E946.6	E950.4	E962.0	E980.4
Thrombin	964.5	E858.2	E934.5	E950.4	E962.0	E980.4
Thrombolysin	964.4	E858.2	E934.4	E950.4	E962.0	E980.4
Thymol	983.0	E864.0	—	E950.7	E962.1	E980.6
Thymus extract	962.9	E858.0	E932.9	E950.4	E962.0	E980.4
Thyroglobulin	962.7	E858.0	E932.7	E950.4	E962.0	E980.4
Thyroid (derivatives) (extract)	962.7	E858.0	E932.7	E950.4	E962.0	E980.4
Thyrolar	962.7	E858.0	E932.7	E950.4	E962.0	E980.4
Thyrotrophin, thyrotropin	977.8	E858.8	E947.8	E950.4	E962.0	E980.4
Thyroxin(e)	962.7	E858.0	E932.7	E950.4	E962.0	E980.4
Tigan	963.0	E858.1	E933.0	E950.4	E962.0	E980.4
Tigloidine	968.0	E855.1	E938.0	E950.4	E962.0	E980.4
Tin (chloride) (dust) (oxide) NEC	985.8	E866.4	—	E950.9	E962.1	E980.9
anti-infectives	961.2	E857	E931.2	E950.4	E962.0	E980.4
Tinactin	976.0	E858.7	E946.0	E950.4	E962.0	E980.4
Tincture, iodine - *see* Iodine	—	—	—	—	—	—
Tindal	969.1	E853.0	E939.1	E950.3	E962.0	E980.3
Titanium (compounds) (vapor)	985.8	E866.4	—	E950.9	E962.1	E980.9
ointment	976.3	E858.7	E946.3	E950.4	E962.0	E980.4
Titroid	962.7	E858.0	E932.7	E950.4	E962.0	E980.4
TMTD - *see* Tetramethylthiuram disulfide	—	—	—	—	—	—
TNT	989.89	E866.8	—	E950.9	E962.1	E980.9
fumes	987.8	E869.8	—	E952.8	E962.2	E982.8
Toadstool	988.1	E865.5	—	E950.9	E962.1	E980.9
Tobacco NEC	989.84	E866.8	—	E950.9	E962.1	E980.9
Indian	988.2	E865.4	—	E950.9	E962.1	E980.9
smoke, second-hand	987.8	E869.4	—	—	—	—

◀ New   ◀▌▌ Revised   ~~deleted~~ Deleted   ● Use Additional Digit(s)

Substance	Poisoning	External Cause (E Code)				
		Accident	Therapeutic Use	Suicide Attempt	Assault	Undetermined
Tocopherol	963.5	E858.1	E933.5	E950.4	E962.0	E980.4
Tocosamine	975.0	E858.6	E945.0	E950.4	E962.0	E980.4
Tofranil	969.05 ◀ⅢⅢ	E854.0	E939.0	E950.3	E962.0	E980.3
Toilet deodorizer	989.89	E866.8	—	E950.9	E962.1	E980.9
Tolazamide	962.3	E858.0	E932.3	E950.4	E962.0	E980.4
Tolazoline	971.3	E855.6	E941.3	E950.4	E962.0	E980.4
Tolbutamide	962.3	E858.0	E932.3	E950.4	E962.0	E980.4
sodium	977.8	E858.8	E947.8	E950.4	E962.0	E980.4
Tolmetin	965.69	E850.6	E935.6	E950.0	E962.0	E980.0
Tolnaftate	976.0	E858.7	E946.0	E950.4	E962.0	E980.4
Tolpropamine	976.1	E858.7	E946.1	E950.4	E962.0	E980.4
Tolserol	968.0	E855.1	E938.0	E950.4	E962.0	E980.4
Toluene (liquid) (vapor)	982.0	E862.4	—	E950.9	E962.1	E980.9
diisocyanate	983.0	E864.0	—	E950.7	E962.1	E980.6
Toluidine	983.0	E864.0	—	E950.7	E962.1	E980.6
vapor	987.8	E869.8	—	E952.8	E962.2	E982.8
Toluol (liquid) (vapor)	982.0	E862.4	—	E950.9	E962.1	E980.9
Tolylene-2,4-diisocyanate	983.0	E864.0	—	E950.7	E962.1	E980.6
Tonics, cardiac	972.1	E858.3	E942.1	E950.4	E962.0	E980.4
Toxaphene (dust) (spray)	989.2	E863.0	—	E950.6	E962.1	E980.7
Toxoids NEC	978.8	E858.8	E948.8	E950.4	E962.0	E980.4
Tractor fuel NEC	981	E862.1	—	E950.9	E962.1	E980.9
Tragacanth	973.3	E858.4	E943.3	E950.4	E962.0	E980.4
Tramazoline	971.2	E855.5	E941.2	E950.4	E962.0	E980.4
Tranquilizers	969.5	E853.9	E939.5	E950.3	E962.0	E980.3
benzodiazepine-based	969.4	E853.2	E939.4	E950.3	E962.0	E980.3
butyrophenone-based	969.2	E853.1	E939.2	E950.3	E962.0	E980.3
major NEC	969.3	E853.8	E939.3	E950.3	E962.0	E980.3
phenothiazine-based	969.1	E853.0	E939.1	E950.3	E962.0	E980.3
specified NEC	969.5	E853.8	E939.5	E950.3	E962.0	E980.3
Trantoin	961.9	E857	E931.9	E950.4	E962.0	E980.4
Tranxene	969.4	E853.2	E939.4	E950.3	E962.0	E980.3
Tranylcypromine (sulfate)	969.01 ◀ⅢⅢ	E854.0	E939.0	E950.3	E962.0	E980.3
Trasentine	975.1	E858.6	E945.1	E950.4	E962.0	E980.4
Travert	974.5	E858.5	E944.5	E950.4	E962.0	E980.4
Trecator	961.8	E857	E931.8	E950.4	E962.0	E980.4
Tretinoin	976.8	E858.7	E946.8	E950.4	E962.0	E980.4
Triacetin	976.0	E858.7	E946.0	E950.4	E962.0	E980.4

◀ New   ◀ⅢⅢ Revised   ~~deleted~~ Deleted   ● Use Additional Digit(s)

Substance	Poisoning	External Cause (E Code)				
		Accident	Therapeutic Use	Suicide Attempt	Assault	Undetermined
Triacetyloleandomycin	960.3	E856	E930.3	E950.4	E962.0	E980.4
Triamcinolone	962.0	E858.0	E932.0	E950.4	E962.0	E980.4
ENT agent	976.6	E858.7	E946.6	E950.4	E962.0	E980.4
ophthalmic preparation	976.5	E858.7	E946.5	E950.4	E962.0	E980.4
topical NEC	976.0	E858.7	E946.0	E950.4	E962.0	E980.4
Triamterene	974.4	E858.5	E944.4	E950.4	E962.0	E980.4
Triaziquone	963.1	E858.1	E933.1	E950.4	E962.0	E980.4
Tribromacetaldehyde	967.3	E852.2	E937.3	E950.2	E962.0	E980.2
Tribromoethanol	968.2	E855.1	E938.2	E950.4	E962.0	E980.4
Tribromomethane	967.3	E852.2	E937.3	E950.2	E962.0	E980.2
Trichlorethane	982.3	E862.4	—	E950.9	E962.1	E980.9
Trichlormethiazide	974.3	E858.5	E944.3	E950.4	E962.0	E980.4
Trichloroacetic acid	983.1	E864.1	—	E950.7	E962.1	E980.6
medicinal (keratolytic)	976.4	E858.7	E946.4	E950.4	E962.0	E980.4
Trichloroethanol	967.1	E852.0	E937.1	E950.2	E962.0	E980.2
Trichloroethylene (liquid) (vapor)	982.3	E862.4	—	E950.9	E962.1	E980.9
anesthetic (gas)	968.2	E855.1	E938.2	E950.4	E962.0	E980.4
Trichloroethyl phosphate	967.1	E852.0	E937.1	E950.2	E962.0	E980.2
Trichlorofluoromethane NEC	987.4	E869.2	—	E952.8	E962.2	E982.8
Trichlorotriethylamine	963.1	E858.1	E933.1	E950.4	E962.0	E980.4
Trichomonacides NEC	961.5	E857	E931.5	E950.4	E962.0	E980.4
Trichomycin	960.1	E856	E930.1	E950.4	E962.0	E980.4
Triclofos	967.1	E852.0	E937.1	E950.2	E962.0	E980.2
Tricresyl phosphate	989.89	E866.8	—	E950.9	E962.1	E980.9
solvent	982.8	E862.4	—	E950.9	E962.1	E980.9
Tricyclamol	966.4	E855.0	E936.4	E950.4	E962.0	E980.4
Tridesilon	976.0	E858.7	E946.0	E950.4	E962.0	E980.4
Tridihexethyl	971.1	E855.4	E941.1	E950.4	E962.0	E980.4
Tridione	966.0	E855.0	E936.0	E950.4	E962.0	E980.4
Triethanolamine NEC	983.2	E864.2	—	E950.7	E962.1	E980.6
detergent	983.2	E861.0	—	E950.7	E962.1	E980.6
trinitrate	972.4	E858.3	E942.4	E950.4	E962.0	E980.4
Triethanomelamine	963.1	E858.1	E933.1	E950.4	E962.0	E980.4
Triethylene melamine	963.1	E858.1	E933.1	E950.4	E962.0	E980.4
Triethylenephosphoramide	963.1	E858.1	E933.1	E950.4	E962.0	E980.4
Triethylenethiophosphoramide	963.1	E858.1	E933.1	E950.4	E962.0	E980.4
Trifluoperazine	969.1	E853.0	E939.1	E950.3	E962.0	E980.3
Trifluperidol	969.2	E853.1	E939.2	E950.3	E962.0	E980.3
Triflupromazine	969.1	E853.0	E939.1	E950.3	E962.0	E980.3

◀ New   ◀▥ Revised   ~~deleted~~ Deleted   ● Use Additional Digit(s)

Substance	Poisoning	External Cause (E Code)				
		Accident	Therapeutic Use	Suicide Attempt	Assault	Undetermined
Trihexyphenidyl	971.1	E855.4	E941.1	E950.4	E962.0	E980.4
Triiodothyronine	962.7	E858.0	E932.7	E950.4	E962.0	E980.4
Trilene	968.2	E855.1	E938.2	E950.4	E962.0	E980.4
Trimeprazine	963.0	E858.1	E933.0	E950.4	E962.0	E980.4
Trimetazidine	972.4	E858.3	E942.4	E950.4	E962.0	E980.4
Trimethadione	966.0	E855.0	E936.0	E950.4	E962.0	E980.4
Trimethaphan	972.3	E858.3	E942.3	E950.4	E962.0	E980.4
Trimethidinium	972.3	E858.3	E942.3	E950.4	E962.0	E980.4
Trimethobenzamide	963.0	E858.1	E933.0	E950.4	E962.0	E980.4
Trimethylcarbinol	980.8	E860.8	—	E950.9	E962.1	E980.9
Trimethylpsoralen	976.3	E858.7	E946.3	E950.4	E962.0	E980.4
Trimeton	963.0	E858.1	E933.0	E950.4	E962.0	E980.4
Trimipramine	969.05 ◀▥	E854.0	E939.0	E950.3	E962.0	E980.3
Trimustine	963.1	E858.1	E933.1	E950.4	E962.0	E980.4
Trinitrin	972.4	E858.3	E942.4	E950.4	E962.0	E980.4
Trinitrophenol	983.0	E864.0	—	E950.7	E962.1	E980.6
Trinitrotoluene	989.89	E866.8	—	E950.9	E962.1	E980.9
fumes	987.8	E869.8	—	E952.8	E962.2	E982.8
Trional	967.8	E852.8	E937.8	E950.2	E962.0	E980.2
Trioxide of arsenic - *see* Arsenic	—	—	—	—	—	—
Trioxsalen	976.3	E858.7	E946.3	E950.4	E962.0	E980.4
Tripelennamine	963.0	E858.1	E933.0	E950.4	E962.0	E980.4
Triperidol	969.2	E853.1	E939.2	E950.3	E962.0	E980.3
Triprolidine	963.0	E858.1	E933.0	E950.4	E962.0	E980.4
Trisoralen	976.3	E858.7	E946.3	E950.4	E962.0	E980.4
Troleandomycin	960.3	E856	E930.3	E950.4	E962.0	E980.4
Trolnitrate (phosphate)	972.4	E858.3	E942.4	E950.4	E962.0	E980.4
Trometamol	963.3	E858.1	E933.3	E950.4	E962.0	E980.4
Tromethamine	963.3	E858.1	E933.3	E950.4	E962.0	E980.4
Tronothane	968.5	E855.2	E938.5	E950.4	E962.0	E980.4
Tropicamide	971.1	E855.4	E941.1	E950.4	E962.0	E980.4
Troxidone	966.0	E855.0	E936.0	E950.4	E962.0	E980.4
Tryparsamide	961.1	E857	E931.1	E950.4	E962.0	E980.4
Trypsin	963.4	E858.1	E933.4	E950.4	E962.0	E980.4
Tryptizol	969.05 ◀▥	E854.0	E939.0	E950.3	E962.0	E980.3
Tuaminoheptane	971.2	E855.5	E941.2	E950.4	E962.0	E980.4
Tuberculin (old)	977.8	E858.8	E947.8	E950.4	E962.0	E980.4
Tubocurare	975.2	E858.6	E945.2	E950.4	E962.0	E980.4
Tubocurarine	975.2	E858.6	E945.2	E950.4	E962.0	E980.4

◀ New　◀▥ Revised　~~deleted~~ Deleted　● Use Additional Digit(s)

Substance	Poisoning	External Cause (E Code)				
		Accident	Therapeutic Use	Suicide Attempt	Assault	Undetermined
Turkish green	969.6	E854.1	E939.6	E950.3	E962.0	E980.3
Turpentine (spirits of) (liquid) (vapor)	982.8	E862.4	—	E950.9	E962.1	E980.9
Tybamate	969.5	E853.8	E939.5	E950.3	E962.0	E980.3
Tyloxapol	975.5	E858.6	E945.5	E950.4	E962.0	E980.4
Tymazoline	971.2	E855.5	E941.2	E950.4	E962.0	E980.4
Typhoid vaccine	978.1	E858.8	E948.1	E950.4	E962.0	E980.4
Typhus vaccine	979.2	E858.8	E949.2	E950.4	E962.0	E980.4
Tyrothricin	976.0	E858.7	E946.0	E950.4	E962.0	E980.4
ENT agent	976.6	E858.7	E946.6	E950.4	E962.0	E980.4
ophthalmic preparation	976.5	E858.7	E946.5	E950.4	E962.0	E980.4
Undecenoic acid	976.0	E858.7	E946.0	E950.4	E962.0	E980.4
Undecylenic acid	976.0	E858.7	E946.0	E950.4	E962.0	E980.4
Unna's boot	976.3	E858.7	E946.3	E950.4	E962.0	E980.4
Uracil mustard	963.1	E858.1	E933.1	E950.4	E962.0	E980.4
Uramustine	963.1	E858.1	E933.1	E950.4	E962.0	E980.4
Urari	975.2	E858.6	E945.2	E950.4	E962.0	E980.4
Urea	974.4	E858.5	E944.4	E950.4	E962.0	E980.4
topical	976.8	E858.7	E946.8	E950.4	E962.0	E980.4
Urethan(e) (antineoplastic)	963.1	E858.1	E933.1	E950.4	E962.0	E980.4
Urginea (maritima) (scilla) - see Squill	—	—	—	—	—	—
Uric acid metabolism agents NEC	974.7	E858.5	E944.7	E950.4	E962.0	E980.4
Urokinase	964.4	E858.2	E934.4	E950.4	E962.0	E980.4
Urokon	977.8	E858.8	E947.8	E950.4	E962.0	E980.4
Urotropin	961.9	E857	E931.9	E950.4	E962.0	E980.4
Urtica	988.2	E865.4	—	E950.9	E962.1	E980.9
Utility gas - see Gas, utility	—	—	—	—	—	—
Vaccine NEC	979.9	E858.8	E949.9	E950.4	E962.0	E980.4
bacterial NEC	978.8	E858.8	E948.8	E950.4	E962.0	E980.4
with	—	—	—	—	—	—
other bacterial component	978.9	E858.8	E948.9	E950.4	E962.0	E980.4
pertussis component	978.6	E858.8	E948.6	E950.4	E962.0	E980.4
viral-rickettsial component	979.7	E858.8	E949.7	E950.4	E962.0	E980.4
mixed NEC	978.9	E858.8	E948.9	E950.4	E962.0	E980.4
BCG	978.0	E858.8	E948.0	E950.4	E962.0	E980.4
cholera	978.2	E858.8	E948.2	E950.4	E962.0	E980.4
diphtheria	978.5	E858.8	E948.5	E950.4	E962.0	E980.4
influenza	979.6	E858.8	E949.6	E950.4	E962.0	E980.4

◀ New   ◀▥ Revised   ~~deleted~~ Deleted   ● Use Additional Digit(s)

Substance	Poisoning	External Cause (E Code)				
		Accident	Therapeutic Use	Suicide Attempt	Assault	Undetermined
Vaccine NEC *(Continued)*						
measles	979.4	E858.8	E949.4	E950.4	E962.0	E980.4
meningococcal	978.8	E858.8	E948.8	E950.4	E962.0	E980.4
mumps	979.6	E858.8	E949.6	E950.4	E962.0	E980.4
paratyphoid	978.1	E858.8	E948.1	E950.4	E962.0	E980.4
pertussis (with diphtheria toxoid) (with tetanus toxoid)	978.6	E858.8	E948.6	E950.4	E962.0	E980.4
plague	978.3	E858.8	E948.3	E950.4	E962.0	E980.4
poliomyelitis	979.5	E858.8	E949.5	E950.4	E962.0	E980.4
poliovirus	979.5	E858.8	E949.5	E950.4	E962.0	E980.4
rabies	979.1	E858.8	E949.1	E950.4	E962.0	E980.4
respiratory syncytial virus	979.6	E858.8	E949.6	E950.4	E962.0	E980.4
rickettsial NEC	979.6	E858.8	E949.6	E950.4	E962.0	E980.4
with	—	—	—	—	—	—
bacterial component	979.7	E858.8	E949.7	E950.4	E962.0	E980.4
pertussis component	978.6	E858.8	E948.6	E950.4	E962.0	E980.4
viral component	979.7	E858.8	E949.7	E950.4	E962.0	E980.4
Rocky Mountain spotted fever	979.6	E858.8	E949.6	E950.4	E962.0	E980.4
rotavirus	979.6	E858.8	E949.6	E950.4	E962.0	E980.4
rubella virus	979.4	E858.8	E949.4	E950.4	E962.0	E980.4
sabin oral	979.5	E858.8	E949.5	E950.4	E962.0	E980.4
smallpox	979.0	E858.8	E949.0	E950.4	E962.0	E980.4
tetanus	978.4	E858.8	E948.4	E950.4	E962.0	E980.4
typhoid	978.1	E858.8	E948.1	E950.4	E962.0	E980.4
typhus	979.2	E858.8	E949.2	E950.4	E962.0	E980.4
viral NEC	979.6	E858.8	E949.6	E950.4	E962.0	E980.4
with	—	—	—	—	—	—
bacterial component	979.7	E858.8	E949.7	E950.4	E962.0	E980.4
pertussis component	978.6	E858.8	E948.6	E950.4	E962.0	E980.4
rickettsial component	979.7	E858.8	E949.7	E950.4	E962.0	E980.4
yellow fever	979.3	E858.8	E949.3	E950.4	E962.0	E980.4
Vaccinia immune globulin (human)	964.6	E858.2	E934.6	E950.4	E962.0	E980.4
Vaginal contraceptives	976.8	E858.7	E946.8	E950.4	E962.0	E980.4
Valethamate	971.1	E855.4	E941.1	E950.4	E962.0	E980.4
Valisone	976.0	E858.7	E946.0	E950.4	E962.0	E980.4
Valium	969.4	E853.2	E939.4	E950.3	E962.0	E980.3
Valmid	967.8	E852.8	E937.8	E950.2	E962.0	E980.2
Vanadium	985.8	E866.4	—	E950.9	E962.1	E980.9
Vancomycin	960.8	E856	E930.8	E950.4	E962.0	E980.4

TABLE OF DRUGS AND CHEMICALS

Substance	Poisoning	External Cause (E Code)				
		Accident	Therapeutic Use	Suicide Attempt	Assault	Undetermined
Vapor (*see also* Gas)	987.9	E869.9	—	E952.9	E962.2	E982.9
kiln (carbon monoxide)	986	E868.8	—	E952.1	E962.2	E982.1
lead - *see* Lead	—	—	—	—	—	—
specified source NEC - (*see also* specific substance)	987.8	E869.8	—	E952.8	E962.2	E982.8
Varidase	964.4	E858.2	E934.4	E950.4	E962.0	E980.4
Varnish	989.89	E861.6	—	E950.9	E962.1	E980.9
cleaner	982.8	E862.9	—	E950.9	E962.1	E980.9
Vaseline	976.3	E858.7	E946.3	E950.4	E962.0	E980.4
Vasodilan	972.5	E858.3	E942.5	E950.4	E962.0	E980.4
Vasodilators NEC	972.5	E858.3	E942.5	E950.4	E962.0	E980.4
coronary	972.4	E858.3	E942.4	E950.4	E962.0	E980.4
Vasopressin	962.5	E858.0	E932.5	E950.4	E962.0	E980.4
Vasopressor drugs	962.5	E858.0	E932.5	E950.4	E962.0	E980.4
Venom, venomous (bite) (sting)	989.5	E905.9	—	E950.9	E962.1	E980.9
arthropod NEC	989.5	E905.5	—	E950.9	E962.1	E980.9
bee	989.5	E905.3	—	E950.9	E962.1	E980.9
centipede	989.5	E905.4	—	E950.9	E962.1	E980.9
hornet	989.5	E905.3	—	E950.9	E962.1	E980.9
lizard	989.5	E905.0	—	E950.9	E962.1	E980.9
marine animals or plants	989.5	E905.6	—	E950.9	E962.1	E980.9
millipede (tropical)	989.5	E905.4	—	E950.9	E962.1	E980.9
plant NEC	989.5	E905.7	—	E950.9	E962.1	E980.9
marine	989.5	E905.6	—	E950.9	E962.1	E980.9
scorpion	989.5	E905.2	—	E950.9	E962.1	E980.9
snake	989.5	E905.0	—	E950.9	E962.1	E980.9
specified NEC	989.5	E905.8	—	E950.9	E962.1	E980.9
spider	989.5	E905.1	—	E950.9	E962.1	E980.9
wasp	989.5	E905.3	—	E950.9	E962.1	E980.9
Ventolin - *see* Salbutamol sulfate	—	—	—	—	—	—
Veramon	967.0	E851	E937.0	E950.1	E962.0	E980.1
Veratrum	—	—	—	—	—	—
album	988.2	E865.4	—	E950.9	E962.1	E980.9
alkaloids	972.6	E858.3	E942.6	E950.4	E962.0	E980.4
viride	988.2	E865.4	—	E950.9	E962.1	E980.9
Verdigris (*see also* Copper)	985.8	E866.4	—	E950.9	E962.1	E980.9
Veronal	967.0	E851	E937.0	E950.1	E962.0	E980.1
Veroxil	961.6	E857	E931.6	E950.4	E962.0	E980.4
Versidyne	965.7	E850.7	E935.7	E950.0	E962.0	E980.0
Viagra	972.5	E858.3	E942.5	E950.4	E962.0	E980.4

◀ New   ◀▥ Revised   ~~deleted~~ Deleted   ● Use Additional Digit(s)

Substance	Poisoning	External Cause (E Code)				
		Accident	Therapeutic Use	Suicide Attempt	Assault	Undetermined
Vienna	—	—	—	—	—	—
green	985.1	E866.3	—	E950.8	E962.1	E980.8
insecticide	985.1	E863.4	—	E950.6	E962.1	E980.7
red	989.89	E866.8	—	E950.9	E962.1	E980.9
pharmaceutical dye	977.4	E858.8	E947.4	E950.4	E962.0	E980.4
Vinbarbital, vinbarbitone	967.0	E851	E937.0	E950.1	E962.0	E980.1
Vinblastine	963.1	E858.1	E933.1	E950.4	E962.0	E980.4
Vincristine	963.1	E858.1	E933.1	E950.4	E962.0	E980.4
Vinesthene, vinethene	968.2	E855.1	E938.2	E950.4	E962.0	E980.4
Vinyl	—	—	—	—	—	—
bital	967.0	E851	E937.0	E950.1	E962.0	E980.1
ether	968.2	E855.1	E938.2	E950.4	E962.0	E980.4
Vioform	961.3	E857	E931.3	E950.4	E962.0	E980.4
topical	976.0	E858.7	E946.0	E950.4	E962.0	E980.4
Viomycin	960.6	E856	E930.6	E950.4	E962.0	E980.4
Viosterol	963.5	E858.1	E933.5	E950.4	E962.0	E980.4
Viper (venom)	989.5	E905.0	—	E950.9	E962.1	E980.9
Viprynium (embonate)	961.6	E857	E931.6	E950.4	E962.0	E980.4
Virugon	961.7	E857	E931.7	E950.4	E962.0	E980.4
Visine	976.5	E858.7	E946.5	E950.4	E962.0	E980.4
Vitamins NEC	963.5	E858.1	E933.5	E950.4	E962.0	E980.4
B_{12}	964.1	E858.2	E934.1	E950.4	E962.0	E980.4
hematopoietic	964.1	E858.2	E934.1	E950.4	E962.0	E980.4
K	964.3	E858.2	E934.3	E950.4	E962.0	E980.4
Vleminckx's solution	976.4	E858.7	E946.4	E950.4	E962.0	E980.4
Voltaren - *see* Diclofenac sodium	—	—	—	—	—	—
Warfarin (potassium) (sodium)	964.2	E858.2	E934.2	E950.4	E962.0	E980.4
rodenticide	989.4	E863.7	—	E950.6	E962.1	E980.7
Wasp (sting)	989.5	E905.3	—	E950.9	E962.1	E980.9
Water	—	—	—	—	—	—
balance agents NEC	974.5	E858.5	E944.5	E950.4	E962.0	E980.4
gas	987.1	E868.1	—	E951.8	E962.2	E981.8
incomplete combustion of - *see* Carbon, monoxide, fuel, utility	—	—	—	—	—	—
hemlock	988.2	E865.4	—	E950.9	E962.1	E980.9
moccasin (venom)	989.5	E905.0	—	E950.9	E962.1	E980.9
Wax (paraffin) (petroleum)	981	E862.3	—	E950.9	E962.1	E980.9
automobile	989.89	E861.2	—	E950.9	E962.1	E980.9
floor	981	E862.0	—	E950.9	E962.1	E980.9
Weed killers NEC	989.4	E863.5	—	E950.6	E962.1	E980.7

◀ New   ◀▥ Revised   ~~deleted~~ Deleted   ● Use Additional Digit(s)

Substance	Poisoning	External Cause (E Code)				
		Accident	Therapeutic Use	Suicide Attempt	Assault	Undetermined
Welldorm	967.1	E852.0	E937.1	E950.2	E962.0	E980.2
White	—	—	—	—	—	—
arsenic - *see* Arsenic	—	—	—	—	—	—
hellebore	988.2	E865.4	—	E950.9	E962.1	E980.9
lotion (keratolytic)	976.4	E858.7	E946.4	E950.4	E962.0	E980.4
spirit	981	E862.0	—	E950.9	E962.1	E980.9
Whitewashes	989.89	E861.6	—	E950.9	E962.1	E980.9
Whole blood	964.7	E858.2	E934.7	E950.4	E962.0	E980.4
Wild	—	—	—	—	—	—
black cherry	988.2	E865.4	—	E950.9	E962.1	E980.9
poisonous plants NEC	988.2	E865.4	—	E950.9	E962.1	E980.9
Window cleaning fluid	989.89	E861.3	—	E950.9	E962.1	E980.9
Wintergreen (oil)	976.3	E858.7	E946.3	E950.4	E962.0	E980.4
Witch hazel	976.2	E858.7	E946.2	E950.4	E962.0	E980.4
Wood	—	—	—	—	—	—
alcohol	980.1	E860.2	—	E950.9	E962.1	E980.9
spirit	980.1	E860.2	—	E950.9	E962.1	E980.9
Woorali	975.2	E858.6	E945.2	E950.4	E962.0	E980.4
Wormseed, American	961.6	E857	E931.6	E950.4	E962.0	E980.4
Xanthine diuretics	974.1	E858.5	E944.1	E950.4	E962.0	E980.4
Xanthocillin	960.0	E856	E930.0	E950.4	E962.0	E980.4
Xanthotoxin	976.3	E858.7	E946.3	E950.4	E962.0	E980.4
Xigris	964.2	E858.2	E934.2	E950.4	E962.0	E980.4
Xylene (liquid) (vapor)	982.0	E862.4	—	E950.9	E962.1	E980.9
Xylocaine (infiltration) (topical)	968.5	E855.2	E938.5	E950.4	E962.0	E980.4
nerve block (peripheral) (plexus)	968.6	E855.2	E938.6	E950.4	E962.0	E980.4
spinal	968.7	E855.2	E938.7	E950.4	E962.0	E980.4
Xylol (liquid) (vapor)	982.0	E862.4	—	E950.9	E962.1	E980.9
Xylometazoline	971.2	E855.5	E941.2	E950.4	E962.0	E980.4
Yellow	—	—	—	—	—	—
fever vaccine	979.3	E858.8	E949.3	E950.4	E962.0	E980.4
jasmine	988.2	E865.4	—	E950.9	E962.1	E980.9
Yew	988.2	E865.4	—	E950.9	E962.1	E980.9
Zactane	965.7	E850.7	E935.7	E950.0	E962.0	E980.0
Zaroxolyn	974.3	E858.5	E944.3	E950.4	E962.0	E980.4
Zephiran (topical)	976.0	E858.7	E946.0	E950.4	E962.0	E980.4
ophthalmic preparation	976.5	E858.7	E946.5	E950.4	E962.0	E980.4
Zerone	980.1	E860.2	—	E950.9	E962.1	E980.9

◀ New　◀▥ Revised　deleted Deleted　● Use Additional Digit(s)

TABLE OF DRUGS AND CHEMICALS

Substance	Poisoning	External Cause (E Code)				
		Accident	Therapeutic Use	Suicide Attempt	Assault	Undetermined
Zinc (compounds) (fumes) (salts) (vapor) NEC	985.8	E866.4	—	E950.9	E962.1	E980.9
anti-infectives	976.0	E858.7	E946.0	E950.4	E962.0	E980.4
antivaricose	972.7	E858.3	E942.7	E950.4	E962.0	E980.4
bacitracin	976.0	E858.7	E946.0	E950.4	E962.0	E980.4
chloride	976.2	E858.7	E946.2	E950.4	E962.0	E980.4
gelatin	976.3	E858.7	E946.3	E950.4	E962.0	E980.4
oxide	976.3	E858.7	E946.3	E950.4	E962.0	E980.4
peroxide	976.0	E858.7	E946.0	E950.4	E962.0	E980.4
pesticides	985.8	E863.4	—	E950.6	E962.1	E980.7
phosphide (rodenticide)	985.8	E863.7	—	E950.6	E962.1	E980.7
stearate	976.3	E858.7	E946.3	E950.4	E962.0	E980.4
sulfate (antivaricose)	972.7	E858.3	E942.7	E950.4	E962.0	E980.4
ENT agent	976.6	E858.7	E946.6	E950.4	E962.0	E980.4
ophthalmic solution	976.5	E858.7	E946.5	E950.4	E962.0	E980.4
topical NEC	976.0	E858.7	E946.0	E950.4	E962.0	E980.4
undecylenate	976.0	E858.7	E946.0	E950.4	E962.0	E980.4
Zovant	964.2	E858.2	E934.2	E950.4	E962.0	E980.4
Zoxazolamine	968.0	E855.1	E938.0	E950.4	E962.0	E980.4
Zygadenus (venenosus)	988.2	E865.4	—	E950.9	E962.1	E980.9

◀ New   ◀▥ Revised   ~~deleted~~ Deleted   ● Use Additional Digit(s)

INDEX TO EXTERNAL CAUSES OF INJURY (E CODE)

This section contains the index to the codes which classify environmental events, circumstances, and other conditions as the cause of injury and other adverse effects. Where a code from the section Supplementary Classification of External Causes of Injury and Poisoning (E800–E998) is applicable, it is intended that the E code shall be used in addition to a code from the main body of the classification, Chapters 1 to 17.

The alphabetic index to the E codes is organized by main terms which describe the accident, circumstance, event, or specific agent which caused the injury or other adverse effect.

Note   Transport accidents (E800–E848) include accidents involving:

> aircraft and spacecraft (E840–E845)
> watercraft (E830–E838)
> motor vehicle (E810–E825)
> railway (E800–E807)
> other road vehicles (E826–E829)

For definitions and examples related to transport accidents - see Supplementary Classification of External Causes of Injury and Poisoning (E800–E999).

The fourth-digit subdivisions for use with categories E800–E848 to identify the injured person are found at the end of this section.

For identifying the place in which an accident or poisoning occurred (circumstances classifiable to categories E850–E869 and E880–E928) - see the listing in this section under "Accident, occurring."

See the Table of Drugs and Chemicals (Section 2 of this volume) for identifying the specific agent involved in drug overdose or a wrong substance given or taken in error, and for intoxication or poisoning by a drug or other chemical substance.

The specific adverse effect, reaction, or localized toxic effect to a correct drug or substance properly administered in therapeutic or prophylactic dosage should be classified according to the nature of the adverse effect (e.g., allergy, dermatitis, tachycardia) listed in Section I of this volume.

A

Abandonment
causing exposure to weather
conditions - *see* Exposure
child, with intent to injure or kill
E968.4
helpless person, infant, newborn
E904.0
with intent to injure or kill E968.4
Abortion, criminal, injury to child
E968.8
Abuse (alleged) (suspected)
adult
by
child E967.4
ex-partner E967.3
ex-spouse E967.3
father E967.0
grandchild E967.7
grandparent E967.6
mother E967.2
non-related caregiver E967.8
other relative E967.7
other specified person E967.1
partner E967.3
sibling E967.5
spouse E967.3
stepfather E967.0
stepmother E967.2
unspecified person E967.9
child
by
boyfriend of parent or guardian
E967.0
child E967.4
father E967.0
female partner of parent or
guardian E967.2
girlfriend of parent or guardian
E967.2
grandchild E967.7
grandparent E967.6
male partner of parent or
guardian E967.0
mother E967.2
non-related caregiver E967.8
other relative E967.7
other specified person(s) E967.1
sibling E967.5
stepfather E967.0
stepmother E967.2
unspecified person E967.9
Accident (to) E928.9
aircraft (in transit) (powered) E841●
at landing, take-off E840●
due to, caused by cataclysm - *see*
categories E908, E909
late effect of E929.1
unpowered (*see also* Collision,
aircraft, unpowered) E842●
while alighting, boarding E843●
amphibious vehicle
on
land - *see* Accident, motor
vehicle
water - *see* Accident, watercraft
animal, ridden NEC E828●
animal-drawn vehicle NEC E827●
balloon (*see also* Collision, aircraft,
unpowered) E842●
caused by, due to
abrasive wheel (metalworking)
E919.3

Accident *(Continued)*
caused by, due to *(Continued)*
animal NEC E906.9
being ridden (in sport or
transport) E828●
avalanche NEC E909.2
band saw E919.4
bench saw E919.4
bore, earth-drilling or mining (land)
(seabed) E919.1
bulldozer E919.7
cataclysmic
earth surface movement or
eruption E909.9
storm E908.9
chain
hoist E919.2
agricultural operations E919.0
mining operations E919.1
saw E920.1
circular saw E919.4
cold (excessive) (*see also* Cold,
exposure to) E901.9
combine E919.0
conflagration - *see* Conflagration
corrosive liquid, substance NEC
E924.1
cotton gin E919.8
crane E919.2
agricultural operations E919.0
mining operations E919.1
cutting or piercing instrument (*see
also* Cut) E920.9
dairy equipment E919.8
derrick E919.2
agricultural operations E919.0
mining operations E919.1
drill E920.1
earth (land) (seabed) E919.1
hand (powered) E920.1
not powered E920.4
metalworking E919.3
woodworking E919.4
earth(-)
drilling machine E919.1
moving machine E919.7
scraping machine E919.7
electric
current (*see also* Electric shock)
E925.9
motor - *see also* Accident,
machine, by type of
machine
current (of) - *see* Electric shock
elevator (building) (grain) E919.2
agricultural operations E919.0
mining operations E919.1
environmental factors NEC E928.9
excavating machine E919.7
explosive material (*see also*
Explosion) E923.9
farm machine E919.0
fire, flames - *see also* Fire
conflagration - *see* Conflagration
firearm missile - *see* Shooting
forging (metalworking) machine
E919.3
forklift (truck) E919.2
agricultural operations E919.0
mining operations E919.1
gas turbine E919.5
harvester E919.0
hay derrick, mower, or rake
E919.0

Accident *(Continued)*
caused by, due to *(Continued)*
heat (excessive) (*see also* Heat)
E900.9
hoist (*see also* Accident, caused by,
due to, lift) E919.2
chain - *see* Accident, caused by,
due to, chain
shaft E919.1
hot
liquid E924.0
caustic or corrosive E924.1
object (not producing fire or
flames) E924.8
substance E924.9
caustic or corrosive E924.1
liquid (metal) NEC E924.0
specified type NEC E924.8
human bite E928.3
ignition - *see* Ignition E919.4
internal combustion engine
E919.5
landslide NEC E909.2
lathe (metalworking) E919.3
turnings E920.8
woodworking E919.4
lift, lifting (appliances) E919.2
agricultural operations
E919.0
mining operations E919.1
shaft E919.1
lightning NEC E907
machine, machinery - *see also*
Accident, machine
drilling, metal E919.3
manufacturing, for manufacture
of steam
beverages E919.8
clothing E919.8
foodstuffs E919.8
paper E919.8
textiles E919.8
milling, metal E919.3
moulding E919.4
power press, metal E919.3
printing E919.8
rolling mill, metal E919.3
sawing, metal E919.3
specified type NEC E919.8
spinning E919.8
weaving E919.8
natural factor NEC E928.9
overhead plane E919.4
plane E920.4
overhead E919.4
powered
hand tool NEC E920.1
saw E919.4
hand E920.1
printing machine E919.8
pulley (block) E919.2
agricultural operations
E919.0
mining operations E919.1
transmission E919.6
radial saw E919.4
radiation - *see* Radiation
reaper E919.0
road scraper E919.7
when in transport under its own
power - *see* categories
E810–E825
roller, coaster E919.8
sander E919.4

E CODES

Accident *(Continued)*
  caused by, due to *(Continued)*
    saw E920.4
      band E919.4
      bench E919.4
      chain E920.1
      circular E919.4
      hand E920.4
        powered E920.1
      powered, except hand E919.4
      radial E919.4
    sawing machine, metal E919.3
    shaft
      hoist E919.1
      lift E919.1
      transmission E919.6
    shears E920.4
      hand E920.4
        powered E920.1
      mechanical E919.3
    shovel E920.4
      steam E919.7
    spinning machine E919.8
    steam - *see also* Burning, steam
      engine E919.5
      shovel E919.7
    thresher E919.0
    thunderbolt NEC E907
    tractor E919.0
      when in transport under its own
        power - *see* categories
        E810–E825
    transmission belt, cable, chain, gear,
      pinion, pulley, shaft E919.6
    turbine (gas) (water driven) E919.5
    under-cutter E919.1
    weaving machine E919.8
    winch E919.2
      agricultural operations E919.0
      mining operations E919.1
  diving E883.0
    with insufficient air supply E913.2
  glider (hang) *(see also* Collision,
    aircraft, unpowered) E842●
  hovercraft
    on
      land - *see* Accident, motor
        vehicle
      water - *see* Accident, watercraft
  ice yacht *(see also* Accident, vehicle
    NEC) E848
  in
    medical, surgical procedure
      as, or due to misadventure - *see*
        Misadventure
      causing an abnormal reaction or
        later complication without
        mention of misadventure - *see*
        Reaction, abnormal
  kite carrying a person *(see also* Collision,
    involving aircraft, unpowered)
    E842●
  land yacht *(see also* Accident, vehicle
    NEC) E848
  late effect of - *see* Late effect
  launching pad E845●
  machine, machinery *(see also* Accident,
    caused by, due to, by specific type
    of machine) E919.9
    agricultural including animal-
      powered premises E919.0
    earth-drilling E919.1
    earth moving or scraping E919.7
    excavating E919.7

Accident *(Continued)*
  machine, machinery *(Continued)*
    involving transport under own
      power on highway or transport
      vehicle - *see* categories E810-
      E825, E840-E845
    lifting (appliances) E919.2
    metalworking E919.3
    mining E919.1
    prime movers, except electric
      motors E919.5
      electric motors - *see* Accident,
        machine, by specific type of
        machine
    recreational E919.8
    specified type NEC E919.8
    transmission E919.6
    watercraft (deck) (engine room)
      (galley) (laundry) (loading)
      E836●
    woodworking or forming E919.4
  motor vehicle (on public highway)
    (traffic) E819●
    due to cataclysm - *see* categories
      E908, E909
    involving
      collision *(see also* Collision, motor
        vehicle) E812●
    nontraffic, not on public highway -
      see categories E820–E825
    not involving collision - *see*
      categories E816–E819
  nonmotor vehicle NEC E829●
    nonroad - *see* Accident, vehicle NEC
    road, except pedal cycle, animal-
      drawn vehicle, or animal being
      ridden E829●
  nonroad vehicle NEC - *see* Accident,
    vehicle NEC
  not elsewhere classifiable involving
    cable car (not on rails) E847
      on rails E829●
    coal car in mine E846
    hand truck - *see* Accident, vehicle
      NEC
    logging car E846
    sled(ge), meaning snow or ice
      vehicle E848
    tram, mine or quarry E846
    truck
      mine or quarry E846
      self-propelled, industrial E846
      station baggage E846
    tub, mine or quarry E846
    vehicle NEC E848
      snow and ice E848
      used only on industrial premises
        E846
    wheelbarrow E848
  occurring (at) (in)
    apartment E849.0
    baseball field, diamond E849.4
    construction site, any E849.3
    dock E849.8
      yard E849.3
    dormitory E849.7
    factory (building) (premises) E849.3
    farm E849.1
      buildings E849.1
      house E849.0
    football field E849.4
    forest E849.8
    garage (place of work) E849.3
      private (home) E849.0

Accident *(Continued)*
  occurring *(Continued)*
    gravel pit E849.2
    gymnasium E849.4
    highway E849.5
    home (private) (residential) E849.0
      institutional E849.7
    hospital E849.7
    hotel E849.6
    house (private) (residential) E849.0
      movie E849.6
      public E849.6
    institution, residential E849.7
    jail E849.7
    mine E849.2
    motel E849.6
    movie house E849.6
    office (building) E849.6
    orphanage E849.7
    park (public) E849.4
      mobile home E849.8
      trailer E849.8
    parking lot or place E849.8
    place
      industrial NEC E849.3
      parking E849.8
      public E849.8
        specified place NEC E849.5
      recreational NEC E849.4
      sport NEC E849.4
    playground (park) (school) E849.4
    prison E849.6
    public building NEC E849.6
    quarry E849.2
    railway
      line NEC E849.8
      yard E849.3
    residence
      home (private) E849.0
    resort (beach) (lake) (mountain)
      (seashore) (vacation) E849.4
    restaurant E849.6
    sand pit E849.2
    school (building) (private) (public)
      (state) E849.6
      reform E849.7
      riding E849.4
    seashore E849.8
      resort E849.4
    shop (place of work) E849.3
      commercial E849.6
    skating rink E849.4
    sports palace E849.4
    stadium E849.4
    store E849.6
    street E849.5
    swimming pool (public) E849.4
      private home or garden E849.0
    tennis court E849.4 public
    theatre, theater E849.6
    trailer court E849.8
    tunnel E849.8
      under construction E849.2
    warehouse E849.3
    yard
      dock E849.3
      industrial E849.3
      private (home) E849.0
      railway E849.3
  off-road type motor vehicle (not on
    public highway) NEC E821●
    on public highway - *see* categories
      E810–E819
  pedal cycle E826●

◄ New   ◄▥ Revised   ~~deleted~~ Deleted   ● Use Additional Digit(s)   ▥ Omit code

Accident (*Continued*)
railway E807●
due to cataclysm - *see* categories E908, E909
involving
burning by engine, locomotive, train (*see also* Explosion, railway engine) E803●
collision (*see also* Collision, railway) E800●
derailment (*see also* Derailment, railway) E802●
explosion (*see also* Explosion, railway engine) E803●
fall (*see also* Fall, from, railway rolling stock) E804●
fire (*see also* Explosion, railway engine) E803●
hitting by, being struck by
object falling in, on, from, rolling stock, train, vehicle E806●
rolling stock, train, vehicle E805●
overturning, railway rolling stock, train, vehicle (*see also* Derailment, railway) E802●
running off rails, railway (*see also* Derailment, railway) E802●
specified circumstances NEC E806●
train or vehicle hit by
avalanche E909.2
falling object (earth, rock, tree) E806●
due to cataclysm - *see* categories E908, E909
landslide E909.2
roller skate E885.1
scooter (nonmotorized) E885.0
skateboard E885.2
ski(ing) E885.3
jump E884.9
lift or tow (with chair or gondola) E847
snow vehicle, motor driven (not on public highway) E820●
on public highway - *see* categories E810–E819
snowboard E885.4
spacecraft E845●
specified cause NEC E928.8
street car E829●
traffic NEC E819●
vehicle NEC (with pedestrian) E848
battery powered
airport passenger vehicle E846
truck (baggage) (mail) E846
powered commercial or industrial (with other vehicle or object within commercial or industrial premises) E846
watercraft E838●
with
drowning or submersion resulting from
accident other than to watercraft E832●
accident to watercraft E830●
injury, except drowning or submersion, resulting from
accident other than to watercraft - *see* categories E833–E838
accident to watercraft E831●

Accident (*Continued*)
watercraft (*Continued*)
due to, caused by cataclysm - *see* categories E908, E909
machinery E836●
Acid throwing E961
Acosta syndrome E902.0
Activity (involving) E030
aerobic and step exercise (class) E009.2
alpine skiing E003.2
animal care NEC E019.9
arts and handcrafts NEC E012.9
athletics NEC E008.9
played
as a team or group NEC E007.9
individually NEC E006.9
baking E015.2
ballet E005.0
barbells E010.2
BASE (Building, Antenna, Span, Earth) jumping E004.2
baseball E007.3
basketball E007.6
bathing (personal) E013.0
beach volleyball E007.7
bike riding E006.4
boogie boarding E002.7
bowling E006.3
boxing E008.0
brass instrument playing E018.3
building and construction E016.2
bungee jumping E004.3
calisthenics E009.1
canoeing (in calm and turbulent water) E002.5
capture the flag E007.8
cardiorespiratory exercise NEC E009.9
caregiving (providing) NEC E014.9
bathing E014.0
lifting E014.1
cellular
communication device E011.1
telephone E011.1
challenge course E009.4
cheerleading E005.4
circuit training E009.3
cleaning
floor E013.4
climbing NEC E004.9
mountain E004.0
rock E004.0
wall climbing E004.0
combatives E008.4
computer
keyboarding E011.0
technology NEC E011.9
confidence course E009.4
construction (building) E016.2
cooking and baking E015.2
cooking and grilling NEC E015.9
cool down exercises E009.1
cricket E007.9
crocheting E012.0
cross country skiing E003.3
dancing (all types) E005.0
digging
dirt E016.0
dirt digging E016.0
dishwashing E015.0
diving (platform) (springboard) E002.1
underwater E002.4

Activity (*Continued*)
dodge ball E007.8
downhill skiing E003.2
drum playing E018.1
dumbbells E010.2
electronic
devices NEC E011.9
hand held interactive E011.1
game playing (using) (with)
interactive device E011.1
keyboard or other stationary device E011.0
elliptical machine E009.0
exercise(s)
machines ((primarily) for)
cardiorespiratory conditioning E009.0
muscle strengthening E010.0
muscle strengthening (non-machine) NEC E010.9
external motion NEC E017.9
rollercoaster E017.0
field hockey E007.4
figure skating (pairs) (singles) E003.0
flag football E007.1
floor mopping and cleaning E013.4
food preparation and clean up E015.0
football (American) NOS E007.0
flag E007.1
tackle E007.0
touch E007.1
four square E007.8
free weights E010.2
frisbee (ultimate) E008.3
furniture
building E012.2
finishing E012.2
repair E012.2
game playing (electronic)
using
interactive device E011.1
keyboard or other stationary device E011.0
gardening E016.1
golf E006.2
grass drills E009.5
grilling and smoking food E015.1
grooming and shearing an animal E019.2
guerilla drills E009.5
gymnastics (rhythmic) E005.2
handball E008.2
handcrafts NEC E012.9
hand held interactive electronic device E011.1
hang gliding E004.4
hiking (on level or elevated terrain) E001.0
hockey (ice) E003.1
field E007.4
horseback riding E006.1
household maintenance NEC E013.9
ice NEC E003.9
dancing E003.0
hockey E003.1
skating E003.0
inline roller skating E006.0
ironing E013.3
judo E008.4

E CODES

Activity *(Continued)*
jumping (off) NEC E004.9 ◀
    BASE (Building, Antenna, Span,
      Earth) E004.2 ◀
    bungee E004.3 ◀
    jacks E009.1 ◀
    rope E006.5 ◀
jumping jacks E009.1 ◀
jumping rope E006.5 ◀
karate E008.4 ◀
kayaking (in calm and turbulent
    water) E002.5 ◀
keyboarding (computer) E011.0 ◀
kickball E007.8 ◀
knitting E012.0 ◀
lacrosse E007.4 ◀
land maintenance NEC E016.9 ◀
landscaping E016.1 ◀
laundry E013.1 ◀
machines (exercise) primarily for
    cardiorespiratory conditioning
    E009.0 ◀
maintenance
    building E016.9 ◀
    household NEC E013.9 ◀
    land E016.9 ◀
    property E016.9 ◀
marching (on level or elevated
    terrain) E001.0 ◀
martial arts E008.4 ◀
microwave oven E015.2 ◀
mopping (floor) E013.4 ◀
mountain climbing E004.0 ◀
milking an animal E019.1 ◀
muscle strengthening
    exercises (non-machine)
      NEC E010.9 ◀
    machines E010.0 ◀
musical keyboard (electronic)
    playing E018.0 ◀
nordic skiing E003.3 ◀
obstacle course E009.4 ◀
oven (microwave) E015.2 ◀
packing up and unpacking in moving
    to a new residence E013.5 ◀
parasailing E002.9 ◀
percussion instrument playing NEC
    E018.1 ◀
personal
    bathing and showering E013.0 ◀
    hygiene NEC E013.8 ◀
    showering E013.0 ◀
physical ◀
    games generally associated with
      school recess, summer camp
      and children 007.8 ◀
    training NEC E009.9 ◀
piano playing E018.0 ◀
pilates E010.3 ◀
platform diving E002.1 ◀
playing musical instrument
    brass instrument E018.3 ◀
    drum E018.1 ◀
    musical keyboard (electronic)
      E018.0 ◀
    percussion instrument NEC
      E018.1 ◀
    piano E018.0 ◀
    string instrument E018.2 ◀
    wind instrument E018.3 ◀
property maintenance NEC E016.9 ◀
pruning (garden and lawn) E016.1 ◀
pull-ups E010.1 ◀
push-ups E010.1 ◀
racquetball E008.2 ◀

Activity *(Continued)*
rafting (in calm and turbulent
    water) E002.5 ◀
raking (leaves) E016.0 ◀
rappelling E004.1 ◀
refereeing a sports activity E029.0 ◀
residential relocation E013.5 ◀
rhythmic
    gymnastics E005.2 ◀
    movement NEC E005.9 ◀
riding
    horseback E006.1 ◀
    rollercoaster E017.0 ◀
rock climbing E004.0 ◀
rollercoaster riding E017.0 ◀
roller skating (inline) E006.0 ◀
rough housing and horseplay E029.2 ◀
rowing (in calm and turbulent
    water) E002.5 ◀
rugby E007.2 ◀
running E001.1 ◀
SCUBA diving E002.4 ◀
sewing E012.1 ◀
shoveling E016.0 ◀
    dirt E016.0 ◀
    snow E016.0 ◀
showering (personal) E013.0 ◀
sit-ups E010.1 ◀
skateboarding E006.0 ◀
skating (ice) E003.0 ◀
    roller E006.0 ◀
skiing (alpine) (downhill) E003.2 ◀
    cross country E003.3 ◀
    nordic E003.3 ◀
sledding (snow) E003.2 ◀
smoking and grilling food E015.1 ◀
snorkeling E002.4 ◀
snow NEC E003.9 ◀
    boarding E003.2 ◀
    shoveling E016.0 ◀
    sledding E003.2 ◀
    tubing E003.2 ◀
soccer E007.5 ◀
softball E007.3 ◀
specified NEC E029.9 ◀
spectator at an event E029.1 ◀
sports NEC E008.9 ◀
sports played as a team or group
    NEC E007.9 ◀
sports played individually NEC
    E006.9 ◀
springboard diving E002.1 ◀
squash E008.2 ◀
stationary bike E009.0 ◀
step (stepping) exercise (class)
    E009.2 ◀
stepper machine E009.0 ◀
stove E015.2 ◀
string instrument playing E018.2 ◀
surfing E002.7 ◀
swimming E002.0 ◀
tackle football E007.0 ◀
tap dancing E005.0 ◀
tennis E008.2 ◀
tobogganing E003.2 ◀
touch football E007.1 ◀
track and field events
    (non-running) E006.6 ◀
    running E001.1 ◀
trampoline E005.3 ◀
treadmill E009.0 ◀
trimming shrubs E016.1 ◀
tubing (in calm and turbulent water)
    E002.5 ◀
    snow E003.2 ◀

Activity *(Continued)*
ultimate frisbee E008.3 ◀
underwater diving E002.4 ◀
unpacking in moving to a new
    residence E013.5 ◀
use of stove, oven and microwave
    oven E015.2 ◀
vacuuming E013.2 ◀
volleyball (beach) (court) E007.7 ◀
wake boarding E002.6 ◀
walking an animal E019.0 ◀
walking (on level or elevated
    terrain) E001.0 ◀
    an animal E019.0 ◀
wall climbing E004.0 ◀
warm up and cool down
    exercises E009.1 ◀
water NEC E002.9 ◀
    aerobics E002.3 ◀
    craft NEC E002.9 ◀
    exercise E002.3 ◀
    polo E002.2 ◀
    skiing E002.6 ◀
    sliding E002.8 ◀
    survival training and testing
      E002.9 ◀
weeding (garden and lawn) E016.1 ◀
wind instrument playing E018.3 ◀
windsurfing E002.7 ◀
wrestling E008.1 ◀
yoga E005.1 ◀
Activity status E000.9 ◀
civilian ◀
    done for
      financial or other compensation
        E000.0 ◀
        pay or income E000.0 ◀
    for income E000.0 ◀
    hobby or leisure E000.8 ◀
    off duty military E000.8 ◀
    military E000.1 ◀
      off duty E000.8 ◀
    recreation E000.8 ◀
    specified NEC E000.8 ◀
    sport not for income E000.8 ◀
    student E000.8 ◀
    volunteer E000.8 ◀
Aeroneurosis E902.1
Aero-otitis media - *see* Effects of, air
    pressure
Aerosinusitis - *see* Effects of, air pressure
After-effect, late - *see* Late effect
Air
    blast
      in
        terrorism E979.2
        war operations E993.9 ◀
    embolism (traumatic) NEC E928.9
      in
        infusion or transfusion E874.1
        perfusion E874.2
    sickness E903
Alpine sickness E902.0
Altitude sickness - *see* Effects of, air
    pressure
Anaphylactic shock, anaphylaxis *(see also*
    Table of Drugs and Chemicals)
    E947.9
    due to bite or sting (venomous) - *see*
      Bite, venomous
Andes disease E902.0
Apoplexy
    heat - *see* Heat
Arachnidism E905.1
Arson E968.0

◀ New   ◀▥ Revised   ~~deleted~~ Deleted   ● Use Additional Digit(s)   ▥ Omit code

E CODES

Asphyxia, asphyxiation
  by
    chemical
      in
        terrorism E979.7
        war operations E997.2
    explosion - *see* Explosion E965.8
    food (bone) (regurgitated food)
      (seed) E911
    foreign object, except food E912
    fumes
      in
        terrorism (chemical weapons)
          E979.7
        war operations E997.2
    gas - *see also* Table of Drugs and
      Chemicals
      in
        terrorism E979.7
        war operations E997.2
      legal
        execution E978
        intervention (tear) E972
      tear E972
    mechanical means (*see also*
      Suffocation) E913.9
  from
    conflagration - *see* Conflagration
    fire - *see also* Fire E899
      in
        terrorism E979.3
        war operations E990.9
    ignition - *see* Ignition
Aspiration
  foreign body - *see* Foreign body,
    aspiration
  mucus, not of newborn (with asphyxia,
    obstruction respiratory passage,
    suffocation) E912
  phlegm (with asphyxia, obstruction
    respiratory passage, suffocation)
    E912
  vomitus (with asphyxia, obstruction
    respiratory passage, suffocation)
    (*see also* Foreign body, aspiration,
    food) E911
Assassination (attempt) (*see also* Assault)
  E968.9
Assault (homicidal) (by) (in) E968.9
  acid E961
    swallowed E962.1
  air gun E968.6
  BB gun E968.6
  bite NEC E968.8
    of human being E968.7
  bomb ((placed in) car or house) E965.8
    antipersonnel E965.5
    letter E965.7
    petrol E965.6
  brawl (hand) (fists) (foot) E960.0
  burning, burns (by fire) E968.0
    acid E961
      swallowed E962.1
    caustic, corrosive substance E961
      swallowed E962.1
    chemical from swallowing caustic,
      corrosive substance NEC
      E962.1
    hot liquid E968.3
    scalding E968.3
    vitriol E961
      swallowed E962.1
  caustic, corrosive substance E961
    swallowed E962.1
  cut, any part of body E966

Assault *(Continued)*
  dagger E966
  drowning E964
  explosives E965.9
    bomb (*see also* Assault, bomb) E965.8
    dynamite E965.8
  fight (hand) (fists) (foot) E960.0
    with weapon E968.9
      blunt or thrown E968.2
      cutting or piercing E966
      firearm - *see* Shooting, homicide
  fire E968.0
  firearm(s) - *see* Shooting, homicide
  garrotting E963
  gunshot (wound) - *see* Shooting,
    homicide
  hanging E963
  injury NEC E968.9
  knife E966
  late effect of E969
  ligature E963
  poisoning E962.9
    drugs or medicinals E962.0
    gas(es) or vapors, except drugs and
      medicinals E962.2
    solid or liquid substances, except
      drugs and medicinals
      E962.1
  puncture, any part of body E966
  pushing
    before moving object, train, vehicle
      E968.5
    from high place E968.1
  rape E960.1
  scalding E968.3
  shooting - *see* Shooting, homicide
  sodomy E960.1
  stab, any part of body E966
  strangulation E963
  submersion E964
  suffocation E963
  transport vehicle E968.5
  violence NEC E968.9
  vitriol E961
    swallowed E962.1
  weapon E968.9
    blunt or thrown E968.2
    cutting or piercing E966
    firearm - *see* Shooting, homicide
  wound E968.9
    cutting E966
    gunshot - *see* Shooting, homicide
    knife E966
    piercing E966
    puncture E966
    stab E966
Attack by animal NEC E906.9
Avalanche E909.2
  falling on or hitting
    motor vehicle (in motion) (on public
      highway) E909.2
    railway train E909.2
Aviators' disease E902.1

B

Barotitis, barodontalgia, berosinusitis,
  barotrauma (otitic) (sinus) - *see*
  Effects of, air pressure
Battered
  baby or child (syndrome) - *see* Abuse,
    child; category E967
  person other than baby or child - *see*
    Assault

Bayonet wound (*see also* Cut, by bayonet)
  E920.3
  in
    legal intervention E974
    terrorism E979.8
    war operations E995.2
Bean in nose E912
Bed set on fire NEC E898.0
Beheading (by guillotine)
  homicide E966
  legal execution E978
Bending, injury in E927.8
Bends E902.0
Bite
  animal NEC E906.5
    other specified (except arthropod)
      E906.3
    venomous NEC E905.9
  arthropod (nonvenomous) NEC E906.4
    venomous - *see* Sting
  black widow spider E905.1
  cat E906.3
  centipede E905.4
  cobra E905.0
  copperhead snake E905.0
  coral snake E905.0
  dog E906.0
  fer de lance E905.0
  gila monster E905.0
  human being
    accidental E928.3
    assault E968.7
  insect (nonvenomous) E906.4
    venomous - *see* Sting
  krait E905.0
  late effect of - *see* Late effect
  lizard E906.2
    venomous E905.0
  mamba E905.0
  marine animal
    nonvenomous E906.3
      snake E906.2
    venomous E905.6
      snake E905.0
  millipede E906.4
    venomous E905.4
  moray eel E906.3
  rat E906.1
  rattlesnake E905.0
  rodent, except rat E906.3
  serpent - *see* Bite, snake
  shark E906.3
  snake (venomous) E905.0
    nonvenomous E906.2
    sea E905.0
  spider E905.1
    nonvenomous E906.4
  tarantula (venomous) E905.1
  venomous NEC E905.9
    by specific animal - *see* category
      E905
  viper E905.0
  water moccasin E905.0
Blast (air)
  in
    terrorism E979.2
      from nuclear explosion E979.5
      underwater E979.0
    war operations E993.9
      from nuclear explosion (*see
        also* War operations,
        injury due to, nuclear
        weapons) E996.0
      underwater E992.9
Blizzard E908.3

Blow E928.9
  by law-enforcing agent, police (on
      duty) E975
    with blunt object (baton)
        (nightstick) (stave)
        (truncheon) E973
Blowing up (see also Explosion) E923.9
Brawl (hand) (fists) (foot) E960.0
Breakage (accidental)
  cable of cable car not on rails E847
  ladder (causing fall) E881.0
  part (any) of
    animal-drawn vehicle E827●
    ladder (causing fall) E881.0
    motor vehicle
      in motion (on public highway)
          E818●
        not on public highway
            E825●
    nonmotor road vehicle, except
        animal-drawn vehicle or pedal
        cycle E829●
    off-road type motor vehicle (not
        on public highway)
        NEC E821●
      on public highway E818●
    pedal cycle E826●
    scaffolding (causing fall) E881.1
    snow vehicle, motor-driven (not on
        public highway) E820●
      on public highway E818●
    vehicle NEC - see Accident, vehicle
Broken
  glass
    fall on E888.0
    injury by E920.8
  power line (causing electric shock)
      E925.1
Bumping against, into (accidentally)
  object (moving) E917.9
    caused by crowd E917.1
      with subsequent fall E917.6
    furniture E917.3
      with subsequent fall E917.7
    in
      running water E917.2
      sports E917.0
        with subsequent fall E917.5
    stationary E917.4
      with subsequent fall E917.8
  person(s) E917.9
    with fall E886.9
      in sports E886.0
    as, or caused by, a crowd E917.1
      with subsequent fall E917.6
    in sports E917.0
      with fall E886.0
Burning, burns (accidental) (by) (from)
    (on) E899
  acid (any kind) E924.1
    swallowed - see Table of Drugs and
        Chemicals
  airgun E928.7 ◀
  bedclothes (see also Fire, specified NEC)
      E898.0
  blowlamp (see also Fire, specified NEC)
      E898.1
  blowtorch (see also Fire, specified NEC)
      E898.1
  boat, ship, watercraft - see categories
      E830, E831, E837
  bonfire (controlled) E897
    uncontrolled E892
  candle (see also Fire, specified NEC)
      E898.1

Burning, burns (Continued)
  caustic liquid, substance E924.1
    swallowed - see Table of Drugs and
        Chemicals
  chemical E924.1
    from swallowing caustic, corrosive
        substance - see Table of Drugs
        and Chemicals
    in
      terrorism E979.7
      war operations E997.2
  cigar(s) or cigarette(s) (see also Fire,
      specified NEC) E898.1
  clothes, clothing, nightdress - see
      Ignition, clothes
    with conflagration - see
        Conflagration
  conflagration - see Conflagration
  corrosive liquid, substance
      E924.1
    swallowed - see Table of Drugs
        and Chemicals
  electric current (see also Electric shock)
      E925.9
  fire, flames (see also Fire) E899
  firearm E928.7 ◀
  flare, Verey pistol E922.8
  heat
    from appliance (electrical) E924.8
    in local application, or packing
        during medical or surgical
        procedure E873.5
  homicide (attempt) (see also Assault,
      burning) E968.0
  hot
    liquid E924.0
      caustic or corrosive E924.1
    object (not producing fire or flames)
        E924.8
    substance E924.9
      caustic or corrosive E924.1
      liquid (metal) NEC E924.0
      specified type NEC E924.8
    tap water E924.2
  ignition - see also Ignition
    clothes, clothing, nightdress - see also
        Ignition, clothes
      with conflagration - see
          Conflagration
    highly inflammable material
        (benzine) (fat) (gasoline)
        (kerosine) (paraffin) (petrol)
        E894
  inflicted by other person
    stated as
      homicidal, intentional (see also
          Assault, burning) E968.0
      undetermined whether
          accidental or intentional
          (see also Burn, stated as
          undetermined whether
          accidental or intentional)
          E988.1
  internal, from swallowed caustic,
      corrosive liquid, substance - see
      Table of Drugs and Chemicals
  in
    terrorism E979.3
      from nuclear explosion E979.5
      petrol bomb E979.3
    war operations (from fire-producing
        device or conventional
        weapon) E990.9
      from nuclear explosion (see
          also War operations,
          injury due to, nuclear
          weapons) E996.2 ◀▥

Burning, burns (Continued)
  in (Continued)
    war operations (Continued)
      incendiary bomb E990.0 ◀
      petrol bomb E990.0
  lamp (see also Fire, specified NEC)
      E898.1
  late effect of NEC E929.4
  lighter (cigar) (cigarette) (see also Fire,
      specified NEC) E898.1
  lightning E907
  liquid (boiling) (hot) (molten)
      E924.0
    caustic, corrosive (external)
        E924.1
      swallowed - see Table of Drugs
          and Chemicals
  local application of externally applied
      substance in medical or surgical
      care E873.5
  machinery - see Accident, machine
  matches (see also Fire, specified NEC)
      E898.1
  medicament, externally applied
      E873.5
  metal, molten E924.0
  object (hot) E924.8
    producing fire or flames - see Fire
  oven (electric) (gas) E924.8
  pipe (smoking) (see also Fire, specified
      NEC) E898.1
  radiation - see Radiation
  railway engine, locomotive, train (see
      also Explosion, railway engine)
      E803●
  self-inflicted (unspecified whether
      accidental or intentional)
      E988.1
    caustic or corrosive substance NEC
        E988.7
    stated as intentional, purposeful
        E958.1
      caustic or corrosive substance
          NEC E958.7
    stated as undetermined whether
        accidental or intentional
        E988.1
      caustic or corrosive substance NEC
          E988.7
  steam E924.0
    pipe E924.8
  substance (hot) E924.9
    boiling or molten E924.0
    caustic, corrosive (external)
        E924.1
      swallowed - see Table of Drugs
          and Chemicals
  suicidal (attempt) NEC E958.1
    caustic substance E958.7
    late effect of E959
  tanning bed E926.2
  therapeutic misadventure
      overdose of radiation E873.2
  torch, welding (see also Fire, specified
      NEC) E898.1
  trash fire (see also Burning, bonfire)
      E897
  vapor E924.0
  vitriol E924.1
  x-rays E926.3
    in medical, surgical procedure - see
        Misadventure, failure, in
        dosage, radiation
        operations
Butted by animal E906.8

◀ New   ◀▥ Revised   ~~deleted~~ Deleted   ● Use Additional Digit(s)   ▥ Omit code

E CODES

C

Cachexia, lead or saturnine E866.0
  from pesticide NEC (see also Table of Drugs and Chemicals) E863.4
Caisson disease E902.2
Capital punishment (any means) E978
Car sickness E903
Casualty (not due to war) NEC E928.9
  terrorism E979.8
  war (see also War operations) E995.9 ◀▥
Cat
  bite E906.3
  scratch E906.8
Cataclysmic (any injury)
  earth surface movement or eruption E909.9
    specified type NEC E909.8
  storm or flood resulting from storm E908.9
    specified type NEC E909.8
Catching fire - see Ignition
Caught
  between
    objects (moving) (stationary and moving) E918
      and machinery - see Accident, machine
  by cable car, not on rails E847
  in
    machinery (moving parts of) - see Accident, machine
    object E918
Cave-in (causing asphyxia, suffocation (by pressure)) (see also Suffocation, due to, cave-in) E913.3
  with injury other than asphyxia or suffocation E916
    with asphyxia or suffocation (see also Suffocation, due to, cave-in) E913.3
  struck or crushed by E916
    with asphyxia or suffocation (see also Suffocation, due to, cave-in) E913.3
Change(s) in air pressure - see also Effects of, air pressure
  sudden, in aircraft (ascent) (descent) (causing aeroneurosis or aviators' disease) E902.1
Chilblains E901.0
  due to manmade conditions E901.1
Choking (on) (any object except food or vomitus) E912
  apple E911
  bone E911
  food, any type (regurgitated) E911
  mucus or phlegm E912
  seed E911
Civil insurrection - see War operations
Cloudburst E908.8
Cold, exposure to (accidental) (excessive) (extreme) (place) E901.9
  causing chilblains or immersion foot E901.0
  due to
    manmade conditions E901.1
    specified cause NEC E901.8
    weather (conditions) E901.0
  late effect of NEC E929.5
  self-inflicted (undetermined whether accidental or intentional) E988.3
    suicidal E958.3
  suicide E958.3

Colic, lead, painters', or saturnine - see category E866
Collapse
  building E916
    burning (uncontrolled fire) E891.8
      in terrorism E979.3
      private E890.8
  dam E909.3
  due to heat - see Heat
  machinery - see Accident, machine or vehicle
  man-made structure E909.3
  postoperative NEC E878.9
  structure
    burning (uncontrolled fire) NEC E891.8
    in terrorism E979.3
Collision (accidental)

Note 80 In the case of collisions between different types of vehicles, persons and objects, priority in classification is in the following order:

> Aircraft
> Watercraft
> Motor vehicle
> Railway vehicle
> Pedal cycle
> Animal-drawn vehicle
> Animal being ridden
> Streetcar or other
>   nonmotor road vehicle
> Other vehicle
> Pedestrian or person using
>   pedestrian conveyance
> Object (except where falling from
>   or set in motion by vehicle, etc.
>   listed above)

In the listing below, the combinations are listed only under the vehicle, etc., having priority. For definitions, see Supplementary Classification of External Causes of Injury and Poisoning (E800–E999).

---

aircraft (with object or vehicle) (fixed) (movable) (moving) E841●
  with
    person (while landing, taking off) (without accident to aircraft) E844●
    powered (in transit) (with unpowered aircraft) E841●
      while landing, taking off E840●
    unpowered E842●
    while landing, taking off E840●
animal being ridden (in sport or transport) E828●
  and
    animal (being ridden) (herded) (unattended) E828●
    nonmotor road vehicle, except pedal cycle or animal-drawn vehicle E828●
    object (fallen) (fixed) (movable) (moving) not falling from or set in motion by vehicle of higher priority E828●
    pedestrian (conveyance or vehicle) E828●
animal-drawn vehicle E827●
  and
    animal (being ridden) (herded) (unattended) E827●

Collision (Continued)
  animal-drawn vehicle (Continued)
    and (Continued)
      nonmotor road vehicle, except pedal cycle E827●
      object (fallen) (fixed) (movable) (moving) not falling from or set in motion by vehicle of higher priority E827●
      pedestrian (conveyance or vehicle) E827●
      streetcar E827●
  motor vehicle (on public highway) (traffic accident) E812●
    after leaving, running off, public highway (without antecedent collision) (without re-entry) E816●
    with antecedent collision on public highway - see categories E810–E815
    with re-entrance collision with another motor vehicle E811●
  and
    abutment (bridge) (overpass) E815●
    animal (herded) (unattended) E815●
      carrying person, property E813●
    animal-drawn vehicle E813●
    another motor vehicle (abandoned) (disabled) (parked) (stalled) (stopped) E812●
      with, involving re-entrance (on same roadway) (across median strip) E811●
    any object, person, or vehicle off the public highway resulting from a noncollision motor vehicle nontraffic accident E816●
    avalanche, fallen or not moving E815●
      falling E909.2
    boundary fence E815●
    culvert E815●
    fallen
      stone E815●
      tree E815●
    guard post or guard rail E815●
    inter-highway divider E815●
    landslide, fallen or not moving E815●
      moving E909.2
    machinery (road) E815●
    nonmotor road vehicle NEC E813●
    object (any object, person, or vehicle off the public highway resulting from a noncollision motor vehicle nontraffic accident) E815●
    off, normally not on, public highway resulting from a noncollision motor vehicle traffic accident E816●
    pedal cycle E813●
    pedestrian (conveyance) E814●
    person (using pedestrian conveyance) E814●

E CODES

Collision *(Continued)*
  vehicle *(Continued)*
    nonmotor *(Continued)*
      nonroad *(Continued)*
        and *(Continued)*
          object (fallen) (fixed) (movable) (moving) not falling from or set in motion by aircraft, animal-drawn vehicle, animal being ridden, motor vehicle, nonmotor road vehicle, pedal cycle, railway train, or streetcar E848
        road, except animal being ridden, animal-drawn vehicle, or pedal cycle E829●
        and
          animal, herded, not being ridden, unattended E829
          another nonmotor road vehicle, except animal being ridden, animal-drawn vehicle, or pedal cycle E829●
          object (fallen) (fixed) (movable) (moving) not falling from or set in motion by, aircraft, animal-drawn vehicle, animal being ridden, motor vehicle, pedal cycle, or railway train E829●
        pedestrian (conveyance) E829●
        person (using pedestrian conveyance) E829●
        vehicle, nonmotor, nonroad E829●
    watercraft E838●
    and
      person swimming or water skiing E838●
    causing
      drowning, submersion E830●
      injury except drowning, submersion E831
Combustion, spontaneous - *see* Ignition
Complication of medical or surgical procedure or treatment
  as an abnormal reaction - *see* Reaction, abnormal
  delayed, without mention of misadventure - *see* Reaction, abnormal
  due to misadventure - *see* Misadventure
Compression
  divers' squeeze E902.2
  trachea by
    food E911
    foreign body, except food E912
Conflagration
  building or structure, except private dwelling (barn) (church) (convalescent or residential home) (factory) (farm outbuilding) (hospital) (hotel) or (institution (educational) (dormitory) (residential)) (school) (shop) (store) (theatre) E891.9

Conflagration *(Continued)*
  building or structure, except private dwelling *(Continued)*
    with or causing (injury due to)
      accident or injury NEC E891.9
        specified circumstance NEC E891.8
      burns, burning E891.3
      carbon monoxide E891.2
      fumes E891.2
      polyvinylchloride (PVC) or similar material E891.1
      smoke E891.2
    causing explosion E891.0
    in terrorism E979.3
  not in building or structure E892
  private dwelling (apartment) (boarding house) (camping place) (caravan) (farmhouse) (home (private)) (house) (lodging house) (private garage) (rooming house) (tenement) E890.9
    with or causing (injury due to)
      accident or injury NEC E890.9
        specified circumstance NEC E890.8
      burns, burning E890.3
      carbon monoxide E890.2
      fumes E890.2
        polyvinylchloride (PVC) or similar material E890.1
      smoke E890.2
    causing explosion E890.0
Constriction, external
  caused by
    hair E928.4
    other object E928.5
Contact with
  dry ice E901.1
  liquid air, hydrogen, nitrogen E901.1
Cramp(s)
  heat - *see* Heat
  swimmers (*see also* category E910) 910.2
    not in recreation or sport E910.3
Cranking (car) (truck) (bus) (engine)
  injury by E917.9
Crash
  aircraft (in transit) (powered) E841●
    at landing, take-off E840●
    in
      terrorism E979.1
      war operations E994.9 ◀▪▪▪▪
    on runway NEC E840●
    stated as
      homicidal E968.8
      suicidal E958.6
      undetermined whether accidental or intentional E988.6
    unpowered E842●
  glider E842●
  motor vehicle - *see also* Accident, motor vehicle
    homicidal E968.5
    suicidal E958.5
    undetermined whether accidental or intentional E988.5
Crushed (accidentally) E928.9
  between
    boat(s), ship(s), watercraft (and dock or pier) (without accident to watercraft) E838●
    after accident to, or collision, watercraft E831●
    objects (moving) (stationary and moving) E918

Crushed *(Continued)*
  by
    avalanche NEC E909.2
    boat, ship, watercraft after accident to, collision, watercraft E831●
    cave-in E916
      with asphyxiation or suffocation (*see also* Suffocation, due to, cave-in) E913.3
    crowd, human stampede E917.1
    falling
      aircraft (*see also* Accident, aircraft) E841●
        in
          terrorism E979.1
          war operations E994.8 ◀▪▪▪▪
      earth, material E916
        with asphyxiation or suffocation (*see also* Suffocation, due to, cave-in) E913.3
      object E916
        on ship, watercraft E838●
        while loading, unloading watercraft E838●
    firearm E928.7 ◀
    landslide NEC E909.2
    lifeboat after abandoning ship E831●
    machinery - *see* Accident, machine
    railway rolling stock, train, vehicle (part of) E805●
    slide trigger mechanism, scope or other part of the gun E928.7 ◀
    street car E829●
    vehicle NEC - *see* Accident, vehicle NEC
  in
    machinery - *see* Accident, machine
    object E918
    transport accident - *see* categories E800–E848
  late effect of NEC E929.9
Cut, cutting (any part of body) (accidental) E920.9
  by
    arrow E920.8
    axe E920.4
    bayonet (*see also* Bayonet wound) E920.3
      in war operations E995.2 ◀
    blender E920.2
    broken glass E920.8
      following fall E888.0
    can opener E920.4
      powered E920.2
    chisel E920.4
    circular saw E919.4
    cutting or piercing instrument - *see also* category E920
      following fall E888.0
      late effect of E929.8
    dagger E920.3
    dart E920.8
    drill - *see* Accident, caused by drill
    edge of stiff paper E920.8
    electric
      beater E920.2
      fan E920.2
      knife E920.2
      mixer E920.2
    firearm component E928.7 ◀
    fork E920.4
    garden fork E920.4

E CODES

Cut, cutting (*Continued*)
  by (*Continued*)
    hand saw or tool (not powered) E920.4
      powered E920.1
    hedge clipper E920.4
      powered E920.1
    hoe E920.4
    ice pick E920.4
    knife E920.3
      electric E920.2
      in war operations E995.2 ◄
    lathe turnings E920.8
    lawn mower E920.4
      powered E920.0
      riding E919.8
    machine - *see* Accident, machine
    meat
      grinder E919.8
      slicer E919.8
    nails E920.8
    needle E920.4
      hypodermic E920.5
    object, edged, pointed, sharp - *see* category E920
    following fall E888.0
    paper cutter E920.4
    piercing instrument - *see also* category E920
    late effect of E929.8
    pitchfork E920.4
    powered
      can opener E920.2
      garden cultivator E920.1
        riding E919.8
      hand saw E920.1
      hand tool NEC E920.1
      hedge clipper E920.1
      household appliance or implement E920.2
      lawn mower (hand) E920.0
        riding E919.8
      rivet gun E920.1
      staple gun E920.1
    rake E920.4
    saw
      circular E919.4
      hand E920.4
    scissors E920.4
    screwdriver E920.4
    sewing machine (electric) (powered) E920.2
      not powered E920.4
    shears E920.4
    shovel E920.4
    slide trigger mechanism, scope or other part of gun E928.7 ◄
    spade E920.4
    splinters E920.8
    sword E920.3
      in war operations E995.2 ◄
    tin can lid E920.8
    wood slivers E920.8
  homicide (attempt) E966
  inflicted by other person
    stated as
      intentional, homicidal E966
      undetermined whether accidental or intentional E986
  late effect of NEC E929.8
  legal
    execution E978
    intervention E974

Cut, cutting (*Continued*)
  self-inflicted (unspecified whether accidental or intentional) E986
    stated as intentional, purposeful E956
    stated as undetermined whether accidental or intentional E986
  suicidal (attempt) E956
  terrorism E979.8
  war operations E995.2 ◄▌▌
Cyclone E908.1

D

Death due to injury occurring one year or more previous - *see* Late effect
Decapitation (accidental circumstances) NEC E928.9
  homicidal E966
  legal execution (by guillotine) E978
Deprivation - *see also* Privation action E913.3
  homicidal intent E968.4
Derailment (accidental)
  railway (rolling stock) (train) (vehicle) (with subsequent collision) E802●
    with
      collision (antecedent) (*see also* Collision, railway) E800●
      explosion (subsequent) (without antecedent collision) E802●
        antecedent collision E803●
      fall (without collision (antecedent)) E802●
      fire (without collision (antecedent)) E802●
  street car E829●
Descent
  parachute (voluntary) (without accident to aircraft) E844●
    due to accident to aircraft - *see* categories E840–E842
Desertion
  child, with intent to injure or kill E968.4
  helpless person, infant, newborn E904.0
    with intent to injure or kill E968.4
Destitution - *see* Privation
Dirty bomb (*see also* War operations, injury due to, nuclear weapons) E996.9 ◄
Disability, late effect or sequela of injury - *see* Late effect
Disease
  Andes E902.0
  aviators' E902.1
  caisson E902.2
  range E902.0
Divers' disease, palsy, paralysis, squeeze E902.0
Dog bite E906.0
Dragged by
  cable car (not on rails) E847
    on rails E829●
  motor vehicle (on highway) E814●
    not on highway, nontraffic accident E825●
  street car E829●
Drinking poison (accidental) - *see* Table of Drugs and Chemicals
Drowning - *see* Submersion
Dust in eye E914

E

Earth falling (on) (with asphyxia or suffocation (by pressure)) (*see also* Suffocation, due to, cave-in) E913.3
  as, or due to, a cataclysm (involving any transport vehicle) - *see* categories E908, E909
  not due to cataclysmic action E913.3
    motor vehicle (in motion) (on public highway) E813●
      not on public highway E825●
    nonmotor road vehicle NEC E829●
    pedal cycle E826●
    railway rolling stock, train, vehicle E806●
    street car E829●
    struck or crushed by E916
      with asphyxiation or suffocation E913.3
      with injury other than asphyxia, suffocation E916
Earthquake (any injury) E909.0
Effect(s) (adverse) of
  air pressure E902.9
    at high altitude E902.9
      in aircraft E902.1
      residence or prolonged visit (causing conditions classifiable to E902.0) E902.0
    due to
      diving E902.2
      specified cause NEC E902.8
    in aircraft E902.1
  cold, excessive (exposure to) (*see also* Cold, exposure to) E901.9
  heat (excessive) (*see also* Heat) E900.9
  hot
    place - *see* Heat
    weather E900.0
  insulation - *see* Heat
  late - *see* Late effect of
  motion E903
  nuclear explosion or weapon
    in
      terrorism E979.5
      war operations ~~(blast) (fireball) (heat) (radiation) (direct) (secondary)~~ (*see also* War operations, injury due to, nuclear weapons) E996.9 ◄
  radiation - *see* Radiation
  terrorism, secondary E979.9
  travel E903
Electric shock, electrocution (accidental) (from exposed wire, faulty appliance, high voltage cable, live rail, open socket) (by) (in) E925.9
  appliance or wiring
    domestic E925.0
    factory E925.2
    farm (building) E925.8
      house E925.0
    home E925.0
    industrial (conductor) (control apparatus) (transformer) E925.2
    outdoors E925.8
    public building E925.8
    residential institution E925.8
    school E925.8
    specified place NEC E925.8
  caused by other person
    stated as
      intentional, homicidal E968.8
      undetermined whether accidental or intentional E988.4

◄ New   ◄▌▌ Revised   ~~deleted~~ Deleted   ● Use Additional Digit(s)   ▒ Omit code

Electric shock, electrocution *(Continued)*
electric power generating plant, distribution station E925.1
electroshock gun (taser) (stun gun) E925.8
caused by other person E968.8
legal intervention E975
stated as accidental E925.8
stated as intentional E968.8
due to legal intervention E975
stated as intentional self-harm (suicidal (attempt)) E958.4
stated as undetermined whether accidental or intentional E988.4
suicide (attempt) E958.4
homicidal (attempt) E968.8
legal execution E978
lightning E907
machinery E925.9
domestic E925.0
factory E925.2
farm E925.8
home E925.0
misadventure in medical or surgical procedure
in electroshock therapy E873.4
self-inflicted (undetermined whether accidental or intentional) E988.4
stated as intentional E958.4
stated as undetermined whether accidental or intentional E988.4
suicidal (attempt) E958.4
transmission line E925.1
Electrocution - *see* Electric shock
Embolism E921.1
air (traumatic) NEC - *see* Air, embolism
Encephalitis
lead or saturnine E866.0
from pesticide NEC E863.4
Entanglement
in
bedclothes, causing suffocation E913.0
wheel of pedal cycle E826●
Entry of foreign body, material, any - *see* Foreign body
Execution, legal (any method) E978
Exertion, excessive physical, from prolonged activity E927.2
Exhaustion
cold - *see* Cold, exposure to
due to excessive exertion E927.8
heat - *see* Heat
Explosion (accidental) (in) (of) (on) E923.9
acetylene E923.2
aerosol can E921.8
aircraft (in transit) (powered) E841●
at landing, take-off E840●
in
terrorism E979.1
war operations ~~E994~~ ◀⊪
from ◀
enemy fire or explosive(s) (device placed on aircraft) E994.0 ◀
own onboard explosives E994.1 ◀
unpowered E842●
air tank (compressed) (in machinery) E921.1
anesthetic gas in operating theatre E923.2

Explosion *(Continued)*
automobile tire NEC E921.8
causing transport accident - *see* categories E810-E825
blasting (cap) (materials) E923.1
boiler (machinery), not on transport vehicle E921.0
steamship - *see* Explosion, watercraft
bomb E923.8
in
terrorism E979.2
war operations E993.8 ◀⊪
after cessation of hostilities E998.1 ◀⊪
atom, hydrogen or nuclear (*see also* War operations, injury due to, nuclear weapons) E996.9 ◀⊪
injury by fragments from E991.9
antipersonnel bomb E991.3
butane E923.2
caused by
other person
stated as
intentional, homicidal - *see* Assault, explosive
undetermined whether accidental or homicidal E985.5
coal gas E923.2
detonator E923.1
dynamite E923.1
explosive (material) NEC E923.9
gas(es) E923.2
missile E923.8
in
terrorism E979.2
war operations E993.1 ◀⊪
injury by fragments from E991.9
antipersonnel bomb E991.3
used in blasting operations E923.1
fire-damp E923.2
fireworks E923.0
gas E923.2
cylinder (in machinery) E921.1
pressure tank (in machinery) E921.1
gasoline (fumes) (tank) not in moving motor vehicle E923.2
grain store (military) (munitions) E923.8
grenade E923.8
in
terrorism E979.2
war operations E993.8 ◀⊪
injury by fragments from E991.4 ◀⊪
homicide (attempt) - *see* Assault, explosive
hot water heater, tank (in machinery) E921.0
in mine (of explosive gases) NEC E923.2
late effect of NEC E929.8
machinery - *see also* Accident, machine
pressure vessel - *see* Explosion, pressure vessel
methane E923.2
missile E923.8
in
terrorism E979.2
war operations E993.1 ◀⊪
injury by fragments from E991.4 ◀⊪

Explosion *(Continued)*
motor vehicle (part of)
in motion (on public highway) E818●
not on public highway E825●
munitions (dump) (factory) E923.8
in
terrorism E979.2
war operations E993.9 ◀⊪
of mine E923.8
in
terrorism
at sea or in harbor E979.0
land E979.2
marine E979.0
war operations
after cessation of hostilities E998.0 ◀⊪
at sea or in harbor E992.2 ◀⊪
land E993.8 ◀⊪
after cessation of hostilities E998.0 ◀⊪
injury by fragments from E991.4 ◀⊪
marine E992.2 ◀⊪
own weapons
in
terrorism (*see also* Suicide) E979.2
war operations E993.7 ◀⊪
injury by fragments from E991.9
antipersonnel bomb E991.3
pressure
cooker E921.8
gas tank (in machinery) E921.1
vessel (in machinery) E921.9
on transport vehicle - *see* categories E800-E848
specified type NEC E921.8
propane E923.2
railway engine, locomotive, train (boiler) (with subsequent collision, derailment, fall) E803●
with
collision (antecedent) (*see also* Collision, railway) E800●
derailment (antecedent) E802●
fire (without antecedent collision or derailment) E803●
secondary fire resulting from - *see* Fire
self-inflicted (unspecified whether accidental or intentional) E985.5
stated as intentional, purposeful E955.5
shell (artillery) E923.8
in
terrorism E979.2
war operations E993.2 ◀⊪
injury by fragments from E991.4 ◀⊪
stated as undetermined whether caused accidentally or purposely inflicted E985.5
steam or water lines (in machinery) E921.0
suicide (attempted) E955.5
terrorism - *see* Terrorism, explosion
torpedo E923.8
in
terrorism E979.0
war operations E992.0 ◀⊪

Explosion (Continued)
   transport accident - *see* categories
     E800–E848
   war operations - *see* War operations,
     explosion
   watercraft (boiler) E837●
     causing drowning, submersion
       (after jumping from
       watercraft) E830●
Exposure (weather) (conditions) (rain)
   (wind) E904.3
   with homicidal intent E968.4
   environmental
     to
       algae bloom E928.6
       blue-green algae bloom
         E928.6
       brown tide E928.6
       cyanobacteria bloom E928.6
       Florida red tide E928.6
       harmful algae
         and toxins E928.6
         bloom E928.6
       pfiesteria piscicida E928.6
       red tide E928.6
   excessive E904.3
     cold (*see also* Cold, exposure to)
       E901.9
       self-inflicted - *see* Cold, exposure
         to, self-inflicted
     heat (*see also* Heat) E900.9
   helpless person, infant, newborn
     due to abandonment or neglect
       E904.0
   noise E928.1
   prolonged in deep-freeze unit or
     refrigerator E901.1
   radiation - *see* Radiation
   resulting from transport accident - *see*
     categories E800–E848
   smoke from, due to
     fire - *see* Fire
     tobacco, second-hand E869.4
   vibration E928.2
External cause status E000.9 ◄
   civilian ◄
     done for ◄
       financial or other
         compensation E000.0 ◄
       pay or income E000.0 ◄
   for income E000.0 ◄
   hobby or leisure E000.8 ◄
     off duty military E000.8 ◄
   military E000.1 ◄
     off duty E000.8 ◄
   recreation E000.8 ◄
   specified NEC E000.8 ◄
   sport not for income E000.8 ◄
   student E000.8 ◄
   volunteer E000.8 ◄

F

Fall, falling (accidental) E888.9
   building E916
     burning E891.8
       private E890.8
   down
     escalator E880.0
     ladder E881.0
       in boat, ship, watercraft
         E833●
     staircase E880.9
     stairs, steps - *see* Fall, from, stairs

Fall, falling (Continued)
   earth (with asphyxia or suffocation (by
     pressure)) (*see also* Earth, falling)
     E913.3
   from, off
     aircraft (at landing, take-off)
       (in-transit) (while alighting,
       boarding) E843●
       resulting from accident to
         aircraft - *see* categories
         E840–E842
     animal (in sport or transport) E828●
     animal-drawn vehicle E827●
     balcony E882
     bed E884.4
     bicycle E826●
     boat, ship, watercraft (into water)
       E832
       after accident to, collision, fire on
         E830●
         and subsequently struck by
           (part of) boat E831●
        and subsequently struck by (part
         of) while alighting, boat
         E838●
       burning, crushed, sinking E830●
        and subsequently struck by
         (part of) boat E831●
     bridge E882
     building E882
       burning (uncontrolled fire) E891.8
        in terrorism E979.3
       private E890.8
     bunk in boat, ship, watercraft
       E834●
       due to accident to watercraft
         E831●
     cable car (not on rails) E847
       on rails E829●
     car - *see* Fall from motor vehicle
       E884.9
     chair E884.2
     cliff E884.1
     commode E884.6
     curb (sidewalk) E880.1
     elevation aboard ship E834●
       due to accident to ship E831●
     embankment E884.9
     escalator E880.0
     fire escape E882
     flagpole E882
     furniture NEC E884.5
     gangplank (into water) (*see also* Fall,
       from, boat) E832●
       to deck, dock E834●
     hammock on ship E834●
       due to accident to watercraft
         E831●
     haystack E884.9
     heelies E885.1
     high place NEC E884.9
       stated as undetermined whether
         accidental or intentional -
         see Jumping, from, high
         place
     horse (in sport or transport) E828●
     in-line skates E885.1
     ladder E881.0
       in boat, ship, watercraft E833●
        due to accident to watercraft
         E831●
     machinery - *see also* Accident,
       machine
       not in operation E884.9

Fall, falling (Continued)
   from, off (Continued)
     motor vehicle (in motion) (on public
       highway) E818●
       not on public highway E825●
        stationary, except while
         alighting, boarding,
         entering, leaving E884.9
        while alighting, boarding,
         entering, leaving E824●
       stationary, except while alighting,
        boarding, entering, leaving
        E884.9
       while alighting, boarding,
        entering, leaving, except
        off-road type motor vehicle
        E817●
        off-road type - *see* Fall, from,
         off-road type motor
         vehicle
     nonmotor road vehicle (while
       alighting, boarding) NEC
       E829●
       stationary, except while alighting,
        boarding, entering, leaving
        E884.9
     off road type motor vehicle (not
       on public highway) NEC
       E821●
       on public highway E818●
        while alighting, boarding,
         entering, leaving
         E817●
       snow vehicle - *see* Fall from snow
        vehicle, motor-driven
     one
       deck to another on ship E834●
        due to accident to ship
         E831●
       level to another NEC E884.9
        boat, ship, or watercraft
         E834●
         due to accident to
          watercraft E831●
     pedal cycle E826●
     playground equipment E884.0
     railway rolling stock, train, vehicle
       (while alighting, boarding)
       E804●
       with
        collision (*see also* Collision,
         railway) E800●
        derailment (*see also*
         Derailment, railway)
         E802●
        explosion (*see also* Explosion,
         railway engine) E803●
     rigging (aboard ship) E834●
       due to accident to watercraft
         E831●
     roller skates E885.1
     scaffolding E881.1
     scooter (nonmotorized) E885.0
     sidewalk (curb) E880.1
       moving E885.9
     skateboard E885.2
     skis E885.3
     snow vehicle, motor-driven (not on
       public highway) E820●
       on public highway E818●
        while alighting, boarding,
         entering, leaving
         E817●
     snowboard E885.4

◄ New   ◄▥ Revised   ~~deleted~~ Deleted   ● Use Additional Digit(s)   ▨ Omit code

E CODES

Fall, falling *(Continued)*
  from, off *(Continued)*
    stairs, steps E880.9
      boat, ship, watercraft E833●
        due to accident to watercraft E831●
      motor bus, motor vehicle - *see* Fall, from, motor vehicle, while alighting, boarding
      street car E829●
    stationary vehicle NEC E884.9
    stepladder E881.0
    street car (while boarding, alighting) E829●
      stationary, except while boarding or alighting E884.9
    structure NEC E882
      burning (uncontrolled fire) E891.8
        in terrorism E979.3
    table E884.9
    toilet E884.6
    tower E882
    tree E884.9
    turret E882
    vehicle NEC - *see also* Accident, vehicle NEC
      stationary E884.9
    viaduct E882
    wall E882
    wheelchair E884.3
    wheelies E885.1
    window E882
  in, on
    aircraft (at landing, take-off) (in-transit) E843●
      resulting from accident to aircraft - *see* categories E840–E842
    boat, ship, watercraft E835●
      due to accident to watercraft E831●
      one level to another NEC E834●
      on ladder, stairs E833●
    cutting or piercing instrument machine E888.0
    deck (of boat, ship, watercraft) E835●
      due to accident to watercraft E831●
    escalator E880.0
    gangplank E835●
    glass, broken E888.0
    knife E888.0
    ladder E881.0
      in boat, ship, watercraft E833●
        due to accident to watercraft E831●
    object
      edged, pointed or sharp E888.0
      other E888.1
    pitchfork E888.0
    railway rolling stock, train, vehicle (while alighting, boarding) E804●
      with
        collision (*see also* Collision, railway) E800●
        derailment (*see also* Derailment, railway) E802●
        explosion (*see also* Explosion, railway engine) E803●

Fall, falling *(Continued)*
  in, on *(Continued)*
    scaffolding E881.1
    scissors E888.0
    staircase, stairs, steps (*see also* Fall, from, stairs) E880.9
    street car E829●
    water transport (*see also* Fall, in, boat) E835●
  into
    cavity E883.9
    dock E883.9
      from boat, ship, watercraft (*see also* Fall, from, boat) E832●
    hold (of ship) E834●
      due to accident to watercraft E831●
    hole E883.9
    manhole E883.2
    moving part of machinery - *see* Accident, machine
    opening in surface NEC E883.9
    pit E883.9
    quarry E883.9
    shaft E883.9
    storm drain E883.2
    tank E883.9
    water (with drowning or submersion) E910.9
    well E883.1
  late effect of NEC E929.3
  object (*see also* Hit by, object, falling) E916
  other E888.8
  over
    animal E885.9
    cliff E884.1
    embankment E884.9
    small object E885.9
  overboard (*see also* Fall, from, boat) E832●
  resulting in striking against object E888.1
    sharp E888.0
  rock E916
  same level NEC E888.9
    aircraft (any kind) E843●
      resulting from accident to aircraft - *see* categories E840–E842
    boat, ship, watercraft E835●
      due to accident to, collision, watercraft E831●
    from
      collision, pushing, shoving, by or with other person(s) E886.9
        as, or caused by, a crowd E917.6
        in sports E886.0
      in-line skates E885.1
      roller skates E885.1
      scooter (nonmotorized) E885.0
      skateboard E885.2
      skis E885.3
      slipping, stumbling, tripping E885.9
      snowboard E885.4
  snowslide E916
    as avalanche E909.2
  stone E916

Fall, falling *(Continued)*
  through
    hatch (on ship) E834●
      due to accident to watercraft E831●
    roof E882
    window E882
    timber E916
  while alighting from, boarding, entering, leaving
    aircraft (any kind) E843●
    motor bus, motor vehicle - *see* Fall, from, motor vehicle, while alighting, boarding
    nonmotor road vehicle NEC E829●
    railway train E804●
    street car E829●
Fallen on by
  animal (horse) (not being ridden) E906.8
    being ridden (in sport or transport) E828●
Fell or jumped from high place, so stated - *see* Jumping, from, high place
Felo-de-se (*see also* Suicide) E958.9
Fever
  heat - *see* Heat
  thermic - *see* Heat
Fight (hand) (fist) (foot) (*see also* Assault, fight) E960.0
Fire (accidental) (caused by great heat from appliance (electrical), hot object, or hot substance) (secondary, resulting from explosion) E899
  conflagration - *see* Conflagration E892
  controlled, normal (in brazier, fireplace, furnace, or stove) (charcoal) (coal) (coke) (electric) (gas) (wood)
    bonfire E897
    brazier, not in building or structure E897
    in building or structure, except private dwelling (barn) (church) (convalescent or residential home) (factory) (farm outbuilding) (hospital) (hotel) (institution (educational) (dormitory) (residential) (private garage) (school) (shop) (store) (theatre) E896
    in private dwelling (apartment) (boarding house) (camping place) (caravan) (farmhouse) (home (private) (house) (lodging house) (rooming house) (tenement) E895
    not in building or structure E897
    trash E897
  forest (uncontrolled) E892
  grass (uncontrolled) E892
  hay (uncontrolled) E892
  homicide (attempt) E968.0
    late effect of E969
  in, of, on, starting in E892
    aircraft (in transit) (powered) E841●
      at landing, take-off E840●
      stationary E892
      unpowered (balloon) (glider) E842●
    balloon E842●
    boat, ship, watercraft - *see* categories E830, E831, E837

◀ New   ◀⫿⫿ Revised   ~~deleted~~ Deleted   ● Use Additional Digit(s)   ▬ Omit code

E CODES

Fire *(Continued)*
  in, of, on, starting in *(Continued)*
    building or structure, except private
        dwelling (barn) (church)
        (convalescent or residential
        home) (factory) (farm
        outbuilding) (hospital) (hotel)
        (institution) (educational)
        (dormitory) (residential))
        (school) (shop) (store) (theatre)
        (see also Conflagration, building
        or structure, except private
        dwelling) E891.9
    forest (uncontrolled) E892
    glider E842●
    grass (uncontrolled) E892
    hay (uncontrolled) E892
    lumber (uncontrolled) E892
    machinery - *see* Accident, machine
    mine (uncontrolled) E892
    motor vehicle (in motion) (on
        public highway) E818●
      not on public highway E825●
      stationary E892
    prairie (uncontrolled) E892
    private dwelling (apartment)
        (boarding house) (camping
        place) (caravan) (farmhouse)
        (home (private)) (house)
        (lodging house) (private
        garage) (rooming house)
        (tenement) *(see also*
        Conflagration, private
        dwelling) E890.9
    railway rolling stock, train, vehicle
        (see also Explosion, railway
        engine) E803●
      stationary E892
    room NEC E898.1
    street car (in motion) E829●
      stationary E892
    terrorism (by fire-producing
        device) E979.3
      fittings or furniture (burning
          building) (uncontrolled
          fire) E979.3
      from nuclear explosion
          E979.5
    transport vehicle, stationary
        NEC E892
    tunnel (uncontrolled) E892
    war operations (by fire-producing
        device or conventional
        weapon) E990.9
      from nuclear explosion *(see
          also* War operations, injury
          due to, nuclear weapons)
          E996.2 ◀
      incendiary bomb E990.0
      petrol bomb E990.0
  late effect of NEC E929.4
  lumber (uncontrolled) E892
  mine (uncontrolled) E892
  prairie (uncontrolled) E892
  self-inflicted (unspecified whether
      accidental or intentional) E988.1
    stated as intentional, purposeful
        E958.1
  specified NEC E898.1
    with
      conflagration - *see* Conflagration
      ignition (of)
        clothing - *see* Ignition, clothes
        highly inflammable material
            (benzine) (fat) (gasoline)
            (kerosene) (paraffin)
            (petrol) E894

Fire *(Continued)*
  started by other person
    stated as
      with intent to injure or kill
          E968.0
      undetermined whether or not
          with intent to injure or kill
          E988.1
  suicide (attempted) E958.1
    late effect of E959
  tunnel (uncontrolled) E892
Fireball effects from nuclear explosion
  in
      terrorism E979.5
      war operations *(see also* War
          operations, injury due to,
          nuclear weapons) E996.2 ◀▥
Fireworks (explosion) E923.0
Flash burns from explosion *(see also*
    Explosion) E923.9
Flood (any injury) (resulting from storm)
    E908.2
  caused by collapse of dam or manmade
      structure E909.3
Forced landing (aircraft) E840●
Foreign body, object or material
    (entrance into (accidental))
  air passage (causing injury) E915
    with asphyxia, obstruction,
        suffocation E912
      food or vomitus E911
    nose (with asphyxia, obstruction,
        suffocation) E912
      causing injury without asphyxia,
          obstruction, suffocation
          E915
  alimentary canal (causing injury)
      (with obstruction) E915
    with asphyxia, obstruction
        respiratory passage,
        suffocation E912
      food E911
    mouth E915
      with asphyxia, obstruction,
          suffocation E912
        food E911
    pharynx E915
      with asphyxia, obstruction,
          suffocation E912
        food E911
  aspiration (with asphyxia, obstruction
      respiratory passage, suffocation)
      E912
    causing injury without asphyxia,
        obstruction respiratory
        passage, suffocation E915
    food (regurgitated) (vomited)
        E911
      causing injury without asphyxia,
          obstruction respiratory
          passage, suffocation E915
    mucus (not of newborn) E912
    phlegm E912
  bladder (causing injury or obstruction)
      E915
  bronchus, bronchi - *see* Foreign body,
      air passages
  conjunctival sac E914
  digestive system - *see* Foreign body,
      alimentary canal
  ear (causing injury or obstruction) E915
  esophagus (causing injury or
      obstruction) *(see also* Foreign
      body, alimentary canal) E915
  eye (any part) E914
  eyelid E914

Foreign body, object or
    material *(Continued)*
  hairball (stomach) (with obstruction)
      E915
  ingestion - *see* Foreign body, alimentary
      canal
  inhalation - *see* Foreign body, aspiration
  intestine (causing injury or obstruction)
      E915
  iris E914
  lacrimal apparatus E914
  larynx - *see* Foreign body, air passage
  late effect of NEC E929.8
  lung - *see* Foreign body, air passage
  mouth - *see* Foreign body, alimentary
      canal, mouth
  nasal passage - *see* Foreign body, air
      passage, nose
  nose - *see* Foreign body, air passage,
      nose
  ocular muscle E914
  operation wound (left in) - *see*
      Misadventure, foreign object
  orbit E914
  pharynx - *see* Foreign body, alimentary
      canal, pharynx
  rectum (causing injury or obstruction)
      E915
  stomach (hairball) (causing injury or
      obstruction) E915
  tear ducts or glands E914
  trachea - *see* Foreign body, air
      passage
  urethra (causing injury or obstruction)
      E915
  vagina (causing injury or obstruction)
      E915
Found dead, injured
  from exposure (to) - *see* Exposure
  on
      public highway E819●
      railway right of way E807●
Fracture (circumstances unknown or
    unspecified) E887
  due to specified external means - *see*
      manner of accident
  late effect of NEC E929.3
  occurring in water transport NEC
      E835●
Freezing - *see* Cold, exposure to
Frostbite E901.0
  due to manmade conditions E901.1
Frozen - *see* Cold, exposure to

G

Garrotting, homicidal (attempted) E963
Gored E906.8
Gunshot wound *(see also* Shooting)
    E922.9

H

Hailstones, injury by E904.3
Hairball (stomach) (with obstruction)
    E915
Hanged himself *(see also* Hanging, self-
    inflicted) E983.0
Hang gliding E842●
Hanging (accidental) E913.8
  caused by other person
    in accidental circumstances
        E913.8

◀ New   ◀▥ Revised   ~~deleted~~ Deleted   ● Use Additional Digit(s)   ▥ Omit code

Hanging *(Continued)*
  caused by other person *(Continued)*
    stated as
      intentional, homicidal E963
      undetermined whether accidental
        or intentional E983.0
  homicide (attempt) E963
  in bed or cradle E913.0
  legal execution E978
  self-inflicted (unspecified whether
    accidental or intentional)
    E983.0
    in accidental circumstances E913.8
    stated as intentional, purposeful
      E953.0
  stated as undetermined whether
    accidental or intentional E983.0
  suicidal (attempt) E953.0
Heat (apoplexy) (collapse) (cramps)
  (effects of) (excessive) (exhaustion)
  (fever) (prostration) (stroke) E900.9
  due to
    manmade conditions (as listed in
      E900.1, except boat, ship,
      watercraft) E900.1
    weather (conditions) E900.0
  from
    electric heating apparatus causing
      burning E924.8
    nuclear explosion
      in
        terrorism E979.5
        war operations *(see also* War
          operations, injury due
          to, nuclear weapons)
          E996.2 ◀▥
    generated in, boiler, engine,
      evaporator, fire room of boat,
      ship, watercraft E838●
    inappropriate in local application or
      packing in medical or surgical
      procedure E873.5
  late effect of NEC E989
Hemorrhage
  delayed following medical or surgical
    treatment without mention of
    misadventure - *see* Reaction,
    abnormal
  during medical or surgical treatment as
    misadventure - *see* Misadventure,
    cut
High
  altitude, effects E902.9
  level of radioactivity, effects - *see*
    Radiation
  pressure effects - *see also* Effects of, air
    pressure
    from rapid descent in water
      (causing caisson or divers'
      disease, palsy, or paralysis)
      E902.2
  temperature, effects - *see* Heat
Hit, hitting (accidental) by
  aircraft (propeller) (without accident to
    aircraft) E844●
    unpowered E842●
  avalanche E909.2
  being thrown against object in or
    part of
      motor vehicle (in motion) (on public
        highway) E818●
        not on public highway E825●
      nonmotor road vehicle NEC
        E829●
      street car E829●

Hit, hitting *(Continued)*
  boat, ship, watercraft
    after fall from watercraft E838●
    damaged, involved in accident
      E831●
    while swimming, water skiing
      E838●
  bullet *(see also* Shooting) E922.9
    from air gun E922.4
    in
      terrorism E979.4
      war operations E991.2
        rubber E991.0
  flare, Verey pistol *(see also* Shooting)
    E922.8
  hailstones E904.3
  landslide E909.2
  law-enforcing agent (on duty) E975
    with blunt object (baton) (night
      stick) (stave) (truncheon)
      E973
  machine - *see* Accident, machine
  missile
    firearm *(see also* Shooting)
      E922.9
    in
      terrorism - *see* Terrorism,
        missile
      war operations - *see* War
        operations, missile
  motor vehicle (on public highway)
    (traffic accident) E814●
    not on public highway, nontraffic
      accident E822●
  nonmotor road vehicle NEC E829●
  object
    falling E916
      from, in, on
        aircraft E844●
          due to accident to aircraft -
            see categories
            E840–E842
          unpowered E842●
        boat, ship, watercraft E838●
          due to accident to
            watercraft E831●
        building E916
          burning E891.8
            in terrorism E979.3
            private E890.8
        cataclysmic
          earth surface movement or
            eruption E909.9
          storm E908.9
        cave-in E916
          with asphyxiation or
            suffocation *(see also*
            Suffocation, due to,
            cave-in) E913.3
        earthquake E909.0
        motor vehicle (in motion)
          (on public highway)
          E818●
          not on public highway
            E825●
          stationary E916
        nonmotor road vehicle NEC
          E829●
        pedal cycle E826●
        railway rolling stock, train,
          vehicle E806●
        street car E829●
        structure, burning NEC
          E891.8
        vehicle, stationary E916

Hit, hitting *(Continued)*
  object *(Continued)*
    moving NEC - *see* Striking against,
      object
    projected NEC - *see* Striking against,
      object
    set in motion by
      compressed air or gas, spring,
        striking, throwing - *see*
        Striking against, object
    explosion - *see* Explosion
    thrown into, on, or towards
      motor vehicle (in motion) (on
        public highway) E818●
      not on public highway E825●
      nonmotor road vehicle NEC
        E829●
      pedal cycle E826●
      street car E829●
    off-road type motor vehicle (not on
      public highway) E821●
    on public highway E814●
    other person(s) E917.9
      with blunt or thrown object
        E917.9
      in sports E917.0
        with subsequent fall E917.5
      intentionally, homicidal E968.2
    as, or caused by, a crowd E917.1
      with subsequent fall E917.6
    in sports E917.0
    pedal cycle E826●
    police (on duty) E975
      with blunt object (baton)
        (nightstick) (stave)
        (truncheon) E973
    railway, rolling stock, train, vehicle
      (part of) E805●
    shot - *see* Shooting
    snow vehicle, motor-driven (not on
      public highway) E820●
      on public highway E814●
    street car E829●
    vehicle NEC - *see* Accident, vehicle
      NEC
Homicide, homicidal (attempt)
  (justifiable) *(see also* Assault) E968.9
Hot
  liquid, object, substance, accident
    caused by - *see also* Accident,
    caused by, hot, by type of
    substance
    late effect of E929.8
  place, effects - *see* Heat
  weather, effects E900.0
Humidity, causing problem E904.3
Hunger E904.1
  resulting from
    abandonment or neglect E904.0
    transport accident - *see* categories
      E800–E848
Hurricane (any injury) E908.0
Hypobarism, hypobaropathy - *see* Effects
  of, air pressure
Hypothermia - *see* Cold, exposure to

I

Ictus
  caloris - *see* Heat
  solaris E900.0
Ignition (accidental)
  anesthetic gas in operating theatre
    E923.2

E CODES

Injury, injured *(Continued)*
  due to *(Continued)*
    war operations - *see* War operations
      occurring after cessation of
        hostilities E998.9 ◀▥
    weapon of mass destruction
      [WMD] E997.3 ◀
  homicidal *(see also* Assault) E968.9
  in, on
    civil insurrection - *see* War
      operations
    fight E960.0
    parachute descent (voluntary)
      (without accident to aircraft)
      E844●
      with accident to aircraft - *see*
        categories E840-E842
    public highway E819●
    railway right of way E807●
    terrorism - *see* Terrorism
    war operations - *see* War operations
  inflicted (by)
    in course of arrest (attempted),
      suppression of disturbance,
      maintenance of order, by law
      enforcing agents - *see* Legal
      intervention
    law-enforcing agent (on duty) - *see*
      Legal intervention
    other person
      stated as
        accidental E928.9
        homicidal, intentional - *see*
          Assault
        undetermined whether
          accidental or intentional -
          see Injury, stated as
          undetermined
    police (on duty) - *see* Legal
      intervention
  late effect of E929.9
  purposely (inflicted) by other
    person(s) - *see* Assault
  self-inflicted (unspecified whether
    accidental or intentional) E988.9
    stated as
      accidental E928.9
      intentionally, purposely E958.9
  specified cause NEC E928.8
  stated as
    undetermined whether accidentally
      or purposely inflicted (by)
      E988.9
      cut (any part of body) E986
      cutting or piercing instrument
        (classifiable to E920) E986
      drowning E984
      explosive(s) (missile) E985.5
      falling from high place E987.9
        manmade structure, except
          residential E987.1
        natural site E987.2
        residential premises E987.0
      hanging E983.0
      knife E986
      late effect of E989
      puncture (any part of body) E986
      shooting - *see* Shooting, stated as
        undetermined whether
        accidental or intentional
      specified means NEC E988.8
      stab (any part of body) E986
      strangulation - *see* Suffocation,
        stated as undetermined
        whether accidental or
        intentional

Injury, injured *(Continued)*
  stated as *(Continued)*
    submersion E984
    suffocation - *see* Suffocation, stated
      as undetermined whether
      accidental or intentional
  to child due to criminal abortion
    E968.8
Insufficient nourishment - *see also* Lack
  of, food
  homicidal intent E968.4
Insulation, effects - *see* Heat
Interruption of respiration by
  food lodged in esophagus E911
  foreign body, except food, in
    esophagus E912
Intervention, legal - *see* Legal
  intervention
Intoxication, drug or poison - *see* Table
  of Drugs and Chemicals
Irradiation - *see* Radiation

J

Jammed (accidentally)
  between objects (moving) (stationary
    and moving) E918
  in object E918
Jumped or fell from high place, so
  stated - *see* Jumping, from, high
  place, stated as
  in undetermined circumstances
Jumping
  before train, vehicle or other moving
    object (unspecified whether
    accidental or intentional)
    E988.0
    stated as
      intentional, purposeful
        E958.0
      suicidal (attempt) E958.0
  from
    aircraft
      by parachute (voluntarily)
        (without accident to
        aircraft) E844●
      due to accident to aircraft - *see*
        categories E840–E842
    boat, ship, watercraft (into water)
      after accident to, fire on,
        watercraft E830●
      and subsequently struck by
        (part of) boat E831●
      burning, crushed, sinking
        E830●
      and subsequently struck by
        (part of) boat E831●
      voluntarily, without accident (to
        boat) with injury other than
        drowning or submersion
        E883.0
    building - *see also* Jumping, from,
      high place
      burning (uncontrolled fire)
        E891.8
      in terrorism E979.3
      private E890.8
    cable car (not on rails) E847
      on rails E829●
    high place
      in accidental circumstances or
        in sport - *see* categories
        E880–E884

Jumping *(Continued)*
  from *(Continued)*
    high place *(Continued)*
      stated as
        with intent to injure self E957.9
          man-made structures NEC
            E957.1
          natural sites E957.2
          residential premises E957.0
        in undetermined
          circumstances E987.9
          man-made structures NEC
            E987.1
          natural sites E987.2
          residential premises E987.0
        suicidal (attempt) E957.9
          man-made structures NEC
            E957.1
          natural sites E957.1
          residential premises E957.0
    motor vehicle (in motion) (on public
      highway) - *see* Fall, from,
      motor vehicle
    nonmotor road vehicle NEC E829●
    street car E829●
    structure - *see also* Jumping, from,
      high place
      burning NEC (uncontrolled fire)
        E891.8
      in terrorism E979.3
  into water
    with injury other than drowning or
      submersion E883.0
    drowning or submersion - *see*
      Submersion
  from, off, watercraft - *see* Jumping,
    from, boat
Justifiable homicide - *see* Assault

K

Kicked by
  animal E906.8
  person(s) (accidentally) E917.9
    with intent to injure or kill E960.0
    as, or caused by a crowd E917.1
      with subsequent fall E917.6
    in fight E960.0
    in sports E917.0
      with subsequent fall E917.5
Kicking against
  object (moving) E917.9
    in sports E917.0
      with subsequent fall E917.5
    stationary E917.4
      with subsequent fall E917.8
  person - *see* Striking against, person
Killed, killing (accidentally) NEC *(see also*
  Injury) E928.9
  in
    action - *see* War operations
    brawl, fight (hand) (fists) (foot)
      E960.0
      by weapon - *see also* Assault
        cutting, piercing E966
        firearm - *see* Shooting,
          homicide
  self
    stated as
      accident E928.9
      suicide - *see* Suicide
    unspecified whether accidental or
      suicidal E988.9

E CODES

Knocked down (accidentally) (by) NEC
E928.9
  animal (not being ridden) E906.8
    being ridden (in sport or transport)
E828●
  blast from explosion (see also
Explosion) E923.9
  crowd, human stampede E917.6
  late effect of - see Late effect
  person (accidentally) E917.9
    in brawl, fight E960.0
    in sports E917.5
  transport vehicle - see vehicle involved
under Hit by
  while boxing E917.5

L

Laceration NEC E928.9
Lack of
  air (refrigerator or closed place),
suffocation by E913.2
  care (helpless person) (infant)
(newborn) E904.0
    homicidal intent E968.4
  food except as result of transport
accident E904.1
    helpless person, infant, newborn
due to abandonment or
neglect E904.0
  water except as result of transport
accident E904.2
    helpless person, infant, newborn
due to abandonment or
neglect E904.0
Landslide E909.2
  falling on, hitting
    motor vehicle (any) (in motion) (on
or off public highway) E909.2
    railway rolling stock, train, vehicle
E909.2
Late effect of
  accident NEC (accident classifiable to
E928.9) E929.9
    specified NEC (accident classifiable
to E910–E928.8) E929.8
  assault E969
  fall, accidental (accident classifiable to
E880–E888) E929.3
  fire, accident caused by (accident
classifiable to E890–E899) E929.4
  homicide, attempt (any means) E969
  injury due to terrorism E999.1
  injury undetermined whether
accidentally or purposely
inflicted (injury classifiable to
E980–E988) E989
  legal intervention (injury classifiable to
E970–E976) E977
  medical or surgical procedure, test or
therapy
    as, or resulting in, or from
      abnormal or delayed reaction or
complication - see Reaction,
abnormal
      misadventure - see Misadventure
  motor vehicle accident (accident
classifiable to E810–E825)
E929.0
  natural or environmental factor,
accident due to (accident
classifiable to E900–E909)
E929.5

Late effect of (Continued)
  poisoning, accidental (accident
classifiable to E850–E858,
E860–E869) E929.2
  suicide, attempt (any means) E959
  transport accident NEC (accident
classifiable to E800–E807,
E826–E838, E840–E848) E929.1
  war operations, injury due to (injury
classifiable to E990–E998)
E999.0
Launching pad accident E845●
Legal
  execution, any method E978
  intervention (by) (injury from)
E976
    baton E973
    bayonet E974
    blow E975
    blunt object (baton) (nightstick)
(stave) (truncheon) E973
    cutting or piercing instrument
E974
    dynamite E971
    execution, any method E973
    explosive(s) (shell) E971
    firearm(s) E970
    gas (asphyxiation) (poisoning)
(tear) E972
    grenade E971
    late effect of E977
    machine gun E970
    manhandling E975
    mortar bomb E971
    nightstick E973
    revolver E970
    rifle E970
    specified means NEC E975
    stabbing E974
    stave E973
    truncheon E973
Lifting, injury in E927.8
Lightning (shock) (stroke) (struck by)
E907
Liquid (noncorrosive) in eye E914
  corrosive E924.1
Loss of control
  motor vehicle (on public highway)
(without antecedent collision)
E816●
    with
      antecedent collision on public
highway - see Collision,
motor vehicle
      involving any object, person or
vehicle not on public
highway E816●
    on public highway - see
Collision, motor vehicle
    not on public highway,
nontraffic accident
E825●
      with antecedent collision -
see Collision, motor
vehicle, not on public
highway
  off-road type motor vehicle (not on
public highway) E821●
    on public highway - see Loss of
control, motor vehicle
  snow vehicle, motor-driven (not on
public highway) E820●
    on public highway - see Loss of
control, motor vehicle

Lost at sea E832●
  with accident to watercraft E830●
  in war operations E995.8 ◄▥
Low
  pressure, effects - see Effects of, air
pressure
  temperature, effects - see Cold
exposure to
Lying before train, vehicle or other
moving object (unspecified
whether accidental or intentional)
E988.0
  stated as intentional, purposeful,
suicidal (attempt) E958.0
Lynching (see also Assault) E968.9

M

Malfunction, atomic power plant in
water transport E838●
Mangled (accidentally) NEC E928.9
Manhandling (in brawl, fight) E960.0
  legal intervention E975
Manslaughter (nonaccidental) - see
Assault
Marble in nose E912
Mauled by animal E906.8
Medical procedure, complication of
  delayed or as an abnormal reaction
without mention of
misadventure - see Reaction,
abnormal
  due to or as a result of misadventure -
see Misadventure
Melting of fittings and furniture in
burning
  in terrorism E979.3
Minamata disease E865.2
Misadventure(s) to patient(s) during
surgical or medical care E876.9
  contaminated blood, fluid, drug or
biological substance (presence of
agents and toxins as listed in
E875) E875.9
    administered (by) NEC E875.9
      infusion E875.0
      injection E875.1
      specified means NEC E875.2
      transfusion E875.0
      vaccination E875.1
  cut, cutting, puncture, perforation or
hemorrhage (accidental)
(inadvertent) (inappropriate)
(during) E870.9
    aspiration of fluid or tissue (by
puncture or catheterization,
except heart) E870.5
    biopsy E870.8
      needle (aspirating) E870.5
    blood sampling E870.5
    catheterization E870.5
      heart E870.6
    dialysis (kidney) E870.2
    endoscopic examination E870.4
    enema E870.7
    infusion E870.1
    injection E870.3
    lumbar puncture E870.5
    needle biopsy E870.5
    paracentesis, abdominal E870.5
    perfusion E870.2
    specified procedure NEC E870.8
    surgical operation E870.0

◄ New   ◄▥ Revised   ~~deleted~~ Deleted   ● Use Additional Digit(s)   ▨ Omit code

E CODES

Misadventure(s) to patient(s) during surgical or medical care (Continued)
cut, cutting, puncture, perforation or hemorrhage (Continued)
 thoracentesis E870.5
 transfusion E870.1
 vaccination E870.3
excessive amount of blood or other fluid during transfusion or infusion E873.0
failure
 in dosage E873.9
 electroshock therapy E873.4
 inappropriate temperature (too hot or too cold) in local application and packing E873.5
 infusion
  excessive amount of fluid E873.0
  incorrect dilution of fluid E873.1
 insulin-shock therapy E873.4
 nonadministration of necessary drug or medicinal E873.6
 overdose - see also Overdose
 radiation, in therapy E873.2
 radiation
  inadvertent exposure of patient (receiving radiation for test or therapy) E873.3
  not receiving radiation for test or therapy - see Radiation
  overdose E873.2
 specified procedure NEC E873.8
 transfusion
  excessive amount of blood E873.0
 mechanical, of instrument or apparatus (during procedure) E874.9
 aspiration of fluid or tissue (by puncture or catheterization, except of heart) E874.4
 biopsy E874.8
  needle (aspirating) E874.4
 blood sampling E874.4
 catheterization E874.4
  heart E874.5
 dialysis (kidney) E874.2
 endoscopic examination E874.3
 enema E874.8
 infusion E874.1
 injection E874.8
 lumbar puncture E874.4
 needle biopsy E874.4
 paracentesis, abdominal E874.4
 perfusion E874.2
 specified procedure NEC E874.8
 surgical operation E874.0
 thoracentesis E874.4
 transfusion E874.1
 vaccination E874.8
 sterile precautions (during procedure) E872.9
 aspiration of fluid or tissue (by puncture or catheterization, except heart) E872.5
 biopsy E872.8
  needle (aspirating) E872.5

Misadventure(s) to patient(s) during surgical or medical care (Continued)
failure (Continued)
 sterile precautions (Continued)
  blood sampling E872.5
  catheterization E872.5
   heart E872.6
  dialysis (kidney) E872.2
  endoscopic examination E872.4
  enema E872.8
  infusion E872.1
  injection E872.3
  lumbar puncture E872.5
  needle biopsy E872.5
  paracentesis, abdominal E872.5
  perfusion E872.2
  removal of catheter or packing E872.8
  specified procedure NEC E872.8
  surgical operation E872.0
  thoracentesis E872.5
  transfusion E872.1
  vaccination E872.3
 suture or ligature during surgical procedure E876.2
 to introduce or to remove tube or instrument E876.4
  foreign object left in body - see Misadventure, foreign object
foreign object left in body (during procedure) E871.9
 aspiration of fluid or tissue (by puncture or catheterization, except heart) E871.5
 biopsy E871.8
  needle (aspirating) E871.5
 blood sampling E871.5
 catheterization E871.5
  heart E871.6
 dialysis (kidney) E871.2
 endoscopic examination E871.4
 enema E871.8
 infusion E871.1
 injection E871.3
 lumbar puncture E871.5
 needle biopsy E871.5
 paracentesis, abdominal E871.5
 perfusion E871.2
 removal of catheter or packing E871.7
 specified procedure NEC E871.8
 surgical operation E871.0
 thoracentesis E871.5
 transfusion E871.1
 vaccination E871.3
hemorrhage - see Misadventure, cut
inadvertent exposure of patient to radiation (being received for test or therapy) E873.3
inappropriate
 operation performed E876.5
 temperature (too hot or too cold) in local application or packing E873.5
infusion - see also Misadventure, by specific type, infusion
 excessive amount of fluid E873.0
 incorrect dilution of fluid E873.1
 wrong fluid E876.1
mismatched blood in transfusion E876.0

Misadventure(s) to patient(s) during surgical or medical care (Continued)
nonadministration of necessary drug or medicinal E873.6
overdose - see also Overdose
 radiation, in therapy E873.2
perforation - see Misadventure, cut
performance of correct operation (procedure) on wrong ◀
 body part E876.7 ◀
 side E876.7 ◀
 site E876.7 ◀
performance of operation (procedure) ◀
 intended for another patient E876.6 ◀
 on patient not scheduled for surgery E876.6 ◀
 on wrong patient E876.6 ◀
performance of inappropriate wrong operation on correct patient E876.5 ◀▥
puncture - see Misadventure, cut
specified type NEC E876.8
 failure
  suture or ligature during surgical operation E876.2
  to introduce or to remove tube or instrument E876.4
   foreign object left in body E871.9
 infusion of wrong fluid E876.1
 performance of inappropriate operation E876.5
 transfusion of mismatched blood E876.0
 wrong
  device implanted into correct surgical site E876.5 ◀
  fluid in infusion E876.1
  placement of endotracheal tube during anesthetic procedure E876.3
  procedure (operation) performed on the correct patient E876.5 ◀
transfusion - see also Misadventure, by specific type, transfusion
 excessive amount of blood E873.0
 mismatched blood E876.0
wrong
 drug given in error - see Table of Drugs and Chemicals
 fluid in infusion E876.1
 placement of endotracheal tube during anesthetic procedure E876.3
Motion (effects) E903
 sickness E903
Mountain sickness E902.0
Mucus aspiration or inhalation, not of newborn (with asphyxia, obstruction respiratory passage, suffocation) E912
Mudslide of cataclysmic nature E909.2
Murder (attempt) (see also Assault) E968.9

N

Nail, injury by E920.8
Needlestick (sewing needle) E920.4
 hypodermic E920.5

◀ New ◀▥ Revised deleted Deleted ● Use Additional Digit(s) ▥ Omit code

E CODES

Neglect - *see also* Privation
  criminal E968.4
  homicidal intent E968.4
Noise (causing injury) (pollution)
  E928.1
Nuclear weapon (*see also* War
  operations, injury due to,
  nuclear weapons) E996.9 ◄

O

Object
  falling
    from, in, on, hitting
      aircraft E844●
        due to accident to aircraft - *see*
          categories E840–E842
      machinery - *see also* Accident,
        machine
      not in operation E916
      motor vehicle (in motion) (on
        public highway) E818●
      not on public highway E825●
      stationary E916
      nonmotor road vehicle NEC
        E829●
      pedal cycle E826●
      person E916
      railway rolling stock, train,
        vehicle E806●
      street car E829●
      watercraft E838●
        due to accident to
          watercraft E831●
  set in motion by
    accidental explosion of pressure
      vessel - *see* category E921
    firearm - *see* category E922
    machine(ry) - *see* Accident,
      machine
    transport vehicle - *see* categories
      E800–E848
  thrown from, in, on, towards
    aircraft E844●
    cable car (not on rails) E847
      on rails E829●
    motor vehicle (in motion) (on public
      highway) E818●
    not on public highway
      E825●
    nonmotor road vehicle NEC E829●
    pedal cycle E826●
    street car E829●
    vehicle NEC - *see* Accident, vehicle
      NEC
Obstruction
  air passages, larynx, respiratory
    passages
    by
      external means NEC - *see*
        Suffocation
      food, any type (regurgitated)
        (vomited) E911
      material or object, except food
        E912
      mucus E912
      phlegm E912
      vomitus E911
  digestive tract, except mouth or
    pharynx
    by
      food, any type E915
      foreign body (any) E915

Obstruction (*Continued*)
  esophagus
    food E911
    foreign body, except food E912
    without asphyxia or obstruction of
      respiratory passage E915
  mouth or pharynx
    by
      food, any type E911
      material or object, except food
        E912
  respiration - *see* Obstruction, air
    passages
Oil in eye E914
Overdose
  anesthetic (drug) - *see* Table of Drugs
    and Chemicals
  drug - *see* Table of Drugs and
    Chemicals
Overexertion E927.9
  from
    lifting E927.8
    maintaining prolonged positions
      E927.1
    holding E927.1
    sitting E927.1
    standing E927.1
    prolonged static position E927.1
    pulling E927.8
    pushing E927.8
    sudden strenuous movement
      E927.0
Overexposure (accidental) (to)
  cold (*see also* Cold, exposure to)
    E901.9
    due to manmade conditions
      E901.1
  heat (*see also* Heat) E900.9
  radiation - *see* Radiation
  radioactivity - *see* Radiation
  sun, except sunburn E900.0
  weather - *see* Exposure
  wind - *see* Exposure
Overheated (*see also* Heat) E900.9
Overlaid E913.0
Overturning (accidental)
  animal-drawn vehicle E827●
  boat, ship, watercraft
    causing
      drowning, submersion E830●
      injury except drowning,
        submersion E831●
  machinery - *see* Accident, machine
  motor vehicle (*see also* Loss of control,
    motor vehicle) E816●
    with antecedent collision on public
      highway - *see* Collision, motor
      vehicle
    not on public highway, nontraffic
      accident E825●
      with antecedent collision - *see*
        Collision, motor vehicle, not
        on public highway
  nonmotor road vehicle NEC E829●
  off-road type motor vehicle - *see* Loss of
    control, off-road type motor
    vehicle
  pedal cycle E826●
  railway rolling stock, train, vehicle
    (*see also* Derailment, railway)
    E802●
  street car E829●
  vehicle NEC - *see* Accident, vehicle
    NEC

P

Palsy, divers' E902.2
Parachuting (voluntary) (without
  accident to aircraft) E844●
  due to accident to aircraft - *see*
    categories E840–E842
Paralysis
  divers' E902.2
  lead or saturnine E866.0
    from pesticide NEC E863.4
Pecked by bird E906.8
Performance of correct operation
  (procedure) on wrong ◄
  body part E876.7 ◄
  side E876.7 ◄
  site E876.7 ◄
Performance of operation
  (procedure) ◄
  intended for another patient
    E876.6 ◄
  on patient not scheduled for
    surgery E876.6 ◄
  on wrong patient E876.6 ◄
Performance of wrong operation on
  correct patient E876.5 ◄
Phlegm aspiration or inhalation (with
  asphyxia, obstruction respiratory
  passage, suffocation) E912
Piercing (*see also* Cut) E920.9
  by slide trigger mechanism, scope
    or other part of gun E928.7 ◄
Pinched
  between objects (moving) (stationary
    and moving) E918
  by slide trigger mechanism, scope
    or other part of gun E928.7 ◄
  in object E918
Pinned under
  machine(ry) - *see* Accident, machine
Place of occurrence of accident - *see*
  Accident (to), occurring (at) (in)
Plumbism E866.0
  from insecticide NEC E863.4
Poisoning (accidental) (by) - *see also* Table
  of Drugs and Chemicals
  carbon monoxide
    generated by
      aircraft in transit E844●
      motor vehicle
        in motion (on public highway)
          E818●
        not on public highway
          E825●
      watercraft (in transit) (not in
        transit) E838●
  caused by injection of poisons or toxins
    into or through skin by plant
    thorns, spines, or other
    mechanism E905.7
  marine or sea plants E905.6
  fumes or smoke due to
    conflagration - *see* Conflagration
    explosion or fire - *see* Fire
    ignition - *see* Ignition
  gas
    in legal intervention E972
    legal execution, by E978
    on watercraft E838●
    used as anesthetic - *see* Table of
      Drugs and Chemicals
  in
    terrorism (chemical weapons) E979.7
    war operations E997.2

◄ New   ◄▥ Revised   ~~deleted~~ Deleted   ● Use Additional Digit(s)   ▨ Omit code

E CODES

Poisoning *(Continued)*
  late effect of - *see* Late effect
  legal
    execution E978
    intervention
      by gas E972
Pressure, external, causing asphyxia,
  suffocation *(see also* Suffocation)
  E913.9
Privation E904.9
  food *(see also* Lack of, food) E904.1
  helpless person, infant, newborn due to
    abandonment or neglect E904.0
  late effect of NEC E929.5
  resulting from transport accident - *see*
    categories E800–E848
  water *(see also* Lack of, water) E904.2
Projected objects, striking against or
  struck by - *see* Striking against,
  object
Prolonged stay in
  high altitude (causing conditions as
    listed in E902.0) E902.0
  weightless environment E928.0
Prostration
  heat - *see* Heat
Pulling, injury in E927.8
Puncture, puncturing *(see also* Cut)
  E920.9
  by
    plant thorns or spines E920.8
      toxic reaction E905.7
      marine or sea plants E905.6
      sea-urchin spine E905.6
Pushing (injury in) (overexertion)
  E927.8
  by other person(s) (accidental) E917.9
    as, or caused by, a crowd, human
      stampede E917.1
      with subsequent fall E917.6
    before moving vehicle or object
      stated as
        intentional, homicidal
          E968.5
        undetermined whether
          accidental or intentional
          E988.8
  from
    high place
      in accidental circumstances -
        see categories E880–E884
      stated as
        intentional, homicidal
          E968.1
        undetermined whether
          accidental or
          intentional E987.9
        man-made structure,
          except residential
          E987.1
        natural site E987.2
        residential E987.0
    motor vehicle *(see also* Fall, from,
      motor vehicle) E818●
      stated as
        intentional, homicidal
          E968.5
        undetermined whether
          accidental or
          intentional E988.8
    in sports E917.0
      with fall E886.0
    with fall E886.9
      in sports E886.0

R

Radiation (exposure to) E926.9
  abnormal reaction to medical test or
    therapy E879.2
  arc lamps E926.2
  atomic power plant (malfunction)
    NEC E926.9
    in water transport E838●
  electromagnetic, ionizing E926.3
  gamma rays E926.3
  in
    terrorism (from or following nuclear
      explosion) (direct) (secondary)
      E979.5
    laser E979.8
    war operations ~~(from or following~~
      ~~nuclear explosion) (direct)~~
      ~~(secondary)~~ *(see also* War
      operations, injury due to,
      nuclear weapons) E996.3 ◄▥
      laser(s) E997.0
    water transport E838●
  inadvertent exposure of patient
    (receiving test or therapy)
    E873.3
  infrared (heaters and lamps)
    E926.1
    excessive heat E900.1
  ionized, ionizing (particles, artificially
    accelerated) E926.8
    electromagnetic E926.3
  isotopes, radioactive - *see* Radiation,
    radioactive isotopes
  laser(s) E926.4
    in
      terrorism E979.8
      war operations E997.0
    misadventure in medical care - *see*
      Misadventure, failure, in
      dosage, radiation
  late effect of NEC E929.8
    excessive heat from - *see* Heat
  light sources (visible) (ultraviolet)
    E926.2
  misadventure in medical or surgical
    procedure - *see* Misadventure,
    failure, in dosage, radiation
  overdose (in medical or surgical
    pacemaker procedure) E873.2
  radar E926.0
  radioactive isotopes E926.5
    atomic power plant malfunction
      E926.5
      in water transport E838●
    misadventure in medical or
      surgical treatment - *see*
      Misadventure, failure, in
      dosage, radiation
  radiobiologicals - *see* Radiation,
    radioactive isotopes
  radiofrequency E926.0
  radiopharmaceuticals - *see* Radiation,
    radioactive isotopes
  radium NEC E926.9
  sun E926.2
    excessive heat from E900.0
  tanning bed E926.2
  welding arc or torch E926.2
    excessive heat from E900.1
  x-rays (hard) (soft) E926.3
    misadventure in medical or
      surgical treatment - *see*
      Misadventure, failure, in
      dosage, radiation

Rape E960.1
Reaction, abnormal to or following
  (medical or surgical procedure)
  E879.9
  amputation (of limbs) E878.5
  anastomosis (arteriovenous) (blood
    vessel) (gastrojejunal) (skin)
    (tendon) (natural, artificial
    material, tissue) E878.2
    external stoma, creation of E878.3
  aspiration (of fluid) E879.4
    tissue E879.8
  biopsy E879.8
  blood
    sampling E879.7
    transfusion
      procedure E879.8
  bypass - *see* Reaction, abnormal,
    anastomosis
  catheterization
    cardiac E879.0
    urinary E879.6
  colostomy E878.3
  cystostomy E878.3
  dialysis (kidney) E879.1
  drugs or biologicals - *see* Table of
    Drugs and Chemicals
  duodenostomy E878.3
  electroshock therapy E879.3
  formation of external stoma E878.3
  gastrostomy E878.3
  graft - *see* Reaction, abnormal,
    anastomosis
  hypothermia E879.8
  implant, implantation (of)
    artificial
      internal device (cardiac
        pacemaker) (electrodes
        in brain) (heart valve
        prosthesis) (orthopedic)
        E878.1
      material or tissue (for
        anastomosis or bypass)
        E878.2
        with creation of external
          stoma E878.3
      natural tissues (for anastomosis or
        bypass) E878.2
      as transplantion - *see* Reaction,
        abnormal, transplant
      with creation of external stoma
        E878.3
  infusion
    procedure E879.8
  injection
    procedure E879.8
  insertion of gastric or duodenal sound
    E879.5
  insulin-shock therapy E879.3
  lumbar puncture E879.4
  perfusion E879.1
  procedures other than surgical
    operation *(see also* Reaction,
    abnormal, by specific type of
    procedure) E879.9
    specified procedure NEC E879.8
  radiological procedure or therapy
    E879.2
  removal of organ (partial) (total)
    NEC E878.6
    with
      anastomosis, bypass or graft
        E878.2
      formation of external stoma
        E878.3

E CODES

Reaction, abnormal to or following *(Continued)*
removal of organ NEC *(Continued)*
with *(Continued)*
implant of artificial internal
device E878.1
transplant(ation)
partial organ E878.4
whole organ E878.0
sampling
blood E879.7
fluid NEC E879.4
tissue E879.8
shock therapy E879.3
surgical operation *(see also* Reaction,
abnormal, by specified type of
operation) E878.9
restorative NEC E878.4
with
anastomosis, bypass or graft
E878.2
formation of external stoma
E878.3
implant(ation) - *see* Reaction,
abnormal, implant
transplantation - *see*
Reaction, abnormal,
transplant
specified operation NEC
E878.8
thoracentesis E879.4
transfusion
procedure E879.8
transplant, transplantation (heart)
(kidney) (liver) E878.0
partial organ E878.4
ureterostomy E878.3
vaccination E879.8
Reduction in
atmospheric pressure - *see also* Effects
of, air pressure
while surfacing from
deep water diving causing
caisson or divers' disease,
palsy or paralysis
E902.2
underground E902.8
Residual (effect) - *see* Late effect
Rock falling on or hitting (accidentally)
motor vehicle (in motion) (on public
highway) E818●
not on public highway E825●
nonmotor road vehicle NEC
E829●
pedal cycle E826●
person E916
railway rolling stock, train, vehicle
E806●
Running off, away
animal (being ridden) (in sport or
transport) E828●
not being ridden E906.8
animal-drawn vehicle E827●
rails, railway *(see also* Derailment)
E802●
roadway
motor vehicle (without antecedent
collision) E816●
nontraffic accident E825●
with antecedent collision - *see*
categories Collision,
motor vehicle, not on
public highway

Running off, away *(Continued)*
roadway *(Continued)*
motor vehicle *(Continued)*
with
antecedent collision - *see*
Collision motor vehicle
subsequent collision
involving any object, person
or vehicle not on
public highway E816●
on public highway E811●
nonmotor road vehicle NEC E829●
pedal cycle E826●
Run over (accidentally) (by)
animal (not being ridden) E906.8
being ridden (in sport or transport)
E828●
animal-drawn vehicle E827●
machinery - *see* Accident, machine
motor vehicle (on public highway) - *see*
Hit by, motor vehicle
nonmotor road vehicle NEC E829●
railway train E805●
street car E829●
vehicle NEC E848

S

Saturnism E866.0
from insecticide NEC E863.4
Scald, scalding (accidental) (by) (from)
(in) E924.0
acid - *see* Scald, caustic
boiling tap water E924.2
caustic or corrosive liquid, substance
E924.1
swallowed - *see* Table of Drugs and
Chemicals
homicide (attempt) - *see* Assault,
burning
inflicted by other person
stated as
intentional or homicidal E968.3
undetermined whether
accidental or intentional
E988.2
late effect of NEC E929.8
liquid (boiling) (hot) E924.0
local application of externally applied
substance in medical or surgical
care E873.5
molten metal E924.0
self-inflicted (unspecified whether
accidental or intentional)
E988.2
stated as intentional, purposeful
E958.2
stated as undetermined whether
accidental or intentional
E988.2
steam E924.0
tap water (boiling) E924.2
transport accident - *see* categories
E800–E848
vapor E924.0
Scratch, cat E906.8
Sea
sickness E903
Self-mutilation - *see* Suicide
Sequelae (of)
in
terrorism E999.1
war operations E999.0

Shock
anaphylactic *(see also* Table of Drugs
and Chemicals) E947.9
due to
bite (venomous) - *see* Bite,
venomous NEC
sting - *see* Sting
electric *(see also* Electric shock) E925.9
from electric appliance or current *(see
also* Electric shock) E925.9
Shooting, shot (accidental(ly)) E922.9
air gun E922.4
BB gun E922.4
hand gun (pistol) (revolver) E922.0
himself *(see also* Shooting, self-
inflicted) E985.4
hand gun (pistol) (revolver) E985.0
military firearm, except hand gun
E985.3
hand gun (pistol) (revolver) E985.0
rifle (hunting) E985.2
military E985.3
shotgun (automatic) E985.1
specified firearm NEC E985.4
Verey pistol E985.4
homicide (attempt) E965.4
air gun E968.6
BB gun E968.6
hand gun (pistol) (revolver) E965.0
military firearm, except hand gun
E965.3
hand gun (pistol) (revolver)
E965.0
paintball gun E965.4
rifle (hunting) E965.2
military E965.3
shotgun (automatic) E965.1
specified firearm NEC E965.4
Verey pistol E965.4
inflicted by other person
in accidental circumstances E922.9
hand gun (pistol) (revolver)
E922.0
military firearm, except hand gun
E922.3
hand gun (pistol) (revolver)
E922.0
rifle (hunting) E922.2
military E922.3
shotgun (automatic) E922.1
specified firearm NEC E922.8
Verey pistol E922.8
stated as
intentional, homicidal E965.4
hand gun (pistol) (revolver)
E965.0
military firearm, except hand
gun E965.3
hand gun (pistol) (revolver)
E965.0
paintball gun E965.4
rifle (hunting) E965.2
military E965.3
shotgun (automatic) E965.1
specified firearm E965.4
Verey pistol E965.4
undetermined whether accidental
or intentional E985.4
air gun E985.6
BB gun E985.6
hand gun (pistol) (revolver)
E985.0
military firearm, except hand
gun E985.3

◀ New   ◀━ Revised   ~~deleted~~ Deleted   ● Use Additional Digit(s)   ▦ Omit code

Shooting, shot *(Continued)*
  inflicted by other person *(Continued)*
    stated as *(Continued)*
      undetermined whether accidental or intentional *(Continued)*
        hand gun (pistol) (revolver) E985.0
        paintball gun E985.7
        rifle (hunting) E985.2
        shotgun (automatic) E985.1
        specified firearm NEC E985.4
        Verey pistol E985.4
  in
    terrorism - *see* Terrorism, shooting
    war operations - *see* War operations, shooting
  legal
    execution E978
    intervention E970
  military firearm, except hand gun E922.3
    hand gun (pistol) (revolver) E922.0
  paintball gun E922.5
  rifle (hunting) E922.2
    military E922.3
  self-inflicted (unspecified whether accidental or intentional) E985.4
    air gun E985.6
    BB gun E985.6
    hand gun (pistol) (revolver) E985.0
    military firearm, except hand gun E985.3
      hand gun (pistol) (revolver) E985.0
    paintball gun E985.7
    rifle (hunting) E985.2
      military E985.3
    shotgun (automatic) E985.1
    specified firearm NEC E985.4
    stated as
      accidental E922.9
        hand gun (pistol) (revolver) E922.0
        military firearm, except hand gun E922.3
          hand gun (pistol) (revolver) E922.0
        paintball gun E922.5
        rifle (hunting) E922.2
          military E922.3
        shotgun (automatic) E922.1
        specified firearm NEC E922.8
        Verey pistol E922.8
      intentional, purposeful E955.4
        hand gun (pistol) (revolver) E955.0
        military firearm, except hand gun E955.3
          hand gun (pistol) (revolver) E955.0
        paintball gun E955.7
        rifle (hunting) E955.2
          military E955.3
        shotgun (automatic) E955.1
        specified firearm NEC E955.4
        Verey pistol E955.4
    shotgun (automatic) E922.1
    specified firearm NEC E922.8

Shooting, shot *(Continued)*
  stated as undetermined whether accidental or intentional E985.4
    hand gun (pistol) (revolver) E985.0
    military firearm, except hand gun E985.3
      hand gun (pistol) (revolver) E985.0
    paintball gun E985.7
    rifle (hunting) E985.2
      military E985.3
    shotgun (automatic) E985.1
    specified firearm NEC E985.4
    Verey pistol E985.4
  suicidal (attempt) E955.4
    air gun E985.6
    BB gun E985.6
    hand gun (pistol) (revolver) E955.0
    military firearm, except hand gun E955.3
      hand gun (pistol) (revolver) E955.0
    paintball gun E955.7
    rifle (hunting) E955.2
      military E955.3
    shotgun (automatic) E955.1
    specified firearm NEC E955.4
    Verey pistol E955.4
  Verey pistol E922.8
Shoving (accidentally) by other person *(see also* Pushing by other person) E917.9
Sickness
  air E903
  alpine E902.0
  car E903
  motion E903
  mountain E902.0
  sea E903
  travel E903
Sinking (accidental)
  boat, ship, watercraft (causing drowning, submersion) E830●
    causing injury except drowning, submersion E831●
Siriasis E900.0
Skydiving E844●
Slashed wrists *(see also* Cut, self-inflicted) E986
Slipping (accidental)
  on
    deck (of boat, ship, watercraft) (icy) (oily) (wet) E835●
    ice E885.9
    ladder of ship E833●
      due to accident to watercraft E831●
    mud E885.9
    oil E885.9
    snow E885.9
    stairs of ship E833●
      due to accident to watercraft E831●
    surface
      slippery E885.9
      wet E885.9
Sliver, wood, injury by E920.8
Smothering, smothered *(see also* Suffocation) E913.9
Smouldering building or structure in terrorism E979.3

Sodomy (assault) E960.1
Solid substance in eye (any part) or adnexa E914
Sound waves (causing injury) E928.1
Splinter, injury by E920.8
Stab, stabbing E966
  accidental - *see* Cut
Starvation E904.1
  helpless person, infant, newborn - *see* Lack of food
  homicidal intent E968.4
  late effect of NEC E929.5
  resulting from accident connected with transport - *see* categories E800–E848
Stepped on
  by
    animal (not being ridden) E906.8
      being ridden (in sport or transport) E828●
    crowd E917.1
    person E917.9
      in sports E917.0
    in sports E917.0
Stepping on
  object (moving) E917.9
    in sports E917.0
      with subsequent fall E917.5
    stationary E917.4
      with subsequent fall E917.8
  person E917.9
    as, or caused by a crowd E917.1
      with subsequent fall E917.6
    in sports E917.0
Sting E905.9
  ant E905.5
  bee E905.3
  caterpillar E905.5
  coral E905.6
  hornet E905.3
  insect NEC E905.5
  jelly fish E905.6
  marine animal or plant E905.6
  nematocysts E905.6
  scorpion E905.2
  sea anemone E905.6
  sea cucumber E905.6
  wasp E905.3
  yellow jacket E905.3
Storm E908.9
  specified type NEC E908.8
Straining, injury in E927.8
Strangling - *see* Suffocation
Strangulation - *see* Suffocation
Strenuous movements (in recreational or other activities) E927.8
Striking against
  bottom (when jumping or diving into water) E883.0
  object (moving) E917.9
    caused by crowd E917.1
      with subsequent fall E917.6
    furniture E917.3
      with subsequent fall E917.7
    in
      running water E917.2
        with drowning or submersion - *see* Submersion
      sports E917.0
        with subsequent fall E917.5
    stationary E917.4
      with subsequent fall E917.8

◀ New   ◀▥ Revised   ~~deleted~~ Deleted   ● Use Additional Digit(s)   ▦ Omit code

E CODES

Striking against *(Continued)*
  person(s) E917.9
    with fall E886.9
      in sports E886.0
    as, or caused by, a crowd E917.1
      with subsequent fall E917.6
      in sports E917.0
        with fall E886.0
Stroke
  heat - *see* Heat
  lightning E907
Struck by - *see also* Hit by
  bullet
    in
      terrorism E979.4
      war operations E991.2
        rubber E991.0
  lightning E907
  missile
    in terrorism - *see* Terrorism, missile
  object
    falling
      from, in, on
        building
          burning (uncontrolled fire)
            in terrorism E979.3
  thunderbolt E907
Stumbling over animal, carpet, curb,
  rug or (small) object (with fall)
  E885.9
  without fall - *see* Striking against, object
Submersion (accidental) E910.8
  boat, ship, watercraft (causing
    drowning, submersion) E830 ●
    causing injury except drowning,
      submersion E831 ●
  by other person
    in accidental circumstances - *see*
      category E910
    intentional, homicidal E964
    stated as undetermined whether
      accidental or intentional E984
  due to
    accident
      machinery - *see* Accident,
        machine
      to boat, ship, watercraft E830 ●
      transport - *see* categories E800-
        E848
    avalanche E909.2
    cataclysmic
      earth surface movement or
        eruption E909.9
      storm E908.9
    cloudburst E908.8
    cyclone E908.1
    fall
      from
        boat, ship, watercraft (not
          involved in accident)
          E832 ●
          burning, crushed E830 ●
          involved in accident,
            collision E830 ●
        gangplank (into water) E832 ●
        overboard NEC E832 ●
    flood E908.2
    hurricane E908.0
    jumping into water E910.8
      from boat, ship, watercraft
        burning, crushed, sinking
          E830 ●
        involved in accident, collision
          E830 ●
        not involved in accident, for
          swim E910.2

Submersion *(Continued)*
  due to *(Continued)*
    jumping into water *(Continued)*
      in recreational activity (without
        diving equipment) E910.2
        with or using diving
          equipment E910.1
      to rescue another person E910.3
    homicide (attempt) E964
  in
    bathtub E910.4
    specified activity, not sport,
      transport or recreational
      E910.3
    sport or recreational activity
      (without diving equipment)
      E910.2
    with or using diving equipment
      E910.1
    water skiing E910.0
    swimming pool NEC E910.8
    terrorism E979.8
    war operations E995.4 ◀▥
      intentional E995.3 ◀
    water transport E832 ●
      due to accident to boat, ship,
        watercraft E830 ●
  landslide E909.2
    overturning boat, ship, watercraft
      E909.2
    sinking boat, ship, watercraft
      E909.2
    submersion boat, ship, watercraft
      E909.2
    tidal wave E909.4
      caused by storm E908.0
    torrential rain E908.2
  late effect of NEC E929.8
  quenching tank E910.8
  self-inflicted (unspecified whether
    accidental or intentional) E984
    in accidental circumstances - *see*
      category E910
    stated as intentional, purposeful
      E954
  stated as undetermined whether
    accidental or intentional
    E984
  suicidal (attempted) E954
  while
    attempting rescue of another person
      E910.3
    engaged in
      marine salvage E910.3
      underwater construction or
        repairs E910.3
    fishing, not from boat E910.2
    hunting, not from boat E910.2
    ice skating E910.2
    pearl diving E910.3
    placing fishing nets E910.3
    playing in water E910.2
    scuba diving E910.1
      nonrecreational E910.3
    skin diving E910.1
    snorkel diving E910.2
    spear fishing underwater E910.1
    surfboarding E910.2
    swimming (swimming pool)
      E910.2
    wading (in water) E910.2
    water skiing E910.0
Sucked
  into
    jet (aircraft) E844 ●

Suffocation (accidental) (by external
  means) (by pressure) (mechanical)
  E913.9
  caused by other person
    in accidental circumstances - *see*
      category E913
    stated as
      intentional, homicidal E963
      undetermined whether accidental
        or intentional E983.9
      by, in
        hanging E983.0
        plastic bag E983.1
        specified means NEC
          E983.8
  due to, by
    avalanche E909.2
    bedclothes E913.0
    bib E913.0
    blanket E913.0
    cave-in E913.3
      caused by cataclysmic earth
        surface movement or
        eruption E909.9
    conflagration - *see* Conflagration
      E983.8
    explosion - *see* Explosion
    falling earth, other substance
      E913.3
    fire - *see* Fire
    food, any type (ingestion)
      (inhalation) (regurgitated)
      (vomited) E911
    foreign body, except food (ingestion)
      (inhalation) E912
    ignition - *see* Ignition
    landslide E909.2
    machine(ry) - *see* Accident,
      machine
    material, object except food entering
      by nose or mouth, ingested,
      inhaled E912
    mucus (aspiration) (inhalation), not
      of newborn E912
    phlegm (aspiration) (inhalation)
      E912
    pillow E913.0
    plastic bag - *see* Suffocation, in,
      plastic bag
    sheet (plastic) E913.0
    specified means NEC E913.8
    vomitus (aspiration) (inhalation)
      E911
  homicidal (attempt) E963
    in war operations E995.3 ◀
  in
    airtight enclosed place E913.2
    baby carriage E913.0
    bed E913.0
    closed place E913.2
    cot, cradle E913.0
    perambulator E913.0
    plastic bag (in accidental
      circumstances) E913.1
      homicidal, purposely inflicted by
        other person E963
      self-inflicted (unspecified
        whether accidental or
        intentional) E983.1
        in accidental circumstances
          E913.1
        intentional, suicidal E953.1
      stated as undetermined whether
        accidentally or purposely
        inflicted E983.1

◀ New   ◀▥ Revised   ~~deleted~~ Deleted   ● Use Additional Digit(s)   ▨ Omit code

E CODES

Suffocation *(Continued)*
  in *(Continued)*
    plastic bag *(Continued)*
      suicidal, purposely self-inflicted
        E953.1
    refrigerator E913.2
    self-inflicted - *see also* Suffocation,
      stated as undetermined whether
      accidental or intentional E953.9
      in accidental circumstances - *see*
        category E913
      stated as intentional, purposeful - *see*
        Suicide, suffocation
    stated as undetermined whether
      accidental or intentional E983.9
      by, in
        hanging E983.0
        plastic bag E983.1
        specified means NEC E983.8
    suicidal - *see* Suicide, suffocation
    war operations E995.3 ◄
Suicide, suicidal (attempted) (by)
    E958.9
  burning, burns E958.1
  caustic substance E958.7
    poisoning E950.7
    swallowed E950.7
  cold, extreme E958.3
  cut (any part of body) E956
  cutting or piercing instrument
    (classifiable to E920) E956
  drowning E954
  electrocution E958.4
  explosive(s) (classifiable to E923)
    E955.5
  fire E958.1
  firearm (classifiable to E922) - *see*
    Shooting, suicidal
  hanging E953.0
  jumping
    before moving object, train, vehicle
      E958.0
    from high place - *see* Jumping,
      from, high place, stated as,
      suicidal
  knife E956
  late effect of E959
  motor vehicle, crashing of E958.5
  poisoning - *see* Table of Drugs and
    Chemicals
  puncture (any part of body) E956
  scald E958.2
  shooting - *see* Shooting, suicidal
  specified means NEC E958.8
  stab (any part of body) E956
  strangulation - *see* Suicide,
    suffocation
  submersion E954
  suffocation E953.9
    by, in
      hanging E953.0
      plastic bag E953.1
      specified means NEC E953.8
  wound NEC E958.9
Sunburn E926.2
Sunstroke E900.0
Supersonic waves (causing injury)
    E928.1
Surgical procedure, complication of
  delayed or as an abnormal reaction
    without mention of
    misadventure, *see* Reaction,
    abnormal
  due to or as a result of misadventure -
    see Misadventure

Swallowed, swallowing
  foreign body - *see* Foreign body,
    alimentary canal
  poison - *see* Table of Drugs and
    Chemicals
  substance
    caustic - *see* Table of Drugs and
      Chemicals drugs
    corrosive - *see* Table of Drugs and
      Chemicals
    poisonous - *see* Table of Drugs and
      Chemicals
Swimmers' cramp (*see also* category
    E910) E910.2
  not in recreation or sport E910.3
Syndrome, battered
  baby or child - *see* Abuse, child
  wife - *see* Assault

T

Tackle in sport E886.0
Terrorism (by) (in) (injury) E979.8
  air blast E979.2
  aircraft burned, destroyed, exploded,
    shot down E979.1
    used as a weapon E979.1
  anthrax E979.6
  asphyxia from
    chemical (weapons) E979.7
    fire, conflagration (caused by fire-
      producing device) E979.3
      from nuclear explosion
        E979.5
    gas or fumes E979.7
  bayonet E979.8
  biological agents E979.6
  blast (air) (effects) E979.2
    from nuclear explosion E979.5
    underwater E979.0
  bomb (antipersonnel) (mortar)
    (explosion) (fragments)
    E979.2
  bullet(s) (from carbine, machine gun,
    pistol, rifle, shotgun)
    E979.4
  burn from
    chemical E979.7
    fire, conflagration (caused by fire-
      producing device) E979.3
      from nuclear explosion E979.5
    gas E979.7
  burning aircraft E979.1
  chemical E979.7
  cholera E979.6
  conflagration E979.3
  crushed by falling aircraft E979.1
  depth-charge E979.0
  destruction of aircraft E979.1
  disability, as sequelae one year or more
    after injury E999.1
  drowning E979.8
  effect
    of nuclear weapon (direct)
      (secondary) E979.5
    secondary NEC E979.9
    sequelae E999.1
  explosion (artillery shell) (breech-
    block) (cannon block) E979.2
    aircraft E979.1
    bomb (antipersonnel) (mortar)
      E979.2
    nuclear (atom) (hydrogen)
      E979.5

Terrorism *(Continued)*
  explosion *(Continued)*
    depth-charge E979.0
    grenade E979.2
    injury by fragments from E979.2
    land-mine E979.2
    marine weapon E979.0
    mine (land) E979.2
      at sea or in harbor E979.0
      marine E979.0
    missile (explosive) NEC E979.2
    munitions (dump) (factory)
      E979.2
    nuclear (weapon) E979.5
      other direct and secondary effects
        of E979.5
    sea-based artillery shell
      E979.0
    torpedo E979.0
  exposure to ionizing radiation from
    nuclear explosion E979.5
  falling aircraft E979.1
  fire or fire-producing device E979.3
  firearms E979.4
  fireball effects from nuclear explosion
    E979.5
  fragments from artillery shell, bomb
    NEC, grenade, guided missile,
    land-mine, rocket, shell, shrapnel
    E979.2
  gas or fumes E979.7
  grenade (explosion) (fragments)
    E979.2
  guided missile (explosion) (fragments)
    E979.2
    nuclear E979.5
  heat from nuclear explosion E979.5
  hot substances E979.3
  hydrogen cyanide E979.7
  land-mine (explosion) (fragments)
    E979.2
  laser(s) E979.8
  late effect of E999.1
  lewisite E979.7
  lung irritant (chemical) (fumes) (gas)
    E979.7
  marine mine E979.0
  mine E979.2
    at sea E979.0
    in harbor E979.0
    land (explosion) (fragments)
      E979.2
    marine E979.0
  missile (explosion) (fragments)
    (guided) E979.2
    marine E979.0
    nuclear weapons E979.5
  mortar bomb (explosion) (fragments)
    E979.2
  mustard gas E979.7
  nerve gas E979.7
  nuclear weapons E979.5
  pellets (shotgun) E979.4
  petrol bomb E979.3
  phosgene E979.7
  piercing object E979.8
  poisoning (chemical) (fumes) (gas)
    E979.7
  radiation, ionizing from nuclear
    explosion E979.5
  rocket (explosion) (fragments)
    E979.2
  saber, sabre E979.8
  sarin E979.7
  screening smoke E979.7

◀ New   ◀▥ Revised   ~~deleted~~ Deleted   ● Use Additional Digit(s)   ▤ Omit code

E CODES

War operations *(Continued)*
  explosion *(Continued)*
    aircraft *(Continued)*
      due to ◀
        enemy fire or explosives
          E994.0 ◀
        own onboard explosives
          E994.1 ◀
    artillery shell E993.2 ◀
    bomb (mortar) E993.2 ◀⃫
      aerial E993.0
      atom *(see also* War operations,
        injury due to, nuclear
        weapons) E996.9 ◀⃫
      hydrogen *(see also* War
        operations, injury due to,
        nuclear weapons) E996.9 ◀⃫
      injury by fragments from
        E991.4 ◀⃫
        antipersonnel E991.3
      nuclear *(see also* War operations,
        injury due to, nuclear
        weapons) E996.9 ◀⃫
    depth charge E992.1 ◀⃫
    injury by fragments from E991.4 ◀⃫
      antipersonnel E991.3
    marine weapon NEC E992.8 ◀⃫
    mine
      at sea or in harbor E992.2 ◀⃫
      land E993.8 ◀⃫
        injury by fragments from
          E991.4 ◀⃫
      marine E992.2 ◀⃫
    missile, guided E993.1 ◀
    mortar E993.2 ◀
    munitions (accidental) (being used
      in war) (dump) (factory)
      E993.9 ◀⃫
      own E993.7
        launch device (autocannons)
          (automatic grenade
          launchers) (missile
          launchers) (small arms)
          E993.7 ◀
    nuclear (weapon) *(see also* War
      operations, injury due to,
      nuclear weapons) E996.9 ◀⃫
    own weapons (accidental) E993.7 ◀⃫
      injury by fragments from E991.9
        antipersonnel E991.3
    sea-based artillery shell E992.3 ◀⃫
    specified NEC E993.8 ◀
    torpedo E992.0 ◀⃫
  exposure to ionizing radiation from
    nuclear explosion *(see also* War
    operations, injury due to, nuclear
    weapons) E996.3 ◀⃫
  falling aircraft E994.8 ◀⃫
  fire or fire-producing device E990.9
    flamethrower E990.1 ◀
    incendiary bomb E990.0 ◀
    incendiary bullet E990.2 ◀
    indirectly caused from conventional
      weapon E990.3 ◀
    petrol bomb E990.0
  fireball effects from nuclear explosion
    E996.2 ◀⃫
  fragments from
    antipersonnel bomb E991.3
    artillery shell ~~bomb NEC, grenade,~~
      ~~guided missile, land mine,~~
      ~~rocket, shell, shrapnel~~
      ~~E991.9~~ E991.4 ◀⃫
    bomb NEC E991.4 ◀
    grenade E991.4 ◀
    guided missile E991.4 ◀

War operations *(Continued)*
  fragments from *(Continued)*
    land mine E991.4 ◀
    rocket E991.4 ◀
    shell E991.4 ◀
    shrapnel E991.9 ◀
  fumes E997.2
  gas E997.2
  grenade (explosion) E993.8 ◀⃫
    fragments, injury by E991.4 ◀⃫
  guided missile (explosion) E993.1 ◀⃫
    fragments, injury by E991.4 ◀⃫
  nuclear *(see also* War operations,
    injury due to, nuclear
    weapons) E996.9 ◀⃫
  heat from nuclear explosion
    E996.2 ◀⃫
  injury due to, ~~but occurring after~~
    ~~cessation of hostilities E998~~
    aerial bomb E993.0 ◀
    air blast E993.9 ◀
    aircraft shot down E994.0 ◀
    artillery shell E993.2 ◀
    blast E993.9 ◀
      wave E993.9 ◀
      wind E993.9 ◀
    bomb E998.8 ◀
    but occurring after cessation of
      hostilities
      explosion of bombs E998.1 ◀
      explosion of mines E998.0 ◀
      specified NEC E998.8 ◀
    conventional warfare E995.9 ◀
      specified form NEC E995.8 ◀
    depth charge E992.1 ◀
    destruction of aircraft E994.9 ◀
      due to ◀
        air to air missile E994.0 ◀
        collision with other aircraft
          E994.2 ◀
        enemy fire or explosives
          E994.0 ◀
        on board explosion
          (explosives) E994.1 ◀
        on board fire E994.3 ◀
        rocket propelled grenade
          [RPG] E994.0 ◀
        small arms fire E994.0 ◀
        surface to air missile E994.0 ◀
      specified NEC E994.8 ◀
    dirty bomb *(see also* War
      operations, injury due to,
      nuclear weapons) E996.9 ◀
    drowning E995.4 ◀
    explosion (direct pressure)
      (indirect pressure)
      (due to) E993.9 ◀
      depth charge E992.1 ◀
      improvised explosive device
        [IED] ◀
        person borne E993.3 ◀
        roadside E993.5 ◀
        specified NEC E993.5 ◀
        transport vehicle (air) (land)
          (water) borne E993.4 ◀
        vehicle (air) (land) (water)
          borne E993.4 ◀
      marine mines (in harbor)
        (at sea) E992.2 ◀
      marine weapons E992.9 ◀
        specified NEC E992.8 ◀
      sea based artillery shell
        E992.3 ◀
      specified NEC E993.8 ◀
      torpedo E992.0 ◀

War operations *(Continued)*
  injury due to, *(Continued)*
    explosion *(Continued)*
      unintentional (of own) ◀
        autocannons E993.7 ◀
        automatic grenade launchers
          E993.7 ◀
        launch device discharge
          E993.7 ◀
        munitions detonation
          (ammunition) (artillery)
          (mortars) E993.6 ◀
        missile launchers E993.7 ◀
        small arms E993.7 ◀
    fragments (from) E991.9 ◀
      artillery E991.8 ◀
      artillery shells E991.4 ◀
      autocannons E991.8 ◀
      automatic grenade launchers
        [AGL] E991.8 ◀
      bombs E991.4 ◀
        antipersonnel E991.3 ◀
      detonation of unexploded
        ordnance [UXO] E991.4 ◀
      grenade E991.4 ◀
      guided missile E991.4 ◀
      improvised explosive device
        [IED] ◀
        person borne E991.5 ◀
        roadside E991.7 ◀
        specified NEC E991.7 ◀
        transport vehicle (air) (land)
          (water) borne E991.6 ◀
        vehicle (air) (land) (water)
          borne E991.6 ◀
      land mine E991.4 ◀
      missile launchers E991.8 ◀
      mortars E991.8 ◀
      munitions (artillery shells)
        (bombs) (grenades)
        (rockets) (shells) E991.4 ◀
      rockets E991.4 ◀
      shells E991.4 ◀
      small arms E991.8 ◀
      specified NEC E991.9 ◀
      weapons (artillery)
        (autocannons) (mortars)
        (small arms) E991.8 ◀
    grenade E993.8 ◀
    guided missile E993.1 ◀
    hand to hand combat,
      unarmed E995.0 ◀
    improvised explosive device
      [IED] ◀
      person borne E993.3 ◀
      roadside E993.5 ◀
      specified NEC E993.5 ◀
      transport vehicle (air) (land)
        (water) borne E993.4 ◀
      vehicle (air) (land) (water) borne
        E993.4 ◀
    inability to surface or obtain air
      E995.4 ◀
    land mine E993.8 ◀
    marine mines (in harbor) (at sea)
      E992.2 ◀
    marine weapons E992.9 ◀
      specified NEC E992.8 ◀
    mortar E993.2 ◀
    nuclear weapons E996.9 ◀
      beta burns E996.3 ◀
      blast debris E996.1 ◀
      blast pressure E996.0 ◀
      burns due to thermal radiation
        E996.2 ◀

◀ New   ◀⃫ Revised   ~~deleted~~ Deleted   ● Use Additional Digit(s)   ▨ Omit code

War operations *(Continued)*
   injury due to, *(Continued)*
      nuclear weapons *(Continued)*
         direct blast effect E996.0 ◄
         fallout exposure E996.3 ◄
         fireball effect E996.2 ◄
         flash burns E996.2 ◄
         heat effect E996.2 ◄
         indirect blast effect E996.1 ◄
         nuclear radiation effects
           E996.3 ◄
         radiation exposure (acute)
           E996.3 ◄
         radiation sickness E996.3 ◄
         secondary effects E996.3 ◄
         specified effects NEC E996.8 ◄
         thermal radiation effect E996.2 ◄
      piercing object E995.2 ◄
      restriction of airway, intentional
         E995.3 ◄
      sea based artillery shell E992.3 ◄
      shrapnel E991.9 ◄
      stave E995.1 ◄
      strangulation E995.3 ◄
      strike by blunt object (baton)
         (nightstick) (stave) E995.1 ◄
      submersion (accidental)
         (unintentional) E995.4 ◄
         intentional E995.3 ◄
      suffocation E995.3 ◄
         accidental E995.4 ◄
      torpedo E992.0 ◄
      underwater blast E992.9 ◄
      weapon of mass destruction
         [WMD] E997.3 ◄
   knife E995.2 ◄
   lacrimator (gas) (chemical) E997.2
   land mine (explosion) E993.8 ◄⫶
      after cessation of hostilities
         E998.0 ◄⫶
      fragments, injury by E991.4 ◄⫶
   laser(s) E997.0
   late effect of E999.0
   lewisite E997.2
   lung irritant (chemical) (fumes)
      (gas) E997.2
   marine mine E992.2 ◄⫶
   mine
      after cessation of hostilities
         E998.0 ◄⫶
      at sea E992.2 ◄⫶

War operations *(Continued)*
   mine *(Continued)*
      in harbor E992.2 ◄⫶
      land (explosion) E993.8 ◄⫶
         fragments, injury by E991.4 ◄⫶
      marine E992.2 ◄⫶
   missile (guided) (explosion) E993.1 ◄⫶
      fragments, injury by E991.4 ◄⫶
      marine E992.8 ◄⫶
      nuclear *(see also* War operations,
         injury due to, nuclear
         weapons) E996.9 ◄⫶
   mortar bomb (explosion) E993.2 ◄⫶
      fragments, injury by E991.4 ◄⫶
   mustard gas E997.2
   nerve gas E997.2
   phosgene E997.2
   piercing object E995.2 ◄
   poisoning (chemical) (fumes) (gas)
      E997.2
   radiation, ionizing from nuclear
      explosion *(see also* War
      operations, injury due to,
      nuclear weapons) E996.3 ◄⫶
   rocket (explosion) E993.8 ◄⫶
      fragments, injury by E991.4 ◄⫶
   saber, sabre E995.2 ◄⫶
   screening smoke E997.8
   shell (aircraft) (artillery) (cannon)
      (land based) (explosion)
      E993.2 ◄⫶
      fragments, injury by E991.4 ◄⫶
      sea-based E992.3 ◄⫶
   shooting E991.2
      after cessation of hostilities
         E998.8 ◄⫶
      bullet(s) E991.2
         rubber E991.0
      pellet(s) (rifle) E991.1
      shrapnel E991.9
   stave E995.2 ◄
   strike by blunt object (baton)
      (nightstick) (stave)
      E995.1 ◄
   submersion E995.4 ◄⫶
      intentional E995.3 ◄
   sword E995.2 ◄
   torpedo E992.0 ◄⫶
   unconventional warfare, except by
      nuclear weapon E997.9
      biological (warfare) E997.1

War operations *(Continued)*
   unconventional warfare *(Continued)*
      gas, fumes, chemicals E997.2
      laser(s) E997.0
      specified type NEC E997.8
   underwater blast E992.9 ◄⫶
   vesicant (chemical) (fumes) (gas)
      E997.2
   weapon burst E993.9 ◄⫶
Washed
   away by flood - *see* Flood
   away by tidal wave - *see* Tidal wave
   off road by storm (transport vehicle)
      E908.9
   overboard E832●
Weapon of mass destruction [WMD]
   E997.3 ◄
Weather exposure - *see also* Exposure
   cold E901.0
   hot E900.0
Weightlessness (causing injury) (effects
   of) (in spacecraft, real or simulated)
   E928.0
Wound (accidental) NEC *(see also* Injury)
   E928.9
   battle *(see also* War operations)
      E995.9 ◄⫶
   bayonet E920.3
      in
         legal intervention E974
         war operations E995.2 ◄⫶
   gunshot - *see* Shooting
   incised - *see* Cut
   saber, sabre E920.3
      in war operations E995.2 ◄⫶
Wrong ◄
   body part, performance of correct
      operation (procedure) on
      E876.7 ◄
   device implanted into correct
      surgical site E876.5 ◄
   patient, performance of operation
      (procedure) on E876.6 ◄
   procedure (operation) performed
      on correct patient E876.5 ◄
   side, performance of correct
      operation (procedure) on
      E876.7 ◄
   site, performance of correct operation
      (procedure) on E876.7 ◄

E CODES

◄ New   ◄⫶ Revised   ~~deleted~~ Deleted   ● Use Additional Digit(s)   ▨ Omit code

PART III

Diseases: Tabular List Volume 1

1. INFECTIOUS AND PARASITIC DISEASES (001–139)

> **Note:** Categories for "late effects" of infectious and parasitic diseases are to be found at 137–139.
>
> **Includes** diseases generally recognized as communicable or transmissible as well as a few diseases of unknown but possibly infectious origin
>
> **Excludes** *acute respiratory infections (460–466)*
> *carrier or suspected carrier of infectious organism (V02.0–V02.9)*
> *certain localized infections*
> *influenza (487.0–487.8, 488, 488.0–488.1)*

INTESTINAL INFECTIOUS DISEASES (001–009)

> **Excludes** *helminthiases (120.0–129)*
> *Diseases or infestations caused by parasitic worms*

● 001 **Cholera**
A serious, often deadly, infectious disease of the small intestine

  001.0 **Due to Vibrio cholerae**

  001.1 **Due to Vibrio cholerae el tor**

  ■001.9 **Cholera, unspecified**

● 002 **Typhoid and paratyphoid fevers**
Caused by Salmonella typhi and Salmonella paratyphi A, B, and C bacteria

  002.0 **Typhoid fever**
  Typhoid (fever) (infection) [any site]

  002.1 **Paratyphoid fever A**

  002.2 **Paratyphoid fever B**

  002.3 **Paratyphoid fever C**

  ■002.9 **Paratyphoid fever, unspecified**

Item 1–1 Salmonella is a bacterium that lives in the intestines of fowl and mammals and can spread to humans through improper food preparation and cooking. Salmonellosis is an infection with the bacterium. Symptoms include diarrhea, fever, and abdominal cramps 12 to 72 hours after infection. The illness usually lasts 4 to 7 days, and most persons recover without treatment. The diarrhea may be so severe that the patient needs to be hospitalized. Patients with immunocompromised systems in chronic, ill health are more likely to have the infection invade their bloodstream with life-threatening results. For example, patients with sickle cell disease are more prone to salmonella osteomyelitis than others.

● 003 **Other salmonella infections**

> **Includes** infection or food poisoning by Salmonella [any serotype]

  003.0 **Salmonella gastroenteritis**
  Salmonellosis

  003.1 **Salmonella septicemia**

● 003.2 **Localized salmonella infections**

  ■003.20 **Localized salmonella infection, unspecified**
  Specified in the documentation as localized, but unspecified as to type

  003.21 **Salmonella meningitis**
  Specified as localized in the meninges

  003.22 **Salmonella pneumonia**
  Specified as localized in the lungs

  003.23 **Salmonella arthritis**
  Specified as localized in the joints

  003.24 **Salmonella osteomyelitis**
  Specified as localized in bone

  ■003.29 **Other**
  Specified as localized (because it is still under localized heading) but does not assign into any of the above codes

INFECTIOUS AND PARASITIC DISEASES (001–139)

■ **003.8**   **Other specified salmonella infections**
Any specified salmonella infection which does NOT assign into any of the above codes (not specified as localized)

■ **003.9**   **Salmonella infection, unspecified**
Unspecified in the documentation as to specific type of salmonella

● **004**   **Shigellosis**
An infectious disease caused by a group of bacteria (Shigella)

Includes   bacillary dysentery

004.0   **Shigella dysenteriae**
Infection by group A Shigella (Schmitz) (Shiga)

004.1   **Shigella flexneri**
Infection by group B Shigella

004.2   **Shigella boydii**
Infection by group C Shigella

004.3   **Shigella sonnei**
Infection by group D Shigella

■ **004.8**   **Other specified shigella infections**

■ **004.9**   **Shigellosis, unspecified**

● **005**   **Other food poisoning (bacterial)**
See Table A, Table of Bacterial Food Poisoning, pg. 1206

Excludes   *salmonella infections (003.0–003.9)*
toxic effect of:
food contaminants (989.7)
noxious foodstuffs (988.0–988.9)

005.0   **Staphylococcal food poisoning**
Staphylococcal toxemia specified as due to food

005.1   **Botulism food poisoning**
Botulism NOS
Food poisoning due to Clostridium botulinum

Excludes   *infant botulism (040.41)*
wound botulism (040.42)

005.2   **Food poisoning due to Clostridium perfringens [C. welchii]**
Enteritis necroticans

005.3   **Food poisoning due to other Clostridia**

005.4   **Food poisoning due to Vibrio parahaemolyticus**

● **005.8**   **Other bacterial food poisoning**

Excludes   *salmonella food poisoning (003.0–003.9)*

005.81   **Food poisoning due to Vibrio vulnificus**

■ **005.89**   **Other bacterial food poisoning**
Food poisoning due to Bacillus cereus

■ **005.9**   **Food poisoning, unspecified**

● **006**   **Amebiasis**
An intestinal illness caused by the microscopic parasite Entamoeba histolytica

Includes   infection due to Entamoeba histolytica

Excludes   *amebiasis due to organisms other than Entamoeba histolytica (007.8)*

006.0   **Acute amebic dysentery without mention of abscess**
Acute amebiasis

006.1   **Chronic intestinal amebiasis without mention of abscess**
Chronic:
amebiasis
amebic dysentery

006.2   **Amebic nondysenteric colitis**

006.3   **Amebic liver abscess**
Hepatic amebiasis

006.4   **Amebic lung abscess**
Amebic abscess of lung (and liver)

006.5   **Amebic brain abscess**
Amebic abscess of brain (and liver) (and lung)

006.6   **Amebic skin ulceration**
Cutaneous amebiasis

■ **006.8**   **Amebic infection of other sites**
Amebic:
appendicitis
balanitis
Ameboma

Excludes   *specific infections by free-living amebae (136.21–136.29)*

■ **006.9**   **Amebiasis, unspecified**
Amebiasis NOS

● **007**   **Other protozoal intestinal diseases**

Includes   protozoal:
colitis
diarrhea
dysentery

007.0   **Balantidiasis**
Infection by Balantidium coli

007.1   **Giardiasis**
Infection by Giardia lamblia
Lambliasis

007.2   **Coccidiosis**
Infection by Isospora belli and Isospora hominis
Isosporiasis

007.3   **Intestinal trichomoniasis**

007.4   **Cryptosporidiosis**
Coding Clinic: 1997, Q4, P30-31

007.5   **Cyclosporiasis**

■ **007.8**   **Other specified protozoal intestinal diseases**
Amebiasis due to organisms other than Entamoeba histolytica

■ **007.9**   **Unspecified protozoal intestinal disease**
Flagellate diarrhea
Protozoal dysentery NOS

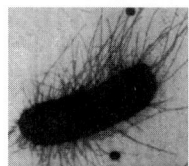

Figure 1–1 Electron micrograph of escherichia coli *(E. coli)* expressing P fimbriae. (From Mandell, Bennett, & Dolin: Principles and Practice of Infectious Diseases, 6th ed. 2005, Churchill Livingstone, An Imprint of Elsevier.)

Item 1–2 *Escherichia coli [E. coli]* is a gram-negative bacterium found in the intestinal tracts of humans and animals and is usually nonpathogenic. Pathogenic strains can cause diarrhea or pyogenic (pus-producing) infections. Can be a threat to food safety.

● **008   Intestinal infections due to other organisms**

    Includes   any condition classifiable to 009.0–009.3 with mention of the responsible organisms

    Excludes   *food poisoning by these organisms (005.0–005.9)*

● **008.0   Escherichia coli [E. coli]**
     Coding Clinic: 1988, Q2, P10

    ■ **008.00   E. coli, unspecified**
        E. coli enteritis NOS

    008.01   Enteropathogenic E. coli

    008.02   Enterotoxigenic E. coli

    008.03   Enteroinvasive E. coli

    008.04   Enterohemorrhagic E. coli

    ■ **008.09   Other intestinal E. coli infections**

   008.1   Arizona group of paracolon bacilli

   008.2   Aerobacter aerogenes
      Enterobacter aerogenes

   008.3   Proteus (mirabilis) (morganii)

● **008.4   Other specified bacteria**

    008.41   Staphylococcus
       Staphylococcal enterocolitis

    008.42   Pseudomonas
       Coding Clinic: 1989, Q2, P10

    008.43   Campylobacter

    008.44   Yersinia enterocolitica

    008.45   Clostridium difficile
       Pseudomembranous colitis

    ■ **008.46   Other anaerobes**
       Anaerobic enteritis NOS
       Bacteroides (fragilis)
       Gram-negative anaerobes

    ■ **008.47   Other gram-negative bacteria**
       Gram-negative enteritis NOS

       Excludes   *gram-negative anaerobes (008.46)*

    ■ **008.49   Other**
       Coding Clinic: 1989, Q2, P10

   ■ **008.5   Bacterial enteritis, unspecified**

● **008.6   Enteritis due to specified virus**

    008.61   Rotavirus

    008.62   Adenovirus

    008.63   Norwalk virus
       Norovirus
       Norwalk-like agent

    ■ **008.64   Other small round viruses [SRV's]**
       Small round virus NOS

    008.65   Calicivirus

    008.66   Astrovirus

    008.67   Enterovirus NEC
       Coxsackie virus
       Echovirus

       Excludes   *poliovirus (045.0–045.9)*

    ■ **008.69   Other viral enteritis**
       Torovirus
       Coding Clinic: 2003, Q1, P10-11

   ■ **008.8   Other organism, not elsewhere classified**
      Viral:
       enteritis NOS
       gastroenteritis

      Excludes   *influenza with involvement of gastrointestinal tract (487.8)*

● **009   Ill-defined intestinal infections**

    Excludes   *diarrheal disease or intestinal infection due to specified organism (001.0–008.8)*
         diarrhea following gastrointestinal surgery (564.4)
         intestinal malabsorption (579.0–579.9)
         ischemic enteritis (557.0–557.9)
         other noninfectious gastroenteritis and colitis (558.1–558.9)
         regional enteritis (555.0–555.9)
         ulcerative colitis (556)

   009.0   Infectious colitis, enteritis, and gastroenteritis
      Colitis (septic)
      Dysentery:
       NOS
       catarrhal
       hemorrhagic
      Enteritis (septic)
      Gastroenteritis (septic)
      Coding Clinic: 1988, Q2, P10

   009.1   Colitis, enteritis, and gastroenteritis of presumed infectious origin

      Excludes   *colitis NOS (558.9)*
         enteritis NOS (558.9)
         gastroenteritis NOS (558.9)
      Coding Clinic: 1999, Q3, P6-7

   009.2   Infectious diarrhea
      Diarrhea:
       dysenteric
       epidemic
      Infectious diarrheal disease NOS

   009.3   Diarrhea of presumed infectious origin

      Excludes   *diarrhea NOS (787.91)*

      Coding Clinic: 1987, Nov-Dec, P7

INFECTIOUS AND PARASITIC DISEASES (001–139)

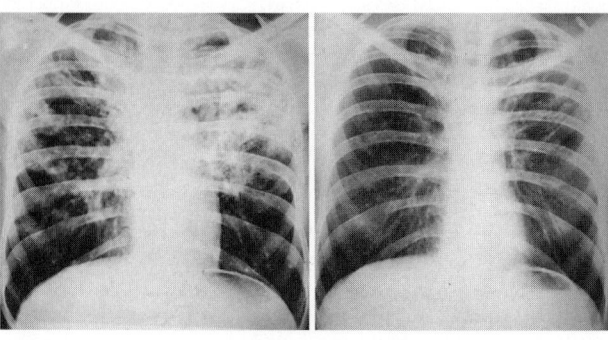

Figure 1–2 Far advanced bilateral pulmonary tuberculosis before and after 8 months of treatment with streptomycin, PAS, and isoniazid. (From Hinshaw HC, Garland LH: Diseases of the Chest, 2nd ed. Philadelphia, WB Saunders, 1963, p. 538.)

Item 1–3 Tuberculosis is a common and deadly infectious disease caused by the *Mycobacterium tuberculosis* organism. The first tuberculosis infection is called the **primary infection** and most commonly attacks the lungs but can affect the central nervous system, lymphatic system, circulatory system, genitourinary system, bones, joints, and even the skin. A **Ghon** lesion is the **initial lesion. A secondary lesion** occurs when the tubercle bacilli are carried to other areas.

TUBERCULOSIS (010–018)

Includes   infection by Mycobacterium tuberculosis (human) (bovine)

Excludes   *congenital tuberculosis (771.2)*
late effects of tuberculosis (137.0–137.4)

The following fifth-digit subclassification is for use with categories 010–018:

> ◻ 0 unspecified
>   1 bacteriological or histological examination not done
>   2 bacteriological or histological examination unknown (at present)
>   3 tubercle bacilli found (in sputum) by microscopy
>   4 tubercle bacilli not found (in sputum) by microscopy, but found by bacterial culture
>   5 tubercle bacilli not found by bacteriological examination, but tuberculosis confirmed histologically
>   6 tubercle bacilli not found by bacteriological or histological examination, but tuberculosis confirmed by other methods [inoculation of animals]

● **010   Primary tuberculous infection**

   Requires fifth digit. See beginning of section 010–018 for codes and definitions.

● **010.0 Primary tuberculous infection**
   [0-6]   **Excludes** *nonspecific reaction to tuberculin skin test without active tuberculosis (795.5)*
   positive PPD (795.5)
   positive tuberculin skin test without active tuberculosis (795.5)

● **010.1 Tuberculous pleurisy in primary progressive**
   [0-6] **tuberculosis**

● ◻ **010.8 Other primary progressive tuberculosis**
   [0-6]   **Excludes** *tuberculous erythema nodosum (017.1)*

● ◻ **010.9 Primary tuberculous infection, unspecified**
   [0-6]

● **011   Pulmonary tuberculosis**

   Requires fifth digit. See beginning of section 010–018 for codes and definitions.

   Use additional code to identify any associated silicosis (502)

● **011.0 Tuberculosis of lung, infiltrative**
   [0-6]

● **011.1 Tuberculosis of lung, nodular**
   [0-6]

● **011.2 Tuberculosis of lung with cavitation**
   [0-6]   *Cavitation = pitting*
   Coding Clinic: 1994, Q4, P36

● **011.3 Tuberculosis of bronchus**
   [0-6]   **Excludes** *isolated bronchial tuberculosis (012.2)*

● **011.4 Tuberculous fibrosis of lung**
   [0-6]

● **011.5 Tuberculous bronchiectasis**
   [0-6]

● **011.6 Tuberculous pneumonia [any form]**
   [0-6]

● **011.7 Tuberculous pneumothorax**
   [0-6]

● ◻ **011.8 Other specified pulmonary tuberculosis**
   [0-6]

● ◻ **011.9 Pulmonary tuberculosis, unspecified**
   [0-6]   Respiratory tuberculosis NOS
   Tuberculosis of lung NOS

● **012   Other respiratory tuberculosis**

   Requires fifth digit. See beginning of section 010–018 for codes and definitions.

   Excludes *respiratory tuberculosis, unspecified (011.9)*

● **012.0 Tuberculous pleurisy**
   [0-6]   Tuberculosis of pleura
   Tuberculous empyema
   Tuberculous hydrothorax

      Excludes *pleurisy with effusion without mention of cause (511.9)*
      tuberculous pleurisy in primary progressive tuberculosis (010.1)

● **012.1 Tuberculosis of intrathoracic lymph nodes**
   [0-6]   Tuberculosis of lymph nodes:
      hilar
      mediastinal
      tracheobronchial
   Tuberculous tracheobronchial adenopathy

      Excludes *that specified as primary (010.0–010.9)*

● **012.2 Isolated tracheal or bronchial tuberculosis**
   [0-6]

● **012.3 Tuberculous laryngitis**
   [0-6]   Tuberculosis of glottis

● ◻ **012.8 Other specified respiratory tuberculosis**
   [0-6]   Tuberculosis of:
      mediastinum
      nasopharynx
      nose (septum)
      sinus [any nasal]

◀ New   ◀▥ Revised   ~~deleted~~ Deleted   ● Use Additional Digit(s)   ◻ Nonspecific Code
● Not first-listed DX   OGCR Official Guidelines   Coding Clinic   Excludes   Includes   Use additional   Code first   Omit code

Item 1–4 *Although it primarily affects the lungs, the bacteria **Mycobacterium tuberculosis** can travel from the pulmonary circulation to virtually any organ in the body, much as a cancer metastasizes to a secondary site. If the immune system becomes compromised by age or disease, what would otherwise be a self-limiting primary tuberculosis in the lungs will develop in other organs. These are known as extrapulmonary sites.*

● **013   Tuberculosis of meninges and central nervous system**

> Requires fifth digit. See beginning of section 010–018 for codes and definitions.

● **013.0   Tuberculous meningitis**
[0-6]   Tuberculosis of meninges (cerebral) (spinal)
> Tuberculous:
>> leptomeningitis
>> meningoencephalitis

>> **Excludes** *tuberculoma of meninges (013.1)*

● **013.1   Tuberculoma of meninges**
[0-6]

● **013.2   Tuberculoma of brain**
[0-6]   Tuberculosis of brain (current disease)

● **013.3   Tuberculous abscess of brain**
[0-6]

● **013.4   Tuberculoma of spinal cord**
[0-6]

● **013.5   Tuberculous abscess of spinal cord**
[0-6]

● **013.6   Tuberculous encephalitis or myelitis**
[0-6]

● ■ **013.8   Other specified tuberculosis of central nervous**
[0-6] **system**

● ■ **013.9   Unspecified tuberculosis of central nervous**
[0-6] **system**
>> Tuberculosis of central nervous system NOS

● **014   Tuberculosis of intestines, peritoneum, and mesenteric glands**

> Requires fifth digit. See beginning of section 010–018 for codes and definitions.

● **014.0   Tuberculous peritonitis**
[0-6]   Tuberculous ascites

● ■ **014.8   Other**
[0-6]   Tuberculosis (of):
>> anus
>> intestine (large) (small)
>> mesenteric glands
>> rectum
>> retroperitoneal (lymph nodes)
> Tuberculous enteritis

● **015   Tuberculosis of bones and joints**

> Requires fifth digit. See beginning of section 010–018 for codes and definitions.

> Use additional code to identify manifestation, as:
>> tuberculous:
>>> arthropathy (711.4)
>>> necrosis of bone (730.8)
>>> osteitis (730.8)
>>> osteomyelitis (730.8)
>>> synovitis (727.01)
>>> tenosynovitis (727.01)

● **015.0   Vertebral column**
[0-6]   Pott's disease

> Use additional code to identify manifestation, as:
>> curvature of spine [Pott's] (737.4)
>> kyphosis (737.4)
>> spondylitis (720.81)

● **015.1   Hip**
[0-6]

● **015.2   Knee**
[0-6]

● **015.5   Limb bones**
[0-6]   Tuberculous dactylitis

● **015.6   Mastoid**
[0-6]   Tuberculous mastoiditis

● ■ **015.7   Other specified bone**
[0-6]

● ■ **015.8   Other specified joint**
[0-6]

● ■ **015.9   Tuberculosis of unspecified bones and joints**
[0-6]

● **016   Tuberculosis of genitourinary system**

> Requires fifth digit. See beginning of section 010–018 for codes and definitions.

● **016.0   Kidney**
[0-6]   Renal tuberculosis

> Use additional code to identify manifestation, as:
>> tuberculous:
>>> nephropathy (583.81)
>>> pyelitis (590.81)
>>> pyelonephritis (590.81)

● **016.1   Bladder**
[0-6]

● **016.2   Ureter**
[0-6]

● ■ **016.3   Other urinary organs**
[0-6]

● **016.4   Epididymis ♂**
[0-6]

● ■ **016.5   Other male genital organs ♂**
[0-6]
> Use additional code to identify manifestation, as:
>> tuberculosis of:
>>> prostate (601.4)
>>> seminal vesicle (608.81)
>>> testis (608.81)

● **016.6   Tuberculous oophoritis and salpingitis ♀**
[0-6]   *Oophoritis = inflammation of ovary*
>> *Salpingitis = inflammation of fallopian tube*

● ■ **016.7   Other female genital organs ♀**
[0-6]   Tuberculous:
>> cervicitis
>> endometritis

● ■ **016.9   Genitourinary tuberculosis, unspecified**
[0-6]

INFECTIOUS AND PARASITIC DISEASES (001–139)

● **017 Tuberculosis of other organs**

> Requires fifth digit. See beginning of section 010–018 for codes and definitions.

● **017.0 Skin and subcutaneous cellular tissue**
[0-6]

Lupus:	Tuberculosis:
exedens	colliquativa
vulgaris	cutis
Scrofuloderma	lichenoides
	papulonecrotica
	verrucosa cutis

> **Excludes** *lupus erythematosus (695.4)*
> *disseminated (710.0)*
> *lupus NOS (710.0)*
> *nonspecific reaction to tuberculin skin test*
> *without active tuberculosis (795.5)*
> *positive PPD (795.5)*
> *positive tuberculin skin test without active*
> *tuberculosis (795.5)*

● **017.1 Erythema nodosum with hypersensitivity reaction in**
[0-6] **tuberculosis**

> Bazin's disease
> Erythema:
> induratum
> nodosum, tuberculous
> Tuberculosis indurativa

> **Excludes** *erythema nodosum NOS (695.2)*

● **017.2 Peripheral lymph nodes**
[0-6]

> Scrofula
> Scrofulous abscess
> Tuberculous adenitis

> **Excludes** *tuberculosis of lymph nodes:*
> *bronchial and mediastinal (012.1)*
> *mesenteric and retroperitoneal (014.8)*
> *tuberculous tracheobronchial adenopathy*
> *(012.1)*

● **017.3 Eye**
[0-6]

> Use additional code to identify manifestation, as:
> tuberculous:
> episcleritis (379.09)
> interstitial keratitis (370.59)
> iridocyclitis, chronic (364.11)
> keratoconjunctivitis (phlyctenular) (370.31)

● **017.4 Ear**
[0-6]

> Tuberculosis of ear
> Tuberculous otitis media

> **Excludes** *tuberculous mastoiditis (015.6)*

● **017.5 Thyroid gland**
[0-6]

● **017.6 Adrenal glands**
[0-6] Addison's disease, tuberculous

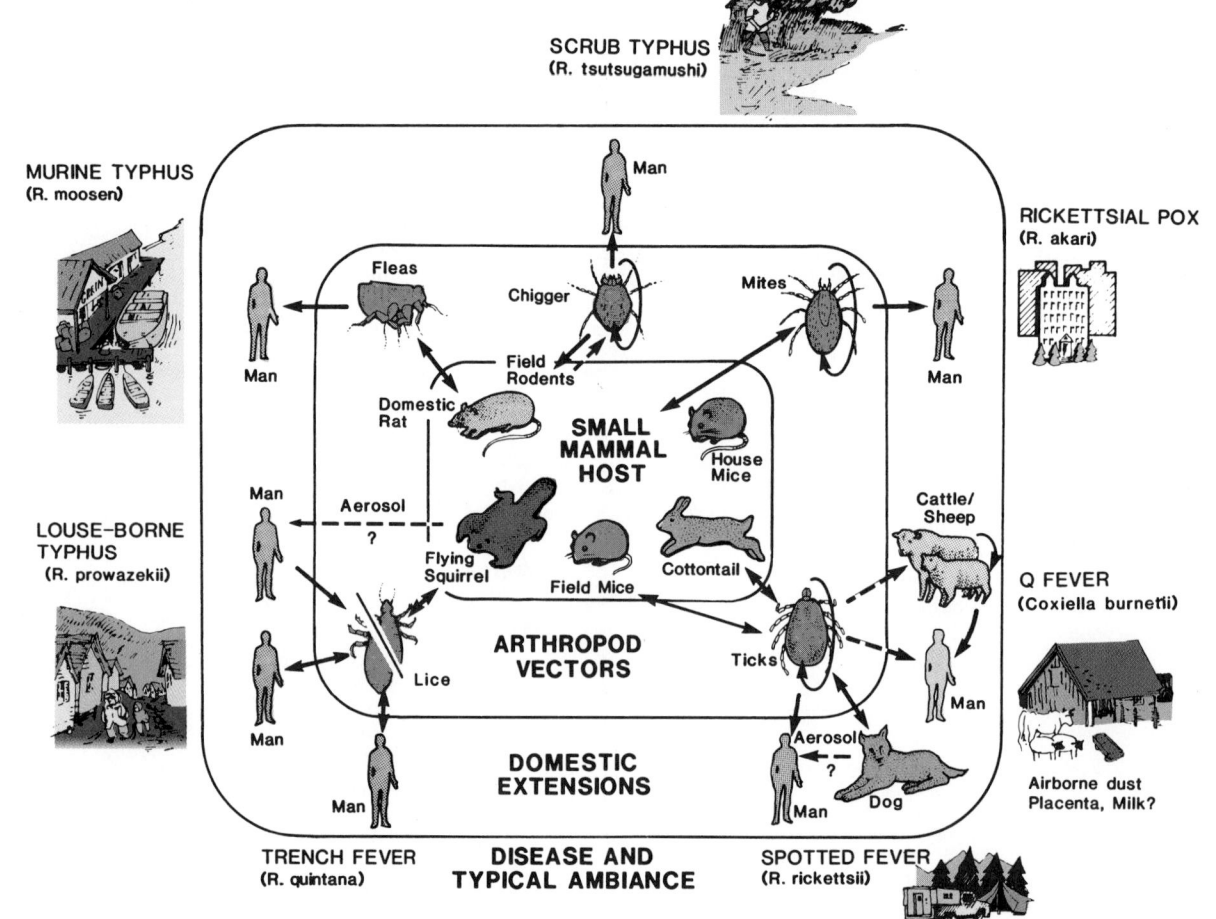

Figure 1-3 Schematic summary of some major interactions between rickettsial organisms and their small animal hosts and arthropod vectors, the participation of domestic animals, and examples of the typical ambiance under which each rickettsial infection is contacted by humans. (From Strickland GT: Hunter's Tropical Medicine, 7th ed. Philadelphia, WB Saunders, 1991, p. 261. Courtesy of Dr. J. K. Frenkel, University of New Mexico, Albuquerque, N.M.)

◄ New   ◄Ⅲ Revised   ~~deleted~~ Deleted   ● Use Additional Digit(s)   ■ Nonspecific Code
● Not first-listed DX   OGCR Official Guidelines   Coding Clinic   Excludes   Includes   Use additional   Code first   Omit code

● **017.7 Spleen**
[0-6]

● **017.8 Esophagus**
[0-6]

● ■ **017.9 Other specified organs**
[0-6]   Use additional code to identify manifestation, as:
tuberculosis of:
endocardium [any valve] (424.91)
myocardium (422.0)
pericardium (420.0)

Item 1–5   Miliary tuberculosis can be a life-threatening condition. If a tuberculous lesion enters a blood vessel, immense dissemination of tuberculous organisms can occur if the immune system is weak. High-risk populations—children under 4 years of age, the elderly, or the immunocompromised—are particularly prone to this type of infection. The lesions will have a millet seed-like appearance on chest x-ray. Bronchial washings and biopsy may aid in diagnosis.

● **018 Miliary tuberculosis**

Requires fifth digit. See beginning of section 010–018 for codes and definitions.

Includes   tuberculosis:
disseminated
generalized
miliary, whether of a single specified site,
multiple sites, or unspecified site
polyserositis

● **018.0 Acute miliary tuberculosis**
[0-6]

● ■ **018.8 Other specified miliary tuberculosis**
[0-6]

● ■ **018.9 Miliary tuberculosis, unspecified**
[0-6]

ZOONOTIC BACTERIAL DISEASES (020–027)

● **020 Plague**
Infectious disease caused by Yersinia pestis bacterium, transmitted by rodent flea bite or handling infected animal

Includes   infection by Yersinia [Pasteurella] pestis

020.0 Bubonic

020.1 Cellulocutaneous

020.2 Septicemic

020.3 Primary pneumonic

020.4 Secondary pneumonic

■ **020.5 Pneumonic, unspecified**

■ **020.8 Other specified types of plague**
Abortive plague
Ambulatory plague
Pestis minor

■ **020.9 Plague, unspecified**

● **021 Tularemia**
Caused by Francisella tularensis bacterium found in rodents, rabbits, and hares; transmitted by contact with infected animal tissues or ticks, biting flies, and mosquitoes

Includes   deerfly fever
infection by Francisella [Pasteurella] tularensis
rabbit fever

021.0 Ulceroglandular tularemia

021.1 Enteric tularemia
Tularemia:
cryptogenic
intestinal
typhoidal

021.2 Pulmonary tularemia
Bronchopneumonic tularemia

021.3 Oculoglandular tularemia

■ **021.8 Other specified tularemia**
Tularemia:
generalized or disseminated
glandular

■ **021.9 Unspecified tularemia**

● **022 Anthrax**
An acute infectious disease caused by the spore-forming Bacillus anthracis; it may occur in humans exposed to infected animals or tissue from infected animals

022.0 Cutaneous anthrax
Malignant pustule

022.1 Pulmonary anthrax
Respiratory anthrax
Wool-sorters' disease

022.2 Gastrointestinal anthrax

022.3 Anthrax septicemia

■ **022.8 Other specified manifestations of anthrax**

■ **022.9 Anthrax, unspecified**

● **023 Brucellosis**
Infectious disease caused by bacterium Brucella. Humans are infected by contact with contaminated animals or animal products. Brucellosis symptoms are similar to flu.

Includes   fever:
Malta
Mediterranean
undulant
Rising and falling

023.0 Brucella melitensis

023.1 Brucella abortus

023.2 Brucella suis

023.3 Brucella canis

■ **023.8 Other brucellosis**
Infection by more than one organism

■ **023.9 Brucellosis, unspecified**

024 Glanders
Infection by:
Actinobacillus mallei
Malleomyces mallei
Pseudomonas mallei
Farcy
Malleus

025 Melioidosis
Infection by:
Malleomyces pseudomallei
Pseudomonas pseudomallei
Whitmore's bacillus
Pseudoglanders

● **026   Rat-bite fever**
> *RBF is an infectious disease caused by Streptobacillus moniliformis or Spirillum minus.*

026.0   Spirillary fever
> Rat-bite fever due to Spirillum minor [S. minus]
> Sodoku

026.1   Streptobacillary fever
> Epidemic arthritic erythema
> Haverhill fever
> Rat-bite fever due to Streptobacillus moniliformis

■ **026.9   Unspecified rat-bite fever**

● **027   Other zoonotic bacterial diseases**

027.0   Listeriosis
> Infection by Listeria monocytogenes
> Septicemia by Listeria monocytogenes

> Use additional code to identify manifestations, as meningitis (320.7)

> Excludes   *congenital listeriosis (771.2)*

027.1   Erysipelothrix infection
> Erysipeloid (of Rosenbach)
> Infection by Erysipelothrix insidiosa [E. rhusiopathiae]
> Septicemia by Erysipelothrix insidiosa [E. rhusiopathiae]

027.2   Pasteurellosis
> Pasteurella pseudotuberculosis infection by Pasteurella multocida [P. septica]
> Mesenteric adenitis by Pasteurella multocida [P. septica]
> Septic infection (cat bite) (dog bite) by Pasteurella multocida [P. septica]

> Excludes   *infection by:*
>   *Francisella [Pasteurella] tularensis (021.0–021.9)*
>   *Yersinia [Pasteurella] pestis (020.0–020.9)*

■ **027.8   Other specified zoonotic bacterial diseases**

■ **027.9   Unspecified zoonotic bacterial disease**

OTHER BACTERIAL DISEASES (030–041)

> Excludes   *bacterial venereal diseases (098.0–099.9)*
>   *bartonellosis (088.0)*

● **030   Leprosy**
> *Also known as Hansen's disease; chronic infectious disease attacking skin, peripheral nerves, and mucous membranes*

> Includes   Hansen's disease
>   infection by Mycobacterium leprae

030.0   Lepromatous [type L]
> Lepromatous leprosy (macular) (diffuse) (infiltrated) (nodular) (neuritic)

030.1   Tuberculoid [type T]
> Tuberculoid leprosy (macular) (maculoanesthetic) (major) (minor) (neuritic)

030.2   Indeterminate [group I]
> Indeterminate [uncharacteristic] leprosy (macular) (neuritic)

030.3   Borderline [group B]
> Borderline or dimorphous leprosy (infiltrated) (neuritic)

■ **030.8   Other specified leprosy**

■ **030.9   Leprosy, unspecified**

● **031   Diseases due to other mycobacteria**

031.0   Pulmonary
> Battey disease
> Infection by Mycobacterium:
>   avium
>   intracellulare [Battey bacillus]
>   kansasii

031.1   Cutaneous
> Buruli ulcer
> Infection by Mycobacterium:
>   marinum [M. balnei]
>   ulcerans

031.2   Disseminated
> Disseminated mycobacterium avium-intracellulare complex (DMAC)
> Mycobacterium avium-intracellulare complex (MAC) bacteremia
> Coding Clinic: 1997, Q4, P31

■ **031.8   Other specified mycobacterial diseases**

■ **031.9   Unspecified diseases due to mycobacteria**
> Atypical mycobacterium infection NOS

● **032   Diphtheria**
> *Highly contagious bacterial disease that results in formation of an adherent membrane in the throat that may lead to suffocation. It may attack the heart and lungs. The exact location is specified in the codes.*

> Includes   infection by Corynebacterium diphtheriae

032.0   Faucial diphtheria
> Membranous angina, diphtheritic

032.1   Nasopharyngeal diphtheria

032.2   Anterior nasal diphtheria

032.3   Laryngeal diphtheria
> Laryngotracheitis, diphtheritic

● **032.8   Other specified diphtheria**

032.81   Conjunctival diphtheria
> Pseudomembranous diphtheritic conjunctivitis

032.82   Diphtheritic myocarditis

032.83   Diphtheritic peritonitis

032.84   Diphtheritic cystitis

032.85   Cutaneous diphtheria

■ **032.89   Other**

■ **032.9   Diphtheria, unspecified**

● **033   Whooping cough**
> *Pertussis (whooping cough) is a highly contagious disease caused by the bacterium Bordetella pertussis and results in a whooping sound.*

> Includes   pertussis

> Use additional code to identify any associated pneumonia (484.3)

033.0   Bordetella pertussis [B. pertussis]

033.1   Bordetella parapertussis [B. parapertussis]

■ **033.8   Whooping cough due to other specified organism**
> Bordetella bronchiseptica [B. bronchiseptica]

■ **033.9   Whooping cough, unspecified organism**

◀ New   ◀▥ Revised   ~~deleted~~ Deleted   ● Use Additional Digit(s)   ■ Nonspecific Code

● Not first-listed DX   OGCR Official Guidelines   Coding Clinic   Excludes   Includes   Use additional   Code first   Omit code

Item 1-6   034.0 is the common **"strep throat"** (sore throat with strep infection). It is grouped in the same three-digit category with scarlet fever. If a patient has both scarlet fever and the strep throat, use both codes. "Streptococcal" must be indicated on the laboratory report to use 034.0; otherwise use 462 for "sore throat" (pharyngitis).

034   Streptococcal sore throat and scarlet fever

034.0   Streptococcal sore throat

Septic:	Streptococcal:
angina	angina
sore throat	laryngitis
	pharyngitis
	tonsillitis

Coding Clinic: 1985, Sept-Oct, P9

034.1   Scarlet fever
Scarlatina

> **Excludes**   *parascarlatina (057.8)*

035   Erysipelas

> **Excludes**   *postpartum or puerperal erysipelas (670.8)* ◀▥

036   Meningococcal infection
Most commonly caused by bacteria Streptococcus pneumoniae and Neisseria meningitidis

036.0   Meningococcal meningitis
Cerebrospinal fever (meningococcal)
Meningitis:
    cerebrospinal
    epidemic

036.1   Meningococcal encephalitis

036.2   Meningococcemia
Meningococcal septicemia

036.3   Waterhouse-Friderichsen syndrome, meningococcal
Meningococcal hemorrhagic adrenalitis
Meningococcic adrenal syndrome
Waterhouse-Friderichsen syndrome NOS

036.4   Meningococcal carditis
   036.40   Meningococcal carditis, unspecified
   036.41   Meningococcal pericarditis
   036.42   Meningococcal endocarditis
   036.43   Meningococcal myocarditis

036.8   Other specified meningococcal infections
   036.81   Meningococcal optic neuritis
   036.82   Meningococcal arthropathy
   036.89   Other

036.9   Meningococcal infection, unspecified
Meningococcal infection NOS

037   Tetanus
Also indexed as "lockjaw." Do not confuse tetanus with tetany, which is severe muscle twitches, cramps, and spasms (781.7).

> **Excludes**   *tetanus:*
>   *complicating:*
>   *abortion (634–638 with .0, 639.0)*
>   *ectopic or molar pregnancy (639.0)*
>   *neonatorum (771.3)*
>   *puerperal (670.8)* ◀▥

038   Septicemia
Blood poisoning/bacteremia, often associated with serious illness.

Note: Use additional code for systemic inflammatory response syndrome (SIRS) (995.91–995.92).

> **Excludes**   *bacteremia (790.7)*
>   *septicemia (sepsis) of newborn (771.81)*

Coding Clinic: 2004, Q2, P16; 1994, Q2, P13; 1993, Q3, P6; 1988, Q2, P12

038.0   Streptococcal septicemia
Coding Clinic: 1996, Q2, P5

038.1   Staphylococcal septicemia
   038.10   Staphylococcal septicemia, unspecified

   038.11   Methicillin susceptible Staphylococcus aureus septicemia
      MSSA septicemia
      Staphylococcus aureus septicemia NOS
      Coding Clinic: 2008, Q4, P69-73; 1998, Q4, P41-42

   038.12   Methicillin resistant Staphylococcus aureus septicemia
      Coding Clinic: 2008, Q4, P69-73

   038.19   Other staphylococcal septicemia

038.2   Pneumococcal septicemia [Streptococcus pneumoniae septicemia]
Coding Clinic: 1996, Q2, P5; 1991, Q1, P13

038.3   Septicemia due to anaerobes
Septicemia due to bacteroides

> **Excludes**   *gas gangrene (040.0)*
>   *that due to anaerobic streptococci (038.0)*

038.4   Septicemia due to other gram-negative organisms
   038.40   Gram-negative organism, unspecified
      Gram-negative septicemia NOS
      Coding Clinic: 2007, Q4, P84-86

   038.41   Hemophilus influenzae [H. influenzae]

   038.42   Escherichia coli [E. coli]
      Coding Clinic: 2003, Q4, P73

   038.43   Pseudomonas

   038.44   Serratia

   038.49   Other

038.8   Other specified septicemias

> **Excludes**   *septicemia (due to):*
>   *anthrax (022.3)*
>   *gonococcal (098.89)*
>   *herpetic (054.5)*
>   *meningococcal (036.2)*
>   *septicemic plague (020.2)*

038.9   Unspecified septicemia
Septicemia NOS

> **Excludes**   *bacteremia NOS (790.7)*

Coding Clinic: 2007, Q4, P96-97; 2005, Q2, P18-20; 2004, Q2, P16; 1999, Q3, P9; Q3, P5-6; 1998, Q1, P5; 1996, Q3, P16; Q2, P6; 1995, Q2, P7

INFECTIOUS AND PARASITIC DISEASES (001–139)

● **039 Actinomycotic infections**

Includes   actinomycotic mycetoma
infection by Actinomycetales, such as
species of Actinomyces, Actinomadura,
Nocardia, Streptomyces
maduromycosis (actinomycotic)
schizomycetoma (actinomycotic)

039.0 Cutaneous
Erythrasma
Trichomycosis axillaris

039.1 Pulmonary
Thoracic actinomycosis

039.2 Abdominal

039.3 Cervicofacial

039.4 Madura foot

Excludes   *madura foot due to mycotic infection (117.4)*

■ **039.8 Of other specified sites**

■ **039.9 Of unspecified site**
Actinomycosis NOS
Maduromycosis NOS
Nocardiosis NOS

Item 1-7 Gas gangrene is a necrotizing subcutaneous infection that will cause tissue death. Patients with poor circulation (e.g., diabetes, peripheral nephropathy) will have low oxygen content in their tissues (hypoxia), which allows the Clostridium bacteria to flourish. Gas gangrene often occurs at the site of a surgical wound or trauma. Onset is sudden and dramatic. Treatment can include debridement, amputation, and/or hyperbaric oxygen treatments.

● **040 Other bacterial diseases**

Excludes   *bacteremia NOS (790.7)*
bacterial infection NOS (041.9)

040.0 Gas gangrene
Gas bacillus infection or gangrene
Infection by Clostridium:
histolyticum
oedematiens
perfringens [welchii]
septicum
sordellii
Malignant edema
Myonecrosis, clostridial
Myositis, clostridial
Coding Clinic: 1995, Q1, P11

040.1 Rhinoscleroma

040.2 Whipple's disease
Intestinal lipodystrophy

040.3 Necrobacillosis
Coding Clinic: 2007, Q4, P84-86

● **040.4 Other specified botulism**
Non-foodborne intoxication due to toxins of
Clostridium botulinum [C. botulinum]

Excludes   *botulism NOS (005.1)*
food poisoning due to toxins of Clostridium botulinum (005.1)

040.41 Infant botulism   P
Coding Clinic: 2007, Q4, P60-61

040.42 Wound botulism
Non-foodborne botulism NOS

Use additional code to identify complicated open wound
Coding Clinic: 2007, Q4, P60-61; 2006, Q2, P7

● **040.8 Other specified bacterial diseases**

040.81 Tropical pyomyositis

040.82 Toxic shock syndrome

Use additional code to identify the organism
Coding Clinic: 2002, Q4, P44

■ **040.89 Other**
Coding Clinic: 1986, Nov-Dec, P7

● **041 Bacterial infection in conditions classified elsewhere and of unspecified site**

Note: This category is provided to be used as an additional code to identify the bacterial agent in diseases classified elsewhere. This category will also be used to classify bacterial infections of unspecified nature or site.
Code the disease first, then the bacterium.

Excludes   *septicemia (038.0–038.9)*
Coding Clinic: 2001, Q2, P12; 1984, July-Aug, P19

● **041.0 Streptococcus**
Gram-positive bacteria that is the primary cause of strep throat

■ **041.00 Streptococcus, unspecified**
Specified in documentation as streptococcus, but unspecified as to Group

041.01 Group A
Specified as Group A
Coding Clinic: 2002, Q1, P3-4

041.02 Group B
Specified as Group B

041.03 Group C
Specified as Group C

041.04 Group D [Enterococcus]
Specified as Group D

041.05 Group G
Specified as Group G

■ **041.09 Other Streptococcus**
Streptococcus that is documented but not specified as Group A, B, C, D, or G

INFECTIOUS AND PARASITIC DISEASES (001–139)

◄ New   ◄▥ Revised   ~~deleted~~ Deleted   ● Use Additional Digit(s)   ■ Nonspecific Code   ● Not first-listed DX   OGCR Official Guidelines   Coding Clinic   Excludes   Includes   Use additional   Code first   Omit code

● **041.1 Staphylococcus**
*"Staph" infections caused by **Staphylococcus aureus**
bacteria and range from common skin infections
(pimples and boils) to serious infection of surgical
wounds, bloodstream infections, and pneumonia.*
Coding Clinic: 1987, Jan-Feb, P14-15

■ **041.10 Staphylococcus, unspecified**
Coding Clinic: 2006, Q2, P15

**041.11 Methicillin susceptible Staphylococcus
aureus**
MSSA
Staphylococcus aureus NOS
Coding Clinic: 2008, Q4, P69-73; 2006, Q2, P16-17; 2003,
Q4, P104-107; 2001, Q2, P11; 1998, Q4, P42-44,
54.55; 1994, Q3, P6

**041.12 Methicillin resistant Staphylococcus
aureus**
Methicillin-resistant staphylococcus
aureus (MRSA)
Coding Clinic: 2008, Q4, P69-73

■ **041.19 Other Staphylococcus**
Coding Clinic: 2008, Q2, P3

041.2 Pneumococcus

041.3 ~~Friedländer's bacillus~~ Klebsiella pneumoniae ◄║
~~Infection by Klebsiella pneumoniae~~
Coding Clinic: 2008, Q4, P148-149

041.4 Escherichia coli [E.coli]
Coding Clinic: 1984, July-Aug, P19

041.5 Hemophilus influenzae [H. influenzae]

041.6 Proteus (mirabilis) (morganii)

041.7 Pseudomonas
Coding Clinic: 1988, Q4, P10

● **041.8 Other specified bacterial infections**

041.81 Mycoplasma
Eaton's agent
Pleuropneumonia-like organisms [PPLO]

041.82 Bacteroides fragilis

041.83 Clostridium perfringens

■ **041.84 Other anaerobes**
Gram-negative anaerobes
Excludes *Helicobacter pylori (041.86)*

041.85 Other gram-negative organisms
Aerobacter aerogenes
Gram-negative bacteria NOS
Mima polymorpha
Serratia
Excludes *gram-negative anaerobes (041.84)*
Coding Clinic: 1994, Q1, P18

041.86 Helicobacter pylori ~~(H. pylori)~~ [H. pylori] ◄║

■ **041.89 Other specified bacteria**
Coding Clinic: 2006, Q2, P7; 2003, Q2, P7-8

■ **041.9 Bacterial infection, unspecified**
Coding Clinic: 1991, Q2, P9

Item 1-8 AIDS (acquired immune deficiency syndrome) is
caused by **HIV** (human immunodeficiency virus). HIV affects
certain white blood cells (T-4 lymphocytes) and destroys the
ability of the cells to fight infections, making patients susceptible
to a host of infectious diseases (e.g., ***Pneumocystis carinii
pneumonia (PCP), Kaposi's sarcoma***, and **lymphoma**).
AIDS-related complex (ARC) is an early stage of AIDS in
which tests for HIV are positive but the symptoms are mild.

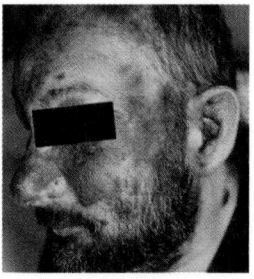

Figure 1-4 Kaposi's sarcoma.
There are large confluent
hyperpigmented patch-stage lesions
with lymphedema. (From Cohen &
Powderly: Infectious Diseases, 2nd
ed. 2004, Mosby, An Imprint of
Elsevier)

OGCR Section I.C.2.a. and b.
If a patient is admitted for an HIV-related condition,
the principal diagnosis should be 042, followed by
additional diagnosis codes for all reported HIV-related
conditions. If a patient with HIV disease is admitted
for an unrelated condition (such as a traumatic injury),
the code for the unrelated condition (e.g., the nature
of injury code) should be the principal diagnosis.
Other diagnoses would be 042 followed by additional
diagnosis codes for all reported HIV-related conditions.

HUMAN IMMUNODEFICIENCY VIRUS (HIV) INFECTION (042)

042 **Human immunodeficiency virus [HIV] disease**
Acquired immune deficiency syndrome
Acquired immunodeficiency syndrome
AIDS
AIDS-like syndrome
AIDS-related complex
ARC
HIV infection, symptomatic

Use additional code(s) to identify all manifestations of
HIV

Use additional code to identify HIV-2 infection (079.53)

Excludes *asymptomatic HIV infection status (V08)
exposure to HIV virus (V01.79)
nonspecific serologic evidence of HIV (795.71)*
Coding Clinic: 2007, Q4, P61-64; 2006, Q3, P14-15; 2004, Q2, P11-12; Q1,
P5; 2003, Q1, P10-11,15; 1999, Q1, P14; 1997, Q4, P30-31; 1994,
Q4, P35-36x2; 1993, Q3, P9; Q1, P20-22; 1990, Q3, P17; 1989,
Q1, P9

N Newborn Age: 0   **P** Pediatric Age: 0–17   **M** Maternity Age: 12–55   **A** Adult Age: 15–124   ♀ Females Only   ♂ Males Only   773

INFECTIOUS AND PARASITIC DISEASES (001–139)

POLIOMYELITIS AND OTHER NON-ARTHROPOD-BORNE VIRAL DISEASES AND PRION DISEASES OF CENTRAL NERVOUS SYSTEM (045–049)

● 045   **Acute poliomyelitis**

Also called infantile paralysis caused by poliovirus, which enters the body orally and infects the intestinal wall and then enters the bloodstream and central nervous system, causing muscle weakness and paralysis.

Excludes *late effects of acute poliomyelitis (138)*

The following fifth-digit subclassification is for use with category 045:

> ■ 0   poliovirus, unspecified type
> 1   poliovirus type I
> 2   poliovirus type II
> 3   poliovirus type III

●■ **045.0   Acute paralytic poliomyelitis specified as bulbar**
[0-3]   Infantile paralysis (acute) specified as bulbar
Poliomyelitis (acute) (anterior) specified as bulbar
Polioencephalitis (acute) (bulbar)
Polioencephalomyelitis (acute) (anterior) (bulbar)

●■ **045.1   Acute poliomyelitis with other paralysis**
[0-3]   Paralysis:
acute atrophic, spinal
infantile, paralytic
Poliomyelitis (acute) with paralysis except bulbar
anterior with paralysis except bulbar
epidemic with paralysis except bulbar

●■ **045.2   Acute nonparalytic poliomyelitis**
[0-3]   Poliomyelitis (acute) specified as nonparalytic
anterior specified as nonparalytic
epidemic specified as nonparalytic

●■ **045.9   Acute poliomyelitis, unspecified**
[0-3]   Infantile paralysis unspecified whether paralytic or nonparalytic
Poliomyelitis (acute) unspecified whether paralytic or nonparalytic
anterior unspecified whether paralytic or nonparalytic
epidemic unspecified whether paralytic or nonparalytic

● 046   **Slow virus infections and prion diseases of central nervous system**

046.0   Kuru

● **046.1   Jakob-Creutzfeldt disease** *(JCD)*

Use additional code to identify dementia: ◄
with behavioral disturbance (294.11) ◄
without behavioral disturbance (294.10) ◄

046.11   Variant Creutzfeldt-Jakob disease
vCJD

■ **046.19   Other and unspecified Creutzfeldt-Jakob disease**
CJD
Familial Creutzfeldt-Jakob disease
Iatrogenic Creutzfeldt-Jakob disease
Jakob-Creutzfeldt disease, unspecified
Sporadic Creutzfeldt-Jakob disease
Subacute spongiform encephalopathy

Excludes *variant Creutzfeldt-Jakob disease (vCJD) (046.11)*

046.2   Subacute sclerosing panencephalitis
Dawson's inclusion body encephalitis
Van Bogaert's sclerosing leukoencephalitis

046.3   Progressive multifocal leukoencephalopathy
Multifocal leukoencephalopathy NOS

● **046.7   Other specified prion diseases of central nervous system**

Excludes *Creutzfeldt-Jakob disease (046.11-046.19)*
Jakob-Creutzfeldt disease (046.11-046.19)
kuru (046.0)
variant Creutzfeldt-Jakob disease (vCJD) (046.11)

046.71   Gerstmann-Sträussler-Scheinker syndrome
GSS syndrome

046.72   Fatal familial insomnia
FFI

■ **046.79   Other and unspecified prion disease of central nervous system**

■ **046.8   Other specified slow virus infection of central nervous system**

■ **046.9   Unspecified slow virus infection of central nervous system**

● 047   **Meningitis due to enterovirus**

Includes   meningitis:
abacterial
aseptic
viral

Excludes *meningitis due to:*
adenovirus (049.1)
arthropod-borne virus (060.0–066.9)
leptospira (100.81)
virus of:
herpes simplex (054.72)
herpes zoster (053.0)
lymphocytic choriomeningitis (049.0)
mumps (072.1)
poliomyelitis (045.0–045.9)
any other infection specifically classified elsewhere

047.0   Coxsackie virus

047.1   ECHO virus
Meningo-eruptive syndrome

■ **047.8   Other specified viral meningitis**

■ **047.9   Unspecified viral meningitis**
Viral meningitis NOS

■ 048   **Other enterovirus diseases of central nervous system**
Boston exanthem

● 049   **Other non-arthropod-borne viral diseases of central nervous system**

Excludes *late effects of viral encephalitis (139.0)*

049.0   Lymphocytic choriomeningitis
Lymphocytic:
meningitis (serous) (benign)
meningoencephalitis (serous) (benign)

049.1   Meningitis due to adenovirus

◄ New   ◄IIII Revised   ~~deleted~~ Deleted   ● Use Additional Digit(s)   ■ Nonspecific Code

● Not first-listed DX   OGCR Official Guidelines   Coding Clinic   Excludes   Includes   Use additional   Code first   Omit code

INFECTIOUS AND PARASITIC DISEASES (001–139)

■**049.8 Other specified non-arthropod-borne viral diseases of central nervous system**

  Encephalitis:

    acute:

      inclusion body

      necrotizing

    epidemic

    lethargica

    Rio Bravo

    von Economo's disease

> **Excludes** *human herpesvirus 6 encephalitis (058.21)*
> *other human herpesvirus encephalitis (058.29)*

■**049.9 Unspecified non-arthropod-borne viral diseases of central nervous system**

  Viral encephalitis NOS

VIRAL DISEASES GENERALLY ACCOMPANIED BY EXANTHEM (050–059) ◀▥

> **Excludes** *arthropod-borne viral diseases (060.0–066.9)*
> *Boston exanthem (048)*

●**050 Smallpox**

  Caused by variola virus and is a serious, contagious, and sometimes fatal infectious disease

  050.0 Variola major

    Hemorrhagic (pustular) smallpox

    Malignant smallpox

    Purpura variolosa

  050.1 Alastrim

    Variola minor

  050.2 Modified smallpox

    Varioloid

  ■**050.9 Smallpox, unspecified**

●**051 Cowpox and paravaccinia**

  ●**051.0 Cowpox and vaccinia not from vaccination**

    Coding Clinic: 2008, Q4, P76-78

    051.01 Cowpox

    051.02 Vaccinia not from vaccination

> **Excludes** *vaccinia (generalized) (from vaccination) (999.0)*

  051.1 Pseudocowpox

    Milkers' node

  051.2 Contagious pustular dermatitis

    Ecthyma contagiosum

    Orf

  ■**051.9 Paravaccinia, unspecified**

●**052 Chickenpox**

  Very contagious disease caused by varicella zoster virus; results in itchy outbreak of skin blisters (varicella). The same virus causes shingles (zoster). The Varicella zoster virus is a member of the herpes virus family.

  052.0 Postvaricella encephalitis

    Postchickenpox encephalitis

  052.1 Varicella (hemorrhagic) pneumonitis

  052.2 Postvaricella myelitis

    Postchickenpox myelitis

  ■**052.7 With other specified complications**

    Coding Clinic: 2002, Q1, P3-4

  ■**052.8 With unspecified complication**

  052.9 Varicella without mention of complication

    Chickenpox NOS

    Varicella NOS

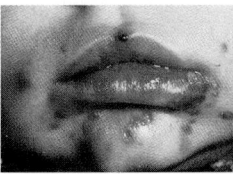

Figure 1–5 Primary herpes simplex in and around the mouth. The infection is usually acquired from siblings or parents and is readily transmitted to other direct contacts. (From Forbes, Jackson: Colour Atlas and Text of Clinical Medicine, International Edition. 2002, Mosby)

Item 1–9 Herpes is a viral disease for which there is no cure. There are two types of the herpes simplex virus: **Type I** causes **cold sores** or **fever blisters,** and **Type II** causes **genital herpes.** The virus can be spread from a sore on the lips to the genitals or from the genitals to the lips.

●**053 Herpes zoster**

  *Also known as **shingles;** caused by same virus as chickenpox. After exposure, the virus lies dormant in nerve tissue and is activated by factors including aging, stress, suppression of the immune system, and certain medication. Begins as a unilateral rash that leads to blisters and sores on skin. Chickenpox NOS is reported with 052.9.*

> **Includes** shingles
> zona

  053.0 With meningitis

  ●**053.1 With other nervous system complications**

    ■**053.10 With unspecified nervous system complication**

    053.11 Geniculate herpes zoster

      Herpetic geniculate ganglionitis

    053.12 Postherpetic trigeminal neuralgia

    053.13 Postherpetic polyneuropathy

    053.14 Herpes zoster myelitis

    ■**053.19 Other**

  ●**053.2 With ophthalmic complications**

    053.20 Herpes zoster dermatitis of eyelid

      Herpes zoster ophthalmicus

    053.21 Herpes zoster keratoconjunctivitis

    053.22 Herpes zoster iridocyclitis

    ■**053.29 Other**

  ●**053.7 With other specified complications**

    053.71 Otitis externa due to herpes zoster

    ■**053.79 Other**

  ■**053.8 With unspecified complication**

  053.9 Herpes zoster without mention of complication

    Herpes zoster NOS

●**054 Herpes simplex**

> **Excludes** *congenital herpes simplex (771.2)*

  054.0 Eczema herpeticum

    Kaposi's varicelliform eruption

  ●**054.1 Genital herpes**

    ■**054.10 Genital herpes, unspecified**

      Herpes progenitalis

      Coding Clinic: 2007, Q4, P61-64; 1985, Jan-Feb, P15-16

    054.11 Herpetic vulvovaginitis ♀

    054.12 Herpetic ulceration of vulva ♀

    054.13 Herpetic infection of penis ♂

    ■**054.19 Other**

INFECTIOUS AND PARASITIC DISEASES (001–139)

054.2 Herpetic gingivostomatitis

054.3 Herpetic meningoencephalitis
Herpes encephalitis   Simian B disease

> **Excludes** *human herpesvirus 6 encephalitis (058.21)*
> *other human herpesvirus encephalitis*
> *(058.29)*

● **054.4 With ophthalmic complications**

■ **054.40 With unspecified ophthalmic complication**

054.41 Herpes simplex dermatitis of eyelid

054.42 Dendritic keratitis

054.43 Herpes simplex disciform keratitis

054.44 Herpes simplex iridocyclitis

■ **054.49 Other**

054.5 Herpetic septicemia

054.6 Herpetic whitlow
Herpetic felon

● **054.7 With other specified complications**

054.71 Visceral herpes simplex

054.72 Herpes simplex meningitis

054.73 Herpes simplex otitis externa

054.74 Herpes simplex myelitis

■ **054.79 Other**

■ **054.8 With unspecified complication**

054.9 Herpes simplex without mention of complication

> **Item 1–10   Rubeola** (055) and **rubella** (056) are medical terms for two different strains of measles. The MMR (measles, mumps, and rubella) vaccination is an attempt to eradicate these childhood diseases.

● **055 Measles**

> **Includes**   morbilli
> rubeola
>
> *The first four combination codes specify condition(s)/*
> *complication(s) manifesting after measles.*

055.0 Postmeasles encephalitis

055.1 Postmeasles pneumonia

055.2 Postmeasles otitis media

● **055.7 With other specified complications**

055.71 Measles keratoconjunctivitis
Measles keratitis

■ **055.79 Other**

■ **055.8 With unspecified complication**

055.9 Measles without mention of complication

● **056 Rubella**

> **Includes**   German measles
> **Excludes**   *congenital rubella (771.0)*

● **056.0 With neurological complications**

■ **056.00 With unspecified neurological complication**

056.01 Encephalomyelitis due to rubella
Encephalitis due to rubella
Meningoencephalitis due to rubella

■ **056.09 Other**

● **056.7 With other specified complications**

056.71 Arthritis due to rubella

■ **056.79 Other**

■ **056.8 With unspecified complications**

056.9 Rubella without mention of complication

● **057 Other viral exanthemata**

057.0 Erythema infectiosum [fifth disease]

■ **057.8 Other specified viral exanthemata**
Dukes (-Filatow) disease   Parascarlatina
Fourth disease   Pseudoscarlatina

> **Excludes**   *exanthema subitum [sixth disease]*
> *(058.10–058.12)*
> *roseola infantum (058.10–058.12)*

■ **057.9 Viral exanthem, unspecified**

● **058 Other human herpesvirus**

> **Excludes**   *congenital herpes (771.2)*
> *cytomegalovirus (078.5)*
> *Epstein-Barr virus (075)*
> *herpes NOS (054.0–054.9)*
> *herpes simplex (054.0–054.9)*
> *herpes zoster (053.0–053.9)*
> *human herpesvirus NOS (054.0–054.9)*
> *human herpesvirus 1 (054.0–054.9)*
> *human herpesvirus 2 (054.0–054.9)*
> *human herpesvirus 3 (052.0–053.9)*
> *human herpesvirus 4 (075)*
> *human herpesvirus 5 (078.5)*
> *varicella (052.0–052.9)*
> *varicella-zoster virus (052.0–053.9)*

● **058.1 Roseola infantum**
Exanthema subitum [sixth disease]

■ **058.10 Roseola infantum, unspecified**   P
Exanthema subitum [sixth disease],
unspecified

**058.11 Roseola infantum due to human
herpesvirus 6**   P
Exanthema subitum [sixth disease]
due to human herpesvirus 6

**058.12 Roseola infantum due to human
herpesvirus 7**   P
Exanthema subitum [sixth disease] due to
human herpesvirus 7

● **058.2 Other human herpesvirus encephalitis**

> **Excludes**   *herpes encephalitis NOS (054.3)*
> *herpes simplex encephalitis (054.3)*
> *human herpesvirus encephalitis NOS*
> *(054.3)*
> *simian B herpes virus encephalitis (054.3)*
>
> Coding Clinic: 2007, Q4, P61-64

058.21 Human herpesvirus 6 encephalitis

058.29 Other human herpesvirus encephalitis
Human herpesvirus 7 encephalitis

● **058.8 Other human herpesvirus infections**

058.81 Human herpesvirus 6 infection

058.82 Human herpesvirus 7 infection

058.89 Other human herpesvirus infection
Human herpesvirus 8 infection
Kaposi's sarcoma-associated herpesvirus
infection
Coding Clinic: 2007, Q4, P61-64

◀ New   ◀ⅢⅢ Revised   ~~deleted~~ Deleted   ● Use Additional Digit(s)   ■ Nonspecific Code

● Not first-listed DX   OGCR Official Guidelines   Coding Clinic   Excludes   Includes   Use additional   Code first   Omit code

● 059 **Other poxvirus infections**

Excludes *contagious pustular dermatitis (051.2)*
cowpox (051.01)
ecthyma contagiosum (051.2)
milker's nodule (051.1)
orf (051.2)
paravaccinia NOS (051.9)
pseudocowpox (051.1)
smallpox (050.0-050.9)
vaccinia (generalized) (from vaccination)
(999.0)
vaccinia not from vaccination (051.02)

Coding Clinic: 2008, Q4, P76-78

● 059.0 **Other orthopoxvirus infections**

■059.00 **Orthopoxvirus infection, unspecified**

059.01 **Monkeypox**

■059.09 **Other orthopoxvirus infection**

● 059.1 **Other parapoxvirus infections**

■059.10 **Parapoxvirus infection, unspecified**

059.11 **Bovine stomatitis**

059.12 **Sealpox**

■059.19 **Other parapoxvirus infections**

● 059.2 **Yatapoxvirus infections**

■059.20 **Yatapoxvirus infection, unspecified**

059.21 **Tanapox**

059.22 **Yaba monkey tumor virus**

■059.8 **Other poxvirus infections**

■059.9 **Poxvirus infections, unspecified**

ARTHROPOD-BORNE VIRAL DISEASES (060–066)

Use additional code to identify any associated meningitis
(321.2)

Excludes *late effects of viral encephalitis (139.0)*

● 060 **Yellow fever**

060.0 **Sylvatic**
Yellow fever:
jungle
sylvan

060.1 **Urban**

■060.9 **Yellow fever, unspecified**

061 **Dengue**
Breakbone fever

Excludes *hemorrhagic fever caused by dengue virus (065.4)*

● 062 **Mosquito-borne viral encephalitis**
*Inflammation of the brain caused most commonly by Herpes
Simplex virus. It may be a complication of Lyme disease
and is often transmitted by mosquitoes, ticks, or rabid
animals.*

062.0 **Japanese encephalitis**
Japanese B encephalitis

062.1 **Western equine encephalitis**

062.2 **Eastern equine encephalitis**

Excludes *Venezuelan equine encephalitis (066.2)*

062.3 **St. Louis encephalitis**

062.4 **Australian encephalitis**
Australian arboencephalitis
Australian X disease
Murray Valley encephalitis

062.5 **California virus encephalitis**
Encephalitis: Encephalitis:
California   Tahyna fever
La Crosse

■062.8 **Other specified mosquito-borne viral encephalitis**
Encephalitis by Ilheus virus

Excludes *West Nile virus (066.40–066.49)*

■062.9 **Mosquito-borne viral encephalitis, unspecified**

● 063 **Tick-borne viral encephalitis**

Includes diphasic meningoencephalitis

063.0 **Russian spring-summer [taiga] encephalitis**

063.1 **Louping ill**

063.2 **Central European encephalitis**

■063.8 **Other specified tick-borne viral encephalitis**
Langat encephalitis
Powassan encephalitis

■063.9 **Tick-borne viral encephalitis, unspecified**

064 **Viral encephalitis transmitted by other and unspecified
arthropods**
Arthropod-borne viral encephalitis, vector unknown
Negishi virus encephalitis

Excludes *viral encephalitis NOS (049.9)*

● 065 **Arthropod-borne hemorrhagic fever**

065.0 **Crimean hemorrhagic fever [CHF Congo virus]**
Central Asian hemorrhagic fever

065.1 **Omsk hemorrhagic fever**

065.2 **Kyasanur Forest disease**

■065.3 **Other tick-borne hemorrhagic fever**

065.4 **Mosquito-borne hemorrhagic fever**
Chikungunya hemorrhagic fever
Dengue hemorrhagic fever

Excludes *Chikungunya fever (066.3)*
dengue (061)
yellow fever (060.0–060.9)

■065.8 **Other specified arthropod-borne hemorrhagic fever**
Mite-borne hemorrhagic fever

■065.9 **Arthropod-borne hemorrhagic fever, unspecified**
Arbovirus hemorrhagic fever NOS

● **066 Other arthropod-borne viral diseases**

  066.0 Phlebotomus fever
    Changuinola fever
    Sandfly fever

  066.1 Tick-borne fever
    Nairobi sheep disease
    Tick fever:
      American mountain
      Colorado
      Kemerovo
      Quaranfil

  066.2 Venezuelan equine fever
    Venezuelan equine encephalitis

■**066.3 Other mosquito-borne fever**
    Fever (viral):   Fever (viral):
      Bunyamwera   Oropouche
      Bwamba   Pixuna
      Chikungunya   Rift valley
      Guama   Ross river
      Mayaro   Wesselsbron
      Mucambo   Zika
      O' Nyong-Nyong
    Excludes *dengue (061)*
      yellow fever (060.0–060.9)

● **066.4 West Nile fever**
  Also indexed as West Nile virus
  Coding Clinic: 2004, Q4, P50-52; 2002, Q4, P44

  ■**066.40 West Nile fever, unspecified**
    West Nile fever NOS
    West Nile fever without complications
    West Nile virus NOS

  066.41 West Nile fever with encephalitis
    West Nile encephalitis
    West Nile encephalomyelitis

  066.42 West Nile fever with other neurologic manifestation
    Use additional code to specify the neurologic manifestation

  066.49 West Nile fever with other complications
    Use additional code to specify the other conditions

■**066.8 Other specified arthropod-borne viral diseases**
    Chandipura fever
    Piry fever

■**066.9 Arthropod-borne viral disease, unspecified**
    Arbovirus infection NOS

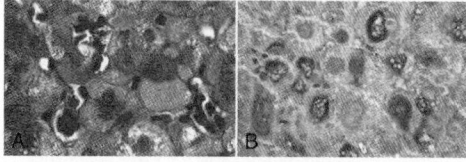

Figure 1-6 Hepatitis B viral infection. **A.** Liver parenchyma showing hepatocytes with diffuse granular cytoplasm, so-called ground glass hepatocytes (H&E). **B.** Immunoperoxidase stains from the same case, showing cytoplasmic inclusions of viral particles. (From Kumar: Robbins and Cotran: Pathologic Basis of Disease, 7th ed. 2005, Saunders, An Imprint of Elsevier)

Item 1-11 Hepatitis A (HAV) was formerly called epidemic, infectious, short-incubation, or acute catarrhal jaundice hepatitis. The primary transmission mode is the oral–fecal route. **Hepatitis B (HBV)** was formerly called long-incubation period, serum, or homologous serum hepatitis. Transmission modes are through blood from infected persons and from body fluids of infected mother to neonate. **Hepatitis C (HCV),** caused by the hepatitis C virus, is primarily transfusion associated. **Hepatitis D (HDV),** also called delta hepatitis, is caused by the hepatitis D virus in patients formerly or currently infected with hepatitis B. **Hepatitis E (HEV)** is also called enterically transmitted non-A, non-B hepatitis. The primary transmission mode is the oral–fecal route, usually through contaminated water.

OTHER DISEASES DUE TO VIRUSES AND CHLAMYDIAE (070–079)

● **070 Viral hepatitis**

  Includes viral hepatitis (acute) (chronic)
  Excludes *cytomegalic inclusion virus hepatitis (078.5)*

The following fifth-digit subclassification is for use with categories 070.2 and 070.3:

> ■ 0 acute or unspecified, without mention of hepatitis delta
> ■ 1 acute or unspecified, with hepatitis delta
>   2 chronic, without mention of hepatitis delta
>   3 chronic, with hepatitis delta

Coding Clinic: 2007, Q2, P6-7x3; 2004, Q4, P52-53

  070.0 Viral hepatitis A with hepatic coma

  070.1 Viral hepatitis A without mention of hepatic coma
    Infectious hepatitis

● **070.2 Viral hepatitis B with hepatic coma**
  [0-3]

● **070.3 Viral hepatitis B without mention of hepatic coma**
  [0-3]   Serum hepatitis
    Coding Clinic: 1993, Q1, P28

● **070.4 Other specified viral hepatitis with hepatic coma**

  ■**070.41 Acute hepatitis C with hepatic coma**

  070.42 Hepatitis delta without mention of active hepatitis B disease with hepatic coma
    Hepatitis delta with hepatitis B carrier state

  070.43 Hepatitis E with hepatic coma

  070.44 Chronic hepatitis C with hepatic coma

  ■**070.49 Other specified viral hepatitis with hepatic coma**

● **070.5 Other specified viral hepatitis without mention of hepatic coma**

◼ **070.51 Acute hepatitis C without mention of hepatic coma**

070.52 Hepatitis delta without mention of active hepatitis B disease or hepatic coma

070.53 Hepatitis E without mention of hepatic coma

070.54 Chronic hepatitis C without mention of hepatic coma
Coding Clinic: 2008, Q4, P120; 2007, Q3, P9; 2006, Q2, P13

◼ **070.59 Other specified viral hepatitis without mention of hepatic coma**

◼ **070.6 Unspecified viral hepatitis with hepatic coma**

Excludes *unspecified viral hepatitis C with hepatic coma (070.71)*

● **070.7 Unspecified viral hepatitis C**

◼ **070.70 Unspecified viral hepatitis C without hepatic coma**
Unspecified viral hepatitis C NOS

◼ **070.71 Unspecified viral hepatitis C with hepatic coma**

◼ **070.9 Unspecified viral hepatitis without mention of hepatic coma**
Viral hepatitis NOS

Excludes *unspecified viral hepatitis C without hepatic coma (070.70)*

071 Rabies
Viral disease affecting central nervous system and transmitted from infected mammals.
Hydrophobia
Lyssa

● **072 Mumps**
An acute, contagious, viral disease that causes painful enlargement of the salivary or parotid glands and is spread by respiratory droplets or direct contact. The following combination codes are specific diseases as an existing complication of mumps.

072.0 Mumps orchitis ♂

072.1 Mumps meningitis

072.2 Mumps encephalitis
Mumps meningoencephalitis

072.3 Mumps pancreatitis

● **072.7 Mumps with other specified complications**

072.71 Mumps hepatitis

072.72 Mumps polyneuropathy

◼ **072.79 Other**

◼ **072.8 Mumps with unspecified complication**

◼ **072.9 Mumps without mention of complication**
Epidemic parotitis
Infectious parotitis

● **073 Ornithosis**

Includes parrot fever
psittacosis

073.0 With pneumonia
Lobular pneumonitis due to ornithosis

◼ **073.7 With other specified complications**

◼ **073.8 With unspecified complication**

◼ **073.9 Ornithosis, unspecified**

● **074 Specific diseases due to Coxsackie virus**

Excludes *Coxsackie virus:*
infection NOS (079.2)
meningitis (047.0)

074.0 Herpangina
Vesicular pharyngitis

074.1 Epidemic pleurodynia
Bornholm disease
Devil's grip
Epidemic:
myalgia
myositis

● **074.2 Coxsackie carditis**

◼ **074.20 Coxsackie carditis, unspecified**

074.21 Coxsackie pericarditis

074.22 Coxsackie endocarditis

074.23 Coxsackie myocarditis
Aseptic myocarditis of newborn

074.3 Hand, foot, and mouth disease
Vesicular stomatitis and exanthem
Check your documentation—this code is HAND, foot, and mouth disease. Code 078.4 is foot and mouth disease.

◼ **074.8 Other specified diseases due to Coxsackie virus**
Acute lymphonodular pharyngitis

075 Infectious mononucleosis
Glandular fever
Pfeiffer's disease
Monocytic angina
Coding Clinic: 2001, Q3, P13-14x2

● **076 Trachoma**

Excludes *late effect of trachoma (139.1)*

076.0 Initial stage
Trachoma dubium

076.1 Active stage
Granular conjunctivitis (trachomatous)
Trachomatous:
follicular conjunctivitis
pannus

◼ **076.9 Trachoma, unspecified**
Trachoma NOS

● **077 Other diseases of conjunctiva due to viruses and Chlamydiae**

Excludes *ophthalmic complications of viral diseases classified elsewhere*

077.0 Inclusion conjunctivitis
Paratrachoma
Swimming pool conjunctivitis

Excludes *inclusion blennorrhea (neonatal) (771.6)*

077.1 Epidemic keratoconjunctivitis
Shipyard eye

077.2 Pharyngoconjunctival fever
Viral pharyngoconjunctivitis

◼ **077.3 Other adenoviral conjunctivitis**
Acute adenoviral follicular conjunctivitis

077.4 Epidemic hemorrhagic conjunctivitis
Apollo:
conjunctivitis
disease
Conjunctivitis due to enterovirus type 70
Hemorrhagic conjunctivitis (acute) (epidemic)

INFECTIOUS AND PARASITIC DISEASES (001–139)

■077.8 **Other viral conjunctivitis**
Newcastle conjunctivitis

●077.9 **Unspecified diseases of conjunctiva due to viruses and Chlamydiae**

    ■077.98 **Due to Chlamydiae**

    ■077.99 **Due to viruses**
        Viral conjunctivitis NOS

●078 **Other diseases due to viruses and Chlamydiae**

    Excludes *viral infection NOS (079.0–079.9)*
                viremia NOS (790.8)

    078.0 **Molluscum contagiosum**

  ●078.1 **Viral warts**
      Viral warts due to human papillomavirus
      Coding Clinic: 1997, Q2, P9

    ■078.10 **Viral warts, unspecified**
        Verruca:
          NOS
          Vulgaris
        Warts (infectious)

    078.11 **Condyloma acuminatum**
        Condyloma NOS
        Genital warts NOS

    078.12 **Plantar wart**
        Verruca plantaris
        Coding Clinic: 2008, Q4, P78-79

    ■078.19 **Other specified viral warts**
        Common wart
        Flat wart
        Verruca plana

    078.2 **Sweating fever**
      Miliary fever
      Sweating disease

    078.3 **Cat-scratch disease**
      Benign lymphoreticulosis (of inoculation)
      Cat-scratch fever

    078.4 **Foot and mouth disease**
      Aphthous fever
      Epizootic:
        aphthae
        stomatitis
      Check your documentation. Code 074.3 is for HAND, foot, and mouth disease.

    078.5 **Cytomegaloviral disease**
      Cytomegalic inclusion disease
      Salivary gland virus disease

      Use additional code to identify manifestation, as:
      cytomegalic inclusion virus:
        hepatitis (573.1)
        pneumonia (484.1)

      Excludes *congenital cytomegalovirus infection (771.1)*
      Coding Clinic: 2003, Q1, P11; 1993, Q3, P13; Q2, P11; Q1, P24; 1989, Q1, P9

    078.6 **Hemorrhagic nephrosonephritis**
      Hemorrhagic fever:
        epidemic
        Korean
        Russian with renal syndrome

    078.7 **Arenaviral hemorrhagic fever**
      Hemorrhagic fever:
        Argentine
        Bolivian
        Junin virus
        Machupo virus

●078.8 **Other specified diseases due to viruses and Chlamydiae**

    Excludes *epidemic diarrhea (009.2)*
               lymphogranuloma venereum (099.1)

    078.81 **Epidemic vertigo**

    078.82 **Epidemic vomiting syndrome**
        Winter vomiting disease

    ■078.88 **Other specified diseases due to Chlamydiae**

    ■078.89 **Other specified diseases due to viruses**
        Epidemic cervical myalgia
        Marburg disease
        ~~Tanapox~~

Item 1–12 Retrovirus develops by copying its RNA, genetic materials, into the DNA, which then produces new virus particles. It is from the Retroviridae virus family.
Human T-cell lymphotropic virus, Type I (HTLV-I) is also called human T-cell leukemia virus, Type I, and is a retrovirus thought to cause T-cell leukemia/lymphoma.
Human T-cell lymphotropic virus, Type II (HTLV-II), is also called human T-cell leukemia virus, Type II, and is a retrovirus associated with hematologic disorders.
HIV-2 is one of the serotypes of HIV and is usually confined to West Africa, whereas HIV-1 is found worldwide.

●079 **Viral and chlamydial infection in conditions classified elsewhere and of unspecified site**

    Note: This category is provided to be used as an additional code to identify the viral agent in diseases classifiable elsewhere. This category will also be used to classify virus infection of unspecified nature or site.

    079.0 **Adenovirus**

    079.1 **ECHO virus**

    079.2 **Coxsackie virus**

    079.3 **Rhinovirus**

    079.4 **Human papillomavirus**
      Coding Clinic: 1997, Q2, P9

  ●079.5 **Retrovirus**

    Excludes *human immunodeficiency virus, type 1 [HIV-1] (042)*
              human T-cell lymphotrophic virus, type III [HTLV-III] (042)
              lymphadenopathy-associated virus [LAV] (042)

    ■079.50 **Retrovirus, unspecified**

    079.51 **Human T-cell lymphotrophic virus, type I [HTLV-I]**

    079.52 **Human T-cell lymphotrophic virus, type II [HTLV-II]**

    079.53 **Human immunodeficiency virus, type 2 [HIV-2]**

    ■079.59 **Other specified retrovirus**

    079.6 **Respiratory syncytial virus (RSV)**
      Coding Clinic: 1996, Q4, P27-28

◀ New   ◀▥ Revised   ~~deleted~~ Deleted   ● Use Additional Digit(s)   ■ Nonspecific Code
● Not first-listed DX   OGCR Official Guidelines   Coding Clinic   Excludes   Includes   Use additional   Code first   Omit code

● **079.8 Other specified viral and chlamydial infections**
Coding Clinic: 1988, Q1, P12; Q1, P12

    079.81 Hantavirus

    079.82 SARS-associated coronavirus
Coding Clinic: 2003, Q4, P46-48

    079.83 Parvovirus B19
Human parvovirus
Parvovirus NOS

      Excludes *erythema infectiosum [fifth disease]*
(057.0)
Coding Clinic: 2007, Q4, P64

    ■**079.88 Other specified chlamydial infection**

    ■**079.89 Other specified viral infection**
Coding Clinic: 1995, Q1, P7

● **079.9 Unspecified viral and chlamydial infections**

    Excludes *viremia NOS (790.8)*
Coding Clinic: 1988, Q4, P10; 1987, Jan-Feb, P16

    ■**079.98 Unspecified chlamydial infection**
Chlamydial infection NOS

    ■**079.99 Unspecified viral infection**
Viral infection NOS
Coding Clinic: 1991, Q2, P8

RICKETTSIOSES AND OTHER ARTHROPOD-BORNE DISEASES (080–088)

    Excludes *arthropod-borne viral diseases (060.0–066.9)*

080 Louse-borne [epidemic] typhus
Typhus (fever):
    classical
    epidemic
      Infecting a large number of individuals at the same time
    exanthematic NOS
    louse-borne

● **081 Other typhus**

    081.0 Murine [endemic] typhus
Typhus (fever):
    endemic
      Restricted to a particular region
    flea-borne

    081.1 Brill's disease
Brill-Zinsser disease
Recrudescent typhus (fever)

    081.2 Scrub typhus
Japanese river fever
Kedani fever
Mite-borne typhus
Tsutsugamushi

    ■**081.9 Typhus, unspecified**
Typhus (fever) NOS

Item 1-13 Rickettsioses are diseases spread from ticks, lice, fleas, or mites to humans.
Typhus is spread to humans chiefly by the fleas of rats.
Endemic identifies a disease as being present in low numbers of humans at all times, whereas **epidemic** identifies a disease as being present in high numbers of humans at a specific time. Morbidity (death) is higher in epidemic diseases.
Brill's disease, also known as **Brill-Zinsser disease,** is spread from human to human by body lice and also from the lice of flying squirrels. **Scrub typhus** is spread in the same ways as Brill's disease.
Malaria is spread to humans by mosquitoes.

● **082 Tick-borne rickettsioses**

    082.0 Spotted fevers
Rocky mountain spotted fever
Sao Paulo fever

    082.1 Boutonneuse fever
African tick typhus
India tick typhus
Kenya tick typhus
Marseilles fever
Mediterranean tick fever

    082.2 North Asian tick fever
Siberian tick typhus

    082.3 Queensland tick typhus

    ● **082.4 Ehrlichiosis**

      ■**082.40 Ehrlichiosis, unspecified**

      082.41 Ehrlichiosis chaffeensis [E. chaffeensis]

      ■**082.49 Other ehrlichiosis**

    ■**082.8 Other specified tick-borne rickettsioses**
Lone star fever
Coding Clinic: 1999, Q4, P19

    ■**082.9 Tick-borne rickettsiosis, unspecified**
Tick-borne typhus NOS

● **083 Other rickettsioses**

    083.0 Q fever

    083.1 Trench fever
Quintan fever
Wolhynian fever

    083.2 Rickettsialpox
Vesicular rickettsiosis

    ■**083.8 Other specified rickettsioses**

    ■**083.9 Rickettsiosis, unspecified**

● **084 Malaria**
Mosquito-borne disease caused by parasite. Left untreated, severe complications and death may result.

    Note: Subcategories 084.0–084.6 exclude the listed conditions with mention of pernicious complications (084.8–084.9).

    Excludes *congenital malaria (771.2)*

    084.0 Falciparum malaria [malignant tertian]
Malaria (fever):
    by Plasmodium falciparum
    subtertian

    084.1 Vivax malaria [benign tertian]
Malaria (fever) by Plasmodium vivax

    084.2 Quartan malaria
Malaria (fever) by Plasmodium malariae
Malariae malaria

    084.3 Ovale malaria
Malaria (fever) by Plasmodium ovale

    ■**084.4 Other malaria**
Monkey malaria

    084.5 Mixed malaria
Malaria (fever) by more than one parasite

    ■**084.6 Malaria, unspecified**
Malaria (fever) NOS

    084.7 Induced malaria
Therapeutically induced malaria

      Excludes *accidental infection from syringe, blood transfusion, etc. (084.0–084.6, above, according to parasite species)*
transmission from mother to child during delivery (771.2)

INFECTIOUS AND PARASITIC DISEASES (001–139)

084.8 Blackwater fever
Hemoglobinuric:
    fever (bilious)
    malaria
Malarial hemoglobinuria

084.9 Other pernicious complications of malaria
Algid malaria
Cerebral malaria

    Use additional code to identify complication, as:
    malarial:
        hepatitis (573.2)
        nephrosis (581.81)

● **085 Leishmaniasis**

085.0 Visceral [kala-azar]
Dumdum fever
Infection by Leishmania:
    donovani
    infantum
Leishmaniasis:
    dermal, post-kala-azar
    Mediterranean
    visceral (Indian)

085.1 Cutaneous, urban
Aleppo boil
Baghdad boil
Delhi boil
Infection by Leishmania tropica (minor)
Leishmaniasis, cutaneous:
    dry form
    late
    recurrent
    ulcerating
Oriental sore

085.2 Cutaneous, Asian desert
Infection by Leishmania tropica major
Leishmaniasis, cutaneous:
    acute necrotizing
    rural
    wet form
    zoonotic form

085.3 Cutaneous, Ethiopian
Infection by Leishmania ethiopica
Leishmaniasis, cutaneous:
    diffuse
    lepromatous

085.4 Cutaneous, American
Chiclero ulcer
Infection by Leishmania mexicana
Leishmaniasis tegumentaria diffusa

085.5 Mucocutaneous (American)
Espundia
Infection by Leishmania braziliensis
Uta

085.9 Leishmaniasis, unspecified

● **086 Trypanosomiasis**
Human African trypanosomiasis (HAT) is transmitted by fly bites that transmit either Trypanosoma brucei gambiense (causes a chronic infection lasting years) or Trypanosoma brucei rhodesiense (causes acute illness lasting several weeks).

Use additional code to identify manifestations, as:
trypanosomiasis:
    encephalitis (323.2)
    meningitis (321.3)

086.0 Chagas' disease with heart involvement
American trypanosomiasis with heart involvement
Infection by Trypanosoma cruzi with heart involvement
Any condition classifiable to 086.2 with heart involvement

086.1 Chagas' disease with other organ involvement
American trypanosomiasis with involvement of organ other than heart
Infection by Trypanosoma cruzi with involvement of organ other than heart
Any condition classifiable to 086.2 with involvement of organ other than heart

086.2 Chagas' disease without mention of organ involvement
American trypanosomiasis
Infection by Trypanosoma cruzi

086.3 Gambian trypanosomiasis
Gambian sleeping sickness
Infection by Trypanosoma gambiense

086.4 Rhodesian trypanosomiasis
Infection by Trypanosoma rhodesiense
Rhodesian sleeping sickness

086.5 African trypanosomiasis, unspecified
Sleeping sickness NOS

086.9 Trypanosomiasis, unspecified

● **087 Relapsing fever**
    Includes   recurrent fever

087.0 Louse-borne

087.1 Tick-borne

087.9 Relapsing fever, unspecified

● **088 Other arthropod-borne diseases**

088.0 Bartonellosis
Carrión's disease
Oroya fever
Verruga peruana

● **088.8 Other specified arthropod-borne diseases**

088.81 Lyme disease
Erythema chronicum migrans
Coding Clinic: 1990, Q3, P14; 1989, Q2, P10

088.82 Babesiosis
Babesiasis

088.89 Other

088.9 Arthropod-borne disease, unspecified

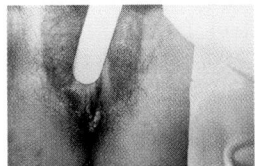

Figure 1–7 *Chance of primary syphilis. (From Mandell, Bennett, & Dolin: Principles and Practice of Infectious Diseases, 6th ed. 2005, Churchill Livingstone, An Imprint of Elsevier)*

Item 1–14 Syphilis, also known as lues, is the most serious of the venereal diseases caused by *Treponema pallidum.* The **primary** stage is characterized by an ulceration known as **chancre,** which usually appears on the genitals but can also develop on the anus, lips, tonsils, breasts, or fingers. Syphilis is easy to cure in its early stages. A single intramuscular injection of penicillin will usually cure a person who has had syphilis for less than a year.

The **secondary** stage is characterized by a rash that can affect any area of the body. **Latent** syphilis is divided into **early,** which is diagnosed within two years of infection, and **late,** which is diagnosed two years or more after infection. Additional doses of penicillin or another antibiotic are needed to treat someone who has had syphilis for longer than a year. For those allergic to penicillin, there are other antibiotic treatments. **Congenital** syphilis is also labeled **early** or **late** based on the time of diagnosis.

SYPHILIS AND OTHER VENEREAL DISEASES (090–099)

> **Excludes** *nonvenereal endemic syphilis (104.0)*
> *urogenital trichomoniasis (131.0)*

● 090 **Congenital syphilis**

   090.0 **Early congenital syphilis, symptomatic**
      Congenital syphilitic:
        choroiditis
        coryza (chronic)
        hepatomegaly
        mucous patches
        periostitis
        splenomegaly
      Syphilitic (congenital):
        epiphysitis
        osteochondritis
        pemphigus
      Any congenital syphilitic condition specified as early or manifest less than two years after birth

   090.1 **Early congenital syphilis, latent**
      Congenital syphilis without clinical manifestations, with positive serological reaction and negative spinal fluid test, less than two years after birth

  ■090.2 **Early congenital syphilis, unspecified**
      Congenital syphilis NOS, less than two years after birth

   090.3 **Syphilitic interstitial keratitis**
      Syphilitic keratitis:
        parenchymatous
        punctata profunda
      > **Excludes** *interstitial keratitis NOS (370.50)*

● 090.4 **Juvenile neurosyphilis**
      Use additional code to identify any associated mental disorder

  ■090.40 **Juvenile neurosyphilis, unspecified**
      Congenital neurosyphilis
      Dementia paralytica juvenilis
      Juvenile:
        general paresis
        tabes
        taboparesis

   090.41 **Congenital syphilitic encephalitis**

   090.42 **Congenital syphilitic meningitis**

  ■090.49 **Other**

■090.5 **Other late congenital syphilis, symptomatic**
      Gumma due to congenital syphilis
      Hutchinson's teeth
      Syphilitic saddle nose
      Any congenital syphilitic condition specified as late or manifest two years or more after birth

   090.6 **Late congenital syphilis, latent**
      Congenital syphilis without clinical manifestations, with positive serological reaction and negative spinal fluid test, two years or more after birth

■090.7 **Late congenital syphilis, unspecified**
      Congenital syphilis NOS, two years or more after birth

■090.9 **Congenital syphilis, unspecified**

● 091 **Early syphilis, symptomatic**

> **Excludes** *early cardiovascular syphilis (093.0–093.9)*
> *early neurosyphilis (094.0–094.9)*

   091.0 **Genital syphilis (primary)**
      Genital chancre

   091.1 **Primary anal syphilis**

  ■091.2 **Other primary syphilis**
      Primary syphilis of:
        breast
        fingers
        lip
        tonsils

   091.3 **Secondary syphilis of skin or mucous membranes**
      Condyloma latum
      Secondary syphilis of:
        anus
        mouth
        pharynx
        skin
        tonsils
        vulva

   091.4 **Adenopathy due to secondary syphilis**
      Syphilitic adenopathy (secondary)
      Syphilitic lymphadenitis (secondary)

INFECTIOUS AND PARASITIC DISEASES (001–139)

Item 1–15 Notice the placement of 091.4 combination code in with the Infectious and Parasitic Disease codes (syphilis). This uveitis does not appear in the eye code section because it is a manifestation of the underlying disease of syphilis.

● 091.5 **Uveitis due to secondary syphilis**
  ■ 091.50 **Syphilitic uveitis, unspecified**
  091.51 **Syphilitic chorioretinitis (secondary)**
  091.52 **Syphilitic iridocyclitis (secondary)**
● 091.6 **Secondary syphilis of viscera and bone**
  091.61 **Secondary syphilitic periostitis**
  091.62 **Secondary syphilitic hepatitis**
    Secondary syphilis of liver
  ■ 091.69 **Other viscera**
091.7 **Secondary syphilis, relapse**
  Secondary syphilis, relapse (treated) (untreated)
● 091.8 **Other forms of secondary syphilis**
  091.81 **Acute syphilitic meningitis (secondary)**
  091.82 **Syphilitic alopecia**
  ■ 091.89 **Other**
■ 091.9 **Unspecified secondary syphilis**

● 092 **Early syphilis, latent**
  Early syphilis is the disease, latent is the characteristic.
  Includes syphilis (acquired) without clinical manifestations, with positive serological reaction and negative spinal fluid test, less than two years after infection
  092.0 **Early syphilis, latent, serological relapse after treatment**
  ■ 092.9 **Early syphilis, latent, unspecified**

● 093 **Cardiovascular syphilis**
  093.0 **Aneurysm of aorta, specified as syphilitic**
    Dilatation of aorta, specified as syphilitic
  093.1 **Syphilitic aortitis**
● 093.2 **Syphilitic endocarditis**
  Check documentation for documentation of a specific valve.
  ■ 093.20 **Valve, unspecified**
    Syphilitic ostial coronary disease
  093.21 **Mitral valve**
  093.22 **Aortic valve**
    Syphilitic aortic incompetence or stenosis
  093.23 **Tricuspid valve**
  093.24 **Pulmonary valve**
● 093.8 **Other specified cardiovascular syphilis**
  093.81 **Syphilitic pericarditis**
  093.82 **Syphilitic myocarditis**
  ■ 093.89 **Other**
■ 093.9 **Cardiovascular syphilis, unspecified**

● 094 **Neurosyphilis**
  Use additional code to identify any associated mental disorder
  094.0 **Tabes dorsalis**
    Locomotor ataxia (progressive)
    Posterior spinal sclerosis (syphilitic)
    Tabetic neurosyphilis
    Use additional code to identify manifestation, as: neurogenic arthropathy [Charcot's joint disease] (713.5)

094.1 **General paresis**
  Dementia paralytica
  General paralysis (of the insane) (progressive)
  Paretic neurosyphilis
  Taboparesis
094.2 **Syphilitic meningitis**
  Meningovascular syphilis
  Excludes *acute syphilitic meningitis (secondary) (091.81)*
094.3 **Asymptomatic neurosyphilis**
● 094.8 **Other specified neurosyphilis**
  094.81 **Syphilitic encephalitis**
  094.82 **Syphilitic Parkinsonism**
  094.83 **Syphilitic disseminated retinochoroiditis**
  094.84 **Syphilitic optic atrophy**
  094.85 **Syphilitic retrobulbar neuritis**
  094.86 **Syphilitic acoustic neuritis**
  094.87 **Syphilitic ruptured cerebral aneurysm**
  ■ 094.89 **Other**
■ 094.9 **Neurosyphilis, unspecified**
  Gumma (syphilitic) of central nervous system NOS
  Syphilis (early) (late) of central nervous system NOS
  Syphiloma of central nervous system NOS

● 095 **Other forms of late syphilis, with symptoms**
  In the late stages, syphilis can damage organs and body systems.
  Includes gumma (syphilitic)
    Destructive lesions of syphilis
    tertiary, or unspecified stage
  095.0 **Syphilitic episcleritis**
  095.1 **Syphilis of lung**
  095.2 **Syphilitic peritonitis**
  095.3 **Syphilis of liver**
  095.4 **Syphilis of kidney**
  095.5 **Syphilis of bone**
  095.6 **Syphilis of muscle**
    Syphilitic myositis
  095.7 **Syphilis of synovium, tendon, and bursa**
    Syphilitic:
    bursitis
    synovitis
  ■ 095.8 **Other specified forms of late symptomatic syphilis**
    Excludes *cardiovascular syphilis (093.0–093.9)*
    neurosyphilis (094.0–094.9)
  ■ 095.9 **Late symptomatic syphilis, unspecified**

096 **Late syphilis, latent**
  Syphilis (acquired) without clinical manifestations, with positive serological reaction and negative spinal fluid test, two years or more after infection

● 097 **Other and unspecified syphilis**
  ■ 097.0 **Late syphilis, unspecified**
  ■ 097.1 **Latent syphilis, unspecified**
    Positive serological reaction for syphilis
  ■ 097.9 **Syphilis, unspecified**
    Syphilis (acquired) NOS
    Excludes *syphilis NOS causing death under two years of age (090.9)*

INFECTIOUS AND PARASITIC DISEASES (001–139)

◀ New   ◀ Revised   ~~deleted~~ Deleted   ● Use Additional Digit(s)   ■ Nonspecific Code   ● Not first-listed DX   OGCR Official Guidelines   Coding Clinic   Excludes   Includes   Use additional   Code first   Omit code

● **098 Gonococcal infections**

STD (sexually transmitted disease) caused by Neisseria gonorrhoeae that flourishes in the warm, moist areas of the reproductive tract. Untreated gonorrhea spreads to other parts of the body, causing inflammation of the testes or prostate or pelvic inflammatory disease (PID).

098.0 Acute, of lower genitourinary tract
Gonococcal:
Bartholinitis (acute)
Female only: Bartholin gland
urethritis (acute)
vulvovaginitis (acute)
Gonorrhea (acute):
NOS
genitourinary (tract) NOS

● **098.1 Acute, of upper genitourinary tract**

■ **098.10 Gonococcal infection (acute) of upper genitourinary tract, site unspecified**

098.11 Gonococcal cystitis (acute)
Gonorrhea (acute) of bladder

098.12 Gonococcal prostatitis (acute) ♂

098.13 Gonococcal epididymo-orchitis (acute) ♂
Gonococcal orchitis (acute)

098.14 Gonococcal seminal vesiculitis (acute) ♂
Gonorrhea (acute) of seminal vesicle

098.15 Gonococcal cervicitis (acute) ♀
Gonorrhea (acute) of cervix

098.16 Gonococcal endometritis (acute) ♀
Gonorrhea (acute) of uterus

098.17 Gonococcal salpingitis, specified as acute ♀

■ **098.19 Other**

098.2 Chronic, of lower genitourinary tract
Gonococcal specified as chronic or with duration of two months or more:
Bartholinitis specified as chronic or with duration of two months or more
urethritis specified as chronic or with duration of two months or more
vulvovaginitis specified as chronic or with duration of two months or more
Gonorrhea specified as chronic or with duration of two months or more:
NOS specified as chronic or with duration of two months or more
genitourinary (tract) specified as chronic or with duration of two months or more
Any condition classifiable to 098.0 specified as chronic or with duration of two months or more

● **098.3 Chronic, of upper genitourinary tract**
Any condition classifiable to 098.1 stated as chronic or with a duration of two months or more

■ **098.30 Chronic gonococcal infection of upper genitourinary tract, site unspecified**

098.31 Gonococcal cystitis, chronic
Any condition classifiable to 098.11, specified as chronic
Gonorrhea of bladder, chronic

098.32 Gonococcal prostatitis, chronic ♂
Any condition classifiable to 098.12, specified as chronic

098.33 Gonococcal epididymo-orchitis, chronic ♂
Any condition classifiable to 098.13, specified as chronic
Chronic gonococcal orchitis

098.34 Gonococcal seminal vesiculitis, chronic ♂
Any condition classifiable to 098.14, specified as chronic
Gonorrhea of seminal vesicle, chronic

098.35 Gonococcal cervicitis, chronic ♀
Any condition classifiable to 098.15, specified as chronic
Gonorrhea of cervix, chronic

098.36 Gonococcal endometritis, chronic ♀
Any condition classifiable to 098.16, specified as chronic

098.37 Gonococcal salpingitis (chronic) ♀

■ **098.39 Other**

● **098.4 Gonococcal infection of eye**

098.40 Gonococcal conjunctivitis (neonatorum)
Neonate = newborn
Gonococcal ophthalmia (neonatorum)

098.41 Gonococcal iridocyclitis

098.42 Gonococcal endophthalmia

098.43 Gonococcal keratitis

■ **098.49 Other**

● **098.5 Gonococcal infection of joint**

098.50 Gonococcal arthritis
Gonococcal infection of joint NOS

098.51 Gonococcal synovitis and tenosynovitis

098.52 Gonococcal bursitis

098.53 Gonococcal spondylitis

■ **098.59 Other**
Gonococcal rheumatism

098.6 Gonococcal infection of pharynx

098.7 Gonococcal infection of anus and rectum
Gonococcal proctitis

● **098.8 Gonococcal infection of other specified sites**

098.81 Gonococcal keratosis (blennorrhagica)

098.82 Gonococcal meningitis

098.83 Gonococcal pericarditis

098.84 Gonococcal endocarditis

■ **098.85 Other gonococcal heart disease**

098.86 Gonococcal peritonitis

■ **098.89 Other**
Gonococcemia
Blood condition

● **099 Other venereal diseases**

099.0 Chancroid
Sexually transmitted infection caused by bacteria (Haemophilus ducreyi).
Bubo (inguinal):
chancroidal
due to Hemophilus ducreyi
Chancre:
Ducrey's simple soft
Ulcus molle (cutis) (skin)

099.1 Lymphogranuloma venereum
Climatic or tropical bubo
(Durand-) Nicolas-Favre disease
Esthiomene
Lymphogranuloma inguinale

099.2 Granuloma inguinale
Donovanosis
Granuloma pudendi (ulcerating)
Granuloma venereum
Pudendal ulcer

099.3 Reiter's disease
Reiter's syndrome
Use additional code for associated:
arthropathy (711.1)
conjunctivitis (372.33)

● **099.4 Other nongonococcal urethritis [NGU]**
■ **099.40 Unspecified**
Nonspecific urethritis

099.41 Chlamydia trachomatis

■ **099.49 Other specified organism**

● **099.5 Other venereal diseases due to Chlamydia trachomatis**
Excludes *Chlamydia trachomatis infection of conjunctiva (076.0–076.9, 077.0, 077.9)*
Lymphogranuloma venereum (099.1)

■ **099.50 Unspecified site**

099.51 Pharynx

099.52 Anus and rectum

099.53 Lower genitourinary sites
Excludes *urethra (099.41)*
Use additional code to specify site of infection, such as:
bladder (595.4)
cervix (616.0)
vagina and vulva (616.11)

■ **099.54 Other genitourinary sites**
Use additional code to specify site of infection, such as:
pelvic inflammatory disease NOS (614.9)
testis and epididymis (604.91)

■ **099.55 Unspecified genitourinary site**

099.56 Peritoneum
Perihepatitis

■ **099.59 Other specified site**

■ **099.8 Other specified venereal diseases**

■ **099.9 Venereal disease, unspecified**

OTHER SPIROCHETAL DISEASES (100–104)

● **100 Leptospirosis**
100.0 Leptospirosis icterohemorrhagica
Leptospiral or spirochetal jaundice (hemorrhagic)
Weil's disease

● **100.8 Other specified leptospiral infections**
100.81 Leptospiral meningitis (aseptic)
■ **100.89 Other**
Fever:
Fort Bragg
pretibial
swamp
Infection by Leptospira:
australis
bataviae
pyrogenes

■ **100.9 Leptospirosis, unspecified**

101 Vincent's angina
Acute necrotizing ulcerative:
gingivitis
stomatitis
Fusospirochetal pharyngitis
Spirochetal stomatitis
Trench mouth
Vincent's:
gingivitis
infection [any site]

● **102 Yaws**
Includes frambesia
pian

102.0 Initial lesions
Chancre of yaws
Frambesia, initial or primary
Initial frambesial ulcer
Mother yaw

102.1 Multiple papillomata and wet crab yaws
Butter yaws
Frambesioma
Pianoma
Plantar or palmar papilloma of yaws

■ **102.2 Other early skin lesions**
Cutaneous yaws, less than five years after infection
Early yaws (cutaneous) (macular) (papular) (maculopapular) (micropapular)
Frambeside of early yaws

102.3 Hyperkeratosis
Ghoul hand
Hyperkeratosis, palmar or plantar (early) (late) due to yaws
Worm-eaten soles

102.4 Gummata and ulcers
Nodular late yaws (ulcerated)
Gummatous frambeside

102.5 Gangosa
Rhinopharyngitis mutilans

102.6 Bone and joint lesions
Goundou of yaws (late)
Gumma, bone of yaws (late)
Gummatous osteitis or periostitis of yaws (late)
Hydrarthrosis of yaws (early) (late)
Osteitis of yaws (early) (late)
Periostitis (hypertrophic) of yaws (early) (late)

■ **102.7 Other manifestations**
Juxta-articular nodules of yaws
Mucosal yaws

102.8 Latent yaws
Yaws without clinical manifestations, with positive serology

■ **102.9 Yaws, unspecified**

● **103 Pinta**
103.0 Primary lesions
Chancre (primary) of pinta [carate]
Papule (primary) of pinta [carate]
Pintid of pinta [carate]

103.1 Intermediate lesions
Erythematous plaques of pinta [carate]
Hyperchromic lesions of pinta [carate]
Hyperkeratosis of pinta [carate]

103.2 Late lesions
Cardiovascular lesions of pinta [carate]
Skin lesions of pinta [carate]:
achromic of pinta [carate]
cicatricial of pinta [carate]
dyschromic of pinta [carate]
Vitiligo of pinta [carate]

103.3 Mixed lesions
Achromic and hyperchromic skin lesions of pinta [carate]

■ **103.9 Pinta, unspecified**

● **104   Other spirochetal infection**
  104.0   Nonvenereal endemic syphilis
          Bejel
          Njovera

  ■**104.8   Other specified spirochetal infections**

          Excludes *relapsing fever (087.0–087.9)*
                      syphilis (090.0–097.9)

  ■**104.9   Spirochetal infection, unspecified**

MYCOSES (110–118)

  Use additional code to identify manifestation, as:
      arthropathy (711.6)
      meningitis (321.0–321.1)
      otitis externa (380.15)

          Excludes *infection by Actinomycetales, such as species of*
                      Actinomyces, Actinomadura, Nocardia,
                      Streptomyces (039.0–039.9)

● **110   Dermatophytosis**
      Also known as tinea or ringworm; condition of scalp, glabrous
      skin, and/or nails. Caused by fungi (dermatophytes).

          Includes infection by species of Epidermophyton,
                      Microsporum, and Trichophyton
                      tinea, any type except those in 111

  110.0   Of scalp and beard
          Kerion
          Sycosis, mycotic
          Trichophytic tinea [black dot tinea], scalp

  110.1   Of nail
          Dermatophytic onychia
          Onychomycosis
          Tinea unguium

  110.2   Of hand
          Tinea manuum

  110.3   Of groin and perianal area
          Dhobie itch
          Eczema marginatum
          Tinea cruris

  110.4   Of foot
          Athlete's foot
          Tinea pedis

  110.5   Of the body
          Herpes circinatus
          Tinea imbricata [Tokelau]

  110.6   Deep seated dermatophytosis
          Granuloma trichophyticum
          Majocchi's granuloma

  ■**110.8   Of other specified sites**

  ■**110.9   Of unspecified site**
          Favus NOS
          Microsporic tinea NOS
          Ringworm NOS

● **111   Dermatomycosis, other and unspecified**
  111.0   Pityriasis versicolor
          Infection by Malassezia [Pityrosporum] furfur
          Tinea flava
          Tinea versicolor

  111.1   Tinea nigra
          Infection by Cladosporium species
          Keratomycosis nigricans
          Microsporosis nigra
          Pityriasis nigra
          Tinea palmaris nigra

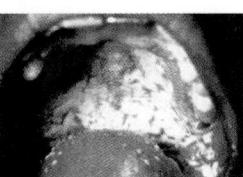

Figure 1-8   Oral candidiasis
(thrush). *(Courtesy of Stephen
Raffanti, MD, MPH.)* (From Mandell,
Bennett, & Dolin: Principles and
Practice of Infectious Diseases, 6th
ed. 2005, Churchill Livingstone, An
Imprint of Elsevier)

Item 1-16   Candidiasis, also called oidiomycosis or moniliasis,
is a fungal infection. It most often appears on moist cutaneous
areas of the body but can also be responsible for a variety of
systemic infections such as endocarditis, meningitis, arthritis, and
myositis. Antifungal medications cure most yeast infections.

  111.2   Tinea blanca
          Infection by Trichosporon (beigelii) cutaneum
          White piedra

  111.3   Black piedra
          Infection by Piedraia hortai

  ■**111.8   Other specified dermatomycoses**

  ■**111.9   Dermatomycosis, unspecified**

● **112   Candidiasis**

          Includes infection by Candida species
                      moniliasis

          Excludes *neonatal monilial infection (771.7)*

  112.0   Of mouth
          Thrush (oral)

  112.1   Of vulva and vagina ♀
          Candidal vulvovaginitis
          Monilial vulvovaginitis
          Coding Clinic: 1994, Q1, P21

  ■**112.2   Of other urogenital sites**
          Candidal balanitis
              Male condition only
          Coding Clinic: 2003, Q4, P105-106; 1996, Q4, P33

  112.3   Of skin and nails
          Candidal intertrigo
          Candidal onychia
          Candidal perionyxis [paronychia]

  112.4   Of lung
          Candidal pneumonia
          Coding Clinic: 1998, Q2, P7

  112.5   Disseminated
          Systemic candidiasis
          Coding Clinic: 1989, Q2, P10

● **112.8   Of other specified sites**
      112.81   Candidal endocarditis
      112.82   Candidal otitis externa
              Otomycosis in moniliasis
      112.83   Candidal meningitis
      112.84   Candidal esophagitis
      112.85   Candidal enteritis
      112.89   Other
              Coding Clinic: 1992, Q1, P17; 1991, Q3, P20

  ■**112.9   Of unspecified site**
          Coding Clinic: 1996, Q4, P33

INFECTIOUS AND PARASITIC DISEASES (001–139)

●114 **Coccidioidomycosis**

    Includes   infection by Coccidioides (immitis)
                 Posada-Wernicke disease

   114.0 **Primary coccidioidomycosis (pulmonary)**
       Acute pulmonary coccidioidomycosis
       Coccidioidomycotic pneumonitis
       Desert rheumatism
       Pulmonary coccidioidomycosis
       San Joaquin Valley fever

   114.1 **Primary extrapulmonary coccidioidomycosis**
       Chancriform syndrome
       Primary cutaneous coccidioidomycosis

   114.2 **Coccidioidal meningitis**

   ■114.3 **Other forms of progressive coccidioidomycosis**
       Coccidioidal granuloma
       Disseminated coccidioidomycosis

   114.4 **Chronic pulmonary coccidioidomycosis**

   ■114.5 **Pulmonary coccidioidomycosis, unspecified**

   ■114.9 **Coccidioidomycosis, unspecified**

Item 1-17 Bird and bat droppings that fall into the soil give rise to a fungus that can spread airborne spores. When inhaled into the lungs, these spores divide and multiply into lesions. Histoplasmosis capsulatum takes three forms: primary (lodged in the lungs only), chronic (resembles TB), and disseminated (infection has moved to other organs). This is an opportunistic infection in immunosuppressed patients.

●115 **Histoplasmosis**
The following fifth-digit subclassification is for use with category 115:

    0 **without mention of manifestation**
    1 **meningitis**
    2 **retinitis**
    3 **pericarditis**
    4 **endocarditis**
    5 **pneumonia**
  ■9 **other**

 ●115.0 **Infection by Histoplasma capsulatum**
[0-5,9]   American histoplasmosis
        Darling's disease
        Reticuloendothelial cytomycosis
        Small form histoplasmosis

 ●115.1 **Infection by Histoplasma duboisii**
[0-5,9]   African histoplasmosis
        Large form histoplasmosis

 ●■115.9 **Histoplasmosis, unspecified**
[0-5,9]   Histoplasmosis NOS

●116 **Blastomycotic infection**
Rare and potentially fatal infections caused by fungus B. dermatitidis inhaled and found in moist soil in temperate climates.

   116.0 **Blastomycosis**
       Blastomycotic dermatitis
       Chicago disease
       Cutaneous blastomycosis
       Disseminated blastomycosis
       Gilchrist's disease
       Infection by Blastomyces [Ajellomyces] dermatitidis
       North American blastomycosis
       Primary pulmonary blastomycosis

   116.1 **Paracoccidioidomycosis**
       Brazilian blastomycosis
       Infection by Paracoccidioides [Blastomyces] brasiliensis
       Lutz-Splendore-Almeida disease
       Mucocutaneous-lymphangitic paracoccidioidomycosis
       Pulmonary paracoccidioidomycosis
       South American blastomycosis
       Visceral paracoccidioidomycosis

   116.2 **Lobomycosis**
       Infections by Loboa [Blastomyces] loboi
       Keloidal blastomycosis
       Lobo's disease

●117 **Other mycoses**

   117.0 **Rhinosporidiosis**
       Infection by Rhinosporidium seeberi

   117.1 **Sporotrichosis**
       Cutaneous sporotrichosis
       Disseminated sporotrichosis
       Infection by Sporothrix [Sporotrichum] schenckii
       Lymphocutaneous sporotrichosis
       Pulmonary sporotrichosis
       Sporotrichosis of the bones

   117.2 **Chromoblastomycosis**
       Chromomycosis
       Infection by Cladosporidium carrionii, Fonsecaea compactum, Fonsecaea pedrosoi, Phialophora verrucosa

   117.3 **Aspergillosis**
       Infection by Aspergillus species, mainly A. fumigatus, A. flavus group, A. terreus group
       Coding Clinic: 1997, Q4, P40

   117.4 **Mycotic mycetomas**
       Infection by various genera and species of Ascomycetes and Deuteromycetes, such as Acremonium [Cephalosporium] falciforme, Neotestudina rosatii, Madurella grisea, Madurella mycetomii, Pyrenochaeta romeroi, Zopfia [Leptosphaeria] senegalensis
       Madura foot, mycotic
       Maduromycosis, mycotic

       Excludes *actinomycotic mycetomas (039.0–039.9)*

   117.5 **Cryptococcosis**
       Busse-Buschke's disease
       European cryptococcosis
       Infection by Cryptococcus neoformans
       Pulmonary cryptococcosis
       Systemic cryptococcosis
       Torula

   117.6 **Allescheriosis [Petriellidosis]**
       Infections by Allescheria [Petriellidium] boydii [Monosporium apiospermum]

       Excludes *mycotic mycetoma (117.4)*

   117.7 **Zygomycosis [Phycomycosis or Mucormycosis]**
       Infection by species of Absidia, Basidiobolus, Conidiobolus, Cunninghamella, Entomophthora, Mucor, Rhizopus, Saksenaea

   117.8 **Infection by dematiacious fungi [Phaehyphomycosis]**
       Infection by dematiacious fungi, such as Cladosporium trichoides [bantianum], Dreschlera hawaiiensis, Phialophora gougerotii, Phialophora jeanselmi

   ■117.9 **Other and unspecified mycoses**
       Coding Clinic: 1995, Q2, P7

INFECTIOUS AND PARASITIC DISEASES (001–139)

118   Opportunistic mycoses
Infection of skin, subcutaneous tissues, and/or organs by
a wide variety of fungi generally considered to be
pathogenic to compromised hosts only (e.g., infection
by species of Alternaria, Dreschlera, Fusarium)

Use additional code to identify manifestation, such as:
keratitis (370.8)

HELMINTHIASES (120–129)

● **120   Schistosomiasis [bilharziasis]**
Parasitic disease (worm induced) that leads to chronic illness

120.0   Schistosoma haematobium
Vesical schistosomiasis NOS

120.1   Schistosoma mansoni
Intestinal schistosomiasis NOS

120.2   Schistosoma japonicum
Asiatic schistosomiasis NOS
Katayama disease or fever

120.3   Cutaneous
Cercarial dermatitis
Infection by cercariae of Schistosoma
Schistosome dermatitis
Swimmers' itch

■ **120.8   Other specified schistosomiasis**
Infection by Schistosoma:
bovis
intercalatum
mattheii
Infection by Schistosoma spindale
Schistosomiasis chestermani

■ **120.9   Schistosomiasis, unspecified**
Blood flukes NOS   Hemic distomiasis

● **121   Other trematode infections**

121.0   Opisthorchiasis
Infection by:
cat liver fluke
Opisthorchis (felineus) (tenuicollis) (viverrini)

121.1   Clonorchiasis
Biliary cirrhosis due to clonorchiasis
Chinese liver fluke disease
Hepatic distomiasis due to Clonorchis sinensis
Oriental liver fluke disease

121.2   Paragonimiasis
Infection by Paragonimus
Lung fluke disease (oriental)
Pulmonary distomiasis

121.3   Fascioliasis
Infection by Fasciola:
gigantica
hepatica
Liver flukes NOS
Sheep liver fluke infection

121.4   Fasciolopsiasis
Infection by Fasciolopsis (buski)
Intestinal distomiasis

121.5   Metagonimiasis
Infection by Metagonimus yokogawai

121.6   Heterophyiasis
Infection by:
Heterophyes heterophyes
Stellantchasmus falcatus

■ **121.8   Other specified trematode infections**
Infection by:
Dicrocoelium dendriticum
Echinostoma ilocanum
Gastrodiscoides hominis

■ **121.9   Trematode infection, unspecified**
Distomiasis NOS
Fluke disease NOS

● **122   Echinococcosis**
*Also known as hydatid disease; caused by Echinococcus
granulosus, E. multilocularis, and E. vogeli tapeworms;
and is contracted from infected food.*

Includes   echinococciasis
hydatid disease
hydatidosis

122.0   Echinococcus granulosus infection of liver

122.1   Echinococcus granulosus infection of lung

122.2   Echinococcus granulosus infection of thyroid

■ **122.3   Echinococcus granulosus infection, other**

■ **122.4   Echinococcus granulosus infection, unspecified**

122.5   Echinococcus multilocularis infection of liver

■ **122.6   Echinococcus multilocularis infection, other**

■ **122.7   Echinococcus multilocularis infection, unspecified**

■ **122.8   Echinococcosis, unspecified, of liver**

■ **122.9   Echinococcosis, other and unspecified**

● **123   Other cestode infection**

123.0   Taenia solium infection, intestinal form
Pork tapeworm (adult) (infection)

123.1   Cysticercosis
Cysticerciasis
Infection by Cysticercus cellulosae [larval form of
Taenia solium]
Coding Clinic: 1997, Q2, P8

123.2   Taenia saginata infection
Beef tapeworm (infection)
Infection by Taeniarhynchus saginatus

■ **123.3   Taeniasis, unspecified**

123.4   Diphyllobothriasis, intestinal
Diphyllobothrium (adult) (latum) (pacificum)
infection
Fish tapeworm (infection)

123.5   Sparganosis [larval diphyllobothriasis]
Infection by:
Diphyllobothrium larvae
Sparganum (mansoni) (proliferum)
Spirometra larvae

123.6   Hymenolepiasis
Dwarf tapeworm (infection)
Hymenolepis (diminuta) (nana) infection
Rat tapeworm (infection)

■ **123.8   Other specified cestode infection**
Diplogonoporus (grandis) infection
Dipylidium (caninum) infection
Dog tapeworm (infection)

■ **123.9   Cestode infection, unspecified**
Tapeworm (infection) NOS

124   Trichinosis
Trichinella spiralis infection
Trichinellosis
Trichiniasis

● **125 Filarial infection and dracontiasis**

 125.0 Bancroftian filariasis
  Chyluria due to Wuchereria bancrofti
  Elephantiasis due to Wuchereria bancrofti
  Infection due to Wuchereria bancrofti
  Lymphadenitis due to Wuchereria bancrofti
  Lymphangitis due to Wuchereria bancrofti
  Wuchereriasis

 125.1 Malayan filariasis
  Brugia filariasis due to Brugia [Wuchereria] malayi
  Chyluria due to Brugia [Wuchereria] malayi
  Elephantiasis due to Brugia [Wuchereria] malayi
  Infection due to Brugia [Wuchereria] malayi
  Lymphadenitis due to Brugia [Wuchereria] malayi
  Lymphangitis due to Brugia [Wuchereria] malayi

 125.2 Loiasis
  Eyeworm disease of Africa
  Loa loa infection

 125.3 Onchocerciasis
  Onchocerca volvulus infection
  Onchocercosis

 125.4 Dipetalonemiasis
  Infection by:
   Acanthocheilonema perstans
   Dipetalonema perstans

 125.5 Mansonella ozzardi infection
  Filariasis ozzardi

 ■**125.6 Other specified filariasis**
  Dirofilaria infection
  Infection by:
   Acanthocheilonema streptocerca
   Dipetalonema streptocerca

 125.7 Dracontiasis
  Guinea-worm infection
  Infection by Dracunculus medinensis

 ■**125.9 Unspecified filariasis**

● **126 Ancylostomiasis and necatoriasis**

 Includes cutaneous larva migrans due to Ancylostoma
  hookworm (disease) (infection)
  uncinariasis

 126.0 Ancylostoma duodenale
 126.1 Necator americanus
 126.2 Ancylostoma braziliense
 126.3 Ancylostoma ceylanicum
 ■**126.8 Other specified Ancylostoma**
 ■**126.9 Ancylostomiasis and necatoriasis, unspecified**
  Creeping eruption NOS
  Cutaneous larva migrans NOS

● **127 Other intestinal helminthiases**

 127.0 Ascariasis
  Ascaridiasis
  Infection by Ascaris lumbricoides
  Roundworm infection

 127.1 Anisakiasis
  Infection by Anisakis larva

 127.2 Strongyloidiasis
  Infection by Strongyloides stercoralis
  Excludes *trichostrongyliasis (127.6)*

 127.3 Trichuriasis
  Infection by Trichuris trichiuria
  Trichocephaliasis
  Whipworm (disease) (infection)

 127.4 Enterobiasis
  Infection by Enterobius vermicularis
  Oxyuriasis
  Oxyuris vermicularis infection
  Pinworm (disease) (infection)
  Threadworm infection

 127.5 Capillariasis
  Infection by Capillaria philippinensis
  Excludes *infection by Capillaria hepatica (128.8)*

 127.6 Trichostrongyliasis
  Infection by Trichostrongylus species

 ■**127.7 Other specified intestinal helminthiasis**
  Infection by:
   Oesophagostomum apiostomum and related
    species
   Ternidens diminutus
   other specified intestinal helminth
  Physalopteriasis

 127.8 Mixed intestinal helminthiasis
  Infection by intestinal helminths classified to more
   than one of the categories 120.0–127.7
  Mixed helminthiasis NOS

 ■**127.9 Intestinal helminthiasis, unspecified**

● **128 Other and unspecified helminthiases**

 128.0 Toxocariasis
  Larva migrans visceralis
  Toxocara (canis) (cati) infection
  Visceral larva migrans syndrome

 128.1 Gnathostomiasis
  Infection by Gnathostoma spinigerum and related
   species

 ■**128.8 Other specified helminthiasis**
  Infection by:
   Angiostrongylus cantonensis
   Capillaria hepatica
   other specified helminth

 ■**128.9 Helminth infection, unspecified**
  Helminthiasis NOS
  Worms NOS

● ■**129 Intestinal parasitism, unspecified**

◄ New ◄▥ Revised ~~deleted~~ Deleted ● Use Additional Digit(s) ■ Nonspecific Code
● Not first-listed DX OGCR Official Guidelines Coding Clinic Excludes Includes Use additional Code first Omit code

Item 1-18 Toxoplasmosis is caused by the protozoa **Toxoplasma gondii,** of which the house cat can be a host. Human infection occurs when contact is made with materials containing the pathogen, such as feces, contaminated soil, or ingestion of infected lamb, goat, or pork. Of the infected, very few have symptoms because a healthy person's immune system keeps the parasite from causing illness. When the immune system is compromised, symptoms may occur. Clinical symptoms include flu-like symptoms, but the disease progresses to include the eyes and the brain in babies.

OTHER INFECTIOUS AND PARASITIC DISEASES (130–136)

● 130 **Toxoplasmosis**

  Includes infection by toxoplasma gondii
              toxoplasmosis (acquired)

  Excludes *congenital toxoplasmosis (771.2)*

  130.0 **Meningoencephalitis due to toxoplasmosis**
        Encephalitis due to acquired toxoplasmosis

  130.1 **Conjunctivitis due to toxoplasmosis**

  130.2 **Chorioretinitis due to toxoplasmosis**
        Focal retinochoroiditis due to acquired toxoplasmosis

  130.3 **Myocarditis due to toxoplasmosis**

  130.4 **Pneumonitis due to toxoplasmosis**

  130.5 **Hepatitis due to toxoplasmosis**

  ■130.7 **Toxoplasmosis of other specified sites**

  130.8 **Multisystemic disseminated toxoplasmosis**
        Toxoplasmosis of multiple sites

  ■130.9 **Toxoplasmosis, unspecified**

● 131 **Trichomoniasis**
      *A common STD caused by a parasite, Trichomonas vaginalis,
      affecting both women and men.*

  Includes infection due to Trichomonas (vaginalis)

● 131.0 **Urogenital trichomoniasis**

  ■131.00 **Urogenital trichomoniasis, unspecified**
         Fluor (vaginalis) trichomonal or due to
           Trichomonas (vaginalis)
         Leukorrhea (vaginalis) trichomonal or due
           to Trichomonas (vaginalis)

  131.01 **Trichomonal vulvovaginitis** ♀
         Vaginitis, trichomonal or due to
           Trichomonas (vaginalis)

  131.02 **Trichomonal urethritis**

  131.03 **Trichomonal prostatitis** ♂

  ■131.09 **Other**

  ■131.8 **Other specified sites**

    Excludes *intestinal (007.3)*

  ■131.9 **Trichomoniasis, unspecified**

● 132 **Pediculosis and phthirus infestation**
      *Infestation of lice, Pediculus humanus, specifically capitis
      infest the head, corporis infest the body-trunk area, and
      pubis infest the pubic region.*

  132.0 **Pediculus capitis [head louse]**

  132.1 **Pediculus corporis [body louse]**

  132.2 **Phthirus pubis [pubic louse]**
        Pediculus pubis

  132.3 **Mixed infestation**
        This is a combination code.
        Infestation classifiable to more than one of the
          categories 132.0–132.2

  ■132.9 **Pediculosis, unspecified**

● 133 **Acariasis**

  133.0 **Scabies**
        Infestation by Sarcoptes scabiei
        Norwegian scabies
        Sarcoptic itch

  ■133.8 **Other acariasis**
        Chiggers
        Infestation by:
          Demodex folliculorum
          Trombicula

  ■133.9 **Acariasis, unspecified**
        Infestation by mites NOS

● 134 **Other infestation**

  134.0 **Myiasis**
        Infestation by:
          Dermatobia (hominis)
          fly larvae
          Gasterophilus (intestinalis)
          maggots
          Oestrus ovis

  ■134.1 **Other arthropod infestation**
        Infestation by:
          chigoe
          Jigger disease
          sand flea
          Scarabiasis
          Tunga penetrans
          Tungiasis

  134.2 **Hirudiniasis**
        Hirudiniasis (external) (internal)
        Leeches (aquatic) (land)

  ■134.8 **Other specified infestations**

  ■134.9 **Infestation, unspecified**
        Infestation (skin) NOS
        Skin parasites NOS

135 **Sarcoidosis**
      *Symptom of an inflammation producing tiny lumps of cells
      (granulomas) in various organs, most commonly the
      lungs and lymph nodes, that affect organ function.*
      Besnier-Boeck-Schaumann disease
      Lupoid (miliary) of Boeck
      Lupus pernio (Besnier)
      Lymphogranulomatosis, benign (Schaumann's)
      Sarcoid (any site):
        NOS
        Boeck
        Darier-Roussy
      Uveoparotid fever

● 136 **Other and unspecified infectious and parasitic diseases**

  136.0 **Ainhum**
        Dactylolysis spontanea

  136.1 **Behçet's syndrome**

● 136.2 **Specific infections by free-living amebae**

  136.21 **Specific infection due to acanthamoeba**
         Use additional code to identify
           manifestation, such as:
           keratitis (370.8)
         Coding Clinic: 2008, Q4, P79-81

  ■136.29 **Other specific infections by free-living
          amebae**
         Meningoencephalitis due to Naegleria
         Coding Clinic: 2008, Q4, P79-81

  136.3 **Pneumocystosis**
        Pneumonia due to Pneumocystis carinii
        Pneumonia due to Pneumocystis jiroveci
        Coding Clinic: 2003, Q1, P15; 1987, Nov-Dec, P5-6

INFECTIOUS AND PARASITIC DISEASES (001–139)

136.4 Psorospermiasis

136.5 Sarcosporidiosis
Infection by Sarcocystis lindemanni

◼ **136.8 Other specified infectious and parasitic diseases**
Candiru infestation

◼ **136.9 Unspecified infectious and parasitic diseases**
Infectious disease NOS
Parasitic disease NOS
Coding Clinic: 1991, Q2, P8

LATE EFFECTS OF INFECTIOUS AND PARASITIC DISEASES (137–139)

Item 1–19 Before you use the late code 137.X, check your documentation. The original problem (tuberculosis, TB) that is causing the current late effect (necrosis) must have been attributable to categories 010–018. A patient who originally had TB of a joint (015.2X) now has a late effect (137.3), which is necrosis of bone (730.8). Because there is no active TB, 015.2X is not coded but serves as an authorization to use the late effect code. Remember to code the manifestation of the late effect, which is the current problem (necrosis).

● **137 Late effects of tuberculosis**
Note: This category is to be used to indicate conditions classifiable to 010–018 as the cause of late effects, which are themselves classified elsewhere. The "late effects" include those specified as such, as sequelae, or as due to old or inactive tuberculosis, without evidence of active disease.

◼ **137.0 Late effects of respiratory or unspecified tuberculosis**

◼ **137.1 Late effects of central nervous system tuberculosis**

◼ **137.2 Late effects of genitourinary tuberculosis**

◼ **137.3 Late effects of tuberculosis of bones and joints**

◼ **137.4 Late effects of tuberculosis of other specified organs**

138 Late effects of acute poliomyelitis
Note: This category is to be used to indicate conditions classifiable to 045 as the cause of late effects, which are themselves classified elsewhere. The "late effects" include conditions specified as such, or as sequelae, or as due to old or inactive poliomyelitis, without evidence of active disease.

● ◼ **139 Late effects of other infectious and parasitic diseases**
Note: This category is to be used to indicate conditions classifiable to categories 001–009, 020–041, 046–136 as the cause of late effects, which are themselves classified elsewhere. The "late effects" include conditions specified as such; they also include sequela of diseases classifiable to the above categories if there is evidence that the disease itself is no longer present.

139.0 Late effects of viral encephalitis
Late effects of conditions classifiable to 049.8–049.9, 062–064

◼ **139.1 Late effects of trachoma**
Late effects of conditions classifiable to 076

◼ **139.8 Late effects of other and unspecified infectious and parasitic diseases**
Coding Clinic: 2006, Q2, P17-18; 1990, Q3, P14

◀ New   ◀▥ Revised   ~~deleted~~ Deleted   ● Use Additional Digit(s)   ◼ Nonspecific Code
● Not first-listed DX   OGCR Official Guidelines   Coding Clinic   Excludes   Includes   Use additional   Code first   Omit code

Item 2-1 Neoplasm: Neo = new, plasm = growth, development, formation. This new growth (mass, tumor) can be malignant or benign, which is confirmed by the pathology report. Do not assign a code to a neoplasm until you review the pathology report. Certain CPT codes will specify benign or malignant lesion, so be certain the diagnosis code supports the procedure code.

2. NEOPLASMS (140–239)

1. Content:
This chapter contains the following broad groups:
140–195 Malignant neoplasms, stated or presumed to be primary, of specified sites, except of lymphatic and hematopoietic tissue
196–198 Malignant neoplasms, stated or presumed to be secondary, of specified sites
199   Malignant neoplasms, without specification of site
200–208 Malignant neoplasms, stated or presumed to be primary, of lymphatic and hematopoietic tissue
209   Neuroendocrine tumors
210–229 Benign neoplasms
230–234 Carcinoma in situ
235–238 Neoplasms of uncertain behavior [see Note, at beginning of section 235–238]
239   Neoplasms of unspecified nature

2. Functional activity
All neoplasms are classified in this chapter, whether or not functionally active. An additional code from Chapter 3 may be used to identify such functional activity associated with any neoplasm, e.g.:
catecholamine-producing malignant pheochromocytoma of adrenal:
code 194.0, additional code 255.6
basophil adenoma of pituitary with Cushing's syndrome:
code 227.3, additional code 255.0

3. Morphology [Histology]
For those wishing to identify the histological type of neoplasms, a comprehensive coded nomenclature, which comprises the morphology rubrics of the ICD-Oncology, is given after the E-code chapter.

4. Malignant neoplasms overlapping site boundaries
Categories 140–195 are for the classification of primary malignant neoplasms according to their point of origin. A malignant neoplasm that overlaps two or more subcategories within a three-digit rubric and whose point of origin cannot be determined should be classified to the subcategory .8 "Other." For example, "carcinoma involving tip and ventral surface of tongue" should be assigned to 141.8. On the other hand, "carcinoma of tip of tongue, extending to involve the ventral surface" should be coded to 141.2, as the point of origin, the tip, is known. Three subcategories (149.8, 159.8, 165.8) have been provided for malignant neoplasms that overlap the boundaries of three-digit rubrics within certain systems. Overlapping malignant neoplasms that cannot be classified as indicated above should be assigned to the appropriate subdivision of category 195 (Malignant neoplasm of other and ill-defined sites).

MALIGNANT NEOPLASM OF LIP, ORAL CAVITY, AND PHARYNX (140–149)

> **Excludes**   carcinoma in situ (230.0)

● **140   Malignant neoplasm of lip**
Malignant neoplasm is a general term used to describe a cancerous growth or tumor.

> **Excludes**   skin of lip (173.0)

140.0 Upper lip, vermilion border
Upper lip: Upper lip:
NOS   lipstick area
external

140.1 Lower lip, vermilion border
Lower lip: Lower lip:
NOS   lipstick area
external

140.3 Upper lip, inner aspect
Upper lip: Upper lip:
buccal aspect   mucosa
frenulum   oral aspect

140.4 Lower lip, inner aspect
Lower lip: Lower lip:
buccal aspect   mucosa
frenulum   oral aspect

■**140.5 Lip, unspecified, inner aspect**
Lip, not specified whether upper or lower:
buccal aspect
frenulum
mucosa
oral aspect

140.6 Commissure of lip
Labial commissure

■**140.8 Other sites of lip**
Malignant neoplasm of contiguous or overlapping sites of lip whose point of origin cannot be determined

■**140.9 Lip, unspecified, vermilion border**
Lip, not specified as upper or lower:
NOS
external
lipstick area

● **141   Malignant neoplasm of tongue**

141.0 Base of tongue
Dorsal surface of base of tongue
Fixed part of tongue NOS
Coding Clinic: 2006, Q4, P88-91

141.1 Dorsal surface of tongue
Anterior two-thirds of tongue, dorsal surface
Dorsal tongue NOS
Midline of tongue

> **Excludes**   dorsal surface of base of tongue (141.0)

141.2 Tip and lateral border of tongue

Figure 2-1 Anatomical structures of the mouth and lips. **A.** Transitional or vermilion borders. Lips are connected to the gums by frenulum. **B.** Dorsal surface. **C.** Ventral surface.

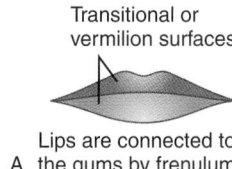

Transitional or vermilion surfaces

Lips are connected to
A the gums by frenulum

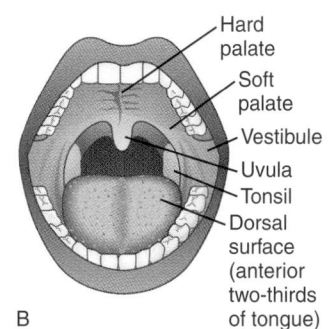

Hard palate
Soft palate
Vestibule
Uvula
Tonsil
Dorsal surface (anterior two-thirds of tongue)
B

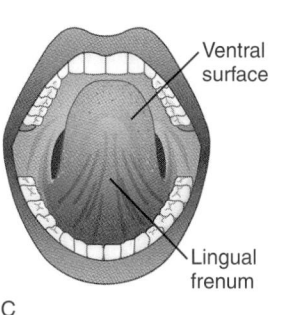

Ventral surface
Lingual frenum
C

NEOPLASMS (140–239)

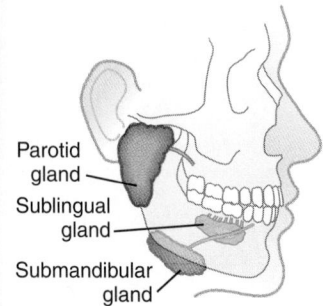

Figure 2-2 Major salivary glands.

Parotid gland

Sublingual gland

Submandibular gland

141.3 Ventral surface of tongue
Anterior two-thirds of tongue, ventral surface
Frenulum linguae

■**141.4 Anterior two-thirds of tongue, part unspecified**
Mobile part of tongue NOS

141.5 Junctional zone
Border of tongue at junction of fixed and mobile
parts at insertion of anterior tonsillar pillar

141.6 Lingual tonsil

■**141.8 Other sites of tongue**
Malignant neoplasm of contiguous or overlapping
sites of tongue whose point of origin cannot
be determined

■**141.9 Tongue, unspecified**
Tongue NOS

●**142 Malignant neoplasm of major salivary glands**

Includes salivary ducts

Excludes *malignant neoplasm of minor salivary glands:*
NOS (145.9)
buccal mucosa (145.0)
soft palate (145.3)
tongue (141.0–141.9)
tonsil, palatine (146.0)

142.0 Parotid gland

142.1 Submandibular gland
Submaxillary gland

142.2 Sublingual gland

■**142.8 Other major salivary glands**
Malignant neoplasm of contiguous or overlapping
sites of salivary glands and ducts whose point
of origin cannot be determined

■**142.9 Salivary gland, unspecified**
Salivary gland (major) NOS

●**143 Malignant neoplasm of gum**

Includes alveolar (ridge) mucosa
gingiva (alveolar) (marginal)
interdental papillae

Excludes *malignant odontogenic neoplasms (170.0–170.1)*

143.0 Upper gum

143.1 Lower gum

■**143.8 Other sites of gum**
Malignant neoplasm of contiguous or overlapping
sites of gum whose point of origin cannot be
determined

■**143.9 Gum, unspecified**

●**144 Malignant neoplasm of floor of mouth**

144.0 Anterior portion
Anterior to the premolar-canine junction

144.1 Lateral portion

■**144.8 Other sites of floor of mouth**
Malignant neoplasm of contiguous or overlapping
sites of floor of mouth whose point of origin
cannot be determined

■**144.9 Floor of mouth, part unspecified**

●**145 Malignant neoplasm of other and unspecified parts of mouth**

Excludes *mucosa of lips (140.0–140.9)*

145.0 Cheek mucosa
Buccal mucosa
Cheek, inner aspect

145.1 Vestibule of mouth
Buccal sulcus (upper) (lower)
Labial sulcus (upper) (lower)

145.2 Hard palate

145.3 Soft palate

Excludes *nasopharyngeal [posterior] [superior]*
surface of soft palate (147.3)
Coding Clinic: 1993, 5th Issue, P16

145.4 Uvula

■**145.5 Palate, unspecified**
Junction of hard and soft palate
Roof of mouth

145.6 Retromolar area

■**145.8 Other specified parts of mouth**
Malignant neoplasm of contiguous or overlapping
sites of mouth whose point of origin cannot
be determined

■**145.9 Mouth, unspecified**
Buccal cavity NOS
Minor salivary gland, unspecified site
Oral cavity NOS

●**146 Malignant neoplasm of oropharynx**

146.0 Tonsil
Tonsil: Tonsil:
NOS   palatine
faucial

Excludes *lingual tonsil (141.6)*
pharyngeal tonsil (147.1)
Coding Clinic: 1987, Sept-Oct, P8

146.1 Tonsillar fossa

146.2 Tonsillar pillars (anterior) (posterior)
Faucial pillar
Glossopalatine fold
Palatoglossal arch
Palatopharyngeal arch

146.3 Vallecula
Anterior and medial surface of the
pharyngoepiglottic fold

146.4 Anterior aspect of epiglottis
Epiglottis, free border [margin]
Glossoepiglottic fold(s)

Excludes *epiglottis:*
NOS (161.1)
suprahyoid portion (161.1)

◀ New ◀️ Revised ~~deleted~~ Deleted ● Use Additional Digit(s) ■ Nonspecific Code
● Not first-listed DX OGCR Official Guidelines Coding Clinic Excludes Includes Use additional Code first Omit code

146.5 Junctional region
Junction of the free margin of the epiglottis, the aryepiglottic fold, and the pharyngoepiglottic fold

146.6 Lateral wall of oropharynx

146.7 Posterior wall of oropharynx

146.8 Other specified sites of oropharynx
Branchial cleft
Malignant neoplasm of contiguous or overlapping sites of oropharynx whose point of origin cannot be determined

146.9 Oropharynx, unspecified
Coding Clinic: 2002, Q2, P6

● **147 Malignant neoplasm of nasopharynx**

147.0 Superior wall
Roof of nasopharynx

147.1 Posterior wall
Adenoid   Pharyngeal tonsil

147.2 Lateral wall
Fossa of Rosenmüller   Pharyngeal recess
Opening of auditory tube

147.3 Anterior wall
Floor of nasopharynx
Nasopharyngeal [posterior] [superior] surface of soft palate
Posterior margin of nasal septum and choanae

147.8 Other specified sites of nasopharynx
Malignant neoplasm of contiguous or overlapping sites of nasopharynx whose point of origin cannot be determined

147.9 Nasopharynx, unspecified
Nasopharyngeal wall NOS

● **148 Malignant neoplasm of hypopharynx**

148.0 Postcricoid region
Behind the cricoid cartilage of neck

148.1 Pyriform sinus
Pyriform fossa

148.2 Aryepiglottic fold, hypopharyngeal aspect
Aryepiglottic fold or interarytenoid fold:
  NOS
  marginal zone

Excludes *aryepiglottic fold or interarytenoid fold, laryngeal aspect (161.1)*

148.3 Posterior hypopharyngeal wall

148.8 Other specified sites of hypopharynx
Malignant neoplasm of contiguous or overlapping sites of hypopharynx whose point of origin cannot be determined

148.9 Hypopharynx, unspecified
Hypopharyngeal wall NOS
Hypopharynx NOS

● **149 Malignant neoplasm of other and ill-defined sites within the lip, oral cavity, and pharynx**

149.0 Pharynx, unspecified

149.1 Waldeyer's ring

149.8 Other
Malignant neoplasms of lip, oral cavity, and pharynx whose point of origin cannot be assigned to any one of the categories 140–148

Excludes *"book leaf" neoplasm [ventral surface of tongue and floor of mouth] (145.8)*

149.9 Ill-defined

MALIGNANT NEOPLASM OF DIGESTIVE ORGANS AND PERITONEUM (150–159)

Excludes *carcinoma in situ (230.1–230.9)*

● **150 Malignant neoplasm of esophagus**

150.0 Cervical esophagus

150.1 Thoracic esophagus

150.2 Abdominal esophagus

Excludes *adenocarcinoma (151.0)*
cardio-esophageal junction (151.0)

150.3 Upper third of esophagus
Proximal third of esophagus

150.4 Middle third of esophagus

150.5 Lower third of esophagus
Distal third of esophagus

Excludes *adenocarcinoma (151.0)*
cardio-esophageal junction (151.0)

150.8 Other specified part
Malignant neoplasm of contiguous or overlapping sites of esophagus whose point of origin cannot be determined

150.9 Esophagus, unspecified

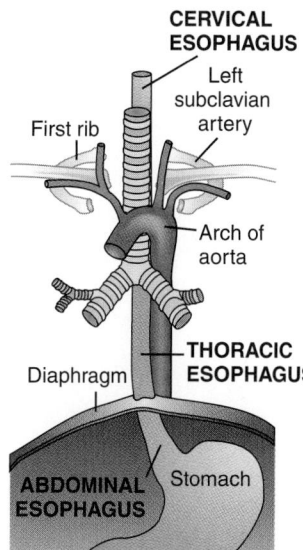

Figure 2–3 The esophagus is the muscular tube that connects the pharynx and the stomach. The 10 inch (25 cm) long esophagus is divided into three parts: **cervical, thoracic,** and **abdominal.**

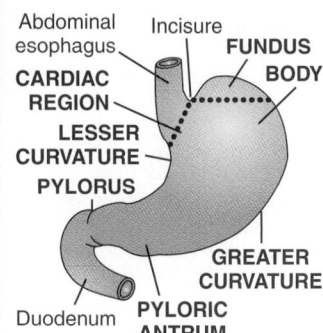

Abdominal esophagus | Incisure
CARDIAC REGION — FUNDUS BODY
LESSER CURVATURE
PYLORUS
Duodenum | PYLORIC ANTRUM | GREATER CURVATURE

Figure 2–4 Parts of the stomach.

Item 2–2 The esophagus opens into the stomach through the **cardiac orifice,** also called the **cardioesophageal junction.** The **cardia** is adjacent to the cardiac orifice. The stomach widens into the **greater** and **lesser curvatures.** The **pyloric antrum** precedes the **pylorus,** which opens to the duodenum.

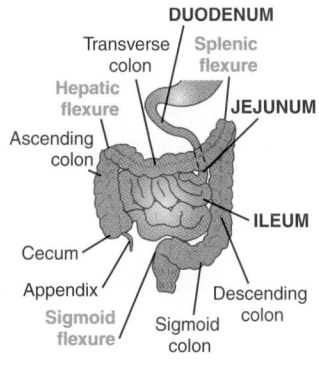

DUODENUM
Transverse colon | Splenic flexure
Hepatic flexure | JEJUNUM
Ascending colon
Cecum | ILEUM
Appendix | Descending colon
Sigmoid flexure | Sigmoid colon

Figure 2–5 Small intestine and colon.

● 151 Malignant neoplasm of stomach

> **Excludes** *benign carcinoid tumor of stomach (209.63)*
> *malignant carcinoid tumor of stomach (209.23)*

151.0 Cardia
   Cardiac orifice
   Cardio-esophageal junction
   Excludes *squamous cell carcinoma (150.2, 150.5)*

151.1 Pylorus
   Prepylorus
   Pyloric canal

151.2 Pyloric antrum
   Antrum of stomach NOS

151.3 Fundus of stomach

151.4 Body of stomach

■151.5 Lesser curvature, unspecified
   Lesser curvature, not classifiable to 151.1–151.4

■151.6 Greater curvature, unspecified
   Greater curvature, not classifiable to 151.0–151.4

■151.8 Other specified sites of stomach
   Anterior wall, not classifiable to 151.0–151.4
   Posterior wall, not classifiable to 151.0–151.4
   Malignant neoplasm of contiguous or overlapping sites of stomach whose point of origin cannot be determined

■151.9 Stomach, unspecified
   Carcinoma ventriculi
   Gastric cancer
   Coding Clinic: 2001, Q2, P17-18; 1988, Q2, P11

● 152 Malignant neoplasm of small intestine, including duodenum

> **Excludes** *benign carcinoid tumor of small intestine and duodenum (209.40-209.43)*
> *malignant carcinoid tumor of small intestine and duodenum (209.00-209.03)*

152.0 Duodenum

152.1 Jejunum

152.2 Ileum
   Excludes *ileocecal valve (153.4)*

152.3 Meckel's diverticulum

■152.8 Other specified sites of small intestine
   Duodenojejunal junction
   Malignant neoplasm of contiguous or overlapping sites of small intestine whose point of origin cannot be determined

■152.9 Small intestine, unspecified

● 153 Malignant neoplasm of colon

> **Excludes** *benign carcinoid tumor of colon (209.50-209.56)*
> *malignant carcinoid tumor of colon (209.10-209.16)*

153.0 Hepatic flexure
   Flexure is a bending in a structure or organ. Note the three flexures illustrated in Figure 2–5. Hepatic = liver, sigmoid = colon, splenic = spleen.

153.1 Transverse colon

153.2 Descending colon
   Left colon
   Coding Clinic: 1995, Q1, P4

153.3 Sigmoid colon
   Sigmoid (flexure)
   Excludes *rectosigmoid junction (154.0)*
   Flexure is a bending in a structure or organ. Note the three flexures illustrated in Figure 2–5. Hepatic = liver, sigmoid = colon, splenic = spleen.

153.4 Cecum
   Ileocecal valve

153.5 Appendix

153.6 Ascending colon
   Right colon

153.7 Splenic flexure
   Flexure is a bending in a structure or organ. Note the three flexures illustrated in Figure 2–5. Hepatic = liver, sigmoid = colon, splenic = spleen.

■153.8 Other specified sites of large intestine
   Malignant neoplasm of contiguous or overlapping sites of colon whose point of origin cannot be determined
   Excludes *ileocecal valve (153.4)*
   rectosigmoid junction (154.0)

■153.9 Colon, unspecified
   Large intestine NOS

● 154 Malignant neoplasm of rectum, rectosigmoid junction, and anus

> **Excludes** *benign carcinoid tumor of rectum (209.57)*
> *malignant carcinoid tumor of rectum (209.17)*

154.0 Rectosigmoid junction
   Colon with rectum
   Rectosigmoid (colon)

154.1 Rectum
   Rectal ampulla

◀ New   ◀▥ Revised   ~~deleted~~ Deleted   ● Use Additional Digit(s)   ■ Nonspecific Code
● Not first-listed DX   OGCR Official Guidelines   Coding Clinic   Excludes   Includes   Use additional   Code first   Omit code

154.2 Anal canal
Anal sphincter

> **Excludes** *skin of anus (172.5, 173.5)*

Coding Clinic: 2001, Q1, P8

■154.3 Anus, unspecified

> **Excludes** *anus:*
> *margin (172.5, 173.5)*
> *skin (172.5, 173.5)*
> *perianal skin (172.5, 173.5)*

■154.8 Other
Anorectum
Cloacogenic zone
Malignant neoplasm of contiguous or overlapping
    sites of rectum, rectosigmoid junction,
    and anus whose point of origin cannot be
    determined

●155 Malignant neoplasm of liver and intrahepatic bile ducts

155.0 Liver, primary
Carcinoma:
    liver, specified as primary
    hepatocellular
    liver cell
Hepatoblastoma

Coding Clinic: 2008, Q4, P82-83

155.1 Intrahepatic bile ducts
Canaliculi biliferi
Interlobular:
    bile ducts
    biliary canals
Intrahepatic:
    biliary passages
    canaliculi
    gall duct

> **Excludes** *hepatic duct (156.1)*

■155.2 Liver, not specified as primary or secondary
Stated as a liver neoplasm, but not specific as to type

●156 Malignant neoplasm of gallbladder and extrahepatic bile ducts
Extrahepatic = outside the liver

156.0 Gallbladder

156.1 Extrahepatic bile ducts
Biliary duct or passage
NOS
Common bile duct
Cystic duct
Hepatic duct
Sphincter of Oddi

156.2 Ampulla of Vater

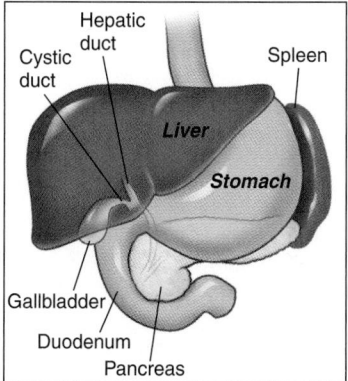

Figure 2–6 Diagram of liver, gallbladder, hepatic duct, pancreas, and spleen. (From Thibodeau and Patton: Anatomy and Physiology, 6th ed. 2007, Mosby)

■156.8 Other specified sites of gallbladder and extrahepatic bile ducts
Malignant neoplasm of contiguous or overlapping
    sites of gallbladder and extrahepatic bile
    ducts whose point of origin cannot be
    determined

■156.9 Biliary tract, part unspecified
Malignant neoplasm involving both intrahepatic
    and extrahepatic bile ducts
Intra = inside; extra = outside

●157 Malignant neoplasm of pancreas
Check documentation for specific site.

157.0 Head of pancreas
Coding Clinic: 2005, Q2, P9-10; 2000, Q4, P39-40

157.1 Body of pancreas

157.2 Tail of pancreas

157.3 Pancreatic duct
Duct of:
    Santorini
    Wirsung

> **Item 2–3** Islets of Langerhans (endocrine producing
> cells comprising 1% to 2% of the pancreatic mass) make
> and secrete hormones that regulate the body's production
> of insulin, glucagon, and stomach acid. Breakdown of the
> insulin-producing cells can cause diabetes mellitus.
> Islet cell tumors can be benign or malignant and
> include glucagonomas, insulinomas, gastrinomas, and
> neuroendocrine tumor. The neoplasm table must be
> consulted for the correct neoplasm code.

157.4 Islets of Langerhans
Islets of Langerhans, any part of pancreas

> Use additional code to identify any functional
>   activity

Coding Clinic: 2007, Q4, P70-72

■157.8 Other specified sites of pancreas
Ectopic pancreatic tissue
Malignant neoplasm of contiguous or overlapping
    sites of pancreas whose point of origin cannot
    be determined

■157.9 Pancreas, part unspecified
Coding Clinic: 1989, Q4, P11

●158 Malignant neoplasm of retroperitoneum and peritoneum

158.0 Retroperitoneum
Periadrenal tissue
Perinephric tissue
Perirenal tissue
Retrocecal tissue

■158.8 Specified parts of peritoneum
Cul-de-sac (of Douglas)
Mesentery
Mesocolon
Omentum
Peritoneum:
    parietal
    pelvic
Rectouterine pouch
Malignant neoplasm of contiguous or overlapping
    sites of retroperitoneum and peritoneum
    whose point of origin cannot be determined

■158.9 Peritoneum, unspecified

NEOPLASMS (140–239)

● 159 **Malignant neoplasm of other and ill-defined sites within the digestive organs and peritoneum**

■ **159.0 Intestinal tract, part unspecified**
Intestine NOS

■ **159.1 Spleen, not elsewhere classified**
Angiosarcoma of spleen
Fibrosarcoma of spleen

> Excludes   *Hodgkin's disease (201.0–201.9)*
> *lymphosarcoma (200.1)*
> *reticulosarcoma (200.0)*

■ **159.8 Other sites of digestive system and intra-abdominal organs**
Malignant neoplasm of digestive organs and peritoneum whose point of origin cannot be assigned to any one of the categories 150–158

> Excludes   *anus and rectum (154.8)*
> *cardio-esophageal junction (151.0)*
> *colon and rectum (154.0)*

■ **159.9 Ill-defined**
Alimentary canal or tract NOS
Gastrointestinal tract NOS

> Excludes   *abdominal NOS (195.2)*
> *intra-abdominal NOS (195.2)*

MALIGNANT NEOPLASM OF RESPIRATORY AND INTRATHORACIC ORGANS (160–165)

> Excludes   *carcinoma in situ (231.0–231.9)*

● 160 **Malignant neoplasm of nasal cavities, middle ear, and accessory sinuses**

160.0 Nasal cavities
Cartilage of nose
Conchae, nasal
Internal nose
Septum of nose
Vestibule of nose

> Excludes   *nasal bone (170.0)*
> *nose NOS (195.0)*
> *olfactory bulb (192.0)*
> *posterior margin of septum and choanae (147.3)*
> *skin of nose (172.3, 173.3)*
> *turbinates (170.0)*

160.1 Auditory tube, middle ear, and mastoid air cells
Antrum tympanicum
Eustachian tube
Tympanic cavity

> Excludes   *auditory canal (external) (172.2, 173.2)*
> *bone of ear (meatus) (170.0)*
> *cartilage of ear (171.0)*
> *ear (external) (skin) (172.2, 173.2)*

160.2 Maxillary sinus
Antrum (Highmore) (maxillary)

160.3 Ethmoidal sinus

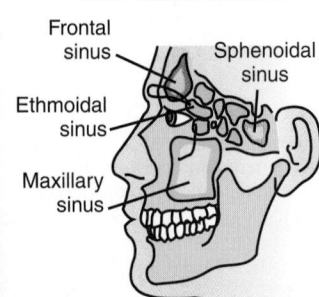

Frontal sinus
Sphenoidal sinus
Ethmoidal sinus
Maxillary sinus

Figure 2–7 Paranasal sinuses. (From Buck CJ: Step-by-Step Medical Coding, 2006 ed. Philadelphia, WB Saunders, 2006.)

160.4 Frontal sinus

160.5 Sphenoidal sinus

■ **160.8 Other**
Malignant neoplasm of contiguous or overlapping sites of nasal cavities, middle ear, and accessory sinuses whose point of origin cannot be determined

■ **160.9 Accessory sinus, unspecified**

● 161 **Malignant neoplasm of larynx**

161.0 Glottis
Intrinsic larynx
Laryngeal commissure (anterior) (posterior)
True vocal cord
> *True vocal cords (lower vocal folds) produce vocalization when air from lungs passes between them. Check your documentation. Code 161.1 is for malignant neoplasm of **false** vocal cords.*
Vocal cord NOS

161.1 Supraglottis
Aryepiglottic fold or interarytenoid fold, laryngeal aspect
Epiglottis (suprahyoid portion) NOS
Extrinsic larynx
False vocal cords
> *False vocal cords (upper vocal folds) are not involved in vocalization. Check your documentation. Code 161.0 is for true vocal cords.*
Posterior (laryngeal) surface of epiglottis
Ventricular bands

> Excludes   *anterior aspect of epiglottis (146.4)*
> *aryepiglottic fold or interarytenoid fold:*
> *NOS (148.2)*
> *hypopharyngeal aspect (148.2)*
> *marginal zone (148.2)*

161.2 Subglottis

161.3 Laryngeal cartilages
Cartilage: Cartilage:
arytenoid   cuneiform
cricoid   thyroid

■ **161.8 Other specified sites of larynx**
Malignant neoplasm of contiguous or overlapping sites of larynx whose point of origin cannot be determined
Coding Clinic: 2007, Q3, P8-9

■ **161.9 Larynx, unspecified**

● 162 **Malignant neoplasm of trachea, bronchus, and lung**

> Excludes   *benign carcinoid tumor of bronchus (209.61)*
> *malignant carcinoid tumor of bronchus (209.21)*

Coding Clinic: 2006, Q3, P7-8

162.0 Trachea
Cartilage of trachea
Mucosa of trachea

162.2 Main bronchus
Carina
Hilus of lung

162.3 Upper lobe, bronchus or lung
Coding Clinic: 2004, Q1, P4-5

162.4 Middle lobe, bronchus or lung

162.5 Lower lobe, bronchus or lung

■ **162.8 Other parts of bronchus or lung**
Malignant neoplasm of contiguous or overlapping sites of bronchus or lung whose point of origin cannot be determined
Coding Clinic: 2006, Q3, P7-8

◀ New   ◀▦ Revised   deleted Deleted   ● Use Additional Digit(s)   ■ Nonspecific Code
● Not first-listed DX   OGCR Official Guidelines   Coding Clinic   Excludes   Includes   Use additional   Code first   Omit code

■162.9 **Bronchus and lung, unspecified**
Coding Clinic: 2006, Q3, P14-15; 1997, Q2, P3; 1996, Q4, P47-48;
1993, Q4, P 36;1988, Q2, P10; 1984, May-June, P11, 14

● 163 **Malignant neoplasm of pleura**
*Pleura are comprised of serous membrane that lines thoracic
cavity (parietal) and covers lungs (visceral).*

163.0 **Parietal pleura**

163.1 **Visceral pleura**

■163.8 **Other specified sites of pleura**
Malignant neoplasm of contiguous or overlapping
sites of pleura whose point of origin cannot
be determined

■163.9 **Pleura, unspecified**

● 164 **Malignant neoplasm of thymus, heart, and mediastinum**

164.0 **Thymus**

Excludes *benign carcinoid tumor of the thymus
(209.62)*
*malignant carcinoid tumor of the thymus
(209.22)*

164.1 **Heart**

Endocardium	Myocardium
Epicardium	Pericardium

Excludes *great vessels (171.4)*

164.2 **Anterior mediastinum**

164.3 **Posterior mediastinum**

■164.8 **Other**
Malignant neoplasm of contiguous or overlapping
sites of thymus, heart, and mediastinum
whose point of origin cannot be determined

■164.9 **Mediastinum, part unspecified**

● 165 **Malignant neoplasm of other and ill-defined sites within
the respiratory system and intrathoracic organs**

■165.0 **Upper respiratory tract, part unspecified**

■165.8 **Other**
Malignant neoplasm of respiratory and
intrathoracic organs whose point of origin
cannot be assigned to any one of the
categories 160–164

■165.9 **Ill-defined sites within the respiratory system**
Respiratory tract NOS

Excludes *intrathoracic NOS (195.1)*
thoracic NOS (195.1)

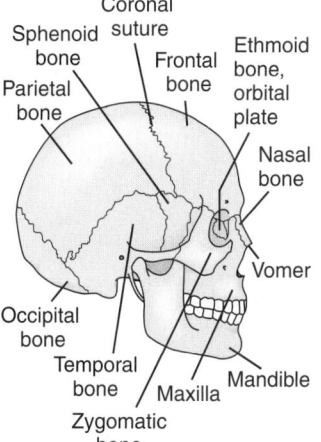

Figure 2–8 Bones of the skull.

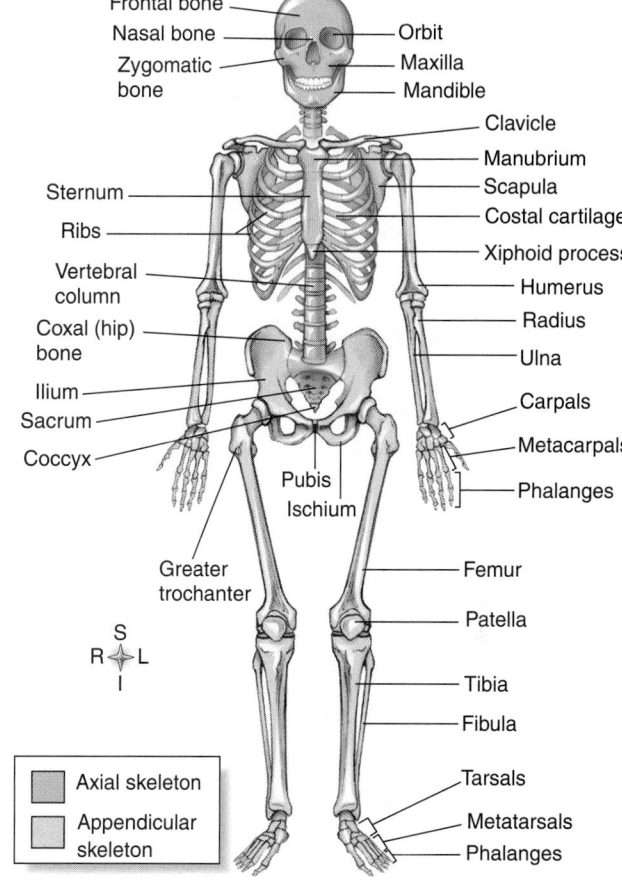

Figure 2–9 Diagram of skeleton of trunk and limbs with bones
labeled. (From Thibodeau and Patton: Anatomy and Physiology,
6th ed. 2007, Mosby)

**MALIGNANT NEOPLASM OF BONE, CONNECTIVE TISSUE, SKIN, AND BREAST
(170–176)**

Excludes *carcinoma in situ:*
breast (233.0)
skin (232.0–232.9)

● 170 **Malignant neoplasm of bone and articular cartilage**

Includes cartilage (articular) (joint)
periosteum

Excludes *bone marrow NOS (202.9)*
cartilage:
ear (171.0)
eyelid (171.0)
larynx (161.3)
nose (160.0)
synovia (171.0–171.9)

170.0 **Bones of skull and face, except mandible**
Mandible = lower jaw

Bone:	Bone:
ethmoid	sphenoid
frontal	temporal
malar	zygomatic
nasal	Maxilla (superior)
occipital	Turbinate
orbital	Upper jaw bone
parietal	Vomer

Excludes *carcinoma, any type except intraosseous or
odontogenic:*
maxilla, maxillary (sinus) (160.2)
upper jaw bone (143.0)
jaw bone (lower) (170.1)

NEOPLASMS (140–239)

170.1 Mandible
Inferior maxilla
Jaw bone NOS
Lower jaw bone

> **Excludes** *carcinoma, any type except intraosseous or*
> *odontogenic:*
> *jaw bone NOS (143.9)*
> *lower (143.1)*
> *upper jaw bone (170.0)*

170.2 Vertebral column, excluding sacrum and coccyx
Spinal column
Spine
Vertebra

> **Excludes** *sacrum and coccyx (170.6)*

170.3 Ribs, sternum, and clavicle
Costal cartilage
Costovertebral joint
Xiphoid process

170.4 Scapula and long bones of upper limb
Acromion   Radius
Bones NOS of upper limb   Ulna
Humerus
Coding Clinic: 1999, Q2, P9

170.5 Short bones of upper limb
Carpal   Scaphoid (of hand)
Cuneiform, wrist   Semilunar or lunate
Metacarpal   Trapezium
Navicular, of hand   Trapezoid
Phalanges of hand   Unciform
Pisiform

170.6 Pelvic bones, sacrum, and coccyx
Coccygeal vertebra   Pubic bone
Ilium   Sacral vertebra
Ischium

170.7 Long bones of lower limb
Bones NOS of lower limb   Fibula
Femur   Tibia

170.8 Short bones of lower limb
Astragalus [talus]   Navicular (of ankle)
Calcaneus   Patella
Cuboid   Phalanges of foot
Cuneiform, ankle   Tarsal
Metatarsal

▪170.9 Bone and articular cartilage, site unspecified

●171 Malignant neoplasm of connective and other soft tissue

> **Includes** blood vessel
> bursa
> fascia
> fat
> ligament, except uterine
> muscle
> peripheral, sympathetic, and parasympathetic
>   nerves and ganglia
> synovia
> tendon (sheath)

> **Excludes** *cartilage (of):*
> *articular (170.0–170.9)*
> *larynx (161.3)*
> *nose (160.0)*
> *connective tissue:*
> *breast (174.0–175.9)*
> *internal organs—code to malignant neoplasm of*
>   *the site [e.g., leiomyosarcoma of stomach,*
>   *151.9]*
> *heart (164.1)*
> *uterine ligament (183.4)*

171.0 Head, face, and neck
Cartilage of:
ear
eyelid
Coding Clinic: 1999, Q2, P6-7

171.2 Upper limb, including shoulder
Arm
Finger
Forearm
Hand

171.3 Lower limb, including hip
Foot
Leg
Popliteal space
> *Popliteal space = popliteal cavity, popliteal fossa.*
> *Depression in posterior aspect of knee (behind*
> *knee).*
Thigh
Toe

171.4 Thorax
Axilla
Diaphragm
Great vessels

> **Excludes** *heart (164.1)*
> *mediastinum (164.2–164.9)*
> *thymus (164.0)*

171.5 Abdomen
Abdominal wall
Hypochondrium

> **Excludes** *peritoneum (158.8)*
> *retroperitoneum (158.0)*

171.6 Pelvis
Buttock
Groin
Inguinal region
Perineum

> **Excludes** *pelvic peritoneum (158.8)*
> *retroperitoneum (158.0)*
> *uterine ligament, any (183.3–183.5)*

▪171.7 Trunk, unspecified
Back NOS
Flank NOS

▪171.8 Other specified sites of connective and other soft tissue
Malignant neoplasm of contiguous or overlapping
   sites of connective tissue whose point of
   origin cannot be determined

▪171.9 Connective and other soft tissue, site unspecified

NEOPLASMS (140–239)

◄ New   ◄▪▪▪ Revised   ~~deleted~~ Deleted   ● Use Additional Digit(s)   ▪ Nonspecific Code
● Not first-listed DX   OGCR Official Guidelines   Coding Clinic   Excludes   Includes   Use additional   Code first   Omit code

Item 2-4 Malignant melanoma is a serious form of skin cancer that affects the melanocytes (pigment-forming cells) and is caused by ultraviolet (UV) rays from the sun that damage skin. It is most commonly seen in the 40- to 60-year-olds with fair skin, blue or green eyes, and red or blond hair who sunburn easily. Melanoma can spread very rapidly and is the most deadly form of skin cancer. It is less common than other types of skin cancer. The rate of melanoma is increasing and currently is the leading cause of death from skin disease.

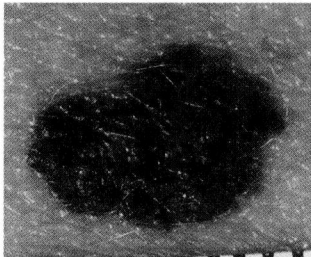

Figure 2-10 Malignant melanoma of skin. (From Goldman: Cecil Textbook of Medicine, 22nd ed. 2004, Saunders)

● **172 Malignant melanoma of skin**

> **Includes**   melanocarcinoma
> melanoma in situ of skin
> melanoma (skin) NOS

> **Excludes**   *skin of genital organs (184.0–184.9, 187.1–187.9)*
> *sites other than skin - code to malignant neoplasm of the site*

172.0 Lip

> **Excludes**   *vermilion border of lip (140.0–140.1, 140.9)*

172.1 Eyelid, including canthus

172.2 Ear and external auditory canal
> Auricle (ear)
> Auricular canal, external
> External [acoustic] meatus
> Pinna

172.3 Other and unspecified parts of face
> Cheek (external)   Forehead
> Chin   Nose, external
> Eyebrow   Temple

172.4 Scalp and neck

172.5 Trunk, except scrotum
> Axilla   Perianal skin
> Breast   Perineum
> Buttock   Umbilicus
> Groin

> **Excludes**   *anal canal (154.2)*
> *anus NOS (154.3)*
> *scrotum (187.7)*

172.6 Upper limb, including shoulder
> Arm   Forearm
> Finger   Hand

172.7 Lower limb, including hip
> Ankle   Leg
> Foot   Popliteal area
> Heel   Thigh
> Knee   Toe

172.8 Other specified sites of skin
> Malignant melanoma of contiguous or overlapping sites of skin whose point of origin cannot be determined

172.9 Melanoma of skin, site unspecified

● **173 Other malignant neoplasm of skin**

> **Includes**   malignant neoplasm of:
> sebaceous glands
> sudoriferous, sudoriparous glands
> sweat glands

> **Excludes**   *Kaposi's sarcoma (176.0–176.9)*
> *malignant melanoma of skin (172.0–172.9)*
> *skin of genital organs (184.0–184.9, 187.1–187.9)*
> Coding Clinic: 2000, Q1, P8; 1996, Q2, P12

173.0 Skin of lip

> **Excludes**   *vermilion border of lip (140.0–140.1, 140.9)*

173.1 Eyelid, including canthus

> **Excludes**   *cartilage of eyelid (171.0)*

173.2 Skin of ear and external auditory canal
> Auricle (ear)
> Auricular canal, external
> External meatus
> Pinna

> **Excludes**   *cartilage of ear (171.0)*

173.3 Skin of other and unspecified parts of face
> Cheek, external
> Chin
> Eyebrow
> Forehead
> Nose, external
> Temple
> Coding Clinic: 2000, Q1, P3

173.4 Scalp and skin of neck

173.5 Skin of trunk, except scrotum
> Axillary fold
> Perianal skin
> Skin of:
> abdominal wall
> anus
> back
> breast
> buttock
> chest wall
> groin
> perineum
> Umbilicus

> **Excludes**   *anal canal (154.2)*
> *anus NOS (154.3)*
> *skin of scrotum (187.7)*
> Coding Clinic: 2001, Q1, P8

173.6 Skin of upper limb, including shoulder
> Arm
> Finger
> Forearm
> Hand

173.7 Skin of lower limb, including hip
> Ankle
> Foot
> Heel
> Knee
> Leg
> Popliteal area
> Thigh
> Toe

173.8 Other specified sites of skin
> Malignant neoplasm of contiguous or overlapping sites of skin whose point of origin cannot be determined

173.9 Skin, site unspecified

NEOPLASMS (140–239)

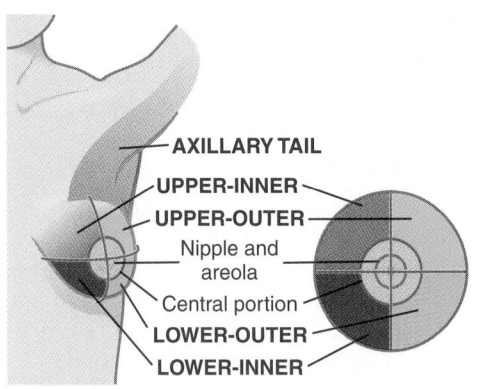

Figure 2–11   Female breast quadrants and axillary tail.

● **174   Malignant neoplasm of female breast**
> *This code is for female breast; see 175 for male breast.*

Includes	breast (female)
	connective tissue
	soft parts
	Paget's disease of:
	breast
	nipple

Use additional code to identify estrogen receptor status (V86.0, V86.1)

Excludes   *skin of breast (172.5, 173.5)*

174.0   Nipple and areola ♀

174.1   Central portion ♀

174.2   Upper-inner quadrant ♀
> Coding Clinic: 1989, Q4, P11

174.3   Lower-inner quadrant ♀
> Coding Clinic: 1989, Q4, P11

174.4   Upper-outer quadrant ♀
> Coding Clinic: 2008, Q4, P152-155; 2004, Q1, P3-4; 1997, Q3, P8; 1984, May-June, P11

174.5   Lower-outer quadrant ♀

174.6   Axillary tail ♀

■ **174.8   Other specified sites of female breast ♀**
> Ectopic sites
> Inner breast
> Lower breast
> Malignant neoplasm of contiguous or overlapping sites of breast whose point of origin cannot be determined
> Midline of breast
> Outer breast
> Upper breast
> Coding Clinic: 1985, July-Aug, P11

■ **174.9   Breast (female), unspecified ♀**
> Coding Clinic: 2005, Q3, P11-12; 1994, Q2, P10x2

● **175   Malignant neoplasm of male breast**

Use additional code to identify estrogen receptor status (V86.0, V86.1)

Excludes   *skin of breast (172.5, 173.5)*

175.0   Nipple and areola ♂

■ **175.9   Other and unspecified sites of male breast ♂**
> Ectopic breast tissue, male

Item 2–5   Kaposi's sarcoma is a cancer that causes patches of abnormal tissue to grow under the skin; in the lining of the mouth, nose, and throat; or in other organs, often beginning and spreading to other organs. Patients who have had organ transplants or patients with AIDS are at high risk for this malignancy.

● **176   Kaposi's sarcoma**

176.0   Skin
> Coding Clinic: 2007, Q4, P61-64

176.1   Soft tissue

Blood vessel	Ligament
Connective tissue	Lymphatic(s) NEC
Fascia	Muscle

> **Excludes**   *lymph glands and nodes (176.5)*

176.2   Palate

176.3   Gastrointestinal sites

176.4   Lung

176.5   Lymph nodes

■ **176.8   Other specified sites**
> Oral cavity NEC

■ **176.9   Unspecified**
> Viscera NOS

MALIGNANT NEOPLASM OF GENITOURINARY ORGANS (179–189)

> **Excludes**   *carcinoma in situ (233.1–233.9)*

■ **179   Malignant neoplasm of uterus, part unspecified ♀**

● **180   Malignant neoplasm of cervix uteri**

Includes	invasive malignancy [carcinoma]
Excludes	*carcinoma in situ (233.1)*

180.0   Endocervix ♀
> *Inside the cervix*
> Cervical canal NOS
> Endocervical canal
> Endocervical gland

180.1   Exocervix ♀
> *Outside the cervix*

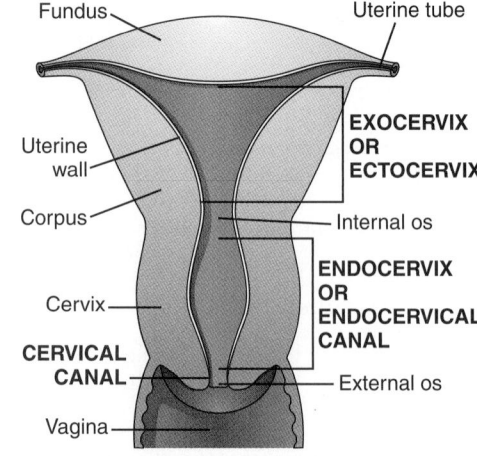

Figure 2–12   Cervix uteri.

■180.8 **Other specified sites of cervix** ♀
Cervical stump
Squamocolumnar junction of cervix
Malignant neoplasm of contiguous or overlapping
sites of cervix uteri whose point of origin
cannot be determined

■180.9 **Cervix uteri, unspecified** ♀

181 **Malignant neoplasm of placenta** ♀
Choriocarcinoma NOS
Chorioepithelioma NOS

> **Excludes** *chorioadenoma (destruens) (236.1)*
> *hydatidiform mole (630)*
> *malignant (236.1)*
> *invasive mole (236.1)*
> *male choriocarcinoma NOS (186.0–186.9)*

●182 **Malignant neoplasm of body of uterus**

> **Excludes** *carcinoma in situ (233.2)*

182.0 **Corpus uteri, except isthmus** ♀
Cornu
Endometrium
Fundus
Myometrium

182.1 **Isthmus** ♀
Lower uterine segment

■182.8 **Other specified sites of body of uterus** ♀
Malignant neoplasm of contiguous or overlapping
sites of body of uterus whose point of origin
cannot be determined

> **Excludes** *uterus NOS (179)*

●183 **Malignant neoplasm of ovary and other uterine adnexa**

> **Excludes** *Douglas' cul-de-sac (158.8)*

183.0 **Ovary** ♀

> Use additional code to identify any functional
> activity
> Coding Clinic: 2007, Q4, P95-96

183.2 **Fallopian tube** ♀
Oviduct
Uterine tube

183.3 **Broad ligament** ♀
Mesovarium
Parovarian region

183.4 **Parametrium** ♀
Uterine ligament NOS
Uterosacral ligament

183.5 **Round ligament** ♀

■183.8 **Other specified sites of uterine adnexa** ♀
Tubo-ovarian
Utero-ovarian
Malignant neoplasm of contiguous or overlapping
sites of ovary and other uterine adnexa whose
point of origin cannot be determined

■183.9 **Uterine adnexa, unspecified** ♀

●184 **Malignant neoplasm of other and unspecified female
genital organs**

> **Excludes** *carcinoma in situ (233.30–233.39)*

184.0 **Vagina** ♀
Gartner's duct   Vaginal vault

184.1 **Labia majora** ♀
Greater vestibular [Bartholin's] gland

184.2 **Labia minora** ♀

184.3 **Clitoris** ♀

■184.4 **Vulva, unspecified** ♀
External female genitalia NOS
Pudendum

■184.8 **Other specified sites of female genital organs** ♀
Malignant neoplasm of contiguous or overlapping
sites of female genital organs whose point of
origin cannot be determined

■184.9 **Female genital organ, site unspecified** ♀
Female genitourinary tract NOS

185 **Malignant neoplasm of prostate** ♂

> **Excludes** *seminal vesicles (187.8)*
> Coding Clinic: 2003, Q3, P13; 1999, Q3, P5; 1994, Q1, P20; 1992, Q3, P7

●186 **Malignant neoplasm of testis**

> Use additional code to identify any functional activity

186.0 **Undescended testis** ♂
Ectopic testis   Retained testis

■186.9 **Other and unspecified testis** ♂
Testis: Testis:
NOS   scrotal
descended

●187 **Malignant neoplasm of penis and other male genital organs**

187.1 **Prepuce** ♂
Foreskin

187.2 **Glans penis** ♂

187.3 **Body of penis** ♂
Corpus cavernosum

■187.4 **Penis, part unspecified** ♂
Skin of penis NOS

187.5 **Epididymis** ♂

187.6 **Spermatic cord** ♂
Vas deferens

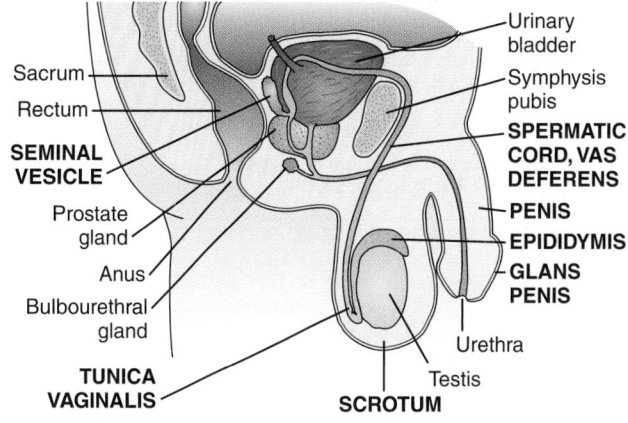

Figure 2–13 Penis and other male genital organs.

187.7 **Scrotum** ♂
Skin of scrotum

■187.8 **Other specified sites of male genital organs** ♂
Seminal vesicle
Tunica vaginalis
Malignant neoplasm of contiguous or overlapping
sites of penis and other male genital organs
whose point of origin cannot be determined

■187.9 **Male genital organ, site unspecified** ♂
Male genital organ or tract NOS

NEOPLASMS (140–239)

● **188 Malignant neoplasm of bladder**

> **Excludes** *carcinoma in situ (233.7)*

188.0 **Trigone of urinary bladder**

188.1 **Dome of urinary bladder**

188.2 **Lateral wall of urinary bladder**

188.3 **Anterior wall of urinary bladder**

188.4 **Posterior wall of urinary bladder**

188.5 **Bladder neck**
Internal urethral orifice

188.6 **Ureteric orifice**

188.7 **Urachus**

■188.8 **Other specified sites of bladder**
Malignant neoplasm of contiguous or overlapping sites of bladder whose point of origin cannot be determined

■188.9 **Bladder, part unspecified**
Bladder wall NOS
Coding Clinic: 2000, Q1, P5

● **189 Malignant neoplasm of kidney and other and unspecified urinary organs**

> **Excludes** *benign carcinoid tumor of kidney (209.64)*
> *malignant carcinoid tumor of kidney (209.24)*

189.0 **Kidney, except pelvis**
Kidney NOS   Kidney parenchyma
Coding Clinic: 2005, Q2, P4-5; 2004, Q2, P4

189.1 **Renal pelvis**
Renal calyces   Ureteropelvic junction

189.2 **Ureter**

> **Excludes** *ureteric orifice of bladder (188.6)*

189.3 **Urethra**

> **Excludes** *urethral orifice of bladder (188.5)*

189.4 **Paraurethral glands**

■189.8 **Other specified sites of urinary organs**
Malignant neoplasm of contiguous or overlapping sites of kidney and other urinary organs whose point of origin cannot be determined

■189.9 **Urinary organ, site unspecified**
Urinary system NOS

MALIGNANT NEOPLASM OF OTHER AND UNSPECIFIED SITES (190–199)

> **Excludes** *carcinoma in situ (234.0–234.9)*

● **190 Malignant neoplasm of eye**

> **Excludes** *carcinoma in situ (234.0)*
> *dark area on retina and choroid (239.81)* ◀
> *eyelid (skin) (172.1, 173.1)*
> *cartilage (171.0)*
> *optic nerve (192.0)*
> *orbital bone (170.0)*
> *retinal freckle (239.81)* ◀

190.0 **Eyeball, except conjunctiva, cornea, retina, and choroid**
Note the use of "except" in this code.
Ciliary body
Crystalline lens
Iris
Sclera
Uveal tract

190.1 **Orbit**
Connective tissue of orbit
Extraocular muscle
Retrobulbar

> **Excludes** *bone of orbit (170.0)*

190.2 **Lacrimal gland**

190.3 **Conjunctiva**

190.4 **Cornea**

190.5 **Retina**

190.6 **Choroid**

190.7 **Lacrimal duct**
Lacrimal sac
Nasolacrimal duct

■190.8 **Other specified sites of eye**
Malignant neoplasm of contiguous or overlapping sites of eye whose point of origin cannot be determined

■190.9 **Eye, part unspecified**

● **191 Malignant neoplasm of brain**

> **Excludes** *cranial nerves (192.0)*
> *retrobulbar area (190.1)*

191.0 **Cerebrum, except lobes and ventricles**
Basal ganglia
Cerebral cortex
Corpus striatum
Globus pallidus
Hypothalamus
Thalamus

191.1 **Frontal lobe**
Coding Clinic: 2005, Q4, P117-119; 1993, Q4, P33

191.2 **Temporal lobe**
Hippocampus
Uncus
Coding Clinic: 2006, Q4, P122-123

191.3 **Parietal lobe**

191.4 **Occipital lobe**

191.5 **Ventricles**
Choroid plexus
Floor of ventricle

191.6 **Cerebellum NOS**
Cerebellopontine angle

191.7 **Brain stem**
Cerebral peduncle
Medulla oblongata
Midbrain
Pons

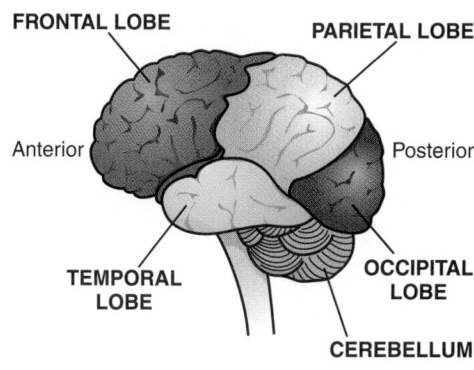

FRONTAL LOBE   PARIETAL LOBE

Anterior   Posterior

TEMPORAL LOBE   OCCIPITAL LOBE

CEREBELLUM

Figure 2–14   The brain.

■191.8 Other parts of brain
Corpus callosum
Tapetum
Malignant neoplasm of contiguous or overlapping sites of brain whose point of origin cannot be determined
Coding Clinic: 2007, Q4, P103-104

■191.9 Brain, unspecified
Cranial fossa NOS
Coding Clinic: 1994, Q2, P8

●192 Malignant neoplasm of other and unspecified parts of nervous system

> **Excludes** *peripheral, sympathetic, and parasympathetic nerves and ganglia (171.0–171.9)*

192.0 Cranial nerves
Olfactory bulb

192.1 Cerebral meninges
Dura (mater)
Falx (cerebelli) (cerebri)
Meninges NOS
Tentorium

192.2 Spinal cord
Cauda equina

192.3 Spinal meninges

■192.8 Other specified sites of nervous system
Malignant neoplasm of contiguous or overlapping sites of other parts of nervous system whose point of origin cannot be determined

■192.9 Nervous system, part unspecified
Nervous system (central) NOS

> **Excludes** *meninges NOS (192.1)*

193 Malignant neoplasm of thyroid gland
Thyroglossal duct

Use additional code to identify any functional activity

●194 Malignant neoplasm of other endocrine glands and related structures

> **Excludes** *islets of Langerhans (157.4)*
> *neuroendocrine tumors (209.00–209.69)*
> *ovary (183.0)*
> *testis (186.0–186.9)*
> *thymus (164.0)*

194.0 Adrenal gland
Adrenal cortex
Adrenal medulla
Suprarenal gland

194.1 Parathyroid gland

194.3 Pituitary gland and craniopharyngeal duct
Craniobuccal pouch
Hypophysis
Rathke's pouch
Sella turcica
Coding Clinic: 1985, July-Aug, P9

194.4 Pineal gland

194.5 Carotid body

194.6 Aortic body and other paraganglia
Coccygeal body
Glomus jugulare
Para-aortic body

■194.8 Other
Pluriglandular involvement NOS

Note: If the sites of multiple involvements are known, they should be coded separately.

■194.9 Endocrine gland, site unspecified

●195 Malignant neoplasm of other and ill-defined sites

> **Includes** malignant neoplasms of contiguous sites, not elsewhere classified, whose point of origin cannot be determined

> **Excludes** *malignant neoplasm:*
> *lymphatic and hematopoietic tissue (200.0–208.9)*
> *secondary sites (196.0–198.8)*
> *unspecified site (199.0–199.1)*

195.0 Head, face, and neck
Cheek NOS
Jaw NOS
Nose NOS
Supraclavicular region NOS
Coding Clinic: 2003, Q4, P107

195.1 Thorax
Axilla
Chest (wall) NOS
Intrathoracic NOS

195.2 Abdomen
Intra-abdominal NOS
Coding Clinic: 1997, Q2, P3

195.3 Pelvis
Groin
Inguinal region NOS
Presacral region
Sacrococcygeal region
Sites overlapping systems within pelvis, as:
rectovaginal (septum)
rectovesical (septum)

195.4 Upper limb

195.5 Lower limb

■195.8 Other specified sites
Back NOS
Flank NOS
Trunk NOS

NEOPLASMS (140–239)

(See Plate 315 on page 85.)

● **196 Secondary and unspecified malignant neoplasm of lymph nodes**

> **Excludes** *any malignant neoplasm of lymph nodes, specified as primary (200.0–202.9)*
> *Hodgkin's disease (201.0–201.9)*
> *lymphosarcoma (200.1)*
> *other forms of lymphoma (202.0–202.9)*
> *reticulosarcoma (200.0)*
> *secondary neuroendocrine tumor of (distant) lymph nodes (209.71)* ◀
>
> Coding Clinic: 1992, Q2, P3-4

196.0 Lymph nodes of head, face, and neck
Cervical   Scalene
Cervicofacial   Supraclavicular
Coding Clinic: 2007, Q3, P8-9

196.1 Intrathoracic lymph nodes
Bronchopulmonary   Mediastinal
Intercostal   Tracheobronchial
Coding Clinic: 2006, Q3, P7-8

196.2 Intra-abdominal lymph nodes
Intestinal   Retroperitoneal
Mesenteric
Coding Clinic: 2003, Q4, P111

196.3 Lymph nodes of axilla and upper limb
Brachial   Infraclavicular
Epitrochlear   Pectoral

196.5 Lymph nodes of inguinal region and lower limb
Femoral   Popliteal
Groin   Tibial

196.6 Intrapelvic lymph nodes
Hypogastric   Obturator
Iliac   Parametrial

■ **196.8 Lymph nodes of multiple sites**

■ **196.9 Site unspecified**
Lymph nodes NOS

● **197 Secondary malignant neoplasm of respiratory and digestive systems**

> **Excludes** *lymph node metastasis (196.0–196.9)*
> *secondary neuroendocrine tumor of liver (209.72)* ◀
> *secondary neuroendocrine tumor of respiratory organs (209.79)* ◀

197.0 Lung
Bronchus
Coding Clinic: 2006, Q1, P4-5; 1999, Q2, P9

197.1 Mediastinum
Coding Clinic: 2006, Q3, P7-8

197.2 Pleura
Coding Clinic: 2008, Q1, P16-17; 2007, Q3, P3; 2003, Q4, P110; 1989, Q4, P11

■ **197.3 Other respiratory organs**
Trachea

197.4 Small intestine, including duodenum

197.5 Large intestine and rectum

197.6 Retroperitoneum and peritoneum
Coding Clinic: 2004, Q2, P4; 1989, Q4, P11

197.7 Liver, specified as secondary
Coding Clinic: 2006, Q1, P4-5; 2005, Q2, P9-10; 1984, May-June, P11

■ **197.8 Other digestive organs and spleen**
Coding Clinic: 1997, Q2, P3

● **198 Secondary malignant neoplasm of other specified sites**

> **Excludes** *lymph node metastasis (196.0–196.9)*
> *secondary neuroendocrine tumor of other specified sites (209.79)* ◀

198.0 Kidney

■ **198.1 Other urinary organs**

198.2 Skin
Skin of breast

198.3 Brain and spinal cord
Coding Clinic: 2007, Q3, P4; 1999, Q3, P7-8; 1984, May-June, P14

■ **198.4 Other parts of nervous system**
Meninges (cerebral) (spinal)

198.5 Bone and bone marrow
Coding Clinic: 2007, Q1, P3-8; 2003, Q4, P110; 1999, Q3, P5; 1989, Q4, P12; 1984, May-June, P14

198.6 Ovary ♀

198.7 Adrenal gland
Suprarenal gland
Coding Clinic: 1988, Q2, P10

● **198.8 Other specified sites**

198.81 Breast

> **Excludes** *skin of breast (198.2)*

198.82 Genital organs

■ **198.89 Other**

> **Excludes** *retroperitoneal lymph nodes (196.2)*
>
> Coding Clinic: 2005, Q2, P4-5; 1997, Q2, P4

● **199 Malignant neoplasm without specification of site**

> **Excludes** *malignant carcinoid tumor of unknown primary site (209.20)*
> *malignant (poorly differentiated) neuroendocrine carcinoma, any site (209.30)* ◀
> *malignant (poorly differentiated) neuroendocrine tumor, any site (209.30)* ◀
> *neuroendocrine carcinoma (high grade), any site (209.30)* ◀

199.0 Disseminated
Carcinomatosis unspecified site (primary) (secondary)
Generalized:
  cancer unspecified site (primary) (secondary)
  malignancy unspecified site (primary) (secondary)
Multiple cancer unspecified site (primary) (secondary)
Coding Clinic: 1989, Q4, P10; 1988, Q2, P11

■ **199.1 Other**
Cancer unspecified site (primary) (secondary)
Carcinoma unspecified site (primary) (secondary)
Malignancy unspecified site (primary) (secondary)
Coding Clinic: 2006, Q3, P14-15; Q1, P4-5

● **199.2 *Malignant neoplasm associated with transplanted organ***

> *Code first complication of transplanted organ (996.80-996.89)*
>
> Use additional code for specific malignancy site ◀
>
> Coding Clinic: 2008, Q4, P82-83

◀ New   ◀▥ Revised   ~~deleted~~ Deleted   ● Use Additional Digit(s)   ■ Nonspecific Code

● Not first-listed DX   OGCR Official Guidelines   Coding Clinic   Excludes   Includes   Use additional   Code first   Omit code

NEOPLASMS (140–239)

Item 2-6 Lymphosarcoma, also known as malignant lymphoma, is a cancer of the lymph system exhibiting abnormal cells encompassing an entire lymph node creating a diffuse pattern without any definite organization. Diffuse pattern lymphoma has a more unfavorable survival outlook than those with a follicular or nodular pattern. Reticulosarcoma is the most common aggressive form of non-Hodgkin's lymphoma.

MALIGNANT NEOPLASM OF LYMPHATIC AND HEMATOPOIETIC TISSUE (200–208)

> **Excludes** *autoimmune lymhoproliferative syndrome*
> *(279.41)*
> *secondary neoplasm of:*
> *bone marrow (198.5)*
> *spleen (197.8)*
> *secondary and unspecified neoplasm of lymph*
> *nodes (196.0–196.9)*

The following fifth-digit subclassification is for use with categories 200–202:

> 0　unspecified site, extranodal and solid organ sites
> 1　lymph nodes of head, face, and neck
> 2　intrathoracic lymph nodes
> 3　intra-abdominal lymph nodes
> 4　lymph nodes of axilla and upper limb
> 5　lymph nodes of inguinal region and lower limb
> 6　intrapelvic lymph nodes
> 7　spleen
> 8　lymph nodes of multiple sites

● **200　Lymphosarcoma and reticulosarcoma and other specified malignant tumors of lymphatic tissue**

> Requires fifth digit. See note before section 200 for codes and definitions.
> Coding Clinic: 2007, Q4, P65-67

● **200.0　Reticulosarcoma**
[0-8]　　Lymphoma (malignant):
　　　　　　histiocytic (diffuse):
　　　　　　　　nodular
　　　　　　　　pleomorphic cell type
　　　　　　reticulum cell type
　　　　　Reticulum cell sarcoma:
　　　　　　NOS
　　　　　　pleomorphic cell type
　　　　Coding Clinic: 2006, Q4, P135-136; 2001, Q3, P12-13

● **200.1　Lymphosarcoma**
[0-8]　　Lymphoblastoma (diffuse)
　　　　　Lymphoma (malignant):
　　　　　　lymphoblastic (diffuse)
　　　　　　lymphocytic (cell type) (diffuse)
　　　　　　lymphosarcoma type
　　　　　Lymphosarcoma:
　　　　　　NOS
　　　　　　diffuse NOS
　　　　　　lymphoblastic (diffuse)
　　　　　　lymphocytic (diffuse)
　　　　　　prolymphocytic

> **Excludes** *lymphosarcoma:*
> *follicular or nodular (202.0)*
> *mixed cell type (200.8)*
> *lymphosarcoma cell leukemia (207.8)*

● **200.2　Burkitt's tumor or lymphoma**
[0-8]　　Malignant lymphoma, Burkitt's type

● **200.3　Marginal zone lymphoma**
[0-8]　　Extranodal marginal zone B-cell lymphoma
　　　　　Mucosa associated lymphoid tissue [MALT]
　　　　　Nodal marginal zone B-cell lymphoma
　　　　　Splenic marginal zone B-cell lymphoma

● **200.4　Mantle cell lymphoma**
[0-8]

● **200.5　Primary central nervous system lymphoma**
[0-8]

● **200.6　Anaplastic large cell lymphoma**
[0-8]

● **200.7　Large cell lymphoma**
[0-8]

●■ **200.8　Other named variants**
[0-8]　　Lymphoma (malignant):
　　　　　　lymphoplasmacytoid type
　　　　　　mixed lymphocytic-histiocytic (diffuse)
　　　　　Lymphosarcoma, mixed cell type (diffuse)
　　　　　Reticulolymphosarcoma (diffuse)

● **201　Hodgkin's disease**
> *Also known as malignant lymphoma/lymphosarcoma and is cancer of the lymphatic system including the lymph nodes and related structures*

> Requires fifth digit. See note before section 200 for codes and definitions.

● **201.0　Hodgkin's paragranuloma**
[0-8]

● **201.1　Hodgkin's granuloma**
[0-8]

● **201.2　Hodgkin's sarcoma**
[0-8]

● **201.4　Lymphocytic-histiocytic predominance**
[0-8]

● **201.5　Nodular sclerosis**
[0-8]　　Hodgkin's disease, nodular sclerosis:
　　　　　　NOS
　　　　　　cellular phase

● **201.6　Mixed cellularity**
[0-8]

● **201.7　Lymphocytic depletion**
[0-8]　　Hodgkin's disease, lymphocytic depletion:
　　　　　　NOS
　　　　　　diffuse fibrosis
　　　　　　reticular type

●■ **201.9　Hodgkin's disease, unspecified**
[0-8]　　Hodgkin's:
　　　　　　disease NOS
　　　　　　lymphoma NOS
　　　　　Malignant:
　　　　　　lymphogranuloma
　　　　　　lymphogranulomatosis

● 202 **Other malignant neoplasms of lymphoid and histiocytic tissue**

> Requires fifth digit. See note before section 200 for codes and definitions.

● 202.0 **Nodular lymphoma**
[0-8]   Brill-Symmers disease
          Lymphoma:
               follicular (giant) (large cell)   ◀▥
               lymphocytic, nodular
          Lymphosarcoma:
               follicular (giant)
               nodular

● 202.1 **Mycosis fungoides**
[0-8]   **Excludes** *peripheral T-cell lymphoma (202.7)*   ◀
          Coding Clinic: 1999, Q2, P7-8; 1992, Q2, P4

● 202.2 **Sézary's disease**
[0-8]   Coding Clinic: 1999, Q2, P7-8

● 202.3 **Malignant histiocytosis**
[0-8]   Histiocytic medullary reticulosis
          Malignant:
               reticuloendotheliosis
               reticulosis

● 202.4 **Leukemic reticuloendotheliosis**
[0-8]   Hairy-cell leukemia

● 202.5 **Letterer-Siwe disease**
[0-8]   Acute:
               differentiated progressive histiocytosis
               histiocytosis X (progressive)
               infantile reticuloendotheliosis
               reticulosis of infancy
          Excludes *Hand-Schüller-Christian disease (277.89)*
                       histiocytosis (acute) (chronic) (277.89)
                       histiocytosis X (chronic) (277.89)

● 202.6 **Malignant mast cell tumors**
[0-8]   Malignant:
               mastocytoma
               mastocytosis
          Mast cell sarcoma
          Systemic tissue mast cell disease
          Excludes *mast cell leukemia (207.8)*

● 202.7 **Peripheral T cell lymphoma**
[0-8]

● ▪202.8 **Other lymphomas**
[0-8]   Lymphoma (malignant):
               NOS
               diffuse
          Excludes *benign lymphoma (229.0)*
          Coding Clinic: 2008, Q4, P82-83; Q1, P16-17; 2007, Q3, P3; 2006,
                       Q4, P135-136; Q2, P20-22; 1993, Q4, P33; 1992, Q2, P3-4

● ▪202.9 **Other and unspecified malignant neoplasms of**
[0-8] **lymphoid and histiocytic tissue**
          Follicular dendritic cell sarcoma
          Interdigitating dendritic cell sarcoma
          Langerhans cell sarcoma
          Malignant neoplasm of bone marrow NOS

● 203 **Multiple myeloma and immunoproliferative neoplasms**
> *Multiple myeloma is cancer of plasma cell (type of white blood cell) and is incurable but treatable disease. Immunoproliferative neoplasm is term for diseases (mostly cancers) in which immune system cells proliferate.*

The following fifth-digit subclassification is for use with category 203:

> **0 without mention of having achieved remission**
> **failed remission**
> **1 in remission**
> **2 in relapse**

Coding Clinic: 2008, Q4, P83-85

● 203.0 **Multiple myeloma**
[0-2]   Kahler's disease   Myelomatosis
          Excludes *solitary myeloma (238.6)*
          Coding Clinic: 2008, Q4, P90-91; 2007, Q2, P9-10; 1999, Q4, P10;
                       1996, Q1, P16

● 203.1 **Plasma cell leukemia**
[0-2]   Plasmacytic leukemia

● ▪203.8 **Other immunoproliferative neoplasms**
[0-2]   Coding Clinic: 1990, Q4, P26

Item 2-7 Leukemia is a cancer (acute or chronic) of the blood-forming tissues of the bone marrow. Blood cells all start out as stem cells. They mature and become red cells, white cells, or platelets. There are three main types of leukocytes (white cells that fight infection): monocytes, lymphocytes, and granulocytes. **Acute monocytic leukemia** (AML) affects monocytes. **Acute lymphoid leukemia** (ALL) affects lymphocytes, and **acute myeloid leukemia** (AML) affects cells that typically develop into white blood cells (not lymphocytes), though it may develop in other blood cells.

● 204 **Lymphoid leukemia**
> **Includes** leukemia: leukemia:
>   lymphatic   lymphocytic
>   lymphoblastic   lymphogenous

The following fifth-digit subclassification is for use with category 204:

> **0 without mention of having achieved remission**
> **failed remission**
> **1 in remission**
> **2 in relapse**

Coding Clinic: 2008, Q4, P83-85

● 204.0 **Acute**
[0-2]   **Excludes** *acute exacerbation of chronic lymphoid leukemia (204.1)*
          Coding Clinic: 1999, Q3, P4, 6-7; 1993, Q3, P4x2; 1985, May-June,
                       P18-19

● 204.1 **Chronic**
[0-2]

● 204.2 **Subacute**
[0-2]

● ▪204.8 **Other lymphoid leukemia**
[0-2]   Aleukemic leukemia:
               lymphatic
               lymphocytic
               lymphoid

● ▪204.9 **Unspecified lymphoid leukemia**
[0-2]

◀ New   ◀▥ Revised   ~~deleted~~ Deleted   ● Use Additional Digit(s)   ▪ Nonspecific Code
● Not first-listed DX   OGCR Official Guidelines   Coding Clinic   Excludes   Includes   Use additional   Code first   Omit code

● **205   Myeloid leukemia**

> **Includes**   leukemia: leukemia:
>   granulocytic   myelomonocytic
>   myeloblastic   myelosclerotic
>   myelocytic   myelosis
>   myelogenous

The following fifth-digit subclassification is for use with category 205:

> **0   without mention of having achieved remission**
>   **failed remission**
> **1   in remission**
> **2   in relapse**

> Coding Clinic: 2008, Q4, P83-85

● **205.0   Acute**
[0-2]   Acute promyelocytic leukemia

> **Excludes**   *acute exacerbation of chronic myeloid
>   leukemia (205.1)*
> Coding Clinic: 2006, Q2, P20-22; 2002, Q1, P11-12; 1993, Q3,
>   P3-4x2

● **205.1   Chronic**
[0-2]   Eosinophilic leukemia
         Neutrophilic leukemia
> Coding Clinic: 2008, Q4, P140-143; 2000, Q1, P6; 1995, Q2, P12;
>   1985, July-Aug, P13

● **205.2   Subacute**
[0-2]

● **205.3   Myeloid sarcoma**
[0-2]   Chloroma
         Granulocytic sarcoma

● ■ **205.8   Other myeloid leukemia**
[0-2]   Aleukemic leukemia:
         granulocytic
         myelogenous
         myeloid
         Aleukemic myelosis

● ■ **205.9   Unspecified myeloid leukemia**
[0-2]   Coding Clinic: 1985, May-June, P18-19

● **206   Monocytic leukemia**

> **Includes**   leukemia:
>   histiocytic
>   monoblastic
>   monocytoid

The following fifth-digit subclassification is for use with category 206:

> **0   without mention of having achieved remission**
>   **failed remission**
> **1   in remission**
> **2   in relapse**

> Coding Clinic: 2008, Q4, P83-85

● **206.0   Acute**
[0-2]   **Excludes**   *acute exacerbation of chronic monocytic
                leukemia (206.1)*

● **206.1   Chronic**
[0-2]

● **206.2   Subacute**
[0-2]

● ■ **206.8   Other monocytic leukemia**
[0-2]   Aleukemic:
         monocytic leukemia
         monocytoid leukemia

● ■ **206.9   Unspecified monocytic leukemia**
[0-2]

● **207   Other specified leukemia**

> **Excludes**   *leukemic reticuloendotheliosis (202.4)
>   plasma cell leukemia (203.1)*

The following fifth-digit subclassification is for use with category 207:

> **0   without mention of having achieved remission**
>   **failed remission**
> **1   in remission**
> **2   in relapse**

> Coding Clinic: 2008, Q4, P83-85

● **207.0   Acute erythremia and erythroleukemia**
[0-2]   Acute erythremic myelosis
         Di Guglielmo's disease
         Erythremic myelosis

● **207.1   Chronic erythremia**
[0-2]   Heilmeyer-Schöner disease

● **207.2   Megakaryocytic leukemia**
[0-2]   Megakaryocytic myelosis
         Thrombocytic leukemia

● ■ **207.8   Other specified leukemia**
[0-2]   Lymphosarcoma cell leukemia

● **208   Leukemia of unspecified cell type**

The following fifth-digit subclassification is for use with category 208:

> **0   without mention of having achieved remission**
>   **failed remission**
> **1   in remission**
> **2   in relapse**

> Coding Clinic: 2008, Q4, P83-85

● ■ **208.0   Acute**
[0-2]   Acute leukemia NOS
         Blast cell leukemia
         Stem cell leukemia

> **Excludes**   *acute exacerbation of chronic unspecified
>   leukemia (208.1)*
> Coding Clinic: 1987, Mar-April, P12

● ■ **208.1   Chronic**
[0-2]   Chronic leukemia NOS

● ■ **208.2   Subacute**
[0-2]   *Somewhat acute, between acute and chronic*
         Subacute leukemia NOS

● ■ **208.8   Other leukemia of unspecified cell type**
[0-2]   Coding Clinic: 1987, Mar-April, P12

● ■ **208.9   Unspecified leukemia**
[0-2]   Leukemia NOS

> **NEUROENDOCRINE TUMORS (209)**

● **209   Neuroendocrine tumors**

> *Code first any associated multiple endocrine neoplasia
>   syndrome (258.01-258.03)*

> Use additional code to identify associated endocrine
>   syndrome, such as:
> carcinoid syndrome (259.2)

> **Excludes**   *benign pancreatic islet cell tumors (211.7)* ◀
>   *malignant pancreatic islet cell tumors (157.4)* ◀
> Coding Clinic: 2008, Q4, P85-90

● **209.0   Malignant carcinoid tumors of the small intestine**

> **209.00   Malignant carcinoid tumor of the small
>   intestine, unspecified portion**

> **209.01   Malignant carcinoid tumor of the
>   duodenum**

NEOPLASMS (140–239)

209.02 Malignant carcinoid tumor of the jejunum

209.03 Malignant carcinoid tumor of the ileum

● **209.1 Malignant carcinoid tumors of the appendix, large intestine, and rectum**

209.10 Malignant carcinoid tumor of the large intestine, unspecified portion
Malignant carcinoid tumor of the colon NOS

209.11 Malignant carcinoid tumor of the appendix

209.12 Malignant carcinoid tumor of the cecum

209.13 Malignant carcinoid tumor of the ascending colon

209.14 Malignant carcinoid tumor of the transverse colon

209.15 Malignant carcinoid tumor of the descending colon

209.16 Malignant carcinoid tumor of the sigmoid colon

209.17 Malignant carcinoid tumor of the rectum

● **209.2 Malignant carcinoid tumors of other and unspecified sites**

209.20 Malignant carcinoid tumor of unknown primary site

209.21 Malignant carcinoid tumor of the bronchus and lung

209.22 Malignant carcinoid tumor of the thymus

209.23 Malignant carcinoid tumor of the stomach
Coding Clinic: 2008, Q4, P85-90

209.24 Malignant carcinoid tumor of the kidney

209.25 Malignant carcinoid tumor of the foregut NOS

209.26 Malignant carcinoid tumor of the midgut NOS

209.27 Malignant carcinoid tumor of the hindgut NOS

■ **209.29 Malignant carcinoid tumors of other sites**

● **209.3 Malignant poorly differentiated neuroendocrine tumors**

209.30 Malignant poorly differentiated neuroendocrine carcinoma, any site ◀▥
High grade neuroendocrine carcinoma, any site
Malignant poorly differentiated neuroendocrine tumor NOS

Excludes *Merkel cell carcinoma (209.31–209.36)* ◀

209.31 Merkel cell carcinoma of the face ◀
Merkel cell carcinoma of the ear ◀
Merkel cell carcinoma of the eyelid, including canthus ◀
Merkel cell carcinoma of the lip ◀

209.32 Merkel cell carcinoma of the scalp and neck ◀

209.33 Merkel cell carcinoma of the upper limb ◀

209.34 Merkel cell carcinoma of the lower limb ◀

209.35 Merkel cell carcinoma of the trunk ◀

209.36 Merkel cell carcinoma of other sites ◀
Merkel cell carcinoma of the buttock ◀
Merkel cell carcinoma of the genitals ◀
Merkel cell carcinoma NOS ◀

● **209.4 Benign carcinoid tumors of the small intestine**

■ **209.40 Benign carcinoid tumor of the small intestine, unspecified portion**

209.41 Benign carcinoid tumor of the duodenum

209.42 Benign carcinoid tumor of the jejunum

209.43 Benign carcinoid tumor of the ileum

● **209.5 Benign carcinoid tumors of the appendix, large intestine, and rectum**

■ **209.50 Benign carcinoid tumor of the large intestine, unspecified portion**
Benign carcinoid tumor of the colon NOS

209.51 Benign carcinoid tumor of the appendix

209.52 Benign carcinoid tumor of the cecum

209.53 Benign carcinoid tumor of the ascending colon

209.54 Benign carcinoid tumor of the transverse colon

209.55 Benign carcinoid tumor of the descending colon

209.56 Benign carcinoid tumor of the sigmoid colon

209.57 Benign carcinoid tumor of the rectum

● **209.6 Benign carcinoid tumors of other and unspecified sites**

■ **209.60 Benign carcinoid tumor of unknown primary site**
Carcinoid tumor NOS
Neuroendocrine tumor NOS

209.61 Benign carcinoid tumor of the bronchus and lung

209.62 Benign carcinoid tumor of the thymus

209.63 Benign carcinoid tumor of the stomach

209.64 Benign carcinoid tumor of the kidney

209.65 Benign carcinoid tumor of the foregut NOS

209.66 Benign carcinoid tumor of the midgut NOS

209.67 Benign carcinoid tumor of the hindgut NOS

■ **209.69 Benign carcinoid tumors of other sites**

● **209.7 Secondary neuroendocrine tumors** ◀
Secondary carcinoid tumors ◀

209.70 Secondary neuroendocrine tumor, unspecified site ◀

209.71 Secondary neuroendocrine tumor of distant lymph nodes ◀
Mesentery metastasis of neuroendocrine tumor ◀

209.72 Secondary neuroendocrine tumor of liver ◀

209.73 Secondary neuroendocrine tumor of bone ◀

209.74 Secondary neuroendocrine tumor of peritoneum ◀

209.75 Secondary Merkel cell carcinoma ◀
Merkel cell carcinoma nodal presentation ◀
Merkel cell carcinoma visceral metastatic presentation ◀
Secondary Merkel cell carcinoma, any site ◀

209.79 Secondary neuroendocrine tumor of other sites ◀

◀ New   ◀▥ Revised   ~~deleted~~ Deleted   ● Use Additional Digit(s)   ■ Nonspecific Code
● Not first-listed DX   OGCR Official Guidelines   Coding Clinic   Excludes   Includes   Use additional   Code first   Omit code

NEOPLASMS (140–239)

<u>**BENIGN NEOPLASMS (210–229)**</u>

Benign neoplasm: Tumor that does not metastasize to other parts of body and is caused by cell overgrowth, differentiating it from cyst or abscess

● **210 Benign neoplasm of lip, oral cavity, and pharynx**

   Excludes *cyst (of):*
                 jaw (526.0–526.2, 526.89)
                 oral soft tissue (528.4)
                 radicular (522.8)

   210.0 Lip
      Frenulum labii
      Lip (inner aspect) (mucosa) (vermilion border)

      Excludes *labial commissure (210.4)*
                    skin of lip (216.0)

   210.1 Tongue
      Lingual tonsil

   210.2 Major salivary glands
      Gland: Gland:
         parotid   submandibular
         sublingual

      Excludes *benign neoplasms of minor salivary glands:*
                    NOS (210.4)
                    buccal mucosa (210.4)
                    lips (210.0)
                    palate (hard) (soft) (210.4)
                    tongue (210.1)
                    tonsil, palatine (210.5)

   210.3 Floor of mouth

   ■ **210.4 Other and unspecified parts of mouth**
      Gingiva
      Gum (upper) (lower)
      Labial commissure
      Oral cavity NOS
      Oral mucosa
      Palate (hard) (soft)
      Uvula

      Excludes *benign odontogenic neoplasms of bone*
                    (213.0–213.1)
                    developmental odontogenic cysts (526.0)
                    mucosa of lips (210.0)
                    nasopharyngeal [posterior] [superior]
                    surface of soft palate (210.7)

   210.5 Tonsil
      Tonsil (faucial) (palatine)

      Excludes *lingual tonsil (210.1)*
                    pharyngeal tonsil (210.7)
                    tonsillar:
                    fossa (210.6)
                    pillars (210.6)

   ■ **210.6 Other parts of oropharynx**
      Branchial cleft or vestiges
      Epiglottis, anterior aspect
      Fauces NOS
      Mesopharynx NOS
      Tonsillar:
         fossa
         pillars
      Vallecula

      Excludes *epiglottis:*
                    NOS (212.1)
                    suprahyoid portion (212.1)

   210.7 Nasopharynx
      Adenoid tissue   Pharyngeal tonsil
      Lymphadenoid tissue   Posterior nasal septum

   210.8 Hypopharynx
      Arytenoid fold   Postcricoid region
      Laryngopharynx   Pyriform fossa

   ■ **210.9 Pharynx, unspecified**
      Throat NOS

● **211 Benign neoplasm of other parts of digestive system**

   Excludes *benign stromal tumors of digestive system*
                 (215.5)

   211.0 Esophagus

   211.1 Stomach
      Body of stomach
      Cardia of stomach
      Fundus of stomach
      Cardiac orifice
      Pylorus

      Excludes *benign carcinoid tumors of the stomach*
                    (209.63)

   211.2 Duodenum, jejunum, and ileum
      Small intestine NOS

      Excludes *ampulla of Vater (211.5)*
                    benign carcinoid tumors of the small
                    intestine (209.40-209.43)
                    ileocecal valve (211.3)

   211.3 Colon
      Appendix   Ileocecal valve
      Cecum   Large intestine NOS

      Excludes *benign carcinoid tumors of the large*
                    intestine (209.50-209.56)
                    rectosigmoid junction (211.4)
                    Coding Clinic: 2005, Q3, P17-18; Q2, P16-17; 2001, Q4, P55-56x2;
                    1995, Q1, P4; 1992, Q3, P11

   211.4 Rectum and anal canal
      Anal canal or sphincter
      Anus NOS
      Rectosigmoid junction

      Excludes *anus:*
                    margin (216.5)
                    perianal skin (216.5)
                    skin (216.5)
                    benign carcinoid tumors of the rectum
                    (209.57)

   211.5 Liver and biliary passages
      Ampulla of Vater   Gallbladder
      Common bile duct   Hepatic duct
      Cystic duct   Sphincter of Oddi

   211.6 Pancreas, except islets of Langerhans

   211.7 Islets of Langerhans
      Islet cell tumor

      Use additional code to identify any functional
         activity

   211.8 Retroperitoneum and peritoneum
      Mesentery   Omentum
      Mesocolon   Retroperitoneal tissue

   ■ **211.9 Other and unspecified site**
      Alimentary tract NOS
      Digestive system NOS
      Gastrointestinal tract NOS
      Intestinal tract NOS
      Intestine NOS
      Spleen, not elsewhere classified

● **212 Benign neoplasm of respiratory and intrathoracic organs**

212.0 Nasal cavities, middle ear, and accessory sinuses

Cartilage of nose
Eustachian tube
Nares
Septum of nose

Sinus: Sinus:
  ethmoidal   maxillary
  frontal   sphenoidal

Excludes *auditory canal (external) (216.2)*
bone of:
ear (213.0)
nose [turbinates] (213.0)
cartilage of ear (215.0)
ear (external) (skin) (216.2)
nose NOS (229.8)
skin (216.3)
olfactory bulb (225.1)
polyp of:
accessory sinus (471.8)
ear (385.30–385.35)
nasal cavity (471.0)
posterior margin of septum and choanae
(210.7)

Coding Clinic: 2000, Q3, P10-11

212.1 Larynx

Cartilage:
  arytenoid
  cricoid
  cuneiform
  thyroid
Epiglottis (suprahyoid portion) NOS
Glottis
Vocal cords (false) (true)

Excludes *epiglottis, anterior aspect (210.6)*
polyp of vocal cord or larynx (478.4)

212.2 Trachea

212.3 Bronchus and lung

Carina
Hilus of lung

Excludes *benign carcinoid tumors of bronchus and*
lung (209.61)

212.4 Pleura

212.5 Mediastinum

212.6 Thymus

Excludes *benign carcinoid tumors of thymus (209.62)*

212.7 Heart

Excludes *great vessels (215.4)*

■**212.8 Other specified sites**

■**212.9 Site unspecified**

Respiratory organ NOS
Upper respiratory tract NOS

Excludes *intrathoracic NOS (229.8)*
thoracic NOS (229.8)

● **213 Benign neoplasm of bone and articular cartilage**

Includes cartilage (articular) (joint)
periosteum

Excludes *cartilage of:*
ear (215.0)
eyelid (215.0)
larynx (212.1)
nose (212.0)
exostosis NOS (726.91)
synovia (215.0–215.9)

213.0 Bones of skull and face

Excludes *lower jaw bone (213.1)*

213.1 Lower jaw bone

213.2 Vertebral column, excluding sacrum and coccyx

213.3 Ribs, sternum, and clavicle

213.4 Scapula and long bones of upper limb

213.5 Short bones of upper limb

213.6 Pelvic bones, sacrum, and coccyx

213.7 Long bones of lower limb

213.8 Short bones of lower limb

■**213.9 Bone and articular cartilage, site unspecified**

● **214 Lipoma**

Slow growing benign tumors (discrete rubbery masses) of
mature fat cells enclosed in a thin fibrous capsule
found in subcutaneous tissues of trunk and proximal
extremities and in internal organs

Includes angiolipoma
fibrolipoma
hibernoma
lipoma (fetal) (infiltrating) (intramuscular)
myelolipoma
myxolipoma

214.0 Skin and subcutaneous tissue of face

■**214.1 Other skin and subcutaneous tissue**

214.2 Intrathoracic organs

214.3 Intra-abdominal organs

214.4 Spermatic cord ♂

■**214.8 Other specified sites**

Coding Clinic: 1994, Q3, P7

■**214.9 Lipoma, unspecified site**

● **215 Other benign neoplasm of connective and other soft tissue**

Includes blood vessel
bursa
fascia
ligament
muscle
peripheral, sympathetic, and parasympathetic
nerves and ganglia
synovia
tendon (sheath)

Excludes *cartilage:*
articular (213.0–213.9)
larynx (212.1)
nose (212.0)
connective tissue of:
breast (217)
internal organ, except lipoma and
hemangioma-code to benign neoplasm
of the site
lipoma (214.0–214.9)

215.0 Head, face, and neck

215.2 Upper limb, including shoulder

215.3 Lower limb, including hip

215.4 Thorax

Excludes *heart (212.7)*
mediastinum (212.5)
thymus (212.6)

215.5 Abdomen

Abdominal wall
Benign stromal tumors of abdomen
Hypochondrium

215.6 Pelvis

Buttock   Inguinal region
Groin   Perineum

Excludes *uterine:*
leiomyoma (218.0–218.9)
ligament, any (221.0)

■**215.7 Trunk, unspecified**
    Back NOS
    Flank NOS

■**215.8 Other specified sites**

■**215.9 Site unspecified**

●**216 Benign neoplasm of skin**

> **Includes**   blue nevus
>   dermatofibroma
>   hydrocystoma
>   pigmented nevus
>   syringoadenoma
>   syringoma

> **Excludes**   *skin of genital organs (221.0–222.9)*

> Coding Clinic: 2000, Q1, P21-22

216.0 Skin of lip
> **Excludes**   *vermilion border of lip (210.0)*

216.1 Eyelid, including canthus
> **Excludes**   *cartilage of eyelid (215.0)*

216.2 Ear and external auditory canal
    Auricle (ear)
    Auricular canal, external
    External meatus
    Pinna
> **Excludes**   *cartilage of ear (215.0)*

■**216.3 Skin of other and unspecified parts of face**
    Cheek, external
    Eyebrow
    Nose, external
    Temple

216.4 Scalp and skin of neck

216.5 Skin of trunk, except scrotum
    Axillary fold
    Perianal skin
    Skin of: Skin of:
      abdominal wall   chest wall
      anus   groin
      back   perineum
      breast
      buttock
    Umbilicus
> **Excludes**   *anal canal (211.4)*
>   *anus NOS (211.4)*
>   *skin of scrotum (222.4)*

216.6 Skin of upper limb, including shoulder

216.7 Skin of lower limb, including hip

■**216.8 Other specified sites of skin**

■**216.9 Skin, site unspecified**

217 Benign neoplasm of breast
Note no gender difference for this code.
    Breast (male) (female)
      connective tissue
      glandular tissue
      soft parts
> **Excludes**   *adenofibrosis (610.2)*
>   *benign cyst of breast (610.0)*
>   *fibrocystic disease (610.1)*
>   *skin of breast (216.5)*
> Coding Clinic: 2000, Q1, P4

●**218 Uterine leiomyoma**
Benign tumors or nodules of the uterine wall
> **Includes**   fibroid (bleeding) (uterine)
>   uterine:
>   fibromyoma
>   myoma

218.0 Submucous leiomyoma of uterus ♀

218.1 Intramural leiomyoma of uterus ♀
    Interstitial leiomyoma of uterus

218.2 Subserous leiomyoma of uterus ♀
    Subperitoneal leiomyoma of uterus

■**218.9 Leiomyoma of uterus, unspecified ♀**
> Coding Clinic: 2003, Q1, P4-5; 1995, Q4, P50

●**219 Other benign neoplasm of uterus**

219.0 Cervix uteri ♀

219.1 Corpus uteri ♀
    Endometrium   Myometrium
    Fundus

■**219.8 Other specified parts of uterus ♀**

■**219.9 Uterus, part unspecified ♀**

220 Benign neoplasm of ovary ♀
    Use additional code to identify any functional activity
    (256.0–256.1)
> **Excludes**   *cyst:*
>   *corpus albicans (620.2)*
>   *corpus luteum (620.1)*
>   *endometrial (617.1)*
>   *follicular (atretic) (620.0)*
>   *graafian follicle (620.0)*
>   *ovarian NOS (620.2)*
>   *retention (620.2)*

Item 2–8   Teratoma: terat = monster, oma = mass, tumor. Alternate terms: dermoid cyst of the ovary, ovarian teratoma. Teratomas are neoplasms and arise from germ cells (ovaries in female and testes in male) and can be benign or malignant. Teratomas have been known to contain hair, nails, and teeth, giving them a bizarre ("monster") appearance.

●**221 Benign neoplasm of other female genital organs**
> **Includes**   adenomatous polyp
>   benign teratoma
> **Excludes**   *cyst:*
>   *epoophoron (752.11)*
>   *fimbrial (752.11)*
>   *Gartner's duct (752.11)*
>   *parovarian (752.11)*

221.0 Fallopian tube and uterine ligaments ♀
    Oviduct
    Parametrium
    Uterine ligament (broad) (round) (uterosacral)
    Uterine tube

221.1 Vagina ♀

221.2 Vulva ♀
    Clitoris
    External female genitalia NOS
    Greater vestibular [Bartholin's] gland
    Labia (majora) (minora)
    Pudendum
> **Excludes**   *Bartholin's (duct) (gland) cyst (616.2)*

■**221.8 Other specified sites of female genital organs ♀**

■**221.9 Female genital organ, site unspecified ♀**
    Female genitourinary tract NOS

NEOPLASMS (140–239)

● **222   Benign neoplasm of male genital organs**

     222.0   Testis ♂

         Use additional code to identify any functional
           activity

     222.1   Penis ♂

         Corpus cavernosum
         Glans penis
         Prepuce

     222.2   Prostate ♂

         Excludes   *adenomatous hyperplasia of prostate*
                       (600.20–600.21)
                prostatic:
                   adenoma (600.20–600.21)
                   enlargement (600.00–600.01)
                   hypertrophy (600.00–600.01)

     222.3   Epididymis ♂

     222.4   Scrotum ♂

         Skin of scrotum

     ■ **222.8   Other specified sites of male genital organs ♂**

         Seminal vesicle
         Spermatic cord

     ■ **222.9   Male genital organ, site unspecified ♂**

         Male genitourinary tract NOS

● **223   Benign neoplasm of kidney and other urinary organs**

     223.0   Kidney, except pelvis

         Kidney NOS

         Excludes   *benign carcinoid tumors of kidney*
                       (209.64)
                renal:
                   calyces (223.1)
                   pelvis (223.1)

     223.1   Renal pelvis

     223.2   Ureter

         Excludes   *ureteric orifice of bladder (223.3)*

     223.3   Bladder

   ● **223.8   Other specified sites of urinary organs**

         223.81   Urethra

              Excludes   *urethral orifice of bladder (223.3)*

       ■ **223.89   Other**

             Paraurethral glands

     ■ **223.9   Urinary organ, site unspecified**

         Urinary system NOS

● **224   Benign neoplasm of eye**

     Excludes   *cartilage of eyelid (215.0)*
             eyelid (skin) (216.1)
             optic nerve (225.1)
             orbital bone (213.0)

     224.0   Eyeball, except conjunctiva, cornea, retina, and choroid

         Ciliary body
         Iris
         Sclera
         Uveal tract

     224.1   Orbit

         Excludes   *bone of orbit (213.0)*

     224.2   Lacrimal gland

     224.3   Conjunctiva

     224.4   Cornea

     224.5   Retina

         Excludes   *hemangioma of retina (228.03)*

     224.6   Choroid

     224.7   Lacrimal duct

         Lacrimal sac
         Nasolacrimal duct

     ■ **224.8   Other specified parts of eye**

     ■ **224.9   Eye, part unspecified**

● **225   Benign neoplasm of brain and other parts of nervous system**

     Excludes   *hemangioma (228.02)*
             neurofibromatosis (237.7)
             peripheral, sympathetic, and parasympathetic
                   nerves and ganglia (215.0–215.9)
             retrobulbar (224.1)

     225.0   Brain

     225.1   Cranial nerves

         Coding Clinic: 2004, Q4, P111-113

     225.2   Cerebral meninges

         Meninges NOS
         Meningioma (cerebral)

     225.3   Spinal cord

         Cauda equina

     225.4   Spinal meninges

         Spinal meningioma

     ■ **225.8   Other specified sites of nervous system**

     ■ **225.9   Nervous system, part unspecified**

         Nervous system (central) NOS

         Excludes   *meninges NOS (225.2)*

   226   Benign neoplasm of thyroid glands

     Use additional code to identify any functional activity

● **227   Benign neoplasm of other endocrine glands and related structures**

     Use additional code to identify any functional activity

     Excludes   *ovary (220)*
             pancreas (211.6)
             testis (222.0)

     227.0   Adrenal gland

         Suprarenal gland

     227.1   Parathyroid gland

     227.3   Pituitary gland and craniopharyngeal duct (pouch)

         Craniobuccal pouch
         Hypophysis
         Rathke's pouch
         Sella turcica

     227.4   Pineal gland

         Pineal body

     227.5   Carotid body

     227.6   Aortic body and other paraganglia

         Coccygeal body
         Glomus jugulare
         Para-aortic body
         Coding Clinic: 1984, Nov-Dec, P17

     ■ **227.8   Other**

     ■ **227.9   Endocrine gland, site unspecified**

◀ New   ◀▮▮▮ Revised   ~~deleted~~ Deleted   ● Use Additional Digit(s)   ■ Nonspecific Code

● Not first-listed DX   OGCR Official Guidelines   Coding Clinic   Excludes   Includes   Use additional   Code first   Omit code

● 228 **Hemangioma and lymphangioma, any site**

    Includes   angioma (benign) (cavernous) (congenital)
                NOS
              cavernous nevus
              glomus tumor
              hemangioma (benign) (congenital)

    Excludes *benign neoplasm of spleen, except hemangioma and*
                lymphangioma (211.9)
              glomus jugulare (227.6)
              nevus:
                NOS (216.0–216.9)
                blue or pigmented (216.0–216.9)
                vascular (757.32)

Item 2–9 **Hemangiomas** are abnormally dense collections of dilated capillaries that occur on the skin or in internal organs. Hemangiomas are both deep and superficial and undergo a rapid growth phase when the size increases rapidly, followed by a rest phase, in which the tumor changes very little, followed by an involutional phase in which the tumor begins to and can disappear altogether. **Lymphangiomas** or cystic hygroma are benign collections of overgrown lymph vessels and, although rare, may occur anywhere but most commonly on the head and neck of children and infants. Visceral organs, lungs, and gastrointestinal tract may also be involved.

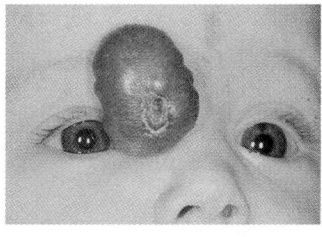

Figure 2–15 Hemangioma of skin and subcutaneous tissue. (From Yanoff: Ophthalmology, 2nd ed. 2004, Mosby, Inc.)

● 228.0 **Hemangioma, any site**
    Coding Clinic: 2001, Q1, P18; 1999, Q2, P9

  ■ **228.00 Of unspecified site**

    228.01 Of skin and subcutaneous tissue
      Coding Clinic: 1988, Q4, P6

    228.02 Of intracranial structures
      Coding Clinic: 1988, Q4, P6; 1985, Jan-Feb, P15

    228.03 Of retina

    228.04 Of intra-abdominal structures
      Peritoneum
      Retroperitoneal tissue
      Coding Clinic: 1988, Q4, P6

  ■ **228.09 Of other sites**
      Systemic angiomatosis
      Coding Clinic: 1991, Q3, P20

  228.1 Lymphangioma, any site
    Congenital lymphangioma
    Lymphatic nevus

● 229 **Benign neoplasm of other and unspecified sites**

  229.0 Lymph nodes

    Excludes *lymphangioma (228.1)*

  ■ **229.8 Other specified sites**
    Intrathoracic NOS
    Thoracic NOS

  ■ **229.9 Site unspecified**

    Includes Bowen's disease
              erythroplasia
              Queyrat's erythroplasia

    Excludes *leukoplakia - see Alphabetic Index*

● 230 **Carcinoma in situ of digestive organs**
    Cancer involving cells in localized tissues that has not spread to nearby tissues

  230.0 Lip, oral cavity, and pharynx
    Gingiva
    Hypopharynx
    Mouth [any part]
    Nasopharynx
    Oropharynx
    Salivary gland or duct
    Tongue

    Excludes *aryepiglottic fold or interarytenoid fold,*
                laryngeal aspect (231.0)
              epiglottis:
                NOS (231.0)
                suprahyoid portion (231.0)
              skin of lip (232.0)

  230.1 Esophagus

  230.2 Stomach
    Body of stomach
    Cardia of stomach
    Fundus of stomach
    Cardiac orifice
    Pylorus

  230.3 Colon
    Appendix
    Cecum
    Ileocecal valve
    Large intestine NOS

    Excludes *rectosigmoid junction (230.4)*

  230.4 Rectum
    Rectosigmoid junction

  230.5 Anal canal
    Anal sphincter

  ■ **230.6 Anus, unspecified**

    Excludes *anus:*
                margin (232.5)
                skin (232.5)
              perianal skin (232.5)

  ■ **230.7 Other and unspecified parts of intestine**
    Duodenum
    Ileum
    Jejunum
    Small intestine NOS

    Excludes *ampulla of Vater (230.8)*

  230.8 Liver and biliary system
    Ampulla of Vater
    Common bile duct
    Cystic duct
    Gallbladder
    Hepatic duct
    Sphincter of Oddi

  ■ **230.9 Other and unspecified digestive organs**
    Digestive organ NOS
    Gastrointestinal tract NOS
    Pancreas
    Spleen

● 231 Carcinoma in situ of respiratory system

    231.0 Larynx

Cartilage:	Epiglottis:
arytenoid	NOS
cricoid	posterior surface
cuneiform	suprahyoid portion
thyroid	Vocal cords (false) (true)

       Excludes *aryepiglottic fold or interarytenoid fold:*
           NOS (230.0)
           hypopharyngeal aspect (230.0)
           marginal zone (230.0)

    231.1 Trachea

    231.2 Bronchus and lung
       Carina
       Hilus of lung

    ■**231.8 Other specified parts of respiratory system**

Accessory sinuses	Nasal cavities
Middle ear	Pleura

       Excludes *ear (external) (skin) (232.2)*
           nose NOS (234.8)
           skin (232.3)

    ■**231.9 Respiratory system, part unspecified**
       Respiratory organ NOS

● 232 Carcinoma in situ of skin

       Includes pigment cells

       Excludes *melanoma in situ of skin (172.0-172.9)*

    232.0 Skin of lip

       Excludes *vermilion border of lip (230.0)*

    232.1 Eyelid, including canthus

    232.2 Ear and external auditory canal

    ■**232.3 Skin of other and unspecified parts of face**

    232.4 Scalp and skin of neck

    232.5 Skin of trunk, except scrotum

Anus, margin	Skin of:
Axillary fold	breast
Perianal skin	buttock
Skin of:	chest wall
abdominal wall	groin
anus	perineum
back	Umbilicus

       Excludes *anal canal (230.5)*
           anus NOS (230.6)
           skin of genital organs (233.30–233.39,
             233.5–233.6)

    232.6 Skin of upper limb, including shoulder

    232.7 Skin of lower limb, including hip

    ■**232.8 Other specified sites of skin**

    ■**232.9 Skin, site unspecified**

● 233 Carcinoma in situ of breast and genitourinary system
    This category incorporates specific male and female
       genitourinary designations (233.0–233.6), while codes
       233.7 and 233.9 apply to either male or female organs.

    233.0 Breast

       Excludes *Paget's disease (174.0–174.9)*
           skin of breast (232.5)

233.1 Cervix uteri ♀
    Adenocarcinoma in situ of cervix
    Cervical intraepithelial glandular neoplasia,
      grade III
    Cervical intraepithelial neoplasia III [CIN III]
    Severe dysplasia of cervix

       Excludes *cervical intraepithelial neoplasia II [CIN II]*
           (622.12)
           cytologic evidence of malignancy without
             histologic confirmation (795.06)
           high grade squamous intraepithelial lesion
             (HGSIL) (795.04)
           moderate dysplasia of cervix (622.12)

      Coding Clinic: 1992, Q3, P7-8; 1991, Q1, P11

■**233.2 Other and unspecified parts of uterus ♀**

● ■**233.3 Other and unspecified female genital organs**
      Coding Clinic: 2007, Q4, P67-68

    ■**233.30 Unspecified female genital organ ♀**

    233.31 Vagina ♀
      Severe dysplasia of vagina
      Vaginal intraepithelial neoplasia
        [VAIN III]

    233.32 Vulva ♀
      Severe dysplasia of vulva
      Vulvar intraepithelial neoplasia
        [VIN III]
      Coding Clinic: 1995, Q1, P8

    233.39 Other female genital organ ♀

    233.4 Prostate ♂

    233.5 Penis ♂

■**233.6 Other and unspecified male genital organs ♂**

    233.7 Bladder

■**233.9 Other and unspecified urinary organs**

● 234 Carcinoma in situ of other and unspecified sites

    234.0 Eye

       Excludes *cartilage of eyelid (234.8)*
           eyelid (skin) (232.1)
           optic nerve (234.8)
           orbital bone (234.8)

■**234.8 Other specified sites**
      Endocrine gland [any]

■**234.9 Site unspecified**
      Carcinoma in situ NOS

NEOPLASMS OF UNCERTAIN BEHAVIOR (235–238)

Note: Categories 235–238 classify by site certain
    histo-morphologically well-defined neoplasms, the
    subsequent behavior of which cannot be predicted
    from the present appearance.

● 235 Neoplasm of uncertain behavior of digestive and
respiratory systems

       Excludes *stromal tumors of uncertain behavior of digestive*
           system (238.1)

    235.0 Major salivary glands
      Gland:
        parotid
        sublingual
        submandibular

       Excludes *minor salivary glands (235.1)*

NEOPLASMS (140–239)

◀ New   ◀■■ Revised   ~~deleted~~ Deleted   ● Use Additional Digit(s)   ■ Nonspecific Code
● Not first-listed DX   OGCR Official Guidelines   Coding Clinic   Excludes   Includes   Use additional   Code first   Omit code

235.1 Lip, oral cavity, and pharynx
Gingiva
Hypopharynx
Minor salivary glands
Mouth
Nasopharynx
Oropharynx
Tongue

> **Excludes**   *aryepiglottic fold or interarytenoid fold,*
>   *laryngeal aspect (235.6)*
>   *epiglottis:*
>   *NOS (235.6)*
>   *suprahyoid portion (235.6)*
>   *skin of lip (238.2)*

235.2 Stomach, intestines, and rectum

235.3 Liver and biliary passages
Ampulla of Vater   Gallbladder
Bile ducts [any]   Liver

235.4 Retroperitoneum and peritoneum

235.5 Other and unspecified digestive organs
Anal: Esophagus
   canal   Pancreas
   sphincter   Spleen
Anus NOS

> **Excludes**   *anus:*
>   *margin (238.2)*
>   *skin (238.2)*
>   *perianal skin (238.2)*

235.6 Larynx

> **Excludes**   *aryepiglottic fold or interarytenoid fold:*
>   *NOS (235.1)*
>   *hypopharyngeal aspect (235.1)*
>   *marginal zone (235.1)*

235.7 Trachea, bronchus, and lung

235.8 Pleura, thymus, and mediastinum

235.9 Other and unspecified respiratory organs
Accessory sinuses
Middle ear
Nasal cavities
Respiratory organ NOS

> **Excludes**   *ear (external) (skin) (238.2)*
>   *nose (238.8)*
>   *skin (238.2)*

● **236 Neoplasm of uncertain behavior of genitourinary organs**

236.0 Uterus ♀

236.1 Placenta ♀
Chorioadenoma (destruens)
Invasive mole
Malignant hydatid(iform) mole

236.2 Ovary ♀
> Use additional code to identify any functional
> activity

236.3 Other and unspecified female genital organs ♀

236.4 Testis ♂
> Use additional code to identify any functional
> activity

236.5 Prostate ♂

236.6 Other and unspecified male genital organs ♂

236.7 Bladder

● **236.9 Other and unspecified urinary organs**

   236.90 Urinary organ, unspecified

   236.91 Kidney and ureter

   236.99 Other

● **237 Neoplasm of uncertain behavior of endocrine glands and nervous system**

237.0 Pituitary gland and craniopharyngeal duct
> Use additional code to identify any functional
> activity

237.1 Pineal gland

237.2 Adrenal gland
Suprarenal gland
> Use additional code to identify any functional
> activity
> *Pair of glands situated on top of or above each kidney*
> *("suprarenal") responsible for regulating stress*
> *response through corticosteroids.*

237.3 Paraganglia
Aortic body
Carotid body
Coccygeal body
Glomus jugulare
Coding Clinic: 1984, Nov-Dec, P17

237.4 Other and unspecified endocrine glands
Parathyroid gland
Thyroid gland

237.5 Brain and spinal cord

237.6 Meninges
Meninges:
   NOS
   cerebral
   spinal

● **237.7 Neurofibromatosis**
> *Disorder of nervous system that causes tumors to grow*
> *around nerves.*
von Recklinghausen's disease

   237.70 Neurofibromatosis, unspecified

   237.71 Neurofibromatosis, type 1 [von Recklinghausen's disease]

   237.72 Neurofibromatosis, type 2 [acoustic neurofibromatosis]

237.9 Other and unspecified parts of nervous system
Cranial nerves

> **Excludes**   *peripheral, sympathetic, and*
>   *parasympathetic nerves and ganglia*
>   *(238.1)*

● **238 Neoplasm of uncertain behavior of other and unspecified sites and tissues**

238.0 Bone and articular cartilage

> **Excludes**   *cartilage:*
>   *ear (238.1)*
>   *eyelid (238.1)*
>   *larynx (235.6)*
>   *nose (235.9)*
>   *synovia (238.1)*
> Coding Clinic: 2004, Q4, P128-129

238.1 Connective and other soft tissue
Peripheral, sympathetic, and parasympathetic
   nerves and ganglia
Stromal tumors of digestive system

> **Excludes**   *cartilage (of):*
>   *articular (238.0)*
>   *larynx (235.6)*
>   *nose (235.9)*
>   *connective tissue of breast (238.3)*

NEOPLASMS (140–239)

238.2 Skin

> **Excludes**   anus NOS (235.5)
> skin of genital organs (236.3, 236.6)
> vermilion border of lip (235.1)

238.3 Breast

> **Excludes**   skin of breast (238.2)

238.4 Polycythemia vera

Primary polycythemia. Secondary polycythemia is 289.0. Check your documentation. Polycythemia is caused by too many red blood cells, which increase thickness of blood (viscosity). This can cause engorgement of the spleen (splenomegaly) with extra RBCs and potential clot formation.

238.5 Histiocytic and mast cells
Mast cell tumor NOS
Mastocytoma NOS

238.6 Plasma cells
Plasmacytoma NOS
Solitary myeloma

● 238.7 Other lymphatic and hematopoietic tissues

> **Excludes**   acute myelogenous leukemia (205.0)
> chronic myelomonocytic leukemia (205.1)
> myelosclerosis NOS (289.89)
> myelosis:
>   NOS (205.9)
>   megakaryocytic (207.2)

Coding Clinic: 2006, Q4, P63-66; 2001, Q3, P13-14; 1997, Q1, P5-6

238.71 Essential thrombocythemia
Essential hemorrhagic thrombocythemia
Essential thrombocytosis
Idiopathic (hemorrhagic) thrombocythemia
Primary thrombocytosis

Coding Clinic: 2006, Q4, P64

238.72 Low grade myelodysplastic syndrome lesions
Refractory anemia (RA)
Refractory anemia with excess blasts-1 (RAEB-1) ◄
Refractory anemia with ringed sideroblasts (RARS)
Refractory cytopenia with multilineage dysplasia (RCMD)
Refractory cytopenia with multilineage dysplasia and ringed sideroblasts (RCMD-RS)

238.73 High grade myelodysplastic syndrome lesions
~~Refractory anemia with excess blasts-1 (RAEB-1)~~
Refractory anemia with excess blasts-2 (RAEB-2)

238.74 Myelodysplastic syndrome with 5q deletion
5q minus syndrome NOS

> **Excludes**   constitutional 5q deletion (758.39)
> high grade myelodysplastic syndrome with 5q deletion (238.73)

238.75 Myelodysplastic syndrome, unspecified

238.76 Myelofibrosis with myeloid metaplasia
Agnogenic myeloid metaplasia
Idiopathic myelofibrosis (chronic)
Myelosclerosis with myeloid metaplasia
Primary myelofibrosis

> **Excludes**   myelofibrosis NOS (289.83)
> myelophthisic anemia (284.2)
> myelophthisis (284.2)
> secondary myelofibrosis (289.83)

● 238.77 *Post-transplant lymphoproliferative disorder (PTLD)*

Code first complications of transplant (996.80-996.89)
Coding Clinic: 2008, Q4, P90-91

238.79 Other lymphatic and hematopoietic tissues
Lymphoproliferative disease (chronic) NO
Megakaryocytic myelosclerosis
Myeloproliferative disease (chronic) NOS
Panmyelosis (acute)

238.8 Other specified sites
Eye
Heart

> **Excludes**   eyelid (skin) (238.2)
> cartilage (238.1)

238.9 Site unspecified

NEOPLASMS OF UNSPECIFIED NATURE (239)

● 239 Neoplasms of unspecified nature

Note: Category 239 classifies by site neoplasms of unspecified morphology and behavior. The term "mass," unless otherwise stated, is not to be regarded as a neoplastic growth.

> **Includes**   "growth" NOS
> neoplasm NOS
> new growth NOS
> tumor NOS

239.0 Digestive system

> **Excludes**   anus:
>   margin (239.2)
>   skin (239.2)
>   perianal skin (239.2)

239.1 Respiratory system

239.2 Bone, soft tissue, and skin

> **Excludes**   anal canal (239.0)
> anus NOS (239.0)
> bone marrow (202.9)
> cartilage:
>   larynx (239.1)
>   nose (239.1)
> connective tissue of breast (239.3)
> skin of genital organs (239.5)
> vermilion border of lip (239.0)

239.3 Breast

> **Excludes**   skin of breast (239.2)

239.4 Bladder

239.5 Other genitourinary organs

239.6 Brain

> **Excludes**   cerebral meninges (239.7)
> cranial nerves (239.7)

239.7 Endocrine glands and other parts of nervous system

> **Excludes**   peripheral, sympathetic, and parasympathetic nerves and ganglia (239.2)

● 239.8 Other specified sites ◄

> **Excludes**   eyelid (skin) (239.2)
> cartilage (239.2)
> great vessels (239.2)
> optic nerve (239.7)

239.81 Retina and choroid ◄
Dark area on retina ◄
Retinal freckle ◄

239.89 Other specified sites ◄

239.9 Site unspecified

◄ New   ◄▥ Revised   ~~deleted~~ Deleted   ● Use Additional Digit(s)   ▧ Nonspecific Code
● Not first-listed DX   OGCR Official Guidelines   Coding Clinic   Excludes   Includes   Use additional   Code first   Omit code

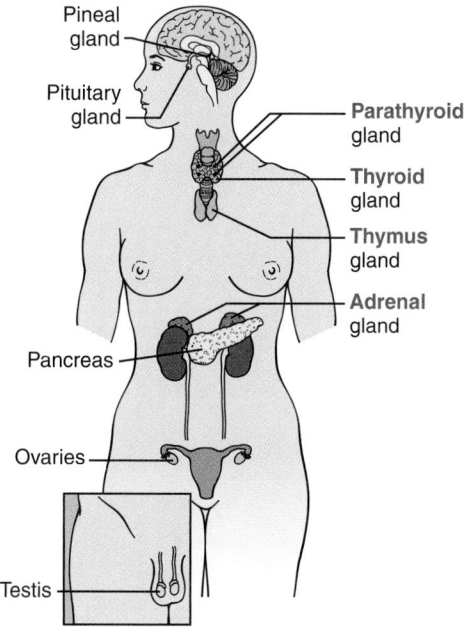

Pineal gland
Pituitary gland
Parathyroid gland
Thyroid gland
Thymus gland
Adrenal gland
Pancreas
Ovaries
Testis

Figure 3–1   The endocrine system. (From Buck CJ: Step-by-Step Medical Coding, 2006 ed. Philadelphia, WB Saunders, 2006.)

Item 3–1   Simple goiter indicates no nodules are present. The most common type of goiter is a **diffuse colloidal,** also called a **nontoxic** or **endemic** goiter. Goiters classifiable to 240.0 or 240.9 are those goiters without mention of nodules.

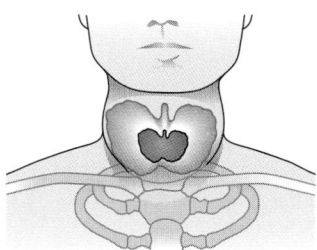

Figure 3–2   Goiter is an enlargement of the thyroid gland.

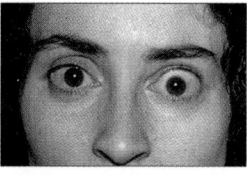

Figure 3–3   Graves' disease. In Graves' disease, exophthalmos often looks more pronounced than it actually is because of the extreme lid retraction that may occur. This patient, for instance, had minimal proptosis of the left eye but marked lid retraction. (Courtesy Dr. HG Scheie. From Yanoff M, Fine BS: Ocular Pathology, ed 5. St. Louis, Mosby, 2002.)

Item 3–2 Thyrotoxicosis is a condition caused by excessive amounts of the thyroid hormone thyroxine production or hyperthyroidism. **Graves' disease is associated with hyperthyroidism** (known as **Basedow's disease** in Europe).

3.   **ENDOCRINE, NUTRITIONAL AND METABOLIC DISEASES, AND IMMUNITY DISORDERS (240–279)**

> **Excludes** *endocrine and metabolic disturbances specific to the fetus and newborn (775.0–775.9)*

Note: All neoplasms, whether functionally active or not, are classified in Chapter 2. Codes in Chapter 3 (i.e., 242.8, 246.0, 251–253, 255–259) may be used to identify such functional activity associated with any neoplasm, or by ectopic endocrine tissue.

DISORDERS OF THYROID GLAND (240–246)

● 240   **Simple and unspecified goiter**

240.0   **Goiter, specified as simple**
Any condition classifiable to 240.9, specified as simple

▪240.9   **Goiter, unspecified**
Enlargement of thyroid   Goiter or struma:
Goiter or struma: hyperplastic
  NOS   nontoxic (diffuse)
  diffuse colloid   parenchymatous
  endemic   sporadic

> **Excludes** *congenital (dyshormonogenic) goiter (246.1)*

● 241   **Nontoxic nodular goiter**

> **Excludes** *adenoma of thyroid (226)*
> *cystadenoma of thyroid (226)*

241.0   **Nontoxic uninodular goiter**
Thyroid nodule
Uninodular goiter (nontoxic)

241.1   **Nontoxic multinodular goiter**
Multinodular goiter (nontoxic)

▪241.9   **Unspecified nontoxic nodular goiter**
Adenomatous goiter
Nodular goiter (nontoxic) NOS
Struma nodosa (simplex)

● 242   **Thyrotoxicosis with or without goiter**

> **Excludes** *neonatal thyrotoxicosis (775.3)*

The following fifth-digit subclassification is for use with category 242:

> **0   without mention of thyrotoxic crisis or storm**
> **1   with mention of thyrotoxic crisis or storm**

● 242.0   **Toxic diffuse goiter**
[0-1]   Basedow's disease
Exophthalmic or toxic goiter NOS
Graves' disease
Primary thyroid hyperplasia

● 242.1   **Toxic uninodular goiter**
[0-1]   Thyroid nodule, toxic or with hyperthyroidism
Uninodular goiter, toxic or with hyperthyroidism

● 242.2   **Toxic multinodular goiter**
[0-1]   Secondary thyroid hyperplasia

● ▪242.3   **Toxic nodular goiter, unspecified**
[0-1]   Adenomatous goiter, toxic or with hyperthyroidism
Nodular goiter, toxic or with hyperthyroidism
Struma nodosa, toxic or with hyperthyroidism
Any condition classifiable to 241.9 specified as toxic or with hyperthyroidism

● 242.4   **Thyrotoxicosis from ectopic thyroid nodule**
[0-1]

242.8 Thyrotoxicosis of other specified origin
[0-1]   Overproduction of thyroid-stimulating hormone [TSH]
Thyrotoxicosis:
    factitia from ingestion of excessive thyroid material

> Use additional E code to identify cause, if drug-induced

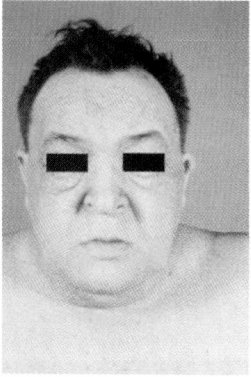

Figure 3–4   Typical appearance of patients with moderately severe primary hypothyroidism or myxedema. (From Larsen: Williams Textbook of Endocrinology, 10th ed. 2003, Saunders, An Imprint of Elsevier)

Item 3–3   Hypothyroidism is a condition in which there are insufficient levels of thyroxine.
Cretinism is congenital hypothyroidism, which can result in mental and physical retardation.

242.9 Thyrotoxicosis without mention of goiter or other
[0-1]   **cause**
Hyperthyroidism NOS
Thyrotoxicosis NOS
Thyrotoxicosis is also known as thyroid storm.

243 Congenital hypothyroidism
Congenital thyroid insufficiency
Cretinism (athyrotic) (endemic)

> Use additional code to identify associated mental retardation

> **Excludes**   *congenital (dyshormonogenic) goiter (246.1)*

244 Acquired hypothyroidism
> **Includes**   athyroidism (acquired)
> hypothyroidism (acquired)
> myxedema (adult) (juvenile)
> thyroid (gland) insufficiency (acquired)

244.0 Postsurgical hypothyroidism

244.1 Other postablative hypothyroidism
Hypothyroidism following therapy, such as irradiation

244.2 Iodine hypothyroidism
Hypothyroidism resulting from administration or ingestion of iodide

> Use additional E code to identify drug

244.3 Other iatrogenic hypothyroidism
Hypothyroidism resulting from:
    P-aminosalicylic acid [PAS]
    Phenylbutazone
    Resorcinol
Iatrogenic hypothyroidism NOS

> Use additional E code to identify drug

244.8 Other specified acquired hypothyroidism
Secondary hypothyroidism NEC
Coding Clinic: 1985, July-Aug, P9

244.9 Unspecified hypothyroidism
Hypothyroidism, primary or NOS
Myxedema, primary or NOS
Coding Clinic: 1999, Q3, P19-20; 1996, Q4, P29

245 Thyroiditis
Inflammation of thyroid gland, results in inability to convert iodine into thyroid hormone. Common types are autoimmune or chronic lymphatic thyroiditis.

245.0 Acute thyroiditis
Abscess of thyroid
Thyroiditis: Thyroiditis:
   nonsuppurative, acute   suppurative
   pyogenic

> Use additional code to identify organism

245.1 Subacute thyroiditis
Thyroiditis: Thyroiditis:
   de Quervain's   granulomatous
   giant cell   viral

245.2 Chronic lymphocytic thyroiditis
Hashimoto's disease   Thyroiditis:
Struma lymphomatosa   autoimmune
                    lymphocytic (chronic)

245.3 Chronic fibrous thyroiditis
Struma fibrosa
Thyroiditis: Thyroiditis:
   invasive (fibrous)   Riedel's
   ligneous

245.4 Iatrogenic thyroiditis
> Use additional E to identify cause

245.8 Other and unspecified chronic thyroiditis
Chronic thyroiditis:
   NOS
   nonspecific

245.9 Thyroiditis, unspecified
Thyroiditis NOS

246 Other disorders of thyroid

246.0 Disorders of thyrocalcitonin secretion
Hypersecretion of calcitonin or thyrocalcitonin

246.1 Dyshormonogenic goiter
Congenital (dyshormonogenic) goiter
Goiter due to enzyme defect in synthesis of thyroid hormone
Goitrous cretinism (sporadic)

246.2 Cyst of thyroid
> **Excludes**   *cystadenoma of thyroid (226)*

246.3 Hemorrhage and infarction of thyroid

246.8 Other specified disorders of thyroid
Abnormality of thyroid-binding globulin
Atrophy of thyroid
Hyper-TBG-nemia
Hypo-TBG-nemia
Coding Clinic: 2006, Q2, P5

246.9 Unspecified disorder of thyroid

◀ New   ◀▥ Revised   ~~deleted~~ Deleted   ● Use Additional Digit(s)   ■ Nonspecific Code
● Not first-listed DX   OGCR Official Guidelines   Coding Clinic   Excludes   Includes   Use additional   Code first   Omit code

DISEASES OF OTHER ENDOCRINE GLANDS (249–259)

OGCR Section I.C.3.a.2
If the type of diabetes mellitus is not documented in the
medical record the default is type II.

● **249 Secondary diabetes mellitus**

Includes diabetes mellitus (due to) (in) (secondary)
(with):
drug-induced or chemical induced
infection

Excludes *gestational diabetes (648.8)*
hyperglycemia NOS (790.29)
neonatal diabetes mellitus (775.1)
nonclinical diabetes (790.29)
Type I diabetes – see category 250
Type II diabetes – see category 250

The following fifth-digit subclassification is for use with
category 249:

> **0 not stated as uncontrolled, or unspecified**
> **1 uncontrolled**

Use additional code to identify any associated insulin
use (V58.67)
Coding Clinic: 2008, Q4, P91-95

● **249.0 Secondary diabetes mellitus without mention of**
[0-1] **complication**
Secondary diabetes mellitus without mention of
complication or manifestation classifiable to
249.1-249.9
Secondary diabetes mellitus NOS

● **249.1 Secondary diabetes mellitus with ketoacidosis**
[0-1] Secondary diabetes mellitus with diabetic
acidosis without mention of coma
Secondary diabetes mellitus with diabetic
ketosis without mention of coma

● **249.2 Secondary diabetes mellitus with**
[0-1] **hyperosmolarity**
Secondary diabetes mellitus with hyperosmolar
(nonketotic) coma

● **249.3 Secondary diabetes mellitus with other coma**
[0-1] Secondary diabetes mellitus with diabetic coma
(with ketoacidosis)
Secondary diabetes mellitus with diabetic
hypoglycemic coma
Secondary diabetes mellitus with insulin coma
NOS

Excludes *secondary diabetes mellitus with*
hyperosmolar coma (249.2)

● **249.4 Secondary diabetes mellitus with renal**
[0-1] **manifestations**
Use additional code to identify manifestation, as:
chronic kidney disease (585.1-585.9)
diabetic nephropathy NOS (583.81)
diabetic nephrosis (581.81)
intercapillary glomerulosclerosis (581.81)
Kimmelstiel-Wilson syndrome (581.81)

● **249.5 Secondary diabetes mellitus with ophthalmic**
[0-1] **manifestations**
Use additional code to identify manifestation, as:
diabetic blindness (369.00-369.9)
diabetic cataract (366.41)
diabetic glaucoma (365.44)
diabetic macular edema (362.07)
diabetic retinal edema (362.07)
diabetic retinopathy (362.01-362.07)

● **249.6 Secondary diabetes mellitus with neurological**
[0-1] **manifestations**
Use additional code to identify manifestation, as:
diabetic amyotrophy (353.5)
diabetic gastroparalysis (536.3)
diabetic gastroparesis (536.3)
diabetic mononeuropathy (354.0-355.9)
diabetic neurogenic arthropathy (713.5)
diabetic peripheral autonomic neuropathy
(337.1)
diabetic polyneuropathy (357.2)
Coding Clinic: 2008, Q4, P91-95

● **249.7 Secondary diabetes mellitus with peripheral**
[0-1] **circulatory disorders**
Use additional code to identify manifestation, as:
diabetic gangrene (785.4)
diabetic peripheral angiopathy (443.81)

● ■ **249.8 Secondary diabetes mellitus with other specified**
[0-1] **manifestations**
Secondary diabetic hypoglycemia in diabetes
mellitus
Secondary hypoglycemic shock in diabetes
mellitus
Use additional code to identify manifestation, as:
any associated ulceration (707.10-707.9)
diabetic bone changes (731.8)

● ■ **249.9 Secondary diabetes mellitus with unspecified**
[0-1] **complication**

● **250 Diabetes mellitus**

Metabolic disease that results in persistent hyperglycemia. The three primary forms of diabetes mellitus are differentiated by patterns of pancreatic failure—type 1, type 2 and 3.

> **Excludes**   *gestational diabetes (648.8)*
> *hyperglycemia NOS (790.29)*
> *neonatal diabetes mellitus (775.1)*
> *nonclinical diabetes (790.29)*
> *secondary diabetes (249.0–249.9)*

The following fifth-digit subclassification is for use with category 250:

> **0   type II or unspecified type, not stated as uncontrolled**
>   Fifth-digit 0 is for use for type II patients, even if the patient requires insulin
>   Use additional code, if applicable, for associated long-term (current) insulin use V58.67
> **1   type I [juvenile type], not stated as uncontrolled**
> **2   type II or unspecified type, uncontrolled**
>   Fifth-digit 2 is for use for type II patients, even if the patient requires insulin
>   Use additional code, if applicable, for associated long-term (current) insulin use V58.67
> **3   type I [juvenile type], uncontrolled**

Coding Clinic: 2006, Q1, P14; 1996, Q3, P5

OGCR   Section I.C.3.a.3

If the documentation in a medical record does not indicate the type of diabetes but does indicate that the patient uses insulin, the appropriate fifth-digit for type II must be used.

● **250.0   Diabetes mellitus without mention of complication**
   [0-3]   Diabetes mellitus without mention of complication or manifestation classifiable to 250.1–250.9
             Diabetes (mellitus) NOS
             Coding Clinic: 2005, Q2, P21-22; Q1, P15; 2004, Q2, P17; 2003, Q4, P105-106, 108-109, P110; Q2, P6-7, 16; Q1, P5; 2002, Q2, P13; Q1, P7-8; 2001, Q2, P16; 1997, Q4, P33; 1994, Q1, P16-17, 21; 1993, Q4, P42; 5th Issue, P15; 1992, Q2, P15; 1990, Q2, P22; 1985, Nov-Dec, P11; Sept-Oct, P11; Mar-April, P12

● **250.1   Diabetes with ketoacidosis**
   [0-3]   Diabetic:
             acidosis without mention of coma
             ketosis without mention of coma
             Coding Clinic: 2006, Q2, P19-20; 2003, Q4, P81-82; 1987, Jan-Feb, P15

● **250.2   Diabetes with hyperosmolarity**
   [0-3]   Hyperosmolar (nonketotic) coma

● **250.3   Diabetes with other coma**
   [0-3]   Diabetic coma (with ketoacidosis)
             Diabetic hypoglycemic coma
             Insulin coma NOS

> **Excludes**   *diabetes with hyperosmolar coma (250.2)*

● **250.4   Diabetes with renal manifestations**
   [0-3]   Use additional code to identify manifestation, as:
             chronic kidney disease (585.1–585.9) diabetic:
                nephropathy NOS (583.81)
                nephrosis (581.81)
                intercapillary glomerulosclerosis (581.81)
                Kimmelstiel-Wilson syndrome (581.81)
             Coding Clinic: 2003, Q1, P20-21; 1987, Sept-Oct, P9

● **250.5   Diabetes with ophthalmic manifestations**
   [0-3]   Use additional code to identify manifestation, as:
             diabetic:
                blindness (369.00–369.9)
                cataract (366.41)
                glaucoma (365.44)
                macular edema (362.07)
                retinal edema (362.07)
                retinopathy (362.01–362.07)
             Coding Clinic: 2005, Q4, P65-67; 1993, Q4, P38; 1985, Sept-Oct, P11

● **250.6   Diabetes with neurological manifestations**
   [0-3]   Use additional code to identify manifestation, as:
             diabetic:
                amyotrophy (353.5)
                gastroparalysis (536.3)
                gastroparesis (536.3)
                mononeuropathy (354.0–355.9)
                neurogenic arthropathy (713.5)
                peripheral autonomic neuropathy (337.1)
                polyneuropathy (357.2)
             Coding Clinic: 2009, Q2, P10; 2008, Q3, P5-6; 2004, Q2, P7; 2003, Q4, P105; 1993, Q2, P6; 5th Issue, P15; 1984, Nov-Dec, P9

● **250.7   Diabetes with peripheral circulatory disorders**
   [0-3]   Use additional code to identify manifestation, as:
             diabetic:
                gangrene (785.4)
                peripheral angiopathy (443.81)
             Coding Clinic: 2004, Q1, P14-15; 2002, Q1, P7-8; 1996, Q1, P10; 1994, Q3, P5; Q2, P17; 1990, Q3, P15; 1986, Mar-April, P12

● ■ **250.8   Diabetes with other specified manifestations**
   [0-3]   Diabetic hypoglycemia NOS
             Hypoglycemic shock NOS

             Use additional code to identify manifestation, as:
                any associated ulceration (707.10–707.9)
                diabetic bone changes (731.8)
             Coding Clinic: 1997, Q4, P43; 1994, Q2, P13

● ■ **250.9   Diabetes with unspecified complication**
   [0-3]   Coding Clinic: 2006, Q1, P14; 1993, Q4, P38; 5th Issue, P15; 5th Issue, P11; 1985, Nov-Dec, P11

● **251 Other disorders of pancreatic internal secretion**

   251.0   Hypoglycemic coma
         Iatrogenic hyperinsulinism
         Non-diabetic insulin coma

         Use additional E code to identify cause, if drug-induced

> **Excludes**   *hypoglycemic coma in diabetes mellitus (249.3, 250.3)*

         Coding Clinic: 1985, Mar-April, P8-9

   ■ **251.1   Other specified hypoglycemia**
         Hyperinsulinism:
           NOS
           ectopic
           functional
         Hyperplasia of pancreatic islet beta cells NOS

> **Excludes**   *hypoglycemia in diabetes mellitus (249.8, 250.8)*
> *hypoglycemia in infant of diabetic mother (775.0)*
> *hypoglycemic coma (251.0)*
> *neonatal hypoglycemia (775.6)*

         Use additional E code to identify cause, if drug-induced
         Coding Clinic: 2003, Q1, P10

◀ New   ◀▥ Revised   ~~deleted~~ Deleted   ● Use Additional Digit(s)   ■ Nonspecific Code
● Not first-listed DX   OGCR Official Guidelines   Coding Clinic   Excludes   Includes   Use additional   Code first   Omit code

251.2 Hypoglycemia, unspecified
    Hypoglycemia:
        NOS
        reactive
        spontaneous

    Excludes *hypoglycemia:*
        with coma (251.0)
        in diabetes mellitus (249.8, 250.8)
        leucine-induced (270.3)
    Coding Clinic: 1985, Mar-April, P8-9

251.3 Postsurgical hypoinsulinemia
    Hypoinsulinemia following complete or partial
        pancreatectomy
    Postpancreatectomy hyperglycemia

    Use additional code to identify (any associated):
        acquired absence of pancreas (V45.79)
        insulin use (V58.67)
        secondary diabetes mellitus (249.00–249.91)

        Excludes *transient hyperglycemia post procedure*
            (790.29)
            transient hypoglycemia post procedure
            (251.2)

251.4 Abnormality of secretion of glucagon
    Hyperplasia of pancreatic islet alpha cells with
        glucagon excess

251.5 Abnormality of secretion of gastrin
    Hyperplasia of pancreatic alpha cells with gastrin
        excess
    Zollinger-Ellison syndrome

251.8 Other specified disorders of pancreatic internal secretion
    Coding Clinic: 1998, Q2, P15

251.9 Unspecified disorder of pancreatic internal secretion
    Islet cell hyperplasia NOS

● **252 Disorders of parathyroid gland**
    Excludes *hungry bone syndrome (275.5)*

● **252.0 Hyperparathyroidism**
    Excludes *ectopic hyperparathyroidism (259.3)*
    Coding Clinic: 2004, Q4, P57-59

    252.00 Hyperparathyroidism, unspecified

    252.01 Primary hyperparathyroidism
        Hyperplasia of parathyroid

    252.02 Secondary hyperparathyroidism, non-renal
        Excludes *secondary hyperparathyroidism (of*
            renal origin) (588.81)

    252.08 Other hyperparathyroidism
        Tertiary hyperparathyroidism

252.1 Hypoparathyroidism
    Parathyroiditis (autoimmune)
    Tetany:
        parathyroid
        parathyroprival

    Excludes *pseudohypoparathyroidism (275.49)*
        pseudopseudohypoparathyroidism (275.49)
        tetany NOS (781.7)
        transitory neonatal hypoparathyroidism
            (775.4)

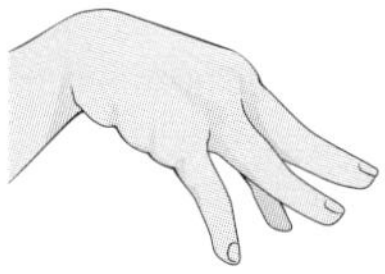

Figure 3–5 Tetany caused by hypoparathyroidism.

Item 3–4 Hyperparathyroidism is an overactive parathyroid gland that secretes excessive parathormone, causing increased levels of circulating calcium. This results in a loss of calcium in the bone (osteoporosis).
Hypoparathyroidism is an underactive parathyroid gland that results in decreased levels of circulating calcium. The primary manifestation is **tetany,** a continuous muscle spasm.

252.8 Other specified disorders of parathyroid gland
    Cyst of parathyroid gland
    Hemorrhage of parathyroid gland

252.9 Unspecified disorder of parathyroid gland

● **253 Disorders of the pituitary gland and its hypothalamic control**
    Includes   the listed conditions whether the disorder is in
            the pituitary or the hypothalamus

    Excludes *Cushing's syndrome (255.0)*

    253.0 Acromegaly and gigantism
        Overproduction of growth hormone

253.1 Other and unspecified anterior pituitary hyperfunction
    Forbes-Albright syndrome

    Excludes *overproduction of:*
        ACTH (255.3)
        thyroid-stimulating hormone [TSH]
            (242.8)
    Coding Clinic: 1985, July-Aug, P9

    253.2 Panhypopituitarism
        Cachexia, pituitary
        Necrosis of pituitary (postpartum)
        Pituitary insufficiency NOS
        Sheehan's syndrome
        Simmonds' disease

        Excludes *iatrogenic hypopituitarism (253.7)*

    253.3 Pituitary dwarfism
        Isolated deficiency of (human) growth hormone
           [HGH]
        Lorain-Levi dwarfism

253.4 Other anterior pituitary disorders
    Isolated or partial deficiency of an anterior
        pituitary hormone, other than growth
        hormone
    Prolactin deficiency
    Coding Clinic: 1985, July-Aug, P9

    253.5 Diabetes insipidus
        Vasopressin deficiency

        Excludes *nephrogenic diabetes insipidus (588.1)*

253.6 Other disorders of neurohypophysis
    Syndrome of inappropriate secretion of antidiuretic
        hormone [ADH]

    Excludes *ectopic antidiuretic hormone secretion*
        (259.3)
    Coding Clinic: 1993, 5th Issue, P8

    253.7 Iatrogenic pituitary disorders
        Hypopituitarism:
           hormone-induced
           hypophysectomy-induced
           postablative
           radiotherapy-induced

        Use additional E code to identify cause

ENDOCRINE, NUTRITIONAL AND METABOLIC DISEASES, AND IMMUNITY DISORDERS (240–279)

ENDOCRINE, NUTRITIONAL AND METABOLIC DISEASES, AND IMMUNITY DISORDERS (240–279)

■253.8 Other disorders of the pituitary and other syndromes of diencephalohypophyseal origin
Abscess of pituitary
Adiposogenital dystrophy
Cyst of Rathke's pouch
Fröhlich's syndrome

Excludes *craniopharyngioma (237.0)*

■253.9 Unspecified
Dyspituitarism

● 254 Diseases of thymus gland

Excludes *aplasia or dysplasia with immunodeficiency (279.2)*
hypoplasia with immunodeficiency (279.2)
myasthenia gravis (358.00–358.01)

254.0 Persistent hyperplasia of thymus
Hypertrophy of thymus

254.1 Abscess of thymus

■254.8 Other specified diseases of thymus gland
Atrophy of thymus
Cyst of thymus

Excludes *thymoma (212.6)*

■254.9 Unspecified disease of thymus gland

● 255 Disorders of adrenal glands

Includes the listed conditions whether the basic disorder is in the adrenals or is pituitary-induced

255.0 Cushing's syndrome
Adrenal hyperplasia due to excess ACTH
Cushing's syndrome:
  NOS
  iatrogenic
  idiopathic
  pituitary-dependent
Ectopic ACTH syndrome
Iatrogenic syndrome of excess cortisol
Overproduction of cortisol

Use additional E code to identify cause, if drug-induced

Excludes *congenital adrenal hyperplasia (255.2)*

● 255.1 Hyperaldosteronism
Coding Clinic: 2003, Q4, P48-50

255.10 Hyperaldosteronism, unspecified
Aldosteronism NOS
Primary aldosteronism, unspecified

Excludes *Conn's syndrome (255.12)*

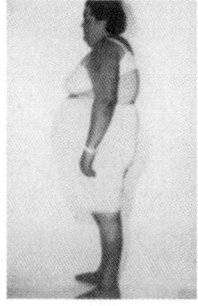

Figure 3–6 Centripetal and generalized obesity and dorsal kyphosis in a 30-year-old woman with Cushing's disease. (From Larsen: Williams Textbook of Endocrinology, 10th ed. 2003, Saunders, An Imprint of Elsevier)

Item 3–5 Hyperadrenalism is overactivity of the adrenal cortex, which secretes corticosterioid hormones. Excessive glucocorticoid hormone results in hyperglycemia (**Cushing's syndrome**), and excessive aldosterone results in **Conn's syndrome. Adrenogenital syndrome** is the result of excessive secretion of androgens, male hormones, which stimulates premature sexual development. **Hypoadrenalism, Addison's disease,** is a condition in which the adrenal glands atrophy.

255.11 Glucocorticoid-remediable aldosteronism
Familial aldosteronism type I

Excludes *Conn's syndrome (255.12)*

255.12 Conn's syndrome

255.13 Bartter's syndrome

■255.14 Other secondary aldosteronism
Coding Clinic: 2006, Q3, P24

255.2 Adrenogenital disorders
Achard-Thiers syndrome
Adrenogenital syndromes, virilizing or feminizing, whether acquired or associated with congenital adrenal hyperplasia consequent on inborn enzyme defects in hormone synthesis
Congenital adrenal hyperplasia
Female adrenal pseudohermaphroditism
Male:
  macrogenitosomia praecox
  sexual precocity with adrenal hyperplasia
Virilization (female) (suprarenal)

Excludes *adrenal hyperplasia due to excess ACTH (255.0)*
isosexual virilization (256.4)

■255.3 Other corticoadrenal overactivity
Acquired benign adrenal androgenic overactivity
Overproduction of ACTH

● 255.4 Corticoadrenal insufficiency

Excludes *tuberculous Addison's disease (017.6)*

Coding Clinic: 2006, Q3, P24; 1985, July-Aug, P8

255.41 Glucocorticoid deficiency
Addisonian crisis
Addison's disease NOS
Adrenal atrophy (autoimmune)
Adrenal calcification
Adrenal crisis
Adrenal hemorrhage
Adrenal infarction
Adrenal insufficiency NOS
Combined glucocorticoid and mineralocorticoid deficiency
Corticoadrenal insufficiency NOS
Coding Clinic: 2007, Q4, P68-70

255.42 Mineralocorticoid deficiency
Hypoaldosteronism

Excludes *combined glucocorticoid and mineralocorticoid deficiency (255.41)*

Coding Clinic: 2006, Q3, P24

■255.5 Other adrenal hypofunction
Adrenal medullary insufficiency

Excludes *Waterhouse-Friderichsen syndrome (meningococcal) (036.3)*

255.6 Medulloadrenal hyperfunction
Catecholamine secretion by pheochromocytoma

■255.8 Other specified disorders of adrenal glands
Abnormality of cortisol-binding globulin
Coding Clinic: 1985, July-Aug, P8

■255.9 Unspecified disorder of adrenal glands

● 256 Ovarian dysfunction

256.0 Hyperestrogenism ♀

■256.1 Other ovarian hyperfunction ♀
Hypersecretion of ovarian androgens
Coding Clinic: 1995, Q3, P15

◀ New   ◀▥ Revised   ~~deleted~~ Deleted   ● Use Additional Digit(s)   ■ Nonspecific Code
● Not first-listed DX   OGCR Official Guidelines   Coding Clinic   Excludes   Includes   Use additional   Code first   Omit code

256.2 Postablative ovarian failure ♀
Ovarian failure:
iatrogenic
postirradiation
postsurgical

Use additional code for states associated with artificial menopause (627.4)

Excludes acquired absence of ovary (V45.77)
asymptomatic age-related (natural) postmenopausal status (V49.81)

Coding Clinic: 2002, Q2, P12-13

● **256.3 Other ovarian failure**

Use additional code for states associated with natural menopause (627.4)

Excludes asymptomatic age-related (natural) postmenopausal status (V49.81)

256.31 Premature menopause ♀ A

256.39 Other ovarian failure ♀
Delayed menarche
Ovarian hypofunction
Primary ovarian failure NOS

256.4 Polycystic ovaries ♀
Isosexual virilization Stein-Leventhal syndrome

256.8 Other ovarian dysfunction ♀

256.9 Unspecified ovarian dysfunction ♀

● **257 Testicular dysfunction**

257.0 Testicular hyperfunction ♂
Hypersecretion of testicular hormones

257.1 Postablative testicular hypofunction ♂
Testicular hypofunction:
iatrogenic
postirradiation
postsurgical

257.2 Other testicular hypofunction
Defective biosynthesis of testicular androgen
Eunuchoidism:
NOS
hypogonadotropic
Failure:
Leydig's cell, adult
seminiferous tubule, adult
Testicular hypogonadism

Excludes azoospermia (606.0)

257.8 Other testicular dysfunction

Excludes androgen insensitivity syndrome (259.50–259.52)

257.9 Unspecified testicular dysfunction ♂

● **258 Polyglandular dysfunction and related disorders**

● **258.0 Polyglandular activity in multiple endocrine adenomatosis**
Multiple endocrine neoplasia [MEN] syndromes

Use additional codes to identify any malignancies and other conditions associated with the syndromes

258.01 Multiple endocrine neoplasia [MEN] type I
Wermer's syndrome
Coding Clinic: 2008, Q4, P85-90; 2007, Q4, P70-72

258.02 Multiple endocrine neoplasia [MEN] type IIA
Sipple's syndrome

258.03 Multiple endocrine neoplasia [MEN] type IIB

258.1 Other combinations of endocrine dysfunction
Lloyd's syndrome
Schmidt's syndrome

258.8 Other specified polyglandular dysfunction

258.9 Polyglandular dysfunction, unspecified

● **259 Other endocrine disorders**

259.0 Delay in sexual development and puberty, not elsewhere classified
Delayed puberty

259.1 Precocious sexual development and puberty, not elsewhere classified P
Sexual precocity:
NOS
constitutional
cryptogenic
idiopathic

259.2 Carcinoid syndrome
Hormone secretion by carcinoid tumors
Coding Clinic: 2008, Q4, P85-90

259.3 Ectopic hormone secretion, not elsewhere classified
Ectopic:
antidiuretic hormone secretion [ADH]
hyperparathyroidism

Excludes ectopic ACTH syndrome (255.0)

259.4 Dwarfism, not elsewhere classified
Dwarfism:
NOS
constitutional

Excludes dwarfism:
achondroplastic (756.4)
intrauterine (759.7)
nutritional (263.2)
pituitary (253.3)
renal (588.0)
progeria (259.8)

● **259.5 Androgen insensitivity syndrome**
Coding Clinic: 2008, Q4, P95-96; 2005, Q4, P53-54

259.50 Androgen insensitivity, unspecified

259.51 Androgen insensitivity syndrome
Complete androgen insensitivity
de Quervain's syndrome
Goldberg-Maxwell Syndrome

259.52 Partial androgen insensitivity
Partial androgen insensitivity syndrome
Reifenstein syndrome

259.8 Other specified endocrine disorders
Pineal gland dysfunction
Progeria
Werner's syndrome

259.9 Unspecified endocrine disorder
Disturbance:
endocrine NOS
hormone NOS
Infantilism NOS

NUTRITIONAL DEFICIENCIES (260–269)

Excludes deficiency anemias (280.0–281.9)

260 Kwashiorkor
Nutritional edema with dyspigmentation of skin and hair

261 Nutritional marasmus
Nutritional atrophy
Severe calorie deficiency
Severe malnutrition NOS
Coding Clinic: 2007, Q4, P96-97; 2006, Q3, P14-15; Q2, P12

ENDOCRINE, NUTRITIONAL AND METABOLIC DISEASES, AND IMMUNITY DISORDERS (240–279)

■262 Other severe protein-calorie malnutrition
Nutritional edema without mention of dyspigmentation of skin and hair
Coding Clinic: 1985, July-Aug, P12-13

● 263 Other and unspecified protein-calorie malnutrition

263.0 Malnutrition of moderate degree
Coding Clinic: 1985, July-Aug, P12-13

263.1 Malnutrition of mild degree
Coding Clinic: 1985, July-Aug, P12-13

263.2 Arrested development following protein-calorie malnutrition
Nutritional dwarfism
Physical retardation due to malnutrition

■263.8 Other protein-calorie malnutrition

■263.9 Unspecified protein-calorie malnutrition
Dystrophy due to malnutrition
Malnutrition (calorie) NOS

> **Excludes** *nutritional deficiency NOS (269.9)*

Coding Clinic: 2006, Q2, P12; 2003, Q4, P109-110; 1984, Nov-Dec, P19

● 264 Vitamin A deficiency

264.0 With conjunctival xerosis

264.1 With conjunctival xerosis and Bitot's spot
Bitot's spot in the young child

264.2 With corneal xerosis

264.3 With corneal ulceration and xerosis

264.4 With keratomalacia

264.5 With night blindness

264.6 With xerophthalmic scars of cornea

■264.7 Other ocular manifestations of vitamin A deficiency
Xerophthalmia due to vitamin A deficiency

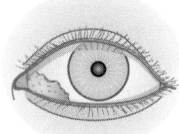

Figure 3-7   Bitot's spot on the conjunctiva.

Item 3-6   Bitot's spots are the result of a buildup of keratin debris found on the superficial surface the conjunctiva; oval, triangular, or irregular in shape; and a sign of vitamin A deficiency and associated with night blindness. The disease may progress to **keratomalacia,** which can result in eventual prolapse of the iris and loss of the lens.

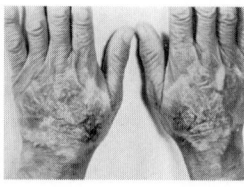

Figure 3-8   The sharply demarcated, characteristic scaling dermatitis of pellagra. (From Kumar: Robbins and Cotran: Pathologic Basis of Disease, 7th ed. 2005, Saunders, An Imprint of Elsevier)

Item 3-7   Pellagra is associated with a deficiency of niacin and its precursor, **tryptophan.** Characteristics of the condition include diarrhea, dermatitis on exposed skin surfaces, dementia, and death. It is prevalent in developing countries where nutrition is inadequate. **Beriberi** is associated with thiamine deficiency.

■264.8 Other manifestations of vitamin A deficiency
Follicular keratosis due to vitamin A deficiency
Xeroderma due to vitamin A deficiency

■264.9 Unspecified vitamin A deficiency
Hypovitaminosis A NOS

● 265 Thiamine and niacin deficiency states

265.0 Beriberi

■265.1 Other and unspecified manifestations of thiamine deficiency
Other vitamin B_1 deficiency states

265.2 Pellagra
Deficiency:
niacin (-tryptophan)
nicotinamide
nicotinic acid
vitamin PP
Pellagra (alcoholic)

● 266 Deficiency of B-complex components

266.0 Ariboflavinosis
Riboflavin [vitamin B_2] deficiency
Coding Clinic: 1986, Sept-Oct, P10

266.1 Vitamin B_6 deficiency
Deficiency:
pyridoxal
pyridoxamine
pyridoxine
Vitamin B_6 deficiency syndrome

> **Excludes** *vitamin B_6-responsive sideroblastic anemia (285.0)*

■266.2 Other B-complex deficiencies
Deficiency:
cyanocobalamin
folic acid
vitamin B_{12}

> **Excludes** *combined system disease with anemia (281.0–281.1)*
> *deficiency anemias (281.0–281.9)*
> *subacute degeneration of spinal cord with anemia (281.0–281.1)*

■266.9 Unspecified vitamin B deficiency

267 Ascorbic acid deficiency
Deficiency of vitamin C
Scurvy

> **Excludes** *scorbutic anemia (281.8)*

● 268 Vitamin D deficiency

> **Excludes** *vitamin D-resistant:*
> *osteomalacia (275.3)*
> *rickets (275.3)*

268.0 Rickets, active

> **Excludes** *celiac rickets (579.0)*
> *renal rickets (588.0)*

●■268.1 *Rickets, late effect*
Any condition specified as due to rickets and stated to be a late effect or sequela of rickets

> *Code first the nature of late effect*

■268.2 Osteomalacia, unspecified
Softening of bone

■268.9 Unspecified vitamin D deficiency
Avitaminosis D

◄ New   ◄▥ Revised   ~~deleted~~ Deleted   ● Use Additional Digit(s)   ■ Nonspecific Code
● Not first-listed DX   OGCR Official Guidelines   Coding Clinic   Excludes   Includes   Use additional   Code first   Omit code

● 269   **Other nutritional deficiencies**

     269.0   Deficiency of vitamin K

         Excludes   *deficiency of coagulation factor due to*
vitamin K deficiency (286.7)
vitamin K deficiency of newborn (776.0)

     ■**269.1   Deficiency of other vitamins**
Deficiency:
     vitamin E
     vitamin P

     ■**269.2   Unspecified vitamin deficiency**
Multiple vitamin deficiency NOS

     269.3   Mineral deficiency, not elsewhere classified
Deficiency:
     calcium, dietary
     iodine

         Excludes   *deficiency:*
calcium NOS (275.40)
potassium (276.8)
sodium (276.1)

     ■**269.8   Other nutritional deficiency**

         Excludes   *adult failure to thrive (783.7)*
failure to thrive in childhood (783.41)
feeding problems (783.31)
newborn (779.31–779.34) ◀▥

     ■**269.9   Unspecified nutritional deficiency**

OTHER METABOLIC AND IMMUNITY DISORDERS (270–279)

Use additional code to identify any associated mental
retardation

● 270   **Disorders of amino-acid transport and metabolism**

         Excludes   *abnormal findings without manifest disease*
(790.0–796.9)
disorders of purine and pyrimidine metabolism
(277.1–277.2)
gout (274.00–274.9) ◀▥

     270.0   Disturbances of amino-acid transport
Cystinosis
Cystinuria
Fanconi (-de Toni) (-Debré) syndrome
Glycinuria (renal)
Hartnup disease

     270.1   Phenylketonuria [PKU]
Hyperphenylalaninemia

     ■**270.2   Other disturbances of aromatic amino-acid**
metabolism
Albinism
Alkaptonuria
Alkaptonuric ochronosis
Disturbances of metabolism of tyrosine and
     tryptophan
Homogentisic acid defects
Hydroxykynureninuria
Hypertyrosinemia
Indicanuria
Kynureninase defects
Oasthouse urine disease
Ochronosis
Tyrosinosis
Tyrosinuria
Waardenburg syndrome

         Excludes   *vitamin B₆-deficiency syndrome (266.1)*

         Coding Clinic: 1999, Q3, P20-21

     270.3   Disturbances of branched-chain amino-acid
metabolism
Disturbances of metabolism of leucine, isoleucine,
     and valine
Hypervalinemia
Intermittent branched-chain ketonuria
Leucine-induced hypoglycemia
Leucinosis
Maple syrup urine disease
     Coding Clinic: 2000, Q3, P8

     270.4   Disturbances of sulphur-bearing amino-acid
metabolism
Cystathioninemia
Cystathioninuria
Disturbances of metabolism of methionine,
     homocystine, and cystathionine
Homocystinuria
Hypermethioninemia
Methioninemia
     Coding Clinic: 2007, Q2, P9; 2004, Q1, P6

     270.5   Disturbances of histidine metabolism
Carnosinemia   Hyperhistidinemia
Histidinemia   Imidazole
                          aminoaciduria

     270.6   Disorders of urea cycle metabolism
Argininosuccinic aciduria
Citrullinemia
Disorders of metabolism of ornithine, citrulline,
     argininosuccinic acid, arginine, and ammonia
Hyperammonemia
Hyperornithinemia

     ■**270.7   Other disturbances of straight-chain amino-acid**
metabolism
Glucoglycinuria
Glycinemia (with methylmalonic acidemia)
Hyperglycinemia
Hyperlysinemia
Pipecolic acidemia
Saccharopinuria
Other disturbances of metabolism of glycine,
     threonine, serine, glutamine, and lysine
     Coding Clinic: 2000, Q3, P8

> **Item 3–8**   Any term ending with "emia" will be a blood
> condition. Any term ending with "uria" will have to do
> with urine. A term ending with "opathy" is a disease
> condition. Check for laboratory work.

     ■**270.8   Other specified disorders of amino-acid metabolism**
Alaninemia   Iminoacidopathy
Ethanolaminuria   Prolinemia
Glycoprolinuria   Prolinuria
Hydroxyprolinemia   Sarcosinemia
Hyperprolinemia

     ■**270.9   Unspecified disorder of amino-acid metabolism**

● 271   **Disorders of carbohydrate transport and metabolism**

         Excludes   *abnormality of secretion of glucagon (251.4)*
diabetes mellitus (249.0–249.9, 250.0–250.9)
hypoglycemia NOS (251.2)
mucopolysaccharidosis (277.5)

     271.0   Glycogenosis
Amylopectinosis
Glucose-6-phosphatase deficiency
Glycogen storage disease
McArdle's disease
Pompe's disease
von Gierke's disease
     Coding Clinic: 1998, Q1, P5-6

271.1 Galactosemia
Galactose-1-phosphate uridyl transferase deficiency
Galactosuria

271.2 Hereditary fructose intolerance
Essential benign fructosuria
Fructosemia

271.3 Intestinal disaccharidase deficiencies and disaccharide malabsorption
Intolerance or malabsorption (congenital) (of):
    glucose-galactose
    lactose
    sucrose-isomaltose

271.4 Renal glycosuria
Renal diabetes

■271.8 Other specified disorders of carbohydrate transport and metabolism
Essential benign pentosuria   Mannosidosis
Fucosidosis   Oxalosis
Glycolic aciduria   Xylosuria
Hyperoxaluria (primary)   Xylulosuria

■271.9 Unspecified disorder of carbohydrate transport and metabolism

● **272 Disorders of lipoid metabolism**

> **Excludes** *localized cerebral lipidoses (330.1)*

272.0 Pure hypercholesterolemia
Familial hypercholesterolemia
Fredrickson Type IIa hyperlipoproteinemia
Hyperbetalipoproteinemia
Hyperlipidemia, Group A
Low-density-lipoid-type [LDL]
    hyperlipoproteinemia
Coding Clinic: 2005, Q4, P68-69

272.1 Pure hyperglyceridemia
Endogenous hyperglyceridemia
Fredrickson Type IV hyperlipoproteinemia
Hyperlipidemia, Group B
Hyperprebetalipoproteinemia
Hypertriglyceridemia, essential
Very-low-density-lipoid-type [VLDL]
    hyperlipoproteinemia
Coding Clinic: 1985, Jan-Feb, P15

272.2 Mixed hyperlipidemia
Broad- or floating-betalipoproteinemia
Combined hyperlipidemia ◄
Elevated cholesterol with elevated
    triglycerides NEC ◄
Fredrickson Type IIb or III hyperlipoproteinemia
Hypercholesterolemia with endogenous
    hyperglyceridemia
Hyperbetalipoproteinemia with
    prebetalipoproteinemia
Tubo-eruptive xanthoma
Xanthoma tuberosum

272.3 Hyperchylomicronemia
Bürger-Grütz syndrome
Fredrickson type I or V hyperlipoproteinemia
Hyperlipidemia, Group D
Mixed hyperglyceridemia

■272.4 Other and unspecified hyperlipidemia
Alpha-lipoproteinemia
~~Combined hyperlipidemia~~
Hyperlipidemia NOS
Hyperlipoproteinemia NOS
Coding Clinic: 2005, Q1, P17

272.5 Lipoprotein deficiencies
Abetalipoproteinemia
Bassen-Kornzweig syndrome
High-density lipoid deficiency
Hypoalphalipoproteinemia
Hypobetalipoproteinemia (familial)

272.6 Lipodystrophy
Barraquer-Simons disease
Progressive lipodystrophy

> Use additional E code to identify cause, if iatrogenic

> **Excludes** *intestinal lipodystrophy (040.2)*

272.7 Lipidoses
Chemically induced lipidosis
Disease:
    Anderson's
    Fabry's
    Gaucher's
    I cell [mucolipidosis I]
    lipoid storage NOS
    Niemann-Pick
    pseudo-Hurler's or mucolipidosis III
    triglyceride storage, Type I or II
    Wolman's or triglyceride storage, Type III
Mucolipidosis II
Primary familial xanthomatosis

> **Excludes** *cerebral lipidoses (330.1)*
> *Tay-Sachs disease (330.1)*

■272.8 Other disorders of lipoid metabolism
Hoffa's disease or liposynovitis prepatellaris
Launois-Bensaude's lipomatosis
Lipoid dermatoarthritis

■272.9 Unspecified disorder of lipoid metabolism

● **273 Disorders of plasma protein metabolism**

> **Excludes** *agammaglobulinemia and*
> *hypogammaglobulinemia (279.0–279.2)*
> *coagulation defects (286.0–286.9)*
> *hereditary hemolytic anemias (282.0–282.9)*

273.0 Polyclonal hypergammaglobulinemia
Hypergammaglobulinemic purpura:
    benign primary
    Waldenström's

273.1 Monoclonal paraproteinemia
Benign monoclonal hypergammaglobulinemia
    [BMH]
Monoclonal gammopathy:
    NOS
    associated with lymphoplasmacytic dyscrasias
    benign
Paraproteinemia:
    benign (familial)
    secondary to malignant or inflammatory disease

■273.2 Other paraproteinemias
Cryoglobulinemic:
    purpura
    vasculitis
Mixed cryoglobulinemia
Coding Clinic: 2008, Q2, P17

273.3 Macroglobulinemia
Macroglobulinemia (idiopathic) (primary)
Waldenström's macroglobulinemia

273.4 Alpha-1-antitrypsin deficiency
AAT deficiency
Coding Clinic: 2004, Q4, P59-60

■273.8 Other disorders of plasma protein metabolism
Abnormality of transport protein
Bisalbuminemia
Coding Clinic: 1998, Q2, P11

■273.9 Unspecified disorder of plasma protein metabolism
Coding Clinic: 1998, Q2, P11

● **274   Gout**
> *Result of accumulation of uric acid caused by either too much production, or insufficient natural removal of uric acid from body. Results in swollen, red, hot, painful, stiff joints. Also called gouty arthritis.*

> **Excludes**   lead gout (984.0–984.9)

● **274.0   Gouty arthropathy** ◀▥

    274.00   Gouty arthropathy, unspecified ◀

    274.01   Acute gouty arthropathy ◀
        Acute gout ◀
        Gout attack ◀
        Gout flare ◀
        Podagra ◀

    274.02   Chronic gouty arthropathy without mention of tophus (tophi) ◀
        Chronic gout ◀

    274.03   Chronic gouty arthropathy with tophus (tophi) ◀
        Chronic tophaceous gout ◀
        Gout with tophi NOS ◀

● **274.1   Gouty nephropathy**

    ■**274.10   Gouty nephropathy, unspecified**
        Coding Clinic: 1985, Nov-Dec, P15

    274.11   Uric acid nephrolithiasis

    ■**274.19   Other**

● **274.8   Gout with other specified manifestations**
> *Tophi = chalky deposit of sodium urate occurring in gout*

    274.81   Gouty tophi of ear

    ■**274.82   Gouty tophi of other sites**
        Gouty tophi of heart

>   **Excludes**   gout with tophi NOS (274.03) ◀
>   gouty arthroplasty with tophi (274.03) ◀

    ■**274.89   Other**
        Use additional code to identify manifestations, as:
        gouty:
          iritis (364.11)
          neuritis (357.4)

    ■**274.9   Gout, unspecified**

● **275   Disorders of mineral metabolism**

> **Excludes**   abnormal findings without manifest disease (790.0–796.9)

    275.0   Disorders of iron metabolism
        Bronzed diabetes
        Hemochromatosis
        Pigmentary cirrhosis (of liver)

>   **Excludes**   anemia:
>   iron deficiency (280.0–280.9)
>   sideroblastic (285.0)

        Coding Clinic: 1997, Q2, P11

    275.1   Disorders of copper metabolism
        Hepatolenticular degeneration
        Wilson's disease

    275.2   Disorders of magnesium metabolism
        Hypermagnesemia
        Hypomagnesemia

    275.3   Disorders of phosphorus metabolism
        Familial hypophosphatemia
        Hypophosphatasia
        Vitamin D-resistant:
          osteomalacia
          rickets

    275.4   Disorders of calcium metabolism

>   **Excludes**   hungry bone syndrome (275.5)
>   parathyroid disorders (252.00–252.9)
>   vitamin D deficiency (268.0–268.9)

    ■**275.40   Unspecified disorder of calcium metabolism**

    275.41   Hypocalcemia
        Coding Clinic: 2007, Q3, P5-6

    275.42   Hypercalcemia
        Coding Clinic: 2003, Q4, P110

    ■**275.49   Other disorders of calcium metabolism**
        Nephrocalcinosis
        Pseudohypoparathyroidism
        Pseudopseudohypoparathyroidism

    275.5   Hungry bone syndrome
        Coding Clinic: 2008, Q4, P96-97

■**275.8   Other specified disorders of mineral metabolism**

■**275.9   Unspecified disorder of mineral metabolism**

● **276   Disorders of fluid, electrolyte, and acid-base balance**

> **Excludes**   diabetes insipidus (253.5)
>   familial periodic paralysis (359.3)

    276.0   Hyperosmolality and/or hypernatremia
        Sodium [Na] excess
        Sodium [Na] overload

    276.1   Hyposmolality and/or hyponatremia
        Sodium [Na] deficiency

    276.2   Acidosis
        Acidosis:
          NOS   metabolic
          lactic   respiratory

>   **Excludes**   diabetic acidosis (249.1, 250.1)

        Coding Clinic: 1987, Jan-Feb, P15

    276.3   Alkalosis
        Alkalosis:
          NOS
          metabolic
          respiratory

    276.4   Mixed acid-base balance disorder
        Hypercapnia with mixed acid-base disorder

> **Item 3–9** Circulating fluid volume is regulated by the amount of water and sodium ingested, excreted by the kidneys into the urine, and lost through the gastrointestinal tract, lungs, and skin. To maintain blood volume within a normal range, the kidneys regulate the amount of water and sodium lost into the urine. Too much **(fluid overload)** or too little fluid volume **(volume depletion)** will affect blood pressure. Severe cases of vomiting, diarrhea, bleeding, and burns (fluid loss through exposed burn surface area) can contribute to fluid loss. Internal body environment must maintain a precise balance (homeostasis) between too much fluid and too little fluid. This complex balancing mechanism is critical to good health.

● **276.5   Volume depletion**

>   **Excludes**   hypovolemic shock:
>   postoperative (998.0)
>   traumatic (958.4)

        Coding Clinic: 2005, Q4, P54-55; Q2, P9-10; 2003, Q1, P5, 20-22; 2002, Q3, P21x2; 1997, Q4, P30-31; 1993, 5th Issue, P1; 1988, Q2, P9-11; 1984, July-Aug, P19-20

    ■**276.50   Volume depletion, unspecified**

    276.51   Dehydration
        Coding Clinic: 2008, Q1, P10-11

    276.52   Hypovolemia
        Depletion of volume of plasma

ENDOCRINE, NUTRITIONAL AND METABOLIC DISEASES, AND IMMUNITY DISORDERS (240–279)

ENDOCRINE, NUTRITIONAL AND METABOLIC DISEASES, AND IMMUNITY DISORDERS (240–279)

276.6 Fluid overload
Fluid retention

> **Excludes** *ascites (789.51–789.59)*
> *localized edema (782.3)*
> Coding Clinic: 2007, Q3, P11; 2006, Q4, P136; 1987, Sept-Oct, P9

276.7 Hyperpotassemia
Hyperkalemia
Potassium [K]:   Potassium [K]:
  excess   overload
  intoxication
Coding Clinic: 2005, Q1, P9-10; 2001, Q2, P12-13

276.8 Hypopotassemia
Hypokalemia
Potassium [K] deficiency

■**276.9 Electrolyte and fluid disorders not elsewhere classified**
Electrolyte imbalance
Hyperchloremia
Hypochloremia

> **Excludes** *electrolyte imbalance:*
> *associated with hyperemesis gravidarum*
> *(643.1)*
> *complicating labor and delivery (669.0)*
> *following abortion and ectopic or molar*
> *pregnancy (634–638 with .4,*
> *639.4)*
> Coding Clinic: 1987, Jan-Feb, P15

●**277 Other and unspecified disorders of metabolism**

●**277.0 Cystic fibrosis**
Fibrocystic disease of the pancreas
Mucoviscidosis
Coding Clinic: 2002, Q4, P45-46; 1994, Q3, P7; 1990, Q3, P18

277.00 Without mention of meconium ileus
Cystic fibrosis NOS
Coding Clinic: 2003, Q2, P12

277.01 With meconium ileus   N
Meconium:
  ileus (of newborn)
  obstruction of intestine in mucoviscidosis

277.02 With pulmonary manifestations
Cystic fibrosis with pulmonary exacerbation

> Use additional code to identify any
> infectious organism present, such as:
> pseudomonas (041.7)
> Coding Clinic: 2002, Q4, P46

277.03 With gastrointestinal manifestations

> **Excludes** *with meconium ileus (277.01)*

■**277.09 With other manifestations**

277.1 Disorders of porphyrin metabolism
Hematoporphyria   Porphyrinuria
Hematoporphyrinuria   Protocoproporphyria
Hereditary coproporphyria   Protoporphyria
Porphyria   Pyrroloporphyria

■**277.2 Other disorders of purine and pyrimidine metabolism**
Hypoxanthine-guanine-phosphoribosyltransferase
deficiency [HG-PRT deficiency]
Lesch-Nyhan syndrome
Xanthinuria

> **Excludes** *gout (274.00–274.9)*   ◀▥
> *orotic aciduric anemia (281.4)*

●**277.3 Amyloidosis**
Disorder resulting from abnormal deposition of
particular protein (amyloid) into tissues.
Coding Clinic: 2006, Q4, P66-67; 1997, Q2, P12-13; 1996, Q1, P16;
1985, July-Aug, P9

■**277.30 Amyloidosis, unspecified**
Amyloidosis NOS

277.31 Familial Mediterranean fever
Benign paroxysmal peritonitis
Hereditary amyloid nephropathy
Periodic familial polyserositis
Recurrent polyserositis

■**277.39 Other amyloidosis**
Hereditary cardiac amyloidosis
Inherited systemic amyloidosis
Neuropathic (Portuguese) (Swiss)
  amyloidosis
Secondary amyloidosis
Coding Clinic: 2009, Q1, P17; 2008, Q2, P8-9

277.4 Disorders of bilirubin excretion
Hyperbilirubinemia:
  congenital
  constitutional
Syndrome:
  Crigler-Najjar
  Dubin-Johnson
  Gilbert's
  Rotor's

> **Excludes** *hyperbilirubinemias specific to the perinatal*
> *period (774.0–774.7)*

277.5 Mucopolysaccharidosis
Gargoylism
Hunter's syndrome
Hurler's syndrome
Lipochondrodystrophy
Maroteaux-Lamy syndrome
Morquio-Brailsford disease
Osteochondrodystrophy
Sanfilippo's syndrome
Scheie's syndrome

■**277.6 Other deficiencies of circulating enzymes**
Hereditary angioedema
Coding Clinic: 2004, Q4, P59-60

277.7 Dysmetabolic syndrome X

> Use additional code for associated manifestation,
> such as:
> cardiovascular disease (414.00–414.07)
> obesity (278.00–278.01)
> Coding Clinic: 2001, Q4, P42

●**277.8 Other specified disorders of metabolism**
Coding Clinic: 2003, Q4, P50-51; 2001, Q2, P18-20

277.81 Primary carnitine deficiency

277.82 Carnitine deficiency due to inborn errors of metabolism

277.83 Iatrogenic carnitine deficiency
Carnitine deficiency due to:
  Hemodialysis
  Valproic acid therapy

277.84 Other secondary carnitine deficiency

277.85 Disorders of fatty acid oxidation
Carnitine palmitoyltransferase deficiencies
  (CPT1, CPT2)
Glutaric aciduria type II (type IIA, IIB, IIC)
Long chain 3-hydroxyacyl CoA
  dehydrogenase deficiency (LCHAD)
Long chain/very long chain acyl CoA
  dehydrogenase deficiency (LCAD,
  VLCAD)
Medium chain acyl CoA dehydrogenase
  deficiency (MCAD)
Short chain acyl CoA dehydrogenase
  deficiency (SCAD)

> **Excludes** *primary carnitine deficiency*
> *(277.81)*
> Coding Clinic: 2004, Q4, P60-61

◀ New   ◀▥ Revised   ~~deleted~~ Deleted   ● Use Additional Digit(s)   ■ Nonspecific Code

● Not first-listed DX   OGCR Official Guidelines   Coding Clinic   Excludes   Includes   Use additional   Code first   Omit code

277.86 Peroxisomal disorders
Adrenomyeloneuropathy
Neonatal adrenoleukodystrophy
Rhizomelic chondrodysplasia punctata
X-linked adrenoleukodystrophy
Zellweger syndrome

Excludes *infantile Refsum disease (356.3)*

Coding Clinic: 2004, Q4, P61-62

277.87 Disorders of mitochondrial metabolism
Kearns-Sayre syndrome
Mitochondrial Encephalopathy, Lactic
Acidosis and Stroke-like episodes
(MELAS syndrome)
Mitochondrial Neurogastrointestinal
Encephalopathy syndrome (MNGIE)
Myoclonus with Epilepsy and with Ragged
Red Fibers (MERRF syndrome)
Neuropathy, Ataxia and Retinitis
Pigmentosa (NARP syndrome)

Use additional code for associated conditions

Excludes *disorders of pyruvate metabolism*
(271.8)
Leber's optic atrophy (377.16)
Leigh's subacute necrotizing
encephalopathy (330.8)
Reye's syndrome (331.81)
Coding Clinic: 2004, Q4, P62-63

277.88 Tumor lysis syndrome ◄
Spontaneous tumor lysis syndrome ◄
Tumor lysis syndrome following ◄
antineoplastic drug therapy ◄

Use additional E code to identify cause, if
drug-induced ◄

◼**277.89 Other specified disorders of metabolism**
Hand-Schüller-Christian disease
Histiocytosis (acute) (chronic)
Histiocytosis X (chronic)

Excludes *histiocytosis:*
acute differentiated progressive
(202.5)
X, acute (progressive) (202.5)

◼**277.9 Unspecified disorder of metabolism**
Enzymopathy NOS
Coding Clinic: 1987, Sept-Oct, P9

● **278 Overweight, obesity and other hyperalimentation**
Excludes *hyperalimentation NOS (783.6)*
poisoning by vitamins NOS (963.5)
polyphagia (783.6)

● **278.0 Overweight and obesity**
Excludes *adiposogenital dystrophy (253.8)*
obesity of endocrine origin NOS (259.9)

Use additional code to identify Body Mass Index
(BMI), if known (V85.0–V85.54)
Coding Clinic: 2005, Q4, P55

◼**278.00 Obesity, unspecified**
Obesity NOS
Coding Clinic: 2001, Q4, P42; 1999, Q1, P5-6

278.01 Morbid obesity
Severe obesity
Coding Clinic: 2006, Q2, P5-6; 2003, Q3, P3-8

278.02 Overweight

278.1 Localized adiposity
Fat pad
Coding Clinic: 2006, Q2, P10-11

278.2 Hypervitaminosis A

278.3 Hypercarotinemia

278.4 Hypervitaminosis D

◼**278.8 Other hyperalimentation**

● **279 Disorders involving the immune mechanism**
● **279.0 Deficiency of humoral immunity**
◼**279.00 Hypogammaglobulinemia, unspecified**
Agammaglobulinemia NOS

279.01 Selective IgA immunodeficiency

279.02 Selective IgM immunodeficiency

◼**279.03 Other selective immunoglobulin**
deficiencies
Selective deficiency of IgG

279.04 Congenital hypogammaglobulinemia
Agammaglobulinemia:
Bruton's type
X-linked

279.05 Immunodeficiency with increased IgM
Immunodeficiency with hyper-IgM:
autosomal recessive
X-linked

279.06 Common variable immunodeficiency
Dysgammaglobulinemia (acquired)
(congenital) (primary)
Hypogammaglobulinemia:
acquired primary
congenital non-sex-linked
sporadic

◼**279.09 Other**
Transient hypogammaglobulinemia of
infancy

● **279.1 Deficiency of cell-mediated immunity**
◼**279.10 Immunodeficiency with predominant T-cell**
defect, unspecified
Coding Clinic: 1987, Sept-Oct, P10; 1985, Mar-April, P7

279.11 DiGeorge's syndrome
Pharyngeal pouch syndrome
Thymic hypoplasia

279.12 Wiskott-Aldrich syndrome

279.13 Nezelof's syndrome
Cellular immunodeficiency with abnormal
immunoglobulin deficiency

◼**279.19 Other**
Excludes *ataxia-telangiectasia (334.8)*
Coding Clinic: 1985, Mar-April, P7

279.2 Combined immunity deficiency
Agammaglobulinemia:
autosomal recessive
Swiss-type
X-linked recessive
Severe combined immunodeficiency [SCID]
Thymic:
alymphoplasia
aplasia or dysplasia with immunodeficiency
Excludes *thymic hypoplasia (279.11)*

◼**279.3 Unspecified immunity deficiency**
● **279.4 Autoimmune disease, not elsewhere classified** ◄▥
~~Autoimmune disease NOS~~

279.41 Autoimmune lymphoproliferative
syndrome ◄
ALPS ◄

279.49 Autoimmune disease, not elsewhere
classified ◄
Autoimmune disease NOS ◄

Excludes *transplant failure or rejection*
(996.80–996.89)
Coding Clinic: 2008, Q3, P5

ENDOCRINE, NUTRITIONAL AND METABOLIC DISEASES, AND IMMUNITY DISORDERS (240–279)

● **279.5 Graft-versus-host disease**

> *Code first underlying cause, such as:*
> complication of blood transfusion (999.89) ◀▥
> complication of transplanted organ ~~(bone marrow)~~ (996.80-996.89) ◀▥

> Use additional code to identify associated
> manifestations, such as:
> desquamative dermatitis (695.89)
> diarrhea (787.91)
> elevated bilirubin (782.4)
> hair loss (704.09)
> Coding Clinic: 2008, Q4, P97-100

● ■ **279.50 *Graft-versus-host disease, unspecified***

● **279.51 *Acute graft-versus-host disease***

● **279.52 *Chronic graft-versus-host disease***

● **279.53 *Acute on chronic graft-versus-host disease***

■ **279.8 Other specified disorders involving the immune mechanism**
> Single complement [C_1-C_9] deficiency or dysfunction

■ **279.9 Unspecified disorder of immune mechanism**
> Coding Clinic: 1996, Q2, P12; 1992, Q3, P13-14

ENDOCRINE, NUTRITIONAL AND METABOLIC DISEASES, AND IMMUNITY DISORDERS (240–279)

◀ New ◀▥ Revised ~~deleted~~ Deleted ● Use Additional Digit(s) ■ Nonspecific Code
● Not first-listed DX OGCR Official Guidelines Coding Clinic Excludes Includes Use additional Code first Omit code

4. DISEASES OF THE BLOOD AND BLOOD-FORMING ORGANS (280–289)

● **280 Iron deficiency anemias**

Disease characterized by decrease in number of red cells (hemoglobin) in blood, diminishing body's ability to carry adequate amounts of oxygen to cells.

Includes   anemia:
     asiderotic
     hypochromic-microcytic
     sideropenic

Excludes   *familial microcytic anemia (282.49)*

280.0 Secondary to blood loss (chronic)
Normocytic anemia due to blood loss

     Excludes   *acute posthemorrhagic anemia (285.1)*

     Coding Clinic: 1993, Q4, P34; 1985, July-Aug, P13

280.1 Secondary to inadequate dietary iron intake

■ **280.8 Other specified iron deficiency anemias**
Paterson-Kelly syndrome
Plummer-Vinson syndrome
Sideropenic dysphagia

■ **280.9 Iron deficiency anemia, unspecified**
Anemia:
     achlorhydric
     chlorotic
     idiopathic hypochromic
     iron [Fe] deficiency NOS

● **281 Other deficiency anemias**

281.0 Pernicious anemia
Anemia:
     Addison's
     Biermer's
     congenital pernicious
Congenital intrinsic factor [Castle's] deficiency

     Excludes   *combined system disease without mention of anemia (266.2)*
         subacute degeneration of spinal cord without mention of anemia (266.2)

■ **281.1 Other vitamin B_{12} deficiency anemia**
Anemia:
     vegan's
     vitamin B_{12} deficiency (dietary)
     due to selective vitamin B_{12} malabsorption with proteinuria
Syndrome:
     Imerslund's
     Imerslund-Gräsbeck

     Excludes   *combined system disease without mention of anemia (266.2)*
         subacute degeneration of spinal cord without mention of anemia (266.2)

281.2 Folate-deficiency anemia
Congenital folate malabsorption
Folate or folic acid deficiency anemia:
     NOS
     dietary
     drug-induced
Goat's milk anemia
Nutritional megaloblastic anemia (of infancy)

     Use additional E code to identify drug

■ **281.3 Other specified megaloblastic anemias, not elsewhere classified**
Combined B_{12} and folate-deficiency anemia

281.4 Protein-deficiency anemia
Amino-acid-deficiency anemia

■ **281.8 Anemia associated with other specified nutritional deficiency**
Scorbutic anemia

■ **281.9 Unspecified deficiency anemia**
Anemia:
     dimorphic
     macrocytic
     megaloblastic NOS
     nutritional NOS
     simple chronic
Coding Clinic: 1984, Sept-Oct, P16

● **282 Hereditary hemolytic anemias**

Genetic condition in which bone marrow is unable to compensate for premature destruction of red blood cells

282.0 Hereditary spherocytosis
Acholuric (familial) jaundice
Congenital hemolytic anemia (spherocytic)
Congenital spherocytosis
Minkowski-Chauffard syndrome
Spherocytosis (familial)

     Excludes   *hemolytic anemia of newborn (773.0–773.5)*

282.1 Hereditary elliptocytosis
Elliptocytosis (congenital)
Ovalocytosis (congenital) (hereditary)

282.2 Anemias due to disorders of glutathione metabolism
Anemia:
     6-phosphogluconic dehydrogenase deficiency
     enzyme deficiency, drug-induced
     erythrocytic glutathione deficiency
     glucose-6-phosphate dehydrogenase [G-6-PD] deficiency
     glutathione-reductase deficiency
     hemolytic nonspherocytic (hereditary), type I
Disorder of pentose phosphate pathway
Favism

■ **282.3 Other hemolytic anemias due to enzyme deficiency**
Anemia:
     hemolytic nonspherocytic (hereditary), type II
     hexokinase deficiency
     pyruvate kinase [PK] deficiency
     triosephosphate isomerase deficiency

● **282.4 Thalassemias**

Hereditary disorders characterized by low production of hemoglobin or excessive destruction of red blood cells

     Excludes   *sickle-cell:*
         disease (282.60–282.69)
         trait (282.5)
     Coding Clinic: 2003, Q4, P51-56

282.41 Sickle-cell thalassemia without crisis
Sickle-cell thalassemia NOS
Thalassemia Hb-S disease without crisis

282.42 Sickle-cell thalassemia with crisis
Sickle-cell thalassemia with vaso-occlusive pain
Thalassemia Hb-S disease with crisis

     Use additional code for type of crisis, such as:
     Acute chest syndrome (517.3)
     Splenic sequestration (289.52)
     Occurs when sickled red blood cells become entrapped in spleen, causing splenomegaly (enlargement) and decreased circulating blood volume.

DISEASES OF THE BLOOD AND BLOOD-FORMING ORGANS (280–289)

■**282.49 Other thalassemia**
    Cooley's anemia
    Hb-Bart's disease
    Hereditary leptocytosis
    Mediterranean anemia (with other
        hemoglobinopathy)
    Microdrepanocytosis
    Thalassemia (alpha) (beta) (intermedia)
        (major) (minima) (minor) (mixed)
        (trait) (with other hemoglobinopathy)
    Thalassemia NOS

282.5 Sickle-cell trait
    Hb-AS genotype
    Hemoglobin S [Hb-S] trait
    Heterozygous:
        hemoglobin S
        Hb-S

    Excludes *that with other hemoglobinopathy*
        (282.60–282.69)
        that with thalassemia (282.49)
    Coding Clinic: 2003, Q4, P51-56

●**282.6 Sickle-cell disease**
    Inherited disease in which red blood cells, normally
        disc-shaped, become crescent shaped. Small blood
        clots form, resulting in painful episodes called
        sickle cell pain crises.
    Sickle-cell anemia

    Excludes *sickle-cell thalassemia (282.41–282.42)*
        sickle-cell trait (282.5)

■**282.60 Sickle-cell disease, unspecified**
    Sickle-cell anemia NOS
    Coding Clinic: 1997, Q2, P11

282.61 Hb-SS disease without crisis
    Coding Clinic: 2007, Q2, P9-10

282.62 Hb-SS disease with crisis
    Hb-SS disease with vaso-occlusive pain
    Sickle-cell crisis NOS

    Use additional code for type of crisis, such
        as:
        Acute chest syndrome (517.3)
        Splenic sequestration (289.52)
    Coding Clinic: 2003, Q4, P51-56; 1998, Q2, P8; 1991, Q2,
    P15

282.63 Sickle-cell/Hb-C disease without crisis
    Hb-S/Hb-C disease without crisis

282.64 Sickle-cell/Hb-C disease with crisis
    Hb-S/Hb-C disease with crisis
    Sickle-cell/Hb-C disease with
        vaso-occlusive pain

    Use additional code for types of crisis,
        such as:
        Acute chest syndrome (517.3)
        Splenic sequestration (289.52)

282.68 Other sickle-cell disease without crisis
    Hb-S/Hb-D disease without crisis
    Hb-S/Hb-E disease without crisis
    Sickle-cell/Hb-D disease without crisis
    Sickle-cell/Hb-E disease without crisis

■**282.69 Other sickle-cell disease with crisis**
    Hb-S/Hb-D disease with crisis
    Hb-S/Hb-E disease with crisis
    Other sickle-cell disease with vaso-occlusive
        pain
    Sickle-cell/Hb-D disease with crisis
    Sickle-cell/Hb-E disease with crisis

    Use additional code for type of crisis, such
        as:
        Acute chest syndrome (517.3)
        Splenic sequestration (289.52)

■**282.7 Other hemoglobinopathies**
    Abnormal hemoglobin NOS
    Congenital Heinz-body anemia
    Disease:
        hemoglobin C [Hb-C]
        hemoglobin D [Hb-D]
        hemoglobin E [Hb-E]
        hemoglobin Zurich [Hb-Zurich]
    Hemoglobinopathy NOS
    Hereditary persistence of fetal hemoglobin
        [HPFH]
    Unstable hemoglobin hemolytic disease

    Excludes *familial polycythemia (289.6)*
        hemoglobin M [Hb-M] disease (289.7)
        high-oxygen-affinity hemoglobin (289.0)

■**282.8 Other specified hereditary hemolytic anemias**
    Stomatocytosis

■**282.9 Hereditary hemolytic anemia, unspecified**
    Hereditary hemolytic anemia NOS

●**283 Acquired hemolytic anemias**
    Also known as autoimmune hemolytic or Coombs positive
        hemolytic anemia. The red blood cells produced are
        healthy but are destroyed when trapped in the spleen by
        infection or certain drugs.

283.0 Autoimmune hemolytic anemias
    Autoimmune hemolytic disease (cold type) (warm
        type)
    Chronic cold hemagglutinin disease
    Cold agglutinin disease or hemoglobinuria
    Hemolytic anemia:
        cold type (secondary) (symptomatic)
        drug-induced
        warm type (secondary) (symptomatic)

    Use additional E code to identify cause, if
        drug-induced

    Excludes *Evans' syndrome (287.32)*
        hemolytic disease of newborn (773.0–773.5)
    Coding Clinic: 2008, Q3, P5

●**283.1 Non-autoimmune hemolytic anemias**

■**283.10 Non-autoimmune hemolytic anemia,**
        unspecified

283.11 Hemolytic-uremic syndrome

■**283.19 Other non-autoimmune hemolytic anemias**
    Hemolytic anemia:
        mechanical
        microangiopathic
        toxic

    Use additional E code to identify cause

283.2 Hemoglobinuria due to hemolysis from external
  causes
    Acute intravascular hemolysis
    Hemoglobinuria:
        from exertion
        march
        paroxysmal (cold) (nocturnal)
        due to other hemolysis
    Marchiafava-Micheli syndrome

    Use additional E code to identify cause

■**283.9 Acquired hemolytic anemia, unspecified**
    Acquired hemolytic anemia NOS
    Chronic idiopathic hemolytic anemia

◀ New   ◀▥ Revised   ~~deleted~~ Deleted   ● Use Additional Digit(s)   ■ Nonspecific Code
● Not first-listed DX   OGCR Official Guidelines   Coding Clinic   Excludes   Includes   Use additional   Code first   Omit code

● **284   Aplastic anemia and other bone marrow failure syndromes**
Coding Clinic: 2006, Q4, P67-69

● **284.0   Constitutional aplastic anemia**
Coding Clinic: 1991, Q1, P14

284.01   Constitutional red blood cell aplasia
Aplasia, (pure) red cell:
congenital
of infants
primary
Blackfan-Diamond syndrome
Familial hypoplastic anemia

■ **284.09   Other constitutional aplastic anemia**
Fanconi's anemia
Pancytopenia with malformations

284.1   Pancytopenia
Marked deficiency of all the blood elements: Red blood cells (erythrocytes), white blood cells (leukocytes), and platelets (thrombocytes). Check laboratory results.

Excludes   *pancytopenia (due to) (with):*
aplastic anemia NOS (284.9)
bone marrow infiltration (284.2)
constitutional red blood cell aplasia (284.01)
drug induced (284.89)
hairy cell leukemia (202.4)
human immunodeficiency virus disease (042)
leukoerythroblastic anemia (284.2)
malformations (284.09)
myelodysplastic syndromes (238.72–238.75)
myeloproliferative disease (238.79)
other constitutional aplastic anemia (284.09)
Coding Clinic: 2005, Q3, P11-12

● **284.2   *Myelophthisis***
Leukoerythroblastic anemia
Myelophthisic anemia

Code first the underlying disorder, such as:
malignant neoplasm of breast (174.0–174.9, 175.0–175.9)
tuberculosis (015.0–015.9)

Excludes   *idiopathic myelofibrosis (238.76)*
myelofibrosis NOS (289.83)
myelofibrosis with myeloid metaplasia (238.76)
primary myelofibrosis (238.76)
secondary myelofibrosis (289.83)

● **284.8   Other specified aplastic anemias**
Coding Clinic: 2007, Q4, P72-73; 2005, Q3, P11-12; 1997, Q1, P5-6; 1991, Q1, P14; 1984, Sept-Oct, P16

284.81   Red cell aplasia (acquired) (adult) (with thymoma)
Red cell aplasia NOS

284.89   Other specified aplastic anemias
Aplastic anemia (due to):
chronic systemic disease
drugs
infection
radiation
toxic (paralytic)

Use additional E code to identify cause
Coding Clinic: 2009, Q1, P17; 2008, Q2, P6

■ **284.9   Aplastic anemia, unspecified**
Anemia:
aplastic (idiopathic) NOS
aregenerative
hypoplastic NOS
nonregenerative
Medullary hypoplasia

Excludes   *refractory anemia (238.72)*

● **285   Other and unspecified anemias**
Coding Clinic: 1990, Q3, P17

285.0   Sideroblastic anemia
Anemia:
hypochromic with iron loading
sideroachrestic
sideroblastic:
acquired
congenital
hereditary
primary
secondary (drug-induced) (due to disease)
sex-linked hypochromic
vitamin B_6-responsive
Pyridoxine-responsive (hypochromic) anemia

Excludes   *refractory sideroblastic anemia (238.72)*

Use additional E code to identify cause, if drug-induced

285.1   Acute posthemorrhagic anemia
Anemia due to acute blood loss

Excludes   *anemia due to chronic blood loss (280.0)*
blood loss anemia NOS (280.0)
Coding Clinic: 2007, Q1, P19; 2004, Q3, P4; 1993, Q4, P34; 1992, Q2, P15-16

● **285.2   Anemia of chronic disease**
Anemia in (due to) (with) chronic illness ◀▥

285.21   Anemia in chronic kidney disease
Anemia in end stage renal disease
Erythropoietin-resistant anemia (EPO resistant anemia)
Coding Clinic: 2000, Q4, P39-40

285.22   Anemia in neoplastic disease

Excludes   *anemia due to antineoplastic chemotherapy (285.3)* ◀
Coding Clinic: 2008, Q2, P6; 2000, Q4, P39-40

OGCR   Section I.C.4.a.2
When assigning code 285.22, Anemia in neoplastic disease, it is also necessary to assign the neoplasm code that is responsible for the anemia. Code 285.22 is for use for anemia that is due to the malignancy, not for anemia due to antineoplastic chemotherapy drugs, which is an adverse effect.

285.29   Anemia of other chronic disease
Anemia in other chronic illness

285.3   Antineoplastic chemotherapy induced anemia ◀
Anemia due to antineoplastic chemotherapy ◀

Excludes   *anemia due to drug NEC – code to type of anemia* ◀
anemia in neoplastic disease (285.22) ◀
aplastic anemia due to antineoplastic chemotherapy (284.89) ◀

■ **285.8   Other specified anemias**
Anemia:
dyserythropoietic (congenital)
dyshematopoietic (congenital)
von Jaksch's
Infantile pseudoleukemia

DISEASES OF THE BLOOD AND BLOOD-FORMING ORGANS (280–289)

■285.9   Anemia, unspecified
    Anemia:
        NOS
        essential
        normocytic, not due to blood loss
        profound
        progressive
        secondary
    Oligocythemia

> **Excludes**   *anemia (due to):*
>   *blood loss:*
>   *acute (285.1)*
>   *chronic or unspecified (280.0)*
>   *iron deficiency (280.0–280.9)*

Coding Clinic: 2009, Q1, P17x2; 2007, Q1, P19; 2002, Q1, P14; 1992, Q2, P15-16; 1985, Mar-April, P13

● 286   Coagulation defects
Can be acquired or genetic and results in inability to control blood clotting. Most common genetic coagulation disorder is hemophilia.
Coding Clinic: 2006, Q2, P17; 1992, Q3, P15

    286.0   Congenital factor VIII disorder
        Antihemophilic globulin [AHG] deficiency
        Factor VIII (functional) deficiency
        Hemophilia:
            NOS
            A
            classical
            familial
            hereditary
        Subhemophilia

> **Excludes**   *factor VIII deficiency with vascular defect (286.4)*

    286.1   Congenital factor IX disorder
        Christmas disease
        Deficiency:
            factor IX (functional)
            plasma thromboplastin component [PTC]
        Hemophilia B

    286.2   Congenital factor XI deficiency
        Hemophilia C
        Plasma thromboplastin antecedent [PTA] deficiency
        Rosenthal's disease

    ■286.3   Congenital deficiency of other clotting factors
        Congenital afibrinogenemia
        Deficiency:
            AC globulin factor:
                I [fibrinogen]
                II [prothrombin]
                V [labile]
                VII [stable]
                X [Stuart-Prower]
                XII [Hageman]
                XIII [fibrin stabilizing]
            Laki-Lorand factor
            proaccelerin
        Disease:
            Owren's
            Stuart-Prower
        Dysfibrinogenemia (congenital)
        Dysprothrombinemia (constitutional)
        Hypoproconvertinemia
        Hypoprothrombinemia (hereditary)
        Parahemophilia

    286.4   von Willebrand's disease
        Angiohemophilia (A) (B)
        Constitutional thrombopathy
        Factor VIII deficiency with vascular defect
        Pseudohemophilia type B
        Vascular hemophilia
        von Willebrand's (-Jürgens') disease

> **Excludes**   *factor VIII deficiency:*
>   *NOS (286.0)*
>   *with functional defect (286.0)*
>   *hereditary capillary fragility (287.8)*

    286.5   Hemorrhagic disorder due to intrinsic circulating anticoagulants
        Antithrombinemia
        Antithromboplastinemia
        Antithromboplastino-genemia
        Hyperheparinemia
        Increase in:
            anti-VIIIa
            anti-IXa
            anti-Xa
            anti-XIa
            antithrombin
        Secondary hemophilia
        Systemic lupus erythematosus [SLE] inhibitor
Coding Clinic: 2004, Q3, P7; 1994, Q1, P22; 1993, 5th Issue, P16; 1992, Q3, P15-16; 1990, Q3, P14

    286.6   Defibrination syndrome
        Afibrinogenemia, acquired
        Consumption coagulopathy
        Diffuse or disseminated intravascular coagulation [DIC syndrome]
        Fibrinolytic hemorrhage, acquired
        Hemorrhagic fibrinogenolysis
        Pathologic fibrinolysis
        Purpura:
            fibrinolytic
            fulminans

> **Excludes**   *that complicating:*
>   *abortion (634–638 with .1, 639.1)*
>   *pregnancy or the puerperium (641.3, 666.3)*
>   *disseminated intravascular coagulation in newborn (776.2)*

    286.7   Acquired coagulation factor deficiency
        Deficiency of coagulation factor due to:
            liver disease
            vitamin K deficiency
        Hypoprothrombinemia, acquired

> **Excludes**   *vitamin K deficiency of newborn (776.0)*

> Use additional E-code to identify cause, if drug-induced

    ■286.9   Other and unspecified coagulation defects
        Defective coagulation NOS
        Deficiency, coagulation factor NOS
        Delay, coagulation
        Disorder:
            coagulation
            hemostasis

> **Excludes**   *abnormal coagulation profile (790.92)*
>   *hemorrhagic disease of newborn (776.0)*
>   *that complicating:*
>   *abortion (634–638 with .1, 639.1)*
>   *pregnancy or the puerperium (641.3, 666.3)*

Coding Clinic: 1999, Q4, P22-23

DISEASES OF THE BLOOD AND BLOOD-FORMING ORGANS (280–289)

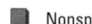

◀ New   ◀▥ Revised   ~~deleted~~ Deleted   ● Use Additional Digit(s)   ■ Nonspecific Code
● Not first-listed DX   OGCR Official Guidelines   Coding Clinic   Excludes   Includes   Use additional   Code first   Omit code

● 287 **Purpura and other hemorrhagic conditions**

> Excludes *hemorrhagic thrombocythemia (238.79)*
> *purpura fulminans (286.6)*

287.0 **Allergic purpura**
Peliosis rheumatica
Purpura:
    anaphylactoid
    autoimmune
    Henoch's
    nonthrombocytopenic:
        hemorrhagic
        idiopathic
    rheumatica
    Schönlein-Henoch
    vascular
Vasculitis, allergic

> Excludes *hemorrhagic purpura (287.39)*
> *purpura annularis telangiectodes (709.1)*

287.1 **Qualitative platelet defects**
Thrombasthenia (hemorrhagic) (hereditary)
Thrombocytasthenia
Thrombocytopathy (dystrophic)
Thrombopathy (Bernard-Soulier)

> Excludes *von Willebrand's disease (286.4)*

■287.2 **Other nonthrombocytopenic purpuras**
Purpura:
    NOS
    senile
    simplex

● 287.3 **Primary thrombocytopenia**
Also known as idiopathic thrombocytopenia, may be
acquired or congenital and is a common cause of
coagulation disorders.

> Excludes *thrombotic thrombocytopenic purpura*
> *(446.6)*
> *transient thrombocytopenia of newborn*
> *(776.1)*
> *Thrombo = clot forming, cyto = cell,*
> *penia = deficiency of: deficiency of*
> *platelets.*

■287.30 **Primary thrombocytopenia unspecified**
Megakaryocytic hypoplasia

287.31 **Immune thrombocytopenic purpura**
Idiopathic thrombocytopenic purpura
Tidal platelet dysgenesis
Coding Clinic: 2005, Q4, P56-57

287.32 **Evans' syndrome**

287.33 **Congenital and hereditary thrombocytopenic**
purpura
Congenital and hereditary
    thrombocytopenia
Thrombocytopenia with absent radii (TAR)
    syndrome

> Excludes *Wiskott-Aldrich syndrome (279.12)*

287.39 **Other primary thrombocytopenia**

287.4 **Secondary thrombocytopenia**
Posttransfusion purpura
Thrombocytopenia (due to):
    dilutional
    drugs
    extracorporeal circulation of blood
    massive blood transfusion
    platelet alloimmunization

Use additional E code to identify cause

> Excludes *heparin-induced thrombocytopenia (HIT)*
> *(289.84)*
> *transient thrombocytopenia of newborn*
> *(776.1)*
> Coding Clinic: 1985, July-Aug, P13; Mar-April, P14

■287.5 **Thrombocytopenia, unspecified**

■287.8 **Other specified hemorrhagic conditions**
Capillary fragility (hereditary)
Vascular pseudohemophilia
Coding Clinic: 1985, Mar-April, P14

■287.9 **Unspecified hemorrhagic conditions**
Hemorrhagic diathesis (familial)

● 288 **Diseases of white blood cells**

> Excludes *leukemia (204.0–208.9)*

● 288.0 **Neutropenia**
Decreased Absolute Neutrophil Count (ANC)

> Use additional code for any associated:
> fever (780.61)
> mucositis (478.11, 528.00–528.09, 538, 616.81)

> Excludes *neutropenic splenomegaly (289.53)*
> *transitory neonatal neutropenia (776.7)*
> Coding Clinic: 2005, Q3, P11-12; 1999, Q3, P6-7; 1996, Q3, P16; Q2,
> P6; 1985, Mar-April, P14

■288.00 **Neutropenia, unspecified**

288.01 **Congenital neutropenia**
Congenital agranulocytosis
Infantile genetic agranulocytosis
Kostmann's syndrome

288.02 **Cyclic neutropenia**
Cyclic hematopoiesis
Periodic neutropenia

288.03 **Drug induced neutropenia**
Use additional E code to identify drug
Coding Clinic: 2006, Q4, P69-73

288.04 **Neutropenia due to infection**

■288.09 **Other neutropenia**
Agranulocytosis
Neutropenia:
    immune
    toxic

288.1 **Functional disorders of polymorphonuclear**
neutrophils
Chronic (childhood) granulomatous disease
Congenital dysphagocytosis
Job's syndrome
Lipochrome histiocytosis (familial)
Progressive septic granulomatosis

288.2 **Genetic anomalies of leukocytes**
Anomaly (granulation) (granulocyte) or syndrome:
    Alder's (-Reilly)
    Chédiak-Steinbrinck (-Higashi)
    Jordan's
    May-Hegglin
    Pelger-Huet
Hereditary:
    hypersegmentation
    hyposegmentation
    leukomelanopathy

288.3 **Eosinophilia**
Eosinophilia
    allergic
    hereditary
    idiopathic
    secondary
Eosinophilic leukocytosis

> Excludes *Löffler's syndrome (518.3)*
> *pulmonary eosinophilia (518.3)*
> Coding Clinic: 2000, Q3, P11

DISEASES OF THE BLOOD AND BLOOD-FORMING ORGANS (280–289)

DISEASES OF THE BLOOD AND BLOOD-FORMING ORGANS (280–289)

288.4 **Hemophagocytic syndromes**
Familial hemophagocytic lymphohistiocytosis
Familial hemophagocytic reticulosis
Hemophagocytic syndrome, infection-associated
Histiocytic syndromes
Macrophage activation syndrome

● 288.5 **Decreased white blood cell count**

> **Excludes** *neutropenia (288.01–288.09)*

■ 288.50 **Leukocytopenia, unspecified**
Decreased leukocytes, unspecified
Decreased white blood cell count,
unspecified
Leukopenia NOS

288.51 **Lymphocytopenia**
Decreased lymphocytes

■ 288.59 **Other decreased white blood cell count**
Basophilic leukopenia
Eosinophilic leukopenia
Monocytopenia
Plasmacytopenia

● 288.6 **Elevated white blood cell count**

> **Excludes** *eosinophilia (288.3)*

■ 288.60 **Leukocytosis, unspecified**
Elevated leukocytes, unspecified
Elevated white blood cell count,
unspecified

288.61 **Lymphocytosis (symptomatic)**
Elevated lymphocytes

288.62 **Leukemoid reaction**
Basophilic leukemoid reaction
Lymphocytic leukemoid reaction
Monocytic leukemoid reaction
Myelocytic leukemoid reaction
Neutrophilic leukemoid reaction

288.63 **Monocytosis (symptomatic)**

> **Excludes** *infectious mononucleosis (075)*

288.64 **Plasmacytosis**

288.65 **Basophilia**

288.66 **Bandemia**
Bandemia without diagnosis of specific
infection

> **Excludes** *confirmed infection – code to*
> *infection*
> *leukemia (204.00–208.9)*
> Coding Clinic: 2007, Q4, P73-74

■ 288.69 **Other elevated white blood cell count**

■ 288.8 **Other specified disease of white blood cells**

> **Excludes** *decreased white blood cell counts*
> *(288.50–288.59)*
> *elevated white blood cell counts*
> *(288.60–288.69)*
> *immunity disorders (279.0–279.9)*
> Coding Clinic: 1987, Mar-April, P12

■ 288.9 **Unspecified disease of white blood cells**

● 289 **Other diseases of blood and blood-forming organs**

289.0 **Polycythemia, secondary**
See 238.4 for primary polycythemia (polycythemia vera)
High-oxygen-affinity hemoglobin
Polycythemia:
acquired
benign
due to:
fall in plasma volume
high altitude
emotional
erythropoietin
hypoxemic
nephrogenous
relative
spurious
stress

> **Excludes** *polycythemia:*
> *neonatal (776.4)*
> *primary (238.4)*
> *vera (238.4)*

289.1 **Chronic lymphadenitis**
Chronic:
adenitis any lymph node, except mesenteric
lymphadenitis any lymph node, except
mesenteric

> **Excludes** *acute lymphadenitis (683)*
> *mesenteric (289.2)*
> *enlarged glands NOS (785.6)*

■ 289.2 **Nonspecific mesenteric lymphadenitis**
Mesenteric lymphadenitis (acute) (chronic)

■ 289.3 **Lymphadenitis, unspecified, except mesenteric**
Coding Clinic: 1992, Q2, P8

289.4 **Hypersplenism**
"Big spleen" syndrome
Dyssplenism
Hypersplenia

> **Excludes** *primary splenic neutropenia (289.53)*

● 289.5 **Other diseases of spleen**

■ 289.50 **Disease of spleen, unspecified**

289.51 **Chronic congestive splenomegaly**

● 289.52 *Splenic sequestration*

> *Code first sickle-cell disease in crisis (282.42,*
> *282.62, 282.64, 282.69)*
> Coding Clinic: 2003, Q4, P51-56

289.53 **Neutropenic splenomegaly**

■ 289.59 **Other**
Lien migrans	Splenic:
Perisplenitis	fibrosis
Splenic:	infarction
abscess	rupture, nontraumatic
atrophy	Splenitis
cyst	Wandering spleen

> **Excludes** *bilharzial splenic fibrosis*
> *(120.0–120.9)*
> *hepatolienal fibrosis (571.5)*
> *splenomegaly NOS (789.2)*

◄ New   ◄▥ Revised   ~~deleted~~ Deleted   ● Use Additional Digit(s)   ■ Nonspecific Code
● Not first-listed DX   OGCR Official Guidelines   Coding Clinic   Excludes   Includes   Use additional   Code first   Omit code

289.6 Familial polycythemia
Familial:
   benign polycythemia
   erythrocytosis

289.7 Methemoglobinemia
Congenital NADH
   [DPNH]-methemoglobin-reductase deficiency
Hemoglobin M [Hb-M] disease
Methemoglobinemia:
   NOS
   acquired (with sulfhemoglobinemia)
   hereditary
   toxic
Stokvis' disease
Sulfhemoglobinemia

   Use additional E code to identify cause

● **289.8 Other specified diseases of blood and blood-forming organs**
Coding Clinic: 2003, Q4, P56-57; 2002, Q1, P16-17; 1987, Mar-April, P12

289.81 Primary hypercoagulable state
Activated protein C resistance
Antithrombin III deficiency
Factor V Leiden mutation
Lupus anticoagulant
Protein C deficiency
Protein S deficiency
Prothrombin gene mutation
Coding Clinic: 2008, Q3, P16-17

289.82 Secondary hypercoagulable state
   Excludes *heparin-induced thrombocytopenia (HIT) (289.84)*
   Coding Clinic: 2008, Q3, P16-17

● **289.83 *Myelofibrosis***
Myelofibrosis NOS
Secondary myelofibrosis

   Code first the underlying disorder, such as:
   malignant neoplasm of breast
      (174.0–174.9, 175.0–175.9)

   Excludes *idiopathic myelofibrosis (238.76)*
   leukoerythroblastic anemia (284.2)
   myelofibrosis with myeloid
      metaplasia (238.76)
   myelophthisic anemia (284.2)
   myelophthisis (284.2)
   primary myelofibrosis (238.76)

   Use additional code for associated therapy-related myelodysplastic syndrome, if applicable (238.72, 238.73)

   Use additional external cause code if due to anti-neoplastic chemotherapy (E933.1)

289.84 Heparin-induced thrombocytopenia (HIT)
Coding Clinic: 2008, Q4, P100-101

■ **289.89 Other specified diseases of blood and blood-forming organs**
Hypergammaglobulinemia
Pseudocholinesterase deficiency

■ **289.9 Unspecified diseases of blood and blood-forming organs**
Blood dyscrasia NOS
Erythroid hyperplasia
Coding Clinic: 1985, Mar-April, P14

DISEASES OF THE BLOOD AND BLOOD-FORMING ORGANS (280–289)

5. MENTAL DISORDERS (290–319)

Item 5-1 Psychosis was a term formerly applied to any mental disorder but is now restricted to disturbances of a great magnitude in which there is a personality disintegration and loss of contact with reality.

PSYCHOSES (290–299)

Excludes *mental retardation (317–319)*

ORGANIC PSYCHOTIC CONDITIONS (290–294)

Includes psychotic organic brain syndrome

Excludes *nonpsychotic syndromes of organic etiology (310.0–310.9)*

psychoses classifiable to 295–298 and without impairment of orientation, comprehension, calculation, learning capacity, and judgment, but associated with physical disease, injury, or condition affecting the brain [e.g., following childbirth] (295.0–298.8)

● **290 Dementias**

Progressive decline in cognition along with a short- and long-term memory loss due to brain damage/disease.

Code first the associated neurological condition

Excludes *dementia due to alcohol (291.0–291.2)*
dementia due to drugs (292.82)
dementia not classified as senile, presenile, or arteriosclerotic (294.10–294.11)
psychoses classifiable to 295–298 occurring in the senium without dementia or delirium (295.0–298.8)
senility with mental changes of nonpsychotic severity (310.1)
transient organic psychotic conditions (293.0–293.9)

290.0 Senile dementia, uncomplicated   A
Senile dementia:
NOS
simple type

Excludes *mild memory disturbances, not amounting to dementia, associated with senile brain disease (310.8)* ◀▥
senile dementia with:
delirium or confusion (290.3)
delusional [paranoid] features (290.20)
depressive features (290.21)
Coding Clinic: 1999, Q4, P4-5; 1994, Q1, P21

● **290.1 Presenile dementia**
Brain syndrome with presenile brain disease

Excludes *arteriosclerotic dementia (290.40–290.43)*
dementia associated with other cerebral conditions (294.10–294.11)

290.10 Presenile dementia, uncomplicated   A
Presenile dementia:
NOS
simple type
Coding Clinic: 1984, Nov-Dec, P20

290.11 Presenile dementia with delirium   A
Presenile dementia with acute confusional state
Coding Clinic: 1984, Nov-Dec, P20

290.12 Presenile dementia with delusional features   A
Presenile dementia, paranoid type
Coding Clinic: 1984, Nov-Dec, P20

290.13 Presenile dementia with depressive features   A
Presenile dementia, depressed type
Coding Clinic: 1984, Nov-Dec, P20

● **290.2 Senile dementia with delusional or depressive features**

Excludes *senile dementia:*
NOS (290.0)
with delirium and/or confusion (290.3)

290.20 Senile dementia with delusional features   A
Senile dementia, paranoid type
Senile psychosis NOS

290.21 Senile dementia with depressive features   A

290.3 Senile dementia with delirium   A
Senile dementia with acute confusional state

Excludes *senile:*
dementia NOS (290.0)
psychosis NOS (290.20)

● **290.4 Vascular dementia**
Multi-infarct dementia or psychosis

Use additional code to identify cerebral atherosclerosis (437.0)

Excludes *suspected cases with no clear evidence of arteriosclerosis (290.9)*

290.40 Vascular dementia, uncomplicated   A
Arteriosclerotic dementia:
NOS
simple type

290.41 Vascular dementia with delirium   A
Arteriosclerotic dementia with acute confusional state

290.42 Vascular dementia with delusions   A
Arteriosclerotic dementia, paranoid type

290.43 Vascular dementia with depressed mood   A
Arteriosclerotic dementia, depressed type

■ **290.8 Other specified senile psychotic conditions**
Presbyophrenic psychosis

■ **290.9 Unspecified senile psychotic condition**   A

● **291 Alcohol-induced mental disorders**

Excludes *alcoholism without psychosis (303.0–303.9)*

291.0 Alcohol withdrawal delirium
Alcoholic delirium
Delirium tremens

Excludes *alcohol withdrawal (291.81)*

291.1 Alcohol-induced persisting amnestic disorder
Alcoholic polyneuritic psychosis
Korsakoff's psychosis, alcoholic
Wernicke-Korsakoff syndrome (alcoholic)

■ **291.2 Alcohol-induced persisting dementia**
Alcoholic dementia NOS
Alcoholism associated with dementia NOS
Chronic alcoholic brain syndrome

◀ New   ◀▥ Revised   ~~deleted~~ Deleted   ● Use Additional Digit(s)   ■ Nonspecific Code
● Not first-listed DX   OGCR Official Guidelines   Coding Clinic   Excludes   Includes   Use additional   Code first   Omit code

291.3 Alcohol-induced psychotic disorder with hallucinations

Alcoholic:

hallucinosis (acute)

psychosis with hallucinosis

Excludes *alcohol withdrawal with delirium (291.0)*

schizophrenia (295.0–295.9) and paranoid

states (297.0–297.9) taking the form

of chronic hallucinosis with clear

consciousness in an alcoholic

291.4 Idiosyncratic alcohol intoxication

Pathologic:

alcohol intoxication

drunkenness

Excludes *acute alcohol intoxication (305.0)*

in alcoholism (303.0)

simple drunkenness (305.0)

291.5 Alcohol-induced psychotic disorder with delusions

Alcoholic:

paranoia

psychosis, paranoid type

Excludes *nonalcoholic paranoid states (297.0–297.9)*

schizophrenia, paranoid type (295.3)

● **291.8 Other specified alcohol-induced mental disorders**

Coding Clinic: 1989, Q2, P9

291.81 Alcohol withdrawal

Alcohol:

abstinence syndrome or symptoms

withdrawal syndrome or symptoms

Excludes *alcohol withdrawal:*

delirium (291.0)

hallucinosis (291.3)

delirium tremens (291.0)

Coding Clinic: 1985, July-Aug, P10

■**291.82 Alcohol induced sleep disorders**

Alcohol induced circadian rhythm sleep

disorders

Alcohol induced hypersomnia

Alcohol induced insomnia

Alcohol induced parasomnia

■**291.89 Other**

Alcohol-induced anxiety disorder

Alcohol-induced mood disorder

Alcohol-induced sexual dysfunction

■**291.9 Unspecified alcohol-induced mental disorders**

Alcoholic:

mania NOS

psychosis NOS

Alcoholism (chronic) with psychosis

Alcohol-related disorder NOS

● **292 Drug-induced mental disorders**

Includes organic brain syndrome associated with

consumption of drugs

Use additional code for any associated drug dependence

(304.0–304.9)

Use additional E code to identify drug

Coding Clinic: 2004, Q3, P8

292.0 Drug withdrawal

Drug:

abstinence syndrome or symptoms

withdrawal syndrome or symptoms

Coding Clinic: 1997, Q1, P12-13

● **292.1 Drug-induced psychotic disorders**

292.11 Drug-induced psychotic disorder with delusions

Paranoid state induced by drugs

292.12 Drug-induced psychotic disorder with hallucinations

Hallucinatory state induced by drugs

Excludes *states following LSD or other*

hallucinogens, lasting only a

few days or less ["bad trips"]

(305.3)

Coding Clinic: 2004, Q3, P8

292.2 Pathological drug intoxication

Drug reaction resulting in brief psychotic states

NOS

idiosyncratic

pathologic

Excludes *expected brief psychotic reactions to*

hallucinogens ["bad trips"] (305.3)

physiological side-effects of drugs (e.g.,

dystonias)

● **292.8 Other specified drug-induced mental disorders**

292.81 Drug-induced delirium

292.82 Drug-induced persisting dementia

Coding Clinic: 2004, Q3, P8

292.83 Drug-induced persisting amnestic disorder

292.84 Drug-induced mood disorder

Depressive state induced by drugs

292.85 Drug induced sleep disorders

Drug induced circadian rhythm sleep

disorder

Drug induced hypersomnia

Drug induced insomnia

Drug induced parasomnia

■**292.89 Other**

Drug-induced anxiety disorder

Drug-induced organic personality

syndrome

Drug-induced sexual dysfunction

Drug intoxication

■**292.9 Unspecified drug-induced mental disorder**

Drug-related disorder NOS

Organic psychosis NOS due to or associated with

drugs

● **293   Transient mental disorders due to conditions classified elsewhere**

> **Includes**   transient organic mental disorders not associated with alcohol or drugs

> *Code first the associated physical or neurological condition*

> **Excludes**   *confusional state or delirium superimposed on senile dementia (290.3)*
> *dementia due to:*
> *alcohol (291.0–291.9)*
> *arteriosclerosis (290.40–290.43)*
> *drugs (292.82)*
> *senility (290.0)*

● **293.0   *Delirium due to conditions classified elsewhere***
Acute:
  confusional state
  infective psychosis
  organic reaction
  posttraumatic organic psychosis
  psycho-organic syndrome
Acute psychosis associated with endocrine, metabolic, or cerebrovascular disorder
Epileptic:
  confusional state
  twilight state
Coding Clinic: 1993, Q3, P11

● **293.1   *Subacute delirium***
Subacute:
  confusional state
  infective psychosis
  organic reaction
  posttraumatic organic psychosis
  psycho-organic syndrome
  psychosis associated with endocrine or metabolic disorder

● **293.8   Other specified transient mental disorders due to conditions classified elsewhere**

  ● **293.81   *Psychotic disorder with delusions in conditions classified elsewhere***
  Transient organic psychotic condition, paranoid type

  ● **293.82   *Psychotic disorder with hallucinations in conditions classified elsewhere***
  Transient organic psychotic condition, hallucinatory type

  ● **293.83   *Mood disorder in conditions classified elsewhere***
  Transient organic psychotic condition, depressive type

  ● **293.84   *Anxiety disorder in conditions classified elsewhere***
  Coding Clinic: 1996, Q4, P29

  ●■ **293.89   *Other***
  Catatonic disorder in conditions classified elsewhere

●■ **293.9   *Unspecified transient mental disorder in conditions classified elsewhere***
Organic psychosis:
  infective NOS
  posttraumatic NOS
  transient NOS
Psycho-organic syndrome

● **294   Persistent mental disorders due to conditions classified elsewhere**

> **Includes**   organic psychotic brain syndromes (chronic), not elsewhere classified

● **294.0   *Amnestic disorder in conditions classified elsewhere***
Korsakoff's psychosis or syndrome (nonalcoholic)

> *Code first underlying condition*

> **Excludes**   *alcoholic:*
> *amnestic syndrome (291.1)*
> *Korsakoff's psychosis (291.1)*

● **294.1   *Dementia in conditions classified elsewhere***
Dementia of the Alzheimer's type

> *Code first any underlying physical condition as:*
> dementia in:
>   Alzheimer's disease (331.0)
>   cerebral lipidoses (330.1)
>   dementia with Lewy bodies (331.82)
>   dementia with Parkinsonism (331.82)
>   epilepsy (345.0–345.9)
>   frontal dementia (331.19)
>   frontotemporal dementia (331.19)
>   general paresis [syphilis] (094.1)
>   hepatolenticular degeneration (275.1)
>   Huntington's chorea (333.4)
>   Jakob-Creutzfeldt disease (046.11–046.19) ◀▥
>   multiple sclerosis (340)
>   Pick's disease of the brain (331.11)
>   polyarteritis nodosa (446.0)
>   syphilis (094.1)

> **Excludes**   *dementia:*
> *arteriosclerotic (290.40–290.43)*
> *presenile (290.10–290.13)*
> *senile (290.0)*
> *epileptic psychosis NOS (294.8)*
Coding Clinic: 1999, Q1, P14; 1985, Sept-Oct, P12

  ● **294.10   *Dementia in conditions classified elsewhere without behavioral disturbance***
  Dementia in conditions classified elsewhere NOS

  ● **294.11   *Dementia in conditions classified elsewhere with behavioral disturbance***
  Aggressive behavior
  Combative behavior
  Violent behavior
  Wandering off
  Coding Clinic: 2000, Q4, P40-41

●■ **294.8   *Other persistent mental disorders due to conditions classified elsewhere***
Amnestic disorder NOS
Dementia NOS
Epileptic psychosis NOS
Mixed paranoid and affective organic psychotic states

> Use additional code for associated epilepsy (345.0–345.9)

> **Excludes**   *mild memory disturbances, not amounting to dementia (310.8)* ◀▥
Coding Clinic: 2003, Q3, P14

●■ **294.9   *Unspecified persistent mental disorders due to conditions classified elsewhere***
Cognitive disorder NOS
Organic psychosis (chronic)
Coding Clinic: 2007, Q2, P5

◀ New   ◀▥ Revised   ~~deleted~~ Deleted   ● Use Additional Digit(s)   ■ Nonspecific Code
● Not first-listed DX   OGCR Official Guidelines   Coding Clinic   Excludes   Includes   Use additional   Code first   Omit code

OTHER PSYCHOSES (295–299)

Use additional code to identify any associated physical disease, injury, or condition affecting the brain with psychoses classifiable to 295–298

● 295   **Schizophrenic disorders**
Personality disorders characterized by multiple mental and behavioral irregularities.

Includes   schizophrenia of the types described in 295.0–295.9 occurring in children

Excludes   *childhood type schizophrenia (299.9)*
infantile autism (299.0)

The following fifth-digit subclassification is for use with category 295:

> ■ 0   **unspecified**
> 1   **subchronic**
> 2   **chronic**
> 3   **subchronic with acute exacerbation**
> 4   **chronic with acute exacerbation**
> 5   **in remission**

● **295.0   Simple type**
[0-5]   Schizophrenia simplex

Excludes   *latent schizophrenia (295.5)*

● **295.1   Disorganized type**
[0-5]   Hebephrenia
Hebephrenic type schizophrenia

● **295.2   Catatonic type**
[0-5]   Catatonic (schizophrenia):
agitation
excitation
excited type
stupor
withdrawn type
Schizophrenic:
catalepsy
catatonia
flexibilitas cerea

● **295.3   Paranoid type**
[0-5]   Paraphrenic schizophrenia

Excludes   *involutional paranoid state (297.2)*
paranoia (297.1)
paraphrenia (297.2)

● **295.4   Schizophreniform disorder**
[0-5]   Oneirophrenia
Schizophreniform:
attack
psychosis, confusional type

Excludes   *acute forms of schizophrenia of:*
catatonic type (295.2)
hebephrenic type (295.1)
paranoid type (295.3)
simple type (295.0)
undifferentiated type (295.8)

● **295.5   Latent schizophrenia**
[0-5]   Latent schizophrenic reaction
Schizophrenia: Schizophrenia:
borderline   prodromal
incipient   pseudoneurotic
prepsychotic   pseudopsychopathic

Excludes   *schizoid personality (301.20–301.22)*

● **295.6   Residual type**
[0-5]   Chronic undifferentiated schizophrenia
Restzustand (schizophrenic)
Schizophrenic residual state
Coding Clinic: 2006, Q4, P76-78

● **295.7   Schizoaffective disorder**
[0-5]   Cyclic schizophrenia
Mixed schizophrenic and affective psychosis
Schizo-affective psychosis
Schizophreniform psychosis, affective type

● ■ **295.8   Other specified types of schizophrenia**
[0-5]   Acute (undifferentiated) schizophrenia
Atypical schizophrenia
Cenesthopathic schizophrenia

Excludes   *infantile autism (299.0)*

● ■ **295.9   Unspecified schizophrenia**
[0-5]   Schizophrenia: Schizophrenia:
NOS   undifferentiated NOS
mixed NOS   undifferentiated type
Schizophrenic reaction NOS
Schizophreniform psychosis NOS
Coding Clinic: 1995, Q3, P6

● 296   **Episodic mood disorders**

Includes   episodic affective disorders

Excludes   *neurotic depression (300.4)*
reactive depressive psychosis (298.0)
reactive excitation (298.1)

Coding Clinic: 1985, Mar-April, P14

The following fifth-digit subclassification is for use with categories 296.0–296.6:

> ■ 0   **unspecified**
> 1   **mild**
> 2   **moderate**
> 3   **severe, without mention of psychotic behavior**
> 4   **severe, specified as with psychotic behavior**
> 5   **in partial or unspecified remission**
> 6   **in full remission**

● **296.0   Bipolar I disorder, single manic episode**
[0-6]   *Manic depressive disorder, characterized by moods that swing between periods of exaggerated euphoria, irritability, or both (manic) and episodes of depression.*
Hypomania (mild) NOS single episode or unspecified
Hypomanic psychosis single episode or unspecified
Mania (monopolar) NOS single episode or unspecified
Manic-depressive psychosis or reaction, single episode or unspecified:
hypomanic, single episode or unspecified
manic, single episode or unspecified

Excludes   *circular type, if there was a previous attack of depression (296.4)*

● **296.1   Manic disorder, recurrent episode**
[0-6]   Any condition classifiable to 296.0, stated to be recurrent

Excludes   *circular type, if there was a previous attack of depression (296.4)*

MENTAL DISORDERS (290–319)

● **296.2 Major depressive disorder, single episode**
[0-6]   Depressive psychosis, single episode or unspecified
Endogenous depression, single episode or unspecified
Involutional melancholia, single episode or unspecified
Manic-depressive psychosis or reaction, depressed type, single episode or unspecified
Monopolar depression, single episode or unspecified
Psychotic depression, single episode or unspecified

> **Excludes** *circular type, if previous attack was of manic type (296.5)*
> *depression NOS (311)*
> *reactive depression (neurotic) (300.4)*
> *psychotic (298.0)*

● **296.3 Major depressive disorder, recurrent episode**
[0-6]   Any condition classifiable to 296.2, stated to be recurrent

> **Excludes** *circular type, if previous attack was of manic type (296.5)*
> *depression NOS (311)*
> *reactive depression (neurotic) (300.4)*
> *psychotic (298.0)*

● **296.4 Bipolar I disorder, most recent episode (or current)**
[0-6] **manic**
Bipolar disorder, now manic
Manic-depressive psychosis, circular type but currently manic

> **Excludes** *brief compensatory or rebound mood swings (296.99)*

● **296.5 Bipolar I disorder, most recent episode (or current)**
[0-6] **depressed**
Bipolar disorder, now depressed
Manic-depressive psychosis, circular type but currently depressed

> **Excludes** *brief compensatory or rebound mood swings (296.99)*

> Coding Clinic: 2006, Q1, P10

● **296.6 Bipolar I disorder, most recent episode (or current)**
[0-6] **mixed**
Manic-depressive psychosis, circular type, mixed

■ **296.7 Bipolar I disorder, most recent episode (or current) unspecified**
Atypical bipolar affective disorder NOS
Manic-depressive psychosis, circular type, current condition not specified as either manic or depressive

● **296.8 Other and unspecified bipolar disorders**

■ **296.80 Bipolar disorder, unspecified**
Bipolar disorder NOS
Manic-depressive:
reaction NOS
syndrome NOS

296.81 Atypical manic disorder

296.82 Atypical depressive disorder

■ **296.89 Other**
Bipolar II disorder
Manic-depressive psychosis, mixed type

● **296.9 Other and unspecified episodic mood disorder**

> **Excludes** *psychogenic affective psychoses (298.0–298.8)*

■ **296.90 Unspecified episodic mood disorder**
Affective psychosis NOS
Melancholia NOS
Mood disorder NOS
Coding Clinic: 1985, Mar-April, P14

■ **296.99 Other specified episodic mood disorder**
Mood swings:
brief compensatory
rebound

● **297 Delusional disorders**

> **Includes** paranoid disorders

> **Excludes** *acute paranoid reaction (298.3)*
> *alcoholic jealousy or paranoid state (291.5)*
> *paranoid schizophrenia (295.3)*

297.0 Paranoid state, simple

297.1 Delusional disorder
Chronic paranoid psychosis
Sander's disease
Systematized delusions

> **Excludes** *paranoid personality disorder (301.0)*

297.2 Paraphrenia
Involutional paranoid state
Late paraphrenia
Paraphrenia (involutional)

297.3 Shared psychotic disorder
Folie à deux
Induced psychosis or paranoid disorder

■ **297.8 Other specified paranoid states**
Paranoia querulans
Sensitiver Beziehungswahn

> **Excludes** *acute paranoid reaction or state (298.3)*
> *senile paranoid state (290.20)*

■ **297.9 Unspecified paranoid state**
Paranoid:
disorder NOS
psychosis NOS
reaction NOS
state NOS

● **298 Other nonorganic psychoses**

> **Includes** psychotic conditions due to or provoked by:
> emotional stress
> environmental factors as major part of etiology

298.0 Depressive type psychosis
Psychogenic depressive psychosis
Psychotic reactive depression
Reactive depressive psychosis

> **Excludes** *manic-depressive psychosis, depressed type (296.2–296.3)*
> *neurotic depression (300.4)*
> *reactive depression NOS (300.4)*

298.1 Excitative type psychosis
Acute hysterical psychosis
Psychogenic excitation
Reactive excitation

> **Excludes** *manic-depressive psychosis, manic type (296.0–296.1)*

◀ New   ◀▥ Revised   ~~deleted~~ Deleted   ● Use Additional Digit(s)   ■ Nonspecific Code
● Not first-listed DX   OGCR Official Guidelines   Coding Clinic   Excludes   Includes   Use additional   Code first   Omit code

298.2 Reactive confusion
Psychogenic confusion
Psychogenic twilight state
> **Excludes** *acute confusional state (293.0)*

298.3 Acute paranoid reaction
Acute psychogenic paranoid psychosis
Bouffée délirante
> **Excludes** *paranoid states (297.0–297.9)*

298.4 Psychogenic paranoid psychosis
Protracted reactive paranoid psychosis

■**298.8 Other and unspecified reactive psychosis**
Brief psychotic disorder
Brief reactive psychosis NOS
Hysterical psychosis
Psychogenic psychosis NOS
Psychogenic stupor
> **Excludes** *acute hysterical psychosis (298.1)*

■**298.9 Unspecified psychosis**
Atypical psychosis
Psychosis NOS
Psychotic disorder NOS
Coding Clinic: 2006, Q3, P22; 1993, Q3, P11

● **299 Pervasive developmental disorders**
> **Excludes** *adult type psychoses occurring in childhood, as:*
> *affective disorders (296.0–296.9)*
> *manic-depressive disorders (296.0–296.9)*
> *schizophrenia (295.0–295.9)*

The following fifth-digit subclassification is for use with category 299:

0	**current or active state**
1	**residual state**

● **299.0 Autistic disorder**
[0-1]   Childhood autism
Infantile psychosis
Kanner's syndrome
> **Excludes** *disintegrative psychosis (299.1)*
> *Heller's syndrome (299.1)*
> *schizophrenic syndrome of childhood (299.9)*

● **299.1 Childhood disintegrative disorder**
[0-1]   Heller's syndrome

Use additional code to identify any associated neurological disorder
> **Excludes** *infantile autism (299.0)*
> *schizophrenic syndrome of childhood (299.9)*

● ■**299.8 Other specified pervasive developmental**
[0-1] **disorders**
Asperger's disorder
Atypical childhood psychosis
Borderline psychosis of childhood
> **Excludes** *simple stereotypes without psychotic disturbance (307.3)*

● ■**299.9 Unspecified pervasive developmental disorder**
[0-1]   Child psychosis NOS
Pervasive developmental disorder NOS
Schizophrenia, childhood type NOS
Schizophrenic syndrome of childhood NOS
> **Excludes** *schizophrenia of adult type occurring in childhood (295.0–295.9)*

Item 5-2   Anxiety is also known as **generalized disorder** and is evidenced by persistent, excessive, and unrealistic worry about everyday things. **Dissociative disorders** are characterized by a persistent disruption in the integration of memory, consciousness, or identity and a lack of mental connectedness to events. **Somatoform disorders** are characterized by unusual physical symptoms in the absence of any known physical pathology and may lead to unnecessary medical treatments.

NEUROTIC DISORDERS, PERSONALITY DISORDERS, AND OTHER NONPSYCHOTIC MENTAL DISORDERS (300–316)

● **300 Anxiety, dissociative and somatoform disorders**

● **300.0 Anxiety states**
> **Excludes** *anxiety in:*
> *acute stress reaction (308.0)*
> *transient adjustment reaction (309.24)*
> *neurasthenia (300.5)*
> *psychophysiological disorders (306.0–306.9)*
> *separation anxiety (309.21)*

■**300.00 Anxiety state, unspecified**
Anxiety:
neurosis
reaction
state (neurotic)
Atypical anxiety disorder

300.01 Panic disorder without agoraphobia
Panic:
attack
state
> **Excludes** *panic disorder with agoraphobia (300.21)*

300.02 Generalized anxiety disorder

■**300.09 Other**

● **300.1 Dissociative, conversion and factitious disorders**
> **Excludes** *adjustment reaction (309.0–309.9)*
> *anorexia nervosa (307.1)*
> *gross stress reaction (308.0–308.9)*
> *hysterical personality (301.50–301.59)*
> *psychophysiologic disorders (306.0–306.9)*

■**300.10 Hysteria, unspecified**

300.11 Conversion disorder
Astasia-abasia, hysterical
Conversion hysteria or reaction
Hysterical:
blindness
deafness
paralysis
Coding Clinic: 1985, Nov-Dec, P15

300.12 Dissociative amnesia
Hysterical amnesia

300.13 Dissociative fugue
Hysterical fugue

300.14 Dissociative identity disorder

■**300.15 Dissociative disorder or reaction, unspecified**

300.16 Factitious disorder with predominantly psychological signs and symptoms
Compensation neurosis
Ganser's syndrome, hysterical

MENTAL DISORDERS (290–319)

■ **300.19 Other and unspecified factitious illness**
Factitious disorder (with combined psychological and physical signs and symptoms) (with predominantly physical signs and symptoms) NOS

Excludes *multiple operations or hospital addiction syndrome (301.51)*

● **300.2 Phobic disorders**
Irrational fear with avoidance of the feared subject, activity, or situation. Divided into 3 types: specific phobias, social phobias, and agoraphobia.

Excludes *anxiety state not associated with a specific situation or object (300.00–300.09)*
obsessional phobias (300.3)

■ **300.20 Phobia, unspecified**
Anxiety-hysteria NOS
Phobia NOS

300.21 Agoraphobia with panic disorder
Fear of:
open spaces with panic attacks
streets with panic attacks
travel with panic attacks
Panic disorder with agoraphobia

Excludes *agoraphobia without panic disorder (300.22)*
panic disorder without agoraphobia (300.01)

300.22 Agoraphobia without mention of panic attacks
Any condition classifiable to 300.21 without mention of panic attacks

300.23 Social phobia
Fear of:
eating in public
public speaking
washing in public

■ **300.29 Other isolated or specific phobias**
Acrophobia
Fear of heights
Animal phobias
Claustrophobia
Fear of closed spaces
Fear of crowds

300.3 Obsessive-compulsive disorders *(OCD)*
Anancastic neurosis
Compulsive neurosis
Obsessional phobia [any]

Excludes *obsessive-compulsive symptoms occurring in:*
endogenous depression (296.2–296.3)
organic states (e.g., encephalitis)
schizophrenia (295.0–295.9)

300.4 Dysthymic disorder
Anxiety depression
Depression with anxiety
Depressive reaction
Neurotic depressive state
Reactive depression

Excludes *adjustment reaction with depressive symptoms (309.0–309.1)*
depression NOS (311)
manic-depressive psychosis, depressed type (296.2–296.3)
reactive depressive psychosis (298.0)

300.5 Neurasthenia
Fatigue neurosis
Nervous debility
Psychogenic:
asthenia
general fatigue

Use additional code to identify any associated physical disorder

Excludes *anxiety state (300.00–300.09)*
neurotic depression (300.4)
psychophysiological disorders (306.0–306.9)
specific nonpsychotic mental disorders following organic brain damage (310.0–310.9)

300.6 Depersonalization disorder
Derealization (neurotic)
Neurotic state with depersonalization episode

Excludes *depersonalization associated with:*
anxiety (300.00–300.09)
depression (300.4)
manic-depressive disorder or psychosis (296.0–296.9)
schizophrenia (295.0–295.9)

300.7 Hypochondriasis
Hypochondriac
Body dysmorphic disorder

Excludes *hypochondriasis in:*
hysteria (300.10–300.19)
manic-depressive psychosis, depressed type (296.2–296.3)
neurasthenia (300.5)
obsessional disorder (300.3)
schizophrenia (295.0–295.9)

● **300.8 Somatoform disorders**

300.81 Somatization disorder
Briquet's disorder
Severe somatoform disorder

300.82 Undifferentiated somatoform disorder
Atypical somatoform disorder
Somatoform disorder NOS

■ **300.89 Other somatoform disorders**
Occupational neurosis, including writers' cramp
Psychasthenia
Psychasthenic neurosis

■ **300.9 Unspecified nonpsychotic mental disorder**
Psychoneurosis NOS

● **301 Personality disorders**
Long-term patterns of thoughts and behaviors causing serious problems with relationships and work.

Includes character neurosis

Use additional code to identify any associated neurosis or psychosis, or physical condition

Excludes *nonpsychotic personality disorder associated with organic brain syndromes (310.0–310.9)*

301.0 Paranoid personality disorder
Fanatic personality
Paranoid personality (disorder)
Paranoid traits

Excludes *acute paranoid reaction (298.3)*
alcoholic paranoia (291.5)
paranoid schizophrenia (295.3)
paranoid states (297.0–297.9)

◀ New   ◀▥ Revised   ~~deleted~~ Deleted   ● Use Additional Digit(s)   ■ Nonspecific Code

● Not first-listed DX   OGCR Official Guidelines   Coding Clinic   Excludes   Includes   Use additional   Code first   Omit code

● **301.1 Affective personality disorder**

    Excludes *affective psychotic disorders (296.0–296.9)*
                  neurasthenia (300.5)
                  neurotic depression (300.4)

    301.10 Affective personality disorder, unspecified

    301.11 Chronic hypomanic personality disorder
          Chronic hypomanic disorder
          Hypomanic personality

    301.12 Chronic depressive personality disorder
          Chronic depressive disorder
          Depressive character or personality

    301.13 Cyclothymic disorder
          Cycloid personality
          Cyclothymia
          Cyclothymic personality

● **301.2 Schizoid personality disorder**

    Excludes *schizophrenia (295.0–295.9)*

    ■**301.20 Schizoid personality disorder, unspecified**

    301.21 Introverted personality

    301.22 Schizotypal personality disorder

301.3 Explosive personality disorder
    Aggressive:
       personality
       reaction
    Aggressiveness
    Emotional instability (excessive)
    Pathological emotionality
    Quarrelsomeness

    Excludes *dyssocial personality (301.7)*
                  hysterical neurosis (300.10–300.19)

301.4 Obsessive-compulsive personality disorder
    Anancastic personality
    Obsessional personality

    Excludes *obsessive-compulsive disorder (300.3)*
                  phobic state (300.20–300.29)

● **301.5 Histrionic personality disorder**

    Excludes *hysterical neurosis (300.10–300.19)*

    ■**301.50 Histrionic personality disorder, unspecified**
          Hysterical personality NOS

    301.51 Chronic factitious illness with physical symptoms
          Hospital addiction syndrome
          Multiple operations syndrome
          Munchausen syndrome

    ■**301.59 Other histrionic personality disorder**
          Personality: Personality:
            emotionally unstable   psychoinfantile
            labile

301.6 Dependent personality disorder
    Asthenic personality
    Inadequate personality
    Passive personality

    Excludes *neurasthenia (300.5)*
                  passive-aggressive personality (301.84)

301.7 Antisocial personality disorder
    Amoral personality
    Asocial personality
    Dyssocial personality
    Personality disorder with predominantly
        sociopathic or asocial manifestation

    Excludes *disturbance of conduct without specifiable*
                  personality disorder (312.0–312.9)
                  explosive personality (301.3)

    Coding Clinic: 1984, Sept-Oct, P16

● **301.8 Other personality disorders**

    301.81 Narcissistic personality disorder

    301.82 Avoidant personality disorder

    301.83 Borderline personality disorder

    301.84 Passive-aggressive personality

    ■**301.89 Other**
          Personality: Personality:
            eccentric   masochistic
            "haltlose" type   psychoneurotic
            immature

          Excludes *psychoinfantile personality (301.59)*

■**301.9 Unspecified personality disorder**
    Pathological personality NOS
    Personality disorder NOS
    Psychopathic:
       constitutional state
       personality (disorder)

● **302 Sexual and gender identity disorders**

    Excludes *sexual disorder manifest in:*
                  organic brain syndrome (290.0–294.9,
                     310.0–310.9)
                  psychosis (295.0–298.9)

    302.0 Ego-dystonic sexual orientation
          Ego-dystonic lesbianism
          Sexual orientation conflict disorder

          Excludes *homosexual pedophilia (302.2)*

    302.1 Zoophilia
          Bestiality

    302.2 Pedophilia

    302.3 Transvestic fetishism

          Excludes *trans-sexualism (302.5)*

    302.4 Exhibitionism

● **302.5 Trans-sexualism**
          Sex reassignment surgery status

          Excludes *transvestism (302.3)*

    ■**302.50 With unspecified sexual history**

    302.51 With asexual history

    302.52 With homosexual history

    302.53 With heterosexual history

    302.6 Gender identity disorder in children
          Check age: adolescents and adults separately classified
            under 302.85.
          Feminism in boys
          Gender identity disorder NOS

          Excludes *gender identity disorder in adult (302.85)*
                  trans-sexualism (302.50–302.53)
                  transvestism (302.3)

● **302.7 Psychosexual dysfunction**

          Excludes *decreased sexual desire NOS (799.81)*
                  impotence of organic origin (607.84)
                  normal transient symptoms from ruptured
                     hymen
                  transient or occasional failures of erection
                     due to fatigue, anxiety, alcohol, or
                     drugs

    ■**302.70 Psychosexual dysfunction, unspecified**
          Sexual dysfunction NOS

    302.71 Hypoactive sexual desire disorder

          Excludes *decreased sexual desire NOS*
                  (799.81)

MENTAL DISORDERS (290–319)

302.72 **With inhibited sexual excitement**
  Female sexual arousal disorder
  Frigidity
  Impotence
  Male erectile disorder

302.73 **Female orgasmic disorder ♀**

302.74 **Male orgasmic disorder ♂**

302.75 **Premature ejaculation ♂**

302.76 **Dyspareunia, psychogenic ♀**

302.79 **With other specified psychosexual dysfunctions**
  Sexual aversion disorder

302.8 **Other specified psychosexual disorders**

302.81 **Fetishism**

302.82 **Voyeurism**

302.83 **Sexual masochism**

302.84 **Sexual sadism**

302.85 **Gender identity disorder in adolescents or adults**
  Use additional code to identify sex reassignment surgery status (302.5)
  Excludes *gender identity disorder NOS (302.6)*
    gender identity disorder in children (302.6)

302.89 **Other**
  Frotteurism
  Nymphomania
  Satyriasis

302.9 **Unspecified psychosexual disorder**
  Paraphilia NOS
  Pathologic sexuality NOS
  Sexual deviation NOS
  Sexual disorder NOS

303 **Alcohol dependence syndrome**
  Use additional code to identify any associated condition, as:
  alcoholic psychoses (291.0–291.9)
  drug dependence (304.0–304.9)
  physical complications of alcohol, such as:
    cerebral degeneration (331.7)
    cirrhosis of liver (571.2)
    epilepsy (345.0–345.9)
    gastritis (535.3)
    hepatitis (571.1)
    liver damage NOS (571.3)
  Excludes *drunkenness NOS (305.0)*
  Coding Clinic: 1995, Q3, P6

The following fifth-digit subclassification is for use with category 303:

  0 unspecified
  1 continuous
  2 episodic
  3 in remission

303.0 **Acute alcoholic intoxication**
[0-3]   Acute drunkenness in alcoholism
  Coding Clinic: 1985, July-Aug, P15

303.9 **Other and unspecified alcohol dependence**
[0-3]   Chronic alcoholism
  Dipsomania
  Coding Clinic: 2002, Q2, P4; Q1, P3-4; 1989, Q2, P9; 1985, Nov-Dec, P14

304 **Drug dependence**
For some "dependence" codes there is a corresponding "abuse" code. There is a point at which drug use crosses from "dependence" to "abuse." Check documentation or query provider for patient status.
  Excludes *nondependent abuse of drugs (305.1–305.9)*

The following fifth-digit subclassification is for use with category 304:

  0 unspecified
  1 continuous
  2 episodic
  3 in remission

304.0 **Opioid type dependence**
[0-3]   Heroin
  Meperidine
  Methadone
  Morphine
  Opium
  Opium alkaloids and their derivatives
  Synthetics with morphine-like effects
  Coding Clinic: 2006, Q2, P7; 1988, Q4, P8

304.1 **Sedative, hypnotic or anxiolytic dependence**
[0-3]   Barbiturates
  Nonbarbiturate sedatives and tranquilizers with a similar effect:
    chlordiazepoxide
    diazepam
    glutethimide
    meprobamate
    methaqualone

304.2 **Cocaine dependence**
[0-3]   Coca leaves and derivatives

304.3 **Cannabis dependence**
[0-3]   *Code 305.2 is for abuse of cannabis.*
  Hashish
  Hemp
  Marihuana

304.4 **Amphetamine and other psychostimulant dependence**
[0-3]   Methylphenidate
  Phenmetrazine

304.5 **Hallucinogen dependence**
[0-3]   Dimethyltryptamine [DMT]
  Lysergic acid diethylamide [LSD] and derivatives
  Mescaline
  Psilocybin

304.6 **Other specified drug dependence**
[0-3]   Absinthe addiction
  Glue sniffing
  Inhalant dependence
  Phencyclidine dependence
  Excludes *tobacco dependence (305.1)*

304.7 **Combinations of opioid type drug with any other**
[0-3]

304.8 **Combinations of drug dependence excluding opioid type drug**
[0-3]   Coding Clinic: 1986, Mar-April, P12

304.9 **Unspecified drug dependence**
[0-3]   Drug addiction NOS
  Drug dependence NOS
  Coding Clinic: 2003, Q4, P103-104

MENTAL DISORDERS (290–319)

◀ New   ◀|||| Revised   ~~deleted~~ Deleted   ● Use Additional Digit(s)   ■ Nonspecific Code
● Not first-listed DX   OGCR Official Guidelines   Coding Clinic   Excludes   Includes   Use additional   Code first   Omit code

● **305 Nondependent abuse of drugs**

  Note: Includes cases where a person, for whom no
  other diagnosis is possible, has come under
  medical care because of the maladaptive effect of
  a drug on which he is not dependent and that he
  has taken on his own initiative *(self-medicating)* to
  the detriment of his health or social functioning.

  Excludes *alcohol dependence syndrome (303.0–303.9)*
  drug dependence (304.0–304.9)
  drug withdrawal syndrome (292.0)
  poisoning by drugs or medicinal substances
  (960.0–979.9)

  The following fifth-digit subclassification is for use with
  codes 305.0, 305.2–305.9:

  ■ **0 unspecified**
  1 continuous
  2 episodic
  3 in remission

● **305.0 Alcohol abuse**
  [0-3]   Drunkenness NOS
          Excessive drinking of alcohol NOS
          "Hangover" (alcohol)
          Inebriety NOS

          Excludes *acute alcohol intoxication in alcoholism*
                    (303.0)
                    alcoholic psychoses (291.0–291.9)
          Coding Clinic: 1996, Q3, P16; 1985, July-Aug, P15

  305.1 Tobacco use disorder   ◀▬
  [0-3]   Tobacco dependence

          Excludes *history of tobacco use (V15.82)*
                    smoking complicating pregnancy (649.0)
                    tobacco use disorder complicating
                    pregnancy (649.0)
          Coding Clinic: 2009, Q1, P8; 1996, Q2, P10; 1984, Nov-Dec, P12

● **305.2 Cannabis abuse**
  [0-3]   *Code 304.3 is for cannabis dependence.*

● **305.3 Hallucinogen abuse**
  [0-3]   Acute intoxication from hallucinogens ["bad
          trips"]
          LSD reaction

● **305.4 Sedative, hypnotic or anxiolytic abuse**
  [0-3]

● **305.5 Opioid abuse**
  [0-3]

● **305.6 Cocaine abuse**
  [0-3]   Coding Clinic: 1993, Q1, P25; Q1, P25; 1988, Q4, P8

● **305.7 Amphetamine or related acting sympathomimetic**
  [0-3]   **abuse**
          Coding Clinic: 2003, Q2, P10,11x2

● **305.8 Antidepressant type abuse**
  [0-3]

● ■ **305.9 Other, mixed, or unspecified drug abuse**
  [0-3]   Caffeine intoxication
          Inhalant abuse
          "Laxative habit"
          Misuse of drugs NOS
          Nonprescribed use of drugs or patent medicinals
          Phencyclidine abuse
          Coding Clinic: 1999, Q3, P20; 1994, Q4, P36

● **306 Physiological malfunction arising from mental factors**

  Includes psychogenic:
            physical symptoms not involving tissue
                damage
            physiological manifestations not involving
                tissue damage

  Excludes *hysteria (300.11–300.19)*
            physical symptoms secondary to a psychiatric
                disorder classified elsewhere
            psychic factors associated with physical conditions
                involving tissue damage classified elsewhere
                (316)
            specific nonpsychotic mental disorders following
                organic brain damage (310.0–310.9)

  306.0 Musculoskeletal
          Psychogenic paralysis
          Psychogenic torticollis

          Excludes *Gilles de la Tourette's syndrome (307.23)*
                    paralysis as hysterical or conversion
                        reaction (300.11)
                    tics (307.20–307.22)

  306.1 Respiratory
          Psychogenic: Psychogenic:
            air hunger   hyperventilation
            cough   yawning
            hiccough

          Excludes *psychogenic asthma (316 and 493.9)*

  306.2 Cardiovascular
          Cardiac neurosis
          Cardiovascular neurosis
          Neurocirculatory asthenia
          Psychogenic cardiovascular disorder

          Excludes *psychogenic paroxysmal tachycardia*
                    (316 and 427.2)
          Coding Clinic: 1985, July-Aug, P14

  306.3 Skin
          Psychogenic pruritus

          Excludes *psychogenic:*
                    alopecia (316 and 704.00)
                    dermatitis (316 and 692.9)
                    eczema (316 and 691.8 or 692.9)
                    urticaria (316 and 708.0–708.9)

  306.4 Gastrointestinal
          Aerophagy
          Cyclical vomiting, psychogenic
          Diarrhea, psychogenic
          Nervous gastritis
          Psychogenic dyspepsia

          Excludes *cyclical vomiting NOS (536.2)*
                    associated with migraine (346.2)
                    globus hystericus (300.11)
                    mucous colitis (316 and 564.9)
                    psychogenic:
                    cardiospasm (316 and 530.0)
                    duodenal ulcer (316 and 532.0–532.9)
                    gastric ulcer (316 and 531.0–531.9)
                    peptic ulcer NOS (316 and 533.0–533.9)
                    vomiting NOS (307.54)
          Coding Clinic: 1989, Q2, P11

MENTAL DISORDERS (290–319)

● **306.5 Genitourinary**

> **Excludes** *enuresis, psychogenic (307.6)*
> *frigidity (302.72)*
> *impotence (302.72)*
> *psychogenic dyspareunia (302.76)*

◾ **306.50 Psychogenic genitourinary malfunction, unspecified**

306.51 Psychogenic vaginismus ♀
Functional vaginismus

306.52 Psychogenic dysmenorrhea ♀

306.53 Psychogenic dysuria

◾ **306.59 Other**

306.6 Endocrine

306.7 Organs of special sense

> **Excludes** *hysterical blindness or deafness (300.11)*
> *psychophysical visual disturbances (368.16)*

◾ **306.8 Other specified psychophysiological malfunction**
Bruxism
Sleep-related bruxism, 327.53
Teeth grinding

◾ **306.9 Unspecified psychophysiological malfunction**
Psychophysiologic disorder NOS
Psychosomatic disorder NOS

● **307 Special symptoms or syndromes, not elsewhere classified**

> **Note:** This category is intended for use if the psychopathology is manifested by a single specific symptom or group of symptoms which is not part of an organic illness or other mental disorder classifiable elsewhere.

> **Excludes** *those due to mental disorders classified elsewhere*
> *those of organic origin*

307.0 Stuttering

> **Excludes** *dysphasia (784.59)*   ◀▥
> *lisping or lalling (307.9)*
> *retarded development of speech (315.31–315.39)*
> *stuttering (fluency disorder) due to late effect of cerebrovascular accident (438.14)*   ◀

307.1 Anorexia nervosa

> **Excludes** *eating disturbance NOS (307.50)*
> *feeding problem (783.3)*
> *of nonorganic origin (307.59)*
> *loss of appetite (783.0)*
> *of nonorganic origin (307.59)*
> Coding Clinic: 2006, Q2, P12; 1989, Q4, P11

● **307.2 Tics**

> **Excludes** *nail-biting or thumb-sucking (307.9)*
> *stereotypes occurring in isolation (307.3)*
> *tics of organic origin (333.3)*

◾ **307.20 Tic disorder, unspecified**
Tic disorder NOS

307.21 Transient tic disorder

307.22 Chronic motor or vocal tic disorder

307.23 Tourette's disorder
Motor-verbal tic disorder

307.3 Stereotypic movement disorder
Body-rocking
Head banging
Spasmus nutans
Stereotypes NOS

> **Excludes** *tics (307.20–307.23)*
> *of organic origin (333.3)*

● **307.4 Specific disorders of sleep of nonorganic origin**

> **Excludes** *narcolepsy (347.00–347.11)*
> *organic hypersomnia (327.10–327.19)*
> *organic insomnia (327.00–327.09)*
> *those of unspecified cause (780.50–780.59)*

◾ **307.40 Nonorganic sleep disorder, unspecified**

307.41 Transient disorder of initiating or maintaining sleep
Adjustment insomnia
Hyposomnia associated with acute or intermittent emotional reactions or conflicts
Insomnia associated with acute or intermittent emotional reactions or conflicts
Sleeplessness associated with acute or intermittent emotional reactions or conflicts

307.42 Persistent disorder of initiating or maintaining sleep
Hyposomnia, insomnia, or sleeplessness associated with:
anxiety
conditioned arousal
depression (major) (minor)
psychosis
Idiopathic insomnia
Paradoxical insomnia
Primary insomnia
Psychophysiological insomnia

307.43 Transient disorder of initiating or maintaining wakefulness
Hypersomnia associated with acute or intermittent emotional reactions or conflicts

307.44 Persistent disorder of initiating or maintaining wakefulness
Hypersomnia associated with depression (major) (minor)
Insufficient sleep syndrome
Primary hypersomnia

> **Excludes** *sleep deprivation (V69.4)*

307.45 Circadian rhythm sleep disorder of nonorganic origin

307.46 Sleep arousal disorder
Night terror disorder
Night terrors
Sleep terror disorder
Sleepwalking
Somnambulism

◾ **307.47 Other dysfunctions of sleep stages or arousal from sleep**
Nightmare disorder
Nightmares:
NOS
REM-sleep type
Sleep drunkenness

307.48 Repetitive intrusions of sleep
Repetitive intrusion of sleep with:
atypical polysomnographic features
environmental disturbances
repeated REM-sleep interruptions

◾ **307.49 Other**
"Short-sleeper"
Subjective insomnia complaint

● **307.5 Other and unspecified disorders of eating**

> **Excludes**   *anorexia:*
> > *nervosa (307.1)*
> > *of unspecified cause (783.0)*
> *overeating, of unspecified cause (783.6)*
> *vomiting:*
> > *NOS (787.03)*
> > *cyclical (536.2)*
> > > *associated with migraine (346.2)*
> > *psychogenic (306.4)*

■ **307.50 Eating disorder, unspecified**
> Eating disorder NOS

307.51 Bulimia nervosa
> Overeating of nonorganic origin

307.52 Pica
> Perverted appetite of nonorganic origin
> *Craving and eating substances such as paint, clay, or dirt to replace a nutritional deficit in the body.*

307.53 Rumination disorder
> Regurgitation, of nonorganic origin, of food with reswallowing
> > **Excludes**   *obsessional rumination (300.3)*

307.54 Psychogenic vomiting

■ **307.59 Other**
> Feeding disorder of infancy or early childhood of nonorganic origin
> Infantile feeding disturbances of nonorganic origin
> Loss of appetite of nonorganic origin

Item 5–3   Enuresis: Bed wetting by children at night. Causes can be either psychological or medical (diabetes, urinary tract infections, or abnormalities). **Encopresis**: Overflow incontinence of bowels sometimes resulting from chronic constipation or fecal impaction. Check the documentation for additional diagnoses.

307.6 Enuresis
> Enuresis (primary) (secondary) of nonorganic origin
> > **Excludes**   *enuresis of unspecified cause (788.3)*

307.7 Encopresis
> Encopresis (continuous) (discontinuous) of nonorganic origin
> > **Excludes**   *encopresis of unspecified cause (787.6)*

● **307.8 Pain disorders related to psychological factors**

■ **307.80 Psychogenic pain, site unspecified**

307.81 Tension headache
> > **Excludes**   *headache:*
> > > *migraine (346.0–346.9)*
> > > *NOS (784.0)*
> > > *syndromes (339.00–339.89)*
> > > *tension type (339.10–339.12)*
> > Coding Clinic: 1985, Nov-Dec, P16

● ■ **307.89 Other**
> *Code first to type or site of pain*
> > **Excludes**   *pain disorder exclusively attributed to psychological factors (307.80)*
> > *psychogenic pain (307.80)*

■ **307.9 Other and unspecified special symptoms or syndromes, not elsewhere classified**
> Communication disorder NOS
> Hair plucking
> Lalling
> Lisping
> Masturbation
> Nail-biting
> Thumb-sucking

● **308 Acute reaction to stress**

> **Includes**   catastrophic stress
> combat fatigue
> gross stress reaction (acute)
> transient disorders in response to exceptional physical or mental stress which usually subside within hours or days

> **Excludes**   *adjustment reaction or disorder (309.0–309.9)*
> *chronic stress reaction (309.1–309.9)*

308.0 Predominant disturbance of emotions
> Anxiety as acute reaction to exceptional [gross] stress
> Emotional crisis as acute reaction to exceptional [gross] stress
> Panic state as acute reaction to exceptional [gross] stress

308.1 Predominant disturbance of consciousness
> Fugues as acute reaction to exceptional [gross] stress

308.2 Predominant psychomotor disturbance
> Agitation states as acute reaction to exceptional [gross] stress
> Stupor as acute reaction to exceptional [gross] stress

■ **308.3 Other acute reactions to stress**
> Acute situational disturbance
> Acute stress disorder
> > **Excludes**   *prolonged posttraumatic emotional disturbance (309.81)*

308.4 Mixed disorders as reaction to stress

■ **308.9 Unspecified acute reaction to stress**

● **309 Adjustment reaction**

> **Includes**   adjustment disorders
> reaction (adjustment) to chronic stress

> **Excludes**   *acute reaction to major stress (308.0–308.9)*
> *neurotic disorders (300.0–300.9)*

309.0 Adjustment disorder with depressed mood
> Grief reaction
> > **Excludes**   *affective psychoses (296.0–296.9)*
> > *neurotic depression (300.4)*
> > *prolonged depressive reaction (309.1)*
> > *psychogenic depressive psychosis (298.0)*

309.1 Prolonged depressive reaction
> > **Excludes**   *affective psychoses (296.0–296.9)*
> > *brief depressive reaction (309.0)*
> > *neurotic depression (300.4)*
> > *psychogenic depressive psychosis (298.0)*

MENTAL DISORDERS (290–319)

● **309.2 With predominant disturbance of other emotions**

  309.21 Separation anxiety disorder

  309.22 Emancipation disorder of adolescence and early adult life

  309.23 Specific academic or work inhibition

  309.24 Adjustment disorder with anxiety

  309.28 Adjustment disorder with mixed anxiety and depressed mood
    Adjustment reaction with anxiety and depression

  ■**309.29 Other**
    Culture shock

309.3 Adjustment disorder with disturbance of conduct
  Conduct disturbance as adjustment reaction
  Destructiveness as adjustment reaction

  Excludes *destructiveness in child (312.9)*
    disturbance of conduct NOS (312.9)
    dyssocial behavior without manifest psychiatric disorder (V71.01–V71.02)
    personality disorder with predominantly sociopathic or asocial manifestations (301.7)

309.4 Adjustment disorder with mixed disturbance of emotions and conduct

● **309.8 Other specified adjustment reactions**

  309.81 Posttraumatic stress disorder
    Chronic posttraumatic stress disorder
    Concentration camp syndrome
    Posttraumatic stress disorder NOS
    Post-Traumatic Stress Disorder (PTSD)

    Excludes *acute stress disorder (308.3)*
      posttraumatic brain syndrome:
      nonpsychotic (310.2)
      psychotic (293.0–293.9)

  309.82 Adjustment reaction with physical symptoms

  309.83 Adjustment reaction with withdrawal
    Elective mutism as adjustment reaction
    Hospitalism (in children) NOS

  ■**309.89 Other**

■**309.9 Unspecified adjustment reaction**
  Adaptation reaction NOS
  Adjustment reaction NOS

● **310 Specific nonpsychotic mental disorders due to brain damage**

  Excludes *neuroses, personality disorders, or other nonpsychotic conditions occurring in a form similar to that seen with functional disorders but in association with a physical condition (300.0–300.9, 301.0–301.9)*

310.0 Frontal lobe syndrome
  Lobotomy syndrome
  Postleucotomy syndrome [state]

  Excludes *postcontusion syndrome (310.2)*

310.1 Personality change due to conditions classified elsewhere
  Cognitive or personality change of other type, of nonpsychotic severity
  Organic psychosyndrome of nonpsychotic severity
  Presbyophrenia NOS
  Senility with mental changes of nonpsychotic severity

  Excludes *memory loss of unknown cause (780.93)*
    mild cognitive impairment (331.83) ◀
    postconcussion syndrome (310.2) ◀
    signs and symptoms involving emotional state (799.21–799.29) ◀

  Coding Clinic: 2005, Q2, P6-7

310.2 Postconcussion syndrome
  Postcontusion syndrome or encephalopathy
  Posttraumatic brain syndrome, nonpsychotic
  Status postcommotio cerebri

  Excludes *any organic psychotic conditions following head injury (293.0–294.0)*
    frontal lobe syndrome (310.0)
    postencephalitic syndrome (310.8)

  Use additional code to identify associated post-traumatic headache, if applicable (339.20-339.22)

■**310.8 Other specified nonpsychotic mental disorders following organic brain damage**
  Mild memory disturbance
  Postencephalitic syndrome
  Other focal (partial) organic psychosyndromes

  Excludes *memory loss of unknown cause (780.93)* ◀

■**310.9 Unspecified nonpsychotic mental disorder following organic brain damage**
  Coding Clinic: 2003, Q4, P103-104

311 Depressive disorder, not elsewhere classified
  Depressive disorder NOS
  Depressive state NOS
  Depression NOS

  Excludes *acute reaction to major stress with depressive symptoms (308.0)*
    affective personality disorder (301.10–301.13)
    affective psychoses (296.0–296.9)
    brief depressive reaction (309.0)
    depressive states associated with stressful events (309.0–309.1)
    disturbance of emotions specific to childhood and adolescence, with misery and unhappiness (313.1)
    mixed adjustment reaction with depressive symptoms (309.4)
    neurotic depression (300.4)
    prolonged depressive adjustment reaction (309.1)
    psychogenic depressive psychosis (298.0)

  Coding Clinic: 2003, Q4, P75-76

● **312 Disturbance of conduct, not elsewhere classified**

  Excludes *adjustment reaction with disturbance of conduct (309.3)*
    drug dependence (304.0–304.9)
    dyssocial behavior without manifest psychiatric disorder (V71.01–V71.02)
    personality disorder with predominantly sociopathic or asocial manifestations (301.7)
    sexual deviations (302.0–302.9)

  The following fifth-digit subclassification is for use with categories 312.0–312.2:

  ■0 unspecified
   1 mild
   2 moderate
   3 severe

● **312.0 Undersocialized conduct disorder, aggressive type**
  [0-3] Aggressive outburst
    Anger reaction
    Unsocialized aggressive disorder

● **312.1 Undersocialized conduct disorder, unaggressive type**
  [0-3] Childhood truancy, unsocialized
    Solitary stealing
    Tantrums

◀ New   ◀▥ Revised   ~~deleted~~ Deleted   ● Use Additional Digit(s)   ■ Nonspecific Code
● Not first-listed DX   OGCR Official Guidelines   Coding Clinic   Excludes   Includes   Use additional   Code first   Omit code

●**312.2 Socialized conduct disorder**
[0-3]   Childhood truancy, socialized
     Group delinquency

> **Excludes**   *gang activity without manifest psychiatric*
>   *disorder (V71.01)*

●**312.3 Disorders of impulse control, not elsewhere classified**

   ■**312.30 Impulse control disorder, unspecified**

   312.31 Pathological gambling

   312.32 Kleptomania *(stealing)*

   312.33 Pyromania *(setting fires)*

   312.34 Intermittent explosive disorder

   312.35 Isolated explosive disorder

   ■**312.39 Other**
        Trichotillomania
        Pulling or twisting hair until it falls out

312.4 Mixed disturbance of conduct and emotions
     Neurotic delinquency

> **Excludes**   *compulsive conduct disorder (312.3)*

●**312.8 Other specified disturbances of conduct, not elsewhere classified**

   312.81 Conduct disorder, childhood onset type

   312.82 Conduct disorder, adolescent onset type

   ■**312.89 Other conduct disorder**
        Conduct disorder of unspecified onset

■**312.9 Unspecified disturbance of conduct**
     Delinquency (juvenile)
     Disruptive behavior disorder NOS

●**313 Disturbance of emotions specific to childhood and adolescence**

> **Excludes**   *adjustment reaction (309.0–309.9)*
>   *emotional disorder of neurotic type (300.0–300.9)*
>   *masturbation, nail-biting, thumb-sucking, and*
>   *other isolated symptoms (307.0–307.9)*

313.0 Overanxious disorder
     Anxiety and fearfulness of childhood and
       adolescence
     Overanxious disorder of childhood and
       adolescence

> **Excludes**   *abnormal separation anxiety (309.21)*
>   *anxiety states (300.00–300.09)*
>   *hospitalism in children (309.83)*
>   *phobic state (300.20–300.29)*

313.1 Misery and unhappiness disorder

> **Excludes**   *depressive neurosis (300.4)*

●**313.2 Sensitivity, shyness, and social withdrawal disorder**

> **Excludes**   *infantile autism (299.0)*
>   *schizoid personality (301.20–301.22)*
>   *schizophrenia (295.0–295.9)*

   313.21 Shyness disorder of childhood
        Sensitivity reaction of childhood or
          adolescence

   313.22 Introverted disorder of childhood
        Social withdrawal of childhood or
          adolescence
        Withdrawal reaction of childhood or
          adolescence

   313.23 Selective mutism

> **Excludes**   *elective mutism as adjustment*
>   *reaction (309.83)*

313.3 Relationship problems
     Sibling jealousy

> **Excludes**   *relationship problems associated with*
>   *aggression, destruction, or other*
>   *forms of conduct disturbance*
>   *(312.0–312.9)*

●**313.8 Other or mixed emotional disturbances of childhood or adolescence**

   313.81 Oppositional defiant disorder

   313.82 Identity disorder
        Identity problem

   313.83 Academic underachievement disorder

   ■**313.89 Other**   P
        Reactive attachment disorder of infancy or
          early childhood

■**313.9 Unspecified emotional disturbance of childhood or adolescence**   P
     Mental disorder of infancy, childhood or
       adolescence NOS

●**314 Hyperkinetic syndrome of childhood**

> **Excludes**   *hyperkinesis as symptom of underlying*
>   *disorder-code the underlying disorder*

●**314.0 Attention deficit disorder** *(ADD)*
     Adult
     Child

   314.00 Without mention of hyperactivity
        Predominantly inattentive type
        Coding Clinic: 1997, Q1, P8-9

   314.01 With hyperactivity
        Attention deficit disorder with
          hyperactivity = ADHD
        Combined type
        Overactivity NOS
        Predominantly hyperactive/impulsive type
        Simple disturbance of attention with
          overactivity
        Coding Clinic: 1997, Q1, P8-9

314.1 Hyperkinesis with developmental delay
     Developmental disorder of hyperkinesis

> Use additional code to identify any associated
>   neurological disorder

314.2 Hyperkinetic conduct disorder
     Hyperkinetic conduct disorder without
       developmental delay

> **Excludes**   *hyperkinesis with significant delays in*
>   *specific skills (314.1)*

■**314.8 Other specified manifestations of hyperkinetic syndrome**

■**314.9 Unspecified hyperkinetic syndrome**
     Hyperkinetic reaction of childhood or adolescence
       NOS
     Hyperkinetic syndrome NOS

●**315 Specific delays in development**

> **Excludes**   *that due to a neurological disorder (320.0–389.9)*

●**315.0 Specific reading disorder**

   ■**315.00 Reading disorder, unspecified**

   315.01 Alexia

   315.02 Developmental dyslexia

   ■**315.09 Other**
        Specific spelling difficulty

MENTAL DISORDERS (290–319)

315.1   **Mathematics disorder**
Dyscalculia

■315.2   **Other specific learning difficulties**
Disorder of written expression

> **Excludes**   *specific arithmetical disorder (315.1)*
> *specific reading disorder (315.00–315.09)*

●315.3   **Developmental speech or language disorder**

315.31   **Expressive language disorder**
Developmental aphasia
Word deafness

> **Excludes**   *acquired aphasia (784.3)*
> *elective mutism (309.83, 313.0,*
> *313.23)*

315.32   **Mixed receptive-expressive language disorder**
Central auditory processing disorder

> **Excludes**   *acquired auditory processing*
> *disorder (388.45)*

Coding Clinic: 2005, Q2, P5-6

315.34   **Speech and language developmental delay due to hearing loss**

Coding Clinic: 2007, Q4, P80-81

■315.39   **Other**
Developmental articulation disorder
Dyslalia
Phonological disorder

> **Excludes**   *lisping and lalling (307.9)*
> *stammering and stuttering (307.0)*

Coding Clinic: 2007, Q3, P9-10

315.4   **Developmental coordination disorder**
Clumsiness syndrome
Dyspraxia syndrome
Specific motor development disorder

315.5   **Mixed development disorder**

Coding Clinic: 2002, Q2, P11

■315.8   **Other specified delays in development**

■315.9   **Unspecified delay in development**
Developmental disorder NOS
Learning disorder NOS

316   **Psychic factors associated with diseases classified elsewhere**
Psychologic factors in physical conditions classified elsewhere

Use additional code to identify the associated physical condition, as:
psychogenic:
asthma (493.9)
dermatitis (692.9)
duodenal ulcer (532.0–532.9)
eczema (691.8, 692.9)
gastric ulcer (531.0–531.9)
mucous colitis (564.9)
paroxysmal tachycardia (427.2)
ulcerative colitis (556)
urticaria (708.0–708.9)
psychosocial dwarfism (259.4)

> **Excludes**   *physical symptoms and physiological*
> *malfunctions, not involving tissue damage,*
> *of mental origin (306.0–306.9)*

MENTAL RETARDATION (317–319)

Use additional code(s) to identify any associated psychiatric or physical condition(s)

317   **Mild mental retardation**
High-grade defect
IQ 50–70
Mild mental subnormality

●318   **Other specified mental retardation**

318.0   **Moderate mental retardation**
IQ 35–49
Moderate mental subnormality

318.1   **Severe mental retardation**
IQ 20–34
Severe mental subnormality

318.2   **Profound mental retardation**
IQ under 20
Profound mental subnormality

■319   **Unspecified mental retardation**
Mental deficiency NOS
Mental subnormality NOS

◄ New   ◄IIII Revised   ~~deleted~~ Deleted   ● Use Additional Digit(s)   ■ Nonspecific Code
● Not first-listed DX   OGCR Official Guidelines   Coding Clinic   Excludes   Includes   Use additional   Code first   Omit code

(See Plate 164 on page 86.)

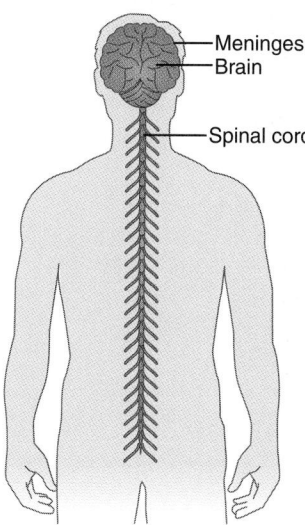

— Meninges
— Brain

— Spinal cord

Figure 6–1 The brain and spinal cord make up the central nervous system.

Item 6–1 The two major classifications of the nervous system are the peripheral nervous system and the central nervous system (CNS). The central nervous system is comprised of the brain and the spinal cord. The peripheral nervous system is comprised of the parasympathetic and sympathetic systems. **Encephalitis** is the swelling of the brain. **Meningitis** is swelling of the covering of the brain, the meninges. Types and causes of brain infections are:

Type	Cause
purulent	bacterial
aseptic/abacterial	viral
chronic meningitis	mycobacterial and fungal

6. DISEASES OF THE NERVOUS SYSTEM AND SENSE ORGANS (320–389)

INFLAMMATORY DISEASES OF THE CENTRAL NERVOUS SYSTEM (320–326)

● **320 Bacterial meningitis**
Infection of cerebrospinal fluid surrounding spinal cord and brain

     Includes   arachnoiditis bacterial
                    leptomeningitis bacterial
                    meningitis bacterial
                    meningoencephalitis bacterial
                    meningomyelitis bacterial
                    pachymeningitis bacterial

     320.0 Hemophilus meningitis
         Meningitis due to Hemophilus influenzae [H. influenzae]

     320.1 Pneumococcal meningitis

     320.2 Streptococcal meningitis

     320.3 Staphylococcal meningitis

● **320.7** *Meningitis in other bacterial diseases classified elsewhere*

     Code first underlying disease as:
         actinomycosis (039.8)
         listeriosis (027.0)
         typhoid fever (002.0)
         whooping cough (033.0–033.9)

     Excludes   *meningitis (in):*
                 epidemic (036.0)
                 gonococcal (098.82)
                 meningococcal (036.0)
                 salmonellosis (003.21)
                 syphilis:
                     NOS (094.2)
                     congenital (090.42)
                     meningovascular (094.2)
                     secondary (091.81)
                 tuberculosis (013.0)

● **320.8 Meningitis due to other specified bacteria**

     320.81 Anaerobic meningitis
         Bacteroides (fragilis)
         Gram-negative anaerobes

     320.82 Meningitis due to gram-negative bacteria, not elsewhere classified
         Aerobacter aerogenes
         Escherichia coli [E. coli]
         Friedlander bacillus
         Klebsiella pneumoniae
         Proteus morganii
         Pseudomonas

         Excludes   *gram-negative anaerobes (320.81)*

     ■**320.89 Meningitis due to other specified bacteria**
         Bacillus pyocyaneus

■**320.9 Meningitis due to unspecified bacterium**

Meningitis:	Meningitis:
bacterial NOS	pyogenic NOS
purulent NOS	suppurative NOS

● **321 Meningitis due to other organisms**

     Includes   arachnoiditis due to organisms other than bacteria
              leptomeningitis due to organisms other than bacteria
              meningitis due to organisms other than bacteria
              pachymeningitis due to organisms other than bacteria

● **321.0** *Cryptococcal meningitis*
     Code first underlying disease (117.5)

● ■**321.1** *Meningitis in other fungal diseases*
     Code first underlying disease (110.0–118)

     Excludes   *meningitis in:*
              candidiasis (112.83)
              coccidioidomycosis (114.2)
              histoplasmosis (115.01, 115.11, 115.91)

DISEASES OF THE NERVOUS SYSTEM AND SENSE ORGANS (320–389)

● **321.2 Meningitis due to viruses not elsewhere classified**

> *Code first* underlying disease, as:
> meningitis due to arbovirus (060.0–066.9)

> **Excludes** *meningitis (due to):*
> *abacterial (047.0–047.9)*
> *adenovirus (049.1)*
> *aseptic NOS (047.9)*
> *Coxsackie (virus) (047.0)*
> *ECHO virus (047.1)*
> *enterovirus (047.0–047.9)*
> *herpes simplex virus (054.72)*
> *herpes zoster virus (053.0)*
> *lymphocytic choriomeningitis virus*
>   *(049.0)*
> *mumps (072.1)*
> *viral NOS (047.9)*
> *meningo-eruptive syndrome (047.1)*

Coding Clinic: 2004, Q4, P50-52

● **321.3 Meningitis due to trypanosomiasis**

> *Code first* underlying disease (086.0–086.9)

● **321.4 Meningitis in sarcoidosis**

> *Code first* underlying disease (135)

● ■ **321.8 Meningitis due to other nonbacterial organisms classified elsewhere**

> *Code first* underlying disease

> **Excludes** *leptospiral meningitis (100.81)*

● **322 Meningitis of unspecified cause**

> **Includes** arachnoiditis with no organism specified as
>   cause
> leptomeningitis with no organism specified as
>   cause
> meningitis with no organism specified as
>   cause
> pachymeningitis with no organism specified
>   as cause

322.0 Nonpyogenic meningitis
Meningitis with clear cerebrospinal fluid

322.1 Eosinophilic meningitis

322.2 Chronic meningitis

■ **322.9 Meningitis, unspecified**

Item 6-2   **Encephalitis** is an inflammation of the brain most often caused by a virus but may also be caused by a bacteria and most commonly transmitted by a mosquito. **Myelitis** is an inflammation of the spinal cord that may disrupt CNS function. Untreated myelitis may rapidly lead to permanent damage to the spinal cord. **Encephalomyelitis** is a general term for an inflammation of the brain and spinal cord.

● **323 Encephalitis, myelitis, and encephalomyelitis**

> **Includes** acute disseminated encephalomyelitis
> meningoencephalitis, except bacterial
> meningomyelitis, except bacterial
> myelitis:
>   ascending
>   transverse

> **Excludes** *acute transverse myelitis NOS (341.20)*
> *acute transverse myelitis in conditions classified*
>   *elsewhere (341.21)*
> *bacterial:*
>   *meningoencephalitis (320.0–320.9)*
>   *meningomyelitis (320.0–320.9)*
> *idiopathic transverse myelitis (341.22)*

Coding Clinic: 2006, Q4, P58-63

● **323.0 Encephalitis, myelitis, and encephalomyelitis in viral diseases classified elsewhere**

> *Code first* underlying disease, as:
> cat-scratch disease (078.3)
> infectious mononucleosis (075)
> ornithosis (073.7)

● **323.01 Encephalitis and encephalomyelitis in viral diseases classified elsewhere**

> **Excludes** *encephalitis (in):*
> *arthropod-borne viral*
>   *(062.0–064)*
> *herpes simplex (054.3)*
> *mumps (072.2)*
> *other viral diseases of central*
>   *nervous system*
>   *(049.8–049.9)*
> *poliomyelitis (045.0–045.9)*
> *rubella (056.01)*
> *slow virus infections of*
>   *central nervous system*
>   *(046.0–046.9)*
> *viral NOS (049.9)*
> *West Nile (066.41)*

● **323.02 Myelitis in viral diseases classified elsewhere**

> **Excludes** *myelitis (in):*
> *herpes simplex (054.74)*
> *herpes zoster (053.14)*
> *other viral diseases of central*
>   *nervous system*
>   *(049.8–049.9)*
> *poliomyelitis (045.0–045.9)*
> *rubella (056.01)*

DISEASES OF THE NERVOUS SYSTEM AND SENSE ORGANS (320–389)

◀ New   ◀ Revised   ~~deleted~~ Deleted   ● Use Additional Digit(s)   ■ Nonspecific Code

● Not first-listed DX   OGCR Official Guidelines   Coding Clinic   Excludes   Includes   Use additional   Code first   Omit code

● **323.1** *Encephalitis, myelitis, and encephalomyelitis in rickettsial diseases classified elsewhere*

　　Code first underlying disease (080–083.9)

● **323.2** *Encephalitis, myelitis, and encephalomyelitis in protozoal diseases classified elsewhere*

　　Code first underlying disease, as:
　　　malaria (084.0–084.9)
　　　trypanosomiasis (086.0–086.9)

● **323.4 Other encephalitis, myelitis, and encephalomyelitis due to infection classified elsewhere**

　　Code first underlying disease

　● **323.41** *Other encephalitis and encephalomyelitis due to infection classified elsewhere*

　　　Excludes *encephalitis (in):*
　　　　　meningococcal (036.1)
　　　　　syphilis:
　　　　　　NOS (094.81)
　　　　　　congenital (090.41)
　　　　　toxoplasmosis (130.0)
　　　　　tuberculosis (013.6)
　　　　　meningoencephalitis due to
　　　　　　free-living ameba [Naegleria]
　　　　　　(136.29)

　● **323.42** *Other myelitis due to infection classified elsewhere*

　　　Excludes *myelitis (in):*
　　　　　syphilis (094.89)
　　　　　tuberculosis (013.6)

● **323.5 Encephalitis, myelitis, and encephalomyelitis following immunization procedures**

　　Use additional E code to identify vaccine

　323.51 Encephalitis and encephalomyelitis following immunization procedures
　　　Encephalitis postimmunization or postvaccinal
　　　Encephalomyelitis postimmunization or postvaccinal

　323.52 Myelitis following immunization procedures
　　　Myelitis postimmunization or postvaccinal

● **323.6 Postinfectious encephalitis, myelitis, and encephalomyelitis**

　　Code first underlying disease

　● **323.61** *Infectious acute disseminated encephalomyelitis (ADEM)*
　　　Acute necrotizing hemorrhagic encephalopathy

　　　Excludes *noninfectious acute disseminated encephalomyelitis (323.81)*

　● **323.62** *Other postinfectious encephalitis and encephalomyelitis*

　　　Excludes *encephalitis:*
　　　　　postchickenpox (052.0)
　　　　　postmeasles (055.0)

　● **323.63** *Postinfectious myelitis*

● **323.7 Toxic encephalitis, myelitis, and encephalomyelitis**

　　Code first underlying cause, as:
　　　carbon tetrachloride (982.1)
　　　hydroxyquinoline derivatives (961.3)
　　　lead (984.0–984.9)
　　　mercury (985.0)
　　　thallium (985.8)

　● **323.71** *Toxic encephalitis and encephalomyelitis*

　● **323.72** *Toxic myelitis*

● **323.8 Other causes of encephalitis, myelitis, and encephalomyelitis**
　　Coding Clinic: 1997, Q2, P8-9

　■**323.81 Other causes of encephalitis and encephalomyelitis**
　　　Noninfectious acute disseminated encephalomyelitis (ADEM)

　■**323.82 Other causes of myelitis**
　　　Transverse myelitis NOS

■**323.9 Unspecified cause of encephalitis, myelitis, and encephalomyelitis**
　　Coding Clinic: 2006, Q1, P8

● **324 Intracranial and intraspinal abscess**
　　Accumulation of pus in either brain or spinal cord

　324.0 Intracranial abscess
　　　Abscess (embolic):
　　　　cerebellar
　　　　cerebral
　　　Abscess (embolic) of brain [any part]:
　　　　epidural
　　　　extradural
　　　　otogenic
　　　　subdural

　　　Excludes *tuberculous (013.3)*

　324.1 Intraspinal abscess
　　　Abscess (embolic) of spinal cord [any part]:
　　　　epidural
　　　　extradural
　　　　subdural

　　　Excludes *tuberculous (013.5)*

　■**324.9 Of unspecified site**
　　　Extradural or subdural abscess NOS

　325 Phlebitis and thrombophlebitis of intracranial venous sinuses
　　　Embolism of cavernous, lateral, or other intracranial or unspecified intracranial venous sinus
　　　Endophlebitis of cavernous, lateral, or other intracranial or unspecified intracranial venous sinus
　　　Phlebitis, septic or suppurative of cavernous, lateral, or other intracranial or unspecified intracranial venous sinus
　　　Thrombophlebitis of cavernous, lateral, or other intracranial or unspecified intracranial venous sinus
　　　Thrombosis of cavernous, lateral, or other intracranial or unspecified intracranial venous sinus

　　　Excludes *that specified as:*
　　　　　complicating pregnancy, childbirth, or the puerperium (671.5)
　　　　　of nonpyogenic origin (437.6)

DISEASES OF THE NERVOUS SYSTEM AND SENSE ORGANS (320–389)

326 Late effects of intracranial abscess or pyogenic infection

> **Note:** This category is to be used to indicate conditions whose primary classification is to 320–325 [excluding 320.7, 321.0–321.8, 323.01–323.42, 323.61–323.72] as the cause of late effects, themselves classifiable elsewhere. The "late effects" include conditions specified as such, or as sequelae, which may occur at any time after the resolution of the causal condition.

> Use additional code to identify condition, as:
> hydrocephalus (331.4)
> paralysis (342.0–342.9, 344.0–344.9)

ORGANIC SLEEP DISORDERS (327)

● **327 Organic sleep disorders**
> *Involve difficulties of sleep at all levels, including difficulty falling or staying asleep, falling asleep at inappropriate times, excessive total sleep time, or abnormal behaviors associated with sleep*

  ● **327.0 Organic disorders of initiating and maintaining sleep [Organic insomnia]**

> **Excludes** *insomnia NOS (780.52)*
> *insomnia not due to a substance or known physiological condition (307.41–307.42)*
> *insomnia with sleep apnea NOS (780.51)*

    ■ **327.00 Organic insomnia, unspecified**

    ● **327.01 *Insomnia due to medical condition classified elsewhere***

> *Code first underlying condition*

> **Excludes** *insomnia due to mental disorder (327.02)*

    ● **327.02 *Insomnia due to mental disorder***

> *Code first mental disorder*

> **Excludes** *alcohol induced insomnia (291.82)*
> *drug induced insomnia (292.85)*

    ■ **327.09 Other organic insomnia**

  ● **327.1 Organic disorder of excessive somnolence [Organic hypersomnia]**

> **Excludes** *hypersomnia NOS (780.54)*
> *hypersomnia not due to a substance or known physiological condition (307.43–307.44)*
> *hypersomnia with sleep apnea NOS (780.53)*

    ■ **327.10 Organic hypersomnia, unspecified**

    327.11 Idiopathic hypersomnia with long sleep time

    327.12 Idiopathic hypersomnia without long sleep time

    327.13 Recurrent hypersomnia
> Kleine-Levin syndrome
> Menstrual related hypersomnia

    ● **327.14 *Hypersomnia due to medical condition classified elsewhere***

> *Code first underlying condition*

> **Excludes** *hypersomnia due to mental disorder (327.15)*

    ● **327.15 *Hypersomnia due to mental disorder***

> *Code first mental disorder*

> **Excludes** *alcohol induced insomnia (291.82)*
> *drug induced insomnia (292.85)*

    ■ **327.19 Other organic hypersomnia**

● **327.2 Organic sleep apnea**
> *Characterized by episodes in which breathing stops during sleep, resulting in a lack of prolonged deep sleep and excessive daytime sleepiness*

> **Excludes** *Cheyne-Stokes breathing (786.04)*
> *hypersomnia with sleep apnea NOS (780.53)*
> *insomnia with sleep apnea NOS (780.51)*
> *sleep apnea in newborn (770.81–770.82)*
> *sleep apnea NOS (780.57)*

  ■ **327.20 Organic sleep apnea, unspecified**

  327.21 Primary central sleep apnea

  327.22 High altitude periodic breathing

  327.23 Obstructive sleep apnea (adult) (pediatric)

  327.24 Idiopathic sleep related nonobstructive alveolar hypoventilation
> Sleep related hypoxia

  327.25 Congenital central alveolar hypoventilation syndrome

  ● **327.26 *Sleep related hypoventilation/hypoxemia in conditions classifiable elsewhere***

> *Code first underlying condition*

  ● **327.27 *Central sleep apnea in conditions classified elsewhere***

> *Code first underlying condition*

  ■ **327.29 Other organic sleep apnea**

● **327.3 Circadian rhythm sleep disorder**
> *Involves one of the sleep/wake regulating hormones. The inability to sleep results from a mismatch between the body's internal clock and the external 24-hour schedule.*
> Organic disorder of sleep wake cycle
> Organic disorder of sleep wake schedule

> **Excludes** *alcohol induced circadian rhythm sleep disorder (291.82)*
> *circadian rhythm sleep disorder of nonorganic origin (307.45)*
> *disruption of 24 hour sleep wake cycle NOS (780.55)*
> *drug induced circadian rhythm sleep disorder (292.85)*

  ■ **327.30 Circadian rhythm sleep disorder, unspecified**

  327.31 Circadian rhythm sleep disorder, delayed sleep phase type

  327.32 Circadian rhythm sleep disorder, advanced sleep phase type

  327.33 Circadian rhythm sleep disorder, irregular sleep-wake type

  327.34 Circadian rhythm sleep disorder, free-running type

  327.35 Circadian rhythm sleep disorder, jet lag type

  327.36 Circadian rhythm sleep disorder, shift work type

  ● **327.37 *Circadian rhythm sleep disorder in conditions classified elsewhere***

> *Code first underlying condition*

  ■ **327.39 Other circadian rhythm sleep disorder**

◄ New   ◄▥ Revised   ~~deleted~~ Deleted   ● Use Additional Digit(s)   ■ Nonspecific Code
● Not first-listed DX   OGCR Official Guidelines   Coding Clinic   Excludes   Includes   Use additional   Code first   Omit code

● 327.4 **Organic parasomnia**

    Excludes *alcohol induced parasomnia (291.82)*
                  drug induced parasomnia (292.85)
                  parasomnia not due to a known
                          physiological condition (307.47)

   ■327.40 **Organic parasomnia, unspecified**

   327.41 **Confusional arousals**

   327.42 **REM sleep behavior disorder**

   327.43 **Recurrent isolated sleep paralysis**

   ●327.44 *Parasomnia in conditions classified elsewhere*

         Code first underlying condition

   ■327.49 **Other organic parasomnia**

● 327.5 **Organic sleep related movement disorders**

    Excludes *restless legs syndrome (333.94)*
                  sleep related movement disorder NOS
                      (780.58)

   327.51 **Periodic limb movement disorder**
        Periodic limb movement sleep disorder

   327.52 **Sleep related leg cramps**

   327.53 **Sleep related bruxism**

   ■327.59 **Other organic sleep related movement disorders**

   327.8 **Other organic sleep disorders**
        Coding Clinic: 2007, Q2, P7-8

Item 6–3   Leukodystrophy is characterized by degeneration and/or failure of the myelin formation of the central nervous system and sometimes of the peripheral nervous system. The disease is inherited and progressive.

HEREDITARY AND DEGENERATIVE DISEASES OF THE CENTRAL NERVOUS SYSTEM (330–337)

    Excludes *hepatolenticular degeneration (275.1)*
                  multiple sclerosis (340)
                  other demyelinating diseases of central nervous
                      system (341.0–341.9)

● 330 **Cerebral degenerations usually manifest in childhood**

    Use additional code to identify associated mental retardation

   330.0 **Leukodystrophy**
        Krabbe's disease
        Leukodystrophy:
           NOS
           globoid cell
           metachromatic
           sudanophilic
        Pelizaeus-Merzbacher disease
        Sulfatide lipidosis

   330.1 **Cerebral lipidoses**
        Amaurotic (familial) idiocy
        Disease:
           Batten
           Jansky-Bielschowsky
           Kufs'
           Spielmeyer-Vogt
           Tay-Sachs
         Gangliosidosis

● 330.2 *Cerebral degeneration in generalized lipidoses*

    Code first underlying disease, as:
        Fabry's disease (272.7)
        Gaucher's disease (272.7)
        Niemann-Pick disease (272.7)
        sphingolipidosis (272.7)

● ■330.3 *Cerebral degeneration of childhood in other diseases classified elsewhere*

    Code first underlying disease, as:
        Hunter's disease (277.5)
        mucopolysaccharidosis (277.5)

   ■330.8 **Other specified cerebral degenerations in childhood**
        Alpers' disease or gray-matter degeneration
        Infantile necrotizing encephalomyelopathy
        Leigh's disease
        Subacute necrotizing encephalopathy or encephalomyelopathy
        Coding Clinic: 1995, Q1, P9

   ■330.9 **Unspecified cerebral degeneration in childhood**

    Item 6–4   Pick's disease is the atrophy of the frontal and temporal lobes, causing dementia; **Alzheimer's** is characterized by a more diffuse cerebral atrophy.

● 331 **Other cerebral degenerations**

    Use additional code, where applicable, to identify dementia:
        with behavioral disturbance (294.11)
        without behavioral disturbance (294.10)

   331.0 **Alzheimer's disease**
        Coding Clinic: 2000, Q4, P40-41; 1999, Q4, P7; 1994, Q2, P10-11; Q1, P21; 1984, Nov-Dec, P20

● 331.1 **Frontotemporal dementia**

   331.11 **Pick's disease**
        Coding Clinic: 2003, Q4, P57-58

   331.19 **Other frontotemporal dementia**
        Frontal dementia
        Coding Clinic: 2003, Q4, P57-58

   331.2 **Senile degeneration of brain**

    Excludes *senility NOS (797)*

   331.3 **Communicating hydrocephalus**
        Secondary normal pressure hydrocephalus

    Excludes *congenital hydrocephalus (742.3)*
              idiopathic normal pressure hydrocephalus (331.5)
              normal pressure hydrocephalus (331.5)
              spina bifida with hydrocephalus (741.0)
        Coding Clinic: 2007, Q4, P74-75; 1985, Sept-Oct, P12

   331.4 **Obstructive hydrocephalus**
        Acquired hydrocephalus NOS

    Excludes *congenital hydrocephalus (742.3)*
              idiopathic normal pressure hydrocephalus (331.5)
              normal pressure hydrocephalus (331.5)
              spina bifida with hydrocephalus (741.0)
        Coding Clinic: 2007, Q4, P74-75; 2003, Q4, P106-107; 1999, Q1, P9-10

DISEASES OF THE NERVOUS SYSTEM AND SENSE ORGANS (320–389)

331.5 Idiopathic normal pressure hydrocephalus (INPH)

Normal pressure hydrocephalus NOS

> **Excludes**   *congenital hydrocephalus (742.3)*
> *secondary normal pressure hydrocephalus (331.3)*
> *spina bifida with hydrocephalus (741.0)*

Coding Clinic: 2007, Q4, P74-75

● **331.7 Cerebral degeneration in diseases classified elsewhere**

Code first underlying disease, as:
alcoholism (303.0–303.9)
beriberi (265.0)
cerebrovascular disease (430–438)
congenital hydrocephalus (741.0, 742.3)
neoplastic disease (140.0–239.9)
myxedema (244.0–244.9)
vitamin B12 deficiency (266.2)

> **Excludes**   *cerebral degeneration in:*
> *Jakob-Creutzfeldt disease (046.11–046.19)* ◄▥
> *progressive multifocal leukoencephalopathy (046.3)*
> *subacute spongiform encephalopathy (046.1)*

● **331.8 Other cerebral degeneration**

331.81 Reye's syndrome   P

331.82 Dementia with Lewy bodies
Dementia with Parkinsonism
Lewy body dementia
Lewy body disease
Coding Clinic: 2003, Q4, P57-58

331.83 Mild cognitive impairment, so stated

> **Excludes**   *altered mental status (780.97)*
> *cerebral degeneration (331.0–331.9)*
> *change in mental status (780.97)*
> *cognitive deficits following (late effects of) cerebral hemorrhage or infarction (438.0)*
> *cognitive impairment due to intracranial or head injury (850–854, 959.01)*
> *cognitive impairment due to late effect of intracranial injury (907.0)*
> *cognitive impairment due to skull fracture (800–801, 803–804)* ◄
> *dementia (290.0–290.43, 294.8)*
> *mild memory disturbance (310.8)*
> *neurologic neglect syndrome (781.8)*
> *personality change, nonpsychotic (310.1)*

Coding Clinic: 2006, Q4, P75-76

■ **331.89 Other**
Cerebral ataxia

■ **331.9 Cerebral degeneration, unspecified**

● **332 Parkinson's disease**

Movement disorder (chronic or progressive); cause unknown, and no cure.

> **Excludes**   *dementia with Parkinsonism (331.82)*

332.0 Paralysis agitans
Parkinsonism or Parkinson's disease:
NOS
idiopathic
primary

332.1 Secondary Parkinsonism
Neuroleptic-induced Parkinsonism
Parkinsonism due to drugs

> Use additional E code to identify drug, if drug-induced

> **Excludes**   *Parkinsonism (in):*
> *Huntington's disease (333.4)*
> *progressive supranuclear palsy (333.0)*
> *Shy-Drager syndrome (333.0)*
> *syphilitic (094.82)*

● **333 Other extrapyramidal disease and abnormal movement disorders**

> **Includes**   other forms of extrapyramidal, basal ganglia, or striatopallidal disease

> **Excludes**   *abnormal movements of head NOS (781.0)*
> *sleep related movement disorders (327.51–327.59)*

■ **333.0 Other degenerative diseases of the basal ganglia**
Atrophy or degeneration:
olivopontocerebellar [Déjérine-Thomas syndrome]
pigmentary pallidal [Hallervorden-Spatz disease] striatonigral
Parkinsonian syndrome associated with:
idiopathic orthostatic hypotension
symptomatic orthostatic hypotension
Progressive supranuclear ophthalmoplegia
Shy-Drager syndrome
Coding Clinic: 1996, Q2, P8-9

■ **333.1 Essential and other specified forms of tremor**
Benign essential tremor
Familial tremor
Medication-induced postural tremor

> Use additional E code to identify drug, if drug-induced

> **Excludes**   *tremor NOS (781.0)*

333.2 Myoclonus
Familial essential myoclonus
Palatal myoclonus   ◄
~~Progressive myoclonic epilepsy~~
~~Unverricht-Lundborg disease~~

> Use additional E code to identify drug, if drug-induced

> **Excludes**   *progressive myoclonic epilepsy (345.1)* ◄
> *Unverricht-Lundborg disease (345.1)* ◄

Coding Clinic: 1997, Q3, P5; 1987, Mar-April, P12

333.3 Tics of organic origin

> **Excludes**   *Gilles de la Tourette's syndrome (307.23)*
> *habit spasm (307.22)*
> *tic NOS (307.20)*

> Use additional E code to identify drug, if drug-induced

◄ New   ◄▥ Revised   ~~deleted~~ Deleted   ● Use Additional Digit(s)   ■ Nonspecific Code

● Not first-listed DX   OGCR Official Guidelines   Coding Clinic   Excludes   Includes   Use additional   Code first   Omit code

DISEASES OF THE NERVOUS SYSTEM AND SENSE ORGANS (320–389)

Item 6–5 Huntington's chorea is an inherited degenerative disorder of the central nervous system and is characterized by ceaseless, jerky movements and progressive cognitive and behavioral deterioration.

333.4 Huntington's chorea

333.5 Other choreas
Hemiballism(us)
Paroxysmal choreo-athetosis

> **Excludes** *Sydenham's or rheumatic chorea (392.0–392.9)*

Use additional E code to identify drug, if drug-induced

333.6 Genetic torsion dystonia
Dystonia:
deformans progressiva
musculorum deformans
(Schwalbe-) Ziehen-Oppenheim disease
Coding Clinic: 2006, Q4, P76-78

333.7 Acquired torsion dystonia
Coding Clinic: 2006, Q4, P76-78

333.71 Athetoid cerebral palsy
Double athetosis (syndrome)
Vogt's disease

> **Excludes** *infantile cerebral palsy (343.0–343.9)*

333.72 Acute dystonia due to drugs
Acute dystonic reaction due to drugs
Neuroleptic-induced acute dystonia

Use additional E code to identify drug

> **Excludes** *blepharospasm due to drugs (333.85)*
> *orofacial dyskinesia due to drugs (333.85)*
> *secondary Parkinsonism (332.1)*
> *subacute dyskinesia due to drugs (333.85)*
> *tardive dyskinesia (333.85)*

333.79 Other acquired torsion dystonia

333.8 Fragments of torsion dystonia

Use additional E code to identify drug, if drug-induced

333.81 Blepharospasm

> **Excludes** *blepharospasm due to drugs (333.85)*

333.82 Orofacial dyskinesia

> **Excludes** *orofacial dyskinesia due to drugs (333.85)*

333.83 Spasmodic torticollis

> **Excludes** *torticollis:*
> *NOS (723.5)*
> *hysterical (300.11)*
> *psychogenic (306.0)*

333.84 Organic writers' cramp

> **Excludes** *psychogenic (300.89)*

333.85 Subacute dyskinesia due to drugs
Blepharospasm due to drugs
Orofacial dyskinesia due to drugs
Tardive dyskinesia

Use additional E code to identify drug

> **Excludes** *acute dystonia due to drugs (333.72)*
> *acute dystonic reaction due to drugs (333.72)*
> *secondary Parkinsonism (332.1)*
> Coding Clinic: 2006, Q4, P76-78

333.89 Other

333.9 Other and unspecified extrapyramidal diseases and abnormal movement disorders

333.90 Unspecified extrapyramidal disease and abnormal movement disorder
Medication-induced movement disorders NOS

Use additional E code to identify drug, if drug-induced

333.91 Stiff-man syndrome

333.92 Neuroleptic malignant syndrome

Use additional E code to identify drug

> **Excludes** *neuroleptic induced Parkinsonism (332.1)*

333.93 Benign shuddering attacks

333.94 Restless legs syndrome (RLS)
Coding Clinic: 2006, Q4, P79

333.99 Other
Neuroleptic-induced acute akathisia

Use additional E code to identify drug, if drug-induced
Coding Clinic: 2004, Q2, P12

334 Spinocerebellar disease
Group of degenerative disorders in which primary symptom is progressive ataxia (jerky, uncoordinated movements)

> **Excludes** *olivopontocerebellar degeneration (333.0)*
> *peroneal muscular atrophy (356.1)*

334.0 Friedreich's ataxia

334.1 Hereditary spastic paraplegia

334.2 Primary cerebellar degeneration
Cerebellar ataxia:
Marie's
Sanger-Brown
Dyssynergia cerebellaris myoclonica
Primary cerebellar degeneration:
NOS
hereditary
sporadic
Coding Clinic: 1987, Mar-April, P9

334.3 Other cerebellar ataxia
Cerebellar ataxia NOS

Use additional E code to identify drug, if drug-induced

334.4 Cerebellar ataxia in diseases classified elsewhere

Code first underlying disease, as:
alcoholism (303.0–303.9)
myxedema (244.0–244.9)
neoplastic disease (140.0–239.9)

334.8 Other spinocerebellar diseases
Ataxia-telangiectasia [Louis-Bar syndrome]
Corticostriatal-spinal degeneration

334.9 Spinocerebellar disease, unspecified

DISEASES OF THE NERVOUS SYSTEM AND SENSE ORGANS (320–389)

● **335   Anterior horn cell disease**

    335.0   Werdnig-Hoffmann disease
        Infantile spinal muscular atrophy
        Progressive muscular atrophy of infancy

  ● **335.1   Spinal muscular atrophy**

      ■ **335.10   Spinal muscular atrophy, unspecified**

      335.11   Kugelberg-Welander disease
           Spinal muscular atrophy:
             familial
             juvenile

      ■ **335.19   Other**
           Adult spinal muscular atrophy

  ● **335.2   Motor neuron disease**

      335.20   Amyotrophic lateral sclerosis   A
           Also listed in the Index as "Lou Gehrig's
             disease" (ALS)
           Motor neuron disease (bulbar) (mixed type)
           Coding Clinic: 1995, Q4, P81

      335.21   Progressive muscular atrophy
           Duchenne-Aran muscular atrophy
           Progressive muscular atrophy (pure)

      335.22   Progressive bulbar palsy

      335.23   Pseudobulbar palsy

      335.24   Primary lateral sclerosis

      ■ **335.29   Other**

  ■ **335.8   Other anterior horn cell diseases**
        Coding Clinic: 2006, Q4, P76-78

  ■ **335.9   Anterior horn cell disease, unspecified**

● **336   Other diseases of spinal cord**

    336.0   Syringomyelia and syringobulbia
        Coding Clinic: 1989, Q1, P10

    336.1   Vascular myelopathies
        Acute infarction of spinal cord (embolic)
           (nonembolic)
        Arterial thrombosis of spinal cord
        Edema of spinal cord
        Hematomyelia
        Subacute necrotic myelopathy

  ● **336.2   *Subacute combined degeneration of spinal cord in diseases classified elsewhere***
        Code first underlying disease, as:
          pernicious anemia (281.0)
          other vitamin B12 deficiency anemia (281.1)
          vitamin B12 deficiency (266.2)

  ● **336.3   *Myelopathy in other diseases classified elsewhere***
        Code first underlying disease, as:
          myelopathy in neoplastic disease (140.0–239.9)

        Excludes   *myelopathy in:*
               intervertebral disc disorder
                  (722.70–722.73)
               spondylosis (721.1, 721.41–721.42,
                  721.91)

      Coding Clinic: 1999, Q3, P5

  ■ **336.8   Other myelopathy**
      Myelopathy:
        drug-induced
        radiation-induced
      Use additional E code to identify cause

■ **336.9   Unspecified disease of spinal cord**
    Cord compression NOS
    Myelopathy NOS

    Excludes   *myelitis (323.02, 323.1, 323.2, 323.42,*
             323.52, 323.63, 323.72, 323.82,
             323.9)
            spinal (canal) stenosis (723.0,
               724.00–724.09)

● **337   Disorders of the autonomic nervous system**

    Includes   disorders of peripheral autonomic,
            sympathetic, parasympathetic, or
            vegetative system

    Excludes   *familial dysautonomia [Riley-Day syndrome]*
            (742.8)

  ● **337.0   Idiopathic peripheral autonomic neuropathy**

      ■ **337.00   Idiopathic peripheral autonomic neuropathy, unspecified**

      337.01   Carotid sinus syndrome
           Carotid sinus syncope
           Coding Clinic: 2008, Q4, P101-102

      ■ **337.09   Other idiopathic peripheral autonomic neuropathy**
           Cervical sympathetic dystrophy or
             paralysis

  ● **337.1   *Peripheral autonomic neuropathy in disorders classified elsewhere***
      Code first underlying disease, as:
        amyloidosis (277.30–277.39)
        diabetes (249.6, 250.6)
      Coding Clinic: 2009, Q2, P10; 1993, Q2, P6; 1984, Nov-Dec, P9

  ● **337.2   Reflex sympathetic dystrophy**

      ■ **337.20   Reflex sympathetic dystrophy, unspecified**
           Complex regional pain syndrome type I,
             unspecified

      337.21   Reflex sympathetic dystrophy of the upper limb
           Complex regional pain syndrome type I of
             the upper limb

      337.22   Reflex sympathetic dystrophy of the lower limb
           Complex regional pain syndrome type I of
             the lower limb

      ■ **337.29   Reflex sympathetic dystrophy of other specified site**
           Complex regional pain syndrome type I of
             other specified site

    337.3   Autonomic dysreflexia
      Use additional code to identify the cause, such as:
        fecal impaction (560.39)
        pressure ulcer (707.00–707.09)
        urinary tract infection (599.0)
      Coding Clinic: 1998, Q4, P37-38

  ■ **337.9   Unspecified disorder of autonomic nervous system**

◀ New   ◀▦ Revised   ~~deleted~~ Deleted   ● Use Additional Digit(s)   ■ Nonspecific Code

● Not first-listed DX   OGCR Official Guidelines   Coding Clinic   Excludes   Includes   Use additional   Code first   Omit code

PAIN (338)

● **338   Pain, not elsewhere classified**

Use additional code to identify:
    pain associated with psychological factors (307.89)

Excludes   *generalized pain (780.96)*
           headache syndromes (339.00-339.89)
           localized pain, unspecified type - code to pain by
             site
           migraines (346.0-346.9)
           pain disorder exclusively attributed to
             psychological factors (307.80)
           vulvar vestibulitis (625.71)
           vulvodynia (625.70-625.79)

338.0   Central pain syndrome
     Déjérine-Roussy syndrome
     Myelopathic pain syndrome
     Thalamic pain syndrome (hyperesthetic)

● **338.1   Acute pain**

    338.11   Acute pain due to trauma
         Coding Clinic: 2007, Q1, P3-8

    338.12   Acute post-thoracotomy pain
         Post-thoracotomy pain NOS

    ■**338.18   Other acute postoperative pain**
         Postoperative pain NOS
         Coding Clinic: 2007, Q2, P13-15; 2003, Q1, P4-5, 8

    ■**338.19   Other acute pain**

        Excludes   *neoplasm related acute pain (338.3)*

        Coding Clinic: 2007, Q2, P13-15

● **338.2   Chronic pain**

       Excludes   *causalgia (355.9)*
                lower limb (355.71)
                upper limb (354.4)
           chronic pain syndrome (338.4)
           myofascial pain syndrome (729.1)
           neoplasm related chronic pain (338.3)
           reflex sympathetic dystrophy
             (337.20–337.29)

     Coding Clinic: 2008, Q3, P4

    338.21   Chronic pain due to trauma

    338.22   Chronic post-thoracotomy pain

    ■**338.28   Other chronic postoperative pain**
         Coding Clinic: 2007, Q2, P13-15

    ■**338.29   Other chronic pain**
         Coding Clinic: 2007, Q2, P13-15

338.3   Neoplasm related pain (acute) (chronic)
     Cancer associated pain
     Pain due to malignancy (primary) (secondary)
     Tumor associated pain
     Coding Clinic: 2007, Q2, P13-15

338.4   Chronic pain syndrome
     Chronic pain associated with significant
       psychosocial dysfunction
     Coding Clinic: 2007, Q2, P13-15

OTHER HEADACHE SYNDROMES (339)

● **339   Other headache syndromes**

       Excludes   *headache:*
               NOS (784.0)
               due to lumbar puncture (349.0)
               migraine (346.0-346.9)
    Coding Clinic: 2008, Q4, P102-109

● **339.0   Cluster headaches and other trigeminal autonomic cephalgias**
     TACS

    ■**339.00   Cluster headache syndrome, unspecified**
         Ciliary neuralgia
         Cluster headache NOS
         Histamine cephalgia
         Lower half migraine
         Migrainous neuralgia

    339.01   Episodic cluster headache

    339.02   Chronic cluster headache

    339.03   Episodic paroxysmal hemicrania
         Paroxysmal hemicrania NOS

    339.04   Chronic paroxysmal hemicrania

    339.05   Short lasting unilateral neuralgiform headache with conjunctival injection and tearing
         SUNCT

    ■**339.09   Other trigeminal autonomic cephalgias**

● **339.1   Tension type headache**

       Excludes   *tension headache NOS (307.81)*
              tension headache related to psychological
                factors (307.81)

    ■**339.10   Tension type headache, unspecified**

    339.11   Episodic tension type headache

    339.12   Chronic tension type headache

● **339.2   Post-traumatic headache**

    ■**339.20   Post-traumatic headache, unspecified**
         Coding Clinic: 2008, Q4, P102-109

    339.21   Acute post-traumatic headache
         Coding Clinic: 2008, Q4, P102-109

    339.22   Chronic post-traumatic headache

● ■**339.3   Drug induced headache, not elsewhere classified**
     Medication overuse headache
     Rebound headache

● **339.4   Complicated headache syndromes**

    339.41   Hemicrania continua

    339.42   New daily persistent headache
         NDPH

    339.43   Primary thunderclap headache

    ■**339.44   Other complicated headache syndrome**

● **339.8   Other specified headache syndromes**

    339.81   Hypnic headache

    339.82   Headache associated with sexual activity
         Orgasmic headache
         Preorgasmic headache

    339.83   Primary cough headache

    339.84   Primary exertional headache

    339.85   Primary stabbing headache

    ■**339.89   Other specified headache syndromes**

DISEASES OF THE NERVOUS SYSTEM AND SENSE ORGANS (320–389)

Item 6-6 Multiple sclerosis (MS) is a nervous system disease affecting the brain and spinal cord by damaging the myelin sheath surrounding and protecting nerve cells. The damage slows down/blocks messages between the brain and body. Symptoms are: visual disturbances, muscle weakness, coordination and balance issues, numbness, prickling, thinking and memory problems. The cause is unknown, though it is thought that it may be an autoimmune disease. It affects women more than men, between 20 and 40 years of age. MS can be mild, but it may cause the loss of ability to write, walk, and speak. There is no cure, but medication may slow or control symptoms.

OTHER DISORDERS OF THE CENTRAL NERVOUS SYSTEM (340–349)

340 Multiple sclerosis *(MS)*
    Disseminated or multiple sclerosis:
      NOS   cord
      brain stem   generalized

● **341 Other demyelinating diseases of central nervous system**

    341.0 Neuromyelitis optica

    341.1 Schilder's disease
        Balo's concentric sclerosis
        Encephalitis periaxialis:
           concentrica [Balo's]
           diffusa [Schilder's]

  ● **341.2 Acute (transverse) myelitis**

      | Excludes | *acute (transverse) myelitis (in) (due to):* |
      following immunization procedures (323.52)
      infection classified elsewhere (323.42)
      postinfectious (323.63)
      protozoal diseases classified elsewhere (323.2)
      rickettsial diseases classified elsewhere (323.1)
      toxic (323.72)
      viral diseases classified elsewhere (323.02)
      transverse myelitis NOS (323.82)

    341.20 Acute (transverse) myelitis NOS

  ● **341.21 *Acute (transverse) myelitis in conditions classified elsewhere***

      Code first underlying condition

    341.22 Idiopathic transverse myelitis

■ **341.8 Other demyelinating diseases of central nervous system**
      Central demyelination of corpus callosum
      Central pontine myelinosis
      Marchiafava (-Bignami) disease
      Coding Clinic: 1987, Nov-Dec, P6

■ **341.9 Demyelinating disease of central nervous system, unspecified**

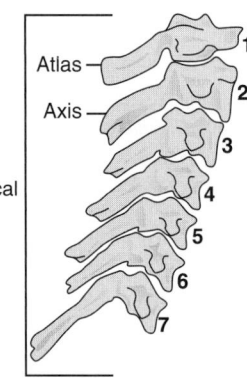

Figure 6–2 Cervical vertebrae.

Atlas — 1
Axis — 2
Cervical — 3, 4, 5, 6, 7

Item 6–7 Hemiplegia is complete paralysis of one side of the body—arm, leg, and trunk. **Hemiparesis** is a generalized weakness or incomplete paralysis of one side of the body. If most activities (eating, writing) are performed with the right hand, the right is the dominant side, and the left is the nondominant side. **Quadriplegia,** also called tetraplegia, is the complete paralysis of all four limbs. **Quadriparesis** is the incomplete paralysis of all four limbs. Nerve damage in C1–C4 is associated with lower limb paralysis, and C5–C7 damage is associated with upper limb paralysis. **Diplegia** is the paralysis of the upper limbs. **Monoplegia** is the complete paralysis of one limb. There are separate codes for upper (344.4x) and lower (344.3x) limb. Dominant, nondominant, or unspecified side becomes the fifth digit. Dominant side (right/left) is the side that a person leads with for movement, such as in writing and sports.
Cauda equina syndrome is due to pressure on the roots of the spinal nerves and causes paresthesia (abnormal sensations).

● **342 Hemiplegia and hemiparesis**
    Note: This category is to be used when hemiplegia (complete) (incomplete) is reported without further specification, or is stated to be old or long-standing but of unspecified cause. The category is also for use in multiple coding to identify these types of hemiplegia resulting from any cause.

    | Excludes | *congenital (343.1)* |
    hemiplegia due to late effect of cerebrovascular accident (438.20–438.22)
    infantile NOS (343.4)

The following fifth-digits are for use with codes 342.0–342.9

> ■ **0 affecting unspecified side**
>   **1 affecting dominant side**
>   **2 affecting nondominant side**

● **342.0 Flaccid hemiplegia**
  [0-2]

● **342.1 Spastic hemiplegia**
  [0-2]

● ■ **342.8 Other specified hemiplegia**
  [0-2]

● ■ **342.9 Hemiplegia, unspecified**
  [0-2]   Coding Clinic: 2006, Q3, P5; 1998, Q4, P87

◀ New   ◀▥ Revised   ~~deleted~~ Deleted   ● Use Additional Digit(s)   ■ Nonspecific Code
● Not first-listed DX   OGCR Official Guidelines   Coding Clinic   Excludes   Includes   Use additional   Code first   Omit code

● **343   Infantile cerebral palsy**

Includes   cerebral:
  palsy NOS
  spastic infantile paralysis
congenital spastic paralysis (cerebral)
Little's disease
paralysis (spastic) due to birth injury:
  intracranial
  spinal

Excludes   *athetoid cerebral palsy (333.71)*
  hereditary cerebral paralysis, such as:
    hereditary spastic paraplegia (334.1)
    Vogt's disease (333.71)
  spastic paralysis specified as noncongenital or
    noninfantile (344.0–344.9)

343.0   Diplegic
  Congenital diplegia
  Congenital paraplegia

343.1   Hemiplegic
  Congenital hemiplegia
  Excludes   *infantile hemiplegia NOS (343.4)*

343.2   Quadriplegic
  Tetraplegic

343.3   Monoplegic

343.4   Infantile hemiplegia
  Infantile hemiplegia (postnatal) NOS

■**343.8   Other specified infantile cerebral palsy**

■**343.9   Infantile cerebral palsy, unspecified**
  Cerebral palsy NOS
  Coding Clinic: 2005, Q4, P89-90

● **344   Other paralytic syndromes**

Note: This category is to be used when the listed
  conditions are reported without further
  specification or are stated to be old or
  long-standing but of unspecified cause. The
  category is also for use in multiple coding to
  identify these conditions resulting from any
  cause.

Includes   paralysis (complete) (incomplete), except as
  classifiable to 342 and 343

Excludes   *congenital or infantile cerebral palsy (343.0–343.9)*
  hemiplegia (342.0–342.9)
    congenital or infantile (343.1, 343.4)

● **344.0   Quadriplegia and quadriparesis**

■**344.00   Quadriplegia, unspecified**
  Coding Clinic: 2003, Q4, P103-104; 1998, Q4, P37-38

344.01   C$_1$-C$_4$, complete

344.02   C$_1$-C$_4$, incomplete

344.03   C$_5$-C$_7$, complete

344.04   C$_5$-C$_7$, incomplete

■**344.09   Other**
  Coding Clinic: 2001, Q1, P12; 1998, Q4, P39-40

344.1   Paraplegia
  Paralysis of both lower limbs
  Paraplegia (lower)
  Coding Clinic: 2003, Q4, P110; 1987, Mar-April, P10-11

344.2   Diplegia of upper limbs
  Diplegia (upper)
  Paralysis of both upper limbs

● **344.3   Monoplegia of lower limb**
  Paralysis of lower limb
  Excludes   *monoplegia of lower limb due to late*
    effect of cerebrovascular accident
    (438.40–438.42)

■**344.30   Affecting unspecified side**

344.31   Affecting dominant side

344.32   Affecting nondominant side

● **344.4   Monoplegia of upper limb**
  Paralysis of upper limb
  Excludes   *monoplegia of upper limb due to late*
    effect of cerebrovascular accident
    (438.30–438.32)

■**344.40   Affecting unspecified side**

344.41   Affecting dominant side

344.42   Affecting nondominant side

■**344.5   Unspecified monoplegia**

● **344.6   Cauda equina syndrome**

344.60   Without mention of neurogenic bladder

344.61   With neurogenic bladder
  Acontractile bladder
  Autonomic hyperreflexia of bladder
  Cord bladder
  Detrusor hyperreflexia
  Coding Clinic: 1987, Mar-April, P10-11

● **344.8   Other specified paralytic syndromes**

344.81   Locked-in state

■**344.89   Other specified paralytic syndrome**
  Coding Clinic: 1999, Q2, P4

■**344.9   Paralysis, unspecified**
  Coding Clinic: 1994, Q3, P4

● **345   Epilepsy and recurrent seizures**

The following fifth-digit subclassification is for use with
categories 345.0, .1, .4–.9:

0   without mention of intractable epilepsy
1   with intractable epilepsy
◄   **pharmacoresistant (pharmacologically**
◄   **resistant)**
◄   **poorly controlled**
◄   **refractory (medically)**
◄   **treatment resistant**

Excludes   *hippocampal sclerosis (348.81)*   ◄
  mesial temporal sclerosis (348.81)   ◄
  progressive myoclonic epilepsy (333.2)   ◄
  temporal sclerosis (348.81)   ◄

● **345.0   Generalized nonconvulsive epilepsy**
  [0-1]   Absences:
    atonic
    typical
  Minor epilepsy
  Petit mal
  Pykno-epilepsy
  Seizures:
    akinetic
    atonic
  Coding Clinic: 2004, Q1, P18; 1992, Q2, P8

● **345.1   Generalized convulsive epilepsy**
  [0-1]   Epileptic seizures:
    clonic
    major epilepsy   Grand mal
    myoclonic   Progressive myoclonic   ◄
    tonic   epilepsy
    tonic-clonic   Unverricht-Lundborg   ◄
                            disease
  Excludes   *convulsions:*
    NOS (780.39)
    infantile (780.39)
    newborn (779.0)
  infantile spasms (345.6)
  Coding Clinic: 1997, Q3, P5; 1994, Q3, P9

DISEASES OF THE NERVOUS SYSTEM AND SENSE ORGANS (320–389)

345.2 Petit mal status
> Epileptic absence status
> *Temporary disturbance of brain function caused by abnormal electrical activity.*

345.3 Grand mal status
> Status epilepticus NOS
> *Grand mal seizure is a generalized tonic-clonic seizure involving the entire body, which involves muscle rigidity, violent muscle contractions, and loss of consciousness.*
>
> > **Excludes** *epilepsia partialis continua (345.7) status:*
> >   *psychomotor (345.7)*
> >   *temporal lobe (345.7)*
>
> Coding Clinic: 2005, Q3, P12-13

● **345.4 Localization-related (focal) (partial) epilepsy and**
[0-1] **epileptic syndromes with complex partial seizures**
> Epilepsy:
> > limbic system
> > partial:
> > > secondarily generalized
> > > with impairment of consciousness
> > > with memory and ideational disturbances
> >
> > psychomotor
> > psychosensory
> > temporal lobe
>
> Epileptic automatism

● **345.5 Localization-related (focal) (partial) epilepsy and**
[0-1] **epileptic syndromes with simple partial seizures**
> Epilepsy:
> > Bravais-Jacksonian NOS
> > focal (motor) NOS
> > Jacksonian NOS
> > motor partial
> > partial NOS
> > > without mention of impairment of consciousness
> >
> > sensory-induced
> > somatomotor
> > somatosensory
> > visceral
> > visual

● **345.6 Infantile spasms**
[0-1]
> Hypsarrhythmia
> Lightning spasms
> Salaam attacks
>
> > **Excludes** *salaam tic (781.0)*
>
> Coding Clinic: 1984, Nov-Dec, P11

● **345.7 Epilepsia partialis continua**
[0-1]
> Kojevnikov's epilepsy

● ■ **345.8 Other forms of epilepsy and recurrent seizures**
[0-1]
> Epilepsy:
> > cursive [running]
> > gelastic
>
> Recurrent seizures NOS
> Seizure disorder NOS

● ■ **345.9 Epilepsy, unspecified**
[0-1]
> Epileptic convulsions, fits, or seizures NOS
> Recurrent seizures NOS
> Seizure disorder NOS
>
> > **Excludes** *convulsion (convulsive) disorder (780.39)*
> >   *convulsive seizure or fit NOS (780.39)*
> >   *recurrent convulsions (780.39)*
>
> Coding Clinic: 2009, Q2, P11; 2008, Q1, P17; 1993, Q1, P24; 1987, Nov-Dec, P12

Item 6-8 Migraine headache is described as an intense pulsing or throbbing pain in one area of the head. It can be accompanied by extreme sensitivity to light (photophoic) and sound and is three times more common in women than in men. Symptoms include nausea and vomiting. Research indicates migraine headaches are caused by inherited abnormalities in genes that control the activities of certain cell populations in the brain.

● **346 Migraine**
> > **Excludes** *headache:*
> >   *NOS (784.0)*
> >   *syndromes (339.00-339.89)*
>
> The following fifth-digit subclassification is for use with category 346:
> Coding Clinic: 2008, Q4, P102-109

> | | |
> |---|---|
> | **0** | **without mention of intractable migraine without mention of status migrainosus** |
> | **1** | **with intractable migraine, so stated, without mention of status migrainosus** |
> | **2** | **without mention of intractable migraine with status migrainosus** |
> | **3** | **with intractable migraine, so stated, with status migrainosus** |

> *Intractable migraine: Not easily cured or managed; relentless pain from a migraine*

● **346.0 Migraine with aura**
[0-3]
> Basilar migraine
> Classic migraine
> Migraine preceded or accompanied by transient focal neurological phenomena
> Migraine triggered seizures
> Migraine with acute-onset aura
> Migraine with aura without headache (migraine equivalents)
> Migraine with prolonged aura
> Migraine with typical aura
> Retinal migraine
>
> > **Excludes** *persistent migraine aura (346.5, 346.6)*

● **346.1 Migraine without aura**
[0-3]
> Common migraine

● **346.2 Variants of migraine, not elsewhere classified**
[0-3]
> Abdominal migraine
> Cyclical vomiting associated with migraine
> Ophthalmoplegic migraine
> Periodic headache syndromes in child or adolescent
>
> > **Excludes** *cyclical vomiting NOS (536.2)*
> >   *psychogenic cyclical vomiting (306.4)*

● **346.3 Hemiplegic migraine**
[0-3]
> Familial migraine
> Sporadic migraine

● **346.4 Menstrual migraine ♀**
[0-3]
> Menstrual headache
> Menstrually related migraine
> Premenstrual headache
> Premenstrual migraine
> Pure menstrual migraine

◀ New   ◀▥ Revised   ~~deleted~~ Deleted   ● Use Additional Digit(s)   ■ Nonspecific Code

● Not first-listed DX   OGCR Official Guidelines   Coding Clinic   Excludes   Includes   Use additional   Code first   Omit code

DISEASES OF THE NERVOUS SYSTEM AND SENSE ORGANS (320–389)

● **346.5** **Persistent migraine aura without cerebral**
[0-3] **infarction**
       Persistent migraine aura NOS

● **346.6** **Persistent migraine aura with cerebral**
[0-3] **infarction**

● **346.7** **Chronic migraine without aura**
[0-3]   Transformed migraine without aura

● ■ **346.8** **Other forms of migraine**
[0-3]

● ■ **346.9** **Migraine, unspecified**
[0-3]   Coding Clinic: 1985, Nov-Dec, P16

● **347** **Cataplexy and narcolepsy**
     Cataplexy is a disorder evidenced by seizures. Narcolepsy is
     difficulty remaining awake during daytime.
     Coding Clinic: 2004, Q4, P74-75

   ● **347.0** **Narcolepsy**

       347.00 **Without cataplexy**
           Narcolepsy NOS

       347.01 **With cataplexy**

   ● **347.1** **Narcolepsy in conditions classified elsewhere**
       Code first underlying condition

      ● **347.10** **Without cataplexy**

      ● **347.11** **With cataplexy**

● **348** **Other conditions of brain**

   348.0 **Cerebral cysts**
       Arachnoid cyst   Porencephaly, acquired
       Porencephalic cyst   Pseudoporencephaly

   348.1 **Anoxic brain damage**
       Brain permanently damaged by lack of oxygen perfusion
       through brain tissues. This is the result of another
       problem, so use an additional E code to identify
       the cause.

       Excludes *that occurring in:*
           abortion (634–638 with .7, 639.8)
           ectopic or molar pregnancy (639.8)
           labor or delivery (668.2, 669.4)
           that of newborn (767.0, 768.0–768.9,
             772.1–772.2)

       Use additional E code to identify cause

   348.2 **Benign intracranial hypertension**
       Pseudotumor cerebri

       Excludes *hypertensive encephalopathy (437.2)*

   ● **348.3** **Encephalopathy, not elsewhere classified**
       A general term for any degenerative brain disease
       Coding Clinic: 2003, Q4, P58-59; 1997, Q3, P5

     ■ **348.30** **Encephalopathy, unspecified**

     348.31 **Metabolic encephalopathy**
       Septic encephalopathy

       Excludes *toxic metabolic encephalopathy*
           (349.82)

     ■ **348.39** **Other encephalopathy**

       Excludes *encephalopathy:*
           alcoholic (291.2)
           hepatic (572.2)
           hypertensive (437.2)
           toxic (349.82)

   348.4 **Compression of brain**
       Compression brain (stem)
       Herniation brain (stem)
       Posterior fossa compression syndrome

   348.5 **Cerebral edema**

   ● **348.8** **Other conditions of brain**   ◄▥
       ~~Cerebral:~~   ~~Cerebral:~~
         ~~calcification~~   ~~fungus~~
       Coding Clinic: 1992, Q3, P8; 1987, Sept-Oct, P9

     348.81 **Temporal sclerosis**   ◄
       Hippocampal sclerosis   ◄
       Mesial temporal sclerosis   ◄

     348.89 **Other conditions of brain**   ◄
       Cerebral: ◄
       calcification   ◄
       fungus   ◄

   ■ **348.9** **Unspecified condition of brain**

● **349** **Other and unspecified disorders of the nervous system**

   349.0 **Reaction to spinal or lumbar puncture**
       Headache following lumbar puncture
       Cerebral spinal fluid (CSF) maintains a specific level
       of pressure inside brain and spinal cord. If
       this pressure does not return to normal after a
       puncture, headache will result.
       Coding Clinic: 1999, Q2, P9-10; 1990, Q3, P18

   349.1 **Nervous system complications from surgically**
       implanted device

       Excludes *immediate postoperative complications*
           (997.00–997.09)
           mechanical complications of nervous system
           device (996.2)

   ■ **349.2** **Disorders of meninges, not elsewhere classified**
       Adhesions, meningeal (cerebral) (spinal)
       Cyst, spinal meninges
       Meningocele, acquired
       Pseudomeningocele, acquired
       Coding Clinic: 2006, Q1, P15-16; 1998, Q2, P18; 1994, Q3, P4; Q1,
           P22-23

   ● **349.3** **Dural tear**
       Coding Clinic: 2008, Q4, P109-110

     349.31 **Accidental puncture or laceration of dura**
       during a procedure
           Incidental (inadvertent) durotomy

     ■ **349.39** **Other dural tear**

   ● **349.8** **Other specified disorders of nervous system**

     349.81 **Cerebrospinal fluid rhinorrhea**

       Excludes *cerebrospinal fluid otorrhea (388.61)*

     349.82 **Toxic encephalopathy**
       Toxic metabolic encephalopathy

       Use additional E code to identify cause

     ■ **349.89** **Other**

   ■ **349.9** **Unspecified disorders of nervous system**
       Disorder of nervous system (central) NOS

DISEASES OF THE NERVOUS SYSTEM AND SENSE ORGANS (320–389)

Item 6-9 The **peripheral nervous system** consists of 31 pairs of spinal nerves, 12 pairs of cranial nerves, and the autonomic nerves, which are divided into the parasympathetic and sympathetic nerves. The cranial nerves are: olfactory (I), optic (II), oculomotor (III), trochlear (IV), trigeminal (V), abducens (VI), facial (VII), vestibulocochlear (VIII), glossopharyngeal (IX), vagus (X), accessory (XI), and hypoglossal (XII).

Item 6-10 Trigeminal neuralgia, tic douloureux, is a pain syndrome diagnosed from the patient's history alone. The condition is characterized by pain and a brief facial spasm or tic. Pain is unilateral and follows the sensory distribution of cranial nerve V, typically radiating to the maxillary (V2) or mandibular (V3) area.

DISORDERS OF THE PERIPHERAL NERVOUS SYSTEM (350–359)

Excludes *diseases of:*
  acoustic [8th] nerve (388.5)
  oculomotor [3rd, 4th, 6th] nerves (378.0–378.9)
  optic [2nd] nerve (377.0–377.9)
  peripheral autonomic nerves (337.0–337.9)
  neuralgia NOS or "rheumatic" (729.2)
  neuritis NOS or "rheumatic" (729.2)
  radiculitis NOS or "rheumatic" (729.2)
  peripheral neuritis in pregnancy (646.4)

● **350 Trigeminal nerve disorders**
   Includes   disorders of 5th cranial nerve
   350.1 Trigeminal neuralgia
       Tic douloureux
       Trifacial neuralgia
       Trigeminal neuralgia NOS
       Excludes *postherpetic (053.12)*
   350.2 Atypical face pain
■ **350.8 Other specified trigeminal nerve disorders**
■ **350.9 Trigeminal nerve disorder, unspecified**

● **351 Facial nerve disorders**
   Includes   disorders of 7th cranial nerve
   Excludes   *that in newborn (767.5)*
   351.0 Bell's palsy
       Facial palsy
   351.1 Geniculate ganglionitis
       Geniculate ganglionitis NOS
       Excludes *herpetic (053.11)*
       Coding Clinic: 2002, Q2, P8

Item 6-11 The most common facial nerve disorder is **Bell's Palsy,** which occurs suddenly and results in facial drooping unilaterally. This disorder is the result of a reaction to a virus that causes the facial nerve in the ear to swell resulting in pressure in the bony canal.

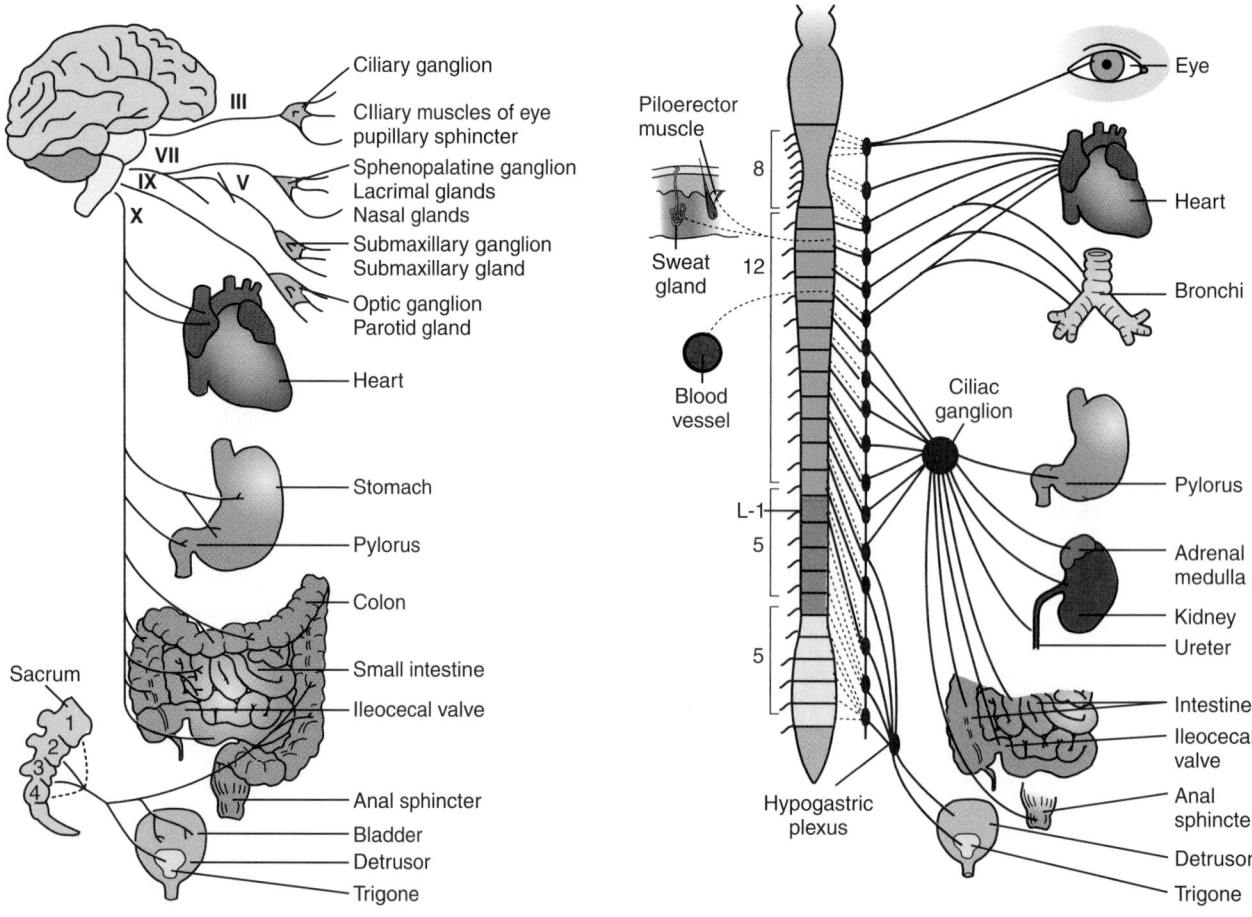

Figure 6–3 A. Parasympathetic nervous system. **B.** Sympathetic nervous system. (From Buck CJ: Step-by-Step Medical Coding, 2nd ed. Philadelphia, WB Saunders, 1998, pp 186 and 187.)

◄ New   ◄▥ Revised   ~~deleted~~ Deleted   ● Use Additional Digit(s)   ■ Nonspecific Code
● Not first-listed DX   OGCR Official Guidelines   Coding Clinic   Excludes   Includes   Use additional   Code first   Omit code

■**351.8 Other facial nerve disorders**
Facial myokymia
Melkersson's syndrome
Coding Clinic: 2002, Q3, P12-13

■**351.9 Facial nerve disorder, unspecified**

●**352 Disorders of other cranial nerves**

352.0 Disorders of olfactory [1st] nerve

352.1 Glossopharyngeal neuralgia
Coding Clinic: 1987, Jan-Feb, P14

■**352.2 Other disorders of glossopharyngeal [9th] nerve**

352.3 Disorders of pneumogastric [10th] nerve
Disorders of vagal nerve

> **Excludes** *paralysis of vocal cords or larynx (478.30–478.34)*

352.4 Disorders of accessory [11th] nerve

352.5 Disorders of hypoglossal [12th] nerve

352.6 Multiple cranial nerve palsies
Collet-Sicard syndrome
Polyneuritis cranialis

■**352.9 Unspecified disorder of cranial nerves**

●**353 Nerve root and plexus disorders**

> **Excludes** *conditions due to:*
> *intervertebral disc disorders (722.0–722.9)*
> *spondylosis (720.0–721.9)*
> *vertebrogenic disorders (723.0–724.9)*

353.0 Brachial plexus lesions
Cervical rib syndrome
Costoclavicular syndrome
Scalenus anticus syndrome
Thoracic outlet syndrome

> **Excludes** *brachial neuritis or radiculitis NOS (723.4)*
> *that in newborn (767.6)*
> Coding Clinic: 2006, Q3, P12

353.1 Lumbosacral plexus lesions

353.2 Cervical root lesions, not elsewhere classified

353.3 Thoracic root lesions, not elsewhere classified

353.4 Lumbosacral root lesions, not elsewhere classified

353.5 Neuralgic amyotrophy
Parsonage-Aldren-Turner syndrome
Phantom limb syndrome: Patients with amputated limbs feel sensations in a limb that no longer exists. There is no separate code for phantom limb pain, and the pain can be part of the syndrome.

> Code first *any associated underlying disease, such as:*
> diabetes mellitus (249.6, 250.6)

353.6 Phantom limb (syndrome)

■**353.8 Other nerve root and plexus disorders**

■**353.9 Unspecified nerve root and plexus disorder**

●**354 Mononeuritis of upper limb and mononeuritis multiplex**

354.0 Carpal tunnel syndrome (CTS)
Of the wrist
Median nerve entrapment
Partial thenar atrophy

■**354.1 Other lesion of median nerve**
Median nerve neuritis

354.2 Lesion of ulnar nerve
Cubital tunnel syndrome
Tardy ulnar nerve palsy

354.3 Lesion of radial nerve
Acute radial nerve palsy
Coding Clinic: 1987, Nov-Dec, P6

354.4 Causalgia of upper limb
Complex regional pain syndrome type II of the upper limb

> **Excludes** *causalgia:*
> *NOS (355.9)*
> *lower limb (355.71)*
> *complex regional pain syndrome type II of the lower limb (355.71)*

354.5 Mononeuritis multiplex
Combinations of single conditions classifiable to 354 or 355

■**354.8 Other mononeuritis of upper limb**

■**354.9 Mononeuritis of upper limb, unspecified**

●**355 Mononeuritis of lower limb**
Coding Clinic: 1989, Q2, P12

355.0 Lesion of sciatic nerve

> **Excludes** *sciatica NOS (724.3)*
> Coding Clinic: 1989, Q2, P12

355.1 Meralgia paresthetica
Lateral cutaneous femoral nerve of thigh compression or syndrome

■**355.2 Other lesion of femoral nerve**

355.3 Lesion of lateral popliteal nerve
Lesion of common peroneal nerve

355.4 Lesion of medial popliteal nerve

355.5 Tarsal tunnel syndrome
Of the ankle

355.6 Lesion of plantar nerve
Morton's metatarsalgia, neuralgia, or neuroma

●**355.7 Other mononeuritis of lower limb**

355.71 Causalgia of lower limb

> **Excludes** *causalgia:*
> *NOS (355.9)*
> *upper limb (354.4)*
> *complex regional pain syndrome type II of the upper limb (354.4)*

■**355.79 Other mononeuritis of lower limb**

■**355.8 Mononeuritis of lower limb, unspecified**

■**355.9 Mononeuritis of unspecified site**
Causalgia NOS
Complex regional pain syndrome NOS

> **Excludes** *causalgia:*
> *lower limb (355.71)*
> *upper limb (354.4)*
> *complex regional pain syndrome:*
> *lower limb (355.71)*
> *upper limb (354.4)*

●**356 Hereditary and idiopathic peripheral neuropathy**
Any disease that affects nervous system and of an unknown cause.

356.0 Hereditary peripheral neuropathy
Déjérine-Sottas disease

356.1 Peroneal muscular atrophy
Charcot-Marie-Tooth disease
Neuropathic muscular atrophy

356.2 Hereditary sensory neuropathy

356.3 Refsum's disease
Heredopathia atactica polyneuritiformis

356.4 Idiopathic progressive polyneuropathy

■**356.8 Other specified idiopathic peripheral neuropathy**
Supranuclear paralysis

■**356.9 Unspecified**

DISEASES OF THE NERVOUS SYSTEM AND SENSE ORGANS (320–389)

● **357 Inflammatory and toxic neuropathy**

  357.0 Acute infective polyneuritis
    Guillain-Barre syndrome
    Postinfectious polyneuritis
    Coding Clinic: 1998, Q2, P12

● **357.1 Polyneuropathy in collagen vascular disease**
    Code first underlying disease, as:
     disseminated lupus erythematosus (710.0)
     polyarteritis nodosa (446.0)
     rheumatoid arthritis (714.0)

● **357.2 Polyneuropathy in diabetes**
    Code first underlying disease (249.6, 250.6)
    Coding Clinic: 2008, Q3, P5-6; 2003, Q4, P105; 1992, Q2, P15

● **357.3 Polyneuropathy in malignant disease**
    Code first underlying disease (140.0–208.9)

● ■ **357.4 Polyneuropathy in other diseases classified elsewhere**
    Code first underlying disease, as:
     amyloidosis (277.30–277.39)
     beriberi (265.0)
     chronic uremia (585.9)
     deficiency of B vitamins (266.0–266.9)
     diphtheria (032.0–032.9)
     hypoglycemia (251.2)
     pellagra (265.2)
     porphyria (277.1)
     sarcoidosis (135)
     uremia NOS (586)

    Excludes polyneuropathy in:
     herpes zoster (053.13)
     mumps (072.72)
    Coding Clinic: 2008, Q2, P8-9; 1998, Q2, P15

  357.5 Alcoholic polyneuropathy

  357.6 Polyneuropathy due to drugs
    Use additional E code to identify drug

■ **357.7 Polyneuropathy due to other toxic agents**
    Use additional E code to identify toxic agent

● ■ **357.8 Other**
    Coding Clinic: 2002, Q4, P47-48; 1998, Q2, P12

  357.81 Chronic inflammatory demyelinating polyneuritis

  357.82 Critical illness polyneuropathy
    Acute motor neuropathy
    Coding Clinic: 2003, Q4, P111

  ■ **357.89 Other inflammatory and toxic neuropathy**

■ **357.9 Unspecified**

● **358 Myoneural disorders**

● **358.0 Myasthenia gravis**
    Acquired and results in fatigable muscle weakness exacerbated by activity and improved with rest. Caused by autoimmune assault against nerve-muscle junction.
    Coding Clinic: 2003, Q4, P59-60

  ■ **358.00 Myasthenia gravis without (acute) exacerbation**

  ■ **358.01 Myasthenia gravis with acute exacerbation**
    Myasthenia gravis in crisis
    Coding Clinic: 2007, Q4, P108-109; 2004, Q4, P139

● **358.1 Myasthenic syndromes in diseases classified elsewhere**
    Eaton-Lambert syndrome from stated cause classified elsewhere
    Code first underlying disease, as:
     botulism (005.1, 040.41–040.42)
     hypothyroidism (244.0–244.9)
     malignant neoplasm (140.0–208.9)
     pernicious anemia (281.0)
     thyrotoxicosis (242.0–242.9)

  358.2 Toxic myoneural disorders
    Use additional E code to identify toxic agent

  358.8 Other specified myoneural disorders

  358.9 Myoneural disorders, unspecified
    Coding Clinic: 2002, Q2, P16

● **359 Muscular dystrophies and other myopathies**
    Excludes idiopathic polymyositis (710.4)

  359.0 Congenital hereditary muscular dystrophy
    Benign congenital myopathy
    Central core disease
    Centronuclear myopathy
    Myotubular myopathy
    Nemaline body disease
    Excludes arthrogryposis multiplex congenita (754.89)

  359.1 Hereditary progressive muscular dystrophy
    Muscular dystrophy:
     NOS
     distal
     Duchenne
     Erb's
     fascioscapulohumeral
     Gower's
     Landouzy-Déjérine
     limb-girdle
     ocular
     oculopharyngeal

Item 6-12 Muscular dystrophies (MD) are a group of rare inherited muscle diseases. Voluntary muscles become progressively weaker. In the late stages of MD, fat and connective tissue replace muscle fibers. In some types of muscular dystrophy, heart muscles, other involuntary muscles, and other organs are affected. **Myopathies** is a general term for neuromuscular diseases in which the muscle fibers dysfunction for any one of many reasons, resulting in muscular weakness.

DISEASES OF THE NERVOUS SYSTEM AND SENSE ORGANS (320–389)

◄ New   ◄═ Revised   deleted Deleted   ● Use Additional Digit(s)   ■ Nonspecific Code
● Not first-listed DX   OGCR Official Guidelines   Coding Clinic   Excludes   Includes   Use additional   Code first   Omit code

● **359.2 Myotonic disorders**

> **Excludes** *periodic paralysis (359.3)*
>
> Coding Clinic: 2007, Q4, P75-77

   359.21 Myotonic muscular dystrophy
> Dystrophia myotonica
> Myotonia atrophica
> Myotonic dystrophy
> Proximal myotonic myopathy (PROMM)
> Steinert's disease

   359.22 Myotonia congenita
> Acetazolamide responsive myotonia
>   congenita
> Dominant form (Thomsen's disease)
> Myotonia levior ◄
> Recessive form (Becker's disease)

   359.23 Myotonic chondrodystrophy
> Congenital myotonic
>   chondrodystrophy
> Schwartz-Jampel disease

   359.24 Drug-induced myotonia
> Use additional E code to identify drug

   359.29 Other specified myotonic disorder
> Myotonia fluctuans
> ~~Myotonia levior~~
> Myotonia permanens
> Paramyotonia congenita
>   (of von Eulenburg)

● **359.3 Periodic paralysis**
> Familial periodic paralysis
> Hyperkalemic periodic paralysis
> Hypokalemic familial periodic paralysis
> Hypokalemic periodic paralysis
> Potassium sensitive periodic paralysis

> **Excludes** *paramyotonia congenita (of von Eulenburg)*
>   *(359.29)*

● **359.4 Toxic myopathy**
> Use additional E code to identify toxic agent

● **359.5 *Myopathy in endocrine diseases classified elsewhere***

> *Code first* underlying disease, as:
> Addison's disease (255.41)
> Cushing's syndrome (255.0)
> hypopituitarism (253.2)
> myxedema (244.0–244.9)
> thyrotoxicosis (242.0–242.9)

● **359.6 *Symptomatic inflammatory myopathy in diseases classified elsewhere***

> *Code first* underlying disease, as:
> amyloidosis (277.30–277.39)
> disseminated lupus erythematosus (710.0)
> malignant neoplasm (140.0–208.9)
> polyarteritis nodosa (446.0)
> rheumatoid arthritis (714.0)
> sarcoidosis (135)
> scleroderma (710.1)
> Sjögren's disease (710.2)

● **359.7 Inflammatory and immune myopathies, NEC** ◄

   359.71 Inclusion body myositis ◄
> IBM ◄

   359.79 Other inflammatory and immune
> **myopathies, NEC** ◄
> Inflammatory myopathy NOS ◄

● ■ **359.8 Other myopathies**
> Coding Clinic: 2002, Q4, P47-48; 1990, Q3, P17

   359.81 Critical illness myopathy
> Acute necrotizing myopathy
> Acute quadriplegic myopathy
> Intensive care (ICU) myopathy
> Myopathy of critical illness

■ **359.89 Other myopathies**

■ **359.9 Myopathy, unspecified**

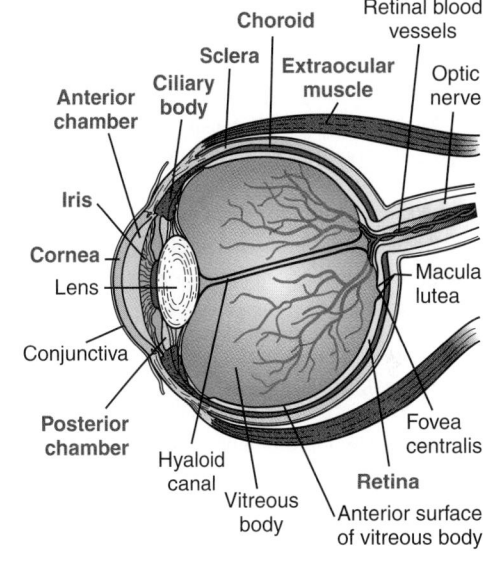

Figure 6–4   Eye and ocular adnexa. (From Buck CJ: Step-by-Step Medical Coding, 2005 ed. Philadelphia, WB Saunders, 2005.)

DISORDERS OF THE EYE AND ADNEXA (360–379)

> Use additional external cause code, if applicable, to identify the cause of the eye condition

● **360 Disorders of the globe**

> **Includes**   disorders affecting multiple structures of eye

● **360.0 Purulent endophthalmitis**

> **Excludes** *bleb associated endophthalmitis (379.63)*

■ **360.00 Purulent endophthalmitis, unspecified**

   360.01 Acute endophthalmitis

   360.02 Panophthalmitis

   360.03 Chronic endophthalmitis

   360.04 Vitreous abscess

● **360.1 Other endophthalmitis**

> **Excludes** *bleb associated endophthalmitis (379.63)*

   360.11 Sympathetic uveitis

   360.12 Panuveitis

   360.13 Parasitic endophthalmitis NOS

   360.14 Ophthalmia nodosa

■ **360.19 Other**
> Phacoanaphylactic endophthalmitis

DISEASES OF THE NERVOUS SYSTEM AND SENSE ORGANS (320–389)

- 360.2 **Degenerative disorders of globe**
  - 360.20 **Degenerative disorder of globe, unspecified**
  - 360.21 **Progressive high (degenerative) myopia**
    Malignant myopia
  - 360.23 **Siderosis**
  - 360.24 **Other metallosis**
    Chalcosis
  - 360.29 **Other**
    Excludes *xerophthalmia (264.7)*
- 360.3 **Hypotony of eye**
  - 360.30 **Hypotony, unspecified**
  - 360.31 **Primary hypotony**
  - 360.32 **Ocular fistula causing hypotony**
  - 360.33 **Hypotony associated with other ocular disorders**
  - 360.34 **Flat anterior chamber**
- 360.4 **Degenerated conditions of globe**
  - 360.40 **Degenerated globe or eye, unspecified**
  - 360.41 **Blind hypotensive eye**
    Atrophy of globe
    Phthisis bulbi
  - 360.42 **Blind hypertensive eye**
    Absolute glaucoma
  - 360.43 **Hemophthalmos, except current injury**
    Excludes *traumatic (871.0–871.9, 921.0–921.9)*
  - 360.44 **Leucocoria**
- 360.5 **Retained (old) intraocular foreign body, magnetic**
  Excludes *current penetrating injury with magnetic foreign body (871.5)*
  retained (old) foreign body of orbit (376.6)
  - 360.50 **Foreign body, magnetic, intraocular, unspecified**
  - 360.51 **Foreign body, magnetic, in anterior chamber**
  - 360.52 **Foreign body, magnetic, in iris or ciliary body**
  - 360.53 **Foreign body, magnetic, in lens**
  - 360.54 **Foreign body, magnetic, in vitreous**
  - 360.55 **Foreign body, magnetic, in posterior wall**
  - 360.59 **Foreign body, magnetic, in other or multiple sites**
- 360.6 **Retained (old) intraocular foreign body, nonmagnetic**
  Retained (old) foreign body:
  NOS
  nonmagnetic
  Excludes *current penetrating injury with (nonmagnetic) foreign body (871.6)*
  retained (old) foreign body in orbit (376.6)
  - 360.60 **Foreign body, intraocular, unspecified**
  - 360.61 **Foreign body in anterior chamber**
  - 360.62 **Foreign body in iris or ciliary body**
  - 360.63 **Foreign body in lens**
  - 360.64 **Foreign body in vitreous**
  - 360.65 **Foreign body in posterior wall**
  - 360.69 **Foreign body in other or multiple sites**
- 360.8 **Other disorders of globe**
  - 360.81 **Luxation of globe**
  - 360.89 **Other**
- 360.9 **Unspecified disorder of globe**

Item 6-13 Retinal detachments and defects are conditions of the eye in which the retina separates from the underlying tissue. Initial detachment may be localized, requiring rapid treatment (medical emergency) to avoid the entire retina from detaching, which leads to vision loss and blindness.

NON-RHEGMATOGENOUS RETINAL DETACHMENT

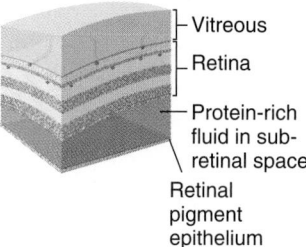

VITREOUS DETACHMENT

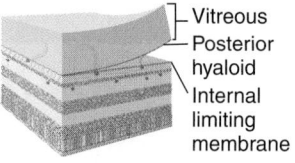

RHEGMATOGENOUS RETINAL DETACHMENT

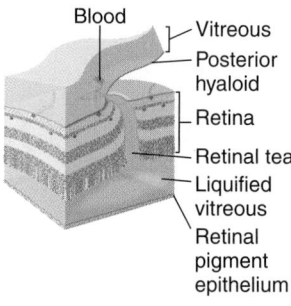

Figure 6–5 Retinal detachment. (From Kumar: Robbins and Cotran: Pathologic Basis of Disease, 7th ed. 2005, Saunders)

- 361 **Retinal detachments and defects**
  - 361.0 **Retinal detachment with retinal defect**
    Rhegmatogenous retinal detachment
    Excludes *detachment of retinal pigment epithelium (362.42–362.43)*
    retinal detachment (serous) (without defect) (361.2)
    Coding Clinic: 1994, Q1, P17
    - 361.00 **Retinal detachment with retinal defect, unspecified**
    - 361.01 **Recent detachment, partial, with single defect**

◄ New   ◄▥ Revised   deleted Deleted   ● Use Additional Digit(s)   ■ Nonspecific Code
● Not first-listed DX   OGCR Official Guidelines   Coding Clinic   Excludes   Includes   Use additional   Code first   Omit code

DISEASES OF THE NERVOUS SYSTEM AND SENSE ORGANS (320–389)

361.02 Recent detachment, partial, with multiple defects

361.03 Recent detachment, partial, with giant tear

361.04 Recent detachment, partial, with retinal dialysis
Dialysis (juvenile) of retina (with detachment)

361.05 Recent detachment, total or subtotal

361.06 Old detachment, partial
Delimited old retinal detachment

361.07 Old detachment, total or subtotal

● **361.1 Retinoschisis and retinal cysts**
Excludes   *juvenile retinoschisis (362.73)*
microcystoid degeneration of retina (362.62)
parasitic cyst of retina (360.13)

■ **361.10 Retinoschisis, unspecified**

361.11 Flat retinoschisis

361.12 Bullous retinoschisis

361.13 Primary retinal cysts

361.14 Secondary retinal cysts

■ **361.19 Other**
Pseudocyst of retina

361.2 Serous retinal detachment
Retinal detachment without retinal defect
Excludes   *central serous retinopathy (362.41)*
retinal pigment epithelium detachment (362.42–362.43)

● **361.3 Retinal defects without detachment**
Excludes   *chorioretinal scars after surgery for detachment (363.30–363.35)*
peripheral retinal degeneration without defect (362.60–362.66)

■ **361.30 Retinal defect, unspecified**
Retinal break(s) NOS

361.31 Round hole of retina without detachment

361.32 Horseshoe tear of retina without detachment
Operculum of retina without mention of detachment

■ **361.33 Multiple defects of retina without detachment**

● **361.8 Other forms of retinal detachment**
361.81 Traction detachment of retina
Traction detachment with vitreoretinal organization

■ **361.89 Other**
Coding Clinic: 1999, Q3, P12

■ **361.9 Unspecified retinal detachment**
Coding Clinic: 1987, Nov–Dec, P10

● **362 Other retinal disorders**
Excludes   *chorioretinal scars (363.30–363.35)*
chorioretinitis (363.0–363.2)

● **362.0 Diabetic retinopathy**
Code first diabetes (249.5, 250.5)

Most common diabetic eye disease and leading cause of blindness in adults. Caused by changes in the blood vessels of retina in which the blood vessels swell and leak fluid into retinal surface.

● **362.01 Background diabetic retinopathy**
Diabetic retinal microaneurysms
Diabetic retinopathy NOS

● **362.02 Proliferative diabetic retinopathy**
Coding Clinic: 1996, Q3, P5

● **362.03 Nonproliferative diabetic retinopathy NOS**

● **362.04 Mild nonproliferative diabetic retinopathy**

● **362.05 Moderate nonproliferative diabetic retinopathy**

● **362.06 Severe nonproliferative diabetic retinopathy**
Coding Clinic: 2005, Q4, P65-67

● **362.07 Diabetic macular edema**
Diabetic retinal edema

Note: Code 362.07 must be used with a code for diabetic retinopathy (362.01–362.06)

● **362.1 Other background retinopathy and retinal vascular changes**
■ **362.10 Background retinopathy, unspecified**
Coding Clinic: 2006, Q1, P12

362.11 Hypertensive retinopathy
OGCR   Section I.C.7.a.6
Two codes are necessary to identify the condition. First assign the code from subcategory 362.11, Hypertensive retinopathy, then the appropriate code from categories 401–405 to indicate the type of hypertension.

362.12 Exudative retinopathy
Coats' syndrome
Coding Clinic: 1999, Q3, P12

362.13 Changes in vascular appearance
Vascular sheathing of retina
Use additional code for any associated atherosclerosis (440.8)

362.14 Retinal microaneurysms NOS

362.15 Retinal telangiectasia

362.16 Retinal neovascularization NOS
Neovascularization:
choroidal
subretinal

■ **362.17 Other intraretinal microvascular abnormalities**
Retinal varices

362.18 Retinal vasculitis
Eales' disease
Retinal:
arteritis
endarteritis
perivasculitis
phlebitis

DISEASES OF THE NERVOUS SYSTEM AND SENSE ORGANS (320–389)

● **362.2　Other proliferative retinopathy**

■ **362.20　Retinopathy of prematurity, unspecified**
　　Retinopathy of prematurity NOS
　　Coding Clinic: 2008, Q4, P110-111

362.21　Retrolental fibroplasia
　　Cicatricial retinopathy of prematurity

362.22　Retinopathy of prematurity, stage 0

362.23　Retinopathy of prematurity, stage 1

362.24　Retinopathy of prematurity, stage 2

362.25　Retinopathy of prematurity, stage 3

362.26　Retinopathy of prematurity, stage 4

362.27　Retinopathy of prematurity, stage 5

■ **362.29　Other nondiabetic proliferative retinopathy**
　　Coding Clinic: 1996, Q3, P5

● **362.3　Retinal vascular occlusion**
　　Blockage in vessel of the retina

■ **362.30　Retinal vascular occlusion, unspecified**

362.31　Central retinal artery occlusion

362.32　Arterial branch occlusion

362.33　Partial arterial occlusion
　　Hollenhorst plaque
　　Retinal microembolism

362.34　Transient arterial occlusion
　　Amaurosis fugax
　　Coding Clinic: 2000, Q1, P16

362.35　Central retinal vein occlusion
　　Coding Clinic: 1993, Q2, P6

362.36　Venous tributary (branch) occlusion

362.37　Venous engorgement
　　Occlusion:
　　　of retinal vein
　　　incipient of retinal vein
　　　partial of retinal vein

● **362.4　Separation of retinal layers**

> **Excludes**　*retinal detachment (serous) (361.2)*
> 　　　*rhegmatogenous (361.00–361.07)*

■ **362.40　Retinal layer separation, unspecified**

362.41　Central serous retinopathy

362.42　Serous detachment of retinal pigment epithelium
　　Exudative detachment of retinal pigment epithelium

362.43　Hemorrhagic detachment of retinal pigment epithelium

> **Item 6-14** Macular degeneration is typically age-related, chronic, and is evidenced by deterioration of the macula (the part of the retina that provides for central field vision), resulting in blurred vision or a blind spot in the center of visual field while not affecting peripheral vision.

● **362.5　Degeneration of macula and posterior pole**

> **Excludes**　*degeneration of optic disc (377.21–377.24)*
> 　　　*hereditary retinal degeneration [dystrophy]*
> 　　　*(362.70–362.77)*

■ **362.50　Macular degeneration (senile), unspecified**

362.51　Nonexudative senile macular degeneration
　　Senile macular degeneration:
　　　atrophic
　　　dry

362.52　Exudative senile macular degeneration
　　Kuhnt-Junius degeneration
　　Senile macular degeneration:
　　　disciform
　　　wet

362.53　Cystoid macular degeneration
　　Cystoid macular edema

362.54　Macular cyst, hole, or pseudohole

362.55　Toxic maculopathy

> Use additional E code to identify drug, if drug induced

362.56　Macular puckering
　　Preretinal fibrosis

362.57　Drusen (degenerative)

● **362.6　Peripheral retinal degenerations**

> **Excludes**　*hereditary retinal degeneration [dystrophy]*
> 　　　*(362.70–362.77)*
> 　　　*retinal degeneration with retinal defect*
> 　　　*(361.00–361.07)*

■ **362.60　Peripheral retinal degeneration, unspecified**

362.61　Paving stone degeneration

362.62　Microcystoid degeneration
　　Blessig's cysts
　　Iwanoff's cysts

362.63　Lattice degeneration
　　Palisade degeneration of retina

362.64　Senile reticular degeneration

362.65　Secondary pigmentary degeneration
　　Pseudoretinitis pigmentosa

362.66　Secondary vitreoretinal degenerations

● **362.7　Hereditary retinal dystrophies**

■ **362.70　Hereditary retinal dystrophy, unspecified**

● **362.71　*Retinal dystrophy in systemic or cerebroretinal lipidoses***

> Code first underlying disease, as:
> 　cerebroretinal lipidoses (330.1)
> 　systemic lipidoses (272.7)

● ■ **362.72　*Retinal dystrophy in other systemic disorders and syndromes***

> Code first underlying disease, as:
> 　Bassen-Kornzweig syndrome (272.5)
> 　Refsum's disease (356.3)

362.73　Vitreoretinal dystrophies
　　Juvenile retinoschisis

362.74　Pigmentary retinal dystrophy
　　Retinal dystrophy, albipunctate
　　Retinitis pigmentosa

■ **362.75　Other dystrophies primarily involving the sensory retina**
　　Progressive cone (-rod) dystrophy
　　Stargardt's disease

362.76　Dystrophies primarily involving the retinal pigment epithelium
　　Fundus flavimaculatus
　　Vitelliform dystrophy

362.77　Dystrophies primarily involving Bruch's membrane
　　Dystrophy:
　　　hyaline
　　　pseudoinflammatory foveal
　　Hereditary drusen

◄ New　◄▥ Revised　~~deleted~~ Deleted　● Use Additional Digit(s)　■ Nonspecific Code
● Not first-listed DX　OGCR Official Guidelines　Coding Clinic　Excludes　Includes　Use additional　Code first　Omit code

● **362.8 Other retinal disorders**

    Excludes *chorioretinal inflammations (363.0–363.2)*
              chorioretinal scars (363.30–363.35)

    362.81 Retinal hemorrhage
        Hemorrhage:
          preretinal
          retinal (deep) (superficial)
          subretinal
        Coding Clinic: 1996, Q4, P43-44

    362.82 Retinal exudates and deposits

    362.83 Retinal edema
        Retinal:
          cotton wool spots
          edema (localized) (macular) (peripheral)

    362.84 Retinal ischemia

    362.85 Retinal nerve fiber bundle defects

    ■**362.89 Other retinal disorders**

■**362.9 Unspecified retinal disorder**

● **363 Chorioretinal inflammations, scars, and other disorders of choroid**

  ● **363.0 Focal chorioretinitis and focal retinochoroiditis**

    Excludes *focal chorioretinitis or retinochoroiditis in:*
              histoplasmosis (115.02, 115.12, 115.92)
              toxoplasmosis (130.2)
              congenital infection (771.2)

    ■**363.00 Focal chorioretinitis, unspecified**
        Focal:
          choroiditis or chorioretinitis NOS
          retinitis or retinochoroiditis NOS

    363.01 Focal choroiditis and chorioretinitis, juxtapapillary

    ■**363.03 Focal choroiditis and chorioretinitis of other posterior pole**

    363.04 Focal choroiditis and chorioretinitis, peripheral

    363.05 Focal retinitis and retinochoroiditis, juxtapapillary
        Neuroretinitis

    363.06 Focal retinitis and retinochoroiditis, macular or paramacular

    ■**363.07 Focal retinitis and retinochoroiditis of other posterior pole**

    363.08 Focal retinitis and retinochoroiditis, peripheral

  ● **363.1 Disseminated chorioretinitis and disseminated retinochoroiditis**

    Excludes *disseminated choroiditis or chorioretinitis in*
              secondary syphilis (091.51)
              neurosyphilitic disseminated retinitis or
                retinochoroiditis (094.83)
              retinal (peri) vasculitis (362.18)

    ■**363.10 Disseminated chorioretinitis, unspecified**
        Disseminated:
          choroiditis or chorioretinitis NOS
          retinitis or retinochoroiditis NOS

    363.11 Disseminated choroiditis and chorioretinitis, posterior pole

    363.12 Disseminated choroiditis and chorioretinitis, peripheral

    363.13 Disseminated choroiditis and chorioretinitis, generalized

        Code first any underlying disease, as:
          tuberculosis (017.3)

    363.14 Disseminated retinitis and retinochoroiditis, metastatic

    363.15 Disseminated retinitis and retinochoroiditis, pigment epitheliopathy
        Acute posterior multifocal placoid pigment
          epitheliopathy

● **363.2 Other and unspecified forms of chorioretinitis and retinochoroiditis**

    Excludes *panophthalmitis (360.02)*
              sympathetic uveitis (360.11)
              uveitis NOS (364.3)

    ■**363.20 Chorioretinitis, unspecified**
        Choroiditis NOS
        Retinitis NOS
        Uveitis, posterior NOS

    363.21 Pars planitis
        Posterior cyclitis

    363.22 Harada's disease

● **363.3 Chorioretinal scars**
    Scar (postinflammatory) (postsurgical)
      (posttraumatic):
      choroid
      retina

    ■**363.30 Chorioretinal scar, unspecified**

    363.31 Solar retinopathy

    ■**363.32 Other macular scars**

    ■**363.33 Other scars of posterior pole**

    363.34 Peripheral scars

    363.35 Disseminated scars

● **363.4 Choroidal degenerations**

    ■**363.40 Choroidal degeneration, unspecified**
        Choroidal sclerosis NOS

    363.41 Senile atrophy of choroid

    363.42 Diffuse secondary atrophy of choroid

    363.43 Angioid streaks of choroid

● **363.5 Hereditary choroidal dystrophies**
    Hereditary choroidal atrophy:
      partial [choriocapillaris]
      total [all vessels]

    ■**363.50 Hereditary choroidal dystrophy or atrophy, unspecified**

    363.51 Circumpapillary dystrophy of choroid, partial

    363.52 Circumpapillary dystrophy of choroid, total
        Helicoid dystrophy of choroid

    363.53 Central dystrophy of choroid, partial
        Dystrophy, choroidal:
          central areolar
          circinate

    363.54 Central choroidal atrophy, total
        Dystrophy, choroidal:
          central gyrate
          serpiginous

    363.55 Choroideremia

    ■**363.56 Other diffuse or generalized dystrophy, partial**
        Diffuse choroidal sclerosis

    ■**363.57 Other diffuse or generalized dystrophy, total**
        Generalized gyrate atrophy, choroid

● **363.6 Choroidal hemorrhage and rupture**

■ **363.61 Choroidal hemorrhage, unspecified**

363.62 Expulsive choroidal hemorrhage

363.63 Choroidal rupture

● **363.7 Choroidal detachment**

■ **363.70 Choroidal detachment, unspecified**

363.71 Serous choroidal detachment

363.72 Hemorrhagic choroidal detachment

■ **363.8 Other disorders of choroid**
Coding Clinic: 2006, Q1, P12

■ **363.9 Unspecified disorder of choroid**

● **364 Disorders of iris and ciliary body**

● **364.0 Acute and subacute iridocyclitis**
Anterior uveitis, acute, subacute
Cyclitis, acute, subacute
Iridocyclitis, acute, subacute
Iritis, acute, subacute

> **Excludes** gonococcal (098.41)
> herpes simplex (054.44)
> herpes zoster (053.22)

■ **364.00 Acute and subacute iridocyclitis, unspecified**

364.01 Primary iridocyclitis

364.02 Recurrent iridocyclitis

364.03 Secondary iridocyclitis, infectious

364.04 Secondary iridocyclitis, noninfectious
Aqueous:
cells
fibrin
flare

364.05 Hypopyon

● **364.1 Chronic iridocyclitis**

> **Excludes** posterior cyclitis (363.21)

■ **364.10 Chronic iridocyclitis, unspecified**

● **364.11 *Chronic iridocyclitis in diseases classified elsewhere***

> *Code first* underlying disease, as:
> sarcoidosis (135)
> tuberculosis (017.3)

> **Excludes** syphilitic iridocyclitis (091.52)

● **364.2 Certain types of iridocyclitis**

> **Excludes** posterior cyclitis (363.21)
> sympathetic uveitis (360.11)

364.21 Fuchs' heterochromic cyclitis

364.22 Glaucomatocyclitic crises

364.23 Lens-induced iridocyclitis

364.24 Vogt-Koyanagi syndrome

■ **364.3 Unspecified iridocyclitis**
Uveitis NOS

● **364.4 Vascular disorders of iris and ciliary body**

364.41 Hyphema
Hemorrhage of iris or ciliary body

364.42 Rubeosis iridis
Neovascularization of iris or ciliary body

● **364.5 Degenerations of iris and ciliary body**

364.51 Essential or progressive iris atrophy

364.52 Iridoschisis

364.53 Pigmentary iris degeneration
Acquired heterochromia of iris
Pigment dispersion syndrome of iris
Translucency of iris

364.54 Degeneration of pupillary margin
Atrophy of sphincter of iris
Ectropion of pigment epithelium of iris

364.55 Miotic cysts of pupillary margin

364.56 Degenerative changes of chamber angle

364.57 Degenerative changes of ciliary body

■ **364.59 Other iris atrophy**
Iris atrophy (generalized) (sector shaped)

● **364.6 Cysts of iris, ciliary body, and anterior chamber**

> **Excludes** miotic pupillary cyst (364.55)
> parasitic cyst (360.13)

364.60 Idiopathic cysts

364.61 Implantation cysts
Epithelial down-growth, anterior chamber
Implantation cysts (surgical) (traumatic)

364.62 Exudative cysts of iris or anterior chamber

364.63 Primary cyst of pars plana

364.64 Exudative cyst of pars plana

● **364.7 Adhesions and disruptions of iris and ciliary body**

> **Excludes** flat anterior chamber (360.34)

■ **364.70 Adhesions of iris, unspecified**
Synechiae (iris) NOS

364.71 Posterior synechiae

364.72 Anterior synechiae

364.73 Goniosynechiae
Peripheral anterior synechiae

364.74 Pupillary membranes
Iris bombé
Pupillary:
occlusion
seclusion

364.75 Pupillary abnormalities
Deformed pupil
Ectopic pupil
Rupture of sphincter, pupil

364.76 Iridodialysis
Coding Clinic: 1985, July-Aug, P16

364.77 Recession of chamber angle

● **364.8 Other disorders of iris and ciliary body**
Coding Clinic: 2007, Q2, P11

364.81 Floppy iris syndrome
Intraoperative floppy iris syndrome (IFIS)

> Use additional E code to identify cause,
> such as:
> sympatholytics [antiadrenergics] causing
> adverse effect in therapeutic use
> (E941.3)
Coding Clinic: 2007, Q4, P77-79

364.82 Plateau iris syndrome
Coding Clinic: 2008, Q4, P112

364.89 Other disorders of iris and ciliary body
Prolapse of iris NOS

> **Excludes** prolapse of iris in recent wound
> (871.1)

■ **364.9 Unspecified disorder of iris and ciliary body**

DISEASES OF THE NERVOUS SYSTEM AND SENSE ORGANS (320–389)

◀ New   ◀▥ Revised   ~~deleted~~ Deleted   ● Use Additional Digit(s)   ■ Nonspecific Code

● Not first-listed DX   OGCR Official Guidelines   Coding Clinic   Excludes   Includes   Use additional   Code first   Omit code

● **365   Glaucoma**

Intraocular pressure (IOP) is too high. IOP is the result of too much aqueous humor because of excess production or inadequate drainage. Leads to optic nerve damage and vision loss.

     Excludes   *blind hypertensive eye [absolute glaucoma] (360.42)*
                   congenital glaucoma (743.20–743.22)

● **365.0   Borderline glaucoma [glaucoma suspect]**

   ■**365.00   Preglaucoma, unspecified**
           Coding Clinic: 1990, Q1, P8

     365.01   Open angle with borderline findings
           Open angle with:
              borderline intraocular pressure
              cupping of optic discs

     365.02   Anatomical narrow angle

     365.03   Steroid responders

   ■**365.04   Ocular hypertension**

● **365.1   Open-angle glaucoma**

   ■**365.10   Open-angle glaucoma, unspecified**
           Wide-angle glaucoma NOS

     365.11   Primary open angle glaucoma
           Chronic simple glaucoma

     365.12   Low tension glaucoma

     365.13   Pigmentary glaucoma

     365.14   Glaucoma of childhood
           Infantile or juvenile glaucoma

     365.15   Residual stage of open angle glaucoma

● **365.2   Primary angle-closure glaucoma**

   ■**365.20   Primary angle-closure glaucoma, unspecified**

     365.21   Intermittent angle-closure glaucoma
           Angle-closure glaucoma:
              interval
              subacute

     365.22   Acute angle-closure glaucoma

     365.23   Chronic angle-closure glaucoma
           Coding Clinic: 1998, Q2, P16

     365.24   Residual stage of angle-closure glaucoma

● **365.3   Corticosteroid-induced glaucoma**

     365.31   Glaucomatous stage

     365.32   Residual stage

● **365.4   Glaucoma associated with congenital anomalies, dystrophies, and systemic syndromes**

   ● *365.41   Glaucoma associated with chamber angle anomalies*

   ● *365.42   Glaucoma associated with anomalies of iris*

   ● ■*365.43   Glaucoma associated with other anterior segment anomalies*

   ● *365.44   Glaucoma associated with systemic syndromes*

       Code first associated disease, as:
         neurofibromatosis (237.7)
         Sturge-Weber (-Dimitri) syndrome (759.6)

● **365.5   Glaucoma associated with disorders of the lens**

     365.51   Phacolytic glaucoma

     365.52   Pseudoexfoliation glaucoma

   ■**365.59   Glaucoma associated with other lens disorders**

● **365.6   Glaucoma associated with other ocular disorders**

   ■**365.60   Glaucoma associated with unspecified ocular disorder**

     365.61   Glaucoma associated with pupillary block

     365.62   Glaucoma associated with ocular inflammations

     365.63   Glaucoma associated with vascular disorders

     365.64   Glaucoma associated with tumors or cysts

     365.65   Glaucoma associated with ocular trauma

● **365.8   Other specified forms of glaucoma**

     365.81   Hypersecretion glaucoma

     365.82   Glaucoma with increased episcleral venous pressure

     365.83   Aqueous misdirection
           Malignant glaucoma
           Coding Clinic: 2002, Q4, P48

   ■**365.89   Other specified glaucoma**
           Coding Clinic: 1998, Q2, P16

   ■**365.9   Unspecified glaucoma**
           Coding Clinic: 2003, Q3, P14; 2001, Q2, P16-17

● **366   Cataract**

     Excludes   *congenital cataract (743.30–743.34)*

● **366.0   Infantile, juvenile, and presenile cataract**

   ■**366.00   Nonsenile cataract, unspecified**
           Coding Clinic: 1987, Mar-April, P9

     366.01   Anterior subcapsular polar cataract

     366.02   Posterior subcapsular polar cataract

     366.03   Cortical, lamellar, or zonular cataract

     366.04   Nuclear cataract

   ■**366.09   Other and combined forms of nonsenile cataract**

● **366.1   Senile cataract**

   ■**366.10   Senile cataract, unspecified**   A
           Coding Clinic: 2003, Q1, P5

     366.11   Pseudoexfoliation of lens capsule   A

     366.12   Incipient cataract   A
           Cataract:
             coronary
             immature NOS
             punctate
           Water clefts

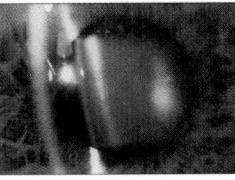

Figure 6–6   Age-related cataract. Nuclear sclerosis and cortical lens opacities are present. (From Yanoff: Ophthalmology, 2nd ed. 2004, Mosby, Inc.)

Item 6–15   Senile cataracts are linked to the aging process. The most common area for the formation of a cataract is the cortical area of the lens. **Polar cataracts** can be either anterior or posterior. **Anterior polar cataracts** are more common and are small, white, capsular cataracts located on the anterior portion of the lens. **Total cataracts,** also called **complete** or **mature,** cause an opacity of all fibers of the lens. **Hypermature** describes a mature cataract with a swollen, milky cortex that covers the entire lens. **Immature,** also called **incipient,** cataracts have a clear cortex and are only slightly opaque. Treatment for all cataracts is the removal of the lens.

DISEASES OF THE NERVOUS SYSTEM AND SENSE ORGANS (320–389)

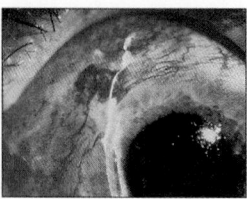

Figure 6–7 Corneal perforation. Preoperative appearance of a patient who has a small, 1.5 mm corneal perforation at the 10 o'clock limbus. *(Courtesy of Dr RK Forster.)* (From Yanoff: Ophthalmology, 2nd ed. 2004, Mosby, Inc.)

366.13 Anterior subcapsular polar senile cataract   A

366.14 Posterior subcapsular polar senile cataract   A

366.15 Cortical senile cataract   A

366.16 Nuclear sclerosis   A
     Cataracta brunescens
     Nuclear cataract
     Coding Clinic: 2007, Q4, P77-79; 1985, Sept-Oct, P11

366.17 Total or mature cataract   A

366.18 Hypermature cataract   A
     Morgagni cataract

366.19 Other and combined forms of senile cataract   A

● 366.2 Traumatic cataract

   366.20 Traumatic cataract, unspecified

   366.21 Localized traumatic opacities
       Vossius' ring

   366.22 Total traumatic cataract

   366.23 Partially resolved traumatic cataract

Item 6–16 Vossius' ring is the result of contusion-type traumatic injury and results in a ring of iris pigment pressed onto the anterior lens capsule.

● 366.3 Cataract secondary to ocular disorders

   366.30 Cataracta complicata, unspecified

   ● 366.31 *Glaucomatous flecks (subcapsular)*
       Code first underlying glaucoma (365.0–365.9)

   ● 366.32 *Cataract in inflammatory disorders*
       Code first underlying condition, as:
         chronic choroiditis (363.0–363.2)

   ● 366.33 *Cataract with neovascularization*
       Code first underlying condition, as:
         chronic iridocyclitis (364.10)

   ● 366.34 *Cataract in degenerative disorders*
       Sunflower cataract
       Code first underlying condition, as:
         chalcosis (360.24)
         degenerative myopia (360.21)
         pigmentary retinal dystrophy (362.74)

● 366.4 Cataract associated with other disorders

   ● 366.41 *Diabetic cataract*
       Code first diabetes (249.5, 250.5)
       Coding Clinic: 1985, Sept-Oct, P11

   ● 366.42 *Tetanic cataract*
       Code first underlying disease as:
         calcinosis (275.40)
         hypoparathyroidism (252.1)

   ● 366.43 *Myotonic cataract*
       Code first underlying disorder (359.21, 359.23)

● 366.44 *Cataract associated with other syndromes*
       Code first underlying condition, as:
         craniofacial dysostosis (756.0)
         galactosemia (271.1)

   366.45 Toxic cataract
       Drug-induced cataract
       Use additional E code to identify drug or other toxic substance
       Coding Clinic: 1995, Q4, P51

   366.46 Cataract associated with radiation and other physical influences
       Use additional E code to identify cause

● 366.5 After-cataract

   366.50 After-cataract, unspecified
       Secondary cataract NOS

   366.51 Soemmering's ring

   366.52 Other after-cataract, not obscuring vision

   366.53 After-cataract, obscuring vision

366.8 Other cataract
     Calcification of lens
     Coding Clinic: 1994, Q1, P16

366.9 Unspecified cataract
     Coding Clinic: 1985, Sept-Oct, P10

● 367 Disorders of refraction and accommodation

   367.0 Hypermetropia
     Far-sightedness
     Hyperopia

   367.1 Myopia
     Near-sightedness

● 367.2 Astigmatism

   367.20 Astigmatism, unspecified

   367.21 Regular astigmatism

   367.22 Irregular astigmatism

● 367.3 Anisometropia and aniseikonia

   367.31 Anisometropia

   367.32 Aniseikonia

367.4 Presbyopia

● 367.5 Disorders of accommodation

   367.51 Paresis of accommodation
     Cycloplegia

   367.52 Total or complete internal ophthalmoplegia

   367.53 Spasm of accommodation

Item 6-17 Disorders of refraction: **Hypermetropia**, or far-sightedness, means focus at a distance is adequate but not on close objects. **Myopia** is near-sightedness or short-sightedness and means the focus on nearby objects is clear but distant objects appear blurred. **Astigmatism** is warping of the curvature of the cornea so light rays entering do not meet a single focal point, resulting in a distorted image. **Anisometropia** is unequal refractive power in which one eye may be myopic (near-sighted) and the other hyperopic (far-sighted). **Presbyopia** is the loss of focus on near objects, which occurs with age because the lens loses elasticity.

DISEASES OF THE NERVOUS SYSTEM AND SENSE ORGANS (320–389)

● **367.8 Other disorders of refraction and accommodation**

    367.81 Transient refractive change

    ■**367.89 Other**
          Drug-induced disorders of refraction and
            accommodation
          Toxic disorders of refraction and
            accommodation

■**367.9 Unspecified disorder of refraction and accommodation**

● **368 Visual disturbances**

> **Excludes** *electrophysiological disturbances (794.11–794.14)*

● **368.0 Amblyopia ex anopsia**

    ■**368.00 Amblyopia, unspecified**

    368.01 Strabismic amblyopia
          Suppression amblyopia

    368.02 Deprivation amblyopia

    368.03 Refractive amblyopia

● **368.1 Subjective visual disturbances**

    ■**368.10 Subjective visual disturbance, unspecified**

    368.11 Sudden visual loss

    368.12 Transient visual loss
          Concentric fading
          Scintillating scotoma

    368.13 Visual discomfort
          Asthenopia
          Eye strain
          Photophobia

    368.14 Visual distortions of shape and size
          Macropsia
          Metamorphopsia
          Micropsia

    ■**368.15 Other visual distortions and entoptic phenomena**
          Photopsia
          Refractive:
            diplopia
            polyopia
          Visual halos

    368.16 Psychophysical visual disturbances
          Prosopagnosia
          Visual:
            agnosia
            disorientation syndrome
            hallucinations
            object agnosia

368.2 Diplopia
    Double vision

● **368.3 Other disorders of binocular vision**

    ■**368.30 Binocular vision disorder, unspecified**

    368.31 Suppression of binocular vision

    368.32 Simultaneous visual perception without fusion

    368.33 Fusion with defective stereopsis

    368.34 Abnormal retinal correspondence

● **368.4 Visual field defects**

    ■**368.40 Visual field defect, unspecified**

    368.41 Scotoma involving central area
          Scotoma:
            central
            centrocecal
            paracentral

    368.42 Scotoma of blind spot area
          Enlarged:
            angioscotoma
            blind spot
          Paracecal scotoma

    368.43 Sector or arcuate defects
          Scotoma:
            arcuate
            Bjerrum
            Seidel

    ■**368.44 Other localized visual field defect**
          Scotoma:
            NOS
            ring
          Visual field defect:
            nasal step
            peripheral

    368.45 Generalized contraction or constriction

    368.46 Homonymous bilateral field defects
          Hemianopsia (altitudinal) (homonymous)
          Quadrant anopia

    368.47 Heteronymous bilateral field defects
          Hemianopsia:
            binasal
            bitemporal

● **368.5 Color vision deficiencies**
    Color blindness

    368.51 Protan defect
          Protanomaly
          Protanopia

    368.52 Deutan defect
          Deuteranomaly
          Deuteranopia

    368.53 Tritan defect
          Tritanomaly
          Tritanopia

    368.54 Achromatopsia
          Monochromatism (cone) (rod)

    368.55 Acquired color vision deficiencies

    ■**368.59 Other color vision deficiencies**

● **368.6 Night blindness**

    ■**368.60 Night blindness, unspecified**

    368.61 Congenital night blindness
          Hereditary night blindness
          Oguchi's disease

    368.62 Acquired night blindness

> **Excludes** *that due to vitamin A deficiency (264.5)*

    368.63 Abnormal dark adaptation curve
          Abnormal threshold of cones or rods
          Delayed adaptation of cones or rods

    ■**368.69 Other night blindness**

■**368.8 Other specified visual disturbances**
    Blurred vision NOS
    Coding Clinic: 2002, Q4, P56

■**368.9 Unspecified visual disturbance**
    Coding Clinic: 2006, Q3, P22

DISEASES OF THE NERVOUS SYSTEM AND SENSE ORGANS (320–389)

● **369 Blindness and low vision**

> **Excludes** *correctable impaired vision due to refractive errors (367.0–367.9)*

> **Note:** Visual impairment refers to a functional limitation of the eye (e.g., limited visual acuity or visual field). It should be distinguished from visual disability, indicating a limitation of the abilities of the individual (e.g., limited reading skills, vocational skills), and from visual handicap, indicating a limitation of personal and socioeconomic independence (e.g., limited mobility, limited employability).

The levels of impairment defined in the table after 369.9 are based on the recommendations of the WHO Study Group on Prevention of Blindness (Geneva, November 6–10, 1972; WHO Technical Report Series 518), and of the International Council of Ophthalmology (1976).

Note that definitions of blindness vary in different settings.

For international reporting, WHO defines blindness as profound impairment. This definition can be applied to blindness of one eye (369.1, 369.6) and to blindness of the individual (369.0).

For determination of benefits in the U.S.A., the definition of legal blindness as severe impairment is often used. This definition applies to blindness of the individual only.

● **369.0 Profound impairment, both eyes**

■ **369.00 Impairment level not further specified**
Blindness:
NOS according to WHO definition
both eyes

■ **369.01 Better eye: total impairment; lesser eye: total impairment**

■ **369.02 Better eye: near-total impairment; lesser eye: not further specified**

■ **369.03 Better eye: near-total impairment; lesser eye: total impairment**

■ **369.04 Better eye: near-total impairment; lesser eye: near-total impairment**

■ **369.05 Better eye: profound impairment; lesser eye: not further specified**

■ **369.06 Better eye: profound impairment; lesser eye: total impairment**

■ **369.07 Better eye: profound impairment; lesser eye: near-total impairment**

■ **369.08 Better eye: profound impairment; lesser eye: profound impairment**

● **369.1 Moderate or severe impairment, better eye, profound impairment lesser eye**

■ **369.10 Impairment level not further specified**
Blindness, one eye, low vision other eye

■ **369.11 Better eye: severe impairment; lesser eye: blind, not further specified**

369.12 Better eye: severe impairment; lesser eye: total impairment

369.13 Better eye: severe impairment; lesser eye: near-total impairment

369.14 Better eye: severe impairment; lesser eye: profound impairment

■ **369.15 Better eye: moderate impairment; lesser eye: blind, not further specified**

369.16 Better eye: moderate impairment; lesser eye: total impairment

369.17 Better eye: moderate impairment; lesser eye: near-total impairment

369.18 Better eye: moderate impairment; lesser eye: profound impairment

● **369.2 Moderate or severe impairment, both eyes**

■ **369.20 Impairment level not further specified**
Low vision, both eyes NOS

■ **369.21 Better eye: severe impairment; lesser eye: not further specified**

369.22 Better eye: severe impairment; lesser eye: severe impairment

■ **369.23 Better eye: moderate impairment; lesser eye: not further specified**

369.24 Better eye: moderate impairment; lesser eye: severe impairment

369.25 Better eye: moderate impairment; lesser eye: moderate impairment

369.3 Unqualified visual loss, both eyes

> **Excludes** *blindness NOS:*
> *legal [U.S.A. definition] (369.4)*
> *WHO definition (369.00)*

369.4 Legal blindness, as defined in U.S.A.
Blindness NOS according to U.S.A. definition

> **Excludes** *legal blindness with specification of impairment level (369.01–369.08, 369.11–369.14, 369.21–369.22)*

● **369.6 Profound impairment, one eye**
Coding Clinic: 2002, Q3, P20-21

■ **369.60 Impairment level not further specified**
Blindness, one eye

■ **369.61 One eye: total impairment; other eye: not specified**

369.62 One eye: total impairment; other eye: near-normal vision

369.63 One eye: total impairment; other eye: normal vision

■ **369.64 One eye: near-total impairment; other eye: not specified**

369.65 One eye: near-total impairment; other eye: near-normal vision

369.66 One eye: near-total impairment; other eye: normal vision

■ **369.67 One eye: profound impairment; other eye: not specified**

369.68 One eye: profound impairment; other eye: near-normal vision

369.69 One eye: profound impairment; other eye: normal vision

● **369.7 Moderate or severe impairment, one eye**

■ **369.70 Impairment level not further specified**
Low vision, one eye

■ **369.71 One eye: severe impairment; other eye: not specified**

369.72 One eye: severe impairment; other eye: near-normal vision

369.73 One eye: severe impairment; other eye: normal vision

■ **369.74 One eye: moderate impairment; other eye: not specified**

369.75 One eye: moderate impairment; other eye: near-normal vision

369.76 One eye: moderate impairment; other eye: normal vision

369.8 Unqualified visual loss, one eye

■ **369.9 Unspecified visual loss**

Classification		Levels of Visual Impairment	Additional Descriptors Which May Be Encountered
"Legal"	WHO	Visual Acuity and/or Visual Field Limitation (Whichever Is Worse)	
	(Near-) normal vision	Range of Normal Vision 20/10 20/13 20/16 20/20 20/25 2.0 1.6 1.25 1.0 0.8	
		Near-Normal Vision 20/30 20/40 20/50 20/60 0.7 0.6 0.5 0.4 0.3	
	Low vision	Moderate Visual Impairment 20/70 20/80 20/100 20/125 20/160 0.25 0.20 0.16 0.12	Moderate low vision
Legal Blindness (U.S.A.) both eyes	Blindness (WHO) one or both eyes	Severe Visual Impairment 20/200 20/250 20/320 20/400 0.10 0.08 0.06 0.05 Visual field: 20 degrees or less	Severe low vision, "Legal" blindness
		Profound Visual Impairment 20/500 20/630 20/800 20/1000 0.04 0.03 0.025 0.02 Count fingers at: less than 3 m (10 ft) Visual field: 10 degrees or less	Profound low vision, Moderate blindness
		Near-Total Visual Impairment Visual acuity: less than 0.02 (20/1000) Count fingers: 1 m (3 ft) or less Hand movements: 5 m (15 ft) or less Light projection, light perception Visual field: 5 degrees or less	Severe blindness, Near-total blindness
		Total Visual Impairment No light perception (NLP)	Total blindness

Visual acuity refers to best achievable acuity with correction.
Non-listed Snellen fractions may be classified by converting to the nearest decimal equivalent, e.g., 10/200 = 0.05, 6/30 = 0.20.
CF (count fingers) without designation of distance, may be classified to profound impairment.
HM (hand motion) without designation of distance, may be classified to near-total impairment.
Visual field measurements refer to the largest field diameter for a 1/100 white test object.

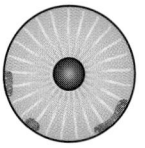

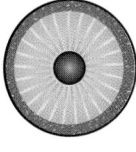

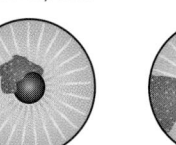

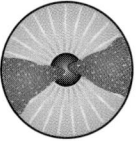

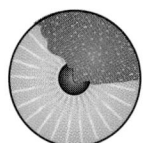

Marginal (catarrhal) ulcer

Ring ulcer

Central corneal ulcer

Rosacea ulcer

Mooren's (rodent) ulcer

Figure 6–8 Corneal ulcers: marginal, ring, central corneal, rosacea, and Mooren's.

Item 6–18 An infected ulcer is usually called a **serpiginous** or **hypopyon** ulcer which is a pus sac in the anterior chamber of the eye.
Marginal ulcers are usually asymptomatic, not primary, and are often superficial and simple. More severe marginal ulcers spread to form a ring ulcer. **Ring** ulcers can extend around the entire corneal periphery.
Central corneal ulcers develop when there is an abrasion to the epithelium and an infection develops in the eroded area.
The **pyocyaneal** ulcer is the most serious corneal infection, which, if left untreated, can lead to loss of the eye.

370 **Keratitis**
● 370.0 **Corneal ulcer**
    Excludes *that due to vitamin A deficiency (264.3)*
  ■370.00 **Corneal ulcer, unspecified**
    370.01 **Marginal corneal ulcer**
    370.02 **Ring corneal ulcer**
    370.03 **Central corneal ulcer**
    370.04 **Hypopyon ulcer**
        Serpiginous ulcer
    370.05 **Mycotic corneal ulcer**
    370.06 **Perforated corneal ulcer**
    370.07 **Mooren's ulcer**
● 370.2 **Superficial keratitis without conjunctivitis**
    Excludes *dendritic [herpes simplex] keratitis (054.42)*
  ■370.20 **Superficial keratitis, unspecified**
    370.21 **Punctate keratitis**
        Thygeson's superficial punctate keratitis
    370.22 **Macular keratitis**
        Keratitis: Keratitis:
          areolar   stellate
          nummular   striate
    370.23 **Filamentary keratitis**
    370.24 **Photokeratitis**
        Snow blindness
        Welders' keratitis
        Coding Clinic: 1996, Q3, P6
● 370.3 **Certain types of keratoconjunctivitis**
    370.31 **Phlyctenular keratoconjunctivitis**
        Phlyctenulosis
        Use additional code for any associated tuberculosis (017.3)
    370.32 **Limbal and corneal involvement in vernal conjunctivitis**
        Use additional code for vernal conjunctivitis (372.13)
  ■370.33 **Keratoconjunctivitis sicca, not specified as Sjögren's**
    Excludes *Sjögren's syndrome (710.2)*
    370.34 **Exposure keratoconjunctivitis**
        Coding Clinic: 1996, Q3, P6
    370.35 **Neurotrophic keratoconjunctivitis**

DISEASES OF THE NERVOUS SYSTEM AND SENSE ORGANS (320–389)

● **370.4 Other and unspecified keratoconjunctivitis**

■ **370.40 Keratoconjunctivitis, unspecified**
Superficial keratitis with conjunctivitis NOS

● *370.44 Keratitis or keratoconjunctivitis in exanthema*
Code first underlying condition (050.0–052.9)

Excludes herpes simplex (054.43)
herpes zoster (053.21)
measles (055.71)

■ **370.49 Other**

Excludes epidemic keratoconjunctivitis
(077.1)

● **370.5 Interstitial and deep keratitis**

■ **370.50 Interstitial keratitis, unspecified**

370.52 Diffuse interstitial keratitis
Cogan's syndrome

370.54 Sclerosing keratitis

370.55 Corneal abscess

■ **370.59 Other**

Excludes disciform herpes simplex keratitis
(054.43)
syphilitic keratitis (090.3)

● **370.6 Corneal neovascularization**

■ **370.60 Corneal neovascularization, unspecified**

370.61 Localized vascularization of cornea

370.62 Pannus (corneal)
Coding Clinic: 2002, Q3, P20-21

370.63 Deep vascularization of cornea

370.64 Ghost vessels (corneal)

● ■ *370.8 Other forms of keratitis*

Code first underlying condition, such as:
Acanthamoeba (136.21)
Fusarium (118)
Coding Clinic: 2008, Q4, P79-81; 1994, Q3, P5

■ **370.9 Unspecified keratitis**

● **371 Corneal opacity and other disorders of cornea**

● **371.0 Corneal scars and opacities**

Excludes that due to vitamin A deficiency (264.6)

■ **371.00 Corneal opacity, unspecified**
Corneal scar NOS

371.01 Minor opacity of cornea
Corneal nebula

371.02 Peripheral opacity of cornea
Corneal macula not interfering with central vision

371.03 Central opacity of cornea
Corneal:
leucoma interfering with central vision
macula interfering with central vision

371.04 Adherent leucoma

● *371.05 Phthisical cornea*

Code first underlying tuberculosis (017.3)

● **371.1 Corneal pigmentations and deposits**

■ **371.10 Corneal deposit, unspecified**

371.11 Anterior pigmentations
Stähli's lines

371.12 Stromal pigmentations
Hematocornea

371.13 Posterior pigmentations
Krukenberg spindle

371.14 Kayser-Fleischer ring

■ **371.15 Other deposits associated with metabolic disorders**

371.16 Argentous deposits

● **371.2 Corneal edema**

■ **371.20 Corneal edema, unspecified**

371.21 Idiopathic corneal edema

371.22 Secondary corneal edema

371.23 Bullous keratopathy

371.24 Corneal edema due to wearing of contact lenses

● **371.3 Changes of corneal membranes**

■ **371.30 Corneal membrane change, unspecified**

371.31 Folds and rupture of Bowman's membrane

371.32 Folds in Descemet's membrane

371.33 Rupture in Descemet's membrane

● **371.4 Corneal degenerations**

■ **371.40 Corneal degeneration, unspecified**

371.41 Senile corneal changes
Arcus senilis   Hassall-Henle bodies

371.42 Recurrent erosion of cornea

Excludes Mooren's ulcer (370.07)

371.43 Band-shaped keratopathy

■ **371.44 Other calcerous degenerations of cornea**

371.45 Keratomalacia NOS

Excludes that due to vitamin A deficiency
(264.4)

371.46 Nodular degeneration of cornea
Salzmann's nodular dystrophy

371.48 Peripheral degenerations of cornea
Marginal degeneration of cornea [Terrien's]

■ **371.49 Other**
Discrete colliquative keratopathy

● **371.5 Hereditary corneal dystrophies**

■ **371.50 Corneal dystrophy, unspecified**

371.51 Juvenile epithelial corneal dystrophy

■ **371.52 Other anterior corneal dystrophies**
Corneal dystrophy:
microscopic cystic
ring-like

371.53 Granular corneal dystrophy

371.54 Lattice corneal dystrophy

371.55 Macular corneal dystrophy

■ **371.56 Other stromal corneal dystrophies**
Crystalline corneal dystrophy

371.57 Endothelial corneal dystrophy
Combined corneal dystrophy
Cornea guttata
Fuchs' endothelial dystrophy

■ **371.58 Other posterior corneal dystrophies**
Polymorphous corneal dystrophy

◀ New   ◀▦ Revised   ~~deleted~~ Deleted   ● Use Additional Digit(s)   ■ Nonspecific Code
● Not first-listed DX   OGCR Official Guidelines   Coding Clinic   Excludes   Includes   Use additional   Code first   Omit code

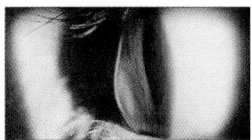

Figure 6-9 Lateral view of the displacement of the cone apex in keratoconus. (From Yanoff: Ophthalmology, 2nd ed. 2004, Mosby, Inc.)

Item 6-19 Keratoconus results in corneal degeneration that begins in childhood, gradually changes the cornea from a round to cone shape, decreasing visual acuity. Treatment includes contact lenses. In severe cases the need for corneal transplant may be the treatment of choice; however, newer technologies may use high frequency radio energy to shrink the edges of the cornea, pulling the central area back to a more normal shape. It can help delay or avoid the need for a corneal transplantation.

● **371.6 Keratoconus**
　■ **371.60 Keratoconus, unspecified**
　371.61 Keratoconus, stable condition
　371.62 Keratoconus, acute hydrops
● **371.7 Other corneal deformities**
　■ **371.70 Corneal deformity, unspecified**
　371.71 Corneal ectasia
　371.72 Descemetocele
　371.73 Corneal staphyloma
● ■ **371.8 Other corneal disorders**
　371.81 Corneal anesthesia and hypoesthesia
　371.82 Corneal disorder due to contact lens

> **Excludes** *corneal edema due to contact lens (371.24)*

　■ **371.89 Other**
> Coding Clinic: 1999, Q3, P12

■ **371.9 Unspecified corneal disorder**

● **372 Disorders of conjunctiva**

> **Excludes** *keratoconjunctivitis (370.3–370.4)*

● **372.0 Acute conjunctivitis**
　■ **372.00 Acute conjunctivitis, unspecified**
　372.01 Serous conjunctivitis, except viral

> **Excludes** *viral conjunctivitis NOS (077.9)*
> Coding Clinic: 2008, Q3, P6-7

　372.02 Acute follicular conjunctivitis
　Conjunctival folliculosis NOS

> **Excludes** *conjunctivitis:*
> *adenoviral (acute follicular) (077.3)*
> *epidemic hemorrhagic (077.4)*
> *inclusion (077.0)*
> *Newcastle (077.8)*
> *epidemic keratoconjunctivitis (077.1)*
> *pharyngoconjunctival fever (077.2)*

　■ **372.03 Other mucopurulent conjunctivitis**
　Catarrhal conjunctivitis

> **Excludes** *blennorrhea neonatorum (gonococcal) (098.40)*
> *neonatal conjunctivitis (771.6)*
> *ophthalmia neonatorum NOS (771.6)*

　372.04 Pseudomembranous conjunctivitis
　Membranous conjunctivitis

> **Excludes** *diphtheritic conjunctivitis (032.81)*

　372.05 Acute atopic conjunctivitis

372.06 Acute chemical conjunctivitis ◄
Acute toxic conjunctivitis ◄

> Use additional E code to identify the chemical or toxic agent ◄
>
> **Excludes** *burn of eye and adnexa* ◄
> *(940.0-940.9)*
> *chemical corrosion injury of* ◄
> *eye (940.2-940.3)*

● **372.1 Chronic conjunctivitis**
　■ **372.10 Chronic conjunctivitis, unspecified**
　372.11 Simple chronic conjunctivitis
　372.12 Chronic follicular conjunctivitis
　372.13 Vernal conjunctivitis
> Coding Clinic: 1996, Q3, P8
　■ **372.14 Other chronic allergic conjunctivitis**
> Coding Clinic: 1996, Q3, P8
　● **372.15 *Parasitic conjunctivitis***

> *Code first underlying disease as:*
> *filariasis (125.0–125.9)*
> *mucocutaneous leishmaniasis (085.5)*

● **372.2 Blepharoconjunctivitis**
　■ **372.20 Blepharoconjunctivitis, unspecified**
　372.21 Angular blepharoconjunctivitis
　372.22 Contact blepharoconjunctivitis
● **372.3 Other and unspecified conjunctivitis**
　■ **372.30 Conjunctivitis, unspecified**
　● **372.31 *Rosacea conjunctivitis***

> *Code first underlying rosacea dermatitis (695.3)*

　● **372.33 *Conjunctivitis in mucocutaneous disease***

> *Code first underlying disease as:*
> *erythema multiforme (695.10–695.19)*
> *Reiter's disease (099.3)*
>
> **Excludes** *ocular pemphigoid (694.61)*

　372.34 Pingueculitis

> **Excludes** *pinguecula (372.51)* ◄
> Coding Clinic: 2008, Q4, P112-113

　■ **372.39 Other**
> Coding Clinic: 2007, Q2, P11
● **372.4 Pterygium**

> **Excludes** *pseudopterygium (372.52)*

　■ **372.40 Pterygium, unspecified**
　372.41 Peripheral pterygium, stationary
　372.42 Peripheral pterygium, progressive
　372.43 Central pterygium
　372.44 Double pterygium
　372.45 Recurrent pterygium

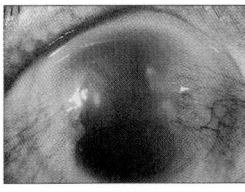

Figure 6-10 Double pterygium. Note both nasal and temporal pterygia in a 57-year-old farmer. (From Yanoff: Ophthalmology, 2nd ed. 2004, Mosby, Inc.)

Item 6-20 Pterygium is Greek for batlike. The condition is characterized by a membrane that extends from the limbus to the center of the cornea and resembles a wing.

DISEASES OF THE NERVOUS SYSTEM AND SENSE ORGANS (320–389)

● 372.5 **Conjunctival degenerations and deposits**
  ■ 372.50 **Conjunctival degeneration, unspecified**
    372.51 **Pinguecula**
      Excludes *pingueculitis (372.34)* ◀
    372.52 **Pseudopterygium**
    372.53 **Conjunctival xerosis**
      Excludes *conjunctival xerosis due to vitamin A deficiency (264.0, 264.1, 264.7)*
    372.54 **Conjunctival concretions**
    372.55 **Conjunctival pigmentations**
      Conjunctival argyrosis
    372.56 **Conjunctival deposits**
● 372.6 **Conjunctival scars**
    372.61 **Granuloma of conjunctiva**
    372.62 **Localized adhesions and strands of conjunctiva**
    372.63 **Symblepharon**
      Extensive adhesions of conjunctiva
    372.64 **Scarring of conjunctiva**
      Contraction of eye socket (after enucleation)
● 372.7 **Conjunctival vascular disorders and cysts**
    372.71 **Hyperemia of conjunctiva**
    372.72 **Conjunctival hemorrhage**
      Hyposphagma
      Subconjunctival hemorrhage
    372.73 **Conjunctival edema**
      Chemosis of conjunctiva
      Subconjunctival edema
    372.74 **Vascular abnormalities of conjunctiva**
      Aneurysm(ata) of conjunctiva
    372.75 **Conjunctival cysts**
● ■ 372.8 **Other disorders of conjunctiva**
    372.81 **Conjunctivochalasis**
      Coding Clinic: 2000, Q4, P41
  ■ 372.89 **Other disorders of conjunctiva**
  ■ 372.9 **Unspecified disorder of conjunctiva**
● 373 **Inflammation of eyelids**
  ● 373.0 **Blepharitis**
      Excludes *blepharoconjunctivitis (372.20–372.22)*
    ■ 373.00 **Blepharitis, unspecified**
    373.01 **Ulcerative blepharitis**
    373.02 **Squamous blepharitis**

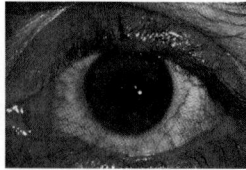

Figure 6–11 Photograph of eyelids with marginal blepharitis. (From Mandell, Bennett, & Dolin: Principles and Practice of Infectious Diseases, 6th ed. 2005, Churchill Livingstone, An Imprint of Elsevier)

Item 6–21 Blepharitis is a common condition in which the eyelid is swollen and yellow scaling and conjunctivitis develop. Usually the hair on the scalp and brow is involved.

● 373.1 **Hordeolum and other deep inflammation of eyelid**
    Bacterial infection (staphylococcus) of sebaceous gland of eyelid (stye)
    373.11 **Hordeolum externum**
      Hordeolum NOS
      Stye
    373.12 **Hordeolum internum**
      Infection of meibomian gland
    373.13 **Abscess of eyelid**
      Furuncle of eyelid
  373.2 **Chalazion**
    Most often caused by accumulation of meibomian gland secretions resulting from blockage of duct.
    Meibomian (gland) cyst
    Excludes *infected meibomian gland (373.12)*
● 373.3 **Noninfectious dermatoses of eyelid**
    373.31 **Eczematous dermatitis of eyelid**
    373.32 **Contact and allergic dermatitis of eyelid**
    373.33 **Xeroderma of eyelid**
    373.34 **Discoid lupus erythematosus of eyelid**
● 373.4 *Infective dermatitis of eyelid of types resulting in deformity*
    Code first underlying disease, as:
      leprosy (030.0–030.9)
      lupus vulgaris (tuberculous) (017.0)
      yaws (102.0–102.9)
● ■ 373.5 *Other infective dermatitis of eyelid*
    Code first underlying disease, as:
      actinomycosis (039.3)
      impetigo (684)
      mycotic dermatitis (110.0–111.9)
      vaccinia (051.0)
      postvaccination (999.0)
    Excludes *herpes:*
      simplex (054.41)
      zoster (053.20)
● 373.6 *Parasitic infestation of eyelid*
    Code first underlying disease, as:
      leishmaniasis (085.0–085.9)
      loiasis (125.2)
      onchocerciasis (125.3)
      pediculosis (132.0)
  ■ 373.8 **Other inflammations of eyelids**
  ■ 373.9 **Unspecified inflammation of eyelid**
● 374 **Other disorders of eyelids**
  ● 374.0 **Entropion and trichiasis of eyelid**
    ■ 374.00 **Entropion, unspecified**
    374.01 **Senile entropion**　　　　　　　　　A
    374.02 **Mechanical entropion**

◀ New   ◀▥ Revised   ~~deleted~~ Deleted   ● Use Additional Digit(s)   ■ Nonspecific Code
● Not first-listed DX   OGCR Official Guidelines   Coding Clinic   Excludes   Includes   Use additional   Code first   Omit code

DISEASES OF THE NERVOUS SYSTEM AND SENSE ORGANS (320–389)

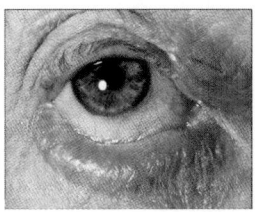

Figure 6–12 Right lower eyelid entropion. Note the inward rotation of the tarsal plate about the horizontal axis and the resultant contact between the mucocutaneous junction and ocular surface. (From Yanoff: Ophthalmology, 2nd ed. 2004, Mosby, Inc.)

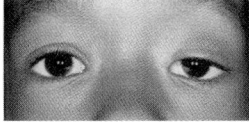

Figure 6–13 Ptosis of eyelid. (From Yanoff: Ophthalmology, 2nd ed. 2004, Mosby, Inc.)

374.03 Spastic entropion

374.04 Cicatricial entropion

374.05 Trichiasis without entropion

● 374.1 Ectropion

◼ 374.10 Ectropion, unspecified

374.11 Senile ectropion   A

374.12 Mechanical ectropion

374.13 Spastic ectropion

374.14 Cicatricial ectropion

● 374.2 Lagophthalmos

◼ 374.20 Lagophthalmos, unspecified

374.21 Paralytic lagophthalmos

374.22 Mechanical lagophthalmos

374.23 Cicatricial lagophthalmos

Item 6-22 Ptosis of eyelid is drooping of the upper eyelid over the pupil when the eyes are fully opened resulting from nerve or muscle damage, which may require surgical correction.

● 374.3 Ptosis of eyelid
        Falling forward, drooping, sagging of eyelid

◼ 374.30 Ptosis of eyelid, unspecified
        Coding Clinic: 1996, Q2, P11

374.31 Paralytic ptosis

374.32 Myogenic ptosis

374.33 Mechanical ptosis

374.34 Blepharochalasis
        Pseudoptosis

● 374.4 Other disorders affecting eyelid function

        Excludes *blepharoclonus (333.81)*
                      blepharospasm (333.81)
                      facial nerve palsy (351.0)
                      third nerve palsy or paralysis
                      (378.51–378.52)
                      tic (psychogenic) (307.20–307.23)
                      organic (333.3)

374.41 Lid retraction or lag

374.43 Abnormal innervation syndrome
        Jaw-blinking
        Paradoxical facial movements

374.44 Sensory disorders

◼ 374.45 Other sensorimotor disorders
        Deficient blink reflex

374.46 Blepharophimosis
        Ankyloblepharon

● 374.5 Degenerative disorders of eyelid and periocular area

◼ 374.50 Degenerative disorder of eyelid, unspecified

● 374.51 *Xanthelasma*
        Xanthoma (planum) (tuberosum) of eyelid
        Code first underlying condition (272.0–272.9)

374.52 Hyperpigmentation of eyelid
        Chloasma
        Dyspigmentation

374.53 Hypopigmentation of eyelid
        Vitiligo of eyelid

374.54 Hypertrichosis of eyelid

374.55 Hypotrichosis of eyelid
        Madarosis of eyelid

◼ 374.56 Other degenerative disorders of skin affecting eyelid

● 374.8 Other disorders of eyelid

374.81 Hemorrhage of eyelid

        Excludes *black eye (921.0)*

374.82 Edema of eyelid
        Hyperemia of eyelid
        Coding Clinic: 2008, Q4, P128-131

374.83 Elephantiasis of eyelid

374.84 Cysts of eyelids
        Sebaceous cyst of eyelid

374.85 Vascular anomalies of eyelid

374.86 Retained foreign body of eyelid

374.87 Dermatochalasis

◼ 374.89 Other disorders of eyelid

◼ 374.9 Unspecified disorder of eyelid

● 375 Disorders of lacrimal system

● 375.0 Dacryoadenitis

◼ 375.00 Dacryoadenitis, unspecified

375.01 Acute dacryoadenitis

375.02 Chronic dacryoadenitis

375.03 Chronic enlargement of lacrimal gland

● 375.1 Other disorders of lacrimal gland

◼ 375.11 Dacryops

◼ 375.12 Other lacrimal cysts and cystic degeneration

375.13 Primary lacrimal atrophy

375.14 Secondary lacrimal atrophy

◼ 375.15 Tear film insufficiency, unspecified
        Dry eye syndrome
        Coding Clinic: 1996, Q3, P6

375.16 Dislocation of lacrimal gland

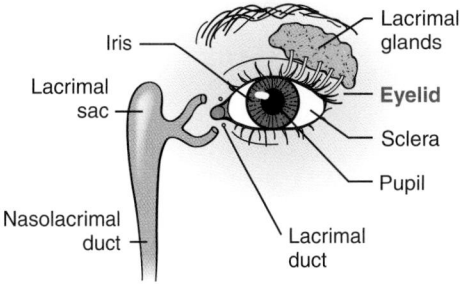

Figure 6–14 Lacrimal apparatus. (From Buck CJ: Step-by-Step Medical Coding. Philadelphia, WB Saunders, 2006, p 302.)

DISEASES OF THE NERVOUS SYSTEM AND SENSE ORGANS (320–389)

- **375.2 Epiphora**
  - **375.20 Epiphora, unspecified as to cause**
  - 375.21 Epiphora due to excess lacrimation
  - 375.22 Epiphora due to insufficient drainage
- **375.3 Acute and unspecified inflammation of lacrimal passages**
  - Excludes *neonatal dacryocystitis (771.6)*
  - **375.30 Dacryocystitis, unspecified**
  - 375.31 Acute canaliculitis, lacrimal
  - 375.32 Acute dacryocystitis
    - Acute peridacryocystitis
  - 375.33 Phlegmonous dacryocystitis
- **375.4 Chronic inflammation of lacrimal passages**
  - 375.41 Chronic canaliculitis
  - 375.42 Chronic dacryocystitis
  - 375.43 Lacrimal mucocele
- **375.5 Stenosis and insufficiency of lacrimal passages**
  - 375.51 Eversion of lacrimal punctum
  - 375.52 Stenosis of lacrimal punctum
  - 375.53 Stenosis of lacrimal canaliculi
  - 375.54 Stenosis of lacrimal sac
  - 375.55 Obstruction of nasolacrimal duct, neonatal
    - Excludes *congenital anomaly of nasolacrimal duct (743.65)*
  - 375.56 Stenosis of nasolacrimal duct, acquired
  - 375.57 Dacryolith
- **375.6 Other changes of lacrimal passages**
  - 375.61 Lacrimal fistula
  - **375.69 Other**
- **375.8 Other disorders of lacrimal system**
  - 375.81 Granuloma of lacrimal passages
  - **375.89 Other**
- **375.9 Unspecified disorder of lacrimal system**

- **376 Disorders of the orbit**
  - **376.0 Acute inflammation of orbit**
    - **376.00 Acute inflammation of orbit, unspecified**
    - 376.01 Orbital cellulitis
      - Abscess of orbit
    - 376.02 Orbital periostitis
    - 376.03 Orbital osteomyelitis
    - 376.04 Tenonitis

- **376.1 Chronic inflammatory disorders of orbit**
  - **376.10 Chronic inflammation of orbit, unspecified**
  - 376.11 Orbital granuloma
    - Pseudotumor (inflammatory) of orbit
  - 376.12 Orbital myositis
  - *376.13 Parasitic infestation of orbit*
    - *Code first* underlying disease, as:
      - hydatid infestation of orbit (122.3, 122.6, 122.9)
      - myiasis of orbit (134.0)
- **376.2 Endocrine exophthalmos**
  - *Code first* underlying thyroid disorder (242.0–242.9)
  - *376.21 Thyrotoxic exophthalmos*
  - *376.22 Exophthalmic ophthalmoplegia*
- **376.3 Other exophthalmic conditions**
  - **376.30 Exophthalmos, unspecified**
  - 376.31 Constant exophthalmos
  - 376.32 Orbital hemorrhage
  - 376.33 Orbital edema or congestion
  - 376.34 Intermittent exophthalmos
  - 376.35 Pulsating exophthalmos
  - 376.36 Lateral displacement of globe
- **376.4 Deformity of orbit**
  - **376.40 Deformity of orbit, unspecified**
  - 376.41 Hypertelorism of orbit
  - 376.42 Exostosis of orbit
  - 376.43 Local deformities due to bone disease
  - 376.44 Orbital deformities associated with craniofacial deformities
  - 376.45 Atrophy of orbit
  - 376.46 Enlargement of orbit
  - 376.47 Deformity due to trauma or surgery
- **376.5 Enophthalmos**
  - **376.50 Enophthalmos, unspecified as to cause**
  - 376.51 Enophthalmos due to atrophy of orbital tissue
  - 376.52 Enophthalmos due to trauma or surgery
- 376.6 Retained (old) foreign body following penetrating wound of orbit
  - Retrobulbar foreign body
- **376.8 Other orbital disorders**
  - 376.81 Orbital cysts
    - Encephalocele of orbit
    - Coding Clinic: 1999, Q3, P13
  - 376.82 Myopathy of extraocular muscles
  - **376.89 Other**
- **376.9 Unspecified disorder of orbit**

Item 6-23 Papilledema is swelling of the optic disc caused by increased intracranial pressure. It is most often bilateral and occurs quickly (hours) or over weeks of time. It is a common symptom of a brain tumor. The term should not be used to describe optic disc swelling with underlying infectious, infiltrative, or inflammatory etiologies.

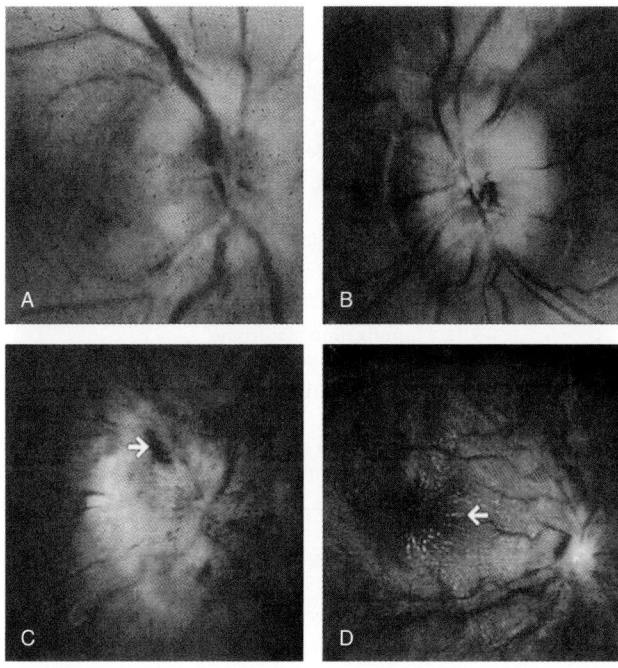

Figure 6–15 Papilledema. (From Behrman: Nelson Textbook of Pediatrics, 17th ed. 2004, Saunders)

- **377 Disorders of optic nerve and visual pathways**
  - **377.0 Papilledema**
    - **377.00 Papilledema, unspecified**
    - **377.01 Papilledema associated with increased intracranial pressure**
    - **377.02 Papilledema associated with decreased ocular pressure**
    - **377.03 Papilledema associated with retinal disorder**
    - **377.04 Foster-Kennedy syndrome**
  - **377.1 Optic atrophy**
    - **377.10 Optic atrophy, unspecified**
    - **377.11 Primary optic atrophy**
      - **Excludes** *neurosyphilitic optic atrophy (094.84)*
    - **377.12 Postinflammatory optic atrophy**
    - **377.13 Optic atrophy associated with retinal dystrophies**
    - **377.14 Glaucomatous atrophy [cupping] of optic disc**

- **377.15 Partial optic atrophy**
  - Temporal pallor of optic disc
- **377.16 Hereditary optic atrophy**
  - Optic atrophy:
    - dominant hereditary
    - Leber's
- **377.2 Other disorders of optic disc**
  - **377.21 Drusen of optic disc**
  - **377.22 Crater-like holes of optic disc**
  - **377.23 Coloboma of optic disc**
  - **377.24 Pseudopapilledema**
- **377.3 Optic neuritis**
  - **Excludes** *meningococcal optic neuritis (036.81)*
  - **377.30 Optic neuritis, unspecified**
  - **377.31 Optic papillitis**
  - **377.32 Retrobulbar neuritis (acute)**
    - **Excludes** *syphilitic retrobulbar neuritis (094.85)*
  - **377.33 Nutritional optic neuropathy**
  - **377.34 Toxic optic neuropathy**
    - Toxic amblyopia
  - **377.39 Other**
    - **Excludes** *ischemic optic neuropathy (377.41)*
- **377.4 Other disorders of optic nerve**
  - **377.41 Ischemic optic neuropathy**
  - **377.42 Hemorrhage in optic nerve sheaths**
  - **377.43 Optic nerve hypoplasia**
    - Coding Clinic: 2006, Q4, P81-82
  - **377.49 Other**
    - Compression of optic nerve
- **377.5 Disorders of optic chiasm**
  - **377.51 Associated with pituitary neoplasms and disorders**
  - **377.52 Associated with other neoplasms**
  - **377.53 Associated with vascular disorders**
  - **377.54 Associated with inflammatory disorders**
- **377.6 Disorders of other visual pathways**
  - **377.61 Associated with neoplasms**
  - **377.62 Associated with vascular disorders**
  - **377.63 Associated with inflammatory disorders**
- **377.7 Disorders of visual cortex**
  - **Excludes** *visual:*
    - *agnosia (368.16)*
    - *hallucinations (368.16)*
    - *halos (368.15)*
  - **377.71 Associated with neoplasms**
  - **377.72 Associated with vascular disorders**
  - **377.73 Associated with inflammatory disorders**
  - **377.75 Cortical blindness**
- **377.9 Unspecified disorder of optic nerve and visual pathways**

DISEASES OF THE NERVOUS SYSTEM AND SENSE ORGANS (320–389)

Item 6-24 Strabismus or esotropia (crossed eyes) is a condition of the extraocular eye muscles, resulting in an inability of the eyes to focus and also affects depth perception.

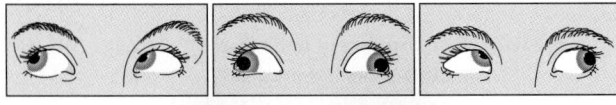

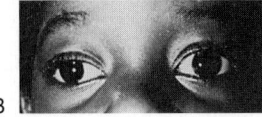

Figure 6–16 A. Image of strabismus. **B.** Exotropia. (**A** from Yanoff: Ophthalmology, 2nd ed. 2004, Mosby, Inc. **B** from Rakel: Textbook of Family Practice, 7th ed. 2007, Saunders)

● **378 Strabismus and other disorders of binocular eye movements**

   Excludes *nystagmus and other irregular eye movements (379.50–379.59)*

● **378.0 Esotropia**
   Convergent concomitant strabismus

   Excludes *intermittent esotropia (378.20–378.22)*

   ■ **378.00 Esotropia, unspecified**

   378.01 Monocular esotropia

   378.02 Monocular esotropia with A pattern

   378.03 Monocular esotropia with V pattern

   ■ **378.04 Monocular esotropia with other noncomitancies**
      Monocular esotropia with X or Y pattern

   378.05 Alternating esotropia

   378.06 Alternating esotropia with A pattern

   378.07 Alternating esotropia with V pattern

   ■ **378.08 Alternating esotropia with other noncomitancies**
      Alternating esotropia with X or Y pattern

● **378.1 Exotropia**
   Misalignment in which one eye deviates outward (away from nose) while other fixates normally
   Divergent concomitant strabismus

   Excludes *intermittent exotropia (378.20, 378.23–378.24)*

   ■ **378.10 Exotropia, unspecified**

   378.11 Monocular exotropia

   378.12 Monocular exotropia with A pattern

   378.13 Monocular exotropia with V pattern

   ■ **378.14 Monocular exotropia with other noncomitancies**
      Monocular exotropia with X or Y pattern

   378.15 Alternating exotropia

   378.16 Alternating exotropia with A pattern

   378.17 Alternating exotropia with V pattern

   ■ **378.18 Alternating exotropia with other noncomitancies**
      Alternating exotropia with X or Y pattern

● **378.2 Intermittent heterotropia**
   Displacement of an organ or part of an organ from normal position

   Excludes *vertical heterotropia (intermittent) (378.31)*

   ■ **378.20 Intermittent heterotropia, unspecified**
      Intermittent:
         esotropia NOS
         exotropia NOS

   378.21 Intermittent esotropia, monocular

   378.22 Intermittent esotropia, alternating

   378.23 Intermittent exotropia, monocular

   378.24 Intermittent exotropia, alternating

● **378.3 Other and unspecified heterotropia**

   ■ **378.30 Heterotropia, unspecified**

   378.31 Hypertropia
      Vertical heterotropia (constant) (intermittent)

   378.32 Hypotropia

   378.33 Cyclotropia

   378.34 Monofixation syndrome
      Microtropia

   378.35 Accommodative component in esotropia

● **378.4 Heterophoria**
   Condition in which one or both eyes wander away from position where both eyes are looking

   ■ **378.40 Heterophoria, unspecified**

   378.41 Esophoria
      Eye deviates inward (toward nose)

   378.42 Exophoria
      Eye deviates outward (toward ear)

   378.43 Vertical heterophoria

   378.44 Cyclophoria

   378.45 Alternating hyperphoria

● **378.5 Paralytic strabismus**

   ■ **378.50 Paralytic strabismus, unspecified**

   378.51 Third or oculomotor nerve palsy, partial

   378.52 Third or oculomotor nerve palsy, total

   378.53 Fourth or trochlear nerve palsy
      Coding Clinic: 2001, Q2, P21

   378.54 Sixth or abducens nerve palsy

   378.55 External ophthalmoplegia
      Coding Clinic: 1989, Q2, P12

   378.56 Total ophthalmoplegia

● **378.6 Mechanical strabismus**

   ■ **378.60 Mechanical strabismus, unspecified**

   378.61 Brown's (tendon) sheath syndrome

   ■ **378.62 Mechanical strabismus from other musculofascial disorders**

   ■ **378.63 Limited duction associated with other conditions**

● **378.7 Other specified strabismus**

   378.71 Duane's syndrome

   378.72 Progressive external ophthalmoplegia

   ■ **378.73 Strabismus in other neuromuscular disorders**

◀ New   ◀▥ Revised   ~~deleted~~ Deleted   ● Use Additional Digit(s)   ■ Nonspecific Code

● Not first-listed DX   OGCR Official Guidelines   Coding Clinic   Excludes   Includes   Use additional   Code first   Omit code

● 378.8 **Other disorders of binocular eye movements**

    Excludes *nystagmus (379.50–379.56)*

    378.81 **Palsy of conjugate gaze**

    378.82 **Spasm of conjugate gaze**

    378.83 **Convergence insufficiency or palsy**

    378.84 **Convergence excess or spasm**

    378.85 **Anomalies of divergence**

    378.86 **Internuclear ophthalmoplegia**

    378.87 **Other dissociated deviation of eye movements**
        Skew deviation

378.9 **Unspecified disorder of eye movements**
    Ophthalmoplegia NOS
    Strabismus NOS
    Coding Clinic: 2001, Q2, P21

● 379   **Other disorders of eye**

● 379.0 **Scleritis and episcleritis**
    Inflammation of white (sclera and episclera) of eye.
    Autoimmune disorders are most common cause.

    Excludes *syphilitic episcleritis (095.0)*

    379.00 **Scleritis, unspecified**
        Episcleritis NOS

    379.01 **Episcleritis periodica fugax**

    379.02 **Nodular episcleritis**

    379.03 **Anterior scleritis**

    379.04 **Scleromalacia perforans**

    379.05 **Scleritis with corneal involvement**
        Scleroperikeratitis

    379.06 **Brawny scleritis**

    379.07 **Posterior scleritis**
        Sclerotenonitis

    379.09 **Other**
        Scleral abscess

● 379.1 **Other disorders of sclera**

    Excludes *blue sclera (743.47)*

    379.11 **Scleral ectasia**
        Scleral staphyloma NOS

    379.12 **Staphyloma posticum**

    379.13 **Equatorial staphyloma**

    379.14 **Anterior staphyloma, localized**

    379.15 **Ring staphyloma**

    379.16 **Other degenerative disorders of sclera**

    379.19 **Other**

● 379.2 **Disorders of vitreous body**

    379.21 **Vitreous degeneration**
        Vitreous:
            cavitation
            detachment
            liquefaction

    379.22 **Crystalline deposits in vitreous**
        Asteroid hyalitis
        Synchysis scintillans

    379.23 **Vitreous hemorrhage**
        Coding Clinic: 1991, Q3, P15-16

    379.24 **Other vitreous opacities**
        Vitreous floaters
        Small clumps of cells that float in vitreous of
         the eye, appearing as black specks or dots
         in field of vision.
        Coding Clinic: 1994, Q1, P16

    379.25 **Vitreous membranes and strands**

    379.26 **Vitreous prolapse**

    379.29 **Other disorders of vitreous**

        Excludes *vitreous abscess (360.04)*

        Coding Clinic: 1999, Q1, P11

● 379.3 **Aphakia and other disorders of lens**

    Excludes *after-cataract (366.50–366.53)*

    379.31 **Aphakia**

        Excludes *cataract extraction status (V45.61)*

    379.32 **Subluxation of lens**
        Coding Clinic: 1994, Q1, P16-17

    379.33 **Anterior dislocation of lens**

    379.34 **Posterior dislocation of lens**

    379.39 **Other disorders of lens**

● 379.4 **Anomalies of pupillary function**

    379.40 **Abnormal pupillary function, unspecified**

    379.41 **Anisocoria**

    379.42 **Miosis (persistent), not due to miotics**

    379.43 **Mydriasis (persistent), not due to mydriatics**

    379.45 **Argyll Robertson pupil, atypical**
        Argyll Robertson phenomenon or pupil,
          nonsyphilitic

        Excludes *Argyll Robertson pupil (syphilitic)*
          (094.89)

    379.46 **Tonic pupillary reaction**
        Adie's pupil or syndrome

    379.49 **Other**
        Hippus
        Pupillary paralysis

● 379.5 **Nystagmus and other irregular eye movements**
    Nystagmus is rapid, involuntary movements of eyes in
     horizontal or vertical direction.

    379.50 **Nystagmus, unspecified**
        Coding Clinic: 2002, Q4, P68; 2001, Q2, P21

    379.51 **Congenital nystagmus**

    379.52 **Latent nystagmus**

    379.53 **Visual deprivation nystagmus**

    379.54 **Nystagmus associated with disorders of the vestibular system**

    379.55 **Dissociated nystagmus**

    379.56 **Other forms of nystagmus**

    379.57 **Deficiencies of saccadic eye movements**
        Abnormal optokinetic response

    379.58 **Deficiencies of smooth pursuit movements**

    379.59 **Other irregularities of eye movements**
        Opsoclonus

DISEASES OF THE NERVOUS SYSTEM AND SENSE ORGANS (320–389)

● 379.6 **Inflammation (infection) of postprocedural bleb**
Postprocedural blebitis

379.60 **Inflammation (infection) of postprocedural bleb, unspecified**

379.61 **Inflammation (infection) of postprocedural bleb, stage 1**

379.62 **Inflammation (infection) of postprocedural bleb, stage 2**
Coding Clinic: 2006, Q4, P82-83

379.63 **Inflammation (infection) of postprocedural bleb, stage 3**
Bleb associated endophthalmitis

■ 379.8 **Other specified disorders of eye and adnexa**

● 379.9 **Unspecified disorder of eye and adnexa**

■ 379.90 **Disorder of eye, unspecified**

379.91 **Pain in or around eye**

379.92 **Swelling or mass of eye**

379.93 **Redness or discharge of eye**

■ 379.99 **Other ill-defined disorders of eye**

Excludes *blurred vision NOS (368.8)*

DISEASES OF THE EAR AND MASTOID PROCESS (380–389)

Use additional external cause code, if applicable, to identify the cause of the ear condition

● 380 **Disorders of external ear**

● 380.0 **Perichondritis and chondritis of pinna**
Chondritis of auricle
Perichondritis of auricle

■ 380.00 **Perichondritis of pinna, unspecified**

380.01 **Acute perichondritis of pinna**

380.02 **Chronic perichondritis of pinna**

380.03 **Chondritis of pinna**
Coding Clinic: 2004, Q4, P75-76

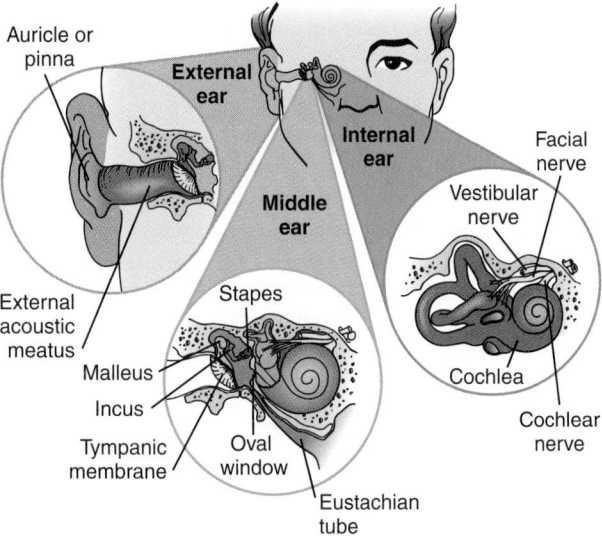

Auricle or pinna
External ear
Internal ear
Middle ear
Facial nerve
Vestibular nerve
External acoustic meatus
Stapes
Malleus
Incus
Tympanic membrane
Oval window
Eustachian tube
Cochlea
Cochlear nerve

● 380.1 **Infective otitis externa**

■ 380.10 **Infective otitis externa, unspecified**
Otitis externa (acute):
NOS
circumscribed
diffuse
hemorrhagica
infective NOS

380.11 **Acute infection of pinna**
Excludes *furuncular otitis externa (680.0)*

380.12 **Acute swimmers' ear**
Beach ear
Tank ear

● ■ 380.13 *Other acute infections of external ear*
Code first underlying disease, as:
erysipelas (035)
impetigo (684)
seborrheic dermatitis (690.10–690.18)
Excludes *herpes simplex (054.73)*
herpes zoster (053.71)

380.14 **Malignant otitis externa**

● 380.15 *Chronic mycotic otitis externa*
Code first underlying disease, as:
aspergillosis (117.3)
otomycosis NOS (111.9)
Excludes *candidal otitis externa (112.82)*

■ 380.16 **Other chronic infective otitis externa**
Chronic infective otitis externa NOS

● 380.2 **Other otitis externa**

380.21 **Cholesteatoma of external ear**
Keratosis obturans of external ear (canal)
Excludes *cholesteatoma NOS (385.30–385.35)*
postmastoidectomy (383.32)

■ 380.22 **Other acute otitis externa**
Acute otitis externa:
actinic
chemical
contact
eczematoid
reactive

■ 380.23 **Other chronic otitis externa**
Chronic otitis externa NOS

● 380.3 **Noninfectious disorders of pinna**

■ 380.30 **Disorder of pinna, unspecified**

380.31 **Hematoma of auricle or pinna**

380.32 **Acquired deformities of auricle or pinna**
Excludes *cauliflower ear (738.7)*
Coding Clinic: 2003, Q3, P12-13

■ 380.39 **Other**
Excludes *gouty tophi of ear (274.81)*

380.4 **Impacted cerumen**
Wax in ear

● 380.5 **Acquired stenosis of external ear canal**
Collapse of external ear canal

■ 380.50 **Acquired stenosis of external ear canal, unspecified as to cause**

380.51 **Secondary to trauma**

380.52 **Secondary to surgery**

380.53 **Secondary to inflammation**

Figure 6–17 Auditory system. (From Buck CJ: Step-by-Step Medical Coding, 2009 ed. Philadelphia, WB Saunders, 2009.)

◀ New   ◀▥ Revised   ~~deleted~~ Deleted   ● Use Additional Digit(s)   ■ Nonspecific Code

● Not first-listed DX   OGCR Official Guidelines   Coding Clinic   Excludes   Includes   Use additional   Code first   Omit code

● **380.8 Other disorders of external ear**

    380.81 Exostosis of external ear canal

    ■**380.89 Other**

■**380.9 Unspecified disorder of external ear**

● **381 Nonsuppurative otitis media and Eustachian tube disorders**
Nonsuppurative: not producing pus.

● **381.0 Acute nonsuppurative otitis media**
Acute tubotympanic catarrh
Otitis media, acute or subacute:
  catarrhal
  exudative
  transudative
  with effusion

    Excludes *otitic barotrauma (993.0)*

    ■**381.00 Acute nonsuppurative otitis media, unspecified**

    381.01 Acute serous otitis media
      Acute or subacute secretory otitis media

    381.02 Acute mucoid otitis media
      Acute or subacute seromucinous otitis media
      Blue drum syndrome

    381.03 Acute sanguinous otitis media

    381.04 Acute allergic serous otitis media

    381.05 Acute allergic mucoid otitis media

    381.06 Acute allergic sanguinous otitis media

● **381.1 Chronic serous otitis media**
Chronic tubotympanic catarrh

    381.10 Chronic serous otitis media, simple or unspecified

    ■**381.19 Other**
      Serosanguinous chronic otitis media

● **381.2 Chronic mucoid otitis media**
Glue ear

    Excludes *adhesive middle ear disease (385.10–385.19)*

    381.20 Chronic mucoid otitis media, simple or unspecified

    ■**381.29 Other**
      Mucosanguinous chronic otitis media

■**381.3 Other and unspecified chronic nonsuppurative otitis media**
Otitis media, chronic: Otitis media, chronic:
  allergic   seromucinous
  exudative   transudative
  secretory   with effusion

■**381.4 Nonsuppurative otitis media, not specified as acute or chronic**
Otitis media: Otitis media:
  allergic   seromucinous
  catarrhal   serous
  exudative   transudative
  mucoid   with effusion
  secretory

● **381.5 Eustachian salpingitis**

    ■**381.50 Eustachian salpingitis, unspecified**

    381.51 Acute Eustachian salpingitis

    381.52 Chronic Eustachian salpingitis

● **381.6 Obstruction of Eustachian tube**
Stenosis of Eustachian tube
Stricture of Eustachian tube

    ■**381.60 Obstruction of Eustachian tube, unspecified**

    381.61 Osseous obstruction of Eustachian tube
      Obstruction of Eustachian tube from cholesteatoma, polyp, or other osseous lesion

    381.62 Intrinsic cartilaginous obstruction of Eustachian tube

    381.63 Extrinsic cartilaginous obstruction of Eustachian tube
      Compression of Eustachian tube

  381.7 Patulous Eustachian tube

● **381.8 Other disorders of Eustachian tube**

    381.81 Dysfunction of Eustachian tube

    ■**381.89 Other**

■**381.9 Unspecified Eustachian tube disorder**

● **382 Suppurative and unspecified otitis media**

● **382.0 Acute suppurative otitis media**
Suppurative: Discharging pus
Otitis media, acute:
  necrotizing NOS
  purulent
  pus-filled

    382.00 Acute suppurative otitis media without spontaneous rupture of ear drum

    382.01 Acute suppurative otitis media with spontaneous rupture of ear drum

● ■**382.02 *Acute suppurative otitis media in diseases classified elsewhere***

    Code first underlying disease, as:
      influenza (487.8)
      scarlet fever (034.1)

    Excludes *postmeasles otitis (055.2)*

  382.1 Chronic tubotympanic suppurative otitis media
Benign chronic suppurative otitis media (with anterior perforation of ear drum)
Chronic tubotympanic disease (with anterior perforation of ear drum)

  382.2 Chronic atticoantral suppurative otitis media
Chronic atticoantral disease (with posterior or superior marginal perforation of ear drum)
Persistent mucosal disease (with posterior or superior marginal perforation of ear drum)

■**382.3 Unspecified chronic suppurative otitis media**
Chronic purulent otitis media

    Excludes *tuberculous otitis media (017.4)*

■**382.4 Unspecified suppurative otitis media**
Purulent otitis media NOS

■**382.9 Unspecified otitis media**
Otitis media:
  NOS
  acute NOS
  chronic NOS

Item 6-25 Mastoiditis is an infection of the portion of the temporal bone of the skull that is behind the ear (mastoid process) caused by an untreated otitis media, leading to an infection of the surrounding structures which may include the brain.

● **383 Mastoiditis and related conditions**

  ● **383.0 Acute mastoiditis**
      Abscess of mastoid
      Empyema of mastoid

    383.00 Acute mastoiditis without complications

    383.01 Subperiosteal abscess of mastoid

    ■ **383.02 Acute mastoiditis with other complications**
        Gradenigo's syndrome

  383.1 Chronic mastoiditis
      Caries of mastoid
      Fistula of mastoid

    Excludes *tuberculous mastoiditis (015.6)*

  ● **383.2 Petrositis**
      Coalescing osteitis of petrous bone
      Inflammation of petrous bone
      Osteomyelitis of petrous bone

    ■ **383.20 Petrositis, unspecified**

    383.21 Acute petrositis

    383.22 Chronic petrositis

  ● **383.3 Complications following mastoidectomy**

    ■ **383.30 Postmastoidectomy complication, unspecified**

    383.31 Mucosal cyst of postmastoidectomy cavity

    383.32 Recurrent cholesteatoma of postmastoidectomy cavity

    383.33 Granulations of postmastoidectomy cavity
        Chronic inflammation of
          postmastoidectomy cavity

  ● **383.8 Other disorders of mastoid**

    383.81 Postauricular fistula

    ■ **383.89 Other**

  ■ **383.9 Unspecified mastoiditis**

● **384 Other disorders of tympanic membrane**

  ● **384.0 Acute myringitis without mention of otitis media**

    ■ **384.00 Acute myringitis, unspecified**
        Acute tympanitis NOS

    384.01 Bullous myringitis
        Myringitis bullosa hemorrhagica

    ■ **384.09 Other**

  384.1 Chronic myringitis without mention of otitis media
      Chronic tympanitis

  ● **384.2 Perforation of tympanic membrane**
      Perforation of ear drum:
        NOS
        persistent posttraumatic
        postinflammatory

    Excludes *otitis media with perforation of tympanic membrane (382.00–382.9)*
        traumatic perforation [current injury] (872.61)

    ■ **384.20 Perforation of tympanic membrane, unspecified**

    384.21 Central perforation of tympanic membrane

    384.22 Attic perforation of tympanic membrane
        Pars flaccida

    ■ **384.23 Other marginal perforation of tympanic membrane**

    384.24 Multiple perforations of tympanic membrane

    384.25 Total perforation of tympanic membrane

● **384.8 Other specified disorders of tympanic membrane**

    384.81 Atrophic flaccid tympanic membrane
        Healed perforation of ear drum

    384.82 Atrophic nonflaccid tympanic membrane

  ■ **384.9 Unspecified disorder of tympanic membrane**

● **385 Other disorders of middle ear and mastoid**

    Excludes *mastoiditis (383.0–383.9)*

  ● **385.0 Tympanosclerosis**

    ■ **385.00 Tympanosclerosis, unspecified as to involvement**

    385.01 Tympanosclerosis involving tympanic membrane only

    385.02 Tympanosclerosis involving tympanic membrane and ear ossicles

    385.03 Tympanosclerosis involving tympanic membrane, ear ossicles, and middle ear

    ■ **385.09 Tympanosclerosis involving other combination of structures**

  ● **385.1 Adhesive middle ear disease**
      Adhesive otitis
      Otitis media: Otitis media:
        chronic adhesive   fibrotic

    Excludes *glue ear (381.20–381.29)*

    ■ **385.10 Adhesive middle ear disease, unspecified as to involvement**

    385.11 Adhesions of drum head to incus

    385.12 Adhesions of drum head to stapes

    385.13 Adhesions of drum head to promontorium

    ■ **385.19 Other adhesions and combinations**

  ● **385.2 Other acquired abnormality of ear ossicles**

    385.21 Impaired mobility of malleus
        Ankylosis of malleus

    ■ **385.22 Impaired mobility of other ear ossicles**
        Ankylosis of ear ossicles, except malleus

    385.23 Discontinuity or dislocation of ear ossicles

    385.24 Partial loss or necrosis of ear ossicles

  ● **385.3 Cholesteatoma of middle ear and mastoid**
      Cholesterosis of (middle) ear
      Epidermosis of (middle) ear
      Keratosis of (middle) ear
      Polyp of (middle) ear

    Excludes *cholesteatoma:*
        external ear canal (380.21)
        recurrent of postmastoidectomy cavity (383.32)

    ■ **385.30 Cholesteatoma, unspecified**

    385.31 Cholesteatoma of attic

    385.32 Cholesteatoma of middle ear

    385.33 Cholesteatoma of middle ear and mastoid
        Coding Clinic: 2000, Q3, P10-11

    385.35 Diffuse cholesteatosis

  ● **385.8 Other disorders of middle ear and mastoid**

    385.82 Cholesterin granuloma

    385.83 Retained foreign body of middle ear
        Coding Clinic: 1987, Nov-Dec, P9

    ■ **385.89 Other**

  ■ **385.9 Unspecified disorder of middle ear and mastoid**

◄ New   ◄▥ Revised   ~~deleted~~ Deleted   ● Use Additional Digit(s)   ■ Nonspecific Code

● Not first-listed DX   OGCR Official Guidelines   Coding Clinic   Excludes   Includes   Use additional   Code first   Omit code

● 386 **Vertiginous syndromes and other disorders of vestibular system**

> **Excludes** *vertigo NOS (780.4)*
>
> Coding Clinic: 1985, Mar-April, P12

● 386.0 **Méniére's disease**
> *Vestibular disorder that produces recurring symptoms including severe and intermittent hearing loss including feeling of ear pressure or pain.*
>
> Endolymphatic hydrops
> Lermoyez's syndrome
> Méniére's syndrome or vertigo

■ 386.00 **Méniére's disease, unspecified**
> Méniére's disease (active)
> Coding Clinic: 1985, Mar-April, P12

386.01 **Active Méniére's disease, cochleovestibular**

386.02 **Active Méniére's disease, cochlear**

386.03 **Active Méniére's disease, vestibular**

386.04 **Inactive Méniére's disease**
> Méniére's disease in remission

● 386.1 **Other and unspecified peripheral vertigo**

> **Excludes** *epidemic vertigo (078.81)*

■ 386.10 **Peripheral vertigo, unspecified**

386.11 **Benign paroxysmal positional vertigo**
> Benign paroxysmal positional nystagmus

386.12 **Vestibular neuronitis**
> Acute (and recurrent) peripheral vestibulopathy

■ 386.19 **Other**
> Aural vertigo   Otogenic vertigo

386.2 **Vertigo of central origin**
> Central positional nystagmus
> Malignant positional vertigo

● 386.3 **Labyrinthitis**
> *Balance disorder that follows a URI or head injury. The inflammatory process affects the labyrinth that houses vestibular system (senses changes in head position) of inner ear.*

■ 386.30 **Labyrinthitis, unspecified**

386.31 **Serous labyrinthitis**
> Diffuse labyrinthitis

386.32 **Circumscribed labyrinthitis**
> Focal labyrinthitis

386.33 **Suppurative labyrinthitis**
> Purulent labyrinthitis

386.34 **Toxic labyrinthitis**

386.35 **Viral labyrinthitis**

● 386.4 **Labyrinthine fistula**

■ 386.40 **Labyrinthine fistula, unspecified**

386.41 **Round window fistula**

386.42 **Oval window fistula**

386.43 **Semicircular canal fistula**

386.48 **Labyrinthine fistula of combined sites**

● 386.5 **Labyrinthine dysfunction**

■ 386.50 **Labyrinthine dysfunction, unspecified**

386.51 **Hyperactive labyrinth, unilateral**

386.52 **Hyperactive labyrinth, bilateral**

386.53 **Hypoactive labyrinth, unilateral**

386.54 **Hypoactive labyrinth, bilateral**

386.55 **Loss of labyrinthine reactivity, unilateral**

386.56 **Loss of labyrinthine reactivity, bilateral**

■ 386.58 **Other forms and combinations**

■ 386.8 **Other disorders of labyrinth**

■ 386.9 **Unspecified vertiginous syndromes and labyrinthine disorders**

● 387 **Otosclerosis**
> *Inherited middle ear spongelike bone growth causing hearing loss because growth prevents vibration from sound waves required for hearing.*

> **Includes** otospongiosis

387.0 **Otosclerosis involving oval window, nonobliterative**

387.1 **Otosclerosis involving oval window, obliterative**

387.2 **Cochlear otosclerosis**
> Otosclerosis involving:
> otic capsule
> round window

■ 387.8 **Other otosclerosis**

■ 387.9 **Otosclerosis, unspecified**

● 388 **Other disorders of ear**

● 388.0 **Degenerative and vascular disorders of ear**

■ 388.00 **Degenerative and vascular disorders, unspecified**

388.01 **Presbyacusis**

388.02 **Transient ischemic deafness**

● 388.1 **Noise effects on inner ear**

■ 388.10 **Noise effects on inner ear, unspecified**

388.11 **Acoustic trauma (explosive) to ear**
> Otitic blast injury

388.12 **Noise-induced hearing loss**

■ 388.2 **Sudden hearing loss, unspecified**

● 388.3 **Tinnitus**
> *Perception of sound in absence of external noise and may affect one or both ears and/or head*

■ 388.30 **Tinnitus, unspecified**

388.31 **Subjective tinnitus**

388.32 **Objective tinnitus**

● 388.4 **Other abnormal auditory perception**

■ 388.40 **Abnormal auditory perception, unspecified**

388.41 **Diplacusis**

388.42 **Hyperacusis**

388.43 **Impairment of auditory discrimination**

388.44 **Recruitment**

388.45 **Acquired auditory processing disorder**
> Auditory processing disorder NOS

> **Excludes** *central auditory processing disorder (315.32)*
>
> Coding Clinic: 2007, Q4, P79

388.5 **Disorders of acoustic nerve**
> Acoustic neuritis
> Degeneration of acoustic or eighth nerve
> Disorder of acoustic or eighth nerve

> **Excludes** *acoustic neuroma (225.1)*
> *syphilitic acoustic neuritis (094.86)*
>
> Coding Clinic: 1987, Mar-April, P8

DISEASES OF THE NERVOUS SYSTEM AND SENSE ORGANS (320–389)

● **388.6 Otorrhea**

◼ **388.60 Otorrhea, unspecified**
Discharging ear NOS

388.61 Cerebrospinal fluid otorrhea

Excludes *cerebrospinal fluid rhinorrhea (349.81)*

◼ **388.69 Other**
Otorrhagia

● **388.7 Otalgia**

◼ **388.70 Otalgia, unspecified**
Earache NOS

388.71 Otogenic pain

388.72 Referred pain
Pain from a diseased area of the body that is not felt directly in that area, but in another part of the body.

◼ **388.8 Other disorders of ear**

◼ **388.9 Unspecified disorder of ear**

● **389 Hearing loss**

● **389.0 Conductive hearing loss**
Conductive deafness

Excludes *mixed conductive and sensorineural hearing loss (389.20–389.22)*

◼ **389.00 Conductive hearing loss, unspecified**

389.01 Conductive hearing loss, external ear

389.02 Conductive hearing loss, tympanic membrane

389.03 Conductive hearing loss, middle ear

389.04 Conductive hearing loss, inner ear

389.05 Conductive hearing loss, unilateral

389.06 Conductive hearing loss, bilateral
Coding Clinic: 2007, Q4, P80-81

389.08 Conductive hearing loss of combined types

● **389.1 Sensorineural hearing loss**
Perceptive hearing loss or deafness

Excludes *abnormal auditory perception (388.40–388.44)*
mixed conductive and sensorineural hearing loss (389.20–389.22)
psychogenic deafness (306.7)
Coding Clinic: 2007, Q4, P80-81; 2006, Q4, P84

◼ **389.10 Sensorineural hearing loss, unspecified**
Coding Clinic: 1993, Q1, P29

389.11 Sensory hearing loss, bilateral

389.12 Neural hearing loss, bilateral

389.13 Neural hearing loss, unilateral

389.14 Central hearing loss

389.15 Sensorineural hearing loss, unilateral

389.16 Sensorineural hearing loss, asymmetrical

389.17 Sensory hearing loss, unilateral

389.18 Sensorineural hearing loss, bilateral

● **389.2 Mixed conductive and sensorineural hearing loss**
Deafness or hearing loss of type classifiable to 389.00–389.08 with type classifiable to 389.10–389.18
Coding Clinic: 2007, Q4, P80-81

389.20 Mixed hearing loss, unspecified

389.21 Mixed hearing loss, unilateral

389.22 Mixed hearing loss, bilateral

389.7 Deaf nonspeaking, not elsewhere classifiable

◼ **389.8 Other specified forms of hearing loss**

◼ **389.9 Unspecified hearing loss**
Deafness NOS
Coding Clinic: 2004, Q1, P15-16

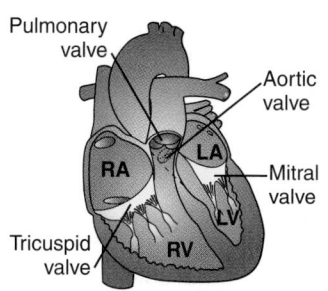

Figure 7-1 Cardiovascular valves.

> **Item 7-1 Rheumatic fever** is the inflammation of the valve(s) of the heart, usually the mitral or aortic, which leads to valve damage. Rheumatic heart inflammations are usually **pericarditis** (sac surrounding heart), **endocarditis** (heart cavity), or **myocarditis** (heart muscle).

7. DISEASES OF THE CIRCULATORY SYSTEM (390–459)

ACUTE RHEUMATIC FEVER (390–392)

390 Rheumatic fever without mention of heart involvement
Arthritis, rheumatic, acute or subacute
Rheumatic fever (active) (acute)
Rheumatism, articular, acute or subacute

> **Excludes** *that with heart involvement (391.0–391.9)*

● **391 Rheumatic fever with heart involvement**

> **Excludes** *chronic heart diseases of rheumatic origin (393–398.99) unless rheumatic fever is also present or there is evidence of recrudescence or activity of the rheumatic process*

391.0 Acute rheumatic pericarditis
Rheumatic:
    fever (active) (acute) with pericarditis
    pericarditis (acute)
Any condition classifiable to 390 with pericarditis

> **Excludes** *that not specified as rheumatic (420.0–420.9)*

391.1 Acute rheumatic endocarditis
Rheumatic:
    endocarditis, acute
    fever (active) (acute) with endocarditis or valvulitis
    valvulitis acute
Any condition classifiable to 390 with endocarditis or valvulitis

391.2 Acute rheumatic myocarditis
Rheumatic fever (active) (acute) with myocarditis
Any condition classifiable to 390 with myocarditis

■ **391.8 Other acute rheumatic heart disease**
Rheumatic:
    fever (active) (acute) with other or multiple types of heart involvement
    pancarditis, acute
Any condition classifiable to 390 with other or multiple types of heart involvement

■ **391.9 Acute rheumatic heart disease, unspecified**
Rheumatic:
    carditis, acute
    fever (active) (acute) with unspecified type of heart involvement
    heart disease, active or acute
Any condition classifiable to 390 with unspecified type of heart involvement

> **Item 7-2 Rheumatic chorea,** also called Sydenham's, juvenile, minor, simple, or St. Vitus' dance, is a major symptom of rheumatic fever and is characterized by ceaseless, involuntary, jerky, purposeless movements.

● **392 Rheumatic chorea**

> **Includes** Sydenham's chorea

> **Excludes** *chorea:*
>   *NOS (333.5)*
>   *Huntington's (333.4)*

392.0 With heart involvement
Rheumatic chorea with heart involvement of any type classifiable to 391

392.9 Without mention of heart involvement

CHRONIC RHEUMATIC HEART DISEASE (393–398)

393 Chronic rheumatic pericarditis
Adherent pericardium, rheumatic
Chronic rheumatic:
    mediastinopericarditis
    myopericarditis

> **Excludes** *pericarditis NOS or not specified as rheumatic (423.0–423.9)*

> **Item 7-3 Mitral stenosis** is the narrowing of the mitral valve separating the left atrium from the left ventricle. **Mitral insufficiency** is the improper closure of the mitral valve which may lead to enlargement (hypertrophy) of the left atrium.

● **394 Diseases of mitral valve**

> **Excludes** *that with aortic valve involvement (396.0–396.9)*

394.0 Mitral stenosis
Mitral (valve):
    obstruction (rheumatic)
    stenosis NOS

394.1 Rheumatic mitral insufficiency
Rheumatic mitral:
    incompetence
    regurgitation

> **Excludes** *that not specified as rheumatic (424.0)*

Coding Clinic: 2005, Q2, P14-15

394.2 Mitral stenosis with insufficiency
Mitral stenosis with incompetence or regurgitation
Coding Clinic: 2007, Q2, P11-12

■ **394.9 Other and unspecified mitral valve diseases**
Mitral (valve):
    disease (chronic)
    failure

Item 7-4 Aortic stenosis is the narrowing of the aortic valve located between the left ventricle and the aorta. **Aortic insufficiency** is the improper closure of the aortic valve which may lead to enlargement (hypertrophy) of the left ventricle.

● **395 Diseases of aortic valve**

> **Excludes** *that not specified as rheumatic (424.1)*
> *that with mitral valve involvement (396.0–396.9)*

395.0 Rheumatic aortic stenosis
Rheumatic aortic (valve) obstruction
Coding Clinic: 1988, Q4, P8

395.1 Rheumatic aortic insufficiency
Rheumatic aortic:
incompetence
regurgitation

395.2 Rheumatic aortic stenosis with insufficiency
Rheumatic aortic stenosis with incompetence or regurgitation

■ **395.9 Other and unspecified rheumatic aortic diseases**
Rheumatic aortic (valve) disease

Item 7-5 Mitral and aortic valve stenosis is the narrowing of these valves, which leads to enlargement (hypertrophy) of the left atrium and left ventricle respectively, while **mitral and aortic insufficiency** is the improper closure of the mitral and aortic valves resulting in the same outcome as stenosis.

● **396 Diseases of mitral and aortic valves**

> **Includes** involvement of both mitral and aortic valves, whether specified as rheumatic or not

396.0 Mitral valve stenosis and aortic valve stenosis
Atypical aortic (valve) stenosis
Mitral and aortic (valve) obstruction (rheumatic)

396.1 Mitral valve stenosis and aortic valve insufficiency

396.2 Mitral valve insufficiency and aortic valve stenosis
Coding Clinic: 2009, Q2, P11; 2000, Q2, P16-17; 1987, Nov-Dec, P8

396.3 Mitral valve insufficiency and aortic valve insufficiency
Mitral and aortic (valve):
incompetence
regurgitation
Coding Clinic: 2009, Q2, P11; Q1, P8; 1995, Q1, P6

396.8 Multiple involvement of mitral and aortic valves
Stenosis and insufficiency of mitral or aortic valve with stenosis or insufficiency, or both, of the other valve

■ **396.9 Mitral and aortic valve diseases, unspecified**

● **397 Diseases of other endocardial structures**
Affects thin serous endothelial tissue that lines inside of heart

397.0 Diseases of tricuspid valve
Tricuspid (valve) (rheumatic):
disease
insufficiency
obstruction
regurgitation
stenosis
Coding Clinic: 2006, Q3, P7; 2000, Q2, P16-17

397.1 Rheumatic diseases of pulmonary valve

> **Excludes** *that not specified as rheumatic (424.3)*

■ **397.9 Rheumatic diseases of endocardium, valve unspecified**
Rheumatic:
endocarditis (chronic)
valvulitis (chronic)

> **Excludes** *that not specified as rheumatic*
> *(424.90–424.99)*

● **398 Other rheumatic heart disease**

398.0 Rheumatic myocarditis
Rheumatic degeneration of myocardium

> **Excludes** *myocarditis not specified as rheumatic*
> *(429.0)*

● **398.9 Other and unspecified rheumatic heart diseases**

■ **398.90 Rheumatic heart disease, unspecified**
Rheumatic:
carditis
heart disease NOS

> **Excludes** *carditis not specified as rheumatic*
> *(429.89)*
> *heart disease NOS not specified as*
> *rheumatic (429.9)*

398.91 Rheumatic heart failure (congestive)
Rheumatic left ventricular failure
Coding Clinic: 2005, Q2, P14-15; 1995, Q1, P6

■ **398.99 Other**

Item 7-6 Hypertension is caused by high arterial blood pressure in the arteries. **Essential, primary,** or **idiopathic** hypertension occurs without identifiable organic cause.
Secondary hypertension is that which has an organic cause.
Malignant hypertension is severely elevated blood pressure.
Benign hypertension is mildly elevated blood pressure.

HYPERTENSIVE DISEASE (401–405)

> **Excludes** *that complicating pregnancy, childbirth, or the*
> *puerperium (642.0–642.9)*
> *that involving coronary vessels (410.00–414.9)*

● **401 Essential hypertension**

> **Includes** high blood pressure
> hyperpiesia
> hyperpiesis
> hypertension (arterial) (essential) (primary)
> (systemic)
> hypertensive vascular:
> degeneration
> disease

> **Excludes** *elevated blood pressure without diagnosis of*
> *hypertension (796.2)*
> *pulmonary hypertension (416.0–416.9)*
> *that involving vessels of:*
> *brain (430–438)*
> *eye (362.11)*

Coding Clinic: 1992, Q2, P5

401.0 Malignant
Coding Clinic: 1993, Q4, P37; 5th Issue, P9-10

401.1 Benign

■ **401.9 Unspecified**
Coding Clinic: 2009, Q1, P6; 2008, Q2, P16; 2005, Q4, P68-69; Q3, P3-9; 2004, Q4, P77-78; 2003, Q4, P105-106,108, 111; Q3, P14-15; Q2, P16; 1997, Q4, P35-37; 1989, Q2, P12; 1987, Sept-Oct, P11

◀ New   ◀▥ Revised   ~~deleted~~ Deleted   ● Use Additional Digit(s)   ■ Nonspecific Code

● Not first-listed DX   OGCR Official Guidelines   Coding Clinic   Excludes   Includes   Use additional   Code first   Omit code

OGCR Section I.C.7.a.2

Heart conditions (425.8, 429.0–429.3, 429.8, 429.9) are assigned to a code from category 402 when a causal relationship is stated (due to hypertension) or implied (hypertensive). Use an additional code from category 428 to identify the type of heart failure in those patients with heart failure. More than one code from category 428 may be assigned if the patient has systolic or diastolic failure and congestive heart failure. The same heart conditions (425.8, 429.0–429.3, 429.8, 429.9) with hypertension, but without a stated causal relationship, are coded separately. Sequence according to the circumstances of the admission/ encounter.

● **402 Hypertensive heart disease**

Includes   hypertensive:
  cardiomegaly
  cardiopathy
  cardiovascular disease
  heart (disease) (failure)
  any condition classifiable to 429.0–429.3, 429.8, 429.9 due to hypertension

Use additional code to specify type of heart failure (428.0–428.43), if known
Coding Clinic: 1993, Q2, P9; 1987, Nov-Dec, P9

● **402.0 Malignant**

  402.00 Without heart failure
    Coding Clinic: 2008, Q4, P177-180

  ■**402.01 With heart failure**

● **402.1 Benign**

  402.10 Without heart failure

  402.11 With heart failure

● **402.9 Unspecified**
  Coding Clinic: 1993, Q2, P9

  ■**402.90 Without heart failure**

  ■**402.91 With heart failure**
    Coding Clinic: 2002, Q4, P52; 1993, Q1, P19-20; 1989, Q2, P12; 1984, Nov-Dec, P18

OGCR Section I.C.7.a.3

Assign codes from category 403, Hypertensive kidney disease, when conditions classified to categories 585–587 are present. Unlike hypertension with heart disease, ICD-9-CM presumes a cause-and-effect relationship and classifies renal failure with hypertension as hypertensive kidney disease.

● **403 Hypertensive chronic kidney disease**

Includes   arteriolar nephritis
  arteriosclerosis of:
    kidney
    renal arterioles
  arteriosclerotic nephritis (chronic) (interstitial)
  hypertensive:
    nephropathy
    renal failure
    uremia (chronic)
  nephrosclerosis
  renal sclerosis with hypertension
  any condition classifiable to 585 with any condition classifiable to 401

Excludes   *acute renal kidney failure (584.5–584.9)* ◀▥
  renal disease stated as not due to hypertension
  renovascular hypertension (405.0–405.9 with fifth-digit 1)
Coding Clinic: 2003, Q1, P20-21; 1992, Q2, P5

The following fifth-digit subclassification is for use with category 403:

> **0 with chronic kidney disease stage I through stage IV, or unspecified**
> Use additional code to identify the stage of chronic kidney disease (585.1–585.4, 585.9)
>
> **1 with chronic kidney disease stage V or end stage renal disease**
> Use additional code to identify the stage of chronic kidney disease (585.5, 585.6)

● **403.0 Malignant**
  [0-1]

● **403.1 Benign**
  [0-1]

●■**403.9 Unspecified**
  [0-1]   Coding Clinic: 2008, Q1, P7-8, 10-11; 2007, Q2, P3; 2006, Q4, P84-86; 2005, Q4, P68-69; 2004, Q1, P14-15; 2001, Q2, P11; 1987, Sept-Oct, P9, 11; 1985, Nov-Dec, P15

OGCR Section I.C.7.a.4

Assign codes from combination category 404 when both hypertensive kidney disease and hypertensive heart disease are stated in the diagnosis. Assume a relationship between the hypertension and the kidney disease, whether or not the condition is so designated. Assign an additional code from category 428, to identify the type of heart failure. More than one code from category 428 may be assigned if the patient has systolic or diastolic failure and congestive heart failure.

● **404 Hypertensive heart and chronic kidney disease**

Includes   disease:
  cardiorenal
  cardiovascular renal
  any condition classifiable to 402 with any condition classifiable to 403

Use additional code to specify type of heart failure (428.0–428.43), if known
Coding Clinic: 2006, Q4, P84-86; 2005, Q4, P68-69

The following fifth-digit subclassification is for use with category 404:

> **0 without heart failure and with chronic kidney disease stage I through stage IV, or unspecified**
> Use additional code to identify the stage of chronic kidney disease (585.1–585.4, 585.9)
>
> **1 with heart failure and with chronic kidney disease stage I through stage IV, or unspecified**
> Use additional code to identify the stage of chronic kidney disease (585.1–585.4, 585.9)
>
> **2 without heart failure and with chronic kidney disease stage V or end stage renal disease**
> Use additional code to identify the stage of chronic kidney disease (585.5, 585.6)
>
> **3 with heart failure and chronic kidney disease stage V or end stage renal disease**
> Use additional code to identify the stage of chronic kidney disease (585.5, 585.6)

● **404.0 Malignant**
  [0-3]

● **404.1 Benign**
  [0-3]

●■**404.9 Unspecified**
  [0-3]

DISEASES OF THE CIRCULATORY SYSTEM (390–459)

● 405 Secondary hypertension

  ● 405.0 Malignant

         405.01 Renovascular

      ■ 405.09 Other

  ● 405.1 Benign

         405.11 Renovascular

      ■ 405.19 Other

  ● 405.9 Unspecified

      ■ 405.91 Renovascular

      ■ 405.99 Other
                  Coding Clinic: 2000, Q3, P4-5; 1987, Sept-Oct, P9, 11

OGCR Section I.C.7.e.1

The codes for acute myocardial infarction (AMI) identify
the site, such as anterolateral wall or true posterior wall.
Subcategories 410.0-410.6 and 410.8 are used for ST
elevation myocardial infarction (STEMI).

ISCHEMIC HEART DISEASE (410–414)

Includes   that with mention of hypertension

Use additional code to identify presence of hypertension
    (401.0–405.9)

● 410 Acute myocardial infarction

  Includes   cardiac infarction
             coronary (artery):
                 embolism
                 occlusion
                 rupture
                 thrombosis
             infarction of heart, myocardium, or ventricle
             rupture of heart, myocardium, or ventricle
             ST elevation (STEMI) and non-ST elevation
                 (NSTEMI) myocardial infarction
             any condition classifiable to 414.1–414.9
                 specified as acute or with a stated
                 duration of 8 weeks or less
     Coding Clinic: 2006, Q2, P9; 1997, Q4, P37; 1994, Q4, P55; 1993, Q4,
        P39-41; 1992, Q1, P10; 1991, Q3, P18; 1986, Nov-Dec, P12

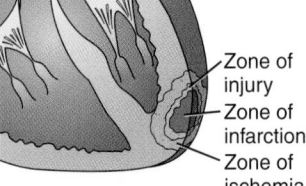

Figure 7–2 Myocardial infarction.

Zone of injury
Zone of infarction
Zone of ischemia

Item 7–7   Myocardial infarction is a sudden decrease in
the coronary artery blood flow that results in death of the heart
muscle. Classifications are based on the affected heart tissue.

The following fifth-digit subclassification is for use with
category 410:

■ 0   episode of care unspecified
      Use when the source document does not contain
      sufficient information for the assignment of
      fifth-digit 1 or 2.
  1   initial episode of care
      Use fifth-digit 1 to designate the first episode of
      care (regardless of facility site) for a newly
      diagnosed myocardial infarction. The
      fifth-digit 1 is assigned regardless of the
      number of times a patient may be transferred
      during the initial episode of care.
  2   subsequent episode of care
      Use fifth-digit 2 to designate an episode of care
      following the initial episode when the patient
      is admitted for further observation, evaluation
      or treatment for a myocardial infarction that
      has received initial treatment, but is still less
      than 8 weeks old.

● 410.0 Of anterolateral wall
  [0-2]   ST elevation myocardial infarction (STEMI) of
          anterolateral wall
      Coding Clinic: 2008, Q4, P69-73; 2001, Q3, P21; 1998, Q3, P15;
         1993, 5th Issue, P14, 17-24

● ■ 410.1 Of other anterior wall
  [0-2]   Infarction:
              anterior (wall) NOS (with contiguous portion of
                  intraventricular septum)
              anteroapical (with contiguous portion of
                  intraventricular septum)
              anteroseptal (with contiguous portion of
                  intraventricular septum)
          ST elevation myocardial infarction (STEMI) of other
              anterior wall
      Coding Clinic: 2003, Q3, P10-11

● 410.2 Of inferolateral wall
  [0-2]   ST elevation myocardial infarction (STEMI) of
          inferolateral wall
      Coding Clinic: 1993, 5th Issue, P17-24

● 410.3 Of inferoposterior wall
  [0-2]   ST elevation myocardial infarction (STEMI) of
          inferoposterior wall

● ■ 410.4 Of other inferior wall
  [0-2]   Infarction:
              diaphragmatic wall NOS (with contiguous
                  portion of intraventricular septum)
              inferior (wall) NOS (with contiguous portion of
                  intraventricular septum)
          ST elevation myocardial infarction (STEMI) of other
              inferior wall
      Coding Clinic: 2006, Q3, P8-9; 2001, Q2, P8-9; 2000, Q1, P7; 1997,
         Q3, P10; 1993, 5th Issue, P13-14x2

DISEASES OF THE CIRCULATORY SYSTEM (390–459)

◄ New   ◀▥ Revised   ~~deleted~~ Deleted   ● Use Additional Digit(s)   ■ Nonspecific Code

● Not first-listed DX   OGCR Official Guidelines   Coding Clinic   Excludes   Includes   Use additional   Code first   Omit code

● ■ **410.5 Of other lateral wall**
[0-2]   Infarction:
        apical-lateral
        basal-lateral
        high lateral
        posterolateral
    ST elevation myocardial infarction (STEMI) of other lateral wall

● **410.6 True posterior wall infarction**
[0-2]   Infarction:
        posterobasal
        strictly posterior
    ST elevation myocardial infarction (STEMI) of true posterior wall

● **410.7 Subendocardial infarction**
[0-2]   Non-ST elevation myocardial infarction (NSTEMI)
    Nontransmural infarction
    Coding Clinic: 2005, Q4, P69-72; Q2, P19-20; 2000, Q1, P7

    OGCR Section I.C.7.e.1
    The ICD-9-CM codes for acute myocardial infarction (AMI) identify the site, such as anterolateral wall or true posterior wall. Subcategories 410.0-410.6 and 410.8 are used for ST elevation myocardial infarction (STEMI). Subcategory 410.7, Subendocardial infarction, is used for non ST elevation myocardial infarction (NSTEMI) and nontransmural MIs.

● ■ **410.8 Of other specified sites**
[0-2]   Infarction of:
        atrium
        papillary muscle
        septum alone
    ST elevation myocardial infarction (STEMI) of other specified sites

● ■ **410.9 Unspecified site**
[0-2]   Acute myocardial infarction NOS
    Coronary occlusion NOS
    Myocardial infarction NOS
    Coding Clinic: 2005, Q2, P18-19; 2002, Q3, P5; 1999, Q4, P9; 1993, 5th Issue, P13

    OGCR Section I.C.7.e.2
    Subcategory 410.9 is the default for the unspecified term acute myocardial infarction. If only STEMI or transmural MI without the site is documented, query the provider as to the site, or assign a code from subcategory 410.9.

● **411 Other acute and subacute forms of ischemic heart disease**
    Coding Clinic: 1994, Q4, P55

411.0 Postmyocardial infarction syndrome
    Dressler's syndrome

411.1 Intermediate coronary syndrome
    Impending infarction
    Preinfarction angina
    Preinfarction syndrome
    Unstable angina

    Excludes *angina (pectoris) (413.9)*
                  decubitus (413.0)
    Coding Clinic: 2005, Q4, P103-106; 2004, Q2, P3-4; 2003, Q1, P12-13; 2001, Q3, P15; Q2, P7-9; 1998, Q4, P85-86; 1996, Q2, P10; 1995, Q2, P18-19; 1993, Q4, P39-40; 5th Issue, P17-24; 1991, Q1, P14; 1989, Q4, P10

● **411.8 Other**

411.81 Acute coronary occlusion without myocardial infarction
    Acute coronary (artery):
        embolism without or not resulting in myocardial infarction
        obstruction without or not resulting in myocardial infarction
        occlusion without or not resulting in myocardial infarction
        thrombosis without or not resulting in myocardial infarction

    Excludes *obstruction without infarction due to atherosclerosis (414.00–414.07)*
               occlusion without infarction due to atherosclerosis (414.00–414.07)
    Coding Clinic: 2001, Q2, P7-8; 1991, Q3, P18; Q1, P14

■ **411.89 Other**
    Coronary insufficiency (acute)
    Subendocardial ischemia
    Coding Clinic: 2001, Q3, P14; 1992, Q1, P9-10; 1991, Q3, P18

Item 7-8 "Old" (healed) myocardial infarction: Code 412 cannot be used if the patient is experiencing current ischemic heart disease symptoms. Recent infarctions still under care cannot be coded to 412. This code is only assigned if infarction has some impact on the current episode of care—essentially, it is a history of (H/O) a past, healed MI. (There is no V code for this status/post MI.)

412 Old myocardial infarction
    Healed myocardial infarction
    Past myocardial infarction diagnosed on ECG [EKG] or other special investigation, but currently presenting no symptoms
    Coding Clinic: 2003, Q2, P10; 2001, Q3, P21; Q2, P9; 1998, Q3, P15; 1993, 5th Issue, P17-24

● **413 Angina pectoris**
    Chest pain/discomfort due to lack of oxygen to heart muscle. Principal symptom of myocardial infarction.

413.0 Angina decubitus
    Nocturnal angina

413.1 Prinzmetal angina
    Variant angina pectoris
    Coding Clinic: 2006, Q3, P23

■ **413.9 Other and unspecified angina pectoris**
    Angina:
        NOS
        cardiac
        equivalent
        of effort
    Anginal syndrome
    Status anginosus
    Stenocardia
    Syncope anginosa

    Excludes *preinfarction angina (411.1)*

    Use additional code(s) for symptoms associated with angina equivalent
    Coding Clinic: 2008, Q2, P16, 2003, Q1, P12-13; 2002, Q3, P4-5; 1995, Q2, P18; 1993, 5th Issue, P17-24; 1991, Q3, P16; 1985, Sept-Oct, P9

DISEASES OF THE CIRCULATORY SYSTEM (390–459)

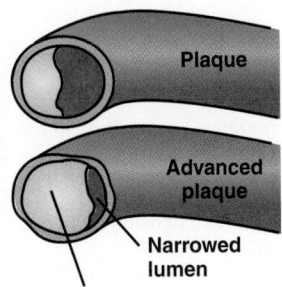

Plaque

Advanced plaque

Narrowed lumen

Atherosclerosis

Figure 7–3 Atherosclerosis. (From Buck CJ: Step-by-Step Medical Coding, 2008 ed. Philadelphia, WB Saunders, 2008.)

Item 7–9 Classification is based on the location of the atherosclerosis. **"Of native coronary artery"** indicates the atherosclerosis is within an original heart artery. **"Of autologous vein bypass graft"** indicates that the atherosclerosis is within a vein graft that was taken from within the patient. **"Of nonautologous biological bypass graft"** indicates the atherosclerosis is within a vessel grafted from other than the patient. **"Of artery bypass graft"** indicates the atherosclerosis is within an artery that was grafted from within the patient.

● **414   Other forms of chronic ischemic heart disease**

   Excludes *arteriosclerotic cardiovascular disease [ASCVD] (429.2)*
       cardiovascular:
        arteriosclerosis or sclerosis (429.2)
        degeneration or disease (429.2)

  ● **414.0 Coronary atherosclerosis**
     Arteriosclerotic heart disease [ASHD]
     Atherosclerotic heart disease
     Coronary (artery):
        arteriosclerosis
        arteritis or endarteritis
        atheroma
        sclerosis
        stricture

     Use additional code, if applicable, to identify chronic total occlusion of coronary artery (414.2)

     Excludes *embolism of graft (996.72)*
        occlusion NOS of graft (996.72)
        thrombus of graft (996.72)

     Coding Clinic: 2002, Q3, P3-9; 1994, Q2, P13, 15; Q1, P6-7; 1993, Q1, P20; 5th Issue, P17-24; 5th Issue, P14; 1984, Nov-Dec, P18

    ■ **414.00 Of unspecified type of vessel, native or graft** A
       Coding Clinic: 2003, Q2, P16; 2001, Q3, P15; 1997, Q3, P15; 1996, Q4, P31

    414.01 Of native coronary artery   A
       Coding Clinic: 2008, Q3, P10-11; Q2, P16; 2006, Q3, P25; 2005, Q4, P68-69; 2004, Q2, P3-4; 2003, Q4, P105-106, 108-109; Q3, P9.10, 14; 2001, Q3, P15-16; Q2, P8-9; 1997, Q3, P15; 1996, Q2, P10; 1995, Q2, P17-19

    414.02 Of autologous biological bypass graft   A
       Coding Clinic: 1995, Q2, P18-19

    414.03 Of nonautologous biological bypass graft   A

    414.04 Of artery bypass graft   A
       Internal mammary artery

    414.05 Of unspecified type of bypass graft   A
       Bypass graft NOS
       Coding Clinic: 1997, Q3, P15; 1996, Q4, P31

    414.06 Of native coronary artery of transplanted heart
       Coding Clinic: 2003, Q4, P60; 2002, Q4, P53-54; Q4, P53-54

    414.07 Of bypass graft (artery) (vein) of transplanted heart   A
       Coding Clinic: 2003, Q4, P60

  ● **414.1 Aneurysm and dissection of heart**
    414.10 Aneurysm of heart (wall)
       Aneurysm (arteriovenous):
         mural
         ventricular

    414.11 Aneurysm of coronary vessels
       Aneurysm (arteriovenous) of coronary vessels
       Coding Clinic: 1999, Q1, P17-18

    414.12 Dissection of coronary artery
       Coding Clinic: 2002, Q4, P54-55

    ■ **414.19 Other aneurysm of heart**
       Arteriovenous fistula, acquired, of heart

  ● **414.2 *Chronic total occlusion of coronary artery***
     Complete occlusion of coronary artery
     Total occlusion of coronary artery

     Code first coronary atherosclerosis (414.00–414.07)

     Excludes *acute coronary occlusion with myocardial infarction (410.00–410.92)*
        acute coronary occlusion without myocardial infarction (411.81)

     Coding Clinic: 2007, Q4, P82

  ● **414.3 *Coronary atherosclerosis due to lipid rich plaque***   A

     Code first coronary atherosclerosis (414.00-414.07)
     Coding Clinic: 2008, Q4, P113

  ■ **414.8 Other specified forms of chronic ischemic heart disease**
     Chronic coronary insufficiency
     Ischemia, myocardial (chronic)
     Any condition classifiable to 410 specified as chronic, or presenting with symptoms after 8 weeks from date of infarction

     Excludes *coronary insufficiency (acute) (411.89)*

     Coding Clinic: 2003, Q2, P10; 2001, Q3, P15-16; 1992, Q1, P10; 1990, Q3, P15; Q2, P19; 1986, Nov-Dec, P12

  ■ **414.9 Chronic ischemic heart disease, unspecified**
     Ischemic heart disease NOS
     Coding Clinic: 2001, Q3, P15-16

◀ New   ◀▥ Revised   ~~deleted~~ Deleted   ● Use Additional Digit(s)   ■ Nonspecific Code

● Not first-listed DX   OGCR Official Guidelines   Coding Clinic   Excludes   Includes   Use additional   Code first   Omit code

DISEASES OF THE CIRCULATORY SYSTEM (390–459)

Item 7-10 Pulmonary heart disease or cor pulmonale is right ventricle hypertrophy or RVH as a result of a respiratory disorder increasing back flow pressure to the right ventricle. Left untreated, cor pulmonale leads to right-heart failure and death.

DISEASES OF PULMONARY CIRCULATION (415–417)

● **415 Acute pulmonary heart disease**

415.0 Acute cor pulmonale

> **Excludes** *cor pulmonale NOS (416.9)*

● **415.1 Pulmonary embolism and infarction**
Pulmonary (artery) (vein):
apoplexy   infarction (hemorrhagic)
embolism   thrombosis

> **Excludes** *chronic pulmonary embolism (416.2)* ◄
> *personal history of pulmonary* ◄
> *embolism (V12.51)*
> *that complicating:*
> *abortion (634–638 with .6, 639.6)*
> *ectopic or molar pregnancy (639.6)*
> *pregnancy, childbirth, or the puerperium (673.0–673.8)*

415.11 Iatrogenic pulmonary embolism and infarction

> Use additional code for associated septic pulmonary embolism, if applicable, 415.12
> Coding Clinic: 1990, Q4, P25

● **415.12 Septic pulmonary embolism**
Septic embolism NOS

> *Code first underlying infection, such as:*
> septicemia (038.0–038.9)

> **Excludes** *septic arterial embolism (449)*
> Coding Clinic: 2007, Q4, P84-86

■ **415.19 Other**
Coding Clinic: 1998, Q2, P8

● **416 Chronic pulmonary heart disease**

416.0 Primary pulmonary hypertension
Idiopathic pulmonary arteriosclerosis
Pulmonary hypertension (essential) (idiopathic) (primary)

416.1 Kyphoscoliotic heart disease

416.2 Chronic pulmonary embolism ◄

> Use additional code, if applicable, for associated long-term (current) use of anticoagulants (V58.61) ◄

> **Excludes** *personal history of pulmonary embolism* ◄
> *(V12.51)* ◄

■ **416.8 Other chronic pulmonary heart diseases**
Pulmonary hypertension, secondary

■ **416.9 Chronic pulmonary heart disease, unspecified**
Chronic cardiopulmonary disease
Cor pulmonale (chronic) NOS

● **417 Other diseases of pulmonary circulation**

417.0 Arteriovenous fistula of pulmonary vessels

> **Excludes** *congenital arteriovenous fistula (747.3)*

417.1 Aneurysm of pulmonary artery

> **Excludes** *congenital aneurysm (747.3)*

■ **417.8 Other specified diseases of pulmonary circulation**
Pulmonary:
arteritis
endarteritis
Rupture of pulmonary vessel
Stricture of pulmonary vessel

■ **417.9 Unspecified disease of pulmonary circulation**

OTHER FORMS OF HEART DISEASE (420–429)

● **420 Acute pericarditis**
Inflammation of the sac surrounding the heart caused by infection. The chest pain is significant on inspiration, and onset is sudden and worst when lying down.

> **Includes** acute:
> mediastinopericarditis
> myopericarditis
> pericardial effusion
> pleuropericarditis
> pneumopericarditis

> **Excludes** *acute rheumatic pericarditis (391.0)*
> *postmyocardial infarction syndrome [Dressler's] (411.0)*

● ■ **420.0 Acute pericarditis in diseases classified elsewhere**

> *Code first underlying disease, as:*
> actinomycosis (039.8)
> amebiasis (006.8)
> chronic uremia (585.9)
> nocardiosis (039.8)
> tuberculosis (017.9)
> uremia NOS (586)

> **Excludes** *pericarditis (acute) (in):*
> *Coxsackie (virus) (074.21)*
> *gonococcal (098.83)*
> *histoplasmosis (115.0–115.9 with fifth-digit 3)*
> *meningococcal infection (036.41)*
> *syphilitic (093.81)*

● **420.9 Other and unspecified acute pericarditis**

■ **420.90 Acute pericarditis, unspecified**
Pericarditis (acute):
NOS
infective NOS
sicca
Coding Clinic: 1989, Q2, P12

420.91 Acute idiopathic pericarditis
Pericarditis, acute:
benign
nonspecific
viral

■ **420.99 Other**
Pericarditis (acute):
pneumococcal
purulent
staphylococcal
streptococcal
suppurative
Pneumopyopericardium
Pyopericardium

> **Excludes** *pericarditis in diseases classified elsewhere (420.0)*

DISEASES OF THE CIRCULATORY SYSTEM (390–459)

● **421 Acute and subacute endocarditis**
Inflammation/infection of lining of heart, affecting heart valves, usually caused by bacterial infection

     421.0 Acute and subacute bacterial endocarditis
        Endocarditis (acute) (chronic) (subacute):
          bacterial
          infective NOS
          lenta
          malignant
          purulent
          septic
          ulcerative
          vegetative
        Infective aneurysm
        Subacute bacterial endocarditis [SBE]

        <u>Use additional</u> code, if desired, to identify infectious organism [e.g., Streptococcus 041.0, Staphylococcus 041.1]
        Coding Clinic: 2008, Q4, P69-73; 2006, Q2, P16-17; 1999, Q1, P12; 1991, Q1, P15

● ■ **421.1 *Acute and subacute infective endocarditis in diseases classified elsewhere***

        Code first underlying disease, as:
          blastomycosis (116.0)
          Q fever (083.0)
          typhoid (fever) (002.0)

        Excludes *endocarditis (in):*
          Coxsackie (virus) (074.22)
          gonococcal (098.84)
          histoplasmosis (115.0–115.9 with
            fifth-digit 4)
          meningococcal infection (036.42)
          monilial (112.81)

    ■ **421.9 Acute endocarditis, unspecified**
        Endocarditis, acute or subacute
        Myoendocarditis, acute or subacute
        Periendocarditis, acute or subacute

        Excludes *acute rheumatic endocarditis (391.1)*

● **422 Acute myocarditis**
An inflammation of the heart muscle due to an infection (viral/bacterial).

        Excludes *acute rheumatic myocarditis (391.2)*

● ■ **422.0 *Acute myocarditis in diseases classified elsewhere***

        Code first underlying disease, as:
          myocarditis (acute):
            influenzal (487.8)
            tuberculous (017.9)

        Excludes *myocarditis (acute) (due to):*
          aseptic, of newborn (074.23)
          Coxsackie (virus) (074.23)
          diphtheritic (032.82)
          meningococcal infection (036.43)
          syphilitic (093.82)
          toxoplasmosis (130.3)

● **422.9 Other and unspecified acute myocarditis**

    ■ **422.90 Acute myocarditis, unspecified**
        Acute or subacute (interstitial) myocarditis

     422.91 Idiopathic myocarditis
        Myocarditis (acute or subacute):
          Fiedler's
          giant cell
          isolated (diffuse) (granulomatous)
          nonspecific granulomatous

     422.92 Septic myocarditis
        Myocarditis, acute or subacute:
          pneumococcal
          staphylococcal

        <u>Use additional</u> code to identify infectious organism [e.g., Staphylococcus 041.1]

        Excludes *myocarditis, acute or subacute:*
          in bacterial diseases classified elsewhere (422.0)
          streptococcal (391.2)

     422.93 Toxic myocarditis

    ■ **422.99 Other**

● **423 Other diseases of pericardium**

        Excludes *that specified as rheumatic (393)*

     423.0 Hemopericardium

     423.1 Adhesive pericardium
        Adherent pericardium
        Fibrosis of pericardium
        Milk spots
        Pericarditis:
          adhesive
          obliterative
        Soldiers' patches

     423.2 Constrictive pericarditis
        Concato's disease
        Pick's disease of heart (and liver)

● **423.3 *Cardiac tamponade***

        Code first the underlying cause
        Coding Clinic: 2007, Q4, P86-87; 2007, Q2, P11-12

■ **423.8 Other specified diseases of pericardium**
        Calcification of pericardium
        Fistula of pericardium
        Coding Clinic: 1989, Q2, P12

■ **423.9 Unspecified disease of pericardium**
        Coding Clinic: 2007, Q2, P11-12

● **424 Other diseases of endocardium**

        Excludes *bacterial endocarditis (421.0–421.9)*
          rheumatic endocarditis (391.1, 394.0–397.9)
          syphilitic endocarditis (093.20–093.24)

     424.0 Mitral valve disorders
        Mitral (valve):
          incompetence NOS of specified cause, except rheumatic
          insufficiency NOS of specified cause, except rheumatic
          regurgitation NOS of specified cause, except rheumatic

        Excludes *mitral (valve):*
          disease (394.9)
          failure (394.9)
          stenosis (394.0)
          the listed conditions:
            specified as rheumatic (394.1)
            unspecified as to cause but with mention of:
              diseases of aortic valve (396.0–396.9)
              mitral stenosis or obstruction (394.2)
        Coding Clinic: 2006, Q3, P7; 2000, Q2, P16-17; 1998, Q3, P11; 1987, Nov-Dec, P8

424.1 Aortic valve disorders
Aortic (valve):
incompetence NOS of specified cause, except
rheumatic
insufficiency NOS of specified cause, except
rheumatic
regurgitation NOS of specified cause, except
rheumatic
stenosis NOS of specified cause, except
rheumatic

Excludes *hypertrophic subaortic stenosis (425.1)*
that specified as rheumatic (395.0–395.9)
that of unspecified cause but with
mention of diseases of mitral valve
(396.0–396.9)
Coding Clinic: 2008, Q4, P177-180; 1988, Q4, P8; 1987, Nov-Dec, P8

424.2 Tricuspid valve disorders, specified as nonrheumatic
Tricuspid valve:
incompetence of specified cause, except rheumatic
insufficiency of specified cause, except
rheumatic
regurgitation of specified cause, except
rheumatic
stenosis of specified cause, except rheumatic

Excludes *rheumatic or of unspecified cause (397.0)*

424.3 Pulmonary valve disorders
Pulmonic:
incompetence NOS
insufficiency NOS
regurgitation NOS
stenosis NOS

Excludes *that specified as rheumatic (397.1)*

● **424.9 Endocarditis, valve unspecified**

■ **424.90 Endocarditis, valve unspecified, unspecified**
cause
Endocarditis (chronic):
NOS
nonbacterial thrombotic
Valvular:
incompetence of unspecified valve,
unspecified cause
insufficiency of unspecified valve,
unspecified cause
regurgitation of unspecified valve,
unspecified cause
stenosis of unspecified valve, unspecified
cause
Valvulitis (chronic)

● ■ **424.91 Endocarditis in diseases classified elsewhere**
Code first underlying disease, as:
atypical verrucous endocarditis
[Libman-Sacks] (710.0)
disseminated lupus erythematosus
(710.0)
tuberculosis (017.9)

Excludes *syphilitic (093.20–093.24)*

■ **424.99 Other**
Any condition classifiable to 424.90 with
specified cause, except rheumatic

Excludes *endocardial fibroelastosis (425.3)*
that specified as rheumatic (397.9)

● **425 Cardiomyopathy**
Disease of the heart muscle resulting in abnormally enlarged,
weakened, thickened, and/or stiffened muscle causing an
inability to pump blood normally and leads to CHF.

Includes myocardiopathy

425.0 Endomyocardial fibrosis

425.1 Hypertrophic obstructive cardiomyopathy
Hypertrophic subaortic stenosis (idiopathic)

425.2 Obscure cardiomyopathy of Africa
Becker's disease
Idiopathic mural endomyocardial disease

425.3 Endocardial fibroelastosis
Elastomyofibrosis

■ **425.4 Other primary cardiomyopathies**
Cardiomyopathy:
NOS
congestive
constrictive
familial
hypertrophic
idiopathic
nonobstructive
obstructive
restrictive
Cardiovascular collagenosis
Coding Clinic: 2007, Q1, P20; 2005, Q2, P14-15; 2000, Q1, P22;
1997, Q4, P54-55; 1990, Q2, P19; 1985, Sept-Oct, P15

425.5 Alcoholic cardiomyopathy
Coding Clinic: 1985, Sept-Oct, P15; July-Aug, P15

● **425.7 *Nutritional and metabolic cardiomyopathy***
Code first underlying disease, as:
amyloidosis (277.30–277.39)
beriberi (265.0)
cardiac glycogenosis (271.0)
mucopolysaccharidosis (277.5)
thyrotoxicosis (242.0–242.9)

Excludes *gouty tophi of heart (274.82)*

● ■ **425.8 *Cardiomyopathy in other diseases classified***
elsewhere
Code first underlying disease, as:
Friedreich's ataxia (334.0)
myotonia atrophica (359.21)
progressive muscular dystrophy (359.1)
sarcoidosis (135)

Excludes *cardiomyopathy in Chagas' disease (086.0)*
Coding Clinic: 1993, Q2, P9

■ **425.9 Secondary cardiomyopathy, unspecified**

● **426 Conduction disorders**
Heart block or atrioventricular block (AV block) caused
by conduction problem resulting in arrhythmias/
dysrhythmias due to lack of electrical impulses being
transmitted normally through heart.

426.0 Atrioventricular block, complete
Third degree atrioventricular block
Coding Clinic: 2006, Q2, P14

DISEASES OF THE CIRCULATORY SYSTEM (390–459)

DISEASES OF THE CIRCULATORY SYSTEM (390–459)

● **426.1 Atrioventricular block, other and unspecified**

◾ **426.10 Atrioventricular block, unspecified**
Atrioventricular [AV] block (incomplete) (partial)

426.11 First degree atrioventricular block
Incomplete atrioventricular block, first degree
Prolonged P-R interval NOS
Coding Clinic: 2006, Q2, P14

426.12 Mobitz (type) II atrioventricular block
Incomplete atrioventricular block:
Mobitz (type) II
second degree, Mobitz (type) II
Coding Clinic: 2006, Q2, P14

◾ **426.13 Other second degree atrioventricular block**
Incomplete atrioventricular block:
Mobitz (type) I [Wenckebach's]
second degree:
NOS
Mobitz (type) I
with 2:1 atrioventricular response [block]
Wenckebach's phenomenon

426.2 Left bundle branch hemiblock
Block:
left anterior fascicular
left posterior fascicular

◾ **426.3 Other left bundle branch block**
Left bundle branch block:
NOS
anterior fascicular with posterior fascicular
complete
main stem

426.4 Right bundle branch block
Coding Clinic: 2000, Q3, P3

● **426.5 Bundle branch block, other and unspecified**

◾ **426.50 Bundle branch block, unspecified**

426.51 Right bundle branch block and left posterior fascicular block

426.52 Right bundle branch block and left anterior fascicular block

◾ **426.53 Other bilateral bundle branch block**
Bifascicular block NOS
Bilateral bundle branch block NOS
Right bundle branch with left bundle branch block (incomplete) (main stem)

426.54 Trifascicular block

◾ **426.6 Other heart block**
Intraventricular block:
NOS
diffuse
myofibrillar
Sinoatrial block
Sinoauricular block

426.7 Anomalous atrioventricular excitation
Atrioventricular conduction:
accelerated
accessory
pre-excitation
Ventricular pre-excitation
Wolff-Parkinson-White syndrome

● **426.8 Other specified conduction disorders**

426.81 Lown-Ganong-Levine syndrome
Syndrome of short P-R interval, normal QRS complexes, and supraventricular tachycardias

426.82 Long QT syndrome
Coding Clinic: 2005, Q4, P72-73

◾ **426.89 Other**
Dissociation:
atrioventricular [AV]
interference
isorhythmic
Nonparoxysmal AV nodal tachycardia

◾ **426.9 Conduction disorder, unspecified**
Heart block NOS
Stokes-Adams syndrome

● **427 Cardiac dysrhythmias**
Abnormality in rate, regularity, or sequence of cardiac activation.

Excludes *that complicating:*
abortion (634–638 with .7, 639.8)
ectopic or molar pregnancy (639.8)
labor or delivery (668.1, 669.4)

427.0 Paroxysmal supraventricular tachycardia
Paroxysmal tachycardia:
atrial [PAT]   junctional
atrioventricular [AV]   nodal

427.1 Paroxysmal ventricular tachycardia
Ventricular tachycardia (paroxysmal)
Coding Clinic: 2008, Q1, P14-15; 2006, Q2, P15-16; 1995, Q3, P9; Q1, P8; 1986, Mar-April, P11-12; 1985, July-Aug, P15

◾ **427.2 Paroxysmal tachycardia, unspecified**
Bouveret-Hoffmann syndrome
Paroxysmal tachycardia:
NOS
essential

● **427.3 Atrial fibrillation and flutter**

427.31 Atrial fibrillation
Most common abnormal heart rhythm (arrhythmia) presenting as irregular, rapid beating (tachycardia) of the heart's upper chamber.
Coding Clinic: 2008, Q4, P134-136; 2005, Q3, P3-9; 2004, Q4, P77-78, 121-122; Q3, P7; 2003, Q4, P93-95, 105-106; Q1, P8; 1999, Q2, P17; 1996, Q2, P7x2; 1995, Q3, P8; 1994, Q1, P22; 1985, July-Aug, P15

427.32 Atrial flutter
Rapid contractions of the upper heart chamber, but regular, rather than irregular, beats.
Coding Clinic: 2003, Q4, P93-95

● **427.4 Ventricular fibrillation and flutter**

427.41 Ventricular fibrillation
Coding Clinic: 2002, Q3, P5

427.42 Ventricular flutter

◾ **427.5 Cardiac arrest**
Cardiorespiratory arrest
Coding Clinic: 2002, Q3, P5; 2000, Q2, P12; 1995, Q3, P9

● **427.6 Premature beats**

◾ **427.60 Premature beats, unspecified**
Ectopic beats
Extrasystoles
Extrasystolic arrhythmia
Premature contractions or systoles NOS

◀ New   ◀▥ Revised   ~~deleted~~ Deleted   ● Use Additional Digit(s)   ◾ Nonspecific Code
● Not first-listed DX   OGCR Official Guidelines   Coding Clinic   Excludes   Includes   Use additional   Code first   Omit code

427.61   Supraventricular premature beats
> Atrial premature beats, contractions, or systoles
> Coding Clinic: 1994, Q1, P20

■**427.69   Other**
> Ventricular premature beats, contractions, or systoles
> Coding Clinic: 1993, Q4, P42-43

●**427.8   Other specified cardiac dysrhythmias**

427.81   Sinoatrial node dysfunction
> Sinus bradycardia:
> > persistent
> > severe
>
> Syndrome:
> > sick sinus
> > tachycardia-bradycardia
>
> **Excludes**   *sinus bradycardia NOS (427.89)*

■**427.89   Other**
> Rhythm disorder:
> > coronary sinus
> > ectopic
> > nodal
>
> Wandering (atrial) pacemaker
>
> **Excludes**   *carotid sinus syncope (337.0)*
> > *neonatal bradycardia (779.81)*
> > *neonatal tachycardia (779.82)*
> > *reflex bradycardia (337.0)*
> > *tachycardia NOS (785.0)*
>
> Coding Clinic: 2000, Q3, P8-9; 1985, July-Aug, P15

■**427.9   Cardiac dysrhythmia, unspecified**
> Arrhythmia (cardiac) NOS
> Coding Clinic: 1989, Q2, P10

●**428   Heart failure**
> Code, if applicable, heart failure due to hypertension first (402.0–402.9, with fifth-digit 1 or 404.0–404.9 with fifth-digit 1 or 3)
>
> **Excludes**   *rheumatic (398.91)*
> > *that complicating:*
> > > *abortion (634–638 with .7, 639.8)*
> > > *ectopic or molar pregnancy (639.8)*
> > > *labor or delivery (668.1, 669.4)*
>
> Coding Clinic: 2005, Q2, P14-15; 2002, Q4, P49-53

Item 7–11 Congestive heart failure (CHF) is a condition in which the left ventricle of the heart cannot pump enough blood to the body. The blood flow from the heart slows or returns to the heart from the venous system back flow resulting in congestion (fluid accumulation) particularly in the abdomen. Most commonly, fluid collects in the lungs and results in shortness of breath, especially when in a reclining position.

■**428.0   Congestive heart failure, unspecified**
> Congestive heart disease
> Right heart failure (secondary to left heart failure)
>
> **Excludes**   *fluid overload NOS (276.6)*
>
> Coding Clinic: 2009, Q1, P6x2; 2008, Q4, P69-73, 177-182; Q3, P12-13x2; 2007, Q3, P11; Q1, P20; 2006, Q3, P7; 2005, Q4, P119-120; Q3, P3-9; Q1, P9; 2004, Q4, P140; Q3, P7; 2003, Q4, P109-110; Q1, P9; 2002, Q4, P52-53; 2001, Q2, P13; 2000, Q4, P47-48; Q2, P16-17; Q1, P22; 1999, Q4, P13-14; Q1, P11, 1998, Q3, P5; 1997, Q4, P54-55; Q3, P10; 1996, Q3, P9; 1991, Q3, P18-20; 1990, Q2, P19; 1989, Q2, P12; 1987, Sept-Oct, P11; 1985, Sept-Oct, P15; Nov-Dec, P14

428.1   Left heart failure
> Acute edema of lung with heart disease NOS or heart failure
> Acute pulmonary edema with heart disease NOS or heart failure
> Cardiac asthma
> Left ventricular failure
> Coding Clinic: 1990, Q2, P19

●**428.2   Systolic heart failure**
> **Excludes**   *combined systolic and diastolic heart failure (428.40–428.43)*

■**428.20   Unspecified**

428.21   Acute
> *Presenting a short and relatively severe episode*

428.22   Chronic
> *Long-lasting, presenting over time*
> Coding Clinic: 2005, Q4, P119-120

428.23   Acute on chronic
> *Combination code. What was a chronic condition now has an acute exacerbation (to make more severe). Because two conditions are now present, the combination code reports both.*
> Coding Clinic: 2009, Q1, P10; 2003, Q1, P9

●**428.3   Diastolic heart failure**
> **Excludes**   *combined systolic and diastolic heart failure (428.40–428.43)*

■**428.30   Unspecified**
> Coding Clinic: 2002, Q4, P52

428.31   Acute

428.32   Chronic
> Coding Clinic: 2008, Q3, P12-13

428.33   Acute on chronic
> Coding Clinic: 2008, Q3, P12; 2007, Q1, P20

●**428.4   Combined systolic and diastolic heart failure**

■**428.40   Unspecified**

428.41   Acute
> Coding Clinic: 2004, Q4, P140

428.42   Chronic

428.43   Acute on chronic
> Coding Clinic: 2006, Q3, P7; 2002, Q4, P52-53

■**428.9   Heart failure, unspecified**
> Cardiac failure NOS
> Heart failure NOS
> Myocardial failure NOS
> Weak heart
> Coding Clinic: 1989, Q2, P10; 1985, Nov-Dec, P14

●**429   Ill-defined descriptions and complications of heart disease**

■**429.0   Myocarditis, unspecified**
> Myocarditis (with mention of arteriosclerosis):
> > NOS (with mention of arteriosclerosis)
> > chronic (interstitial) (with mention of arteriosclerosis)
> > fibroid (with mention of arteriosclerosis)
> > senile (with mention of arteriosclerosis)
>
> Use additional code to identify presence of arteriosclerosis
>
> **Excludes**   *acute or subacute (422.0–422.9)*
> > *rheumatic (398.0)*
> > > *acute (391.2)*
> > *that due to hypertension (402.0–402.9)*

DISEASES OF THE CIRCULATORY SYSTEM (390–459)

429.1 Myocardial degeneration
Degeneration of heart or myocardium (with mention of arteriosclerosis):
  fatty (with mention of arteriosclerosis)
  mural (with mention of arteriosclerosis)
  muscular (with mention of arteriosclerosis)
Myocardial (with mention of arteriosclerosis):
  degeneration (with mention of arteriosclerosis)
  disease (with mention of arteriosclerosis)

Use additional code to identify presence of arteriosclerosis

Excludes *that due to hypertension (402.0–402.9)*

429.2 Cardiovascular disease, unspecified
Arteriosclerotic cardiovascular disease [ASCVD]
Cardiovascular arteriosclerosis
Cardiovascular:
  degeneration (with mention of arteriosclerosis)
  disease (with mention of arteriosclerosis)
  sclerosis (with mention of arteriosclerosis)

Use additional code to identify presence of arteriosclerosis

Excludes *that due to hypertension (402.0–402.9)*

429.3 Cardiomegaly
Cardiac:
  dilatation
  hypertrophy
Ventricular dilatation

Excludes *that due to hypertension (402.0–402.9)*

429.4 Functional disturbances following cardiac surgery
Cardiac insufficiency following cardiac surgery or due to prosthesis
Heart failure following cardiac surgery or due to prosthesis
Postcardiotomy syndrome
Postvalvulotomy syndrome

Excludes *cardiac failure in the immediate postoperative period (997.1)*

Coding Clinic: 2002, Q2, P12-13

429.5 Rupture of chordae tendineae

429.6 Rupture of papillary muscle

● 429.7 Certain sequelae of myocardial infarction, not elsewhere classified
Use additional code to identify the associated myocardial infarction:
  with onset of 8 weeks or less (410.00–410.92)
  with onset of more than 8 weeks (414.8)

Excludes *congenital defects of heart (745, 746)*
coronary aneurysm (414.11)
disorders of papillary muscle (429.6, 429.81)
postmyocardial infarction syndrome (411.0)
rupture of chordae tendineae (429.5)

429.71 Acquired cardiac septal defect   A
Excludes *acute septal infarction (410.00–410.92)*

429.79 Other   A
Mural thrombus (atrial) (ventricular) acquired, following myocardial infarction
Coding Clinic: 1992, Q1, P10

● 429.8 Other ill-defined heart diseases
429.81 Other disorders of papillary muscle
Papillary muscle:
  atrophy
  degeneration
  dysfunction
  incompetence
  incoordination
  scarring

429.82 Hyperkinetic heart disease

429.83 Takotsubo syndrome
Broken heart syndrome
Reversible left ventricular dysfunction following sudden emotional stress
Stress induced cardiomyopathy
Transient left ventricular apical ballooning syndrome
Coding Clinic: 2006, Q4, P87

429.89 Other
Carditis
Excludes *that due to hypertension (402.0–402.9)*
Coding Clinic: 2006, Q2, P18-19; 2005, Q3, P14; 1992, Q1, P10

429.9 Heart disease, unspecified
Heart disease (organic) NOS
Morbus cordis NOS

Excludes *that due to hypertension (402.0–402.9)*
Coding Clinic: 2009, Q1, P10x2; 1993, Q1, P19-20

CEREBROVASCULAR DISEASE (430–438)

Includes with mention of hypertension (conditions classifiable to 401–405)

Use additional code to identify presence of hypertension

Excludes *any condition classifiable to 430–434, 436, 437 occurring during pregnancy, childbirth, or the puerperium, or specified as puerperal (674.0)*
iatrogenic cerebrovascular infarction or hemorrhage (997.02)

OGCR Section I.C.7.a.5
First assign codes from 430-438, Cerebrovascular disease, then the appropriate hypertension code from categories 401-405.

430 Subarachnoid hemorrhage
Meningeal hemorrhage
Ruptured:
  berry aneurysm
  (congenital) cerebral aneurysm NOS

Excludes *syphilitic ruptured cerebral aneurysm (094.87)*
Coding Clinic: 2000, Q3, P16; 1991, Q3, P15-16

431 Intracerebral hemorrhage
Hemorrhage (of):
  basilar
  bulbar
  cerebellar
  cerebral
  cerebromeningeal
  cortical
  internal capsule
  intrapontine
  pontine
  subcortical
  ventricular
Rupture of blood vessel in brain
Coding Clinic: 2007, Q3, P4; 1997, Q3, P11

◀ New   ◀||| Revised   ~~deleted~~ Deleted   ● Use Additional Digit(s)   ■ Nonspecific Code
● Not first-listed DX   OGCR Official Guidelines   Coding Clinic   Excludes   Includes   Use additional   Code first   Omit code

DISEASES OF THE CIRCULATORY SYSTEM (390–459)

● **432 Other and unspecified intracranial hemorrhage**

     432.0 Nontraumatic extradural hemorrhage
         Nontraumatic epidural hemorrhage

     432.1 Subdural hemorrhage
         Subdural hematoma, nontraumatic

     ▢**432.9 Unspecified intracranial hemorrhage**
         Intracranial hemorrhage NOS

● **433 Occlusion and stenosis of precerebral arteries**

     The following fifth-digit subclassification is for use with category 433:

> **0 without mention of cerebral infarction**
> **1 with cerebral infarction**

     Includes   embolism of basilar, carotid, and vertebral arteries
                   narrowing of basilar, carotid, and vertebral arteries
                   obstruction of basilar, carotid, and vertebral arteries
                   thrombosis of basilar, carotid, and vertebral arteries

     Excludes   *insufficiency NOS of precerebral arteries (435.0–435.9)*

     Use additional code, if applicable, to identify status post administration of tPA (rtPA) in a different facility within the last 24 hours prior to admission to current facility (V45.88)
     Coding Clinic: 1995, Q2, P16; 1993, Q4, P38-39

●   **433.0 Basilar artery**
     [0-1]

●   **433.1 Carotid artery**
     [0-1]   Coding Clinic: 2006, Q1, P17; 2002, Q1, P7-8, 10-11; 2000, Q1, P16; 1995, Q2, P16

●   **433.2 Vertebral artery**
     [0-1]

●   **433.3 Multiple and bilateral**
     [0-1]   Coding Clinic: 2006, Q1, P17; 2002, Q1, P10-11

● ▢**433.8 Other specified precerebral artery**
     [0-1]

● ▢**433.9 Unspecified precerebral artery**
     [0-1]   Precerebral artery NOS

● **434 Occlusion of cerebral arteries**

     The following fifth-digit subclassification is for use with category 434:

> **0 without mention of cerebral infarction**
> **1 with cerebral infarction**

     Use additional code, if applicable, to identify status post administration of tPA (rtPA) in a different facility within the last 24 hours prior to admission to current facility (V45.88)
     Coding Clinic: 2007, Q3, P12; 1995, Q2, P16; 1993, Q4, P38-39

●   **434.0 Cerebral thrombosis**
     [0-1]   Thrombosis of cerebral arteries

●   **434.1 Cerebral embolism**
     [0-1]   Coding Clinic: 1997, Q3, P11

● ▢**434.9 Cerebral artery occlusion, unspecified**
     [0-1]   Coding Clinic: 2008, Q4, P102-109; 2007, Q1, P23-24; 2004, Q4, P77-78; 1998, Q4, P87; 1996, Q2, P5

OGCR Section I.C.7.b
The terms stroke and CVA are often used interchangeably to refer to a cerebral vascular infarction. The terms stroke, CVA, and cerebral infarction NOS are all indexed to the default code 434.91, Cerebral artery occlusion, unspecified, with infarction. Code 436, Acute, but ill-defined, cerebrovascular disease, should not be used when the documentation states stroke or CVA.

● **435 Transient cerebral ischemia**

     Includes   cerebrovascular insufficiency (acute) with transient focal neurological signs and symptoms
                   insufficiency of basilar, carotid, and vertebral arteries
                   spasm of cerebral arteries

     Excludes   *acute cerebrovascular insufficiency NOS (437.1)*
                   that due to any condition classifiable to 433 (433.0–433.9)

     435.0 Basilar artery syndrome

     435.1 Vertebral artery syndrome

     435.2 Subclavian steal syndrome

     435.3 Vertebrobasilar artery syndrome

     ▢**435.8 Other specified transient cerebral ischemias**

     ▢**435.9 Unspecified transient cerebral ischemia**
         Impending cerebrovascular accident
         Intermittent cerebral ischemia
         Transient ischemic attack [TIA]
         Coding Clinic: 1985, Nov-Dec, P12

     436 Acute, but ill-defined, cerebrovascular disease
         Apoplexy, apoplectic:
             NOS
             attack
             cerebral
             seizure
         Cerebral seizure

     Excludes   *any condition classifiable to categories 430–435*
                   cerebrovascular accident (434.91)
                   CVA (ischemic) (434.91)
                      embolic (434.11)
                      hemorrhagic (430, 431, 432.0–432.9)
                      thrombotic (434.01)
                   postoperative cerebrovascular accident (997.02)
                   stroke (ischemic) (434.91)
                      embolic (434.11)
                      hemorrhagic (430, 431, 432.0–432.9)
                      thrombotic (434.01)
     Coding Clinic: 2004, Q4, P77-78; 1999, Q4, P3-4; 1993, Q4, P38-39; Q1, P27

OGCR Section I.C.7.b
The terms stroke and CVA are often used interchangeably to refer to a cerebral vascular infarction. The terms stroke, CVA, and cerebral infarction NOS are all indexed to the default code 434.91, Cerebral artery occlusion, unspecified, with infarction. Code 436, Acute, but ill-defined, cerebrovascular disease, should not be used when the documentation states stroke or CVA.

● **437 Other and ill-defined cerebrovascular disease**

     437.0 Cerebral atherosclerosis   A
         Atheroma of cerebral arteries
         Cerebral arteriosclerosis

     ▢**437.1 Other generalized ischemic cerebrovascular disease**
         Acute cerebrovascular insufficiency NOS
         Cerebral ischemia (chronic)
         Coding Clinic: 2009, Q1, P10

     437.2 Hypertensive encephalopathy

N   Newborn Age: 0   P   Pediatric Age: 0–17   M   Maternity Age: 12–55   A   Adult Age: 15–124   ♀   Females Only   ♂   Males Only

437.3 **Cerebral aneurysm, nonruptured**
Internal carotid artery, intracranial portion
Internal carotid artery NOS

> **Excludes** *congenital cerebral aneurysm, nonruptured (747.81)*
> *internal carotid artery, extracranial portion (442.81)*

Coding Clinic: 2009, Q2, P11

437.4 **Cerebral arteritis**
Coding Clinic: 1999, Q4, P21-22

437.5 **Moyamoya disease**

437.6 **Nonpyogenic thrombosis of intracranial venous sinus**

> **Excludes** *pyogenic (325)*

437.7 **Transient global amnesia**

437.8 **Other**

437.9 **Unspecified**
Cerebrovascular disease or lesion NOS

> **OGCR** Section I.C.7.d.3
> Assign code V12.54, Transient ischemic attack (TIA), and cerebral infarction without residual deficits (and not a code from category 438) as an additional code for history of cerebrovascular disease when no neurologic deficits are present.

Coding Clinic: 2009, Q1, P16; 1986, Nov-Dec, P12

438 **Late effects of cerebrovascular disease**

> **Note:** This category is to be used to indicate conditions in 430–437 as the cause of late effects. The "late effects" include conditions specified as such, or as sequelae, which may occur at any time after the onset of the causal condition.

> **Excludes** *personal history of:*
> *cerebral infarction without residual deficits (V12.54)*
> *PRIND (Prolonged reversible ischemic neurologic deficit) (V12.54)*
> *RIND (Reversible ischemic neurological deficit) (V12.54)*
> *transient ischemic attack (TIA) (V12.54)*

Coding Clinic: 2006, Q3, P3-4, 6; 1999, Q4, P6-8x2; Q4, P4-5; 1994, Q1, P22-23; 1993, Q1, P27

438.0 **Cognitive deficits**
Coding Clinic: 2007, Q2, P5

438.1 **Speech and language deficits**

438.10 **Speech and language deficit, unspecified**

438.11 **Aphasia**
Coding Clinic: 2003, Q4, P105-106; 1997, Q4, P35-37

438.12 **Dysphasia**
Coding Clinic: 1999, Q4, P9; Q4, P3-4

438.13 **Dysarthria** ◄

438.14 **Fluency disorder** ◄
Stuttering ◄

438.19 **Other speech and language deficits**

438.2 **Hemiplegia/hemiparesis**
Coding Clinic: 2005, Q1, P13

438.20 **Hemiplegia affecting unspecified side**
Coding Clinic: 2007, Q4, P92-95; 2003, Q4, P105-106; 1999, Q4, P9; Q4, P3-4

438.21 **Hemiplegia affecting dominant side**

438.22 **Hemiplegia affecting nondominant side**
Coding Clinic: 2003, Q4, P105; 2002, Q1, P16

438.3 **Monoplegia of upper limb**

438.30 **Monoplegia of upper limb affecting unspecified side**

438.31 **Monoplegia of upper limb affecting dominant side**

438.32 **Monoplegia of upper limb affecting nondominant side**

438.4 **Monoplegia of lower limb**

438.40 **Monoplegia of lower limb affecting unspecified side**

438.41 **Monoplegia of lower limb affecting dominant side**

438.42 **Monoplegia of lower limb affecting nondominant side**

438.5 **Other paralytic syndrome**

> Use additional code to identify type of paralytic syndrome, such as:
> locked-in state (344.81)
> quadriplegia (344.00–344.09)

> **Excludes** *late effects of cerebrovascular accident with:*
> *hemiplegia/hemiparesis (438.20–438.22)*
> *monoplegia of lower limb (438.40–438.42)*
> *monoplegia of upper limb (438.40–438.42)*

438.50 **Other paralytic syndrome affecting unspecified side**

438.51 **Other paralytic syndrome affecting dominant side**

438.52 **Other paralytic syndrome affecting nondominant side**

438.53 **Other paralytic syndrome, bilateral**
Coding Clinic: 1998, Q4, P39-40

438.6 **Alterations of sensations**

> Use additional code to identify the altered sensation

Coding Clinic: 2002, Q4, P56

438.7 **Disturbances of vision**

> Use additional code to identify the visual disturbance

Coding Clinic: 2002, Q4, P56

438.8 **Other late effects of cerebrovascular disease**
Coding Clinic: 2005, Q1, P13; 2002, Q4, P56

438.81 **Apraxia**

438.82 **Dysphagia**

> Use additional code to identify the type of dysphagia, if known (787.20–787.29)

Coding Clinic: 2007, Q4, P92-95

438.83 **Facial weakness**
Facial droop

438.84 **Ataxia**

438.85 **Vertigo**
Coding Clinic: 2002, Q4, P56

438.89 **Other late effects of cerebrovascular disease**

> Use additional code to identify the late effect

Coding Clinic: 2009, Q2, P11; 2005, Q1, P13; 1998, Q4, P39-40

438.9 **Unspecified late effects of cerebrovascular disease**

DISEASES OF THE CIRCULATORY SYSTEM (390–459)

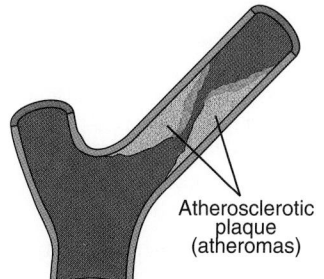

Figure 7-4 Atherosclerotic plaque.

Atherosclerotic
plaque
(atheromas)

DISEASES OF ARTERIES, ARTERIOLES, AND CAPILLARIES (440–449)

● **440 Atherosclerosis**
Disease in which fatty deposits form on walls of arteries

Includes arteriolosclerosis
arteriosclerosis (obliterans) (senile)
arteriosclerotic vascular disease
atheroma
degeneration:
arterial
arteriovascular
vascular
endarteritis deformans or obliterans
senile:
arteritis
endarteritis

Excludes *atheroembolism (445.01–445.89)*
atherosclerosis of bypass graft of the extremities (440.30–440.32)

440.0 Of aorta A
Coding Clinic: 1993, Q2, P7-8; 1988, Q4, P8

440.1 Of renal artery A

Excludes *atherosclerosis of renal arterioles (403.00–403.91)*

● **440.2 Of native arteries of the extremities**

Use additional code, if applicable, to identify chronic total occlusion of artery of the extremities (440.4)

Excludes *atherosclerosis of bypass graft of the extremities (440.30–440.32)*
Coding Clinic: 1994, Q3, P5; 1990, Q3, P15

▪**440.20 Atherosclerosis of the extremities, unspecified** A

440.21 Atherosclerosis of the extremities with intermittent claudication A

440.22 Atherosclerosis of the extremities with rest pain A
Any condition classifiable to 440.21

440.23 Atherosclerosis of the extremities with ulceration A
Any condition classifiable to 440.21–440.22
Use additional code for any associated ulceration (707.10–707.9)

440.24 Atherosclerosis of the extremities with gangrene
Any condition classifiable to 440.21, 440.22, and 440.23 with ischemic gangrene 785.4
Use additional code for any associated ulceration (707.10–707.9)

Excludes *gas gangrene 040.0*
Coding Clinic: 2003, Q4, P109-110; Q3, P14x2; 1995, Q1, P11; 1994, Q3, P5

▪**440.29 Other** A
Coding Clinic: 1995, Q1, P11

● **440.3 Of bypass graft of the extremities**

Excludes *atherosclerosis of native artery of the extremity (440.21–440.24)*
embolism [occlusion NOS] [thrombus] of graft (996.74)

▪**440.30 Of unspecified graft** A
440.31 Of autologous vein bypass graft A
440.32 Of nonautologous vein bypass graft A

● **440.4 Chronic total occlusion of artery of the extremities**
Complete occlusion of artery of the extremities
Total occlusion of artery of the extremities

Code first atherosclerosis of arteries of the extremities (440.20–440.29, 440.30–440.32)

Excludes *acute occlusion of artery of extremity (444.21–444.22)*
Coding Clinic: 2007, Q4, P82-83

▪**440.8 Of other specified arteries** A

Excludes *basilar (433.0)*
carotid (433.1)
cerebral (437.0)
coronary (414.00–414.07)
mesenteric (557.1)
precerebral (433.0–433.9)
pulmonary (416.0)
vertebral (433.2)

▪**440.9 Generalized and unspecified atherosclerosis** A
Arteriosclerotic vascular disease NOS

Excludes *arteriosclerotic cardiovascular disease [ASCVD] (429.2)*

● **441 Aortic aneurysm and dissection**

Excludes *syphilitic aortic aneurysm (093.0)*
traumatic aortic aneurysm (901.0, 902.0)

● **441.0 Dissection of aorta**
Coding Clinic: 1989, Q4, P10

▪**441.00 Unspecified site**
441.01 Thoracic
Coding Clinic: 2009, Q1, P16; 2007, Q4, P86-87

441.02 Abdominal
441.03 Thoracoabdominal
441.1 Thoracic aneurysm, ruptured
Coding Clinic: 1994, Q2, P15

441.2 Thoracic aneurysm without mention of rupture
Coding Clinic: 1992, Q3, P10-11

441.3 Abdominal aneurysm, ruptured

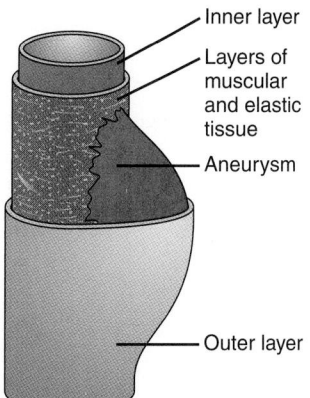

Inner layer
Layers of muscular and elastic tissue
Aneurysm
Outer layer

Figure 7-5 An aneurysm is an enclosed swelling on the wall of the vessel.

Item 7-12 Rupture is the tearing of the aneurysm.

441.4 Abdominal aneurysm without mention of rupture
Coding Clinic: 2000, Q4, P63-64; 1999, Q1, P15-17x2; 1992, Q3, P10-11

441.5 Aortic aneurysm of unspecified site, ruptured
Rupture of aorta NOS

441.6 Thoracoabdominal aneurysm, ruptured

441.7 Thoracoabdominal aneurysm, without mention of rupture
Coding Clinic: 2006, Q2, P16-17

441.9 Aortic aneurysm of unspecified site without mention of rupture
Aneurysm
Dilatation of aorta
Hyaline necrosis of aorta
Coding Clinic: 1992, Q3, P10-11

442 Other aneurysm

Includes	aneurysm (ruptured) (cirsoid) (false) (varicose) aneurysmal varix

Excludes	arteriovenous aneurysm or fistula:
	   acquired (447.0)
	   congenital (747.60–747.69)
	   traumatic (900.0–904.9)

442.0 Of artery of upper extremity

442.1 Of renal artery

442.2 Of iliac artery
Coding Clinic: 1999, Q1, P16-17

442.3 Of artery of lower extremity
Aneurysm:
   femoral artery
   popliteal artery
Coding Clinic: 2008, Q2, P13; 2002, Q3, P24-27; 1999, Q1, P16

442.8 Of other specified artery

442.81 Artery of neck
Aneurysm of carotid artery (common) (external) (internal, extracranial portion)

Excludes	internal carotid artery, intracranial portion (437.3)

442.82 Subclavian artery

442.83 Splenic artery

442.84 Other visceral artery
Aneurysm:
   celiac artery
   gastroduodenal artery
   gastroepiploic artery
   hepatic artery
   pancreaticoduodenal artery
   superior mesenteric artery

442.89 Other
Aneurysm: Aneurysm:
   mediastinal artery   spinal artery

Excludes	cerebral (nonruptured) (437.3)
	   congenital (747.81)
	   ruptured (430)
	coronary (414.11)
	heart (414.10)
	pulmonary (417.1)

442.9 Of unspecified site

443 Other peripheral vascular disease

443.0 Raynaud's syndrome
Resulting from a diminishing oxygen supply to fingers, toes, nose, and ears when exposed to temperature changes or stress with symptoms of pallor, numbness, and feeling cold
Raynaud's:
   disease
   phenomenon (secondary)
Use additional code to identify gangrene (785.4)

443.1 Thromboangiitis obliterans [Buerger's disease]
Inflammatory occlusive disease resulting in poor circulation to legs, feet, and sometimes hands due to progressive inflammatory narrowing of the small arteries
Presenile gangrene

443.2 Other arterial dissection

Excludes	dissection of aorta (441.00–441.03) dissection of coronary arteries (414.12)
Coding Clinic: 2002, Q4, P54-55

443.21 Dissection of carotid artery

443.22 Dissection of iliac artery

443.23 Dissection of renal artery

443.24 Dissection of vertebral artery

443.29 Dissection of other artery

443.8 Other specified peripheral vascular diseases

443.81 Peripheral angiopathy in diseases classified elsewhere

Code first underlying disease, as:
   diabetes mellitus (249.7, 250.7)
Coding Clinic: 2004, Q1, P14-15; 1996, Q1, P10

443.82 Erythromelalgia
Coding Clinic: 2005, Q4, P73-74

443.89 Other
Acrocyanosis
Acroparesthesia:
   simple [Schultze's type]
   vasomotor [Nothnagel's type]
Erythrocyanosis

Excludes	chilblains (991.5)
	   frostbite (991.0–991.3)
	   immersion foot (991.4)

Coding Clinic: 2007, Q4, P124

443.9 Peripheral vascular disease, unspecified
Intermittent claudication NOS
Peripheral:
   angiopathy NOS
   vascular disease NOS
Spasm of artery

Excludes	atherosclerosis of the arteries of the extremities (440.20–440.22) spasm of cerebral artery (435.0–435.9)

◀ New   ◀ Revised   ~~deleted~~ Deleted   ● Use Additional Digit(s)   ■ Nonspecific Code
● Not first-listed DX   OGCR Official Guidelines   Coding Clinic   Excludes   Includes   Use additional   Code first   Omit code

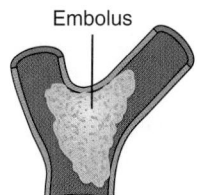

Embolus

Figure 7-6 An arterial embolus.

Item 7-13 An **embolus** is a mass of undissolved matter present in the blood that is transported by the blood current. A **thrombus** is a blood clot that occludes or shuts off a vessel. When a thrombus is dislodged, it becomes an embolus.

● **444　Arterial embolism and thrombosis**

> **Includes**　infarction:
> 　　　embolic
> 　　　thrombotic
> 　　　occlusion

> **Excludes**　*atheroembolism (445.01–445.89)*
> 　　　*septic arterial embolism (449)*
> 　　　*that complicating:*
> 　　　　*abortion (634–638 with .6, 639.6)*
> 　　　　*ectopic or molar pregnancy (639.6)*
> 　　　　*pregnancy, childbirth, or the puerperium*
> 　　　　*(673.0–673.8)*

> Coding Clinic: 2003, Q1, P16-18x2; 1992, Q2, P10-11

444.0　Of abdominal aorta
Aortic bifurcation syndrome
Aortoiliac obstruction
Leriche's syndrome
Saddle embolus
Coding Clinic: 1990, Q4, P27

444.1　Of thoracic aorta
Embolism or thrombosis of aorta (thoracic)

● **444.2　Of arteries of the extremities**

444.21　Upper extremity
Coding Clinic: 1990, Q3, P16

444.22　Lower extremity
Arterial embolism or thrombosis:
　femoral　　　　popliteal
　peripheral NOS

> **Excludes**　*iliofemoral (444.81)*

Coding Clinic: 2007, Q4, P84-86; 2003, Q3, P10

● **444.8　Of other specified artery**

444.81　Iliac artery
Coding Clinic: 2003, Q1, P16-17

■**444.89　Other**

> **Excludes**　*basilar (433.0)*
> 　　*carotid (433.1)*
> 　　*cerebral (434.0–434.9)*
> 　　*coronary (410.00–410.92)*
> 　　*mesenteric (557.0)*
> 　　*ophthalmic (362.30–362.34)*
> 　　*precerebral (433.0–433.9)*
> 　　*pulmonary (415.19)*
> 　　*renal (593.81)*
> 　　*retinal (362.30–362.34)*
> 　　*vertebral (433.2)*

■**444.9　Of unspecified artery**

● **445　Atheroembolism**

> **Includes**　Atherothrombotic microembolism
> 　　　Cholesterol embolism

> Coding Clinic: 2002, Q4, P57-58

● **445.0　Of extremities**

445.01　Upper extremity

445.02　Lower extremity

● **445.8　Of other sites**

445.81　Kidney

> Use additional code for any associated acute
> ~~renal~~ kidney failure or chronic kidney
> disease (584, 585)　　　　　◄▥

■**445.89　Other site**

● **446　Polyarteritis nodosa and allied conditions**

446.0　Polyarteritis nodosa
Disseminated necrotizing periarteritis
Necrotizing angiitis
Panarteritis (nodosa)
Periarteritis (nodosa)

446.1　Acute febrile mucocutaneous lymph node syndrome [MCLS]
Kawasaki disease

● **446.2　Hypersensitivity angiitis**

> **Excludes**　*antiglomerular basement membrane disease*
> 　　*without pulmonary hemorrhage*
> 　　*(583.89)*

■**446.20　Hypersensitivity angiitis, unspecified**

446.21　Goodpasture's syndrome
Antiglomerular basement membrane
　antibody-mediated nephritis with
　pulmonary hemorrhage

> Use additional code to identify renal
> disease (583.81)

■**446.29　Other specified hypersensitivity angiitis**
Coding Clinic: 1995, Q1, P3

446.3　Lethal midline granuloma
Malignant granuloma of face

446.4　Wegener's granulomatosis
Necrotizing respiratory granulomatosis
Wegener's syndrome
Coding Clinic: 2000, Q3, P11

446.5　Giant cell arteritis
Cranial arteritis
Horton's disease
Temporal arteritis

446.6　Thrombotic microangiopathy
Moschcowitz's syndrome
Thrombotic thrombocytopenic purpura

446.7　Takayasu's disease
Aortic arch arteritis
Pulseless disease

DISEASES OF THE CIRCULATORY SYSTEM (390–459)

● **447   Other disorders of arteries and arterioles**

    447.0   Arteriovenous fistula, acquired
       Arteriovenous aneurysm, acquired

       Excludes   *cerebrovascular (437.3)*
           coronary (414.19)
           pulmonary (417.0)
           surgically created arteriovenous shunt or
             fistula:
             complication (996.1, 996.61–996.62)
             status or presence (V45.11)
           traumatic (900.0–904.9)

    447.1   Stricture of artery
       Coding Clinic: 1993, Q2, P8; 1987, Jan-Feb, P14

    447.2   Rupture of artery
       Erosion of artery
       Fistula, except arteriovenous of artery
       Ulcer of artery

       Excludes   *traumatic rupture of artery (900.0–904.9)*

    447.3   Hyperplasia of renal artery
       Fibromuscular hyperplasia of renal artery

    447.4   Celiac artery compression syndrome
       Celiac axis syndrome
       Marable's syndrome

    447.5   Necrosis of artery

    ■**447.6   Arteritis, unspecified**
       Aortitis NOS
       Endarteritis NOS

       Excludes   *arteritis, endarteritis:*
           aortic arch (446.7)
           cerebral (437.4)
           coronary (414.00–414.07)
           deformans (440.0–440.9)
           obliterans (440.0–440.9)
           pulmonary (417.8)
           senile (440.0–440.9)
         polyarteritis NOS (446.0)
         syphilitic aortitis (093.1)
       Coding Clinic: 1999, Q4, P21-22

    ■**447.8   Other specified disorders of arteries and arterioles**
       Fibromuscular hyperplasia of arteries, except
          renal

    ■**447.9   Unspecified disorders of arteries and arterioles**

● **448   Disease of capillaries**

    448.0   Hereditary hemorrhagic telangiectasia
       Rendu-Osler-Weber disease

    448.1   Nevus, non-neoplastic
       Nevus:
          araneus
          senile
          spider
          stellar

       Excludes   *neoplastic (216.0–216.9)*
           port wine (757.32)
           strawberry (757.32)

    ■**448.9   Other and unspecified capillary diseases**
       Capillary:
          hemorrhage
          hyperpermeability
          thrombosis

       Excludes   *capillary fragility (hereditary) (287.8)*

449   Septic arterial embolism

       Code first underlying infection, such as:
       infective endocarditis (421.0)
       lung abscess (513.0)

       Use additional code to identify the site of the embolism
          (433.0–433.9, 444.0–444.9)

       Excludes   *septic pulmonary embolism (415.12)*
       Coding Clinic: 2007, Q4, P84-86

DISEASES OF VEINS AND LYMPHATICS, AND OTHER DISEASES OF CIRCULATORY SYSTEM (451–459)

● **451   Phlebitis and thrombophlebitis**
       Inflammation of vein with infiltration of walls (phlebitis)
          and, usually, formation of clot (thrombus) in vein
          (thrombophlebitis)

       Includes   endophlebitis
          inflammation, vein
          periphlebitis
          suppurative phlebitis

       Use additional E code to identify drug if drug-induced

       Excludes   *that complicating:*
          abortion (634–638 with .7, 639.8)
          ectopic or molar pregnancy (639.8)
          pregnancy, childbirth, or the puerperium
             (671.0–671.9)
          that due to or following:
          implant or catheter device (996.61–996.62)
          infusion, perfusion, or transfusion (999.2)
       Coding Clinic: 2004, Q4, P78-80; 1993, Q1, P26; 1992, Q1, P15-16

    451.0   Of superficial vessels of lower extremities
       Saphenous vein (greater) (lesser)

    ● **451.1   Of deep vessels of lower extremities**
       Coding Clinic: 1991, Q3, P16

       451.11   Femoral vein (deep) (superficial)

       ■**451.19   Other**
          Femoropopliteal vein
          Popliteal vein
          Tibial vein

    ■**451.2   Of lower extremities, unspecified**
       Coding Clinic: 2004, Q4, P78-80

    ● **451.8   Of other sites**

       Excludes   *intracranial venous sinus (325)*
          nonpyogenic (437.6)
          portal (vein) (572.1)

       451.81   Iliac vein

       451.82   Of superficial veins of upper extremities
          Antecubital vein
          Basilic vein
          Cephalic vein

       451.83   Of deep veins of upper extremities
          Brachial vein
          Radial vein
          Ulnar vein

       ■**451.84   Of upper extremities, unspecified**

       ■**451.89   Other**
          Axillary vein
          Jugular vein
          Subclavian vein
          Thrombophlebitis of breast (Mondor's
            disease)

    ■**451.9   Of unspecified site**

    452   Portal vein thrombosis
       Portal (vein) obstruction

       Excludes   *hepatic vein thrombosis (453.0)*
          phlebitis of portal vein (572.1)

◄ New   ◄■ Revised   ~~deleted~~ Deleted   ● Use Additional Digit(s)   ■ Nonspecific Code
● Not first-listed DX   OGCR Official Guidelines   Coding Clinic   Excludes   Includes   Use additional   Code first   Omit code

DISEASES OF THE CIRCULATORY SYSTEM (390–459)

● **453   Other venous embolism and thrombosis**

> **Excludes**   *that complicating:*
> *abortion (634–638 with .7, 639.8)*
> *ectopic or molar pregnancy (639.8)*
> *pregnancy, childbirth, or the puerperium*
> *(671.0–671.9)*
> ~~*that with inflammation, phlebitis, and*~~
> ~~*thrombophlebitis (451.0–451.9)*~~
>
> Coding Clinic: 2004, Q4, P78-80; 1992, Q1, P15-16

453.0   Budd-Chiari syndrome
> Hepatic vein thrombosis

453.1   Thrombophlebitis migrans
> *"White leg" is the other term used to describe a*
> *migrating thrombus.*

453.2   Of inferior vena cava ◀▥

453.3   Of renal vein

● **453.4   Acute ~~V~~venous embolism and thrombosis of deep vessels of lower extremity** ◀▥

▪ **453.40   Acute ~~V~~venous embolism and thrombosis of unspecified deep vessels of lower extremity** ◀▥
> Deep vein thrombosis NOS
> DVT NOS

453.41   Acute ~~V~~venous embolism and thrombosis of deep vessels of proximal lower extremity ◀▥
> Femoral
> Iliac
> Popliteal
> Thigh
> Upper leg NOS
> Coding Clinic: 2004, Q4, P78-80

453.42   Acute ~~V~~venous embolism and thrombosis of deep vessels of distal lower extremity ◀▥
> Calf
> Lower leg NOS
> Peroneal
> Tibial

● **453.5   Chronic venous embolism and thrombosis of deep vessels of lower extremity** ◀

> Use additional code, if applicable, for associated long-term (current) use of anticoagulants (V58.61) ◀
>
> **Excludes**   *personal history of venous thrombosis and embolism (V12.51)* ◀

453.50   Chronic venous embolism and thrombosis of unspecified deep vessels of lower extremity ◀

453.51   Chronic venous embolism and thrombosis of deep vessels of proximal lower extremity ◀

453.52   Chronic venous embolism and thrombosis of deep vessels of distal lower extremity ◀

453.6   Venous embolism and thrombosis of superficial vessels of lower extremity ◀
> Saphenous vein (greater) (lesser) ◀

● **453.7   Chronic venous embolism and thrombosis of other specified vessels** ◀

> Use additional code, if applicable, for associated long-term (current) use of anticoagulants (V58.61) ◀
>
> **Excludes**   *personal history of venous thrombosis and embolism (V12.51)* ◀

453.71   Chronic venous embolism and thrombosis of superficial veins of upper extremity ◀
> Antecubital vein ◀
> Basilic vein ◀
> Cephalic vein ◀

453.72   Chronic venous embolism and thrombosis of deep veins of upper extremity ◀
> Brachial vein ◀
> Radial vein ◀
> Ulnar vein ◀

453.73   Chronic venous embolism and thrombosis of upper extremity, unspecified ◀

453.74   Chronic venous embolism and thrombosis of axillary veins ◀

453.75   Chronic venous embolism and thrombosis of subclavian veins ◀

453.76   Chronic venous embolism and thrombosis of internal jugular veins ◀

453.77   Chronic venous embolism and thrombosis of other thoracic veins ◀
> Brachiocephalic (innominate) ◀
> Superior vena cava ◀

453.79   Chronic venous embolism and thrombosis of other specified veins ◀

● **453.8   Acute venous embolism and thrombosis ⊖of other specified veins** ◀▥

> **Excludes**   *cerebral (434.0–434.9)*
> *coronary (410.00–410.92)*
> *intracranial venous sinus (325)*
>   *nonpyogenic (437.6)*
> *mesenteric (557.0)*
> *portal (452)*
> *precerebral (433.0–433.9)*
> *pulmonary (415.19)*
>
> Coding Clinic: 2004, Q4, P78-80; 1992, Q1, P15-16

453.81   Acute venous embolism and thrombosis of superficial veins of upper extremity ◀
> Antecubital vein ◀
> Basilic vein ◀
> Cephalic vein ◀

453.82   Acute venous embolism and thrombosis of deep veins of upper extremity ◀
> Brachial vein ◀
> Radial vein ◀
> Ulnar vein ◀

453.83   Acute venous embolism and thrombosis of upper extremity, unspecified ◀

453.84   Acute venous embolism and thrombosis of axillary veins ◀

453.85   Acute venous embolism and thrombosis of subclavian veins ◀

453.86   Acute venous embolism and thrombosis of internal jugular veins ◀

453.87   Acute venous embolism and thrombosis of other thoracic veins ◀
> Brachiocephalic (innominate) ◀
> Superior vena cava ◀

453.89   Acute venous embolism and thrombosis of other specified veins ◀

▪ **453.9   Of unspecified site**
> Embolism of vein
> Thrombosis (vein)

Item 7–14 Varicose/Varicosities (varix = singular, varices = plural): Enlarged, engorged, tortuous, twisted vascular vessels (veins, arteries, lymphatics). As such, the condition can present in various parts of the body, although the most familiar locations are the lower extremities. A common complication of varices is thrombophlebitis. Varicosities of the anus and rectum are called hemorrhoids. There are additional codes for esophageal, sublingual (under the tongue), scrotal, pelvic, vulval, and nasal varices as well.

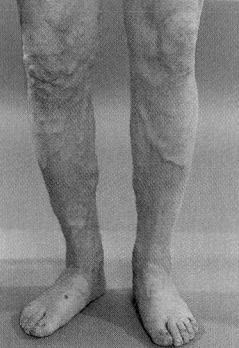

Figure 7–7 Varicose veins of the legs. (From Goldman: Cecil Medicine, 23rd ed. 2008, Saunders)

● **454 Varicose veins of lower extremities**

  Excludes *that complicating pregnancy, childbirth, or the puerperium (671.0)*

  454.0 With ulcer   A
      Varicose ulcer (lower extremity, any part)
      Varicose veins with ulcer of lower extremity [any part] or of unspecified site
      Any condition classifiable to 454.9 with ulcer or specified as ulcerated
      Coding Clinic: 1999, Q4, P18

  454.1 With inflammation   A
      Stasis dermatitis
      Varicose veins with inflammation of lower extremity [any part] or of unspecified site
      Any condition classifiable to 454.9 with inflammation or specified as inflamed
      Coding Clinic: 1991, Q2, P20

  454.2 With ulcer and inflammation   A
      Varicose veins with ulcer and inflammation of lower extremity [any part] or of unspecified site
      Any condition classifiable to 454.9 with ulcer and inflammation
      Coding Clinic: 2004, Q3, P5-6; 1991, Q2, P20

  ■**454.8 With other complications**
      Edema
      Pain
      Swelling
      Coding Clinic: 2002, Q4, P58-60

  454.9 Asymptomatic varicose veins   A
      Phlebectasia of lower extremity [any part] or of unspecified site
      Varicose veins NOS
      Varicose veins of lower extremity [any part] or of unspecified site
      Varix of lower extremity [any part] or of unspecified site

● **455 Hemorrhoids**

  Includes hemorrhoids (anus) (rectum)
        piles
        varicose veins, anus or rectum

  Excludes *that complicating pregnancy, childbirth, or the puerperium (671.8)*

  455.0 Internal hemorrhoids without mention of complication
      Coding Clinic: 2005, Q3, P17

  455.1 Internal thrombosed hemorrhoids

  ■**455.2 Internal hemorrhoids with other complication**
      Internal hemorrhoids:
          bleeding
          prolapsed
          strangulated
          ulcerated
      Coding Clinic: 2005, Q3, P17; 2003, Q1, P8

  455.3 External hemorrhoids without mention of complication
      Coding Clinic: 2007, Q1, P13

  455.4 External thrombosed hemorrhoids

  ■**455.5 External hemorrhoids with other complication**
      External hemorrhoids:
          bleeding
          prolapsed
          strangulated
          ulcerated
      Coding Clinic: 2005, Q3, P17; 2003, Q1, P8

  ■**455.6 Unspecified hemorrhoids without mention of complication**
      Hemorrhoids NOS

  ■**455.7 Unspecified thrombosed hemorrhoids**
      Thrombosed hemorrhoids, unspecified whether internal or external

  ■**455.8 Unspecified hemorrhoids with other complication**
      Hemorrhoids, unspecified whether internal or external:
          bleeding
          prolapsed
          strangulated
          ulcerated

  455.9 Residual hemorrhoidal skin tags
      Skin tags, anus or rectum

● **456 Varicose veins of other sites**

  456.0 Esophageal varices with bleeding

  456.1 Esophageal varices without mention of bleeding

● **456.2 Esophageal varices in diseases classified elsewhere**
      Code first underlying disease, as:
          cirrhosis of liver (571.0–571.9)
          portal hypertension (572.3)

    ● *456.20 With bleeding*
        Coding Clinic: 1985, Nov-Dec, P14

    ● *456.21 Without mention of bleeding*
        Coding Clinic: 2005, Q3, P15-16; 2002, Q2, P4

  456.3 Sublingual varices

  456.4 Scrotal varices ♂
      Varicocele

  456.5 Pelvic varices
      Varices of broad ligament

  456.6 Vulval varices ♀
      Varices of perineum

      Excludes *that complicating pregnancy, childbirth, or the puerperium (671.1)*

  ■**456.8 Varices of other sites**
      Varicose veins of nasal septum (with ulcer)

      Excludes *placental varices (656.7)*
            retinal varices (362.17)
            varicose ulcer of unspecified site (454.0)
            varicose veins of unspecified site (454.9)
      Coding Clinic: 2002, Q2, P4

◄ New   ◄▥ Revised   d̶e̶l̶e̶t̶e̶d̶ Deleted   ● Use Additional Digit(s)   ■ Nonspecific Code
● Not first-listed DX   OGCR Official Guidelines   Coding Clinic   Excludes   Includes   Use additional   Code first   Omit code

● **457   Noninfectious disorders of lymphatic channels**

     457.0   Postmastectomy lymphedema syndrome   A
         Elephantiasis due to mastectomy
         Obliteration of lymphatic vessel due to mastectomy
         Coding Clinic: 2002, Q2, P12-13

     ■**457.1   Other lymphedema**
         Elephantiasis (nonfilarial) NOS
         Lymphangiectasis
         Lymphedema:
            acquired (chronic)
            praecox
            secondary
         Obliteration, lymphatic vessel

         Excludes   *elephantiasis (nonfilarial):*
               congenital (757.0)
               eyelid (374.83)
               vulva (624.8)
         Coding Clinic: 2004, Q3, P5-6

     457.2   Lymphangitis
         Lymphangitis:
            NOS
            chronic
            subacute

         Excludes   *acute lymphangitis (682.0–682.9)*

     ■**457.8   Other noninfectious disorders of lymphatic channels**
         Chylocele (nonfilarial)
         Chylous:
            ascites
            cyst
         Lymph node or vessel:
            fistula
            infarction
            rupture

         Excludes   *chylocele:*
               filarial (125.0–125.9)
               tunica vaginalis (nonfilarial) (608.84)
         Coding Clinic: 2004, Q1, P5; 2003, Q3, P16-17

     ■**457.9   Unspecified noninfectious disorder of lymphatic channels**

● **458   Hypotension**
     Subnormal arterial blood pressure

     Includes   hypopiesis

     Excludes   *cardiovascular collapse (785.50)*
               maternal hypotension syndrome (669.2)
               shock (785.50–785.59)
               Shy-Drager syndrome (333.0)
     Coding Clinic: 1994, Q3, P9; 1993, 5th Issue, P6-7

     458.0   Orthostatic hypotension
         Hypotension:
            orthostatic (chronic)
            postural
            Moving from sitting or reclining position to standing position precipitates sudden drop in blood pressure.
         Coding Clinic: 2000, Q3, P8-9

     458.1   Chronic hypotension
         Permanent idiopathic hypotension

     458.2   Iatrogenic hypotension
         Coding Clinic: 2002, Q3, P12; 1993, Q4, P41-42

       458.21   Hypotension of hemodialysis
            Intra-dialytic hypotension
            Coding Clinic: 2003, Q4, P60-61

       458.29   Other iatrogenic hypotension
            Postoperative hypotension
            Coding Clinic: 1993, Q4, P41-42

     ■**458.8   Other specified hypotension**
         Coding Clinic: 1997. Q4, P37

     ■**458.9   Hypotension, unspecified**
         Hypotension (arterial) NOS

● **459   Other disorders of circulatory system**

     ■**459.0   Hemorrhage, unspecified**
         Rupture of blood vessel NOS
         Spontaneous hemorrhage NEC

         Excludes   *hemorrhage:*
               gastrointestinal NOS (578.9)
               in newborn NOS (772.9)
               nontraumatic hematoma of soft tissue (729.92)
               secondary or recurrent following trauma (958.2)
               traumatic rupture of blood vessel (900.0–904.9)
         Coding Clinic: 1999, Q4, P18

     ●**459.1   Postphlebitic syndrome**
         Chronic venous hypertension due to deep vein thrombosis

         Excludes   *chronic venous hypertension without deep vein thrombosis (459.30–459.39)*
         Coding Clinic: 2002, Q4, P58-60; 1991, Q2, P20

       459.10   Postphlebitic syndrome without complications
            Asymptomatic postphlebitic syndrome
            Postphlebitic syndrome NOS

       459.11   Postphlebitic syndrome with ulcer

       459.12   Postphlebitic syndrome with inflammation

       459.13   Postphlebitic syndrome with ulcer and inflammation

       ■**459.19   Postphlebitic syndrome with other complication**

     459.2   Compression of vein
         Stricture of vein
         Vena cava syndrome (inferior) (superior)

     ●**459.3   Chronic venous hypertension (idiopathic)**
         Stasis edema

         Excludes   *chronic venous hypertension due to deep vein thrombosis (459.10–459.19)*
               varicose veins (454.0–454.9)
         Coding Clinic: 2002, Q4, P58-60

       459.30   Chronic venous hypertension without complications
            Asymptomatic chronic venous hypertension
            Chronic venous hypertension NOS

       459.31   Chronic venous hypertension with ulcer

       459.32   Chronic venous hypertension with inflammation

       459.33   Chronic venous hypertension with ulcer and inflammation

       ■**459.39   Chronic venous hypertension with other complication**

     ●**459.8   Other specified disorders of circulatory system**

       ■**459.81   Venous (peripheral) insufficiency, unspecified**
            Chronic venous insufficiency NOS

            Use additional code for any associated ulceration (707.10–707.9)
            Coding Clinic: 2004, Q3, P5-6; 1991, Q2, P20

       ■**459.89   Other**
            Collateral circulation (venous), any site
            Phlebosclerosis
            Venofibrosis

     ■**459.9   Unspecified circulatory system disorder**

DISEASES OF THE CIRCULATORY SYSTEM (390–459)

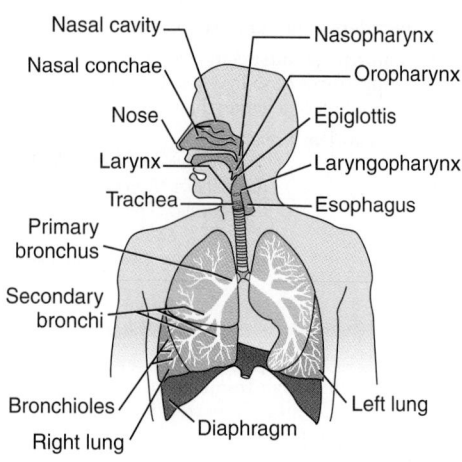

Figure 8–1 Respiratory system. (From Buck CJ: Step-by-Step Medical Coding, 2006 ed. Philadelphia, WB Saunders, 2006.)

8. DISEASES OF THE RESPIRATORY SYSTEM (460–519)

Use additional code to identify infectious organism

ACUTE RESPIRATORY INFECTIONS (460–466)

Excludes *pneumonia and influenza (480.0–488)*

460 Acute nasopharyngitis [common cold]
Coryza (acute)
Nasal catarrh, acute

Nasopharyngitis:	Rhinitis:
NOS	acute
acute	infective
infective NOS	

Excludes *nasopharyngitis, chronic (472.2)*
pharyngitis:
acute or unspecified (462)
chronic (472.1)
rhinitis:
allergic (477.0–477.9)
chronic or unspecified (472.0)
sore throat:
acute or unspecified (462)
chronic (472.1)
Coding Clinic: 1988, Q1, P12

● **461 Acute sinusitis**
Code to specific sinus if indicated in documentation.

Includes abscess, acute, of sinus (accessory) (nasal)
empyema, acute, of sinus (accessory) (nasal)
infection, acute, of sinus (accessory) (nasal)
inflammation, acute, of sinus (accessory) (nasal)
suppuration, acute, of sinus (accessory) (nasal)

Excludes *chronic or unspecified sinusitis (473.0–473.9)*

461.0 Maxillary
Acute antritis

461.1 Frontal

461.2 Ethmoidal

461.3 Sphenoidal

■ **461.8 Other acute sinusitis**
Acute pansinusitis

■ **461.9 Acute sinusitis, unspecified**
Acute sinusitis NOS

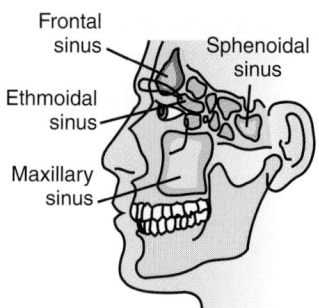

Figure 8–2 Paranasal sinuses. (From Buck CJ: Step-by-Step Medical Coding, 2006 ed. Philadelphia, WB Saunders, 2006.)

Item 8-1 Pharyngitis is painful inflammation of the pharynx (sore throat). Ninety percent of the infections are caused by a virus with the remaining being bacterial and rarely a fungus (candidiasis). Other irritants such as pollutants, chemicals, or smoke may cause similar symptoms.

462 Acute pharyngitis
Acute sore throat NOS
Pharyngitis (acute):
NOS
gangrenous
infective
phlegmonous
pneumococcal
staphylococcal
suppurative
ulcerative
Sore throat (viral) NOS
Viral pharyngitis

Excludes *abscess:*
peritonsillar [quinsy] (475)
pharyngeal NOS (478.29)
retropharyngeal (478.24)
chronic pharyngitis (472.1)
infectious mononucleosis (075)
that specified as (due to):
Coxsackie (virus) (074.0)
gonococcus (098.6)
herpes simplex (054.79)
influenza (487.1)
septic (034.0)
streptococcal (034.0)
Coding Clinic: 1985, Sept-Oct, P9

463 Acute tonsillitis
Inflammation of pharyngeal tonsils caused by virus/bacteria

Tonsillitis (acute):	Tonsillitis (acute):
NOS	septic
follicular	staphylococcal
gangrenous	suppurative
infective	ulcerative
pneumococcal	viral

Excludes *chronic tonsillitis (474.0)*
hypertrophy of tonsils (474.1)
peritonsillar abscess [quinsy] (475)
sore throat:
acute or NOS (462)
septic (034.0)
streptococcal tonsillitis (034.0)
Coding Clinic: 1984, Nov-Dec, P16

◀ New   ◀▥ Revised   ~~deleted~~ Deleted   ● Use Additional Digit(s)   ■ Nonspecific Code
● Not first-listed DX   OGCR Official Guidelines   Coding Clinic   Excludes   Includes   Use additional   Code first   Omit code

Item 8-2   Laryngitis is an inflammation of the larynx (voice box) resulting in hoarse voice or the complete loss of the voice. **Tracheitis** is an inflammation of the trachea (often following a URI) commonly caused by *staphylococcus aureus* resulting in inspiratory stridor (crowing sound on inspiration) and a croup like cough.

● **464   Acute laryngitis and tracheitis**

    Excludes   *that associated with influenza (487.1)*
        that due to Streptococcus (034.0)

● **464.0   Acute laryngitis**
    Laryngitis (acute):
      NOS
      edematous
      Hemophilus influenzae [H. influenzae]
      pneumococcal
      septic
      suppurative
      ulcerative

      Excludes   *chronic laryngitis (476.0–476.1)*
          influenzal laryngitis (487.1)

    464.00   Without mention of obstruction

    464.01   With obstruction

● **464.1   Acute tracheitis**
    Tracheitis (acute):   Tracheitis (acute):
      NOS   viral
      catarrhal

      Excludes   *chronic tracheitis (491.8)*

    464.10   Without mention of obstruction

    464.11   With obstruction

● **464.2   Acute laryngotracheitis**
    Laryngotracheitis (acute)
    Tracheitis (acute) with laryngitis (acute)

      Excludes   *chronic laryngotracheitis (476.1)*

    464.20   Without mention of obstruction

    464.21   With obstruction

● **464.3   Acute epiglottitis**
    Viral epiglottitis

      Excludes   *epiglottitis, chronic (476.1)*

    464.30   Without mention of obstruction

    464.31   With obstruction

  464.4   Croup
    Croup syndrome

● **464.5   Supraglottitis, unspecified**

    464.50   Without mention of obstruction
       Coding Clinic: 2001, Q4, P42-43

    464.51   With obstruction

● **465   Acute upper respiratory infections of multiple or unspecified sites**

    Excludes   *upper respiratory infection due to:*
        influenza (487.1)
        Streptococcus (034.0)

  465.0   Acute laryngopharyngitis

■ **465.8   Other multiple sites**
    Multiple URI
    Coding Clinic: 2007, Q4, P84-86

■ **465.9   Unspecified site**
    Acute URI NOS
    Upper respiratory infection (acute)
    Coding Clinic: 1990, Q1, P19

● **466   Acute bronchitis and bronchiolitis**

    Includes   that with:
        bronchospasm
        obstruction

  466.0   Acute bronchitis
    Inflammation/irritation of bronchial tubes lasting 2-3 weeks, which is most commonly caused by a virus
    Bronchitis, acute or   Bronchitis, acute or
      subacute: subacute:
      fibrinous   septic
      membranous   viral
      pneumococcal   with tracheitis
      purulent
    Croupous bronchitis
    Tracheobronchitis, acute

    Excludes   *acute bronchitis with chronic obstructive pulmonary disease (491.22)*
    Coding Clinic: 2004, Q4, P81-82,137; Q1, P3; 2002, Q4, P46; 1996, Q4, P27-28; 1993, 5th Issue, P4x2; 1991, Q3, P17-18; 1988, Q1, P12

  OGCR Section I.C.8.b.1

  Acute bronchitis, 466.0, is due to an infectious organism. When acute bronchitis is documented with COPD, code 491.22, Obstructive chronic bronchitis with acute bronchitis, should be assigned. It is not necessary to also assign code 466.0. If a medical record documents acute bronchitis with COPD with acute exacerbation, only code 491.22 should be assigned. The acute bronchitis included in code 491.22 supersedes the acute exacerbation. If a medical record documents COPD with acute exacerbation without mention of acute bronchitis, only code 491.21 should be assigned.

● **466.1   Acute bronchiolitis**
    Bronchiolitis (acute)
    Capillary pneumonia
    Coding Clinic: 1988, Q1, P12

    466.11   Acute bronchiolitis due to respiratory syncytial virus (RSV)
       Coding Clinic: 2005, Q1, P10; 1996, Q4, P27-28

    ■ **466.19   Acute bronchiolitis due to other infectious organisms**

       Use additional code to identify organism

OTHER DISEASES OF THE UPPER RESPIRATORY TRACT (470–478)

---

  470   Deviated nasal septum
    Deflected septum (nasal) (acquired)

    Excludes   *congenital (754.0)*

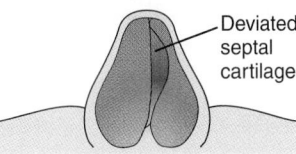

Deviated septal cartilage

Figure 8–3   Deviated nasal septum.

Item 8-3   A deviated nasal septum is the displacement of the septal cartilage that separates the nares. This displacement causes obstructed air flow through the nasal passages. A child can be born with this displacement (congenital), or the condition may be acquired through trauma, such as a sports injury. Symptoms include nasal block, sinusitis, and related secondary infections. Septoplasty is surgical repair of this condition.

Item 8-4   Nasal polyps are an abnormal growth of tissue (tumor) projecting from a mucous membrane and attached to the surface by a narrow elongated stalk (pedunculated). Nasal polyps usually originate in the ethmoid sinus but also may occur in the maxillary sinus. Symptoms are nasal block, sinusitis, anosmia, and secondary infections.

DISEASES OF THE RESPIRATORY SYSTEM (460–519)

● **471 Nasal polyps**

     Excludes *adenomatous polyps (212.0)*

     471.0 Polyp of nasal cavity
        Polyp:
          choanal
          nasopharyngeal

     471.1 Polypoid sinus degeneration
        Woakes' syndrome or ethmoiditis

     ■**471.8 Other polyp of sinus**
        Polyp of sinus:
          accessory
          ethmoidal
          maxillary
          sphenoidal

     ■**471.9 Unspecified nasal polyp**
        Nasal polyp NOS

● **472 Chronic pharyngitis and nasopharyngitis**

     472.0 Chronic rhinitis
        Ozena
        Rhinitis: Rhinitis:
          NOS   obstructive
          atrophic   purulent
          granulomatous   ulcerative
          hypertrophic

        Excludes *allergic rhinitis (477.0–477.9)*

     472.1 Chronic pharyngitis
        Chronic sore throat
        Pharyngitis: Pharyngitis:
          atrophic   hypertrophic
          granular (chronic)

     472.2 Chronic nasopharyngitis

        Excludes *acute or unspecified nasopharyngitis (460)*

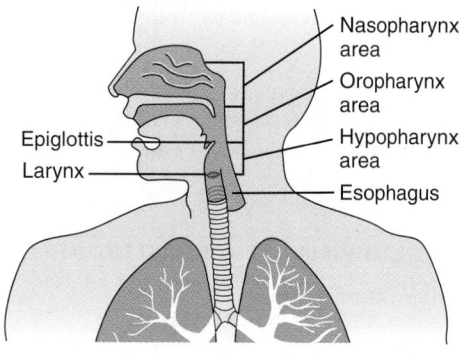

Nasopharynx area
Oropharynx area
Hypopharynx area
Esophagus
Epiglottis
Larynx

Figure 8–4   The pharynx.

Item 8–5   The **pharynx** is the passage for both food and air between the mouth and the esophagus and is divided into three areas: nasopharynx, oropharynx, and hypopharynx. The hypopharynx branches into the esophagus and the voice box.

● **473 Chronic sinusitis**

     Includes   abscess (chronic) of sinus (accessory) (nasal)
                   empyema (chronic) of sinus (accessory) (nasal)
                   infection (chronic) of sinus (accessory) (nasal)
                   suppuration (chronic) of sinus (accessory) (nasal)

     Excludes *acute sinusitis (461.0–461.9)*

     473.0 Maxillary
        Antritis (chronic)

     473.1 Frontal

     473.2 Ethmoidal

        Excludes *Woakes' ethmoiditis (471.1)*

     473.3 Sphenoidal

     ■**473.8 Other chronic sinusitis**
        Pansinusitis (chronic)

     ■**473.9 Unspecified sinusitis (chronic)**
        Sinusitis (chronic) NOS

● **474 Chronic disease of tonsils and adenoids**

   ● **474.0 Chronic tonsillitis and adenoiditis**

        Excludes *acute or unspecified tonsillitis (463)*

       474.00 Chronic tonsillitis
          Coding Clinic: 1984, Nov-Dec, P16

       474.01 Chronic adenoiditis

       474.02 Chronic tonsillitis and adenoiditis

   ● **474.1 Hypertrophy of tonsils and adenoids**
        Enlargement of tonsils or adenoids
        Hyperplasia of tonsils or adenoids
        Hypertrophy of tonsils or adenoids

        Excludes *that with:*
              adenoiditis (474.01)
              adenoiditis and tonsillitis (474.02)
              tonsillitis (474.00)

       474.10 Tonsils with adenoids
          Coding Clinic: 2005, Q2, P16

       474.11 Tonsils alone
          Coding Clinic: 1984, Nov-Dec, P16

       474.12 Adenoids alone

     474.2 Adenoid vegetations

     ■**474.8 Other chronic disease of tonsils and adenoids**
        Amygdalolith
        Calculus, tonsil
        Cicatrix of tonsil (and adenoid)
        Tonsillar tag
        Ulcer, tonsil

     ■**474.9 Unspecified chronic disease of tonsils and adenoids**
        Disease (chronic) of tonsils (and adenoids)

  475 Peritonsillar abscess
        Abscess of tonsil
        Peritonsillar cellulitis
        Quinsy

     Excludes *tonsillitis:*
          acute or NOS (463)
          chronic (474.0)

● **476 Chronic laryngitis and laryngotracheitis**

476.0 Chronic laryngitis

Laryngitis:	Laryngitis:
catarrhal	sicca
hypertrophic	

476.1 Chronic laryngotracheitis

Laryngitis, chronic, with tracheitis (chronic)

Tracheitis, chronic, with laryngitis

Excludes *chronic tracheitis (491.8)*
laryngitis and tracheitis, acute or
unspecified (464.00–464.51)

● **477 Allergic rhinitis**

Includes allergic rhinitis (nonseasonal) (seasonal)
hay fever
spasmodic rhinorrhea

Excludes *allergic rhinitis with asthma (bronchial) (493.0)*

477.0 Due to pollen
Pollinosis

477.1 Due to food

477.2 Due to animal (cat) (dog) hair and dander

■ **477.8 Due to other allergen**

■ **477.9 Cause unspecified**
Coding Clinic: 1997, Q2, P9-10

● **478 Other diseases of upper respiratory tract**

478.0 Hypertrophy of nasal turbinates

● **478.1 Other diseases of nasal cavity and sinuses**

Excludes *varicose ulcer of nasal septum (456.8)*

Coding Clinic: 1995, Q4, P50; 1990, Q1, P8

478.11 Nasal mucositis (ulcerative)

Use additional E code to identify adverse
effects of therapy, such as:
antineoplastic and immunosuppressive
drugs (E930.7, E933.1)
radiation therapy (E879.2)
Coding Clinic: 2006, Q4, P88-91

■ **478.19 Other disease of nasal cavity and sinuses**
Abscess of nose (septum)
Cyst or mucocele of sinus (nasal)
Necrosis of nose (septum)
Rhinolith
Ulcer of nose (septum)

● **478.2 Other diseases of pharynx, not elsewhere classified**

■ **478.20 Unspecified disease of pharynx**

478.21 Cellulitis of pharynx or nasopharynx

478.22 Parapharyngeal abscess

478.24 Retropharyngeal abscess

478.25 Edema of pharynx or nasopharynx

478.26 Cyst of pharynx or nasopharynx

■ **478.29 Other**
Abscess of pharynx or nasopharynx

Excludes *ulcerative pharyngitis (462)*

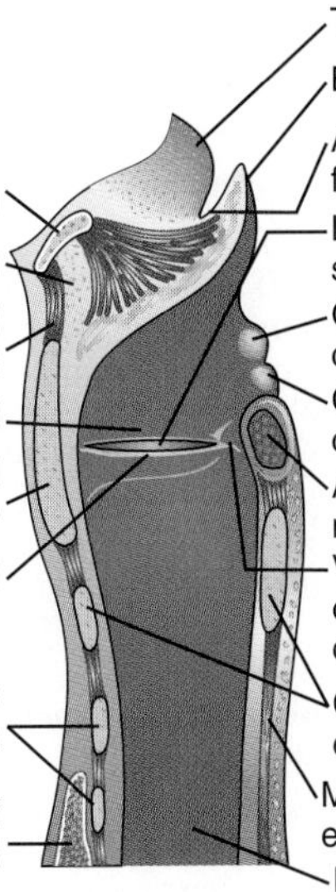

Figure 8–5   Coronal section of the larynx.

Item 8–6 The **larynx** extends from the tongue to the trachea and is divided into an upper and lower portion separated by folds. The framework of the larynx is cartilage composed of the single cricoid, thyroid, and epiglottic cartilages, and the paired arytenoid, cuneiform, and corniculate cartilages.

● **478.3 Paralysis of vocal cords or larynx**

■ **478.30 Paralysis, unspecified**
Laryngoplegia
Paralysis of glottis

478.31 Unilateral, partial

478.32 Unilateral, complete

478.33 Bilateral, partial

478.34 Bilateral, complete

478.4 Polyp of vocal cord or larynx

Excludes *adenomatous polyps (212.1)*

■ **478.5 Other diseases of vocal cords**
Abscess of vocal cords
Cellulitis of vocal cords
Granuloma of vocal cords
Leukoplakia of vocal cords
Chorditis (fibrinous) (nodosa) (tuberosa)
Singers' nodes

478.6 Edema of larynx
Edema (of):
glottis
subglottic
supraglottic

DISEASES OF THE RESPIRATORY SYSTEM (460–519)

- 478.7 **Other diseases of larynx, not elsewhere classified**
  - 478.70 **Unspecified disease of larynx**
  - 478.71 **Cellulitis and perichondritis of larynx**
  - 478.74 **Stenosis of larynx**
  - 478.75 **Laryngeal spasm**
    Laryngismus (stridulus)
  - 478.79 **Other**
    Abscess of larynx
    Necrosis of larynx
    Obstruction of larynx
    Pachyderma of larynx
    Ulcer of larynx
    > **Excludes** *ulcerative laryngitis (464.00–464.01)*
    Coding Clinic: 1991, Q3, P20

- 478.8 **Upper respiratory tract hypersensitivity reaction, site unspecified**
  > **Excludes** *hypersensitivity reaction of lower respiratory tract, as:*
  > *extrinsic allergic alveolitis (495.0–495.9)*
  > *pneumoconiosis (500–505)*

- 478.9 **Other and unspecified diseases of upper respiratory tract**
  Abscess of trachea
  Cicatrix of trachea

PNEUMONIA AND INFLUENZA (480–488)

> **Excludes** *pneumonia:*
> *allergic or eosinophilic (518.3)*
> *aspiration:*
> *NOS (507.0)*
> *newborn (770.18)*
> *solids and liquids (507.0–507.8)*
> *congenital (770.0)*
> *lipoid (507.1)*
> *passive (514)*
> *rheumatic (390)*
> *ventilator-associated (997.31)*

Item 8-7 Pneumonia is an infection of the lungs, caused by a variety of microorganisms, including viruses, most commonly the *Streptococcus pneumoniae* (pneumococcus) bacteria, fungi, and parasites. Pneumonia occurs when the immune system is weakened, often by a URI or influenza.

- 480 **Viral pneumonia**
  - 480.0 **Pneumonia due to adenovirus**
  - 480.1 **Pneumonia due to respiratory syncytial virus**
    Coding Clinic: 1996, Q4, P27-28; 1988, Q1, P12
  - 480.2 **Pneumonia due to parainfluenza virus**
  - 480.3 **Pneumonia due to SARS-associated coronavirus**
    Coding Clinic: 2003, Q4, P46-48
  - 480.8 **Pneumonia due to other virus not elsewhere classified**
    > **Excludes** *congenital rubella pneumonitis (771.0)*
    > *influenza with pneumonia, any form (487.0)*
    > *pneumonia complicating viral diseases classified elsewhere (484.1–484.8)*
  - 480.9 **Viral pneumonia, unspecified**
    Coding Clinic: 1998, Q3, P5

- 481 **Pneumococcal pneumonia [Streptococcus pneumoniae pneumonia]**
  Lobar pneumonia, organism unspecified
  Coding Clinic: 1998, Q2, P7; 1991, Q1, P13; 1988, Q1, P13; 1985, Mar-April, P6

- 482 **Other bacterial pneumonia**
  - 482.0 **Pneumonia due to Klebsiella pneumoniae**
  - 482.1 **Pneumonia due to Pseudomonas**
  - 482.2 **Pneumonia due to Hemophilus influenzae [H. influenzae]**
    Coding Clinic: 2005, Q2, P19-20; 1993, Q4, P39
  - 482.3 **Pneumonia due to Streptococcus**
    > **Excludes** *Streptococcus pneumoniae pneumonia (481)*
    Coding Clinic: 1988, Q1, P13
    - 482.30 **Streptococcus, unspecified**
    - 482.31 **Group A**
    - 482.32 **Group B**
    - 482.39 **Other Streptococcus**
  - 482.4 **Pneumonia due to Staphylococcus**
    Coding Clinic: 1991, Q3, P16-17
    - 482.40 **Pneumonia due to Staphylococcus, unspecified**
    - 482.41 **Methicillin susceptible pneumonia due to Staphylococcus aureus**
      MSSA pneumonia
      Pneumonia due to Staphylococcus aureus NOS
      Coding Clinic: 2008, Q4, P69-73
    - 482.42 **Methicillin resistant pneumonia due to Staphylococcus aureus**
      Coding Clinic: 2008, Q4, P69-73
    - 482.49 **Other Staphylococcus pneumonia**
  - 482.8 **Pneumonia due to other specified bacteria**
    > **Excludes** *pneumonia complicating infectious disease classified elsewhere (484.1–484.8)*
    Coding Clinic: 1988, Q3, P11
    - 482.81 **Anaerobes**
      Bacteroides (melaninogenicus)
      Gram-negative anaerobes
    - 482.82 **Escherichia coli [E. coli]**
    - 482.83 **Other gram-negative bacteria**
      Gram-negative pneumonia NOS
      Proteus
      Serratia marcescens
      > **Excludes** *gram-negative anaerobes (482.81)*
      > *Legionnaires' disease (482.84)*
      Coding Clinic: 1998, Q2, P5; 1994, Q3, P9; 1993, Q4, P39
    - 482.84 **Legionnaires' disease**
    - 482.89 **Other specified bacteria**
      Coding Clinic: 1998, Q2, P6; 1997, Q2, P6; 1994, Q1, P17-18
  - 482.9 **Bacterial pneumonia unspecified**
    Coding Clinic: 1998, Q2, P4, 6X2; 1997, Q2, P6; 1994, Q1, P17-18

- 483 **Pneumonia due to other specified organism**
  - 483.0 **Mycoplasma pneumoniae**
    Eaton's agent
    Pleuropneumonia-like organisms [PPLO]
    Coding Clinic: 1987, Nov-Dec, P5-6
  - 483.1 **Chlamydia**
  - 483.8 **Other specified organism**

◄ New ◄═ Revised ~~deleted~~ Deleted ● Use Additional Digit(s) ■ Nonspecific Code

● Not first-listed DX   OGCR Official Guidelines   Coding Clinic   Excludes   Includes   Use additional   Code first   Omit code

● **484 Pneumonia in infectious diseases classified elsewhere**
> **Excludes** *influenza with pneumonia, any form (487.0)*

● **484.1 Pneumonia in cytomegalic inclusion disease**
> *Code first* underlying disease, as: (078.5)

● **484.3 Pneumonia in whooping cough**
> *Code first* underlying disease, as: (033.0–033.9)

● **484.5 Pneumonia in anthrax**
> *Code first* underlying disease (022.1)

● **484.6 Pneumonia in aspergillosis**
> *Code first* underlying disease (117.3)
> Coding Clinic: 1997, Q4, P40

● ■**484.7 Pneumonia in other systemic mycoses**
> *Code first* underlying disease
> **Excludes** *pneumonia in:*
> *candidiasis (112.4)*
> *coccidioidomycosis (114.0)*
> *histoplasmosis (115.0–115.9 with fifth-digit 5)*

● ■**484.8 Pneumonia in other infectious diseases classified elsewhere**
> *Code first* underlying disease, as:
> Q fever (083.0)
> typhoid fever (002.0)
> **Excludes** *pneumonia in:*
> *actinomycosis (039.1)*
> *measles (055.1)*
> *nocardiosis (039.1)*
> *ornithosis (073.0)*
> *Pneumocystis carinii (136.3)*
> *salmonellosis (003.22)*
> *toxoplasmosis (130.4)*
> *tuberculosis (011.6)*
> *tularemia (021.2)*
> *varicella (052.1)*

■**485 Bronchopneumonia, organism unspecified**
Bronchopneumonia: Pneumonia:
hemorrhagic lobular
terminal segmental
Pleurobronchopneumonia
> **Excludes** *bronchiolitis (acute) (466.11–466.19)*
> *chronic (491.8)*
> *lipoid pneumonia (507.1)*

■**486 Pneumonia, organism unspecified**
> **Excludes** *hypostatic or passive pneumonia (514)*
> *influenza with pneumonia, any form (487.0)*
> *inhalation or aspiration pneumonia due to foreign materials (507.0–507.8)*
> *pneumonitis due to fumes and vapors (506.0)*
> Coding Clinic: 2008, Q4, P140-143; 2006, Q2, P20; 1999, Q4, P6; Q3, P9; 1998, Q3, P7; Q2, P4-5; Q1, P8; 1997, Q3, P9; 1995, Q4, P52; 1994, Q1, P17-18; 1993, Q3, P9; Q1, P21; 1985, Mar-April, P6

●**487 Influenza**
Influenza caused by unspecified influenza virus ◀
A contagious viral respiratory illness which if left untreated may lead to death.
> **Excludes** *Hemophilus influenzae [H. influenzae]:*
> *infection NOS (041.5)*
> *influenza due to 2009 H1N1 [swine] influenza virus (488.1)* ◀
> *influenza due to identified avian influenza virus (488.0)* ◀
> *influenza due to identified novel H1N1 influenza virus (488.1)* ◀
> *laryngitis (464.00–464.01)*
> *meningitis (320.0)*

487.0 With pneumonia
Influenza with pneumonia, any form
Influenzal:
bronchopneumonia
pneumonia
> Use additional code to identify the type of pneumonia (480.0–480.9, 481, 482.0–482.9, 483.0–483.8, 485)
> Coding Clinic: 2005, Q2, P18-19

■**487.1 With other respiratory manifestations**
Influenza NOS
Influenzal:
laryngitis
pharyngitis
respiratory infection (upper) (acute)
> Coding Clinic: 2005, Q2, P18-19; 1999, Q4, P26; 1987, Jan-Feb, P16

■**487.8 With other manifestations**
Encephalopathy due to influenza
Influenza with involvement of gastrointestinal tract
> **Excludes** *"intestinal flu" [viral gastroenteritis] (008.8)*

●**488 Influenza due to certain identified ~~avian~~ influenza viruses** ◀
> Note: ~~Influenza caused by influenza viruses that normally infect only birds and, less commonly, other animals~~
> **Excludes** *influenza caused by ~~other~~ unspecified influenza viruses (487.0–487.8)* ◀
> Coding Clinic: 2007, Q4, P87-88

488.0 Influenza due to identified avian influenza virus ◀
Avian influenza ◀
Bird flu ◀
Influenza A/H5N1 ◀

488.1 Influenza due to identified novel H1N1 influenza virus ◀
2009 H1N1 [swine] influenza virus ◀
Novel 2009 influenza H1NI ◀
Novel H1N1 influenza ◀
Novel influenza A/H1N1 ◀
Swine flu ◀

CHRONIC OBSTRUCTIVE PULMONARY DISEASE AND ALLIED CONDITIONS (490–496)

■**490 Bronchitis, not specified as acute or chronic**
Bronchitis NOS: Bronchitis NOS:
catarrhal with tracheitis NOS
Tracheobronchitis NOS
> **Excludes** *bronchitis:*
> *allergic NOS (493.9)*
> *asthmatic NOS (493.9)*
> *due to fumes and vapors (506.0)*

Item 8-8 Chronic bronchitis is usually defined as being present in any patient who has persistent cough with sputum production for at least three months in at least two consecutive years. **Simple chronic bronchitis** is marked by a productive cough but no pathological airflow obstruction. **Chronic obstructive pulmonary disease (COPD)** is a group of conditions—bronchitis, emphysema, asthma, bronchiectasis, allergic alveolitis—marked by dyspnea. **Catarrhal** bronchitis is an acute form of bronchitis marked by profuse mucus and pus production (**mucopurulent** discharge). **Croupous** bronchitis, also known as pseudomembranous, fibrinous, plastic, exudative, or membranous, is marked by a violent cough and dyspnea.

DISEASES OF THE RESPIRATORY SYSTEM (460–519)

● **491 Chronic bronchitis**

> **Excludes** *chronic obstructive asthma (493.2)*

491.0 Simple chronic bronchitis
> Catarrhal bronchitis, chronic
> Smokers' cough

491.1 Mucopurulent chronic bronchitis
> Bronchitis (chronic) (recurrent):
>> fetid   purulent
>> mucopurulent
> Coding Clinic: 1988, Q2, P11

● **491.2 Obstructive chronic bronchitis**
> Bronchitis:
>> emphysematous
>> obstructive (chronic) (diffuse)
> Bronchitis with:
>> chronic airway obstruction
>> emphysema
>
>> **Excludes** *asthmatic bronchitis (acute) (NOS) 493.9*
>>> *chronic obstructive asthma 493.2*
> Coding Clinic: 2004, Q4, P81-82; 2002, Q3, P18, 19x2; 1991, Q2,
> P21; 1984, Nov-Dec, P17

491.20 Without exacerbation
> Emphysema with chronic bronchitis
> Coding Clinic: 1997, Q3, P9

491.21 With (acute) exacerbation
> Acute exacerbation of chronic obstructive
>> pulmonary disease [COPD]
> Decompensated chronic obstructive
>> pulmonary disease [COPD]
> Decompensated chronic obstructive
>> pulmonary disease [COPD] with
>> exacerbation
>
>> **Excludes** *chronic obstructive asthma with*
>>> *acute exacerbation 493.22*
> Coding Clinic: 2004, Q1, P3; 1996, Q2, P10; 1993, 5th
> Issue, P5x2

491.22 With acute bronchitis
> Coding Clinic: 2006, Q3, P20; 2004, Q4, P80-81; Q1, P3

> **OGCR** Section I.C.8.b.1
>> When acute bronchitis, 466.0, is
>> documented with COPD, code 491.22
>> should be assigned. It is not necessary to
>> also assign code 466.0. If a medical record
>> documents acute bronchitis with COPD
>> with acute exacerbation, only code 491.22
>> should be assigned. The acute bronchitis
>> included in code 491.22 supersedes the
>> acute exacerbation. If a medical record
>> documents COPD with acute exacerbation
>> without mention of acute bronchitis, only
>> code 491.21 should be assigned.

■ **491.8 Other chronic bronchitis**
> Chronic: Chronic:
>> tracheitis   tracheobronchitis

■ **491.9 Unspecified chronic bronchitis**
> Coding Clinic: 1991, Q3, P17-18

● **492 Emphysema**
> Coding Clinic: 1991, Q2, P21; 1984, Nov-Dec, P19

492.0 Emphysematous bleb
> Giant bullous emphysema
> Ruptured emphysematous bleb
> Tension pneumatocele
> Vanishing lung

■ **492.8 Other emphysema**
> Emphysema (lung or   Emphysema (lung or
>> pulmonary):   pulmonary):
>> NOS   panacinar
>> centriacinar   panlobular
>> centrilobular   unilateral
>> obstructive   vesicular
> MacLeod's syndrome
> Swyer-James syndrome
> Unilateral hyperlucent lung
>
>> **Excludes** *emphysema:*
>>> *with chronic bronchitis 491.20–491.22)*
>>> *compensatory (518.2)*
>>> *due to fumes and vapors (506.4)*
>>> *interstitial (518.1)*
>>>> *newborn (770.2)*
>>> *mediastinal (518.1)*
>>> *surgical (subcutaneous) (998.81)*
>>> *traumatic (958.7)*
> Coding Clinic: 2008, Q4, P174-175; 1993, Q4, P41; 5th Issue, P4

● **493 Asthma**

> **Excludes** *wheezing NOS (786.07)*
> Coding Clinic: 2003, Q4, P62, 137; 1991, Q1, P13; 1985, July-Aug, P8

The following fifth-digit subclassification is for use with
category 493.0–493.2, 493.9:

> | 0 | unspecified |
> |---|---|
> | 1 | with status asthmaticus |
> | 2 | with (acute) exacerbation |

● **493.0 Extrinsic asthma**
[0-2]
> Asthma:
>> allergic with stated cause
>> atopic
>> childhood
>> hay
>> platinum
> Hay fever with asthma
>
>> **Excludes** *asthma:*
>>> *allergic NOS (493.9)*
>>> *detergent (507.8)*
>>> *miners' (500)*
>>> *wood (495.8)*
> Coding Clinic: 1990, Q2, P20

Item 8-9   Asthma is a bronchial condition marked by airway
obstruction, hyper-responsiveness, and inflammation. **Extrinsic**
asthma, also known as allergic asthma, is characterized by the
same symptoms that occur with exposure to allergens and is
divided into the following types: **atopic, occupational, and
allergic bronchopulmonary aspergillosis. Intrinsic**
asthma occurs in patients who have no history of allergy or
sensitivities to allergens and is divided into the following types:
nonreaginic and pharmacologic. Status asthmaticus
is the most severe form of asthma attack and can last for days
or weeks.

DISEASES OF THE RESPIRATORY SYSTEM (460–519)

● **493.1 Intrinsic asthma**
[0-2]   Late-onset asthma
            Coding Clinic: 1990, Q2, P20

● **493.2 Chronic obstructive asthma**
[0-2]   Asthma with chronic obstructive pulmonary
                disease [COPD]
            Chronic asthmatic bronchitis

            Excludes   *acute bronchitis (466.0)*
                         chronic obstructive bronchitis
                             (491.20–491.22)
            Coding Clinic: 2009, Q1, P16; 2006, Q3, P20; 2003, Q4, P108; 1993,
                5th Issue, P4; 1991, Q2, P21; 1990, Q2, P20

● **493.8 Other forms of asthma**

        493.81 Exercise induced bronchospasm
                Coding Clinic: 2003, Q4, P62

        493.82 Cough variant asthma
                Coding Clinic: 2003, Q4, P62

● ■ **493.9 Asthma, unspecified**
[0-2]   Asthma (bronchial) (allergic NOS)
            Bronchitis:
                allergic
                asthmatic
            Coding Clinic: 2004, Q4, P137; 2003, Q4, P108-109; Q1, P9; 1999,
                Q4, P25; 1997, Q4, P39-40; Q1, P7; 1996, Q3, P20; 1993,
                Q4, P32; 1992, Q1, P15; 1990, Q2, P20; 1984, Nov-Dec, P17

● **494 Bronchiectasis**
        Bronchiectasis (fusiform) (postinfectious) (recurrent)
        Bronchiolectasis

        Excludes   *congenital (748.61)*
                     tuberculous bronchiectasis (current disease) (011.5)

        494.0 Bronchiectasis without acute exacerbation

        494.1 Bronchiectasis with acute exacerbation

● **495 Extrinsic allergic alveolitis**

        Includes   allergic alveolitis and pneumonitis due to
                     inhaled organic dust particles of fungal,
                     thermophilic actinomycete, or other
                     origin

        495.0 Farmers' lung

        495.1 Bagassosis

        495.2 Bird-fanciers' lung
                Budgerigar-fanciers' disease or lung
                Pigeon-fanciers' disease or lung

        495.3 Suberosis
                Cork-handlers' disease or lung

        495.4 Malt workers' lung
                Alveolitis due to Aspergillus clavatus

        495.5 Mushroom workers' lung

        495.6 Maple bark-strippers' lung
                Alveolitis due to Cryptostroma corticale

        495.7 "Ventilation" pneumonitis
                Allergic alveolitis due to fungal, thermophilic
                    actinomycete, and other organisms growing
                    in ventilation [air conditioning] systems

    ■ **495.8 Other specified allergic alveolitis and pneumonitis**
                Cheese-washers' lung
                Coffee workers' lung
                Fish-meal workers' lung
                Furriers' lung
                Grain-handlers' disease or lung
                Pituitary snuff-takers' disease
                Sequoiosis or red-cedar asthma
                Wood asthma

    ■ **495.9 Unspecified allergic alveolitis and pneumonitis**
                Alveolitis, allergic (extrinsic)
                Hypersensitivity pneumonitis

■ **496 Chronic airway obstruction, not elsewhere classified**
        Chronic:
            nonspecific lung disease
            obstructive lung disease
            obstructive pulmonary disease [COPD] NOS

        Note: This code is not to be used with any code from
            categories 491–493.

        Excludes   *chronic obstructive lung disease [COPD] specified*
                         (as) (with):
                     allergic alveolitis (495.0–495.9)
                     asthma (493.2)
                     bronchiectasis (494.0–494.1)
                     bronchitis (491.20–491.22)
                         with emphysema (491.20–491.22)
                     decompensated (491.21)
                     emphysema (492.0–492.8)
        Coding Clinic: 2009, Q1, P16; 2006, Q3, P20; 2003, Q4, P109-110; 2000, Q2,
            P15; 1994, Q1, P19; 1993, Q4, P 43; 1992, Q2, P16-17; 1991, Q2,
            P21; 1988, Q2, P12

        OGCR Section I.C.8.a.2
        Code 496 is a nonspecific code that should only be used
        when the documentation in a medical record does not
        specify the type of COPD being treated.

**PNEUMOCONIOSES AND OTHER LUNG DISEASES DUE TO
EXTERNAL AGENTS (500–508)**

500 Coal workers' pneumoconiosis   A
        Anthracosilicosis   Coal workers' lung
        Anthracosis   Miners' asthma
        Black lung disease

501 Asbestosis   A

■ **502 Pneumoconiosis due to other silica or silicates**
        Pneumoconiosis due to talc
        Silicotic fibrosis (massive) of lung
        Silicosis (simple) (complicated)

■ **503 Pneumoconiosis due to other inorganic dust**
        Aluminosis (of lung)
        Bauxite fibrosis (of lung)
        Berylliosis
        Graphite fibrosis (of lung)
        Siderosis
        Stannosis

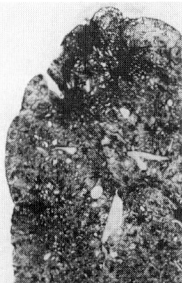

Figure 8–6 Progressive massive
fibrosis superimposed on coal workers'
pneumoconiosis. The large, blackened scars
are located principally in the upper lobe.
(From Cotran R, Kumar V, Collins T: Robbins
Pathologic Basis of Disease, 6th ed.
Philadelphia, WB Saunders, 1999, p 730.
Courtesy of Dr. Warner Laquer, Dr. Jerome
Kleinerman, and the National Institute of
Occupational Safety and Health,
Morgantown, WV.)

Item 8–10 Pneumoconiosis refers to a lung condition
resulting from exposure to inorganic or organic airborne
particles, such as coal dust or moldy hay, as well as chemical
fumes and vapors, such as insecticides. In this condition, the
lungs retain the airborne particles.

N Newborn Age: 0   **P** Pediatric Age: 0–17   **M** Maternity Age: 12–55   **A** Adult Age: 15–124   ♀ Females Only   ♂ Males Only

DISEASES OF THE RESPIRATORY SYSTEM (460–519)

504 **Pneumonopathy due to inhalation of other dust**
Byssinosis
Cannabinosis
Flax-dressers' disease

> **Excludes** *allergic alveolitis (495.0–495.9)*
> *asbestosis (501)*
> *bagassosis (495.1)*
> *farmers' lung (495.0)*

505 **Pneumoconiosis, unspecified**

506 **Respiratory conditions due to chemical fumes and vapors**

Use additional E code to identify cause

506.0 **Bronchitis and pneumonitis due to fumes and vapors**
Chemical bronchitis (acute)
Coding Clinic: 2008, Q3, P6-7

506.1 **Acute pulmonary edema due to fumes and vapors**
Chemical pulmonary edema (acute)

> **Excludes** *acute pulmonary edema NOS (518.4)*
> *chronic or unspecified pulmonary edema (514)*

506.2 **Upper respiratory inflammation due to fumes and vapors**
Coding Clinic: 2005, Q3, P10

506.3 **Other acute and subacute respiratory conditions due to fumes and vapors**

506.4 **Chronic respiratory conditions due to fumes and vapors**
Emphysema (diffuse) (chronic) due to inhalation of chemical fumes and vapors
Obliterative bronchiolitis (chronic) (subacute) due to inhalation of chemical fumes and vapors
Pulmonary fibrosis (chronic) due to inhalation of chemical fumes and vapors

506.9 **Unspecified respiratory conditions due to fumes and vapors**
Silo-fillers' disease

507 **Pneumonitis due to solids and liquids**

> **Excludes** *fetal aspiration pneumonitis (770.18)*

Coding Clinic: 1993, Q2, P9-10

507.0 **Due to inhalation of food or vomitus**
Aspiration pneumonia (due to):
NOS   milk
food (regurgitated)   saliva
gastric secretions   vomitus
Coding Clinic: 2008, Q1, P18-19; Q1, P18-19; 1991, Q3, P16-17; 1989, Q1, P10

507.1 **Due to inhalation of oils and essences**
Lipoid pneumonia (exogenous)

> **Excludes** *endogenous lipoid pneumonia (516.8)*

Coding Clinic: 1991, Q3, P16-17

507.8 **Due to other solids and liquids**
Detergent asthma
Coding Clinic: 1991, Q3, P16-17

508 **Respiratory conditions due to other and unspecified external agents**

Use additional E code to identify cause

508.0 **Acute pulmonary manifestations due to radiation**
Radiation pneumonitis

508.1 **Chronic and other pulmonary manifestations due to radiation**
Fibrosis of lung following radiation

508.8 **Respiratory conditions due to other specified external agents**

508.9 **Respiratory conditions due to unspecified external agent**

OTHER DISEASES OF RESPIRATORY SYSTEM (510–519)

510 **Empyema**

Use additional code to identify infectious organism (041.0–041.9)

> **Excludes** *abscess of lung (513.0)*

510.0 **With fistula**
Fistula:
bronchocutaneous
bronchopleural
hepatopleural
mediastinal
pleural
thoracic
Any condition classifiable to 510.9 with fistula

510.9 **Without mention of fistula**
Abscess:
pleura
thorax
Empyema (chest) (lung) (pleura)
Fibrinopurulent pleurisy
Pleurisy:
purulent
septic
seropurulent
suppurative
Pyopneumothorax
Pyothorax
Coding Clinic: 2007, Q4, P109-113; 1994, Q3, P6

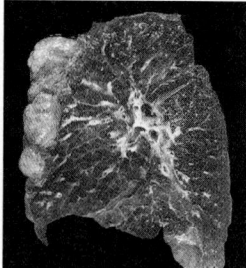

Figure 8–7 Bullous emphysema with large subpleural bullae *(upper left)*. (From Kumar: Robbins and Cotran: Pathologic Basis of Disease, 7th ed. 2005, Saunders, An Imprint of Elsevier)

Item 8–11 **Empyema** is a condition in which pus accumulates in a body cavity. Empyema **with fistula** occurs when the pus passes from one cavity to another organ or structure.

● **511 Pleurisy**
Occurs when double membrane (pleura) lining chest cavity and lung surface becomes inflamed causing sharp pain on inspiration and expiration.

> **Excludes** *pleurisy with mention of tuberculosis, current disease (012.0)*

511.0 Without mention of effusion or current tuberculosis
Adhesion, lung or pleura
Calcification of pleura
Pleurisy (acute) (sterile):
    diaphragmatic
    fibrinous
    interlobar
Pleurisy:
    NOS
    pneumococcal
    staphylococcal
    streptococcal
Thickening of pleura
Coding Clinic: 1994, Q3, P5

■**511.1 With effusion, with mention of a bacterial cause other than tuberculosis**
Pleurisy with effusion (exudative) (serous):
    pneumococcal
    staphylococcal
    streptococcal
    other specified nontuberculous bacterial cause

● **511.8 Other specified forms of effusion, except tuberculous**

> **Excludes** *traumatic (860.2–860.5, 862.29, 862.39)*

Coding Clinic: 2008, Q1, P16-17; 1997, Q1, P10

511.81 Malignant pleural effusion

> *Code first malignant neoplasm, if known*

Coding Clinic: 2008, Q4, P113-114

■**511.89 Other specified forms of effusion, except tuberculous**
Encysted pleurisy
Hemopneumothorax
Hemothorax
Hydropneumothorax
Hydrothorax

■**511.9 Unspecified pleural effusion**
Pleural effusion NOS
Pleurisy:
    exudative
    serofibrinous
    serous
    with effusion NOS
Coding Clinic: 2003, Q2, P7-8; 1991, Q3, P19-20; 1989, Q4, P11; 1988, Q1, P9

● **512 Pneumothorax**
Collapsed lung

512.0 Spontaneous tension pneumothorax
Tension pneumothorax (most serious type) occurs when air (positive pressure) collects in the pleural space

512.1 Iatrogenic pneumothorax
Postoperative pneumothorax
Coding Clinic: 2003, Q3, P19

■**512.8 Other spontaneous pneumothorax**
Pneumothorax: Pneumothorax:
    NOS   chronic
    acute

> **Excludes** *pneumothorax:*
>   *congenital (770.2)*
>   *traumatic (860.0–860.1, 860.4–860.5)*
>   *tuberculous, current disease (011.7)*

Coding Clinic: 1993, Q2, P3

● **513 Abscess of lung and mediastinum**

513.0 Abscess of lung
Abscess (multiple) of lung
Gangrenous or necrotic pneumonia
Pulmonary gangrene or necrosis
Coding Clinic: 2007, Q4, P84-86; 2005, Q2, P14-15; 1998, Q2, P7

513.1 Abscess of mediastinum

514 Pulmonary congestion and hypostasis
Hypostatic:
    bronchopneumonia
    pneumonia
Passive pneumonia
Pulmonary congestion (chronic) (passive)
Pulmonary edema:
    NOS
    chronic

> **Excludes** *acute pulmonary edema:*
>   *NOS (518.4)*
>   *with mention of heart disease or failure (428.1)*
>   *hypostatic pneumonia due to or specified as a specific type of pneumonia - code to the type of pneumonia (480.0–480.9, 481, 482.0–482.9, 483.0–483.8, 485, 486, 487.0)*

Coding Clinic: 1998, Q2, P6-7

515 Postinflammatory pulmonary fibrosis
Cirrhosis of lung chronic or unspecified
Fibrosis of lung (atrophic) (confluent) (massive) (perialveolar) (peribronchial) chronic or unspecified
Induration of lung chronic or unspecified

● **516 Other alveolar and parietoalveolar pneumonopathy**

516.0 Pulmonary alveolar proteinosis

● **516.1 Idiopathic pulmonary hemosiderosis**
Essential brown induration of lung

> *Code first underlying disease (275.0)*

516.2 Pulmonary alveolar microlithiasis

516.3 Idiopathic fibrosing alveolitis
Alveolar capillary block
Diffuse (idiopathic) (interstitial) pulmonary fibrosis
Hamman-Rich syndrome

■**516.8 Other specified alveolar and parietoalveolar pneumonopathies**
Endogenous lipoid pneumonia
Interstitial pneumonia (desquamative) (lymphoid)

> **Excludes** *lipoid pneumonia, exogenous or unspecified (507.1)*

Coding Clinic: 2006, Q2, P20; 1992, Q1, P12

■**516.9 Unspecified alveolar and parietoalveolar pneumonopathy**

● **517 Lung involvement in conditions classified elsewhere**

> **Excludes** *rheumatoid lung (714.81)*

● **517.1 Rheumatic pneumonia**

> *Code first underlying disease (390)*

● **517.2 Lung involvement in systemic sclerosis**

> *Code first underlying disease (710.1)*

● **517.3 Acute chest syndrome**

> *Code first sickle-cell disease in crisis (282.42, 282.62, 282.64, 282.69)*

Coding Clinic: 2003, Q4, P51-56; 1998, Q2, P8

DISEASES OF THE RESPIRATORY SYSTEM (460–519)

● ■ **517.8 Lung involvement in other diseases classified elsewhere**

> Code first underlying disease, as:
> amyloidosis (277.30–277.39)
> polymyositis (710.4)
> sarcoidosis (135)
> Sjögren's disease (710.2)
> systemic lupus erythematosus (710.0)

Excludes syphilis (095.1)

Coding Clinic: 2003, Q2, P7-8

● **518 Other diseases of lung**

518.0 Pulmonary collapse
Atelectasis
Collapse of lung
Middle lobe syndrome

Excludes atelectasis:
congenital (partial) (770.5)
primary (770.4)
tuberculous, current disease (011.8)

Coding Clinic: 1990, Q4, P25

518.1 Interstitial emphysema
Mediastinal emphysema

Excludes surgical (subcutaneous) emphysema (998.81)
that in fetus or newborn (770.2)
traumatic emphysema (958.7)

518.2 Compensatory emphysema

518.3 Pulmonary eosinophilia
Eosinophilic asthma
Löffler's syndrome
Pneumonia:
allergic
eosinophilic
Tropical eosinophilia

■ **518.4 Acute edema of lung, unspecified**
Acute pulmonary edema NOS
Pulmonary edema, postoperative

Excludes pulmonary edema:
acute, with mention of heart disease or failure (428.1)
chronic or unspecified (514)
due to external agents (506.0–508.9)

518.5 Pulmonary insufficiency following trauma and surgery
Adult respiratory distress syndrome
Pulmonary insufficiency following:
shock
surgery
trauma
Shock lung

Excludes adult respiratory distress syndrome associated with other conditions (518.82)
pneumonia:
aspiration (507.0)
hypostatic (514)
respiratory failure in other conditions (518.81, 518.83–518.84)

Coding Clinic: 2004, Q4, P139

518.6 Allergic bronchopulmonary aspergillosis
Coding Clinic: 1997, Q4, P39-40

518.7 Transfusion related acute lung injury (TRALI)
Coding Clinic: 2006, Q4, P91-92

● ■ **518.8 Other diseases of lung**

518.81 Acute respiratory failure
Respiratory failure NOS

Excludes acute and chronic respiratory failure (518.84)
acute respiratory distress (518.82)
chronic respiratory failure (518.83)
respiratory arrest (799.1)
respiratory failure, newborn (770.84)

Coding Clinic: 2009, Q2, P13; 2008, Q1, P18-19; 2007, Q3, P7-8; 2005, Q2, P19-20; Q1, P3-8; 2004, Q4, P139; 2003, Q2, P21-22; Q1, P15; 1993, Q1, P25; 1991, Q3, P14; 1990, Q4, P25; 1987, Nov-Dec, P5-6

■ **518.82 Other pulmonary insufficiency, not elsewhere classified**
Acute respiratory distress
Acute respiratory insufficiency
Adult respiratory distress syndrome NEC

Excludes adult respiratory distress syndrome associated with trauma or surgery (518.5)
pulmonary insufficiency following trauma or surgery (518.5)
respiratory distress:
NOS (786.09)
newborn (770.89)
syndrome, newborn (769)
shock lung (518.5)

Coding Clinic: 2003, Q4, P105-106; 1995, Q1, P7; 1991, Q2, P21

518.83 Chronic respiratory failure
Coding Clinic: 2003, Q4, P103-104, 111

518.84 Acute and chronic respiratory failure
Acute on chronic respiratory failure

■ **518.89 Other diseases of lung, not elsewhere classified**
Broncholithiasis
Calcification of lung
Lung disease NOS
Pulmolithiasis

Coding Clinic: 1988, Q4, P6; 1987, Nov-Dec, P8; 1986, Sept-Oct, P10

● **519 Other diseases of respiratory system**

● **519.0 Tracheostomy complications**
These complications do not appear in the usual complication range of 996–999.

■ **519.00 Tracheostomy complication, unspecified**

519.01 Infection of tracheostomy

Use additional code to identify type of infection, such as:
abscess or cellulitis of neck (682.1)
septicemia (038.0–038.9)

Use additional code to identify organism (041.00–041.9)
Coding Clinic: 1998, Q4, P41-42

519.02 Mechanical complication of tracheostomy
Tracheal stenosis due to tracheostomy

519.09 Other tracheostomy complications
Hemorrhage due to tracheostomy
Tracheoesophageal fistula due to tracheostomy

◀ New   ◀▥ Revised   ~~deleted~~ Deleted   ● Use Additional Digit(s)   ■ Nonspecific Code

● Not first-listed DX   OGCR Official Guidelines   Coding Clinic   Excludes   Includes   Use additional   Code first   Omit code

DISEASES OF THE RESPIRATORY SYSTEM (460–519)

● **519.1 Other diseases of trachea and bronchus, not elsewhere classified**
Coding Clinic: 2002, Q3, P18

  519.11 Acute bronchospasm
     Bronchospasm NOS

     Excludes *acute bronchitis with bronchospasm*
(466.0)
asthma (493.00–493.92)
exercise induced bronchospasm
(493.81)

     Coding Clinic: 2006, Q4, P92-93

  ■**519.19 Other diseases of trachea and bronchus**
     Calcification of bronchus or trachea
     Stenosis of bronchus or trachea
     Ulcer of bronchus or trachea

519.2 Mediastinitis

■**519.3 Other diseases of mediastinum, not elsewhere classified**
     Fibrosis of mediastinum
     Hernia of mediastinum
     Retraction of mediastinum

519.4 Disorders of diaphragm
     Diaphragmitis
     Paralysis of diaphragm
     Relaxation of diaphragm

     Excludes *congenital defect of diaphragm (756.6)*
diaphragmatic hernia (551–553 with .3)
congenital (756.6)

■**519.8 Other diseases of respiratory system, not elsewhere classified**
     Coding Clinic: 1989, Q4, P12

■**519.9 Unspecified disease of respiratory system**
     Respiratory disease (chronic) NOS

DISEASES OF THE RESPIRATORY SYSTEM (460–519)

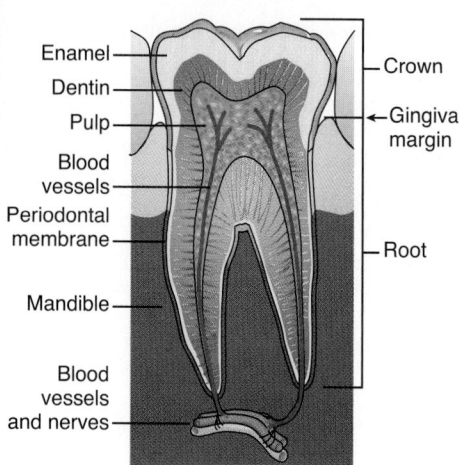

Enamel
Dentin
Pulp
Blood vessels
Periodontal membrane
Mandible
Blood vessels and nerves

Crown
Gingival margin
Root

Figure 9–1
Anatomy of a tooth.

Item 9–1 Anodontia is the congenital absence of teeth. **Hypodontia** is partial anodontia. **Oligodontia** is the congenital absence of some teeth, whereas **supernumerary** is having more teeth than the normal number. **Mesiodens** are small extra teeth that often appear in pairs, although single small teeth are not uncommon.

9. DISEASES OF THE DIGESTIVE SYSTEM (520–579)

DISEASES OF ORAL CAVITY, SALIVARY GLANDS, AND JAWS (520–529)

● **520 Disorders of tooth development and eruption**

520.0 Anodontia
Absence of teeth (complete) (congenital) (partial)
Hypodontia
Oligodontia

> **Excludes** *acquired absence of teeth (525.10–525.19)*

520.1 Supernumerary teeth
Distomolar
Fourth molar
Mesiodens
Paramolar
Supplemental teeth

> **Excludes** *supernumerary roots (520.2)*

520.2 Abnormalities of size and form
Concrescence of teeth
Fusion of teeth
Gemination of teeth
Dens evaginatus
Dens in dente
Dens invaginatus
Enamel pearls
Macrodontia
Microdontia
Peg-shaped [conical] teeth
Supernumerary roots
Taurodontism
Tuberculum paramolare

> **Excludes** *that due to congenital syphilis (090.5)*
> *tuberculum Carabelli, which is regarded as a normal variation*

520.3 Mottled teeth
Dental fluorosis
Mottling of enamel
Nonfluoride enamel opacities

520.4 Disturbances of tooth formation
Aplasia and hypoplasia of cementum
Dilaceration of tooth
Enamel hypoplasia (neonatal) (postnatal) (prenatal)
Horner's teeth
Hypocalcification of teeth
Regional odontodysplasia
Turner's tooth

> **Excludes** *Hutchinson's teeth and mulberry molars in congenital syphilis (090.5)*
> *mottled teeth (520.3)*

520.5 Hereditary disturbances in tooth structure, not elsewhere classified
Amelogenesis imperfecta
Dentinogenesis imperfecta
Odontogenesis imperfecta
Dentinal dysplasia
Shell teeth

520.6 Disturbances in tooth eruption
Teeth:
embedded
impacted
natal
neonatal
prenatal
primary [deciduous]:
persistent
shedding, premature
Tooth eruption:
late
obstructed
premature

> **Excludes** *exfoliation of teeth (attributable to disease of surrounding tissues) (525.0–525.19)*
> Coding Clinic: 2006, Q1, P18; 2005, Q2, P15-16; 2004, Q1, P17

520.7 Teething syndrome

■ **520.8 Other specified disorders of tooth development and eruption**
Color changes during tooth formation
Pre-eruptive color changes

> **Excludes** *posteruptive color changes (521.7)*

■ **520.9 Unspecified disorder of tooth development and eruption**

◀ New ◀▦ Revised ~~deleted~~ Deleted ● Use Additional Digit(s) ■ Nonspecific Code
● Not first-listed DX OGCR Official Guidelines Coding Clinic Excludes Includes Use additional Code first Omit code

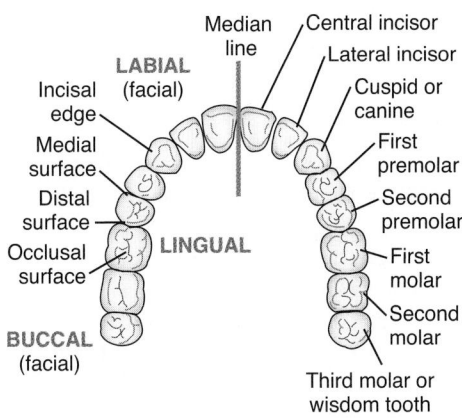

Figure 9–2 The permanent teeth within the dental arch.

Item 9–2 Each dental arch (jaw) normally contains 16 teeth. Tooth decay or **dental caries** is a disease of the enamel, dentin, and cementum of the tooth and can result in a cavity.

● 521 **Diseases of hard tissues of teeth**

  ● 521.0 **Dental caries**

    ■521.00 **Dental caries, unspecified**

    521.01 **Dental caries limited to enamel**
      Initial caries
      White spot lesion

    521.02 **Dental caries extending into dentin**

    521.03 **Dental caries extending into pulp**

    521.04 **Arrested dental caries**

    521.05 **Odontoclasia**
      Infantile melanodontia
      Melanodontoclasia

      Excludes *internal and external resorption of teeth (521.40–521.49)*

    521.06 **Dental caries pit and fissure**
      Primary dental caries, pit and fissure origin

    521.07 **Dental caries of smooth surface**
      Primary dental caries, smooth surface origin

    521.08 **Dental caries of root surface**
      Primary dental caries, root surface

    ■521.09 **Other dental caries**
      Coding Clinic: 2002, Q3, P14

  ● 521.1 **Excessive attrition (approximal wear) (occlusal wear)**

    ■521.10 **Excessive attrition, unspecified**

    521.11 **Excessive attrition, limited to enamel**

    521.12 **Excessive attrition, extending into dentine**

    521.13 **Excessive attrition, extending into pulp**

    521.14 **Excessive attrition, localized**

    521.15 **Excessive attrition, generalized**

● 521.2 **Abrasion**
  Abrasion of teeth:
    dentifrice
    habitual
    occupational
    ritual
    traditional
  Wedge defect NOS of teeth

  ■521.20 **Abrasion, unspecified**

  521.21 **Abrasion, limited to enamel**

  521.22 **Abrasion, extending into dentine**

  521.23 **Abrasion, extending into pulp**

  521.24 **Abrasion, localized**

  521.25 **Abrasion, generalized**

● 521.3 **Erosion**
  Erosion of teeth:
    NOS
    due to:
      medicine
      persistent vomiting
    idiopathic
    occupational

  ■521.30 **Erosion, unspecified**

  521.31 **Erosion, limited to enamel**

  521.32 **Erosion, extending into dentine**

  521.33 **Erosion, extending into pulp**

  521.34 **Erosion, localized**

  521.35 **Erosion, generalized**

● 521.4 **Pathological resorption**

  ■521.40 **Pathological resorption, unspecified**

  521.41 **Pathological resorption, internal**

  521.42 **Pathological resorption, external**

  ■521.49 **Other pathological resorption**
    Internal granuloma of pulp

  521.5 **Hypercementosis**
    Cementation hyperplasia

  521.6 **Ankylosis of teeth**

  521.7 **Intrinsic posteruptive color changes**
    Staining [discoloration] of teeth:
      NOS
      due to:
        drugs
        metals
        pulpal bleeding

      Excludes *accretions [deposits] on teeth (523.6)*
          extrinsic color changes (523.6)
          pre-eruptive color changes (520.8)

● 521.8 **Other specified diseases of hard tissues of teeth**

  521.81 **Cracked tooth**

      Excludes *asymptomatic craze lines in enamel - omit code*
          broken tooth due to trauma (873.63, 873.73)
          fractured tooth due to trauma (873.63, 873.73)

  ■521.89 **Other specified diseases of hard tissues of teeth**
    Irradiated enamel
    Sensitive dentin

  ■521.9 **Unspecified disease of hard tissues of teeth**

● **522 Diseases of pulp and periapical tissues**

522.0 Pulpitis
Pulpal:
  abscess
  polyp
Pulpitis:
  acute
  chronic (hyperplastic) (ulcerative)
  suppurative

522.1 Necrosis of the pulp
Pulp gangrene

522.2 Pulp degeneration
Denticles   Pulp calcifications
Pulp stones

522.3 Abnormal hard tissue formation in pulp
Secondary or irregular dentin

522.4 Acute apical periodontitis of pulpal origin

522.5 Periapical abscess without sinus
Abscess:
  dental
  dentoalveolar
Excludes *periapical abscess with sinus (522.7)*

522.6 Chronic apical periodontitis
Apical or periapical granuloma
Apical periodontitis NOS

522.7 Periapical abscess with sinus
Fistula:
  alveolar process
  dental

522.8 Radicular cyst
Cyst:
  apical (periodontal)
  periapical
  radiculodental
  residual radicular
Excludes *lateral developmental or lateral periodontal*
            cyst (526.0)

■**522.9 Other and unspecified diseases of pulp and**
       periapical tissues

Item 9–3 Acute gingivitis, also known as orilitis or
ulitis, is the short-term, severe inflammation of the gums
(gingiva) caused by bacteria. **Chronic gingivitis** is
persistent inflammation of the gums. When the gingivitis
moves into the periodontium it is called periodontitis, also
known as paradentitis.

● **523 Gingival and periodontal diseases**

●**523.0 Acute gingivitis**
Excludes *acute necrotizing ulcerative gingivitis (101)*
            herpetic gingivostomatitis (054.2)

523.00 Acute gingivitis, plaque induced
Acute gingivitis NOS

523.01 Acute gingivitis, non-plaque induced

●**523.1 Chronic gingivitis**
Gingivitis (chronic):
  desquamative
  hyperplastic
  simple marginal
  ulcerative
Excludes *herpetic gingivostomatitis (054.2)*

523.10 Chronic gingivitis, plaque induced
Chronic gingivitis NOS
Gingivitis NOS

523.11 Chronic gingivitis, non-plaque induced

●**523.2 Gingival recession**
Gingival recession (postinfective) (postoperative)

■**523.20 Gingival recession, unspecified**

523.21 Gingival recession, minimal

523.22 Gingival recession, moderate

523.23 Gingival recession, severe

523.24 Gingival recession, localized

523.25 Gingival recession, generalized

●**523.3 Aggressive and acute periodontitis**
Acute:
  pericementitis
  pericoronitis
Excludes *acute apical periodontitis (522.4)*
            periapical abscess (522.5, 522.7)

■**523.30 Aggressive periodontitis, unspecified**

523.31 Aggressive periodontitis, localized
Periodontal abscess

523.32 Aggressive periodontitis, generalized

523.33 Acute periodontitis

●**523.4 Chronic periodontitis**
Chronic pericoronitis
Pericementitis (chronic)
Periodontitis:
  NOS
  complex
  simplex
Excludes *chronic apical periodontitis (522.6)*

■**523.40 Chronic periodontitis, unspecified**

523.41 Chronic periodontitis, localized

523.42 Chronic periodontitis, generalized

523.5 Periodontosis

523.6 Accretions on teeth
Dental calculus:
  subgingival
  supragingival
Deposits on teeth:
  betel
  materia alba
  soft
  tartar
  tobacco
Extrinsic discoloration of teeth
Excludes *intrinsic discoloration of teeth (521.7)*

■**523.8 Other specified periodontal diseases**
Giant cell:
  epulis
  peripheral granuloma
Gingival:
  cysts
  enlargement NOS
  fibromatosis
Gingival polyp
Periodontal lesions due to traumatic occlusion
Peripheral giant cell granuloma
Excludes *leukoplakia of gingiva (528.6)*

■**523.9 Unspecified gingival and periodontal disease**
Coding Clinic: 2002, Q3, P14

◀ New   ◀▥ Revised   ~~deleted~~ Deleted   ● Use Additional Digit(s)   ■ Nonspecific Code
● Not first-listed DX   OGCR Official Guidelines   Coding Clinic   Excludes   Includes   Use additional   Code first   Omit code

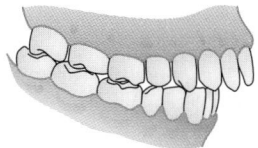

Figure 9–3 Dentofacial malocclusion.

Item 9-4 Hyperplasia is a condition of overdevelopment, whereas **hypoplasia** is a condition of underdevelopment. **Macrogenia** is overdevelopment of the chin, whereas microgenia is underdevelopment of the chin.

● 524 **Dentofacial anomalies, including malocclusion**

● 524.0 **Major anomalies of jaw size**

> **Excludes** *hemifacial atrophy or hypertrophy (754.0)*
> *unilateral condylar hyperplasia or*
> *hypoplasia of mandible*

▪524.00 **Unspecified anomaly**

524.01 **Maxillary hyperplasia**

524.02 **Mandibular hyperplasia**

524.03 **Maxillary hypoplasia**

524.04 **Mandibular hypoplasia**

524.05 **Macrogenia**

524.06 **Microgenia**

524.07 **Excessive tuberosity of jaw**
Entire maxillary tuberosity

▪524.09 **Other specified anomaly**

● 524.1 **Anomalies of relationship of jaw to cranial base**

▪524.10 **Unspecified anomaly**
Prognathism   Retrognathism

524.11 **Maxillary asymmetry**

▪524.12 **Other jaw asymmetry**

▪524.19 **Other specified anomaly**

● 524.2 **Anomalies of dental arch relationship**
Anomaly of dental arch

> **Excludes** *hemifacial atrophy or hypertrophy (754.0)*
> *soft tissue impingement (524.81–524.82)*
> *unilateral condylar hyperplasia or*
> *hypoplasia of mandible (526.89)*

▪524.20 **Unspecified anomaly of dental arch relationship**

524.21 **Malocclusion, Angle's class I**
Neutro-occlusion

524.22 **Malocclusion, Angle's class II**
Disto-occlusion Division I
Disto-occlusion Division II

524.23 **Malocclusion, Angle's class III**
Mesio-occlusion

524.24 **Open anterior occlusal relationship**
Anterior open bite

524.25 **Open posterior occlusal relationship**
Posterior open bite

524.26 **Excessive horizontal overlap**
Excessive horizontal overjet

524.27 **Reverse articulation**
Anterior articulation
Crossbite
Posterior articulation

524.28 **Anomalies of interarch distance**
Excessive interarch distance
Inadequate interarch distance

524.29 **Other anomalies of dental arch relationship**
Other anomalies of dental arch

● 524.3 **Anomalies of tooth position of fully erupted teeth**

> **Excludes** *impacted or embedded teeth with abnormal*
> *position of such teeth or adjacent teeth*
> *(520.6)*

Coding Clinic: 2004, Q1, P17

▪524.30 **Unspecified anomaly of tooth position**
Diastema of teeth NOS
Displacement of teeth NOS
Transposition of teeth NOS

524.31 **Crowding of teeth**

524.32 **Excessive spacing of teeth**

524.33 **Horizontal displacement of teeth**
Tipped teeth
Tipping of teeth

524.34 **Vertical displacement of teeth**
Extruded tooth
Infraeruption of teeth
Intruded tooth
Supraeruption of teeth

524.35 **Rotation of tooth/teeth**

524.36 **Insufficient interocclusal distance of teeth (ridge)**
Lack of adequate intermaxillary vertical dimension

524.37 **Excessive interocclusal distance of teeth**
Excessive intermaxillary vertical dimension
Loss of occlusal vertical dimension

524.39 **Other anomalies of tooth position**

▪524.4 **Malocclusion, unspecified**

● 524.5 **Dentofacial functional abnormalities**

▪524.50 **Dentofacial functional abnormality, unspecified**

524.51 **Abnormal jaw closure**

524.52 **Limited mandibular range of motion**

524.53 **Deviation in opening and closing of the mandible**

524.54 **Insufficient anterior guidance**
Insufficient anterior occlusal guidance

524.55 **Centric occlusion maximum intercuspation discrepancy**
Centric occlusion of teeth discrepancy

524.56 **Non-working side interference**
Balancing side interference

524.57 **Lack of posterior occlusal support**

▪524.59 **Other dentofacial functional abnormalities**
Abnormal swallowing
Mouth breathing
Sleep postures
Tongue, lip, or finger habits

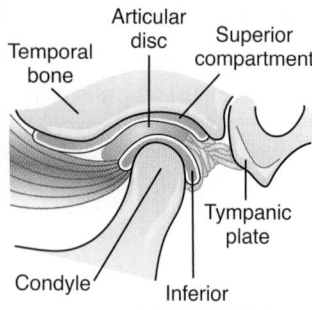

Figure 9-4
Temporomandibular joint.

Item 9-5 Dysfunction of the temporomandibular joint is termed **temporomandibular joint (TMJ) syndrome** and is characterized by pain and tenderness/spasm of the muscles of mastication, joint noise, and in the later stages, limited mandibular movement.

● 524.6 **Temporomandibular joint disorders**

> **Excludes** *current temporomandibular joint:*
> *dislocation (830.0–830.1)*
> *strain (848.1)*

■ 524.60 **Temporomandibular joint disorders, unspecified**
Temporomandibular joint-pain-dysfunction syndrome [TMJ]

524.61 **Adhesions and ankylosis (bony or fibrous)**

524.62 **Arthralgia of temporomandibular joint**

524.63 **Articular disc disorder (reducing or nonreducing)**

524.64 **Temporomandibular joint sounds on opening and/or closing the jaw**

■ 524.69 **Other specified temporomandibular joint disorders**

● 524.7 **Dental alveolar anomalies**

■ 524.70 **Unspecified alveolar anomaly**

524.71 **Alveolar maxillary hyperplasia**

524.72 **Alveolar mandibular hyperplasia**

524.73 **Alveolar maxillary hypoplasia**

524.74 **Alveolar mandibular hypoplasia**

524.75 **Vertical displacement of alveolus and teeth**
Extrusion of alveolus and teeth

524.76 **Occlusal plane deviation**

■ 524.79 **Other specified alveolar anomaly**

● 524.8 **Other specified dentofacial anomalies**

524.81 **Anterior soft tissue impingement**

524.82 **Posterior soft tissue impingement**

■ 524.89 **Other specified dentofacial anomalies**

■ 524.9 **Unspecified dentofacial anomalies**

● 525 **Other diseases and conditions of the teeth and supporting structures**

525.0 **Exfoliation of teeth due to systemic causes**

● 525.1 **Loss of teeth due to trauma, extraction, or periodontal disease**

> *Code first class of edentulism (525.40–525.44, 525.50–525.54)*

● ■ 525.10 *Acquired absence of teeth, unspecified*
Tooth extraction status, NOS

● 525.11 *Loss of teeth due to trauma*
Check for E code assignment.

● 525.12 *Loss of teeth due to periodontal disease*

● 525.13 *Loss of teeth due to caries*

● ■ 525.19 *Other loss of teeth*

● 525.2 **Atrophy of edentulous alveolar ridge**

■ 525.20 **Unspecified atrophy of edentulous alveolar ridge**
Atrophy of the mandible NOS
Atrophy of the maxilla NOS

525.21 **Minimal atrophy of the mandible**

525.22 **Moderate atrophy of the mandible**

525.23 **Severe atrophy of the mandible**

525.24 **Minimal atrophy of the maxilla**

525.25 **Moderate atrophy of the maxilla**

525.26 **Severe atrophy of the maxilla**

525.3 **Retained dental root**

● 525.4 **Complete edentulism**

> Use additional code to identify cause of edentulism (525.10–525.19)

■ 525.40 **Complete edentulism, unspecified**
Edentulism NOS

525.41 **Complete edentulism, class I**

525.42 **Complete edentulism, class II**

525.43 **Complete edentulism, class III**

525.44 **Complete edentulism, class IV**

● 525.5 **Partial edentulism**

> Use additional code to identify cause of edentulism (525.10–525.19)

■ 525.50 **Partial edentulism, unspecified**

525.51 **Partial edentulism, class I**

525.52 **Partial edentulism, class II**

525.53 **Partial edentulism, class III**

525.54 **Partial edentulism, class IV**

● 525.6 **Unsatisfactory restoration of tooth**
Defective bridge, crown, fillings
Defective dental restoration

> **Excludes** *dental restoration status (V45.84)*
> *unsatisfactory endodontic treatment (526.61–526.69)*

■ 525.60 **Unspecified unsatisfactory restoration of tooth**
Unspecified defective dental restoration

525.61 **Open restoration margins**
Dental restoration failure of marginal integrity
Open margin on tooth restoration

525.62 **Unrepairable overhanging of dental restorative materials**
Overhanging of tooth restoration

525.63 **Fractured dental restorative material without loss of material**

> **Excludes** *cracked tooth (521.81)*
> *fractured tooth (873.63, 873.73)*

525.64 **Fractured dental restorative material with loss of material**

> **Excludes** *cracked tooth (521.81)*
> *fractured tooth (873.63, 873.73)*

525.65 Contour of existing restoration of tooth biologically incompatible with oral health
Dental restoration failure of periodontal anatomical integrity
Unacceptable contours of existing restoration
Unacceptable morphology of existing restoration

525.66 Allergy to existing dental restorative material
Use additional code to identify the specific type of allergy

525.67 Poor aesthetics of existing restoration
Dental restoration aesthetically inadequate or displeasing

525.69 Other unsatisfactory restoration of existing tooth

● **525.7 Endosseous dental implant failure**

525.71 Osseointegration failure of dental implant
Failure of dental implant due to infection
Failure of dental implant due to unintentional loading
Failure of dental implant osseointegration due to premature loading
Failure of dental implant to osseointegrate prior to intentional prosthetic loading
Hemorrhagic complications of dental implant placement
Iatrogenic osseointegration failure of dental implant
Osseointegration failure of dental implant due to complications of systemic disease
Osseointegration failure of dental implant due to poor bone quality
Pre-integration failure of dental implant NOS
Pre-osseointegration failure of dental implant

525.72 Post-osseointegration biological failure of dental implant
Failure of dental implant due to lack of attached gingiva
Failure of dental implant due to occlusal trauma (caused by poor prosthetic design)
Failure of dental implant due to parafunctional habits
Failure of dental implant due to periodontal infection (peri-implantitis)
Failure of dental implant due to poor oral hygiene
Failure of dental implant to osseointegrate following intentional prosthetic loading
Iatrogenic post-osseointegration failure of dental implant
Post-osseointegration failure of dental implant due to complications of systemic disease

525.73 Post-osseointegration mechanical failure of dental implant
Failure of dental prosthesis causing loss of dental implant
Fracture of dental implant
Mechanical failure of dental implant NOS

Excludes   *cracked tooth (521.81)*
fractured dental restorative material with loss of material (525.64)
fractured dental restorative material without loss of material (525.63)
fractured tooth (873.63, 873.73)

525.79 Other endosseous dental implant failure
Dental implant failure NOS

525.8 Other specified disorders of the teeth and supporting structures
Enlargement of alveolar ridge NOS
Irregular alveolar process

525.9 Unspecified disorder of the teeth and supporting structures

● **526 Diseases of the jaws**

526.0 Developmental odontogenic cysts
Cyst:
  dentigerous
  eruption
  follicular
  lateral developmental
  lateral periodontal
  primordial
Keratocyst

Excludes   *radicular cyst (522.8)*

526.1 Fissural cysts of jaw
Cyst:
  globulomaxillary
  incisor canal
  median anterior maxillary
  median palatal
  nasopalatine
  palatine of papilla

Excludes   *cysts of oral soft tissues (528.4)*

526.2 Other cysts of jaws

Cyst of jaw:	Cyst of jaw:
NOS	hemorrhagic
aneurysmal	traumatic

526.3 Central giant cell (reparative) granuloma

Excludes   *peripheral giant cell granuloma (523.8)*

526.4 Inflammatory conditions
Abscess of jaw (acute) (chronic) (suppurative)
Osteitis of jaw (acute) (chronic) (suppurative)
Osteomyelitis (neonatal) of jaw (acute) (chronic) (suppurative)
Periostitis of jaw (acute) (chronic) (suppurative)
Sequestrum of jaw bone

Excludes   *alveolar osteitis (526.5)*
osteonecrosis of jaw (733.45)

526.5 Alveolitis of jaw
Alveolar osteitis
Dry socket

● **526.6 Periradicular pathology associated with previous endodontic treatment**

526.61 Perforation of root canal space

526.62 Endodontic overfill

526.63 Endodontic underfill

526.69 Other periradicular pathology associated with previous endodontic treatment

● **526.8 Other specified diseases of the jaws**

526.81 Exostosis of jaw
Torus mandibularis
Torus palatinus

526.89 Other
Cherubism
Fibrous dysplasia of jaw(s)
Latent bone cyst of jaw(s)
Osteoradionecrosis of jaw(s)
Unilateral condylar hyperplasia or hypoplasia of mandible

526.9 Unspecified disease of the jaws

DISEASES OF THE DIGESTIVE SYSTEM (520–579)

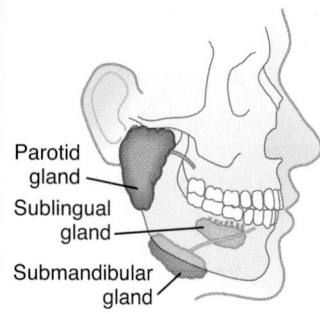

Figure 9–5 Major salivary glands.

Parotid gland

Sublingual gland

Submandibular gland

Item 9–6 Atrophy is wasting away of a tissue or organ, whereas **hypertrophy** is overdevelopment or enlargement of a tissue or organ. **Sialoadenitis** is salivary gland inflammation. **Parotitis** is the inflammation of the parotid gland. In the epidemic form, parotitis is also known as mumps. **Sialolithiasis** is the formation of calculus within a salivary gland. **Mucocele** is a polyp composed of mucus.

● **527 Diseases of the salivary glands**

527.0 Atrophy

527.1 Hypertrophy

527.2 Sialoadenitis

    Parotitis: Sialoangitis
       NOS   Sialodochitis
       allergic
       toxic

    Excludes *epidemic or infectious parotitis (072.0–072.9)*
                   uveoparotid fever (135)

527.3 Abscess

527.4 Fistula

    Excludes *congenital fistula of salivary gland (750.24)*

527.5 Sialolithiasis

    Calculus of salivary gland or duct
    Stone of salivary gland or duct
    Sialodocholithiasis

527.6 Mucocele

    Mucous:
       extravasation cyst of salivary gland
       retention cyst of salivary gland
    Ranula

527.7 Disturbance of salivary secretion

    Hyposecretion
    Ptyalism
    Sialorrhea
    Xerostomia

■**527.8 Other specified diseases of the salivary glands**

    Benign lymphoepithelial lesion of salivary gland
    Sialectasia
    Sialosis
    Stenosis of salivary duct
    Stricture of salivary duct

■**527.9 Unspecified disease of the salivary glands**

Item 9–7 Stomatitis is the inflammation of the oral mucosa. **Cancrum oris,** also known as **noma** or **gangrenous stomatitis,** begins as an ulcer of the gingiva and results in a progressive gangrenous process. Mucositis is the inflammation of the mucous membranes lining the digestive tract from the mouth to the anus. It is a common side effect of chemotherapy and of radiotherapy that involves any part of the digestive tract.

● **528 Diseases of the oral soft tissues, excluding lesions specific for gingiva and tongue**

● **528.0 Stomatitis and mucositis (ulcerative)**

    Excludes *Stevens-Johnson syndrome (695.13)*
                stomatitis:
                  acute necrotizing ulcerative (101)
                  aphthous (528.2)
                  cellulitis and abscess of mouth (528.3)
                  diphtheritic stomatitis (032.0)
                  epizootic stomatitis (078.4)
                  gangrenous (528.1)
                  gingivitis (523.0–523.1)
                  herpetic (054.2)
                  oral thrush (112.0)
                  Vincent's (101)
    Coding Clinic: 1999, Q2, P9

■**528.00 Stomatitis and mucositis, unspecified**

    Mucositis NOS
    Ulcerative mucositis NOS
    Ulcerative stomatitis NOS
    Vesicular stomatitis NOS

528.01 Mucositis (ulcerative) due to antineoplastic therapy

    Use additional E code to identify adverse effects of therapy, such as:
       antineoplastic and immunosuppressive drugs (E930.7, E933.1)
       radiation therapy (E879.2)
    Coding Clinic: 2006, Q4, P88-91

528.02 Mucositis (ulcerative) due to other drugs

    Use additional E code to identify drug

■**528.09 Other stomatitis and mucositis (ulcerative)**

528.1 Cancrum oris

    Gangrenous stomatitis
    Noma

528.2 Oral aphthae

    Aphthous stomatitis
    Canker sore
    Periadenitis mucosa necrotica recurrens
    Recurrent aphthous ulcer
    Stomatitis herpetiformis

    Excludes *herpetic stomatitis (054.2)*

528.3 Cellulitis and abscess

    Cellulitis of mouth (floor)
    Ludwig's angina
    Oral fistula

    Excludes *abscess of tongue (529.0)*
                cellulitis or abscess of lip (528.5)
                fistula (of):
                   dental (522.7)
                   lip (528.5)
                gingivitis (523.00–523.11)

◀ New   ◀▦ Revised   ~~deleted~~ Deleted   ● Use Additional Digit(s)   ■ Nonspecific Code

● Not first-listed DX   OGCR Official Guidelines   Coding Clinic   Excludes   Includes   Use additional   Code first   Omit code

528.4 Cysts
    Dermoid cyst of mouth
    Epidermoid cyst of mouth
    Epstein's pearl of mouth
    Lymphoepithelial cyst of mouth
    Nasoalveolar cyst of mouth
    Nasolabial cyst of mouth

> **Excludes**   *cyst:*
>   *gingiva (523.8)*
>   *tongue (529.8)*

528.5 Diseases of lips
    Abscess of lip(s)
    Cellulitis of lip(s)
    Fistula of lip(s)
    Hypertrophy of lip(s)
    Cheilitis:
        NOS
        angular
    Cheilodynia
    Cheilosis

> **Excludes**   *actinic cheilitis (692.79)*
>   *congenital fistula of lip (750.25)*
>   *leukoplakia of lips (528.6)*

Coding Clinic: 1986, Sept-Oct, P10

528.6 Leukoplakia of oral mucosa, including tongue
    Considered precancerous and evidenced by thickened
        white patches of epithelium on mucous membranes
    Leukokeratosis of oral mucosa
    Leukoplakia of:
        gingiva
        lips
        tongue

> **Excludes**   *carcinoma in situ (230.0, 232.0)*
>   *leukokeratosis nicotina palati (528.79)*

● 528.7 Other disturbances of oral epithelium, including tongue

> **Excludes**   *carcinoma in situ (230.0, 232.0)*
>   *leukokeratosis NOS (702.8)*

528.71 Minimal keratinized residual ridge mucosa
    Minimal keratinization of alveolar ridge
        mucosa

528.72 Excessive keratinized residual ridge mucosa
    Excessive keratinization of alveolar ridge
        mucosa

■528.79 Other disturbances of oral epithelium, including tongue
    Erythroplakia of mouth or tongue
    Focal epithelial hyperplasia of mouth or
        tongue
    Leukoedema of mouth or tongue
    Leukokeratosis nicotina palati
    Other oral epithelium disturbances

528.8 Oral submucosal fibrosis, including of tongue

■528.9 Other and unspecified diseases of the oral soft tissues
    Cheek and lip biting
    Denture sore mouth
    Denture stomatitis
    Melanoplakia
    Papillary hyperplasia of palate
    Eosinophilic granuloma of oral mucosa
    Irritative hyperplasia of oral mucosa
    Pyogenic granuloma of oral mucosa
    Ulcer (traumatic) of oral mucosa

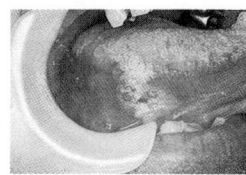

Figure 9–6 Oral leukoplakia and associated squamous carcinoma. (From Feldman: Sleisenger & Fordtran's Gastrointestinal and Liver Disease, 8th ed. 2006, Saunders, An Imprint of Elsevier)

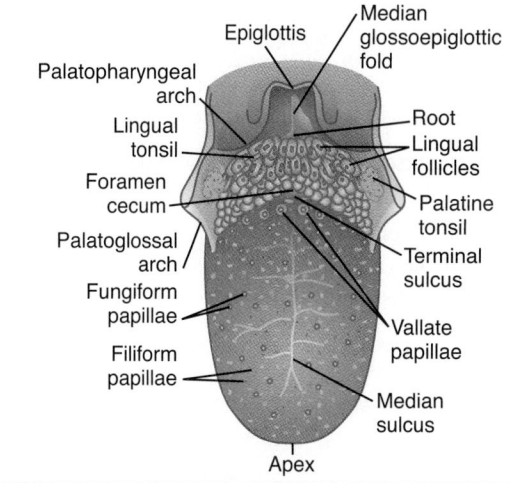

Figure 9–7 Structure of the tongue.

● 529 Diseases and other conditions of the tongue

529.0 Glossitis
    Abscess of tongue
    Ulceration (traumatic) of tongue

> **Excludes**   *glossitis:*
>   *benign migratory (529.1)*
>   *Hunter's (529.4)*
>   *median rhomboid (529.2)*
>   *Moeller's (529.4)*

529.1 Geographic tongue
    Benign migratory glossitis
    Glossitis areata exfoliativa

529.2 Median rhomboid glossitis

529.3 Hypertrophy of tongue papillae
    Black hairy tongue
    Coated tongue
    Hypertrophy of foliate papillae
    Lingua villosa nigra

529.4 Atrophy of tongue papillae
    Bald tongue
    Glazed tongue
    Glossitis:
        Hunter's
        Moeller's
    Glossodynia exfoliativa
    Smooth atrophic tongue

529.5 Plicated tongue
    Fissured tongue   Scrotal tongue
    Furrowed tongue

> **Excludes**   *fissure of tongue, congenital (750.13)*

529.6 Glossodynia
    Glossopyrosis   Painful tongue

> **Excludes**   *glossodynia exfoliativa (529.4)*

DISEASES OF THE DIGESTIVE SYSTEM (520–579)

■529.8 **Other specified conditions of the tongue**
Atrophy (of) tongue
Crenated (of) tongue
Enlargement (of) tongue
Hypertrophy (of) tongue
Glossocele
Glossoptosis

> **Excludes** *erythroplasia of tongue (528.79)*
> *leukoplakia of tongue (528.6)*
> *macroglossia (congenital) (750.15)*
> *microglossia (congenital) (750.16)*
> *oral submucosal fibrosis (528.8)*

■529.9 **Unspecified condition of the tongue**

DISEASES OF ESOPHAGUS, STOMACH, AND DUODENUM (530–538)

●530 **Diseases of esophagus**

> **Excludes** *esophageal varices (456.0–456.2)*

530.0 **Achalasia and cardiospasm**
Achalasia (of cardia)
Aperistalsis of esophagus
Megaesophagus

> **Excludes** *congenital cardiospasm (750.7)*

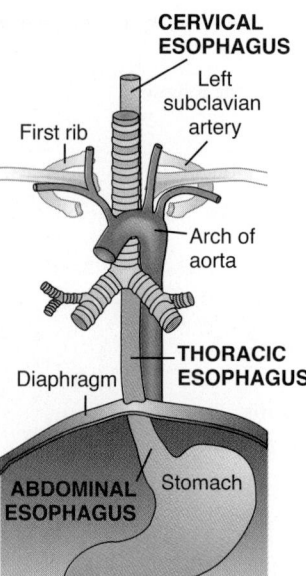

CERVICAL ESOPHAGUS
Left subclavian artery
First rib
Arch of aorta
Diaphragm
THORACIC ESOPHAGUS
ABDOMINAL ESOPHAGUS
Stomach

Figure 9–8 The esophagus is the muscular tube that connects the pharynx and the stomach. The 10 inch (25 cm) long esophagus is divided into three parts: **cervical, thoracic,** and **abdominal.**

Item 9–8 Achalasia is a condition in which the smooth muscle fibers of the esophagus do not relax. Most frequently, this condition occurs at the esophagogastric sphincter. **Cardiospasm,** also known as **megaesophagus,** is achalasia of the thoracic esophagus.

Item 9–9 Dyskinesia is difficulty in moving, and **diverticulum** is a sac or pouch.

●530.1 **Esophagitis**
Esophagitis: Esophagitis:
chemical   postoperative
peptic   regurgitant

> Use additional E code to identify cause, if induced by chemical

> **Excludes** *tuberculous esophagitis (017.8)*

Coding Clinic: 1985, Sept-Oct, P9

■530.10 **Esophagitis, unspecified**
Esophagitis NOS
Coding Clinic: 2005, Q3, P17-18

530.11 **Reflux esophagitis**
Coding Clinic: 1995, Q4, P82

530.12 **Acute esophagitis**

530.13 **Eosinophilic esophagitis**
Coding Clinic: 2008, Q4, P115-116

■530.19 **Other esophagitis**
Abscess of esophagus
Coding Clinic: 2001, Q3, P15

●530.2 **Ulcer of esophagus**
Ulcer of esophagus
fungal
peptic
Ulcer of esophagus due to ingestion of:
aspirin
chemicals
medicines

> Use additional E code to identify cause, if induced by chemical or drug

530.20 **Ulcer of esophagus without bleeding**
Ulcer of esophagus NOS

530.21 **Ulcer of esophagus with bleeding**

> **Excludes** *bleeding esophageal varices (456.0, 456.20)*

530.3 **Stricture and stenosis of esophagus**
Compression of esophagus
Obstruction of esophagus

> **Excludes** *congenital stricture of esophagus (750.3)*

Coding Clinic: 2001, Q2, P4; 1997, Q2, P3; 1988, Q1, P13

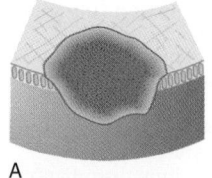
A

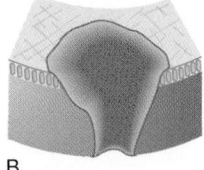
B

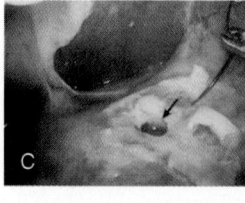
C

Figure 9–9 **A.** Ulcer. **B.** Perforated ulcer. **C.** Laparoscopic view of a perforated duodenal ulcer *(arrow)* with fibrinous exudate on the adjacent peritoneum. (**C** from Feldman: Sleisenger & Fordtran's Gastrointestinal and Liver Disease, 8th ed. 2006, Saunders, An Imprint of Elsevier)

Item 9–10 Gastric ulcers are lesions of the stomach that result in the death of the tissue and a defect of the surface. **Perforated ulcers** are those in which the lesion penetrates the gastric wall, leaving a hole. **Peptic ulcers** are lesions of the stomach or the duodenum. **Peptic** refers to the gastric juice, pepsin.

◄ New   ◄▥ Revised   ~~deleted~~ Deleted   ● Use Additional Digit(s)   ■ Nonspecific Code
● Not first-listed DX   OGCR Official Guidelines   Coding Clinic   Excludes   Includes   Use additional   Code first   Omit code

530.4 Perforation of esophagus
Rupture of esophagus

> **Excludes** *traumatic perforation of esophagus (862.22, 862.32, 874.4–874.5)*

530.5 Dyskinesia of esophagus
Corkscrew esophagus
Curling esophagus
Esophagospasm
Spasm of esophagus

> **Excludes** *cardiospasm (530.0)*

Coding Clinic: 1988, Q1, P13; 1984, Nov-Dec, P19

530.6 Diverticulum of esophagus, acquired
Diverticulum, acquired:
    epiphrenic
    pharyngoesophageal
    pulsion
    subdiaphragmatic
    traction
    Zenker's (hypopharyngeal)
Esophageal pouch, acquired
Esophagocele, acquired

> **Excludes** *congenital diverticulum of esophagus (750.4)*

Coding Clinic: 1985, Mar-April, P15

530.7 Gastroesophageal laceration-hemorrhage syndrome
Mallory-Weiss syndrome

● 530.8 Other specified disorders of esophagus

    530.81 Esophageal reflux
        Gastroesophageal reflux

>   **Excludes** *reflux esophagitis (530.11)*

        Coding Clinic: 2001, Q2, P4; 1995, Q1, P7

    530.82 Esophageal hemorrhage

>   **Excludes** *hemorrhage due to esophageal varices (456.0–456.2)*

        Coding Clinic: 2005, Q1, P17-18

    530.83 Esophageal leukoplakia

    530.84 Tracheoesophageal fistula

>   **Excludes** *congenital tracheoesophageal fistula (750.3)*

    530.85 Barrett's esophagus
        Coding Clinic: 2003, Q4, P63

    530.86 Infection of esophagostomy
        Use additional code to specify infection
        Coding Clinic: 2004, Q4, P83

    530.87 Mechanical complication of esophagostomy
        Malfunction of esophagostomy
        Coding Clinic: 2004, Q4, P83

    ■530.89 Other

>   **Excludes** *Paterson-Kelly syndrome (280.8)*

■530.9 Unspecified disorder of esophagus

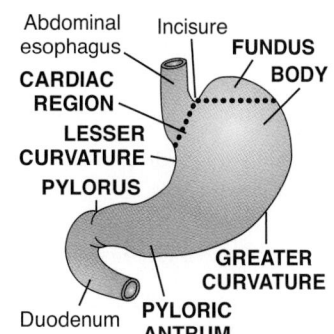

Figure 9–10 Parts of the stomach.

Labels: Abdominal esophagus, Incisure, FUNDUS, BODY, CARDIAC REGION, LESSER CURVATURE, PYLORUS, Duodenum, GREATER CURVATURE, PYLORIC ANTRUM

Item 9–11 **Esophageal reflux** is the return flow of the contents of the stomach to the esophagus and is referred to as GERD and/or "heartburn." **Gastroesophageal reflux** is the return flow of the contents of the stomach and duodenum to the esophagus. **Esophageal leukoplakia** are white areas on the mucous membrane of the esophagus for which no specific cause can be identified.

● 531 Gastric ulcer

> **Includes** ulcer (peptic):
>   prepyloric
>   pylorus
>   stomach

Use additional E code to identify drug, if drug-induced

> **Excludes** *peptic ulcer NOS (533.0–533.9)*

Coding Clinic: 1990, Q4, P27

The following fifth-digit subclassification is for use with category 531:

0	without mention of obstruction
1	with obstruction

● 531.0 Acute with hemorrhage
[0-1]   Coding Clinic: 1984, Nov-Dec, P15

● 531.1 Acute with perforation
[0-1]

● 531.2 Acute with hemorrhage and perforation
[0-1]

● 531.3 Acute without mention of hemorrhage or
[0-1] perforation

● 531.4 Chronic or unspecified with hemorrhage
[0-1]

● 531.5 Chronic or unspecified with perforation
[0-1]

● 531.6 Chronic or unspecified with hemorrhage and
[0-1] perforation

● 531.7 Chronic without mention of hemorrhage or
[0-1] perforation

● ■531.9 Unspecified as acute or chronic, without mention of
[0-1] hemorrhage or perforation

DISEASES OF THE DIGESTIVE SYSTEM (520–579)

● **532 Duodenal ulcer**

> **Includes** erosion (acute) of duodenum
> ulcer (peptic):
>> duodenum
>> postpyloric
>
> Use additional E code to identify drug, if drug-induced
>
> **Excludes** *peptic ulcer NOS (533.0–533.9)*
>
> Coding Clinic: 1990, Q4, P27

The following fifth-digit subclassification is for use with category 532:

> 0 without mention of obstruction
> 1 with obstruction

● **532.0 Acute with hemorrhage**
  [0-1]

● **532.1 Acute with perforation**
  [0-1]

● **532.2 Acute with hemorrhage and perforation**
  [0-1]

● **532.3 Acute without mention of hemorrhage or**
  [0-1] **perforation**

● **532.4 Chronic or unspecified with hemorrhage**
  [0-1]

● **532.5 Chronic or unspecified with perforation**
  [0-1]

● **532.6 Chronic or unspecified with hemorrhage and**
  [0-1] **perforation**

● **532.7 Chronic without mention of hemorrhage or**
  [0-1] **perforation**

●■ **532.9 Unspecified as acute or chronic, without mention of**
  [0-1] **hemorrhage or perforation**

● **533 Peptic ulcer, site unspecified**

> **Includes** gastroduodenal ulcer NOS
> peptic ulcer NOS
> stress ulcer NOS
>
> Use additional E code to identify drug, if drug-induced
>
> **Excludes** *peptic ulcer:*
>> *duodenal (532.0–532.9)*
>> *gastric (531.0–531.9)*
>
> Coding Clinic: 1990, Q4, P27

The following fifth-digit subclassification is for use with category 533:

> 0 without mention of obstruction
> 1 with obstruction

● **533.0 Acute with hemorrhage**
  [0-1]

● **533.1 Acute with perforation**
  [0-1]

● **533.2 Acute with hemorrhage and perforation**
  [0-1]

● **533.3 Acute without mention of hemorrhage and**
  [0-1] **perforation**

● **533.4 Chronic or unspecified with hemorrhage**
  [0-1]

● **533.5 Chronic or unspecified with perforation**
  [0-1]

● **533.6 Chronic or unspecified with hemorrhage and**
  [0-1] **perforation**

● **533.7 Chronic without mention of hemorrhage or**
  [0-1] **perforation**
       Coding Clinic: 1989, Q2, P16

●■ **533.9 Unspecified as acute or chronic, without mention of**
  [0-1] **hemorrhage or perforation**

● **534 Gastrojejunal ulcer**

> **Includes** ulcer (peptic) or erosion:
>> anastomotic
>> gastrocolic
>> gastrointestinal
>> gastrojejunal
>> jejunal
>> marginal
>> stomal
>
> **Excludes** *primary ulcer of small intestine (569.82)*
>
> Coding Clinic: 1990, Q4, P27

The following fifth-digit subclassification is for use with category 534:

> 0 without mention of obstruction
> 1 with obstruction

● **534.0 Acute with hemorrhage**
  [0-1]

● **534.1 Acute with perforation**
  [0-1]

● **534.2 Acute with hemorrhage and perforation**
  [0-1]

● **534.3 Acute without mention of hemorrhage or**
  [0-1] **perforation**

● **534.4 Chronic or unspecified with hemorrhage**
  [0-1]

● **534.5 Chronic or unspecified with perforation**
  [0-1]

● **534.6 Chronic or unspecified with hemorrhage and**
  [0-1] **perforation**

● **534.7 Chronic without mention of hemorrhage or**
  [0-1] **perforation**

●■ **534.9 Unspecified as acute or chronic, without mention of**
  [0-1] **hemorrhage or perforation**

> **Item 9–12 Gastritis** is a severe inflammation of the stomach. **Atrophic gastritis** is a chronic inflammation of the stomach that results in destruction of the cells of the mucosa of the stomach. Duodenitis is an inflammation of the duodenum, the first section of the small intestine.

● **535 Gastritis and duodenitis**
       Coding Clinic: 2007, Q2, P13; 2005, Q3, P17-18

The following fifth-digit subclassification is for use with category 535:

> 0 without mention of hemorrhage
> 1 with hemorrhage

● **535.0 Acute gastritis**
  [0-1]   Coding Clinic: 1992, Q2, P8-9; 1986, Nov-Dec, P9

● **535.1 Atrophic gastritis**
  [0-1]   Gastritis:
              atrophic-hyperplastic   chronic (atrophic)
              Coding Clinic: 1994, Q1, P18

● **535.2 Gastric mucosal hypertrophy**
  [0-1]   Hypertrophic gastritis

● **535.3 Alcoholic gastritis**
  [0-1]

◀ New   ◀▥ Revised   deleted Deleted   ● Use Additional Digit(s)   ■ Nonspecific Code
● Not first-listed DX   OGCR Official Guidelines   Coding Clinic   Excludes   Includes   Use additional   Code first   Omit code

DISEASES OF THE DIGESTIVE SYSTEM (520–579)

● ■**535.4 Other specified gastritis**
    [0-1]   Gastritis:
             allergic
             bile induced
             irritant
             superficial
             toxic

          Excludes   *eosinophilic gastritis (535.7)*

          Coding Clinic: 1990, Q4, P27

● ■**535.5 Unspecified gastritis and gastroduodenitis**
    [0-1]   Coding Clinic: 2005, Q3, P17-18; 1999, Q4, P25-26; 1992, Q3, P15

● ■**535.6 Duodenitis**
    [0-1]   Coding Clinic: 2005, Q3, P17-18

● ■**535.7 Eosinophilic gastritis 1**
    [0-1]   Coding Clinic: 2008, Q4, P115-116

         Item 9–13   Achlorhydria, also known as gastric anacidity, is the absence of gastric acid. **Gastroparesis** is paralysis of the stomach.

● **536 Disorders of function of stomach**

        Excludes   *functional disorders of stomach specified as psychogenic (306.4)*

  536.0 Achlorhydria

  536.1 Acute dilatation of stomach
        Acute distention of stomach

  536.2 Persistent vomiting
        Cyclical vomiting
        Habit vomiting
        Persistent vomiting [not of pregnancy]
        Uncontrollable vomiting

          Excludes   *bilious emesis (vomiting) (787.04)* ◀
                     excessive vomiting in pregnancy (643.0–643.9)
                     vomiting of fecal matter (569.87) ◀
                     vomiting NOS (787.03)
                       cyclical, associated with migraine (346.2)

● **536.3 *Gastroparesis***
        Gastroparalysis

        Code first underlying disease, such as:
          diabetes mellitus (249.6, 250.6)
          Coding Clinic: 2004, Q2, P7-8x2; 2001, Q2, P4

● **536.4 Gastrostomy complications**

    ■**536.40 Gastrostomy complication, unspecified**

    536.41 Infection of gastrostomy

          Use additional code to identify type of
            infection, such as:
             abscess or cellulitis of abdomen (682.2)
             septicemia (038.0–038.9)

          Use additional code to identify organism
            (041.00–041.9)
          Coding Clinic: 1998, Q4, P42-44

    536.42 Mechanical complication of gastrostomy

    ■**536.49 Other gastrostomy complications**
          Coding Clinic: 1998, Q4, P42-44

  ■**536.8 Dyspepsia and other specified disorders of function of stomach**

        Achylia gastrica   Hyperchlorhydria
        Hourglass contraction   Hypochlorhydria
          of stomach   Indigestion
        Hyperacidity   Tachygastria

          Excludes   *achlorhydria (536.0)*
                      heartburn (787.1)
          Coding Clinic: 1993, Q2, P6; 1989, Q2, P16; 1984, Nov-Dec, P9

■**536.9 Unspecified functional disorder of stomach**
        Functional gastrointestinal:
          disorder
          disturbance
          irritation
        Coding Clinic: 2007, Q1, P19

● **537 Other disorders of stomach and duodenum**

  537.0 Acquired hypertrophic pyloric stenosis
        Constriction of pylorus, acquired or adult
        Obstruction of pylorus, acquired or adult
        Stricture of pylorus, acquired or adult

          Excludes   *congenital or infantile pyloric stenosis (750.5)*
          Coding Clinic: 2001, Q2, P17-18; 1985, Jan-Feb, P14-15

  537.1 Gastric diverticulum
          Excludes   *congenital diverticulum of stomach (750.7)*

  537.2 Chronic duodenal ileus

■**537.3 Other obstruction of duodenum**
        Cicatrix of duodenum
          Cicatrix = scar
        Stenosis of duodenum
          Stenosis = narrowing
        Stricture of duodenum
          Stricture = narrowing
        Volvulus of duodenum
          Volvulus = twisting/knotting

          Excludes   *congenital obstruction of duodenum (751.1)*

  537.4 Fistula of stomach or duodenum
        Gastrocolic fistula
        Gastrojejunocolic fistula

  537.5 Gastroptosis

  537.6 Hourglass stricture or stenosis of stomach
        Cascade stomach

          Excludes   *congenital hourglass stomach (750.7)*
                     hourglass contraction of stomach (536.8)

● **537.8 Other specified disorders of stomach and duodenum**

    537.81 Pylorospasm
          Excludes   *congenital pylorospasm (750.5)*

    537.82 Angiodysplasia of stomach and duodenum without mention of hemorrhage
          Coding Clinic: 2007, Q2, P9; 1996, Q3, P10

    537.83 Angiodysplasia of stomach and duodenum with hemorrhage
          Coding Clinic: 2007, Q2, P9

    537.84 Dieulafoy lesion (hemorrhagic) of stomach and duodenum
          Coding Clinic: 2002, Q4, P60-61

    ■**537.89 Other**
        Gastric or duodenal:
          prolapse
          rupture
        Intestinal metaplasia of gastric mucosa
        Passive congestion of stomach

          Excludes   *diverticula of duodenum (562.00–562.01)*
                     gastrointestinal hemorrhage (578.0–578.9)
          Coding Clinic: 2005, Q3, P15-16

■**537.9 Unspecified disorder of stomach and duodenum**

  538 Gastrointestinal mucositis (ulcerative)

        Use additional E code to identify adverse effects of
          therapy, such as:
        antineoplastic and immunosuppressive drugs (E930.7, E933.1)
        radiation therapy (E879.2)

          Excludes   *mucositis (ulcerative) of mouth and oral soft tissue (528.00–528.09)*

DISEASES OF THE DIGESTIVE SYSTEM (520–579)

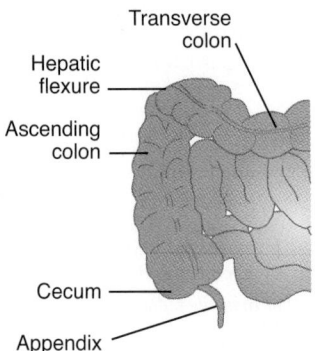

Figure 9–11 Acute appendicitis is the inflammation of the appendix, usually associated with obstruction. Most often this is a disease of adolescents and young adults.

APPENDICITIS (540–543)

● **540 Acute appendicitis**

540.0 With generalized peritonitis
Appendicitis (acute) with: perforation, peritonitis (generalized), rupture:
 fulminating
 gangrenous
 obstructive
Cecitis (acute) with: perforation, peritonitis (generalized), rupture
Rupture of appendix

> **Excludes** *acute appendicitis with peritoneal abscess (540.1)*
> Coding Clinic: 1984, Nov-Dec, P19

540.1 With peritoneal abscess
Abscess of appendix
 With generalized peritonitis
Coding Clinic: 1984, Nov-Dec, P19

540.9 Without mention of peritonitis
Acute:
 appendicitis without mention of perforation, peritonitis, or rupture:
  fulminating
  gangrenous
  inflamed
  obstructive
 cecitis without mention of perforation, peritonitis, or rupture
Coding Clinic: 2001, Q1, P15-16; 1997, Q4, P52

■ **541 Appendicitis, unqualified**
Coding Clinic: 1990, Q2, P26

■ **542 Other appendicitis**
Appendicitis:
 chronic relapsing
 recurrent
 subacute

> **Excludes** *hyperplasia (lymphoid) of appendix (543.0)*
> Coding Clinic: 2001, Q1, P15-16

● **543 Other diseases of appendix**

543.0 Hyperplasia of appendix (lymphoid)

■ **543.9 Other and unspecified diseases of appendix**
Appendicular or appendiceal:
 colic
 concretion
 fistula
Diverticulum of appendix
Fecalith of appendix
Intussusception of appendix
Mucocele of appendix
Stercolith of appendix

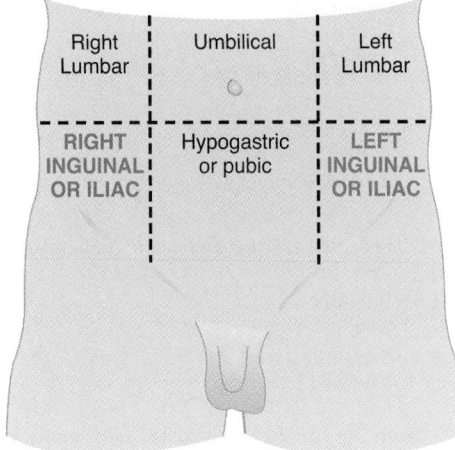

Figure 9–12 Inguinal hernias are those that are located in the inguinal or iliac areas of the abdomen.

Item 9–14 Hernias of the groin are the most common type, accounting for 80 percent of all hernias. There are two major types of inguinal hernias: indirect (oblique) affecting men only and direct. **Indirect inguinal hernias** result when the intestines emerge through the abdominal wall in an indirect fashion through the inguinal canal. **Direct inguinal hernias** penetrate through the abdominal wall in a direct fashion. **Femoral hernias** occur at the femoral ring where the femoral vessels enter the thigh and is most common in women. An abdominal wall hernia is also called a ventral or epigastric hernia and occurs in both sexes. Classification is based on location of the hernia and whether there is obstruction or gangrene.

HERNIA OF ABDOMINAL CAVITY (550–553)

> **Includes** hernia:
> acquired
> congenital, except diaphragmatic or hiatal

● **550 Inguinal hernia**

> **Includes** bubonocele
> inguinal hernia (direct) (double) (indirect) (oblique) (sliding)
> scrotal hernia

The following fifth-digit subclassification is for use with category 550:

> ■ **0** unilateral or unspecified (not specified as recurrent)
> **Unilateral NOS**
> **1** unilateral or unspecified, recurrent
> **2** bilateral (not specified as recurrent)
> **Bilateral NOS**
> **3** bilateral, recurrent

● **550.0 Inguinal hernia, with gangrene**
[0-3] Inguinal hernia with gangrene (and obstruction)

● **550.1 Inguinal hernia, with obstruction, without mention**
[0-3] **of gangrene**
 Inguinal hernia with mention of incarceration, irreducibility, or strangulation

● **550.9 Inguinal hernia, without mention of obstruction or**
[0-3] **gangrene**
 Inguinal hernia NOS
 Coding Clinic: 2003, Q3, P10-11; 2003, Q1, P4; 1985, Nov-Dec, P12; 1984, May-June, P11

◀ New   ◀▥ Revised   d̶e̶l̶e̶t̶e̶d̶ Deleted   ● Use Additional Digit(s)   ■ Nonspecific Code
● Not first-listed DX   OGCR Official Guidelines   Coding Clinic   Excludes   Includes   Use additional   Code first   Omit code

● **551   Other hernia of abdominal cavity, with gangrene**

> **Includes**   that with gangrene (and obstruction)

● **551.0   Femoral hernia with gangrene**

▪ **551.00   Unilateral or unspecified (not specified as recurrent)**
> Femoral hernia NOS with gangrene

551.01   Unilateral or unspecified, recurrent

551.02   Bilateral (not specified as recurrent)

551.03   Bilateral, recurrent

551.1   Umbilical hernia with gangrene
> Parumbilical hernia specified as gangrenous

● **551.2   Ventral hernia with gangrene**

▪ **551.20   Ventral, unspecified, with gangrene**

551.21   Incisional, with gangrene
> Hernia:
>> postoperative specified as gangrenous
>> recurrent, ventral specified as gangrenous

▪ **551.29   Other**
> Epigastric hernia specified as gangrenous

551.3   Diaphragmatic hernia with gangrene
> Hernia:
>> hiatal (esophageal) (sliding) specified as gangrenous
>> paraesophageal specified as gangrenous
> Thoracic stomach specified as gangrenous

> **Excludes**   *congenital diaphragmatic hernia (756.6)*

▪ **551.8   Hernia of other specified sites, with gangrene**
> Any condition classifiable to 553.8 if specified as gangrenous

▪ **551.9   Hernia of unspecified site, with gangrene**
> Any condition classifiable to 553.9 if specified as gangrenous

● **552   Other hernia of abdominal cavity, with obstruction, but without mention of gangrene**

> **Excludes**   *that with mention of gangrene (551.0–551.9)*

● **552.0   Femoral hernia with obstruction**
> Femoral hernia specified as incarcerated, irreducible, strangulated, or causing obstruction

▪ **552.00   Unilateral or unspecified (not specified as recurrent)**

552.01   Unilateral or unspecified, recurrent

552.02   Bilateral (not specified as recurrent)

552.03   Bilateral, recurrent

552.1   Umbilical hernia with obstruction
> Parumbilical hernia specified as incarcerated, irreducible, strangulated, or causing obstruction

Item 9-15   Ventral, epigastric, or incisional hernia occurs on the abdominal surface caused by musculature weakness or a tear at a previous surgical site and is evidenced by a bulge that changes in size, becoming larger with exertion. An **incarcerated** hernia is one in which the intestines become trapped in the hernia. A **strangulated** hernia is one in which the blood supply to the intestines is lost. Hiatal hernia occurs when a loop of the stomach protrudes upward through the small opening in the diaphragm through which the esophagus passes, leaving the abdominal cavity and entering the chest. It occurs in both sexes.

● **552.2   Ventral hernia with obstruction**
> Ventral hernia specified as incarcerated, irreducible, strangulated, or causing obstruction

▪ **552.20   Ventral, unspecified, with obstruction**

552.21   Incisional, with obstruction
> Hernia:
>> postoperative specified as incarcerated, irreducible, strangulated, or causing obstruction
>> recurrent, ventral specified as incarcerated, irreducible, strangulated, or causing obstruction
> Coding Clinic: 2003, Q3, P11

▪ **552.29   Other**
> Epigastric hernia specified as incarcerated, irreducible, strangulated, or causing obstruction

552.3   Diaphragmatic hernia with obstruction
> Hernia:
>> hiatal (esophageal) (sliding) specified as incarcerated, irreducible, strangulated, or causing obstruction
>> paraesophageal specified as incarcerated, irreducible, strangulated, or causing obstruction
> Thoracic stomach specified as incarcerated, irreducible, strangulated, or causing obstruction

> **Excludes**   *congenital diaphragmatic hernia (756.6)*

▪ **552.8   Hernia of other specified sites, with obstruction**
> Any condition classifiable to 553.8 if specified as incarcerated, irreducible, strangulated, or causing obstruction

> **Excludes**   *hernia due to adhesion with obstruction (560.81)*
> Coding Clinic: 2004, Q1, P10-11

▪ **552.9   Hernia of unspecified site, with obstruction**
> Any condition classifiable to 553.9 if specified as incarcerated, irreducible, strangulated, or causing obstruction

DISEASES OF THE DIGESTIVE SYSTEM (520–579)

● 553 **Other hernia of abdominal cavity without mention of obstruction or gangrene**

> **Excludes** *the listed conditions with mention of:*
> *gangrene (and obstruction) (551.0–551.9)*
> *obstruction (552.0–552.9)*

● 553.0 **Femoral hernia**

▪ 553.00 **Unilateral or unspecified (not specified as recurrent)**
Femoral hernia NOS

553.01 **Unilateral or unspecified, recurrent**

553.02 **Bilateral (not specified as recurrent)**

553.03 **Bilateral, recurrent**

553.1 **Umbilical hernia**
Parumbilical hernia

● 553.2 **Ventral hernia**

▪ 553.20 **Ventral, unspecified**
Coding Clinic: 2006, Q2, P10-11; 2003, Q3, P6-7; 1996, Q3, P15

553.21 **Incisional**
Hernia:
postoperative
recurrent, ventral
Coding Clinic: 2003, Q3, P6

▪ 553.29 **Other**
Hernia:
epigastric
spigelian

553.3 **Diaphragmatic hernia**
Hernia:
hiatal (esophageal) (sliding)
paraesophageal
Thoracic stomach

> **Excludes** *congenital:*
> *diaphragmatic hernia (756.6)*
> *hiatal hernia (750.6)*
> *esophagocele (530.6)*
Coding Clinic: 2001, Q2, P6; 2000, Q1, P6

▪ 553.8 **Hernia of other specified sites**
Hernia:
ischiatic
ischiorectal
lumbar
obturator
pudendal
retroperitoneal
sciatic
Other abdominal hernia of specified site

> **Excludes** *vaginal enterocele (618.6)*

▪ 553.9 **Hernia of unspecified site**
Enterocele
Epiplocele
Hernia:
NOS
interstitial
intestinal
intra-abdominal
Rupture (nontraumatic)
Sarcoepiplocele

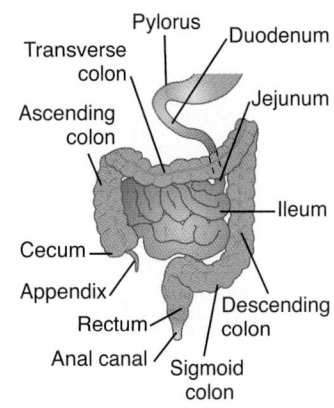

Figure 9–13 Small and large intestines.

Pylorus
Duodenum
Transverse colon
Jejunum
Ascending colon
Ileum
Cecum
Appendix
Descending colon
Rectum
Anal canal
Sigmoid colon

Item 9–16 Crohn's disease, also known as **regional enteritis,** is a chronic inflammatory disease of the intestines. Classification is based on location in the small (duodenum, ileum, jejunum) or large (cecum, colon, rectum, anal canal) intestine.

NONINFECTIOUS ENTERITIS AND COLITIS (555–558)

● 555 **Regional enteritis**

> **Includes**   Crohn's disease
> Granulomatous enteritis

> **Excludes** *ulcerative colitis (556)*

555.0 **Small intestine**
Ileitis:
regional
segmental
terminal
Regional enteritis or Crohn's disease of:
duodenum
ileum
jejunum

555.1 **Large intestine**
Colitis:
granulomatous
regional
transmural
Regional enteritis or Crohn's disease of:
colon
large bowel
rectum
Coding Clinic: 1999, Q3, P8

555.2 **Small intestine with large intestine**
Regional ileocolitis
Coding Clinic: 2003, Q1, P18

▪ 555.9 **Unspecified site**
Crohn's disease NOS
Regional enteritis NOS
Coding Clinic: 2009, Q1, P20; 2005, Q2, P11-12; 1999, Q3, P8-9; 1997, Q4, P37; Q2, P3; 1996, Q1, P13; 1988, Q2, P9-10

◀ New   ◀▦ Revised   ~~deleted~~ Deleted   ● Use Additional Digit(s)   ▪ Nonspecific Code
● Not first-listed DX   OGCR Official Guidelines   Coding Clinic   Excludes   Includes   Use additional   Code first   Omit code

Item 9–17 **Ulcerative colitis** attacks the colonic mucosa and forms abscesses. The disease involves the intestines. Classification is based on the location:
Enterocolitis: large and small intestine
Ileocolitis: ileum and colon
Proctitis: rectum
Proctosigmoiditis: sigmoid colon and rectum

● 556 **Ulcerative colitis**

556.0 Ulcerative (chronic) enterocolitis

556.1 Ulcerative (chronic) ileocolitis

556.2 Ulcerative (chronic) proctitis

556.3 Ulcerative (chronic) proctosigmoiditis

556.4 Pseudopolyposis of colon

556.5 Left-sided ulcerative (chronic) colitis

556.6 Universal ulcerative (chronic) colitis
Pancolitis

■**556.8 Other ulcerative colitis**

■**556.9 Ulcerative colitis, unspecified**
Ulcerative enteritis NOS
Coding Clinic: 2003, Q1, P10-11

● 557 **Vascular insufficiency of intestine**

Excludes *necrotizing enterocolitis of the newborn (777.50–777.53)*

557.0 Acute vascular insufficiency of intestine
Acute:
hemorrhagic enterocolitis
ischemic colitis, enteritis, or enterocolitis
massive necrosis of intestine
Bowel infarction
Embolism of mesenteric artery
Fulminant enterocolitis
Hemorrhagic necrosis of intestine
Infarction of appendices epiploicae
Intestinal gangrene
Intestinal infarction (acute) (agnogenic)
(hemorrhagic) (nonocclusive)
Mesenteric infarction (embolic) (thrombotic)
Necrosis of intestine
Terminal hemorrhagic enteropathy
Thrombosis of mesenteric artery
Coding Clinic: 2008, Q2, P15-16

557.1 Chronic vascular insufficiency of intestine
Angina, abdominal
Chronic ischemic colitis, enteritis, or enterocolitis
Ischemic stricture of intestine
Mesenteric:
angina
artery syndrome (superior)
vascular insufficiency
Coding Clinic: 1996, Q3, P9-10; 1986, Nov-Dec, P11; 1985, Sept-Oct, P9

■**557.9 Unspecified vascular insufficiency of intestine**
Alimentary pain due to vascular insufficiency
Ischemic colitis, enteritis, or enterocolitis NOS

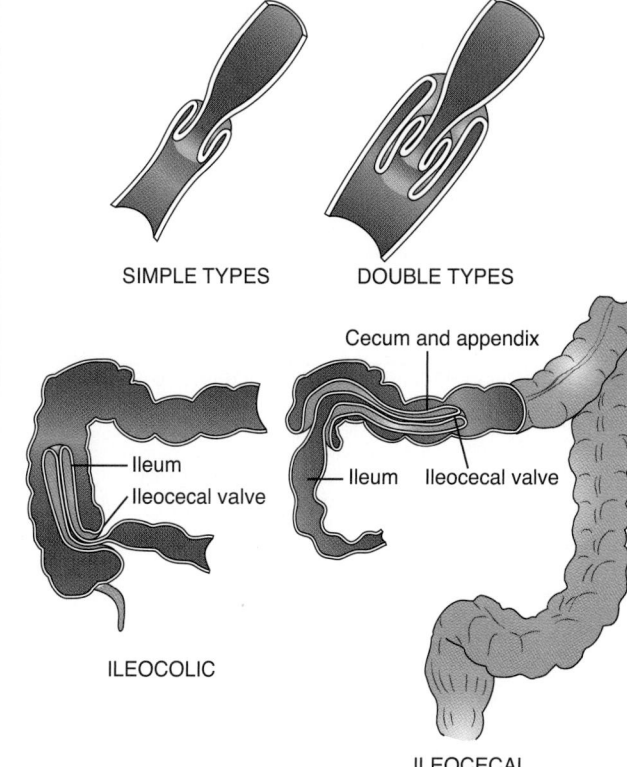

SIMPLE TYPES   DOUBLE TYPES

Cecum and appendix

Ileum
Ileocecal valve

Ileum   Ileocecal valve

ILEOCOLIC

ILEOCECAL

Figure 9–14 Types of intussusception.

● 558 **Other and unspecified noninfectious gastroenteritis and colitis**

Excludes *infectious:*
colitis, enteritis, or gastroenteritis (009.0–009.1)
diarrhea (009.2–009.3)

558.1 Gastroenteritis and colitis due to radiation
Radiation enterocolitis

558.2 Toxic gastroenteritis and colitis
Use additional E code to identify cause
Coding Clinic: 2008, Q2, P10-11

558.3 Allergic gastroenteritis and colitis
Use additional code to identify type of food allergy (V15.01–V15.05)
Coding Clinic: 2008, Q4, P115-116; 2003, Q1, P12

● **558.4 Eosinophilic gastroenteritis and colitis**

558.41 Eosinophilic gastroenteritis
Eosinophilic enteritis
Coding Clinic: 2008, Q4, P115-116

558.42 Eosinophilic colitis
Coding Clinic: 2008, Q4, P115-116

■**558.9 Other and unspecified noninfectious gastroenteritis and colitis**
Colitis, NOS, dietetic, or noninfectious
Enteritis, NOS, dietetic, or noninfectious
Gastroenteritis, NOS, dietetic, or noninfectious
Ileitis, NOS, dietetic or noninfectious
Jejunitis, NOS, dietetic, or noninfectious
Sigmoiditis, NOS, dietetic, or noninfectious
Coding Clinic: 2008, Q2, P10-11; Q1, P10-12; 1999, Q3, P4-7; 1987, Nov-Dec, P7-8; 1984, July-Aug, P19-20

DISEASES OF THE DIGESTIVE SYSTEM (520–579)

Item 9–18 Intussusception is the prolapse (telescoping) of a part of the intestine into another adjacent part of the intestine. Intussusception may be enteric (ileoileal, jejunoileal, jejunojejunal), colic (colocolic), or intracolic (ileocecal, ileocolic).

Item 9–19 Volvulus is the twisting of a segment of the intestine, resulting in obstruction. Paralytic ileus is paralysis of the intestine. It need not be a complete paralysis, but it must prohibit the passage of food through the intestine and lead to intestinal blockage. It is a common aftermath of some types of surgery.

OTHER DISEASES OF INTESTINES AND PERITONEUM (560–569)

● 560   **Intestinal obstruction without mention of hernia**

     Excludes   *duodenum (537.2–537.3)*
         inguinal hernia with obstruction (550.1)
         intestinal obstruction complicating hernia
           (552.0–552.9)
         mesenteric:
           embolism (557.0)
           infarction (557.0)
           thrombosis (557.0)
         neonatal intestinal obstruction (277.01,
           777.1–777.2, 777.4)

     560.0 Intussusception
         Intussusception (colon) (intestine) (rectum)
         Invagination of intestine or colon

         Excludes   *intussusception of appendix (543.9)*

         Coding Clinic: 1998, Q4, P82-83

     560.1 Paralytic ileus
         Adynamic ileus
         Ileus (of intestine) (of bowel) (of colon)
         Paralysis of intestine or colon

         Excludes   *gallstone ileus (560.31)*

         Coding Clinic: 1987, Jan-Feb, P13-14

     560.2 Volvulus
         Knotting of intestine, bowel, or colon
         Strangulation of intestine, bowel, or colon
         Torsion of intestine, bowel, or colon
         Twist of intestine, bowel, or colon

● **560.3 Impaction of intestine**

     ■ **560.30 Impaction of intestine, unspecified**
         Impaction of colon

     560.31 Gallstone ileus
         Obstruction of intestine by gallstone

     ■ **560.39 Other**
         Concretion of intestine
         Enterolith
         Fecal impaction
         Coding Clinic: 1998, Q4, P37-38

● **560.8 Other specified intestinal obstruction**

     560.81 Intestinal or peritoneal adhesions with obstruction (postoperative) (postinfection)

         Excludes   *adhesions without obstruction*
            (568.0)
         Coding Clinic: 1995, Q3, P6; 1987, Nov-Dec, P9

     ■ **560.89 Other**
         Acute pseudo-obstruction of intestine
         Mural thickening causing obstruction

         Excludes   *ischemic stricture of intestine*
            (557.1)
         Coding Clinic: 1997, Q2, P3

■ **560.9 Unspecified intestinal obstruction**
     Enterostenosis
     Obstruction of intestine or colon
     Occlusion of intestine or colon
     Stenosis of intestine or colon
     Stricture of intestine or colon

     Excludes   *congenital stricture or stenosis of intestine*
         (751.1–751.2)

Item 9–20 Diverticula of the intestines are acquired herniations of the mucosa. Diverticulum (singular): Pocket or pouch that bulges outward through a weak spot (herniation) in the colon. Diverticula (plural). **Diverticulosis** is the condition of having diverticula. **Diverticulitis** is inflammation of these pouches or herniations. Classification is based on location (small intestine or colon) and whether it occurs with or without hemorrhage.

● 562   **Diverticula of intestine**

     Use additional code to identify any associated:
     peritonitis (567.0–567.9)

     Excludes   *congenital diverticulum of colon (751.5)*
         diverticulum of appendix (543.9)
         Meckel's diverticulum (751.0)

● **562.0 Small intestine**

     562.00 Diverticulosis of small intestine (without mention of hemorrhage)
         Diverticulosis:
           duodenum without mention of
             diverticulitis
           ileum without mention of diverticulitis
           jejunum without mention of diverticulitis

     562.01 Diverticulitis of small intestine (without mention of hemorrhage)
         Diverticulitis (with diverticulosis):
           duodenum
           ileum
           jejunum
           small intestine

     562.02 Diverticulosis of small intestine with hemorrhage

     562.03 Diverticulitis of small intestine with hemorrhage

● **562.1 Colon**

     562.10 Diverticulosis of colon (without mention of hemorrhage)
         Diverticulosis without mention of
           diverticulitis:
           NOS
           intestine (large) without mention of
             diverticulitis
         Diverticular disease (colon) without
           mention of diverticulitis
         Coding Clinic: 2005, Q3, P17-18; 2002, Q3, P14-15

     562.11 Diverticulitis of colon without mention of hemorrhage
         Diverticulitis (with diverticulosis):
           NOS
           colon
           intestine (large)
         Coding Clinic: 1996, Q1, P13-14

     562.12 Diverticulosis of colon with hemorrhage

     562.13 Diverticulitis of colon with hemorrhage

● **564   Functional digestive disorders, not elsewhere classified**

Excludes *functional disorders of stomach (536.0–536.9)*
those specified as psychogenic (306.4)

● **564.0 Constipation**

Excludes *psychogenic constipation (306.4)*

■564.00 Constipation, unspecified

564.01 Slow transit constipation

564.02 Outlet dysfunction constipation

■564.09 Other constipation

564.1 Irritable bowel syndrome
Irritable colon
Spastic colon

564.2 Postgastric surgery syndromes
Dumping syndrome
Jejunal syndrome
Postgastrectomy syndrome
Postvagotomy syndrome

Excludes *malnutrition following gastrointestinal*
surgery (579.3)
postgastrojejunostomy ulcer (534.0–534.9)
Coding Clinic: 1995, Q1, P11

564.3 Vomiting following gastrointestinal surgery
Vomiting (bilious) following gastrointestinal
surgery

■**564.4 Other postoperative functional disorders**
Diarrhea following gastrointestinal surgery

Excludes *colostomy and enterostomy complications*
(569.60–569.69)

564.5 Functional diarrhea

Excludes *diarrhea:*
NOS (787.91)
psychogenic (306.4)
Coding Clinic: 1988, Q2, P9-10

564.6 Anal spasm
Proctalgia fugax

564.7 Megacolon, other than Hirschsprung's
Dilatation of colon

Excludes *megacolon:*
congenital [Hirschsprung's] (751.3)
toxic (556)

● **564.8 Other specified functional disorders of intestine**

Excludes *malabsorption (579.0–579.9)*

564.81 Neurogenic bowel
Coding Clinic: 2001, Q1, P12

■**564.89 Other functional disorders of intestine**
Atony of colon

■**564.9 Unspecified functional disorder of intestine**

Item 9–21   A **fissure** is a groove in the surface, whereas a
fistula is an abnormal passage. An abscess is an accumulation
of pus in a tissue cavity resulting from a bacterial or parasitic
infection.

● **565   Anal fissure and fistula**

565.0 Anal fissure

Excludes *anal sphincter tear (healed) (non-traumatic)*
(old) (569.43)
traumatic (863.89, 863.99)

565.1 Anal fistula
Fistula:
anorectal
rectal
rectum to skin

Excludes *fistula of rectum to internal organs - see*
Alphabetic Index
ischiorectal fistula (566)
rectovaginal fistula (619.1)
Coding Clinic: 2007, Q1, P13

566   Abscess of anal and rectal regions

Abscess:	Cellulitis:
ischiorectal	anal
perianal	perirectal
perirectal	rectal
	Ischiorectal fistula

Coding Clinic: 1999, Q3, P8-9

● **567   Peritonitis and retroperitoneal infections**

Excludes *peritonitis:*
benign paroxysmal (277.31)
pelvic, female (614.5, 614.7)
periodic familial (277.31)
puerperal (670.8)
with or following:
abortion (634–638 with .0, 639.0)
appendicitis (540.0–540.1)
ectopic or molar pregnancy (639.0)

● *567.0 Peritonitis in infectious diseases classified elsewhere*

Code first underlying disease

Excludes *peritonitis:*
gonococcal (098.86)
syphilitic (095.2)
tuberculous (014.0)

567.1 Pneumococcal peritonitis

Item 9-22 Peritonitis is an inflammation of the lining
(peritoneum) of the abdominal cavity and surface of the intestines.
Retroperitoneal infections occur between the posterior
parietal peritoneum and posterior abdominal wall where the
kidneys, adrenal glands, ureters, duodenum, ascending colon,
descending colon, pancreas, and the large vessels and nerves
are located. Both are caused by bacteria, parasites, injury,
bleeding, or diseases such as systemic lupus erythematosus.

DISEASES OF THE DIGESTIVE SYSTEM (520–579)

● **567.2 Other suppurative peritonitis**
Coding Clinic: 2005, Q4, P74-77; 1998, Q2, P19-20; 1996, Q1, P13-14; 1987, Jan-Feb, P14-15

  567.21 Peritonitis (acute) generalized
Pelvic peritonitis, male

  567.22 Peritoneal abscess

Abscess (of):	Abscess (of):
abdominopelvic	retrocecal
mesenteric	subdiaphragmatic
omentum	subhepatic
peritoneum	subphrenic

  567.23 Spontaneous bacterial peritonitis

> **Excludes** *bacterial peritonitis NOS (567.29)*

  ■**567.29 Other suppurative peritonitis**
Subphrenic peritonitis
Coding Clinic: 2001, Q2, P11-12; 1999, Q3, P9; 1995, Q3, P5

● **567.3 Retroperitoneal infections**

  567.31 Psoas muscle abscess

  ■**567.38 Other retroperitoneal abscess**
Coding Clinic: 2005, Q4, P74-77; 1998, Q2, P19-20

  ■**567.39 Other retroperitoneal infections**

● **567.8 Other specified peritonitis**

  567.81 Choleperitonitis
Peritonitis due to bile

  567.82 Sclerosing mesenteritis
Fat necrosis of peritoneum
(Idiopathic) sclerosing mesenteric fibrosis
Mesenteric lipodystrophy
Mesenteric panniculitis
Retractile mesenteritis
Coding Clinic: 2005, Q4, P74-77

  ■**567.89 Other specified peritonitis**
Chronic proliferative peritonitis
Mesenteric saponification
Peritonitis due to urine

■**567.9 Unspecified peritonitis**

Peritonitis:	Peritonitis:
NOS	of unspecified cause

Coding Clinic: 2004, Q1, P10-11

● **568 Other disorders of peritoneum**

  568.0 Peritoneal adhesions (postoperative) (postinfection)

Adhesions (of):	Adhesions (of):
abdominal (wall)	mesenteric
diaphragm	omentum
intestine	stomach
male pelvis	

Adhesive bands

> **Excludes** *adhesions:*
> *pelvic, female (614.6)*
> *with obstruction:*
> *duodenum (537.3)*
> *intestine (560.81)*

Coding Clinic: 2003, Q3, P7&11; 1995, Q3, P7; 1985, Sept-Oct, P11

● **568.8 Other specified disorders of peritoneum**

  568.81 Hemoperitoneum (nontraumatic)

  568.82 Peritoneal effusion (chronic)

> **Excludes** *ascites NOS (789.51–789.59)*

■**568.89 Other**

Peritoneal:	Peritoneal:
cyst	granuloma

■**568.9 Unspecified disorder of peritoneum**

● **569 Other disorders of intestine**

  569.0 Anal and rectal polyp
Anal and rectal polyp NOS

> **Excludes** *adenomatous anal and rectal polyp (211.4)*

  569.1 Rectal prolapse

Procidentia:	Prolapse:
anus (sphincter)	anal canal
rectum (sphincter)	rectal mucosa
Proctoptosis	

> **Excludes** *prolapsed hemorrhoids (455.2, 455.5)*

  569.2 Stenosis of rectum and anus
Stricture of anus (sphincter)

  569.3 Hemorrhage of rectum and anus

> **Excludes** *gastrointestinal bleeding NOS (578.9)*
> *melena (578.1)*

Coding Clinic: 2005, Q3, P17

● **569.4 Other specified disorders of rectum and anus**

  569.41 Ulcer of anus and rectum
Solitary ulcer of anus (sphincter) or rectum (sphincter)
Stercoral ulcer of anus (sphincter) or rectum (sphincter)

  569.42 Anal or rectal pain
Coding Clinic: 2003, Q1, P8; 1996, Q1, P13

  569.43 Anal sphincter tear (healed) (old)
Tear of anus, nontraumatic

Use additional code for any associated fecal incontinence (787.6)

> **Excludes** *anal fissure (565.0)*
> *anal sphincter tear (healed) (old)*
> *complicating delivery (654.8)*

  569.44 Dysplasia of anus
Anal intraepithelial neoplasia I and II (AIN I and II) (histologically confirmed)
Dysplasia of anus NOS
Mild and moderate dysplasia of anus (histologically confirmed)

> **Excludes** *abnormal results from anal cytologic examination without histologic confirmation (796.70-796.79)*
> *anal intraepithelial neoplasia III (230.5, 230.6)*
> *carcinoma in situ of anus (230.5, 230.6)*
> *HGSIL of anus (796.74)*
> *severe dysplasia of anus (230.5, 230.6)*

Coding Clinic: 2008, Q4, P117-119

◄ New   ◄▬ Revised   ~~deleted~~ Deleted   ● Use Additional Digit(s)   ■ Nonspecific Code
● Not first-listed DX   OGCR Official Guidelines   Coding Clinic   Excludes   Includes   Use additional   Code first   Omit code

■569.49 **Other**
Granuloma of rectum (sphincter)
Rupture of rectum (sphincter)
Hypertrophy of anal papillae
Proctitis NOS

Excludes *fistula of rectum to:*
internal organs - see Alphabetic
Index
skin (565.1)
hemorrhoids (455.0–455.9)
incontinence of sphincter ani
(787.6)

569.5 **Abscess of intestine**

Excludes *appendiceal abscess (540.1)*

Coding Clinic: 1996, Q1, P13-14

● 569.6 **Colostomy and enterostomy complications**

■569.60 **Colostomy and enterostomy complication, unspecified**

569.61 **Infection of colostomy and enterostomy**
Use additional code to specify type of infection, such as:
abscess or cellulitis of abdomen (682.2)
septicemia (038.0–038.9)
Use additional code to identify organism (041.00–041.9)

569.62 **Mechanical complication of colostomy and enterostomy**
Malfunction of colostomy and enterostomy
Coding Clinic: 2005, Q2, P11-12; 2003, Q1, P10

■569.69 **Other complication**
Fistula   Prolapse
Hernia

● 569.7 **Complications of intestinal pouch** ◄

569.71 **Pouchitis** ◄
Inflammation of internal ileoanal pouch ◄

569.79 **Other complications of intestinal pouch** ◄

● 569.8 **Other specified disorders of intestine**

569.81 **Fistula of intestine, excluding rectum and anus**
Fistula:
abdominal wall
enterocolic
enteroenteric
ileorectal

Excludes *fistula of intestine to internal*
organs - see Alphabetic Index
persistent postoperative fistula
(998.6)

Coding Clinic: 1999, Q3, P8

569.82 **Ulceration of intestine**
Primary ulcer of intestine
Ulceration of colon

Excludes *that with perforation (569.83)*

569.83 **Perforation of intestine**

569.84 **Angiodysplasia of intestine (without mention of hemorrhage)**
Coding Clinic: 1996, Q3, P9-10

569.85 **Angiodysplasia of intestine with hemorrhage**
Coding Clinic: 1996, Q3, P9-10

569.86 **Dieulafoy lesion (hemorrhagic) of intestine**
Coding Clinic: 2002, Q4, P60-61

569.87 **Vomiting of fecal matter** ◄

■569.89 **Other**
Enteroptosis   Pericolitis
Granuloma of intestine   Perisigmoiditis
Prolapse of intestine   Visceroptosis

Excludes *gangrene of intestine, mesentery,*
or omentum (557.0)
hemorrhage of intestine NOS
(578.9)
obstruction of intestine
(560.0–560.9)

■569.9 **Unspecified disorder of intestine**

OTHER DISEASES OF DIGESTIVE SYSTEM (570–579)

570 **Acute and subacute necrosis of liver**
Acute hepatic failure
Acute or subacute hepatitis, not specified as infective
Necrosis of liver (acute) (diffuse) (massive) (subacute)
Parenchymatous degeneration of liver
Yellow atrophy (liver) (acute) (subacute)

Excludes *icterus gravis of newborn (773.0–773.2)*
serum hepatitis (070.2–070.3)
that with:
abortion (634–638 with .7, 639.8)
ectopic or molar pregnancy (639.8)
pregnancy, childbirth, or the puerperium
(646.7)
viral hepatitis (070.0–070.9)
Coding Clinic: 2005, Q2, P9-10; 2000, Q1, P22

● 571 **Chronic liver disease and cirrhosis**

571.0 **Alcoholic fatty liver**   A

571.1 **Acute alcoholic hepatitis**   A
Acute alcoholic liver disease
Coding Clinic: 2002, Q2, P4

571.2 **Alcoholic cirrhosis of liver**   A
Florid cirrhosis
Laennec's cirrhosis (alcoholic)
Coding Clinic: 2007, Q3, P9; Q2, P6-7x2; 2002, Q2, P4; Q1, P3; 1985, Nov-Dec, P14

■571.3 **Alcoholic liver damage, unspecified**   A

● 571.4 **Chronic hepatitis**

Excludes *viral hepatitis (acute) (chronic)*
(070.0–070.9)

■571.40 **Chronic hepatitis, unspecified**

571.41 **Chronic persistent hepatitis**

571.42 **Autoimmune hepatitis**
Coding Clinic: 2008, Q4, P120

■571.49 **Other**
Chronic hepatitis:
active
aggressive
Recurrent hepatitis
Coding Clinic: 1999, Q3, P19

DISEASES OF THE DIGESTIVE SYSTEM (520–579)

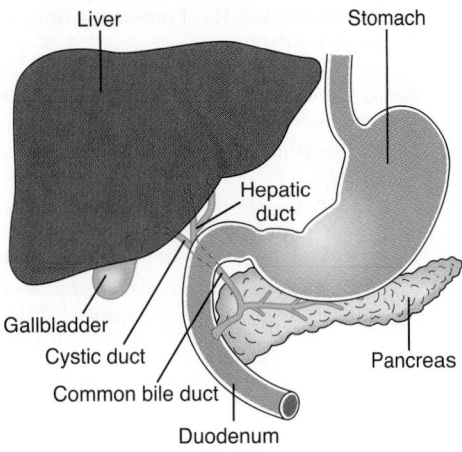

Figure 9–15 Liver and bile ducts.

Item 9–23 Cirrhosis is the progressive fibrosis of the liver resulting in loss of liver function. The main causes of cirrhosis of the liver are alcohol abuse, chronic hepatitis (inflammation of the liver), biliary disease, and excessive amounts of iron. **Alcoholic cirrhosis of the liver** is also called portal, Laënnec's, or fatty nutritional cirrhosis.

571.5 Cirrhosis of liver without mention of alcohol

Cirrhosis of liver:	Cirrhosis of liver:
NOS	micronodular
cryptogenic	posthepatitic
macronodular	postnecrotic

Healed yellow atrophy (liver)
Portal cirrhosis

Code first, if applicable, viral hepatitis (acute) (chronic) (070.0-070.9)
Coding Clinic: 2007, Q3, P9

571.6 Biliary cirrhosis
Chronic nonsuppurative destructive cholangitis
Cirrhosis:
cholangitic
cholestatic

■**571.8 Other chronic nonalcoholic liver disease**
Chronic yellow atrophy (liver)
Fatty liver, without mention of alcohol
Coding Clinic: 1996, Q2, P12

■**571.9 Unspecified chronic liver disease without mention of alcohol**

●**572 Liver abscess and sequelae of chronic liver disease**

572.0 Abscess of liver
Excludes *amebic liver abscess (006.3)*

572.1 Portal pyemia
Phlebitis of portal vein
Portal thrombophlebitis
Pylephlebitis
Pylethrombophlebitis

572.2 Hepatic ~~coma~~ encephalopathy   ◀▥
~~Hepatic encephalopathy~~
Hepatic coma   ◀
Hepatocerebral intoxication
Portal-systemic encephalopathy
Excludes *hepatic coma associated with viral hepatitis - see category 070*
Coding Clinic: 2007, Q2, P6; 2005, Q2, P9-10; 2002, Q1, P3; 1995, Q3, P14

572.3 Portal hypertension
Coding Clinic: 2005, Q3, P15-16

572.4 Hepatorenal syndrome
Excludes *that following delivery (674.8)*
Coding Clinic: 1992, Q3, P15

■**572.8 Other sequelae of chronic liver disease**

●**573 Other disorders of liver**
Excludes *amyloid or lardaceous degeneration of liver (277.39)*
congenital cystic disease of liver (751.62)
glycogen infiltration of liver (271.0)
hepatomegaly NOS (789.1)
portal vein obstruction (452)

573.0 Chronic passive congestion of liver

●**573.1 Hepatitis in viral diseases classified elsewhere**
Code first underlying disease, as:
Coxsackie virus disease (074.8)
cytomegalic inclusion virus disease (078.5)
infectious mononucleosis (075)
Excludes *hepatitis (in):*
mumps (072.71)
viral (070.0–070.9)
yellow fever (060.0–060.9)

●■**573.2 Hepatitis in other infectious diseases classified elsewhere**
Code first underlying disease, as:
malaria (084.9)
Excludes *hepatitis in:*
late syphilis (095.3)
secondary syphilis (091.62)
toxoplasmosis (130.5)

■**573.3 Hepatitis, unspecified**
Toxic (noninfectious) hepatitis
Use additional E code to identify cause
Coding Clinic: 1998, Q3, P4; 1990, Q4, P26

573.4 Hepatic infarction

■**573.8 Other specified disorders of liver**
Hepatoptosis

■**573.9 Unspecified disorder of liver**

●**574 Cholelithiasis**
Presence or formation of gallstones
Coding Clinic: 1990, Q1, P19

The following fifth-digit subclassification is for use with category 574:

0	**without mention of obstruction**
1	**with obstruction**

Check documentation for acute/chronic gallbladder/common bile duct either with or without obstruction.

●**574.0 Calculus of gallbladder with acute cholecystitis**
[0-1]   Biliary calculus with acute cholecystitis
Calculus of cystic duct with acute cholecystitis
Cholelithiasis with acute cholecystitis
Any condition classifiable to 574.2 with acute cholecystitis
Coding Clinic: 1996, Q4, P32; 1984, Nov-Dec, P18

◀ New   ◀▥ Revised   ~~deleted~~ Deleted   ● Use Additional Digit(s)   ■ Nonspecific Code
● Not first-listed DX   OGCR Official Guidelines   Coding Clinic   Excludes   Includes   Use additional   Code first   Omit code

●■**574.1 Calculus of gallbladder with other cholecystitis**
[0-1]   Biliary calculus with cholecystitis
      Calculus of cystic duct with cholecystitis
      Cholelithiasis with cholecystitis
      Cholecystitis with cholelithiasis NOS
      Any condition classifiable to 574.2 with
        cholecystitis (chronic)
      Coding Clinic: 2003, Q1, P5; 1999, Q3, P9; 1996, Q4, P69; Q2,
      P13-15; Q1, P7

●**574.2 Calculus of gallbladder without mention of**
[0-1] **cholecystitis**
      Biliary:
        calculus NOS
        colic NOS
      Calculus of cystic duct
      Cholelithiasis NOS
      Colic (recurrent) of gallbladder
      Gallstone (impacted)
      Coding Clinic: 1995, Q4, P51-52; 1988, Q1, P14

●**574.3 Calculus of bile duct with acute cholecystitis**
[0-1]   Calculus of bile duct [any] with acute cholecystitis
      Choledocholithiasis with acute cholecystitis
      Any condition classifiable to 574.5 with acute
        cholecystitis

●■**574.4 Calculus of bile duct with other cholecystitis**
[0-1]   Calculus of bile duct [any] with cholecystitis
        (chronic)
      Choledocholithiasis with cholecystitis (chronic)
      Any condition classifiable to 574.5 with
        cholecystitis (chronic)
      Coding Clinic: 1996, Q1, P7

●**574.5 Calculus of bile duct without mention of**
[0-1] **cholecystitis**
      Calculus of: Choledocholithiasis
        bile duct [any]   Hepatic:
        common duct   colic (recurrent)
        hepatic duct   lithiasis
      Coding Clinic: 1996, Q2, P13-15; 1994, Q3, P11

●**574.6 Calculus of gallbladder and bile duct with acute**
[0-1] **cholecystitis**
      Any condition classifiable to 574.0 and 574.3

●**574.7 Calculus of gallbladder and bile duct with other**
[0-1] **cholecystitis**
      Any condition classifiable to 574.1 and 574.4

●**574.8 Calculus of gallbladder and bile duct with acute and**
[0-1] **chronic cholecystitis**
      Any condition classifiable to 574.6 and 574.7
      Coding Clinic: 1996, Q4, P32

●**574.9 Calculus of gallbladder and bile duct without**
[0-1] **cholecystitis**
      Any condition classifiable to 574.2 and 574.5

●**575 Other disorders of gallbladder**
      Cholecystitis is chronic or acute inflammation of gallbladder.

    575.0 Acute cholecystitis
      Abscess of gallbladder without mention of calculus
      Angiocholecystitis without mention of calculus
      Cholecystitis without mention of calculus:
        emphysematous (acute)
        gangrenous
        suppurative
      Empyema of gallbladder without mention of
        calculus
      Gangrene of gallbladder without mention of
        calculus

      Excludes   *that with:*
         acute and chronic cholecystitis (575.12)
         choledocholithiasis (574.3)
         choledocholithiasis and cholelithiasis
           (574.6)
         cholelithiasis (574.0)
      Coding Clinic: 1991, Q3, P17-18

●**575.1 Other cholecystitis**
      Cholecystitis without mention of calculus:
        NOS without mention of calculus
        chronic without mention of calculus

      Excludes   *that with:*
         choledocholithiasis (574.4)
         choledocholithiasis and cholelithiasis
           (574.8)
         cholelithiasis (574.1)
      Coding Clinic: 1991, Q3, P17-18

    ■**575.10 Cholecystitis, unspecified**
      Cholecystitis NOS

    575.11 Chronic cholecystitis

    575.12 Acute and chronic cholecystitis
      Coding Clinic: 1997, Q4, P52; 1996, Q4, P32

    575.2 Obstruction of gallbladder
      Occlusion of cystic duct or gallbladder without
        mention of calculus
      Stenosis of cystic duct or gallbladder without
        mention of calculus
      Stricture of cystic duct or gallbladder without
        mention of calculus

    575.3 Hydrops of gallbladder
      Mucocele of gallbladder

    575.4 Perforation of gallbladder
      Rupture of cystic duct or gallbladder

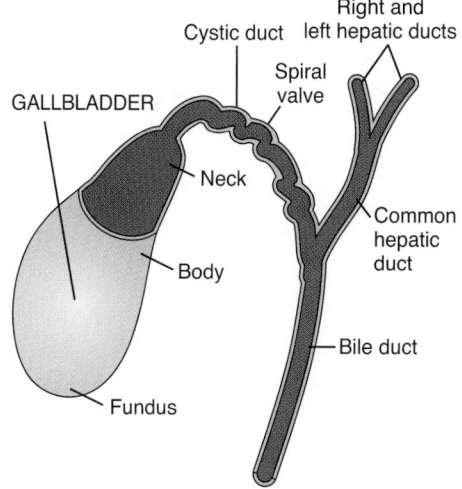

Figure 9–16   Gallbladder and bile ducts.

DISEASES OF THE DIGESTIVE SYSTEM (520–579)

575.5 Fistula of gallbladder

    Fistula: Fistula:
       cholecystoduodenal   cholecystoenteric

575.6 Cholesterolosis of gallbladder

    Strawberry gallbladder

■575.8 Other specified disorders of gallbladder

    Adhesions (of) cystic duct gallbladder
    Atrophy (of) cystic duct gallbladder
    Cyst (of) cystic duct gallbladder
    Hypertrophy (of) cystic duct gallbladder
    Nonfunctioning (of) cystic duct gallbladder
    Ulcer (of) cystic duct gallbladder
    Biliary dyskinesia

> **Excludes** *Hartmann's pouch of intestine (V44.3)*
>   *nonvisualization of gallbladder (793.3)*
> Coding Clinic: 1989, Q2, P13

■575.9 Unspecified disorder of gallbladder

●576 Other disorders of biliary tract

> **Excludes** *that involving the:*
>   *cystic duct (575.0–575.9)*
>   *gallbladder (575.0–575.9)*

576.0 Postcholecystectomy syndrome

    Coding Clinic: 1988, Q1, P10

576.1 Cholangitis

    Cholangitis: Cholangitis:
      NOS   recurrent
      acute   sclerosing
      ascending   secondary
      chronic   stenosing
      primary   suppurative
    Coding Clinic: 1999, Q2, P13-14; 1995, Q2, P7

576.2 Obstruction of bile duct

    Occlusion of bile duct, except cystic duct, without
        mention of calculus
    Stenosis of bile duct, except cystic duct, without
        mention of calculus
    Stricture of bile duct, except cystic duct, without
        mention of calculus

> **Excludes** *congenital (751.61)*
>   *that with calculus (574.3–574.5 with*
>   *fifth-digit 1)*
> Coding Clinic: 2003, Q3, P17-18; 2001, Q1, P8-9; 1999, Q2, P13-14

576.3 Perforation of bile duct

    Rupture of bile duct, except cystic duct

576.4 Fistula of bile duct

    Choledochoduodenal fistula

576.5 Spasm of sphincter of Oddi

■576.8 Other specified disorders of biliary tract

    Adhesions of bile duct [any]
    Atrophy of bile duct [any]
    Cyst of bile duct [any]
    Hypertrophy of bile duct [any]
    Stasis of bile duct [any]
    Ulcer of bile duct [any]

> **Excludes** *congenital choledochal cyst (751.69)*
> Coding Clinic: 2003, Q3, P17-18; 1999, Q2, P14

■576.9 Unspecified disorder of biliary tract

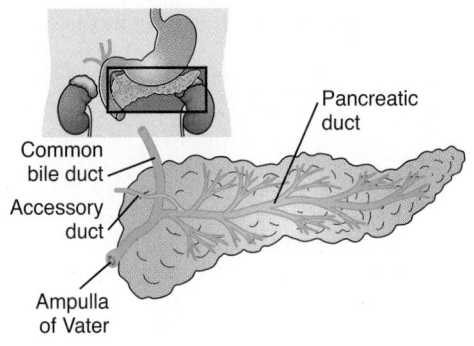

Figure 9–17 Pancreatic ductal system.

●577 Diseases of pancreas

    Pancreatitis is inflammatory process that may be acute or
    chronic.

577.0 Acute pancreatitis

    Abscess of pancreas
    Necrosis of pancreas:
      acute
      infective
    Pancreatitis:
      NOS
      acute (recurrent)
      apoplectic
      hemorrhagic
      subacute
      suppurative

> **Excludes** *mumps pancreatitis (072.3)*
> Coding Clinic: 1999, Q3, P9; 1998, Q2, P19-20; 1996, Q2, P13-15;
>   1989, Q2, P9

577.1 Chronic pancreatitis

    Chronic pancreatitis: Pancreatitis:
      NOS   painless
      infectious   recurrent
      interstitial   relapsing
    Coding Clinic: 2001, Q1, P8-9; 1996, Q2, P13-15; 1994, Q3, P11

577.2 Cyst and pseudocyst of pancreas

■577.8 Other specified diseases of pancreas

    Atrophy of pancreas
    Calculus of pancreas
    Cirrhosis of pancreas
    Fibrosis of pancreas
    Pancreatic:
      infantilism
      necrosis:
        NOS
        aseptic
        fat
    Pancreatolithiasis

> **Excludes** *fibrocystic disease of pancreas*
>   *(277.00–277.09)*
>   *islet cell tumor of pancreas (211.7)*
>   *pancreatic steatorrhea (579.4)*
> Coding Clinic: 2001, Q1, P8-9

■577.9 Unspecified disease of pancreas

◄ New   ◄▦ Revised   ~~deleted~~ Deleted   ● Use Additional Digit(s)   ■ Nonspecific Code

● Not first-listed DX   OGCR Official Guidelines   Coding Clinic   Excludes   Includes   Use additional   Code first   Omit code

● 578   **Gastrointestinal hemorrhage**

> **Excludes**   *that with mention of:*
> *angiodysplasia of stomach and duodenum*
> *(537.83)*
> *angiodysplasia of intestine (569.85)*
> *diverticulitis, intestine:*
> *large (562.13)*
> *small (562.03)*
> *diverticulosis, intestine:*
> *large (562.12)*
> *small (562.02)*
> *gastritis and duodenitis (535.0–535.6)*
> *ulcer:*
> *duodenal, gastric, gastrojejunal, or peptic*
> *(531.00–534.91)*
> Coding Clinic: 2007, Q2, P13; 1992, Q2, P9-10; Q2, P8-9

     578.0   Hematemesis
         Vomiting of blood
         Coding Clinic: 2002, Q2, P4

     578.1   Blood in stool
         Melena

> **Excludes**   *melena of the newborn (772.4, 777.3)*
> *occult blood (792.1)*
> Coding Clinic: 2006, Q2, P17; 1992, Q2, P8-9

   ■ **578.9   Hemorrhage of gastrointestinal tract, unspecified**
         Gastric hemorrhage   Intestinal hemorrhage
         Coding Clinic: 2008, Q2, P15-16; 2006, Q4, P91-92; 2005, Q3,
              P17-18; 1986, Nov-Dec, P9; 1985, Sept-Oct, P9

● 579   **Intestinal malabsorption**

     579.0   Celiac disease

Celiac:	Gee (-Herter) disease
crisis	Gluten enteropathy
infantilism	Idiopathic steatorrhea
rickets	Nontropical sprue

     579.1   Tropical sprue
         Sprue:
            NOS
            tropical
         Tropical steatorrhea

     579.2   Blind loop syndrome
         Postoperative blind loop syndrome

   ■ **579.3   Other and unspecified postsurgical nonabsorption**
         Hypoglycemia following gastrointestinal surgery
         Malnutrition following gastrointestinal surgery
         Coding Clinic: 2003, Q4, P104-105

     579.4   Pancreatic steatorrhea

   ■ **579.8   Other specified intestinal malabsorption**
         Enteropathy:
            exudative
            protein-losing
         Steatorrhea (chronic)
         Coding Clinic: 2003, Q1, P12

   ■ **579.9   Unspecified intestinal malabsorption**
         Malabsorption syndrome NOS
         Coding Clinic: 2004, Q4, P57-59

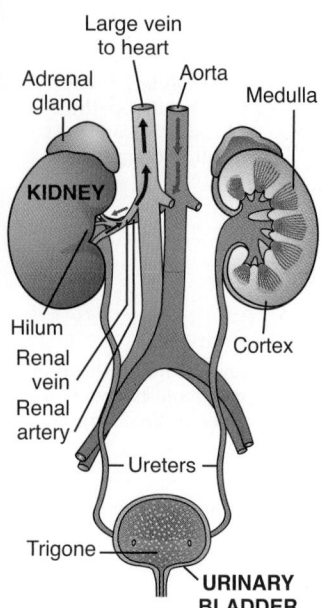

Figure 10-1 Kidneys within the urinary system.

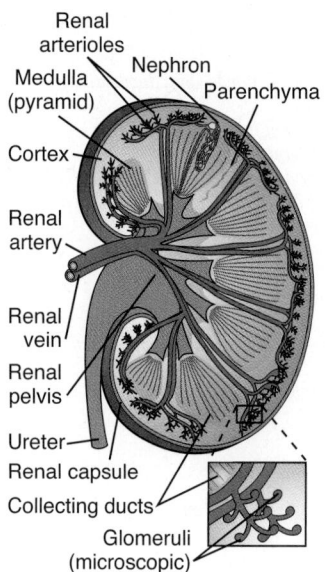

Figure 10-2 Kidney cross section.

Item 10-1 Glomerulonephritis is nephritis accompanied by inflammation of the glomeruli of the kidney, resulting in the degeneration of the glomeruli and the nephrons.
Acute glomerulonephritis primarily affects children and young adults and is usually a result of a streptococcal infection.
Proliferative glomerulonephritis is the acute form of the disease resulting from a streptococcal infection.
Rapidly progressive glomerulonephritis, also known as **crescentic** or **malignant glomerulonephritis,** is the acute form of the disease, which leads quickly to rapid and progressive decline in renal function.

Item 10-2 Nephrotic syndrome (NS) is marked by massive proteinuria (protein in the urine) and water retention. Patients with NS are particularly vulnerable to staphylococcal and pneumococcal infections. NS with lesion of proliferative glomerulonephritis results from a streptococcal infection. NS with lesion of membranous glomerulonephritis results in thickening of the capillary walls. NS with lesion of minimal change glomerulonephritis is usually a benign disorder that occurs mostly in children and requires electron microscopy (biopsy) to verify changes in the glomeruli.

10.   DISEASES OF THE GENITOURINARY SYSTEM (580–629)

NEPHRITIS, NEPHROTIC SYNDROME, AND NEPHROSIS (580–589)

> **Excludes** *hypertensive chronic kidney disease (403.00–403.91, 404.00–404.93)*

● **580   Acute glomerulonephritis**

> **Includes**   acute nephritis

580.0 With lesion of proliferative glomerulonephritis
Acute (diffuse) proliferative glomerulonephritis
Acute poststreptococcal glomerulonephritis

580.4 With lesion of rapidly progressive glomerulonephritis
Acute nephritis with lesion of necrotizing glomerulitis

● **580.8 With other specified pathological lesion in kidney**

> ● **580.81 *Acute glomerulonephritis in diseases classified elsewhere***
>
> > *Code first underlying disease, as:*
> > infectious hepatitis (070.0–070.9)
> > mumps (072.79)
> > subacute bacterial endocarditis (421.0)
> > typhoid fever (002.0)

■ **580.89 Other**
Glomerulonephritis, acute, with lesion of:
exudative nephritis
interstitial (diffuse) (focal) nephritis

■ **580.9 Acute glomerulonephritis with unspecified pathological lesion in kidney**
Glomerulonephritis: specified as acute
NOS specified as acute
hemorrhagic specified as acute
Nephritis specified as acute
Nephropathy specified as acute

◀ New   ◀▥ Revised   ~~deleted~~ Deleted   ● Use Additional Digit(s)   ■ Nonspecific Code
● Not first-listed DX   OGCR Official Guidelines   Coding Clinic   Excludes   Includes   Use additional   Code first   Omit code

● **581   Nephrotic syndrome**

   581.0   With lesion of proliferative glomerulonephritis

   581.1   With lesion of membranous glomerulonephritis
           Epimembranous nephritis
           Idiopathic membranous glomerular disease
           Nephrotic syndrome with lesion of:
               focal glomerulosclerosis
               sclerosing membranous glomerulonephritis
               segmental hyalinosis

   **581.2   With lesion of membranoproliferative
           glomerulonephritis**
           Nephrotic syndrome with lesion (of):
               endothelial glomerulonephritis
               hypocomplementemic glomerulonephritis
                   persistent glomerulonephritis
               lobular glomerulonephritis
               mesangiocapillary glomerulonephritis
               mixed membranous and proliferative
                   glomerulonephritis

   581.3   With lesion of minimal change glomerulonephritis
           Foot process disease
           Lipoid nephrosis
           Minimal change:
               glomerular disease
               glomerulitis
               nephrotic syndrome
           Coding Clinic: 2007, Q1, P23

● **581.8   With other specified pathological lesion in
           kidney**

   ● *581.81   Nephrotic syndrome in diseases classified
               elsewhere*

           Code first underlying disease, as:
               amyloidosis (277.30–277.39)
               diabetes mellitus (249.4, 250.4)
               malaria (084.9)
               polyarteritis (446.0)
               systemic lupus erythematosus (710.0)

           Excludes *nephrosis in epidemic hemorrhagic
                       fever (078.6)*

   ■ **581.89   Other**
           Glomerulonephritis with edema and
               lesion of:
               exudative nephritis
               interstitial (diffuse) (focal) nephritis

   ■ **581.9   Nephrotic syndrome with unspecified pathological
           lesion in kidney**
           Glomerulonephritis with edema NOS
           Nephritis:
               nephrotic NOS
               with edema NOS
           Nephrosis NOS
           Renal disease with edema NOS

Item 10–3   Chronic glomerulonephritis (GN) persists
over a period of years, with remissions and exacerbation.
**Chronic   GN   with   lesion   of   proliferative
glomerulonephritis** results from a streptococcal infection.
**Chronic   GN   with   lesion   of   membranous
glomerulonephritis,** also known as membranous
nephropathy, is characterized by deposits along the epithelial
side of the basement membrane.
**Chronic GN with lesion of membranoproliferative
glomerulonephritis** (MPGN) is a group of disorders
characterized by alterations in the basement membranes of the
kidney and the glomerular cells.
**Chronic GN with lesion of rapidly progressive
glomerulonephritis** is characterized by necrosis, endothelial
proliferation, and mesangial proliferation. The condition is
marked by rapid and progressive decline in renal function.

● **582   Chronic glomerulonephritis**

   Includes   chronic nephritis

   582.0   With lesion of proliferative glomerulonephritis
           Chronic (diffuse) proliferative glomerulonephritis

   582.1   With lesion of membranous glomerulonephritis
           Chronic glomerulonephritis:
               membranous
               sclerosing
           Focal glomerulosclerosis
           Segmental hyalinosis
           Coding Clinic: 1984, Sept-Oct, P16

   **582.2   With lesion of membranoproliferative
           glomerulonephritis**
           Chronic glomerulonephritis:
               endothelial
               hypocomplementemic persistent
               lobular
               membranoproliferative
               mesangiocapillary
               mixed membranous and proliferative

   **582.4   With lesion of rapidly progressive
           glomerulonephritis**
           Chronic nephritis with lesion of necrotizing
               glomerulitis

● **582.8   With other specified pathological lesion in kidney**

   ● *582.81   Chronic glomerulonephritis in diseases
               classified elsewhere*

           Code first underlying disease, as:
               amyloidosis (277.30–277.39)
               systemic lupus erythematosus (710.0)

   ■ **582.89   Other**
           Chronic glomerulonephritis with lesion of:
               exudative nephritis
               interstitial (diffuse) (focal) nephritis

   ■ **582.9   Chronic glomerulonephritis with unspecified
           pathological lesion in kidney**
           Glomerulonephritis: specified as chronic
               NOS specified as chronic
               hemorrhagic specified as chronic
           Nephritis specified as chronic
           Nephropathy specified as chronic
           Coding Clinic: 2001, Q2, P12

DISEASES OF THE GENITOURINARY SYSTEM (580–629)

Item 10–4 Nephritis (inflammation) or **nephropathy** (disease) **with lesion of proliferative glomerulonephritis** results from a streptococcal infection.

Nephritis (inflammation) or **nephropathy** (disease) **with lesion of membranous glomerulonephritis** is characterized by deposits along the epithelial side of the basement membrane.

Nephritis (inflammation) or **nephropathy** (disease) **with lesion of membranoproliferative glomerulonephritis** is characterized by alterations in the basement membranes of the kidney and the glomerular cells.

Nephritis (inflammation) or **nephropathy** (disease) **with lesion of rapidly progressive glomerulonephritis** is characterized by rapid and progressive decline in renal function.

Nephritis (inflammation) or **nephropathy** (disease) **with lesion of renal cortical necrosis** is characterized by death of the cortical tissues.

Nephritis (inflammation) or **nephropathy** (disease) **with lesion of renal medullary necrosis** is characterized by death of the tissues that collect urine.

● **583 Nephritis and nephropathy, not specified as acute or chronic**

Includes   "renal disease" so stated, not specified as acute or chronic but with stated pathology or cause

583.0   With lesion of proliferative glomerulonephritis
Proliferative:
glomerulonephritis (diffuse) NOS
nephritis NOS
nephropathy NOS

583.1   With lesion of membranous glomerulonephritis
Membranous:
glomerulonephritis NOS
nephritis NOS
Membranous nephropathy NOS

583.2   With lesion of membranoproliferative glomerulonephritis
Membranoproliferative:
glomerulonephritis NOS
nephritis NOS
nephropathy NOS
Nephritis NOS, with lesion of:
hypocomplementemic persistent
glomerulonephritis
lobular glomerulonephritis
mesangiocapillary glomerulonephritis
mixed membranous and proliferative
glomerulonephritis

583.4   With lesion of rapidly progressive glomerulonephritis
Necrotizing or rapidly progressive:
glomerulitis NOS
glomerulonephritis NOS
nephritis NOS
nephropathy NOS
Nephritis, unspecified, with lesion of necrotizing
glomerulitis

583.6   With lesion of renal cortical necrosis
Nephritis NOS with (renal) cortical necrosis
Nephropathy NOS with (renal) cortical necrosis
Renal cortical necrosis NOS

583.7   With lesion of renal medullary necrosis
Nephritis NOS with (renal) medullary [papillary]
necrosis
Nephropathy NOS with (renal) medullary
[papillary] necrosis

● **583.8 With other specified pathological lesion in kidney**

● *583.81 Nephritis and nephropathy, not specified as acute or chronic, in diseases classified elsewhere*

Code first underlying disease, as:
amyloidosis (277.30–277.39)
diabetes mellitus (249.4, 250.4)
gonococcal infection (098.19)
Goodpasture's syndrome (446.21)
systemic lupus erythematosus (710.0)
tuberculosis (016.0)

Excludes   *gouty nephropathy (274.10)*
syphilitic nephritis (095.4)
Coding Clinic: 2003, Q2, P7

■ **583.89 Other**
Glomerulitis with lesion of:
exudative nephritis
interstitial nephritis
Glomerulonephritis with lesion of:
exudative nephritis
interstitial nephritis
Nephritis with lesion of:
exudative nephritis
interstitial nephritis
Nephropathy with lesion of:
exudative nephritis
interstitial nephritis
Renal disease with lesion of:
exudative nephritis
interstitial nephritis

■ **583.9 With unspecified pathological lesion in kidney**
Glomerulitis NOS   Nephritis NOS
Glomerulonephritis NOS   Nephropathy NOS

Excludes   *nephropathy complicating pregnancy, labor,*
or the puerperium (642.0–642.9,
646.2)
renal disease NOS with no stated cause
(593.9)
Coding Clinic: 1994, Q4, P35

Item 10–5   Decreased blood flow is the usual cause of **acute renal failure** that offers a good prognosis for recovery. **Chronic renal failure** is usually the result of long-standing kidney disease and is a very serious condition that generally results in death.

● **584 Acute ~~renal~~ kidney failure**   ◀▥

Includes   Acute renal failure   ◀

Excludes   *following labor and delivery (669.3)*
posttraumatic (958.5)
that complicating:
abortion (634–638 with .3, 639.3)
ectopic or molar pregnancy (639.3)
Coding Clinic: 1992, Q2, P5x2

584.5   Acute kidney failure ~~W~~with lesion of tubular necrosis   ◀▥
Lower nephron nephrosis
Renal failure with (acute) tubular necrosis
Tubular necrosis:
NOS
acute

584.6   Acute kidney failure ~~W~~with lesion of renal cortical necrosis   ◀▥

584.7   Acute kidney failure ~~W~~with lesion of renal medullary [papillary] necrosis   ◀▥
Necrotizing renal papillitis

■ **584.8 Acute kidney failure ~~W~~with other specified pathological lesion in kidney**   ◀▥

◀ New   ◀▥ Revised   ~~deleted~~ Deleted   ● Use Additional Digit(s)   ■ Nonspecific Code
● Not first-listed DX   OGCR Official Guidelines   Coding Clinic   Excludes   Includes   Use additional   Code first   Omit code

DISEASES OF THE GENITOURINARY SYSTEM (580–629)

■**584.9 Acute kidney failure ~~renal~~, unspecified** ◄▥
  Acute kidney injury (nontraumatic)
  Excludes *traumatic kidney injury (866.00-866.13)*
  Coding Clinic: 2008, Q4, P192-193; 2007, Q4, P96-97; 2005, Q2, P18-19; 2003, Q2, P7; 2003, Q1, P22; 2002, Q3, P21x2, 28x2; 2001, Q2, P14x2; 2000, Q3, P9; 2000, Q1, P22; 1996, Q3, P9; 1993, Q4, P34

  OGCR Section I.C.10.a.1
  The ICD-9-CM classifies CKD based on severity. The severity of CKD is designated by stages I-V. Stage II, code 585.2, equates to mild CKD; stage III, code 585.3, equates to moderate CKD; and stage IV, code 585.4, equates to severe CKD. Code 585.6, End stage renal disease (ESRD), is assigned when the provider has documented end-stage-renal disease (ESRD). If both a stage of CKD and ESRD are documented, assign code 585.6 only.

●**585 Chronic kidney disease (CKD)**
  Includes Chronic uremia
  Code first hypertensive chronic kidney disease, if applicable, (403.00–403.91, 404.00–404.93)
  Use additional code to identify:
    kidney transplant status, if applicable (V42.0)
    manifestation as:
      uremic:
        neuropathy (357.4)
        pericarditis (420.0)

  585.1 Chronic kidney disease, Stage I
  585.2 Chronic kidney disease, Stage II (mild)
  585.3 Chronic kidney disease, Stage III (moderate)
    Coding Clinic: 2005, Q4, P68-69
  585.4 Chronic kidney disease, Stage IV (severe)
  585.5 Chronic kidney disease, Stage V
    Excludes *chronic kidney disease, stage V requiring chronic dialysis (585.6)*
  585.6 End stage renal disease
    Chronic kidney disease, stage V requiring chronic dialysis
    Coding Clinic: 2008, Q4, P193; Q1, P7-8; 2007, Q4, P84-86; Q3, P5-6; Q3, P11; 2006, Q4, P136; 2004, Q1, P5
  585.9 Chronic kidney disease, unspecified
    Chronic renal disease
    Chronic renal failure NOS
    Chronic renal insufficiency
    Coding Clinic: 2008, Q1, P7-8, 19; 2007, Q2, P3; 2006, Q4, P84-86; 2003, Q4, P60-61,111-112; 2001, Q2, P11-13x2; Q1, P3; 2000, Q4, P39-40; 1998, Q4, P54-55; Q3, P6-7; Q2, P20-21; 1996, Q3, P9; 1995, Q2, P10; 1987, Sept-Oct, P10; 1985, Nov-Dec, P15

■**586 Renal failure, unspecified**
  Includes Uremia NOS
  Excludes *following labor and delivery (669.3)*
    posttraumatic renal failure (958.5)
    that complicating:
      abortion (634–638 with .3, 639.3)
      ectopic or molar pregnancy (639.3)
    uremia:
      extrarenal (788.9)
      prerenal (788.9)
  Coding Clinic: 1998, Q3, P6; 1984, Sept-Oct, P16

■**587 Renal sclerosis, unspecified**
  ~~Atrophy of kidney~~
  Includes Atrophy of kidney ◄
    Contracted kidney
    Renal:
      cirrhosis
      fibrosis

●**588 Disorders resulting from impaired renal function**
  588.0 Renal osteodystrophy
    Azotemic osteodystrophy
    Phosphate-losing tubular disorders
    Renal:
      dwarfism
      infantilism
      rickets
  588.1 Nephrogenic diabetes insipidus
    Excludes *diabetes insipidus NOS (253.5)*
  588.8 Other specified disorders resulting from impaired renal function
    Excludes *secondary hypertension (405.0–405.9)*
    Coding Clinic: 2004, Q4, P57-59
    588.81 Secondary hyperparathyroidism (of renal origin)
      Secondary hyperparathyroidism NOS
    588.89 Other specified disorders resulting from impaired renal function
      Hypokalemic nephropathy
  ■**588.9 Unspecified disorder resulting from impaired renal function**

●**589 Small kidney of unknown cause**
  589.0 Unilateral small kidney
  589.1 Bilateral small kidneys
  ■**589.9 Small kidney, unspecified**

OTHER DISEASES OF URINARY SYSTEM (590–599)

●**590 Infections of kidney**
  Use additional code to identify organism, such as Escherichia coli [E. coli] (041.4)
  ●**590.0 Chronic pyelonephritis**
    Chronic pyelitis
    Chronic pyonephrosis
    Code, if applicable, any causal condition first
    590.00 Without lesion of renal medullary necrosis
    590.01 With lesion of renal medullary necrosis
  ●**590.1 Acute pyelonephritis**
    Acute pyelitis
    Acute pyonephrosis
    590.10 Without lesion of renal medullary necrosis
    590.11 With lesion of renal medullary necrosis
  590.2 Renal and perinephric abscess
    Abscess:
      kidney
      nephritic
      perirenal
    Carbuncle of kidney
  590.3 Pyeloureteritis cystica
    Infection of renal pelvis and ureter
    Ureteritis cystica
    Cystica is an infection of the urinary bladder.

DISEASES OF THE GENITOURINARY SYSTEM (580–629)

DISEASES OF THE GENITOURINARY SYSTEM (580–629)

- ● **590.8 Other pyelonephritis or pyonephrosis, not specified as acute or chronic**
  - ■ **590.80 Pyelonephritis, unspecified**
    Pyelitis NOS
    Pyelonephritis NOS
    Coding Clinic: 1997, Q4, P40
  - ● **590.81 Pyelitis or pyelonephritis in diseases classified elsewhere**
    Code first underlying disease, as:
    tuberculosis (016.0)
- ■ **590.9 Infection of kidney, unspecified**
  Excludes *urinary tract infection NOS (599.0)*

591 Hydronephrosis
Hydrocalycosis
Hydronephrosis
Hydroureteronephrosis
Excludes *congenital hydronephrosis (753.29)*
hydroureter (593.5)
Coding Clinic: 1998, Q2, P9

- ● **592 Calculus of kidney and ureter**
  Excludes *nephrocalcinosis (275.49)*
  - **592.0 Calculus of kidney**
    Nephrolithiasis NOS
    Renal calculus or stone
    Staghorn calculus
    Stone in kidney
    Excludes *uric acid nephrolithiasis (274.11)*
    Coding Clinic: 2000, Q1, P4; 1993, Q2, P3
  - **592.1 Calculus of ureter**
    Ureteric stone
    Ureterolithiasis
    Coding Clinic: 1998, Q2, P9; 1991, Q1, P11
  - ■ **592.9 Urinary calculus, unspecified**
    Coding Clinic: 1997, Q4, P40

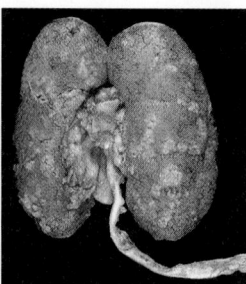

Figure 10–3 Acute pyelonephritis. Cortical surface exhibits grayish white areas of inflammation and abscess formation. (From Kumar: Robbins and Cotran: Pathologic Basis of Disease, 7th ed. 2005, Saunders, An Imprint of Elsevier)

Item 10-6 Pyelonephritis is an infection of the kidneys and ureters and may be chronic or acute in one or both kidneys.

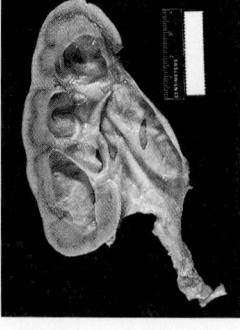

Figure 10–4 Hydronephrosis of the kidney, with marked dilatation of pelvis and calyces and thinning of renal parenchyma. (From Kumar: Robbins and Cotran: Pathologic Basis of Disease, 7th ed. 2005, Saunders, An Imprint of Elsevier)

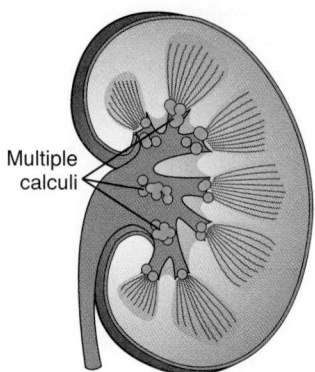

Figure 10–5 Multiple urinary calculi.

Multiple calculi

- ● **593 Other disorders of kidney and ureter**
  - **593.0 Nephroptosis**
    Floating kidney   Mobile kidney
  - **593.1 Hypertrophy of kidney**
  - **593.2 Cyst of kidney, acquired**
    Cyst (multiple) (solitary) of kidney, not congenital
    Peripelvic (lymphatic) cyst
    Excludes *calyceal or pyelogenic cyst of kidney (591)*
    congenital cyst of kidney (753.1)
    polycystic (disease of) kidney (753.1)
  - **593.3 Stricture or kinking of ureter**
    Angulation of ureter (postoperative)
    Constriction of ureter (postoperative)
    Stricture of pelviureteric junction
    Coding Clinic: 1994, Q3, P8
  - ■ **593.4 Other ureteric obstruction**
    Idiopathic retroperitoneal fibrosis
    Occlusion NOS of ureter
    Excludes *that due to calculus (592.1)*
    Coding Clinic: 1997, Q2, P4
  - **593.5 Hydroureter**
    Excludes *congenital hydroureter (753.22)*
    hydroureteronephrosis (591)
  - **593.6 Postural proteinuria**
    Benign postural proteinuria
    Orthostatic proteinuria
    Excludes *proteinuria NOS (791.0)*
  - ● **593.7 Vesicoureteral reflux**
    Occurs when urine flows from bladder back into ureters
    - ■ **593.70 Unspecified or without reflux nephropathy**
    - **593.71 With reflux nephropathy, unilateral**
    - **593.72 With reflux nephropathy, bilateral**
    - ■ **593.73 With reflux nephropathy NOS**
  - ● **593.8 Other specified disorders of kidney and ureter**
    - **593.81 Vascular disorders of kidney**
      Renal (artery):
      embolism
      hemorrhage
      thrombosis
      Renal infarction
    - **593.82 Ureteral fistula**
      Intestinoureteral fistula
      Excludes *fistula between ureter and female genital tract (619.0)*

◄ New   ◄═ Revised   ~~deleted~~ Deleted   ● Use Additional Digit(s)   ■ Nonspecific Code
● Not first-listed DX   OGCR Official Guidelines   Coding Clinic   Excludes   Includes   Use additional   Code first   Omit code

■593.89 **Other**
Adhesions, kidney or ureter
Periureteritis
Polyp of ureter
Pyelectasia
Ureterocele

Excludes *tuberculosis of ureter (016.2)*
ureteritis cystica (590.3)
Coding Clinic: 1984, Nov-Dec, P17

■593.9 **Unspecified disorder of kidney and ureter**
Acute renal disease
Acute renal insufficiency
Renal disease NOS
Salt-losing nephritis or syndrome

Excludes *chronic renal insufficiency (585.9)*
cystic kidney disease (753.1)
nephropathy, so stated (583.0–583.9)
renal disease:
arising in pregnancy or the puerperium
(642.1–642.2, 642.4–642.7, 646.2)
not specified as acute or chronic, but
with stated pathology or cause
(583.0–583.9)
Coding Clinic: 2005, Q4, P79-80; 1998, Q2, P9

● 594 **Calculus of lower urinary tract**

594.0 **Calculus in diverticulum of bladder**

■594.1 **Other calculus in bladder**
Urinary bladder stone

Excludes *staghorn calculus (592.0)*

594.2 **Calculus in urethra**

■594.8 **Other lower urinary tract calculus**
Coding Clinic: 1985, Jan-Feb, P16

■594.9 **Calculus of lower urinary tract, unspecified**

Excludes *calculus of urinary tract NOS (592.9)*

● 595 **Cystitis**
A general term used to describe an infection of the bladder and
irritations in the lower urinary tract

Excludes *prostatocystitis (601.3)*

Use additional code to identify organism, such as
Escherichia coli [E. coli] (041.4)

595.0 **Acute cystitis**

Excludes *trigonitis (595.3)*

Coding Clinic: 1999, Q2, P15-16; 1984, Nov-Dec, P15

595.1 **Chronic interstitial cystitis**
Describes an ongoing infection of the kidney glomeruli
and tubules
Hunner's ulcer
Panmural fibrosis of bladder
Submucous cystitis

■595.2 **Other chronic cystitis**
Chronic cystitis NOS
Subacute cystitis

Excludes *trigonitis (595.3)*

595.3 **Trigonitis**
Inflammation of triangular area of bladder (where
ureters and urethra come together)
Follicular cystitis
Trigonitis (acute) (chronic)
Urethrotrigonitis

● 595.4 *Cystitis in diseases classified elsewhere*
Code first underlying disease, as:
actinomycosis (039.8)
amebiasis (006.8)
bilharziasis (120.0–120.9)
Echinococcus infestation (122.3, 122.6)

Excludes *cystitis:*
diphtheritic (032.84)
gonococcal (098.11, 098.31)
monilial (112.2)
trichomonal (131.09)
tuberculous (016.1)

● 595.8 **Other specified types of cystitis**

595.81 **Cystitis cystica**

595.82 **Irradiation cystitis**
Use additional E code to identify cause

■595.89 **Other**
Abscess of bladder
Cystitis:
bullous
emphysematous
glandularis

■595.9 **Cystitis, unspecified**

● 596 **Other disorders of bladder**
Use additional code to identify urinary incontinence
(625.6, 788.30–788.39)

596.0 **Bladder neck obstruction**
Contracture (acquired) of bladder neck or
vesicourethral orifice
Obstruction (acquired) of bladder neck or
vesicourethral orifice
Stenosis (acquired) of bladder neck or
vesicourethral orifice

Excludes *congenital (753.6)*

Coding Clinic: 2002, Q3, P28; 2001, Q2, P14; 1994, Q3, P12

596.1 **Intestinovesical fistula**
Passage between bladder and the intestine
Fistula:　　　　　　　　Fistula:
enterovesical　　　　　　vesicoenteric
vesicocolic　　　　　　　vesicorectal

596.2 **Vesical fistula, not elsewhere classified**
Fistula:　　　　　　　　Fistula:
bladder NOS　　　　　　vesicocutaneous
urethrovesical　　　　　vesicoperineal

Excludes *fistula between bladder and female genital*
tract (619.0)

596.3 **Diverticulum of bladder**
Formation of a sac from a herniation of the wall of the
bladder
Diverticulitis of bladder
Diverticulum (acquired) (false) of bladder

Excludes *that with calculus in diverticulum of*
bladder (594.0)

596.4 **Atony of bladder**
Diminished tone of bladder muscle
High compliance bladder
Hypotonicity of bladder
Inertia of bladder

Excludes *neurogenic bladder (596.54)*

DISEASES OF THE GENITOURINARY SYSTEM (580–629)

● **596.5 Other functional disorders of bladder**

> **Excludes** *cauda equina syndrome with neurogenic bladder (344.61)*

596.51 Hypertonicity of bladder
Hyperactivity
Overactive bladder

596.52 Low bladder compliance

596.53 Paralysis of bladder

596.54 Neurogenic bladder NOS
Coding Clinic: 2001, Q1, P12

596.55 Detrusor sphincter dyssynergia

■**596.59 Other functional disorder of bladder**
Detrusor instability
Coding Clinic: 1995, Q4, P72-73

596.6 Rupture of bladder, nontraumatic

596.7 Hemorrhage into bladder wall
Hyperemia of bladder

> **Excludes** *acute hemorrhagic cystitis (595.0)*

■**596.8 Other specified disorders of bladder**
Calcified
Contracted
Hemorrhage
Hypertrophy

> **Excludes** *cystocele, female (618.01–618.02, 618.09, 618.2–618.4)*
> *hernia or prolapse of bladder, female (618.01–618.02, 618.09, 618.2–618.4)*

■**596.9 Unspecified disorder of bladder**

● **597 Urethritis, not sexually transmitted, and urethral syndrome**
Inflammation of urethra caused by bacteria or virus

> **Excludes** *nonspecific urethritis, so stated (099.4)*

597.0 Urethral abscess
Abscess of:
bulbourethral gland
Cowper's gland
Littré's gland
Abscess:
periurethral
urethral (gland)
Periurethral cellulitis

> **Excludes** *urethral caruncle (599.3)*

● **597.8 Other urethritis**

■**597.80 Urethritis, unspecified**

597.81 Urethral syndrome NOS

■**597.89 Other**
Adenitis, Skene's glands
Cowperitis
Meatitis, urethral
Ulcer, urethra (meatus)
Verumontanitis

> **Excludes** *trichomonal (131.02)*

● **598 Urethral stricture**
Narrowing of lumen of urethra caused by scarring from an infection or injury, which results in functional obstruction

> **Includes** pinhole meatus
> stricture of urinary meatus

Use additional code to identify urinary incontinence (625.6, 788.30–788.39)

> **Excludes** *congenital stricture of urethra and urinary meatus (753.6)*

● **598.0 Urethral stricture due to infection**

■**598.00 Due to unspecified infection**

● *598.01 Due to infective diseases classified elsewhere*

> *Code first underlying disease, as:*
> gonococcal infection (098.2)
> schistosomiasis (120.0–120.9)
> syphilis (095.8)

598.1 Traumatic urethral stricture
Stricture of urethra:
late effect of injury
postobstetric

> **Excludes** *postoperative following surgery on genitourinary tract (598.2)*

598.2 Postoperative urethral stricture
Postcatheterization stricture of urethra
Coding Clinic: 1997, Q3, P6

■**598.8 Other specified causes of urethral stricture**
Coding Clinic: 1984, Nov-Dec, P9

■**598.9 Urethral stricture, unspecified**

● **599 Other disorders of urethra and urinary tract**

■**599.0 Urinary tract infection, site not specified**

> **Excludes** *Candidiasis of urinary tract (112.2)*
> *urinary tract infection of newborn (771.82)*

Use additional code to identify organism, such as Escherichia coli [E. coli] (041.4)
Coding Clinic: 2005, Q3, P12-13; 2004, Q2, P13; 1999, Q4, P6; Q2, P15-16; 1998, Q1, P5; 1996, Q4, P33; 1995, Q2, P7; 1994, Q1, P21; 1992, Q1, P13; 1988, Q4, P10; 1984, Nov-Dec, P15; July-Aug, P19

599.1 Urethral fistula
Fistula:
urethroperineal
urethrorectal
Urinary fistula NOS

> **Excludes** *fistula:*
> *urethroscrotal (608.89)*
> *urethrovaginal (619.0)*
> *urethrovesicovaginal (619.0)*
> Coding Clinic: 1997, Q3, P6

599.2 Urethral diverticulum

599.3 Urethral caruncle
Polyp of urethra

599.4 Urethral false passage

599.5 Prolapsed urethral mucosa
Prolapse of urethra
Urethrocele

> **Excludes** *urethrocele, female (618.03, 618.09, 618.2–618.4)*

● **599.6 Urinary obstruction**
Use additional code to identify urinary
incontinence (625.6, 788.30–788.39)
Excludes *obstructive nephropathy NOS (593.89)*
Coding Clinic: 2005, Q4, P80-81

◼ **599.60 Urinary obstruction, unspecified**
Obstructive uropathy NOS
Urinary (tract) obstruction NOS

◼ **599.69 Urinary obstruction, not elsewhere classified**
Code, if applicable, any causal condition first,
such as:
hyperplasia of prostate (600.0–600.9 with
fifth-digit 1)

● **599.7 Hematuria**
Hematuria (benign) (essential)
Excludes *hemoglobinuria (791.2)*
Coding Clinic: 2008, Q4, P121; 2000, Q1, P5; 1995, Q3, P8; 1993, Q1,
P26; 5th Issue, P16; 1985, Nov-Dec, P15

◼ **599.70 Hematuria, unspecified**

599.71 Gross hematuria

599.72 Microscopic hematuria

● **599.8 Other specified disorders of urethra and urinary tract**
Use additional code to identify urinary
incontinence (625.6, 788.30–788.39)
Excludes *symptoms and other conditions classifiable*
to 788.0–788.2, 788.4–788.9,
791.0–791.9

599.81 Urethral hypermobility

599.82 Intrinsic (urethral) sphincter deficiency [ISD]

599.83 Urethral instability

◼ **599.84 Other specified disorders of urethra**
Rupture of urethra (nontraumatic)
Urethral:
cyst
granuloma
Coding Clinic: 2009, Q1, P20

◼ **599.89 Other specified disorders of urinary tract**

◼ **599.9 Unspecified disorder of urethra and urinary tract**

(See Plates 366B, 387 on pages 87 and 89.)

DISEASES OF MALE GENITAL ORGANS (600–608)

● **600 Hyperplasia of prostate**
Benign prostatic hyperplasia (BPH) and is an enlargement of
prostate gland usually occurring with age and causing
obstructed urine flow
Includes Enlarged prostate
Coding Clinic: 2005, Q3, P20; 2003, Q4, P63-64; 2002, Q3, P28; 1994, Q3,
P12-13; 1992, Q3, P7; 1986, Sept-Oct, P12; Nov-Dec, P10; 1984,
Nov-Dec, P9

● **600.0 Hypertrophy (benign) of prostate**
Benign prostatic hypertrophy
Enlargement of prostate
Smooth enlarged prostate
Soft enlarged prostate
Coding Clinic: 2003, Q1, P6; 2001, Q2, P14

600.00 Hypertrophy (benign) of prostate without
urinary obstruction and other lower urinary
tract symptoms (LUTS) ♂ A
Hypertrophy (benign) of prostate NOS

600.01 Hypertrophy (benign) of prostate with
urinary obstruction and other lower urinary
tract symptoms (LUTS) ♂ A
Hypertrophy (benign) of prostate with
urinary retention

Use additional code to identify symptoms:
incomplete bladder emptying (788.21)
nocturia (788.43)
straining on urination (788.65)
urinary frequency (788.41)
urinary hesitancy (788.64)
urinary incontinence (788.30–788.39)
urinary obstruction (599.69)
urinary retention (788.20)
urinary urgency (788.63)
weak urinary stream (788.62)
Coding Clinic: 2006, Q4, P93-95

● **600.1 Nodular prostate**
Hard, firm prostate
Multinodular prostate
Excludes *malignant neoplasm of prostate (185)*

600.10 Nodular prostate without urinary
obstruction ♂ A
Nodular prostate NOS

600.11 Nodular prostate with urinary obstruction ♂ A
Nodular prostate with urinary retention

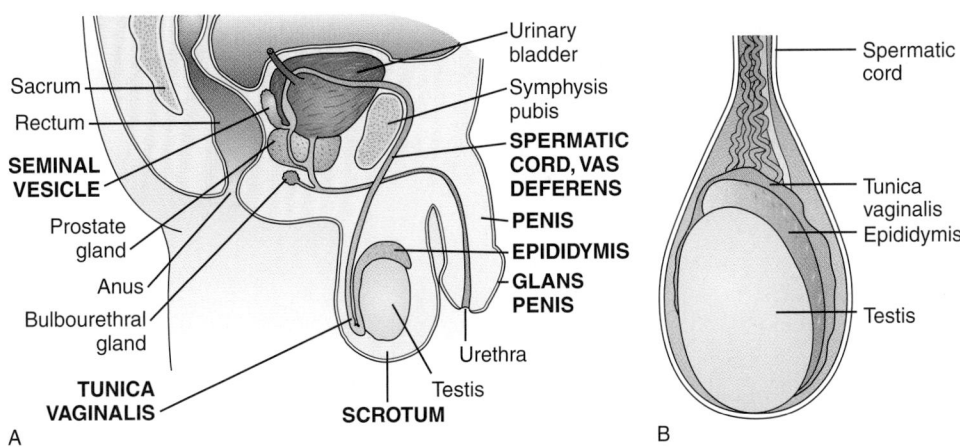

Figure 10–6 A. Male genital system. **B.** Testis.

DISEASES OF THE GENITOURINARY SYSTEM (580–629)

DISEASES OF THE GENITOURINARY SYSTEM (580–629)

● **600.2 Benign localized hyperplasia of prostate**
Adenofibromatous hypertrophy of prostate
Adenoma of prostate
Fibroadenoma of prostate
Fibroma of prostate
Myoma of prostate
Polyp of prostate

> **Excludes** *benign neoplasms of prostate (222.2)*
> *hypertrophy of prostate (600.00–600.01)*
> *malignant neoplasm of prostate (185)*

600.20 Benign localized hyperplasia of prostate without urinary obstruction and other lower urinary tract symptoms (LUTS) ♂   A
Benign localized hyperplasia of prostate NOS

600.21 Benign localized hyperplasia of prostate with urinary obstruction and other lower urinary tract symptoms (LUTS) ♂   A
Benign localized hyperplasia of prostate with urinary retention

> Use additional code to identify symptoms:
> incomplete bladder emptying (788.21)
> nocturia (788.43)
> straining on urination (788.65)
> urinary frequency (788.41)
> urinary hesitancy (788.64)
> urinary incontinence (788.30–788.39)
> urinary obstruction (599.69)
> urinary retention (788.20)
> urinary urgency (788.63)
> weak urinary stream (788.62)

600.3 Cyst of prostate ♂   A

● **600.9 Hyperplasia of prostate, unspecified**
Median bar
Prostatic obstruction NOS

■ **600.90 Hyperplasia of prostate, unspecified, without urinary obstruction and other lower urinary tract symptoms (LUTS) ♂**   A
Hyperplasia of prostate NOS

■ **600.91 Hyperplasia of prostate, unspecified, with urinary obstruction and other lower urinary tract symptoms (LUTS) ♂**   A
Hyperplasia of prostate, unspecified, with urinary retention

> Use additional code to identify symptoms:
> incomplete bladder emptying (788.21)
> nocturia (788.43)
> straining on urination (788.65)
> urinary frequency (788.41)
> urinary hesitancy (788.64)
> urinary incontinence (788.30–788.39)
> urinary obstruction (599.69)
> urinary retention (788.20)
> urinary urgency (788.63)
> weak urinary stream (788.62)

● **601 Inflammatory diseases of prostate**

> Use additional code to identify organism, such as Staphylococcus (041.1), or Streptococcus (041.0)

601.0 Acute prostatitis ♂   A

601.1 Chronic prostatitis ♂   A

601.2 Abscess of prostate ♂   A

601.3 Prostatocystitis ♂   A

● **601.4 *Prostatitis in diseases classified elsewhere* ♂**   A

> *Code first* underlying disease, as:
> actinomycosis (039.8)   syphilis (095.8)
> blastomycosis (116.0)   tuberculosis (016.5)

> **Excludes** *prostatitis:*
> *gonococcal (098.12, 098.32)*
> *monilial (112.2)*
> *trichomonal (131.03)*

■ **601.8 Other specified inflammatory diseases of prostate ♂** A
Prostatitis:
cavitary   granulomatous
diverticular

■ **601.9 Prostatitis, unspecified ♂**   A
Prostatitis NOS

● **602 Other disorders of prostate**

602.0 Calculus of prostate ♂   A
Prostatic stone

602.1 Congestion or hemorrhage of prostate ♂   A

602.2 Atrophy of prostate ♂   A

602.3 Dysplasia of prostate ♂
Prostatic intraepithelial neoplasia I (PIN I)
Prostatic intraepithelial neoplasia II (PIN II)

> **Excludes** *prostatic intraepithelial neoplasia III (PIN III) (233.4)*

■ **602.8 Other specified disorders of prostate ♂**   A
Fistula of prostate
Infarction of prostate
Stricture of prostate
Periprostatic adhesions

■ **602.9 Unspecified disorder of prostate ♂**   A

● **603 Hydrocele**

> **Includes** hydrocele of spermatic cord, testis, or tunica vaginalis

> **Excludes** *congenital (778.6)*

603.0 Encysted hydrocele

603.1 Infected hydrocele

> Use additional code to identify organism

■ **603.8 Other specified types of hydrocele**

■ **603.9 Hydrocele, unspecified**

◀ New   ◀▥ Revised   ~~deleted~~ Deleted   ● Use Additional Digit(s)   ■ Nonspecific Code
● Not first-listed DX   OGCR Official Guidelines   Coding Clinic   Excludes   Includes   Use additional   Code first   Omit code

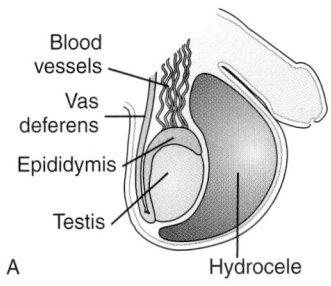
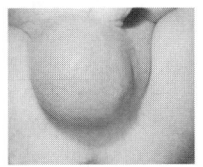

Blood vessels
Vas deferens
Epididymis
Testis
Hydrocele

A   B

Figure 10–7 **A.** Hydrocele. **B.** Newborn with large right hydrocele. (**B** from Behrman: Nelson Textbook of Pediatrics, 17th ed. 2004, Saunders, An Imprint of Elsevier)

Item 10–7 **Hydrocele** is a sac of fluid accumulating in the testes membrane.

● **604 Orchitis and epididymitis**

*An inflammation of one or both testes as a result of mumps or other infection, trauma, or metastasis. **Epididymitis** is an inflammation of the epididymis (the tubular structure that connects testicle with vas deferens).*

Use additional code to identify organism such as Escherichia coli [E. coli] (041.4), Staphylococcus (041.1), or Streptococcus (041.0)

604.0 Orchitis, epididymitis, and epididymo-orchitis, with abscess ♂
Abscess of epididymis or testis

● **604.9 Other orchitis, epididymitis, and epididymo-orchitis, without mention of abscess**

▉ **604.90 Orchitis and epididymitis, unspecified ♂**

● **604.91 Orchitis and epididymitis in diseases classified elsewhere ♂**

Code first underlying disease, as:
diphtheria (032.89)
filariasis (125.0–125.9)
syphilis (095.8)

Excludes *orchitis:*
gonococcal (098.13, 098.33)
mumps (072.0)
tuberculous (016.5)
tuberculous epididymitis (016.4)

▉ **604.99 Other ♂**

605 Redundant prepuce and phimosis ♂
Adherent prepuce
Paraphimosis
Phimosis (congenital)
Tight foreskin
Coding Clinic: 2008, Q3, P9

Item 10-8 Male infertility is the inability of the female sex partner to conceive after one year of unprotected intercourse. **Azoospermia** is no sperm ejaculated and **oligospermia** is few sperm ejaculated—both resulting in infertility. Extratesticular causes such as injury, infections, radiation, and chemotherapy may also cause male infertility.

● **606 Infertility, male**
Coding Clinic: 1996, Q2, P9

606.0 Azoospermia ♂   A
Absolute infertility
Infertility due to:
germinal (cell) aplasia
spermatogenic arrest (complete)

606.1 Oligospermia ♂   A
Infertility due to:
germinal cell desquamation
hypospermatogenesis
incomplete spermatogenic arrest

606.8 Infertility due to extratesticular causes ♂   A
Infertility due to:
drug therapy
infection
obstruction of efferent ducts
radiation
systemic disease

▉ **606.9 Male infertility, unspecified ♂**   A

● **607 Disorders of penis**
Excludes *phimosis (605)*

607.0 Leukoplakia of penis ♂
Kraurosis of penis
Excludes *carcinoma in situ of penis (233.5)*
erythroplasia of Queyrat (233.5)

607.1 Balanoposthitis ♂
Balanitis
Use additional code to identify organism

▉ **607.2 Other inflammatory disorders of penis ♂**
Abscess of corpus cavernosum or penis
Boil of corpus cavernosum or penis
Carbuncle of corpus cavernosum or penis
Cellulitis of corpus cavernosum or penis
Cavernitis (penis)
Use additional code to identify organism
Excludes *herpetic infection (054.13)*

607.3 Priapism ♂
Painful erection

DISEASES OF THE GENITOURINARY SYSTEM (580–629)

● **607.8 Other specified disorders of penis**

   607.81 Balanitis xerotica obliterans ♂
      Induratio penis plastica

   607.82 Vascular disorders of penis ♂
      Embolism of corpus cavernosum or penis
      Hematoma (nontraumatic) of corpus cavernosum or penis
      Hemorrhage of corpus cavernosum or penis
      Thrombosis of corpus cavernosum or penis

   607.83 Edema of penis ♂

   607.84 Impotence of organic origin ♂   **A**
      Excludes *nonorganic (302.72)*
      Coding Clinic: 1985, July-Aug, P9

   607.85 Peyronie's disease ♂
      Coding Clinic: 2003, Q4, P64-65

   ■**607.89 Other** ♂
      Atrophy of corpus cavernosum or penis
      Fibrosis of corpus cavernosum or penis
      Hypertrophy of corpus cavernosum or penis
      Ulcer (chronic) of corpus cavernosum or penis

  ■**607.9 Unspecified disorder of penis** ♂

● **608 Other disorders of male genital organs**

   608.0 Seminal vesiculitis ♂
      Abscess of seminal vesicle
      Cellulitis of seminal vesicle
      Vesiculitis (seminal)
      Use additional code to identify organism
      Excludes *gonococcal infection (098.14, 098.34)*

   608.1 Spermatocele ♂

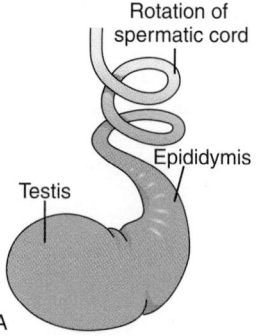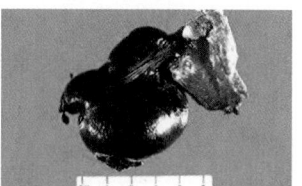

Figure 10–8 A. Torsion of testis. **B.** Torsion of the testis. (**B** from Kumar: Robbins and Cotran: Pathologic Basis of Disease, 7th ed. 2005, Saunders, An Imprint of Elsevier)

Rotation of spermatic cord — Epididymis — Testis — A — B

Item 10–9 Seminal vesiculitis is an inflammation of the seminal vesicle. Spermatocele is a benign cystic accumulation of sperm arising from the head of the epididymis. Torsion of the testis is a medical emergency occurring most commonly in boys 7 to 12 years of age and results from a congenital abnormality of the covering of the testis allowing the testis to twist within its sac and cutting off the blood supply to the testis.

● **608.2 Torsion of testis**
      Coding Clinic: 2006, Q4, P95-96

  ■**608.20 Torsion of testis, unspecified** ♂

   608.21 Extravaginal torsion of spermatic cord ♂

   608.22 Intravaginal torsion of spermatic cord ♂
      Torsion of spermatic cord NOS

   608.23 Torsion of appendix testis ♂

   608.24 Torsion of appendix epididymis ♂

  608.3 Atrophy of testis ♂

■**608.4 Other inflammatory disorders of male genital organs** ♂
   Abscess of scrotum, spermatic cord, testis [except abscess], tunica vaginalis, or vas deferens
   Boil of scrotum, spermatic cord, testis [except abscess], tunica vaginalis, or vas deferens
   Carbuncle of scrotum, spermatic cord, testis [except abscess], tunica vaginalis, or vas deferens
   Cellulitis of scrotum, spermatic cord, testis [except abscess], tunica vaginalis, or vas deferens
   Vasitis
   Use additional code to identify organism
   Excludes *abscess of testis (604.0)*

● **608.8 Other specified disorders of male genital organs**

  ● *608.81 Disorders of male genital organs in diseases classified elsewhere* ♂
     Code first underlying disease, as:
     filariasis (125.0–125.9)
     tuberculosis (016.5)

   608.82 Hematospermia ♂

   608.83 Vascular disorders ♂
     Hematoma (nontraumatic) of seminal vesicle, spermatic cord, testis, scrotum, tunica vaginalis, or vas deferens
     Hemorrhage of seminal vesicle, spermatic cord, testis, scrotum, tunica vaginalis, or vas deferens
     Thrombosis of seminal vesicle, spermatic cord, testis, scrotum, tunica vaginalis, or vas deferens
     Hematocele NOS, male
     Coding Clinic: 2003, Q4, P110

   608.84 Chylocele of tunica vaginalis ♂

   608.85 Stricture ♂
     Stricture of: Stricture of:
      spermatic cord   vas deferens
      tunica vaginalis

   608.86 Edema ♂

   608.87 Retrograde ejaculation ♂

  ■**608.89 Other** ♂
     Atrophy of seminal vesicle, spermatic cord, testis, scrotum tunica vaginalis, or vas deferens
     Fibrosis of seminal vesicle, spermatic cord, testis, scrotum tunica vaginalis, or vas deferens
     Hypertrophy of seminal vesicle, spermatic cord, testis, scrotum tunica vaginalis, or vas deferens
     Ulcer of seminal vesicle, spermatic cord, testis, scrotum tunica vaginalis, or vas deferens
     Excludes *atrophy of testis (608.3)*

■**608.9 Unspecified disorder of male genital organs** ♂

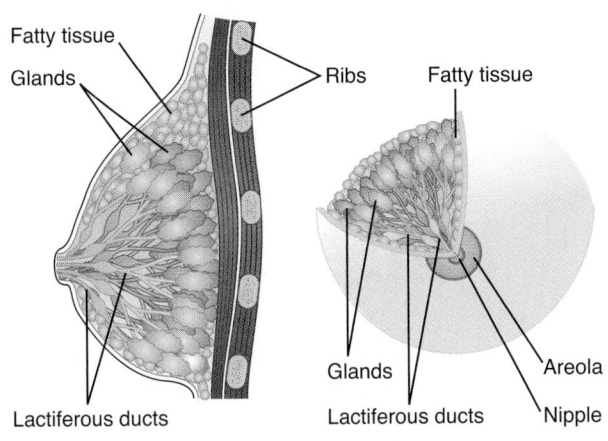

Fatty tissue
Glands
Ribs
Fatty tissue
Glands
Areola
Lactiferous ducts
Lactiferous ducts
Nipple

Figure 10-9 Breast.

DISORDERS OF BREAST (610–612)

● **610 Benign mammary dysplasias**
Benign lumpiness of the breast.

610.0 Solitary cyst of breast
Cyst (solitary) of breast

610.1 Diffuse cystic mastopathy   A
Chronic cystic mastitis
Cystic breast
Fibrocystic disease of breast
Coding Clinic: 2006, Q2, P10

610.2 Fibroadenosis of breast
Fibroadenosis of   Fibroadenosis of
breast: breast:
NOS   diffuse
chronic   periodic
cystic   segmental

610.3 Fibrosclerosis of breast

610.4 Mammary duct ectasia
Comedomastitis
Duct ectasia
Mastitis:
periductal
plasma cell

■ **610.8 Other specified benign mammary dysplasias**
Mazoplasia
Sebaceous cyst of breast
Coding Clinic: 2009, Q2, P8

■ **610.9 Benign mammary dysplasia, unspecified**

● **611 Other disorders of breast**

Excludes *that associated with lactation or the puerperium
(675.0–676.9)*

611.0 Inflammatory disease of breast
Abscess (acute) (chronic) (nonpuerperal) of:
areola
breast
Mammillary fistula
Mastitis (acute) (subacute) (nonpuerperal):
NOS
infective
retromammary
submammary

Excludes *carbuncle of breast (680.2)
chronic cystic mastitis (610.1)
neonatal infective mastitis (771.5)
thrombophlebitis of breast [Mondor's
disease] (451.89)*

611.1 Hypertrophy of breast
Gynecomastia
Hypertrophy of breast:
NOS
massive pubertal

Excludes *breast engorgement in newborn (778.7)
disproportion of reconstructed breast
(612.1)*

611.2 Fissure of nipple

● **611.3 Fat necrosis of breast**
Fat necrosis (segmental) of breast

Code first breast necrosis due to breast graft (996.79)

611.4 Atrophy of breast

611.5 Galactocele

611.6 Galactorrhea not associated with childbirth
Excessive or spontaneous flow of milk
Coding Clinic: 1985, July-Aug, P9

● **611.7 Signs and symptoms in breast**

611.71 Mastodynia
Pain in breast

611.72 Lump or mass in breast
Coding Clinic: 2003, Q2, P3-5

■ **611.79 Other**
Induration of breast
Inversion of nipple
Nipple discharge
Retraction of nipple

● **611.8 Other specified disorders of breast**
Coding Clinic: 2008, Q4, P121-122

611.81 Ptosis of breast   A

Excludes *ptosis of native breast in relation to
reconstructed breast (612.1)*

611.82 Hypoplasia of breast   A
Micromastia

Excludes *congenital absence of breast
(757.6)
hypoplasia of native breast in
relation to reconstructed
breast (612.1)*

611.83 Capsular contracture of breast implant   A

■ **611.89 Other specified disorders of breast**
Hematoma (nontraumatic) of breast
Infarction of breast
Occlusion of breast duct
Subinvolution of breast (postlactational)
(postpartum)

■ **611.9 Unspecified breast disorder**

● **612 Deformity and disproportion of reconstructed breast**
Coding Clinic: 2008, Q4, P123

612.0 Deformity of reconstructed breast   A
Contour irregularity in reconstructed breast
Excess tissue in reconstructed breast
Misshapen reconstructed breast

612.1 Disproportion of reconstructed breast   A
Breast asymmetry between native breast and
reconstructed breast
Disproportion between native breast and
reconstructed breast

DISEASES OF THE GENITOURINARY SYSTEM (580–629)

(See Plate 366A on page 87.)

Item 10-10   **Salpingitis** is an infection of one or both fallopian tubes. **Oophoritis** is an infection of one or both ovaries.

INFLAMMATORY DISEASE OF FEMALE PELVIC ORGANS (614–616)

Use additional code to identify organism, such as Staphylococcus (041.1), or Streptococcus (041.0)

Excludes *that associated with pregnancy, abortion, childbirth, or the puerperium (630–676.9)*

● **614 Inflammatory disease of ovary, fallopian tube, pelvic cellular tissue, and peritoneum**

Excludes *endometritis (615.0–615.9)*
major infection following delivery (670.0–670.8) ◀▥
that complicating:
    abortion (634–638 with .0, 639.0)
    ectopic or molar pregnancy (639.0)
    pregnancy or labor (646.6)

614.0 Acute salpingitis and oophoritis ♀
Any condition classifiable to 614.2, specified as acute or subacute

614.1 Chronic salpingitis and oophoritis ♀
Hydrosalpinx
Salpingitis:
   follicularis
   isthmica nodosa
Any condition classifiable to 614.2, specified as chronic

◼**614.2 Salpingitis and oophoritis not specified as acute, subacute, or chronic ♀**
Abscess (of):
   fallopian tube
   ovary
   tubo-ovarian
Oophoritis
Perioophoritis
Perisalpingitis
Pyosalpinx
Salpingitis
Salpingo-oophoritis
Tubo-ovarian inflammatory disease

Excludes *gonococcal infection (chronic) (098.37)*
acute (098.17)
tuberculous (016.6)

614.3 Acute parametritis and pelvic cellulitis ♀
Acute inflammatory pelvic disease
Any condition classifiable to 614.4, specified as acute

614.4 Chronic or unspecified parametritis and pelvic cellulitis ♀
Abscess (of):
   broad ligament chronic or NOS
   parametrium chronic or NOS
   pelvis, female chronic or NOS
   pouch of Douglas chronic or NOS
Chronic inflammatory pelvic disease
Pelvic cellulitis, female

Excludes *tuberculous (016.7)*

614.5 Acute or unspecified pelvic peritonitis, female ♀

614.6 Pelvic peritoneal adhesions, female (postoperative) (postinfection) ♀
Adhesions:
   peritubal
   tubo-ovarian

Use additional code to identify any associated infertility (628.2)
Coding Clinic: 2003, Q3, P6-7; Q1, P4-5; 1995, Q3, P7

◼**614.7 Other chronic pelvic peritonitis, female ♀**

Excludes *tuberculous (016.7)*

◼**614.8 Other specified inflammatory disease of female pelvic organs and tissues ♀**

◼**614.9 Unspecified inflammatory disease of female pelvic organs and tissues ♀**
Pelvic infection or inflammation, female NOS
Pelvic inflammatory disease [PID]

● **615 Inflammatory diseases of uterus, except cervix**

Excludes *following delivery (670.0–670.8)* ◀▥
hyperplastic endometritis (621.30–621.35) ◀▥
that complicating:
   abortion (634–638 with .0, 639.0)
   ectopic or molar pregnancy (639.0)
   pregnancy or labor (646.6)

615.0 Acute ♀
Any condition classifiable to 615.9, specified as acute or subacute

615.1 Chronic ♀
Any condition classifiable to 615.9, specified as chronic

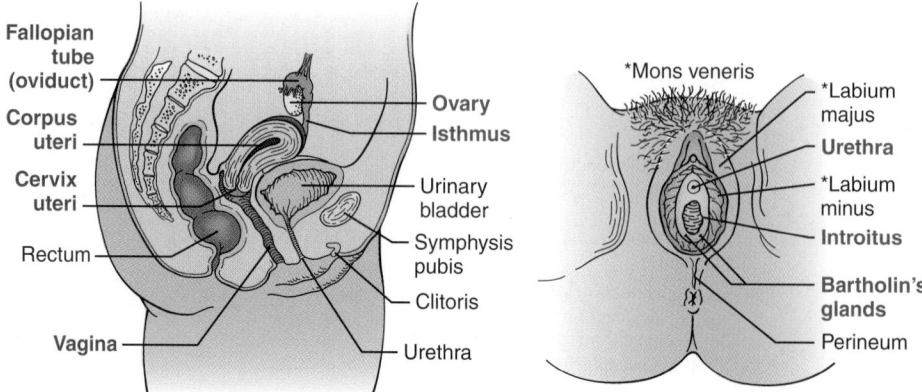

Figure 10–10 **A.** Female genital system. **B.** External female genital system. (From Buck CJ: Step-by-Step Medical Coding, 2006 ed. Philadelphia, WB Saunders, 2006.)

A   Female Genital System   B   *The three parts of the **vulva**

◀ New   ◀▥ Revised   ~~deleted~~ Deleted   ● Use Additional Digit(s)   ◼ Nonspecific Code
● Not first-listed DX   OGCR Official Guidelines   Coding Clinic   Excludes   Includes   Use additional   Code first   Omit code

◼ **615.9 Unspecified inflammatory disease of uterus ♀**

Endometritis	Perimetritis
Endomyometritis	Pyometra
Metritis	Uterine abscess
Myometritis	

● **616   Inflammatory disease of cervix, vagina, and vulva**

> **Excludes** *that complicating:*
> *abortion (634–638 with .0, 639.0)*
> *ectopic or molar pregnancy (639.0)*
> *pregnancy, childbirth, or the puerperium*
> *(646.6)*

616.0 Cervicitis and endocervicitis ♀

Cervicitis with or without mention of erosion or
  ectropion
Endocervicitis with or without mention of erosion
  or ectropion
Nabothian (gland) cyst or follicle

> **Excludes** *erosion or ectropion without mention of*
> *cervicitis (622.0)*

● **616.1 Vaginitis and vulvovaginitis**

> **Excludes** *vulvar vestibulitis (625.71)*

◼ **616.10 Vaginitis and vulvovaginitis, unspecified ♀**

Vaginitis:
  NOS
  postirradiation
Vulvitis NOS
Vulvovaginitis NOS

> Use additional code to identify organism,
> such as Escherichia coli [E. coli]
> (041.4), Staphylococcus (041.1), or
> Streptococcus (041.0)

> **Excludes** *noninfective leukorrhea (623.5)*
> *postmenopausal or senile vaginitis*
> *(627.3)*

● **616.11 Vaginitis and vulvovaginitis in diseases
classified elsewhere ♀**

> *Code first underlying disease, as:*
> pinworm vaginitis (127.4)

> **Excludes** *herpetic vulvovaginitis (054.11)*
> *monilial vulvovaginitis (112.1)*
> *trichomonal vaginitis or*
> *vulvovaginitis (131.01)*

616.2 Cyst of Bartholin's gland ♀

Cysts filled with liquid or semisolid material.
Bartholin's duct cyst

616.3 Abscess of Bartholin's gland ♀

Localized collection of pus
Vulvovaginal gland abscess

◼ **616.4 Other abscess of vulva ♀**

Abscess of vulva
Carbuncle of vulva
Furuncle of vulva

● **616.5 Ulceration of vulva**

616.50 Ulceration of vulva, unspecified ♀

Ulcer NOS of vulva

● **616.51 Ulceration of vulva in diseases classified
elsewhere ♀**

> *Code first underlying disease, as:*
> Behçet's syndrome (136.1)
> tuberculosis (016.7)

> **Excludes** *vulvar ulcer (in):*
> *gonococcal (098.0)*
> *herpes simplex (054.12)*
> *syphilitic (091.0)*

● **616.8 Other specified inflammatory diseases of cervix,
vagina, and vulva**

> **Excludes** *noninflammatory disorders of:*
> *cervix (622.0–622.9)*
> *vagina (623.0–623.9)*
> *vulva (624.0–624.9)*

**616.81 Mucositis (ulcerative) of cervix, vagina, and
vulva ♀**

> Use additional E code to identify adverse
> effects of therapy, such as:
> antineoplastic and immunosuppressive
> drugs (E930.7, E933.1)
> radiation therapy (E879.2)

◼ **616.89 Other inflammatory disease of cervix, vagina
and vulva ♀**

Caruncle, vagina or labium
Ulcer, vagina

◼ **616.9 Unspecified inflammatory disease of cervix, vagina,
and vulva ♀**

OTHER DISORDERS OF FEMALE GENITAL TRACT (617–629)

● **617   Endometriosis**

Coding Clinic: 1995, Q1, P7

617.0 Endometriosis of uterus ♀

Adenomyosis
Endometriosis:
  cervix
  internal
  myometrium

> **Excludes** *stromal endometriosis (236.0)*

Coding Clinic: 1992, Q3, P7-8

617.1 Endometriosis of ovary ♀

Chocolate cyst of ovary
Endometrial cystoma of ovary

617.2 Endometriosis of fallopian tube ♀

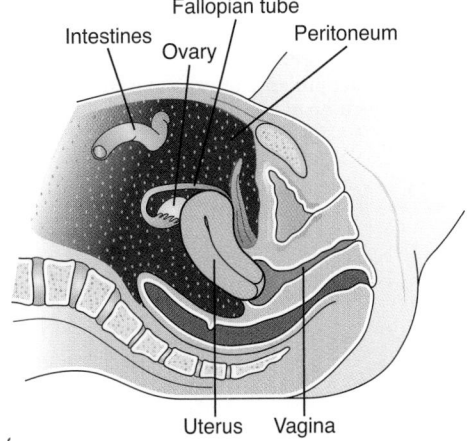

Figure 10–11 Sites of potential endometrial implants.

Item 10–11 Endometriosis is a condition for which no clear
cause has been identified. Endometrial tissue is expelled from the
uterus into the abdominal cavity and can implant onto a variety
of organs. Classification is based on the site of implant of the
endometrial tissue.

DISEASES OF THE GENITOURINARY SYSTEM (580–629)

617.3 Endometriosis of pelvic peritoneum ♀
 Endometriosis:
  broad ligament
  cul-de-sac (Douglas')
  parametrium
  round ligament

617.4 Endometriosis of rectovaginal septum and vagina ♀

617.5 Endometriosis of intestine ♀
 Endometriosis:
  appendix
  colon
  rectum

617.6 Endometriosis in scar of skin ♀

■**617.8 Endometriosis of other specified sites ♀**
 Endometriosis:
  bladder
  lung
  umbilicus
  vulva

■**617.9 Endometriosis, site unspecified ♀**

●**618 Genital prolapse**

 Use additional code to identify urinary incontinence
 (625.6, 788.31, 788.33–788.39)

 Excludes *that complicating pregnancy, labor, or delivery*
  (654.4)

●**618.0 Prolapse of vaginal walls without mention of uterine prolapse**

  Excludes *that with uterine prolapse (618.2–618.4)*
   enterocele (618.6)
   vaginal vault prolapse following
    hysterectomy (618.5)
  Coding Clinic: 2004, Q4, P83-85

 ■**618.00 Unspecified prolapse of vaginal walls ♀**
  Vaginal prolapse NOS

 618.01 Cystocele, midline ♀
  Cystocele NOS

 618.02 Cystocele, lateral ♀
  Paravaginal

 618.03 Urethrocele ♀

 618.04 Rectocele ♀
  Proctocele

 618.05 Perineocele ♀

 ■**618.09 Other prolapse of vaginal walls without mention of uterine prolapse ♀**
  Cystourethrocele

618.1 Uterine prolapse without mention of vaginal wall prolapse ♀
 Descensus uteri
 Uterine prolapse:
  NOS
  complete
  first degree
  second degree
  third degree

  Excludes *that with mention of cystocele, urethrocele,*
   or rectocele (618.2–618.4)

618.2 Uterovaginal prolapse, incomplete ♀

618.3 Uterovaginal prolapse, complete ♀

■**618.4 Uterovaginal prolapse, unspecified ♀**

618.5 Prolapse of vaginal vault after hysterectomy ♀

618.6 Vaginal enterocele, congenital or acquired ♀
 Pelvic enterocele, congenital or acquired

618.7 Old laceration of muscles of pelvic floor ♀

●**618.8 Other specified genital prolapse**

 618.81 Incompetence or weakening of pubocervical tissue ♀

 618.82 Incompetence or weakening of rectovaginal tissue ♀

 618.83 Pelvic muscle wasting ♀
  Disuse atrophy of pelvic muscles and anal sphincter

 618.84 Cervical stump prolapse ♀

 ■**618.89 Other specified genital prolapse ♀**

■**618.9 Unspecified genital prolapse ♀**

●**619 Fistula involving female genital tract**

 Excludes *vesicorectal and intestinovesical fistula (596.1)*

619.0 Urinary-genital tract fistula, female ♀
 Fistula:
  cervicovesical
  ureterovaginal
  urethrovaginal
  urethrovesicovaginal
  uteroureteric
  uterovesical
  vesicocervicovaginal
  vesicovaginal

619.1 Digestive-genital tract fistula, female ♀
 Fistula: Fistula:
  intestinouterine rectovulval
  intestinovaginal sigmoidovaginal
  rectovaginal   uterorectal

619.2 Genital tract-skin fistula, female ♀
 Fistula:
  uterus to abdominal wall
  vaginoperineal

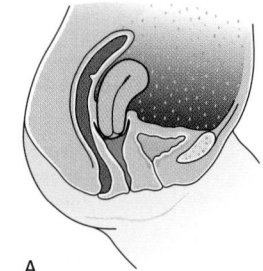 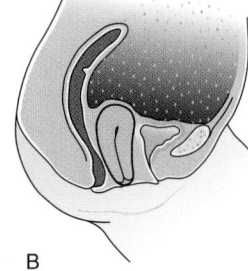 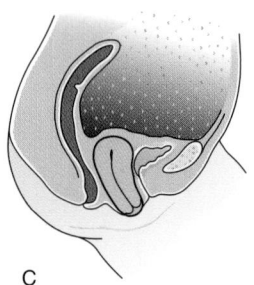

Figure 10–12 Three stages of uterine prolapse.
A. Uterus is prolapsed. **B.** Vagina and uterus are prolapsed (incomplete uterovaginal prolapse).
C. Vagina and uterus are completely prolapsed and are exposed through the external genitalia (complete uterovaginal prolapse).

A   B   C

DISEASES OF THE GENITOURINARY SYSTEM (580–629)

◀ New ◀▥ Revised ~~deleted~~ Deleted ● Use Additional Digit(s) ■ Nonspecific Code
● Not first-listed DX OGCR Official Guidelines Coding Clinic Excludes Includes Use additional Code first Omit code

■**619.8 Other specified fistulas involving female genital tract** ♀

    Fistula:
        cervix
        cul-de-sac (Douglas')
        uterus
        vagina

■**619.9 Unspecified fistula involving female genital tract** ♀

● **620 Noninflammatory disorders of ovary, fallopian tube, and broad ligament**

    Excludes   *hydrosalpinx (614.1)*

    620.0 Follicular cyst of ovary ♀
        Cyst of graafian follicle

    620.1 Corpus luteum cyst or hematoma ♀
        Corpus luteum hemorrhage or rupture
        Lutein cyst

    ■**620.2 Other and unspecified ovarian cyst** ♀
        Cyst of ovary:
            NOS
            corpus albicans
            retention NOS
            serous
            theca-lutein
        Simple cystoma of ovary

        Excludes   *cystadenoma (benign) (serous) (220)*
                    developmental cysts (752.0)
                    neoplastic cysts (220)
                    polycystic ovaries (256.4)
                    Stein-Leventhal syndrome (256.4)

    620.3 Acquired atrophy of ovary and fallopian tube ♀
        Senile involution of ovary

    620.4 Prolapse or hernia of ovary and fallopian tube ♀
        Displacement of ovary and fallopian tube
        Salpingocele

    620.5 Torsion of ovary, ovarian pedicle, or fallopian tube ♀
        Torsion:
            accessory tube
            hydatid of Morgagni

    620.6 Broad ligament laceration syndrome ♀
        Masters-Allen syndrome

    620.7 Hematoma of broad ligament ♀
        Hematocele, broad ligament

    ■**620.8 Other noninflammatory disorders of ovary, fallopian tube, and broad ligament** ♀
        Cyst of broad ligament or fallopian tube
        Polyp of broad ligament or fallopian tube
        Infarction of ovary or fallopian tube
        Rupture of ovary or fallopian tube
        Hematosalpinx of ovary or fallopian tube

        Excludes   *hematosalpinx in ectopic pregnancy (639.2)*
                    peritubal adhesions (614.6)
                    torsion of ovary, ovarian pedicle, or fallopian tube (620.5)

    ■**620.9 Unspecified noninflammatory disorder of ovary, fallopian tube, and broad ligament** ♀

● **621 Disorders of uterus, not elsewhere classified**

    621.0 Polyp of corpus uteri ♀
        Polyp:
            endometrium
            uterus NOS

        Excludes   *cervical polyp NOS (622.7)*

    621.1 Chronic subinvolution of uterus ♀

        Excludes   *puerperal (674.8)*

    621.2 Hypertrophy of uterus ♀
        Bulky or enlarged uterus

        Excludes   *puerperal (674.8)*

● **621.3 Endometrial hyperplasia**

    ~~Hyperplasia (adenomatous) (cystic) (glandular) of endometrium~~

    ~~Hyperplastic endometritis~~

    Coding Clinic: 2004, Q4, P85-86

    ■**621.30 Endometrial hyperplasia, unspecified** ♀
        Endometrial hyperplasia NOS
        Hyperplasia (adenomatus) (cystic) (glandular) of endometrium ◄
        Hyperplastic endometritis ◄

    621.31 Simple endometrial hyperplasia without atypia ♀

        Excludes   *benign endometrial hyperplasia (621.34)* ◄

    621.32 Complex endometrial hyperplasia without atypia ♀

        Excludes   *benign endometrial hyperplasia (621.34)* ◄

    621.33 Endometrial hyperplasia with atypia ♀

        Excludes   *endometrial intraepithelial neoplasia [EIN] (621.35)* ◄

    621.34 Benign endometrial hyperplasia ◄

    621.35 Endometrial intraepithelial neoplasia [EIN] ◄

        Excludes   *malignant neoplasm of endometrium with endometrial intraepithelial neoplasia [EIN] (182.0)* ◄

    621.4 Hematometra ♀
        Hemometra

        Excludes   *that in congenital anomaly (752.2–752.3)*

    621.5 Intrauterine synechiae ♀
        Adhesions of uterus   Band(s) of uterus

    621.6 Malposition of uterus ♀
        Anteversion of uterus
        Retroflexion of uterus
        Retroversion of uterus

        Excludes   *malposition complicating pregnancy, labor, or delivery (654.3–654.4)*
                    prolapse of uterus (618.1–618.4)

    621.7 Chronic inversion of uterus ♀

        Excludes   *current obstetrical trauma (665.2)*
                    prolapse of uterus (618.1–618.4)

    ■**621.8 Other specified disorders of uterus, not elsewhere classified** ♀
        Atrophy, acquired of uterus
        Cyst of uterus
        Fibrosis NOS of uterus
        Old laceration (postpartum) of uterus
        Ulcer of uterus

        Excludes   *bilharzial fibrosis (120.0–120.9)*
                    endometriosis (617.0)
                    fistulas (619.0–619.8)
                    inflammatory diseases (615.0–615.9)

    ■**621.9 Unspecified disorder of uterus** ♀

● **622 Noninflammatory disorders of cervix**

    Excludes   *abnormality of cervix complicating pregnancy, labor, or delivery (654.5–654.6)*
                    fistula (619.0–619.8)

    622.0 Erosion and ectropion of cervix ♀
        Eversion of cervix
        Ulcer of cervix

        Excludes   *that in chronic cervicitis (616.0)*

DISEASES OF THE GENITOURINARY SYSTEM (580–629)

● **622.1 Dysplasia of cervix (uteri)**

> **Excludes** *abnormal results from cervical cytologic examination without histologic confirmation (795.00–795.09)*
> *carcinoma in situ of cervix (233.1)*
> *cervical intraepithelial neoplasia III [CIN III] (233.1)*
> *HGSIL of cervix (795.04)*
> Coding Clinic: 2004, Q4, P86-88; 1991, Q1, P11

■ **622.10 Dysplasia of cervix, unspecified ♀**
Anaplasia of cervix
Cervical atypism
Cervical dysplasia NOS

622.11 Mild dysplasia of cervix ♀
Cervical intraepithelial neoplasia I [CIN I]

622.12 Moderate dysplasia of cervix ♀
Cervical intraepithelial neoplasia II [CIN II]

> **Excludes** *carcinoma in situ of cervix (233.1)*
> *cervical intraepithelial neoplasia III [CIN III] (233.1)*
> *severe dysplasia (233.1)*

622.2 Leukoplakia of cervix (uteri) ♀

> **Excludes** *carcinoma in situ of cervix (233.1)*

622.3 Old laceration of cervix ♀
Adhesions of cervix
Band(s) of cervix
Cicatrix (postpartum) of cervix

> **Excludes** *current obstetrical trauma (665.3)*

622.4 Stricture and stenosis of cervix ♀
Atresia (acquired) of cervix
Contracture of cervix
Occlusion of cervix
Pinpoint os uteri

> **Excludes** *congenital (752.49)*
> *that complicating labor (654.6)*

622.5 Incompetence of cervix ♀

> **Excludes** *complicating pregnancy (654.5)*
> *that affecting fetus or newborn (761.0)*

622.6 Hypertrophic elongation of cervix ♀

622.7 Mucous polyp of cervix ♀
Polyp NOS of cervix

> **Excludes** *adenomatous polyp of cervix (219.0)*

■ **622.8 Other specified noninflammatory disorders of cervix ♀**
Atrophy (senile) of cervix
Cyst of cervix
Fibrosis of cervix
Hemorrhage of cervix

> **Excludes** *endometriosis (617.0)*
> *fistula (619.0–619.8)*
> *inflammatory diseases (616.0)*

■ **622.9 Unspecified noninflammatory disorder of cervix ♀**

● **623 Noninflammatory disorders of vagina**

> **Excludes** *abnormality of vagina complicating pregnancy, labor, or delivery (654.7)*
> *congenital absence of vagina (752.49)*
> *congenital diaphragm or bands (752.49)*
> *fistulas involving vagina (619.0–619.8)*

623.0 Dysplasia of vagina ♀
Mild and moderate dysplasia of vagina
Vaginal intraepithelial neoplasia I and II [VAIN I and II]

> **Excludes** *abnormal results from vaginal cytological examination without histologic confirmation (795.10-795.19)*
> *carcinoma in situ of vagina (233.31)*
> *HGSIL of vagina (795.14)*
> *severe dysplasia of vagina (233.31)*
> *vaginal intraepithelial neoplasia III [VAIN III] (233.31)*

623.1 Leukoplakia of vagina ♀

623.2 Stricture or atresia of vagina ♀
Adhesions (postoperative) (postradiation) of vagina
Occlusion of vagina
Stenosis, vagina

> Use additional E code to identify any external cause

> **Excludes** *congenital atresia or stricture (752.49)*

623.3 Tight hymenal ring ♀
Rigid hymen acquired or congenital
Tight hymenal ring acquired or congenital
Tight introitus acquired or congenital

> **Excludes** *imperforate hymen (752.42)*

623.4 Old vaginal laceration ♀

> **Excludes** *old laceration involving muscles of pelvic floor (618.7)*

623.5 Leukorrhea, not specified as infective ♀
Leukorrhea NOS of vagina
Vaginal discharge NOS

> **Excludes** *trichomonal (131.00)*

623.6 Vaginal hematoma ♀

> **Excludes** *current obstetrical trauma (665.7)*

623.7 Polyp of vagina ♀

■ **623.8 Other specified noninflammatory disorders of vagina ♀**
Cyst of vagina
Hemorrhage of vagina

■ **623.9 Unspecified noninflammatory disorder of vagina ♀**

● **624   Noninflammatory disorders of vulva and perineum**

> **Excludes** *abnormality of vulva and perineum complicating pregnancy, labor, or delivery (654.8)*
> *condyloma acuminatum (078.11)* ◀▥▥
> *fistulas involving:*
> *perineum - see Alphabetic Index*
> *vulva (619.0–619.8)*
> *vulval varices (456.6)*
> *vulvar involvement in skin conditions (690–709.9)*

● **624.0   Dystrophy of vulva**

> **Excludes** *carcinoma in situ of vulva (233.32)*
> *severe dysplasia of vulva (233.32)*
> *vulvar intraepithelial neoplasia III [VIN III] (233.32)*

624.01   Vulvar intraepithelial neoplasia I [VIN I] ♀
Mild dysplasia of vulva

624.02   Vulvar intraepithelial neoplasia II [VIN II] ♀
Moderate dysplasia of vulva
Coding Clinic: 2007, Q4, P90-91

■ **624.09   Other dystrophy of vulva ♀**
Kraurosis of vulva
Leukoplakia of vulva

624.1   Atrophy of vulva ♀

624.2   Hypertrophy of clitoris ♀

> **Excludes** *that in endocrine disorders (255.2, 256.1)*

624.3   Hypertrophy of labia ♀
Hypertrophy of vulva NOS

624.4   Old laceration or scarring of vulva ♀

624.5   Hematoma of vulva ♀

> **Excludes** *that complicating delivery (664.5)*

624.6   Polyp of labia and vulva ♀

■ **624.8   Other specified noninflammatory disorders of vulva and perineum ♀**
Cyst of vulva
Edema of vulva
Stricture of vulva
Coding Clinic: 2003, Q1, P13-14; 1995, Q1, P8

■ **624.9   Unspecified noninflammatory disorder of vulva and perineum ♀**

● **625   Pain and other symptoms associated with female genital organs**

625.0   Dyspareunia ♀
Painful intercourse/coitus

> **Excludes** *psychogenic dyspareunia (302.76)*

625.1   Vaginismus ♀
Colpospasm
Vulvismus

> **Excludes** *psychogenic vaginismus (306.51)*

625.2   Mittelschmerz ♀
Intermenstrual pain
Ovulation pain

625.3   Dysmenorrhea ♀
Painful menstruation

> **Excludes** *psychogenic dysmenorrhea (306.52)*

Coding Clinic: 1994, Q2, P12

625.4   Premenstrual tension syndromes ♀
Menstrual molimen
Premenstrual dysphoric disorder
Premenstrual syndrome
Premenstrual tension NOS

> **Excludes** *menstrual migraine (346.4)*

Coding Clinic: 2003, Q4, P116

625.5   Pelvic congestion syndrome ♀
Congestion-fibrosis syndrome
Taylor's syndrome

625.6   Stress incontinence, female ♀

> **Excludes** *mixed incontinence (788.33)*
> *stress incontinence, male (788.32)*

● **625.7   Vulvodynia**
Coding Clinic: 2008, Q4, P124

■ **625.70   Vulvodynia, unspecified ♀**
Vulvodynia NOS

625.71   Vulvar vestibulitis ♀

■ **625.79   Other vulvodynia ♀**

■ **625.8   Other specified symptoms associated with female genital organs ♀**
Coding Clinic: 1985, Nov-Dec, P16

■ **625.9   Unspecified symptom associated with female genital organs ♀**
Coding Clinic: 2006, Q4, P109-110; 1994, Q2, P12; 1985, Nov-Dec, P16

● **626   Disorders of menstruation and other abnormal bleeding from female genital tract**

> **Excludes** *menopausal and premenopausal bleeding (627.0)*
> *pain and other symptoms associated with menstrual cycle (625.2–625.4)*
> *postmenopausal bleeding (627.1)*

626.0   Absence of menstruation ♀
Amenorrhea (primary) (secondary)
Coding Clinic: 1985, July-Aug, P9

626.1   Scanty or infrequent menstruation ♀
Hypomenorrhea
Oligomenorrhea

626.2   Excessive or frequent menstruation ♀
Heavy periods   Menorrhagia
Menometrorrhagia   Polymenorrhea

> **Excludes** *premenopausal (627.0)*
> *that in puberty (626.3)*

Coding Clinic: 2006, Q4, P97-98; 2004, Q4, P88-90; 1994, Q2, P12

626.3   Puberty bleeding ♀
Excessive bleeding associated with onset of menstrual periods
Pubertal menorrhagia

626.4   Irregular menstrual cycle ♀
Irregular: Irregular:
bleeding NOS   periods
menstruation

626.5   Ovulation bleeding ♀
Regular intermenstrual bleeding

626.6   Metrorrhagia ♀
Bleeding unrelated to menstrual cycle
Irregular intermenstrual bleeding

626.7   Postcoital bleeding ♀

■ **626.8   Other ♀**
Dysfunctional or functional uterine hemorrhage NOS
Menstruation: Menstruation:
retained   suppression of

■ **626.9   Unspecified ♀**

DISEASES OF THE GENITOURINARY SYSTEM (580–629)

● **627   Menopausal and postmenopausal disorders**

> **Excludes**   *asymptomatic age-related (natural) postmenopausal status (V49.81)*

    627.0   Premenopausal menorrhagia ♀
       Excessive bleeding associated with onset of menopause
       Menorrhagia: Menorrhagia:
          climacteric   preclimacteric
          menopausal

    627.1   Postmenopausal bleeding ♀

    627.2   Symptomatic menopausal or female climacteric states ♀
       Symptoms, such as flushing, sleeplessness, headache, lack of concentration, associated with the menopause

    627.3   Postmenopausal atrophic vaginitis ♀
       Senile (atrophic) vaginitis

    627.4   Symptomatic states associated with artificial menopause ♀
       Postartificial menopause syndromes
       Any condition classifiable to 627.1, 627.2, or 627.3 which follows induced menopause

    ■**627.8   Other specified menopausal and postmenopausal disorders ♀**

> **Excludes**   *premature menopause NOS (256.31)*

    ■**627.9   Unspecified menopausal and postmenopausal disorder ♀**

● **628   Infertility, female**

> **Includes**   primary and secondary sterility

       Coding Clinic: 1996, Q2, P9; 1995, Q1, P7

    628.0   Associated with anovulation ♀
       Anovulatory cycle
       Use additional code for any associated Stein-Leventhal syndrome (256.4)

    ●**628.1   *Of pituitary-hypothalamic origin* ♀**

> *Code first underlying disease, as:*
>   adiposogenital dystrophy (253.8)
>   anterior pituitary disorder (253.0–253.4)

    628.2   Of tubal origin ♀
       Infertility associated with congenital anomaly of tube
       Tubal: Tubal:
          block   stenosis
          occlusion
       Use additional code for any associated peritubal adhesions (614.6)

    628.3   Of uterine origin ♀
       Infertility associated with congenital anomaly of uterus
       Nonimplantation
       Use additional code for any associated tuberculous endometritis (016.7)

    628.4   Of cervical or vaginal origin ♀
       Infertility associated with:
          anomaly or cervical mucus
          congenital structural anomaly
          dysmucorrhea

    ■**628.8   Of other specified origin ♀**

    ■**628.9   Of unspecified origin ♀**

● **629   Other disorders of female genital organs**

    629.0   Hematocele, female, not elsewhere classified ♀

> **Excludes**   *hematocele or hematoma:*
>   *broad ligament (620.7)*
>   *fallopian tube (620.8)*
>   *that associated with ectopic pregnancy*
>   *(633.00–633.91)*
>   *uterus (621.4)*
>   *vagina (623.6)*
>   *vulva (624.5)*

    629.1   Hydrocele, canal of Nuck ♀
       Cyst of canal of Nuck (acquired)

> **Excludes**   *congenital (752.41)*

    ●**629.2   Female genital multilation status**
       Female circumcision status
       Female genital cutting

    ■**629.20   Female genital mutilation status, unspecified ♀**
       Female genital cutting status, unspecified
       Female genital mutilation status NOS

    629.21   Female genital mutilation Type I status ♀
       Clitorectomy status
       Female genital cutting Type I status

    629.22   Female genital mutilation Type II status ♀
       Clitorectomy with excision of labia minora status
       Female genital cutting Type II status
       Coding Clinic: 2004, Q4, P88-90

    629.23   Female genital mutilation Type III status ♀
       Female genital cutting Type III status
       Infibulation status

    ■**629.29   Other female genital mutilation status ♀**
       Female genital cutting Type IV status
       Female genital mutilation Type IV status
       Other female genital cutting status

    ●**629.8   Other specified disorders of female genital organs**

    629.81   Habitual aborter without current pregnancy ♀

> **Excludes**   *habitual aborter with current pregnancy (646.3)*

       Coding Clinic: 2006, Q4, P98

    ■**629.89   Other specified disorders of female genital organs ♀**

    ■**629.9   Unspecified disorder of female genital organs ♀**

◀ New   ◀◀◀ Revised   ~~deleted~~ Deleted   ● Use Additional Digit(s)   ■ Nonspecific Code
● Not first-listed DX   OGCR Official Guidelines   Coding Clinic   Excludes   Includes   Use additional   Code first   Omit code

(See Plate 375 on page 88.)

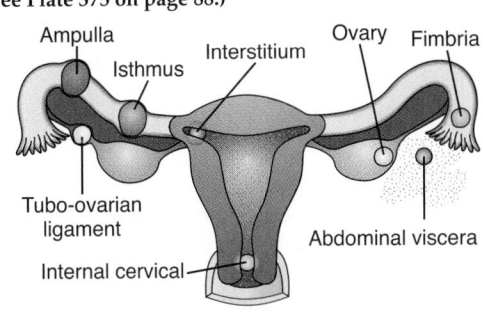

Figure 11–1 Implantation sites of ectopic pregnancy.

Item 11–1 Ectopic pregnancy most often occurs in the fallopian tube. Pregnancy outside the uterus may end in a life-threatening rupture.

Item 11–2 A hydatidiform mole is a benign tumor of the placenta. The tumor secretes a hormone, chorionic gonadotropic hormone (CGH), that indicates a positive pregnancy test.

OGCR Section I.C.11.a
Chapter 11 codes have sequencing priority over codes from other chapters. Additional codes from other chapters may be used in conjunction with chapter 11 codes to further specify conditions. Should the provider document that the pregnancy is incidental to the encounter, then code V22.2 should be used in place of any chapter 11 codes. It is the provider's responsibility to state that the condition being treated is not affecting the pregnancy. Chapter 11 codes are to be used only on the maternal record, never on the record of the newborn.

11. COMPLICATIONS OF PREGNANCY, CHILDBIRTH, AND THE PUERPERIUM (630–679)

ECTOPIC AND MOLAR PREGNANCY (630–633)

Use additional code from category 639 to identify any complications

630 Hydatidiform mole ♀ M
Trophoblastic disease NOS
Vesicular mole

> **Excludes** *chorioadenoma (destruens) (236.1)*
> *chorionepithelioma (181)*
> *malignant hydatidiform mole (236.1)*

631 Other abnormal product of conception ♀ M
Blighted ovum
Mole:
 NOS
 carneous
 fleshy
 stone

632 Missed abortion ♀ M
Early fetal death before completion of 22 weeks' gestation with retention of dead fetus
Retained products of conception, not following spontaneous or induced abortion or delivery

> **Excludes** *failed induced abortion (638.0–638.9)*
> *fetal death (intrauterine) (late) (656.4)*
> *missed delivery (656.4)*
> *that with abnormal product of conception (630, 631)*

Coding Clinic: 2001, Q1, P5

● 633 Ectopic pregnancy

> **Includes** ruptured ectopic pregnancy

Coding Clinic: 2002, Q4, P61-62

● 633.0 Abdominal pregnancy
Intraperitoneal pregnancy

 633.00 Abdominal pregnancy without intrauterine pregnancy ♀ M

 633.01 Abdominal pregnancy with intrauterine pregnancy ♀ M

● 633.1 Tubal pregnancy
Fallopian pregnancy
Rupture of (fallopian) tube due to pregnancy
Tubal abortion

 633.10 Tubal pregnancy without intrauterine pregnancy ♀ M

 633.11 Tubal pregnancy with intrauterine pregnancy ♀ M

● 633.2 Ovarian pregnancy

 633.20 Ovarian pregnancy without intrauterine pregnancy ♀ M

 633.21 Ovarian pregnancy with intrauterine pregnancy ♀ M

● 633.8 Other ectopic pregnancy
Pregnancy:
 cervical
 combined
 cornual
 intraligamentous
 mesometric
 mural

 633.80 Other ectopic pregnancy without intrauterine pregnancy ♀ M

 633.81 Other ectopic pregnancy with intrauterine pregnancy ♀ M

● 633.9 Unspecified ectopic pregnancy

 633.90 Unspecified ectopic pregnancy without intrauterine pregnancy ♀ M

 633.91 Unspecified ectopic pregnancy with intrauterine pregnancy ♀ M

OTHER PREGNANCY WITH ABORTIVE OUTCOME (634–639)

The following fourth digit subdivisions are for use with categories 634–638:

0 Complicated by genital tract and pelvic infection
  Endometritis
  Salpingo-oophoritis
  Sepsis NOS
  Septicemia NOS
  Any condition classifiable to 639.0, with condition classifiable to 634–638

  Excludes *urinary tract infection (634–638 with .7)*

1 Complicated by delayed or excessive hemorrhage
  Afibrinogenemia
  Defibrination syndrome
  Intravascular hemolysis
  Any condition classifiable to 639.1, with condition classifiable to 634–638

2 Complicated by damage to pelvic organs and tissues
  Laceration, perforation, or tear of:
    bladder
    uterus
  Any condition classifiable to 639.2, with condition classifiable to 634–638

3 Complicated by renal failure
  Oliguria
  Uremia
  Any condition classifiable to 639.3, with condition classifiable to 634–638

4 Complicated by metabolic disorder
  Electrolyte imbalance with conditions classifiable to 634–638

5 Complicated by shock
  Circulatory collapse
  Shock (postoperative) (septic)
  Any condition classifiable to 639.5, with condition classifiable to 634–638

6 Complicated by embolism
  Embolism:
    NOS
    amniotic fluid
    pulmonary
  Any condition classifiable to 639.6, with condition classifiable to 634–638

7 With other specified complications
  Cardiac arrest or failure
  Urinary tract infection
  Any condition classifiable to 639.8, with condition classifiable to 634–638

8 With unspecified complications

9 Without mention of complication

OGCR Section I.C.10.k.1
Fifth-digits are required for abortion categories 634-637. Fifth-digit 1, incomplete, indicates that all of the products of conception have not been expelled from the uterus. Fifth-digit 2, complete, indicates that all products of conception have been expelled from the uterus.

OGCR Section I.C.10.k.5
Subsequent admissions for retained products of conception following a spontaneous or legally induced abortion are assigned the appropriate code from category 634, Spontaneous abortion, or 635 Legally induced abortion, with a fifth digit of "1" (incomplete). This advice is appropriate even when the patient was discharged previously with a discharge diagnosis of complete abortion.

634 Spontaneous abortion

Requires fifth digit to identify stage:

  0 unspecified
  1 incomplete
  2 complete

  Includes   miscarriage
                    spontaneous abortion

634.0 Complicated by genital tract and pelvic [0-2] **infection** ♀   M

634.1 Complicated by delayed or excessive hemorrhage ♀ M
[0-2]   Coding Clinic: 2003, Q1, P6

634.2 Complicated by damage to pelvic organs or [0-2] **tissues** ♀   M

634.3 Complicated by renal failure ♀   M
[0-2]

634.4 Complicated by metabolic disorder ♀   M
[0-2]

634.5 Complicated by shock ♀   M
[0-2]

634.6 Complicated by embolism ♀   M
[0-2]

634.7 With other specified complications ♀   M
[0-2]

634.8 With unspecified complication ♀   M
[0-2]

634.9 Without mention of complication ♀   M
[0-2]

635 Legally induced abortion

Requires fifth digit to identify stage:

  0 unspecified
  1 incomplete
  2 complete

  Includes   abortion or termination of pregnancy:
                    elective
                    legal
                    therapeutic

  Excludes *menstrual extraction or regulation (V25.3)*

635.0 Complicated by genital tract and pelvic [0-2] **infection** ♀   M

635.1 Complicated by delayed or excessive hemorrhage ♀ M
[0-2]

635.2 Complicated by damage to pelvic organs or [0-2] **tissues** ♀   M

635.3 Complicated by renal failure ♀   M
[0-2]

635.4 Complicated by metabolic disorder ♀   M
[0-2]

635.5 Complicated by shock ♀   M
[0-2]

635.6 Complicated by embolism ♀   M
[0-2]

635.7 With other specified complications ♀   M
[0-2]

635.8 With unspecified complication ♀   M
[0-2]

635.9 Without mention of complication ♀   M
[0-2]   Coding Clinic: 1994, Q2, P14

◀ New   ⬅ Revised   deleted Deleted   ● Use Additional Digit(s)   ■ Nonspecific Code
● Not first-listed DX   OGCR Official Guidelines   Coding Clinic   Excludes   Includes   Use additional   Code first   Omit code

● **636 Illegally induced abortion**

Requires fifth digit to identify stage:

> ■ 0 unspecified
> 1 incomplete
> 2 complete

Includes abortion:
> criminal
> illegal
> self-induced

● **636.0** Complicated by genital tract and pelvic
[0-2]   infection ♀   M
● **636.1** Complicated by delayed or excessive hemorrhage ♀ M
[0-2]
● **636.2** Complicated by damage to pelvic organs or
[0-2]   tissues ♀   M
● **636.3** Complicated by renal failure ♀   M
[0-2]
● **636.4** Complicated by metabolic disorder ♀   M
[0-2]
● **636.5** Complicated by shock ♀   M
[0-2]
● **636.6** Complicated by embolism ♀   M
[0-2]
● ■**636.7** With other specified complications ♀   M
[0-2]
● ■**636.8** With unspecified complication ♀   M
[0-2]
● **636.9** Without mention of complication ♀   M
[0-2]

● **637 Unspecified abortion**

Requires following fifth digit to identify stage:
Coding Clinic: 1994, Q2, P14

> ■ 0 unspecified
> 1 incomplete
> 2 complete

Includes abortion NOS
> retained products of conception following
> abortion, not classifiable elsewhere

● ■**637.0** Complicated by genital tract and pelvic
[0-2]   infection ♀   M
● ■**637.1** Complicated by delayed or excessive hemorrhage ♀ M
[0-2]
● ■**637.2** Complicated by damage to pelvic organs or
[0-2]   tissues ♀   M
● ■**637.3** Complicated by renal failure ♀   M
[0-2]
● ■**637.4** Complicated by metabolic disorder ♀   M
[0-2]
● ■**637.5** Complicated by shock ♀   M
[0-2]
● ■**637.6** Complicated by embolism ♀   M
[0-2]
● ■**637.7** With other specified complications ♀   M
[0-2]
● ■**637.8** With unspecified complication ♀   M
[0-2]
● ■**637.9** Without mention of complication ♀   M
[0-2]

● **638 Failed attempted abortion**

Includes failure of attempted induction of (legal)
> abortion

Excludes *incomplete abortion (634.0–637.9)*

638.0 Complicated by genital tract and pelvic
infection ♀   M
638.1 Complicated by delayed or excessive
hemorrhage ♀   M
638.2 Complicated by damage to pelvic organs or
tissues ♀   M
638.3 Complicated by renal failure ♀   M
638.4 Complicated by metabolic disorder ♀   M
638.5 Complicated by shock ♀   M
638.6 Complicated by embolism ♀   M
■**638.7** With other specified complications ♀   M
■**638.8** With unspecified complication ♀   M
638.9 Without mention of complication ♀   M

● **639 Complications following abortion and ectopic and molar
pregnancies**

Note: This category is provided for use when it is
required to classify separately the complications
classifiable to the fourth digit level in categories
634–638; for example:
a) when the complication itself was responsible
for an episode of medical care, the abortion,
ectopic or molar pregnancy itself having been
dealt with at a previous episode
b) when these conditions are immediate
complications of ectopic or molar pregnancies
classifiable to 630–633 where they cannot be
identified at fourth digit level.

OGCR Section I.C.10.k.3

Code 639 is to be used for all complications following
abortion. Code 639 cannot be assigned with codes from
categories 634-638.

639.0 Genital tract and pelvic infection ♀   M
Endometritis following conditions classifiable to
630–638
Parametritis following conditions classifiable to
630–638
Pelvic peritonitis following conditions classifiable
to 630–638
Salpingitis following conditions classifiable to
630–638
Salpingo-oophoritis following conditions
classifiable to 630–638
Sepsis NOS following conditions classifiable to
630–638
Septicemia NOS following conditions classifiable
to 630–638

Excludes *urinary tract infection (639.8)*

639.1 Delayed or excessive hemorrhage ♀   M
Afibrinogenemia following conditions classifiable
to 630–638
Defibrination syndrome following conditions
classifiable to 630–638
Intravascular hemolysis following conditions
classifiable to 630–638

COMPLICATIONS OF PREGNANCY, CHILDBIRTH, AND THE PUERPERIUM (630–679)

639.2 Damage to pelvic organs and tissues ♀　　M
Laceration, perforation, or tear of:
　bladder following conditions classifiable to
　　630–638
　bowel following conditions classifiable to
　　630–638
　broad ligament following conditions classifiable
　　to 630–638
　cervix following conditions classifiable to
　　630–638
　periurethral tissue following conditions
　　classifiable to 630–638
　uterus following conditions classifiable to
　　630–638
　vagina following conditions classifiable to
　　630–638

639.3 ~~Renal~~ Kidney failure ♀　　M ◀▥
Oliguria following conditions classifiable to 630–638
Renal (kidney):　　　　　　　　　　　　　◀▥
　failure (acute) following conditions classifiable
　　to 630–638
　shutdown following conditions classifiable to
　　630–638
　tubular necrosis following conditions classifiable
　　to 630–638
Uremia following conditions classifiable to 630–638

639.4 Metabolic disorders ♀　　M
Electrolyte imbalance following conditions
　classifiable to 630–638

639.5 Shock ♀　　M
Circulatory collapse following conditions
　classifiable to 630–638
Shock (postoperative) (septic) following conditions
　classifiable to 630–638

639.6 Embolism ♀　　M
Embolism:
　NOS following conditions classifiable to 630–638
　air following conditions classifiable to 630–638
　amniotic fluid following conditions classifiable
　　to 630–638
　blood-clot following conditions classifiable to
　　630–638
　fat following conditions classifiable to 630–638
　pulmonary following conditions classifiable to
　　630–638
　pyemic following conditions classifiable to
　　630–638
　septic following conditions classifiable to 630–638
　soap following conditions classifiable to 630–638

**■639.8 Other specified complications following abortion or
ectopic and molar pregnancy ♀**　　M
Acute yellow atrophy or necrosis of liver following
　conditions classifiable to 630–638
Cardiac arrest or failure following conditions
　classifiable to 630–638
Cerebral anoxia following conditions classifiable to
　630–638
Urinary tract infection following conditions
　classifiable to 630–638

**■639.9 Unspecified complication following abortion or
ectopic and molar pregnancy ♀**　　M
Complication(s) not further specified following
　conditions classifiable to 630–638

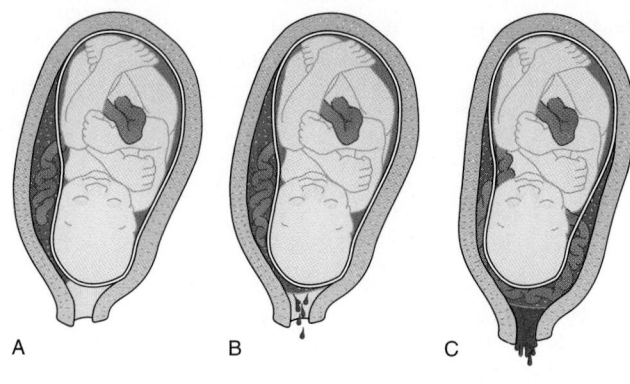

Figure 11–2　A. Marginal placenta previa. **B.** Partial placenta previa. **C.** Total placenta previa.

Item 11–3 Placenta previa is a condition in which the opening of the cervix is obstructed by the displaced placenta. The three types, marginal, partial, and total, are varying degrees of placenta displacement. Placenta abruption is the premature breaking away of the placenta from the site of the uterine implant before the delivery of the fetus.

OGCR Section I.C.10.k.2

A code from categories 640-648 and 651-659 may be used as additional codes with an abortion code to indicate the complication leading to the abortion. Fifth digit 3 is assigned with codes from these categories when used with an abortion code because the other fifth digits will not apply. Codes from the 660-669 series are not to be used for complications of abortion.

COMPLICATIONS MAINLY RELATED TO PREGNANCY (640–649)

Includes　the listed conditions even if they arose or were
　　　　　　present during labor, delivery, or the
　　　　　　puerperium

The following fifth-digit subclassification is for use with categories 640–649 to denote the current episode of care:

**0　unspecified as to episode of care or not applicable
1　delivered, with or without mention of antepartum
　　condition**
　　　Antepartum condition with delivery
　　　Delivery NOS (with mention of antepartum
　　　　complication during current episode of care)
　　　Intrapartum
　　　　obstetric condition (with mention of antepartum
　　　　　complication during current episode of care)
　　　Pregnancy, delivered (with mention of antepartum
　　　　complication during current episode of care)
2　delivered, with mention of postpartum complication
　　　Delivery with mention of puerperal complication
　　　　during current episode of care
3　antepartum condition or complication
　　　Antepartum obstetric condition, not delivered
　　　　during the current episode of care
4　postpartum condition or complication
　　　Postpartum or puerperal obstetric condition or
　　　　complication following delivery that occurred:
　　　　during previous episode of care
　　　　outside hospital, with subsequent admission for
　　　　　observation or care

◀ New　　◀▥ Revised　　~~deleted~~ Deleted　　● Use Additional Digit(s)　　■ Nonspecific Code
● Not first-listed DX　　OGCR Official Guidelines　　Coding Clinic　　Excludes　　Includes　　Use additional　　Code first　　Omit code

● **640 Hemorrhage in early pregnancy**

Requires fifth digit; valid digits are in [brackets] under each code. See beginning of section 640–649 for definitions.

     Includes   hemorrhage before completion of 22 weeks' gestation

● **640.0 Threatened abortion** ♀   M
[0,1,3]

● ■ **640.8 Other specified hemorrhage in early pregnancy** ♀   M
[0,1,3]

● ■ **640.9 Unspecified hemorrhage in early pregnancy** ♀   M
[0,1,3]

● **641 Antepartum hemorrhage, abruptio placentae, and placenta previa**

Requires fifth digit; valid digits are in [brackets] under each code. See beginning of section 640–649 for definitions.

● **641.0 Placenta previa without hemorrhage** ♀   M
[0,1,3]   Low implantation of placenta without hemorrhage
Placenta previa noted:
    during pregnancy without hemorrhage
    before labor (and delivered by cesarean delivery)
      without hemorrhage

● **641.1 Hemorrhage from placenta previa** ♀   M
[0,1,3]   Low-lying placenta NOS or with hemorrhage
      (intrapartum)
Placenta previa:
    incomplete NOS or with hemorrhage
      (intrapartum)
    marginal NOS or with hemorrhage
      (intrapartum)
    partial NOS or with hemorrhage (intrapartum)
    total NOS or with hemorrhage (intrapartum)

     Excludes   *hemorrhage from vasa previa (663.5)*

● **641.2 Premature separation of placenta** ♀   M
[0,1,3]   Ablatio placentae
    Abruptio placentae
    Accidental antepartum hemorrhage
    Couvelaire uterus
    Detachment of placenta (premature)
    Premature separation of normally implanted
      placenta

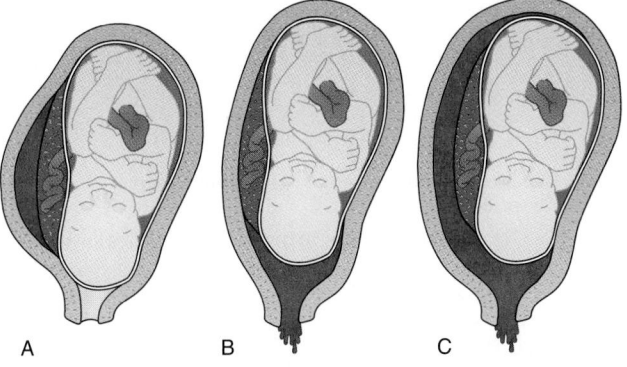

A   B   C

Figure 11–3   Abruptio placentae is classified according to the grade of separation of the placenta from the uterine wall. **A.** Mild separation in which hemorrhage is internal. **B.** Moderate separation in which there is external hemorrhage. **C.** Severe separation in which there is external hemorrhage and extreme separation.

● **641.3 Antepartum hemorrhage associated with coagulation**
[0,1,3] **defects** ♀   M
    Antepartum or intrapartum hemorrhage associated
      with:
      afibrinogenemia
      hyperfibrinolysis
      hypofibrinogenemia

     Excludes   *coagulation defects not associated with*
                   antepartum hemorrhage (649.3)

● ■ **641.8 Other antepartum hemorrhage** ♀   M
[0,1,3]   Antepartum or intrapartum hemorrhage associated
      with:
      trauma
      uterine leiomyoma

● ■ **641.9 Unspecified antepartum hemorrhage** ♀   M
[0,1,3]   Hemorrhage:
      antepartum NOS
      intrapartum NOS
      of pregnancy NOS

● **642 Hypertension complicating pregnancy, childbirth, and the puerperium**

Requires fifth digit; valid digits are in [brackets] under each code. See beginning of section 640–649 for definitions.

● **642.0 Benign essential hypertension complicating**
[0-4] **pregnancy, childbirth, and the puerperium** ♀   M
    Hypertension:
      benign essential specified as complicating,
        or as a reason for obstetric care during
        pregnancy, childbirth, or the puerperium
      chronic NOS specified as complicating, or as a
        reason for obstetric care during pregnancy,
        childbirth, or the puerperium
      essential specified as complicating, or as a
        reason for obstetric care during pregnancy,
        childbirth, or the puerperium
      pre-existing NOS specified as complicating,
        or as a reason for obstetric care during
        pregnancy, childbirth, or the puerperium

● **642.1 Hypertension secondary to renal disease,**
[0-4] **complicating pregnancy, childbirth, and the**
      puerperium ♀   M
    Hypertension secondary to renal disease, specified
      as complicating, or as a reason for obstetric
      care during pregnancy, childbirth, or the
      puerperium

● **642.2 Other pre-existing hypertension complicating**
[0-4] **pregnancy, childbirth, and the puerperium** ♀   M
    Hypertensive:
      chronic kidney disease specified as
        complicating, or as a reason for obstetric
        care during pregnancy, childbirth, or the
        puerperium
      heart and chronic kidney disease specified as
        complicating, or as a reason for obstetric
        care during pregnancy, childbirth, or the
        puerperium
      heart disease specified as complicating, or as a
        reason for obstetric care during pregnancy,
        childbirth, or the puerperium
    Malignant hypertension specified as complicating,
      or as a reason for obstetric care during
      pregnancy, childbirth, or the puerperium

● **642.3 Transient hypertension of pregnancy** ♀   M
[0-4]   Gestational hypertension
    Transient hypertension, so described, in pregnancy,
      childbirth, or the puerperium

COMPLICATIONS OF PREGNANCY, CHILDBIRTH, AND THE PUERPERIUM (630–679)

OGCR Section I.C.7.a.8

Assign code 796.2, Elevated blood pressure reading without diagnosis of hypertension, unless patient has an established diagnosis of hypertension. Assign code 642.3x for transient hypertension of pregnancy.

● **642.4 Mild or unspecified pre-eclampsia** ♀   M
[0-4]   Hypertension in pregnancy, childbirth, or the puerperium, not specified as pre-existing, with either albuminuria or edema, or both; mild or unspecified
Pre-eclampsia:
   NOS
   mild
Toxemia (pre-eclamptic):
   NOS
   mild

Excludes *albuminuria in pregnancy, without mention of hypertension (646.2)*
edema in pregnancy, without mention of hypertension (646.1)

● **642.5 Severe pre-eclampsia** ♀   M
[0-4]   Hypertension in pregnancy, childbirth, or the puerperium, not specified as pre-existing, with either albuminuria or edema, or both; specified as severe
Pre-eclampsia, severe
Toxemia (pre-eclamptic), severe

● **642.6 Eclampsia** ♀   M
[0-4]   Toxemia:
   eclamptic
   with convulsions

● **642.7 Pre-eclampsia or eclampsia superimposed on pre-**
[0-4] **existing hypertension** ♀   M
Conditions classifiable to 642.4–642.6, with conditions classifiable to 642.0–642.2

● ■ **642.9 Unspecified hypertension complicating pregnancy,**
[0-4] **childbirth, or the puerperium** ♀   M
Hypertension NOS, without mention of albuminuria or edema, complicating pregnancy, childbirth, or the puerperium
Coding Clinic: 2009, Q1, P18

● **643 Excessive vomiting in pregnancy**
Requires fifth digit; valid digits are in [brackets] under each code. See beginning of section 640–649 for definitions.

Includes hyperemesis arising during pregnancy
vomiting:
   persistent arising during pregnancy
   vicious arising during pregnancy
   hyperemesis gravidarum

● **643.0 Mild hyperemesis gravidarum** ♀   M
[0,1,3]   Hyperemesis gravidarum, mild or unspecified, starting before the end of the 22nd week of gestation

● **643.1 Hyperemesis gravidarum with metabolic**
[0,1,3] **disturbance** ♀   M
Hyperemesis gravidarum, starting before the end of the 22nd week of gestation, with metabolic disturbance, such as:
   carbohydrate depletion
   dehydration
   electrolyte imbalance

● **643.2 Late vomiting of pregnancy** ♀   M
[0,1,3]   Excessive vomiting starting after 22 completed weeks of gestation

● ■ **643.8 Other vomiting complicating pregnancy** ♀   M
[0,1,3]   Vomiting due to organic disease or other cause, specified as complicating pregnancy, or as a reason for obstetric care during pregnancy

Use additional code to specify cause

● ■ **643.9 Unspecified vomiting of pregnancy** ♀   M
[0,1,3]   Vomiting as a reason for care during pregnancy, length of gestation unspecified

● **644 Early or threatened labor**
Requires fifth digit; valid digits are in [brackets] under each code. See beginning of section 640–649 for definitions.

● **644.0 Threatened premature labor** ♀   M
[0,3]   Premature labor after 22 weeks, but before 37 completed weeks of gestation without delivery

Excludes *that occurring before 22 completed weeks of gestation (640.0)*

● ■ **644.1 Other threatened labor** ♀   M
[0,3]   False labor:
   NOS without delivery
   after 37 completed weeks of gestation without delivery
Threatened labor NOS without delivery

● **644.2 Early onset of delivery** ♀   M
[0-1]   Onset (spontaneous) of delivery before 37 completed weeks of gestation
Premature labor with onset of delivery before 37 completed weeks of gestation
Coding Clinic: 1991, Q2, P16

OGCR Section I.C.10.k.4

When an attempted termination of pregnancy results in a liveborn fetus assign code 644.21 with an appropriate code from category V27, Outcome of Delivery. The procedure code for the attempted termination of pregnancy should also be assigned.

● **645 Late pregnancy**
Requires fifth digit; valid digits are in [brackets] under each code. See beginning of section 640–649 for definitions.
Coding Clinic: 2000, Q1, P17-18

● **645.1 Post term pregnancy** ♀   M
[0,1,3]   Pregnancy over 40 completed weeks to 42 completed weeks gestation

● **645.2 Prolonged pregnancy** ♀   M
[0,1,3]   Pregnancy which has advanced beyond 42 completed weeks of gestation

● **646 Other complications of pregnancy, not elsewhere classified**

Use additional code(s) to further specify complication

Requires fifth digit; valid digits are in [brackets] under each code. See beginning of section 640–649 for definitions.

● **646.0 Papyraceous fetus** ♀   M
[0,1,3]

● **646.1 Edema or excessive weight gain in pregnancy,**
[0-4] **without mention of hypertension** ♀   M
Gestational edema
Maternal obesity syndrome

Excludes *that with mention of hypertension (642.0–642.9)*

● ■ **646.2 Unspecified renal disease in pregnancy, without** M
[0-4] **mention of hypertension** ♀

   Albuminuria in pregnancy or the puerperium,
      without mention of hypertension
   Nephropathy NOS in pregnancy or the
      puerperium, without mention of
      hypertension
   Renal disease NOS in pregnancy or the
      puerperium, without mention of
      hypertension
   Uremia in pregnancy or the puerperium, without
      mention of hypertension
   Gestational proteinuria in pregnancy or
      the puerperium, without mention of
      hypertension

   Excludes *that with mention of hypertension*
                (642.0–642.9)

● **646.3 Habitual aborter** ♀ M
[0,1,3] **Excludes** *with current abortion (634.0–634.9)*
                     without current pregnancy (629.81)

● **646.4 Peripheral neuritis in pregnancy** ♀ M
[0-4]

● **646.5 Asymptomatic bacteriuria in pregnancy** ♀ M
[0-4]

● **646.6 Infections of genitourinary tract in** M
[0-4] **pregnancy** ♀
   Conditions classifiable to 590, 595, 597, 599.0, 616
      complicating pregnancy, childbirth, or the
      puerperium
   Conditions classifiable to 614.0–614.5, 614.7–614.9,
      615 complicating pregnancy or labor

   Excludes *major puerperal infection (670.0–670.8)* ◀

   Coding Clinic: 2004, Q4, P88-90

   OGCR Section I.C.2.g.
   During pregnancy, childbirth or the puerperium,
   a patient admitted (or presenting for a health
   care encounter) because of an HIV-related illness
   should receive a principal diagnosis code of
   647.6X, Other specified infectious and parasitic
   diseases in the mother classifiable elsewhere, but
   complicating the pregnancy, childbirth or the
   puerperium, followed by 042 and the code(s) for
   the HIV-related illness(es). Codes from Chapter
   15 always take sequencing priority. Patients with
   asymptomatic HIV infection status admitted (or
   presenting for a health care encounter) during
   pregnancy, childbirth, or the puerperium should
   receive codes of 647.6X and V08.

● **646.7 Liver disorders in pregnancy** ♀ M
[0,1,3] Acute yellow atrophy of liver (obstetric) (true) of
            pregnancy
         Icterus gravis of pregnancy
         Necrosis of liver of pregnancy

   Excludes *hepatorenal syndrome following delivery*
                (674.8)
                viral hepatitis (647.6)

● ■ **646.8 Other specified complications of pregnancy** ♀ M
[0-4] Fatigue during pregnancy
       Herpes gestationis
       Insufficient weight gain of pregnancy
       Coding Clinic: 1998, Q3, P16; 1985, Jan-Feb, P15-16

● ■ **646.9 Unspecified complication of pregnancy** ♀ M
[0,1,3]

● **647 Infectious and parasitic conditions in the mother**
      classifiable elsewhere, but complicating pregnancy,
      childbirth, or the puerperium

   Use additional code(s) to further specify complication

   Requires fifth digit; valid digits are in [brackets] under
      each code. See beginning of section 640–649 for
      definitions.

   Includes the listed conditions when complicating
               the pregnant state, aggravated by the
               pregnancy, or when a main reason for
               obstetric care

   Excludes *those conditions in the mother known or suspected*
                to have affected the fetus (655.0–655.9)

● **647.0 Syphilis** ♀ M
[0-4] Conditions classifiable to 090–097

● **647.1 Gonorrhea** ♀ M
[0-4] Conditions classifiable to 098

● ■ **647.2 Other venereal diseases** ♀ M
[0-4] Conditions classifiable to 099

● **647.3 Tuberculosis** ♀ M
[0-4] Conditions classifiable to 010–018

● **647.4 Malaria** ♀ M
[0-4] Conditions classifiable to 084

● **647.5 Rubella** ♀ M
[0-4] Conditions classifiable to 056

● ■ **647.6 Other viral diseases** ♀ M
[0-4] Conditions classifiable to 042, 050-055, 057-079,
          795.05, 795.15, 796.75
       Coding Clinic: 1985, Jan-Feb, P15-16

● ■ **647.8 Other specified infectious and parasitic** M
[0-4] **diseases** ♀

● ■ **647.9 Unspecified infection or infestation** ♀ M
[0-4]

● **648 Other current conditions in the mother classifiable**
      elsewhere, but complicating pregnancy, childbirth,
      or the puerperium

   Use additional code(s) to identify the condition

   Requires fifth digit; valid digits are in [brackets] under
      each code. See beginning of section 640–649 for
      definitions.

   Includes the listed conditions when complicating
               the pregnant state, aggravated by the
               pregnancy, or when a main reason for
               obstetric care

   Excludes *those conditions in the mother known or suspected*
                to have affected the fetus (655.0–655.9)

● **648.0 Diabetes mellitus** ♀ M
[0-4] Conditions classifiable to 249, 250

   Excludes *gestational diabetes (648.8)*

● **648.1 Thyroid dysfunction** ♀ M
[0-4] Conditions classifiable to 240–246

● **648.2 Anemia** ♀ M
[0-4] Conditions classifiable to 280–285
       Coding Clinic: 2002, Q1, P14

● **648.3 Drug dependence** ♀ M
[0-4] Conditions classifiable to 304
       Coding Clinic: 1998, Q2, P13-14; 1988, Q4, P8

COMPLICATIONS OF PREGNANCY, CHILDBIRTH, AND THE PUERPERIUM (630–679)

● **648.4 Mental disorders** ♀   M
[0-4]   Conditions classifiable to 290–303, 305.0,
305.2–305.9, 306–316, 317–319
Coding Clinic: 1998, Q2, P13-14

● **648.5 Congenital cardiovascular disorders** ♀   M
[0-4]   Conditions classifiable to 745–747

● ■ **648.6 Other cardiovascular diseases** ♀   M
[0-4]   Conditions classifiable to 390–398, 410–429

> **Excludes**   *cerebrovascular disorders in the puerperium*
> *(674.0)*
> *peripartum cardiomyopathy (674.5)*
> *venous complications (671.0–671.9)*
Coding Clinic: 1998, Q3, P11

● **648.7 Bone and joint disorders of back, pelvis, and lower**
[0-4]   **limbs** ♀   M
    Conditions classifiable to 720–724, and those
classifiable to 711–719 or 725–738, specified as
affecting the lower limbs

● **648.8 Abnormal glucose tolerance** ♀   M
[0-4]   Conditions classifiable to 790.21–790.29
Gestational diabetes

> Use **additional** code, if applicable, for associated
> long-term (current) insulin use V58.67
Coding Clinic: 2004, Q4, P53-56

● ■ **648.9 Other current conditions classifiable elsewhere** ♀   M
[0-4]   Conditions classifiable to 440–459, 795.01–795.04,
795.06, 795.10–795.14, 795.16, 796.70–796.74,
796.76
Nutritional deficiencies [conditions classifiable to
260–269]
Coding Clinic: 2009, Q1, P17; 2006, Q3, P14; 2004, Q4, P88-90;
2002, Q1, P14-15; 1984, Nov-Dec, P18

649 Other conditions or status of the mother complicating
pregnancy, childbirth, or the puerperium

> Requires fifth digit; valid digits are in [brackets] under
> each code. See beginning of section 640-649 for
> definitions.

● **649.0 Tobacco use disorder complicating pregnancy,**
[0-4]   **childbirth, or the puerperium** ♀   M
    Smoking complicating pregnancy, childbirth, or
the puerperium

● **649.1 Obesity complicating pregnancy, childbirth, or the**
[0-4]   **puerperium** ♀   M

> Use **additional** code to identify the obesity (278.00,
> 278.01)

● **649.2 Bariatric surgery status complicating pregnancy,**
[0-4]   **childbirth, or the puerperium** ♀   M
    Gastric banding status complicating pregnancy,
childbirth, or the puerperium
Gastric bypass status for obesity complicating
pregnancy, childbirth, or the puerperium
Obesity surgery status complicating pregnancy,
childbirth, or the puerperium

● **649.3 Coagulation defects complicating pregnancy,**
[0-4]   **childbirth, or the puerperium** ♀   M
    Conditions classifiable to 286, 287, 289 ◀▥

> Use **additional** code to identify the specific
> coagulation defect (286.0–286.9, 287.0–287.9,
> 289.0–289.9) ◀▥

> **Excludes**   *coagulation defects causing antepartum*
> *hemorrhage (641.3)*

● **649.4 Epilepsy complicating pregnancy, childbirth, or the**
[0-4]   **puerperium** ♀   M
    Conditions classifiable to 345

> Use **additional** code to identify the specific type of
> epilepsy (345.00–345.91)

> **Excludes**   *eclampsia (642.6)*

● **649.5 Spotting complicating pregnancy** ♀   M
[0,1,3]   **Excludes**   *antepartum hemorrhage (641.0–641.9)*
> *hemorrhage in early pregnancy*
> *(640.0–640.9)*

● **649.6 Uterine size date discrepancy** ♀   M
[0-4]   **Excludes**   *suspected problem with fetal growth not*
> *found (V89.04)*

● **649.7 Cervical shortening** ♀   M
[0,1,3]   **Excludes**   *suspected cervical shortening not found*
> *(V89.05)*
Coding Clinic: 2008, Q4, P124-125

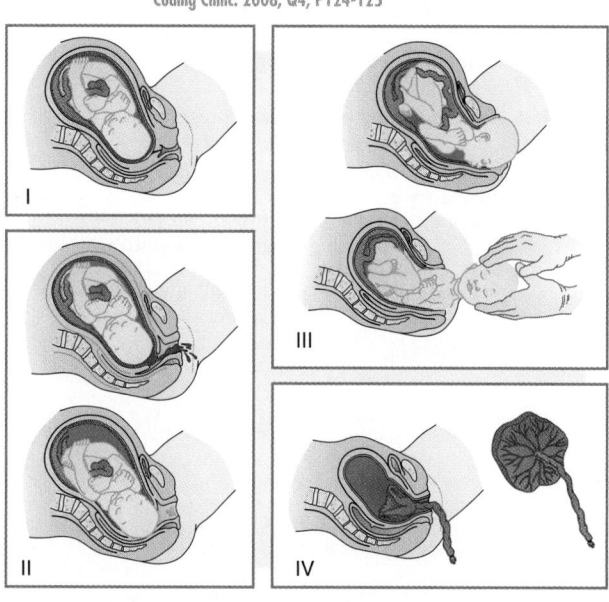

Figure 11–4   The four stages of normal delivery: **I.** Lightening,
which occurs 2 to 4 weeks before birth, at which time the fetus turns
with head toward the vagina. **II.** Regular contractions begin, the
amniotic sac ruptures, and dilation is complete. **III.** Delivery of the
head and rotation. **IV.** Expulsion of placenta.

OGCR   **Section I.C.10.h.1**

Code 650 is for use in cases when a woman is admitted
for a full-term normal delivery and delivers a single,
healthy infant without any complications antepartum,
during the delivery, or postpartum during the delivery
episode. Code 650 is always a principal diagnosis.
It is not to be used if any other code from chapter 11
is needed to describe a current complication of the
antenatal, delivery, or perinatal period. Additional codes
from other chapters may be used with code 650 if they
are not related to or are in any way complicating the
pregnancy.

OGCR   **Section I.C.10.h.2**

Code 650 may be used if the patient had a complication
at some point during her pregnancy, but the complication
is not present at the time of the admission for delivery.

◀ New   ◀▥ Revised   ~~deleted~~ Deleted   ● Use Additional Digit(s)   ■ Nonspecific Code

● Not first-listed DX   **OGCR**   Official Guidelines   Coding Clinic   Excludes   Includes   Use additional   Code first   Omit code

NORMAL DELIVERY, AND OTHER INDICATIONS FOR CARE IN PREGNANCY, LABOR, AND DELIVERY (650–659)

The following fifth-digit subclassification is for use with categories 651–659 to denote the current episode of care:

> 0 unspecified as to episode of care or not applicable
> 1 delivered, with or without mention of antepartum condition
> 2 delivered, with mention of postpartum complication
> 3 antepartum condition or complication
> 4 postpartum condition or complication

650 Normal delivery ♀   M
Delivery requiring minimal or no assistance, with or without episiotomy, without fetal manipulation [e.g., rotation version] or instrumentation [forceps] of a spontaneous, cephalic, vaginal, full-term, single, live-born infant. This code is for use as a single diagnosis code and is not to be used with any other code in the range 630–676.

Use additional code to indicate outcome of delivery (V27.0)

Excludes breech delivery (assisted) (spontaneous) NOS (652.2)
delivery by vacuum extractor, forceps, cesarean section, or breech extraction, without specified complication (669.5–669.7)
Coding Clinic: 2002, Q2, P10; 2001, Q3, P12; 2000, Q3, P5

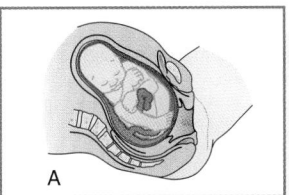
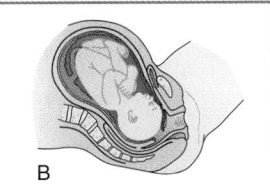
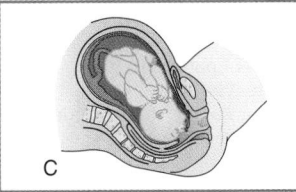
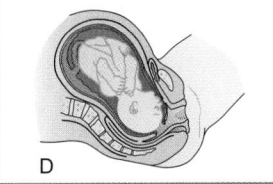
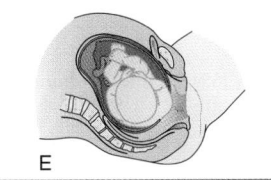

Figure 11–5 Five types of malposition and malpresentation of the fetus: **A.** Breech. **B.** Vertex. **C.** Face. **D.** Brow. **E.** Shoulder.

651 Multiple gestation
Requires fifth digit; valid digits are in [brackets] under each code. See beginning of section 650–659 for definitions.
Excludes fetal conjoined twins (678.1)

651.0 Twin pregnancy ♀   M
[0,1,3]   **Excludes** fetal conjoined twins (678.1)
Coding Clinic: 2006, Q3, P16-18; 1992, Q3, P10

651.1 Triplet pregnancy ♀   M
[0,1,3]

651.2 Quadruplet pregnancy ♀   M
[0,1,3]

651.3 Twin pregnancy with fetal loss and retention of one   M
[0,1,3] fetus ♀

651.4 Triplet pregnancy with fetal loss and retention of   M
[0,1,3] one or more fetus(es) ♀

651.5 Quadruplet pregnancy with fetal loss and retention   M
[0,1,3] of one or more fetus(es) ♀

651.6 Other multiple pregnancy with fetal loss and   M
[0,1,3] retention of one or more fetus(es) ♀

651.7 Multiple gestation following (elective) fetal   M
[0,1,3] reduction ♀
Fetal reduction of multiple fetuses reduced to single fetus
Coding Clinic: 2006, Q3, P16-18; 2005, Q4, P81

651.8 Other specified multiple gestation ♀   M
[0,1,3]

651.9 Unspecified multiple gestation ♀   M
[0,1,3]

652 Malposition and malpresentation of fetus
Requires fifth digit; valid digits are in [brackets] under each code. See beginning of section 650–659 for definitions.
Code first any associated obstructed labor (660.0)
Coding Clinic: 1995, Q3, P10

652.0 Unstable lie ♀   M
[0,1,3]

652.1 Breech or other malpresentation successfully   M
[0,1,3] converted to cephalic presentation ♀
Cephalic version NOS

652.2 Breech presentation without mention of version ♀   M
[0,1,3] Breech delivery (assisted) (spontaneous) NOS
Buttocks presentation
Complete breech
Frank breech
Excludes footling presentation (652.8)
incomplete breech (652.8)

652.3 Transverse or oblique presentation ♀   M
[0,1,3] Oblique lie
Transverse lie
Excludes transverse arrest of fetal head (660.3)

652.4 Face or brow presentation ♀   M
[0,1,3] Mentum presentation

COMPLICATIONS OF PREGNANCY, CHILDBIRTH, AND THE PUERPERIUM (630–679)

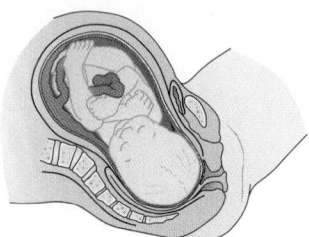

Figure 11–6 Hydrocephalic fetus causing disproportion.

● **652.5 High head at term ♀**   M
[0,1,3]   Failure of head to enter pelvic brim

● **652.6 Multiple gestation with malpresentation of one**
[0,1,3]   **fetus or more ♀**   M

● **652.7 Prolapsed arm ♀**   M
[0,1,3]

● ■ **652.8 Other specified malposition or malpresentation ♀**   M
[0,1,3]   Compound presentation

● ■ **652.9 Unspecified malposition or malpresentation ♀**   M
[0,1,3]

● **653 Disproportion**

Requires fifth digit; valid digits are in [brackets] under each code. See beginning of section 650–659 for definitions.

Code first any associated obstructed labor (660.1)

Coding Clinic: 1995, Q3, P10

● **653.0 Major abnormality of bony pelvis, not further**
[0,1,3]   **specified ♀**   M
      Pelvic deformity NOS

● **653.1 Generally contracted pelvis ♀**   M
[0,1,3]   Contracted pelvis NOS

● **653.2 Inlet contraction of pelvis ♀**   M
[0,1,3]   Inlet contraction (pelvis)

● **653.3 Outlet contraction of pelvis ♀**   M
[0,1,3]   Outlet contraction (pelvis)

● **653.4 Fetopelvic disproportion ♀**   M
[0,1,3]   Cephalopelvic disproportion NOS
      Disproportion of mixed maternal and fetal origin, with normally formed fetus

● **653.5 Unusually large fetus causing disproportion ♀**   M
[0,1,3]   Disproportion of fetal origin with normally formed fetus
      Fetal disproportion NOS

      Excludes *that when the reason for medical care was concern for the fetus (656.6)*

● **653.6 Hydrocephalic fetus causing disproportion ♀**   M
[0,1,3]
      Excludes *that when the reason for medical care was concern for the fetus (655.0)*

● ■ **653.7 Other fetal abnormality causing disproportion ♀**   M
[0,1,3]   Fetal: Fetal:
     ascites   sacral teratoma
     hydrops   tumor
     myelomeningocele

      Excludes *conjoined twins causing disporportion (678.1)*

● ■ **653.8 Disproportion of other origin ♀**   M
[0,1,3]   **Excludes** *shoulder (girdle) dystocia (660.4)*

● ■ **653.9 Unspecified disproportion ♀**   M
[0,1,3]

● **654 Abnormality of organs and soft tissues of pelvis**

Requires fifth digit; valid digits are in [brackets] under each code. See beginning of section 650–659 for definitions.

Includes   the listed conditions during pregnancy, childbirth, or the puerperium

Code first any associated obstructed labor (660.2)

Excludes *trauma to perineum and vulva complicating current delivery (664.0–664.9)*

Coding Clinic: 1995, Q3, P10

● **654.0 Congenital abnormalities of uterus ♀**   M
[0-4]   Double uterus
      Uterus bicornis

● **654.1 Tumors of body of uterus ♀**   M
[0-4]   Uterine fibroids
      Coding Clinic: 1994, Q2, P14

● **654.2 Previous cesarean delivery ♀**   M
[0,1,3]   Uterine scar from previous cesarean delivery

● **654.3 Retroverted and incarcerated gravid uterus ♀**   M
[0-4]

● ■ **654.4 Other abnormalities in shape or position of**
[0-4]   **gravid uterus and of neighboring structures ♀**   M
      Cystocele
      Pelvic floor repair
      Pendulous abdomen
      Prolapse of gravid uterus
      Rectocele
      Rigid pelvic floor

● **654.5 Cervical incompetence ♀**   M
[0-4]   Presence of Shirodkar suture with or without mention of cervical incompetence

● ■ **654.6 Other congenital or acquired abnormality of**
[0-4]   **cervix ♀**   M
      Cicatricial cervix
      Polyp of cervix
      Previous surgery to cervix
      Rigid cervix (uteri)
      Stenosis or stricture of cervix
      Tumor of cervix

● **654.7 Congenital or acquired abnormality of vagina ♀**   M
[0-4]   Previous surgery to vagina
      Septate vagina
      Stenosis of vagina (acquired) (congenital)
      Stricture of vagina
      Tumor of vagina

● **654.8 Congenital or acquired abnormality of vulva ♀**   M
[0-4]   Anal sphincter tear (healed) (old) complicating delivery
      Fibrosis of perineum
      Persistent hymen
      Previous surgery to perineum or vulva
      Rigid perineum
      Tumor of vulva

      Excludes *anal sphincter tear (healed) (old) not associated with delivery (569.43)*
                varicose veins of vulva (671.1)

      Coding Clinic: 2003, Q1, P14

● ■ **654.9 Other and unspecified ♀**   M
[0-4]   Uterine scar NEC

COMPLICATIONS OF PREGNANCY, CHILDBIRTH, AND THE PUERPERIUM (630–679)

◀ New   ◀▥ Revised   ~~deleted~~ Deleted   ● Use Additional Digit(s)   ■ Nonspecific Code

● Not first-listed DX   OGCR Official Guidelines   Coding Clinic   Excludes   Includes   Use additional   Code first   Omit code

OGCR   Section I.C.10.a.2

In cases when in utero surgery is performed on the fetus, a code from category 655 should be assigned identifying the fetal condition. Procedure code 75.36, Correction of fetal defect, should be assigned on the hospital inpatient record. No code from Chapter 15, the perinatal codes, should be used on the mother's record to identify fetal conditions. Surgery performed in utero on a fetus is still to be coded as an obstetric encounter.

● 655   **Known or suspected fetal abnormality affecting management of mother**

   Requires fifth digit; valid digits are in [brackets] under each code. See beginning of section 650–659 for definitions.

   Includes   the listed conditions in the fetus as a reason for observation or obstetrical care of the mother, or for termination of pregnancy

● 655.0   **Central nervous system malformation in fetus** ♀   M
   [0,1,3]   Fetal or suspected fetal:
      anencephaly
      hydrocephalus
      spina bifida (with myelomeningocele)

● 655.1   **Chromosomal abnormality in fetus** ♀   M
   [0,1,3]

● 655.2   **Hereditary disease in family possibly affecting**
   [0,1,3]   **fetus** ♀   M

● 655.3   **Suspected damage to fetus from viral disease in the**
   [0,1,3]   **mother** ♀   M
      Suspected damage to fetus from maternal rubella

●■ 655.4   **Suspected damage to fetus from other disease in the**
   [0,1,3]   **mother** ♀   M
      Suspected damage to fetus from maternal:
         alcohol addiction
         listeriosis
         toxoplasmosis

● 655.5   **Suspected damage to fetus from drugs** ♀   M
   [0,1,3]

● 655.6   **Suspected damage to fetus from radiation** ♀   M
   [0,1,3]

● 655.7   **Decreased fetal movements** ♀   M
   [0,1,3]   Coding Clinic: 1997, Q4, P41

●■ 655.8   **Other known or suspected fetal abnormality, not**
   [0,1,3]   **elsewhere classified** ♀   M
      Suspected damage to fetus from:
         environmental toxins
         intrauterine contraceptive device
      Coding Clinic: 2006, Q3, P16-18x2

●■ 655.9   **Unspecified** ♀   M
   [0,1,3]

● 656   **Other known or suspected fetal and placental problems affecting management of mother**

   Requires fifth digit; valid digits are in [brackets] under each code. See beginning of section 650–659 for definitions.

   Excludes   *fetal hematologic conditions (678.0)*
      suspected placental problems not found (V89.02)

● 656.0   **Fetal-maternal hemorrhage** ♀   M
   [0,1,3]   Leakage (microscopic) of fetal blood into maternal circulation

● 656.1   **Rhesus isoimmunization** ♀   M
   [0,1,3]   Anti-D [Rh] antibodies
      Rh incompatibility

●■ 656.2   **Isoimmunization from other and unspecified blood-**
   [0,1,3]   **group incompatibility** ♀   M
      ABO isoimmunization
      Coding Clinic: 2006, Q4, P135

● 656.3   **Fetal distress** ♀   M
   [0,1,3]   Fetal metabolic acidemia

      Excludes   *abnormal fetal acid-base balance (656.8)*
         abnormality in fetal heart rate or rhythm (659.7)
         fetal bradycardia (659.7)
         fetal tachycardia (659.7)
         meconium in liquor (656.8)

● 656.4   **Intrauterine death** ♀   M
   [0,1,3]   Fetal death:
         NOS
         after completion of 22 weeks' gestation
         late
      Missed delivery

      Excludes   *missed abortion (632)*

● 656.5   **Poor fetal growth** ♀   M
   [0,1,3]   "Light-for-dates"
      "Placental insufficiency"
      "Small-for-dates"

● 656.6   **Excessive fetal growth** ♀   M
   [0,1,3]   "Large-for-dates"

●■ 656.7   **Other placental conditions** ♀   M
   [0,1,3]   Abnormal placenta
      Placental infarct

      Excludes   *placental polyp (674.4)*
         placentitis (658.4)

●■ 656.8   **Other specified fetal and placental problems** ♀   M
   [0,1,3]   Abnormal acid-base balance
      Intrauterine acidosis
      Lithopedian
      Meconium in liquor
      Subchorionic hematoma

●■ 656.9   **Unspecified fetal and placental problem** ♀   M
   [0,1,3]

● 657   **Polyhydramnios** ♀   M
   [0,1,3]   Hydramnios

   Requires fifth digit; valid digits are in [brackets] under each code. See beginning of section 650–659 for definitions.

   Use 0 as fourth digit for category 657

   Excludes   *suspected polyhydramnios not found (V89.01)*

   Coding Clinic: 2006, Q3, P16-18

● **658 Other problems associated with amniotic cavity and membranes**

> Requires fifth digit; valid digits are in [brackets] under each code. See beginning of section 650–659 for definitions.

> **Excludes** *amniotic fluid embolism (673.1)*
> *suspected problems with amniotic cavity and membranes not found (V89.01)*

● **658.0 Oligohydramnios ♀**   M
[0,1,3]   Oligohydramnios without mention of rupture of membranes
             Coding Clinic: 2006, Q3, P16-18

● **658.1 Premature rupture of membranes ♀**   M
[0,1,3]   Rupture of amniotic sac less than 24 hours prior to the onset of labor
             Coding Clinic: 2001, Q1, P5; 1998, Q4, P76-77

● **658.2 Delayed delivery after spontaneous or unspecified**
[0,1,3] **rupture of membranes ♀**   M
             Prolonged rupture of membranes NOS
             Rupture of amniotic sac 24 hours or more prior to the onset of labor

● **658.3 Delayed delivery after artificial rupture of**
[0,1,3] **membranes ♀**   M

● **658.4 Infection of amniotic cavity ♀**   M
[0,1,3]   Amnionitis
             Chorioamnionitis
             Membranitis
             Placentitis

● ■ **658.8 Other ♀**   M
[0,1,3]   Amnion nodosum
             Amniotic cyst

● ■ **658.9 Unspecified ♀**   M
[0,1,3]

● **659 Other indications for care or intervention related to labor and delivery, not elsewhere classified**

> Requires fifth digit; valid digits are in [brackets] under each code. See beginning of section 650–659 for definitions.

● **659.0 Failed mechanical induction ♀**   M
[0,1,3]   Failure of induction of labor by surgical or other instrumental methods

● **659.1 Failed medical or unspecified induction ♀**   M
[0,1,3]   Failed induction NOS
             Failure of induction of labor by medical methods, such as oxytocic drugs

● ■ **659.2 Maternal pyrexia during labor, unspecified ♀**   M
[0,1,3]

● **659.3 Generalized infection during labor ♀**   M
[0,1,3]   Septicemia during labor

● **659.4 Grand multiparity ♀**   M
[0,1,3]   **Excludes** *supervision only, in pregnancy (V23.3)*
                          without current pregnancy (V61.5)

● **659.5 Elderly primigravida ♀**   M
[0,1,3]   First pregnancy in a woman who will be 35 years of age or older at expected date of delivery
             Excludes *supervision only, in pregnancy (V23.81)*
             Coding Clinic: 2001, Q3, P12

● ■ **659.6 Elderly multigravida ♀**   M
[0,1,3]   Second or more pregnancy in a woman who will be 35 years of age or older at expected date of delivery
             Excludes *elderly primigravida (659.5)*
                          supervision only, in pregnancy (V23.82)
             Coding Clinic: 2001, Q3, P12

● ■ **659.7 Abnormality in fetal heart rate or rhythm ♀**   M
[0,1,3]   Depressed fetal heart tones
             Fetal:
                bradycardia
                tachycardia
             Fetal heart rate decelerations
             Non-reassuring fetal heart rate or rhythm
             Coding Clinic: 1998, Q4, P47-48

● ■ **659.8 Other specified indications for care or intervention**
[0,1,3] **related to labor and delivery ♀**   M
             Pregnancy in a female less than 16 years of age at expected date of delivery
             Very young maternal age
             Coding Clinic: 2001, Q3, P12

● ■ **659.9 Unspecified indication for care or intervention**
[0,1,3] **related to labor and delivery ♀**   M

OGCR Section I.C.10.k.2
Codes from the 660-669 series are not to be used for complications of abortion.

COMPLICATIONS OCCURRING MAINLY IN THE COURSE OF LABOR AND DELIVERY (660–669)

> The following fifth-digit subclassification is for use with categories 660–669 to denote the current episode of care:

> ■ **0 unspecified as to episode of care or not applicable**
> **1 delivered, with or without mention of antepartum condition**
> **2 delivered, with mention of postpartum complication**
> **3 antepartum condition or complication**
> **4 postpartum condition or complication**

● **660 Obstructed labor**

> Requires fifth digit; valid digits are in [brackets] under each code. See beginning of section 660–669 for definitions.
> Coding Clinic: 1995, Q3, P10

● **660.0 Obstruction caused by malposition of fetus at onset**
[0,1,3] **of labor ♀**   M
             Any condition classifiable to 652, causing obstruction during labor
             Use additional code from 652.0–652.9 to identify condition
             Coding Clinic: 1995, Q3, P10

● **660.1 Obstruction by bony pelvis ♀**   M
[0,1,3]   Any condition classifiable to 653, causing obstruction during labor
             Use additional code from 653.0–653.9 to identify condition
             Coding Clinic: 1995, Q3, P10

◄ New   ◄◖ Revised   ~~deleted~~ Deleted   ● Use Additional Digit(s)   ■ Nonspecific Code
● Not first-listed DX   OGCR Official Guidelines   Coding Clinic   Excludes   Includes   Use additional   Code first   Omit code

● **660.2 Obstruction by abnormal pelvic soft tissues** ♀   **M**
[0,1,3]   Prolapse of anterior lip of cervix
     Any condition classifiable to 654, causing
       obstruction during labor

     Use additional code from 654.0–654.9 to identify
       condition
     Coding Clinic: 1995, Q3, P10

● **660.3 Deep transverse arrest and persistent occipito-**
[0,1,3] **posterior position** ♀   **M**

● **660.4 Shoulder (girdle) dystocia** ♀   **M**
[0,1,3]   Impacted shoulders

● **660.5 Locked twins** ♀   **M**
[0,1,3]

● ■ **660.6 Failed trial of labor, unspecified** ♀   **M**
[0,1,3]   Failed trial of labor, without mention of condition
       or suspected condition

● ■ **660.7 Failed forceps or vacuum extractor, unspecified** ♀   **M**
[0,1,3]   Application of ventouse or forceps, without
       mention of condition

● ■ **660.8 Other causes of obstructed labor** ♀   **M**
[0,1,3]   Use additional code to identify condition

● ■ **660.9 Unspecified obstructed labor** ♀   **M**
[0,1,3]   Dystocia:
       NOS
       fetal NOS
       maternal NOS

● **661 Abnormality of forces of labor**

     Requires fifth digit; valid digits are in [brackets] under
     each code. See beginning of section 660–669 for
     definitions.

● **661.0 Primary uterine inertia** ♀   **M**
[0,1,3]   Failure of cervical dilation
     Hypotonic uterine dysfunction, primary
     Prolonged latent phase of labor
     Coding Clinic: 1985, July-Aug, P11

● **661.1 Secondary uterine inertia** ♀   **M**
[0,1,3]   Arrested active phase of labor
     Hypotonic uterine dysfunction, secondary
     Coding Clinic: 1985, July-Aug, P11

● ■ **661.2 Other and unspecified uterine inertia** ♀   **M**
[0,1,3]   Atony of uterus without hemorrhage
     Desultory labor
     Irregular labor
     Poor contractions
     Slow slope active phase of labor

     Excludes *atony of uterus with hemorrhage (666.1)*
       postpartum atony of uterus without
       hemorrhage (669.8)
     Coding Clinic: 1985, July-Aug, P11

● **661.3 Precipitate labor** ♀   **M**
[0,1,3]

● **661.4 Hypertonic, incoordinate, or prolonged uterine**
[0,1,3] **contractions** ♀   **M**
     Cervical spasm
     Contraction ring (dystocia)
     Dyscoordinate labor
     Hourglass contraction of uterus
     Hypertonic uterine dysfunction
     Incoordinate uterine action
     Retraction ring (Bandl's) (pathological)
     Tetanic contractions
     Uterine dystocia NOS
     Uterine spasm

● ■ **661.9 Unspecified abnormality of labor** ♀   **M**
[0,1,3]

● **662 Long labor**

     Requires fifth digit; valid digits are in [brackets] under
     each code. See beginning of section 660–669 for
     definitions.

● **662.0 Prolonged first stage** ♀   **M**
[0,1,3]

● ■ **662.1 Prolonged labor, unspecified** ♀   **M**
[0,1,3]

● **662.2 Prolonged second stage** ♀   **M**
[0,1,3]

● **662.3 Delayed delivery of second twin, triplet, etc.** ♀   **M**
[0,1,3]

● **663 Umbilical cord complications**

     Requires fifth digit; valid digits are in [brackets] under
     each code. See beginning of section 660–669 for
     definitions.

● **663.0 Prolapse of cord** ♀   **M**
[0,1,3]   Presentation of cord

● **663.1 Cord around neck, with compression** ♀   **M**
[0,1,3]   Cord tightly around neck

● ■ **663.2 Other and unspecified cord entanglement, with**
[0,1,3] **compression** ♀   **M**
     Entanglement of cords of twins in mono-amniotic
       sac
     Knot in cord (with compression)

● ■ **663.3 Other and unspecified cord entanglement, without**
[0,1,3] **mention of compression** ♀   **M**
     Coding Clinic: 2003, Q2, P9

● **663.4 Short cord** ♀   **M**
[0,1,3]

● **663.5 Vasa previa** ♀   **M**
[0,1,3]

● **663.6 Vascular lesions of cord** ♀   **M**
[0,1,3]   Bruising of cord
     Hematoma of cord
     Thrombosis of vessels of cord

● ■ **663.8 Other umbilical cord complications** ♀   **M**
[0,1,3]   Velamentous insertion of umbilical cord

● ■ **663.9 Unspecified umbilical cord complication** ♀   **M**
[0,1,3]

● **664 Trauma to perineum and vulva during delivery**

     Requires fifth digit; valid digits are in [brackets] under
     each code. See beginning of section 660–669 for
     definitions.

     Includes   damage from instruments
       that from extension of episiotomy
     Coding Clinic: 2008, Q4, P192; 1992, Q1, P10-11

● **664.0 First-degree perineal laceration** ♀   **M**
[0,1,4]   Perineal laceration, rupture, or tear involving:
     fourchette
     hymen
     labia vulva
     skin
     vagina
     Coding Clinic: 1984, Nov-Dec, P10

● **664.1 Second-degree perineal laceration** ♀   **M**
[0,1,4]   Perineal laceration, rupture, or tear (following
       episiotomy) involving:
     pelvic floor
     perineal muscles
     vaginal muscles

     Excludes *that involving anal sphincter (664.2)*
     Coding Clinic: 2008, Q4, P192; 1984, Nov-Dec, P10

COMPLICATIONS OF PREGNANCY, CHILDBIRTH, AND THE PUERPERIUM (630–679)

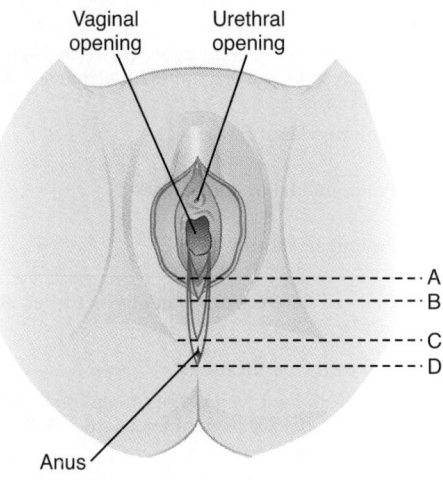

Vaginal opening Urethral opening

Anus

Figure 11–7 Perineal lacerations: **A.** First-degree is laceration of superficial tissues. **B.** Second-degree is limited to the pelvic floor and may involve the perineal or vaginal muscles. **C.** Third-degree involves the anal sphincter. **D.** Fourth-degree involves anal or rectal mucosa.

● **664.2 Third-degree perineal laceration ♀**   M
[0,1,4]   Perineal laceration, rupture, or tear (following episiotomy) involving:
     anal sphincter
     rectovaginal septum
     sphincter NOS

     Excludes   *anal sphincter tear during delivery not associated with third-degree perineal laceration (664.6)*
       that with anal or rectal mucosal laceration (664.3)
     Coding Clinic: 1984, Nov-Dec, P10

● **664.3 Fourth-degree perineal laceration ♀**   M
[0,1,4]   Perineal laceration, rupture, or tear as classifiable to 664.2 and involving also:
     anal mucosa
     rectal mucosa
     Coding Clinic: 1984, Nov-Dec, P10

● ■**664.4 Unspecified perineal laceration ♀**   M
[0,1,4]   Central laceration

● **664.5 Vulval and perineal hematoma ♀**   M
[0,1,4]   Coding Clinic: 1984, Nov-Dec, P10

● **664.6 Anal sphincter tear complicating delivery, not**
[0,1,4] **associated with third-degree perineal laceration ♀**   M

     Excludes   *third-degree perineal laceration (664.2)*
     Coding Clinic: 2007, Q4, P88-90

● ■**664.8 Other specified trauma to perineum and vulva ♀**   M
[0,1,4]   Coding Clinic: 2007, Q4, P125

● ■**664.9 Unspecified trauma to perineum and vulva ♀**   M
[0,1,4]

● **665 Other obstetrical trauma**
     Requires fifth digit; valid digits are in [brackets] under each code. See beginning of section 660–669 for definitions.
     Includes   damage from instruments

● **665.0 Rupture of uterus before onset of labor ♀**   M
[0,1,3]

● **665.1 Rupture of uterus during labor ♀**   M
[0,1]   Rupture of uterus NOS

● **665.2 Inversion of uterus ♀**   M
[0,2,4]

● **665.3 Laceration of cervix ♀**   M
[0,1,4]   Coding Clinic: 1984, Nov-Dec, P10

● **665.4 High vaginal laceration ♀**   M
[0,1,4]   Laceration of vaginal wall or sulcus without mention of perineal laceration
     Coding Clinic: 1984, Nov-Dec, P10

● ■**665.5 Other injury to pelvic organs ♀**   M
[0,1,4]   Injury to:
     bladder
     urethra
     Coding Clinic: 1984, Nov-Dec, P10, 12

● **665.6 Damage to pelvic joints and ligaments ♀**   M
[0,1,4]   Avulsion of inner symphyseal cartilage
     Damage to coccyx
     Separation of symphysis (pubis)

● **665.7 Pelvic hematoma ♀**   M
[0-2,4]   Hematoma of vagina
     Coding Clinic: 1984, Nov-Dec, P10

● ■**665.8 Other specified obstetrical trauma ♀**   M
[0-4]

● ■**665.9 Unspecified obstetrical trauma ♀**   M
[0-4]

● **666 Postpartum hemorrhage**
     Requires fifth digit; valid digits are in [brackets] under each code. See beginning of section 660–669 for definitions.

● **666.0 Third-stage hemorrhage ♀**   M
[0,2,4]   Hemorrhage associated with retained, trapped, or adherent placenta
     Retained placenta NOS
     Coding Clinic: 1988, Q1, P14

● ■**666.1 Other immediate postpartum hemorrhage ♀**   M
[0,2,4]   Atony of uterus with hemorrhage
     Hemorrhage within the first 24 hours following delivery of placenta
     Postpartum atony of uterus with hemorrhage
     Postpartum hemorrhage (atonic) NOS

     Excludes   *atony of uterus without hemorrhage (661.2)*
       postpartum atony of uterus without hemorrhage (669.8)
     Coding Clinic: 1988, Q1, P14

● **666.2 Delayed and secondary postpartum**
[0,2,4] **hemorrhage ♀**   M
     Hemorrhage:
       after the first 24 hours following delivery
       associated with retained portions of placenta or membranes
     Postpartum hemorrhage specified as delayed or secondary
     Retained products of conception NOS, following delivery
     Coding Clinic: 1988, Q1, P14

● **666.3 Postpartum coagulation defects ♀**   M
[0,2,4]   Postpartum:
     afibrinogenemia
     fibrinolysis

◀ New   ◀▥ Revised   ~~deleted~~ Deleted   ● Use Additional Digit(s)   ■ Nonspecific Code
● Not first-listed DX   OGCR Official Guidelines   Coding Clinic   Excludes   Includes   Use additional   Code first   Omit code

● **667   Retained placenta without hemorrhage**

> Requires fifth digit; valid digits are in [brackets] under each code. See beginning of section 660–669 for definitions.

● **667.0   Retained placenta without hemorrhage** ♀   **M**
[0,2,4]   Placenta accreta without hemorrhage
Retained placenta:
   NOS without hemorrhage
   total without hemorrhage
Coding Clinic: 1988, Q1, P14

● **667.1   Retained portions of placenta or membranes,**
[0,2,4]   **without hemorrhage** ♀   **M**
   Retained products of conception following delivery, without hemorrhage
Coding Clinic: 1988, Q1, P14

● **668   Complications of the administration of anesthetic or other sedation in labor and delivery**

> Use additional code(s) to further specify complication

> Requires fifth digit; valid digits are in [brackets] under each code. See beginning of section 660–669 for definitions.

Includes   complications arising from the administration of a general or local anesthetic, analgesic, or other sedation in labor and delivery

Excludes   *reaction to spinal or lumbar puncture (349.0)*
spinal headache (349.0)

● **668.0   Pulmonary complications** ♀   **M**
[0-4]   Inhalation [aspiration] of stomach contents or secretions following anesthesia or other sedation in labor or delivery
Mendelson's syndrome following anesthesia or other sedation in labor or delivery
Pressure collapse of lung following anesthesia or other sedation in labor or delivery

● **668.1   Cardiac complications** ♀   **M**
[0-4]   Cardiac arrest or failure following anesthesia or other sedation in labor and delivery

● **668.2   Central nervous system complications** ♀   **M**
[0-4]   Cerebral anoxia following anesthesia or other sedation in labor and delivery

● ■ **668.8   Other complications of anesthesia or other sedation**
[0-4]   **in labor and delivery** ♀   **M**
Coding Clinic: 1999, Q2, P9-10

● ■ **668.9   Unspecified complication of anesthesia and other**
[0-4]   **sedation** ♀   **M**

● **669   Other complications of labor and delivery, not elsewhere classified**

> Requires fifth digit; valid digits are in [brackets] under each code. See beginning of section 660–669 for definitions.

● **669.0   Maternal distress** ♀   **M**
[0-4]   Metabolic disturbance in labor and delivery

● **669.1   Shock during or following labor and**
[0-4]   **delivery** ♀   **M**
   Obstetric shock

● **669.2   Maternal hypotension syndrome** ♀   **M**
[0-4]

● **669.3   Acute** ~~renal~~ **kidney failure following labor and**
[0,2,4]   **delivery** ♀   **M** ◀||||

● ■ **669.4   Other complications of obstetrical surgery and**
[0-4]   **procedures** ♀   **M**
   Cardiac:
      arrest following cesarean or other obstetrical surgery or procedure, including delivery NOS
      failure following cesarean or other obstetrical surgery or procedure, including delivery NOS
   Cerebral anoxia following cesarean or other obstetrical surgery or procedure, including delivery NOS

Excludes   *complications of obstetrical surgical wounds (674.1–674.3)*

● **669.5   Forceps or vacuum extractor delivery without**
[0,1]   **mention of indication** ♀   **M**
   Delivery by ventouse, without mention of indication

● **669.6   Breech extraction, without mention of indication** ♀ **M**
[0,1]   **Excludes**   *breech delivery NOS (652.2)*

● **669.7   Cesarean delivery, without mention of indication** ♀ **M**
[0,1]   Coding Clinic: 2001, Q1, P11-12

● ■ **669.8   Other complications of labor and delivery** ♀   **M**
[0-4]   Coding Clinic: 2006, Q4, P135

● ■ **669.9   Unspecified complication of labor and delivery** ♀   **M**
[0-4]

COMPLICATIONS OF THE PUERPERIUM (670–677)

Note: Categories 671 and 673–676 include the listed conditions even if they occur during pregnancy or childbirth.

The following fifth-digit subclassification is for use with categories 670–676 to denote the current episode of care:

> ■ **0**   unspecified as to episode of care or not applicable
> **1**   delivered, with or without mention of antepartum condition
> **2**   delivered, with mention of postpartum complication
> **3**   antepartum condition or complication
> **4**   postpartum condition or complication

● **670   Major puerperal infection** ♀
~~[0,2,4]   Use 0 as fourth digit for category 670~~
~~Puerperal:~~
   ~~endometritis~~
   ~~fever (septic)~~
   ~~pelvic:~~
      ~~cellulitis~~
      ~~sepsis~~
   ~~peritonitis~~
   ~~pyemia~~
   ~~salpingitis~~
   ~~septicemia~~

> Requires fifth digit; valid digits are in [brackets] under each code. See beginning of section 670–676 for definitions.

Excludes   *infection following abortion (639.0)*
minor genital tract infection following delivery (646.6)
puerperal fever NOS (672)
puerperal pyrexia NOS (672)
puerperal pyrexia of unknown origin (672)
urinary tract infection following delivery (646.6)

670.0   Major puerperal infection, unspecified ♀   **M** ◀
[0,2,4]   ◀

670.1   Puerperal endometritis ♀   **M** ◀
[0,2,4]   ◀

COMPLICATIONS OF PREGNANCY, CHILDBIRTH, AND THE PUERPERIUM (630–679)

670.2 Puerperal sepsis♀ M◀
[0,2,4]   Puerperal pyemia ◀

670.3 Puerperal septic thrombophlebitis♀ M◀
[0,2,4]

670.8 Other major puerperal infection♀ M◀
[0,2,4]   Puerperal:
     pelvic cellulitis ◀
     peritonitis ◀
     salpingitis ◀
   Coding Clinic: 2007, Q3, P10

● **671 Venous complications in pregnancy and the puerperium**

   Excludes *personal history of venous complications prior*
       to pregnancy, such as: ◀
         thrombophlebitis (V12.52) ◀
         thrombosis and embolism (V12.51) ◀

   Requires fifth digit; valid digits are in [brackets] under each code. See beginning of section 670–676 for definitions.

● **671.0 Varicose veins of legs♀** M
[0-4]   Varicose veins NOS

● **671.1 Varicose veins of vulva and perineum♀** M
[0-4]

● **671.2 Superficial thrombophlebitis♀** M
[0-4]   Phlebitis NOS ◀
     Thrombophlebitis (superficial)
     Thrombosis NOS ◀

● **671.3 Deep phlebothrombosis, antepartum♀** M
[0,1,3]   Deep-vein thrombosis, antepartum

   Use additional code to identify the deep vein thrombosis (453.40-453.42, 453.50-453.52, 453.72-453.79, 453.82-453.89) ◀

   Use additional code for long term (current) use of anticoagulants, if applicable (V58.61) ◀

● **671.4 Deep phlebothrombosis, postpartum♀** M
[0,2,4]   Deep-vein thrombosis, postpartum
     Pelvic thrombophlebitis, postpartum
     Phlegmasia alba dolens (puerperal)

   Use additional code to identify the deep vein thrombosis (453.40-453.42, 453.50-453.52, 453.72-453.79, 453.82-453.89) ◀

   Use additional code for long term (current) use of anticoagulants, if applicable (V58.61) ◀

● ■ **671.5 Other phlebitis and thrombosis♀** M
[0-4]   Cerebral venous thrombosis
     Thrombosis of intracranial venous sinus

● ■ **671.8 Other venous complications♀** M
[0-4]   Hemorrhoids

● ■ **671.9 Unspecified venous complication♀** M
[0-4]   ~~Phlebitis NOS~~
     ~~Thrombosis NOS~~

● **672 Pyrexia of unknown origin during the**
[0,2,4] **puerperium♀** M
   Postpartum fever NOS
   Puerperal fever NOS
   Puerperal pyrexia NOS

   Requires fifth digit; valid digits are in [brackets] under each code. See beginning of section 670–676 for definitions.

   Use 0 as fourth digit for category 672

● **673 Obstetrical pulmonary embolism**

   Requires fifth digit; valid digits are in [brackets] under each code. See beginning of section 670–676 for definitions.

   Includes pulmonary emboli in pregnancy, childbirth, or the puerperium, or specified as puerperal

   Excludes *embolism following abortion (639.6)*

● **673.0 Obstetrical air embolism♀** M
[0-4]

● **673.1 Amniotic fluid embolism♀** M
[0-4]

● **673.2 Obstetrical blood-clot embolism♀** M
[0-4]   Puerperal pulmonary embolism NOS

● **673.3 Obstetrical pyemic and septic**
[0-4] **embolism♀** M

● ■ **673.8 Other pulmonary embolism♀** M
[0-4]   Fat embolism

● **674 Other and unspecified complications of the puerperium, not elsewhere classified**

   Requires fifth digit; valid digits are in [brackets] under each code. See beginning of section 670–676 for definitions.

● **674.0 Cerebrovascular disorders in the**
[0-4] **puerperium♀** M
   Any condition classifiable to 430–434, 436–437 occurring during pregnancy, childbirth, or the puerperium, or specified as puerperal

   Excludes *intracranial venous sinus thrombosis (671.5)*

● **674.1 Disruption of cesarean wound♀** M
[0,2,4]   Dehiscence or disruption of uterine wound

   Excludes *uterine rupture before onset of labor (665.0)*
     uterine rupture during labor (665.1)

● **674.2 Disruption of perineal wound♀** M
[0,2,4]   Breakdown of perineum
     Disruption of wound of:
       episiotomy
       perineal laceration
     Secondary perineal tear
   Coding Clinic: 1997, Q1, P9-10

● ■ **674.3 Other complications of obstetrical surgical**
[0,2,4] **wounds♀** M
   Hematoma of cesarean section or perineal wound
   Hemorrhage of cesarean section or perineal wound
   Infection of cesarean section or perineal wound

   Excludes *damage from instruments in delivery (664.0–665.9)*

● **674.4 Placental polyp♀** M
[0,2,4]

● **674.5 Peripartum cardiomyopathy♀** M
[0-4]   Postpartum cardiomyopathy
   Coding Clinic: 2003, Q4, P65

● ■ **674.8 Other♀** M
[0,2,4]   Hepatorenal syndrome, following delivery
     Postpartum:
       subinvolution of uterus
       uterine hypertrophy
   Coding Clinic: 1998, Q3, P16

● ■ **674.9 Unspecified♀** M
[0,2,4]   Sudden death of unknown cause during the puerperium

◀ New   ◀▥ Revised   ~~deleted~~ Deleted   ● Use Additional Digit(s)   ■ Nonspecific Code
● Not first-listed DX   OGCR Official Guidelines   Coding Clinic   Excludes   Includes   Use additional   Code first   Omit code

● **675 Infections of the breast and nipple associated with childbirth**

> Requires fifth digit; valid digits are in [brackets] under each code. See beginning of section 670–676 for definitions.

> **Includes**   the listed conditions during pregnancy, childbirth, or the puerperium

● **675.0 Infections of nipple ♀**   **M**
[0-4]   Abscess of nipple

● **675.1 Abscess of breast ♀**   **M**
[0-4]   Abscess:
　　　　　　　mammary
　　　　　　　subareolar
　　　　　　　submammary
　　　　　　Mastitis:
　　　　　　　purulent
　　　　　　　retromammary
　　　　　　　submammary

● **675.2 Nonpurulent mastitis ♀**   **M**
[0-4]   Lymphangitis of breast
　　　　　　Mastitis:
　　　　　　　NOS
　　　　　　　interstitial
　　　　　　　parenchymatous

● ■ **675.8 Other specified infections of the breast and**
[0-4]   **nipple ♀**   **M**

● ■ **675.9 Unspecified infection of the breast and nipple ♀** **M**
[0-4]

● **676 Other disorders of the breast associated with childbirth and disorders of lactation**

> Requires fifth digit; valid digits are in [brackets] under each code. See beginning of section 670–676 for definitions.

> **Includes**   the listed conditions during pregnancy, the puerperium, or lactation

● **676.0 Retracted nipple ♀**   **M**
[0-4]

● **676.1 Cracked nipple ♀**   **M**
[0-4]   Fissure of nipple

● **676.2 Engorgement of breasts ♀**   **M**
[0-4]

● ■ **676.3 Other and unspecified disorder of breast ♀**   **M**
[0-4]

● **676.4 Failure of lactation ♀**   **M**
[0-4]   Agalactia

● **676.5 Suppressed lactation ♀**   **M**
[0-4]

● **676.6 Galactorrhea ♀**   **M**
[0-4]   **Excludes**   galactorrhea not associated with childbirth
　　　　　　　　　　　　(611.6)
　　　　　　 Coding Clinic: 1985, July-Aug, P9

● ■ **676.8 Other disorders of lactation ♀**   **M**
[0-4]   Galactocele

● ■ **676.9 Unspecified disorder of lactation ♀**   **M**
[0-6]

OGCR Section I.C.10.j.1-3
Code 677, Late effect of complication of pregnancy, childbirth, and the puerperium is for use in those cases when an initial complication of a pregnancy develops a sequelae requiring care or treatment at a future date. This code may be used at any time after the initial postpartum period and like all late effect codes, is to be sequenced following the code describing the sequelae of the complication.

■ **677 Late effect of complication of pregnancy, childbirth, and the puerperium ♀**

> **Note:** This category is to be used to indicate conditions in 632–648.9 and 651–676.9 as the cause of the late effect, themselves classifiable elsewhere. The "late effects " include conditions specified as such, or as sequelae, which may occur at any time after the puerperium.

> *Code first* any sequelae

> Coding Clinic: 1997, Q1, P9-10

OTHER MATERNAL AND FETAL COMPLICATIONS (678-679)

The following fifth-digit subclassification is for use with categories 678-679 to denote the current episode of care:

> 0   unspecified as to episode of care or not applicable
> 1   delivered, with or without mention of antepartum condition
> 2   delivered, with mention of postpartum complication
> 3   antepartum condition or complication
> 4   postpartum condition or complication

● **678 Other fetal conditions**

> Requires fifth digit; valid digits are in [brackets] under each code. See beginning of section 678-679 for definitions.
> Coding Clinic: 2008, Q4, P125-127

● **678.0 Fetal hematologic conditions ♀**   **M**
[0,1,3]   Fetal anemia
　　　　　　Fetal thrombocytopenia
　　　　　　Fetal twin to twin transfusion

> **Excludes**   fetal and neonatal hemorrhage
　　　　　　　　　　(772.0-772.9)
　　　　　　　　fetal hematologic disorders affecting
　　　　　　　　　　newborn (776.0-776.9)
　　　　　　　　fetal-maternal hemorrhage
　　　　　　　　　　(656.00-656.03)
　　　　　　　　isoimmunization incompatibility
　　　　　　　　　　(656.10-656.13, 656.20-656.23)

● **678.1 Fetal conjoined twins ♀**   **M**
[0,1,3]

● **679 Complications of in utero procedures**

> Requires fifth digit; valid digits are in [brackets] under each code. See beginning of section 678-679 for definitions.
> Coding Clinic: 2008, Q4, P127-128

● **679.0 Maternal complications from in utero procedure ♀** **M**
[0-4]   **Excludes**   maternal history of in utero procedure
　　　　　　　　　　　　　during previous pregnancy (V23.86)

● **679.1 Fetal complications from in utero procedure ♀**   **M**
[0-4]   Fetal complications from amniocentesis

> **Excludes**   newborn affected by in utero procedure
　　　　　　　　　　(760.61-760.64)

COMPLICATIONS OF PREGNANCY, CHILDBIRTH, AND THE PUERPERIUM (630–679)

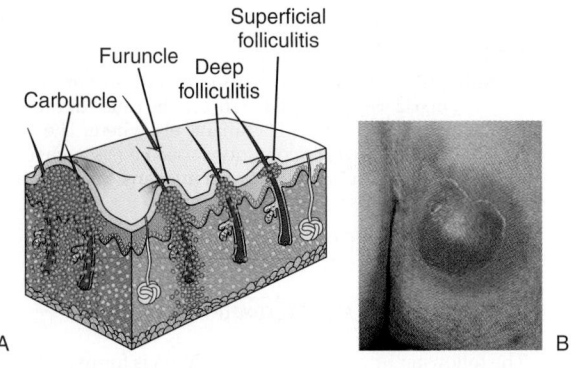

Figure 12–1   Furuncle, also known as a boil, is a staphylococcal infection. The organism enters the body through a hair follicle and so furuncles usually appear in hairy areas of the body. A cluster of furuncles is known as a carbuncle and involves infection into the deep subcutaneous fascia. These usually appear on the back and neck. (**B** from Habif: Clinical Dermatology, 4th ed. 2004, Mosby)

12. DISEASES OF THE SKIN AND SUBCUTANEOUS TISSUE (680–709)

INFECTIONS OF SKIN AND SUBCUTANEOUS TISSUE (680–686)

Excludes   *certain infections of skin classified under "Infectious and Parasitic Diseases," such as:*
erysipelas (035)
erysipeloid of Rosenbach (027.1)
herpes:
    simplex (054.0–054.9)
    zoster (053.0–053.9)
molluscum contagiosum (078.0)
viral warts (078.10–078.19) ◄

● **680   Carbuncle and furuncle**

    Includes   boil
                   furunculosis

680.0   Face
    Ear [any part]   Nose (septum)
    Face [any part, except eye]   Temple (region)
    Excludes   *eyelid (373.13)*
                   lacrimal apparatus (375.31)
                   orbit (376.01)

680.1   Neck

680.2   Trunk
    Abdominal wall
    Back [any part, except buttocks]
    Breast
    Chest wall
    Flank
    Groin
    Pectoral region
    Perineum
    Umbilicus
    Excludes   *buttocks (680.5)*
                   external genital organs:
                     female (616.4)
                     male (607.2, 608.4)

680.3   Upper arm and forearm
    Arm [any part, except hand]
    Axilla
    Shoulder

680.4   Hand
    Finger [any]   Wrist
    Thumb

680.5   Buttock
    Anus   Gluteal region

680.6   Leg, except foot
    Ankle   Knee
    Hip   Thigh

680.7   Foot
    Heel
    Toe

■**680.8   Other specified sites**
    Head [any part, except face]
    Scalp
    Excludes   *external genital organs:*
                   female (616.4)
                   male (607.2, 608.4)

■**680.9   Unspecified site**
    Boil NOS   Furuncle NOS
    Carbuncle NOS

Item 12-1   Cellulitis is an acute spreading bacterial infection below the surface of the skin characterized by redness (erythema), warmth, swelling, pain, fever, chills, and enlarged lymph nodes ("swollen glands"). **Abscess** is a localized collection of pus in tissues or organs and is a sign of infection resulting in swelling and inflammation. **Onychia** is an inflammation of the tissue surrounding the nail with pus accumulation and loss of the nail, resulting from microscopic pathogens entering through small wounds. **Paronychia** is a nail disease also known as felon or whitlow and is a bacterial or fungal infection.

● **681   Cellulitis and abscess of finger and toe**
    Includes   that with lymphangitis
    Use additional code to identify organism, such as:
         Staphylococcus (041.1)

● **681.0   Finger**
    681.00   Cellulitis and abscess, unspecified
    681.01   Felon
         Pulp abscess   Whitlow
         Excludes   *herpetic whitlow (054.6)*
    681.02   Onychia and paronychia of finger
         Panaritium of finger
         Perionychia of finger

● **681.1   Toe**
    ■**681.10   Cellulitis and abscess, unspecified**
         Coding Clinic: 2005, Q1, P14
    681.11   Onychia and paronychia of toe
         Panaritium of toe
         Perionychia of toe

■**681.9   Cellulitis and abscess of unspecified digit**
    Infection of nail NOS

◄ New   ◄◄ Revised   ~~deleted~~ Deleted   ● Use Additional Digit(s)   ■ Nonspecific Code
● Not first-listed DX   OGCR Official Guidelines   Coding Clinic   Excludes   Includes   Use additional   Code first   Omit code

● **682   Other cellulitis and abscess**

> **Includes**   abscess (acute) (with lymphangitis) except of
> finger or toe
> cellulitis (diffuse) (with lymphangitis) except
> of finger or toe
> lymphangitis, acute (with lymphangitis)
> except of finger or toe

Use additional code to identify organism, such as:
Staphylococcus (041.1)

> **Excludes**   *lymphangitis (chronic) (subacute) (457.2)*

682.0   Face
> *This code reports forehead but not head (682.8).*
>
> | | |
> |---|---|
> | Cheek, external | Nose, external |
> | Chin | Submandibular |
> | Forehead | Temple (region) |
>
> **Excludes**   *ear [any part] (380.10–380.16)*
> *eyelid (373.13)*
> *lacrimal apparatus (375.31)*
> *lip (528.5)*
> *mouth (528.3)*
> *nose (internal) (478.1)*
> *orbit (376.01)*

682.1   Neck

682.2   Trunk
> Abdominal wall
> Back [any part, except buttock]
> *Buttocks see 682.5*
> Chest wall
> Flank
> Groin
> Pectoral region
> Perineum
> Umbilicus, except newborn
>
> **Excludes**   *anal and rectal regions (566)*
> *breast:*
> *NOS (611.0)*
> *puerperal (675.1)*
> *external genital organs:*
> *female (616.3–616.4)*
> *male (604.0, 607.2, 608.4)*
> *umbilicus, newborn (771.4)*
>
> Coding Clinic: 1993, Q1, P26

682.3   Upper arm and forearm
> Arm [any part, except hand]
> Axilla
> Shoulder
>
> **Excludes**   *hand (682.4)*
>
> Coding Clinic: 2003, Q2, P7-8; 1998, Q4, P42-44

682.4   Hand, except fingers and thumb
> Wrist
>
> **Excludes**   *finger and thumb (681.00–681.02)*

682.5   Buttock
> Gluteal region
>
> **Excludes**   *anal and rectal regions (566)*

682.6   Leg, except foot
> Ankle
> Hip
> Knee
> Thigh
> Coding Clinic: 2009, Q1, P18x2; 2004, Q3, P5-6; 2003, Q4, P108;
> 1995, Q1, P3

682.7   Foot, except toes
> Heel
>
> **Excludes**   *toe (681.10–681.11)*

■**682.8   Other specified sites**
> Head [except face]
> Scalp
>
> **Excludes**   *face (682.0)*

■**682.9   Unspecified site**
> Abscess NOS
> Cellulitis NOS
> Lymphangitis, acute NOS
>
> **Excludes**   *lymphangitis NOS (457.2)*

683   Acute lymphadenitis
> *Short term inflammation of lymph nodes which can be*
> *regionalized to involve a given area of lymph system or*
> *systemic involvement*
>
> Abscess (acute) lymph gland or node, except mesenteric
> Adenitis, acute lymph gland or node, except mesenteric
> Lymphadenitis, acute lymph gland or node, except
> mesenteric
>
> Use additional code to identify organism such as
> Staphylococcus (041.1)
>
> **Excludes**   *enlarged glands NOS (785.6)*
> *lymphadenitis:*
> *chronic or subacute, except mesenteric (289.1)*
> *mesenteric (acute) (chronic) (subacute) (289.2)*
> *unspecified (289.3)*

684   Impetigo
> *Contagious skin infection caused by streptococcus or*
> *staphylococcus aureus that produces blisters or sores on*
> *the face and hands*
>
> Impetiginization of other dermatoses
> Impetigo (contagiosa) [any site] [any organism]:
> bullous neonatorum
> circinate
> simplex
> Pemphigus neonatorum
>
> **Excludes**   *impetigo herpetiformis (694.3)*

● **685   Pilonidal cyst**
> **Includes**   fistula, coccygeal or pilonidal
> sinus, coccygeal or pilonidal

685.0   With abscess

685.1   Without mention of abscess

● **686   Other local infections of skin and subcutaneous tissue**
> Use additional code to identify any infectious organism
> (041.0–041.8)

● **686.0   Pyoderma**
> Dermatitis:
> purulent
> septic
> suppurative

■**686.00   Pyoderma, unspecified**

686.01   Pyoderma gangrenosum
> Coding Clinic: 1997, Q4, P42

■**686.09   Other pyoderma**

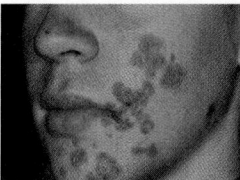

Figure 12–2   Impetigo. A thick,
honey-yellow adherent crust covers
the entire eroded surface. (From
Habif: Clinical Dermatology, 4th ed.
2004, Mosby, Inc.)

Item 12–2   Pilonidal cyst, also called a coccygeal cyst, is
the result of a disorder called pilonidal disease. The cyst usually
contains hair and pus.

DISEASES OF THE SKIN AND SUBCUTANEOUS TISSUE (680–709)

686.1 Pyogenic granuloma
Granuloma:
   septic
   suppurative
   telangiectaticum

> **Excludes** *pyogenic granuloma of oral mucosa (528.9)*

686.8 Other specified local infections of skin and subcutaneous tissue
Bacterid (pustular)
Dermatitis vegetans
Ecthyma
Perlèche

> **Excludes** *dermatitis infectiosa eczematoides (690.8)*
> *panniculitis (729.30–729.39)*

686.9 Unspecified local infection of skin and subcutaneous tissue
Fistula of skin NOS
Skin infection NOS

> **Excludes** *fistula to skin from internal organs—see Alphabetic Index*

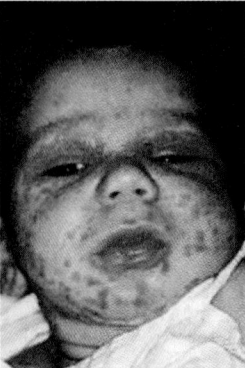

Figure 12–3 Seborrheic dermatitis. (From Cohen BA: Atlas of Pediatric Dermatology. St. Louis, Mosby, 1993.)

Item 12–3 Seborrheic dermatitis is characterized by greasy, scaly, red patches and is associated with oily skin and scalp.

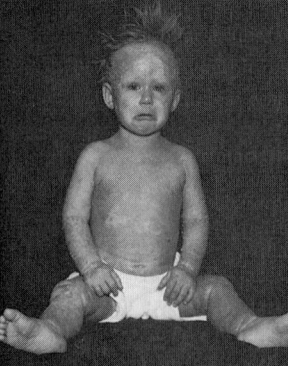

Figure 12–4 Atopic dermatitis. (From Moschella SL, Hurley HJ: Dermatology, 2nd ed. Philadelphia, WB Saunders, 1985, p 336.)

Item 12–4 Atopic dermatitis, also known as atopic eczema, infantile eczema, disseminated neurodermatitis, flexural eczema, and *prurigo diathesique* (Besnier), is characterized by intense itching and is often hereditary.

OTHER INFLAMMATORY CONDITIONS OF SKIN AND SUBCUTANEOUS TISSUE (690–698)

> **Excludes** *panniculitis (729.30–729.39)*

● **690 Erythematosquamous dermatosis**

> **Excludes** *eczematous dermatitis of eyelid (373.31)*
> *parakeratosis variegata (696.2)*
> *psoriasis (696.0–696.1)*
> *seborrheic keratosis (702.11–702.19)*

● **690.1 Seborrheic dermatitis**

▪ **690.10 Seborrheic dermatitis, unspecified**
Seborrheic dermatitis NOS

690.11 Seborrhea capitis   P
Cradle cap

690.12 Seborrheic infantile dermatitis   P

▪ **690.18 Other seborrheic dermatitis**

▪ **690.8 Other erythematosquamous dermatosis**

● **691 Atopic dermatitis and related conditions**

691.0 Diaper or napkin rash
Ammonia dermatitis
Diaper or napkin:
   dermatitis
   erythema
   rash
Psoriasiform napkin eruption

▪ **691.8 Other atopic dermatitis and related conditions**
Atopic dermatitis
Besnier's prurigo
Eczema:
   atopic
   flexural
   intrinsic (allergic)
Neurodermatitis:
   atopic
   diffuse (of Brocq)

● **692 Contact dermatitis and other eczema**

> **Includes** dermatitis:
>   NOS
>   contact
>   occupational
>   venenata
> eczema (acute) (chronic):
>   NOS
>   allergic
>   erythematous
>   occupational

> **Excludes** *allergy NOS (995.3)*
> *contact dermatitis of eyelids (373.32)*
> *dermatitis due to substances taken internally (693.0–693.9)*
> *eczema of external ear (380.22)*
> *perioral dermatitis (695.3)*
> *urticarial reactions (708.0–708.9, 995.1)*

692.0 Due to detergents

692.1 Due to oils and greases

692.2 Due to solvents
Dermatitis due to solvents of:
   chlorocompound group
   cyclohexane group
   ester group
   glycol group
   hydrocarbon group
   ketone group

DISEASES OF THE SKIN AND SUBCUTANEOUS TISSUE (680–709)

◀ New   ◀▥ Revised   ~~deleted~~ Deleted   ● Use Additional Digit(s)   ▪ Nonspecific Code
● Not first-listed DX   OGCR Official Guidelines   Coding Clinic   Excludes   Includes   Use additional   Code first   Omit code

692.3 Due to drugs and medicines in contact with skin
Dermatitis (allergic) (contact) due to:
  arnica
  fungicides
  iodine
  keratolytics
  mercurials
  neomycin
  pediculocides
  phenols
  scabicides
  any drug applied to skin
Dermatitis medicamentosa due to drug applied to skin

Use additional E code to identify drug

Excludes *allergy NOS due to drugs (995.27)*
dermatitis due to ingested drugs (693.0)
dermatitis medicamentosa NOS (693.0)

■692.4 Due to other chemical products
Dermatitis due to: Dermatitis due to:
  acids   insecticide
  adhesive plaster   nylon
  alkalis   plastic
  caustics   rubber
  dichromate
Coding Clinic: 2008, Q3, P6-7; 1989, Q2, P16

692.5 Due to food in contact with skin
Dermatitis, contact, due to:
  cereals
  fish
  flour
  fruit
  meat
  milk

Excludes *dermatitis due to:*
dyes (692.89)
ingested foods (693.1)
preservatives (692.89)

692.6 Due to plants [except food]
Dermatitis due to:
  lacquer tree [Rhus verniciflua]
  poison:
    ivy [Rhus toxicodendron]
    oak [Rhus diversiloba]
    sumac [Rhus venenata]
    vine [Rhus radicans]
  primrose [Primula]
  ragweed [Senecio jacobae]
  other plants in contact with the skin

Excludes *allergy NOS due to pollen (477.0)*
nettle rash (708.8)

● 692.7 Due to solar radiation

Excludes *sunburn due to other ultraviolet radiation*
exposure (692.82)

■692.70 Unspecified dermatitis due to sun

692.71 Sunburn
First degree sunburn
See codes 692.76 and 692.77 for second and third degrees.
Sunburn NOS

692.72 Acute dermatitis due to solar radiation
Berloque dermatitis
Photoallergic response
Phototoxic response
Polymorphous light eruption
Acute solar skin damage NOS

Excludes *sunburn (692.71, 692.76–692.77)*

Use additional E code to identify drug, if drug induced

692.73 Actinic reticuloid and actinic granuloma

■692.74 Other chronic dermatitis due to solar radiation
Chronic solar skin damage NOS
Solar elastosis

Excludes *actinic [solar] keratosis (702.0)*

692.75 Disseminated superficial actinic porokeratosis (DSAP)

692.76 Sunburn of second degree

692.77 Sunburn of third degree

■692.79 Other dermatitis due to solar radiation
Hydroa aestivale
Photodermatitis (due to sun)
Photosensitiveness (due to sun)
Solar skin damage NOS

● 692.8 Due to other specified agents

692.81 Dermatitis due to cosmetics

■692.82 Dermatitis due to other radiation
Infrared rays
Light, except from sun
Radiation NOS
Tanning bed
Ultraviolet rays, except from sun
X-rays

Excludes *that due to solar radiation*
(692.70–692.79)
Coding Clinic: 2000, Q3, P5

692.83 Dermatitis due to metals
Jewelry

692.84 Due to animal (cat) (dog) dander
Due to animal (cat) (dog) hair
Coding Clinic: 2004, Q4, P90-91

■692.89 Other
Dermatitis due to:
  cold weather
  dyes
  hot weather
  preservatives

Excludes *allergy (NOS) (rhinitis) due to*
animal hair or dander (477.2)
allergy to dust (477.8)
sunburn (692.71, 692.76–692.77)

■692.9 Unspecified cause
Dermatitis:
  NOS
  contact NOS
  venenata NOS
Eczema NOS

● 693 Dermatitis due to substances taken internally

Excludes *adverse effect NOS of drugs and medicines*
(995.20)
allergy NOS (995.3)
contact dermatitis (692.0–692.9)
urticarial reactions (708.0–708.9, 995.1)

693.0 Due to drugs and medicines
Dermatitis medicamentosa NOS

Use additional E code to identify drug

Excludes *that due to drugs in contact with skin*
(692.3)
Coding Clinic: 2007, Q2, P9-10

693.1 Due to food

■693.8 Due to other specified substances taken internally

■693.9 Due to unspecified substance taken internally

Excludes *dermatitis NOS (692.9)*

DISEASES OF THE SKIN AND SUBCUTANEOUS TISSUE (680–709)

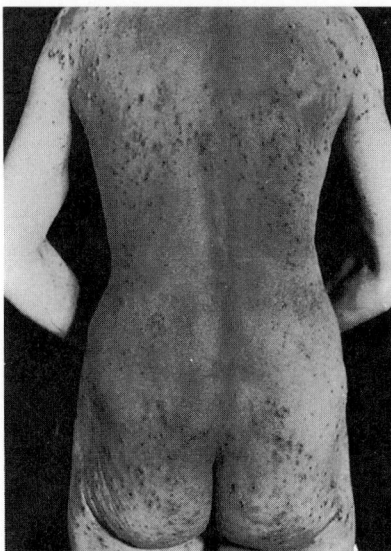

Figure 12–5   Dermatitis herpetiformis. (From Arnold HL, Odom RB, James WD: Andrews' Diseases of the Skin, Clinical Dermatology, 8th ed. Philadelphia, WB Saunders, 1990, p 553.)

Item 12–5   **Dermatitis herpetiformis,** also known as Duhring's disease, is a systemic disease characterized by small blisters (3 to 5 mm) and occasionally large bullae (+5 mm).

● **694   Bullous dermatoses**

    694.0   Dermatitis herpetiformis
         Dermatosis herpetiformis
         Duhring's disease
         Hydroa herpetiformis

         Excludes   *herpes gestationis (646.8)*
                 dermatitis herpetiformis:
                   juvenile (694.2)
                   senile (694.5)

    694.1   Subcorneal pustular dermatosis
         Sneddon-Wilkinson disease or syndrome

    694.2   Juvenile dermatitis herpetiformis
         Juvenile pemphigoid

    694.3   Impetigo herpetiformis

    694.4   Pemphigus
         Pemphigus:
            NOS
            erythematosus
            foliaceus
            malignant
            vegetans
            vulgaris

         Excludes   *pemphigus neonatorum (684)*

    694.5   Pemphigoid
         Benign pemphigus NOS
         Bullous pemphigoid
         Herpes circinatus bullosus
         Senile dermatitis herpetiformis

● **694.6   Benign mucous membrane pemphigoid**
         Cicatricial pemphigoid
         Mucosynechial atrophic bullous dermatitis

    694.60   Without mention of ocular involvement

    694.61   With ocular involvement
         Ocular pemphigus

■ **694.8   Other specified bullous dermatoses**
         Excludes   *herpes gestationis (646.8)*

■ **694.9   Unspecified bullous dermatoses**

● **695   Erythematous conditions**

    695.0   Toxic erythema
         Erythema venenatum

● **695.1   Erythema multiforme**
     Use additional code to identify associated manifestations, such as:
         arthropathy associated with dermatological disorders (713.3)
         conjunctival edema (372.73)
         conjunctivitis (372.04, 372.33)
         corneal scars and opacities (371.00-371.05)
         corneal ulcer (370.00-370.07)
         edema of eyelid (374.82)
         inflammation of eyelid (373.8)
         keratoconjunctivitis sicca (370.33)
         mechanical lagophthalmos (374.22)
         mucositis (478.11, 528.00, 538, 616.81)
         stomatitis (528.00)
         symblepharon (372.63)
     Use additional E-code to identify drug, if drug-induced
     Use additional code to identify percentage of skin exfoliation (695.50–695.59)

         Excludes   *(staphylococcal) scalded skin syndrome (695.81)*
         Coding Clinic: 2008, Q4, P128-131

■ **695.10   Erythema multiforme, unspecified**
         Erythema iris
         Herpes iris

    695.11   Erythema multiforme minor

    695.12   Erythema multiforme major

    695.13   Stevens-Johnson syndrome

    695.14   Stevens-Johnson syndrome-toxic epidermal necrolysis overlap syndrome
         SJS-TEN overlap syndrome
         Coding Clinic: 2008, Q4, P128-131

    695.15   Toxic epidermal necrolysis
         Lyell's syndrome

■ **695.19   Other erythema multiforme**

    695.2   Erythema nodosum
         Excludes   *tuberculous erythema nodosum (017.1)*

    695.3   Rosacea
         Acne:
            erythematosa
            rosacea
         Perioral dermatitis
         Rhinophyma

    695.4   Lupus erythematosus
         See 710.0 for designated as systemic lupus erythematosus (SLE).
         Lupus:
            erythematodes (discoid)
            erythematosus (discoid), not disseminated

         Excludes   *lupus (vulgaris) NOS (017.0)*
                 systemic [disseminated] lupus erythematosus (710.0)

DISEASES OF THE SKIN AND SUBCUTANEOUS TISSUE (680–709)

◀ New   ◀▥ Revised   ~~deleted~~ Deleted   ● Use Additional Digit(s)   ■ Nonspecific Code
● Not first-listed DX   OGCR Official Guidelines   Coding Clinic   Excludes   Includes   Use additional   Code first   Omit code

● **695.5 Exfoliation due to erythematous conditions according to extent of body surface involved**

Code first erythematous condition causing exfoliation, such as:
  Ritter's disease (695.81)
  (Staphylococcal) scalded skin syndrome (695.81)
  Stevens-Johnson syndrome (695.13)
  Stevens-Johnson syndrome-toxic epidermal necrolysis overlap syndrome (695.14)
  toxic epidermal necrolysis (695.15)

   695.50 Exfoliation due to erythematous condition involving less than 10 percent of body surface
      Exfoliation due to erythematous condition NOS

   695.51 Exfoliation due to erythematous condition involving 10-19 percent of body surface

   695.52 Exfoliation due to erythematous condition involving 20-29 percent of body surface

   695.53 Exfoliation due to erythematous condition involving 30-39 percent of body surface
      Coding Clinic: 2008, Q4, P128-131

   695.54 Exfoliation due to erythematous condition involving 40-49 percent of body surface

   695.55 Exfoliation due to erythematous condition involving 50-59 percent of body surface

   695.56 Exfoliation due to erythematous condition involving 60-69 percent of body surface

   695.57 Exfoliation due to erythematous condition involving 70-79 percent of body surface

   695.58 Exfoliation due to erythematous condition involving 80-89 percent of body surface

   695.59 Exfoliation due to erythematous condition involving 90 percent or more of body surface

● **695.8 Other specified erythematous conditions**

   695.81 Ritter's disease
      Dermatitis exfoliativa neonatorum
      (Staphylococcal) Scalded skin syndrome
      Use additional code to identify percentage of skin exfoliation (695.50-695.59)

   ■**695.89 Other**
      Erythema intertrigo
      Intertrigo
      Pityriasis rubra (Hebra)
      Excludes *mycotic intertrigo (111.0–111.9)*
      Coding Clinic: 1986, Sept-Oct, P10

■ **695.9 Unspecified erythematous condition**
   Erythema NOS
   Erythroderma (secondary)

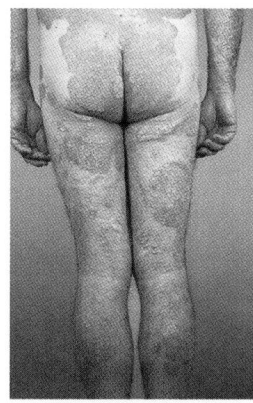

Figure 12–6 Erythematous plaques with silvery scales in a patient with psoriasis. (From Goldman: Cecil Textbook of Medicine, 22nd ed. 2004, Saunders)

Item 12–6 Psoriasis is a chronic, recurrent inflammatory skin disease characterized by small patches covered with thick silvery scales. **Parapsoriasis** is a treatment-resistant erythroderma. **Pityriasis rosea** is characterized by a herald patch that is a single large lesion and that usually appears on the trunk and is followed by scattered, smaller lesions.

● **696 Psoriasis and similar disorders**

   696.0 Psoriatic arthropathy

   ■**696.1 Other psoriasis**
      Acrodermatitis continua
      Dermatitis repens
      Psoriasis:
        NOS
        any type, except arthropathic
      Excludes *psoriatic arthropathy (696.0)*
      Coding Clinic: 1996, Q2, P12

   696.2 Parapsoriasis
      Parakeratosis variegata
      Parapsoriasis lichenoides chronica
      Pityriasis lichenoides et varioliformis

   696.3 Pityriasis rosea
      Pityriasis circinata (et maculata)

   696.4 Pityriasis rubra pilaris
      Devergie's disease
      Lichen ruber acuminatus
      Excludes *pityriasis rubra (Hebra) (695.89)*

   ■**696.5 Other and unspecified pityriasis**
      Pityriasis:
        NOS
        alba
        streptogenes
      Excludes *pityriasis:*
        simplex (690.18)
        versicolor (111.0)

   ■**696.8 Other**

DISEASES OF THE SKIN AND SUBCUTANEOUS TISSUE (680–709)

● 697   **Lichen**

> **Excludes**   *lichen:*
> > *obtusus corneus (698.3)*
> > *pilaris (congenital) (757.39)*
> > *ruber acuminatus (696.4)*
> > *sclerosus et atrophicus (701.0)*
> > *scrofulosus (017.0)*
> > *simplex chronicus (698.3)*
> > *spinulosus (congenital) (757.39)*
> > *urticatus (698.2)*

697.0   Lichen planus
> Lichen:
> > planopilaris
> > ruber planus

697.1   Lichen nitidus
> Pinkus' disease

■ **697.8   Other lichen, not elsewhere classified**
> Lichen:
> > ruber moniliforme
> > striata

■ **697.9   Lichen, unspecified**

● 698   **Pruritus and related conditions**

> **Excludes**   *pruritus specified as psychogenic (306.3)*

698.0   Pruritus ani
> Perianal itch

698.1   Pruritus of genital organs

698.2   Prurigo
> Lichen urticatus
> Prurigo: Prurigo:
> > NOS   mitis
> > Hebra's   simplex
> Urticaria papulosa (Hebra)
>
> > **Excludes**   *prurigo nodularis (698.3)*

698.3   Lichenification and lichen simplex chronicus
> Hyde's disease
> Neurodermatitis (circumscripta) (local)
> Prurigo nodularis
>
> > **Excludes**   *neurodermatitis, diffuse (of Brocq) (691.8)*

698.4   Dermatitis factitia [artefacta]
> Dermatitis ficta
> Neurotic excoriation
>
> > Use additional code to identify any associated mental disorder

■ **698.8   Other specified pruritic conditions**
> Pruritus:
> > hiemalis
> > senilis
> Winter itch

■ **698.9   Unspecified pruritic disorder**
> Itch NOS
> Pruritus NOS

Item 12-7   Scleroderma means hard skin. It is a group of diseases that causes abnormal growth of connective tissues that support the skin and organs. There are two types: localized scleroderma affecting the skin and systemic scleroderma affecting blood vessels and internal organs and the skin. **Keratoderma** is characterized by firm horny papules that have a cobblestone appearance. **Keratoderma climactericum,** also known as endocrine keratoderma, is hyperkeratosis located on the palms and soles.

OTHER DISEASES OF SKIN AND SUBCUTANEOUS TISSUE (700–709)

> **Excludes**   *conditions confined to eyelids (373.0–374.9)*
> > *congenital conditions of skin, hair, and nails (757.0–757.9)*

700   **Corns and callosities**
> Callus
> Clavus

● 701   **Other hypertrophic and atrophic conditions of skin**

> **Excludes**   *dermatomyositis (710.3)*
> > *hereditary edema of legs (757.0)*
> > *scleroderma (generalized) (710.1)*

701.0   Circumscribed scleroderma
> Addison's keloid
> Dermatosclerosis, localized
> Lichen sclerosus et atrophicus
> Morphea
> Scleroderma, circumscribed or localized

701.1   Keratoderma, acquired
> Acquired:
> > ichthyosis
> > keratoderma palmaris et plantaris
> Elastosis perforans serpiginosa
> Hyperkeratosis:
> > NOS
> > follicularis in cutem penetrans
> > palmoplantaris climacterica
> Keratoderma:
> > climactericum
> > tylodes, progressive
> Keratosis (blennorrhagica)
>
> > **Excludes**   *Darier's disease [keratosis follicularis]*
> > > *(congenital) (757.39)*
> > > *keratosis:*
> > > > *arsenical (692.4)*
> > > > *gonococcal (098.81)*

701.2   Acquired acanthosis nigricans
> Keratosis nigricans

701.3 Striae atrophicae
Atrophic spots of skin
Atrophoderma maculatum
Atrophy blanche (of Milian)
Degenerative colloid atrophy
Senile degenerative atrophy
Striae distensae

701.4 Keloid scar
Cheloid
Hypertrophic scar
Keloid
Coding Clinic: 1995, Q3, P14

701.5 Other abnormal granulation tissue
Excessive granulation

701.8 Other specified hypertrophic and atrophic conditions of skin
Acrodermatitis atrophicans chronica
Atrophia cutis senilis
Atrophoderma neuriticum
Confluent and reticulate papillomatosis
Cutis laxa senilis
Elastosis senilis
Folliculitis ulerythematosa reticulata
Gougerot-Carteaud syndrome or disease
Coding Clinic: 2008, Q1, P7-8

701.9 Unspecified hypertrophic and atrophic conditions of skin
Atrophoderma

● **702 Other dermatoses**

Excludes *carcinoma in situ (232.0–232.9)*

702.0 Actinic keratosis

● **702.1 Seborrheic keratosis**

    702.11 Inflamed seborrheic keratosis

    702.19 Other seborrheic keratosis
      Seborrheic keratosis NOS

702.8 Other specified dermatoses

● **703 Diseases of nail**

Excludes *congenital anomalies (757.5)*
onychia and paronychia (681.02, 681.11)

703.0 Ingrowing nail
Ingrowing nail with infection
Unguis incarnatus

Excludes *infection, nail NOS (681.9)*

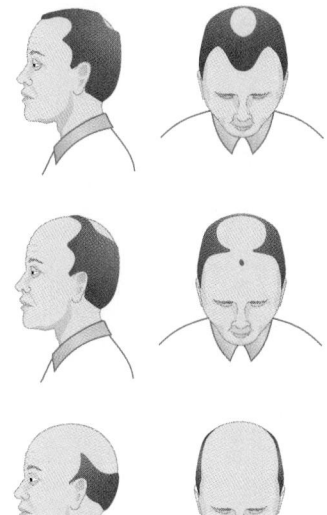

Figure 12–7 Male pattern alopecia.

Item 12-8 **Alopecia** is lack of hair and takes many forms. The most common is male pattern alopecia, also known as **androgenetic alopecia. Telogen effluvium** is early and excessive loss of hair resulting from a trauma to the hair follicle (fever, drugs, surgery, etc.).

703.8 Other specified diseases of nail
Dystrophia unguium
Hypertrophy of nail
Koilonychia
Leukonychia (punctata) (striata)
Onychauxis
Onychogryposis
Onycholysis

703.9 Unspecified disease of nail

● **704 Diseases of hair and hair follicles**

Excludes *congenital anomalies (757.4)*

● **704.0 Alopecia**

Excludes *madarosis (374.55)*
syphilitic alopecia (091.82)

704.00 Alopecia, unspecified
Baldness   Loss of hair

    704.01 Alopecia areata
Ophiasis

    704.02 Telogen effluvium

704.09 Other
Folliculitis decalvans
Hypotrichosis:
    NOS
    postinfectional NOS
Pseudopelade

DISEASES OF THE SKIN AND SUBCUTANEOUS TISSUE (680–709)

704.1 Hirsutism
Excessive growth of hair
Hypertrichosis:
  NOS
  lanuginosa, acquired
Polytrichia

> **Excludes** *hypertrichosis of eyelid (374.54)*

704.2 Abnormalities of the hair
Atrophic hair
Clastothrix
Fragilitas crinium
Trichiasis:
  NOS
  cicatrical
Trichorrhexis (nodosa)

> **Excludes** *trichiasis of eyelid (374.05)*

Coding Clinic: 2004, Q4, P91-92

704.3 Variations in hair color
Canities (premature)
Grayness, hair (premature)
Heterochromia of hair
Poliosis:
  NOS
  circumscripta, acquired

704.8 Other specified diseases of hair and hair follicles
Folliculitis:
  NOS
  abscedens et suffodiens
  pustular
Perifolliculitis:
  NOS
  capitis abscedens et suffodiens
  scalp
Sycosis:
  NOS
  barbae [not parasitic]
  lupoid
  vulgaris

704.9 Unspecified disease of hair and hair follicles

705 Disorders of sweat glands

705.0 Anhidrosis
Hypohidrosis   Oligohidrosis

705.1 Prickly heat
Heat rash   Sudamina
Miliaria rubra (tropicalis)

705.2 Focal hyperhidrosis

> **Excludes** *generalized (secondary) hyperhidrosis (780.8)*

705.21 Primary focal hyperhidrosis
Focal hyperhidrosis NOS
Hyperhidrosis NOS
Hyperhidrosis of:
  axilla   palms
  face   soles

705.22 Secondary focal hyperhidrosis
Frey's syndrome

705.8 Other specified disorders of sweat glands

705.81 Dyshidrosis
Cheiropompholyx
Pompholyx

705.82 Fox-Fordyce disease

705.83 Hidradenitis
Hidradenitis suppurativa

705.89 Other
Bromhidrosis   Granulosis rubra nasi
Chromhidrosis   Urhidrosis

> **Excludes** *hidrocystoma (216.0–216.9)*
> *generalized hyperhidrosis (780.8)*

705.9 Unspecified disorder of sweat glands
Disorder of sweat glands NOS

706 Diseases of sebaceous glands

706.0 Acne varioliformis
Acne:
  frontalis
  necrotica

706.1 Other acne
Acne:
  NOS
  conglobata
  cystic
  pustular
  vulgaris
Blackhead
Comedo

> **Excludes** *acne rosacea (695.3)*

706.2 Sebaceous cyst
Atheroma, skin
Keratin cyst
Wen

706.3 Seborrhea

> **Excludes** *seborrhea:*
> *capitis (690.11)*
> *sicca (690.18)*
> *seborrheic*
> *dermatitis (690.10)*
> *keratosis (702.11–702.19)*

706.8 Other specified diseases of sebaceous glands
Asteatosis (cutis)
Xerosis cutis

706.9 Unspecified disease of sebaceous glands

◀ New   ◀ Revised   ~~deleted~~ Deleted   ● Use Additional Digit(s)   ■ Nonspecific Code
● Not first-listed DX   OGCR Official Guidelines   Coding Clinic   Excludes   Includes   Use additional   Code first   Omit code

● **707　Chronic ulcer of skin**

> **Includes**　non-infected sinus of skin
> non-healing ulcer
>
> **Excludes**　*varicose ulcer (454.0, 454.2)*

● **707.0　Pressure ulcer**
> Bed sore
> Decubitus ulcer
> Plaster ulcer
>
> Use additional code to identify pressure ulcer
> stage (707.20–707.25)
> Coding Clinic: 2004, Q4, P92-93; Q1, P14-15; 2003, Q4, P110; 1999,
> Q4, P20; 1996, Q1, P15; 1990, Q3, P15; 1987, Nov-Dec, P9

▪ **707.00　Unspecified site**

707.01　Elbow

707.02　Upper back
> Shoulder blades

707.03　Lower back
> Coccyx
> Sacrum
> Coding Clinic: 2008, Q3, P17; 2005, Q1, P16

707.04　Hip

707.05　Buttock

707.06　Ankle

707.07　Heel
> Coding Clinic: 2005, Q1, P16

▪ **707.09　Other site**
> Head
> Coding Clinic: 2008, Q3, P17

● **707.1　Ulcer of lower limbs, except pressure ulcer**
> Ulcer, chronic, of lower limb:
> neurogenic of lower limb
> trophic of lower limb
> *Code if applicable, any causal condition first:*
> atherosclerosis of the extremities with ulceration
> (440.23)
> chronic venous hypertension with ulcer (459.31)
> chronic venous hypertension with ulcer and
> inflammation (459.33)
> diabetes mellitus (249.80–249.81, 250.80–250.83)
> postphlebitic syndrome with ulcer (459.11)
> postphlebitic syndrome with ulcer and
> inflammation (459.13)
> Coding Clinic: 2004, Q1, P14-15; 1999, Q4, P15; 1996, Q1, P10

▪ **707.10　Ulcer of lower limb, unspecified**
> Coding Clinic: 2004, Q3, P5-6

707.11　Ulcer of thigh

707.12　Ulcer of calf

707.13　Ulcer of ankle

707.14　Ulcer of heel and midfoot
> Plantar surface of midfoot

707.15　Ulcer of other part of foot
> Toes

707.19　Ulcer of other part of lower limb

● **707.2　Pressure ulcer stages**
> *Code first site of pressure ulcer (707.00-707.09)*
> Coding Clinic: 2008, Q4, P132-134

● ▪ **707.20　*Pressure ulcer, unspecified stage***
> Healing pressure ulcer NOS
> Healing pressure ulcer, unspecified stage

● **707.21　*Pressure ulcer stage I***
> Healing pressure ulcer, stage I
> Pressure pre-ulcer skin changes limited to
> persistent focal erythema

● **707.22　*Pressure ulcer stage II***
> Healing pressure ulcer, stage II
> Pressure ulcer with abrasion, blister, partial
> thickness skin loss involving
> epidermis and/or dermis

● **707.23　*Pressure ulcer stage III***
> Healing pressure ulcer, stage III
> Pressure ulcer with full thickness skin loss
> involving damage or necrosis of
> subcutaneous tissue

● **707.24　*Pressure ulcer stage IV***
> Healing pressure ulcer, stage IV
> Pressure ulcer with necrosis of soft tissues
> through to underlying muscle, tendon,
> or bone

● **707.25　*Pressure ulcer, unstageable***

▪ **707.8　Chronic ulcer of other specified sites**
> Ulcer, chronic, of other specified sites:
> neurogenic of other specified sites
> trophic of other specified sites

▪ **707.9　Chronic ulcer of unspecified site**
> Chronic ulcer NOS　　　Tropical ulcer NOS
> Trophic ulcer NOS　　　Ulcer of skin NOS

● **708　Urticaria**

> **Excludes**　*edema:*
> *angioneurotic (995.1)*
> *Quincke's (995.1)*
> *hereditary angioedema (277.6)*
> *urticaria:*
> *giant (995.1)*
> *papulosa (Hebra) (698.2)*
> *pigmentosa (juvenile) (congenital) (757.33)*

708.0　Allergic urticaria
> Coding Clinic: 1984, May-June, P11

708.1　Idiopathic urticaria

708.2　Urticaria due to cold and heat
> Thermal urticaria

708.3　Dermatographic urticaria
> Dermatographia
> Factitial urticaria

708.4　Vibratory urticaria

708.5　Cholinergic urticaria
> Coding Clinic: 1995, Q4, P50

▪ **708.8　Other specified urticaria**
> Nettle rash
> Urticaria:
> chronic
> recurrent periodic

▪ **708.9　Urticaria, unspecified**
> Hives NOS

DISEASES OF THE SKIN AND SUBCUTANEOUS TISSUE (680–709)

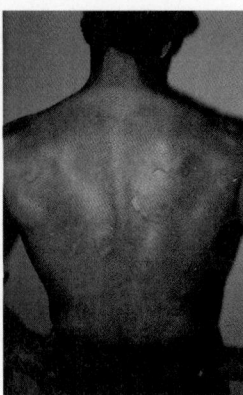

Figure 12–8 Urticaria (hives). *(Courtesy of David Effron, MD.)* (From Marx: Rosen's Emergency Medicine: Concepts and Clinical Practice, 6th ed. 2006, Mosby, Inc.)

Item 12–9 Urticaria is a vascular reaction in which wheals surrounded by a red halo appear and cause severe itching. The causes of urticaria or hives are extensive and varied (e.g., food, heat, cold, drugs, stress, infections). Dyschromia is any disorder of the pigmentation of the skin or hair.

709 Other disorders of skin and subcutaneous tissue

709.0 Dyschromia

> **Excludes** *albinism (270.2)*
> *pigmented nevus (216.0–216.9)*
> *that of eyelid (374.52–374.53)*

709.00 Dyschromia, unspecified

709.01 Vitiligo

709.09 Other

709.1 Vascular disorders of skin
Angioma serpiginosum
Purpura (primary) annularis telangiectodes

709.2 Scar conditions and fibrosis of skin
Adherent scar (skin)
Cicatrix
Disfigurement (due to scar)
Fibrosis, skin NOS
Scar NOS

> **Excludes** *keloid scar (701.4)*

Coding Clinic: 1984, Nov-Dec, P19

709.3 Degenerative skin disorders
Calcinosis:
circumscripta
cutis
Colloid milium
Degeneration, skin
Deposits, skin
Senile dermatosis NOS
Subcutaneous calcification

709.4 Foreign body granuloma of skin and subcutaneous tissue

> **Excludes** *residual foreign body without granuloma of skin and subcutaneous tissue (729.6)*
> *that of muscle (728.82)*

709.8 Other specified disorders of skin
Epithelial hyperplasia
Menstrual dermatosis
Vesicular eruption
Coding Clinic: 1987, Nov-Dec, P6

709.9 Unspecified disorder of skin and subcutaneous tissue
Dermatosis NOS

◀ New   ◀▥ Revised   ~~deleted~~ Deleted   ● Use Additional Digit(s)   ■ Nonspecific Code   ● Not first-listed DX   OGCR Official Guidelines   Coding Clinic   Excludes   Includes   Use additional   Code first   Omit code

13. DISEASES OF THE MUSCULOSKELETAL SYSTEM AND CONNECTIVE TISSUE (710–739)

Use additional external cause code, if applicable, to identify the cause of the musculoskeletal condition

The following fifth-digit subclassification is for use with categories 711–712, 715–716, 718–719, and 730:

▨0 site unspecified
  1 **shoulder region**
     Acromioclavicular joint(s)
     Clavicle
     Glenohumeral joint(s)
     Scapula
     Sternoclavicular joint(s)
  2 **upper arm**
     Elbow joint
     Humerus
  3 **forearm**
     Radius
     Ulna
     Wrist joint
  4 **hand**
     Carpus
     Metacarpus
     Phalanges [fingers]
  5 **pelvic region and thigh**
     Buttock
     Femur
     Hip (joint)
  6 **lower leg**
     Fibula
     Knee joint
     Patella
     Tibia
  7 **ankle and foot**
     Ankle joint
     Digits [toes]
     Metatarsus
     Phalanges, foot
     Tarsus
     Other joints in foot
▨8 **other specified sites**
     Head
     Neck
     Ribs
     Skull
     Trunk
     Vertebral column
▨9 **multiple sites**

ARTHROPATHIES AND RELATED DISORDERS (710–719)

Excludes *disorders of spine (720.0–724.9)*

● **710 Diffuse diseases of connective tissue**

Includes all collagen diseases whose effects are not mainly confined to a single system

Excludes *those affecting mainly the cardiovascular system, i.e., polyarteritis nodosa and allied conditions (446.0–446.7)*

710.0 Systemic lupus erythematosus
  Autoimmune inflammatory connective tissue disease of unknown cause that occurs most often in women. See 695.4 for nonsystemic.
  Disseminated lupus erythematosus
  Libman-Sacks disease

  Use additional code to identify manifestation, as:
     endocarditis (424.91)
     nephritis (583.81)
        chronic (582.81)
     nephrotic syndrome (581.81)

  Excludes *lupus erythematosus (discoid) NOS (695.4)*

  Coding Clinic: 2003, Q2, P7x2; 1997, Q2, P8-9; 1987, Sept-Oct, P8

710.1 Systemic sclerosis
  Acrosclerosis
  CRST syndrome
  Progressive systemic sclerosis
  Scleroderma

  Use additional code to identify manifestation, as:
     lung involvement (517.2)
     myopathy (359.6)

  Excludes *circumscribed scleroderma (701.0)*

710.2 Sicca syndrome
  Keratoconjunctivitis sicca
  Sjögren's disease

710.3 Dermatomyositis
  Poikilodermatomyositis
  Polymyositis with skin involvement

710.4 Polymyositis

710.5 Eosinophilia myalgia syndrome
  Toxic oil syndrome

  Use additional E code to identify drug, if drug induced

▨**710.8 Other specified diffuse diseases of connective tissue**
  Multifocal fibrosclerosis (idiopathic) NEC
  Systemic fibrosclerosing syndrome
  Coding Clinic: 1987, Mar-April, P12

▨**710.9 Unspecified diffuse connective tissue disease**
  Collagen disease NOS

● **711   Arthropathy associated with infections**
Abnormality of a joint

Includes   arthritis associated with conditions classifiable
below
arthropathy associated with conditions
classifiable below
polyarthritis associated with conditions
classifiable below
polyarthropathy associated with conditions
classifiable below

Excludes   *rheumatic fever (390)*

Coding Clinic: 1992, Q1, P16-17

The following fifth-digit subclassification is for use with
category 711; valid digits are in [brackets] under each code.
See list at beginning of chapter for definitions:

> ■0   site unspecified
> 1   shoulder region
> 2   upper arm
> 3   forearm
> 4   hand
> 5   pelvic region and thigh
> 6   lower leg
> 7   ankle and foot
> ■8   other specified sites
> ■9   multiple sites

● **711.0   Pyogenic arthritis**
[0-9]   Arthritis or polyarthritis (due to):
coliform [Escherichia coli]
Hemophilus influenzae [H. influenzae]
pneumococcal
Pseudomonas
staphylococcal
streptococcal
Pyarthrosis

Use additional code to identify infectious organism
(041.0–041.8)
Coding Clinic: 1992, Q1, P16-17; 1991, Q1, P15

● ● **711.1   Arthropathy associated with Reiter's disease and**
[0-9]   *nonspecific urethritis*

Code first *underlying disease, as:*
nonspecific urethritis (099.4)
Reiter's disease (099.3)

● ● **711.2   Arthropathy in Behçet's syndrome**
[0-9]   Code first *underlying disease (136.1)*

● ● **711.3   Postdysenteric arthropathy**
[0-9]   Code first *underlying disease, as:*
dysentery (009.0)
enteritis, infectious (008.0–009.3)
paratyphoid fever (002.1–002.9)
typhoid fever (002.0)

Excludes   *salmonella arthritis (003.23)*

● ● ■ **711.4   Arthropathy associated with other bacterial**
[0-9]   *diseases*

Code first *underlying disease, as:*
diseases classifiable to 010–040, 090–099, except
as in 711.1, 711.3, and 713.5
leprosy (030.0–030.9)
tuberculosis (015.0–015.9)

Excludes   *gonococcal arthritis (098.50)*
meningococcal arthritis (036.82)

● ● ■ **711.5   Arthropathy associated with other viral diseases**
[0-9]   Code first *underlying disease, as:*
diseases classifiable to 045–049, 050–079, 480, 487
O'nyong-nyong (066.3)

Excludes   *that due to rubella (056.71)*

● ● **711.6   Arthropathy associated with mycoses**
[0-9]   Code first *underlying disease (110.0–118)*

● ● **711.7   Arthropathy associated with helminthiasis**
[0-9]   Code first *underlying disease, as:*
filariasis (125.0–125.9)

● ● ■ **711.8   Arthropathy associated with other infectious and**
[0-9]   *parasitic diseases*

Code first *underlying disease, as:*
diseases classifiable to 080–088, 100–104,
130–136

Excludes   *arthropathy associated with sarcoidosis
(713.7)*

Coding Clinic: 1990, Q3, P14

● ■ **711.9   Unspecified infective arthritis**
[0-9]   Infective arthritis or polyarthritis (acute) (chronic)
(subacute) NOS

● **712   Crystal arthropathies**

Includes   crystal-induced arthritis and synovitis

Excludes   *gouty arthropathy (274.00–274.03)* ◀▭

The following fifth-digit subclassification is for use with
category 712; valid digits are in [brackets] under each code.
See list at beginning of chapter for definitions:

> ■0   site unspecified
> 1   shoulder region
> 2   upper arm
> 3   forearm
> 4   hand
> 5   pelvic region and thigh
> 6   lower leg
> 7   ankle and foot
> ■8   other specified sites
> ■9   multiple sites

● ● **712.1   Chondrocalcinosis due to dicalcium phosphate**
[0-9]   *crystals*
Chondrocalcinosis due to dicalcium phosphate
crystals (with other crystals)

Code first *underlying disease (275.49)*

● ● **712.2   Chondrocalcinosis due to pyrophosphate crystals**
[0-9]   Code first *underlying disease (275.49)*

● ● ■ **712.3   Chondrocalcinosis, unspecified**
[0-9]   Code first *underlying disease (275.49)*

● ■ **712.8   Other specified crystal arthropathies**
[0-9]

● ■ **712.9   Unspecified crystal arthropathy**
[0-9]

◀   New   ◀▥   Revised   ~~deleted~~   Deleted   ●   Use Additional Digit(s)   ■   Nonspecific Code

●   Not first-listed DX   OGCR   Official Guidelines   Coding Clinic   Excludes   Includes   Use additional   Code first   Omit code

● **713 Arthropathy associated with other disorders classified elsewhere**

> **Includes** arthritis associated with conditions classifiable below
> arthropathy associated with conditions classifiable below
> polyarthritis associated with conditions classifiable below
> polyarthropathy associated with conditions classifiable below

●■ **713.0 *Arthropathy associated with other endocrine and metabolic disorders***

> *Code first* underlying disease, as:
> acromegaly (253.0)
> hemochromatosis (275.0)
> hyperparathyroidism (252.00–252.08)
> hypogammaglobulinemia (279.00–279.09)
> hypothyroidism (243–244.9)
> lipoid metabolism disorder (272.0–272.9)
> ochronosis (270.2)

> **Excludes** *arthropathy associated with:*
> *amyloidosis (713.7)*
> *crystal deposition disorders, except gout (712.1–712.9)*
> *diabetic neuropathy (713.5)*
> *gouty arthropathy (274.00–274.03)* ◄

● **713.1 *Arthropathy associated with gastrointestinal conditions other than infections***

> *Code first* underlying disease, as:
> regional enteritis (555.0–555.9)
> ulcerative colitis (556)

● **713.2 *Arthropathy associated with hematological disorders***

> *Code first* underlying disease, as:
> hemoglobinopathy (282.4–282.7)
> hemophilia (286.0–286.2)
> leukemia (204.0–208.9)
> malignant reticulosis (202.3)
> multiple myelomatosis (203.0)

> **Excludes** *arthropathy associated with Henoch-Schönlein purpura (713.6)*

● **713.3 *Arthropathy associated with dermatological disorders***

> *Code first* underlying disease, as:
> erythema multiforme (695.10–695.19)
> erythema nodosum (695.2)

> **Excludes** *psoriatic arthropathy (696.0)*

● **713.4 *Arthropathy associated with respiratory disorders***

> *Code first* underlying disease, as:
> diseases classifiable to 490–519

> **Excludes** *arthropathy associated with respiratory infections (711.0, 711.4–711.8)*

● **713.5 *Arthropathy associated with neurological disorders***

> Charcot's arthropathy associated with diseases classifiable elsewhere
> Neuropathic arthritis associated with diseases classifiable elsewhere

> *Code first* underlying disease, as:
> neuropathic joint disease [Charcot's joints]:
> NOS (094.0)
> diabetic (249.6, 250.6)
> syringomyelic (336.0)
> tabetic [syphilitic] (094.0)

● **713.6 *Arthropathy associated with hypersensitivity reaction***

> *Code first* underlying disease, as:
> Henoch-Schönlein purpura (287.0)
> serum sickness (999.5)

> **Excludes** *allergic arthritis NOS (716.2)*

●■ **713.7 *Other general diseases with articular involvement***

> *Code first* underlying disease, as:
> amyloidosis (277.30–277.39)
> familial Mediterranean fever (277.31)
> sarcoidosis (135)
> Coding Clinic: 1997, Q2, P12-13

●■ **713.8 *Arthropathy associated with other conditions classifiable elsewhere***

> *Code first* underlying disease, as:
> conditions classifiable elsewhere except as in 711.1–711.8, 712, and 713.0–713.7

Item 13-1 Rheumatoid arthritis (RA) is a chronic systemic inflammatory disease of undetermined etiology involving primarily the synovial membranes and articular structures of multiple joints. The disease is often progressive and results in pain, stiffness, and swelling of joints. In late stages, deformity, ankylosis, and other **inflammatory polyarthropathies** develop.

● **714 Rheumatoid arthritis and other inflammatory polyarthropathies**

> **Excludes** *rheumatic fever (390)*
> *rheumatoid arthritis of spine NOS (720.0)*

714.0 Rheumatoid arthritis
> Arthritis or polyarthritis:
> atrophic
> rheumatic (chronic)

> Use additional code to identify manifestation, as:
> myopathy (359.6)
> polyneuropathy (357.1)

> **Excludes** *juvenile rheumatoid arthritis NOS (714.30)*

> Coding Clinic: 2006, Q2, P20; 1995, Q4, P51

DISEASES OF THE MUSCULOSKELETAL SYSTEM AND CONNECTIVE TISSUE (710–739)

714.1 Felty's syndrome
　　Rheumatoid arthritis with splenoadenomegaly and leukopenia

■714.2 Other rheumatoid arthritis with visceral or systemic involvement
　　Rheumatoid carditis

●714.3 Juvenile chronic polyarthritis

■714.30 Polyarticular juvenile rheumatoid arthritis, chronic or unspecified
　　Juvenile rheumatoid arthritis NOS
　　Still's disease

714.31 Polyarticular juvenile rheumatoid arthritis, acute

714.32 Pauciarticular juvenile rheumatoid arthritis

714.33 Monoarticular juvenile rheumatoid arthritis

714.4 Chronic postrheumatic arthropathy
　　Chronic rheumatoid nodular fibrositis
　　Jaccoud's syndrome

●714.8 Other specified inflammatory polyarthropathies

714.81 Rheumatoid lung
　　Caplan's syndrome
　　Diffuse interstitial rheumatoid disease of lung
　　Fibrosing alveolitis, rheumatoid

■714.89 Other

■714.9 Unspecified inflammatory polyarthropathy
　　Inflammatory polyarthropathy or polyarthritis NOS
　　Excludes polyarthropathy NOS (716.5)

●715 Osteoarthrosis and allied disorders
　　Degenerative joint disease with breaking down the cartilage causing pain, swelling, and reduced motion in the joints, affecting any joint.

　　Note: Localized, in the subcategories below, includes bilateral involvement of the same site.

　　Includes arthritis or polyarthritis:
　　　　degenerative
　　　　hypertrophic
　　　　degenerative joint disease
　　　　osteoarthritis

　　Excludes Marie-Strümpell spondylitis (720.0)
　　　　osteoarthrosis [osteoarthritis] of spine (721.0–721.9)

The following fifth-digit subclassification is for use with category 715; valid digits are in [brackets] under each code. See list at beginning of chapter for definitions:

> ■0　site unspecified
> 　1　shoulder region
> 　2　upper arm
> 　3　forearm
> 　4　hand
> 　5　pelvic region and thigh
> 　6　lower leg
> 　7　ankle and foot
> ■8　other specified sites
> ■9　multiple sites

●715.0 Osteoarthrosis, generalized
[0,4,9]　Degenerative joint disease, involving multiple joints
　　Primary generalized hypertrophic osteoarthrosis
　　Coding Clinic: 1995, Q2, P5

●715.1 Osteoarthrosis, localized, primary
[0-8]　Localized osteoarthropathy, idiopathic

●715.2 Osteoarthrosis, localized, secondary
[0-8]　Coxae malum senilis

●■715.3 Osteoarthrosis, localized, not specified whether
[0-8]　**primary or secondary**
　　Otto's pelvis
　　Coding Clinic: 2004, Q2, P15; 2003, Q2, P18; 1995, Q2, P5

●■715.8 Osteoarthrosis involving, or with mention of more
[0,9]　**than one site, but not specified as generalized**
　　Coding Clinic: 1995, Q2, P5

●■715.9 Osteoarthrosis, unspecified whether generalized or
[0-8]　**localized**
　　Coding Clinic: 2003, Q2, P18; 1997, Q2, P12-13; 1996, Q1, P16; 1995, Q2, P5

●716 Other and unspecified arthropathies

　　Excludes cricoarytenoid arthropathy (478.79)

The following fifth-digit subclassification is for use with category 716; valid digits are in [brackets] under each code. See list at beginning of chapter for definitions:

> ■0　site unspecified
> 　1　shoulder region
> 　2　upper arm
> 　3　forearm
> 　4　hand
> 　5　pelvic region and thigh
> 　6　lower leg
> 　7　ankle and foot
> ■8　other specified sites
> ■9　multiple sites

●716.0 Kaschin-Beck disease
[0-9]　Endemic polyarthritis

●716.1 Traumatic arthropathy
[0-9]　Coding Clinic: 2009, Q2, P13; 2002, Q1, P9-10

●716.2 Allergic arthritis
[0-9]　**Excludes** arthritis associated with Henoch-Schönlein purpura or serum sickness (713.6)

●716.3 Climacteric arthritis ♀
[0-9]　Menopausal arthritis

●716.4 Transient arthropathy
[0-9]　**Excludes** palindromic rheumatism (719.3)

●■716.5 Unspecified polyarthropathy or polyarthritis
[0-9]

●■716.6 Unspecified monoarthritis
[0-8]　Coxitis

●■716.8 Other specified arthropathy
[0-9]

●■716.9 Arthropathy, unspecified
[0-9]　Arthritis (acute) (chronic) (subacute)
　　Arthropathy (acute) (chronic) (subacute)
　　Articular rheumatism (chronic)
　　Inflammation of joint NOS

◀ New　◀▥ Revised　d̶e̶l̶e̶t̶e̶d̶ Deleted　● Use Additional Digit(s)　■ Nonspecific Code
● Not first-listed DX　OGCR Official Guidelines　Coding Clinic　Excludes　Includes　Use additional　Code first　Omit code

⬤ **717 Internal derangement of knee**

> **Includes** degeneration of articular cartilage or meniscus of knee
> rupture, old of articular cartilage or meniscus of knee
> tear, old of articular cartilage or meniscus of knee

> **Excludes** *acute derangement of knee (836.0–836.6)*
> *ankylosis (718.5)*
> *contracture (718.4)*
> *current injury (836.0–836.6)*
> *deformity (736.4–736.6)*
> *recurrent dislocation (718.3)*

717.0 Old bucket handle tear of medial meniscus
> Old bucket handle tear of unspecified cartilage

717.1 Derangement of anterior horn of medial meniscus

717.2 Derangement of posterior horn of medial meniscus

▪**717.3 Other and unspecified derangement of medial meniscus**
> Degeneration of internal semilunar cartilage

⬤ **717.4 Derangement of lateral meniscus**

> ▪**717.40 Derangement of lateral meniscus, unspecified**

> **717.41 Bucket handle tear of lateral meniscus**

> **717.42 Derangement of anterior horn of lateral meniscus**

> **717.43 Derangement of posterior horn of lateral meniscus**

> ▪**717.49 Other**

717.5 Derangement of meniscus, not elsewhere classified
> Congenital discoid meniscus
> Cyst of semilunar cartilage
> Derangement of semilunar cartilage NOS

717.6 Loose body in knee
> Joint mice, knee
> Rice bodies, knee (joint)

717.7 Chondromalacia of patella
> Chondromalacia patellae
> Degeneration [softening] of articular cartilage of patella
> Coding Clinic: 1985, July-Aug, P14; 1984, Nov-Dec, P9

⬤ **717.8 Other internal derangement of knee**

> **717.81 Old disruption of lateral collateral ligament**

> **717.82 Old disruption of medial collateral ligament**

> **717.83 Old disruption of anterior cruciate ligament**

> **717.84 Old disruption of posterior cruciate ligament**

> ▪**717.85 Old disruption of other ligaments of knee**
> Capsular ligament of knee

> ▪**717.89 Other**
> Old disruption of ligaments of knee NOS

▪**717.9 Unspecified internal derangement of knee**
> Derangement NOS of knee

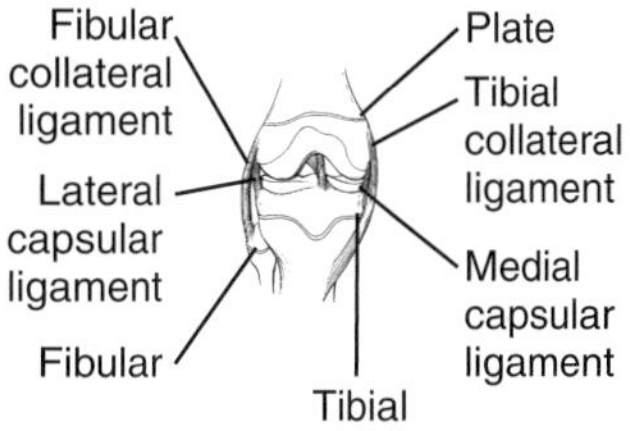

Figure 13–1 Collateral and cruciate ligament of knee. (From DeLee: DeLee and Drez's Orthopaedic Sports Medicine, 2nd ed. 2002, Saunders)

⬤ **718 Other derangement of joint**

> **Excludes** *current injury (830.0–848.9)*
> *jaw (524.60–524.69)*

The following fifth-digit subclassification is for use with category 718; valid digits are in [brackets] under each code. See list at beginning of chapter for definitions:

> ▪0 site unspecified
> 1 shoulder region
> 2 upper arm
> 3 forearm
> 4 hand
> 5 pelvic region and thigh
> 6 lower leg
> 7 ankle and foot
> ▪8 other specified sites
> ▪9 multiple sites

⬤ **718.0 Articular cartilage disorder**
[0-5,7-9] Meniscus:
> disorder
> rupture, old
> tear, old
> Old rupture of ligament(s) of joint NOS

> **Excludes** *articular cartilage disorder:*
> *in ochronosis (270.2)*
> *knee (717.0–717.9)*
> *chondrocalcinosis (275.49)*
> *metastatic calcification (275.40)*

⬤ **718.1 Loose body in joint**
[0-5,7-9] Joint mice

> **Excludes** *knee (717.6)*

> Coding Clinic: 2001, Q2, P14-15

⬤ **718.2 Pathological dislocation**
[0-9] Dislocation or displacement of joint, not recurrent and not current

⬤ **718.3 Recurrent dislocation of joint**
[0-9] Coding Clinic: 1987, Nov-Dec, P7

⬤ **718.4 Contracture of joint**
[0-9] Coding Clinic: 1998, Q4, P39-40

⬤ **718.5 Ankylosis of joint**
[0-9] Ankylosis of joint (fibrous) (osseous)

> **Excludes** *spine (724.9)*
> *stiffness of joint without mention of ankylosis (719.5)*

> Coding Clinic: 1995, Q1, P10

● ■**718.6 Unspecified intrapelvic protrusion of acetabulum**
[0,5]   Protrusio acetabuli, unspecified

● **718.7 Developmental dislocation of joint**
[0-9]
Excludes *congenital dislocation of joint (754.0–755.8)*
traumatic dislocation of joint (830–839)

● ■**718.8 Other joint derangement, not elsewhere classified**
[0-9]   Flail joint (paralytic)
Instability of joint

Excludes *deformities classifiable to 736 (736.0–736.9)*

Coding Clinic: 2000, Q2, P14-15

● ■**718.9 Unspecified derangement of joint**
[0-5,7-9]   **Excludes** *knee (717.9)*

● **719 Other and unspecified disorders of joint**
Excludes *jaw (524.60–524.69)*

The following fifth-digit subclassification is for use with codes 719.0–719.6, 719.8–719.9; valid digits are in [brackets] under each code. See list at beginning of chapter for definitions:

> ■0 site unspecified
> 1 shoulder region
> 2 upper arm
> 3 forearm
> 4 hand
> 5 pelvic region and thigh
> 6 lower leg
> 7 ankle and foot
> ■8 other specified sites
> ■9 multiple sites

● **719.0 Effusion of joint**
[0-9]   Hydrarthrosis
Swelling of joint, with or without pain

Excludes *intermittent hydrarthrosis (719.3)*

● **719.1 Hemarthrosis**
[0-9]   **Excludes** *current injury (840.0–848.9)*

● **719.2 Villonodular synovitis**
[0-9]

● **719.3 Palindromic rheumatism**
[0-9]   Hench-Rosenberg syndrome
Intermittent hydrarthrosis

● **719.4 Pain in joint**
[0-9]   Arthralgia
Coding Clinic: 2001, Q1, P3-4

● **719.5 Stiffness of joint, not elsewhere classified**
[0-9]

● ■**719.6 Other symptoms referable to joint**
[0-9]   Joint crepitus
Snapping hip
Coding Clinic: 2007, Q2, P7; 1984, Sept-Oct, P15-16

719.7 Difficulty in walking
Excludes *abnormality of gait (781.2)*
Coding Clinic: 2004, Q2, P15

● ■**719.8 Other specified disorders of joint**
[0-9]   Calcification of joint
Fistula of joint

Excludes *temporomandibular joint-pain-dysfunction syndrome [Costen's syndrome] (524.60)*

● ■**719.9 Unspecified disorder of joint**
[0-9]

Item 13-2 Ankylosis or arthrokleisis is a consolidation of a joint due to disease, injury, or surgical procedure. Spondylosis is the degeneration of the vertebral processes and formation of osteophytes and commonly occurs with age. **Spondylitis** or ankylosing spondylitis is a type of arthritis that affects the spine or backbone causing back pain and stiffness.

DORSOPATHIES (720–724)

Excludes *curvature of spine (737.0–737.9)*
osteochondrosis of spine (juvenile) (732.0) adult (732.8)

● **720 Ankylosing spondylitis and other inflammatory spondylopathies**

720.0 Ankylosing spondylitis
Rheumatoid arthritis of spine NOS
Spondylitis:
Marie-Strümpell
rheumatoid

720.1 Spinal enthesopathy
Disorder of peripheral ligamentous or muscular attachments of spine
Romanus lesion

720.2 Sacroiliitis, not elsewhere classified
Inflammation of sacroiliac joint NOS

● **720.8 Other inflammatory spondylopathies**

● **720.81 Inflammatory spondylopathies in diseases classified elsewhere**
Code first underlying disease, as:
tuberculosis (015.0)

■**720.89 Other**

■**720.9 Unspecified inflammatory spondylopathy**
Spondylitis NOS

● **721 Spondylosis and allied disorders**
Coding Clinic: 1989, Q2, P14

721.0 Cervical spondylosis without myelopathy
Cervical or cervicodorsal:
arthritis
osteoarthritis
spondylarthritis

721.1 Cervical spondylosis with myelopathy
Anterior spinal artery compression syndrome
Spondylogenic compression of cervical spinal cord
Vertebral artery compression syndrome

721.2 Thoracic spondylosis without myelopathy
Thoracic:
arthritis
osteoarthritis
spondylarthritis

721.3 Lumbosacral spondylosis without myelopathy
Lumbar or lumbosacral:
arthritis
osteoarthritis
spondylarthritis
Coding Clinic: 2002, Q4, P107-108

● **721.4 Thoracic or lumbar spondylosis with myelopathy**

721.41 Thoracic region
Spondylogenic compression of thoracic spinal cord

721.42 Lumbar region
Spondylogenic compression of lumbar spinal cord

◀ New   ◀‖‖ Revised   ~~deleted~~ Deleted   ● Use Additional Digit(s)   ■ Nonspecific Code
● Not first-listed DX   OGCR Official Guidelines   Coding Clinic   Excludes   Includes   Use additional   Code first   Omit code

721.5 Kissing spine
Baastrup's syndrome

721.6 Ankylosing vertebral hyperostosis

721.7 Traumatic spondylopathy
Kümmell's disease or spondylitis

■ **721.8 Other allied disorders of spine**

● **721.9 Spondylosis of unspecified site**

721.90 Without mention of myelopathy
Spinal:
arthritis (deformans) (degenerative)
(hypertrophic)
osteoarthritis NOS
Spondylarthrosis NOS

721.91 With myelopathy
Spondylogenic compression of spinal cord
NOS

● **722 Intervertebral disc disorders**
Coding Clinic: 1989, Q2, P14

722.0 Displacement of cervical intervertebral disc without myelopathy
Neuritis (brachial) or radiculitis due to
displacement or rupture of cervical
intervertebral disc
Any condition classifiable to 722.2 of the cervical or
cervicothoracic intervertebral disc
Coding Clinic: 1988, Q1, P10

● **722.1 Displacement of thoracic or lumbar intervertebral disc without myelopathy**

722.10 Lumbar intervertebral disc without myelopathy
Lumbago or sciatica due to displacement of
intervertebral disc
Neuritis or radiculitis due to displacement
or rupture of lumbar intervertebral
disc
Any condition classifiable to 722.2 of the
lumbar or lumbosacral intervertebral
disc
Coding Clinic: 2008, Q4, P183-184; 2007, Q1, P9; 2003, Q3,
P12; Q1, P7; 2002, Q4, P107-108; 1994, Q3, P14

722.11 Thoracic intervertebral disc without myelopathy
Any condition classifiable to 722.2 of
thoracic intervertebral disc

■ **722.2 Displacement of intervertebral disc, site unspecified, without myelopathy**
Discogenic syndrome NOS
Herniation of nucleus pulposus NOS
Intervertebral disc NOS:
extrusion
prolapse
protrusion
rupture
Neuritis or radiculitis due to displacement or
rupture of intervertebral disc
Coding Clinic: 1988, Q1, P10

● **722.3 Schmorl's nodes**

■ **722.30 Unspecified region**

722.31 Thoracic region

722.32 Lumbar region

■ **722.39 Other**

722.4 Degeneration of cervical intervertebral disc
Degeneration of cervicothoracic intervertebral disc

● **722.5 Degeneration of thoracic or lumbar intervertebral disc**

722.51 Thoracic or thoracolumbar intervertebral disc

722.52 Lumbar or lumbosacral intervertebral disc
Coding Clinic: 2006, Q2, P18; 2004, Q4, P129-133

■ **722.6 Degeneration of intervertebral disc, site unspecified**
Degenerative disc disease NOS
Narrowing of intervertebral disc or space NOS

● **722.7 Intervertebral disc disorder with myelopathy**

■ **722.70 Unspecified region**

722.71 Cervical region

722.72 Thoracic region

722.73 Lumbar region

● **722.8 Postlaminectomy syndrome**

■ **722.80 Unspecified region**

722.81 Cervical region

722.82 Thoracic region

722.83 Lumbar region
Coding Clinic: 1997, Q2, P15x2

● **722.9 Other and unspecified disc disorder**
Calcification of intervertebral cartilage or disc
Discitis

■ **722.90 Unspecified region**
Coding Clinic: 1984, Nov-Dec, P19

722.91 Cervical region

722.92 Thoracic region

722.93 Lumbar region

● **723 Other disorders of cervical region**

Excludes *conditions due to:*
intervertebral disc disorders (722.0–722.9)
spondylosis (721.0–721.9)
Coding Clinic: 1989, Q2, P14

723.0 Spinal stenosis of cervical region
Coding Clinic: 2003, Q4, P99-101

723.1 Cervicalgia
Pain in neck

723.2 Cervicocranial syndrome
Barré-Liéou syndrome
Posterior cervical sympathetic syndrome

723.3 Cervicobrachial syndrome (diffuse)
Coding Clinic: 1985, Nov-Dec, P12

723.4 Brachia neuritis or radiculitis NOS
Cervical radiculitis
Radicular syndrome of upper limbs

■ **723.5 Torticollis, unspecified**
Contracture of neck

Excludes *congenital (754.1)*
due to birth injury (767.8)
hysterical (300.11)
ocular torticollis (781.93)
psychogenic (306.0)
spasmodic (333.83)
traumatic, current (847.0)
Coding Clinic: 2001, Q2, P21; 1995, Q1, P7

723.6 Panniculitis specified as affecting neck

723.7 Ossification of posterior longitudinal ligament in cervical region

DISEASES OF THE MUSCULOSKELETAL SYSTEM AND CONNECTIVE TISSUE (710–739)

■ **723.8 Other syndromes affecting cervical region**
Cervical syndrome NEC
Klippel's disease
Occipital neuralgia
Coding Clinic: 2000, Q1, P7-8

■ **723.9 Unspecified musculoskeletal disorders and symptoms referable to neck**
Cervical (region) disorder NOS

● **724 Other and unspecified disorders of back**
Excludes collapsed vertebra (code to cause, e.g., osteoporosis, 733.00–733.09)
conditions due to:
intervertebral disc disorders (722.0–722.9)
spondylosis (721.0–721.9)
Coding Clinic: 1989, Q2, P14

● **724.0 Spinal stenosis, other than cervical**
■ **724.00 Spinal stenosis, unspecified region**
724.01 Thoracic region
724.02 Lumbar region
Coding Clinic: 2008, Q4, P109-110; 2007, Q4, P116-120; Q1, P20-21; 1999, Q4, P13-14; 1994, Q3, P14
■ **724.09 Other**
724.1 Pain in thoracic spine
724.2 Lumbago
Low back pain
Low back syndrome
Lumbalgia
Coding Clinic: 2007, Q2, P13-15; 1985, Nov-Dec, P12
724.3 Sciatica
Neuralgia or neuritis of sciatic nerve
Excludes specified lesion of sciatic nerve (355.0)
Coding Clinic: 1989, Q2, P12
■ **724.4 Thoracic or lumbosacral neuritis or radiculitis, unspecified**
Radicular syndrome of lower limbs
Coding Clinic: 1999, Q2, P3-4
■ **724.5 Backache, unspecified**
Vertebrogenic (pain) syndrome NOS
724.6 Disorders of sacrum
Ankylosis, lumbosacral or sacroiliac (joint)
Instability, lumbosacral or sacroiliac (joint)
● **724.7 Disorders of coccyx**
■ **724.70 Unspecified disorder of coccyx**
724.71 Hypermobility of coccyx
■ **724.79 Other**
Coccygodynia
■ **724.8 Other symptoms referable to back**
Ossification of posterior longitudinal ligament NOS
Panniculitis specified as sacral or affecting back
■ **724.9 Other unspecified back disorders**
Ankylosis of spine NOS
Compression of spinal nerve root NEC
Spinal disorder NOS
Excludes sacroiliitis (720.2)

Item 13-3 **Polymyalgia rheumatica** is a syndrome characterized by aching and morning stiffness and is related to aging and hereditary predisposition.

RHEUMATISM, EXCLUDING THE BACK (725–729)

Includes disorders of muscles and tendons and their attachments, and of other soft tissues

725 Polymyalgia rheumatica

● **726 Peripheral enthesopathies and allied syndromes**
Note: Enthesopathies are disorders of peripheral ligamentous or muscular attachments.
Excludes spinal enthesopathy (720.1)
726.0 Adhesive capsulitis of shoulder
● **726.1 Rotator cuff syndrome of shoulder and allied disorders**
■ **726.10 Disorders of bursae and tendons in shoulder region, unspecified**
Rotator cuff syndrome NOS
Supraspinatus syndrome NOS
Coding Clinic: 2001, Q2, P12
726.11 Calcifying tendinitis of shoulder
726.12 Bicipital tenosynovitis
■ **726.19 Other specified disorders**
Excludes complete rupture of rotator cuff, nontraumatic (727.61)
Coding Clinic: 2002, Q1, P9-10
■ **726.2 Other affections of shoulder region, not elsewhere classified**
Periarthritis of shoulder
Scapulohumeral fibrositis
● **726.3 Enthesopathy of elbow region**
■ **726.30 Enthesopathy of elbow, unspecified**
726.31 Medial epicondylitis
726.32 Lateral epicondylitis
Epicondylitis NOS   Tennis elbow
Golfers' elbow
726.33 Olecranon bursitis
Bursitis of elbow
■ **726.39 Other**
726.4 Enthesopathy of wrist and carpus
Bursitis of hand or wrist
Periarthritis of wrist
726.5 Enthesopathy of hip region
Bursitis of hip   Psoas tendinitis
Gluteal tendinitis   Trochanteric tendinitis
Iliac crest spur
● **726.6 Enthesopathy of knee**
■ **726.60 Enthesopathy of knee, unspecified**
Bursitis of knee NOS
726.61 Pes anserinus tendinitis or bursitis
726.62 Tibial collateral ligament bursitis
Pellegrini-Stieda syndrome
726.63 Fibular collateral ligament bursitis
726.64 Patellar tendinitis
726.65 Prepatellar bursitis
Coding Clinic: 2006, Q2, P15
■ **726.69 Other**
Bursitis:
infrapatellar
subpatellar

DISEASES OF THE MUSCULOSKELETAL SYSTEM AND CONNECTIVE TISSUE (710–739)

◄ New   ⬅ Revised   deleted Deleted   ● Use Additional Digit(s)   ■ Nonspecific Code
● Not first-listed DX   OGCR Official Guidelines   Coding Clinic   Excludes   Includes   Use additional   Code first   Omit code

● **726.7 Enthesopathy of ankle and tarsus**

■ **726.70 Enthesopathy of ankle and tarsus, unspecified**
Metatarsalgia NOS

> **Excludes** *Morton's metatarsalgia (355.6)*

726.71 Achilles bursitis or tendinitis

726.72 Tibialis tendinitis
Tibialis (anterior) (posterior) tendinitis

726.73 Calcaneal spur

■ **726.79 Other**
Peroneal tendinitis

■ **726.8 Other peripheral enthesopathies**

● **726.9 Unspecified enthesopathy**

■ **726.90 Enthesopathy of unspecified site**
Capsulitis NOS   Tendinitis NOS
Periarthritis NOS

■ **726.91 Exostosis of unspecified site**
Bone spur NOS
Coding Clinic: 2001, Q2, P13-15

Item 13-4 Synovitis is an inflammation of a synovial membrane resulting in pain on motion and is characterized by fluctuating swelling due to effusion in a synovial sac. **Tenosynovitis** is an inflammation of a tendon sheath and occurs most commonly in the wrists, hands, and feet. Bursitis is inflammation of a bursa (fluid filled sac) caused by repetitive use, trauma, infection, or systemic inflammatory disease. Bursae act as protectors and facilitate movement between bones and overlapping muscles (deep bursae) or between bones and tendons/skin (superficial bursae).

● **727 Other disorders of synovium, tendon, and bursa**

● **727.0 Synovitis and tenosynovitis**

■ **727.00 Synovitis and tenosynovitis, unspecified**
Synovitis NOS
Tenosynovitis NOS

● *727.01 Synovitis and tenosynovitis in diseases classified elsewhere*

> *Code first* underlying disease, as:
> tuberculosis (015.0–015.9)

> **Excludes** *crystal-induced (275.49)*
> *gonococcal (098.51)*
> *gouty (274.00–274.03)* ◄▥
> *syphilitic (095.7)*

727.02 Giant cell tumor of tendon sheath

727.03 Trigger finger (acquired)

727.04 Radial styloid tenosynovitis
de Quervain's disease

■ **727.05 Other tenosynovitis of hand and wrist**

727.06 Tenosynovitis of foot and ankle

■ **727.09 Other**

727.1 Bunion

■ **727.2 Specific bursitides often of occupational origin**
Beat:
elbow
hand
knee
Chronic crepitant synovitis of wrist
Miners':
elbow
knee

■ **727.3 Other bursitis**
Bursitis NOS

> **Excludes** *bursitis:*
> *gonococcal (098.52)*
> *subacromial (726.19)*
> *subcoracoid (726.19)*
> *subdeltoid (726.19)*
> *syphilitic (095.7)*
> *"frozen shoulder" (726.0)*

● **727.4 Ganglion and cyst of synovium, tendon, and bursa**

■ **727.40 Synovial cyst, unspecified**

> **Excludes** *that of popliteal space (727.51)*
> Coding Clinic: 1997, Q2, P6

727.41 Ganglion of joint

727.42 Ganglion of tendon sheath

■ **727.43 Ganglion, unspecified**

■ **727.49 Other**
Cyst of bursa

● **727.5 Rupture of synovium**

■ **727.50 Rupture of synovium, unspecified**

727.51 Synovial cyst of popliteal space
Baker's cyst (knee)

■ **727.59 Other**

● **727.6 Rupture of tendon, nontraumatic**

■ **727.60 Nontraumatic rupture of unspecified tendon**

727.61 Complete rupture of rotator cuff

727.62 Tendons of biceps (long head)

727.63 Extensor tendons of hand and wrist

727.64 Flexor tendons of hand and wrist

727.65 Quadriceps tendon

727.66 Patellar tendon

727.67 Achilles tendon

■ **727.68 Other tendons of foot and ankle**

■ **727.69 Other**

● **727.8 Other disorders of synovium, tendon, and bursa**

727.81 Contracture of tendon (sheath)
Short Achilles tendon (acquired)

727.82 Calcium deposits in tendon and bursa
Calcification of tendon NOS
Calcific tendinitis NOS

> **Excludes** *peripheral ligamentous or muscular*
> *attachments (726.0–726.9)*

727.83 Plica syndrome
Plica knee

■ **727.89 Other**
Abscess of bursa or tendon

> **Excludes** *xanthomatosis localized to tendons*
> *(272.7)*
> Coding Clinic: 1989, Q2, P15; 1985, July-Aug, P14; 1984, Nov-Dec, P9

■ **727.9 Unspecified disorder of synovium, tendon, and bursa**

● **728 Disorders of muscle, ligament, and fascia**

> **Excludes** *enthesopathies (726.0–726.9)*
> *muscular dystrophies (359.0–359.1)*
> *myoneural disorders (358.00–358.9)*
> *myopathies (359.2–359.9)*
> *nontraumatic hematoma of muscle (729.92)*
> *old disruption of ligaments of knee (717.81–717.89)*

728.0 Infective myositis
Myositis:
purulent
suppurative

> **Excludes** *myositis:*
> *epidemic (074.1)*
> *interstitial (728.81)*
> *myoneural disorder (358.00–358.9)*
> *syphilitic (095.6)*
> *tropical (040.81)*

● **728.1 Muscular calcification and ossification**

■ **728.10 Calcification and ossification, unspecified**
Massive calcification (paraplegic)

728.11 Progressive myositis ossificans

728.12 Traumatic myositis ossifications
Myositis ossificans (circumscripta)

728.13 Postoperative heterotopic calcification

■ **728.19 Other**
Polymyositis ossificans

728.2 Muscular wasting and disuse atrophy, not elsewhere classified
Amyotrophia NOS
Myofibrosis

> **Excludes** *neuralgic amyotrophy (353.5)*
> *pelvic muscle wasting and disuse atrophy (618.83)*
> *progressive muscular atrophy (335.0–335.9)*

■ **728.3 Other specific muscle disorders**
Arthrogryposis
Immobility syndrome (paraplegic)

> **Excludes** *arthrogryposis multiplex congenita (754.89)*
> *stiff-man syndrome (333.91)*

728.4 Laxity of ligament

728.5 Hypermobility syndrome

728.6 Contracture of palmar fascia   A
Dupuytren's contracture

● **728.7 Other fibromatoses**

728.71 Plantar fascial fibromatosis
Contracture of plantar fascia
Plantar fasciitis (traumatic)

■ **728.79 Other**
Garrod's or knuckle pads
Nodular fasciitis
Pseudosarcomatous Fibromatosis (proliferative) (subcutaneous)

● **728.8 Other disorders of muscle, ligament, and fascia**

728.81 Interstitial myositis

728.82 Foreign body granuloma of muscle
Talc granuloma of muscle

728.83 Rupture of muscle, nontraumatic

728.84 Diastasis of muscle
Diastasis recti (abdomen)

> **Excludes** *diastasis recti complicating pregnancy, labor, and delivery (665.8)*

728.85 Spasm of muscle

728.86 Necrotizing fasciitis
Use additional code to identify:
infectious organism (041.00–041.89)
gangrene (785.4), if applicable

728.87 Muscle weakness (generalized)

> **Excludes** *generalized weakness (780.79)*

Coding Clinic: 2005, Q1, P13

728.88 Rhabdomyolysis
Coding Clinic: 2003, Q4, P66-67; 2001, Q2, P14

■ **728.89 Other**
Eosinophilic fasciitis
Use additional E code to identify drug, if drug induced
Coding Clinic: 2006, Q3, P13; 2002, Q3, P28; 2001, Q2, P15

■ **728.9 Unspecified disorder of muscle, ligament, and fascia**

● **729 Other disorders of soft tissues**

> **Excludes** *acroparesthesia (443.89)*
> *carpal tunnel syndrome (354.0)*
> *disorders of the back (720.0–724.9)*
> *entrapment syndromes (354.0–355.9)*
> *palindromic rheumatism (719.3)*
> *periarthritis (726.0–726.9)*
> *psychogenic rheumatism (306.0)*

Coding Clinic: 1984, Nov-Dec, P17

■ **729.0 Rheumatism, unspecified and fibrositis**

■ **729.1 Myalgia and myositis, unspecified**
Fibromyositis NOS
Coding Clinic: 1984, Nov-Dec, P17

■ **729.2 Neuralgia, neuritis, and radiculitis, unspecified**

> **Excludes** *brachia radiculitis (723.4)*
> *cervical radiculitis (723.4)*
> *lumbosacral radiculitis (724.4)*
> *mononeuritis (354.0–355.9)*
> *radiculitis due to intervertebral disc involvement (722.0–722.2, 722.7)*
> *sciatica (724.3)*

● **729.3 Panniculitis, unspecified**
Inflammation of adipose tissue of heel pad

■ **729.30 Panniculitis, unspecified site**
Weber-Christian disease

729.31 Hypertrophy of fat pad, knee
Hypertrophy of infrapatellar fat pad

■ **729.39 Other site**

Excludes *panniculitis specified as (affecting):*
back (724.8)
neck (723.6)
sacral (724.8)

■ **729.4 Fasciitis, unspecified**

Excludes *necrotizing fasciitis (728.86)*
nodular fasciitis (728.79)
Coding Clinic: 1994, Q2, P13

729.5 Pain in limb
Coding Clinic: 2007, Q2, P13-15

729.6 Residual foreign body in soft tissue

Excludes *foreign body granuloma:*
muscle (728.82)
skin and subcutaneous tissue (709.4)

● **729.7 Nontraumatic compartment syndrome**

Excludes *compartment syndrome NOS (958.90)*
traumatic compartment syndrome
(958.90–958.99)

Code first, if applicable, postprocedural complication
(998.89)

729.71 Nontraumatic compartment syndrome of upper extremity
Nontraumatic compartment syndrome of shoulder, arm, forearm, wrist, hand and fingers
Coding Clinic: 2006, Q4, P100-102

729.72 Nontraumatic compartment syndrome of lower extremity
Nontraumatic compartment syndrome of hip, buttock, thigh, leg, foot and toes

729.73 Nontraumatic compartment syndrome of abdomen

■ **729.79 Nontraumatic compartment syndrome of other sites**

● **729.8 Other musculoskeletal symptoms referable to limbs**

729.81 Swelling of limb
Coding Clinic: 1988, Q4, P6

729.82 Cramp

■ **729.89 Other**

Excludes *abnormality of gait (781.2)*
tetany (781.7)
transient paralysis of limb (781.4)
Coding Clinic: 1988, Q4, P12

● **729.9 Other and unspecified disorders of soft tissue**
Coding Clinic: 2008, Q4, P134-136

■ **729.90 Disorders of soft tissue, unspecified**

729.91 Post-traumatic seroma

Excludes *seroma complicating a procedure*
(998.13)

729.92 Nontraumatic hematoma of soft tissue
Nontraumatic hematoma of muscle

■ **729.99 Other disorders of soft tissue**
Polyalgia

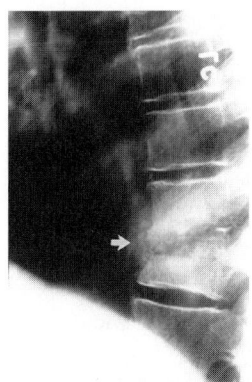

Figure 13-2 Osteomyelitis of the spine. A lateral view of the lower thoracic spine demonstrates destruction of the disk space *(arrow)* as well as destruction of the adjoining vertebral bodies. (From Mettler: Essentials of Radiology, 2nd ed. 2005, Saunders, An Imprint of Elsevier)

Item 13–5 **Osteomyelitis** is an inflammation of the bone. **Acute osteomyelitis** is a rapidly destructive, pus-producing infection capable of causing severe bone destruction. **Chronic osteomyelitis** can remain long after the initial acute episode has passed and may lead to a recurrence of the acute phase. **Brodie's abscess** is an encapsulated focal abscess that must be surgically drained. Periostitis is an inflammation of the periosteum, a dense membrane composed of fibrous connective tissue that closely wraps all bone, except those with articulating surfaces in joints, which are covered by synovial membranes.

OSTEOPATHIES, CHONDROPATHIES, AND ACQUIRED MUSCULOSKELETAL DEFORMITIES (730–739)

● **730 Osteomyelitis, periostitis, and other infections involving bone**

Excludes *jaw (526.4–526.5)*
petrous bone (383.2)

Use additional code to identify organism, such as: Staphylococcus (041.1)
Coding Clinic: 1997, Q4, P43; 1993, 5th Issue, P3

The following fifth-digit subclassification is for use with category 730; valid digits are in [brackets] under each code. See list at beginning of chapter for definitions:

> ■ 0 site unspecified
> 1 shoulder region
> 2 upper arm
> 3 forearm
> 4 hand
> 5 pelvic region and thigh
> 6 lower leg
> 7 ankle and foot
> ■ 8 other specified sites
> ■ 9 multiple sites

● **730.0 Acute osteomyelitis**
[0-9]　Abscess of any bone except accessory sinus, jaw, or mastoid
Acute or subacute osteomyelitis, with or without mention of periostitis

Use additional code to identify major osseous defect, if applicable (731.3)
Coding Clinic: 2004, Q1, P14-15; 2002, Q1, P3-4

DISEASES OF THE MUSCULOSKELETAL SYSTEM AND CONNECTIVE TISSUE (710–739)

730.1 Chronic osteomyelitis
[0-9]
Brodie's abscess
Chronic or old osteomyelitis, with or without mention of periostitis
Sequestrum
Sclerosing osteomyelitis of Garré

Use additional code to identify major osseous defect, if applicable (731.3)

Excludes *aseptic necrosis of bone (733.40–733.49)*

Coding Clinic: 2000, Q3, P4

730.2 Unspecified osteomyelitis
[0-9]
Osteitis or osteomyelitis NOS, with or without mention of periostitis

Use additional code to identify major osseous defect, if applicable (731.3)

730.3 Periostitis without mention of osteomyelitis
[0-9]
Abscess of periosteum, without mention of osteomyelitis
Periostosis, without mention of osteomyelitis

Excludes *that in secondary syphilis (091.61)*

730.7 *Osteopathy resulting from poliomyelitis*
[0-9]
Code first underlying disease (045.0–045.9)

730.8 *Other infections involving bone in disease classified elsewhere*
[0-9]
Code first underlying disease, as:
    tuberculosis (015.0–015.9)
    typhoid fever (002.0)

Excludes *syphilitis of bone NOS (095.5)*

730.9 Unspecified infection of bone
[0-9]

731 Osteitis deformans and osteopathies associated with other disorders classified elsewhere
Also known as Paget's Disease; chronic disorder that results in enlarged and deformed bones. The excessive breakdown and formation of bone tissue causes bones to weaken and results in bone pain, arthritis, deformities, and fractures. Osteopathy describes bone pathologies of unknown cause.

731.0 Osteitis deformans without mention of bone tumor
Paget's disease of bone
Coding Clinic: 1994, Q2, P6-7

731.1 *Osteitis deformans in diseases classified elsewhere*
Code first underlying disease, as:
    malignant neoplasm of bone (170.0–170.9)

731.2 Hypertrophic pulmonary osteoarthropathy
Bamberger-Marie disease

731.3 Major osseous defects
Code first underlying disease, if known, such as:
    aseptic necrosis (733.40–733.49)
    malignant neoplasm of bone (170.0–170.9)
    osteomyelitis (730.00–730.29)
    osteoporosis (733.00–733.09)
    peri-prosthetic osteolysis (996.45)
Coding Clinic: 2006, Q4, P103-104

731.8 *Other bone involvement in diseases classified elsewhere*
Code first underlying disease, as:
    diabetes mellitus (249.8, 250.8)

Use additional code to specify bone condition, such as:
    acute osteomyelitis (730.00–730.09)
Coding Clinic: 2004, Q1, P14-115; 1997, Q4, P43

732 Osteochondropathies

732.0 Juvenile osteochondrosis of spine
Juvenile osteochondrosis (of):
    marginal or vertebral ephiphysis (of Scheuermann) spine NOS
Vertebral epiphysitis

Excludes *adolescent postural kyphosis (737.0)*

732.1 Juvenile osteochondrosis of hip and pelvis
Coxa plana
Ischiopubic synchondrosis (of van Neck)
Osteochondrosis (juvenile) of:
    acetabulum
    head of femur (of Legg-Calvé-Perthes)
    iliac crest (of Buchanan)
    symphysis pubis (of Pierson)
Pseudocoxalgia

732.2 Nontraumatic slipped upper femoral epiphysis
Slipped upper femoral epiphysis NOS

732.3 Juvenile osteochondrosis of upper extremity
Osteochondrosis (juvenile) of:
    capitulum of humerus (of Panner)
    carpal lunate (of Kienbock)
    hand NOS
    head of humerus (of Haas)
    heads of metacarpals (of Mauclaire)
    lower ulna (of Burns)
    radial head (of Brailsford)
    upper extremity NOS

732.4 Juvenile osteochondrosis of lower extremity, excluding foot
Osteochondrosis (juvenile) of:
    lower extremity NOS
    primary patellar center (of Köhler)
    proximal tibia (of Blount)
    secondary patellar center (of Sinding-Larsen)
    tibial tubercle (of Osgood-Schlatter)
Tibia vara

732.5 Juvenile osteochondrosis of foot
Calcaneal apophysitis
Epiphysitis, os calcis
Osteochondrosis (juvenile) of:
    astragalus (of Diaz)
    calcaneum (of Sever)
    foot NOS
    metatarsal:
        second (of Freiberg)
        fifth (of Iselin)
    os tibiale externum (of Haglund)
    tarsal navicular (of Köhler)

732.6 Other juvenile osteochondrosis
Apophysitis specified as juvenile, of other site, or site NOS
Epiphysitis specified as juvenile, of other site, or site NOS
Osteochondritis specified as juvenile, of other site, or site NOS
Osteochondrosis specified as juvenile, of other site, or site NOS

732.7 Osteochondritis dissecans

732.8 Other specified forms of osteochondropathy
Adult osteochondrosis of spine

◀ New   ⫷ Revised   ~~deleted~~ Deleted   ● Use Additional Digit(s)   ■ Nonspecific Code

● Not first-listed DX   OGCR Official Guidelines   Coding Clinic   Excludes   Includes   Use additional   Code first   Omit code

732.9 Unspecified osteochondropathy
Apophysitis
NOS
not specified as adult or juvenile, of unspecified site
Epiphysitis
NOS
not specified as adult or juvenile, of unspecified site
Osteochondritis
NOS
not specified as adult or juvenile, of unspecified site
Osteochondrosis
NOS
not specified as adult or juvenile, of unspecified site

● **733 Other disorders of bone and cartilage**
Excludes *bone spur (726.91)*
cartilage of, or loose body in, joint (717.0–717.9, 718.0–718.9)
giant cell granuloma of jaw (526.3)
osteitis fibrosa cystica generalisata (252.01)
osteomalacia (268.2)
polyostotic fibrous dysplasia of bone (756.54)
prognathism, retrognathism (524.1)
xanthomatosis localized to bone (272.7)

● **733.0 Osteoporosis**
Condition of excessive skeletal fragility (porous bone) resulting in bone fractures
Use additional code to identify:
major osseous defect, if applicable (731.3)
personal history of pathologic (healed) fracture (V13.51)
Coding Clinic: 1993, Q4, P25-26

733.00 Osteoporosis, unspecified
Wedging of vertebra NOS
Coding Clinic: 2007, Q4, P91-92; Q1, P22; 2001, Q3, P19; 1998, Q2, P12

733.01 Senile osteoporosis
Postmenopausal osteoporosis
Coding Clinic: 2007, Q1, P3-8

733.02 Idiopathic osteoporosis

733.03 Disuse osteoporosis

733.09 Other
Drug-induced osteoporosis
Use additional E code to identify drug
Coding Clinic: 2003, Q4, P108-109

● **733.1 Pathologic fracture**
Chronic fracture
Spontaneous fracture ◀
Excludes *stress fracture (733.93–733.95)*
traumatic fractures (800–829)
Coding Clinic: 1986, Nov-Dec, P10; 1985, Nov-Dec, P16

733.10 Pathologic fracture, unspecified site

733.11 Pathologic fracture of humerus

733.12 Pathologic fracture of distal radius and ulna
Wrist NOS

733.13 Pathologic fracture of vertebrae
Collapse of vertebra NOS
Coding Clinic: 2008, Q3, P4; 2007, Q1, P3-8,22; 1999, Q3, P5

733.14 Pathologic fracture of neck of femur
Femur NOS
Hip NOS
Coding Clinic: 2001, Q1, P10-11; 1996, Q1, P16; 1993, Q4, P25-26

733.15 Pathologic fracture of other specified part of femur
Coding Clinic: 1998, Q2, P12; 1994, Q2, P6-7

733.16 Pathologic fracture of tibia and fibula
Ankle NOS

733.19 Pathologic fracture of other specified site

● **733.2 Cyst of bone**
733.20 Cyst of bone (localized), unspecified

733.21 Solitary bone cyst
Unicameral bone cyst

733.22 Aneurysmal bone cyst

733.29 Other
Fibrous dysplasia (monostotic)
Excludes *cyst of jaw (526.0–526.2, 526.89)*
osteitis fibrosa cystica (252.01)
polyostotic fibrous dysplasia of bone (756.54)

733.3 Hyperostosis of skull
Hyperostosis interna frontalis
Leontiasis ossium

● **733.4 Aseptic necrosis of bone**
Use additional code to identify major osseous defect, if applicable (731.3)
Excludes *osteochondropathies (732.0–732.9)*
Coding Clinic: 2007, Q4, P116-120

733.40 Aseptic necrosis of bone, site unspecified

733.41 Head of humerus

733.42 Head and neck of femur
Femur NOS
Excludes *Legg-Calvé-Perthes disease (732.1)*

733.43 Medial femoral condyle

733.44 Talus

733.45 Jaw
Use additional E code to identify drug, if drug-induced
Excludes *osteoradionecrosis of jaw (526.89)*
Coding Clinic: 2007, Q4, P91-92

733.49 Other

733.5 Osteitis condensans
Piriform sclerosis of ilium

733.6 Tietze's disease
Costochondral junction syndrome
Costochondritis

733.7 Algoneurodystrophy
Disuse atrophy of bone
Sudeck's atrophy

● **733.8 Malunion and nonunion of fracture**
733.81 Malunion of fracture
Fracture ends do not heal together correctly.

733.82 Nonunion of fracture
Total failure of fracture healing
Pseudoarthrosis (bone)
Coding Clinic: 1994, Q2, P7; 1987, Jan-Feb, P13; 1984, Nov-Dec, P18

● **733.9 Other and unspecified disorders of bone and cartilage**
Coding Clinic: 2008, Q4, P136-137

733.90 Disorder of bone and cartilage, unspecified

733.91 Arrest of bone development or growth
Epiphyseal arrest

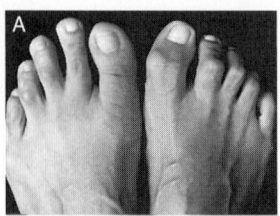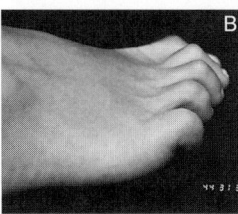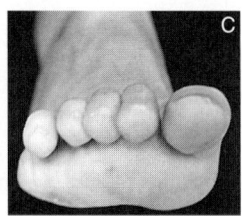

Figure 13-3 **A.** Claw toes, right foot, secondary to medial and lateral plantar nerve laceration. **B.** Metatarsophalangeal joints of second and third toes could not be flexed to neutral position and none could be flexed past neutral. **C.** Extension posture of claw toes increases plantar pressure on metatarsal heads. (From Canale: Campbell's Operative Orthopaedics, 10th ed. 2003, Mosby, Inc.)

733.92 Chondromalacia
Chondromalacia:
NOS
localized, except patella
systemic
tibial plateau
Excludes *chondromalacia of patella (717.7)*

733.93 Stress fracture of tibia or fibula
Stress reaction of tibia or fibula
Use additional external cause code(s) to identify the cause of the stress fracture

733.94 Stress fracture of the metatarsals
Stress reaction of metatarsals
Use additional external cause code(s) to identify the cause of the stress fracture
Coding Clinic: 2001, Q4, P48-49

733.95 Stress fracture of other bone
Stress reaction of other bone
Use additional external cause code(s) to identify the cause of the stress fracture
Excludes *stress fracture of:*
femoral neck (733.96)
fibula (733.93)
metatarsals (733.94)
pelvis (733.98)
shaft of femur (733.97)
tibia (733.93)

733.96 Stress fracture of femoral neck
Stress reaction of femoral neck
Use additional external cause code(s) to identify the cause of the stress fracture

733.97 Stress fracture of shaft of femur
Stress reaction of shaft of femur
Use additional external cause code(s) to identify the cause of the stress fracture

733.98 Stress fracture of pelvis
Stress reaction of pelvis
Use additional external cause code(s) to identify the cause of the stress fracture

733.99 Other
Diaphysitis
Hypertrophy of bone
Relapsing polychondritis
Coding Clinic: 2000, Q3, P4; 1987, Jan-Feb, P14

734 Flat foot
Pes planus (acquired)
Talipes planus (acquired)
Excludes *congenital (754.61)*
rigid flat foot (754.61)
spastic (everted) flat foot (754.61)

Item 13-6 Claw toe is caused by a contraction of the flexor tendon producing a flexion deformity characterized by hyperextension of the big toe.

Figure 13-4 Hallux valgus or bunion.

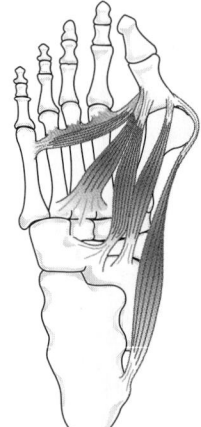

Item 13-7 Hallux valgus, or bunion, is a bursa usually found along the medial aspect of the big toe. It is most often attributed to heredity or poorly fitted shoes.

Item 13-8 Hallux valgus or bunion is a sometimes painful structural deformity caused by an inflammation of the bursal sac at the base of the metatarsophalangeal joint (big toe). **Hallus varus** is a deviation of the great toe to the inner side of the foot or away from the next toe.

Item 13-9 Cubitus valgus is a deformity of the elbow resulting in an increased carrying angle in which the arm extends at the side and the palm faces forward, which results in the forearm and hand extended at greater than 15 degrees. Cubitus varus is a deformity of the elbow resulting in the arm extended at the side and the palm facing forward so that the forearm and hand are held at less than 5 degrees, decreasing the carrying angle.

735 Acquired deformities of toe
Excludes *congenital (754.60–754.69, 755.65–755.66)*
735.0 Hallux valgus (acquired)
735.1 Hallux varus (acquired)
735.2 Hallux rigidus
735.3 Hallux malleus
735.4 Other hammer toe (acquired)
735.5 Claw toe (acquired)
Coding Clinic: 2007, Q4, P123
735.8 Other acquired deformities of toe
735.9 Unspecified acquired deformity of toe

736 Other acquired deformities of limbs
Excludes *congenital (754.3–755.9)*
736.0 Acquired deformities of forearm, excluding fingers
736.00 Unspecified deformity
Deformity of elbow, forearm, hand, or wrist (acquired) NOS

◀ New　◀▥ Revised　deleted Deleted　● Use Additional Digit(s)　■ Nonspecific Code
● Not first-listed DX　OGCR Official Guidelines　Coding Clinic　Excludes　Includes　Use additional　Code first　Omit code

736.01　Cubitus valgus (acquired)

736.02　Cubitus varus (acquired)

736.03　Valgus deformity of wrist (acquired)

736.04　Varus deformity of wrist (acquired)

736.05　Wrist drop (acquired)

736.06　Claw hand (acquired)

736.07　Club hand (acquired)

■736.09　Other

736.1　Mallet finger

● 736.2　Other acquired deformities of finger

■736.20　Unspecified deformity
　　　　　Deformity of finger (acquired) NOS

736.21　Boutonniere deformity

736.22　Swan-neck deformity

■736.29　Other
　　　　　Excludes *trigger finger (727.03)*
　　　　　Coding Clinic: 2005, Q2, P7; 1989, Q2, P13

● 736.3　Acquired deformities of hip
　　　　　Coding Clinic: 2008, Q2, P3-4

■736.30　Unspecified deformity
　　　　　Deformity of hip (acquired) NOS

736.31　Coxa valga (acquired)

736.32　Coxa vara (acquired)

■736.39　Other

● 736.4　Genu valgum or varum (acquired)

736.41　Genu valgum (acquired)

736.42　Genu varum (acquired)

736.5　Genu recurvatum (acquired)

■736.6　Other acquired deformities of knee
　　　　　Deformity of knee (acquired) NOS

● 736.7　Other acquired deformities of ankle and foot
　　　　　Excludes *deformities of toe (acquired) (735.0–735.9)*
　　　　　　　　　　pes planus (acquired) (734)

■736.70　Unspecified deformity of ankle and foot, acquired

736.71　Acquired equinovarus deformity
　　　　　Clubfoot, acquired
　　　　　Excludes *clubfoot not specified as acquired (754.5–754.7)*

736.72　Equinus deformity of foot, acquired

736.73　Cavus deformity of foot
　　　　　Excludes *that with claw foot (736.74)*

736.74　Claw foot, acquired

736.75　Cavovarus deformity of foot, acquired

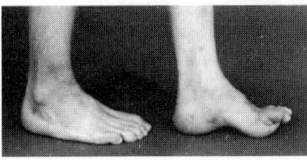

Figure 13–5 Supination and cavus deformity of forefoot. *(Courtesy Jay Cummings, MD.)* (From Canale: Campbell's Operative Orthopaedics, 10th ed. 2003, Mosby, Inc.)

Item 13–10　Equinus foot is a term referring to the hoof of a horse. The deformity is usually congenital or spastic. Talipes equinovarus is referred to as clubfoot. The foot tends to be smaller than normal, with the heel pointing downward and the forefoot turning inward. The heel cord (Achilles tendon) is tight, causing the heel to be drawn up toward the leg.

■736.76　Other calcaneus deformity

■736.79　Other
　　　　　Acquired:
　　　　　　pes not elsewhere classified
　　　　　　talipes not elsewhere classified

● 736.8　Acquired deformities of other parts of limbs

736.81　Unequal leg length (acquired)
　　　　　Coding Clinic: 1995, Q1, P10

■736.89　Other
　　　　　Deformity (acquired):
　　　　　　arm or leg, not elsewhere classified
　　　　　　shoulder
　　　　　Coding Clinic: 2008, Q2, P5-6

■736.9　Acquired deformity of limb, site unspecified
　　　　　Coding Clinic: 2008, Q2, P3-4

● 737　Curvature of spine
　　　　　Excludes *congenital (754.2)*

737.0　Adolescent postural kyphosis
　　　　　Excludes *osteochondrosis of spine (juvenile) (732.0)*
　　　　　　　　　　adult (732.8)

● ■737.1　Kyphosis (acquired)

737.10　Kyphosis (acquired) (postural)

737.11　Kyphosis due to radiation

737.12　Kyphosis, postlaminectomy

■737.19　Other
　　　　　Excludes *that associated with conditions classifiable elsewhere (737.41)*
　　　　　Coding Clinic: 2007, Q1, P20-21

Item 13–11　Kyphosis is an abnormal curvature of the spine. **Senile kyphosis** is a result of disc degeneration causing ossification (turning to bone). **Adolescent** or **juvenile kyphosis** is also known as **Scheuermann's disease,** a condition in which the discs of the lower thoracic spine herniate, causing the disc space to narrow and the spine to tilt forward. This condition is attributed to poor posture. Lordosis or swayback is an abnormal curvature of the spine resulting in an inward curve of the lumbar spine just above the buttocks. Scoliosis causes a sideways curve to the spine. The curves are S- or C-shaped, and it is most commonly acquired in late childhood and early teen years, when growth is fast.

Item 13–12　Spondylolisthesis is a condition caused by the slipping forward of one disc over another.

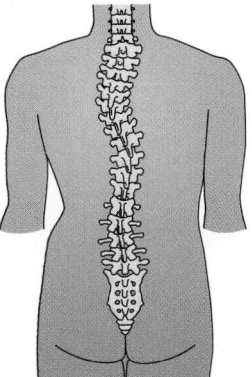

Figure 13–6 Scoliosis is a lateral curvature of the spine.

DISEASES OF THE MUSCULOSKELETAL SYSTEM AND CONNECTIVE TISSUE (710–739)

DISEASES OF THE MUSCULOSKELETAL SYSTEM AND CONNECTIVE TISSUE (710–739)

● **737.2 Lordosis (acquired)**
  Abnormal increase in normal curvature of lumbar spine (sway back)

    737.20 Lordosis (acquired) (postural)

    737.21 Lordosis, postlaminectomy

    737.22 Other postsurgical lordosis

    ■**737.29 Other**
        Excludes *that associated with conditions classifiable elsewhere (737.42)*

● **737.3 Kyphoscoliosis and scoliosis**

    737.30 Scoliosis [and kyphoscoliosis], idiopathic
        Coding Clinic: 2003, Q3, P19x2

    737.31 Resolving infantile idiopathic scoliosis

    737.32 Progressive infantile idiopathic scoliosis
        Coding Clinic: 2002, Q3, P12

    737.33 Scoliosis due to radiation

    737.34 Thoracogenic scoliosis

    ■**737.39 Other**
        Excludes *that associated with conditions classifiable elsewhere (737.43)*
        that in kyphoscoliotic heart disease (416.1)
        Coding Clinic: 2002, Q2, P16

● **737.4 Curvature of spine associated with other conditions**
    Code first associated condition, as:
    Charcot-Marie-Tooth disease (356.1)
    mucopolysaccharidosis (277.5)
    neurofibromatosis (237.7)
    osteitis deformans (731.0)
    osteitis fibrosa cystica (252.01)
    osteoporosis (733.00–733.09)
    poliomyelitis (138)
    tuberculosis [Pott's curvature] (015.0)

    ● ■**737.40 *Curvature of spine, unspecified***

    ● **737.41 *Kyphosis***

    ● **737.42 *Lordosis***

    ● **737.43 *Scoliosis***

■**737.8 Other curvatures of spine**

■**737.9 Unspecified curvature of spine**
    Curvature of spine (acquired) (idiopathic) NOS
    Hunchback, acquired
    Excludes *deformity of spine NOS (738.5)*

● **738 Other acquired deformity**
    Excludes *congenital (754.0–756.9, 758.0–759.9)*
    dentofacial anomalies (524.0–524.9)

    738.0 Acquired deformity of nose
    Deformity of nose (acquired)
    Overdevelopment of nasal bones
    Excludes *deflected or deviated nasal septum (470)*

● **738.1 Other acquired deformity of head**

    ■**738.10 Unspecified deformity**

    738.11 Zygomatic hyperplasia

    738.12 Zygomatic hypoplasia

    ■**738.19 Other specified deformity**
        Coding Clinic: 2006, Q1, P6-7; 2003, Q2, P13

738.2 Acquired deformity of neck

738.3 Acquired deformity of chest and rib
    Deformity:
    chest (acquired)
    rib (acquired)
    Pectus:
    carinatum, acquired
    excavatum, acquired

738.4 Acquired spondylolisthesis
    Degenerative spondylolisthesis
    Spondylolysis, acquired
    Excludes *congenital (756.12)*
    Coding Clinic: 2007, Q4, P116-120

■**738.5 Other acquired deformity of back or spine**
    Deformity of spine NOS
    Excludes *curvature of spine (737.0–737.9)*
    Coding Clinic: 2007, Q4, P116-120

738.6 Acquired deformity of pelvis
    Pelvic obliquity
    Excludes *intrapelvic protrusion of acetabulum (718.6)*
    that in relation to labor and delivery (653.0–653.4, 653.8–653.9)

738.7 Cauliflower ear

■**738.8 Acquired deformity of other specified site**
    Deformity of clavicle
    Coding Clinic: 2001, Q2, P14-15

■**738.9 Acquired deformity of unspecified site**

● **739 Nonallopathic lesions, not elsewhere classified**
    Includes segmental dysfunction
    somatic dysfunction
    Coding Clinic: 1995, Q4, P51; 1990, Q1, P18

    739.0 Head region
    Occipitocervical region

    739.1 Cervical region
    Cervicothoracic region

    739.2 Thoracic region
    Thoracolumbar region

    739.3 Lumbar region
    Lumbosacral region

    739.4 Sacral region
    Sacrococcygeal region
    Sacroiliac region

    739.5 Pelvic region
    Hip region
    Pubic region

    739.6 Lower extremities

    739.7 Upper extremities
    Acromioclavicular region
    Sternoclavicular region

    739.8 Rib cage
    Costochondral region
    Costovertebral region
    Sternochondral region

    739.9 Abdomen and other

◄ New ◄ Revised ~~deleted~~ Deleted ● Use Additional Digit(s) ■ Nonspecific Code
● Not first-listed DX OGCR Official Guidelines Coding Clinic Excludes Includes Use additional Code first Omit code

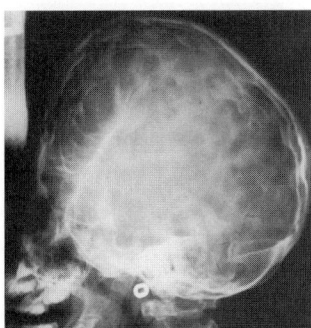

Figure 14-1 Generalized craniosynostosis in a 4-year-old girl without symptoms or signs of increased intracranial pressure. (From Bell WE, McCormick WF: Increased Intracranial Pressure in Children, 2nd ed. Philadelphia, WB Saunders, 1978, p 116.)

Item 14-1 **Anencephalus** is a congenital deformity of the cranial vault. **Craniosynostosis**, also known as craniostenosis and stenocephaly, signifies any form of congenital deformity of the skull that results from the premature closing of the sutures of the skull. **Iniencephaly** is a deformity in which the head and neck are flexed backward to a great extent and the head is very large in comparison to the shortened body.

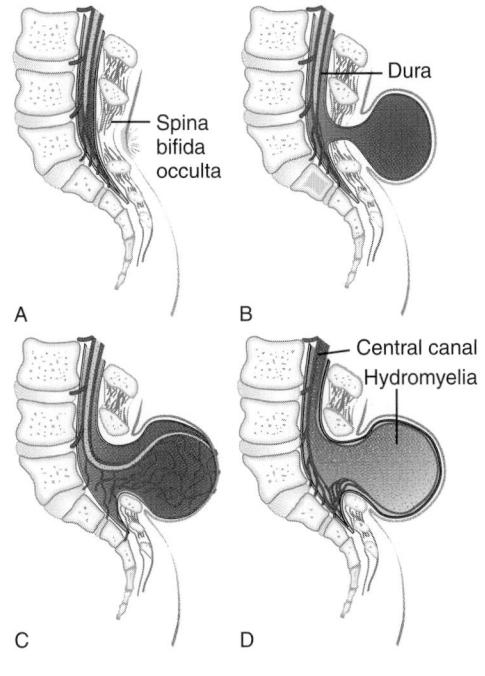

Figure 14-2 **A.** Spina bifida occulta. **B.** Meningocele. **C.** Myelomeningocele. **D.** Myelocystocele (syringomyelocele) or hydromyelia.

Item 14-2 **Spina bifida** is a midline spinal defect in which one or more vertebrae fail to fuse, leaving an opening in the vertebral canal. When the defect is not visible, it is called spina bifida occulta, and when it is visible, it is called spina bifida cystica.

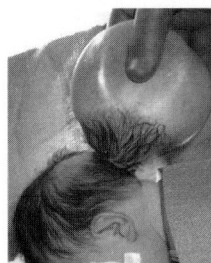

Figure 14-3 An infant with a large occipital encephalocele. The large skin-covered encephalocele is visible. (From Townsend: Sabiston Textbook of Surgery, 17th ed. 2004, Saunders, An Imprint of Elsevier)

14. CONGENITAL ANOMALIES (740–759)

● **740 Anencephalus and similar anomalies**

740.0 Anencephalus
Acrania
Amyelencephalus
Hemianencephaly
Hemicephaly

740.1 Craniorachischisis

740.2 Iniencephaly

● **741 Spina bifida**

Excludes spina bifida occulta (756.17)
Coding Clinic: 1994, Q3, P7

The following fifth-digit subclassification is for use with category 741:

> 0 **unspecified region**
> 1 **cervical region**
> 2 **dorsal (thoracic) region**
> 3 **lumbar region**

● **741.0 With hydrocephalus**
[0-3] Arnold-Chiari syndrome, type II
Any condition classifiable to 741.9 with any condition classifiable to 742.3
Chiari malformation, type II
Coding Clinic: 1997, Q4, P51; 1987, Sept-Oct, P10

● **741.9 Without mention of hydrocephalus**
[0-3] Hydromeningocele (spinal)
Hydromyelocele
Meningocele (spinal)
Meningomyelocele
Myelocele
Myelocystocele
Rachischisis
Spina bifida (aperta)
Syringomyelocele
Coding Clinic: 1987, Sept-Oct, P10

● **742 Other congenital anomalies of nervous system**

Excludes congenital central alveolar hypoventilation syndrome (327.25)

742.0 Encephalocele
Sac-like protrusions of brain and membranes visible through an opening in various locations in skull
Encephalocystocele
Encephalomyelocele
Hydroencephalocele
Hydromeningocele, cranial
Meningocele, cerebral
Meningoencephalocele

742.1 Microcephalus
Describes head size that measures significantly below normal based on standardized charts for age and sex
Hydromicrocephaly
Micrencephaly

742.2 Reduction deformities of brain
Absence of part of brain
Agenesis of part of brain
Agyria
Aplasia of part of brain
Arhinencephaly
Holoprosencephaly
Hypoplasia of part of brain
Microgyria
Coding Clinic: 2003, Q3, P15-16

N Newborn Age: 0   **P** Pediatric Age: 0–17   **M** Maternity Age: 12–55   **A** Adult Age: 15–124   ♀ Females Only   ♂ Males Only   **1015**

CONGENITAL ANOMALIES (740–759)

742.3 Congenital hydrocephalus

An accumulation of cerebrospinal fluid in ventricles resulting in swelling and enlargement

Aqueduct of Sylvius:
  anomaly
  obstruction, congenital
  stenosis
Atresia of foramina of Magendie and Luschka
Hydrocephalus in newborn

Excludes *hydrocephalus:*
  acquired (331.3–331.4)
  due to congenital toxoplasmosis (771.2)
  with any condition classifiable to 741.9 (741.0)

Coding Clinic: 2005, Q4, P82-83

742.4 Other specified anomalies of brain

Congenital cerebral cyst
Macroencephaly
Macrogyria
Megalencephaly
Multiple anomalies of brain NOS
Porencephaly
Ulegyria

Coding Clinic: 1999, Q1, P9-10; 1992, Q3, P12

742.5 Other specified anomalies of spinal cord

742.51 Diastematomyelia

742.53 Hydromyelia
  Hydrorhachis

742.59 Other
  Amyelia
  Atelomyelia
  Congenital anomaly of spinal meninges
  Defective development of cauda equina
  Hypoplasia of spinal cord
  Myelatelia
  Myelodysplasia

Coding Clinic: 1991, Q2, P14; 1989, Q1, P10

742.8 Other specified anomalies of nervous system

Agenesis of nerve
Displacement of brachial plexus
Familial dysautonomia
Jaw-winking syndrome
Marcus-Gunn syndrome
Riley-Day syndrome

Excludes *neurofibromatosis (237.7)*

742.9 Unspecified anomaly of brain, spinal cord, and nervous system

Anomaly of brain, nervous system, and spinal cord
Congenital, of brain, nervous system, and spinal cord:
  disease of brain, nervous system, and spinal cord
  lesion of brain, nervous system, and spinal cord
Deformity of brain, nervous system, and spinal cord

743 Congenital anomalies of eye

743.0 Anophthalmos

Absence of eye and optic pit

743.00 Clinical anophthalmos, unspecified
  Agenesis
  Congenital absence of eye
  Anophthalmos NOS

743.03 Cystic eyeball, congenital

743.06 Cryptophthalmos

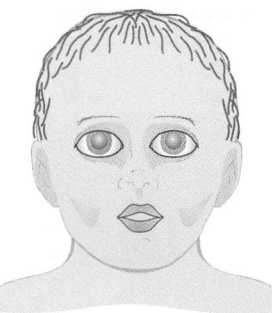

Figure 14–4 Bilateral congenital **hydrophthalmia,** in which the eyes are very large in comparison to the other facial features due to glaucoma.

743.1 Microphthalmos

Partial absence of eye and optic pit
Dysplasia of eye
Hypoplasia of eye
Rudimentary eye

743.10 Microphthalmos, unspecified

743.11 Simple microphthalmos

743.12 Microphthalmos associated with other anomalies of eye and adnexa

743.2 Buphthalmos

Also known as Sturge-Weber Syndrome and is congenital syndrome characterized by a port-wine nevus covering portions of face and cranium
Glaucoma:
  congenital
  newborn
Hydrophthalmos

Excludes *glaucoma of childhood (365.14)*
  traumatic glaucoma due to birth injury (767.8)

743.20 Buphthalmos, unspecified

743.21 Simple buphthalmos

743.22 Buphthalmos associated with other ocular anomalies
  Keratoglobus, congenital, associated with buphthalmos
  Megalocornea associated with buphthalmos

743.3 Congenital cataract and lens anomalies

Excludes *infantile cataract (366.00–366.09)*

743.30 Congenital cataract, unspecified

743.31 Capsular and subcapsular cataract

743.32 Cortical and zonular cataract

743.33 Nuclear cataract

743.34 Total and subtotal cataract, congenital

743.35 Congenital aphakia
  Congenital absence of lens

743.36 Anomalies of lens shape
  Microphakia
  Spherophakia

743.37 Congenital ectopic lens

743.39 Other

743.4 Coloboma and other anomalies of anterior segment

743.41 Anomalies of corneal size and shape
  Microcornea

Excludes *that associated with buphthalmos (743.22)*

743.42 Corneal opacities, interfering with vision, congenital

■743.43 **Other corneal opacities, congenital**

■743.44 **Specified anomalies of anterior chamber, chamber angle, and related structures**
Anomaly:
    Axenfeld's
    Peters'
    Rieger's

743.45 **Aniridia**
Coding Clinic: 2002, Q3, P20-21

■743.46 **Other specified anomalies of iris and ciliary body**
Anisocoria, congenital
Atresia of pupil
Coloboma of iris
Corectopia

■743.47 **Specified anomalies of sclera**

■743.48 **Multiple and combined anomalies of anterior segment**

■743.49 **Other**

● 743.5 **Congenital anomalies of posterior segment**

743.51 **Vitreous anomalies**
Congenital vitreous opacity

743.52 **Fundus coloboma**

743.53 **Chorioretinal degeneration, congenital**

743.54 **Congenital folds and cysts of posterior segment**

743.55 **Congenital macular changes**

■743.56 **Other retinal changes, congenital**
Coding Clinic: 1999, Q3, P12

■743.57 **Specified anomalies of optic disc**
Coloboma of optic disc (congenital)

743.58 **Vascular anomalies**
Congenital retinal aneurysm

■743.59 **Other**

● 743.6 **Congenital anomalies of eyelids, lacrimal system, and orbit**

743.61 **Congenital ptosis**

743.62 **Congenital deformities of eyelids**
Ablepharon
Absence of eyelid
Accessory eyelid
Congenital:
    ectropion
    entropion
Coding Clinic: 2000, Q1, P22-23

■743.63 **Other specified congenital anomalies of eyelid**
Absence, agenesis, of cilia

■743.64 **Specified congenital anomalies of lacrimal gland**

■743.65 **Specified congenital anomalies of lacrimal passages**
Absence, agenesis of:
    lacrimal apparatus
    punctum lacrimale
Accessory lacrimal canal

■743.66 **Specified congenital anomalies of orbit**

■743.69 **Other**
Accessory eye muscles

■743.8 **Other specified anomalies of eye**

Excludes *congenital nystagmus (379.51)*
ocular albinism (270.2)
optic nerve hypoplasia (377.43)
retinitis pigmentosa (362.74)

■743.9 **Unspecified anomaly of eye**
Congenital:
    anomaly NOS of eye [any part]
    deformity NOS of eye [any part]

● 744 **Congenital anomalies of ear, face, and neck**

Excludes *anomaly of:*
cervical spine (754.2, 756.10–756.19)
larynx (748.2–748.3)
nose (748.0–748.1)
parathyroid gland (759.2)
thyroid gland (759.2)
cleft lip (749.10–749.25)

● ■744.0 **Anomalies of ear causing impairment of hearing**

Excludes *congenital deafness without mention of cause (380.0–389.9)*

■744.00 **Unspecified anomaly of ear with impairment of hearing**

744.01 **Absence of external ear**
Absence of:
    auditory canal (external)
    auricle (ear) (with stenosis or atresia of auditory canal)

■744.02 **Other anomalies of external ear with impairment of hearing**
Atresia or stricture of auditory canal (external)

744.03 **Anomaly of middle ear, except ossicles**
Atresia or stricture of osseous meatus (ear)

744.04 **Anomalies of ear ossicles**
Fusion of ear ossicles

744.05 **Anomalies of inner ear**
Congenital anomaly of:
    membranous labyrinth
    organ of Corti

■744.09 **Other**
Absence of ear, congenital

744.1 **Accessory auricle**
Accessory tragus
Polyotia
Preauricular appendage
Supernumerary:
    ear
    lobule

● 744.2 **Other specified anomalies of ear**

Excludes *that with impairment of hearing (744.00–744.09)*

744.21 **Absence of ear lobe, congenital**

744.22 **Macrotia**
Enlarged ear

744.23 **Microtia**
Abnormally small ear

■744.24 **Specified anomalies of Eustachian tube**
Absence of Eustachian tube

■744.29 **Other**
Bat ear
Darwin's tubercle
Pointed ear
Prominence of auricle
Ridge ear

Excludes *preauricular sinus (744.46)*

■744.3 **Unspecified anomaly of ear**
Congenital:
    anomaly NOS of ear, NEC
    deformity NOS of ear, NEC

CONGENITAL ANOMALIES (740–759)

● **744.4 Branchial cleft cyst or fistula; preauricular sinus**

    744.41 Branchial cleft sinus or fistula
        Branchial:
           sinus (external) (internal)
           vestige

    744.42 Branchial cleft cyst

    744.43 Cervical auricle

    744.46 Preauricular sinus or fistula

    744.47 Preauricular cyst

    ■**744.49 Other**
        Fistula (of):
           auricle, congenital
           cervicoaural

  744.5 Webbing of neck
    Pterygium colli

● **744.8 Other specified anomalies of face and neck**

    744.81 Macrocheilia
        Hypertrophy of lip, congenital

    744.82 Microcheilia

    744.83 Macrostomia
        Abnormally large mouth

    744.84 Microstomia

    ■**744.89 Other**
        Excludes *congenital fistula of lip (750.25)*
               musculoskeletal anomalies
                 (754.0–754.1, 756.0)

■**744.9 Unspecified anomalies of face and neck**
    Congenital:
        anomaly NOS of face [any part] or neck [any
           part]
        deformity NOS of face [any part] or neck [any
           part]

● **745 Bulbus cordis anomalies and anomalies of cardiac septal closure**

  745.0 Common truncus
    Absent septum between aorta and pulmonary
        artery
    Communication (abnormal) between aorta and
        pulmonary artery
    Aortic septal defect
    Common aortopulmonary trunk
    Persistent truncus arteriosus

● **745.1 Transposition of great vessels**

    745.10 Complete transposition of great vessels
        Transposition of great vessels:
           NOS
           classical

    745.11 Double outlet right ventricle
        Dextrotransposition of aorta
        Incomplete transposition of great vessels
        Origin of both great vessels from right
           ventricle
        Taussig-Bing syndrome or defect

    745.12 Corrected transposition of great vessels

    ■**745.19 Other**

  745.2 Tetralogy of Fallot
    Fallot's pentalogy
    Ventricular septal defect with pulmonary stenosis
        or atresia, dextroposition of aorta, and
        hypertrophy of right ventricle
      Excludes *Fallot's triad (746.09)*

  745.3 Common ventricle
    Cor triloculare biatriatum
    Single ventricle

  745.4 Ventricular septal defect
    Eisenmenger's defect or complex
    Gerbode defect
    Interventricular septal defect
    Left ventricular-right atrial communication
    Roger's disease
      Excludes *common atrioventricular canal type*
               (745.69)
               single ventricle (745.3)

  745.5 Ostium secundum type atrial septal defect
    Defect: Patent or persistent:
      atrium secundum   foramen ovale
      fossa ovalis   ostium secundum
    Lutembacher's syndrome

● **745.6 Endocardial cushion defects**

    ■**745.60 Endocardial cushion defect, unspecified type**

    745.61 Ostium primum defect
        Persistent ostium primum

    ■**745.69 Other**
        Absence of atrial septum
        Atrioventricular canal type ventricular
           septal defect
        Common atrioventricular canal
        Common atrium

  745.7 Cor biloculare
    Absence of atrial and ventricular septa

■**745.8 Other**

■**745.9 Unspecified defect of septal closure**
    Septal defect NOS

● **746 Other congenital anomalies of heart**
    Excludes *endocardial fibroelastosis (425.3)*
    Coding Clinic: 2004, Q3, P4-5

● **746.0 Anomalies of pulmonary valve**
    Excludes *infundibular or subvalvular pulmonic*
               stenosis (746.83)
               tetralogy of Fallot (745.2)

    ■**746.00 Pulmonary valve anomaly, unspecified**

    746.01 Atresia, congenital
        Congenital absence of pulmonary valve

    746.02 Stenosis, congenital
        Coding Clinic: 2004, Q1, P16-17

    ■**746.09 Other**
        Congenital insufficiency of pulmonary
           valve
        Fallot's triad or trilogy

  746.1 Tricuspid atresia and stenosis, congenital
    Absence of tricuspid valve

  746.2 Ebstein's anomaly

  746.3 Congenital stenosis of aortic valve
    Congenital aortic stenosis
      Excludes *congenital:*
               subaortic stenosis (746.81)
               supravalvular aortic stenosis (747.22)
      Coding Clinic: 1988, Q4, P8

  746.4 Congenital insufficiency of aortic valve
    Bicuspid aortic valve
    Congenital aortic insufficiency

746.5　Congenital mitral stenosis
　　　Fused commissure of mitral valve
　　　Parachute deformity of mitral valve
　　　Supernumerary cusps of mitral valve
　　　Coding Clinic: 2007, Q3, P3

746.6　Congenital mitral insufficiency

746.7　Hypoplastic left heart syndrome
　　　Atresia, or marked hypoplasia, of aortic orifice or
　　　　valve, with hypoplasia of ascending aorta and
　　　　defective development of left ventricle (with
　　　　mitral valve atresia)

● **746.8　Other specified anomalies of heart**

　　746.81　Subaortic stenosis
　　　　　Coding Clinic: 2007, Q3, P3

　　746.82　Cor triatriatum

　　746.83　Infundibular pulmonic stenosis
　　　　　Subvalvular pulmonic stenosis

　　746.84　Obstructive anomalies of heart, NEC
　　　　　Shone's syndrome
　　　　　Uhl's disease

　　　　　Use additional code for associated
　　　　　　anomalies, such as:
　　　　　　coarctation of aorta (747.10)
　　　　　　congenital mitral stenosis (746.5)
　　　　　　subaortic stenosis (746.81)

　　746.85　Coronary artery anomaly
　　　　　Anomalous origin or communication of
　　　　　　coronary artery
　　　　　Arteriovenous malformation of coronary
　　　　　　artery
　　　　　Coronary artery:
　　　　　　absence
　　　　　　arising from aorta or pulmonary trunk
　　　　　　single

　　746.86　Congenital heart block
　　　　　Complete or incomplete atrioventricular
　　　　　　[AV] block

　　746.87　Malposition of heart and cardiac apex
　　　　　Abdominal heart
　　　　　Dextrocardia
　　　　　Ectopia cordis
　　　　　Levocardia (isolated)
　　　　　Mesocardia

　　　　　Excludes *dextrocardia with complete*
　　　　　　transposition of viscera
　　　　　　(759.3)

　　■**746.89　Other**
　　　　　Atresia of cardiac vein
　　　　　Hypoplasia of cardiac vein
　　　　　Congenital:
　　　　　　cardiomegaly
　　　　　　diverticulum, left ventricle
　　　　　　pericardial defect
　　　　　Coding Clinic: 2000, Q3, P3; 1999, Q1, P11; 1995, Q1, P8

■**746.9　Unspecified anomaly of heart**
　　　Congenital:
　　　　anomaly of heart NOS
　　　　heart disease NOS

● **747　Other congenital anomalies of circulatory system**

　747.0　Patent ductus arteriosus *(PDA)*
　　　　Patent ductus Botalli
　　　　Persistent ductus arteriosus

● **747.1　Coarctation of aorta**

　　747.10　Coarctation of aorta (preductal) (postductal)
　　　　　Hypoplasia of aortic arch
　　　　　Coding Clinic: 2007, Q3, P3; 1999, Q1, P11; 1988, Q4, P8

　　747.11　Interruption of aortic arch

● **747.2　Other anomalies of aorta**

　　■**747.20　Anomaly of aorta, unspecified**

　　747.21　Anomalies of aortic arch
　　　　　Anomalous origin, right subclavian artery
　　　　　Dextroposition of aorta
　　　　　Double aortic arch
　　　　　Kommerell's diverticulum
　　　　　Overriding aorta
　　　　　Persistent:
　　　　　　convolutions, aortic arch
　　　　　　right aortic arch
　　　　　Vascular ring

　　　　　Excludes *hypoplasia of aortic arch (747.10)*

　　　　　Coding Clinic: 2003, Q1, P15-16

　　747.22　Atresia and stenosis of aorta
　　　　　Absence of aorta
　　　　　Aplasia of aorta
　　　　　Hypoplasia of aorta
　　　　　Stricture of aorta
　　　　　Supra (valvular)-aortic stenosis

　　　　　Excludes *congenital aortic (valvular) stenosis*
　　　　　　or stricture, so stated (746.3)
　　　　　　hypoplasia of aorta in hypoplastic
　　　　　　left heart syndrome (746.7)

　　　　　Coding Clinic: 1988, Q4, P8

　　■**747.29　Other**
　　　　　Aneurysm of sinus of Valsalva
　　　　　Congenital:　　　　　　Congenital:
　　　　　　aneurysm of aorta　　　dilation of aorta

　747.3　Anomalies of pulmonary artery
　　　　Agenesis of pulmonary artery
　　　　Anomaly of pulmonary artery
　　　　Atresia of pulmonary artery
　　　　Coarctation of pulmonary artery
　　　　Hypoplasia of pulmonary artery
　　　　Stenosis of pulmonary artery
　　　　Pulmonary arteriovenous aneurysm
　　　　Coding Clinic: 2004, Q1, P16-17; 1994, Q1, P15

● **747.4　Anomalies of great veins**

　　■**747.40　Anomaly of great veins, unspecified**
　　　　　Anomaly NOS of:　　　Anomaly NOS of:
　　　　　　pulmonary veins　　　vena cava

　　747.41　Total anomalous pulmonary venous
　　　　　connection
　　　　　Total anomalous pulmonary venous return
　　　　　　[TAPVR]:
　　　　　　subdiaphragmatic
　　　　　　supradiaphragmatic

　　747.42　Partial anomalous pulmonary venous
　　　　　connection
　　　　　Partial anomalous pulmonary venous
　　　　　　return

CONGENITAL ANOMALIES (740–759)

747.49 Other anomalies of great veins
Absence of vena cava (inferior) (superior)
Congenital stenosis of vena cava (inferior)
(superior)
Persistent:
left posterior cardinal vein
left superior vena cava
Scimitar syndrome
Transposition of pulmonary veins NOS

747.5 Absence or hypoplasia of umbilical artery
Single umbilical artery

● **747.6 Other anomalies of peripheral vascular system**
Absence of artery or vein, NEC
Anomaly of artery or vein, NEC
Atresia of artery or vein, NEC
Arteriovenous aneurysm (peripheral)
Arteriovenous malformation of the peripheral
vascular system
Congenital: Congenital:
aneurysm (peripheral)   stricture, artery
phlebectasia   varix
Multiple renal arteries

Excludes anomalies of:
cerebral vessels (747.81)
pulmonary artery (747.3)
congenital retinal aneurysm (743.58)
hemangioma (228.00–228.09)
lymphangioma (228.1)

**747.60 Anomaly of the peripheral vascular system,
unspecified site**

747.61 Gastrointestinal vessel anomaly
Coding Clinic: 1996, Q3, P10

747.62 Renal vessel anomaly

747.63 Upper limb vessel anomaly

747.64 Lower limb vessel anomaly

**747.69 Anomalies of other specified sites of
peripheral vascular system**

● **747.8 Other specified anomalies of circulatory system**

747.81 Anomalies of cerebrovascular system
Arteriovenous malformation of brain
Cerebral arteriovenous aneurysm,
congenital
Congenital anomalies of cerebral vessels

Excludes ruptured cerebral (arteriovenous)
aneurysm (430)
Coding Clinic: 1985, Jan-Feb, P15

747.82 Spinal vessel anomaly
Arteriovenous malformation of spinal
vessel
Coding Clinic: 1995, Q3, P5-6

747.83 Persistent fetal circulation   N
Persistent pulmonary hypertension
Primary pulmonary hypertension of
newborn
Coding Clinic: 2002, Q4, P62-63

747.89 Other
Aneurysm, congenital, specified site not
elsewhere classified

Excludes congenital aneurysm:
coronary (746.85)
peripheral (747.6)
pulmonary (747.3)
retinal (743.58)

747.9 Unspecified anomaly of circulatory system

● **748 Congenital anomalies of respiratory system**

Excludes congenital central alveolar hypoventilation
syndrome (327.25)
congenital defect of diaphragm (756.6)

748.0 Choanal atresia
Atresia of nares (anterior) (posterior)
Congenital stenosis of nares (anterior) (posterior)

748.1 Other anomalies of nose
Absent nose
Accessory nose
Cleft nose
Deformity of wall of nasal sinus
Congenital:
deformity of nose
notching of tip of nose
perforation of wall of nasal sinus

Excludes congenital deviation of nasal septum (754.0)

748.2 Web of larynx
Web of larynx: Web of larynx:
NOS   subglottic
glottic

748.3 Other anomalies of larynx, trachea, and bronchus
Absence or agenesis of:
bronchus
larynx
trachea
Anomaly (of):   Anomaly (of):
cricoid cartilage   thyroid cartilage
epiglottis   tracheal cartilage
Atresia (of):   Atresia (of):
epiglottis   larynx
glottis   trachea
Cleft thyroid, cartilage, congenital
Congenital:
dilation, trachea
stenosis:
larynx
trachea
tracheocele
Diverticulum:
bronchus
trachea
Fissure of epiglottis
Laryngocele
Posterior cleft of cricoid cartilage (congenital)
Rudimentary tracheal bronchus
Stridor, laryngeal, congenital
Coding Clinic: 1999, Q1, P14

748.4 Congenital cystic lung
Disease, lung:
cystic, congenital
polycystic, congenital
Honeycomb lung, congenital

Excludes acquired or unspecified cystic lung (518.89)

748.5 Agenesis, hypoplasia, and dysplasia of lung
Absence of lung (fissures) (lobe)
Aplasia of lung
Hypoplasia of lung (lobe)
Sequestration of lung

● **748.6 Other anomalies of lung**

748.60 Anomaly of lung, unspecified

748.61 Congenital bronchiectasis

748.69 Other
Accessory lung (lobe)
Azygos lobe (fissure), lung

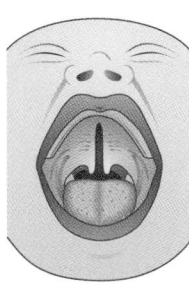

Figure 14–5   Cleft palate.

748.8 Other specified anomalies of respiratory system
Abnormal communication between pericardial and pleural sacs
Anomaly, pleural folds
Atresia of nasopharynx
Congenital cyst of mediastinum

748.9 Unspecified anomaly of respiratory system
Anomaly of respiratory system NOS

● **749 Cleft palate and cleft lip**

● **749.0 Cleft palate**

749.00 Cleft palate, unspecified

749.01 Unilateral, complete

749.02 Unilateral, incomplete
Cleft uvula

749.03 Bilateral, complete

749.04 Bilateral, incomplete

● **749.1 Cleft lip**
Cheiloschisis   Harelip
Congenital fissure of lip   Labium leporinum

749.10 Cleft lip, unspecified

749.11 Unilateral, complete

749.12 Unilateral, incomplete

749.13 Bilateral, complete

749.14 Bilateral, incomplete

● **749.2 Cleft palate with cleft lip**
Cheilopalatoschisis

749.20 Cleft palate with cleft lip, unspecified

749.21 Unilateral, complete

749.22 Unilateral, incomplete

749.23 Bilateral, complete
Coding Clinic: 1996, Q1, P14

749.24 Bilateral, incomplete

749.25 Other combinations

● **750 Other congenital anomalies of upper alimentary tract**
Excludes *dentofacial anomalies (524.0–524.9)*

750.0 Tongue tie
Ankyloglossia

● **750.1 Other anomalies of tongue**

750.10 Anomaly of tongue, unspecified

750.11 Aglossia

750.12 Congenital adhesions of tongue

750.13 Fissure of tongue
Bifid tongue
Double tongue

750.15 Macroglossia
Congenital hypertrophy of tongue

750.16 Microglossia
Hypoplasia of tongue

750.19 Other

● **750.2 Other specified anomalies of mouth and pharynx**

750.21 Absence of salivary gland

750.22 Accessory salivary gland

750.23 Atresia, salivary gland
Imperforate salivary duct

750.24 Congenital fistula of salivary gland

750.25 Congenital fistula of lip
Congenital (mucus) lip pits

750.26 Other specified anomalies of mouth
Absence of uvula

750.27 Diverticulum of pharynx
Pharyngeal pouch

750.29 Other specified anomalies of pharynx
Imperforate pharynx

750.3 Tracheoesophageal fistula, esophageal atresia and stenosis
Absent esophagus
Atresia of esophagus
Congenital:
esophageal ring
stenosis of esophagus
stricture of esophagus
Congenital fistula:
esophagobronchial
esophagotracheal
Imperforate esophagus
Webbed esophagus

750.4 Other specified anomalies of esophagus
Dilatation, congenital, of esophagus
Displacement, congenital, of esophagus
Diverticulum of esophagus
Duplication of esophagus
Esophageal pouch
Giant esophagus

Excludes *congenital hiatus hernia (750.6)*

750.5 Congenital hypertrophic pyloric stenosis
Congenital or infantile:
constriction of pylorus
hypertrophy of pylorus
spasm of pylorus
stenosis of pylorus
stricture of pylorus

750.6 Congenital hiatus hernia
Displacement of cardia through esophageal hiatus

Excludes *congenital diaphragmatic hernia (756.6)*

Item 14-3 A muscle thickening and pyloric stenosis overgrows the pyloric sphincter, resulting in a narrowing of the outlet between the stomach and small intestine. Infants with pyloric stenosis have projectile vomiting, leading to dehydration and electrolyte imbalance.

Figure 14–6   Pyloric stenosis.

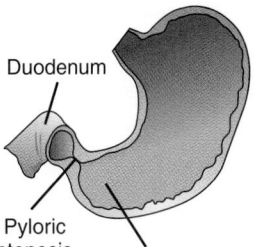

Duodenum
Pyloric stenosis
Pyloric part of stomach

CONGENITAL ANOMALIES (740–759)

■750.7 **Other specified anomalies of stomach**
　　Congenital:
　　　　cardiospasm
　　　　hourglass stomach
　　Displacement of stomach
　　Diverticulum of stomach, congenital
　　Duplication of stomach
　　Megalogastria
　　Microgastria
　　Transposition of stomach

■750.8 **Other specified anomalies of upper alimentary tract**

■750.9 **Unspecified anomaly of upper alimentary tract**
　　Congenital:
　　　　anomaly NOS of upper alimentary tract [any
　　　　　　part, except tongue]
　　　　deformity NOS of upper alimentary tract [any
　　　　　　part, except tongue]

● **751 Other congenital anomalies of digestive system**

　751.0 Meckel's diverticulum
　　Meckel's diverticulum (displaced) (hypertrophic)
　　Persistent:
　　　　omphalomesenteric duct
　　　　vitelline duct
　　Coding Clinic: 2004, Q1, P10-11

　751.1 Atresia and stenosis of small intestine　　　　P
　　Atresia of:
　　　　duodenum
　　　　ileum
　　　　intestine NOS
　　Congenital:
　　　　absence of small intestine or intestine NOS
　　　　obstruction of small intestine or intestine NOS
　　　　stenosis of small intestine or intestine NOS
　　　　stricture of small intestine or intestine NOS
　　Imperforate jejunum

　**751.2 Atresia and stenosis of large intestine, rectum, and
　　anal canal**　　　　P
　　Absence:
　　　　anus (congenital)
　　　　appendix, congenital
　　　　large instestine, congenital
　　　　rectum
　　Atresia of:
　　　　anus
　　　　colon
　　　　rectum
　　Congenital or infantile:
　　　　obstruction of large intestine
　　　　occlusion of anus
　　　　stricture of anus
　　Imperforate:
　　　　anus
　　　　rectum
　　Stricture of rectum, congenital
　　Coding Clinic: 1998, Q2, P16-17

■**751.3 Hirschsprung's disease and other congenital
　　functional disorders of colon**
　　*Absence of ganglion cells in distal colon resulting in
　　　　functional obstruction.*
　　Aganglionosis
　　Congenital dilation of colon
　　Congenital megacolon
　　Macrocolon

　751.4 Anomalies of intestinal fixation
　　Congenital adhesions:
　　　　omental, anomalous
　　　　peritoneal
　　Jackson's membrane
　　Malrotation of colon
　　Rotation of cecum or colon:
　　　　failure of
　　　　incomplete
　　　　insufficient
　　Universal mesentery
　　Coding Clinic: 1985, Sept-Oct, P11

■**751.5 Other anomalies of intestine**
　　Congenital diverticulum,　　Megaloappendix
　　　　colon　　　　　　　　Megaloduodenum
　　Dolichocolon　　　　　　Microcolon
　　Duplication of:　　　　　Persistent cloaca
　　　　anus　　　　　　　　Transposition of:
　　　　appendix　　　　　　　appendix
　　　　cecum　　　　　　　　colon
　　　　intestine　　　　　　　intestine
　　Ectopic anus
　　Coding Clinic: 2002, Q3, P11; 2001, Q3, P8-9

● **751.6 Anomalies of gallbladder, bile ducts, and liver**

　■**751.60 Unspecified anomaly of gallbladder, bile
　　　ducts, and liver**

　　751.61 Biliary atresia　　　　　　　　　　P
　　　Congenital:
　　　　　absence of bile duct (common) or passage
　　　　　hypoplasia of bile duct (common) or
　　　　　　　passage
　　　　　obstruction of bile duct (common) or
　　　　　　　passage
　　　　　stricture of bile duct (common) or
　　　　　　　passage
　　　Coding Clinic: 1987, Sept-Oct, P8

　　751.62 Congenital cystic disease of liver
　　　Congenital polycystic disease of liver
　　　Fibrocystic disease of liver

　■**751.69 Other anomalies of gallbladder, bile ducts,
　　　and liver**
　　　Absence of:
　　　　　gallbladder, congenital
　　　　　liver (lobe)
　　　Accessory:
　　　　　hepatic ducts
　　　　　liver
　　　Congenital:
　　　　　choledochal cyst
　　　　　hepatomegaly
　　　Duplication of:　　　　　Duplication of:
　　　　　biliary duct　　　　　　gallbladder
　　　　　cystic duct　　　　　　liver
　　　Floating:　　　　　　　　Floating:
　　　　　gallbladder　　　　　　liver
　　　Intrahepatic gallbladder
　　　Coding Clinic: 1987, Sept-Oct, P8

　751.7 Anomalies of pancreas
　　Absence of pancreas
　　Accessory pancreas
　　Agenesis of pancreas
　　Annular pancreas
　　Ectopic pancreatic tissue
　　Hypoplasia of pancreas
　　Pancreatic heterotopia

　　　Excludes *diabetes mellitus (249.0–249.9,
　　　　　　(250.0–250.9)
　　　　　fibrocystic disease of pancreas
　　　　　　(277.00–277.09)
　　　　　neonatal diabetes mellitus (775.1)*

751.8 Other specified anomalies of digestive system
Absence (complete) (partial) of alimentary tract NOS
Duplication of digestive organs NOS
Malposition, congenital of digestive organs NOS

> **Excludes** *congenital diaphragmatic hernia (756.6)*
> *congenital hiatus hernia (750.6)*

751.9 Unspecified anomaly of digestive system
Congenital:
anomaly NOS of digestive system NOS
deformity NOS of digestive system NOS

752 Congenital anomalies of genital organs

> **Excludes** *syndromes associated with anomalies in the*
> *number and form of chromosomes*
> *(758.0–758.9)*

752.0 Anomalies of ovaries ♀
Absence, congenital, of ovary
Accessory ovary
Ectopic ovary
Streak of ovary

752.1 Anomalies of fallopian tubes and broad ligaments

752.10 Unspecified anomaly of fallopian tubes and broad ligaments ♀

752.11 Embryonic cyst of fallopian tubes and broad ligaments ♀
Cyst:
epoophoron
fimbrial
parovarian
Coding Clinic: 1985, Sept-Oct, P13

752.19 Other ♀
Absence of fallopian tube or broad ligament
Accessory fallopian tube or broad ligament
Atresia of fallopian tube or broad ligament

752.2 Doubling of uterus ♀
Didelphic uterus
Doubling of uterus [any degree] (associated with doubling of cervix and vagina)

752.3 Other anomalies of uterus ♀
Absence, congenital, of uterus
Agenesis of uterus
Aplasia of uterus
Bicornuate uterus
Uterus unicornis
Uterus with only one functioning horn
Coding Clinic: 2006, Q3, P18-19

752.4 Anomalies of cervix, vagina, and external female genitalia

752.40 Unspecified anomaly of cervix, vagina, and external female genitalia ♀

752.41 Embryonic cyst of cervix, vagina, and external female genitalia ♀
Cyst of:
canal of Nuck, congenital
Gartner's duct
vagina, embryonal
vulva, congenital

752.42 Imperforate hymen ♀

752.49 Other anomalies of cervix, vagina, and external female genitalia ♀
Absence of cervix, clitoris, vagina, or vulva
Agenesis of cervix, clitoris, vagina, or vulva
Congenital stenosis or stricture of:
cervical canal
vagina

> **Excludes** *double vagina associated with total duplication (752.2)*

Coding Clinic: 2006, Q3, P18-19

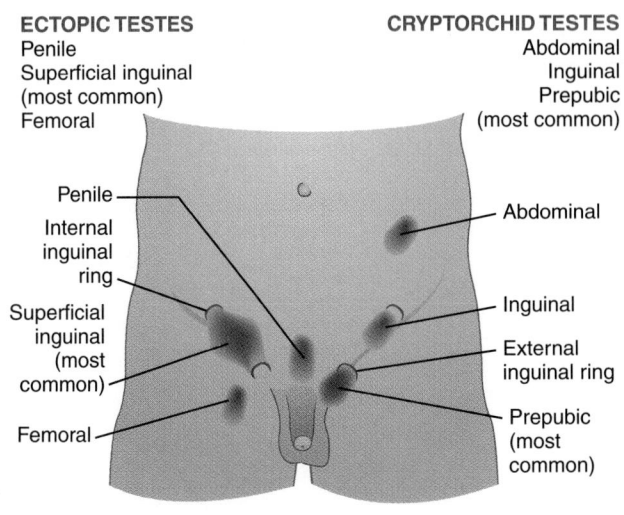

ECTOPIC TESTES
Penile
Superficial inguinal (most common)
Femoral

CRYPTORCHID TESTES
Abdominal
Inguinal
Prepubic (most common)

Figure 14–7 Undescended testes and the positions of the testes in various types of cryptorchidism or abnormal paths of descent.

Item 14–4 Testes form in the abdomen of the male and only descend into the scrotum during normal embryonic development. "Ectopic" testes are out of their normal place or "retained" (left behind) in the abdomen. Crypto (hidden) orchism (testicle) is a major risk factor for testicular cancer.

752.5 Undescended and retractile testicle

752.51 Undescended testis ♂
Cryptorchism
Ectopic testis

752.52 Retractile testis ♂

752.6 Hypospadias and epispadias and other penile anomalies

752.61 Hypospadias ♂
Coding Clinic: 2003, Q4, P67-68; 1997, Q3, P6; Q3, P6; 1996, Q4, P34-35

752.62 Epispadias ♂
Anaspadias

752.63 Congenital chordee ♂
Coding Clinic: 1996, Q4, P34-35

752.64 Micropenis ♂

752.65 Hidden penis ♂

752.69 Other penile anomalies ♂

752.7 Indeterminate sex and pseudohermaphroditism
Condition in which internal reproductive organs are opposite external physical characteristics.
Gynandrism
Hermaphroditism
Ovotestis
Pseudohermaphroditism (male) (female)
Pure gonadal dysgenesis

> **Excludes** *androgen insensitivity (259.50–259.52)*
> *pseudohermaphroditism:*
> *female, with adrenocortical disorder (255.2)*
> *male, with gonadal disorder (257.8)*
> *with specified chromosomal anomaly (758.0–758.9)*
> *testicular feminization syndrome (259.50–259.52)*

CONGENITAL ANOMALIES (740–759)

● **752.8 Other specified anomalies of genital organs**

> **Excludes** *congenital hydrocele (778.6)*
> *penile anomalies (752.61–752.69)*
> *phimosis or paraphimosis (605)*

    752.81 Scrotal transposition ♂
       Coding Clinic: 2003, Q4, P67-68

    ■**752.89 Other specified anomalies of genital organs**
       Check Index for V codes for acquired or
          congenital.
       Absence of:
         prostate
         spermatic cord
         vas deferens
       Anorchism
       Aplasia (congenital) of:
         prostate
         round ligament
         testicle
       Atresia of:
         ejaculatory duct
         vas deferens
       Fusion of testes
       Hypoplasia of testis
       Monorchism
       Polyorchism

  ■**752.9 Unspecified anomaly of genital organs**
     Congenital:
       anomaly NOS of genital organ, NEC
       deformity NOS of genital organ, NEC

● **753 Congenital anomalies of urinary system**

  753.0 Renal agenesis and dysgenesis
     Atrophy of kidney:
       congenital
       infantile
     Congenital absence of kidney(s)
     Hypoplasia of kidney(s)

● **753.1 Cystic kidney disease**

> **Excludes** *acquired cyst of kidney (593.2)*

  ■**753.10 Cystic kidney disease, unspecified**

    753.11 Congenital single renal cyst

  ■**753.12 Polycystic kidney, unspecified type**
       PKD (polycystic kidney disease)

    753.13 Polycystic kidney, autosomal dominant

    753.14 Polycystic kidney, autosomal recessive

    753.15 Renal dysplasia

    753.16 Medullary cystic kidney
       Nephronophthisis

    753.17 Medullary sponge kidney

  ■**753.19 Other specified cystic kidney disease**
       Multicystic kidney

● **753.2 Obstructive defects of renal pelvis and ureter**

  ■**753.20 Unspecified obstructive defect of renal pelvis and ureter**

    753.21 Congenital obstruction of ureteropelvic junction

    753.22 Congenital obstruction of ureterovesical junction
       Adynamic ureter
       Congenital hydroureter

    753.23 Congenital ureterocele

  ■**753.29 Other**

■**753.3 Other specified anomalies of kidney**
    Accessory kidney
    Congenital:
      calculus of kidney
      displaced kidney
    Discoid kidney
    Double kidney with double pelvis
    Ectopic kidney
    Fusion of kidneys
    Giant kidney
    Horseshoe kidney
    Hyperplasia of kidney
    Lobulation of kidney
    Malrotation of kidney
    Trifid kidney (pelvis)
    Coding Clinic: 2007, Q1, P23

■**753.4 Other specified anomalies of ureter**
    Absent ureter
    Accessory ureter
    Deviaton of ureter
    Displaced ureteric orifice
    Double ureter
    Ectopic ureter
    Implantation, anomalous, of ureter

753.5 Exstrophy of urinary bladder
    Ectopia vesicae
    Extroversion of bladder

753.6 Atresia and stenosis of urethra and bladder neck
    Congenital obstruction:
      bladder neck
      urethra
    Congenital stricture of:
      urethra (valvular)
      urinary meatus
      vesicourethral orifice
    Imperforate urinary meatus
    Impervious urethra
    Urethral valve formation

753.7 Anomalies of urachus
    Cyst (of) urachus
    Fistula (of) urachus
    Patent (of) urachus
    Persistent umbilical sinus

■**753.8 Other specified anomalies of bladder and urethra**
    Absence, congenital of:
      bladder
      urethra
    Accessory:
      bladder
      urethra
    Congenital:
      diverticulum of bladder
      hernia of bladder
    Congenital urethrorectal fistula
    Congenital prolapse of:
      bladder (mucosa)
      urethra
    Double:
      urethra
      urinary meatus

■**753.9 Unspecified anomaly of urinary system**
    Congenital:
      anomaly NOS of urinary system [any part, except urachus]
      deformity NOS of urinary system [any part, except urachus]

◄ New   ◄▥ Revised   ~~deleted~~ Deleted   ● Use Additional Digit(s)   ■ Nonspecific Code

● Not first-listed DX   OGCR Official Guidelines   Coding Clinic   Excludes   Includes   Use additional   Code first   Omit code

● **754   Certain congenital musculoskeletal deformities**

Includes   nonteratogenic deformities which are
considered to be due to intrauterine
malposition and pressure

754.0 Of skull, face, and jaw
Asymmetry of face
Compression facies
Depressions in skull
Deviation of nasal septum, congenital
Dolichocephaly
Plagiocephaly
Potter's facies
Squashed or bent nose, congenital

Excludes   dentofacial anomalies (524.0–524.9)
syphilitic saddle nose (090.5)

754.1 Of sternocleidomastoid muscle
Congenital sternomastoid torticollis
Congenital wryneck
Contracture of sternocleidomastoid (muscle)
Sternomastoid tumor

754.2 Of spine
Congenital postural:
lordosis
scoliosis

● **754.3 Congenital dislocation of hip**

754.30 Congenital dislocation of hip, unilateral
Congenital dislocation of hip NOS

754.31 Congenital dislocation of hip, bilateral

754.32 Congenital subluxation of hip, unilateral
Congenital flexion deformity, hip or thigh
Predislocation status of hip at birth
Preluxation of hip, congenital

754.33 Congenital subluxation of hip, bilateral

**754.35 Congenital dislocation of one hip with
subluxation of other hip**

● **754.4 Congenital genu recurvatum and bowing of long
bones of leg**

754.40 Genu recurvatum
*Hyperextension of knee resulting from
hypermobility*

**754.41 Congenital dislocation of knee (with genu
recurvatum)**

754.42 Congenital bowing of femur

754.43 Congenital bowing of tibia and fibula

■**754.44 Congenital bowing of unspecified long bones
of leg**

● **754.5 Varus deformities of feet**
*Foot deformity (pes equino varus) also known as club
foot in which there is an inward angulation of
distal segment of a bone or joint*

Excludes   acquired (736.71, 736.75, 736.79)

754.50 Talipes varus
Congenital varus deformity of foot,
unspecified
Pes varus

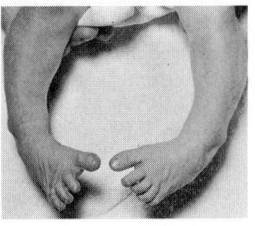

Figure 14–8 Mild to moderate inbowing of the lower leg. (From Jones KL: Smith's Recognizable Patterns of Human Malformation, 4th ed. Philadelphia, Saunders, 1988, p 671.)

754.51 Talipes equinovarus
Equinovarus (congenital)

754.52 Metatarsus primus varus

754.53 Metatarsus varus

■**754.59 Other**
Talipes calcaneovarus

● **754.6 Valgus deformities of feet**
Inward angulation

Excludes   valgus deformity of foot (acquired) (736.79)

754.60 Talipes valgus
Congenital valgus deformity of foot,
unspecified

754.61 Congenital pes planus
Congenital rocker bottom flat foot
Flat foot, congenital

Excludes   pes planus (acquired) (734)

754.62 Talipes calcaneovalgus

■**754.69 Other**
Talipes:
equinovalgus
planovalgus

● **754.7 Other deformities of feet**

Excludes   acquired (736.70–736.79)

■**754.70 Talipes, unspecified**
Congenital deformity of foot NOS

754.71 Talipes cavus
Cavus foot (congenital)

■**754.79 Other**
Asymmetric talipes
Talipes:
calcaneus
equinus

● **754.8 Other specified nonteratogenic anomalies**

754.81 Pectus excavatum
Congenital funnel chest

754.82 Pectus carinatum
Congenital pigeon chest [breast]

■**754.89 Other**
Club hand (congenital)
Congenital:
deformity of chest wall
dislocation of elbow
Generalized flexion contractures of lower
limb joints, congenital
Spade-like hand (congenital)

CONGENITAL ANOMALIES (740–759)

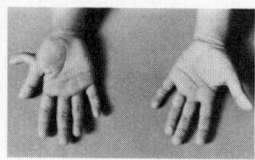

Figure 14–9 Polydactyly, congenital duplicated thumb. (From DeLee: DeLee and Drez's Orthopaedic Sports Medicine, 2nd ed. 2003, Saunders, An Imprint of Elsevier)

- **755 Other congenital anomalies of limbs**

  Excludes *those deformities classifiable to 754.0–754.8*

  - **755.0 Polydactyly**

    Also known as hyperdactyly, consists of duplicate fingers or toes

    - **755.00 Polydactyly, unspecified digits**
      Supernumerary digits

    - **755.01 Of fingers**
      Accessory fingers

    - **755.02 Of toes**
      Accessory toes

  - **755.1 Syndactyly**
    Symphalangy
    Webbing of digits

    - **755.10 Of multiple and unspecified sites**

    - **755.11 Of fingers without fusion of bone**

    - **755.12 Of fingers with fusion of bone**

    - **755.13 Of toes without fusion of bone**

    - **755.14 Of toes with fusion of bone**

  - **755.2 Reduction deformities of upper limb**

    - **755.20 Unspecified reduction deformity of upper limb**
      Ectromelia NOS of upper limb
      Gross hypoplasia or aplasia of one or more long bones of one or more limbs
      Hemimelia NOS of upper limb
      Absence of one-half of long bone
      Shortening of arm, congenital

    - **755.21 Transverse deficiency of upper limb**
      Amelia of upper limb
      Congenital absence of:
        fingers, all (complete or partial)
        forearm, including hand and fingers
        upper limb, complete
      Congenital amputation of upper limb
      Transverse hemimelia of upper limb

    - **755.22 Longitudinal deficiency of upper limb, NEC**
      Phocomelia NOS of upper limb
      Absence/shortening of long bones primarily as a result of thalidomide
      Rudimentary arm

    - **755.23 Longitudinal deficiency, combined, involving humerus, radius, and ulna (complete or incomplete)**
      Congenital absence of arm and forearm (complete or incomplete) with or without metacarpal deficiency and/or phalangeal deficiency, incomplete
      Phocomelia, complete, of upper limb

  - **755.24 Longitudinal deficiency, humeral, complete or partial (with or without distal deficiencies, incomplete)**
    Congenital absence of humerus (with or without absence of some [but not all] distal elements)
    Proximal phocomelia of upper limb

  - **755.25 Longitudinal deficiency, radioulnar, complete or partial (with or without distal deficiencies, incomplete)**
    Congenital absence of radius and ulna (with or without absence of some [but not all] distal elements)
    Distal phocomelia of upper limb

  - **755.26 Longitudinal deficiency, radial, complete or partial (with or without distal deficiencies, incomplete)**
    Agenesis of radius
    Congenital absence of radius (with or without absence of some [but not all] distal elements)

  - **755.27 Longitudinal deficiency, ulnar, complete or partial (with or without distal deficiencies, incomplete)**
    Agenesis of ulna
    Congenital absence of ulna (with or without absence of some [but not all] distal elements)

  - **755.28 Longitudinal deficiency, carpals or metacarpals, complete or partial (with or without incomplete phalangeal deficiency)**

  - **755.29 Longitudinal deficiency, phalanges, complete or partial**
    Absence of finger, congenital
    Aphalangia of upper limb, terminal, complete or partial

    Excludes *terminal deficiency of all five digits (755.21)*
    transverse deficiency of phalanges (755.21)

  - **755.3 Reduction deformities of lower limb**

    - **755.30 Unspecified reduction deformity of lower limb**
      Ectromelia NOS of lower limb
      Hemimelia NOS of lower limb
      Shortening of leg, congenital

    - **755.31 Transverse deficiency of lower limb**
      Amelia of lower limb
      Congenital absence of:
        foot
        leg, including foot and toes
        lower limb, complete
        toes, all, complete
      Transverse hemimelia of lower limb

    - **755.32 Longitudinal deficiency of lower limb, NEC**
      Phocomelia NOS of lower limb

    - **755.33 Longitudinal deficiency, combined, involving femur, tibia, and fibula (complete or incomplete)**
      Congenital absence of thigh and (lower) leg (complete or incomplete) with or without metacarpal deficiency and/or phalangeal deficiency, incomplete
      Phocomelia, complete, of lower limb

◀ New   ◀▥ Revised   ~~deleted~~ Deleted   ● Use Additional Digit(s)   ■ Nonspecific Code

● Not first-listed DX   OGCR Official Guidelines   Coding Clinic   Excludes   Includes   Use additional   Code first   Omit code

755.34 **Longitudinal deficiency, femoral, complete or partial (with or without distal deficiencies, incomplete)**
Congenital absence of femur (with or without absence of some [but not all] distal elements)
Proximal phocomelia of lower limb

755.35 **Longitudinal deficiency, tibiofibular, complete or partial (with or without distal deficiencies, incomplete)**
Congenital absence of tibia and fibula (with or without absence of some [but not all] distal elements)
Distal phocomelia of lower limb

755.36 **Longitudinal deficiency, tibia, complete or partial (with or without distal deficiencies, incomplete)**
Agenesis of tibia
Congenital absence of tibia (with or without absence of some [but not all] distal elements)

755.37 **Longitudinal deficiency, fibular, complete or partial (with or without distal deficiencies, incomplete)**
Agenesis of fibula
Congenital absence of fibula (with or without absence of some [but not all] distal elements)

755.38 **Longitudinal deficiency, tarsals or metatarsals, complete or partial (with or without incomplete phalangeal deficiency)**

755.39 **Longitudinal deficiency, phalanges, complete or partial**
Absence of toe, congenital
Aphalangia of lower limb, terminal, complete or partial
Excludes *terminal deficiency of all five digits (755.31)*
transverse deficiency of phalanges (755.31)

755.4 **Reduction deformities, unspecified limb**
Absence, congenital (complete or partial) of limb NOS
Amelia of unspecified limb
Ectromelia of unspecified limb
Hemimelia of unspecified limb
Phocomelia of unspecified limb

755.5 **Other anomalies of upper limb, including shoulder girdle**

755.50 **Unspecified anomaly of upper limb**

755.51 **Congenital deformity of clavicle**

755.52 **Congenital elevation of scapula**
Sprengel's deformity

755.53 **Radioulnar synostosis**

755.54 **Madelung's deformity**

755.55 **Acrocephalosyndactyly**
Apert's syndrome

755.56 **Accessory carpal bones**

755.57 **Macrodactylia (fingers)**

755.58 **Cleft hand, congenital**
Lobster-claw hand

755.59 **Other**
Cleidocranial dysostosis
Cubitus:
valgus, congenital
varus, congenital
Excludes *club hand (congenital) (754.89)*
congenital dislocation of elbow (754.89)

755.6 **Other anomalies of lower limb, including pelvic girdle**

755.60 **Unspecified anomaly of lower limb**

755.61 **Coxa valga, congenital**

755.62 **Coxa vara, congenital**

755.63 **Other congenital deformity of hip (joint)**
Congenital anteversion of femur (neck)
Excludes *congenital dislocation of hip (754.30–754.35)*

755.64 **Congenital deformity of knee (joint)**
Congenital:
absence of patella
genu valgum [knock-knee]
genu varum [bowleg]
Rudimentary patella
Coding Clinic: 1985, July-Aug, P14; 1984, Nov-Dec, P9

755.65 **Macrodactylia of toes**

755.66 **Other anomalies of toes**
Congenital:
hallux valgus
hallux varus
hammer toe

755.67 **Anomalies of foot, NEC**
Astragaloscaphoid synostosis
Calcaneonavicular bar
Coalition of calcaneus
Talonavicular synostosis
Tarsal coalitions

755.69 **Other**
Congenital:
angulation of tibia
deformity (of):
ankle (joint)
sacroiliac (joint)
fusion of sacroiliac joint

755.8 **Other specified anomalies of unspecified limb**

755.9 **Unspecified anomaly of unspecified limb**
Congenital:
anomaly NOS of unspecified limb
deformity NOS of unspecified limb
Excludes *reduction deformity of unspecified limb (755.4)*

CONGENITAL ANOMALIES (740–759)

● **756 Other congenital musculoskeletal anomalies**

> **Excludes** *congenital myotonic chondrodystrophy (359.23)*
> *those deformities classifiable to 754.0–754.8*

756.0 Anomalies of skull and face bones
Absence of skull bones
Acrocephaly
Congenital deformity of forehead
Craniosynostosis
Crouzon's disease
Hypertelorism
Imperfect fusion of skull
Oxycephaly
Platybasia
Premature closure of cranial sutures
Tower skull
Trigonocephaly

> **Excludes** *acrocephalosyndactyly [Apert's syndrome]*
> *(755.55)*
> *dentofacial anomalies (524.0–524.9)*
> *skull defects associated with brain*
> *anomalies, such as:*
> *anencephalus (740.0)*
> *encephalocele (742.0)*
> *hydrocephalus (742.3)*
> *microcephalus (742.1)*
>
> Coding Clinic: 1998, Q3, P9-10; 1996, Q3, P15

● **756.1 Anomalies of spine**

■ **756.10 Anomaly of spine, unspecified**

756.11 Spondylolysis, lumbosacral region
Prespondylolisthesis (lumbosacral)

756.12 Spondylolisthesis

756.13 Absence of vertebra, congenital

756.14 Hemivertebra

756.15 Fusion of spine [vertebra], congenital

756.16 Klippel-Feil syndrome

756.17 Spina bifida occulta

> **Excludes** *spina bifida (aperta) (741.0–741.9)*

■ **756.19 Other**
Platyspondylia
Supernumerary vertebra

756.2 Cervical rib
Supernumerary rib in the cervical region

■ **756.3 Other anomalies of ribs and sternum**
Congenital absence of:
rib
sternum
Congenital:
fissure of sternum
fusion of ribs
Sternum bifidum

> **Excludes** *nonteratogenic deformity of chest wall*
> *(754.81–754.89)*

756.4 Chondrodystrophy
Skeletal dysplasia (dwarfism) is caused by genetic
mutations affecting hyaline cartilage capping long
bones and vertebrae
Achondroplasia   Enchondromatosis
Chondrodystrophia (fetalis)   Ollier's disease
Dyschondroplasia

> **Excludes** *congenital myotonic chondrodystrophy*
> *(359.23)*
> *lipochondrodystrophy [Hurler's syndrome]*
> *(277.5)*
> *Morquio's disease (277.5)*
>
> Coding Clinic: 2002, Q2, P16-17; 1987, Sept-Oct, P10

● **756.5 Osteodystrophies**
Defective bone development; most commonly caused
by renal disease or disturbances in calcium and
phosphorus metabolism

■ **756.50 Osteodystrophy, unspecified**

756.51 Osteogenesis imperfecta
Fragilitas ossium
Osteopsathyrosis

756.52 Osteopetrosis

756.53 Osteopoikilosis

756.54 Polyostotic fibrous dysplasia of bone

756.55 Chondroectodermal dysplasia
Ellis-van Creveld syndrome

756.56 Multiple epiphyseal dysplasia

■ **756.59 Other**
Albright (-McCune)-Sternberg syndrome

756.6 Anomalies of diaphragm
Absence of diaphragm
Congenital hernia:
diaphragmatic
foramen of Morgagni
Eventration of diaphragm

> **Excludes** *congenital hiatus hernia (750.6)*

● **756.7 Anomalies of abdominal wall**

■ **756.70 Anomaly of abdominal wall, unspecified**

756.71 Prune belly syndrome
Eagle-Barrett syndrome
Prolapse of bladder mucosa

756.72 Omphalocele ◄
Exomphalos ◄

756.73 Gastroschisis ◄

■ **756.79 Other congenital anomalies of abdominal wall**
~~Exomphalos~~   ~~Omphalocele~~
~~Gastroschisis~~

> **Excludes** *umbilical hernia (551–553 with .1)*

● **756.8 Other specified anomalies of muscle, tendon, fascia, and connective tissue**

756.81 Absence of muscle and tendon
Absence of muscle (pectoral)

756.82 Accessory muscle

756.83 Ehlers-Danlos syndrome

■ **756.89 Other**
Amyotrophia congenita
Congenital shortening of tendon
Coding Clinic: 1999, Q3, P16-17

■ **756.9 Other and unspecified anomalies of musculoskeletal system**
Congenital:
anomaly NOS of musculoskeletal system, NEC
deformity NOS of musculoskeletal system, NEC

● **757 Congenital anomalies of the integument**

> **Includes** anomalies of skin, subcutaneous tissue, hair, nails, and breast

> **Excludes** *hemangioma (228.00–228.09)*
> *pigmented nevus (216.0–216.9)*

757.0 Hereditary edema of legs
Congenital lymphedema
Hereditary trophedema
Milroy's disease

◄ New   ◄▦ Revised   ~~deleted~~ Deleted   ● Use Additional Digit(s)   ■ Nonspecific Code
● Not first-listed DX   OGCR Official Guidelines   Coding Clinic   Excludes   Includes   Use additional   Code first   Omit code

CONGENITAL ANOMALIES (740–759)

757.1 Ichthyosis congenita
Congenital ichthyosis
Harlequin fetus
Ichthyosiform erythroderma

757.2 Dermatoglyphic anomalies
Abnormal palmar creases

● **757.3 Other specified anomalies of skin**

    757.31 Congenital ectodermal dysplasia

    757.32 Vascular hamartomas
        Birthmarks
        Port-wine stain
        Strawberry nevus

    757.33 Congenital pigmentary anomalies of skin
        Congenital poikiloderma
        Urticaria pigmentosa
        Xeroderma pigmentosum
        Excludes *albinism (270.2)*

    ■**757.39 Other**
        Accessory skin tags, congenital
        Congenital scar
        Epidermolysis bullosa
        Keratoderma (congenital)
        Excludes *pilonidal cyst (685.0–685.1)*

■**757.4 Specified anomalies of hair**
Congenital:
  alopecia
  atrichosis
  beaded hair
  hypertrichosis
  monilethrix
Persistent lanugo

■**757.5 Specified anomalies of nails**
Anonychia
Congenital:
  clubnail
  koilonychia
  leukonychia
  onychauxis
  pachyonychia

■**757.6 Specified congenital anomalies of breast**
Congenital absent breast or nipple
Accessory breast or nipple
Supernumerary breast or nipple
    Excludes *absence of pectoral muscle (756.81)*
              hypoplasia of breast (611.82)
              micromastia (611.82)

■**757.8 Other specified anomalies of the integument**

■**757.9 Unspecified anomaly of the integument**
Congenital:
  anomaly NOS of integument
  deformity NOS of integument

● **758 Chromosomal anomalies**
  Includes syndromes associated with anomalies in the
         number and form of chromosomes

  Use additional codes for conditions associated with the
    chromosomal anomalies

758.0 Down's syndrome
Mongolism
Translocation Down's syndrome
Trisomy:
  21 or 22
  G

758.1 Patau's syndrome
Trisomy:
  13
  D$_1$

758.2 Edward's syndrome
Trisomy:
  18
  E$_3$

● **758.3 Autosomal deletion syndromes**
  Coding Clinic: 2004, Q4, P93-95; 1995, Q2, P6-7, 11

    758.31 Cri-du-chat syndrome
        Deletion 5p

    758.32 Velo-cardio-facial syndrome
        Deletion 22q11.2

    ■**758.33 Other microdeletions**
        Miller-Dieker syndrome
        Smith-Magenis syndrome

    ■**758.39 Other autosomal deletions**

758.4 Balanced autosomal translocation in normal individual

■**758.5 Other conditions due to autosomal anomalies**
Accessory autosomes NEC

758.6 Gonadal dysgenesis
Ovarian dysgenesis
Turner's syndrome
XO syndrome
    Excludes *pure gonadal dysgenesis (752.7)*

758.7 Klinefelter's syndrome ♂
XXY syndrome

● **758.8 Other conditions due to chromosome anomalies**

    ■**758.81 Other conditions due to sex chromosome anomalies**

    ■**758.89 Other**

■**758.9 Conditions due to anomaly of unspecified chromosome**

● **759 Other and unspecified congenital anomalies**

759.0 Anomalies of spleen
Aberrant spleen   Congenital splenomegaly
Absent spleen   Ectopic spleen
Accessory spleen   Lobulation of spleen

759.1 Anomalies of adrenal gland
Aberrant adrenal gland
Absent adrenal gland
Accessory adrenal gland
    Excludes *adrenogenital disorders (255.2)*
              congenital disorders of steroid metabolism
                (255.2)

■**759.2 Anomalies of other endocrine glands**
Absent parathyroid gland
Accessory thyroid gland
Persistent thyroglossal or thyrolingual duct
Thyroglossal (duct) cyst
    Excludes *congenital:*
        goiter (246.1)
        hypothyroidism (243)

759.3 Situs inversus
Situs inversus or transversus:
  abdominalis
  thoracis
Transposition of viscera:
  abdominal
  thoracic
    Excludes *dextrocardia without mention of complete transposition (746.87)*

759.4 Conjoined twins
Craniopagus
Dicephalus
Pygopagus
Thoracopagus
Xiphopagus

759.5 **Tuberous sclerosis**
  Bourneville's disease
  Epiloia

■759.6 **Other hamartoses, NEC**
  Syndrome:
    Peutz-Jeghers
    Sturge-Weber (-Dimitri)
    von Hippel-Lindau
    Excludes *neurofibromatosis (237.7)*
    Coding Clinic: 1992, Q3, P11

759.7 **Multiple congenital anomalies, so described**
  Congenital:
    anomaly, multiple NOS
    deformity, multiple NOS

●759.8 **Other specified anomalies**

  759.81 **Prader-Willi syndrome**

  759.82 **Marfan syndrome**
    Coding Clinic: 1993, Q3, P11

  759.83 **Fragile X syndrome**

■759.89 **Other**
    Index directs coder to this code for Noonan's
      syndrome.
    Congenital malformation syndromes
      affecting multiple systems, NEC
    Laurence-Moon-Biedl syndrome
    Coding Clinic: 2008, Q3, P3-4; 2006, Q3, P21; 2005, Q2,
      P17; 2004, Q2, P12; 2001, Q1, P3; 1999, Q3,
      P17-19x2; 1998, Q3, P8; 1987, Sept-Oct, P9; 1985,
      Sept-Oct, P11

■759.9 **Congenital anomaly, unspecified**

◀ New   ◀▥ Revised   deleted Deleted   ● Use Additional Digit(s)   ■ Nonspecific Code
● Not first-listed DX   OGCR Official Guidelines   Coding Clinic   Excludes   Includes   Use additional   Code first   Omit code

15.   CERTAIN CONDITIONS ORIGINATING IN THE PERINATAL PERIOD (760–779)

Includes   conditions which have their origin in the perinatal period, before birth through the first 28 days after birth, even though death or morbidity occurs later

Use additional code(s) to further specify condition

MATERNAL CAUSES OF PERINATAL MORBIDITY AND MORTALITY (760–763)

● **760   Fetus or newborn affected by maternal conditions which may be unrelated to present pregnancy**

Includes   the listed maternal conditions only when specified as a cause of mortality or morbidity of the fetus or newborn

Excludes   *maternal endocrine and metabolic disorders affecting fetus or newborn (775.0–775.9)*
Coding Clinic: 1992, Q2, P12

760.0   Maternal hypertensive disorders
Fetus or newborn affected by maternal conditions classifiable to 642

760.1   Maternal renal and urinary tract diseases
Fetus or newborn affected by maternal conditions classifiable to 580–599

760.2   Maternal infections
Fetus or newborn affected by maternal infectious disease classifiable to 001–136 and 487, but fetus or newborn not manifesting that disease

Excludes   *congenital infectious diseases (771.0–771.8) maternal genital tract and other localized infections (760.8)*

■ **760.3   Other chronic maternal circulatory and respiratory diseases**
Fetus or newborn affected by chronic maternal conditions classifiable to 390–459, 490–519, 745–748

760.4   Maternal nutritional disorders
Fetus or newborn affected by:
    maternal disorders classifiable to 260–269
    maternal malnutrition NOS

Excludes   *fetal malnutrition (764.10–764.29)*

760.5   Maternal injury
Fetus or newborn affected by maternal conditions classifiable to 800–995

● **760.6   Surgical operation on mother and fetus**

Excludes   *cesarean section for present delivery (763.4) damage to placenta from amniocentesis, cesarean section, or surgical induction (762.1)*
Coding Clinic: 2008, Q4, P137-138

760.61   Newborn affected by amniocentesis

Excludes   *fetal complications from amniocentesis (679.1)*

760.62   Newborn affected by other in utero procedure

Excludes   *fetal complications of in utero procedure (679.1)*

760.63   Newborn affected by other surgical operations on mother during pregnancy

Excludes   *newborn affected by previous surgical procedure on mother not associated with pregnancy (760.64)*

760.64   Newborn affected by previous surgical procedure on mother not associated with pregnancy

● **760.7   Noxious influences affecting fetus or newborn via placenta or breast milk**
Fetus or newborn affected by noxious substance transmitted via placenta or breast milk

Excludes   *anesthetic and analgesic drugs administered during labor and delivery (763.5) drug withdrawal syndrome in newborn (779.5)*
Coding Clinic: 1991, Q3, P21

■ **760.70   Unspecified noxious substance**
Fetus or newborn affected by:
    drug NEC

760.71   Alcohol
Fetal alcohol syndrome

760.72   Narcotics

760.73   Hallucinogenic agents

760.74   Anti-infectives
Antibiotics
Antifungals

760.75   Cocaine
Coding Clinic: 1994, Q3, P6; 1992, Q2, P12

760.76   Diethylstilbestrol [DES]

760.77   Anticonvulsants   N
Carbamazepine
Phenobarbital
Phenytoin
Valproic acid
Coding Clinic: 2005, Q4, P82-83

760.78   Antimetabolic agents   N
Methotrexate
Retinoic acid
Statins
Coding Clinic: 2005, Q4, P82-83

■ **760.79   Other**
Fetus or newborn affected by:
    immune sera transmitted via placenta or breast milk
    medicinal agents NEC transmitted via placenta or breast milk
    toxic substance NEC transmitted via placenta or breast milk

CERTAIN CONDITIONS ORIGINATING IN THE PERINATAL PERIOD (760–779)

760.8 Other specified maternal conditions affecting fetus or newborn
Maternal genital tract and other localized infection affecting fetus or newborn, but fetus or newborn not manifesting that disease

> **Excludes** *maternal urinary tract infection affecting fetus or newborn (760.1)*

760.9 Unspecified maternal condition affecting fetus or newborn

● **761 Fetus or newborn affected by maternal complications of pregnancy**

> **Includes** the listed maternal conditions only when specified as a cause of mortality or morbidity of the fetus or newborn

761.0 Incompetent cervix

761.1 Premature rupture of membranes

761.2 Oligohydramnios
Scant volume of amniotic fluid

> **Excludes** *that due to premature rupture of membranes (761.1)*

761.3 Polyhydramnios
Overabundance of amniotic fluid
Hydramnios (acute) (chronic)

761.4 Ectopic pregnancy
Pregnancy:
abdominal
intraperitoneal
tubal

761.5 Multiple pregnancy
Triplet (pregnancy)
Twin (pregnancy)

761.6 Maternal death

761.7 Malpresentation before labor
Breech presentation before labor
External version before labor
Oblique lie before labor
Transverse lie before labor
Unstable lie before labor

761.8 Other specified maternal complications of pregnancy affecting fetus or newborn
Spontaneous abortion, fetus

761.9 Unspecified maternal complication of pregnancy affecting fetus or newborn

● **762 Fetus or newborn affected by complications of placenta, cord, and membranes**

> **Includes** the listed maternal conditions only when specified as a cause of mortality or morbidity in the fetus or newborn

762.0 Placenta previa   N

762.1 Other forms of placental separation and hemorrhage   N
Abruptio placentae
Antepartum hemorrhage
Damage to placenta from amniocentesis, cesarean section, or surgical induction
Maternal blood loss
Premature separation of placenta
Rupture of marginal sinus

762.2 Other and unspecified morphological and functional abnormalities of placenta   N
Placental:
dysfunction
infarction
insufficiency

762.3 Placental transfusion syndromes   N
Placental and cord abnormality resulting in twin-to-twin or other transplacental transfusion

> Use additional code to indicate resultant condition in ~~fetus or~~ newborn:
> fetal blood loss (772.0)
> polycythemia neonatorum (776.4)

762.4 Prolapsed cord   N
Cord presentation

762.5 Other compression of umbilical cord   N
Cord around neck
Entanglement of cord
Knot in cord
Torsion of cord
Coding Clinic: 2003, Q2, P9

762.6 Other and unspecified conditions of umbilical cord N
Short cord
Thrombosis of umbilical cord
Varices of umbilical cord
Velamentous insertion of umbilical cord
Vasa previa

> **Excludes** *infection of umbilical cord (771.4)*
> *single umbilical artery (747.5)*

762.7 Chorioamnionitis   N
Amnionitis
Membranitis
Placentitis

762.8 Other specified abnormalities of chorion and amnion N

762.9 Unspecified abnormality of chorion and amnion   N

● **763 Fetus or newborn affected by other complications of labor and delivery**

> **Includes** the listed conditions only when specified as a cause of mortality or morbidity in the fetus or newborn

> **Excludes** *newborn affected by surgical procedures on mother (760.61-760.64)*

763.0 Breech delivery and extraction   N

763.1 Other malpresentation, malposition, and disproportion during labor and delivery   N
Fetus or newborn affected by:
abnormality of bony pelvis
contracted pelvis
persistent occipitoposterior position
shoulder presentation
transverse lie
conditions classifiable to 652, 653, and 660

763.2 Forceps delivery   N
Fetus or newborn affected by forceps extraction

763.3 Delivery by vacuum extractor   N

763.4 Cesarean delivery   N

> **Excludes** *placental separation or hemorrhage from cesarean section (762.1)*

763.5 Maternal anesthesia and analgesia   N
Reactions and intoxications from maternal opiates and tranquilizers during labor and delivery

> **Excludes** *drug withdrawal syndrome in newborn (779.5)*

763.6 Precipitate delivery   N
Rapid second stage

763.7 Abnormal uterine contractions   N
Fetus or newborn affected by:
contraction ring
hypertonic labor
hypotonic uterine dysfunction
uterine inertia or dysfunction
conditions classifiable to 661, except 661.3

CERTAIN CONDITIONS ORIGINATING IN THE PERINATAL PERIOD (760–779)

● **763.8 Other specified complications of labor and delivery affecting fetus or newborn**

     763.81 Abnormality in fetal heart rate or rhythm before the onset of labor   N

     763.82 Abnormality in fetal heart rate or rhythm during labor   N
         Coding Clinic: 1998, Q4, P46-47

     ■**763.83 Abnormality in fetal heart rate or rhythm, unspecified as to time of onset**   N

     763.84 Meconium passage during delivery   N

         Excludes *meconium aspiration (770.11, 770.12)*
                meconium staining (779.84)
         Coding Clinic: 2005, Q4, P83-89

     763.89 Other specified complications of labor and delivery affecting fetus or newborn   N
         Fetus or newborn affected by:
            abnormality of maternal soft tissues
            destructive operation on live fetus to facilitate delivery
            induction of labor (medical)
            other conditions classifiable to 650–669
            other procedures used in labor and delivery

■**763.9 Unspecified complication of labor and delivery affecting fetus or newborn**   N

OTHER CONDITIONS ORIGINATING IN THE PERINATAL PERIOD (764–779)

The following fifth-digit subclassification is for use with category 764 and codes 765.0 and 765.1 to denote birthweight:

■0	unspecified [weight]
1	less than 500 grams
2	500–749 grams
3	750–999 grams
4	1,000–1,249 grams
5	1,250–1,499 grams
6	1,500–1,749 grams
7	1,750–1,999 grams
8	2,000–2,499 grams
9	2,500 grams and over

● **764 Slow fetal growth and fetal malnutrition**

     Requires fifth digit. See beginning of section 764–779 for codes and definitions.
     Coding Clinic: 2009, Q1, P7; 2004, Q3, P4-5; 1994, Q1, P15; 1989, Q2, P15

     OGCR Section I.C.15.i
     The 5th digit assignment for category 764 codes is based on the recorded birth weight and estimated gestational age

● **764.0 "Light-for-dates" without mention of fetal**
   [0-9]   **malnutrition**   N
         Infants underweight for gestational age
         "Small-for-dates"

● **764.1 "Light-for-dates" with signs of fetal malnutrition**   N
   [0-9]   Infants "light-for-dates" classifiable to 764.0, who in addition show signs of fetal malnutrition, such as dry peeling skin and loss of subcutaneous tissue

● **764.2 Fetal malnutrition without mention of**
   [0-9]   **"light-for-dates"**   N
         Infants, not underweight for gestational age, showing signs of fetal malnutrition, such as dry peeling skin and loss of subcutaneous tissue
         Intrauterine malnutrition

● ■**764.9 Fetal growth retardation, unspecified**   N
   [0-9]   Intrauterine growth retardation
         Coding Clinic: 1997, Q1, P6

● **765 Disorders relating to short gestation and low birthweight**

     Requires fifth digit. See beginning of section 764–779 for codes and definitions.

     Includes   the listed conditions, without further specification, as causes of mortality, morbidity, or additional care, in fetus or newborn
     Coding Clinic: 2002, Q4, P63-64; 1994, Q1, P15; 1991, Q2, P19, 1989, Q2, P15

● **765.0 Extreme immaturity**   N
   [0-9]   **Note:** Usually implies a birthweight of less than 1,000 grams

         Use additional code for weeks of gestation (765.20–765.29)
         Coding Clinic: 2009, Q1, P12; 2004, Q3, P4-5; 2001, Q4, P50-51

         OGCR Section I.C.15.i
         Providers utilize different criteria in determining prematurity. A code for prematurity should not be assigned unless it is documented. The 5th digit assignment for codes from subcategory 765.0 should be based on the recorded birth weight and estimated gestational age.

● ■**765.1 Other preterm infants**   N
   [0-9]   Prematurity NOS
         Prematurity or small size, not classifiable to 765.0 or as "light-for-dates" in 764
         Note: Usually implies birthweight of 1,000–2,499 grams

         Use additional code for weeks of gestation (765.20–765.29)
         Coding Clinic: 2009, Q1, P12; 2008, Q4, P138-140; 2004, Q3, P4-5; 2002, Q4, P64; 1997, Q1, P6; 1994, Q1, P14

         OGCR Section I.C.15.i
         Providers utilize different criteria in determining prematurity. A code for prematurity should not be assigned unless it is documented. The 5th digit assignment for codes from subcategory 765.1 should be based on the recorded birth weight and estimated gestational age.

● **765.2 Weeks of gestation**
     Coding Clinic: 2004, Q3, P4-5

     OGCR Section I.C.15.i
     A code from subcategory 765.2, Weeks of gestation, should be assigned as an additional code with category 764 and codes from 765.0 and 765.1 to specify weeks of gestation as documented by the provider in the record.

     ■**765.20 Unspecified weeks of gestation**   N

     765.21 Less than 24 completed weeks of gestation   N

     765.22 24 weeks of gestation   N

     765.23 25–26 weeks of gestation   N
         Coding Clinic: 2009, Q1, P6

     765.24 27–28 weeks of gestation   N

     765.25 29–30 weeks of gestation   N

     765.26 31–32 weeks of gestation   N
         Coding Clinic: 2008, Q4, P138-140

     765.27 33–34 weeks of gestation   N

     765.28 35–36 weeks of gestation   N
         Coding Clinic: 2002, Q4, P64

     765.29 37 or more weeks of gestation   N

CERTAIN CONDITIONS ORIGINATING IN THE PERINATAL PERIOD (760–779)

● **766 Disorders relating to long gestation and high birthweight**

    Includes   the listed conditions, without further specification, as causes of mortality, morbidity, or additional care, in fetus or newborn

    766.0 Exceptionally large baby   N

        Note: Usually implies a birthweight of 4,500 grams or more.

    ■**766.1 Other "heavy-for-dates" infants**   N

        Other fetus or infant "heavy-" or "large-for-dates" regardless of period of gestation

    ● **766.2 Late infant, not "heavy-for-dates"**

        Coding Clinic: 2006, Q2, P12-13; 2003, Q4, P69

        766.21 Post-term infant   N

            Infant with gestation period over 40 completed weeks to 42 completed weeks

            Coding Clinic: 2009, Q1, P6; 2006, Q2, P12-13

        766.22 Prolonged gestation of infant   N

            Infant with gestation period over 42 completed weeks

            Postmaturity NOS

            Coding Clinic: 2009, Q1, P6; 2006, Q2, P12-13

● **767 Birth trauma**

    767.0 Subdural and cerebral hemorrhage   N

        Subdural and cerebral hemorrhage, whether described as due to birth trauma or to intrapartum anoxia or hypoxia

        Subdural hematoma (localized)

        Tentorial tear

        Use additional code to identify cause

        Excludes   *intraventricular hemorrhage (772.10–772.14)*

                subarachnoid hemorrhage (772.2)

    ● **767.1 Injuries to scalp**

        Coding Clinic: 2003, Q4, P69-70

        767.11 Epicranial subaponeurotic hemorrhage (massive)   N

            Subgaleal hemorrhage

        ■**767.19 Other injuries to scalp**   N

            Caput succedaneum

            Cephalhematoma

            Chignon (from vacuum extraction)

    767.2 Fracture of clavicle   N

    ■**767.3 Other injuries to skeleton**   N

        Fracture of:

            long bones

            skull

        Excludes   *congenital dislocation of hip (754.30–754.35)*

                fracture of spine, congenital (767.4)

    767.4 Injury to spine and spinal cord   N

        Dislocation of spine or spinal cord due to birth trauma

        Fracture of spine or spinal cord due to birth trauma

        Laceration of spine or spinal cord due to birth trauma

        Rupture of spine or spinal cord due to birth trauma

    767.5 Facial nerve injury   N

        Facial palsy

    767.6 Injury to brachial plexus   N

        Palsy or paralysis:

            brachial

            Erb (-Duchenne)

            Klumpke (-Déjérine)

    ■**767.7 Other cranial and peripheral nerve injuries**   N

        Phrenic nerve paralysis

    ■**767.8 Other specified birth trauma**   N

        Eye damage

        Hematoma of:

            liver (subcapsular)

            testes

            vulva

        Rupture of:

            liver

            spleen

        Scalpel wound

        Traumatic glaucoma

        Excludes   *hemorrhage classifiable to 772.0–772.9*

    ■**767.9 Birth trauma, unspecified**   N

        Birth injury NOS

● **768 Intrauterine hypoxia and birth asphyxia**

    Use only when associated with newborn morbidity classifiable elsewhere

    Excludes   *acidemia NOS of newborn (775.81)*

            acidosis NOS of newborn (775.81)

            cerebral ischemia NOS (779.2)

            hypoxia NOS of newborn (770.88)

            mixed metabolic and respiratory acidosis of newborn (775.81)

            respiratory arrest of newborn (770.87)

    ■**768.0 Fetal death from asphyxia or anoxia before onset of labor or at unspecified time**   N

    768.1 Fetal death from asphyxia or anoxia during labor   N

    768.2 Fetal distress before onset of labor, in liveborn infant   N

        Fetal metabolic acidemia before onset of labor, in liveborn infant

    768.3 Fetal distress first noted during labor and delivery, in liveborn infant   N

        Fetal metabolic acidemia first noted during labor and delivery, in liveborn infant

    ■**768.4 Fetal distress, unspecified as to time of onset, in liveborn infant**   N

        Fetal metabolic acidemia unspecified as to time of onset, in liveborn infant

        Coding Clinic: 1986, Nov-Dec, P10

    768.5 Severe birth asphyxia   N

        Birth asphyxia with neurologic involvement

        Excludes   *hypoxic-ischemic encephalopathy (HIE) (768.70–768.73)* ◀━

    768.6 Mild or moderate birth asphyxia   N

        Other specified birth asphyxia (without mention of neurologic involvement)

        Excludes   *hypoxic-ischemic encephalopathy (HIE) (768.70–768.73)* ◀━

    ● **768.7 Hypoxic-ischemic encephalopathy (HIE)**   N ◀━

        Coding Clinic: 2006, Q4, P104-106

        768.70 Hypoxic-ischemic encephalopathy, unspecified   ◀

        768.71 Mild hypoxic-ischemic encephalopathy   ◀

        768.72 Moderate hypoxic-ischemic encephalopathy   ◀

        768.73 Severe hypoxic-ischemic encephalopathy   ◀

    ■**768.9 Unspecified birth asphyxia in liveborn infant**   N

        Anoxia NOS, in liveborn infant

        Asphyxia NOS, in liveborn infant

◀ New   ◀━ Revised   ~~deleted~~ Deleted   ● Use Additional Digit(s)   ■ Nonspecific Code

● Not first-listed DX   OGCR Official Guidelines   Coding Clinic   Excludes   Includes   Use additional   Code first   Omit code

769 Respiratory distress syndrome   N
Cardiorespiratory distress syndrome of newborn
Hyaline membrane disease (pulmonary)
Idiopathic respiratory distress syndrome [IRDS or RDS]
of newborn
Pulmonary hypoperfusion syndrome

> **Excludes** *transient tachypnea of newborn (770.6)*

Coding Clinic: 1989, Q1, P10

● **770 Other respiratory conditions of fetus and newborn**

770.0 Congenital pneumonia   N
Infective pneumonia acquired prenatally

> **Excludes** *pneumonia from infection acquired after birth (480.0–486)*

Coding Clinic: 2005, Q1, P10-11

● **770.1 Fetal and newborn aspiration**

> **Excludes** *aspiration of postnatal stomach contents (770.85, 770.86)*
> *meconium passage during delivery (763.84)*
> *meconium staining (779.84)*

Coding Clinic: 2005, Q4, P83-89

770.10 Fetal and newborn aspiration, unspecified   N

770.11 Meconium aspiration without respiratory symptoms   N
Meconium aspiration NOS

770.12 Meconium aspiration with respiratory symptoms   N
Meconium aspiration pneumonia
Meconium aspiration pneumonitis
Meconium aspiration syndrome NOS

> Use additional code to identify any secondary pulmonary hypertension (416.8), if applicable

770.13 Aspiration of clear amniotic fluid without respiratory symptoms   N
Aspiration of clear amniotic fluid NOS

770.14 Aspiration of clear amniotic fluid with respiratory symptoms   N
Aspiration of clear amniotic fluid with pneumonia
Aspiration of clear amniotic fluid with pneumonitis

> Use additional code to identify any secondary pulmonary hypertension (416.8), if applicable

770.15 Aspiration of blood without respiratory symptoms   N
Aspiration of blood NOS

770.16 Aspiration of blood with respiratory symptoms   N
Aspiration of blood with pneumonia
Aspiration of blood with pneumonitis

> Use additional code to identify any secondary pulmonary hypertension (416.8), if applicable

770.17 Other fetal and newborn aspiration without respiratory symptoms   N

770.18 Other fetal and newborn aspiration with respiratory symptoms   N
Other aspiration pneumonia
Other aspiration pneumonitis

> Use additional code to identify any secondary pulmonary hypertension (416.8), if applicable

770.2 Interstitial emphysema and related conditions   N
Pneumomediastinum originating in the perinatal period
Pneumopericardium originating in the perinatal period
Pneumothorax originating in the perinatal period

770.3 Pulmonary hemorrhage   N
Hemorrhage:
alveolar (lung) originating in the perinatal period
intra-alveolar (lung) originating in the perinatal period
massive pulmonary originating in the perinatal period

770.4 Primary atelectasis   N
Failure of lungs to expand properly at birth
Pulmonary immaturity NOS

■**770.5 Other and unspecified atelectasis**   N
Atelectasis:
NOS originating in the perinatal period
partial originating in the perinatal period
secondary originating in the perinatal period
Pulmonary collapse originating in the perinatal period

770.6 Transitory tachypnea of newborn   N
Idiopathic tachypnea of newborn
Wet lung syndrome

> **Excludes** *respiratory distress syndrome (769)*

Coding Clinic: 1993, Q3, P7x2; 1989, Q1, P10

770.7 Chronic respiratory disease arising in the perinatal period   N
Bronchopulmonary dysplasia
Interstitial pulmonary fibrosis of prematurity
Wilson-Mikity syndrome
Coding Clinic: 1991, Q2, P19; 1986, Nov-Dec, P11-12

● ■**770.8 Other respiratory problems after birth**

> **Excludes** *mixed metabolic and respiratory acidosis of newborn (775.81)*

Coding Clinic: 2005, Q4, P83-89; 2002, Q4, P65-66; 1998, Q2, P10; 1996, Q2, P10-11

770.81 Primary apnea of newborn   N
Apneic spells of newborn NOS
Essential apnea of newborn
Sleep apnea of newborn

770.82 Other apnea of newborn   N
Obstructive apnea of newborn

770.83 Cyanotic attacks of newborn   N

770.84 Respiratory failure of newborn   N

> **Excludes** *respiratory distress syndrome (769)*

770.85 Aspiration of postnatal stomach contents without respiratory symptoms   N
Aspiration of postnatal stomach contents NOS

770.86 Aspiration of postnatal stomach contents with respiratory symptoms   N
Aspiration of postnatal stomach contents with pneumonia
Aspiration of postnatal stomach contents with pneumonitis

> Use additional code to identify any secondary pulmonary hypertension (416.8), if applicable

770.87 Respiratory arrest of newborn   N

770.88 Hypoxemia of newborn   N
Hypoxia NOS, in liveborn infant

■**770.89 Other respiratory problems after birth**   N

■**770.9 Unspecified respiratory condition of fetus and newborn**   N

CERTAIN CONDITIONS ORIGINATING IN THE PERINATAL PERIOD (760–779)

● **771 Infections specific to the perinatal period**

Includes   infections acquired before or during birth or
                via the umbilicus or during the first 28
                days after birth

Excludes   *congenital pneumonia (770.0)*
                congenital syphilis (090.0–090.9)
                infant botulism (040.41)
                maternal infectious disease as a cause of mortality
                or morbidity in fetus or newborn, but fetus
                or newborn not manifesting the disease
                (760.2)
                ophthalmia neonatorum due to gonococcus
                (098.40)
                other infections not specifically classified to this
                category
                Coding Clinic: 2005, Q1, P10

771.0 Congenital rubella   N
         Congenital rubella pneumonitis

771.1 Congenital cytomegalovirus infection   N
         Congenital cytomegalic inclusion disease

■**771.2 Other congenital infections**   N
         Congenital: Congenital:
           herpes simplex   toxoplasmosis
           listeriosis   tuberculosis
           malaria

771.3 Tetanus neonatorum   N
         Tetanus omphalitis

         Excludes   *hypocalcemic tetany (775.4)*

771.4 Omphalitis of the newborn   N
         Infection: Infection:
           navel cord   umbilical stump

         Excludes   *tetanus omphalitis (771.3)*

771.5 Neonatal infective mastitis   N

         Excludes   *noninfective neonatal mastitis (778.7)*

771.6 Neonatal conjunctivitis and dacryocystitis   N
         Ophthalmia neonatorum NOS

         Excludes   *ophthalmia neonatorum due to gonococcus*
                        (098.40)

771.7 Neonatal Candida infection   N
         Neonatal moniliasis
         Thrush in newborn

● ■**771.8 Other infections specific to the perinatal period**
         Use additional code to identify organism
         (041.00–041.9)

         771.81 Septicemia [sepsis] of newborn   N
                  Use additional code to identify
                     severe sepsis (995.92) and any
                     associated acute organ dysfunction,
                     if applicable
                  OGCR Section I.C.15.j
                  771.81 should be assigned with a secondary
                  code from category 041, Bacterial infections
                  in conditions classified elsewhere and of
                  unspecified site, to identify the organism.

771.82 Urinary tract infection of newborn   N
771.83 Bacteremia of newborn   N
■**771.89 Other infections specific to the perinatal
          period**   N
          Intra-amniotic infection of fetus NOS
          Infection of newborn NOS
          Coding Clinic: 2005, Q1, P10

● **772 Fetal and neonatal hemorrhage**

Excludes   *fetal hematologic conditions complicating*
                pregnancy (678.0)   ◄
                hematological disorders of fetus and newborn
                (776.0–776.9)

772.0 Fetal blood loss affecting newborn   N ◄▥
         Fetal blood loss from:
           cut end of co-twin's cord
           placenta
           ruptured cord
           vasa previa
         Fetal exsanguination
         Fetal hemorrhage into:
           co-twin
           mother's circulation

● **772.1 Intraventricular hemorrhage**
         Intraventricular hemorrhage from any perinatal
         cause
         Coding Clinic: 1992, Q3, P8; 1988, Q4, P8

         ■**772.10 Unspecified grade**   N
         772.11 Grade I   N
                  Bleeding into germinal matrix
         772.12 Grade II   N
                  Bleeding into ventricle
         772.13 Grade III   N
                  Bleeding with enlargement of ventricle
                  Coding Clinic: 2001, Q4, P50-51
         772.14 Grade IV   N
                  Bleeding into cerebral cortex

772.2 Subarachnoid hemorrhage   N
         Subarachnoid hemorrhage from any perinatal
         cause

         Excludes   *subdural and cerebral hemorrhage (767.0)*

772.3 Umbilical hemorrhage after birth   N
         Slipped umbilical ligature

772.4 Gastrointestinal hemorrhage   N

         Excludes   *swallowed maternal blood (777.3)*

772.5 Adrenal hemorrhage   N

772.6 Cutaneous hemorrhage   N
         Bruising in fetus or newborn
         Ecchymoses in fetus or newborn
         Petechiae in fetus or newborn
         Superficial hematoma in fetus or newborn

■**772.8 Other specified hemorrhage of fetus or newborn** N

         Excludes   *hemorrhagic disease of newborn (776.0)*
                        pulmonary hemorrhage (770.3)

■**772.9 Unspecified hemorrhage of newborn**   N

● **773 Hemolytic disease of fetus or newborn, due to isoimmunization**

Also known as erythroblastosis fetalis as a result of Rh blood factor incompatibilities between mother (Rh negative) and fetus (Rh positive)

773.0 Hemolytic disease due to Rh isoimmunization N
 Anemia due to RH:
  antibodies
  isoimmunization
  maternal/fetal incompatibility
 Erythroblastosis (fetalis) due to RH:
  antibodies
  isoimmunization
  maternal/fetal incompatibility
 Hemolytic disease (fetus) (newborn) due to RH:
  antibodies
  isoimmunization
  maternal/fetal incompatibility
 Jaundice due to RH:
  antibodies
  isoimmunization
  maternal/fetal incompatibility
 Rh hemolytic disease
 Rh isoimmunization

773.1 Hemolytic disease due to ABO isoimmunization N
 ABO hemolytic disease
 ABO isoimmunization
 Anemia due to ABO:
  antibodies
  isoimmunization
  maternal/fetal incompatibility
 Erythroblastosis (fetalis) due to ABO:
  antibodies
  isoimmunization
  maternal/fetal incompatibility
 Hemolytic disease (fetus) (newborn) due to ABO:
  antibodies
  isoimmunization
  maternal/fetal incompatibility
 Jaundice due to ABO:
  antibodies
  isoimmunization
  maternal/fetal incompatibility
 Coding Clinic: 2003, Q2, P14-15; 1992, Q3, P8-9

■**773.2 Hemolytic disease due to other and unspecified isoimmunization** N
 Erythroblastosis (fetalis) (neonatorum) NOS
 Hemolytic disease (fetus) (newborn) NOS
 Jaundice or anemia due to other and unspecified blood-group incompatibility
 Coding Clinic: 1994, Q1, P13

773.3 Hydrops fetalis due to isoimmunization N

 Use additional code, if desired, to identify type of isoimmunization (773.0–773.2)

773.4 Kernicterus due to isoimmunization N

 Use additional code, if desired, to identify type of isoimmunization (773.0–773.2)

773.5 Late anemia due to isoimmunization N

● **774 Other perinatal jaundice**

● **774.0 *Perinatal jaundice from hereditary hemolytic anemias*** N

 Code first underlying disease (282.0–282.9)

■**774.1 Perinatal jaundice from other excessive hemolysis** N
 Fetal or neonatal jaundice from:
  bruising
  drugs or toxins transmitted from mother
  infection
  polycythemia
  swallowed maternal blood

 Use additional code to identify cause

 Excludes *jaundice due to isoimmunization (773.0–773.2)*

774.2 Neonatal jaundice associated with preterm delivery N
 Hyperbilirubinemia of prematurity
 Jaundice due to delayed conjugation associated with preterm delivery
 Coding Clinic: 1994, Q1, P13; 1991, Q3, P21

● **774.3 Neonatal jaundice due to delayed conjugation from other causes**

 ■**774.30 Neonatal jaundice due to delayed conjugation, cause unspecified** N

 ● **774.31 *Neonatal jaundice due to delayed conjugation in diseases classified elsewhere*** N

  Code first underlying diseases, as:
   congenital hypothyroidism (243)
   Crigler-Najjar syndrome (277.4)
   Gilbert's syndrome (277.4)

 ■**774.39 Other** N
  Jaundice due to delayed conjugation from causes, such as:
   breast milk inhibitors
   delayed development of conjugating system

774.4 Perinatal jaundice due to hepatocellular damage N
 Fetal or neonatal hepatitis
 Giant cell hepatitis
 Inspissated bile syndrome

● ■**774.5 *Perinatal jaundice from other causes*** N

 Code first underlying cause, as:
  congenital obstruction of bile duct (751.61)
  galactosemia (271.1)
  mucoviscidosis (277.00–277.09)

■**774.6 Unspecified fetal and neonatal jaundice** N
 Icterus neonatorum
 Neonatal hyperbilirubinemia (transient)
 Physiologic jaundice NOS in newborn

 Excludes *that in preterm infants (774.2)*

 Coding Clinic: 1994, Q1, P13

774.7 Kernicterus not due to isoimmunization N
 Bilirubin encephalopathy
 Kernicterus of newborn NOS

 Excludes *kernicterus due to isoimmunization (773.4)*

CERTAIN CONDITIONS ORIGINATING IN THE PERINATAL PERIOD (760–779)

● **775 Endocrine and metabolic disturbances specific to the fetus and newborn**

> **Includes** transitory endocrine and metabolic disturbances caused by the infant's response to maternal endocrine and metabolic factors, its removal from them, or its adjustment to extrauterine existence

775.0 Syndrome of "infant of a diabetic mother" N
Maternal diabetes mellitus affecting fetus or newborn (with hypoglycemia)
Coding Clinic: 2004, Q1, P7-8x3

775.1 Neonatal diabetes mellitus N
Diabetes mellitus syndrome in newborn infant

775.2 Neonatal myasthenia gravis N

775.3 Neonatal thyrotoxicosis N
Neonatal hyperthyroidism (transient)

775.4 Hypocalcemia and hypomagnesemia of newborn N
Cow's milk hypocalcemia
Hypocalcemic tetany, neonatal
Neonatal hypoparathyroidism
Phosphate-loading hypocalcemia

■**775.5 Other transitory neonatal electrolyte disturbances** N
Dehydration, neonatal
Coding Clinic: 2008, Q4, P139-140; 2005, Q1, P9-10

775.6 Neonatal hypoglycemia N
> **Excludes** infant of mother with diabetes mellitus (775.0)

775.7 Late metabolic acidosis of newborn N

● **775.8 Other neonatal endocrine and metabolic disturbances**

■**775.81 Other acidosis of newborn** N
Acidemia NOS of newborn
Acidosis of newborn NOS
Mixed metabolic and respiratory acidosis of newborn

■**775.89 Other neonatal endocrine and metabolic disturbances** N
Amino-acid metabolic disorders described as transitory

■**775.9 Unspecified endocrine and metabolic disturbances specific to the fetus and newborn** N

● **776 Hematological disorders of newborn** ◀▥

> **Includes** disorders specific to the ~~fetus or~~ newborn though possibly originating in utero
> **Excludes** fetal hematologic conditions (678.0)

776.0 Hemorrhagic disease of newborn N
Hemorrhagic diathesis of newborn
Vitamin K deficiency of newborn
> **Excludes** fetal or neonatal hemorrhage (772.0–772.9)

776.1 Transient neonatal thrombocytopenia N
Lack of sufficient numbers of circulating thrombocytes (platelets)
Neonatal thrombocytopenia due to:
exchange transfusion
idiopathic maternal thrombocytopenia
isoimmunization

776.2 Disseminated intravascular coagulation in newborn N

■**776.3 Other transient neonatal disorders of coagulation** N
Transient coagulation defect, newborn

776.4 Polycythemia neonatorum N
Excess number of thrombocytes (platelets)
Plethora of newborn
Polycythemia due to:
donor twin transfusion
maternal-fetal transfusion

776.5 Congenital anemia N
Anemia following fetal blood loss
> **Excludes** anemia due to isoimmunization (773.0–773.2, 773.5)
> hereditary hemolytic anemias (282.0–282.9)

776.6 Anemia of prematurity N

776.7 Transient neonatal neutropenia N
Isoimmune neutropenia
Low levels of granulocytic neutrophilic white blood cells
Maternal transfer neutropenia
> **Excludes** congenital neutropenia (nontransient) (288.01)

■**776.8 Other specified transient hematological disorders** N

■**776.9 Unspecified hematological disorder specific to ~~fetus or~~ newborn** N ◀▥

● **777 Perinatal disorders of digestive system**

> **Includes** disorders specific to the fetus and newborn
> **Excludes** intestinal obstruction classifiable to 560.0–560.9

777.1 Meconium obstruction N
Congenital fecaliths
Stoney feces formations
Delayed passage of meconium
Meconium ileus NOS
Meconium plug syndrome
> **Excludes** meconium ileus in cystic fibrosis (277.01)

777.2 Intestinal obstruction due to inspissated milk N
Being thickened, dried, or made less fluid

777.3 Hematemesis and melena due to swallowed maternal blood N
Swallowed blood syndrome in newborn
> **Excludes** that not due to swallowed maternal blood (772.4)

777.4 Transitory ileus of newborn N
> **Excludes** Hirschsprung's disease (751.3)

● **777.5 Necrotizing enterocolitis in newborn**
~~Pseudomembranous enterocolitis in newborn~~

■**777.50 Necrotizing enterocolitis in newborn, unspecified** N
Necrotizing enterocolitis in newborn, NOS

777.51 Stage I necrotizing enterocolitis in newborn N
Necrotizing enterocolitis without pneumatosis, without perforation ◀

777.52 Stage II necrotizing enterocolitis in newborn N
Necrotizing enterocolitis with pneumatosis, without perforation

777.53 Stage III necrotizing enterocolitis in newborn N
Necrotizing enterocolitis with perforation
Necrotizing enterocolitis with pneumatosis and perforation
Coding Clinic: 2008, Q4, P138-140

777.6 Perinatal intestinal perforation N
Meconium peritonitis

■**777.8 Other specified perinatal disorders of digestive system** N

■**777.9 Unspecified perinatal disorder of digestive system** N

◀ New   ◀▥ Revised   ~~deleted~~ Deleted   ● Use Additional Digit(s)   ■ Nonspecific Code
● Not first-listed DX   OGCR Official Guidelines   Coding Clinic   Excludes   Includes   Use additional   Code first   Omit code

● **778 Conditions involving the integument and temperature regulation of fetus and newborn**

778.0 Hydrops fetalis not due to isoimmunization N
Idiopathic hydrops
Severe, life-threatening problem of edema (swelling) in fetus and newborn

Excludes *hydrops fetalis due to isoimmunization (773.3)*

778.1 Sclerema neonatorum N

778.2 Cold injury syndrome of newborn N

■**778.3 Other hypothermia of newborn** N

■**778.4 Other disturbances of temperature regulation of newborn** N
Dehydration fever in newborn
Environmentally induced pyrexia
Hyperthermia in newborn
Transitory fever of newborn

■**778.5 Other and unspecified edema of newborn** N
Edema neonatorum

778.6 Congenital hydrocele
Congenital hydrocele of tunica vaginalis

778.7 Breast engorgement in newborn N
Noninfective mastitis of newborn

Excludes *infective mastitis of newborn (771.5)*

■**778.8 Other specified conditions involving the integument of fetus and newborn** N
Urticaria neonatorum
Skin rash

Excludes *impetigo neonatorum (684)*
pemphigus neonatorum (684)

■**778.9 Unspecified condition involving the integument and temperature regulation of fetus and newborn** N

● **779 Other and ill-defined conditions originating in the perinatal period**

779.0 Convulsions in newborn N
Fits in newborn
Seizures in newborn
Coding Clinic: 1984, Nov-Dec, P11

■**779.1 Other and unspecified cerebral irritability in newborn** N

779.2 Cerebral depression, coma, and other abnormal cerebral signs N
Cerebral ischemia NOS of newborn
CNS dysfunction in newborn NOS

Excludes *cerebral ischemia due to birth trauma (767.0)*
intrauterine cerebral ischemia (768.2–768.9)
intraventricular hemorrhage (772.10–772.14)

● **779.3 Disorder of stomach function and ~~F~~feeding problems in newborn** N ◀
~~Regurgitation of food in newborn~~
~~Slow feeding in newborn~~
~~Vomiting in newborn~~
Coding Clinic: 1989, Q2, P15

779.31 Feeding problems in newborn ◀
Slow feeding in newborn ◀

Excludes *feeding problem in child over 28 days old (783.3)* ◀

779.32 Bilious vomiting in newborn ◀

Excludes *bilious vomiting in child over 28 days old (787.04)* ◀

779.33 Other vomiting in newborn ◀
Regurgitation of food in newborn ◀

Excludes *vomiting in child over 28 days old (536.2, 787.01-787.03, 787.04)* ◀

779.34 Failure to thrive in newborn ◀

Excludes *failure to thrive in child over 28 days old (783.41)* ◀

779.4 Drug reactions and intoxications specific to newborn N
Gray syndrome from chloramphenicol administration in newborn

Excludes *fetal alcohol syndrome (760.71)*
reactions and intoxications from maternal opiates and tranquilizers (763.5)

779.5 Drug withdrawal syndrome in newborn N
Drug withdrawal syndrome in infant of dependent mother

Excludes *fetal alcohol syndrome (760.71)*
Coding Clinic: 1994, Q3, P6

779.6 Termination of pregnancy (fetus) N
Fetal death due to:
induced abortion
termination of pregnancy

Excludes *spontaneous abortion (fetus) (761.8)*

779.7 Periventricular leukomalacia
Coding Clinic: 2001, Q4, P50-51

● ■**779.8 Other specified conditions originating in the perinatal period**
Coding Clinic: 2006, Q1, P18; 2002, Q4, P67; 1994, Q1, P15

779.81 Neonatal bradycardia N

Excludes *abnormality in fetal heart rate or rhythm complicating labor and delivery (763.81–763.83)*
bradycardia due to birth asphyxia (768.5–768.9)

779.82 Neonatal tachycardia N

Excludes *abnormality in fetal heart rate or rhythm complicating labor and delivery (763.81–763.83)*

779.83 Delayed separation of umbilical cord N
Coding Clinic: 2003, Q4, P71

779.84 Meconium staining N

Excludes *meconium aspiration (770.11, 770.12)*
meconium passage during delivery (763.84)
Coding Clinic: 2005, Q4, P83-89x2

779.85 Cardiac arrest of newborn N

■**779.89 Other specified conditions originating in the perinatal period** N

Use additional code to specify condition
Coding Clinic: 2005, Q2, P15-16; Q1, P9

OGCR Section I.C.15.a.2
If the index does not provide a specific code for a perinatal condition, assign code 779.89 followed by the code from another chapter that specifies the condition.

■**779.9 Unspecified condition originating in the perinatal period** N
Congenital debility NOS
Stillbirth NEC

CERTAIN CONDITIONS ORIGINATING IN THE PERINATAL PERIOD (760–779)

N Newborn Age: 0   **P** Pediatric Age: 0–17   **M** Maternity Age: 12–55   **A** Adult Age: 15–124   ♀ Females Only   ♂ Males Only

1039

16. SYMPTOMS, SIGNS, AND ILL-DEFINED CONDITIONS (780–799)

This section includes symptoms, signs, abnormal results of laboratory or other investigative procedures, and ill-defined conditions regarding which no diagnosis classifiable elsewhere is recorded.

Signs and symptoms that point rather definitely to a given diagnosis are assigned to some category in the preceding part of the classification. In general, categories 780–796 include the more ill-defined conditions and symptoms that point with perhaps equal suspicion to two or more diseases or to two or more systems of the body, and without the necessary study of the case to make a final diagnosis. Practically all categories in this group could be designated as "not otherwise specified," or as "unknown etiology," or as "transient." The Alphabetic Index should be consulted to determine which symptoms and signs are to be allocated here and which to more specific sections of the classification; the residual subcategories numbered .9 are provided for other relevant symptoms which cannot be allocated elsewhere in the classification.

The conditions and signs or symptoms included in categories 780–796 consist of: (a) cases for which no more specific diagnosis can be made even after all facts bearing on the case have been investigated; (b) signs or symptoms existing at the time of initial encounter that proved to be transient and whose causes could not be determined; (c) provisional diagnoses in a patient who failed to return for further investigation or care; (d) cases referred elsewhere for investigation or treatment before the diagnosis was made; (e) cases in which a more precise diagnosis was not available for any other reason; (f) certain symptoms which represent important problems in medical care and which it might be desired to classify in addition to a known cause.

SYMPTOMS (780–789)

● **780   General symptoms**

  ● **780.0   Alteration of consciousness**

     Excludes   *alteration of consciousness due to:* ◀
         intracranial injuries (850.0–854.19) ◀
         skull fractures (800.00–801.99, ◀
           803.00–804.99)
         coma:
           diabetic (249.2–249.3, 250.2–250.3)
           hepatic (572.2)
           originating in the perinatal period
            (779.2)

     780.01   Coma
         Coding Clinic: 1996, Q3, P16

     780.02   Transient alteration of awareness

     780.03   Persistent vegetative state

     ■ **780.09   Other**
         Drowsiness   Somnolence
         Semicoma   Stupor
                             Unconsciousness

   780.1   Hallucinations
     Hallucinations:
       NOS
       auditory
       gustatory
       olfactory
       tactile

     Excludes   *those associated with mental disorders, as*
         functional psychoses (295.0–298.9)
         organic brain syndromes (290.0–294.9,
           310.0–310.9)
         visual hallucinations (368.16)

   780.2   Syncope and collapse
     Blackout   (Near) (Pre)syncope
     Fainting   Vasovagal attack

     Excludes   *carotid sinus syncope (337.0)*
         heat syncope (992.1)
         neurocirculatory asthenia (306.2)
         orthostatic hypotension (458.0)
         shock NOS (785.50)
     Coding Clinic: 2002, Q1, P6; 2000, Q3, P12; 1995, Q4, P50-51; Q3, P14; 1992, Q3, P16; 1990, Q1, P9; 1985, Nov-Dec, P12

● **780.3   Convulsions**

     Excludes   *convulsions:*
         epileptic (345.10–345.91)
         in newborn (779.0)
     Coding Clinic: 1984, Nov-Dec, P11

     780.31   Febrile convulsions (simple), unspecified
         Febrile seizures NOS
         Coding Clinic: 2005, Q3, P12-13; 1987, Nov-Dec, P11

     780.32   Complex febrile convulsions
         Febrile seizure:
           atypical
           complex
           complicated

         Excludes   *status epilepticus (345.3)*
         Coding Clinic: 2006, Q4, P106-107

     ■ **780.39   Other convulsions**
         Convulsive disorder NOS
         Fits NOS
         Recurrent convulsions NOS
         Seizure NOS
         Seizures NOS
         Coding Clinic: 2008, Q1, P17; 2006, Q3, P22; 2004, Q4, P50-52; 2003, Q1, P7; 1998, Q4, P39-40; 1997, Q2, P8; Q1, P12-13; 1994, Q3, P9; 1993, Q1, P24; 1987, Nov-Dec, P12; 1985, July-Aug, P10; 1984, May-June, P14

   780.4   Dizziness and giddiness
     Light-headedness
     Vertigo NOS

     Excludes   *Méniére's disease and other specified*
         vertiginous syndromes
         (386.0–386.9)
     Coding Clinic: 2003, Q2, P11; 2000, Q3, P12; 1997, Q2, P9-10; 1991, Q2, P17

● **780.5   Sleep disturbances**

     Excludes   *circadian rhythm sleep disorders*
         (327.30–327.39)
         organic hypersomnia (327.10–327.19)
         organic insomnia (327.00–327.09)
         organic sleep apnea (327.20–327.29)
         organic sleep related movement disorders
         (327.51–327.59)
         parasomnias (327.40–327.49)
         that of nonorganic origin (307.40–307.49)

     ■ **780.50   Sleep disturbance, unspecified**

     ■ **780.51   Insomnia with sleep apnea, unspecified**
         Coding Clinic: 1993, Q1, P28-29

     ■ **780.52   Insomnia, unspecified**

     ■ **780.53   Hypersomnia with sleep apnea, unspecified**
         Coding Clinic: 1993, Q1, P28-29

     ■ **780.54   Hypersomnia, unspecified**

     780.55   Disruptions of 24 hour sleep wake cycle, unspecified

     780.56   Dysfunctions associated with sleep stages or arousal from sleep

◀ New   ◀▦ Revised   ~~deleted~~ Deleted   ● Use Additional Digit(s)   ■ Nonspecific Code

● Not first-listed DX   OGCR Official Guidelines   Coding Clinic   Excludes   Includes   Use additional   Code first   Omit code

780.57 Unspecified sleep apnea
> Coding Clinic: 2001, Q1, P6-7; 1997, Q1, P5; 1993, Q1, P28-29

780.58 Sleep related movement disorder, unspecified
> **Excludes** *restless legs syndrome (333.94)*
>
> Coding Clinic: 2004, Q4, P95-96

780.59 Other

● **780.6 Fever and other physiologic disturbances of temperature regulation**
> **Excludes** *effects of reduced environmental temperature (991.0-991.9)*
> *effects of heat and light (992.0-992.9)*
> *fever, chills or hypothermia associated with confirmed infection – code to infection*
>
> Coding Clinic: 2008, Q4, P140-143; 2005, Q3, P16-17; 2000, Q3, P13; 1991, Q2, P8x2; 1990, Q1, P8; 1985, July-Aug, P13

780.60 Fever, unspecified
Chills with fever
Fever NOS
Fever of unknown origin (FUO)
Hyperpyrexia NOS
Pyrexia NOS
Pyrexia of unknown origin
> **Excludes** *chills without fever (780.64)*
> *neonatal fever (778.4)*
> *pyrexia of unknown origin (during):*
>   *in newborn (778.4)*
>   *labor (659.2)*
>   *the puerperium (672)*

● **780.61 Fever presenting with conditions classified elsewhere**
> *Code first* underlying condition when associated fever is present, such as with:
> leukemia (conditions classifiable to 204-208)
>   neutropenia (288.00-288.09)
>   sickle-cell disease (282.60-282.69)
>
> Coding Clinic: 2008, Q4, P140-143

780.62 Postprocedural fever
> **Excludes** *postvaccination fever (780.63)*

780.63 Postvaccination fever
Postimmunization fever

780.64 Chills (without fever)
Chills NOS
> **Excludes** *chills with fever (780.60)*

780.65 Hypothermia not associated with low environmental temperature
> **Excludes** *hypothermia:*
> *associated with low environmental temperature (991.6)*
> *due to anesthesia (995.89)*
> *of newborn (778.2, 778.3)*

● **780.7 Malaise and fatigue**
> **Excludes** *debility, unspecified (799.3)*
> *fatigue (during):*
>   *combat (308.0–308.9)*
>   *heat (992.6)*
>   *pregnancy (646.8)*
> *neurasthenia (300.5)*
> *senile asthenia (797)*

780.71 Chronic fatigue syndrome
> Coding Clinic: 1998, Q4, P48-49

780.72 Functional quadriplegia
Complete immobility due to severe physical disability or frailty
> **Excludes** *hysterical paralysis (300.11)*
> *immobility syndrome (728.3)*
> *neurologic quadriplegia (344.00-344.09)*
> *quadriplegia NOS (344.00)*
>
> Coding Clinic: 2008, Q4, P143

780.79 Other malaise and fatigue
Asthenia NOS
Lethargy
Postviral (asthenic) syndrome
Tiredness
> Coding Clinic: 2004, Q4, P77-78; 2000, Q1, P6

780.8 Generalized hyperhidrosis
Diaphoresis
Excessive sweating
Secondary hyperhidrosis
> **Excludes** *focal (localized) (primary) (secondary) hyperhidrosis (705.21–705.22)*
> *Frey's syndrome (705.22)*

● **780.9 Other general symptoms**
> **Excludes** *hypothermia:*
>   *NOS (accidental) (991.6)*
>   *due to anesthesia (995.89)*
> *memory disturbance as part of a pattern of mental disorder*
> *of newborn (778.2–778.3)*
>
> Coding Clinic: 2002, Q4, P67-68

780.91 Fussy infant (baby)   P

780.92 Excessive crying of infant (baby)   N
> **Excludes** *excessive crying of child, adolescent or adult (780.95)*
>
> Coding Clinic: 2005, Q4, P89-90

780.93 Memory loss
Amnesia (retrograde)
Memory loss NOS
> **Excludes** *memory loss due to:* ◄
>   *intracranial injuries (850.0–854.19)* ◄
>   *skull fractures (800.00–801.99, 803.00–804.99)* ◄
> *mild memory disturbance due to organic brain damage (310.8)* ◄
> *transient global amnesia (437.7)*
>
> Coding Clinic: 2003, Q4, P71

780.94 Early satiety
> Coding Clinic: 2003, Q4, P72

780.95 Excessive crying of child, adolescent, or adult
> **Excludes** *excessive crying of infant (baby) (780.92)*
>
> Coding Clinic: 2005, Q4, P89-90

780.96 Generalized pain
Pain NOS

780.97 Altered mental status
Change in mental status
> **Excludes** *altered level of consciousness (780.01–780.09)*
> *altered mental status due to known condition - code to condition*
> *delirium NOS (780.09)*
>
> Coding Clinic: 2006, Q4, P107-108; 1993, Q3, P11

780.99 Other general symptoms
> Coding Clinic: 2003, Q4, P103-104; 1999, Q4, P10; 1985, Nov-Dec, P12

SYMPTOMS, SIGNS, AND ILL-DEFINED CONDITIONS (780–799)

● 781 Symptoms involving nervous and musculoskeletal systems

> **Excludes** depression NOS (311)
>> disorders specifically relating to:
>>> back (724.0–724.9)
>>> hearing (388.0–389.9)
>>> joint (718.0–719.9)
>>> limb (729.0–729.9)
>>> neck (723.0–723.9)
>>> vision (368.0–369.9)
>> pain in limb (729.5)

781.0 Abnormal involuntary movements
Abnormal head movements
Fasciculation
Spasms NOS
Tremor NOS

> **Excludes** abnormal reflex (796.1)
> chorea NOS (333.5)
> infantile spasms (345.60–345.61)
> spastic paralysis (342.1, 343.0–344.9)
> specified movement disorders classifiable to 333 (333.0–333.9)
> that of nonorganic origin (307.2–307.3)

781.1 Disturbances of sensation of smell and taste
Anosmia   Parosmia
Parageusia

781.2 Abnormality of gait
Gait:
    ataxic
    paralytic
    spastic
    staggering

> **Excludes** ataxia:
>> NOS (781.3)
>> difficulty in walking (719.7)
>> locomotor (progressive) (094.0)

> Coding Clinic: 2005, Q2, P6-7; 2004, Q2, P15

781.3 Lack of coordination
Ataxia NOS
Muscular incoordination

> **Excludes** ataxic gait (781.2)
> cerebellar ataxia (334.0–334.9)
> difficulty in walking (719.7)
> vertigo NOS (780.4)

> Coding Clinic: 2004, Q4, P50-52; 1997, Q3, P12-13

781.4 Transient paralysis of limb
Monoplegia, transient NOS

> **Excludes** paralysis (342.0–344.9)

781.5 Clubbing of fingers

781.6 Meningismus
Dupre's syndrome   Meningism
> Coding Clinic: 2000, Q3, P13

781.7 Tetany
Carpopedal spasm

> **Excludes** tetanus neonatorum (771.3)
> tetany:
>> hysterical (300.11)
>> newborn (hypocalcemic) (775.4)
>> parathyroid (252.1)
>> psychogenic (306.0)

781.8 Neurologic neglect syndrome
Asomatognosia   Left-sided neglect
Hemi-akinesia   Sensory extinction
Hemi-inattention   Sensory neglect
Hemispatial neglect   Visuospatial neglect

781.9 Other symptoms involving nervous and musculoskeletal systems

781.91 Loss of height

> **Excludes** osteoporosis (733.00–733.09)

781.92 Abnormal posture

781.93 Ocular torticollis
> Coding Clinic: 2002, Q4, P68; Q4, P68

781.94 Facial weakness
Facial droop

> **Excludes** facial weakness due to late effect of cerebrovascular accident (438.83)

> Coding Clinic: 2003, Q4, P72

781.99 Other symptoms involving nervous and musculoskeletal systems

● 782 Symptoms involving skin and other integumentary tissue

> **Excludes** symptoms relating to breast (611.71–611.79)

782.0 Disturbance of skin sensation
Anesthesia of skin
Burning or prickling sensation
Hyperesthesia
Hypoesthesia
Numbness
Paresthesia
Tingling

782.1 Rash and other nonspecific skin eruption
Exanthem

> **Excludes** vesicular eruption (709.8)

782.2 Localized superficial swelling, mass, or lump
Subcutaneous nodules

> **Excludes** localized adiposity (278.1)

782.3 Edema
Anasarca
Dropsy
Localized edema NOS

> **Excludes** ascites (789.51–789.59)
> edema of:
>> newborn NOS (778.5)
>> pregnancy (642.0–642.9, 646.1)
> fluid retention (276.6)
> hydrops fetalis (773.3, 778.0)
> hydrothorax (511.81–511.89)
> nutritional edema (260, 262)

> Coding Clinic: 2000, Q2, P18

782.4 Jaundice, unspecified, not of newborn
Cholemia NOS
Icterus NOS

> **Excludes** due to isoimmunization (773.0–773.2, 773.4)
> jaundice in newborn (774.0–774.7)

782.5 Cyanosis

> **Excludes** newborn (770.83)

● 782.6 Pallor and flushing

782.61 Pallor

782.62 Flushing
Excessive blushing

782.7 Spontaneous ecchymoses
Petechiae

> **Excludes** ecchymosis in fetus or newborn (772.6)
> purpura (287.0–287.9)

◀ New   ◀▦ Revised   ~~deleted~~ Deleted   ● Use Additional Digit(s)   ■ Nonspecific Code

 Not first-listed DX   OGCR Official Guidelines   Coding Clinic   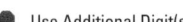 Excludes   Includes   Use additional   Code first   Omit code

SYMPTOMS, SIGNS, AND ILL-DEFINED CONDITIONS (780–799)

782.8 Changes in skin texture
Induration of skin
Thickening of skin

782.9 Other symptoms involving skin and integumentary tissues

783 Symptoms concerning nutrition, metabolism, and development

783.0 Anorexia
Loss of appetite

> **Excludes**   *anorexia nervosa (307.1)*
> *loss of appetite of nonorganic origin (307.59)*

783.1 Abnormal weight gain

> **Excludes**   *excessive weight gain in pregnancy (646.1)*
> *obesity (278.00)*
> *morbid (278.01)*

783.2 Abnormal loss of weight and underweight
Use additional code to identify Body Mass Index (BMI), if known (V85.0–V85.54)

783.21 Loss of weight

783.22 Underweight

783.3 Feeding difficulties and mismanagement
Feeding problem (elderly) (infant)

> **Excludes**   *feeding disturbance or problems:*
> *in newborn (779.31–779.34)* ◀||||
> *of nonorganic origin (307.50–307.59)*

Coding Clinic: 1997, Q3, P12-13; 1994, Q2, P10-11

783.4 Lack of expected normal physiological development in childhood

> **Excludes**   *delay in sexual development and puberty (259.0)*
> *gonadal dysgenesis (758.6)*
> *pituitary dwarfism (253.31–779.34)*
> *slow fetal growth and fetal malnutrition (764.00–764.99)*
> *specific delays in mental development (315.0–315.9)*

Coding Clinic: 1997, Q3, P5

783.40 Lack of normal physiological development, unspecified
Inadequate development
Lack of development

783.41 Failure to thrive   P
Failure to gain weight

> **Excludes**   *failure to thrive in newborn (779.34)* ◀

Coding Clinic: 2003, Q1, P12

783.42 Delayed milestones   P
Late talker
Late walker

783.43 Short stature
Growth failure
Growth retardation
Lack of growth
Physical retardation
Coding Clinic: 2004, Q2, P3

783.5 Polydipsia
Excessive thirst

783.6 Polyphagia
Excessive eating
Hyperalimentation NOS

> **Excludes**   *disorders of eating of nonorganic origin (307.50–307.59)*

783.7 Adult failure to thrive   A

783.9 Other symptoms concerning nutrition, metabolism, and development
Hypometabolism

> **Excludes**   *abnormal basal metabolic rate (794.7)*
> *dehydration (276.51)*
> *other disorders of fluid, electrolyte, and acid-base balance (276.0–276.9)*

Coding Clinic: 2004, Q2, P3

784 Symptoms involving head and neck

> **Excludes**   *encephalopathy NOS (348.30)*
> *specific symptoms involving neck classifiable to 723 (723.0–723.9)*

784.0 Headache
Facial pain
Pain in head NOS

> **Excludes**   *atypical face pain (350.2)*
> *migraine (346.0–346.9)*
> *tension headache (307.81)*

Coding Clinic: 2006, Q3, P22; Q2, P17-18; 2000, Q3, P13; 1992, Q3, P14; 1990, Q1, P9

784.1 Throat pain

> **Excludes**   *dysphagia (787.20–787.29)*
> *neck pain (723.1)*
> *sore throat (462)*
> *chronic (472.1)*

784.2 Swelling, mass, or lump in head and neck
Space-occupying lesion, intracranial NOS
Coding Clinic: 2003, Q1, P8

784.3 Aphasia

> **Excludes**   *aphasia due to late effects of cerebrovascular disease (438.11)*
> *developmental aphasia (315.31)*

Coding Clinic: 2004, Q4, P77-78; 1998, Q4, P87; 1997, Q3, P12-13

784.4 Voice ~~disturbance~~ and resonance disorders ◀||||

784.40 Voice ~~disturbance~~ and resonance disorder, unspecified ◀||||

784.41 Aphonia
Loss of voice

784.42 Dysphonia ◀
Hoarseness ◀

784.43 Hypernasality ◀

784.44 Hyponasality ◀

784.49 Other voice and resonance disorders ◀||||
Change in voice
~~Dysphonia~~
~~Hoarseness~~
~~Hypernasality~~
~~Hyponasality~~

784.5 Other speech disturbance ◀||||
~~Dysarthria~~
~~Dysphasia~~
~~Slurred speech~~

> **Excludes**   *speech disorder due to late effect of cerebrovascular accident (438.10–438.19)* ◀
> *stammering and stuttering (307.0)*
> *that of nonorganic origin (307.0, 307.9)*

784.51 Dysarthria ◀

> **Excludes**   *dysarthria due to late effect of cerebrovascular accident (438.13)* ◀

SYMPTOMS, SIGNS, AND ILL-DEFINED CONDITIONS (780–799)

784.59 Other speech disturbance ◄
     Dysphasia ◄
     Slurred speech ◄
     Speech disturbance NOS ◄

● **784.6 Other symbolic dysfunction**

     Excludes   *developmental learning delays*
                    (315.0–315.9)

   ■ **784.60 Symbolic dysfunction, unspecified**

   784.61 Alexia and dyslexia
     Alexia (with agraphia)
     Loss of ability to read

   ■ **784.69 Other**
     Acalculia
     Difficulty performing simple mathematical tasks
     Agnosia
     Loss of ability to recognize objects, persons, sounds, shapes, or smells
     Agraphia NOS
     Apraxia
     Loss of the ability to execute or carry out movements

784.7 Epistaxis
     Hemorrhage from nose
     Nosebleed
     Coding Clinic: 2004, Q3, P7; 1995, Q1, P5

784.8 Hemorrhage from throat

     Excludes   *hemoptysis (786.3)*
                  Spitting blood

● **784.9 Other symptoms involving head and neck**

   784.91 Postnasal drip

   ■ **784.99 Other symptoms involving head and neck**
     Choking sensation
     Feeling of foreign body in throat
     Halitosis
     Bad breath
     Mouth breathing
     Sneezing

       Excludes   *foreign body in throat (933.0)*

● **785 Symptoms involving cardiovascular system**

     Excludes   *heart failure NOS (428.9)*

■ **785.0 Tachycardia, unspecified**
     Rapid heart beat

     Excludes   *neonatal tachycardia (779.82)*
                  paroxysmal tachycardia (427.0–427.2)
     Coding Clinic: 2003, Q2, P11

785.1 Palpitations
     Awareness of heart beat

     Excludes   *specified dysrhythmias (427.0–427.9)*

785.2 Undiagnosed cardiac murmurs
     Heart murmur NOS

■ **785.3 Other abnormal heart sounds**
     Cardiac dullness, increased or decreased
     Friction fremitus, cardiac
     Precordial friction

785.4 Gangrene
     Gangrene:
       NOS
       spreading cutaneous
     Gangrenous cellulitis
     Phagedena
     Rapidly spreading destructive ulceration of soft tissue

     Code first any associated underlying condition

     Excludes   *gangrene of certain sites–see Alphabetic Index*
                  gangrene with atherosclerosis of the extremities (440.24)
                  gas gangrene (040.0)
     Coding Clinic: 2004, Q1, P14-15; 1994, Q3, P5; 1990, Q3, P15; 1986, Mar-April, P12

● **785.5 Shock without mention of trauma**

   ■ **785.50 Shock, unspecified**
     Failure of peripheral circulation
     Resulting in significant blood pressure drop

   785.51 Cardiogenic shock
     Coding Clinic: 2008, Q4, P180-182; 2005, Q3, P14

   ● **785.52 *Septic shock***
     Endotoxic
     Gram-negative

     Code first:
       systemic inflammatory response syndrome due to infectious process with organ dysfunction (995.92)
     Coding Clinic: 2005, Q3, P23; Q2, P18-20x2; 2003, Q4, P73,79-81

   ■ **785.59 Other**
     Shock:
       hypovolemic
       Decreased blood volume

     Excludes   *shock (due to):*
                  anesthetic (995.4)
                  anaphylactic (995.0)
                  due to serum (999.4)
                  electric (994.8)
                  following abortion (639.5)
                  lightning (994.0)
                  obstetrical (669.1)
                  postoperative (998.0)
                  traumatic (958.4)
     Coding Clinic: 2008, Q4, P97-100

785.6 Enlargement of lymph nodes
     Lymphadenopathy
     "Swollen glands"

     Excludes   *lymphadenitis (chronic) (289.1–289.3)*
                  acute (683)

■ **785.9 Other symptoms involving cardiovascular system**
     Bruit (arterial)   Weak pulse

● **786 Symptoms involving respiratory system and other chest symptoms**

   ● **786.0 Dyspnea and respiratory abnormalities**

     ■ **786.00 Respiratory abnormality, unspecified**

     786.01 Hyperventilation

       Excludes   *hyperventilation, psychogenic (306.1)*

     786.02 Orthopnea

     786.03 Apnea

       Excludes   *apnea of newborn (770.81, 770.82)*
                  sleep apnea (780.51, 780.53, 780.57)
     Coding Clinic: 1998, Q2, P10

◄ New   ◄▥ Revised   ~~deleted~~ Deleted   ● Use Additional Digit(s)   ■ Nonspecific Code
● Not first-listed DX   OGCR Official Guidelines   Coding Clinic   Excludes   Includes   Use additional   Code first   Omit code

786.04 Cheyne-Stokes respiration
Abnormal pattern of breathing with gradually increasing and decreasing tidal volume with some periods of apnea

786.05 Shortness of breath
Coding Clinic: 1999, Q4, P25; Q1, P6

786.06 Tachypnea
Excludes *transitory tachypnea of newborn (770.6)*

786.07 Wheezing
Excludes *asthma (493.00–493.92)*

◼**786.09 Other**
Respiratory:
distress
insufficiency
Excludes *respiratory distress:*
following trauma and surgery (518.5)
newborn (770.89)
respiratory failure (518.81, 518.83–518.84)
newborn (770.84)
syndrome (newborn) (769)
adult (518.5)
Coding Clinic: 1990, Q1, P9

786.1 Stridor
Excludes *congenital laryngeal stridor (748.3)*

786.2 Cough
Excludes *cough:*
psychogenic (306.1)
smokers' (491.0)
with hemorrhage (786.3)
Coding Clinic: 1995, Q4, P50; 1990, Q1, P8

786.3 Hemoptysis
Cough with hemorrhage
Pulmonary hemorrhage NOS
Excludes *pulmonary hemorrhage of newborn (770.3)*
Coding Clinic: 2006, Q2, P17

786.4 Abnormal sputum
Abnormal:
amount of sputum
color of sputum
odor of sputum
Excessive sputum

●**786.5 Chest pain**

◼**786.50 Chest pain, unspecified**
Coding Clinic: 2007, Q1, P19; 2006, Q2, P7-8; 2003, Q1, P6-7; 2002, Q1, P4-5; 1999, Q4, P25-26; 1993, Q1, P25

786.51 Precordial pain
Coding Clinic: 1984, May-June, P11

786.52 Painful respiration
Pain:
anterior chest wall
pleuritic
Pleurodynia
Excludes *epidemic pleurodynia (074.1)*
Coding Clinic: 1984, Nov-Dec, P17

◼**786.59 Other**
Discomfort in chest
Pressure in chest
Tightness in chest
Excludes *pain in breast (611.71)*
Coding Clinic: 2007, Q1, P19; 2002, Q1, P6

786.6 Swelling, mass, or lump in chest
Excludes *lump in breast (611.72)*

786.7 Abnormal chest sounds
Abnormal percussion, chest
Friction sounds, chest
Rales
Wet rattling, clicking, crackling sounds on auscultation
Tympany, chest
Excludes *wheezing (786.07)*

786.8 Hiccough
Excludes *psychogenic hiccough (306.1)*

◼**786.9 Other symptoms involving respiratory system and chest**
Breath-holding spell

●**787 Symptoms involving digestive system**
Excludes *constipation (564.0–564.9)*
pylorospasm (537.81)
congenital (750.5)

●**787.0 Nausea and vomiting**
Emesis
Excludes *hematemesis NOS (578.0)*
vomiting:
bilious, following gastrointestinal surgery (564.3)
cyclical (536.2)
associated with migraine (346.2)
psychogenic (306.4)
excessive, in pregnancy (643.0–643.9)
fecal matter (569.87) ◄
habit (536.2)
of newborn (779.32, 779.33) ◄
persistent (536.2) ◄
psychogenic NOS (307.54)

787.01 Nausea with vomiting
Concurrent conditions
Coding Clinic: 2003, Q1, P5

787.02 Nausea alone
Separate condition
Coding Clinic: 2000, Q3, P12; 1997, Q2, P9-10

787.03 Vomiting alone
Separate condition
Coding Clinic: 1985, Mar-April, P11

787.04 Bilious emesis ◄
Bilious vomiting ◄
Excludes *bilious emesis (vomiting) in newborn (779.32)* ◄

787.1 Heartburn
Pyrosis
Waterbrash
Excludes *dyspepsia or indigestion (536.8)*
Coding Clinic: 2001, Q2, P6

●**787.2 Dysphagia**
Code first, if applicable, dysphagia due to late effect of cerebrovascular accident (438.82)
Coding Clinic: 2007, Q3, P8-9; 2003, Q4, P103-104, 109-110; 2001, Q2, P4-6; 1993, 5th Issue, P16; 1986, Nov-Dec, P10

787.20 Dysphagia, unspecified
Difficulty in swallowing NOS

787.21 Dysphagia, oral phase

787.22 Dysphagia, oropharyngeal phase
Coding Clinic: 2007, Q4, P92-95

787.23 Dysphagia, pharyngeal phase

787.24 Dysphagia, pharyngoesophageal phase

787.29 Other dysphagia
Cervical dysphagia
Neurogenic dysphagia

SYMPTOMS, SIGNS, AND ILL-DEFINED CONDITIONS (780–799)

787.3 Flatulence, eructation, and gas pain
Abdominal distention (gaseous)
Bloating
Tympanites (abdominal) (intestinal)

> **Excludes** *aerophagy (306.4)*

787.4 Visible peristalsis
Hyperperistalsis

787.5 Abnormal bowel sounds
Absent bowel sounds
Hyperactive bowel sounds

787.6 Incontinence of feces
Encopresis NOS
Incontinence of sphincter ani

> **Excludes** *that of nonorganic origin (307.7)*

Coding Clinic: 1997, Q1, P9-10

787.7 Abnormal feces
Bulky stools

> **Excludes** *abnormal stool content (792.1)*
> *melena:*
> *NOS (578.1)*
> *newborn (772.4, 777.3)*

● **787.9 Other symptoms involving digestive system**

> **Excludes** *gastrointestinal hemorrhage (578.0–578.9)*
> *intestinal obstruction (560.0–560.9)*
> *specific functional digestive disorders:*
> *esophagus (530.0–530.9)*
> *stomach and duodenum (536.0–536.9)*
> *those not elsewhere classified*
> *(564.0–564.9)*

787.91 Diarrhea
Diarrhea NOS
Coding Clinic: 2008, Q4, P97-100

787.99 Other
Change in bowel habits
Tenesmus (rectal)

● **788 Symptoms involving urinary system**

> **Excludes** *hematuria (599.70–599.72)*
> *nonspecific findings on examination of the urine*
> *(791.0–791.9)*
> *small kidney of unknown cause (589.0–589.9)*
> *uremia NOS (586)*
> *urinary obstruction (599.60, 599.69)*

788.0 Renal colic
Colic (recurrent) of:
kidney
ureter
Coding Clinic: 2004, Q3, P8

788.1 Dysuria
Painful urination
Strangury

● **788.2 Retention of urine**

> *Code first, if applicable, hyperplasia of prostate*
> *(600.0–600.9 with fifth-digit 1)*
> Coding Clinic: 2003, Q3, P13; 1994, Q1, P20; 1986, Sept-Oct, P12

■ **788.20 Retention of urine, unspecified**
Coding Clinic: 2006, Q4, P93-95; 2004, Q2, P18; 2003, Q3,
P12; Q1, P6; 1996, Q3, P10-11; 1994, Q3, P13

788.21 Incomplete bladder emptying

■ **788.29 Other specified retention of urine**

● **788.3 Urinary incontinence**

> **Excludes** *functional urinary incontinence (788.91)*
> *that of nonorganic origin (307.6)*
> *urinary incontinence associated with*
> *cognitive impairment (788.91)*
> *Code, if applicable, any causal condition first,*
> *such as:*
> *congenital ureterocele (753.23)*
> *genital prolapse (618.00–618.9)*
> *hyperplasia of prostate (600.0–600.9 with*
> *fifth-digit 1)*
> Coding Clinic: 2005, Q3, P20

■ **788.30 Urinary incontinence, unspecified**
Enuresis NOS
Coding Clinic: 2009, Q1, P18; 1995, Q4, P72-73

788.31 Urge incontinence
Coding Clinic: 2000, Q1, P19-20

788.32 Stress incontinence, male ♂

> **Excludes** *stress incontinence, female (625.6)*

Coding Clinic: 1995, Q4, P72-73

788.33 Mixed incontinence (female) (male)
Urge and stress

788.34 Incontinence without sensory awareness

788.35 Post-void dribbling

788.36 Nocturnal enuresis

788.37 Continuous leakage

788.38 Overflow incontinence
Coding Clinic: 2004, Q4, P96

■ **788.39 Other urinary incontinence**

● **788.4 Frequency of urination and polyuria**

> *Code first, if applicable, hyperplasia of prostate*
> *(600.0–600.9 with fifth-digit 1)*

788.41 Urinary frequency
Frequency of micturition

788.42 Polyuria

788.43 Nocturia

788.5 Oliguria and anuria
Deficient secretion of urine
Suppression of urinary secretion

> **Excludes** *that complicating:*
> *abortion (634–638 with .3, 639.3)*
> *ectopic or molar pregnancy (639.3)*
> *pregnancy, childbirth, or the puerperium*
> *(642.0–642.9, 646.2)*

● **788.6 Other abnormality of urination**

> *Code first, if applicable, hyperplasia of prostate*
> *(600.0–600.9 with fifth-digit 1)*

788.61 Splitting of urinary stream
Intermittent urinary stream

788.62 Slowing of urinary stream
Weak stream

788.63 Urgency of urination

> **Excludes** *urge incontinence (788.31, 788.33)*

Coding Clinic: 2003, Q4, P74

788.64 Urinary hesitancy

788.65 Straining on urination

■ **788.69 Other**

◄ New   ⬅ Revised   ~~deleted~~ Deleted   ● Use Additional Digit(s)   ■ Nonspecific Code

● Not first-listed DX   OGCR Official Guidelines   Coding Clinic   Excludes   Includes   Use additional   Code first   Omit code

SYMPTOMS, SIGNS, AND ILL-DEFINED CONDITIONS (780–799)

788.7 Urethral discharge
Penile discharge
Urethrorrhea

788.8 Extravasation of urine
Leakage, discharge

● **788.9 Other symptoms involving urinary system**
Coding Clinic: 2005, Q1, P12-13

788.91 Functional urinary incontinence
Urinary incontinence due to cognitive
impairment, or severe physical
disability or immobility

| Excludes | *urinary incontinence due to physiologic condition (788.30-788.39)* |

Coding Clinic: 2008, Q4, P144-145

■ **788.99 Other symptoms involving urinary system**
Extrarenal uremia
Vesical:
pain
tenesmus

● **789 Other symptoms involving abdomen and pelvis**
The following fifth-digit subclassification is to be used for
codes 789.0, 789.3, 789.4, 789.6

> ■ 0   unspecified site
>   1   right upper quadrant
>   2   left upper quadrant
>   3   right lower quadrant
>   4   left lower quadrant
>   5   periumbilic
>   6   epigastric
> ■ 7   generalized
> ■ 9   other specified site
>   multiple sites

| Excludes | *symptoms referable to genital organs: female (625.0–625.9) male (607.0–608.9) psychogenic (302.70–302.79)* |

● **789.0 Abdominal pain**
[0-7,9]   ~~Colic:~~
     ~~NOS~~
     ~~infantile~~
     Cramps, abdominal

| ~~Excludes~~ | ~~renal colic (788.0)~~ |

Coding Clinic: 2002, Q1, P5; 1995, Q1, P3; 1990, Q2, P26

789.1 Hepatomegaly
Enlargement of liver

789.2 Splenomegaly
Enlargement of spleen

● **789.3 Abdominal or pelvic swelling, mass, or lump**
[0-7,9]   Diffuse or generalized swelling or mass:
     abdominal NOS
     umbilical

| Excludes | *abdominal distention (gaseous) (787.3) ascites (789.51–789.59)* |

● **789.4 Abdominal rigidity**
[0-7,9]

● **789.5 Ascites**
Fluid in peritoneal cavity
Coding Clinic: 2008, Q1, P16-18; 2007, Q4, P95-96; 2005, Q2, P8; 1989, Q4, P11

● **789.51 *Malignant ascites***
Code first malignancy, such as:
malignant neoplasm of ovary (183.0)
secondary malignant neoplasm of
retroperitoneum and peritoneum
(197.6)
Coding Clinic: 2008, Q1, P16-17

■ **789.59 Other ascites**

● **789.6 Abdominal tenderness**
[0-7,9]   Rebound tenderness

789.7 Colic ◄
Colic NOS ◄
Infantile colic ◄

| Excludes | *colic in adult and child over 12 months old (789.0)* ◄ *renal colic (788.0)* ◄ |

■ **789.9 Other symptoms involving abdomen and pelvis**
Umbilical: Umbilical:
  bleeding   discharge

NONSPECIFIC ABNORMAL FINDINGS (790–796)

● **790 Nonspecific findings on examination of blood**

| Excludes | *abnormality of: platelets (287.0–287.9) thrombocytes (287.0–287.9) white blood cells (288.00–288.9)* |

● **790.0 Abnormality of red blood cells**

| Excludes | *anemia: congenital (776.5) newborn, due to isoimmunization (773.0–773.2, 773.5) of premature infant (776.6) other specified types (280.0–285.9) hemoglobin disorders (282.5–282.7) polycythemia: familial (289.6) neonatorum (776.4) secondary (289.0) vera (238.4)* |

790.01 Precipitous drop in hematocrit
Drop in hematocrit
Drop in hemoglobin ◄
Decrease in red blood cells

■ **790.09 Other abnormality of red blood cells**
Abnormal red cell morphology NOS
Abnormal red cell volume NOS
Anisocytosis
Red blood cells of unequal size
Poikilocytosis
Red blood cells of abnormal shape

■ **790.1 Elevated sedimentation rate**

● **790.2 Abnormal glucose**

| Excludes | *diabetes mellitus (249.00–249.91, 250.00–250.93) dysmetabolic syndrome X (277.7) gestational diabetes (648.8) glycosuria (791.5) hypoglycemia (251.2) that complicating pregnancy, childbirth, or the puerperium (648.8)* |

Coding Clinic: 2003, Q4, P74-75

790.21 Impaired fasting glucose
Elevated fasting glucose

790.22 Impaired glucose tolerance test (oral)
Elevated glucose tolerance test

SYMPTOMS, SIGNS, AND ILL-DEFINED CONDITIONS (780–799)

790.29 Other abnormal glucose
  Abnormal glucose NOS
  Abnormal non-fasting glucose
  Hyperglycemia NOS
  Pre-diabetes NOS
  Coding Clinic: 2005, Q2, P21-22; 2004, Q4, P53-56

790.3 Excessive blood level of alcohol
  Elevated blood-alcohol

790.4 Nonspecific elevation of levels of transaminase or lactic acid dehydrogenase [LDH]

790.5 Other nonspecific abnormal serum enzyme levels
  Abnormal serum level of:
    acid phosphatase
    alkaline phosphatase
    amylase
    lipase
  Excludes *deficiency of circulating enzymes (277.6)*

790.6 Other abnormal blood chemistry
  Abnormal blood levels of:
    cobalt
    copper
    iron
    lead
    lithium
    magnesium
    mineral
    zinc
  Excludes *abnormality of electrolyte or acid-base*
             balance (276.0–276.9)
             hypoglycemia NOS (251.2)
             lead poisoning (984.0–984.9)
             specific finding indicating abnormality of:
               amino-acid transport and metabolism
                 (270.0–270.9)
               carbohydrate transport and metabolism
                 (271.0–271.9)
               lipid metabolism (272.0–272.9)
             uremia NOS (586)

790.7 Bacteremia
  Excludes *bacteremia of newborn (771.83)*
             septicemia (038)
  Use additional code to identify organism (041)
  Coding Clinic: 2003, Q2, P7-8

790.8 Viremia, unspecified
  Coding Clinic: 1988, Q4, P10

790.9 Other nonspecific findings on examination of blood

  790.91 Abnormal arterial blood gases

  790.92 Abnormal coagulation profile
    Abnormal or prolonged:
      bleeding time
      coagulation time
      partial thromboplastin time [PTT]
      prothrombin time [PT]
    Excludes *coagulation (hemorrhagic) disorders*
               (286.0–286.9)
    Coding Clinic: 1994, Q1, P22

  790.93 Elevated prostate specific antigen [PSA] ♂   A

  790.94 Euthyroid sick syndrome

  790.95 Elevated C-reactive protein (CRP)
    Coding Clinic: 2004, Q4, P96-97

  790.99 Other

791 Nonspecific findings on examination of urine
  Excludes *hematuria NOS (599.70–599.72)*
             specific findings indicating abnormality of:
               amino-acid transport and metabolism
                 (270.0–270.9)
               carbohydrate transport and metabolism
                 (271.0–271.9)

  791.0 Proteinuria
    Albuminuria
    Bence-Jones proteinuria
    Excludes *postural proteinuria (593.6)*
               that arising during pregnancy or the
                 puerperium (642.0–642.9, 646.2)

  791.1 Chyluria
    White milky urine
    Excludes *filarial (125.0–125.9)*

  791.2 Hemoglobinuria

  791.3 Myoglobinuria

  791.4 Biliuria

  791.5 Glycosuria
    Excludes *renal glycosuria (271.4)*

  791.6 Acetonuria
    Ketonuria

  791.7 Other cells and casts in urine

  791.9 Other nonspecific findings on examination of urine
    Crystalluria
    Elevated urine levels of:
      17-ketosteroids
      catecholamines
      indolacetic acid
      vanillylmandelic acid [VMA]
    Melanuria
    Coding Clinic: 2005, Q1, P12

792 Nonspecific abnormal findings in other body substances
  Excludes *that in chromosomal analysis (795.2)*

  792.0 Cerebrospinal fluid

  792.1 Stool contents
    Abnormal stool color
    Fat in stool
    Mucus in stool
    Occult blood
    Pus in stool
    Excludes *blood in stool [melena] (578.1)*
               newborn (772.4, 777.3)
    Coding Clinic: 1992, Q2, P9-10; Q2, P9

  792.2 Semen ♂
    Abnormal spermatozoa
    Excludes *azoospermia (606.0)*
               oligospermia (606.1)

  792.3 Amniotic fluid ♀   M

  792.4 Saliva
    Excludes *that in chromosomal analysis (795.2)*

  792.5 Cloudy (hemodialysis) (peritoneal) dialysis effluent

  792.9 Other nonspecific abnormal findings in body substances
    Peritoneal fluid
    Pleural fluid
    Synovial fluid
    Vaginal fluids

● **793 Nonspecific (abnormal) findings on radiological and other examination of body structure** ◀━

     Includes   nonspecific abnormal findings of:
         thermography
         ultrasound examination [echogram]
         x-ray examination

     Excludes   *abnormal results of function studies and radioisotope scans (794.0–794.9)*

   793.0 Skull and head

         Excludes   *nonspecific abnormal echoencephalogram (794.01)*

         Coding Clinic: 2006, Q3, P22

   793.1 Lung field
       Coin lesion lung
       Shadow, lung

■ **793.2 Other intrathoracic organ**
       Abnormal:
         echocardiogram
         heart shadow
         ultrasound cardiogram
       Mediastinal shift

   793.3 Biliary tract
       Nonvisualization of gallbladder

   793.4 Gastrointestinal tract

   793.5 Genitourinary organs
       Filling defect:
         bladder
         kidney
         ureter

   793.6 Abdominal area, including retroperitoneum

   793.7 Musculoskeletal system

● **793.8 Breast**

     ■ **793.80 Abnormal mammogram, unspecified**

     793.81 Mammographic microcalcification

         Excludes   *mammographic calcification (793.89)*
                 mammographic calculus (793.89)

     793.82 Inconclusive mammogram ◀
       Dense breasts NOS ◀
       Inconclusive mammogram NEC ◀
       Inconclusive mammography due to
         dense breasts ◀
       Inconclusive mammography NEC ◀

     ■ **793.89 Other (abnormal) findings on radiological examination of breast** ◀━
       Mammographic calcification
       Mammographic calculus

● **793.9 Other**

     Excludes   *abnormal finding by radioisotope localization of placenta (794.9)*

     793.91 Image test inconclusive due to excess body fat

       Use additional code to identify Body Mass Index (BMI), if known (V85.0–V85.54)
       Coding Clinic: 2006, Q4, P109-110

     ■ **793.99 Other nonspecific (abnormal) findings on radiological and other examinations of body structure** ◀━
       Abnormal:
         placental finding by x-ray or ultrasound
           method
         radiological findings in skin and
           subcutaneous tissue

● **794 Nonspecific abnormal results of function studies**

     Includes   radioisotope:
         scans
         uptake studies
       scintiphotography

● **794.0 Brain and central nervous system**

     ■ **794.00 Abnormal function study, unspecified**

     794.01 Abnormal echoencephalogram

     794.02 Abnormal electroencephalogram [EEG]

     794.09 Other
       Abnormal brain scan

● **794.1 Peripheral nervous system and special senses**

     ■ **794.10 Abnormal response to nerve stimulation, unspecified**

     794.11 Abnormal retinal function studies
       Abnormal electroretinogram [ERG]

     794.12 Abnormal electro-oculogram [EOG]

     794.13 Abnormal visually evoked potential

     794.14 Abnormal oculomotor studies

     794.15 Abnormal auditory function studies
       Coding Clinic: 2004, Q1, P15-16

     794.16 Abnormal vestibular function studies

     794.17 Abnormal electromyogram [EMG]
         Excludes   *that of eye (794.14)*

     ■ **794.19 Other**

   794.2 Pulmonary
       Abnormal lung scan
       Reduced:
         ventilatory capacity
         vital capacity

● **794.3 Cardiovascular**

     ■ **794.30 Abnormal function study, unspecified**

     794.31 Abnormal electrocardiogram [ECG] [EKG]

         Excludes   *long QT syndrome (426.82)*

         Coding Clinic: 1985, Mar-April, P13

     ■ **794.39 Other**
       Abnormal:
         ballistocardiogram
         phonocardiogram
         vectorcardiogram

   794.4 Kidney
       Abnormal renal function test

   794.5 Thyroid
       Abnormal thyroid:
         scan
         uptake

   ■ **794.6 Other endocrine function study**

   794.7 Basal metabolism
       Abnormal basal metabolic rate [BMR]

   794.8 Liver
       Abnormal liver scan

   ■ **794.9 Other**
       Bladder
       Pancreas
       Placenta
       Spleen

SYMPTOMS, SIGNS, AND ILL-DEFINED CONDITIONS (780–799)

● **795   Other and nonspecific abnormal cytological, histological, immunological, and DNA test findings**

> **Excludes**   *abnormal cytologic smear of anus and anal HPV (796.70-796.79)*
> *nonspecific abnormalities of red blood cells (790.01–790.09)*
>
> Coding Clinic: 2002, Q4, P69-70

● **795.0   Abnormal Papanicolaou smear of cervix and cervical HPV**

> Abnormal thin preparation smear of cervix
> Abnormal cervical cytology
>
> > **Excludes**   *abnormal cytologic smear of vagina and vaginal HPV (795.10-795.19)*
> > *carcinoma in situ ~~in situ~~ of cervix (233.1)* ◀▥
> > *cervical intraepithelial neoplasia I (CIN I) (622.11)*
> > *cervical intraepithelial neoplasia II (CIN II) (622.12)*
> > *cervical intraepithelial neoplasia III (CIN III) (233.1)*
> > *dysplasia (histologically confirmed) of cervix (uteri) NOS (622.10)*
> > *mild cervical dysplasia (histologically confirmed) (622.11)*
> > *moderate cervical dysplasia (histologically confirmed) (622.12)*
> > *severe cervical dysplasia (histologically confirmed) (233.1)*
> >
> > Coding Clinic: 2008, Q4, P145-148; 2004, Q4, P97-99

> ▣ **795.00   Abnormal glandular Papanicolaou smear of cervix ♀**
>
> > Atypical endocervical cells NOS
> > Atypical endometrial cells NOS
> > Atypical cervical glandular cells NOS

> **795.01   Papanicolaou smear of cervix with atypical squamous cells of undetermined significance (ASC-US) ♀**
>
> > Coding Clinic: 2006, Q2, P3,4

> **795.02   Papanicolaou smear of cervix with atypical squamous cells cannot exclude high grade squamous intraepithelial lesion (ASC-H) ♀**

> **795.03   Papanicolaou smear of cervix with low grade squamous intraepithelial lesion (LGSIL) ♀**

> **795.04   Papanicolaou smear of cervix with high grade squamous intraepithelial lesion (HGSIL) ♀**

> **795.05   Cervical high risk human papillomavirus (HPV) DNA test positive ♀**

> **795.06   Papanicolaou smear of cervix with cytologic evidence of malignancy ♀**

> **795.07   Satisfactory cervical smear but lacking transformation zone ♀**

> **795.08   Unsatisfactory cervical cytology smear ♀**
>
> > Inadequate cervical cytology sample
> > Coding Clinic: 2006, Q2, P3,4

> ▣ **795.09   Other abnormal Papanicolaou smear of cervix and cervical HPV ♀**
>
> > Cervical low risk human papillomavirus (HPV) DNA test positive
> >
> > Use additional code for associated human papillomavirus (079.4)
> >
> > > **Excludes**   *encounter for Papanicolaou cervical smear to confirm findings of recent normal smear following initial abnormal smear (V72.32)*

● **795.1   Abnormal Papanicolaou smear of vagina and vaginal HPV**

> Abnormal thin preparation smear of vagina NOS
> Abnormal vaginal cytology NOS
>
> Use additional code to identify acquired absence of uterus and cervix, if applicable (V88.01-V88.03)
>
> > **Excludes**   *abnormal cytologic smear of cervix and cervical HPV (795.00-795.09)*
> > *carcinoma in situ of vagina (233.31)*
> > *carcinoma in situ of vulva (233.32)*
> > *dysplasia (histologically confirmed) of vagina NOS (623.0, 233.31)*
> > *dysplasia (histologically confirmed) of vulva NOS (624.01, 624.02, 233.32)*
> > *mild vaginal dysplasia (histologically confirmed) (623.0)*
> > *mild vulvar dysplasia (histologically confirmed) (624.01)*
> > *moderate vaginal dysplasia (histologically confirmed) (623.0)*
> > *moderate vulvar dysplasia (histologically confirmed) (624.02)*
> > *severe vaginal dysplasia (histologically confirmed) (233.31)*
> > *severe vulvar dysplasia (histologically confirmed) (233.32)*
> > *vaginal intraepithelial neoplasia I (VAIN I) (623.0)*
> > *vaginal intraepithelial neoplasia II (VAIN II) (623.0)*
> > *vaginal intraepithelial neoplasia III (VAIN III) (233.31)*
> > *vulvar intraepithelial neoplasia I (VIN I) (624.01)*
> > *vulvar intraepithelial neoplasia II (VIN II) (624.02)*
> > *vulvar intraepithelial neoplasia III (VIN III) (233.32)*
> >
> > Coding Clinic: 2008, Q4, P145-148

> **795.10   Abnormal glandular Papanicolaou smear of vagina ♀**
>
> > Atypical vaginal glandular cells NOS

> **795.11   Papanicolaou smear of vagina with atypical squamous cells of undetermined significance (ASC-US) ♀**

> **795.12   Papanicolaou smear of vagina with atypical squamous cells cannot exclude high grade squamous intraepithelial lesion (ASC-H) ♀**

> **795.13   Papanicolaou smear of vagina with low grade squamous intraepithelial lesion (LGSIL) ♀**

> **795.14   Papanicolaou smear of vagina with high grade squamous intraepithelial lesion (HGSIL) ♀**

> **795.15   Vaginal high risk human papillomavirus (HPV) DNA test positive ♀**
>
> > **Excludes**   *condyloma acuminatum (078.11)*
> > *genital warts (078.11)*

> **795.16   Papanicolaou smear of vagina with cytologic evidence of malignancy ♀**
>
> > Coding Clinic: 2004, Q2, P11

> **795.18   Unsatisfactory vaginal cytology smear ♀**
>
> > Inadequate vaginal cytology sample

> ▣ **795.19   Other abnormal Papanicolaou smear of vagina and vaginal HPV ♀**
>
> > Vaginal low risk human papillomavirus (HPV) DNA test positive
> >
> > Use additional code for associated human papillomavirus (079.4)

795.2 **Nonspecific abnormal findings on chromosomal analysis**
Abnormal karyotype

795.3 **Nonspecific positive culture findings**
Positive culture findings in:
nose
sputum
throat
wound

Excludes *that of:*
blood (790.7–790.8)
urine (791.9)

795.31 **Nonspecific positive findings for anthrax**
Positive findings by nasal swab
Coding Clinic: 2002, Q4, P70

795.39 **Other nonspecific positive culture findings**

Excludes *colonization status*
(V02.0–V02.9) ◄

795.4 **Other nonspecific abnormal histological findings**

795.5 **Nonspecific reaction to tuberculin skin test without active tuberculosis**
Abnormal result of Mantoux test
PPD positive
Tuberculin (skin test):
positive
reactor

795.6 **False positive serological test for syphilis**
False positive Wassermann reaction

795.7 **Other nonspecific immunological findings**

Excludes *abnormal tumor markers (795.81–795.89)*
elevated prostate specific antigen [PSA]
(790.93)
elevated tumor associated antigens
(795.81–795.89)
isoimmunization, in pregnancy
(656.1–656.2)
affecting fetus or newborn (773.0–773.2)

795.71 **Nonspecific serologic evidence of human immunodeficiency virus [HIV]**
Inconclusive human immunodeficiency virus [HIV] test (adult) (infant)

Note: This code is ONLY to be used when a test finding is reported as nonspecific. Asymptomatic positive findings are coded to V08. If any HIV infection symptom or condition is present, see code 042. Negative findings are not coded.

Excludes *acquired immunodeficiency*
syndrome [AIDS] (042)
asymptomatic human
immunodeficiency virus
[HIV] infection status (V08)
HIV infection, symptomatic (042)
human immunodeficiency virus
[HIV] disease (042)
positive (status) NOS (V08)

OGCR Section I.C.2.e.
Patients with inconclusive HIV serology, but no definitive diagnosis or manifestations of the illness, may be assigned code 795.71, Inconclusive serologic test for Human Immunodeficiency Virus [HIV].

795.79 **Other and unspecified nonspecific immunological findings**
Raised antibody titer
Raised level of immunoglobulins

Coding Clinic: 1993, Q2, P6

795.8 **Abnormal tumor markers**
Elevated tumor associated antigens [TAA]
Elevated tumor specific antigens [TSA]

Excludes *elevated prostate specific antigen*
[PSA] (790.93)
Coding Clinic: 2006, Q4, P111-112; 1993, Q1, P21-22; 1992, Q2, P11

795.81 **Elevated carcinoembryonic antigen [CEA]**

795.82 **Elevated cancer antigen 125 [CA 125]** ♀

795.89 **Other abnormal tumor markers**

796 **Other nonspecific abnormal findings**

796.0 **Nonspecific abnormal toxicological findings**
Abnormal levels of heavy metals or drugs in blood, urine, or other tissue

Excludes *excessive blood level of alcohol (790.3)*
Coding Clinic: 1997, Q1, P16

796.1 **Abnormal reflex**

796.2 **Elevated blood pressure reading without diagnosis of hypertension**

Note: This category is to be used to record an episode of elevated blood pressure in a patient in whom no formal diagnosis of hypertension has been made, or as an incidental finding.
Coding Clinic: 2003, Q2, P11; 1993, 5th Issue, P6-7

OGCR Section I.C.7.a.8
Assign code 796.2, Elevated blood pressure reading without diagnosis of hypertension, unless patient has an established diagnosis of hypertension. Assign code 642.3x for transient hypertension of pregnancy.

796.3 **Nonspecific low blood pressure reading**

796.4 **Other abnormal clinical findings**
Coding Clinic: 1995, Q3, P13

796.5 **Abnormal finding on antenatal screening** ♀   M

796.6 **Abnormal findings on neonatal screening**   N

Excludes *nonspecific serologic evidence of human*
immunodeficiency virus [HIV]
(795.71)
Coding Clinic: 2004, Q4, P99-100

796.7 **Abnormal cytologic smear of anus and anal HPV**

Excludes *abnormal cytologic smear of cervix and*
cervical HPV (795.00-795.09)
abnormal cytologic smear of vagina and
vaginal HPV (795.10-795.19)
anal intraepithelial neoplasia I (AIN I)
(569.44)
anal intraepithelial neoplasia II (AIN II)
(569.44)
anal intraepithelial neoplasia III (AIN III)
(230.5, 230.6)
carcinoma in situ of anus (230.5, 230.6)
dysplasia (histologically confirmed) of
anus NOS (569.44)
mild anal dysplasia (histologically
confirmed) (569.44)
moderate anal dysplasia (histologically
confirmed) (569.44)
severe anal dysplasia (histologically
confirmed) (569.44) (230.5, 230.6) ◄
Coding Clinic: 2008, Q4, P117-119

796.70 **Abnormal glandular Papanicolaou smear of anus**
Atypical anal glandular cells NOS

796.71 **Papanicolaou smear of anus with atypical squamous cells of undetermined significance (ASC-US)**

SYMPTOMS, SIGNS, AND ILL-DEFINED CONDITIONS (780–799)

796.72 Papanicolaou smear of anus with atypical squamous cells cannot exclude high grade squamous intraepithelial lesion (ASC-H)

796.73 Papanicolaou smear of anus with low grade squamous intraepithelial lesion (LGSIL)

796.74 Papanicolaou smear of anus with high grade squamous intraepithelial lesion (HGSIL)

796.75 Anal high risk human papillomavirus (HPV) DNA test positive

796.76 Papanicolaou smear of anus with cytologic evidence of malignancy

796.77 Satisfactory anal smear but lacking transformation zone

796.78 Unsatisfactory anal cytology smear
Inadequate anal cytology sample

796.79 Other abnormal Papanicolaou smear of anus and anal HPV
Anal low risk human papillomavirus (HPV) DNA test positive

Use additional code for associated human papillomavirus (079.4)

796.9 Other

ILL-DEFINED AND UNKNOWN CAUSES OF MORBIDITY AND MORTALITY (797–799)

797 Senility without mention of psychosis
Frailty
Old age
Senescence
Senile asthenia
Senile:
debility
exhaustion

Excludes *senile psychoses (290.0–290.9)*

798 Sudden death, cause unknown

798.0 Sudden infant death syndrome *(SIDS)*   P
Cot death
Crib death
Sudden death of nonspecific cause in infancy

798.1 *Instantaneous death*

798.2 *Death occurring in less than 24 hours from onset of symptoms, not otherwise explained*
Death known not to be violent or instantaneous, for which no cause could be discovered
Died without sign of disease

798.9 *Unattended death*
Death in circumstances where the body of the deceased was found and no cause could be discovered
Found dead

799 Other ill-defined and unknown causes of morbidity and mortality

799.0 Asphyxia and hypoxemia

Excludes *asphyxia and hypoxemia (due to):*
carbon monoxide (986)
hypercapnia (786.09)
inhalation of food or foreign body (932–934.9)
newborn (768.0–768.9)
traumatic (994.7)
Coding Clinic: 2005, Q4, P90; 1990, Q1, P20

799.01 Asphyxia

799.02 Hypoxemia
Coding Clinic: 2006, Q2, P24,25

799.1 Respiratory arrest
Cardiorespiratory failure

Excludes *cardiac arrest (427.5)*
failure of peripheral circulation (785.50)
respiratory distress:
NOS (786.09)
acute (518.82)
following trauma or surgery (518.5)
newborn (770.89)
syndrome (newborn) (769)
adult (following trauma or surgery) (518.5)
other (518.82)
respiratory failure (518.81, 518.83–518.84)
newborn (770.84)
respiratory insufficiency (786.09)
acute (518.82)

799.2 ~~Nervousness~~ Signs and symptoms involving emotional state   ◀▥
"Nerves"

Excludes *anxiety (293.84, 300.00-300.09)* ◀
depression (311) ◀

799.21 Nervousness ◀
Nervous ◀

799.22 Irritability ◀
Irritable ◀

799.23 Impulsiveness ◀
Impulsive ◀

Excludes *impulsive neurosis (300.3)* ◀

799.24 Emotional lability ◀

799.25 Demoralization and apathy ◀
Apathetic ◀

799.29 Other signs and symptoms involving emotional state ◀

799.3 Debility, unspecified

Excludes *asthenia (780.79)*
nervous debility (300.5)
neurasthenia (300.5)
senile asthenia (797)
Coding Clinic: 1997, Q3, P11-12

799.4 Cachexia
Wasting disease
Code first underlying condition, if known
Coding Clinic: 2006, Q3, P14-15x2; 1990, Q3, P17

799.8 Other ill-defined conditions

799.81 Decreased libido   A
Decreased sexual desire

Excludes *psychosexual dysfunction with inhibited sexual desire (302.71)*
Coding Clinic: 2003, Q4, P75-76; Q4, P75-76

799.82 Apparent life threatening event in infant ◀
ALTE ◀
Apparent life threatening event in newborn and infant ◀

Use additional code(s) for associated signs and symptoms ◀

Excludes *signs and symptoms associated with a confirmed diagnosis- code to confirmed diagnosis* ◀

799.89 Other ill-defined conditions

799.9 Other unknown and unspecified cause
Undiagnosed disease, not specified as to site or system involved
Unknown cause of morbidity or mortality
Coding Clinic: 1998, Q1, P4; 1990, Q1, P22

SYMPTOMS, SIGNS, AND ILL-DEFINED CONDITIONS (780–799)

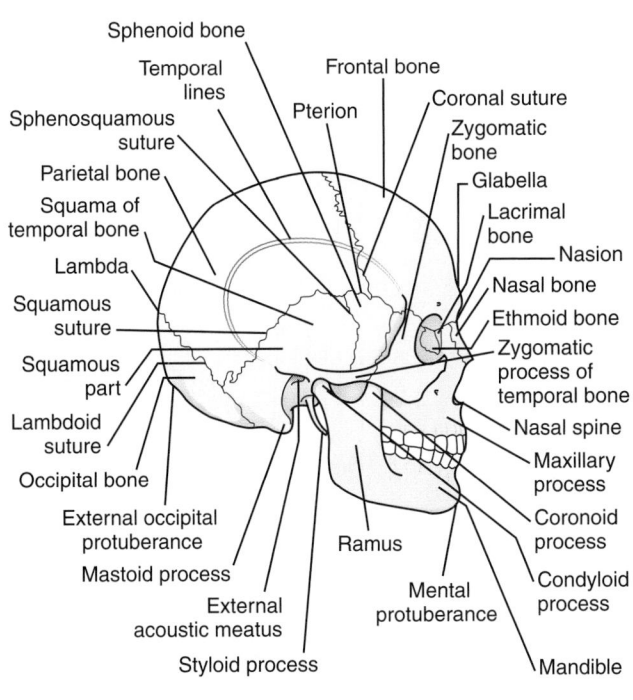

Figure 17–1 Lateral view of skull.

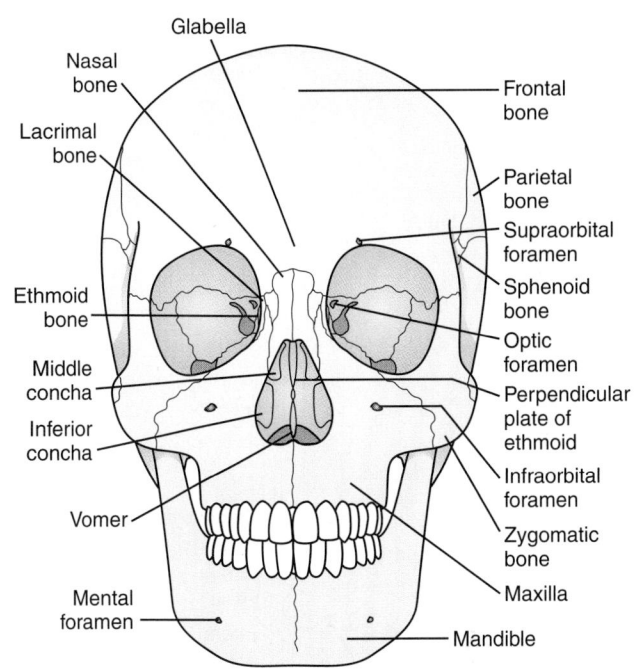

Figure 17–2 Frontal view of skull.

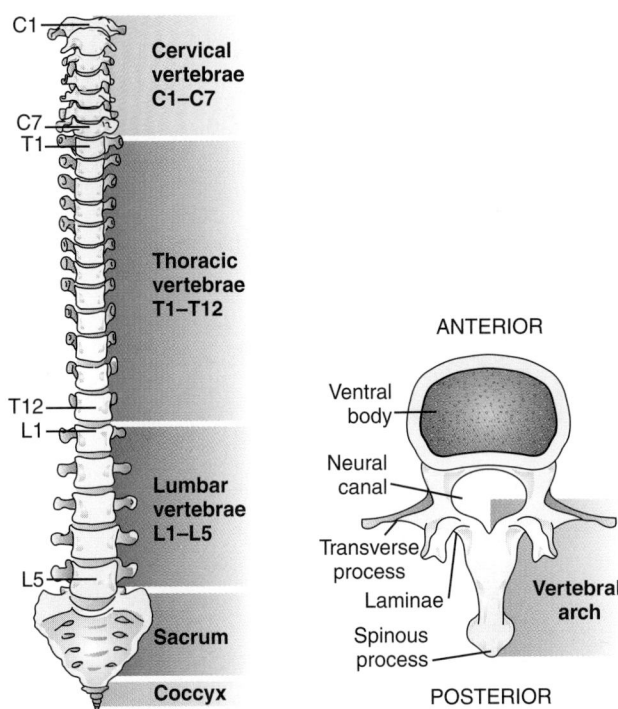

Figure 17–3 Anterior view of vertebral column.

Figure 17–4 Vertebra viewed from above.

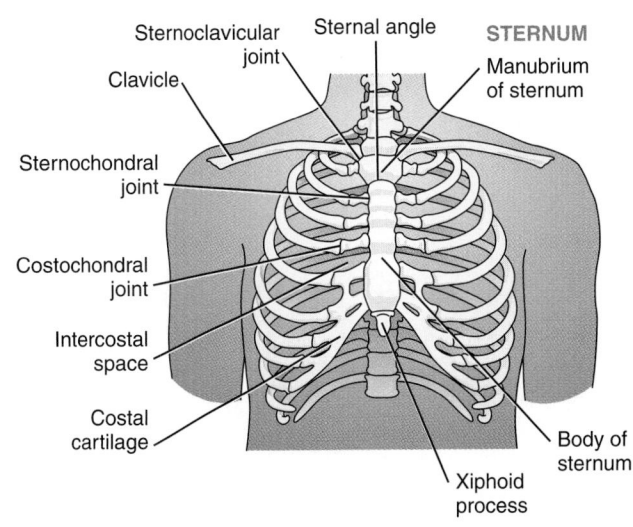

Figure 17–5 Anterior view of rib cage.

INJURY AND POISONING (800–999)

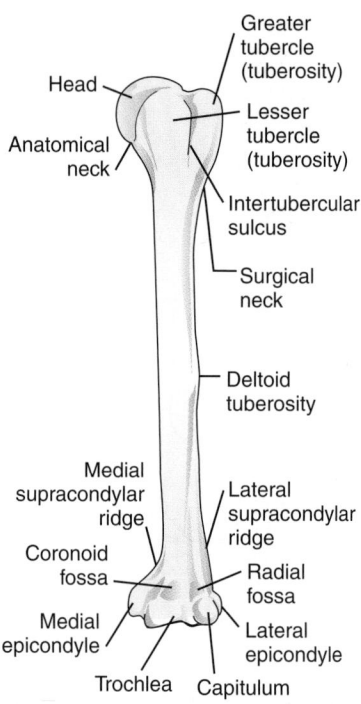

Figure 17–6 Anterior aspect of left humerus.

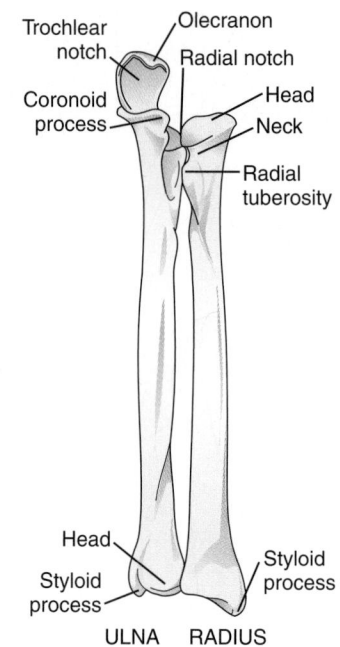

Figure 17–7 Anterior aspect of left radius and ulna.

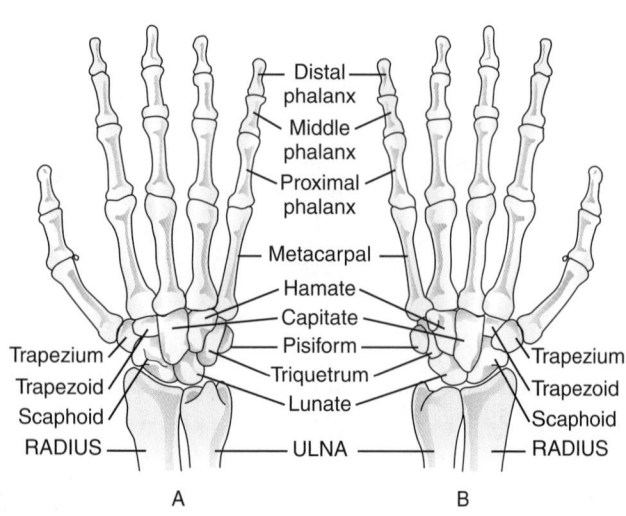

Figure 17–8 Right hand and wrist: **A.** Dorsal surface. **B.** Palmar surface.

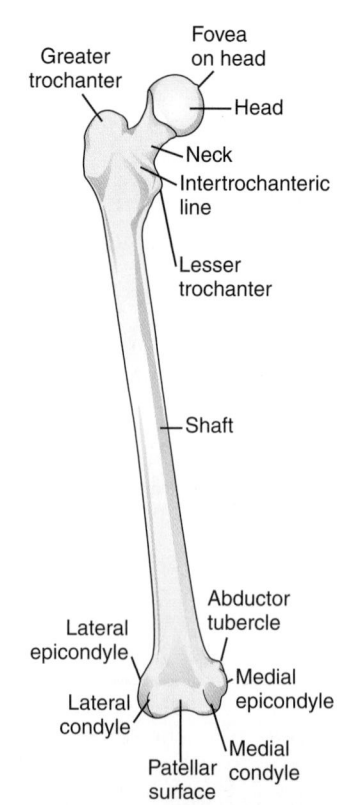

Figure 17–9 Anterior aspect of right femur.

◀ New   ◀▭ Revised   ~~deleted~~ Deleted   ● Use Additional Digit(s)   ■ Nonspecific Code

● Not first-listed DX   OGCR Official Guidelines   Coding Clinic   Excludes   Includes   Use additional   Code first   Omit code

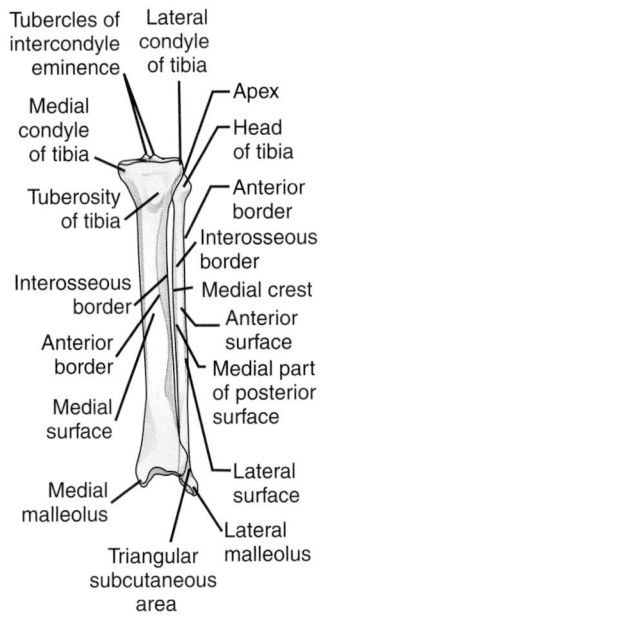

Figure 17–10 Anterior aspect of left tibia and fibula.

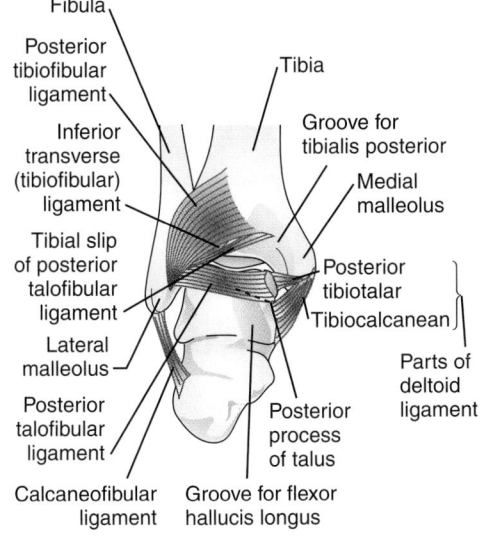

Figure 17–11 Posterior aspect of the left ankle joint.

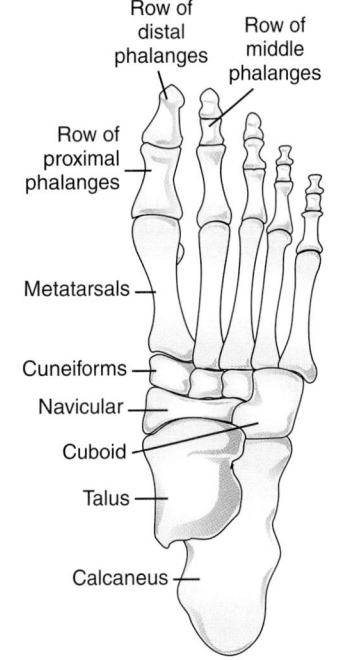

Figure 17–12 Right foot viewed from above.

OGCR Section I.C.17.a

When coding injuries, assign separate codes for each injury unless a combination code is provided, in which case the combination code is assigned. Multiple injury codes are provided in ICD-9-CM, but should not be assigned unless information for a more specific code is not available. These codes are not to be used for normal, healing surgical wounds or to identify complications of surgical wounds.

The code for the most serious injury, as determined by the provider and the focus of treatment, is sequenced first.

1) **Superficial injuries:** Superficial injuries such as abrasions or contusions are not coded when associated with more severe injuries of the same site.

2) **Primary injury with damage to nerves/blood vessels:** When a primary injury results in minor damage to peripheral nerves or blood vessels, the primary injury is sequenced first with additional code(s) from categories 950-957, Injury to nerves and spinal cord, and/or 900-904, Injury to blood vessels. When the primary injury is to the blood vessels or nerves, that injury should be sequenced first.

INJURY AND POISONING (800–999)

17. INJURY AND POISONING (800–999)

Use E code(s) to identify the cause and intent of the injury or poisoning (E800–E999)

Note:

1. The principle of multiple coding of injuries should be followed wherever possible. Combination categories for multiple injuries are provided for use when there is insufficient detail as to the nature of the individual conditions, or for primary tabulation purposes when it is more convenient to record a single code; otherwise, the component injuries should be coded separately.

   Where multiple sites of injury are specified in the titles, the word "with" indicates involvement of both sites, and the word "and" indicates involvement of either or both sites. The word "finger" includes thumb.

2. Categories for "late effect" of injuries are to be found at 905–909.

FRACTURES (800–829)

Excludes *malunion (733.81)*
nonunion (733.82)
pathologic or spontaneous fracture (733.10–733.19)
stress fracture (733.93–733.95)

The terms "condyle," "coronoid process," "ramus," and "symphysis" indicate the portion of the bone fractured, not the name of the bone involved.

The descriptions "closed" and "open" used in the fourth-digit subdivisions include the following terms:

closed (with or without delayed healing):
    comminuted
    depressed
    elevated
    fissured
    fracture NOS
    greenstick
    impacted
    linear
    simple
    slipped epiphysis
    spiral
open (with or without delayed healing):
    compound
    infected
    missile
    puncture
    with foreign body

Note: A fracture not indicated as closed or open should be classified as closed.

FRACTURE OF SKULL (800–804)

Includes traumatic brain injury due to fracture of skull ◀

The following fifth-digit subclassification is for use with the appropriate codes in categories 800, 801, 803, and 804:

> 0 unspecified state of consciousness
> 1 with no loss of consciousness
> 2 with brief [less than one hour] loss of consciousness
> 3 with moderate [1–24 hours] loss of consciousness
> 4 with prolonged [more than 24 hours] loss of consciousness and return to pre-existing conscious level
> 5 with prolonged [more than 24 hours] loss of consciousness, without return to pre-existing conscious level
>   Use fifth-digit 5 to designate when a patient is unconscious and dies before regaining consciousness, regardless of the duration of the loss of consciousness
> 6 with loss of consciousness of unspecified duration
> 9 with concussion, unspecified

● **800 Fracture of vault of skull**

Requires fifth digit. See beginning of section 800–804 for codes and definitions.

Includes frontal bone
parietal bone

● **800.0 Closed without mention of intracranial injury**
[0-6,9]

● **800.1 Closed with cerebral laceration and contusion**
[0-6,9]

● **800.2 Closed with subarachnoid, subdural, and extradural**
[0-6,9] **hemorrhage**

● ■ **800.3 Closed with other and unspecified intracranial**
[0-6,9] **hemorrhage**

● ■ **800.4 Closed with intracranial injury of other and**
[0-6,9] **unspecified nature**

● **800.5 Open without mention of intracranial injury**
[0-6,9]

● **800.6 Open with cerebral laceration and contusion**
[0-6,9]

● **800.7 Open with subarachnoid, subdural, and extradural**
[0-6,9] **hemorrhage**

● ■ **800.8 Open with other and unspecified intracranial**
[0-6,9] **hemorrhage**

● ■ **800.9 Open with intracranial injury of other and**
[0-6,9] **unspecified nature**

◀ New   ◀▥ Revised   ~~deleted~~ Deleted   ● Use Additional Digit(s)   ■ Nonspecific Code
● Not first-listed DX   OGCR Official Guidelines   Coding Clinic   Excludes   Includes   Use additional   Code first   Omit code

● **801   Fracture of base of skull**

Requires fifth digit. See beginning of section 800–804 for codes and definitions.

Includes   fossa:
anterior
middle
posterior
occiput bone
orbital roof
sinus:
ethmoid
frontal
sphenoid bone
temporal bone

● **801.0   Closed without mention of intracranial**
[0-6,9]   **injury**

● **801.1   Closed with cerebral laceration and contusion**
[0-6,9]   Coding Clinic: 1996, Q4, P36.37

● **801.2   Closed with subarachnoid, subdural, and extradural**
[0-6,9]   **hemorrhage**

● ■ **801.3   Closed with other and unspecified intracranial**
[0-6,9]   **hemorrhage**

● ■ **801.4   Closed with intracranial injury of other and**
[0-6,9]   **unspecified nature**

● **801.5   Open without mention of intracranial injury**
[0-6,9]

● **801.6   Open with cerebral laceration and contusion**
[0-6,9]

● **801.7   Open with subarachnoid, subdural, and extradural**
[0-6,9]   **hemorrhage**

● ■ **801.8   Open with other and unspecified intracranial**
[0-6,9]   **hemorrhage**

● ■ **801.9   Open with intracranial injury of other and**
[0-6,9]   **unspecified nature**

● **802   Fracture of face bones**

802.0   Nasal bones, closed

802.1   Nasal bones, open

● **802.2   Mandible, closed**
Inferior maxilla
Lower jaw (bone)

■ **802.20   Unspecified site**

802.21   Condylar process

802.22   Subcondylar

802.23   Coronoid process

■ **802.24   Ramus, unspecified**

802.25   Angle of jaw

802.26   Symphysis of body

802.27   Alveolar border of body

■ **802.28   Body, other and unspecified**

■ **802.29   Multiple sites**

● **802.3   Mandible, open**

■ **802.30   Unspecified site**

802.31   Condylar process

802.32   Subcondylar

802.33   Coronoid process

■ **802.34   Ramus, unspecified**

802.35   Angle of jaw

802.36   Symphysis of body

802.37   Alveolar border of body

■ **802.38   Body, other and unspecified**

■ **802.39   Multiple sites**

802.4   Malar and maxillary bones, closed
Superior maxilla
Upper jaw (bone)
Zygoma
Zygomatic arch

802.5   Malar and maxillary bones, open

802.6   Orbital floor (blow-out), closed

802.7   Orbital floor (blow-out), open

■ **802.8   Other facial bones, closed**
Alveolus
Orbit:
NOS
part other than roof or floor
Palate

Excludes   *orbital:*
floor (802.6)
roof (801.0–801.9)

■ **802.9   Other facial bones, open**

● **803   Other and unqualified skull fractures**

Requires fifth digit. See beginning of section 800–804 for codes and definitions.

Includes   skull NOS
skull multiple NOS

● **803.0   Closed without mention of intracranial injury**
[0-6,9]

● **803.1   Closed with cerebral laceration and contusion**
[0-6,9]

● **803.2   Closed with subarachnoid, subdural, and extradural**
[0-6,9]   **hemorrhage**

● ■ **803.3   Closed with other and unspecified intracranial**
[0-6,9]   **hemorrhage**

● ■ **803.4   Closed with intracranial injury of other and**
[0-6,9]   **unspecified nature**

● **803.5   Open without mention of intracranial injury**
[0-6,9]

● **803.6   Open with cerebral laceration and contusion**
[0-6,9]

● **803.7   Open with subarachnoid, subdural, and extradural**
[0-6,9]   **hemorrhage**

● ■ **803.8   Open with other and unspecified intracranial**
[0-6,9]   **hemorrhage**

● ■ **803.9   Open with intracranial injury of other and**
[0-6,9]   **unspecified nature**

INJURY AND POISONING (800–999)

● **804   Multiple fractures involving skull or face with other bones**

     Requires fifth digit. See beginning of section 800–804 for codes and definitions.

● **804.0   Closed without mention of intracranial injury**
    [0-6,9]

● **804.1   Closed with cerebral laceration and contusion**
    [0-6,9]   Coding Clinic: 2006, Q1, P6-7

● **804.2   Closed with subarachnoid, subdural, and extradural**
    [0-6,9]   **hemorrhage**

● ■ **804.3   Closed with other and unspecified intracranial**
    [0-6,9]   **hemorrhage**

● ■ **804.4   Closed with intracranial injury of other and**
    [0-6,9]   **unspecified nature**

● **804.5   Open without mention of intracranial injury**
    [0-6,9]

● **804.6   Open with cerebral laceration and contusion**
    [0-6,9]

● **804.7   Open with subarachnoid, subdural, and extradural**
    [0-6,9]   **hemorrhage**

● ■ **804.8   Open with other and unspecified intracranial**
    [0-6,9]   **hemorrhage**

● ■ **804.9   Open with intracranial injury of other and**
    [0-6,9]   **unspecified nature**

FRACTURE OF NECK AND TRUNK (805–809)

● **805   Fracture of vertebral column without mention of spinal cord injury**

     Includes   neural arch
                     spine
                     spinous process
                     transverse process
                     vertebra
     Coding Clinic: 1985, Nov-Dec, P16

The following fifth-digit subclassification is for use with codes 805.0–805.1:

> ■ **0**   cervical vertebra, unspecified level
>   **1**   first cervical vertebra
>   **2**   second cervical vertebra
>   **3**   third cervical vertebra
>   **4**   fourth cervical vertebra
>   **5**   fifth cervical vertebra
>   **6**   sixth cervical vertebra
>   **7**   seventh cervical vertebra
> ■ **8**   multiple cervical vertebrae

● **805.0   Cervical, closed**
    [0-8]   Atlas
             Axis

● **805.1   Cervical, open**
    [0-8]

805.2   Dorsal [thoracic], closed

805.3   Dorsal [thoracic], open

805.4   Lumbar, closed
     Coding Clinic: 2007, Q1, P3-8

805.5   Lumbar, open

805.6   Sacrum and coccyx, closed

805.7   Sacrum and coccyx, open

■ **805.8   Unspecified, closed**

■ **805.9   Unspecified, open**

● **806   Fracture of vertebral column with spinal cord injury**

     Includes   any condition classifiable to 805 with:
                     complete or incomplete transverse lesion (of cord)
                     hematomyelia
                     injury to:
                         cauda equina
                         nerve
                     paralysis
                     paraplegia
                     quadriplegia
                     spinal concussion

● **806.0   Cervical, closed**

■ **806.00 C_1-C_4 level with unspecified spinal cord injury**
       Cervical region NOS with spinal cord injury NOS

   806.01 C_1-C_4 level with complete lesion of cord

   806.02 C_1-C_4 level with anterior cord syndrome

   806.03 C_1-C_4 level with central cord syndrome

■ **806.04 C_1-C_4 level with other specified spinal cord injury**
       C_1-C_4 level with:
          incomplete spinal cord lesion NOS
          posterior cord syndrome

■ **806.05 C_5-C_7 level with unspecified spinal cord injury**

   806.06 C_5-C_7 level with complete lesion of cord

   806.07 C_5-C_7 level with anterior cord syndrome

   806.08 C_5-C_7 level with central cord syndrome

■ **806.09 C_5-C_7 level with other specified spinal cord injury**
       C_5-C_7 level with:
          incomplete spinal cord lesion NOS
          posterior cord syndrome

● **806.1   Cervical, open**

■ **806.10 C_1-C_4 level with unspecified spinal cord injury**

   806.11 C_1-C_4 level with complete lesion of cord

   806.12 C_1-C_4 level with anterior cord syndrome

   806.13 C_1-C_4 level with central cord syndrome

■ **806.14 C_1-C_4 level with other specified spinal cord injury**
       C_1-C_4 level with:
          incomplete spinal cord lesion NOS
          posterior cord syndrome

■ **806.15 C_5-C_7 level with unspecified spinal cord injury**

   806.16 C_5-C_7 level with complete lesion of cord

   806.17 C_5-C_7 level with anterior cord syndrome

   806.18 C_5-C_7 level with central cord syndrome

■ **806.19 C_5-C_7 level with other specified spinal cord injury**
       C_5-C_7 level with:
          incomplete spinal cord lesion NOS
          posterior cord syndrome

◀ New   ◀▥ Revised   ~~deleted~~ Deleted   ● Use Additional Digit(s)   ■ Nonspecific Code
● Not first-listed DX   OGCR Official Guidelines   Coding Clinic   Excludes   Includes   Use additional   Code first   Omit code

● **806.2 Dorsal [thoracic], closed**

■ 806.20 T_1-T_6 level with unspecified spinal cord injury
Thoracic region NOS with spinal cord injury NOS

806.21 T_1-T_6 level with complete lesion of cord

806.22 T_1-T_6 level with anterior cord syndrome

806.23 T_1-T_6 level with central cord syndrome

■ 806.24 T_1-T_6 level with other specified spinal cord injury
T_1-T_6 level with:
incomplete spinal cord lesion NOS
posterior cord syndrome

■ 806.25 T_7-T_{12} level with unspecified spinal cord injury

806.26 T_7-T_{12} level with complete lesion of cord

806.27 T_7-T_{12} level with anterior cord syndrome

806.28 T_7-T_{12} level with central cord syndrome

■ 806.29 T_7-T_{12} level with other specified spinal cord injury
T_7-T_{12} level with:
incomplete spinal cord lesion NOS
posterior cord syndrome

● **806.3 Dorsal [thoracic], open**

■ 806.30 T_1-T_6 level with unspecified spinal cord injury

806.31 T_1-T_6 level with complete lesion of cord

806.32 T_1-T_6 level with anterior cord syndrome

806.33 T_1-T_6 level with central cord syndrome

■ 806.34 T_1-T_6 level with other specified spinal cord injury
T_1-T_6 level with:
incomplete spinal cord lesion NOS
posterior cord syndrome

■ 806.35 T_7-T_{12} level with unspecified spinal cord injury

806.36 T_7-T_{12} level with complete lesion of cord

806.37 T_7-T_{12} level with anterior cord syndrome

806.38 T_7-T_{12} level with central cord syndrome

■ 806.39 T_7-T_{12} level with other specified spinal cord injury
T_7-T_{12} level with:
incomplete spinal cord lesion NOS
posterior cord syndrome

806.4 **Lumbar, closed**
Coding Clinic: 1999, Q4, P11-13

806.5 **Lumbar, open**

● **806.6 Sacrum and coccyx, closed**

■ 806.60 With unspecified spinal cord injury

806.61 With complete cauda equina lesion

■ 806.62 With other cauda equina injury

■ 806.69 With other spinal cord injury

● **806.7 Sacrum and coccyx, open**

■ 806.70 With unspecified spinal cord injury

806.71 With complete cauda equina lesion

■ 806.72 With other cauda equina injury

■ 806.79 With other spinal cord injury

■ **806.8 Unspecified, closed**

■ **806.9 Unspecified, open**

● **807 Fracture of rib(s), sternum, larynx, and trachea**

The following fifth-digit subclassification is for use with codes 807.0–807.1:

■ 0 rib(s), unspecified
1 one rib
2 two ribs
3 three ribs
4 four ribs
5 five ribs
6 six ribs
7 seven ribs
8 eight or more ribs
■ 9 multiple ribs, unspecified

● **807.0 Rib(s), closed**
[0-9]

● **807.1 Rib(s), open**
[0-9]

807.2 **Sternum, closed**

807.3 **Sternum, open**

807.4 **Flail chest**
Unstable chest due to sternum and/or rib fracture

807.5 **Larynx and trachea, closed**
Hyoid bone
Thyroid cartilage
Trachea

807.6 **Larynx and trachea, open**

● **808 Fracture of pelvis**

808.0 **Acetabulum, closed**

808.1 **Acetabulum, open**

808.2 **Pubis, closed**
Coding Clinic: 2008, Q1, P9-10

808.3 **Pubis, open**

● **808.4 Other specified part, closed**

808.41 **Ilium**

808.42 **Ischium**

■ 808.43 **Multiple pelvic fractures with disruption of pelvic circle**
Coding Clinic: 2008, Q1, P9-10

■ 808.49 **Other**
Innominate bone
Pelvic rim

● **808.5 Other specified part, open**

808.51 **Ilium**

808.52 **Ischium**

■ 808.53 **Multiple pelvic fractures with disruption of pelvic circle**

■ 808.59 **Other**

■ **808.8 Unspecified, closed**

■ **808.9 Unspecified, open**

● **809 Ill-defined fractures of bones of trunk**

Includes   bones of trunk with other bones except those of skull and face
multiple bones of trunk

Excludes   *multiple fractures of:*
pelvic bones alone (808.0–808.9)
ribs alone (807.0–807.1, 807.4)
ribs or sternum with limb bones (819.0–819.1, 828.0–828.1)
skull or face with other bones (804.0–804.9)

809.0 **Fracture of bones of trunk, closed**

809.1 **Fracture of bones of trunk, open**

INJURY AND POISONING (800–999)

FRACTURE OF UPPER LIMB (810–819)

● 810 Fracture of clavicle

Includes collar bone
interligamentous part of clavicle

The following fifth-digit subclassification is for use with category 810:

■ 0 **unspecified part**
Clavicle NOS
1 **sternal end of clavicle**
2 **shaft of clavicle**
3 **acromial end of clavicle**

● 810.0 **Closed**
[0-3]

● 810.1 **Open**
[0-3]

● 811 Fracture of scapula

Includes shoulder blade

The following fifth-digit subclassification is for use with category 811:

■ 0 **unspecified part**
1 **acromial process**
Acromion (process)
2 **coracoid process**
3 **glenoid cavity and neck of scapula**
■ 9 **other**

● 811.0 **Closed**
[0-3,9]

● 811.1 **Open**
[0-3,9]

● 812 Fracture of humerus

● 812.0 **Upper end, closed**

■ 812.00 **Upper end, unspecified part**
Proximal end
Shoulder

812.01 **Surgical neck**
Neck of humerus NOS

812.02 **Anatomical neck**

812.03 **Greater tuberosity**

■ 812.09 **Other**
Head
Upper epiphysis

● 812.1 **Upper end, open**

■ 812.10 **Upper end, unspecified part**

812.11 **Surgical neck**

812.12 **Anatomical neck**

812.13 **Greater tuberosity**

■ 812.19 **Other**

● 812.2 **Shaft or unspecified part, closed**

■ 812.20 **Unspecified part of humerus**
Humerus NOS
Upper arm NOS

812.21 **Shaft of humerus**
Coding Clinic: 2005, Q4, P127-129; 1999, Q3, P14-15

● 812.3 **Shaft or unspecified part, open**

■ 812.30 **Unspecified part of humerus**

812.31 **Shaft of humerus**

● 812.4 **Lower end, closed**
Distal end of humerus
Elbow

■ 812.40 **Lower end, unspecified part**

812.41 **Supracondylar fracture of humerus**

812.42 **Lateral condyle**
External condyle

812.43 **Medial condyle**
Internal epicondyle

■ 812.44 **Condyle(s), unspecified**
Articular process NOS
Lower epiphysis

■ 812.49 **Other**
Multiple fractures of lower end
Trochlea

● 812.5 **Lower end, open**

■ 812.50 **Lower end, unspecified part**

812.51 **Supracondylar fracture of humerus**

812.52 **Lateral condyle**

812.53 **Medial condyle**

■ 812.54 **Condyle(s), unspecified**

■ 812.59 **Other**

● 813 Fracture of radius and ulna

● 813.0 **Upper end, closed**
Proximal end

■ 813.00 **Upper end of forearm, unspecified**

813.01 **Olecranon process of ulna**

813.02 **Coronoid process of ulna**

813.03 **Monteggia's fracture**

■ 813.04 **Other and unspecified fractures of proximal end of ulna (alone)**
Multiple fractures of ulna, upper end

813.05 **Head of radius**

813.06 **Neck of radius**

■ 813.07 **Other and unspecified fractures of proximal end of radius (alone)**
Multiple fractures of radius, upper end

813.08 **Radius with ulna, upper end [any part]**

● 813.1 **Upper end, open**

■ 813.10 **Upper end of forearm, unspecified**

813.11 **Olecranon process of ulna**

813.12 **Coronoid process of ulna**

813.13 **Monteggia's fracture**

■ 813.14 **Other and unspecified fractures of proximal end of ulna (alone)**

813.15 **Head of radius**

813.16 **Neck of radius**

■ 813.17 **Other and unspecified fractures of proximal end of radius (alone)**

813.18 **Radius with ulna, upper end [any part]**

● 813.2 **Shaft, closed**

■ 813.20 **Shaft, unspecified**

813.21 **Radius (alone)**

813.22 **Ulna (alone)**

813.23 **Radius with ulna**

● 813.3 **Shaft, open**

■ 813.30 **Shaft, unspecified**

813.31 **Radius (alone)**

◀ New   ◀▥ Revised   deleted Deleted   ● Use Additional Digit(s)   ■ Nonspecific Code
● Not first-listed DX   OGCR Official Guidelines   Coding Clinic   Excludes   Includes   Use additional   Code first   Omit code

813.32 Ulna (alone)

813.33 Radius with ulna

● 813.4 **Lower end, closed**
Distal end

■ 813.40 **Lower end of forearm, unspecified**

813.41 **Colles' fracture**
Smith's fracture

■ 813.42 **Other fractures of distal end of radius (alone)**
Dupuytren's fracture, radius
Radius, lower end

813.43 **Distal end of ulna (alone)**
Ulna: Ulna:
head   lower epiphysis
lower end   styloid process

813.44 **Radius with ulna, lower end**
Coding Clinic: 2007, Q1, P3-8

813.45 **Torus fracture of radius (alone)**   ◀▥

Excludes *torus fracture of radius
and ulna (813.47)*   ◀
Coding Clinic: 2002, Q4, P70-71

813.46 **Torus fracture of ulna (alone)**   ◀

Excludes *torus fracture of radius and ulna
(813.47)*   ◀

813.47 **Torus fracture of radius and ulna**   ◀

● 813.5 **Lower end, open**

■ 813.50 **Lower end of forearm, unspecified**

813.51 **Colles' fracture**

■ 813.52 **Other fractures of distal end of radius
(alone)**

813.53 **Distal end of ulna (alone)**

813.54 **Radius with ulna, lower end**

● 813.8 **Unspecified part, closed**

■ 813.80 **Forearm, unspecified**

■ 813.81 **Radius (alone)**
Coding Clinic: 1998, Q2, P19

■ 813.82 **Ulna (alone)**

■ 813.83 **Radius with ulna**

● 813.9 **Unspecified part, open**

■ 813.90 **Forearm, unspecified**

■ 813.91 **Radius (alone)**

■ 813.92 **Ulna (alone)**

■ 813.93 **Radius with ulna**

● 814 **Fracture of carpal bone(s)**

The following fifth-digit subclassification is for use with
category 814:

■ 0 **carpal bone, unspecified**
Wrist NOS
1 **navicular [scaphoid] of wrist**
2 **lunate [semilunar] bone of wrist**
3 **triquetral [cuneiform] bone of wrist**
4 **pisiform**
5 **trapezium bone [larger multangular]**
6 **trapezoid bone [smaller multangular]**
7 **capitate bone [os magnum]**
8 **hamate [unciform] bone**
■ 9 **other**

● 814.0 **Closed**
[0-9]

● 814.1 **Open**
[0-9]

● 815 **Fracture of metacarpal bone(s)**

Includes hand [except finger]
metacarpus

The following fifth-digit subclassification is for use with
category 815:

■ 0 **metacarpal bone(s), site unspecified**
1 **base of thumb [first] metacarpal**
Bennett's fracture
2 **base of other metacarpal bone(s)**
3 **shaft of metacarpal bone(s)**
4 **neck of metacarpal bone(s)**
■ 9 **multiple sites of metacarpus**

● 815.0 **Closed**
[0-4,9]   Coding Clinic: 1994, Q2, P6

● 815.1 **Open**
[0-4,9]

● 816 **Fracture of one or more phalanges of hand**

Includes finger(s)
thumb

The following fifth-digit subclassification is for use with
category 816:

■ 0 **phalanx or phalanges, unspecified**
1 **middle or proximal phalanx or phalanges**
2 **distal phalanx or phalanges**
■ 3 **multiple sites**

● 816.0 **Closed**
[0-3]

● 816.1 **Open**
[0-3]   Coding Clinic: 2003, Q4, P76-78

● 817 **Multiple fractures of hand bones**

Includes metacarpal bone(s) with phalanx or phalanges
of same hand

817.0 **Closed**

817.1 **Open**

● 818 **Ill-defined fractures of upper limb**

Includes arm NOS
multiple bones of same upper limb

Excludes *multiple fractures of:*
*metacarpal bone(s) with phalanx or phalanges
(817.0–817.1)*
phalanges of hand alone (816.0–816.1)
radius with ulna (813.0–813.9)

■ 818.0 **Closed**

■ 818.1 **Open**

OGCR Section I.C.17.b.3
Multiple fracture category 819 classifies bilateral
fractures of both upper limbs, but without any detail at
the fourth-digit level other than open and closed type of
fractures.

● 819 **Multiple fractures involving both upper limbs, and upper
limb with rib(s) and sternum**

Includes arm(s) with rib(s) or sternum
both arms [any bones]

819.0 **Closed**

819.1 **Open**

INJURY AND POISONING (800–999)

FRACTURE OF LOWER LIMB (820–829)

● **820 Fracture of neck of femur**

  ● **820.0 Transcervical fracture, closed**

    ■ **820.00 Intracapsular section, unspecified**

    820.01 Epiphysis (separation) (upper)
      Transepiphyseal
      Fracture and separation across growth plate

    820.02 Midcervical section
      Transcervical NOS
      Coding Clinic: 2003, Q3, P12-13

    820.03 Base of neck
      Cervicotrochanteric section

    ■ **820.09 Other**
      Head of femur
      Subcapital

  ● **820.1 Transcervical fracture, open**

    ■ **820.10 Intracapsular section, unspecified**

    820.11 Epiphysis (separation) (upper)

    820.12 Midcervical section

    820.13 Base of neck

    820.19 Other

  ● **820.2 Pertrochanteric fracture, closed**

    ■ **820.20 Trochanteric section, unspecified**
      Trochanter:
        NOS
        greater
        lesser

    820.21 Intertrochanteric section
      Coding Clinic: 1994, Q2, P6; 1984, May-June, P11

    820.22 Subtrochanteric section

  ● **820.3 Pertrochanteric fracture, open**

    ■ **820.30 Trochanteric section, unspecified**

    820.31 Intertrochanteric section

    820.32 Subtrochanteric section

  ■ **820.8 Unspecified part of neck of femur, closed**
    Hip NOS
    Neck of femur NOS
    Coding Clinic: 1994, Q2, P9; 1985, Nov-Dec, P16

  ■ **820.9 Unspecified part of neck of femur, open**

● **821 Fracture of other and unspecified parts of femur**

  ● **821.0 Shaft or unspecified part, closed**

    ■ **821.00 Unspecified part of femur**
      Thigh   Upper leg
      Excludes *hip NOS (820.8)*

    821.01 Shaft
      Coding Clinic: 2007, Q1, P3-8; 1999, Q1, P5

  ● **821.1 Shaft or unspecified part, open**

    ■ **821.10 Unspecified part of femur**

    821.11 Shaft

  ● **821.2 Lower end, closed**
    Distal end

    ■ **821.20 Lower end, unspecified part**

    821.21 Condyle, femoral

    821.22 Epiphysis, lower (separation)

    821.23 Supracondylar fracture of femur

    ■ **821.29 Other**
      Multiple fractures of lower end

  ● **821.3 Lower end, open**

    ■ **821.30 Lower end, unspecified part**

    821.31 Condyle, femoral

    821.32 Epiphysis, lower (separation)

    821.33 Supracondylar fracture of femur

    ■ **821.39 Other**

● **822 Fracture of patella**

  822.0 Closed

  822.1 Open

● **823 Fracture of tibia and fibula**

  Excludes *Dupuytren's fracture (824.4–824.5)*
      ankle (824.4–824.5)
      radius (813.42, 813.52)
      Pott's fracture (824.4–824.5)
      that involving ankle (824.0–824.9)

The following fifth-digit subclassification is for use with category 823:

> 0 tibia alone
> 1 fibula alone
> 2 fibula with tibia

  ● **823.0 Upper end, closed**
    [0-2]   Head
        Proximal end
        Tibia:
          condyles
          tuberosity

  ● **823.1 Upper end, open**
    [0-2]

  ● **823.2 Shaft, closed**
    [0-2]

  ● **823.3 Shaft, open**
    [0-2]

  ● **823.4 Torus fracture**
    [0-2]   Coding Clinic: 2002, Q4, P70-71

  ● ■ **823.8 Unspecified part, closed**
    [0-2]   Lower leg NOS
      Coding Clinic: 1997, Q1, P8

  ● ■ **823.9 Unspecified part, open**
    [0-2]

● **824 Fracture of ankle**

  824.0 Medial malleolus, closed]
    Tibia involving:
      ankle
      malleolus
    Coding Clinic: 2004, Q1, P9

  824.1 Medial malleolus, open

  824.2 Lateral malleolus, closed
    Fibula involving:
      ankle
      malleolus
    Coding Clinic: 2002, Q2, P3

  824.3 Lateral malleolus, open

  824.4 Bimalleolar, closed
    Dupuytren's fracture, fibula
    Pott's fracture

  824.5 Bimalleolar, open

  824.6 Trimalleolar, closed
    Lateral and medial malleolus with anterior or
      posterior lip of tibia

  824.7 Trimalleolar, open

◄ New   ◄▥ Revised   ~~deleted~~ Deleted   ● Use Additional Digit(s)   ■ Nonspecific Code
● Not first-listed DX   OGCR Official Guidelines   Coding Clinic   Excludes   Includes   Use additional   Code first   Omit code

▪824.8   **Unspecified, closed**
     Ankle NOS
     Coding Clinic: 2000, Q3, P12; 1994, Q2, P7

▪824.9   **Unspecified, open**

● **825   Fracture of one or more tarsal and metatarsal bones**

    ▪825.0   **Fracture of calcaneus, closed**
        Heel bone
        Os calcis

    825.1   **Fracture of calcaneus, open**

    ● 825.2   **Fracture of other tarsal and metatarsal bones, closed**

       ▪825.20   **Unspecified bone(s) of foot [except toes]**
           Instep

       825.21   **Astragalus**
           Talus

       825.22   **Navicular [scaphoid], foot**

       825.23   **Cuboid**

       825.24   **Cuneiform, foot**

       825.25   **Metatarsal bone(s)**

       ▪825.29   **Other**
           Tarsal with metatarsal bone(s) only

           Excludes   *calcaneus (825.0)*

           Coding Clinic: 1994, Q2, P5

    ● 825.3   **Fracture of other tarsal and metatarsal bones, open**

       ▪825.30   **Unspecified bone(s) of foot [except toes]**

       825.31   **Astragalus**

       825.32   **Navicular [scaphoid], foot**

       825.33   **Cuboid**

       825.34   **Cuneiform, foot**

       825.35   **Metatarsal bone(s)**

       ▪825.39   **Other**

● **826   Fracture of one or more phalanges of foot**

    Includes   toe(s)

    826.0   **Closed**

    826.1   **Open**

● **827   Other, multiple, and ill-defined fractures of lower limb**

    Includes   leg NOS
               multiple bones of same lower limb

    Excludes   *multiple fractures of:*
               ankle bones alone (824.4–824.9)
               phalanges of foot alone (826.0–826.1)
               tarsal with metatarsal bones (825.29, 825.39)
               tibia with fibula (823.0–823.9 with fifth-digit 2)

    827.0   **Closed**

    827.1   **Open**

● **828   Multiple fractures involving both lower limbs, lower with upper limb, and lower limb(s) with rib(s) and sternum**

    Includes   arm(s) with leg(s) [any bones]
               both legs [any bones]
               leg(s) with rib(s) or sternum

    OGCR   Section I.C.17.b.3
    Multiple fracture category 828 classifies bilateral
    fractures of both upper limbs, but without any detail at
    the fourth-digit level other than open and closed type of
    fractures.

    828.0   **Closed**

    828.1   **Open**

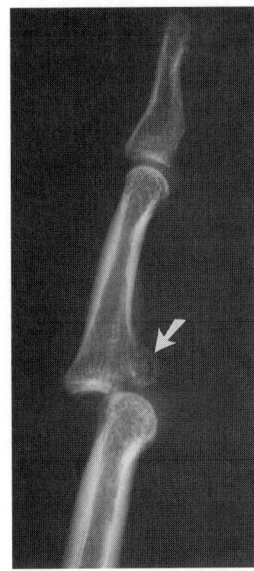
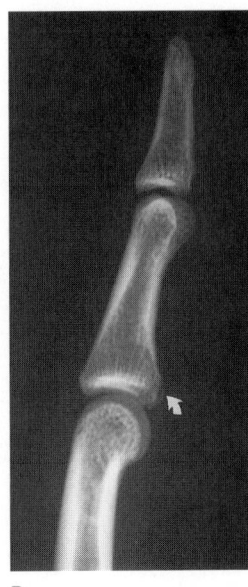

    A   B

Figure 17-13   Dislocation including displacement and subluxation. (From Grainger & Allison's Diagnostic Radiology: A Textbook of Medical Imaging, 4th ed. 2001, Churchill Livingstone)

● **829   Fracture of unspecified bones**

    ▪829.0   **Unspecified bone, closed**

    ▪829.1   **Unspecified bone, open**

DISLOCATION (830–839)

    Includes   displacement
               subluxation
               Out of position

    Excludes   *congenital dislocation (754.0–755.8)*
               pathological dislocation (718.2)
               recurrent dislocation (718.3)

The descriptions "closed" and "open," used in the fourth-digit subdivisions, include the following terms:
    closed:
       complete
       dislocation NOS
       partial
       simple
       uncomplicated
    open:
       compound
       infected
       with foreign body

Note: A dislocation not indicated as closed or open should be classified as closed.

● **830   Dislocation of jaw**

    Includes   jaw (cartilage) (meniscus)
               mandible
               maxilla (inferior)
               temporomandibular (joint)

    830.0   **Closed dislocation**

    830.1   **Open dislocation**

INJURY AND POISONING (800–999)

● 831 **Dislocation of shoulder**

Excludes *sternoclavicular joint (839.61, 839.71)*
sternum (839.61, 839.71)

The following fifth-digit subclassification is for use with category 831:

■ 0 **shoulder, unspecified**
    Humerus NOS
  1 **anterior dislocation of humerus**
  2 **posterior dislocation of humerus**
  3 **inferior dislocation of humerus**
  4 **acromioclavicular (joint)**
    Clavicle
■ 9 **other**
    Scapula

● 831.0 **Closed dislocation**
[0-4,9]   Coding Clinic: 1987, Nov-Dec, P7

● 831.1 **Open dislocation**
[0-4,9]

● 832 **Dislocation of elbow**

The following fifth-digit subclassification is for use with ~~category 832~~ subcategories 832.0 and 832.1: ◄▥

■ 0 **elbow unspecified**
  1 **anterior dislocation of elbow**
  2 **posterior dislocation of elbow**
  3 **medial dislocation of elbow**
  4 **lateral dislocation of elbow**
■ 9 **other**

● 832.0 **Closed dislocation**
[0-4,9]

● 832.1 **Open dislocation**
[0-4,9]

832.2 **Nursemaid's elbow** ◄
    Subluxation of radial head ◄

● 833 **Dislocation of wrist**

The following fifth-digit subclassification is for use with category 833:

■ 0 **wrist, unspecified part**
    Carpal (bone)
    Radius, distal end
  1 **radioulnar (joint), distal**
  2 **radiocarpal (joint)**
  3 **midcarpal (joint)**
  4 **carpometacarpal (joint)**
  5 **metacarpal (bone), proximal end**
■ 9 **other**
    Ulna, distal end

● 833.0 **Closed dislocation**
[0-5,9]

● 833.1 **Open dislocation**
[0-5,9]

● 834 **Dislocation of finger**

Includes finger(s)
phalanx of hand
thumb

The following fifth-digit subclassification is for use with category 834:

■ 0 **finger, unspecified part**
  1 **metacarpophalangeal (joint)**
    Metacarpal (bone), distal end
  2 **interphalangeal (joint), hand**

● 834.0 **Closed dislocation**
[0-2]

● 834.1 **Open dislocation**
[0-2]

● 835 **Dislocation of hip**

The following fifth-digit subclassification is for use with category 835:

■ 0 **dislocation of hip, unspecified**
  1 **posterior dislocation**
  2 **obturator dislocation**
■ 3 **other anterior dislocation**

● 835.0 **Closed dislocation**
[0-3]

● 835.1 **Open dislocation**
[0-3]

● 836 **Dislocation of knee**

Excludes *dislocation of knee:*
old or pathological (718.2)
recurrent (718.3)
internal derangement of knee joint (717.0–717.5, 717.8–717.9)
old tear of cartilage or meniscus of knee (717.0–717.5, 717.8–717.9)

836.0 **Tear of medial cartilage or meniscus of knee, current**
    Bucket handle tear:
    NOS current injury
    medial meniscus current injury

836.1 **Tear of lateral cartilage or meniscus of knee, current**

■ 836.2 **Other tear of cartilage or meniscus of knee, current**
    Tear of:
      cartilage (semilunar) current injury, not specified as medial or lateral
      meniscus current injury, not specified as medial or lateral

836.3 **Dislocation of patella, closed**

836.4 **Dislocation of patella, open**

INJURY AND POISONING (800–999)

● 836.5   Other dislocation of knee, closed

  ■ 836.50   Dislocation of knee, unspecified

    836.51   Anterior dislocation of tibia, proximal end
          Posterior dislocation of femur, distal end

    836.52   Posterior dislocation of tibia, proximal end
          Anterior dislocation of femur, distal end

    836.53   Medial dislocation of tibia, proximal end

    836.54   Lateral dislocation of tibia, proximal end

    836.59   Other

● 836.6   Other dislocation of knee, open

  ■ 836.60   Dislocation of knee, unspecified

    836.61   Anterior dislocation of tibia, proximal end

    836.62   Posterior dislocation of tibia, proximal end

    836.63   Medial dislocation of tibia, proximal end

    836.64   Lateral dislocation of tibia, proximal end

  ■ 836.69   Other

● 837   Dislocation of ankle

Includes	astragalus	scaphoid, foot
	fibula, distal end	tibia, distal end
	navicular, foot	

   837.0   Closed dislocation

   837.1   Open dislocation

● 838   Dislocation of foot

The following fifth-digit subclassification is for use with category 838:

  ■ **0   foot, unspecified**
     1   tarsal (bone), joint unspecified
     2   midtarsal (joint)
     3   tarsometatarsal (joint)
     4   metatarsal (bone), joint unspecified
     5   metatarsophalangeal (joint)
     6   interphalangeal (joint), foot
  ■ **9   other**
       Phalanx of foot
       Toe(s)

● 838.0   Closed dislocation
[0-6,9]

● 838.1   Open dislocation
[0-6,9]

● 839   Other, multiple, and ill-defined dislocations
     Coding Clinic: 1995, Q4, P51

 ● 839.0   Cervical vertebra, closed
       Cervical spine
       Neck

  ■ 839.00   Cervical vertebra, unspecified

    839.01   First cervical vertebra

    839.02   Second cervical vertebra

    839.03   Third cervical vertebra

    839.04   Fourth cervical vertebra

    839.05   Fifth cervical vertebra

    839.06   Sixth cervical vertebra

    839.07   Seventh cervical vertebra

  ■ 839.08   Multiple cervical vertebrae

● 839.1   Cervical vertebra, open

  ■ 839.10   Cervical vertebra, unspecified

    839.11   First cervical vertebra

    839.12   Second cervical vertebra

    839.13   Third cervical vertebra

    839.14   Fourth cervical vertebra

    839.15   Fifth cervical vertebra

    839.16   Sixth cervical vertebra

    839.17   Seventh cervical vertebra

  ■ 839.18   Multiple cervical vertebrae

● 839.2   Thoracic and lumbar vertebra, closed

    839.20   Lumbar vertebra

    839.21   Thoracic vertebra
          Dorsal [thoracic] vertebra

● 839.3   Thoracic and lumbar vertebra, open

    839.30   Lumbar vertebra

    839.31   Thoracic vertebra

● 839.4   Other vertebra, closed

  ■ 839.40   Vertebra, unspecified site
          Spine NOS

    839.41   Coccyx

    839.42   Sacrum
          Sacroiliac (joint)

  ■ 839.49   Other

● 839.5   Other vertebra, open

  ■ 839.50   Vertebra, unspecified site

    839.51   Coccyx

    839.52   Sacrum

  ■ 839.59   Other

● 839.6   Other location, closed

    839.61   Sternum
          Sternoclavicular joint

  ■ 839.69   Other
          Pelvis

● 839.7   Other location, open

    839.71   Sternum

  ■ 839.79   Other

■ 839.8   Multiple and ill-defined, closed
     Arm
     Back
     Hand
     Multiple locations, except fingers or toes alone
     Other ill-defined locations
     Unspecified location

■ 839.9   Multiple and ill-defined, open

SPRAINS AND STRAINS OF JOINTS AND ADJACENT MUSCLES (840–848)

Includes   avulsion of joint capsule, ligament, muscle, tendon
hemarthrosis of joint capsule, ligament, muscle, tendon
Bleeding into joint space
laceration of joint capsule, ligament, muscle, tendon
rupture of joint capsule, ligament, muscle, tendon
sprain of joint capsule, ligament, muscle, tendon
strain of joint capsule, ligament, muscle, tendon
tear of joint capsule, ligament, muscle, tendon

Excludes   *laceration of tendon in open wounds (880–884 and 890–894 with .2)*

● **840   Sprains and strains of shoulder and upper arm**
Sprains are an injury to ligaments when one or more is stretched/torn and strains are caused by twisting or pulling a muscle(s) or tendon.

840.0   Acromioclavicular (joint) (ligament)

840.1   Coracoclavicular (ligament)

840.2   Coracohumeral (ligament)

840.3   Infraspinatus (muscle) (tendon)

840.4   Rotator cuff (capsule)

Excludes   *complete rupture of rotator cuff, nontraumatic (727.61)*

840.5   Subscapularis (muscle)

840.6   Supraspinatus (muscle) (tendon)

840.7   Superior glenoid labrum lesion
SLAP lesion
Coding Clinic: 2001, Q4, P52

■840.8   Other specified sites of shoulder and upper arm

■840.9   Unspecified site of shoulder and upper arm
Arm NOS
Shoulder NOS

● **841   Sprains and strains of elbow and forearm**

841.0   Radial collateral ligament

841.1   Ulnar collateral ligament

841.2   Radiohumeral (joint)

841.3   Ulnohumeral (joint)

■841.8   Other specified sites of elbow and forearm

■841.9   Unspecified site of elbow and forearm
Elbow NOS

● **842   Sprains and strains of wrist and hand**

● 842.0   Wrist

■842.00   Unspecified site

842.01   Carpal (joint)

842.02   Radiocarpal (joint) (ligament)

■842.09   Other
Radioulnar joint, distal

● 842.1   Hand

■842.10   Unspecified site

842.11   Carpometacarpal (joint)

842.12   Metacarpophalangeal (joint)

842.13   Interphalangeal (joint)

■842.19   Other
Midcarpal (joint)

● **843   Sprains and strains of hip and thigh**

843.0   Iliofemoral (ligament)

843.1   Ischiocapsular (ligament)

■843.8   Other specified sites of hip and thigh

■843.9   Unspecified site of hip and thigh
Hip NOS
Thigh NOS

● **844   Sprains and strains of knee and leg**

844.0   Lateral collateral ligament of knee

844.1   Medial collateral ligament of knee

844.2   Cruciate ligament of knee

844.3   Tibiofibular (joint) (ligament), superior

■844.8   Other specified sites of knee and leg

■844.9   Unspecified site of knee and leg
Knee NOS
Leg NOS

● **845   Sprains and strains of ankle and foot**

● 845.0   Ankle

■845.00   Unspecified site
Coding Clinic: 2002, Q2, P3

845.01   Deltoid (ligament), ankle
Internal collateral (ligament), ankle

845.02   Calcaneofibular (ligament)

845.03   Tibiofibular (ligament), distal
Coding Clinic: 2004, Q1, P9

■845.09   Other
Achilles tendon

● 845.1   Foot

■845.10   Unspecified site

845.11   Tarsometatarsal (joint) (ligament)

845.12   Metatarsophalangeal (joint)

845.13   Interphalangeal (joint), toe

■845.19   Other

● **846   Sprains and strains of sacroiliac region**

846.0   Lumbosacral (joint) (ligament)

846.1   Sacroiliac ligament

846.2   Sacrospinatus (ligament)

846.3   Sacrotuberous (ligament)

■846.8   Other specified sites of sacroiliac region

■846.9   Unspecified site of sacroiliac region

● **847   Sprains and strains of other and unspecified parts of back**

Excludes   *lumbosacral (846.0)*

847.0   Neck
Anterior longitudinal (ligament), cervical
Atlanto-axial (joints)
Atlanto-occipital (joints)
Whiplash injury

Excludes   *neck injury NOS (959.09)*
thyroid region (848.2)

847.1   Thoracic

847.2   Lumbar

847.3   Sacrum
Sacrococcygeal (ligament)

847.4   Coccyx

■847.9   Unspecified site of back
Back NOS

◀ New   ◀▥ Revised   ~~deleted~~ Deleted   ● Use Additional Digit(s)   ■ Nonspecific Code
● Not first-listed DX   OGCR Official Guidelines   Coding Clinic   Excludes   Includes   Use additional   Code first   Omit code

● 848 **Other and ill-defined sprains and strains**

848.0 **Septal cartilage of nose**

848.1 **Jaw**
Temporomandibular (joint) (ligament)

848.2 **Thyroid region**
Cricoarytenoid (joint) (ligament)
Cricothyroid (joint) (ligament)
Thyroid cartilage

848.3 **Ribs**
Chondrocostal (joint) without mention of injury to sternum
Costal cartilage without mention of injury to sternum

● 848.4 **Sternum**
■ 848.40 **Unspecified site**

848.41 **Sternoclavicular (joint) (ligament)**

848.42 **Chondrosternal (joint)**

■ 848.49 **Other**
Xiphoid cartilage

848.5 **Pelvis**
Symphysis pubis
Excludes *that in childbirth (665.6)*

■ 848.8 **Other specified sites of sprains and strains**

■ 848.9 **Unspecified site of sprain and strain**

INTRACRANIAL INJURY, EXCLUDING THOSE WITH SKULL FRACTURE (850–854)

Includes traumatic brain injury without skull fracture

Excludes *intracranial injury with skull fracture (800–801 and 803–804, except .0 and .5)*
open wound of head without intracranial injury (870.0–873.9)
skull fracture alone (800–801 and 803–804 with .0, .5)

Note: The description "with open intracranial wound," used in the fourth-digit subdivisions, includes those specified as open or with mention of infection or foreign body.

The following fifth-digit subclassification is for use with categories 851–854:

■ 0 **unspecified state of consciousness**
1 **with no loss of consciousness**
2 **with brief [less than one hour] loss of consciousness**
3 **with moderate [1–24 hours] loss of consciousness**
4 **with prolonged [more than 24 hours] loss of consciousness and return to pre-existing conscious level**
5 **with prolonged [more than 24 hours] loss of consciousness without return to pre-existing conscious level**
    Use fifth-digit 5 to designate when a patient is unconscious and dies before regaining consciousness, regardless of the duration of the loss of consciousness
■ 6 **with loss of consciousness of unspecified duration**
■ 9 **with concussion, unspecified**

● 850 **Concussion**
Includes commotio cerebri
Excludes *concussion with:*
cerebral laceration or contusion (851.0–851.9)
cerebral hemorrhage (852–853)
head injury NOS (959.01)
Coding Clinic: 1993, Q1, P22-23

850.0 **With no loss of consciousness**
Concussion with mental confusion or disorientation, without loss of consciousness
Coding Clinic: 1992, Q2, P5-6

● 850.1 **With brief loss of consciousness**
Loss of consciousness for less than one hour
Coding Clinic: 2003, Q4, P76; 1999, Q1, P10; 1992, Q2, P5-6

850.11 **With loss of consciousness of 30 minutes or less**

850.12 **With loss of consciousness from 31 to 59 minutes**

850.2 **With moderate loss of consciousness**
Loss of consciousness for 1–24 hours

850.3 **With prolonged loss of consciousness and return to pre-existing conscious level**
Loss of consciousness for more than 24 hours with complete recovery

850.4 **With prolonged loss of consciousness, without return to pre-existing conscious level**

■ 850.5 **With loss of consciousness of unspecified duration**

■ 850.9 **Concussion, unspecified**

● 851 **Cerebral laceration and contusion**
Cerebral lacerations are tears in brain tissue. Cerebral contusions are bruises on brain.
Requires fifth digit. See beginning of section 850–854 for codes and definitions.
Coding Clinic: 1993, Q1, P22-23

● 851.0 **Cortex (cerebral) contusion without mention of open**
[0-6,9] **intracranial wound**

● 851.1 **Cortex (cerebral) contusion with open intracranial**
[0-6,9] **wound**

● 851.2 **Cortex (cerebral) laceration without mention of open**
[0-6,9] **intracranial wound**

● 851.3 **Cortex (cerebral) laceration with open intracranial**
[0-6,9] **wound**

● 851.4 **Cerebellar or brain stem contusion without mention**
[0-6,9] **of open intracranial wound**

● 851.5 **Cerebellar or brain stem contusion with open**
[0-6,9] **intracranial wound**

● 851.6 **Cerebellar or brain stem laceration without mention**
[0-6,9] **of open intracranial wound**

● 851.7 **Cerebellar or brain stem laceration with open**
[0-6,9] **intracranial wound**

● ■ 851.8 **Other and unspecified cerebral laceration and**
[0-6,9] **contusion, without mention of open intracranial wound**
Brain (membrane) NOS
Coding Clinic: 1996, Q4, P36.37

● ■ 851.9 **Other and unspecified cerebral laceration and**
[0-6,9] **contusion, with open intracranial wound**

INJURY AND POISONING (800–999)

● 852   **Subarachnoid, subdural, and extradural hemorrhage, following injury**

> Requires fifth digit. See beginning of section 850–854 for codes and definitions.

> **Excludes**   *cerebral contusion or laceration (with hemorrhage) (851.0–851.9)*

● 852.0   **Subarachnoid hemorrhage following injury without**
[0-6,9]   **mention of open intracranial wound**
> Middle meningeal hemorrhage following injury
> Coding Clinic: 1991, Q3, P15-16

● 852.1   **Subarachnoid hemorrhage following injury with**
[0-6,9]   **open intracranial wound**
> Coding Clinic: 1991, Q3, P15-16

● 852.2   **Subdural hemorrhage following injury without**
[0-6,9]   **mention of open intracranial wound**
> Coding Clinic: 2007, Q4, P105-107; 1996, Q4, P43-44

● 852.3   **Subdural hemorrhage following injury with open**
[0-6,9]   **intracranial wound**

● 852.4   **Extradural hemorrhage following injury without**
[0-6,9]   **mention of open intracranial wound**
> Epidural hematoma following injury

● 852.5   **Extradural hemorrhage following injury with open**
[0-6,9]   **intracranial wound**

● 853   **Other and unspecified intracranial hemorrhage following injury**

> Requires fifth digit. See beginning of section 850–854 for codes and definitions.

● ▪853.0   **Without mention of open intracranial wound**
[0-6,9]   Cerebral compression due to injury
> Intracranial hematoma following injury
> Traumatic cerebral hemorrhage
> Coding Clinic: 1990, Q3, P14

● ▪853.1   **With open intracranial wound**
[0-6,9]

● 854   **Intracranial injury of other and unspecified nature**

> Requires fifth digit. See beginning of section 850-854 for codes and definitions.

> **Includes**   injury:
>   brain ~~injury~~ NOS   ◀⃪⃟
>   cavernous sinus
>   intracranial ~~injury~~   ◀⃪⃟
>   traumatic brain NOS   ◀

> **Excludes**   *any condition classifiable to 850–853*
> *head injury NOS (959.01)*
> Coding Clinic: 1999, Q1, P10; 1992, Q2, P5-6

● ▪854.0   **Without mention of open intracranial wound**
[0-6,9]
> Coding Clinic: 2005, Q2, P6-7

● ▪854.1   **With open intracranial wound**
[0-6,9]

Item 17-1   **Pneumothorax** is a collection of gas (positive air pressure) in the pleural space resulting in the lung collapsing. A tension pneumothorax is life-threatening and is a result of air in the pleural space causing a displacement in the mediastinal structures and cardiopulmonary function compromise. A traumatic pneumothorax results from blunt or penetrating injury that disrupts the parietal/visceral pleura. **Hemothorax** is blood or bloody fluid in the pleural cavity as a result of traumatic blood vessel rupture or inflammation of the lungs from pneumonia.

INTERNAL INJURY OF THORAX, ABDOMEN, AND PELVIS (860–869)

> **Includes**   blast injuries of internal organs
>   blunt trauma of internal organs
>   bruise of internal organs
>   concussion injuries (except cerebral) of internal organs
>   crushing of internal organs
>   hematoma of internal organs
>   laceration of internal organs
>   puncture of internal organs
>   tear of internal organs
>   traumatic rupture of internal organs

> **Excludes**   *concussion NOS (850.0–850.9)*
> *flail chest (807.4)*
> *foreign body entering through orifice (930.0–939.9)*
> *injury to blood vessels (901.0–902.9)*

> **Note:**   The description "with open wound," used in the fourth-digit subdivisions, includes those with mention of infection or foreign body.

● 860   **Traumatic pneumothorax and hemothorax**

860.0   **Pneumothorax without mention of open wound into thorax**
> Coding Clinic: 1993, Q2, P4-5

860.1   **Pneumothorax with open wound into thorax**
> Coding Clinic: 1995, Q3, P17; 1993, Q2, P4-5

860.2   **Hemothorax without mention of open wound into thorax**

860.3   **Hemothorax with open wound into thorax**
> Coding Clinic: 1995, Q3, P17

860.4   **Pneumohemothorax without mention of open wound into thorax**

860.5   **Pneumohemothorax with open wound into thorax**
> Coding Clinic: 1995, Q3, P17

● 861   **Injury to heart and lung**

> **Excludes**   *injury to blood vessels of thorax (901.0–901.9)*
> Coding Clinic: 1992, Q1, P9-10

● 861.0   **Heart, without mention of open wound into thorax**

▪861.00   **Unspecified injury**

861.01   **Contusion**
> Cardiac contusion
> Myocardial contusion

861.02   **Laceration without penetration of heart chambers**

861.03   **Laceration with penetration of heart chambers**

● 861.1   Heart, with open wound into thorax
- ■861.10   Unspecified injury
-   861.11   Contusion
-   861.12   Laceration without penetration of heart chambers
-   861.13   Laceration with penetration of heart chambers

● 861.2   Lung, without mention of open wound into thorax
- ■861.20   Unspecified injury
-   861.21   Contusion
-   861.22   Laceration

● 861.3   Lung, with open wound into thorax
- ■861.30   Unspecified injury
-   861.31   Contusion
-   861.32   Laceration

● 862   Injury to other and unspecified intrathoracic organs

> **Excludes**   *injury to blood vessels of thorax (901.0–901.9)*

-   862.0   Diaphragm, without mention of open wound into cavity
-   862.1   Diaphragm, with open wound into cavity
- ● 862.2   Other specified intrathoracic organs, without mention of open wound into cavity
  -   862.21   Bronchus
  -   862.22   Esophagus
  - ■862.29   Other
    - Pleura
    - Thymus gland
- ● 862.3   Other specified intrathoracic organs, with open wound into cavity
  -   862.31   Bronchus
  -   862.32   Esophagus
  - ■862.39   Other
- ■862.8   Multiple and unspecified intrathoracic organs, without mention of open wound into cavity
  - Crushed chest
  - Multiple intrathoracic organs
- ■862.9   Multiple and unspecified intrathoracic organs, with open wound into cavity

● 863   Injury to gastrointestinal tract

Trauma to any structure from the stomach to the anus

> **Excludes**   *anal sphincter laceration during delivery (664.2)*
> *bile duct (868.0–868.1 with fifth-digit 2)*
> *gallbladder (868.0–868.1 with fifth-digit 2)*

-   863.0   Stomach, without mention of open wound into cavity
-   863.1   Stomach, with open wound into cavity
- ● 863.2   Small intestine, without mention of open wound into cavity
  - ■863.20   Small intestine, unspecified site
  -   863.21   Duodenum
  - ■863.29   Other

● 863.3   Small intestine, with open wound into cavity
- ■863.30   Small intestine, unspecified site
-   863.31   Duodenum
- ■863.39   Other

● 863.4   Colon or rectum, without mention of open wound into cavity
- ■863.40   Colon, unspecified site
-   863.41   Ascending [right] colon
-   863.42   Transverse colon
-   863.43   Descending [left] colon
-   863.44   Sigmoid colon
-   863.45   Rectum
- ■863.46   Multiple sites in colon and rectum
- ■863.49   Other

● 863.5   Colon or rectum, with open wound into cavity
- ■863.50   Colon, unspecified site
-   863.51   Ascending [right] colon
-   863.52   Transverse colon
-   863.53   Descending [left] colon
-   863.54   Sigmoid colon
-   863.55   Rectum
- ■863.56   Multiple sites in colon and rectum
- ■863.59   Other

● 863.8   Other and unspecified gastrointestinal sites, without mention of open wound into cavity
- ■863.80   Gastrointestinal tract, unspecified site
-   863.81   Pancreas, head
-   863.82   Pancreas, body
-   863.83   Pancreas, tail
- ■863.84   Pancreas, multiple and unspecified sites
-   863.85   Appendix
- ■863.89   Other
  - Intestine NOS

● 863.9   Other and unspecified gastrointestinal sites, with open wound into cavity
- ■863.90   Gastrointestinal tract, unspecified site
-   863.91   Pancreas, head
-   863.92   Pancreas, body
-   863.93   Pancreas, tail
- ■863.94   Pancreas, multiple and unspecified sites
-   863.95   Appendix
- ■863.99   Other

INJURY AND POISONING (800–999)

● 864 **Injury to liver**

The following fifth-digit subclassification is for use with category 864:

> ■ 0 **unspecified injury**
> 1 **hematoma and contusion**
> 2 **laceration, minor**
>   Laceration involving capsule only, or without significant involvement of hepatic parenchyma [i.e., less than 1 cm deep]
> 3 **laceration, moderate**
>   Laceration involving parenchyma but without major disruption of parenchyma [i.e., less than 10 cm long and less than 3 cm deep]
> 4 **laceration, major**
>   Laceration with significant disruption of hepatic parenchyma [i.e., 10 cm long and 3 cm deep]
>   Multiple moderate lacerations, with or without hematoma
>   Stellate lacerations of liver
> ■ 5 **laceration, unspecified**
> ■ 9 **other**

● **864.0 Without mention of open wound into**
[0-5,9] **cavity**

● **864.1 With open wound into cavity**
[0-5,9]

● 865 **Injury to spleen**

The following fifth-digit subclassification is for use with category 865:

> ■ 0 **unspecified injury**
> 1 **hematoma without rupture of capsule**
> 2 **capsular tears, without major disruption of parenchyma**
> 3 **laceration extending into parenchyma**
> 4 **massive parenchymal disruption**
> ■ 9 **other**

● **865.0 Without mention of open wound into**
[0-4,9] **cavity**

● **865.1 With open wound into cavity**
[0-4,9]

● 866 **Injury to kidney**

The following fifth-digit subclassification is for use with category 866:

> ■ 0 **unspecified injury**
> 1 **hematoma without rupture of capsule**
> 2 **laceration**
> 3 **complete disruption of kidney parenchyma**

> **Excludes** *acute kidney injury (nontraumatic) (584.9)*

● **866.0 Without mention of open wound into cavity**
[0-3] Coding Clinic: 2008, Q4, P192-193

● **866.1 With open wound into cavity**
[0-3]

● 867 **Injury to pelvic organs**

> **Excludes** *injury during delivery (664.0–665.9)*

867.0 Bladder and urethra, without mention of open wound into cavity
Coding Clinic: 2009, Q1, P8; 1985, Nov-Dec, P15; 1984, Nov-Dec, P15

867.1 Bladder and urethra, with open wound into cavity
Coding Clinic: 1984, Nov-Dec, P12

867.2 Ureter, without mention of open wound into cavity

867.3 Ureter, with open wound into cavity

867.4 Uterus, without mention of open wound into cavity ♀

867.5 Uterus, with open wound into cavity ♀

■ **867.6 Other specified pelvic organs, without mention of open wound into cavity**
    Fallopian tube
    Ovary
    Prostate
    Seminal vesicle
    Vas deferens

■ **867.7 Other specified pelvic organs, with open wound into cavity**

■ **867.8 Unspecified pelvic organ, without mention of open wound into cavity**

■ **867.9 Unspecified pelvic organ, with open wound into cavity**

● 868 **Injury to other intra-abdominal organs**

The following fifth-digit subclassification is for use with category 868:

> ■ 0 **unspecified intra-abdominal organ**
> 1 **adrenal gland**
> 2 **bile duct and gallbladder**
> 3 **peritoneum**
> 4 **retroperitoneum**
> ■ 9 **other and multiple intra-abdominal organs**

● **868.0 Without mention of open wound into cavity**
[0-4,9]

● **868.1 With open wound into cavity**
[0-4,9]

● 869 **Internal injury to unspecified or ill-defined organs**

> **Includes** internal injury NOS
>   multiple internal injury NOS

■ **869.0 Without mention of open wound into cavity**

■ **869.1 With open wound into cavity**

◀ New   ◀▦ Revised   ~~deleted~~ Deleted   ● Use Additional Digit(s)   ■ Nonspecific Code
● Not first-listed DX   OGCR Official Guidelines   Coding Clinic   Excludes   Includes   Use additional   Code first   Omit code

INJURY AND POISONING (800–999)

OPEN WOUNDS (870–897)

Includes   animal bite
avulsion
cut
laceration
puncture wound
traumatic amputation

Excludes   *burn (940.0–949.5)*
crushing (925–929.9)
puncture of internal organs (860.0–869.1)
superficial injury (910.0–919.9)
that incidental to:
    dislocation (830.0–839.9)
    fracture (800.0–829.1)
    internal injury (860.0–869.1)
    intracranial injury (851.0–854.1)

Note: The description "complicated" used in the fourth-digit subdivisions includes those with mention of delayed healing, delayed treatment, foreign body, or infection.

Use additional code to identify infection

OPEN WOUND OF HEAD, NECK, AND TRUNK (870–879)

● **870   Open wound of ocular adnexa**

    870.0   Laceration of skin of eyelid and periocular area

    870.1   Laceration of eyelid, full-thickness, not involving lacrimal passages

    870.2   Laceration of eyelid involving lacrimal passages

    870.3   Penetrating wound of orbit, without mention of foreign body

    870.4   Penetrating wound of orbit with foreign body

       Excludes   *retained (old) foreign body in orbit (376.6)*

    ■870.8   Other specified open wounds of ocular adnexa

    ■870.9   Unspecified open wound of ocular adnexa

● **871   Open wound of eyeball**

      Excludes   *2nd cranial nerve [optic] injury (950.0–950.9)*
                            3rd cranial nerve [oculomotor] injury (951.0)

    871.0   Ocular laceration without prolapse of intraocular tissue
       Coding Clinic: 1996, Q3, P7

    871.1   Ocular laceration with prolapse or exposure of intraocular tissue

    871.2   Rupture of eye with partial loss of intraocular tissue

    871.3   Avulsion of eye
       Traumatic enucleation

    ■871.4   Unspecified laceration of eye

    871.5   Penetration of eyeball with magnetic foreign body

       Excludes   *retained (old) magnetic foreign body in globe (360.50–360.59)*

    871.6   Penetration of eyeball with (nonmagnetic) foreign body

       Excludes   *retained (old) (nonmagnetic) foreign body in globe (360.60–360.69)*

    ■871.7   Unspecified ocular penetration

    ■871.9   Unspecified open wound of eyeball

● **872   Open wound of ear**

    ● 872.0   **External ear, without mention of complication**

       ■872.00   External ear, unspecified site

       872.01   Auricle, ear
          Pinna

       872.02   Auditory canal

    ● 872.1   **External ear, complicated**

       ■872.10   External ear, unspecified site

       872.11   Auricle, ear

       872.12   Auditory canal

    ● 872.6   **Other specified parts of ear, without mention of complication**

       872.61   Ear drum
          Drumhead
          Tympanic membrane

       872.62   Ossicles

       872.63   Eustachian tube

       872.64   Cochlea

       ■872.69   Other and multiple sites

    ● 872.7   **Other specified parts of ear, complicated**

       872.71   Ear drum

       872.72   Ossicles

       872.73   Eustachian tube

       872.74   Cochlea

       ■872.79   Other and multiple sites

    ■872.8   **Ear, part unspecified, without mention of complication**
       Ear NOS

    ■872.9   **Ear, part unspecified, complicated**

● **873   Other open wound of head**

    873.0   Scalp, without mention of complication

    873.1   Scalp, complicated

    ● 873.2   **Nose, without mention of complication**

       ■873.20   Nose, unspecified site

       873.21   Nasal septum

       873.22   Nasal cavity

       873.23   Nasal sinus

       ■873.29   Multiple sites

    ● 873.3   **Nose, complicated**

       ■873.30   Nose, unspecified site

       873.31   Nasal septum

       873.32   Nasal cavity

       873.33   Nasal sinus

       ■873.39   Multiple sites

    ● 873.4   **Face, without mention of complication**

       ■873.40   Face, unspecified site

       873.41   Cheek

       873.42   Forehead
          Eyebrow
          Coding Clinic: 1996, Q4, P43-44

       873.43   Lip

       873.44   Jaw

       ■873.49   Other and multiple sites

INJURY AND POISONING (800–999)

● 873.5 **Face, complicated**

■ 873.50 **Face, unspecified site**

873.51 **Cheek**

873.52 **Forehead**

873.53 **Lip**

873.54 **Jaw**

■ 873.59 **Other and multiple sites**

● 873.6 **Internal structures of mouth, without mention of complication**

■ 873.60 **Mouth, unspecified site**

873.61 **Buccal mucosa**

873.62 **Gum (alveolar process)**

873.63 **Tooth (broken) (fractured) (due to trauma)**

> **Excludes** *cracked tooth (521.81)*
>
> Coding Clinic: 2004, Q1, P17

873.64 **Tongue and floor of mouth**

873.65 **Palate**

■ 873.69 **Other and multiple sites**

● 873.7 **Internal structures of mouth, complicated**

■ 873.70 **Mouth, unspecified site**

873.71 **Buccal mucosa**

873.72 **Gum (alveolar process)**

873.73 **Tooth (broken) (fractured) (due to trauma)**

> **Excludes** *cracked tooth (521.81)*
>
> Coding Clinic: 2004, Q1, P17

873.74 **Tongue and floor of mouth**

873.75 **Palate**

■ 873.79 **Other and multiple sites**

■ 873.8 **Other and unspecified open wound of head without mention of complication**
Head NOS

■ 873.9 **Other and unspecified open wound of head, complicated**

● 874 **Open wound of neck**

● 874.0 **Larynx and trachea, without mention of complication**

874.00 **Larynx with trachea**

874.01 **Larynx**

874.02 **Trachea**

● 874.1 **Larynx and trachea, complicated**

874.10 **Larynx with trachea**

874.11 **Larynx**

874.12 **Trachea**

874.2 **Thyroid gland, without mention of complication**

874.3 **Thyroid gland, complicated**

874.4 **Pharynx, without mention of complication**
Cervical esophagus

874.5 **Pharynx, complicated**

■ 874.8 **Other and unspecified parts, without mention of complication**
Nape of neck   Throat NOS
Supraclavicular region

■ 874.9 **Other and unspecified parts, complicated**

● 875 **Open wound of chest (wall)**

> **Excludes** *open wound into thoracic cavity (860.0–862.9)*
> *traumatic pneumothorax and hemothorax (860.1, 860.3, 860.5)*
>
> Coding Clinic: 1995, Q3, P17

875.0 **Without mention of complication**

875.1 **Complicated**

● 876 **Open wound of back**

> **Includes** loin
> lumbar region

> **Excludes** *open wound into thoracic cavity (860.0–862.9)*
> *traumatic pneumothorax and hemothorax (860.1, 860.3, 860.5)*
>
> Coding Clinic: 1995, Q3, P17

876.0 **Without mention of complication**
Coding Clinic: 1993, Q2, P4-5

876.1 **Complicated**

● 877 **Open wound of buttock**

> **Includes** sacroiliac region

877.0 **Without mention of complication**

877.1 **Complicated**

● 878 **Open wound of genital organs (external), including traumatic amputation**

> **Excludes** *injury during delivery (664.0–665.9)*
> *internal genital organs (867.0–867.9)*

878.0 **Penis, without mention of complication** ♂

878.1 **Penis, complicated** ♂

878.2 **Scrotum and testes, without mention of complication** ♂

878.3 **Scrotum and testes, complicated** ♂

878.4 **Vulva, without mention of complication** ♀
Labium (majus) (minus)

878.5 **Vulva, complicated** ♀

878.6 **Vagina, without mention of complication** ♀

878.7 **Vagina, complicated** ♀

■ 878.8 **Other and unspecified parts, without mention of complication**

■ 878.9 **Other and unspecified parts, complicated**

● 879 **Open wound of other and unspecified sites, except limbs**

879.0 **Breast, without mention of complication**

879.1 **Breast, complicated**

879.2 **Abdominal wall, anterior, without mention of complication**
Abdominal wall NOS   Pubic region
Epigastric region   Umbilical region
Hypogastric region

879.3 **Abdominal wall, anterior, complicated**

879.4 **Abdominal wall, lateral, without mention of complication**
Flank   Iliac (region)
Groin   Inguinal region
Hypochondrium

879.5 **Abdominal wall, lateral, complicated**

■ 879.6 **Other and unspecified parts of trunk, without mention of complication**
Pelvic region   Trunk NOS
Perineum

■879.7 **Other and unspecified parts of trunk, complicated**

■879.8 **Open wound(s) (multiple) of unspecified site(s) without mention of complication**
    Multiple open wounds NOS
    Open wound NOS

■879.9 **Open wound(s) (multiple) of unspecified site(s), complicated**

OPEN WOUND OF UPPER LIMB (880–887)

● 880 **Open wound of shoulder and upper arm**
The following fifth-digit subclassification is for use with category 880:

> 0 shoulder region
> 1 scapular region
> 2 axillary region
> 3 upper arm
> ■9 multiple sites

● 880.0 **Without mention of complication**
[0-3,9]

● 880.1 **Complicated**
[0-3,9]   Coding Clinic: 2006, Q2, P7

● 880.2 **With tendon involvement**
[0-3,9]

● 881 **Open wound of elbow, forearm, and wrist**
The following fifth-digit subclassification is for use with category 881:

> 0 forearm
> 1 elbow
> 2 wrist

● 881.0 **Without mention of complication**
[0-2]

● 881.1 **Complicated**
[0-2]

● 881.2 **With tendon involvement**
[0-2]

● 882 **Open wound of hand except finger(s) alone**
882.0 **Without mention of complication**
882.1 **Complicated**
   Coding Clinic: 2008, Q4, P149-152
882.2 **With tendon involvement**

● 883 **Open wound of finger(s)**
Includes   fingernail
     thumb (nail)
883.0 **Without mention of complication**
Avulsion of fingernail reported with this code
883.1 **Complicated**
883.2 **With tendon involvement**

● 884 **Multiple and unspecified open wound of upper limb**
Includes   arm NOS
     multiple sites of one upper limb
     upper limb NOS
■884.0 **Without mention of complication**
■884.1 **Complicated**
■884.2 **With tendon involvement**

● 885 **Traumatic amputation of thumb (complete) (partial)**
Includes   thumb(s) (with finger(s) of either hand)
885.0 **Without mention of complication**
   Coding Clinic: 2003, Q1, P7
885.1 **Complicated**

● 886 **Traumatic amputation of other finger(s) (complete) (partial)**
Includes   finger(s) of one or both hands, without mention of thumb(s)
886.0 **Without mention of complication**
886.1 **Complicated**

● 887 **Traumatic amputation of arm and hand (complete) (partial)**
887.0 **Unilateral, below elbow, without mention of complication**
887.1 **Unilateral, below elbow, complicated**
887.2 **Unilateral, at or above elbow, without mention of complication**
887.3 **Unilateral, at or above elbow, complicated**
■887.4 **Unilateral, level not specified, without mention of complication**
■887.5 **Unilateral, level not specified, complicated**
887.6 **Bilateral [any level], without mention of complication**
    One hand and other arm
887.7 **Bilateral [any level], complicated**

OPEN WOUND OF LOWER LIMB (890–897)

● 890 **Open wound of hip and thigh**
890.0 **Without mention of complication**
890.1 **Complicated**
890.2 **With tendon involvement**

● 891 **Open wound of knee, leg [except thigh], and ankle**
Includes   leg NOS
     multiple sites of leg, except thigh
Excludes   *that of thigh (890.0–890.2)*
     with multiple sites of lower limb (894.0–894.2)
891.0 **Without mention of complication**
891.1 **Complicated**
   Coding Clinic: 2008, Q4, P69-73
891.2 **With tendon involvement**

● 892 **Open wound of foot except toe(s) alone**
Includes   heel
892.0 **Without mention of complication**
892.1 **Complicated**
   Coding Clinic: 1985, Sept-Oct, P10
892.2 **With tendon involvement**

● 893 **Open wound of toe(s)**
Includes   toenail
893.0 **Without mention of complication**
893.1 **Complicated**
   Coding Clinic: 2008, Q4, P69-73
893.2 **With tendon involvement**

INJURY AND POISONING (800–999)

● **894 Multiple and unspecified open wound of lower limb**

    Includes   lower limb NOS
                 multiple sites of one lower limb, with thigh

   ■ **894.0 Without mention of complication**

   ■ **894.1 Complicated**

   ■ **894.2 With tendon involvement**

● **895 Traumatic amputation of toe(s) (complete) (partial)**

    Includes   toe(s) of one or both feet

   895.0 Without mention of complication

   895.1 Complicated

● **896 Traumatic amputation of foot (complete) (partial)**

   896.0 Unilateral, without mention of complication

   896.1 Unilateral, complicated

   896.2 Bilateral, without mention of complication

     Excludes *one foot and other leg (897.6–897.7)*

   896.3 Bilateral, complicated

● **897 Traumatic amputation of leg(s) (complete) (partial)**

   897.0 Unilateral, below knee, without mention of complication

   897.1 Unilateral, below knee, complicated

   897.2 Unilateral, at or above knee, without mention of complication

   897.3 Unilateral, at or above knee, complicated

   ■ **897.4 Unilateral, level not specified, without mention of complication**

   ■ **897.5 Unilateral, level not specified, complicated**

   897.6 Bilateral [any level], without mention of complication
         One foot and other leg

   897.7 Bilateral [any level], complicated

INJURY TO BLOOD VESSELS (900–904)

    Includes arterial hematoma of blood vessel, secondary to other injuries, e.g., fracture or open wound
             avulsion of blood vessel, secondary to other injuries, e.g., fracture or open wound
             cut of blood vessel, secondary to other injuries, e.g., fracture or open wound
             laceration of blood vessel, secondary to other injuries, e.g., fracture or open wound
             rupture of blood vessel, secondary to other injuries, e.g., fracture or open wound
             traumatic aneurysm or fistula (arteriovenous) of blood vessel, secondary to other injuries, e.g., fracture or open wound

    Excludes *accidental puncture or laceration during medical procedure (998.2)*
             intracranial hemorrhage following injury (851.0–854.1)

● **900 Injury to blood vessels of head and neck**

   ● **900.0 Carotid artery**

     ■ **900.00 Carotid artery, unspecified**

     900.01 Common carotid artery

     900.02 External carotid artery

     900.03 Internal carotid artery

   900.1 Internal jugular vein

   ● **900.8 Other specified blood vessels of head and neck**

     900.81 External jugular vein
        Jugular vein NOS

     ■ **900.82 Multiple blood vessels of head and neck**

     ■ **900.89 Other**

   ■ **900.9 Unspecified blood vessel of head and neck**

● **901 Injury to blood vessels of thorax**

    Excludes *traumatic hemothorax (860.2–860.5)*

   901.0 Thoracic aorta

   901.1 Innominate and subclavian arteries

   901.2 Superior vena cava

   901.3 Innominate and subclavian veins

   ● **901.4 Pulmonary blood vessels**

     ■ **901.40 Pulmonary vessel(s), unspecified**

     901.41 Pulmonary artery

     901.42 Pulmonary vein

   ● **901.8 Other specified blood vessels of thorax**

     901.81 Intercostal artery or vein

     901.82 Internal mammary artery or vein

     901.83 Multiple blood vessels of thorax

     ■ **901.89 Other**
        Azygos vein
        Hemiazygos vein

   ■ **901.9 Unspecified blood vessel of thorax**

● **902 Injury to blood vessels of abdomen and pelvis**

   902.0 Abdominal aorta

   ● **902.1 Inferior vena cava**

     ■ **902.10 Inferior vena cava, unspecified**

     902.11 Hepatic veins

     ■ **902.19 Other**

   ● **902.2 Celiac and mesenteric arteries**

     ■ **902.20 Celiac and mesenteric arteries, unspecified**

     902.21 Gastric artery

     902.22 Hepatic artery

     902.23 Splenic artery

     ■ **902.24 Other specified branches of celiac axis**

     902.25 Superior mesenteric artery (trunk)

     902.26 Primary branches of superior mesenteric artery
        Ileo-colic artery

     902.27 Inferior mesenteric artery

     ■ **902.29 Other**

◀ New   ◀▥ Revised   ~~deleted~~ Deleted   ● Use Additional Digit(s)   ■ Nonspecific Code

● Not first-listed DX   OGCR Official Guidelines   Coding Clinic   Excludes   Includes   Use additional   Code first   Omit code

● 902.3   **Portal and splenic veins**

     902.31   **Superior mesenteric vein and primary subdivisions**
              Ileo-colic vein

     902.32   **Inferior mesenteric vein**

     902.33   **Portal vein**

     902.34   **Splenic vein**

     ■902.39   **Other**
              Cystic vein
              Gastric vein

● 902.4   **Renal blood vessels**

     ■902.40   **Renal vessel(s), unspecified**

     902.41   **Renal artery**

     902.42   **Renal vein**

     ■902.49   **Other**
              Suprarenal arteries

● 902.5   **Iliac blood vessels**

     ■902.50   **Iliac vessel(s), unspecified**

     902.51   **Hypogastric artery**

     902.52   **Hypogastric vein**

     902.53   **Iliac artery**

     902.54   **Iliac vein**

     902.55   **Uterine artery ♀**

     902.56   **Uterine vein ♀**

     ■902.59   **Other**

● 902.8   **Other specified blood vessels of abdomen and pelvis**

     902.81   **Ovarian artery ♀**

     902.82   **Ovarian vein ♀**

     ■902.87   **Multiple blood vessels of abdomen and pelvis**

     ■902.89   **Other**

■ 902.9   **Unspecified blood vessel of abdomen and pelvis**

● 903   **Injury to blood vessels of upper extremity**

  ● 903.0   **Axillary blood vessels**

     ■903.00   **Axillary vessel(s), unspecified**

     903.01   **Axillary artery**

     903.02   **Axillary vein**

   903.1   **Brachial blood vessels**

   903.2   **Radial blood vessels**

   903.3   **Ulnar blood vessels**

   903.4   **Palmar artery**

   903.5   **Digital blood vessels**

   ■903.8   **Other specified blood vessels of upper extremity**
          Multiple blood vessels of upper extremity

   ■903.9   **Unspecified blood vessel of upper extremity**

● 904   **Injury to blood vessels of lower extremity and unspecified sites**

   904.0   **Common femoral artery**
          Femoral artery above profunda origin
          Profunda = deep and posterior

   904.1   **Superficial femoral artery**

   904.2   **Femoral veins**

   904.3   **Saphenous veins**
          Saphenous vein (greater) (lesser)

● 904.4   **Popliteal blood vessels**

     ■904.40   **Popliteal vessel(s), unspecified**

     904.41   **Popliteal artery**

     904.42   **Popliteal vein**

● 904.5   **Tibial blood vessels**

     ■904.50   **Tibial vessel(s), unspecified**

     904.51   **Anterior tibial artery**

     904.52   **Anterior tibial vein**

     904.53   **Posterior tibial artery**

     904.54   **Posterior tibial vein**

   904.6   **Deep plantar blood vessels**

   ■904.7   **Other specified blood vessels of lower extremity**
          Multiple blood vessels of lower extremity

   ■904.8   **Unspecified blood vessel of lower extremity**

   ■904.9   **Unspecified site**
          Injury to blood vessel NOS

LATE EFFECTS OF INJURIES, POISONINGS, TOXIC EFFECTS, AND OTHER EXTERNAL CAUSES (905–909)

Note: These categories are to be used to indicate conditions classifiable to 800–999 as the cause of late effects, which are themselves classified elsewhere. The "late effects" include those specified as such, or as sequelae, which may occur at any time after the acute injury.

● 905   **Late effects of musculoskeletal and connective tissue injuries**

   ■905.0   **Late effect of fracture of skull and face bones**
          Late effect of injury classifiable to 800–804
          Coding Clinic: 1997, Q3, P12-13

   ■905.1   **Late effect of fracture of spine and trunk without mention of spinal cord lesion**
          Late effect of injury classifiable to 805, 807–809
          Coding Clinic: 2007, Q1, P20-21

   ■905.2   **Late effect of fracture of upper extremities**
          Late effect of injury classifiable to 810–819

   ■905.3   **Late effect of fracture of neck of femur**
          Late effect of injury classifiable to 820

   ■905.4   **Late effect of fracture of lower extremities**
          Late effect of injury classifiable to 821–827
          Coding Clinic: 1995, Q1, P10; 1994, Q2, P7

   ■905.5   **Late effect of fracture of multiple and unspecified bones**
          Late effect of injury classifiable to 828–829

   ■905.6   **Late effect of dislocation**
          Late effect of injury classifiable to 830–839

   ■905.7   **Late effect of sprain and strain without mention of tendon injury**
          Late effect of injury classifiable to 840–848, except tendon injury

   ■905.8   **Late effect of tendon injury**
          Late effect of tendon injury due to:
             open wound [injury classifiable to 880–884 with .2, 890–894 with .2]
             sprain and strain [injury classifiable to 840–848]
          Coding Clinic: 1989, Q2, P15; Q2, P13

   ■905.9   **Late effect of traumatic amputation**
          Late effect of injury classifiable to 885–887, 895–897

          Excludes   *late amputation stump complication (997.60–997.69)*

INJURY AND POISONING (800–999)

● **906 Late effects of injuries to skin and subcutaneous tissues**

◾ **906.0 Late effect of open wound of head, neck, and trunk**
Late effect of injury classifiable to 870–879

◾ **906.1 Late effect of open wound of extremities without mention of tendon injury**
Late effect of injury classifiable to 880–884, 890–894 except .2
Coding Clinic: 1993, 5th Issue, P3

◾ **906.2 Late effect of superficial injury**
Late effect of injury classifiable to 910–919

◾ **906.3 Late effect of contusion**
Late effect of injury classifiable to 920–924

◾ **906.4 Late effect of crushing**
Late effect of injury classifiable to 925–929

◾ **906.5 Late effect of burn of eye, face, head, and neck**
Late effect of injury classifiable to 940–941
Coding Clinic: 2004, Q4, P75-76

◾ **906.6 Late effect of burn of wrist and hand**
Late effect of injury classifiable to 944

◾ **906.7 Late effect of burn of other extremities**
Late effect of injury classifiable to 943 or 945

◾ **906.8 Late effect of burns of other specified sites**
Late effect of injury classifiable to 942, 946–947

◾ **906.9 Late effect of burn of unspecified site**
Late effect of injury classifiable to 948–949

OGCR Section I.C.17.c.7
Encounters for the treatment of the late effects of burns (i.e., scars or joint contractures) should be coded to the residual condition (sequelae) followed by the appropriate late effect code (906.5-906.9). A late effect E code may also be used, if desired.

● **907 Late effects of injuries to the nervous system**

◾ **907.0 Late effect of intracranial injury without mention of skull fracture**
Late effect of injury classifiable to 850–854
Coding Clinic: 2008, Q4, P102-109; 2003, Q4, P103-104; 1987, Nov-Dec, P12

◾ **907.1 Late effect of injury to cranial nerve**
Late effect of injury classifiable to 950–951

◾ **907.2 Late effect of spinal cord injury**
Late effect of injury classifiable to 806, 952
Coding Clinic: 2003, Q4, P103-104; 1998, Q4, P37-38; 1994, Q3, P4

◾ **907.3 Late effect of injury to nerve root(s), spinal plexus(es), and other nerves of trunk**
Late effect of injury classifiable to 953–954
Coding Clinic: 2007, Q2, P13-15

◾ **907.4 Late effect of injury to peripheral nerve of shoulder girdle and upper limb**
Late effect of injury classifiable to 955

◾ **907.5 Late effect of injury to peripheral nerve of pelvic girdle and lower limb**
Late effect of injury classifiable to 956

◾ **907.9 Late effect of injury to other and unspecified nerve**
Late effect of injury classifiable to 957

● **908 Late effects of other and unspecified injuries**

◾ **908.0 Late effect of internal injury to chest**
Late effect of injury classifiable to 860–862

◾ **908.1 Late effect of internal injury to intra-abdominal organs**
Late effect of injury classifiable to 863–866, 868

◾ **908.2 Late effect of internal injury to other internal organs**
Late effect of injury classifiable to 867 or 869

◾ **908.3 Late effect of injury to blood vessel of head, neck, and extremities**
Late effect of injury classifiable to 900, 903–904

◾ **908.4 Late effect of injury to blood vessel of thorax, abdomen, and pelvis**
Late effect of injury classifiable to 901–902

◾ **908.5 Late effect of foreign body in orifice**
Late effect of injury classifiable to 930–939

◾ **908.6 Late effect of certain complications of trauma**
Late effect of complications classifiable to 958

◾ **908.9 Late effect of unspecified injury**
Late effect of injury classifiable to 959
Coding Clinic: 2000, Q3, P4

● **909 Late effects of other and unspecified external causes**

◾ **909.0 Late effect of poisoning due to drug, medicinal or biological substance**
Late effect of conditions classifiable to 960–979

Excludes Late effect of adverse effect of drug, medicinal or biological substance (909.5)
Coding Clinic: 2003, Q4, P103-104; 1984, Sept-Oct, P16

◾ **909.1 Late effect of toxic effects of nonmedical substances**
Late effect of conditions classifiable to 980–989

◾ **909.2 Late effect of radiation**
Late effect of conditions classifiable to 990
Coding Clinic: 1984, Nov-Dec, P19

◾ **909.3 Late effect of complications of surgical and medical care**
Late effect of conditions classifiable to 996–999
Coding Clinic: 1993, Q1, P29

◾ **909.4 Late effect of certain other external causes**
Late effect of conditions classifiable to 991–994

◾ **909.5 Late effect of adverse effect of drug, medicinal or biological substance**

Excludes late effect of poisoning due to drug, medicinal or biological substances (909.0)

◾ **909.9 Late effect of other and unspecified external causes**

◀ New   ◀ Revised   deleted Deleted   ● Use Additional Digit(s)   ◾ Nonspecific Code

● Not first-listed DX   OGCR Official Guidelines   Coding Clinic   Excludes   Includes   Use additional   Code first   Omit code

SUPERFICIAL INJURY (910–919)

> **Excludes** *burn (blisters) (940.0–949.5)*
> *contusion (920–924.9)*
> *foreign body:*
>   *granuloma (728.82)*
>   *inadvertently left in operative wound (998.4)*
>   *residual, in soft tissue (729.6)*
>   *insect bite, venomous (989.5)*
>   *open wound with incidental foreign body*
>   *(870.0–897.7)*

● **910   Superficial injury of face, neck, and scalp except eye**

> **Includes**   cheek   lip
>   ear   nose
>   gum   throat

> **Excludes** *eye and adnexa (918.0–918.9)*

910.0   **Abrasion or friction burn without mention of infection**

910.1   **Abrasion or friction burn, infected**

910.2   **Blister without mention of infection**

910.3   **Blister, infected**

910.4   **Insect bite, nonvenomous, without mention of infection**

910.5   **Insect bite, nonvenomous, infected**

910.6   **Superficial foreign body (splinter) without major open wound and without mention of infection**

910.7   **Superficial foreign body (splinter) without major open wound, infected**

■910.8   **Other and unspecified superficial injury of face, neck, and scalp without mention of infection**

■910.9   **Other and unspecified superficial injury of face, neck, and scalp, infected**

● **911   Superficial injury of trunk**

> **Includes**   abdominal wall   interscapular region
>   anus   labium (majus) (minus)
>   back   penis
>   breast   perineum
>   buttock   scrotum
>   chest wall   testis
>   flank   vagina
>   groin   vulva

> **Excludes** *hip (916.0–916.9)*
> *scapular region (912.0–912.9)*

911.0   **Abrasion or friction burn without mention of infection**
      Coding Clinic: 2001, Q3, P10

911.1   **Abrasion or friction burn, infected**

911.2   **Blister without mention of infection**

911.3   **Blister, infected**

911.4   **Insect bite, nonvenomous, without mention of infection**

911.5   **Insect bite, nonvenomous, infected**

911.6   **Superficial foreign body (splinter) without major open wound and without mention of infection**

911.7   **Superficial foreign body (splinter) without major open wound, infected**

■911.8   **Other and unspecified superficial injury of trunk without mention of infection**

■911.9   **Other and unspecified superficial injury of trunk, infected**

● **912   Superficial injury of shoulder and upper arm**

> **Includes**   axilla
>   scapular region

912.0   **Abrasion or friction burn without mention of infection**

912.1   **Abrasion or friction burn, infected**

912.2   **Blister without mention of infection**

912.3   **Blister, infected**

912.4   **Insect bite, nonvenomous, without mention of infection**

912.5   **Insect bite, nonvenomous, infected**

912.6   **Superficial foreign body (splinter) without major open wound and without mention of infection**

912.7   **Superficial foreign body (splinter) without major open wound, infected**

■912.8   **Other and unspecified superficial injury of shoulder and upper arm without mention of infection**

■912.9   **Other and unspecified superficial injury of shoulder and upper arm, infected**

● **913   Superficial injury of elbow, forearm, and wrist**

913.0   **Abrasion or friction burn without mention of infection**

913.1   **Abrasion or friction burn, infected**

913.2   **Blister without mention of infection**

913.3   **Blister, infected**

913.4   **Insect bite, nonvenomous, without mention of infection**

913.5   **Insect bite, nonvenomous, infected**

913.6   **Superficial foreign body (splinter) without major open wound and without mention of infection**

913.7   **Superficial foreign body (splinter) without major open wound, infected**

■913.8   **Other and unspecified superficial injury of elbow, forearm, and wrist without mention of infection**

■913.9   **Other and unspecified superficial injury of elbow, forearm, and wrist, infected**

● **914   Superficial injury of hand(s) except finger(s) alone**

914.0   **Abrasion or friction burn without mention of infection**

914.1   **Abrasion or friction burn, infected**

914.2   **Blister without mention of infection**

914.3   **Blister, infected**

914.4   **Insect bite, nonvenomous, without mention of infection**

914.5   **Insect bite, nonvenomous, infected**

914.6   **Superficial foreign body (splinter) without major open wound and without mention of infection**

914.7   **Superficial foreign body (splinter) without major open wound, infected**

■914.8   **Other and unspecified superficial injury of hand without mention of infection**

■914.9   **Other and unspecified superficial injury of hand, infected**

● **915 Superficial injury of finger(s)**

Includes   fingernail
               thumb (nail)

915.0 Abrasion or friction burn without mention of infection

915.1 Abrasion or friction burn, infected

915.2 Blister without mention of infection

915.3 Blister, infected

915.4 Insect bite, nonvenomous, without mention of infection

915.5 Insect bite, nonvenomous, infected

915.6 Superficial foreign body (splinter) without major open wound and without mention of infection

915.7 Superficial foreign body (splinter) without major open wound, infected

■**915.8 Other and unspecified superficial injury of fingers without mention of infection**
Coding Clinic: 2001, Q3, P10

■**915.9 Other and unspecified superficial injury of fingers, infected**

● **916 Superficial injury of hip, thigh, leg, and ankle**

916.0 Abrasion or friction burn without mention of infection
Coding Clinic: 2000, Q4, P61

916.1 Abrasion or friction burn, infected

916.2 Blister without mention of infection

916.3 Blister, infected

916.4 Insect bite, nonvenomous, without mention of infection

916.5 Insect bite, nonvenomous, infected

916.6 Superficial foreign body (splinter) without major open wound and without mention of infection

916.7 Superficial foreign body (splinter) without major open wound, infected

■**916.8 Other and unspecified superficial injury of hip, thigh, leg, and ankle without mention of infection**

■**916.9 Other and unspecified superficial injury of hip, thigh, leg, and ankle, infected**

● **917 Superficial injury of foot and toe(s)**

Includes   heel
               toenail

917.0 Abrasion or friction burn without mention of infection

917.1 Abrasion or friction burn, infected

917.2 Blister without mention of infection

917.3 Blister, infected

917.4 Insect bite, nonvenomous, without mention of infection

917.5 Insect bite, nonvenomous, infected

917.6 Superficial foreign body (splinter) without major open wound and without mention of infection

917.7 Superficial foreign body (splinter) without major open wound, infected

■**917.8 Other and unspecified superficial injury of foot and toes without mention of infection**
Coding Clinic: 2003, Q1, P13

■**917.9 Other and unspecified superficial injury of foot and toes, infected**
Coding Clinic: 2003, Q1, P13

● **918 Superficial injury of eye and adnexa**

Excludes   *burn (940.0–940.9)*
               foreign body on external eye (930.0–930.9)

918.0 Eyelids and periocular area
Abrasion
Insect bite
Superficial foreign body (splinter)

918.1 Cornea
Corneal abrasion
Superficial laceration

Excludes   *corneal injury due to contact lens (371.82)*

918.2 Conjunctiva

■**918.9 Other and unspecified superficial injuries of eye**
Eye (ball) NOS

● **919 Superficial injury of other, multiple, and unspecified sites**

Excludes   *multiple sites classifiable to the same three-digit category (910.0–918.9)*

■**919.0 Abrasion or friction burn without mention of infection**

■**919.1 Abrasion or friction burn, infected**

■**919.2 Blister without mention of infection**

■**919.3 Blister, infected**

■**919.4 Insect bite, nonvenomous, without mention of infection**

■**919.5 Insect bite, nonvenomous, infected**

■**919.6 Superficial foreign body (splinter) without major open wound and without mention of infection**

■**919.7 Superficial foreign body (splinter) without major open wound, infected**

■**919.8 Other and unspecified superficial injury without mention of infection**

■**919.9 Other and unspecified superficial injury, infected**

CONTUSION WITH INTACT SKIN SURFACE (920–924)

Includes   bruise without fracture or open wound
               hematoma without fracture or open wound

Excludes   *concussion (850.0–850.9)*
               hemarthrosis (840.0–848.9)
               internal organs (860.0–869.1)
               that incidental to:
                   crushing injury (925–929.9)
                   dislocation (830.0–839.9)
                   fracture (800.0–829.1)
                   internal injury (860.0–869.1)
                   intracranial injury (850.0–854.1)
                   nerve injury (950.0–957.9)
                   open wound (870.0–897.7)

920 Contusion of face, scalp, and neck except eye(s)

Cheek	Mandibular joint area
Ear (auricle)	Nose
Gum	Throat
Lip	

● **921 Contusion of eye and adnexa**

■**921.0 Black eye, NOS**

921.1 Contusion of eyelids and periocular area

921.2 Contusion of orbital tissues

921.3 Contusion of eyeball
Coding Clinic: 1985, July-Aug, P16

■**921.9 Unspecified contusion of eye**
Injury of eye NOS

◀ New   ◀▥ Revised   ~~deleted~~ Deleted   ● Use Additional Digit(s)   ■ Nonspecific Code

● Not first-listed DX   OGCR Official Guidelines   Coding Clinic   Excludes   Includes   Use additional   Code first   Omit code

INJURY AND POISONING (800–999)

● **922 Contusion of trunk**

     922.0 Breast

     922.1 Chest wall

     922.2 Abdominal wall
         Flank
         Groin

● **922.3 Back**

         922.31 Back

             Excludes *interscapular region (922.33)*

             Coding Clinic: 1999, Q3, P14-15

         922.32 Buttock

         922.33 Interscapular region

             Excludes *scapular region (923.01)*

     922.4 Genital organs
         Labium (majus) (minus)   Testis
         Penis   Vagina
         Perineum   Vulva
         Scrotum

     ■**922.8 Multiple sites of trunk**

     ■**922.9 Unspecified part**
         Trunk NOS

● **923 Contusion of upper limb**

    ● **923.0 Shoulder and upper arm**

         923.00 Shoulder region

         923.01 Scapular region

         923.02 Axillary region

         923.03 Upper arm

        ■**923.09 Multiple sites**

    ● **923.1 Elbow and forearm**

         923.10 Forearm

         923.11 Elbow

    ● **923.2 Wrist and hand(s), except finger(s) alone**

         923.20 Hand(s)

         923.21 Wrist

     923.3 Finger
         Fingernail
         Thumb (nail)

     ■**923.8 Multiple sites of upper limb**

     ■**923.9 Unspecified part of upper limb**
         Arm NOS

● **924 Contusion of lower limb and of other and unspecified sites**

    ● **924.0 Hip and thigh**

         924.00 Thigh
             Coding Clinic: 2009, Q1, P10x2

         924.01 Hip

    ● **924.1 Knee and lower leg**

         924.10 Lower leg

         924.11 Knee

    ● **924.2 Ankle and foot, excluding toe(s)**

         924.20 Foot
             Heel

         924.21 Ankle

     924.3 Toe
         Toenail

     ■**924.4 Multiple sites of lower limb**

     ■**924.5 Unspecified part of lower limb**
         Leg NOS

     ■**924.8 Multiple sites, not elsewhere classified**
         Coding Clinic: 2003, Q1, P7

     ■**924.9 Unspecified site**

CRUSHING INJURY (925–929)

Use additional code to identify any associated injuries, such as:
fractures (800–829)
internal injuries (860.0–869.1)
intracranial injury (850.0–854.1)

● **925 Crushing injury of face, scalp, and neck**
     Cheek
     Ear
     Larynx
     Pharynx
     Throat
     Coding Clinic: 2003, Q4, P76-78

     925.1 Crushing injury of face and scalp
         Cheek
         Ear

     925.2 Crushing injury of neck
         Larynx
         Throat
         Pharynx

● **926 Crushing injury of trunk**
     Coding Clinic: 2003, Q4, P76-78

     926.0 External genitalia
         Labium (majus) (minus)
         Penis
         Scrotum
         Testis
         Vulva

    ● **926.1 Other specified sites**

         926.11 Back

         926.12 Buttock

        ■**926.19 Other**
         Breast

     ■**926.8 Multiple sites of trunk**

     ■**926.9 Unspecified site**
         Trunk NOS

● **927 Crushing injury of upper limb**

    ● **927.0 Shoulder and upper arm**

         927.00 Shoulder region

         927.01 Scapular region

         927.02 Axillary region

         927.03 Upper arm

        ■**927.09 Multiple sites**

    ● **927.1 Elbow and forearm**

         927.10 Forearm

         927.11 Elbow

    ● **927.2 Wrist and hand(s), except finger(s) alone**

         927.20 Hand(s)

         927.21 Wrist

     927.3 Finger(s)
         Coding Clinic: 2003, Q4, P76-78

     ■**927.8 Multiple sites of upper limb**

     ■**927.9 Unspecified site**
         Arm NOS

INJURY AND POISONING (800–999)

● **928 Crushing injury of lower limb**
    Coding Clinic: 2003, Q4, P76-78

  ● **928.0 Hip and thigh**

    928.00 Thigh

    928.01 Hip

  ● **928.1 Knee and lower leg**

    928.10 Lower leg

    928.11 Knee

  ● **928.2 Ankle and foot, excluding toe(s) alone**

    928.20 Foot
        Heel

    928.21 Ankle

  928.3 Toe(s)

  ■ **928.8 Multiple sites of lower limb**

  ■ **928.9 Unspecified site**
      Leg NOS

● **929 Crushing injury of multiple and unspecified sites**
    Coding Clinic: 2003, Q4, P76-78

  ■ **929.0 Multiple sites, not elsewhere classified**

  ■ **929.9 Unspecified site**

EFFECTS OF FOREIGN BODY ENTERING THROUGH ORIFICE (930–939)

    Excludes *foreign body:*
        granuloma (728.82)
        inadvertently left in operative wound (998.4, 998.7)
        in open wound (800–839, 851–897)
        residual, in soft tissues (729.6)
        superficial without major open wound (910–919 with .6 or .7)

● **930 Foreign body on external eye**

    Excludes *foreign body in penetrating wound of:*
        eyeball (871.5–871.6)
           retained (old) (360.5–360.6)
        ocular adnexa (870.4)
           retained (old) (376.6)

  930.0 Corneal foreign body

  930.1 Foreign body in conjunctival sac

  930.2 Foreign body in lacrimal punctum

  ■ **930.8 Other and combined sites**

  ■ **930.9 Unspecified site**
      External eye NOS

931 Foreign body in ear
    Auditory canal
    Auricle

932 Foreign body in nose
    Nasal sinus
    Nostril

● **933 Foreign body in pharynx and larynx**

  933.0 Pharynx
    Nasopharynx
    Throat NOS

  933.1 Larynx
    Asphyxia due to foreign body
    Choking due to:
      food (regurgitated)
      phlegm

● **934 Foreign body in trachea, bronchus, and lung**

  934.0 Trachea

  934.1 Main bronchus

  ■ **934.8 Other specified parts**
    Bronchioles
    Lung

  ■ **934.9 Respiratory tree, unspecified**
    Inhalation of liquid or vomitus, lower respiratory tract NOS

● **935 Foreign body in mouth, esophagus, and stomach**

  935.0 Mouth

  935.1 Esophagus
    Coding Clinic: 1988, Q1, P13

  935.2 Stomach
    Coding Clinic: 1985, Jan-Feb, P14-15

936 Foreign body in intestine and colon

937 Foreign body in anus and rectum
    Rectosigmoid (junction)

■ **938 Foreign body in digestive system, unspecified**
    Alimentary tract NOS
    Swallowed foreign body

● **939 Foreign body in genitourinary tract**

  939.0 Bladder and urethra

  939.1 Uterus, any part ♀

    Excludes *intrauterine contraceptive device:*
        complications from (996.32, 996.65)
        presence of (V45.51)

  939.2 Vulva and vagina ♀

  939.3 Penis ♂

■ **939.9 Unspecified site**

◀ New   ◀▥ Revised   ~~deleted~~ Deleted   ● Use Additional Digit(s)   ■ Nonspecific Code

● Not first-listed DX   OGCR Official Guidelines   Coding Clinic   Excludes   Includes   Use additional   Code first   Omit code

INJURY AND POISONING (800–999)

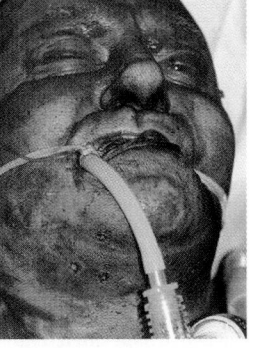
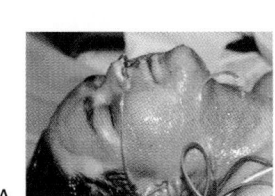

A   B

Figure 17–14   A. 2nd degree burn. **B.** 3rd degree burn. (From Cummings: Otolaryngology: Head & Neck Surgery, 4th ed. 2005, Mosby)

BURNS (940–949)

OGCR Section I.C.17.c
Current burns (940-948) are classified by depth, extent and by agent (E code). Burns are classified by depth as first degree (erythema), second degree (blistering), and third degree (full-thickness involvement).

OGCR Section I.C.17.c.1
Sequence first the code that reflects the highest degree of burn when more than one burn is present.

OGCR Section I.C.17.c.2
Classify burns of the same local site (three-digit category level, 940-947) but of different degrees to the subcategory identifying the highest degree recorded in the diagnosis.

Includes   burns from:
         electrical heating appliance
         electricity
         flame
         hot object
         lightning
         radiation
         chemical burns (external) (internal)
         scalds

Excludes   *friction burns (910–919 with .0, .1)*
              sunburn (692.71, 692.76–692.77)

● 940   **Burn confined to eye and adnexa**

    940.0   Chemical burn of eyelids and periocular area

    ▪940.1   Other burns of eyelids and periocular area

    940.2   Alkaline chemical burn of cornea and conjunctival sac

    940.3   Acid chemical burn of cornea and conjunctival sac

    ▪940.4   Other burn of cornea and conjunctival sac

    940.5   Burn with resulting rupture and destruction of eyeball

    ▪940.9   Unspecified burn of eye and adnexa

● 941   **Burn of face, head, and neck**

    Excludes   *mouth (947.0)*

    The following fifth-digit subclassification is for use with category 941:

    > ▪0   face and head, unspecified site
    > 1   ear [any part]
    > 2   eye (with other parts of face, head, and neck)
    > 3   lip(s)
    > 4   chin
    > 5   nose (septum)
    > 6   scalp [any part]
    >   Temple (region)
    > 7   forehead and cheek
    > 8   neck
    > ▪9   multiple sites [except with eye] of face, head, and neck

  ●▪941.0   Unspecified degree
        [0-9]

  ●941.1   Erythema [first degree]
        [0-9]   Coding Clinic: 2005, Q3, P10-11

  ●941.2   Blisters, epidermal loss [second degree]
        [0-9]

  ●941.3   Full-thickness skin loss [third degree NOS]
        [0-9]

  ●941.4   Deep necrosis of underlying tissues [deep third
        [0-9]   degree] without mention of loss of a body part

  ●941.5   Deep necrosis of underlying tissues [deep third
        [0-9]   degree] with loss of a body part

● 942   **Burn of trunk**

    Excludes   *scapular region (943.0–943.5 with fifth-digit 6)*

    The following fifth-digit subclassification is for use with category 942:

    > ▪0   trunk, unspecified site
    > 1   breast
    > 2   chest wall, excluding breast and nipple
    > 3   abdominal wall
    >   Flank
    >   Groin
    > 4   back [any part]
    >   Buttock
    >   Interscapular region
    > 5   genitalia
    >   Labium (majus) (minus)   Scrotum
    >   Penis   Testis
    >   Perineum   Vulva
    > ▪9   other and multiple sites of trunk

  ●▪942.0   Unspecified degree
        [0-5,9]

  ●942.1   Erythema [first degree]
        [0-5,9]

  ●942.2   Blisters, epidermal loss [second degree]
        [0-5,9]   Coding Clinic: 1984, Nov-Dec, P13

  ●942.3   Full-thickness skin loss [third degree NOS]
        [0-5,9]

  ●942.4   Deep necrosis of underlying tissues [deep third
        [0-5,9]   degree] without mention of loss of a body part

  ●942.5   Deep necrosis of underlying tissues [deep third
        [0-5,9]   degree] with loss of a body part

INJURY AND POISONING (800–999)

● **943   Burn of upper limb, except wrist and hand**

The following fifth-digit subclassification is for use with category 943:

> ■ 0   upper limb, unspecified site
>   1   forearm
>   2   elbow
>   3   upper arm
>   4   axilla
>   5   shoulder
>   6   scapular region
> ■ 9   multiple sites of upper limb, except wrist and hand

● ■ **943.0   Unspecified degree**
[0-6,9]

● **943.1   Erythema [first degree]**
[0-6,9]

● **943.2   Blisters, epidermal loss [second degree]**
[0-6,9]

● **943.3   Full-thickness skin loss [third degree NOS]**
[0-6,9]

● **943.4   Deep necrosis of underlying tissues [deep third**
[0-6,9]   **degree] without mention of loss of a body part**

● **943.5   Deep necrosis of underlying tissues [deep third**
[0-6,9]   **degree] with loss of a body part**

● **944   Burn of wrist(s) and hand(s)**

The following fifth-digit subclassification is for use with category 944:

> ■ 0   hand, unspecified site
>   1   single digit [finger (nail)] other than thumb
>   2   thumb (nail)
>   3   two or more digits, not including thumb
>   4   two or more digits including thumb
>   5   palm
>   6   back of hand
>   7   wrist
> ■ 8   multiple sites of wrist(s) and hand(s)

● ■ **944.0   Unspecified degree**
[0-8]

● **944.1   Erythema [first degree]**
[0-8]

● **944.2   Blisters, epidermal loss [second degree]**
[0-8]

● **944.3   Full-thickness skin loss [third degree NOS]**
[0-8]

● **944.4   Deep necrosis of underlying tissues [deep third**
[0-8]   **degree] without mention of loss of a body part**

● **944.5   Deep necrosis of underlying tissues [deep third**
[0-8]   **degree] with loss of a body part**

● **945   Burn of lower limb(s)**

The following fifth-digit subclassification is for use with category 945:

> ■ 0   lower limb [leg], unspecified site
>   1   toe(s) (nail)
>   2   foot
>   3   ankle
>   4   lower leg
>   5   knee
>   6   thigh [any part]
> ■ 9   multiple sites of lower limb(s)

● ■ **945.0   Unspecified degree**
[0-6, 9]   ◄▥

● **945.1   Erythema [first degree]**
[0-6, 9]   ◄▥

● **945.2   Blisters, epidermal loss [second degree]**
[0-6, 9]   ◄▥

● **945.3   Full-thickness skin loss [third degree NOS]**
[0-6, 9]   ◄▥

● **945.4   Deep necrosis of underlying tissues [deep third**
[0-6, 9]   **degree] without mention of loss of a body part**   ◄▥

● **945.5   Deep necrosis of underlying tissues [deep third**
[0-6, 9]   **degree] with loss of a body part**   ◄▥

● **946   Burns of multiple specified sites**

Documented as multiple sites but not specified as to location

Includes   burns of sites classifiable to more than one three-digit category in 940–945

Excludes   *multiple burns NOS (949.0–949.5)*

■ **946.0   Unspecified degree**

946.1   Erythema [first degree]

946.2   Blisters, epidermal loss [second degree]

946.3   Full-thickness skin loss [third degree NOS]

946.4   Deep necrosis of underlying tissues [deep third degree] without mention of loss of a body part

946.5   Deep necrosis of underlying tissues [deep third degree] with loss of a body part

OGCR Section I.C.17.c.5
When coding burns, assign separate codes for each burn site. Category 946 should only be used if the location of the burns are not documented.

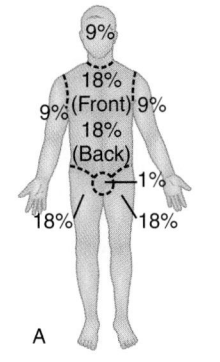

Figure 17–15 Rule of nines: percentages of total body area. (From Marx: Rosen's Emergency Medicine: Concepts and Clinical Practice, 6th ed. 2006, Mosby)

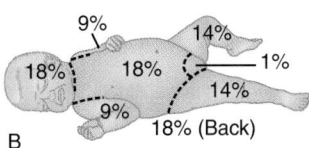

● 947   **Burn of internal organs**

    Includes burns from chemical agents (ingested)

    947.0 **Mouth and pharynx**
        Gum
        Tongue

    947.1 **Larynx, trachea, and lung**

    947.2 **Esophagus**

    947.3 **Gastrointestinal tract**
        Colon
        Rectum
        Small intestine
        Stomach

    947.4 **Vagina and uterus** ♀

    ■**947.8** **Other specified sites**

    ■**947.9** **Unspecified site**

OGCR Section I.C.17.c.6
Fourth-digit identifies percentage of **total body surface** involved in a burn (all degrees). **Fifth-digit** identifies the percentage of body surface involved in **third-degree burn** with zero (0) assigned when less than 10 percent or when no body surface is involved in a third-degree burn.
    Category 948 is based on the classic "rule of nines" in estimating body surface involved: head and neck are assigned nine percent, each arm nine percent, each leg 18 percent, the anterior trunk 18 percent, posterior trunk 18 percent, and genitalia one percent.

● 948   **Burns classified according to extent of body surface involved**

    Excludes *sunburn (692.71, 692.76–692.77)*

    Note: This category is to be used when the site of the burn is unspecified, or with categories 940–947 when the site is specified.
    Coding Clinic: 1984, Nov-Dec, P13

The following fifth-digit subclassification is for use with category 948 to indicate the percent of body surface with third degree burn; valid digits are in [brackets] under each code:

> 0 less than 10 percent or unspecified
> 1 10–19%
> 2 20–29%
> 3 30–39%
> 4 40–49%
> 5 50–59%
> 6 60–69%
> 7 70–79%
> 8 80–89%
> 9 90% or more of body surface

● **948.0** **Burn [any degree] involving less than 10 percent of**
    [0] **body surface**

● **948.1** **10–19 percent of body surface**
    [0-1] Coding Clinic: 1984, Nov-Dec, P13

● **948.2** **20–29 percent of body surface**
    [0-2] Coding Clinic: 1984, Nov-Dec, P13

● **948.3** **30–39 percent of body surface**
    [0-3]

● **948.4** **40–49 percent of body surface**
    [0-4]

● **948.5** **50–59 percent of body surface**
    [0-5]

● **948.6** **60–69 percent of body surface**
    [0-6]

● **948.7** **70–79 percent of body surface**
    [0-7]

● **948.8** **80–89 percent of body surface**
    [0-8]

● **948.9** **90 percent or more of body surface**
    [0-9]

OGCR Section I.C.17.c.5
When coding burns, assign separate codes for each burn site. Category 949, Burn, unspecified, is extremely vague and should rarely be used.

● 949   **Burn, unspecified**

    Includes burn NOS
              multiple burns NOS

    Excludes *burn of unspecified site but with statement of the extent of body surface involved (948.0–948.9)*

    ■**949.0** **Unspecified degree**

    ■**949.1** **Erythema [first degree]**

    ■**949.2** **Blisters, epidermal loss [second degree]**

    ■**949.3** **Full-thickness skin loss [third degree NOS]**

    ■**949.4** **Deep necrosis of underlying tissues [deep third degree] without mention of loss of a body part**

    ■**949.5** **Deep necrosis of underlying tissues [deep third degree] with loss of a body part**

INJURY AND POISONING (800–999)

INJURY TO NERVES AND SPINAL CORD (950–957)

Includes division of nerve
lesion in continuity (with open wound)
traumatic neuroma (with open wound)
traumatic transient paralysis (with open
wound)

Excludes *accidental puncture or laceration during medical
procedure (998.2)*

● **950 Injury to optic nerve and pathways**

950.0 Optic nerve injury
Second cranial nerve

950.1 Injury to optic chiasm

950.2 Injury to optic pathways

950.3 Injury to visual cortex

■**950.9 Unspecified**
Traumatic blindness NOS

● **951 Injury to other cranial nerve(s)**

951.0 Injury to oculomotor nerve
Third cranial nerve

951.1 Injury to trochlear nerve
Fourth cranial nerve

951.2 Injury to trigeminal nerve
Fifth cranial nerve

951.3 Injury to abducens nerve
Sixth cranial nerve

951.4 Injury to facial nerve
Seventh cranial nerve

951.5 Injury to acoustic nerve
Auditory nerve
Eighth cranial nerve
Traumatic deafness NOS

951.6 Injury to accessory nerve
Eleventh cranial nerve

951.7 Injury to hypoglossal nerve
Twelfth cranial nerve

■**951.8 Injury to other specified cranial nerves**
Glossopharyngeal [9th cranial] nerve
Olfactory [1st cranial] nerve
Pneumogastric [10th cranial] nerve
Traumatic anosmia NOS
Vagus [10th cranial] nerve

■**951.9 Injury to unspecified cranial nerve**

● **952 Spinal cord injury without evidence of spinal bone injury**

● **952.0 Cervical**

■**952.00 C_1-C_4 level with unspecified spinal cord injury**
Spinal cord injury, cervical region NOS

952.01 C_1-C_4 level with complete lesion of spinal cord

952.02 C_1-C_4 level with anterior cord syndrome

952.03 C_1-C_4 level with central cord syndrome

■**952.04 C_1-C_4 level with other specified spinal cord injury**
Incomplete spinal cord lesion at C_1-C_4 level:
NOS
with posterior cord syndrome

■**952.05 C_5-C_7 level with unspecified spinal cord injury**

952.06 C_5-C_7 level with complete lesion of spinal cord

952.07 C_5-C_7 level with anterior cord syndrome

952.08 C_5-C_7 level with central cord syndrome

■**952.09 C_5-C_7 level with other specified spinal cord injury**
Incomplete spinal cord lesion at C_5-C_7 level:
NOS
with posterior cord syndrome

● **952.1 Dorsal [thoracic]**

■**952.10 T_1-T_6 level with unspecified spinal cord injury**
Spinal cord injury, thoracic region NOS

952.11 T_1-T_6 level with complete lesion of spinal cord

952.12 T_1-T_6 level with anterior cord syndrome

952.13 T_1-T_6 level with central cord syndrome

■**952.14 T_1-T_6 level with other specified spinal cord injury**
Incomplete spinal cord lesion at T_1-T_6 level:
NOS
with posterior cord syndrome

■**952.15 T_7-T_{12} level with unspecified spinal cord injury**

952.16 T_7-T_{12} level with complete lesion of spinal cord

952.17 T_7-T_{12} level with anterior cord syndrome

952.18 T_7-T_{12} level with central cord syndrome

■**952.19 T_7-T_{12} level with other specified spinal cord injury**
Incomplete spinal cord lesion at T_7-T_{12} level:
NOS
with posterior cord syndrome

952.2 Lumbar

952.3 Sacral

952.4 Cauda equina

■**952.8 Multiple sites of spinal cord**

■**952.9 Unspecified site of spinal cord**

● **953 Injury to nerve roots and spinal plexus**

953.0 Cervical root

953.1 Dorsal root

953.2 Lumbar root

953.3 Sacral root

953.4 Brachial plexus

953.5 Lumbosacral plexus

■**953.8 Multiple sites**

■**953.9 Unspecified site**

● **954 Injury to other nerve(s) of trunk, excluding shoulder and pelvic girdles**

954.0 Cervical sympathetic

■**954.1 Other sympathetic**
Celiac ganglion or plexus　　Splanchnic nerve(s)
Inferior mesenteric plexus　　Stellate ganglion

■**954.8 Other specified nerve(s) of trunk**

■**954.9 Unspecified nerve of trunk**

◀ New　　◀▥ Revised　　deleted Deleted　　● Use Additional Digit(s)　　■ Nonspecific Code
● Not first-listed DX　　OGCR Official Guidelines　　Coding Clinic　　Excludes　　Includes　　Use additional　　Code first　　Omit code

● 955 **Injury to peripheral nerve(s) of shoulder girdle and upper limb**

  955.0 Axillary nerve

  955.1 Median nerve

  955.2 Ulnar nerve

  955.3 Radial nerve

  955.4 Musculocutaneous nerve

  955.5 Cutaneous sensory nerve, upper limb

  955.6 Digital nerve

  ■955.7 Other specified nerve(s) of shoulder girdle and upper limb

  ■955.8 Multiple nerves of shoulder girdle and upper limb

  ■955.9 Unspecified nerve of shoulder girdle and upper limb

● 956 **Injury to peripheral nerve(s) of pelvic girdle and lower limb**

  956.0 Sciatic nerve

  956.1 Femoral nerve

  956.2 Posterior tibial nerve

  956.3 Peroneal nerve

  956.4 Cutaneous sensory nerve, lower limb

  ■956.5 Other specified nerve(s) of pelvic girdle and lower limb

  ■956.8 Multiple nerves of pelvic girdle and lower limb

  ■956.9 Unspecified nerve of pelvic girdle and lower limb

● 957 **Injury to other and unspecified nerves**

  957.0 Superficial nerves of head and neck

  ■957.1 Other specified nerve(s)

  ■957.8 Multiple nerves in several parts
      Multiple nerve injury NOS

  ■957.9 Unspecified site
      Nerve injury NOS

CERTAIN TRAUMATIC COMPLICATIONS AND UNSPECIFIED INJURIES (958–959)

● 958 **Certain early complications of trauma**

  Excludes *adult respiratory distress syndrome (518.5)*
      flail chest (807.4)
      post-traumatic seroma (729.91)
      shock lung (518.5)
      that occurring during or following medical procedures (996.0–999.9)

  958.0 **Air embolism**
      Pneumathemia

    Excludes *that complicating:*
        abortion (634–638 with .6, 639.6)
        ectopic or molar pregnancy (639.6)
        pregnancy, childbirth, or the puerperium (673.0)

  958.1 **Fat embolism**

    Excludes *that complicating:*
        abortion (634–638 with .6, 639.6)
        pregnancy, childbirth, or the puerperium (673.8)

  958.2 **Secondary and recurrent hemorrhage**

  958.3 **Posttraumatic wound infection, not elsewhere classified**

    Excludes *infected open wounds - code to complicated open wound of site*
    Coding Clinic: 1993, 5th Issue, P3; 1985, Sept-Oct, P10; 1984, Nov-Dec, P20

    OGCR Section I.C.17.c.4
    Assign code 958.3 as an additional code for any documented infected burn site.

  958.4 **Traumatic shock**
      Shock (immediate) (delayed) following injury

    Excludes *shock:*
        anaphylactic (995.0)
          due to serum (999.4)
        anesthetic (995.4)
        electric (994.8)
        following abortion (639.5)
        lightning (994.0)
        nontraumatic NOS (785.50)
        obstetric (669.1)
        postoperative (998.0)

  958.5 **Traumatic anuria**
      Crush syndrome
      Renal failure following crushing

    Excludes *that due to a medical procedure (997.5)*

  958.6 **Volkmann's ischemic contracture**
      Posttraumatic muscle contracture

  958.7 **Traumatic subcutaneous emphysema**

    Excludes *subcutaneous emphysema resulting from a procedure (998.81)*

  ■958.8 **Other early complications of trauma**
      Coding Clinic: 1992, Q2, P13

● ■958.9 **Traumatic compartment syndrome**

    Excludes *nontraumatic compartment syndrome (729.71–729.79)*

  ■958.90 Compartment syndrome, unspecified

  958.91 Traumatic compartment syndrome of upper extremity
      Traumatic compartment syndrome of shoulder, arm, forearm, wrist, hand, and fingers

  958.92 Traumatic compartment syndrome of lower extremity
      Traumatic compartment syndrome of hip, buttock, thigh, leg, foot, and toes

  958.93 Traumatic compartment syndrome of abdomen
      Coding Clinic: 2006, Q4, P100-102

  ■958.99 Traumatic compartment syndrome of other sites

● **959 Injury, other and unspecified**

     Includes   injury NOS

     Excludes   *injury NOS of:*
            blood vessels (900.0–904.9)
            eye (921.0–921.9)
            internal organs (860.0–869.1)
            intracranial sites (854.0–854.1)
            nerves (950.0–951.9, 953.0–957.9)
            spinal cord (952.0–952.9)

       Coding Clinic: 1984, Nov-Dec, P9

● **959.0 Head, face, and neck**

     ■ **959.01 Head injury, unspecified**

         Excludes   *concussion (850.0–850.9)*
                 with head injury NOS
                     (850.0–850.9)
                 head injury NOS with loss of
                     consciousness (850.1–850.5)
                 specified head injuries
                     (850.0–854.1)

           Coding Clinic: 2008, Q4, P102-109; 1999, Q1, P10

     959.09 Injury of face and neck

● **959.1 Trunk**

     Excludes   *scapular region (959.2)*

     ■ **959.11 Other injury of chest wall**

     ■ **959.12 Other injury of abdomen**

     959.13 Fracture of corpus cavernosum penis ♂

     959.14 Other injury of external genitals

     ■ **959.19 Other injury of other sites of trunk**
           Injury of trunk NOS

   959.2 Shoulder and upper arm
         Axilla
         Scapular region

   959.3 Elbow, forearm, and wrist
         Coding Clinic: 1997, Q1, P8

   959.4 Hand, except finger

   959.5 Finger
         Fingernail
         Thumb (nail)

   959.6 Hip and thigh
         Upper leg

   959.7 Knee, leg, ankle, and foot

■ **959.8 Other specified sites, including multiple**

     Excludes   *multiple sites classifiable to the same*
                four-digit category (959.0–959.7)

■ **959.9 Unspecified site**
      Coding Clinic: 1984, Nov-Dec, P9

OGCR   Section I.C.17.e.1

Poisoning: An **error** was made in drug prescription or in the administration of the drug by provider, nurse, patient, or other person, use the appropriate poisoning code from the 960-979 series. If an overdose of a drug was **intentionally** taken or administered and resulted in drug toxicity, it would be coded as a poisoning (960-979 series). If a **nonprescribed** drug or medicinal agent was taken in combination with a correctly prescribed and properly administered drug, any drug toxicity or other reaction resulting from the interaction of the two drugs would be classified as a poisoning.

When a reaction results from the interaction of a drug(s) and alcohol, this would be classified as poisoning.

Sequencing of poisoning: When coding a poisoning or reaction to the improper use of a medication (e.g., wrong dose, wrong substance, wrong route of administration) the poisoning code is sequenced first, followed by a code for the manifestation. If there is also a diagnosis of drug abuse or dependence to the substance, the abuse or dependence is coded as an additional code.

See Section I.C.3.a.6.b. if poisoning is the result of insulin pump malfunctions and Section I.C.19 for general use of E-codes.

POISONING BY DRUGS, MEDICINAL AND BIOLOGICAL SUBSTANCES (960–979)

     Includes   overdose of these substances
                wrong substance given or taken in error

     Excludes   *adverse effects ["hypersensitivity," "reaction,"*
                etc.] of correct substance properly
                administered. Such cases are to be classified
                according to the nature of the adverse effect,
                such as:
                adverse effect NOS (995.20)
                allergic lymphadenitis (289.3)
                aspirin gastritis (535.4)
                blood disorders (280.0–289.9)
                dermatitis:
                   contact (692.0–692.9)
                   due to ingestion (693.0–693.9)
                nephropathy (583.9)
                [The drug giving rise to the adverse effect may be
                   identified by use of categories E930–E949.]
                drug dependence (304.0–304.9)
                drug reaction and poisoning affecting the newborn
                   (760.0–779.9)
                nondependent abuse of drugs (305.0–305.9)
                pathological drug intoxication (292.2)

     Use additional code to specify the effects of the poisoning

● **960 Poisoning by antibiotics**

     Excludes   *antibiotics:*
                ear, nose, and throat (976.6)
                eye (976.5)
                local (976.0)

     960.0 Penicillins
         Ampicillin
         Carbenicillin
         Cloxacillin
         Penicillin G

960.1 Antifungal antibiotics
    Amphotericin B
    Griseofulvin
    Nystatin
    Trichomycin
    Excludes *preparations intended for topical use
    (976.0–976.9)*

960.2 Chloramphenicol group
    Chloramphenicol
    Thiamphenicol

960.3 Erythromycin and other macrolides
    Oleandomycin
    Spiramycin

960.4 Tetracycline group
    Doxycycline
    Minocycline
    Oxytetracycline

960.5 Cephalosporin group
    Cephalexin   Cephaloridine
    Cephaloglycin   Cephalothin

960.6 Antimycobacterial antibiotics
    Cycloserine
    Kanamycin
    Rifampin
    Streptomycin

960.7 Antineoplastic antibiotics
    Actinomycin such as:
      Bleomycin   Dactinomycin
      Cactinomycin   Daunorubicin
                         Mitomycin

■**960.8 Other specified antibiotics**

■**960.9 Unspecified antibiotic**

● **961 Poisoning by other anti-infectives**
    Excludes *anti-infectives:*
        ear, nose, and throat (976.6)
        eye (976.5)
        local (976.0)

961.0 Sulfonamides
    Sulfadiazine
    Sulfafurazole
    Sulfamethoxazole

961.1 Arsenical anti-infectives

961.2 Heavy metal anti-infectives
    Compounds of: Compounds of:
      antimony   lead
      bismuth   mercury
    Excludes *mercurial diuretics (974.0)*

961.3 Quinoline and hydroxyquinoline derivatives
    Chiniofon
    Diiodohydroxyquin
    Excludes *antimalarial drugs (961.4)*

**961.4 Antimalarials and drugs acting on other blood
protozoa**
    Chloroquine
    Cycloguanil
    Primaquine
    Proguanil [chloroguanide]
    Pyrimethamine
    Quinine

■**961.5 Other antiprotozoal drugs**
    Emetine

961.6 Anthelmintics
    Hexylresorcinol   Thiabendazole
    Piperazine

961.7 Antiviral drugs
    Methisazone
    Excludes *amantadine (966.4)*
        cytarabine (963.1)
        idoxuridine (976.5)

■**961.8 Other antimycobacterial drugs**
    Ethambutol
    Ethionamide
    Isoniazid
    Para-aminosalicylic acid derivatives
    Sulfones

■**961.9 Other and unspecified anti-infectives**
    Flucytosine
    Nitrofuran derivatives

● **962 Poisoning by hormones and synthetic substitutes**
    Excludes *oxytocic hormones (975.0)*

962.0 Adrenal cortical steroids
    Cortisone derivatives
    Desoxycorticosterone derivatives
    Fluorinated corticosteroids

962.1 Androgens and anabolic congeners
    Methandriol
    Nandrolone
    Oxymetholone
    Testosterone

962.2 Ovarian hormones and synthetic substitutes
    Contraceptives, oral
    Estrogens
    Estrogens and progestogens, combined
    Progestogens

962.3 Insulins and antidiabetic agents
    Acetohexamide
    Biguanide derivatives, oral
    Chlorpropamide
    Glucagon
    Insulin
    Phenformin
    Sulfonylurea derivatives, oral
    Tolbutamide

962.4 Anterior pituitary hormones
    Corticotropin
    Gonadotropin
    Somatotropin [growth hormone]

962.5 Posterior pituitary hormones
    Vasopressin
    Excludes *oxytocic hormones (975.0)*

962.6 Parathyroid and parathyroid derivatives

962.7 Thyroid and thyroid derivatives
    Dextrothyroxin
    Levothyroxine sodium
    Liothyronine
    Thyroglobulin

962.8 Antithyroid agents
    Iodides
    Thiouracil
    Thiourea

■**962.9 Other and unspecified hormones and synthetic
substitutes**

● 963   **Poisoning by primarily systemic agents**

    963.0   **Antiallergic and antiemetic drugs**

Antihistamines	Diphenylpyraline
Chlorpheniramine	Thonzylamine
Diphenhydramine	Tripelennamine

       Excludes   *phenothiazine-based tranquilizers (969.1)*

    963.1   **Antineoplastic and immunosuppressive drugs**

       Azathioprine
       Busulfan
       Chlorambucil
       Cyclophosphamide
       Cytarabine
       Fluorouracil
       Mercaptopurine
       thio-TEPA

       Excludes   *antineoplastic antibiotics (960.7)*

    963.2   **Acidifying agents**

    963.3   **Alkalizing agents**

    963.4   **Enzymes, not elsewhere classified**
       Penicillinase

    963.5   **Vitamins, not elsewhere classified**
       Vitamin A
       Vitamin D

       Excludes   *nicotinic acid (972.2)*
                   vitamin K (964.3)

   ■ 963.8   **Other specified systemic agents**
       Heavy metal antagonists

   ■ 963.9   **Unspecified systemic agent**

● 964   **Poisoning by agents primarily affecting blood constituents**

    964.0   **Iron and its compounds**
       Ferric salts
       Ferrous sulfate and other ferrous salts

    964.1   **Liver preparations and other antianemic agents**
       Folic acid

    964.2   **Anticoagulants**
       Coumarin
       Heparin
       Phenindione
       Warfarin sodium
       Coding Clinic: 1994, Q1, P22

    964.3   **Vitamin K [phytonadione]**

    964.4   **Fibrinolysis-affecting drugs**
       Aminocaproic acid
       Streptodornase
       Streptokinase
       Urokinase

    964.5   **Anticoagulant antagonists and other coagulants**
       Hexadimethrine
       Protamine sulfate

    964.6   **Gamma globulin**

    964.7   **Natural blood and blood products**

Blood plasma	Packed red cells
Human fibrinogen	Whole blood

       Excludes   *transfusion reactions (999.4–999.8)*

   ■ 964.8   **Other specified agents affecting blood constituents**
       Macromolecular blood substitutes
       Plasma expanders

   ■ 964.9   **Unspecified agents affecting blood constituents**

● 965   **Poisoning by analgesics, antipyretics, and antirheumatics**

    Use additional code to identify:
       drug dependence (304.0–304.9)
       nondependent abuse (305.0–305.9)

   ● 965.0   **Opiates and related narcotics**

     ■ 965.00   **Opium (alkaloids), unspecified**
       Coding Clinic: 2007, Q3, P7-8

      965.01   **Heroin**
       Diacetylmorphine

      965.02   **Methadone**

     ■ 965.09   **Other**
       Codeine [methylmorphine]
       Meperidine [pethidine]
       Morphine
       Coding Clinic: 2007, Q3, P7-8

    965.1   **Salicylates**
       Acetylsalicylic acid [aspirin]
       Salicylic acid salts
       Coding Clinic: 1984, Nov-Dec, P15

    965.4   **Aromatic analgesics, not elsewhere classified**
       Acetanilid
       Paracetamol [acetaminophen]
       Phenacetin [acetophenetidin]

    965.5   **Pyrazole derivatives**
       Aminophenazone [aminopyrine]
       Phenylbutazone

   ● 965.6   **Antirheumatics [antiphlogistics]**

       Excludes   *salicylates (965.1)*
                   steroids (962.0–962.9)

      965.61   **Propionic acid derivatives**
       Fenoprofen
       Flurbiprofen
       Ibuprofen
       Ketoprofen
       Naproxen
       Oxaprozin
       Coding Clinic: 1998, Q4, P42-44

     ■ 965.69   **Other antirheumatics**
       Gold salts
       Indomethacin

   ■ 965.7   **Other non-narcotic analgesics**
       Pyrabital

   ■ 965.8   **Other specified analgesics and antipyretics**
       Pentazocine

   ■ 965.9   **Unspecified analgesic and antipyretic**

● 966   **Poisoning by anticonvulsants and anti-Parkinsonism drugs**

    966.0   **Oxazolidine derivatives**
       Paramethadione
       Trimethadione

    966.1   **Hydantoin derivatives**
       Phenytoin

    966.2   **Succinimides**
       Ethosuximide
       Phensuximide

   ■ 966.3   **Other and unspecified anticonvulsants**
       Primidone

       Excludes   *barbiturates (967.0)*
                   sulfonamides (961.0)

    966.4   **Anti-Parkinsonism drugs**
       Amantadine
       Ethopropazine [profenamine]
       Levodopa [L-dopa]

◀ New   ◀▥ Revised   ~~deleted~~ Deleted   ● Use Additional Digit(s)   ■ Nonspecific Code

● Not first-listed DX   OGCR Official Guidelines   Coding Clinic   Excludes   Includes   Use additional   Code first   Omit code

● 967 **Poisoning by sedatives and hypnotics**

> Use additional code to identify:
> drug dependence (304.0–304.9)
> nondependent abuse (305.0–305.9)

  967.0 **Barbiturates**
  Amobarbital [amylobarbitone]
  Barbital [barbitone]
  Butabarbital [butabarbitone]
  Pentobarbital [pentobarbitone]
  Phenobarbital [phenobarbitone]
  Secobarbital [quinalbarbitone]

  > **Excludes** *thiobarbiturate anesthetics (968.3)*

  967.1 **Chloral hydrate group**

  967.2 **Paraldehyde**

  967.3 **Bromine compounds**
  Bromide
  Carbromal (derivatives)

  967.4 **Methaqualone compounds**

  967.5 **Glutethimide group**

  967.6 **Mixed sedatives, not elsewhere classified**

  ■967.8 **Other sedatives and hypnotics**

  ■967.9 **Unspecified sedative or hypnotic**
  Sleeping: Sleeping:
    drug NOS   tablet NOS
    pill NOS

● 968 **Poisoning by other central nervous system depressants and anesthetics**

> Use additional code to identify:
> drug dependence (304.0–304.9)
> nondependent abuse (305.0–305.9)

  968.0 **Central nervous system muscle-tone depressants**
  Chlorphenesin (carbamate)
  Mephenesin
  Methocarbamol

  968.1 **Halothane**

  ■968.2 **Other gaseous anesthetics**
  Ether
  Halogenated hydrocarbon derivatives, except halothane
  Nitrous oxide

  968.3 **Intravenous anesthetics**
  Ketamine
  Methohexital [methohexitone]
  Thiobarbiturates, such as thiopental sodium

  ■968.4 **Other and unspecified general anesthetics**

  968.5 **Surface [topical] and infiltration anesthetics**
  Cocaine   Procaine
  Lidocaine [lignocaine]   Tetracaine
  Coding Clinic: 1993, Q1, P25

  968.6 **Peripheral nerve- and plexus-blocking anesthetics**

  968.7 **Spinal anesthetics**

  ■968.9 **Other and unspecified local anesthetics**

● 969 **Poisoning by psychotropic agents**

> Use additional code to identify:
> drug dependence (304.0–304.9)
> nondependent abuse (305.0–305.9)

  ● 969.0 **Antidepressants** ◀▥
  ~~Amitriptyline~~
  ~~Imipramine~~
  ~~Monoamine oxidase [MAO] inhibitors~~

    969.00 **Antidepressant, unspecified** ◀

    969.01 **Monoamine oxidase inhibitors** ◀
    MAOI ◀

    969.02 **Selective serotonin and norepinephrine reuptake inhibitors** ◀
    SSNRI antidepressants ◀

    969.03 **Selective serotonin reuptake inhibitors** ◀
    SSRI antidepressants

    969.04 **Tetracyclic antidepressants** ◀

    969.05 **Tricyclic antidepressants** ◀

    969.09 **Other antidepressants** ◀
    Coding Clinic: 2007, Q3, P7-8; 1991, Q3, P14

  969.1 **Phenothiazine-based tranquilizers**
  Chlorpromazine
  Fluphenazine
  Prochlorperazine
  Promazine

  969.2 **Butyrophenone-based tranquilizers**
  Haloperidol   Trifluperidol
  Spiperone

  ■969.3 **Other antipsychotics, neuroleptics, and major tranquilizers**

  969.4 **Benzodiazepine-based tranquilizers**
  Chlordiazepoxide   Lorazepam
  Diazepam   Medazepam
  Flurazepam   Nitrazepam
  Coding Clinic: 1991, Q3, P14

  ■969.5 **Other tranquilizers**
  Hydroxyzine
  Meprobamate

  969.6 **Psychodysleptics [hallucinogens]**
  Cannabis (derivatives)
  Lysergide [LSD]
  Marihuana (derivatives)
  Marijuana
  Mescaline
  Psilocin
  Psilocybin

  ● 969.7 **Psychostimulants** ◀▥
  ~~Amphetamine~~
  ~~Caffeine~~

  > **Excludes** *central appetite depressants (977.0)*

    969.70 **Psychostimulant, unspecified** ◀

    969.71 **Caffeine** ◀

    969.72 **Amphetamines** ◀
    Methamphetamines ◀

    969.73 **Methylphenidate** ◀

    969.79 **Other psychostimulants** ◀
    Coding Clinic: 2003, Q2, P11

  ■969.8 **Other specified psychotropic agents**

  ■969.9 **Unspecified psychotropic agent**

● 970 **Poisoning by central nervous system stimulants**

  970.0 **Analeptics**
  Lobeline
  Nikethamide

  970.1 **Opiate antagonists**
  Levallorphan
  Nalorphine
  Naloxone

  ■970.8 **Other specified central nervous system stimulants**

  ■970.9 **Unspecified central nervous system stimulant**

● 971 **Poisoning by drugs primarily affecting the autonomic nervous system**

INJURY AND POISONING (800–999)

971.0 **Parasympathomimetics [cholinergics]**
    Acetylcholine
    Anticholinesterase:
        organophosphorus
        reversible
    Pilocarpine

971.1 **Parasympatholytics [anticholinergics and antimuscarinics] and spasmolytics**
    Atropine
    Homatropine
    Hyoscine [scopolamine]
    Quaternary ammonium derivatives
    Excludes *papaverine (972.5)*

971.2 **Sympathomimetics [adrenergics]**
    Epinephrine [adrenalin]
    Levarterenol [noradrenalin]

971.3 **Sympatholytics [antiadrenergics]**
    Phenoxybenzamine
    Tolazoline hydrochloride

971.9 **Unspecified drug primarily affecting autonomic nervous system**

● 972 **Poisoning by agents primarily affecting the cardiovascular system**

972.0 **Cardiac rhythm regulators**
    Practolol
    Procainamide
    Propranolol
    Quinidine
    Excludes *lidocaine (968.5)*

972.1 **Cardiotonic glycosides and drugs of similar action**
    Digitalis glycosides
    Digoxin
    Strophanthins

972.2 **Antilipemic and antiarteriosclerotic drugs**
    Clofibrate
    Nicotinic acid derivatives

972.3 **Ganglion-blocking agents**
    Pentamethonium bromide

972.4 **Coronary vasodilators**
    Dipyridamole
    Nitrates [nitroglycerin]
    Nitrites

972.5 **Other vasodilators**
    Cyclandelate
    Diazoxide
    Papaverine
    Excludes *nicotinic acid (972.2)*

972.6 **Other antihypertensive agents**
    Clonidine
    Guanethidine
    Rauwolfia alkaloids
    Reserpine

972.7 **Antivaricose drugs, including sclerosing agents**
    Sodium morrhuate
    Zinc salts

972.8 **Capillary-active drugs**
    Adrenochrome derivatives
    Metaraminol

972.9 **Other and unspecified agents primarily affecting the cardiovascular system**

● 973 **Poisoning by agents primarily affecting the gastrointestinal system**

973.0 **Antacids and antigastric secretion drugs**
    Aluminum hydroxide
    Magnesium trisilicate
    Coding Clinic: 2003, Q1, P19

973.1 **Irritant cathartics**
    Bisacodyl
    Castor oil
    Phenolphthalein

973.2 **Emollient cathartics**
    Dioctyl sulfosuccinates

973.3 **Other cathartics, including intestinal atonia drugs**
    Magnesium sulfate

973.4 **Digestants**
    Pancreatin   Pepsin
    Papain

973.5 **Antidiarrheal drugs**
    Kaolin
    Pectin
    Excludes *anti-infectives (960.0–961.9)*

973.6 **Emetics**

973.8 **Other specified agents primarily affecting the gastrointestinal system**

973.9 **Unspecified agent primarily affecting the gastrointestinal system**

● 974 **Poisoning by water, mineral, and uric acid metabolism drugs**

974.0 **Mercurial diuretics**
    Chlormerodrin
    Mercaptomerin
    Mersalyl

974.1 **Purine derivative diuretics**
    Theobromine
    Theophylline
    Excludes *aminophylline [theophylline*
                   ethylenediamine] (975.7)
            caffeine (969.71) ◀▥

974.2 **Carbonic acid anhydrase inhibitors**
    Acetazolamide

974.3 **Saluretics**
    Benzothiadiazides
    Chlorothiazide group

974.4 **Other diuretics**
    Ethacrynic acid
    Furosemide

974.5 **Electrolytic, caloric, and water-balance agents**

974.6 **Other mineral salts, not elsewhere classified**

974.7 **Uric acid metabolism drugs**
    Allopurinol
    Colchicine
    Probenecid

● 975 **Poisoning by agents primarily acting on the smooth and skeletal muscles and respiratory system**

975.0 **Oxytocic agents**
    Ergot alkaloids
    Oxytocin
    Prostaglandins

975.1 **Smooth muscle relaxants**
    Adiphenine
    Metaproterenol [orciprenaline]
    Excludes *papaverine (972.5)*

975.2 **Skeletal muscle relaxants**

975.3 **Other and unspecified drugs acting on muscles**

975.4 **Antitussives**
    Dextromethorphan
    Pipazethate

975.5 **Expectorants**
Acetylcysteine
Guaifenesin
Terpin hydrate

975.6 **Anti-common cold drugs**

975.7 **Antiasthmatics**
Aminophylline [theophylline ethylenediamine]

■975.8 **Other and unspecified respiratory drugs**

● 976 **Poisoning by agents primarily affecting skin and mucous membrane, ophthalmological, otorhinolaryngological, and dental drugs**

976.0 **Local anti-infectives and anti-inflammatory drugs**

976.1 **Antipruritics**

976.2 **Local astringents and local detergents**

976.3 **Emollients, demulcents, and protectants**

976.4 **Keratolytics, keratoplastics, other hair treatment drugs and preparations**

976.5 **Eye anti-infectives and other eye drugs**
Idoxuridine

976.6 **Anti-infectives and other drugs and preparations for ear, nose, and throat**

976.7 **Dental drugs topically applied**

> **Excludes** *anti-infectives (976.0)*
> *local anesthetics (968.5)*

■976.8 **Other agents primarily affecting skin and mucous membrane**
Spermicides [vaginal contraceptives]

■976.9 **Unspecified agent primarily affecting skin and mucous membrane**

● 977 **Poisoning by other and unspecified drugs and medicinal substances**

977.0 **Dietetics**
Central appetite depressants

977.1 **Lipotropic drugs**

977.2 **Antidotes and chelating agents, not elsewhere classified**

977.3 **Alcohol deterrents**

977.4 **Pharmaceutical excipients**
Pharmaceutical adjuncts

■977.8 **Other specified drugs and medicinal substances**
Contrast media used for diagnostic x-ray procedures
Diagnostic agents and kits

■977.9 **Unspecified drug or medicinal substance**
Coding Clinic: 1986, Mar-April, P12

● 978 **Poisoning by bacterial vaccines**

978.0 **BCG**

978.1 **Typhoid and paratyphoid**

978.2 **Cholera**

978.3 **Plague**

978.4 **Tetanus**

978.5 **Diphtheria**

978.6 **Pertussis vaccine, including combinations with a pertussis component**

■978.8 **Other and unspecified bacterial vaccines**

978.9 **Mixed bacterial vaccines, except combinations with a pertussis component**

● 979 **Poisoning by other vaccines and biological substances**

> **Excludes** *gamma globulin (964.6)*

979.0 **Smallpox vaccine**

979.1 **Rabies vaccine**

979.2 **Typhus vaccine**

979.3 **Yellow fever vaccine**

979.4 **Measles vaccine**

979.5 **Poliomyelitis vaccine**

■979.6 **Other and unspecified viral and rickettsial vaccines**
Mumps vaccine

979.7 **Mixed viral-rickettsial and bacterial vaccines, except combinations with a pertussis component**

> **Excludes** *combinations with a pertussis component (978.6)*

■979.9 **Other and unspecified vaccines and biological substances**

OGCR Section I.C.17.e.3
When a harmful substance is ingested or comes in contact with a person, this is classified as a toxic effect. The toxic effect codes are in categories 980-989. A toxic effect code should be sequenced first, followed by the code(s) that identify the result of the toxic effect. An external cause code from categories E860-E869 for accidental exposure, codes E950.6 or E950.7 for intentional self-harm, category E962 for assault, or categories E980-E982, for undetermined, should also be assigned to indicate intent.

TOXIC EFFECTS OF SUBSTANCES CHIEFLY NONMEDICINAL AS TO SOURCE (980–989)

> **Excludes** *burns from chemical agents (ingested) (947.0–947.9)*
> *localized toxic effects indexed elsewhere (001.0–799.9)*
> *respiratory conditions due to external agents (506.0–508.9)*

Use additional code to specify the nature of the toxic effect

● 980 **Toxic effect of alcohol**

980.0 **Ethyl alcohol**
Denatured alcohol
Ethanol
Grain alcohol

Use additional code to identify any associated:
acute alcohol intoxication (305.0)
in alcoholism (303.0)
drunkenness (simple) (305.0)
pathological (291.4)
Coding Clinic: 1996, Q3, P16; 1991, Q3, P14

980.1 **Methyl alcohol**
Methanol
Wood alcohol

980.2 **Isopropyl alcohol**
Dimethyl carbinol
Isopropanol
Rubbing alcohol

980.3 **Fusel oil**
Alcohol:
amyl
butyl
propyl

■980.8 **Other specified alcohols**

■980.9 **Unspecified alcohol**

INJURY AND POISONING (800–999)

981 Toxic effect of petroleum products
  Benzine
  Gasoline
  Kerosene
  Paraffin wax
  Petroleum:
    ether
    naphtha
    spirit

● 982 Toxic effect of solvents other than petroleum based

  982.0 Benzene and homologues

  982.1 Carbon tetrachloride

  982.2 Carbon disulfide
    Carbon bisulfide

  ■**982.3 Other chlorinated hydrocarbon solvents**
    Tetrachloroethylene
    Trichloroethylene

    Excludes *chlorinated hydrocarbon preparations other*
              than solvents (989.2)
    Coding Clinic: 2008, Q3, P6, 7x2

  982.4 Nitroglycol

  ■**982.8 Other nonpetroleum-based solvents**
    Acetone

● 983 Toxic effect of corrosive aromatics, acids, and caustic alkalis

  983.0 Corrosive aromatics
    Carbolic acid or phenol
    Cresol

  983.1 Acids
    Acid:
      hydrochloric
      nitric
      sulfuric

  983.2 Caustic alkalis
    Lye
    Potassium hydroxide
    Sodium hydroxide

  ■**983.9 Caustic, unspecified**

● 984 Toxic effect of lead and its compounds (including fumes)

    Includes that from all sources except medicinal
              substances

  984.0 Inorganic lead compounds
    Lead dioxide
    Lead salts

  984.1 Organic lead compounds
    Lead acetate
    Tetraethyl lead

  ■**984.8 Other lead compounds**

  ■**984.9 Unspecified lead compound**

● 985 Toxic effect of other metals

    Includes that from all sources except medicinal
              substances

  985.0 Mercury and its compounds
    Minamata disease

  985.1 Arsenic and its compounds

  985.2 Manganese and its compounds

  985.3 Beryllium and its compounds

  985.4 Antimony and its compounds

  985.5 Cadmium and its compounds

  985.6 Chromium

  ■**985.8 Other specified metals**
    Brass fumes
    Copper salts
    Iron compounds
    Nickel compounds

  ■**985.9 Unspecified metal**

986 Toxic effect of carbon monoxide

● 987 Toxic effect of other gases, fumes, or vapors

  987.0 Liquefied petroleum gases
    Butane
    Propane

  ■**987.1 Other hydrocarbon gas**

  987.2 Nitrogen oxides
    Nitrogen dioxide
    Nitrous fumes

  987.3 Sulfur dioxide

  987.4 Freon
    Dichloromonofluoromethane

  987.5 Lacrimogenic gas
    Bromobenzyl cyanide
    Chloroacetophenone
    Ethyliodoacetate

  987.6 Chlorine gas

  987.7 Hydrocyanic acid gas

  ■**987.8 Other specified gases, fumes, or vapors**
    Phosgene
    Polyester fumes

  ■**987.9 Unspecified gas, fume, or vapor**
    Coding Clinic: 2005, Q3, P10-11

● 988 Toxic effect of noxious substances eaten as food

    Excludes *allergic reaction to food, such as:*
              gastroenteritis (558.3)
              rash (692.5, 693.1)
              food poisoning (bacterial) (005.0–005.9)

              toxic effects of food contaminants, such as:
              aflatoxin and other mycotoxin (989.7)
              mercury (985.0)

  988.0 Fish and shellfish

  988.1 Mushrooms

  988.2 Berries and other plants

  ■**988.8 Other specified noxious substances eaten as food**

  ■**988.9 Unspecified noxious substance eaten as food**

● **989   Toxic effect of other substances, chiefly nonmedicinal as to source**

   989.0   Hydrocyanic acid and cyanides
      Potassium cyanide
      Sodium cyanide

      Excludes   *gas and fumes (987.7)*

   989.1   Strychnine and salts

   989.2   Chlorinated hydrocarbons
      Aldrin
      Chlordane
      DDT
      Dieldrin

      Excludes   *chlorinated hydrocarbon solvents (982.0–982.3)*

   989.3   Organophosphate and carbamate
      Carbaryl   Parathion
      Dichlorvos   Phorate
      Malathion   Phosdrin

  ■**989.4   Other pesticides, not elsewhere classified**
      Mixtures of insecticides

   989.5   Venom
      Bites of venomous snakes, lizards, and spiders
      Tick paralysis

   989.6   Soaps and detergents

   989.7   Aflatoxin and other mycotoxin [food contaminants]

● **989.8   Other substances, chiefly nonmedicinal as to source**

   989.81   Asbestos

      Excludes   *asbestosis (501)*
                 exposure to asbestos (V15.84)

   989.82   Latex

   989.83   Silicone

      Excludes   *silicone used in medical devices, implants and grafts (996.00–996.79)*

   989.84   Tobacco

   989.89   Other

  ■**989.9   Unspecified substance, chiefly nonmedicinal as to source**

OTHER AND UNSPECIFIED EFFECTS OF EXTERNAL CAUSES (990–995)

■**990   Effects of radiation, unspecified**
      Complication of:
        phototherapy
        radiation therapy
      Radiation sickness

      Excludes   *specified adverse effects of radiation. Such conditions are to be classified according to the nature of the adverse effect, as:*
          burns (940.0–949.5)
          dermatitis (692.7–692.8)
          leukemia (204.0–208.9)
          pneumonia (508.0)
          sunburn (692.71, 692.76–692.77)
          [The type of radiation giving rise to the adverse effect may be identified by use of the E codes.]

● **991   Effects of reduced temperature**

   991.0   Frostbite of face

   991.1   Frostbite of hand

   991.2   Frostbite of foot

  ■**991.3   Frostbite of other and unspecified sites**

   991.4   Immersion foot
      Trench foot

   991.5   Chilblains
      Erythema pernio
      Perniosis

   991.6   Hypothermia
      Hypothermia (accidental)

      Excludes   *hypothermia following anesthesia (995.89)*
          hypothermia not associated with low environmental temperature (780.65)

  ■**991.8   Other specified effects of reduced temperature**

  ■**991.9   Unspecified effect of reduced temperature**
      Effects of freezing or excessive cold NOS

● **992   Effects of heat and light**

      Excludes   *burns (940.0–949.5)*
          diseases of sweat glands due to heat (705.0–705.9)
          malignant hyperpyrexia following anesthesia (995.86)
          sunburn (692.71, 692.76–692.77)

   992.0   Heat stroke and sunstroke
      Heat apoplexy
      Heat pyrexia
      Ictus solaris
      Siriasis
      Thermoplegia

   992.1   Heat syncope
      Heat collapse

   992.2   Heat cramps

   992.3   Heat exhaustion, anhydrotic
      Heat prostration due to water depletion

      Excludes   *that associated with salt depletion (992.4)*

   992.4   Heat exhaustion due to salt depletion
      Heat prostration due to salt (and water) depletion

  ■**992.5   Heat exhaustion, unspecified**
      Heat prostration NOS

   992.6   Heat fatigue, transient

   992.7   Heat edema

  ■**992.8   Other specified heat effects**

  ■**992.9   Unspecified**

● **993   Effects of air pressure**

   993.0   Barotrauma, otitic
      Aero-otitis media
      Effects of high altitude on ears

   993.1   Barotrauma, sinus
      Aerosinusitis
      Effects of high altitude on sinuses

  ■**993.2   Other and unspecified effects of high altitude**
      Alpine sickness
      Andes disease
      Anoxia due to high altitude
      Hypobaropathy
      Mountain sickness

INJURY AND POISONING (800–999)

993.3 **Caisson disease**
Bends
Compressed-air disease
Decompression sickness
Divers' palsy or paralysis

993.4 **Effects of air pressure caused by explosion**

■ 993.8 **Other specified effects of air pressure**

■ 993.9 **Unspecified effect of air pressure**

● 994 **Effects of other external causes**

> **Excludes** *certain adverse effects not elsewhere classified (995.0–995.8)*

994.0 **Effects of lightning**
Shock from lightning
Struck by lightning NOS

> **Excludes** *burns (940.0–949.5)*

994.1 **Drowning and nonfatal submersion**
Bathing cramp
Immersion

994.2 **Effects of hunger**
Deprivation of food
Starvation

994.3 **Effects of thirst**
Deprivation of water

994.4 **Exhaustion due to exposure**

994.5 **Exhaustion due to excessive exertion**
Exhaustion due to overexertion

994.6 **Motion sickness**
Air sickness
Seasickness
Travel sickness

994.7 **Asphyxiation and strangulation**
Suffocation (by):
bedclothes
cave-in
constriction
mechanical
plastic bag
pressure
strangulation

> **Excludes** *asphyxia from:*
> *carbon monoxide (986)*
> *inhalation of food or foreign body (932–934.9)*
> *other gases, fumes, and vapors (987.0–987.9)*

994.8 **Electrocution and nonfatal effects of electric current**
Shock from electric current
Shock from electroshock gun (taser)

> **Excludes** *electric burns (940.0–949.5)*

■ 994.9 **Other effects of external causes**
Effects of:
abnormal gravitational [G] forces or states
weightlessness

● 995 **Certain adverse effects not elsewhere classified**

> **Excludes** *complications of surgical and medical care (996.0–999.9)*

> Coding Clinic: 2008, Q1, P12-13

■ 995.0 **Other anaphylactic shock**
Allergic shock NOS or due to adverse effect of correct medicinal substance properly administered
Anaphylactic reaction NOS or due to adverse effect of correct medicinal substance properly administered
Anaphylaxis NOS or due to adverse effect of correct medicinal substance properly administered

> **Excludes** *anaphylactic reaction to serum (999.4)*
> *anaphylactic shock due to adverse food reaction (995.60–995.69)*

Use additional E code to identify external cause, such as:
adverse effects of correct medicinal substance properly administered [E930–E949]

995.1 **Angioneurotic edema**
Giant urticaria

> **Excludes** *urticaria:*
> *due to serum (999.5)*
> *other specified (698.2, 708.0–708.9, 757.33)*

● 995.2 **Other and unspecified adverse effect of drug, medicinal and biological substance (due) to correct medicinal substance properly administered**
Adverse effect to correct medicinal substance properly administered
Allergic reaction to correct medicinal substance properly administered
Hypersensitivity to correct medicinal substance properly administered
Idiosyncrasy due to correct medicinal substance properly administered
Drug:
hypersensitivity NOS
reaction NOS

> **Excludes** *pathological drug intoxication (292.2)*

> Coding Clinic: 2006, Q4, P112-113; 1997, Q2, P12; 1995, Q3, P13; 1992, Q3, P16-17

■ 995.20 **Unspecified adverse effect of unspecified drug, medicinal and biological substance**

995.21 **Arthus phenomenon**
Arthus reaction
Hypersensitivity reaction resulting from immune complex reactions

■ 995.22 **Unspecified adverse effect of anesthesia**

■ 995.23 **Unspecified adverse effect of insulin**

995.24 **Failed moderate sedation during procedure** ◀
Failed conscious sedation during procedure ◀

■ 995.27 **Other drug allergy**
Drug allergy NOS
Drug hypersensitivity NOS

■ 995.29 **Unspecified adverse effect of other drug, medicinal and biological substance**

■995.3 Allergy, unspecified
Allergic reaction NOS
Hypersensitivity NOS
Idiosyncrasy NOS

> **Excludes** *allergic reaction NOS to correct medicinal*
> *substance properly administered*
> *(995.27)*
> *allergy to existing dental restorative*
> *materials (525.66)*
> *specific types of allergic reaction, such as:*
> *allergic diarrhea (558.3)*
> *dermatitis (691.0–693.9)*
> *hayfever (477.0–477.9)*

995.4 Shock due to anesthesia
Shock due to anesthesia in which the correct
substance was properly administered

> **Excludes** *complications of anesthesia in labor or*
> *delivery (668.0–668.9)*
> *overdose or wrong substance given*
> *(968.0–969.9)*
> *postoperative shock NOS (998.0)*
> *specified adverse effects of anesthesia*
> *classified elsewhere, such as:*
> *anoxic brain damage (348.1)*
> *hepatitis (070.0–070.9), etc.*
> *unspecified adverse effect of anesthesia*
> *(995.22)*

● 995.5 Child maltreatment syndrome

Use additional code(s), if applicable, to identify
any associated injuries

Use additional E code to identify:
nature of abuse (E960–E968)
perpetrator (E967.0–E967.9)
Coding Clinic: 1998, Q1, P11; 1984, Sept-Oct, P16; 1984, Nov-Dec, P9

■995.50 Child abuse, unspecified   P

995.51 Child emotional/psychological abuse   P

995.52 Child neglect (nutritional)   P

> Use additional code to identify intent of
> neglect (E904.0,E968.4)

995.53 Child sexual abuse   P

995.54 Child physical abuse   P
Battered baby or child syndrome

> **Excludes** *Shaken infant syndrome (995.55)*

> Coding Clinic: 1999, Q3, P14-15

995.55 Shaken infant syndrome   P

> Use additional code(s) to identify any
> associated injuries
> Coding Clinic: 1996, Q4, P43-44

■995.59 Other child abuse and neglect   P
Multiple forms of abuse

> Use additional code to identify intent of
> neglect (E904.0,E968.4)

● 995.6 Anaphylactic shock due to adverse food reaction
Anaphylactic reaction due to food
Anaphylactic shock due to nonpoisonous foods

■995.60 Due to unspecified food

995.61 Due to peanuts

995.62 Due to crustaceans

995.63 Due to fruits and vegetables

995.64 Due to tree nuts and seeds
> Coding Clinic: 2008, Q1, P12-13

995.65 Due to fish

995.66 Due to food additives

995.67 Due to milk products

995.68 Due to eggs

■995.69 Due to other specified food

**995.7 Other adverse food reactions, not elsewhere
classified**

> Use additional code to identify the type of
> reaction, such as:
> hives (708.0)
> wheezing (786.07)

> **Excludes** *anaphylactic shock due to adverse food*
> *reaction (995.6)*
> *asthma (493.0, 493.9)*
> *dermatitis due to food (693.1)*
> *in contact with the skin (692.5)*
> *gastroenteritis and colitis due to food*
> *(558.3)*
> *rhinitis due to food (477.1)*

**● 995.8 Other specified adverse effects, not elsewhere
classified**

■995.80 Adult maltreatment, unspecified   A
Abused person NOS

> Use additional code to identify:
> any associated injury
> nature of abuse (E960–E968)
> perpetrator (E967.0–E967.9)

995.81 Adult physical abuse   A
Battered:
person syndrome NEC
man
spouse
woman

> Use additional code to identify:
> any associated injury
> nature of abuse (E960–E968)
> perpetrator (E967.0–E967.9)
> Coding Clinic: 1996, Q4, P43-44; 1984, Sept-Oct, P16

995.82 Adult emotional/psychological abuse   A

> Use additional E code to identify
> perpetrator (E967.0–E967.9)

995.83 Adult sexual abuse   A

> Use additional code to identify:
> any associated injury
> perpetrator (E967.0–E967.9)

995.84 Adult neglect (nutritional)   A

> Use additional code to identify:
> intent of neglect (E904.0–E968.4)
> perpetrator (E967.0–E967.9)

■995.85 Other adult abuse and neglect   A
Multiple forms of abuse and neglect

> Use additional code to identify:
> any associated injury
> intent of neglect (E904.0, E968.4)
> nature of abuse (E960–E968)
> perpetrator (E967.0–E967.9)

995.86 Malignant hyperthermia
Malignant hyperpyrexia due to anesthesia
*Extremely high body temperature—greater
than 106° F or 41.1° C*

■995.89 Other
Hypothermia due to anesthesia
> Coding Clinic: 2004, Q2, P18; 2003, Q3, P12

INJURY AND POISONING (800—999)

● 995.9 **Systemic inflammatory response syndrome (SIRS)**
   Coding Clinic: 2006, Q4, P113-116; 2005, Q3, P23; 2004, Q2, P16; 2002, Q4, P71-73

   ■ 995.90 **Systemic inflammatory response syndrome, unspecified SIRS NOS**

● 995.91 *Sepsis*
   Systemic inflammatory response syndrome due to infectious process without acute organ dysfunction

   Code first underlying infection

   Excludes *sepsis with acute organ dysfunction (995.92)*
   sepsis with multiple organ dysfunction (995.92)
   severe sepsis (995.92)
   Coding Clinic: 2008, Q4, P69-73; 2007, Q4, P84-86; 2004, Q2, P16

   OGCR Section I.C.1.b.2.12
   Only one code from subcategory 995.9 should be assigned. Therefore, when a non-infectious condition leads to an infection resulting in sepsis or severe sepsis, assign either code 995.91 or 995.92. Do not additionally assign code 995.93, Systemic inflammatory response syndrome due to non-infectious process without acute organ dysfunctiion, or 995.94, Systemic inflammatory response syndrome with acute organ dysfunction.

● 995.92 *Severe sepsis*
   Sepsis with acute organ dysfunction
   Sepsis with multiple organ dysfunction (MOD)
   Systemic inflammatory response syndrome due to infectious process with acute organ dysfunction

   Code first underlying infection

   Use additional code to specify acute organ dysfunction, such as:
   acute ~~renal~~ kidney failure (584.5–584.9)   ◄▥
   acute respiratory failure (518.81)
   critical illness myopathy (359.81)
   critical illness polyneuropathy (357.82)
   disseminated intravascular coagulopathy (DIC) syndrome (286.6)
   encephalopathy (348.31)
   hepatic failure (570)
   septic shock (785.52)
   Coding Clinic: 2007, Q4, P96-97; 2005, Q2, P18-20x2; 2004, Q2, P16; 2003, Q4, P73, 79-81

● 995.93 *Systemic inflammatory response syndrome due to noninfectious process without acute organ dysfunction*

   Code first underlying conditions, such as:
   acute pancreatitis (577.0)
   trauma

   Excludes *systemic inflammatory response syndrome due to noninfectious process with acute organ dysfunction (995.94)*

   OGCR Section I.C.19.a.7
   An external cause code(s) may be used with codes 995.93 if trauma was the initiating insult that precipitated the SIRS. The external cause(s) code should correspond to the most serious injury resulting from the trauma. The external cause code(s) should only be assigned if the trauma necessitated the admission in which the patient also developed SIRS. If a patient is admitted with SIRS but the trauma has been treated previously, the external cause codes should not be used.

● 995.94 *Systemic inflammatory response syndrome due to non-infectious process with acute organ dysfunction*

   Code first underlying conditions, such as:
   acute pancreatitis (577.0)
   trauma

   Use additional code to specify acute organ dysfunction, such as:
   acute ~~renal~~ kidney failure (584.5–584.9)   ◄▥
   acute respiratory failure (518.81)
   critical illness myopathy (359.81)
   critical illness polyneuropathy (357.82)
   disseminated intravascular coagulopathy (DIC) syndrome (286.6)
   encephalopathy (348.31)
   hepatic failure (570)

   Excludes *severe sepsis (995.92)*

   Coding Clinic: 2005, Q2, P19-20

◄ New   ◄▥ Revised   ~~deleted~~ Deleted   ● Use Additional Digit(s)   ■ Nonspecific Code
● Not first-listed DX   OGCR Official Guidelines   Coding Clinic   Excludes   Includes   Use additional   Code first   Omit code

OGCR Section I.C.19.a.7

An external cause code(s) may be used with codes 995.94 if trauma was the initiating insult that precipitated the SIRS. The external cause(s) code should correspond to the most serious injury resulting from the trauma. The external cause code(s) should only be assigned if the trauma necessitated the admission in which the patient also developed SIRS. If a patient is admitted with SIRS but the trauma has been treated previously, the external cause codes should not be used.

COMPLICATIONS OF SURGICAL AND MEDICAL CARE, NOT ELSEWHERE CLASSIFIED (996–999)

Excludes *adverse effects of medicinal agents (001.0–799.9, 995.0–995.8)*
burns from local applications and irradiation (940.0–949.5)
complications of:
   conditions for which the procedure was performed
   surgical procedures during abortion, labor, and delivery (630–676.9)
poisoning and toxic effects of drugs and chemicals (960.0–989.9)
postoperative conditions in which no complications are present, such as:
   artificial opening status (V44.0–V44.9)
   closure of external stoma (V55.0–V55.9)
   fitting of prosthetic device (V52.0–V52.9)
specified complications classified elsewhere:
   anesthetic shock (995.4)
   electrolyte imbalance (276.0–276.9)
   postlaminectomy syndrome (722.80–722.83)
   postmastectomy lymphedema syndrome (457.0)
   postoperative psychosis (293.0–293.9)
any other condition classified elsewhere in the Alphabetic Index when described as due to a procedure

● **996 Complications peculiar to certain specified procedures**

Includes complications, not elsewhere classified, in the use of artificial substitutes [e.g., Dacron, metal, Silastic, Teflon] or natural sources [e.g., bone] involving:
   anastomosis (internal)
   graft (bypass) (patch)
   implant
   internal device:
      catheter
      electronic
      fixation
      prosthetic
   reimplant
   transplant

Excludes *accidental puncture or laceration during procedure (998.2)*
capsular contracture of breast implant (611.83)
complications of internal anastomosis of:
   gastrointestinal tract (997.4)
   urinary tract (997.5)
endosseous dental implant failures (525.71–525.79)
intraoperative floppy iris syndrome (IFIS) (364.81)
mechanical complication of respirator (V46.14)
other specified complications classified elsewhere, such as:
   hemolytic anemia (283.1)
   functional cardiac disturbances (429.4)
   serum hepatitis (070.2–070.3)

● **996.0 Mechanical complication of cardiac device, implant, and graft**

Breakdown (mechanical)	Obstruction, mechanical
Displacement	Perforation
Leakage	Protrusion

Coding Clinic: 2007, Q3, P7-8

■ **996.00 Unspecified device, implant, and graft**

996.01 Due to cardiac pacemaker (electrode)
Coding Clinic: 2006, Q2, P15-16; 1999, Q2, P11-12

996.02 Due to heart valve prosthesis
Coding Clinic: 1999, Q2, P4

996.03 Due to coronary bypass graft

Excludes *atherosclerosis of graft (414.02, 414.03)*
embolism [occlusion NOS] [thrombus] of graft (996.72)

Coding Clinic: 1993, Q4, P40-41

996.04 Due to automatic implantable cardiac defibrillator
Coding Clinic: 2005, Q2, P3

■ **996.09 Other**
Coding Clinic: 1993, Q2, P9

INJURY AND POISONING (800–999)

◼ **996.1 Mechanical complication of other vascular device, implant, and graft**
     Mechanical complications involving:
         aortic (bifurcation) graft (replacement)
         arteriovenous:
            dialysis catheter
            fistula surgically created
            shunt surgically created
         balloon (counterpulsation) device, intra-aortic
         carotid artery bypass graft
         femoral-popliteal bypass graft
         umbrella device, vena cava

     Excludes   *atherosclerosis of biological graft*
                 (440.30–440.32)
            embolism [occlusion NOS] [thrombus] of
                 (biological) (synthetic) graft (996.74)
            peritoneal dialysis catheter (996.56)
     Coding Clinic: 2006, Q1, P10-11; 2005, Q2, P8; 2002, Q1, P13; 1995,
         Q1, P3

996.2 Mechanical complication of nervous system device, implant, and graft
     Mechanical complications involving:
         dorsal column stimulator
         electrodes implanted in brain [brain
            "pacemaker"]
         peripheral nerve graft
         ventricular (communicating) shunt
     Coding Clinic: 1987, Sept-Oct, P10

● **996.3 Mechanical complication of genitourinary device, implant, and graft**

   ◼ **996.30 Unspecified device, implant, and graft**

   996.31 Due to urethral [indwelling] catheter

   996.32 Due to intrauterine contraceptive device ♀

   ◼ **996.39 Other**
       Cystostomy catheter
       Prosthetic reconstruction of vas deferens
       Repair (graft) of ureter without mention of
         resection

       Excludes   *complications due to:*
                external stoma of urinary tract
                   (997.5)
                internal anastomosis of urinary
                   tract (997.5)

● **996.4 Mechanical complication of internal orthopedic device, implant, and graft**
     Mechanical complications involving:
         external (fixation) device utilizing internal
            screw(s), pin(s) or other methods of
            fixation
         grafts of bone, cartilage, muscle, or tendon
         internal (fixation) device such as nail, plate,
            rod, etc.

     Use additional code to identify prosthetic
         joint with mechanical complication
         (V43.60–V43.69)

     Excludes   *complications of external orthopedic device,*
                such as:
                pressure ulcer due to cast
                   (707.00–707.09)
     Coding Clinic: 2005, Q4, P91-93, 110-112; 1999, Q2, P10-11; 1998,
         Q2, P19; 1996, Q2, P11; 1985, Nov-Dec, P11; 1984, Nov-Dec,
         P18

996.40 Unspecified mechanical complication of internal orthopedic device, implant, and graft

996.41 Mechanical loosening of prosthetic joint
     Aseptic loosening
     Coding Clinic: 2005, Q4, P91-93

996.42 Dislocation of prosthetic joint
     Instability of prosthetic joint
     Subluxation of prosthetic joint

996.43 ~~Prosthetic joint implant failure~~ ◀▥
     Broken prosthetic joint implant
     Breakage (fracture) of prosthetic joint

996.44 Peri-prosthetic fracture around prosthetic joint
     Coding Clinic: 2005, Q4, P91-93

996.45 Peri-prosthetic osteolysis
     Use additional code to identify major
         osseous defect, if applicable (731.3)
     Coding Clinic: 2006, Q4, P103-104

996.46 Articular bearing surface wear of prosthetic joint

◼ **996.47 Other mechanical complication of prosthetic joint implant**
     Mechanical complication of prosthetic joint
         NOS
     Prosthetic joint implant failure NOS   ◀

◼ **996.49 Other mechanical complication of other internal orthopedic device, implant, and graft**
     Breakage of internal fixation device in
         bone
     Dislocation of internal fixation device in
         bone

     Excludes   *mechanical complication of*
                prosthetic joint implant
                (996.41–996.46)

● **996.5 Mechanical complication of other specified prosthetic device, implant, and graft**
     Mechanical complications involving:
         prosthetic implant in:
            bile duct
            breast
            chin
            orbit of eye
         nonabsorbable surgical material NOS
         other graft, implant, and internal device, not
            elsewhere classified

996.51 Due to corneal graft

◼ **996.52 Due to graft of other tissue, not elsewhere classified**
     Skin graft failure or rejection

     Excludes   *failure of artificial skin graft*
                (996.55)
            failure of decellularized allodermis
                (996.55)
            sloughing of temporary skin
                allografts or xenografts
                (pigskin)- omit code
     Coding Clinic: 1996, Q1, P10; 1990, Q3, P15

996.53 Due to ocular lens prosthesis

     Excludes   *contact lenses—code to condition*
     Coding Clinic: 2000, Q1, P9-10

◀ New   ◀▥ Revised   ~~deleted~~ Deleted   ● Use Additional Digit(s)   ◼ Nonspecific Code

● Not first-listed DX   OGCR Official Guidelines   Coding Clinic   Excludes   Includes   Use additional   Code first   Omit code

996.54 Due to breast prosthesis
Breast capsule (prosthesis)
Mammary implant
Coding Clinic: 1998, Q2, P14; 1992, Q3, P4-5

996.55 Due to artificial skin graft and decellularized allodermis
Dislodgement
Displacement
Failure
Non-adherence
Poor incorporation
Shearing
Coding Clinic: 1998, Q4, P52-53

996.56 Due to peritoneal dialysis catheter

Excludes *mechanical complication of arteriovenous dialysis catheter (996.1)*
Coding Clinic: 1998, Q4, P54

996.57 Due to insulin pump
Coding Clinic: 2003, Q4, P81-82

OGCR Section I.C.3.a.6.a

An underdose of insulin due to an insulin pump failure should be assigned 996.57, Mechanical complication due to insulin pump, as the principal or first listed code, followed by the appropriate diabetes mellitus code based on documentation.

OGCR Section I.C.3.a.6.b

The principal or first listed code for an encounter due to an insulin pump malfunction resulting in an overdose of insulin, should also be 996.57, Mechanical complication due to insulin pump, followed by 962.3, Poisoning by insulins and antidiabetic agents, and the appropriate diabetes mellitus code based on documentation.

996.59 Due to other implant and internal device, not elsewhere classified
Nonabsorbable surgical material NOS
Prosthetic implant in:
    bile duct
    chin
    orbit of eye
Coding Clinic: 1999, Q2, P13-14; 1997, Q3, P7; 1994, Q3, P7x2

● **996.6 Infection and inflammatory reaction due to internal prosthetic device, implant, and graft**
Infection (causing obstruction) due to (presence of) any device, implant, and graft classifiable to 996.0–996.5
Inflammation due to (presence of) any device, implant, and graft classifiable to 996.0–996.5

Use additional code to identify specified infections
Coding Clinic: 2008, Q2, P9-10; 1987, Jan-Feb, P14-15

996.60 Due to unspecified device, implant and graft

996.61 Due to cardiac device, implant and graft
Cardiac pacemaker or defibrillator:
    electrode(s), lead(s)
    pulse generator
    subcutaneous pocket
Coronary artery bypass graft
Heart valve prosthesis

996.62 Due to vascular device, implant and graft
Arterial graft
Arteriovenous fistula or shunt
Infusion pump
Vascular catheter (arterial) (dialysis) (peripheral venous)

Excludes *infection due to:*
central venous catheter (999.31)
Hickman catheter (999.31)
peripherally inserted central catheter (PICC) (999.31)
portacath (port-a-cath) (999.31)
triple lumen catheter (999.31)
umbilical venous catheter (999.31)
Coding Clinic: 2007, Q4, P84-86; 2004, Q2, P16; Q1, P5; 2003, Q4, P111-112; Q2, P7-8; 1994, Q2, P13

996.63 Due to nervous system device, implant and graft
Electrodes implanted in brain
Peripheral nerve graft
Spinal canal catheter
Ventricular (communicating) shunt (catheter)

996.64 Due to indwelling urinary catheter

Use additional code to identify specified infections, such as:
    cystitis (595.0–595.9)
    sepsis (038.0–038.9)
Coding Clinic: 1993, Q3, P6

996.65 Due to other genitourinary device, implant and graft
Intrauterine contraceptive device
Coding Clinic: 2000, Q1, P15-16

996.66 Due to internal joint prosthesis

Use additional code to identify infected prosthetic joint (V43.60–V43.69)
Coding Clinic: 2008, Q2, P3-5x3; 2007, Q2, P8-9; 2005, Q4, P110-112; 1991, Q2, P18

996.67 Due to other internal orthopedic device, implant and graft
Bone growth stimulator (electrode)
Internal fixation device (pin) (rod) (screw)

996.68 Due to peritoneal dialysis catheter
Exit-site infection or inflammation
Coding Clinic: 2001, Q2, P11; 1998, Q4, P55

996.69 Due to other internal prosthetic device, implant, and graft
Breast prosthesis
Ocular lens prosthesis
Prosthetic orbital implant
Coding Clinic: 2008, Q2, P9-11; 2003, Q4, P108; 1998, Q4, P52-53

INJURY AND POISONING (800–999)

● **996.7 Other complications of internal (biological) (synthetic) prosthetic device, implant, and graft**
Complication NOS due to (presence of) any device, implant, and graft classifiable to 996.0–996.5
occlusion NOS
Embolism due to (presence of) any device, implant, and graft classifiable to 996.0–996.5
Fibrosis due to (presence of) any device, implant, and graft classifiable to 996.0–996.5
Hemorrhage due to (presence of) any device, implant, and graft classifiable to 996.0–996.5
Pain due to (presence of) any device, implant, and graft classifiable to 996.0–996.5
Stenosis due to (presence of) any device, implant, and graft classifiable to 996.0–996.5
Thrombus due to (presence of) any device, implant, and graft classifiable to 996.0–996.5

Use additional code to identify complication, such as:
pain due to presence of device, implant or graft (338.18–338.19, 338.28–338.29)
venous embolism and thrombosis (453.2–453.9) ◄

Excludes *disruption (dehiscence) of internal suture material (998.31)*
transplant rejection (996.8)
Coding Clinic: 2007, Q2, P13-15; 2004, Q2, P7-8; 1989, Q1, P9&10; 1984, Nov-Dec, P18

■**996.70 Due to unspecified device, implant, and graft**

996.71 Due to heart valve prosthesis
Coding Clinic: 2008, Q2, P9-10

996.72 Due to other cardiac device, implant, and graft
Cardiac pacemaker or defibrillator: electrode(s), lead(s)
subcutaneous pocket
Coronary artery bypass (graft)
Excludes *occlusion due to atherosclerosis (414.00–414.07)*
Coding Clinic: 2008, Q3, P10-11; 2006, Q3, P8-9, 25; 2001, Q3, P20

996.73 Due to renal dialysis device, implant, and graft
Coding Clinic: 1991, Q2, P18

■**996.74 Due to vascular device, implant, and graft**
Excludes *occlusion of biological graft due to atherosclerosis (440.30–440.32)*
Coding Clinic: 2003, Q1, P16-18x2; 2000, Q1, P10

996.75 Due to nervous system device, implant, and graft

996.76 Due to genitourinary device, implant, and graft
Coding Clinic: 2009, Q1, P13; 2000, Q1, P15-16

996.77 Due to internal joint prosthesis
Use additional code to identify prosthetic joint (V43.60–V43.69)

■**996.78 Due to other internal orthopedic device, implant, and graft**
Coding Clinic: 2003, Q2, P14

■**996.79 Due to other internal prosthetic device, implant, and graft**
Coding Clinic: 2004, Q2, P7; 2001, Q1, P8-9; 1995, Q3, P14; 1992, Q3, P4-5

● **996.8 Complications of transplanted organ**
Transplant failure or rejection

Use additional code to identify nature of complication, such as:
cytomegalovirus [CMV] infection (078.5)
graft-versus-host disease (279.50-279.53)
malignancy associated with organ transplant (199.2)
post-transplant lymphoproliferative disorder (PTLD) (238.77)
Coding Clinic: 2003, Q1, P11; 2002, Q4, P53-54; 2001, Q3, P12-13; 1993, Q2, P11; Q1, P24

OGCR Section I.C.17.f.1.a
Transplant complications other than kidney: Codes under subcategory 996.8, Complications of transplanted organ, are for use for both complications and rejection of transplanted organs. A transplant complication code is only assigned if the complication affects the function of the transplanted organ. Two codes are required to fully describe a transplant complication, the appropriate code from subcategory 996.8 and a secondary code that identifies the complication. Pre-existing conditions or conditions that develop after the transplant are not coded as complications unless they affect the function of the transplanted organs.
See I.C.18.d.3) for transplant organ removal status
See I.C.2.i for malignant neoplasm associated with transplanted organ.

■**996.80 Transplanted organ, unspecified**

996.81 Kidney
Coding Clinic: 2008, Q4, P82-83; 2003, Q3, P16-17; 1998, Q3, P6x2&7; 1994, Q3, P8; Q2, P9; 1993, Q4, P32-33; Q1, P24-25

996.82 Liver
Coding Clinic: 2008, Q4, P82-83, 97-100; 2003, Q3, P16x2&17; 1998, Q3, P4

996.83 Heart
Coding Clinic: 2003, Q3, P16; 2002, Q4, P53-54; 2001, Q3, P13-14x2; 1998, Q3, P5; 1993, Q3, P13

996.84 Lung
Coding Clinic: 2003, Q2, P12; 1998, Q3, P5

996.85 Bone marrow
Coding Clinic: 2008, Q4, P90-91

996.86 Pancreas

996.87 Intestine
Coding Clinic: 2000, Q4, P47-48

■**996.89 Other specified transplanted organ**
Coding Clinic: 1994, Q3, P5

● **996.9 Complications of reattached extremity or body part**

■**996.90 Unspecified extremity**

996.91 Forearm

996.92 Hand

996.93 Finger(s)

■**996.94 Upper extremity, other and unspecified**

996.95 Foot and toe(s)

■**996.96 Lower extremity, other and unspecified**

■**996.99 Other specified body part**

● 997   **Complications affecting specified body systems, not elsewhere classified**

Use additional code to identify complication

Excludes *the listed conditions when specified as:*
  causing shock (998.0)
  complications of:
    anesthesia:
      adverse effect (001.0–799.9, 995.0–995.8)
      in labor or delivery (668.0–668.9)
      poisoning (968.0–969.9)
    implanted device or graft (996.0–996.9)
    obstetrical procedures (669.0–669.4)
    reattached extremity (996.90–996.96)
    transplanted organ (996.80–996.89)

Coding Clinic: 1995, Q2, P7; 1993, Q2, P9-10; 1992, Q1, P13

● 997.0   **Nervous system complications**

▪ 997.00   **Nervous system complication, unspecified**

997.01   **Central nervous system complication**
  Anoxic brain damage
  Cerebral hypoxia

  Excludes *Cerebrovascular hemorrhage or infarction (997.02)*

  Coding Clinic: 2007, Q1, P22-23; 2006, Q1, P15-16

997.02   **Iatrogenic cerebrovascular infarction or hemorrhage**
  Postoperative stroke
  Coding Clinic: 2006, Q3, P6; 2004, Q2, P8-9

  OGCR Section I.C.7.c

  A cerebrovascular hemorrhage or infarction that occurs as a result of medical intervention is coded to 997.02. Documentation should clearly specify cause-and-effect relationship between the medical intervention and the cerebrovascular accident in order to assign this code. A secondary code from the code range 430-432 or from a code from subcategories 433 or 434 with a fifth digit of "1" should also be used to identify the type of hemorrhage or infarct.

▪ 997.09   **Other nervous system complications**

997.1   **Cardiac complications**
  Cardiac:
    arrest during or resulting from a procedure
    insufficiency during or resulting from a procedure
  Cardiorespiratory failure during or resulting from a procedure
  Heart failure during or resulting from a procedure

  Excludes *the listed conditions as long-term effects of cardiac surgery or due to the presence of cardiac prosthetic device (429.4)*

  Coding Clinic: 2008, Q4, P177-180; 2000, Q2, P12; 1994, Q3, P9; Q1, P20; 1993, Q4, P37, 39-43; 5th Issue, P6-7

997.2   **Peripheral vascular complications**
  Phlebitis or thrombophlebitis during or resulting from a procedure

  Excludes *the listed conditions due to:*
    implant or catheter device (996.62)
    infusion, perfusion, or transfusion (999.2)
    complications affecting blood vessels (997.71–997.79)

  Coding Clinic: 2003, Q1, P6-7; 2002, Q3, P24-27; 1993, Q1, P26

● 997.3   **Respiratory complications**

  Excludes *iatrogenic [postoperative] pneumothorax (512.1)*
    iatrogenic pulmonary embolism (415.11)
    Mendelson's syndrome in labor and delivery (668.0)
      Aspiration into the lungs of gastric contents following vomiting or regurgitation
    specified complications classified elsewhere, such as:
      adult respiratory distress syndrome (518.5)
      pulmonary edema, postoperative (518.4)
      respiratory insufficiency, acute, postoperative (518.5)
      shock lung (518.5)
      tracheostomy complications (519.00–519.09)
      transfusion related acute lung injury (TRALI) (518.7)

  Coding Clinic: 1997, Q1, P10; 1993, Q4, P 43; Q2, P9-10; Q2, P3-4; 1990, Q4, P25x2; 1989, Q1, P10

997.31   **Ventilator associated pneumonia**
  Ventilator associated pneumonitis ◀

  Use additional code to identify organism

  Coding Clinic: 2008, Q4, P148-149; 2006, Q2, P25

▪ 997.39   **Other respiratory complications**
  Mendelson's syndrome resulting from a procedure

  Pneumonia (aspiration) resulting from a procedure

997.4   **Digestive system complications**
  Complications of:
    intestinal (internal) anastomosis and bypass, not elsewhere classified, except that involving urinary tract
  Hepatic failure specified as due to a procedure
  Hepatorenal syndrome specified as due to a procedure
    Acute renal failure occurring along with cirrhosis or fulminant liver failure associated with portal hypertension
  Intestinal obstruction NOS specified as due to a procedure

  Excludes *specified gastrointestinal complications classified elsewhere, such as:*
    blind loop syndrome (579.2)
    colostomy or enterostomy complications (569.60–569.69)
    complications of intestinal pouch (569.71–569.79) ◀
    gastrojejunal ulcer (534.0–534.9)
    gastrostomy complications (536.40–536.49)
    infection of esophagostomy (530.86)
    infection of external stoma (569.61)
    mechanical complication of esophagostomy (530.87)
    pelvic peritoneal adhesions, female (614.6)
    peritoneal adhesions (568.0)
    peritoneal adhesions with obstruction (560.81)
    postcholecystectomy syndrome (576.0)
    postgastric surgery syndromes (564.2) ◀
    pouchitis (569.71) ◀
    vomiting following gastrointestinal surgery (564.3)

  Coding Clinic: 2003, Q1, P18; 2001, Q2, P4-6x2; 1999, Q3, P4-5; Q2, P14; 1997, Q3, P7; Q1, P11; 1995, Q3, P7, 16; Q2, P7; 1993, Q1, P26; 1992, Q3, P15; 1989, Q2, P15; 1988, Q1, P14; 1987, Nov-Dec, P9; 1985, Sept-Oct, P11; Mar-April, P11

INJURY AND POISONING (800–999)

997.5   Urinary complications

Complications of:
> external stoma of urinary tract
> internal anastomosis and bypass of urinary tract, including that involving intestinal tract

Oliguria or anuria specified as due to procedure

Renal (kidney):
> failure (acute) specified as due to procedure
> insufficiency (acute) specified as due to procedure
> Tubular necrosis (acute) specified as due to procedure

> **Excludes**   *specified complications classified elsewhere, such as:*
> > *postoperative stricture of:*
> > > *ureter (593.3)*
> > > *urethra (598.2)*

> Coding Clinic: 2003, Q3, P13; 1996, Q3, P10-11,15; 1995, Q4, P72-73; 1994, Q1, P20; 1992, Q1, P13; 1989, Q2, P16

● 997.6   Amputation stump complication

> **Excludes**   *admission for treatment for a current traumatic amputation - code to complicated traumatic amputation*
> > *phantom limb (syndrome) (353.6)*

> Coding Clinic: 1996, Q4, P45-46

■ 997.60   Unspecified complication

997.61   Neuroma of amputation stump

997.62   Infection (chronic)

> Use additional code to identify the organism

> Coding Clinic: 2005, Q1, P14-15; 2003, Q3, P14; 1996, Q4, P45-46

■ 997.69   Other

> Coding Clinic: 2005, Q1, P15

● 997.7   Vascular complications of other vessels

> **Excludes**   *peripheral vascular complications (997.2)*

997.71   Vascular complications of mesenteric artery

> Coding Clinic: 2001, Q4, P53

997.72   Vascular complications of renal artery

■ 997.79   Vascular complications of other vessels

● 997.9   Complications affecting other specified body systems, not elsewhere classified

> **Excludes**   *specified complications classified elsewhere, such as:*
> > *broad ligament laceration syndrome (620.6)*
> > *postartificial menopause syndrome (627.4)*
> > *postoperative stricture of vagina (623.2)*

> Coding Clinic: 1994, Q1, P16; 1993, Q4, P41-42

997.91   Hypertension

> **Excludes**   *Essential hypertension (401.0–401.9)*

■ 997.99   Other

> Vitreous touch syndrome

> Coding Clinic: 1994, Q2, P12; Q1, P17; Q1, P16-17

● 998   Other complications of procedures, NEC

998.0   Postoperative shock

Collapse NOS during or resulting from a surgical procedure

Shock (endotoxic) (hypovolemic) (septic) during or resulting from a surgical procedure

> **Excludes**   *shock:*
> > *anaphylactic due to serum (999.4)*
> > *anesthetic (995.4)*
> > *electric (994.8)*
> > *following abortion (639.5)*
> > *obstetric (669.1)*
> > *traumatic (958.4)*

● 998.1   Hemorrhage or hematoma or seroma complicating a procedure

> **Excludes**   *hemorrhage, hematoma or seroma:*
> > *complicating cesarean section or puerperal perineal wound (674.3)*
> > *due to implanted device or graft (996.70–996.79)*

> Coding Clinic: 2003, Q3, P13; 1993, Q1, P26; 1992, Q2, P15-16; 1987, Sept-Oct, P8

998.11   Hemorrhage complicating a procedure

> Coding Clinic: 2003, Q3, P13; Q1, P4; 1997, Q4, P52; Q1, P10; 1994, Q1, P19-20

998.12   Hematoma complicating a procedure

> Coding Clinic: 2006, Q3, P12; 2003, Q1, P6-7; 2002, Q3, P24-25; 1994, Q1, P20

998.13   Seroma complicating a procedure

> *Pocket of clear serous fluid that sometimes develops in the body after surgery*

> Coding Clinic: 1996, Q4, P46

998.2   Accidental puncture or laceration during a procedure

Accidental perforation by catheter or other instrument during a procedure on:
> blood vessel
> nerve
> organ

> **Excludes**   *iatrogenic [postoperative] pneumothorax (512.1)*
> > *puncture or laceration caused by implanted device intentionally left in operation wound (996.0–996.5)*
> > *specified complications classified elsewhere, such as:*
> > > *broad ligament laceration syndrome (620.6)*
> > > *dural tear (349.31)*
> > > *incidental durotomy (349.31)*
> > > *trauma from instruments during delivery (664.0–665.9)*

> Coding Clinic: 2007, Q2, P11-12; 2006, Q1, P15; 2002, Q3, P24-27; 1994, Q3, P6; 1994, Q1, P17; 1990, Q3, P17-18; 1984, Nov-Dec, P12

● **998.3 Disruption of wound**
Dehiscence of operation wound
Splitting open
Disruption of any suture materials or other closure
method
Rupture of operation wound

> **Excludes** *disruption of:*
> *amputation of stump (997.69)*
> *cesarean wound (674.1)*
> *perineal wound, puerperal (674.2)*
> Coding Clinic: 2008, Q4, P149-152; 2002, Q4, P73; 1993, Q1, P19

998.30 Disruption of wound, unspecified
Disruption of wound NOS

**998.31 Disruption of internal operation surgical
wound**
Disruption or dehiscence of closure of:
fascia, superficial or muscular
internal organ
muscle or muscle flap
ribs or rib cage
skull or craniotomy
sternum or sternotomy
tendon or ligament
Deep disruption or dehiscence of
operation wound NOS

> **Excludes** *complications of internal*
> *anastomosis of:*
> *gastrointestinal tract (997.4)*
> *urinary tract (997.5)*

**998.32 Disruption of external operation (surgical)
wound**
Disruption of operation wound NOS
Disruption or dehiscence of closure of:
cornea
mucosa
skin
subcutaneous tissue
Full-thickness skin disruption or
dehiscence
Superficial disruption or dehiscence
of operation wound
Coding Clinic: 2006, Q1, P8; 2005, Q1, P11; 2003, Q4,
P104-107

**998.33 Disruption of traumatic injury wound
repair**
Disruption or dehiscence of closure of
traumatic laceration (external)
(internal)

**998.4 Foreign body accidentally left during a
procedure**
Adhesions due to foreign body accidentally left
in operative wound or body cavity during a
procedure
Obstruction due to foreign body accidentally left
in operative wound or body cavity during a
procedure
Perforation due to foreign body accidentally left
in operative wound or body cavity during a
procedure

> **Excludes** *obstruction or perforation caused by*
> *implanted device intentionally left in*
> *body (996.0–996.5)*
> Coding Clinic: 2009, Q1, P13; 1989, Q1, P9

● **998.5 Postoperative infection**

> **Excludes** *bleb associated endophthalmitis (379.63)*
> *infection due to:*
> *implanted device (996.60–996.69)*
> *infusion, perfusion, or transfusion*
> *(999.31–999.39)*
> *postoperative obstetrical wound infection*
> *(674.3)*
> Coding Clinic: 1996, Q4, P45-46; 1995, Q2, P7; 1994, Q3, P6; 1987,
> Jan-Feb, P13-14

998.51 Infected postoperative seroma
Use additional code to identify organism
Coding Clinic: 1996, Q4, P46

■ **998.59 Other postoperative infection**
Abscess: postoperative
intra-abdominal postoperative
stitch postoperative
subphrenic postoperative
wound postoperative
Septicemia postoperative

Use additional code to identify infection
Coding Clinic: 2006, Q2, P23-24; 2004, Q4, P75-76; 2003,
Q4, P104-107; 1995, Q3, P5; Q2, P7, 11; 1993,
Q1, P19

> **OGCR** Section I.C.1.b.10.b
> Sepsis due to postprocedural infection:
> In cases of postprocedural sepsis, the
> complication code, such as code 998.59,
> Other postoperative infection, or 674.3x,
> Other complications of obstetrical surgical
> wounds should be coded first followed
> by the appropriate sepsis codes (systemic
> infection code and either code 995.91 or
> 995.92). An additional code(s) for any acute
> organ dysfunction should also be assigned
> for cases of severe sepsis.

998.6 Persistent postoperative fistula
Coding Clinic: 1987, Jan-Feb, P14

**998.7 Acute reaction to foreign substance accidentally left
during a procedure**
Peritonitis:
aseptic
chemical

● **998.8 Other specified complications of procedures, not
elsewhere classified**
Coding Clinic: 1993, 5th Issue, P8, 15; 1989, Q1, P9; 1987,
Jan-Feb, P13

**998.81 Emphysema (subcutaneous) (surgical)
resulting from a procedure**

**998.82 Cataract fragments in eye following cataract
surgery**

998.83 Non-healing surgical wound
Coding Clinic: 1996, Q4, P47

■ **998.89 Other specified complications**
Coding Clinic: 2009, Q2, P13x2, 15; 2006, Q3, P9-10; 2005,
Q3, P16-17; 1999, Q3, P13; 1998, Q2, P16

■ **998.9 Unspecified complication of procedure, not
elsewhere classified**
Postoperative complication NOS

> **Excludes** *complication NOS of obstetrical surgery or*
> *procedure (669.4)*
> Coding Clinic: 1993, Q4, P41-42

INJURY AND POISONING (800–999)

● **999   Complications of medical care, not elsewhere classified**

> **Includes**   complications, not elsewhere classified, of:
> > dialysis (hemodialysis) (peritoneal) (renal)
> > extracorporeal circulation
> > hyperalimentation therapy
> > immunization
> > infusion
> > inhalation therapy
> > injection
> > inoculation
> > perfusion
> > transfusion
> > vaccination
> > ventilation therapy

> Use additional code, where applicable, to identify specific complication

> **Excludes**   *specified complications classified elsewhere such as:*
> > *complications of implanted device (996.0–996.9)*
> > *contact dermatitis due to drugs (692.3)*
> > *dementia dialysis (294.8)*
> > > *transient (293.9)*
> > *dialysis disequilibrium syndrome (276.0–276.9)*
> > *poisoning and toxic effects of drugs and chemicals (960.0–989.9)*
> > *postvaccinal encephalitis (323.51)*
> > *water and electrolyte imbalance (276.0–276.9)*

999.0   Generalized vaccinia

> **Excludes**   *vaccinia not from vaccine (051.02)*

999.1   Air embolism

> Air embolism to any site following infusion, perfusion, or transfusion

> **Excludes**   *embolism specified as:*
> > *complicating:*
> > > *abortion (634–638 with .6, 639.6)*
> > > *ectopic or molar pregnancy (639.6)*
> > > *pregnancy, childbirth, or the puerperium (673.0)*
> > *due to implanted device (996.7)*
> > *traumatic (958.0)*

■ **999.2   Other vascular complications**

> Phlebitis following infusion, perfusion, or transfusion
> Thromboembolism following infusion, perfusion, or transfusion
> Thrombophlebitis following infusion, perfusion, or transfusion

> **Excludes**   *extravasation of vesicant drugs (999.81, 999.82)*
> > *the listed conditions when specified as:*
> > > *due to implanted device (996.61–996.62, 996.72–996.74)*
> > > *postoperative NOS (997.2, 997.71–997.79)*

> Coding Clinic: 1997, Q2, P5

● **999.3   Other infection**

> Infection following infusion, injection, transfusion, or vaccination
> Sepsis following infusion, injection, transfusion, or vaccination
> Septicemia following infusion, injection, transfusion, or vaccination

> Use additional code to identify the specified infection, such as:
> > septicemia (038.0–038.9)

> **Excludes**   *the listed conditions when specified as:*
> > *due to implanted device (996.60–996.69)*
> > *postoperative NOS (998.51–998.59)*

> Coding Clinic: 2001, Q2, P11-12; 1987, Jan-Feb, P14-15

999.31   Infection due to central venous catheter

> Catheter-related bloodstream infection (CRBSI) NOS
> Infection due to:
> > Hickman catheter
> > peripherally inserted central catheter (PICC)
> > portacath (port-a-cath)
> > triple lumen catheter
> > umbilical venous catheter

> **Excludes**   *infection due to:*
> > *arterial catheter (996.62)*
> > *catheter NOS (996.69)*
> > *peripheral venous catheter (996.62)*
> > *urinary catheter (996.64)*

> Coding Clinic: 2008, Q4, P69-73, 192-193; 2007, Q4, P96-97

999.39   Infection following other infusion, injection, transfusion, or vaccination

999.4   Anaphylactic shock due to serum

> Anaphylactic reaction due to serum

> **Excludes**   *shock:*
> > *allergic NOS (995.0)*
> > *anaphylactic:*
> > > *NOS (995.0)*
> > > *due to drugs and chemicals (995.0)*

■ **999.5   Other serum reaction**

> Intoxication by serum
> Protein sickness
> Serum rash
> Serum sickness
> Urticaria due to serum

> **Excludes**   *serum hepatitis (070.2–070.3)*

999.6   ABO incompatibility reaction

> Incompatible blood transfusion
> Reaction to blood group incompatibility in infusion or transfusion

> **Excludes**   *minor blood group antigens reactions (Duffy) (E) (K(ell)) (Kidd) (Lewis) (M) (N) (P) (S) (999.89)*   ◄

999.7   Rh incompatibility reaction

> Reactions due to Rh factor in infusion or transfusion

◄ New   ◄═ Revised   ~~deleted~~ Deleted   ● Use Additional Digit(s)   ■ Nonspecific Code
● Not first-listed DX   OGCR Official Guidelines   Coding Clinic   Excludes   Includes   Use additional   Code first   Omit code

● **999.8 Other infusion and transfusion reaction**

     Excludes *postoperative shock (998.0)*
                     transfusion related acute lung injury
                           (TRALI) (518.7)
       Coding Clinic: 2008, Q4, P152-155; 2000, Q3, P9

     999.81 Extravasation of vesicant chemotherapy
           Infiltration of vesicant chemotherapy
           Coding Clinic: 2008, Q4, P152-155

     999.82 Extravasation of other vesicant agent
           Infiltration of other vesicant agent

■ **999.88 Other infusion reaction**

■ **999.89 Other transfusion reaction**
           Transfusion reaction NOS

           Use additional code to identify
               graft-versus-host reaction (279.5)

■ **999.9 Other and unspecified complications of medical care, not elsewhere classified**
     Complications, not elsewhere classified, of:
       electroshock therapy   ultrasound therapy
       inhalation therapy   ventilation therapy
     Unspecified misadventure of medical care

     Excludes *unspecified complication of:*
                 phototherapy (990)
                 radiation therapy (990)
                 ventilator associated pneumonia (997.31)
     Coding Clinic: 2006, Q2, P25; 2003, Q1, P19; 1997, Q2, P5; 1994, Q3, P9

INJURY AND POISONING (800–999)

SUPPLEMENTARY CLASSIFICATION OF FACTORS INFLUENCING HEALTH STATUS AND CONTACT WITH HEALTH SERVICES (V01–V89)

This classification is provided to deal with occasions when circumstances other than a disease or injury classifiable to categories 001–999 (the main part of ICD) are recorded as "diagnoses" or "problems." This can arise mainly in three ways:

a) When a person who is not currently sick encounters the health services for some specific purpose, such as to act as a donor of an organ or tissue, to receive prophylactic vaccination, or to discuss a problem which is in itself not a disease or injury. This will be a fairly rare occurrence among hospital inpatients, but will be relatively more common among hospital outpatients and patients of family practitioners, health clinics, etc.

b) When a person with a known disease or injury, whether it is current or resolving, encounters the health care system for a specific treatment of that disease or injury (e.g., dialysis for renal disease; chemotherapy for malignancy; cast change).

c) When some circumstance or problem is present which influences the person's health status but is not in itself a current illness or injury. Such factors may be elicited during population surveys, when the person may or may not be currently sick, or be recorded as an additional factor to be borne in mind when the person is receiving care for some current illness or injury classifiable to categories 001–999.

In the latter circumstances the V code should be used only as a supplementary code and should not be the one selected for use in primary, single cause tabulations. Examples of these circumstances are a personal history of certain diseases, or a person with an artificial heart valve in situ.

OGCR Section I.C.18.b

V codes are for use in any healthcare setting as either a first listed (principal diagnosis code in the inpatient setting) or secondary code, depending on the circumstances of the encounter. Certain V codes may only be used as first listed, others only as secondary codes.

PERSONS WITH POTENTIAL HEALTH HAZARDS RELATED TO COMMUNICABLE DISEASES (V01–V06)

Excludes *family history of infectious and parasitic diseases (V18.8)*
personal history of infectious and parasitic diseases (V12.0)

OGCR Section I.C.18.d.1

Category V01 indicates contact with or exposure to communicable diseases. These codes are for patients who do not show any sign or symptom of a disease but have been exposed to it by close personal contact with an infected individual or are in an area where a disease is epidemic. These codes may be used as a first listed code to explain an encounter for testing, or, more commonly, as a secondary code to identify a potential risk.

● **V01 Contact with or exposure to communicable diseases**
Coding Clinic: 2001, Q1, P10

V01.0 Cholera
Conditions classifiable to 001

V01.1 Tuberculosis
Conditions classifiable to 010–018

V01.2 Poliomyelitis
Conditions classifiable to 045

V01.3 Smallpox
Conditions classifiable to 050

V01.4 Rubella
Conditions classifiable to 056

V01.5 Rabies
Conditions classifiable to 071

V01.6 Venereal diseases
Conditions classifiable to 090–099
Coding Clinic: 2007, Q4, P124-125x2

● **V01.7 Other viral diseases**
Conditions classifiable to 042–078, and V08, except as above

V01.71 Varicella

V01.79 Other viral diseases
Coding Clinic: 1992, Q2, P11

● **V01.8 Other communicable diseases**
Conditions classifiable to 001–136, except as above

V01.81 Anthrax

V01.82 Exposure to SARS-associated coronavirus
Coding Clinic: 2003, Q4, P46-48

V01.83 Escherichia coli (E. coli)

V01.84 Meningococcus

V01.89 Other communicable diseases

V01.9 Unspecified communicable disease

● **V02 Carrier or suspected carrier of infectious diseases**
Includes Colonization status

V02.0 Cholera

V02.1 Typhoid

V02.2 Amebiasis

V02.3 Other gastrointestinal pathogens

V02.4 Diphtheria

● **V02.5 Other specified bacterial diseases**

V02.51 Group B streptococcus
Coding Clinic: 2006, Q3, P14; 2002, Q1, P14-15; 1998, Q4, P56; 1994, Q3, P4

V02.52 Other streptococcus

V02.53 Methicillin susceptible Staphylococcus aureus
MSSA colonization
Coding Clinic: 2008, Q4, P69-73

V02.54 Methicillin resistant Staphylococcus aureus
MRSA colonization
Coding Clinic: 2008, Q4, P69-73

V02.59 Other specified bacterial diseases
Meningococcal
Staphylococcal

● **V02.6 Viral hepatitis**

V02.60 Viral hepatitis carrier, unspecified

V02.61 Hepatitis B carrier

V02.62 Hepatitis C carrier

V02.69 Other viral hepatitis carrier

V02.7 Gonorrhea

V02.8 Other venereal diseases

V02.9 Other specified infectious organism
Coding Clinic: 1994, Q4, P36; 1993, Q1, P22

New   Revised   deleted Deleted   ● Use Additional Digit(s)   Nonspecific Code   ❶ First Listed   First Listed or Additional
❷ Additional Only   Not first-listed DX   OGCR Official Guidelines   Coding Clinic   Excludes   Includes   Use additional   Code first

V01-V89

OGCR Section I.C.18.d.2
Categories V03-V06 are for encounters for inoculations and vaccinations. They indicate that a patient is being seen to receive a prophylactic inoculation against a disease. The injection itself must be represented by the appropriate procedure code. A code from V03-V06 may be used as a secondary code if the inoculation is given as a routine part of preventive health care, such as a well-baby visit.

● V03   Need for prophylactic vaccination and inoculation against bacterial diseases

> **Excludes**   *vaccination not carried out (V64.00–V64.09)*
> *vaccines against combinations of diseases (V06.0–V06.9)*

🦠 V03.0   Cholera alone

🦠 V03.1   Typhoid-paratyphoid alone [TAB]

🦠 V03.2   Tuberculosis [BCG]

🦠 V03.3   Plague

🦠 V03.4   Tularemia

🦠 V03.5   Diphtheria alone

🦠 V03.6   Pertussis alone

🦠 V03.7   Tetanus toxoid alone

● V03.8   Other specified vaccinations against single bacterial diseases

     🦠 V03.81   Hemophilus influenza, type B [Hib]

     🦠 V03.82   Streptococcus pneumoniae [pneumococcus]

     🦠 V03.89   Other specified vaccination
          Coding Clinic: 2000, Q2, P9

🦠 V03.9   Unspecified single bacterial disease

● V04   Need for prophylactic vaccination and inoculation against certain diseases

> **Excludes**   *vaccines against combinations of diseases (V06.0–V06.9)*

🦠 V04.0   Poliomyelitis

🦠 V04.1   Smallpox

🦠 V04.2   Measles alone

🦠 V04.3   Rubella alone

🦠 V04.4   Yellow fever

🦠 V04.5   Rabies

🦠 V04.6   Mumps alone

🦠 V04.7   Common cold

● V04.8   Other viral diseases

     🦠 V04.81   Influenza

     🦠 V04.82   Respiratory syncytial virus (RSV)
          Coding Clinic: 2009, Q1, P5; 2001, Q1, P4

     🦠 V04.89   Other viral diseases
          Coding Clinic: 2007, Q2, P11

● V05   Need for prophylactic vaccination and inoculation against single diseases

> **Excludes**   *vaccines against combinations of diseases (V06.0–V06.9)*

🦠 V05.0   Arthropod-borne viral encephalitis

🦠 V05.1   Other arthropod-borne viral diseases

🦠 V05.2   Leishmaniasis

🦠 V05.3   Viral hepatitis

🦠 V05.4   Varicella
        Chicken pox

🦠 V05.8   Other specified disease
        Coding Clinic: 2001, Q1, P4; 1991, Q3, P20-21

🦠 V05.9   Unspecified single disease

● V06   Need for prophylactic vaccination and inoculation against combinations of diseases

> **Note:** Use additional single vaccination codes from categories V03–V05 to identify any vaccinations not included in a combination code.

🦠 V06.0   Cholera with typhoid-paratyphoid [cholera TAB]

🦠 V06.1   Diphtheria-tetanus-pertussis, combined [DTP] [DTaP]
        Coding Clinic: 1998, Q3, P13-14

🦠 V06.2   Diphtheria-tetanus-pertussis with typhoid-paratyphoid [DTP TAB]

🦠 V06.3   Diphtheria-tetanus-pertussis with poliomyelitis [DTP+polio]

🦠 V06.4   Measles-mumps-rubella [MMR]

🦠 V06.5   Tetanus-diphtheria [Td] [DT]

🦠 V06.6   Streptococcus pneumoniae [pneumococcus] and influenza

🦠 V06.8   Other combinations

> **Excludes**   *multiple single vaccination codes (V03.0–V05.9)*
> Coding Clinic: 1994, Q1, P19

🦠 V06.9   Unspecified combined vaccine

PERSONS WITH NEED FOR ISOLATION, OTHER POTENTIAL HEALTH HAZARDS AND PROPHYLACTIC MEASURES (V07–V09)

● V07   Need for isolation and other prophylactic measures

> **Excludes**   *prophylactic organ removal (V50.41–V50.49)*

🦠 V07.0   Isolation
        Admission to protect the individual from his surroundings or for isolation of individual after contact with infectious diseases

🦠 V07.1   Desensitization to allergens

🦠 V07.2   Prophylactic immunotherapy
        Administration of:
           antivenin
           immune sera [gamma globulin]
           RhoGAM
           tetanus antitoxin

N Newborn Age: 0   **P** Pediatric Age: 0–17   **M** Maternity Age: 12–55   **A** Adult Age: 15–124   ♀ Females Only   ♂ Males Only   **1107**

V01-V89

● V07.3   **Other prophylactic chemotherapy**

   V07.31   **Prophylactic fluoride administration**

   V07.39   **Other prophylactic chemotherapy**

      Excludes   *maintenance chemotherapy following disease (V58.11)*

❷ V07.4   Hormone replacement therapy (postmenopausal) ♀

● V07.5   **Prophylactic use of agents affecting estrogen receptors and estrogen levels**

      Code first, if applicable:

      malignant neoplasm of breast (174.0-174.9, 175.0-175.9)

      malignant neoplasm of prostate (185)

      Use additional code, if applicable, to identify:

      estrogen receptor positive status (V86.0)

      family history of breast cancer (V16.3)

      genetic susceptibility to cancer (V84.01-V84.09)

      personal history of breast cancer (V10.3)

      personal history of prostate cancer (V10.46)

      postmenopausal status (V49.81)

      Excludes   *hormone replacement therapy (postmenopausal) (V07.4)*

   ❷ V07.51   Prophylactic use of selective estrogen receptor modulators (SERMs)

      Prophylactic use of:

      raloxifene (Evista)

      tamoxifen (Nolvadex)

      toremifene (Fareston)

   ❷ V07.52   Prophylactic use of aromatase inhibitors

      Prophylactic use of:

      anastrozole (Arimidex)

      ~~exemestar~~ exemestane (Aromasin) ◀▥

      letrozole (Femara)

   ❷ ▪V07.59   Prophylactic use of other agents affecting estrogen receptors and estrogen levels

      Prophylactic use of:

      estrogen receptor downregulators

      fulvestrant (Faslodex)

      gonadotropin-releasing hormone (GnRH) agonist

      goserelin acetate (Zoladex)

      leuprolide acetate (leuprorelin) (Lupron)

      megestrol acetate (Megace)

   V07.8   **Other specified prophylactic measure**

      Coding Clinic: 1992, Q1, P11

   ▪V07.9   **Unspecified prophylactic measure**

OGCR Section I.C.2.d

V08, Asymptomatic human immunodeficiency virus [HIV] infection, is to be applied when the patient without any documentation of symptoms is listed as being "HIV positive," "known HIV," "HIV test positive," or similar terminology. Do not use this code if the term "AIDS" is used or if the patient is treated for any HIV-related illness or is described as having any condition(s) resulting from HIV positive status; use 042 in these cases.

V08   Asymptomatic human immunodeficiency virus [HIV] infection status

      HIV positive NOS

      Note: This code is ONLY to be used when NO HIV infection symptoms or conditions are present. If any HIV infection symptoms or conditions are present, see code 042.

      Excludes   *AIDS (042)*

         human immunodeficiency virus [HIV] disease (042)

         exposure to HIV (V01.79)

         nonspecific serologic evidence of HIV (795.71)

         symptomatic human immunodeficiency virus [HIV] infection (042)

      Coding Clinic: 2004, Q2, P11; 1999, Q2, P8

● V09   **Infection with drug-resistant microorganisms**

      Note: This category is intended for use as an additional code for infectious conditions classified elsewhere to indicate the presence of drug-resistance of the infectious organism.

      Coding Clinic: 2008, Q4, P69-73

   ❷ V09.0   Infection with microorganisms resistant to penicillins

      Coding Clinic: 2006, Q2, P16-17; 2003, Q4, P104-107; 1994, Q3, P4

   ❷ V09.1   Infection with microorganisms resistant to cephalosporins and other B-lactam antibiotics

   ❷ V09.2   Infection with microorganisms resistant to macrolides

   ❷ V09.3   Infection with microorganisms resistant to tetracyclines

   ❷ V09.4   Infection with microorganisms resistant to aminoglycosides

   ● V09.5   **Infection with microorganisms resistant to quinolones and fluoroquinolones**

      ❷ V09.50   Without mention of resistance to multiple quinolones and fluoroquinoles

      ❷ V09.51   With resistance to multiple quinolones and fluoroquinoles

   ❷ V09.6   Infection with microorganisms resistant to sulfonamides

   ● V09.7   **Infection with microorganisms resistant to other specified antimycobacterial agents**

      Excludes   *Amikacin (V09.4)*

         Kanamycin (V09.4)

         Streptomycin [SM] (V09.4)

      ❷ V09.70   Without mention of resistance to multiple antimycobacterial agents

      ❷ V09.71   With resistance to multiple antimycobacterial agents

---

◀ New   ◀▥ Revised   ~~deleted~~ Deleted   ● Use Additional Digit(s)   ▪ Nonspecific Code   ❶ First Listed   First Listed or Additional

❷ Additional Only   ● Not first-listed DX   **OGCR** Official Guidelines   Coding Clinic   Excludes   Includes   Use additional   Code first

● **V09.8 Infection with microorganisms resistant to other specified drugs**

    Vancomycin (glycopeptide) intermediate staphylococcus aureus (VISA/GISA)

    Vancomycin (glycopeptide) resistant enterococcus (VRE)

    Vancomycin (glycopeptide) resistant staphylococcus aureus (VRSA/GRSA)

    ❷ **V09.80 Without mention of resistance to multiple drugs**

    ❷ **V09.81 With resistance to multiple drugs**

● **V09.9 Infection with drug-resistant microorganisms, unspecified**

    Drug resistance NOS

    ❷ **V09.90 Without mention of multiple drug resistance**

    ❷ **V09.91 With multiple drug resistance**

    Multiple drug resistance NOS

PERSONS WITH POTENTIAL HEALTH HAZARDS RELATED TO PERSONAL AND FAMILY HISTORY (V10–V19)

Excludes *obstetric patients where the possibility that the fetus might be affected is the reason for observation or management during pregnancy (655.0–655.9)*

OGCR Section I.C.2.d

When a primary malignancy has been previously excised or eradicated from its site and there is no further treatment directed to that site and there is no evidence of any existing primary malignancy, a code from category V10 should be used to indicate the former site of the malignancy. Any mention of extension, invasion, or metastasis to another site is coded as a secondary malignant neoplasm to that site. The secondary site may be the principal or first-listed with the V10 code used as a secondary code.

● **V10 Personal history of malignant neoplasm**

~~*Code first any continuing functional activity, such as:*~~
   ~~carcinoid syndrome (259.2)~~
   Coding Clinic: 1994, Q2, P8

OGCR Section I.C.18.d.3

Personal history codes explain a patient's past medical condition that no longer exists and is not receiving any treatment, but that has the potential for recurrence, and therefore may require continued monitoring.

● **V10.0 Gastrointestinal tract**

    History of conditions classifiable to 140–159

    Excludes *personal history of malignant carcinoid tumor (V10.91)* ◀
            personal history of malignant neuroendocrine tumor (V10.91) ◀

    🐾**V10.00 Gastrointestinal tract, unspecified**

    🐾**V10.01 Tongue**

    🐾**V10.02 Other and unspecified oral cavity and pharynx**

    🐾**V10.03 Esophagus**

    🐾**V10.04 Stomach**

    🐾**V10.05 Large intestine**
        Coding Clinic: 1999, Q3, P7-8; 1995, Q1, P3-4

    🐾**V10.06 Rectum, rectosigmoid junction, and anus**

    🐾**V10.07 Liver**

    🐾**V10.09 Other**
        Coding Clinic: 2003, Q4, P111

● **V10.1 Trachea, bronchus, and lung**

    History of conditions classifiable to 162

    Excludes *personal history of malignant carcinoid tumor (V10.91)* ◀
            personal history of malignant neuroendocrine tumor (V10.91) ◀

    🐾**V10.11 Bronchus and lung**

    🐾**V10.12 Trachea**

● **V10.2 Other respiratory and intrathoracic organs**

    History of conditions classifiable to 160, 161, 163–165

    🐾**V10.20 Respiratory organ, unspecified**

    🐾**V10.21 Larynx**
        Coding Clinic: 2003, Q4, P108,110

    🐾**V10.22 Nasal cavities, middle ear, and accessory sinuses**

    🐾**V10.29 Other**

🐾● **V10.3 Breast**

    History of conditions classifiable to 174 and 175
    Coding Clinic: 2007, Q3, P4; Q1, P3-8; 2003, Q2, P3-5; 2001, Q4, P66; 1997, Q4, P50; 1995, Q4, P53; 1990, Q1, P21

● **V10.4 Genital organs**

    History of conditions classifiable to 179–187

    🐾**V10.40 Female genital organ, unspecified ♀**

    🐾**V10.41 Cervix uteri ♀**
        Coding Clinic: 2007, Q4, P99-101

    🐾**V10.42 Other parts of uterus ♀**

    🐾**V10.43 Ovary ♀**

    🐾**V10.44 Other female genital organs ♀**

    🐾**V10.45 Male genital organ, unspecified ♂**

    🐾**V10.46 Prostate ♂**
        Coding Clinic: 2009, Q1, P5; 1994, Q2, P12; 1984, May-June, P10

    🐾**V10.47 Testis ♂**

    🐾**V10.48 Epididymis ♂**

    🐾**V10.49 Other male genital organs ♂**

● **V10.5 Urinary organs**

    History of conditions classifiable to 188 and 189
    Coding Clinic: 1995, Q2, P8

    🐾**V10.50 Urinary organ, unspecified**

    🐾**V10.51 Bladder**
        Coding Clinic: 1995, Q2, P8;1985, July-Aug, P16

    🐾**V10.52 Kidney**

        Excludes *renal pelvis (V10.53)*
        Coding Clinic: 2004, Q2, P4

    🐾**V10.53 Renal pelvis**

    🐾**V10.59 Other**

● **V10.6 Leukemia**

    Conditions classifiable to 204–208

    Excludes *leukemia in remission (204–208)*

    Coding Clinic: 1992, Q2, P13; 1985, May-June, P8-9

    🐾**V10.60 Leukemia, unspecified**

    🐾**V10.61 Lymphoid leukemia**

    🐾**V10.62 Myeloid leukemia**

    🐾**V10.63 Monocytic leukemia**

    🐾**V10.69 Other**

N Newborn Age: 0   **P** Pediatric Age: 0–17   **M** Maternity Age: 12–55   **A** Adult Age: 15–124   ♀ Females Only   ♂ Males Only   **1109**

V01-V89

● **V10.7 Other lymphatic and hematopoietic neoplasms**
Conditions classifiable to 200–203

> **Excludes** *listed conditions in 200–203 in remission*
> Coding Clinic: 1985, May-June, P8-9

🔲 **V10.71 Lymphosarcoma and reticulosarcoma**

🔲 **V10.72 Hodgkin's disease**

🔲 **V10.79 Other**

● **V10.8 Personal history of malignant neoplasm of other sites**
History of conditions classifiable to 170–173, 190–195

> **Excludes** *personal history of malignant carcinoid tumor (V10.91)* ◄
> *personal history of malignant neuroendocrine tumor (V10.91)* ◄

🔲 **V10.81 Bone**
Coding Clinic: 2003, Q2, P13

🔲 **V10.82 Malignant melanoma of skin**

🔲 **V10.83 Other malignant neoplasm of skin**

🔲 **V10.84 Eye**

🔲 **V10.85 Brain**
Coding Clinic: 2001, Q1, P6-7

🔲 **V10.86 Other parts of nervous system**

> **Excludes** *peripheral, sympathetic, and parasympathetic nerves (V10.89)*

🔲 **V10.87 Thyroid**

🔲 **V10.88 Other endocrine glands and related structures**

🔲 **V10.89 Other**

● **V10.9 Other and U̶unspecified personal history of malignant neoplasm**

🔲 **V10.90 Personal history of unspecified malignant neoplasm** ◄
Personal history of malignant neoplasm NOS ◄

> **Excludes** *personal history of malignant carcinoid tumor (V10.91)* ◄
> *personal history of malignant neuroendocrine tumor (V10.91)* ◄
> *personal history of Merkel cell carcinoma (V10.91)* ◄

🔲 **V10.91 Personal history of malignant neuroendocrine tumor** ◄
Personal history of malignant carcinoid tumor NOS ◄
Personal history of malignant neuroendocrine tumor NOS ◄
Personal history of Merkel cell carcinoma NOS ◄

> *Code first any continuing functional activity, such as:*
> carcinoid syndrome (259.2) ◄

● **V11 Personal history of mental disorder**

🔲 **V11.0 Schizophrenia**

> **Excludes** *that in remission (295.0–295.9 with fifth-digit 5)*
> Coding Clinic: 1995, Q3, P6

🔲 **V11.1 Affective disorders**
Personal history of manic-depressive psychosis

> **Excludes** *that in remission (296.0–296.6 with fifth-digit 5, 6)*

🔲 **V11.2 Neurosis**

🔲 **V11.3 Alcoholism**

🔲 **V11.8 Other mental disorders**

🔲 **V11.9 Unspecified mental disorder**

● **V12 Personal history of certain other diseases**
Coding Clinic: 2005, Q4, P94-100; 1992, Q3, P11

● **V12.0 Infectious and parasitic diseases**

> **Excludes** *personal history of infectious diseases specific to a body system*

🔲 **V12.00 Unspecified infectious and parasitic disease**

🔲 **V12.01 Tuberculosis**

🔲 **V12.02 Poliomyelitis**

🔲 **V12.03 Malaria**

🔲 **V12.04 Methicillin resistant Staphylococcus aureus**
MRSA
Coding Clinic: 2008, Q4, P69-73

🔲 **V12.09 Other**

🔲 **V12.1 Nutritional deficiency**

🔲 **V12.2 Endocrine, metabolic, and immunity disorders**

> **Excludes** *history of allergy (V14.0–V14.9, V15.01–V15.09)*
> Coding Clinic: 2007, Q3, P5-6

🔲 **V12.3 Diseases of blood and blood-forming organs**

● **V12.4 Disorders of nervous system and sense organs**

🔲 **V12.40 Unspecified disorder of nervous system and sense organs**

🔲 **V12.41 Benign neoplasm of the brain**

🔲 **V12.42 Infections of the central nervous system**
Encephalitis
Meningitis

🔲 **V12.49 Other disorders of nervous system and sense organs**
Coding Clinic: 1998, Q4, P59-60

● **V12.5 Diseases of circulatory system**

> **Excludes** *old myocardial infarction (412)*
> *postmyocardial infarction syndrome (411.0)*

🔲 **V12.50 Unspecified circulatory disease**

🔲 **V12.51 Venous thrombosis and embolism**
Pulmonary embolism
Coding Clinic: 2006, Q3, P12; 2003, Q4, P108; 2002, Q1, P15-16

🔲 **V12.52 Thrombophlebitis**

🔲 **V12.53 Sudden cardiac arrest**
Sudden cardiac death successfully resuscitated
Coding Clinic: 2007, Q4, P99-101

◄ New   ⬅ Revised   ~~deleted~~ Deleted   ● Use Additional Digit(s)   🔲 Nonspecific Code   ❶ First Listed   🔲 First Listed or Additional
❷ Additional Only   ● Not first-listed DX   OGCR Official Guidelines   Coding Clinic   Excludes   Includes   Use additional   Code first

V12.54 Transient ischemic attack (TIA), and cerebral infarction without residual deficits
Prolonged reversible ischemic neurological deficit (PRIND)
Reversible ischemic neurologic deficit (RIND)
Stroke NOS without residual deficits

> **Excludes** *history of traumatic brain injury (V15.52)*
> *late effects of cerebrovascular disease (438.0–438.9)*

Coding Clinic: 2007, Q4, P99-101; 2007, Q2, P3

OGCR Section I.C.7.d.3
Assign code V12.54, Transient ischemic attack (TIA), and cerebral infarction without residual deficits (and not a code from category 438) as an additional code for history of cerebrovascular disease when no neurologic deficits are present.

V12.59 Other
Coding Clinic: 2007, Q2, P3; 1997, Q4, P35-37

● **V12.6 Diseases of respiratory system**
> **Excludes** *tuberculosis (V12.01)*

V12.60 Unspecified disease of respiratory system

V12.61 Pneumonia (recurrent)

V12.69 Other diseases of respiratory system

● **V12.7 Diseases of digestive system**
Coding Clinic: 1995, Q1, P3; 1992, Q3, P11; 1989, Q2, P16

V12.70 Unspecified digestive disease

V12.71 Peptic ulcer disease

V12.72 Colonic polyps
Coding Clinic: 2002, Q3, P14-15

V12.79 Other

● **V13 Personal history of other diseases**

● **V13.0 Disorders of urinary system**

V13.00 Unspecified urinary disorder

V13.01 Urinary calculi

V13.02 Urinary (tract) infection

V13.03 Nephrotic syndrome

V13.09 Other
Coding Clinic: 1996, Q2, P7x2

V13.1 Trophoblastic disease ♀
> **Excludes** *supervision during a current pregnancy (V23.1)*

● **V13.2 Other genital system and obstetric disorders**
> **Excludes** *supervision during a current pregnancy of a woman with poor obstetric history (V23.0–V23.9)*
> *habitual aborter (646.3)*
> *without current pregnancy (629.81)*

V13.21 Personal history of pre-term labor ♀
> **Excludes** *current pregnancy with history of pre-term labor (V23.41)*

V13.22 Personal history of cervical dysplasia ♀
Personal history of conditions classifiable to 622.10–622.12
> **Excludes** *personal history of malignant neoplasm of cervix uteri (V10.41)*
Coding Clinic: 2007, Q4, P99-101

V13.29 Other genital system and obstetric disorders ♀

V13.3 Diseases of skin and subcutaneous tissue

V13.4 Arthritis

● **V13.5 Other musculoskeletal disorders**

V13.51 Pathologic fracture
Healed pathologic fracture
> **Excludes** *personal history of traumatic fracture (V15.51)*

V13.52 Stress fracture
Healed stress fracture
> **Excludes** *personal history of traumatic fracture (V15.51)*

V13.59 Other musculoskeletal disorders

● **V13.6 Congenital malformations**

V13.61 Hypospadias ♂

V13.69 Other congenital malformations
Coding Clinic: 2004, Q1, P16-17

V13.7 Perinatal problems
> **Excludes** *low birth weight status (V21.30–V21.35)*

V13.8 Other specified diseases

V13.9 Unspecified disease

● **V14 Personal history of allergy to medicinal agents**

V14.0 Penicillin

V14.1 Other antibiotic agent

V14.2 Sulfonamides

V14.3 Other anti-infective agent

V14.4 Anesthetic agent

V14.5 Narcotic agent

V14.6 Analgesic agent

V14.7 Serum or vaccine

V14.8 Other specified medicinal agents

V14.9 Unspecified medicinal agent

● **V15 Other personal history presenting hazards to health**
> **Excludes** *personal history of drug therapy (V87.41–V87.49)*

● **V15.0 Allergy, other than to medicinal agents**
> **Excludes** *allergy to food substance used as base for medicinal agent (V14.0–V14.9)*

V15.01 Allergy to peanuts

V15.02 Allergy to milk products
> **Excludes** *lactose intolerance (271.3)*
Coding Clinic: 2003, Q1, P12

V15.03 Allergy to eggs

V15.04 Allergy to seafood
Seafood (octopus) (squid) ink
Shellfish

V15.05 Allergy to other foods
Food additives
Nuts other than peanuts

V15.06 Allergy to insects and arachnids
Bugs
Insect bites and stings
Spiders

V15.07 Allergy to latex
Latex sensitivity

V15.08 Allergy to radiographic dye
Contrast media used for diagnostic x-ray procedures

V15.09 Other allergy, other than to medicinal agents

N Newborn Age: 0   **P** Pediatric Age: 0–17   **M** Maternity Age: 12–55   **A** Adult Age: 15–124   ♀ Females Only   ♂ Males Only   1111

V01-V89

❷ **V15.1 Surgery to heart and great vessels**

    Excludes *replacement by transplant or*
                other means (V42.1–V42.2,
                V43.2–V43.4)

    Coding Clinic: 2004, Q1, P16-17

● **V15.2 Surgery to other organs**

    Excludes *replacement by transplant or other*
                means (V42.0–V43.8)

    ❷ **V15.21 Personal history of undergoing in utero**
            procedure during pregnancy ♀

    ❷ **V15.22 Personal history of undergoing in utero**
            procedure while a fetus

    ❷■ **V15.29 Surgery to other organs**

❷ **V15.3 Irradiation**

    Previous exposure to therapeutic or other
    ionizing radiation

● **V15.4 Psychological trauma**

    Excludes *history of condition classifiable to*
                290–316 (V11.0–V11.9)

    ❷ **V15.41 History of physical abuse**
            Rape
            Coding Clinic: 1999, Q3, P15

    ❷ **V15.42 History of emotional abuse**
            Neglect
            Coding Clinic: 1999, Q3, P15

    ❷ **V15.49 Other**
            Coding Clinic: 1999, Q3, P15

● **V15.5 Injury**

    ❷ **V15.51 Traumatic fracture**
            Healed traumatic fracture

        Excludes *personal history of pathologic*
                    and stress fracture
                    (V13.51, V13.52)

    ❷ **V15.52 History of traumatic brain injury** ◀

        Excludes *personal history of*
                    cerebrovascular accident
                    (cerebral infarction)
                    without residual
                    deficits (V12.54) ◀

    ❷■ **V15.59 Other injury**

❷ **V15.6 Poisoning**

■ **V15.7 Contraception**

    Excludes *current contraceptive management*
                (V25.0–V25.4)
             presence of intrauterine contraceptive
                device as incidental finding
                (V45.5)

● **V15.8 Other specified personal history presenting**
    hazards to health

    Excludes *contact with and (suspected)*
                exposure to:
                aromatic compounds and dyes
                  (V87.11-V87.19)
                arsenic and other metals
                  (V87.01-V87.09)
                molds (V87.31)

    ❷ **V15.80 History of failed moderate sedation** ◀
            History of failed conscious sedation ◀

    ❷ **V15.81 Noncompliance with medical**
            treatment

        Excludes *noncompliance with renal*
                    dialysis (V45.12)
        Coding Clinic: 2007, Q3, P11; 2006, Q4, P136; 2003,
            Q2, P7-8; 2001, Q2, P13; 1999, Q2, P17; Q1,
            P13-14; 1997, Q2, P11; 1996, Q3, P9

❷ **V15.82 History of tobacco use**

    Excludes *tobacco dependence (305.1)*

    Coding Clinic: 2009, Q1, P15

❷ **V15.83 Underimmunization status** ◀
        Delinquent immunization status ◀
        Lapsed immunization schedule
            status ◀

❷ **V15.84 Contact with and (suspected) exposure to**
        ~~Exposure to~~ **asbestos** ◀▥

❷ **V15.85 Contact with and (suspected) exposure to**
        ~~Exposure to~~ **potentially hazardous body**
        fluids ◀▥

❷ **V15.86 Contact with and (suspected) exposure to**
        ~~Exposure to~~ **lead** ◀▥

❷ **V15.87 History of extracorporeal membrane**
        oxygenation [ECMO]

◍❷ **V15.88 History of fall**
        At risk for falling
        Coding Clinic: 2005, Q4, P94-100

❷ **V15.89 Other**

        Excludes *contact with and (suspected)*
                    exposure to other
                    potentially hazardous
                    chemicals (V87.2)
                contact with and (suspected)
                    exposure to other
                    potentially hazardous
                    substances (V87.39)
        Coding Clinic: 2008, Q3, P6-7; 2007, Q3, P6; 1990,
            Q1, P21

❷ **V15.9 Unspecified personal history presenting hazards**
    to health

    OGCR Section I.C.18.d.3

    Family history codes are for use when a patient has
    a family member(s) who has had a particular disease
    that causes the patient to be at higher risk of also
    contracting the disease.

● **V16 Family history of malignant neoplasm**
    Coding Clinic: 1985, Nov-Dec, P13

◍ **V16.0 Gastrointestinal tract**
    Family history of condition classifiable to
    140–159
    Coding Clinic: 1999, Q1, P4

◍ **V16.1 Trachea, bronchus, and lung**
    Family history of condition classifiable to 162

◍ **V16.2 Other respiratory and intrathoracic organs**
    Family history of condition classifiable to
    160–161, 163–165

◍ **V16.3 Breast**
    Family history of condition classifiable to 174
    Coding Clinic: 2004, Q4, P106-107; 2003, Q2, P3-5; 2000, Q2,
    P8-9; 1995, Q4, P61; 1992, Q1, P11; 1990, Q1, P21

● **V16.4 Genital organs**
    Family history of condition classifiable to
    179–187

    ◍ **V16.40 Genital organ, unspecified**

    ◍ **V16.41 Ovary**

    ◍ **V16.42 Prostate**

    ◍ **V16.43 Testis**

    ◍ **V16.49 Other**
            Coding Clinic: 2006, Q2, P3,4

◀ New   ◀▥ Revised   ~~deleted~~ Deleted   ● Use Additional Digit(s)   ■ Nonspecific Code   ❶ First Listed   ◍ First Listed or Additional
❷ Additional Only   ● Not first-listed DX   OGCR Official Guidelines   Coding Clinic   Excludes   Includes   Use additional   Code first

● **V16.5   Urinary organs**
      Family history of condition classifiable to
          188–189

   V16.51   Kidney

   V16.52   Bladder

   V16.59   Other

V16.6   Leukemia
      Family history of condition classifiable to
          204–208

**V16.7   Other lymphatic and hematopoietic
     neoplasms**
      Family history of condition classifiable to
          200–203

V16.8   Other specified malignant neoplasm
      Family history of other condition classifiable to
          140–199

V16.9   Unspecified malignant neoplasm

● **V17   Family history of certain chronic disabling diseases**
      Coding Clinic: 1985, Nov-Dec, P13

V17.0   Psychiatric condition

> **Excludes**   *family history of mental retardation
>   (V18.4)*

V17.1   Stroke (cerebrovascular)

V17.2   Other neurological diseases
      Epilepsy
      Huntington's chorea

V17.3   Ischemic heart disease

● **V17.4   Other cardiovascular diseases**
      Coding Clinic: 2004, Q1, P6-7

   **V17.41   Family history of sudden cardiac death
           (SCD)**

> **Excludes**   *family history of ischemic heart
>   disease (V17.3)
>   family history of myocardial
>   infarction (V17.3)*

   **V17.49   Family history of other cardiovascular
           diseases**
           Family history of cardiovascular
             disease NOS

V17.5   Asthma

V17.6   Other chronic respiratory conditions

V17.7   Arthritis

● **V17.8   Other musculoskeletal diseases**

   V17.81   Osteoporosis

   V17.89   Other musculoskeletal diseases

● **V18   Family history of certain other specific conditions**
      Coding Clinic: 1985, Nov-Dec, P13

V18.0   Diabetes mellitus
      Coding Clinic: 2005, Q2, P21; 2004, Q1, P8

● **V18.1   Other endocrine and metabolic diseases**

   **V18.11   Multiple endocrine neoplasia [MEN]
           syndrome**

   V18.19   Other endocrine and metabolic diseases

V18.2   Anemia

V18.3   Other blood disorders

V18.4   Mental retardation

● **V18.5   Digestive disorders**

   V18.51   Colonic polyps

> **Excludes**   *family history of malignant
>   neoplasm of
>   gastrointestinal
>   tract (V16.0)*

   V18.59   Other digestive disorders

● **V18.6   Kidney diseases**

   V18.61   Polycystic kidney

   V18.69   Other kidney diseases

V18.7   Other genitourinary diseases

V18.8   Infectious and parasitic diseases

V18.9   Genetic disease carrier

● **V19   Family history of other conditions**
      Coding Clinic: 1985, Nov-Dec, P13

V19.0   Blindness or visual loss

V19.1   Other eye disorders

V19.2   Deafness or hearing loss

V19.3   Other ear disorders

V19.4   Skin conditions

V19.5   Congenital anomalies

V19.6   Allergic disorders

V19.7   Consanguinity

V19.8   Other condition

PERSONS ENCOUNTERING HEALTH SERVICES IN CIRCUMSTANCES RELATED TO REPRODUCTION AND DEVELOPMENT (V20–V29)

● **V20   Health supervision of infant or child**

   ❶ **V20.0   Foundling**   P

   ❶ **V20.1   Other healthy infant or child receiving care**   P
      Medical or nursing care supervision of healthy
         infant in cases of:
      maternal illness, physical or psychiatric
      socioeconomic adverse condition at home
      too many children at home preventing or
         interfering with normal care
      Coding Clinic: 2000, Q1, P25; 1993, Q4, P36; 1989, Q3, P14

   ❶ **V20.2   Routine infant or child health check**   P
      Developmental testing of infant or child
      Immunizations appropriate for age
      ~~Initial and subsequent routine newborn check~~
      Health check for child over 28 days old   ◀
      Routine vision and hearing testing

> **Excludes**   *health check for child under 29 days old*   ◀
>   *(V20.31–V20.32)*
>   *newborn health supervision (V20.31–*   ◀
>   *V20.32)*
>   *special screening for developmental*   ◀
>   *handicaps (V79.3)*

      Use additional code(s) to identify:
      Special screening examination(s) performed
         (V73.0–V82.9)
      Coding Clinic: 2009, Q1, P15; 2004, Q1, P15-16x2

● **V20.3   Newborn health supervision**   ◀
      Health check for child under 29 days old   ◀

> **Excludes**   *health check for child over 28 days*   ◀
>   *old (V20.2)*

   ❶ **V20.31   Health supervision for newborn
           under 8 days old**   N ◀
           Health check for newborn under
             8 days old   ◀

   ❶ **V20.32   Health supervision for newborn
           8 to 28 days old**   N ◀
           Health check for newborn
             8 to 28 days old   ◀
           Newborn weight check   ◀

● **V21   Constitutional states in development**

   ❷ **V21.0   Period of rapid growth in childhood**

   ❷ **V21.1   Puberty**

   ❷ **V21.2   Other adolescence**

N Newborn Age: 0   **P** Pediatric Age: 0–17   **M** Maternity Age: 12–55   **A** Adult Age: 15–124   ♀ Females Only   ♂ Males Only   **1113**

V01-V89

● **V21.3 Low birth weight status**

     Excludes *history of perinatal problems (V13.7)*

   ❷ **V21.30 Low birth weight status, unspecified**

   ❷ **V21.31 Low birth weight status, less than 500 grams**

   ❷ **V21.32 Low birth weight status, 500–999 grams**

   ❷ **V21.33 Low birth weight status, 1000–1499 grams**

   ❷ **V21.34 Low birth weight status, 1500–1999 grams**

   ❷ **V21.35 Low birth weight status, 2000–2500 grams**

❷ **V21.8 Other specified constitutional states in development**

❷ **V21.9 Unspecified constitutional state in development**

● **V22 Normal pregnancy**

     Excludes *pregnancy examination or test, pregnancy unconfirmed (V72.40)*

     Coding Clinic: 2007, Q4, P124-125

     OGCR Section I.C.11.b.1

     For routine outpatient prenatal visits when no complications are present codes V22.0, Supervision of normal first pregnancy, and V22.1, Supervision of other normal pregnancy, should be used as the first-listed diagnoses. These codes should not be used in conjunction with chapter 11 codes.

❶ **V22.0 Supervision of normal first pregnancy** ♀

     Coding Clinic: 1999, Q3, P16; 1990, Q1, P10; 1984, Nov-Dec, P18

❶ **V22.1 Supervision of other normal pregnancy** ♀

     Coding Clinic: 1999, Q3, P16; 1990, Q1, P10

❷ **V22.2 Pregnant state, incidental** ♀

     Pregnant state NOS

     Coding Clinic: 1998, Q2, P13-14; 1994, Q2, P14

     OGCR Section I.C.11.b.2

     For prenatal outpatient visits for patients with high-risk pregnancies, a code from category V23, Supervision of high-risk pregnancy, should be used as the principal or first-listed diagnosis. Secondary chapter 11 codes may be used in conjunction with these codes if appropriate.

● **V23 Supervision of high-risk pregnancy**

     Coding Clinic: 1990, Q1, P10

❖ **V23.0 Pregnancy with history of infertility** ♀   **M**

❖ **V23.1 Pregnancy with history of trophoblastic disease** ♀   **M**

     Pregnancy with history of:
        hydatidiform mole
        vesicular mole

     Excludes *that without current pregnancy (V13.1)*

❖ **V23.2 Pregnancy with history of abortion** ♀   **M**

     Pregnancy with history of conditions classifiable to 634–638

     Excludes *habitual aborter:*
         care during pregnancy (646.3)
         that without current pregnancy (629.81)

❖ **V23.3 Grand multiparity** ♀   **M**

     Excludes *care in relation to labor and delivery (659.4)*
         that without current pregnancy (V61.5)

● **V23.4 Pregnancy with other poor obstetric history**

     Pregnancy with history of other conditions classifiable to 630–676

   ❖ **V23.41 Pregnancy with history of pre-term labor** ♀   **M**

   ❖ **V23.49 Pregnancy with other poor obstetric history** ♀   **M**

❖ **V23.5 Pregnancy with other poor reproductive history** ♀   **M**

     Pregnancy with history of stillbirth or neonatal death

❖ **V23.7 Insufficient prenatal care** ♀   **M**

     History of little or no prenatal care

● **V23.8 Other high-risk pregnancy**

     Coding Clinic: 1998, Q4, P50-51

   ❖ **V23.81 Elderly primigravida** ♀   **M**

     First pregnancy in a woman who will be 35 years of age or older at expected date of delivery

     Excludes *elderly primigravida complicating pregnancy (659.5)*

     Coding Clinic: 1998, Q4, P58

   ❖ **V23.82 Elderly multigravida** ♀   **M**

     Second or more pregnancy in a woman who will be 35 years of age or older at expected date of delivery

     Excludes *elderly multigravida complicating pregnancy (659.6)*

   ❖ **V23.83 Young primigravida** ♀   **M**

     First pregnancy in a female less than 16 years old at expected date of delivery

     Excludes *young primigravida complicating pregnancy (659.8)*

   ❖ **V23.84 Young multigravida** ♀   **M**

     Second or more pregnancy in a female less than 16 years old at expected date of delivery

     Excludes *young multigravida complicating pregnancy (659.8)*

   ❖ **V23.85 Pregnancy resulting from assisted reproductive technology** ♀   **M A**

     Pregnancy resulting from in vitro fertilization

   ❖ **V23.86 Pregnancy with history of in utero procedure during previous pregnancy** ♀   **M**

     Excludes *management of pregnancy affected by in utero procedure during current pregnancy (679.0–679.1)* ◀▥

   ❖ **V23.89 Other high-risk pregnancy** ♀   **M**

     Coding Clinic: 2006, Q3, P14

❖ **V23.9 Unspecified high-risk pregnancy** ♀   **M**

◀ New   ◀▥ Revised   ~~deleted~~ Deleted   ● Use Additional Digit(s)   ▩ Nonspecific Code   ❶ First Listed   ❖ First Listed or Additional
   ❷ Additional Only   ● Not first-listed DX   OGCR Official Guidelines   Coding Clinic   Excludes   Includes   Use additional   Code first

OGCR Section I.C.18.d.8

> The follow-up codes (V24, V67 and V89), are used to explain continuing surveillance following completed treatment of a disease, condition, or injury. They imply that the condition has been fully treated and no longer exists. They should not be confused with aftercare codes that explain current treatment for a healing condition or its sequelae. Follow-up codes may be used in conjunction with history codes to provide the full picture of the healed condition and its treatment. The follow-up code is sequenced first, followed by the history code. A follow-up code may be used to explain repeated visits. Should a condition be found to have recurred on the follow-up visit, then the diagnosis code should be used in place of the follow-up code.

● **V24 Postpartum care and examination**

❶ V24.0 Immediately after delivery ♀   **M**
  Care and observation in uncomplicated cases
  Coding Clinic: 2006, Q3, P11

  OGCR Section I.C.10.i.5

  > When the mother delivers outside the hospital prior to admission and is admitted for routine postpartum care and no complications are noted, code V24.0, Postpartum care and examination immediately after delivery, should be assigned as the principal diagnosis.

❶ V24.1 Lactating mother ♀
  Supervision of lactation

❶ V24.2 Routine postpartum follow-up ♀

● **V25 Encounter for contraceptive management**

● **V25.0 General counseling and advice**

  V25.01 Prescription of oral contraceptives ♀

  V25.02 Initiation of other contraceptive measures
    Fitting of diaphragm
    Prescription of foams, creams, or other agents
    Coding Clinic: 1997, Q3, P7

  V25.03 Encounter for emergency contraceptive counseling and prescription
    Encounter for postcoital contraceptive counseling and prescription

  V25.04 Counseling and instruction in natural family planning to avoid pregnancy
    Coding Clinic: 2007, Q4, P99-101

  V25.09 Other
    Family planning advice

V25.1 Insertion of intrauterine contraceptive device ♀

V25.2 Sterilization
  Admission for interruption of fallopian tubes or vas deferens

V25.3 Menstrual extraction ♀
  Menstrual regulation

● **V25.4 Surveillance of previously prescribed contraceptive methods**
  Checking, reinsertion, or removal of contraceptive device
  Repeat prescription for contraceptive method
  Routine examination in connection with contraceptive maintenance

  Excludes *presence of intrauterine contraceptive device as incidental finding (V45.5)*

  V25.40 Contraceptive surveillance, unspecified

  V25.41 Contraceptive pill ♀

  V25.42 Intrauterine contraceptive device ♀
    Checking, reinsertion, or removal of intrauterine device

  V25.43 Implantable subdermal contraceptive ♀

  V25.49 Other contraceptive method
    Coding Clinic: 1997, Q3, P7

V25.5 Insertion of implantable subdermal contraceptive ♀

V25.8 Other specified contraceptive management
  Postvasectomy sperm count

  Excludes *sperm count following sterilization reversal (V26.22)*
  sperm count for fertility testing (V26.21)

  Coding Clinic: 1996, Q3, P9

V25.9 Unspecified contraceptive management

● **V26 Procreative management**

V26.0 Tuboplasty or vasoplasty after previous sterilization
  Coding Clinic: 1995, Q2, P10

V26.1 Artificial insemination ♀

● **V26.2 Investigation and testing**

  Excludes *postvasectomy sperm count (V25.8)*

  Coding Clinic: 1996, Q2, P9; 1985, Nov-Dec, P15

  V26.21 Fertility testing
    Fallopian insufflation
    Sperm count for fertility testing

    Excludes *genetic counseling and testing (V26.31–V26.39)*

  V26.22 Aftercare following sterilization reversal
    Fallopian insufflation following sterilization reversal
    Sperm count following sterilization reversal

  V26.29 Other investigation and testing

● V26.3 Genetic counseling and testing

> **Excludes** *fertility testing (V26.21)*
> *nonprocreative genetic screening*
> *(V82.71, V82.79)*
> Coding Clinic: 2006, Q4, P117; 2005, Q4, P94-100

OGCR Section I.C.18.d.3
> If the purpose of the encounter is genetic
> counseling associated with procreative
> management, a code from subcategory V26.3
> should be assigned as the first-listed code,
> followed by a code from category V84, Genetic
> susceptibility to disease. Additional codes
> should be assigned for any applicable family or
> personal history.

  ✇ **V26.31** Testing of female genetic disease carrier status ♀

  ✇ **V26.32** Other genetic testing of female ♀
> Use additional code to identify
> habitual aborter (629.81, 646.3)

  ✇ **V26.33** Genetic counseling

  ✇ **V26.34** Testing of male for genetic disease carrier status ♂

  ✇ **V26.35** Encounter for testing of male partner of habitual aborter ♂

  ✇ **V26.39** Other genetic testing of male ♂

● V26.4 General counseling and advice

  ✇ **V26.41** Procreative counseling and advice using natural family planning
> Coding Clinic: 2007, Q4, P99-101

  ✇ **V26.42** Encounter for fertility preservation counseling ◄
> Encounter for fertility preservation
> counseling prior to cancer
> therapy ◄
> Encounter for fertility preservation
> counseling prior to surgical
> removal of gonads ◄

  ✇ **V26.49** Other procreative management counseling and advice

● V26.5 Sterilization status

  ❷ **V26.51** Tubal ligation status ♀
> **Excludes** *infertility not due to*
> *previous tubal ligation*
> *(628.0–628.9)*

  ❷ **V26.52** Vasectomy status ♂

● V26.8 Other specified procreative management

  ❶ **V26.81** Encounter for assisted reproductive fertility procedure cycle ♀
> Patient undergoing in vitro
> fertilization cycle
> Use additional code to identify the
> type of infertility
> **Excludes** *pre-cycle diagnosis and*
> *testing - code to reason*
> *for encounter*
> Coding Clinic: 2007, Q4, P99-101

  ✇ **V26.82** Encounter for fertility preservation procedure ◄
> Encounter for fertility preservation
> procedure prior to cancer
> therapy ◄
> Encounter for fertility preservation
> procedure prior to surgical
> removal of gonads ◄

  ✇ **V26.89** Other specified procreative management

✇ **V26.9** Unspecified procreative management

OGCR Section I.C.10.h.3
> V27.0, Single liveborn, is the only outcome of delivery
> code appropriate for use with 650.

OGCR Section I.C.10.k.4
> When an attempted termination of pregnancy
> results in a liveborn fetus assign code 644.21 with
> an appropriate code from category V27, Outcome
> of Delivery. The procedure code for the attempted
> termination of pregnancy should also be assigned.

OGCR Section I.C.11.b.5
> An outcome of delivery code, V27.0-V27.9, should be
> included on every maternal record when a delivery
> has occurred. These codes are not to be used on
> subsequent records or on the newborn record.

● V27 Outcome of delivery
> **Note:** This category is intended for the coding of the
> outcome of delivery on the mother's record.
> Coding Clinic: 1991, Q2, P16

  ❷ **V27.0** Single liveborn ♀   M
> Coding Clinic: 2008, Q4, P192; 2005, Q4, P81; 2003, Q2, P9;
> 2002, Q2, P10; 2000, Q3, P5; 1998, Q4, P76-77

  ❷ **V27.1** Single stillborn ♀   M
> Coding Clinic: 2001, Q1, P11-12

  ❷ **V27.2** Twins, both liveborn ♀   M
> Coding Clinic: 1992, Q3, P10

  ❷ **V27.3** Twins, one liveborn and one stillborn ♀   M

  ❷ **V27.4** Twins, both stillborn ♀   M

  ❷ **V27.5** Other multiple birth, all liveborn ♀   M

  ❷ **V27.6** Other multiple birth, some liveborn ♀   M

  ❷ **V27.7** Other multiple birth, all stillborn ♀   M

  ❷ **V27.9** Unspecified outcome of delivery ♀   M
> routine prenatal care (V22.0–V23.9)

● V28 Encounter for antenatal screening of mother
> **Excludes** *abnormal findings on screening - code to*
> *findings*
> *suspected fetal conditions affecting management*
> *of pregnancy (655.00–655.93,*
> *656.00–656.93, 657.00–657.03,*
> *658.00–658.93)*
> *suspected fetal conditions not found*
> *(V89.01-V89.09)*

OGCR Section I.C.18.d.5
> See V73-V82 to report special screening examinations.

  ✇ **V28.0** Screening for chromosomal anomalies by amniocentesis ♀   M

  ✇ **V28.1** Screening for raised alpha-fetoprotein levels in amniotic fluid ♀   M

  ✇ **V28.2** Other screening based on amniocentesis ♀   M

  ✇ **V28.3** Encounter for routine screening for malformation using ultrasonics ♀
> Encounter for routine fetal ultrasound NOS
> **Excludes** *encounter for fetal anatomic survey*
> *(V28.81)*
> *genetic counseling and testing*
> *(V26.31–V26.39)*

  ✇ **V28.4** Screening for fetal growth retardation using ultrasonics ♀

  ✇ **V28.5** Screening for isoimmunization ♀

  ✇ **V28.6** Screening for Streptococcus B ♀   M

◄ New   ◄◄ Revised   deleted Deleted   ● Use Additional Digit(s)   ■ Nonspecific Code   ❶ First Listed   ✇ First Listed or Additional
❷ Additional Only   ● Not first-listed DX   OGCR Official Guidelines   Coding Clinic   Excludes   Includes   Use additional   Code first

V01-V89

● **V28.8 Other specified antenatal screening**
Coding Clinic: 1999, Q3, P16

    ⚕**V28.81 Encounter for fetal anatomic survey** ♀   **M**

    ⚕**V28.82 Encounter for screening for risk of pre-term labor** ♀   **M**

    ⚕**V28.89 Other specified antenatal screening** ♀   **M**
         Chorionic villus sampling
         Genomic screening
         Nuchal translucency testing
         Proteomic screening

⚕**V28.9 Unspecified antenatal screening** ♀

OGCR Section I.C.15.d.1
Assign a code from category V29 to identify those instances when a healthy newborn is evaluated for a suspected condition that is determined after study not to be present. Do not use a code from category V29 when the patient has identified signs or symptoms of a suspected problem; in such cases, code the sign or symptom. A code from category V29 may also be assigned as a principal code for readmissions or encounters when the V30 code no longer applies. Codes from category V29 are for use only for healthy newborns and infants for which no condition after study is found to be present.

OGCR Section I.C.15.d.2
A V29 code is to be used as a secondary code after the V30.

OGCR Section I.C.18.d.6
Observation codes V29, V71 and V89 are for use in very limited circumstances when a person is being observed for a suspected condition that is ruled out. The observation codes are not for use if an injury or illness or any signs or symptoms related to the suspected condition are present. In such cases the diagnosis/symptom code is used with the corresponding E code to identify any external cause. The observation codes are to be used as principal diagnosis only. The only exception to this is when the principal diagnosis is required to be a code from the V30, Live born infant, category. Then the V29 observation code is sequenced after the V30 code. Additional codes may be used in addition to the observation code but only if they are unrelated to the suspected condition being observed.

● **V29 Observation and evaluation of newborns for suspected condition not found**

    Note: This category is to be used for newborns, within the neonatal period (the first 28 days of life), who are suspected of having an abnormal condition resulting from exposure from the mother or the birth process, but without signs or symptoms, and which, after examination and observation, is found not to exist.

    Excludes *suspected fetal conditions not found (V89.01–V89.09)*
    Coding Clinic: 2000, Q1, P25-26

⚕**V29.0 Observation for suspected infectious condition**   **N**
Coding Clinic: 2001, Q1, P10

⚕**V29.1 Observation for suspected neurological condition**   **N**

⚕**V29.2 Observation for suspected respiratory condition**   **N**

⚕**V29.3 Observation for suspected genetic or metabolic condition**   **N**
Coding Clinic: 2005, Q2, P21; 2004, Q1, P8; 1998, Q4, P59

⚕**V29.8 Observation for other specified suspected condition**   **N**
Coding Clinic: 2003, Q2, P15-16

⚕**V29.9 Observation for unspecified suspected condition**   **N**
Coding Clinic: 2002, Q1, P6-7

LIVEBORN INFANTS ACCORDING TO TYPE OF BIRTH (V30–V39)

OGCR Section I.C.15.b
When coding the birth of an infant, assign a code from categories V30-V39, according to the type of birth. A code from this series is assigned as a principal diagnosis, and assigned only once to a newborn at the time of birth.

OGCR Section I.C.15.c
If the newborn is transferred to another institution, the V30 series is not used at the receiving hospital.

Note: These categories are intended for the coding of liveborn infants who are consuming health care [e.g., crib or bassinet occupancy].

The following fourth-digit subdivisions are for use with categories V30–V39:

> **0 Born in hospital**
> **1 Born before admission to hospital**
> **2 Born outside hospital and not hospitalized**

The following two fifths-digits are for use with the fourth-digit .0, Born in hospital:

> **0 delivered without mention of cesarean delivery**
> **1 delivered by cesarean delivery**

❶ ● **V30 Single liveborn**   **N**
Coding Clinic: 2006, Q3, P10-11; 2005, Q4, P83-89; Q2, P21; 2004, Q1, P8, 16; 2003, Q4, P67-68; Q2, P9; 2001, Q4, P50-51; 2000, Q1, P25-26; 1998, Q4, P46-47, 59; 1994, Q3, P4; 1993, Q4, P36

❶ ● **V31 Twin, mate liveborn**   **N**
Coding Clinic: 1992, Q3, P10

❶ ● **V32 Twin, mate stillborn**   **N**

❶ ● **V33 Twin, unspecified**   **N**

❶ ● **V34 Other multiple, mates all liveborn**   **N**

❶ ● **V35 Other multiple, mates all stillborn**   **N**

❶ ● **V36 Other multiple, mates live- and stillborn**   **N**

❶ ● **V37 Other multiple, unspecified**   **N**

❶ ● **V39 Unspecified**   **N**

PERSONS WITH A CONDITION INFLUENCING THEIR HEALTH STATUS (V40–V49)

    Note: These categories are intended for use when these conditions are recorded as "diagnoses" or "problems."

● **V40 Mental and behavioral problems**

    ■**V40.0 Problems with learning**

    ■**V40.1 Problems with communication [including speech]**

    ■**V40.2 Other mental problems**

    ■**V40.3 Other behavioral problems**

    ■**V40.9 Unspecified mental or behavioral problem**

N Newborn Age: 0   **P** Pediatric Age: 0–17   **M** Maternity Age: 12–55   **A** Adult Age: 15–124   ♀ Females Only   ♂ Males Only   **1117**

V01-V89

● **V41   Problems with special senses and other special functions**

◻ **V41.0   Problems with sight**

◻ **V41.1   Other eye problems**

◻ **V41.2   Problems with hearing**

◻ **V41.3   Other ear problems**

◻ **V41.4   Problems with voice production**

◻ **V41.5   Problems with smell and taste**

◻ **V41.6   Problems with swallowing and mastication**

◻ **V41.7   Problems with sexual function**

> **Excludes**   *marital problems (V61.10)*
> *psychosexual disorders (302.0–302.9)*

◻ **V41.8   Other problems with special functions**

◻ **V41.9   Unspecified problem with special functions**

● **V42   Organ or tissue replaced by transplant**

> **Includes**   homologous or heterologous (animal) (human) transplant organ status
> Coding Clinic: 1998, Q3, P5

> **OGCR**   Section I.C.17.f.2.a
>
> Transplant complications other than kidney: Codes under subcategory 996.8, Complications of transplanted organ, are for use for both complications and rejection of transplanted organs. A transplant complication code is only assigned if the complication affects the function of the transplanted organ. Two codes are required to fully describe a transplant complication, the appropriate code from subcategory 996.8 and a secondary code that identifies the complication.
>
> Pre-existing conditions or conditions that develop after the transplant are not coded as complications unless they affect the function of the transplanted organs.
>
> See I.C.18.d.3) for transplant organ removal status.
>
> See I.C.2.i for malignant neoplasm associated with transplanted organ.

❷ **V42.0   Kidney**

> Coding Clinic: 2008, Q1, P10-13; 2003, Q1, P10-11; 2001, Q3, P12-13; 1994, Q2, P9x2

> **OGCR**   Section I.C.17.f.2.b
>
> Patients who have undergone kidney transplant may still have some form of chronic kidney disease (CKD) because the kidney transplant may not fully restore kidney function. Code 996.81 should be assigned for documented complications of a kidney transplant, such as transplant failure or rejection or other transplant complication. Code 996.81 should not be assigned for post kidney transplant patients who have chronic kidney (CKD) unless a transplant complication such as transplant failure or rejection is documented. If the documentation is unclear as to whether the patient has a complication of the transplant, query the provider. For patients with CKD following a kidney transplant, but who do not have a complication such as failure or rejection, see section I.C.10.a.2, Chronic kidney disease and kidney transplant status.

❷ **V42.1   Heart**

> Coding Clinic: 2003, Q3, P16; 2001, Q3, P13-14x2; 1994, Q2, P13

❷ **V42.2   Heart valve**

❷ **V42.3   Skin**

❷ **V42.4   Bone**

❷ **V42.5   Cornea**

❷ **V42.6   Lung**

❷ **V42.7   Liver**

● **V42.8   Other specified organ or tissue**

❷ **V42.81   Bone marrow**

❷ **V42.82   Peripheral stem cells**

❷ **V42.83   Pancreas**

> Coding Clinic: 2003, Q1, P10-11; 2001, Q2, P16

❷ **V42.84   Intestines**

> Coding Clinic: 2000, Q4, P47-48

❷ **V42.89   Other**

❷ **V42.9   Unspecified organ or tissue**

● **V43   Organ or tissue replaced by other means**

> **Includes**   organ or tissue assisted by other means
> replacement of organ by:
> artificial device
> mechanical device
> prosthesis

> **Excludes**   *cardiac pacemaker in situ (V45.01)*
> *fitting and adjustment of prosthetic device (V52.0–V52.9)*
> *renal dialysis status (V45.11)*

❷ **V43.0   Eye globe**

❷ **V43.1   Lens**

> Pseudophakos

● **V43.2   Heart**

❷ **V43.21   Heart assist device**

⌖ **V43.22   Fully implantable artificial heart**

❷ **V43.3   Heart valve**

> Coding Clinic: 2006, Q3, P7; 2002, Q3, P13-15

❷ **V43.4   Blood vessel**

❷ **V43.5   Bladder**

● **V43.6   Joint**

> Coding Clinic: 1991, Q1, P15

❷ **V43.60   Unspecified joint**

❷ **V43.61   Shoulder**

❷ **V43.62   Elbow**

❷ **V43.63   Wrist**

❷ **V43.64   Hip**

> Coding Clinic: 2009, Q1, P15; 2008, Q2, P3-5; 2006, Q3, P4-5; 2005, Q4, P83-89, 110-112; 2004, Q2, P15

❷ **V43.65   Knee**

> Coding Clinic: 2006, Q3, P5

❷ **V43.66   Ankle**

❷ **V43.69   Other**

❷ **V43.7   Limb**

● **V43.8   Other organ or tissue**

❷ **V43.81   Larynx**

❷ **V43.82   Breast**

❷ **V43.83   Artificial skin**

❷ **V43.89   Other**

● V44   **Artificial opening status**

     Excludes   *artificial openings requiring attention or management (V55.0–V55.9)*

   ❷ V44.0   **Tracheostomy**
       Coding Clinic: 2003, Q4, P103-104, 107, 111; 2001, Q1, P6-7

   ❷ V44.1   **Gastrostomy**
       Coding Clinic: 2003, Q4, P103-104, 107-108, 110; 2001, Q1, P12; 1998, Q4, P42-44; 1997, Q3, P12-13; 1993, Q1, P26

   ❷ V44.2   **Ileostomy**
       Coding Clinic: 1988, Q2, P9-10

   ❷ V44.3   **Colostomy**
       Coding Clinic: 2003, Q4, P110

   ❷ V44.4   **Other artificial opening of gastrointestinal tract**

   ● V44.5   **Cystostomy**

     ❷ V44.50   **Cystostomy, unspecified**

     ❷ V44.51   **Cutaneous-vesicostomy**

     ❷ V44.52   **Appendico-vesicostomy**

     ❷ V44.59   **Other cystostomy**

   ❷ V44.6   **Other artificial opening of urinary tract**
       Nephrostomy
       Ureterostomy
       Urethrostomy

   ❷ V44.7   **Artificial vagina**

   ❷ V44.8   **Other artificial opening status**

   ❷ V44.9   **Unspecified artificial opening status**

● V45   **Other postprocedural states**

     Excludes   *aftercare management (V51–V58.9)*
       malfunction or other complication-code to condition

   ● V45.0   **Cardiac device in situ**

     Excludes   *artificial heart (V43.22)*
       heart assist device (V43.21)
       Coding Clinic: 1994, Q2, P10x2; 1993, 5th Issue, P12

     ❷ V45.00   **Unspecified cardiac device**

     ❷ V45.01   **Cardiac pacemaker**

     ❷ V45.02   **Automatic implantable cardiac defibrillator**

     ❷ V45.09   **Other specified cardiac device**
       Carotid sinus pacemaker in situ

   ● V45.1   **Renal dialysis status**

     Excludes   *admission for dialysis treatment or session (V56.0)*
       Coding Clinic: 2008, Q1, P7-8; 2007, Q4, P84-86; Q3, P11; 2006, Q4, P136; 2004, Q1, P22,23; 2001, Q2, P12-13; 1987, Sept-Oct, P8; Jan-Feb, P15

     ❷ V45.11   **Renal dialysis status**
       Hemodialysis status
       Patient requiring intermittent renal dialysis
       Peritoneal dialysis status
       Presence of arterial-venous shunt (for dialysis)
       Coding Clinic: 2008, Q4, P193; 2004, Q1, P23

     ❷ V45.12   **Noncompliance with renal dialysis**
       Coding Clinic: 2006, Q4, P136

   ❷ V45.2   **Presence of cerebrospinal fluid drainage device**
       Cerebral ventricle (communicating) shunt, valve, or device in situ

     Excludes   *malfunction (996.2)*
       Coding Clinic: 2003, Q4, P106-107

   ❷ V45.3   **Intestinal bypass or anastomosis status**

     Excludes   *bariatric surgery status (V45.86)*
       gastric bypass status (V45.86)
       obesity surgery status (V45.86)

   ❷ V45.4   **Arthrodesis status**
       Coding Clinic: 1984, Nov-Dec, P18

   ● V45.5   **Presence of contraceptive device**

     Excludes   *checking, reinsertion, or removal of device (V25.42)*
       complication from device (996.32)
       insertion of device (V25.1)

     ❷ V45.51   **Intrauterine contraceptive device** ♀

     ❷ V45.52   **Subdermal contraceptive implant**
       Coding Clinic: 1995, Q3, P14

     ❷ V45.59   **Other**

   ● V45.6   **States following surgery of eye and adnexa**

     Excludes   *aphakia (379.31)*
       artificial:
       eye globe (V43.0)

     ❷ V45.61   **Cataract extraction status**
       Use additional code for associated artificial lens status (V43.1)

     ❷ V45.69   **Other states following surgery of eye and adnexa**
       Coding Clinic: 2001, Q2, P16-17

   ● V45.7   **Acquired absence of organ**

     ❷⚕ V45.71   **Acquired absence of breast and nipple**

       Excludes   *congenital absence of breast and nipple (757.6)* ◀
       Coding Clinic: 2001, Q4, P66; 1997, Q4, P50

     ❷⚕ V45.72   **Acquired absence of intestine (large) (small)**

     ❷⚕ V45.73   **Acquired absence of kidney**

     ❷⚕ V45.74   **Other parts of urinary tract**
       Bladder

     ❷⚕ V45.75   **Stomach**

     ❷⚕ V45.76   **Lung**

     ❷⚕ V45.77   **Genital organs**

       Excludes   *acquired absence of cervix and uterus (V88.01–V88.03)*
       female genital mutilation status (629.20–629.29)
       Coding Clinic: 2003, Q1, P13-14x2

     ❷⚕ V45.78   **Eye**

     ❷⚕ V45.79   **Other acquired absence of organ**

N Newborn Age: 0   **P** Pediatric Age: 0–17   **M** Maternity Age: 12–55   **A** Adult Age: 15–124   ♀ Females Only   ♂ Males Only   **1119**

V01-V89

● **V45.8 Other postprocedural status**

❷ **V45.81 Aortocoronary bypass status**
Coding Clinic: 2003, Q4, P105-106; 2001, Q3, P15; 1997, Q3, P16

❷ **V45.82 Percutaneous transluminal coronary angioplasty status**
Coding Clinic: 1995, Q2, P18

❷ **V45.83 Breast implant removal status**

❷ **V45.84 Dental restoration status**
Dental crowns status
Dental fillings status

❷ **V45.85 Insulin pump status**

❷ **V45.86 Bariatric surgery status**
Gastric banding status
Gastric bypass status for obesity
Obesity surgery status

Excludes *bariatric surgery status complicating pregnancy, childbirth or the puerperium (649.2)*
intestinal bypass or anastomosis status (V45.3)
Coding Clinic: 2009, Q2, P13

❷ **V45.87 Transplanted organ removal status**
Transplanted organ previously removed due to complication, failure, rejection or infection

Excludes *encounter for removal of transplanted organ – code to complication of transplanted organ (996.80–996.89)*

❷ **V45.88 Status post administration of tPA (rtPA) in a different facility within the last 24 hours prior to admission to the current facility**

Code first condition requiring tPA administration, such as:
acute cerebral infarction (433.0–433.9 with fifth-digit 1, 434.0–434.9 with fifth digit 1)
acute myocardial infarction (410.00–410.92)

❷ **V45.89 Other**
Presence of neuropacemaker or other electronic device

Excludes *artificial heart valve in situ (V43.3)*
vascular prosthesis in situ (V43.4)
Coding Clinic: 1995, Q1, P11

● **V46 Other dependence on machines and devices**

❷ **V46.0 Aspirator**

● **V46.1 Respirator [Ventilator]**
Iron lung
Coding Clinic: 2005, Q4, P94-100; 2004, Q4, P100-101

❷ **V46.11 Dependence on respirator, status**
Coding Clinic: 2003, Q4, P104-105; 2001, Q1, P12

❶ **V46.12 Encounter for respirator dependence during power failure**

❶ **V46.13 Encounter for weaning from respirator [ventilator]**

❷ **V46.14 Mechanical complication of respirator [ventilator]**
Mechanical failure of respirator [ventilator]

❷ **V46.2 Supplemental oxygen**
Long-term oxygen therapy

❷ **V46.3 Wheelchair dependence**
Wheelchair confinement status

Code first cause of dependence, such as:
muscular dystrophy (359.1)
obesity (278.00, 278.01)

❷ **V46.8 Other enabling machines**
Hyperbaric chamber
Possum [Patient-Operated-Selector-Mechanism]

Excludes *cardiac pacemaker (V45.0)*
kidney dialysis machine (V45.11)

■ **V46.9 Unspecified machine dependence**

● **V47 Other problems with internal organs**

■ **V47.0 Deficiencies of internal organs**

■ **V47.1 Mechanical and motor problems with internal organs**

■ **V47.2 Other cardiorespiratory problems**
Cardiovascular exercise intolerance with pain (with):
at rest
less than ordinary activity
ordinary activity

■ **V47.3 Other digestive problems**

■ **V47.4 Other urinary problems**

■ **V47.5 Other genital problems**

■ **V47.9 Unspecified**

● V48 Problems with head, neck, and trunk
  ◾ V48.0 Deficiencies of head
      Excludes *deficiencies of ears, eyelids, and nose (V48.8)*
  ◾ V48.1 Deficiencies of neck and trunk
  ◾ V48.2 Mechanical and motor problems with head
  ◾ V48.3 Mechanical and motor problems with neck and trunk
  ◾ V48.4 Sensory problem with head
  ◾ V48.5 Sensory problem with neck and trunk
  ◾ V48.6 Disfigurements of head
  ◾ V48.7 Disfigurements of neck and trunk
  ◾ V48.8 Other problems with head, neck, and trunk
  ◾ V48.9 Unspecified problem with head, neck, or trunk

● V49 Other conditions influencing health status
  ◾ V49.0 Deficiencies of limbs
  ◾ V49.1 Mechanical problems with limbs
  ◾ V49.2 Motor problems with limbs
  ◾ V49.3 Sensory problems with limbs
  ◾ V49.4 Disfigurements of limbs
  ◾ V49.5 Other problems of limbs
  ● V49.6 Upper limb amputation status
      Coding Clinic: 1998, Q4, P42-44
    V49.60 Unspecified level
    V49.61 Thumb
    V49.62 Other finger(s)
        Coding Clinic: 2005, Q2, P7
    V49.63 Hand
    V49.64 Wrist
        Disarticulation of wrist
    V49.65 Below elbow
    V49.66 Above elbow
        Disarticulation of elbow
    V49.67 Shoulder
        Disarticulation of shoulder
  ● V49.7 Lower limb amputation status
      Coding Clinic: 2006, Q3, P5; 1998, Q4, P42-44
    V49.70 Unspecified level
    V49.71 Great toe
    V49.72 Other toe(s)
    V49.73 Foot
    V49.74 Ankle
        Disarticulation of ankle
    V49.75 Below knee
    V49.76 Above knee
        Disarticulation of knee
        Coding Clinic: 2005, Q2, P14
    V49.77 Hip
        Disarticulation of hip

● V49.8 Other specified conditions influencing health status
  V49.81 Asymptomatic postmenopausal status (age-related) (natural) ♀   A
      Excludes *menopausal and premenopausal disorders (627.0–627.9)*
                    postsurgical menopause (256.2)
                    premature menopause (256.31)
                    symptomatic menopause (627.0–627.9)
      Coding Clinic: 2000, Q4, P53-54
  ❷ V49.82 Dental sealant status
  ❷ V49.83 Awaiting organ transplant status
      Coding Clinic: 2004, Q4, P101
  V49.84 Bed confinement status
      Coding Clinic: 2005, Q4, P94-100
  ❷ V49.85 Dual sensory impairment
      Blindness with deafness
      Combined visual hearing impairment
      Code first:
          hearing impairment (389.00–389.9)
          visual impairment (369.00–369.9)
      Coding Clinic: 2007, Q4, P99-101
  V49.89 Other specified conditions influencing health status
◾ V49.9 Unspecified

PERSONS ENCOUNTERING HEALTH SERVICES FOR SPECIFIC PROCEDURES AND AFTERCARE (V50–V59)

Note: Categories V51–V58 are intended for use to indicate a reason for care in patients who may have already been treated for some disease or injury not now present, or who are receiving care to consolidate the treatment, to deal with residual states, or to prevent recurrence.

Excludes *follow-up examination for medical surveillance following treatment (V67.0–V67.9)*

● V50 Elective surgery for purposes other than remedying health states
  V50.0 Hair transplant
  V50.1 Other plastic surgery for unacceptable cosmetic appearance
      Breast augmentation or reduction
      Face-lift
      Excludes *encounter for breast reduction (611.1)*
                    plastic surgery following healed injury or operation (V51.0–V51.8)
  V50.2 Routine or ritual circumcision ♂
      Circumcision in the absence of significant medical indication
  V50.3 Ear piercing

N Newborn Age: 0   **P** Pediatric Age: 0–17   **M** Maternity Age: 12–55   **A** Adult Age: 15–124   ♀ Females Only   ♂ Males Only   1121

V01-V89

● **V50.4 Prophylactic organ removal**

  Excludes *organ donations (V59.0–V59.9)*
                  therapeutic organ removal-code to
                  condition

  🔲**V50.41 Breast**
     Coding Clinic: 2004, Q4, P106-107

  🔲**V50.42 Ovary ♀**

  🔲**V50.49 Other**

    OGCR Section I.C.18.d.14

    For encounters specifically for prophylactic removal of breasts, ovaries, or another organ due to a genetic susceptibility to cancer or a family history of cancer, the principal or first listed code should be a code from subcategory V50.4, Prophylactic organ removal, followed by the appropriate genetic susceptibility code and the appropriate family history code.

🔲**V50.8 Other**

🔲**V50.9 Unspecified**

● **V51 Aftercare involving the use of plastic surgery**
  Plastic surgery following healed injury or operation

  Includes plastic surgery following healed injury or
               operation

  Excludes *cosmetic plastic surgery (V50.1)*
             plastic surgery as treatment for current
                 condition or injury - code to condition or
                 injury
             repair of scar tissue - code to scar

  ❶ **V51.0 Encounter for breast reconstruction following mastectomy**   A

    Excludes *deformity and disproportion*
               of reconstructed breast
               (612.0–612.1)

  🔲**V51.8 Other aftercare involving the use of plastic surgery**

● **V52 Fitting and adjustment of prosthetic device and implant**

  Includes removal of device

  Excludes *malfunction or complication of prosthetic device*
                 (996.0–996.7)
             status only, without need for care
                 (V43.0–V43.8)

🔲**V52.0 Artificial arm (complete) (partial)**

🔲**V52.1 Artificial leg (complete) (partial)**

🔲**V52.2 Artificial eye**

🔲**V52.3 Dental prosthetic device**

🔲**V52.4 Breast prosthesis and implant ♀**
  Elective implant exchange (different material) (different size)
  Removal of tissue expander without synchronous insertion of permanent implant

  Excludes *admission for initial breast implant*
                 insertion for breast augmentation
                 (V50.1)
                 complications of breast implant (996.54,
                 996.69, 996.79)
                 encounter for breast reconstruction
                 following mastectomy (V51.0)
    Coding Clinic: 1995, Q4, P80.81

🔲**V52.8 Other specified prosthetic device**
  Coding Clinic: 2002, Q3, P12; Q2, P16-17

🔲**V52.9 Unspecified prosthetic device**

● **V53 Fitting and adjustment of other device**

  Includes removal of device
            replacement of device

  Excludes *status only, without need for care*
                 (V45.0–V45.8)

● **V53.0 Devices related to nervous system and special senses**

  🔲**V53.01 Fitting and adjustment of cerebral ventricle (communicating) shunt**
    Coding Clinic: 1997, Q4, P51

  🔲**V53.02 Neuropacemaker (brain) (peripheral nerve) (spinal cord)**

  🔲**V53.09 Fitting and adjustment of other devices related to nervous system and special senses**
    Auditory substitution device
    Visual substitution device
    Coding Clinic: 1999, Q2, P3-4

🔲**V53.1 Spectacles and contact lenses**

🔲**V53.2 Hearing aid**

● **V53.3 Cardiac device**
  Reprogramming
  Coding Clinic: 1992, Q3, P3

  🔲**V53.31 Cardiac pacemaker**

    Excludes *mechanical complication*
               of cardiac pacemaker
               (996.01)
    Coding Clinic: 2002, Q1, P3; 1984, Nov-Dec, P18

  🔲**V53.32 Automatic implantable cardiac defibrillator**
    Coding Clinic: 2005, Q3, P3-9

  🔲**V53.39 Other cardiac device**
    Coding Clinic: 2008, Q2, P9-10; 2007, Q1, P20

🔲**V53.4 Orthodontic devices**

● **V53.5 Other gastrointestinal appliance and device** ◀

  Excludes *colostomy (V55.3)*
             ileostomy (V55.2)
             other artifical opening of digestive tract
               (V55.4)

  🔲**V53.50 Fitting and adjustment of intestinal appliance and device** ◀

  🔲**V53.51 Fitting and adjustment of gastric lap band** ◀

  🔲**V53.59 Fitting and adjustment of other gastrointestinal appliance and device** ◀

🔲**V53.6 Urinary devices**
  Urinary catheter

  Excludes *cystostomy (V55.5)*
             nephrostomy (V55.6)
             ureterostomy (V55.6)
             urethrostomy (V55.6)

🔲**V53.7 Orthopedic devices**
  Orthopedic:
    brace
    cast
    corset
    shoes

  Excludes *other orthopedic aftercare (V54)*

🔲**V53.8 Wheelchair**

V01-V89

● **V53.9 Other and unspecified device**
Coding Clinic: 2003, Q2, P6-7

   ◍ **V53.90 Unspecified device**

   ◍ **V53.91 Fitting and adjustment of insulin pump**
      Insulin pump titration

   ◍ **V53.99 Other device**
     Coding Clinic: 2009, Q2, P17

● **V54 Other orthopedic aftercare**
   Excludes *fitting and adjustment of orthopedic devices (V53.7)*
     malfunction of internal orthopedic device (996.40–996.49)
     other complication of nonmechanical nature (996.60–996.79)

● **V54.0 Aftercare involving internal fixation device**
   Excludes *malfunction of internal orthopedic device (996.40–996.49)*
     other complication of nonmechanical nature (996.60–996.79)
     removal of external fixation device (V54.89)

   ◍ **V54.01 Encounter for removal of internal fixation device**

   ◍ **V54.02 Encounter for lengthening/adjustment of growth rod**

   ◍ **V54.09 Other aftercare involving internal fixation device**
     Coding Clinic: 2009, Q1, P15

● **V54.1 Aftercare for healing traumatic fracture**
   Excludes *aftercare following joint replacement (V54.81)*
     aftercare for amputation stump (V54.89)

   ◍ **V54.10 Aftercare for healing traumatic fracture of arm, unspecified**

   ◍ **V54.11 Aftercare for healing traumatic fracture of upper arm**

   ◍ **V54.12 Aftercare for healing traumatic fracture of lower arm**
     Coding Clinic: 2007, Q1, P3-8

   ◍ **V54.13 Aftercare for healing traumatic fracture of hip**
     Coding Clinic: 2009, Q1, P15; 2007, Q1, P3-8; 2003, Q4, P103-105

   ◍ **V54.14 Aftercare for healing traumatic fracture of leg, unspecified**

   ◍ **V54.15 Aftercare for healing traumatic fracture of upper leg**
     Excludes *aftercare for healing traumatic fracture of hip (V54.13)*
     Coding Clinic: 2006, Q3, P6

   ◍ **V54.16 Aftercare for healing traumatic fracture of lower leg**
     Coding Clinic: 2009, Q1, P14

   ◍ **V54.17 Aftercare for healing traumatic fracture of vertebrae**

   ◍ **V54.19 Aftercare for healing traumatic fracture of other bone**
     Coding Clinic: 2005, Q1, P13

● **V54.2 Aftercare for healing pathologic fracture**
   Excludes *aftercare following joint replacement (V54.81)*

   ◍ **V54.20 Aftercare for healing pathologic fracture of arm, unspecified**

   ◍ **V54.21 Aftercare for healing pathologic fracture of upper arm**

   ◍ **V54.22 Aftercare for healing pathologic fracture of lower arm**

   ◍ **V54.23 Aftercare for healing pathologic fracture of hip**

   ◍ **V54.24 Aftercare for healing pathologic fracture of leg, unspecified**

   ◍ **V54.25 Aftercare for healing pathologic fracture of upper leg**
     Excludes *aftercare for healing pathologic fracture of hip (V54.23)*

   ◍ **V54.26 Aftercare for healing pathologic fracture of lower leg**

   ◍ **V54.27 Aftercare for healing pathologic fracture of vertebrae**
     Coding Clinic: 2008, Q3, P4; 2003, Q4, P108-109

   ◍ **V54.29 Aftercare for healing pathologic fracture of other bone**

● **V54.8 Other orthopedic aftercare**
   Coding Clinic: 2001, Q3, P19; 1999, Q4, P5x2; 1990, Q1, P10, 20

   ◍ **V54.81 Aftercare following joint replacement**
     Use additional code to identify joint replacement site (V43.60–V43.69)
     Coding Clinic: 2009, Q1, P14; 2006, Q3, P4; 2004, Q3, P12; Q2, P15

   ◍ **V54.89 Other orthopedic aftercare**
     Aftercare for healing fracture NOS
     Coding Clinic: 2007, Q2, P8-9

   ◍ **V54.9 Unspecified orthopedic aftercare**

● **V55 Attention to artificial openings**
   Includes adjustment or repositioning of catheter
     closure
     passage of sounds or bougies
     reforming
     removal or replacement of catheter
     toilet or cleansing
   Excludes *complications of external stoma (519.00–519.09, 569.60–569.69, 997.4, 997.5)*
     status only, without need for care (V44.0–V44.9)
   Coding Clinic: 1995, Q3, P13

   ◍ **V55.0 Tracheostomy**

   ◍ **V55.1 Gastrostomy**
     Coding Clinic: 1999, Q4, P9; 1997, Q3, P7-8; 1996, Q1, P14; 1995, Q3, P13

   ◍ **V55.2 Ileostomy**

   ◍ **V55.3 Colostomy**
     Coding Clinic: 2009, Q1, P14; 2005, Q2, P4-5; 1997, Q3, P9-10

   ◍ **V55.4 Other artificial opening of digestive tract**
     Coding Clinic: 2005, Q2, P14; 2003, Q1, P10

   ◍ **V55.5 Cystostomy**

   ◍ **V55.6 Other artificial opening of urinary tract**
     Nephrostomy
     Ureterostomy
     Urethrostomy

   ◍ **V55.7 Artificial vagina**

   ◍ **V55.8 Other specified artificial opening**

   ◍ **V55.9 Unspecified artificial opening**

N Newborn Age: 0   **P** Pediatric Age: 0–17   **M** Maternity Age: 12–55   **A** Adult Age: 15–124   ♀ Females Only   ♂ Males Only   **1123**

V01-V89

● **V56 Encounter for dialysis and dialysis catheter care**

    Use additional code to identify the associated condition

    Excludes *dialysis preparation-code to condition*

    Coding Clinic: 1993, Q1, P29

❶ **V56.0 Extracorporeal dialysis**

    Dialysis (renal) NOS

    Excludes *dialysis status (V45.11)*

    Coding Clinic: 2005, Q4, P77-79; 2004, Q1, P23; 2000, Q4, P39-40; 1998, Q3, P6; Q2, P20-21; 1993, Q4, P34

🔹 **V56.1 Fitting and adjustment of extracorporeal dialysis catheter**

    Removal or replacement of catheter
    Toilet or cleansing

    Use additional code for any concurrent extracorporeal dialysis (V56.0)

    Coding Clinic: 1998, Q2, P20-21

🔹 **V56.2 Fitting and adjustment of peritoneal dialysis catheter**

    Use additional code for any concurrent peritoneal dialysis (V56.8)

    Coding Clinic: 1998, Q4, P55

● **V56.3 Encounter for adequacy testing for dialysis**

🔹 **V56.31 Encounter for adequacy testing for hemodialysis**

🔹 **V56.32 Encounter for adequacy testing for peritoneal dialysis**

    Peritoneal equilibration test

🔹 **V56.8 Other dialysis**

    Peritoneal dialysis
    Coding Clinic: 1998, Q4, P55

● **V57 Care involving use of rehabilitation procedures**

    Use additional code to identify underlying condition

    Coding Clinic: 2002, Q1, P18-19; 1997, Q3, P12

❶ **V57.0 Breathing exercises**

❶ **V57.1 Other physical therapy**

    Therapeutic and remedial exercises, except breathing
    Coding Clinic: 2006, Q3, P4; 2004, Q2, P15; 2002, Q4, P56; 1999, Q4, P5

● **V57.2 Occupational therapy and vocational rehabilitation**

❶ **V57.21 Encounter for occupational therapy**
    Coding Clinic: 1999, Q4, P7

❶ **V57.22 Encounter for vocational therapy**

❶ **V57.3 Speech-language therapy**   ◀▥
    Coding Clinic: 1997, Q4, P35-37

❶ **V57.4 Orthoptic training**

● **V57.8 Other specified rehabilitation procedure**

❶ **V57.81 Orthotic training**
    Gait training in the use of artificial limbs

❶ **V57.89 Other**
    Multiple training or therapy
    Coding Clinic: 2007, Q4, P92-95; 2006, Q3, P6; 2003, Q4, P105-106, 108-109; Q2, P16; 2002, Q1, P16; 2001, Q3, P21; 1997, Q3, P11-13

❶ **V57.9 Unspecified rehabilitation procedure**

OGCR Section I.C.2.e.2

If a patient admission/encounter is solely for the administration of chemotherapy, immunotherapy or radiation therapy assign code V58.0, Encounter for radiation therapy, or V58.11, Encounter for antineoplastic chemotherapy, or V58.12, Encounter for antineoplastic immunotherapy as the first-listed or principal diagnosis. If a patient receives more than one of these therapies during the same admission more than one of these codes may be assigned, in any sequence.

● **V58 Encounter for other and unspecified procedures and aftercare**

    Excludes *convalescence and palliative care (V66.0–V66.9)*

❶ **V58.0 Radiotherapy**

    Encounter or admission for radiotherapy

    Excludes *encounter for radioactive implant-code to condition*
    radioactive iodine therapy-code to condition

    Coding Clinic: 1994, Q2, P10x2; 1993, Q4, P 36; 1987, Jan-Feb, P13

● **V58.1 Encounter for chemotherapy and immunotherapy for neoplastic conditions**

    Encounter or admission for chemotherapy

    Excludes *chemotherapy and immunotherapy for nonneoplastic conditions-code to condition*

    Coding Clinic: 2005, Q4, P94-100; 2004, Q1, P13-14; 2003, Q2, P16-17; 2000, Q1, P23; 1993, Q4, P34, 36; Q3, P4x5; 1992, Q2, P16-17; 1991, Q2, P17; 1987, Sept-Oct, P8

❶ **V58.11 Encounter for antineoplastic chemotherapy**
    Coding Clinic: 2008, Q4, P82-83, 152-155; 2007, Q4, P103-104; 2006, Q2, P20-22; 2004, Q1, P13-14

❶ **V58.12 Encounter for antineoplastic immunotherapy**
    Coding Clinic: 2004, Q1, P13-14

■ **V58.2 Blood transfusion, without reported diagnosis**
    Coding Clinic: 1994, Q1, P22

● **V58.3 Attention to dressings and sutures**

    Change or removal of wound packing

    Excludes *attention to drains (V58.49)*
    planned postoperative wound closure (V58.41)

    Coding Clinic: 2006, Q4, P117-118; 2005, Q2, P14

🔹 **V58.30 Encounter for change or removal of nonsurgical wound dressing**
    Encounter for change or removal of wound dressing NOS

🔹 **V58.31 Encounter for change or removal of surgical wound dressing**

🔹 **V58.32 Encounter for removal of sutures**
    Encounter for removal of staples

◀ New   ◀▥ Revised   ~~deleted~~ Deleted   ● Use Additional Digit(s)   ■ Nonspecific Code   ❶ First Listed   🔹 First Listed or Additional
❷ Additional Only   ● Not first-listed DX   OGCR Official Guidelines   Coding Clinic   Excludes   Includes   Use additional   Code first

● **V58.4   Other aftercare following surgery**

    Note: Codes from this subcategory should be used in conjunction with other aftercare codes to fully identify the reason for the aftercare encounter.

      Excludes   *aftercare following sterilization reversal surgery (V26.22)*
                attention to artificial openings (V55.0–V55.9)
                orthopedic aftercare (V54.0–V54.9)

      Coding Clinic: 1999, Q4, P8-9

⌀ **V58.41   Encounter for planned post-operative wound closure**

      Excludes   *disruption of operative wound (998.31–998.32)*
                encounter for dressings and suture aftercare (V58.30–V58.32)

      Coding Clinic: 1999, Q4, P15

⌀ **V58.42   Aftercare following surgery for neoplasm**
      Conditions classifiable to 140–239

⌀ **V58.43   Aftercare following surgery for injury and trauma**
      Conditions classifiable to 800–999

      Excludes   *aftercare for healing traumatic fracture (V54.10–V54.19)*

      Coding Clinic: 2007, Q2, P8-9; 1987, Nov-Dec, P9

⌀ **V58.44   Aftercare following organ transplant**
      Use additional code to identify the organ transplanted (V42.0–V42.9)
      Coding Clinic: 2004, Q4, P101

⌀ **V58.49   Other specified aftercare following surgery**
      Change or removal of drains
      Coding Clinic: 1996, Q1, P8-9x2

■ **V58.5   Orthodontics**

      Excludes   *fitting and adjustment of orthodontic device (V53.4)*

      OGCR   Section I.C.18.d.3

      This subcategory (V58.6) indicates a patient's continuous use of a prescribed drug (including such things as aspirin therapy) for the long-term treatment of a condition or for prophylactic use. It is not for use for patients who have addictions to drugs. This subcategory is not for use of medications for detoxification or maintenance programs to prevent withdrawal symptoms in patients with drug dependence (e.g., methadone maintenance for opiate dependence). Assign the appropriate code for the drug dependence instead.

      Assign a code from subcategory V58.6 if the patient is receiving a medication for an extended period as a prophylactic measure (such as for the prevention of deep vein thrombosis) or as treatment of a chronic condition (such as arthritis) or a disease requiring a lengthy course of treatment (such as cancer). Do not assign a code from subcategory V58.6 for medication being administered for a brief period of time to treat an acute illness or injury (such as a course of antibiotics to treat acute bronchitis).

● **V58.6   Long-term (current) drug use**

      Excludes   *drug abuse (305.00–305.93)*
                drug abuse and dependence complicating pregnancy (648.3–648.4)
                drug dependence (304.00–304.93)
                hormone replacement therapy (postmenopausal) (V07.4)
                prophylactic use of agents affecting estrogen receptors and estrogen levels (V07.51–V07.59)

❷ **V58.61   Long-term (current) use of anticoagulants**

      Excludes   *long-term (current) use of aspirin (V58.66)*

      Coding Clinic: 2008, Q4, P134-136; 2006, Q3, P13; 2004, Q3, P7; 2003, Q4, P108; 2003, Q1, P11-12; 2002, Q3, P13-16; Q1, P16

❷ **V58.62   Long-term (current) use of antibiotics**
      Coding Clinic: 1998, Q4, P59-60

❷ **V58.63   Long-term (current) use of antiplatelets/ antithrombotics**

      Excludes   *long-term (current) use of aspirin (V58.66)*

❷ **V58.64   Long-term (current) use of non-steroidal anti-inflammatories (NSAID)**

      Excludes   *long-term (current) use of aspirin (V58.66)*

❷ **V58.65   Long-term (current) use of steroids**

❷ **V58.66   Long-term (current) use of aspirin**
      Coding Clinic: 2004, Q4, P102-103; 2003, Q1, P11-12

❷ **V58.67   Long-term (current) use of insulin**
      Coding Clinic: 2004, Q4, P53-56

❷ **V58.69   Long-term (current) use of other medications**
      Long term current use of methadone
      Long term current use of opiate analgesic
      Other high-risk medications
      Coding Clinic: 2004, Q2, P10; Q1, P13-14; 2003, Q1, P11-12; 2000, Q2, P8-9; 1999, Q3, 13-14; 1996, Q3, P20; Q2, P7x2; 1995, Q4, P51,61

N Newborn Age: 0   **P** Pediatric Age: 0–17   **M** Maternity Age: 12–55   **A** Adult Age: 15–124   ♀ Females Only   ♂ Males Only   **1125**

V01-V89

● **V58.7 Aftercare following surgery to specified body systems, not elsewhere classified**

> **Note:** Codes from this subcategory should be used in conjunction with other aftercare codes to fully identify the reason for the aftercare encounter.

> **Excludes** *aftercare following organ transplant (V58.44)*
> *aftercare following surgery for neoplasm (V58.42)*
> Coding Clinic: 2003, Q4, P104-105

V58.71 Aftercare following surgery of the sense organs, NEC
> Conditions classifiable to 360–379, 380–389

V58.72 Aftercare following surgery of the nervous system, NEC
> Conditions classifiable to 320–359

> **Excludes** *aftercare following surgery of the sense organs, NEC (V58.71)*

V58.73 Aftercare following surgery of the circulatory system, NEC
> Conditions classifiable to 390–459
> Coding Clinic: 2009, Q2, P17

V58.74 Aftercare following surgery of the respiratory system, NEC
> Conditions classifiable to 460–519

V58.75 Aftercare following surgery of the teeth, oral cavity and digestive system, NEC
> Conditions classifiable to 520–579
> Coding Clinic: 2005, Q2, P14

V58.76 Aftercare following surgery of the genitourinary system, NEC
> Conditions classifiable to 580–629

> **Excludes** *aftercare following sterilization reversal (V26.22)*
> Coding Clinic: 2005, Q1, P11,12

V58.77 Aftercare following surgery of the skin and subcutaneous tissue, NEC
> Conditions classifiable to 680–709

V58.78 Aftercare following surgery of the musculoskeletal system, NEC
> Conditions classifiable to 710–739

> **Excludes** *orthopedic aftercare (V54.01–V54.9)*

● **V58.8 Other specified procedures and aftercare**
> Coding Clinic: 1994, Q2, P8x2

V58.81 Fitting and adjustment of vascular catheter
> Removal or replacement of catheter
> Toilet or cleansing

> **Excludes** *complications of renal dialysis (996.73)*
> *complications of vascular catheter (996.74)*
> *dialysis preparation—code to condition*
> *encounter for dialysis (V56.0–V56.8)*
> *fitting and adjustment of dialysis catheter (V56.1)*

V58.82 Fitting and adjustment of non-vascular catheter NEC
> Removal or replacement of catheter
> Toilet or cleansing

> **Excludes** *fitting and adjustment of peritoneal dialysis catheter (V56.2)*
> *fitting and adjustment of urinary catheter (V53.6)*

V58.83 Encounter for therapeutic drug monitoring
> Use additional code for any associated long-term (current) drug use (V58.61–V58.69)

> **Excludes** *blood-drug testing for medicolegal reasons (V70.4)*
> Coding Clinic: 2004, Q2, P10-11; Q1, P13-14; 2002, Q3, P13-16

V58.89 Other specified aftercare
> Coding Clinic: 2003, Q4, P106-107; 1998, Q4, P59-60

■ **V58.9 Unspecified aftercare**

OGCR Section I.C.18.d.9

Category V59 is the donor codes. They are used for living individuals who are donating blood or other body tissue. These codes are only for individuals donating for others, not for self donations. They are not for use to identify cadaveric donations.

● **V59 Donors**

> **Excludes** *examination of potential donor (V70.8)*
> *self-donation of organ or tissue--code to condition*
> Coding Clinic: 2008, Q2, P8-9; 1995, Q4, P50x2

● **V59.0 Blood**
> Coding Clinic: 1990, Q1, P9-10

❶ **V59.01 Whole blood**

❶ **V59.02 Stem cells**
> Coding Clinic: 1995, Q4, P51

❶ **V59.09 Other**

❶ **V59.1 Skin**

❶ **V59.2 Bone**

❶ **V59.3 Bone marrow**
> Coding Clinic: 1985, Jan-Feb, P15

❶ **V59.4 Kidney**

❶ **V59.5 Cornea**

❶ **V59.6 Liver**

● **V59.7 Egg (oocyte) (ovum)**

❶ **V59.70 Egg (oocyte) (ovum) donor, unspecified ♀**

❶ **V59.71 Egg (oocyte) (ovum) donor, under age 35, anonymous recipient ♀**
> Egg donor, under age 35 NOS

❶ **V59.72 Egg (oocyte) (ovum) donor, under age 35, designated recipient ♀**

❶ **V59.73 Egg (oocyte) (ovum) donor, age 35 and over, anonymous recipient ♀**
> Egg donor, age 35 and over NOS

❶ **V59.74 Egg (oocyte) (ovum) donor, age 35 and over, designated recipient ♀**

❶ **V59.8 Other specified organ or tissue**
> Coding Clinic: 2002, Q3, P20-21

❶ **V59.9 Unspecified organ or tissue**

◄ New   ◀▥ Revised   deleted Deleted   ● Use Additional Digit(s)   ■ Nonspecific Code   ❶ First Listed   First Listed or Additional
❷ Additional Only   ● Not first-listed DX   OGCR Official Guidelines   Coding Clinic   Excludes   Includes   Use additional   Code first

PERSONS ENCOUNTERING HEALTH SERVICES IN OTHER CIRCUMSTANCES (V60–V69)

● **V60 Housing, household, and economic circumstances**

❷ **V60.0 Lack of housing**
Hobos
Social migrants
Tramps
Transients
Vagabonds

❷ **V60.1 Inadequate housing**
Lack of heating
Restriction of space
Technical defects in home preventing adequate care

❷ **V60.2 Inadequate material resources**
Economic problem
Poverty NOS

❷ **V60.3 Person living alone**

❷ **V60.4 No other household member able to render care**
Person requiring care (has) (is):
     family member too handicapped, ill, or otherwise unsuited to render care
     partner temporarily away from home
     temporarily away from usual place of abode

     Excludes *holiday relief care (V60.5)*

❷ **V60.5 Holiday relief care**
Provision of health care facilities to a person normally cared for at home, to enable relatives to take a vacation

❷ **V60.6 Person living in residential institution**
Boarding school resident

● **V60.8 Other specified housing or economic circumstances**

❷ **V60.81 Foster case (status)**

❷ **V60.89 Other specified housing or economic circumstances**

❷ **V60.9 Unspecified housing or economic circumstance**

● **V61 Other family circumstances**

Includes   when these circumstances or fear of them, affecting the person directly involved or others, are mentioned as the reason, justified or not, for seeking or receiving medical advice or care

● **V61.0 Family disruption**

◐ **V61.01 Family disruption due to family member on military deployment**
Individual or family affected by other family member being on deployment

     Excludes *family disruption due to family member on non-military extended absence from home (V61.08)*

◐ **V61.02 Family disruption due to return of family member from military deployment**
Individual or family affected by other family member having returned from deployment (current or past conflict)

◐ **V61.03 Family disruption due to divorce or legal separation**

◐ **V61.04 Family disruption due to parent-child estrangement**

     Excludes *other family estrangement (V61.09)*

◐ **V61.05 Family disruption due to child in welfare custody**

◐ **V61.06 Family disruption due to child in foster care or in care of non-parental family member**

◐ **V61.07 Family disruption due to death of family member**

     Excludes *bereavement (V62.82)*

◐ **V61.08 Family disruption due to other extended absence of family member**

     Excludes *family disruption due to family member on military deployment (V61.01)*

◐■ **V61.09 Other family disruption**
Family estrangement NOS

● **V61.1 Counseling for marital and partner problems**

     Excludes *problems related to:*
         psychosexual disorders (302.0–302.9)
         sexual function (V41.7)

◐ **V61.10 Counseling for marital and partner problems, unspecified**
Marital conflict
Marital relationship problem
Partner conflict
Partner relationship problem

◐ **V61.11 Counseling for victim of spousal and partner abuse**

     Excludes *encounter for treatment of current injuries due to abuse (995.80–995.85)*

◐ **V61.12 Counseling for perpetrator of spousal and partner abuse**

● **V61.2 Parent-child problems**

◐ **V61.20 Counseling for parent-child problem, unspecified**
Concern about behavior of child
Parent-child conflict
Parent-child relationship problem

◐ **V61.21 Counseling for victim of child abuse**
Child battering
Child neglect

     Excludes *current injuries due to abuse (995.50–995.59)*

◐ **V61.22 Counseling for perpetrator of parental child abuse**

     Excludes *counseling for non-parental abuser (V62.83)*

◐ **V61.23 Counseling for parent-biological child problem**
Concern about behavior of biological child
Parent-biological child conflict
Parent-biological child relationship problem

◐ **V61.24 Counseling for parent-adopted child problem**
Concern about behavior of adopted child
Parent-adopted child conflict
Parent-adopted child relationship problem

N Newborn Age: 0   **P** Pediatric Age: 0–17   **M** Maternity Age: 12–55   **A** Adult Age: 15–124   ♀ Females Only   ♂ Males Only   **1127**

V01-V89

V61.25 Counseling for parent (guardian)-foster child problem ◄

    Concern about behavior of foster child ◄

    Parent (guardian)-foster child conflict ◄

    Parent (guardian)-foster child relationship problem ◄

V61.29 Other parent-child problems ◄▥

    ~~Problem concerning adopted or foster child~~

    Coding Clinic: 1999, Q3, P16

V61.3 Problems with aged parents or in-laws

● **V61.4** Health problems within family

  V61.41 Alcoholism in family

  V61.42 Substance abuse in family ◄

  V61.49 Other

    Care of sick or handicapped person in family or household

    Presence of sick or handicapped person in family or household

V61.5 Multiparity

V61.6 Illegitimacy or illegitimate pregnancy ♀   M

V61.7 Other unwanted pregnancy ♀   M

V61.8 Other specified family circumstances

    Problems with family members NEC

    Sibling relationship problem

    Coding Clinic: 1994, Q1, P21

V61.9 Unspecified family circumstance

● **V62** Other psychosocial circumstances

  Includes   those circumstances or fear of them, affecting the person directly involved or others, mentioned as the reason, justified or not, for seeking or receiving medical advice or care

  Excludes   *previous psychological trauma (V15.41–V15.49)*

❷ **V62.0** Unemployment

  Excludes   *circumstances when main problem is economic inadequacy or poverty (V60.2)*

❷ **V62.1** Adverse effects of work environment

● **V62.2** Other occupational circumstances or maladjustment

  ❷ **V62.21** Personal current military deployment status   A

    Individual (civilian or military) currently deployed in theater or in support of military war, peacekeeping and humanitarian operations

  ❷ **V62.22** Personal history of return from military deployment   A

    Individual (civilian or military) with past history of military war, peacekeeping and humanitarian deployment (current or past conflict)

  ❷ **V62.29** Other occupational circumstances or maladjustment   A

    Career choice problem

    Dissatisfaction with employment

    Occupational problem

❷ **V62.3** Educational circumstances

    Academic problem

    Dissatisfaction with school environment

    Educational handicap

❷ **V62.4** Social maladjustment

    Acculturation problem

    Cultural deprivation

    Political, religious, or sex discrimination

    Social:

      isolation

      persecution

❷ **V62.5** Legal circumstances

    Imprisonment

    Legal investigation

    Litigation

    Prosecution

❷ **V62.6** Refusal of treatment for reasons of religion or conscience

● **V62.8** Other psychological or physical stress, not elsewhere classified

  ❷ **V62.81** Interpersonal problems, not elsewhere classified

    Relational problem NOS

  ❷ **V62.82** Bereavement, uncomplicated

    Excludes   *bereavement as adjustment reaction (309.0)*

        family disruption due to death of family member (V61.07) ◄

  ❷ **V62.83** Counseling for perpetrator of physical/sexual abuse

    Excludes   *counseling for perpetrator of parental child abuse (V61.22)*

        counseling for perpetrator of spousal and partner abuse (V61.12)

  ❷ **V62.84** Suicidal ideation

    Excludes   *suicidal tendencies (300.9)*

    Coding Clinic: 2005, Q4, P94-100

  ❷ **V62.89** Other

    Borderline intellectual functioning

    Life circumstance problems

    Phase of life problems

    Religious or spiritual problem

❷ **V62.9** Unspecified psychosocial circumstance

● **V63** Unavailability of other medical facilities for care

V63.0 Residence remote from hospital or other health care facility

V63.1 Medical services in home not available

  Excludes   *no other household member able to render care (V60.4)*

  Coding Clinic: 2001, Q4, P67; Q1, P12

V63.2 Person awaiting admission to adequate facility elsewhere

  Coding Clinic: 1994, Q1, P22-23

V63.8 Other specified reasons for unavailability of medical facilities

    Person on waiting list undergoing social agency investigation

V63.9 Unspecified reason for unavailability of medical facilities

◄ New   ◄▥ Revised   ~~deleted~~ Deleted   ● Use Additional Digit(s)   ■ Nonspecific Code   ❶ First Listed   First Listed or Additional

❷ Additional Only   ● Not first-listed DX   OGCR Official Guidelines   Coding Clinic   Excludes   Includes   Use additional   Code first

● **V64 Persons encountering health services for specific procedures, not carried out**

● **V64.0 Vaccination not carried out**

❷ **V64.00 Vaccination not carried out, unspecified reason**

❷ **V64.01 Vaccination not carried out because of acute illness**

❷ **V64.02 Vaccination not carried out because of chronic illness or condition**

❷ **V64.03 Vaccination not carried out because of immune compromised state**

❷ **V64.04 Vaccination not carried out because of allergy to vaccine or component**

❷ **V64.05 Vaccination not carried out because of caregiver refusal**
Guardian refusal
Parent refusal

Excludes *vaccination not carried out because of caregiver refusal for religious reasons (V64.07)*
Coding Clinic: 2007, Q1, P12

❷ **V64.06 Vaccination not carried out because of patient refusal**

❷ **V64.07 Vaccination not carried out for religious reasons**

❷ **V64.08 Vaccination not carried out because patient had disease being vaccinated against**

❷ **V64.09 Vaccination not carried out for other reason**

❷ **V64.1 Surgical or other procedure not carried out because of contraindication**
Coding Clinic: 1993, 5th Issue, P9-10; 1985, Mar-April, P13; 1984, May-June, P11

❷ **V64.2 Surgical or other procedure not carried out because of patient's decision**
Coding Clinic: 2001, Q2, P8-9; 1999, Q1, P13-14; 1987, Jan-Feb, P13; 1985, July-Aug, P14

❷ **V64.3 Procedure not carried out for other reasons**

● **V64.4 Closed surgical procedure converted to open procedure**

❷ **V64.41 Laparoscopic surgical procedure converted to open procedure**
Coding Clinic: 1997, Q4, P52

❷ **V64.42 Thoracoscopic surgical procedure converted to open procedure**

❷ **V64.43 Arthroscopic surgical procedure converted to open procedure**

● **V65 Other persons seeking consultation**

◐ **V65.0 Healthy person accompanying sick person**
Boarder
Coding Clinic: 1993, Q4, P36

● **V65.1 Person consulting on behalf of another person**
Advice or treatment for nonattending third party

Excludes *concern (normal) about sick person in family (V61.41–V61.49)*

◐ **V65.11 Pediatric pre-birth visit for expectant ~~mother~~ parent(s)♀**　　**M** ◀▥
Pre-adoption visit for adoptive parent(s)　　◀

◐ **V65.19 Other person consulting on behalf of another person**

◐ **V65.2 Person feigning illness**
Malingerer
Peregrinating patient
Coding Clinic: 1999, Q3, P20

◐ **V65.3 Dietary surveillance and counseling**
Dietary surveillance and counseling (in):
NOS
colitis
diabetes mellitus
food allergies or intolerance
gastritis
hypercholesterolemia
hypoglycemia
obesity

Use additional code to identify Body Mass Index (BMI), if known (V85.0–V85.54)

● **V65.4 Other counseling, not elsewhere classified**
Health:
advice
education
instruction

Excludes *counseling (for):*
contraception (V25.40–V25.49)
genetic (V26.31–V26.39)
on behalf of third party (V65.11–V65.19)
procreative management (V26.41–V26.49)

◐ **V65.40 Counseling NOS**

◐ **V65.41 Exercise counseling**

◐ **V65.42 Counseling on substance use and abuse**

◐ **V65.43 Counseling on injury prevention**

◐ **V65.44 Human immunodeficiency virus [HIV] counseling**
Coding Clinic: 1994, Q4, P35x3

OGCR Section I.C.1.h
When a patient returns to be informed of HIV test results use V65.44 if the results of the test are negative.

◐ **V65.45 Counseling on other sexually transmitted diseases**

◐ **V65.46 Encounter for insulin pump training**

◐ **V65.49 Other specified counseling**
Coding Clinic: 2000, Q2, P8-9

◐ **V65.5 Person with feared complaint in whom no diagnosis was made**
Feared condition not demonstrated
Problem was normal state
"Worried well"
Coding Clinic: 1984, July-Aug, P20

◐ **V65.8 Other reasons for seeking consultation**
Excludes *specified symptoms*
Coding Clinic: 1992, Q3, P4

◐ **V65.9 Unspecified reason for consultation**

● **V66 Convalescence and palliative care**

❶ **V66.0 Following surgery**

❶ **V66.1 Following radiotherapy**

❶ **V66.2 Following chemotherapy**

❶ **V66.3 Following psychotherapy and other treatment for mental disorder**

❶ **V66.4 Following treatment of fracture**

❶ **V66.5 Following other treatment**

❶ **V66.6 Following combined treatment**

V01-V89

❷ **V66.7   Encounter for palliative care**
End-of-life care
Hospice care
Terminal care

Code first underlying disease

Coding Clinic: 2008, Q3, P13-14; 2005, Q2, P9-10; 2003, Q4, P107; 1996, Q4, P47-48

❶ **V66.9   Unspecified convalescence**

Coding Clinic: 1999, Q4, P8

OGCR   Section I.C.18.d.8

The follow-up codes, V24 and V67, are used to explain continuing surveillance following completed treatment of a disease, condition, or injury. They imply that the condition has been fully treated and no longer exists. They should not be confused with aftercare codes that explain current treatment for a healing condition or its sequelae. Follow-up codes may be used in conjunction with history codes to provide the full picture of the healed condition and its treatment. The follow-up code is sequenced first, followed by the history code. A follow-up code may be used to explain repeated visits. Should a condition be found to have recurred on the follow-up visit, then the diagnosis code should be used in place of the follow-up code.

● **V67   Follow-up examination**

Includes   surveillance only following completed treatment

Excludes   *surveillance of contraception (V25.40–V25.49)*

Coding Clinic: 2009, Q1, P14; 2003, Q2, P5

● **V67.0   Following surgery**

Coding Clinic: 1997, Q4, P50; 1995, Q1, P4; 1992, Q3, P11; 1985, July-Aug, P16

🗞 **V67.00   Following surgery, unspecified**

🗞 **V67.01   Follow-up vaginal pap smear ♀**
Vaginal pap smear, status-post hysterectomy for malignant condition

Use additional code to identify:
acquired absence of uterus (V88.01–V88.03)
personal history of malignant neoplasm (V10.40–V10.44)

Excludes   *vaginal pap smear status-post hysterectomy for non-malignant condition (V76.47)*

🗞 **V67.09   Following other surgery**

Excludes   *sperm count following sterilization reversal (V26.22)*
sperm count for fertility testing (V26.21)

Coding Clinic: 2008, Q3, P6; 2003, Q3, P16; 2002, Q3, P14-15; 1995, Q4, P53; Q2, P8; 1993, Q4, P32; 1992, Q3, P11; 1984, May-June, P10

🗞 **V67.1   Following radiotherapy**

Coding Clinic: 1985, July-Aug, P16

🗞 **V67.2   Following chemotherapy**
Cancer chemotherapy follow-up

Coding Clinic: 1985, July-Aug, P16

🗞 **V67.3   Following psychotherapy and other treatment for mental disorder**

🗞 **V67.4   Following treatment of healed fracture**

Excludes   *current (healing) fracture aftercare (V54.0–V54.9)*

Coding Clinic: 2009, Q1, P14

● **V67.5   Following other treatment**

🗞 **V67.51   Following completed treatment with high-risk medication, not elsewhere classified**

Excludes   *long-term (current) drug use (V58.61–V58.69)*

Coding Clinic: 1999, Q1, P5-6x2; 1990, Q1, P18

🗞 **V67.59   Other**

🗞 **V67.6   Following combined treatment**

🗞 **V67.9   Unspecified follow-up examination**

● **V68   Encounters for administrative purposes**

● **V68.0   Issue of medical certificates**

Excludes   *encounter for general medical examination (V70.0–V70.9)*

❶ **V68.01   Disability examination**

Use additional code(s) to identify:
specific examination(s), screening and testing performed (V72.0–V82.9)

Coding Clinic: 2007, Q4, P99-101

❶ **V68.09   Other issue of medical certificates**

❶ **V68.1   Issue of repeat prescriptions**
Issue of repeat prescription for:
appliance
glasses
medications

Excludes   *repeat prescription for contraceptives (V25.41–V25.49)*

❶ **V68.2   Request for expert evidence**

● **V68.8   Other specified administrative purpose**

❶ **V68.81   Referral of patient without examination or treatment**

❶ **V68.89   Other**

❶ **V68.9   Unspecified administrative purpose**

● **V69   Problems related to lifestyle**

🗞 **V69.0   Lack of physical exercise**

🗞 **V69.1   Inappropriate diet and eating habits**

Excludes   *anorexia nervosa (307.1)*
bulimia (783.6)
malnutrition and other nutritional deficiencies (260–269.9)
other and unspecified eating disorders (307.50–307.59)

🗞 **V69.2   High-risk sexual behavior**

🗞 **V69.3   Gambling and betting**

Excludes   *pathological gambling (312.31)*

🗞 **V69.4   Lack of adequate sleep**
Sleep deprivation

Excludes   *insomnia (780.52)*

Coding Clinic: 2004, Q4, P104

🗞 **V69.5   Behavioral insomnia of childhood**   P

🗞 **V69.8   Other problems related to lifestyle**
Self-damaging behavior

🗞 **V69.9   Problem related to lifestyle, unspecified**

PERSONS WITHOUT REPORTED DIAGNOSIS ENCOUNTERED DURING EXAMINATION AND INVESTIGATION OF INDIVIDUALS AND POPULATIONS (V70–V82)

Note: Nonspecific abnormal findings disclosed at the time of these examinations are classifiable to categories 790–796.

● **V70 General medical examination**

Use additional code(s) to identify any special screening examination(s) performed (V73.0–V82.9)
Coding Clinic: 1993, Q1, P28; 1985, Nov-Dec, P13

❶ **V70.0 Routine general medical examination at a health care facility**
Health checkup

Excludes   *health checkup of infant or child over 28 days old (V20.2)* ◀▥
health supervision of newborn 8 to 28 days old (V20.32) ◀
health supervision of newborn under 8 days old (V20.31) ◀
pre-procedural general physical examination (V72.83)

❶ **V70.1 General psychiatric examination, requested by the authority**

❶ **V70.2 General psychiatric examination, other and unspecified**

❶ **V70.3 Other medical examination for administrative purposes**
General medical examination for:
admission to old age home
adoption
camp
driving license
immigration and naturalization
insurance certification
marriage
prison
school admission
sports competition

Excludes   *attendance for issue of medical certificates (V68.0)*
pre-employment screening (V70.5)
Coding Clinic: 2008, Q3, P6

❶ **V70.4 Examination for medicolegal reasons**
Blood-alcohol tests
Blood-drug tests
Paternity testing

Excludes   *examination and observation following:*
accidents (V71.3, V71.4)
assault (V71.6)
rape (V71.5)

❶ **V70.5 Health examination of defined subpopulations**
Armed forces personnel
Inhabitants of institutions
Occupational health examinations
Pre-employment screening
Preschool children
Prisoners
Prostitutes
Refugees
School children
Students

❶ **V70.6 Health examination in population surveys**

Excludes   *special screening (V73.0–V82.9)*

⚕❷ **V70.7 Examination of participant in clinical trial**
Examination of participant or control in clinical research
Coding Clinic: 2006, Q2, P5-6

❶ **V70.8 Other specified general medical examinations**
Examination of potential donor of organ or tissue

❶ **V70.9 Unspecified general medical examination**

OGCR   Section I.C.18.d.6

Observation codes V29, V71 and V89 are for use in very limited circumstances when a person is being observed for a suspected condition that is ruled out. The observation codes are not for use if an injury or illness or any signs or symptoms related to the suspected condition are present. In such cases the diagnosis/symptom code is used with the corresponding E code to identify any external cause. The observation codes are to be used as principal diagnosis only. The only exception to this is when the principal diagnosis is required to be a code from the V30, Live born infant, category. Then the V29 observation code is sequenced after the V30 code. Additional codes may be used in addition to the observation code but only if they are unrelated to the suspected condition being observed.

● **V71 Observation and evaluation for suspected conditions not found**

Note: This category is to be used when persons without a diagnosis are suspected of having an abnormal condition, without signs or symptoms, which requires study, but after examination and observation, is found not to exist. This category is also for use for administrative and legal observation status.

Excludes   *suspected maternal and fetal conditions not found (V89.01–V89.09)*
Coding Clinic: 1990, Q1, P19; 1985, Nov-Dec, P10, 13

● **V71.0 Observation for suspected mental condition**

❶ **V71.01 Adult antisocial behavior**   A
Dyssocial behavior or gang activity in adult without manifest psychiatric disorder

❶ **V71.02 Childhood or adolescent antisocial behavior**
Dyssocial behavior or gang activity in child or adolescent without manifest psychiatric disorder

❶ **V71.09 Other suspected mental condition**

❶ **V71.1 Observation for suspected malignant neoplasm**
Coding Clinic: 1990, Q1, P21

❶ **V71.2 Observation for suspected tuberculosis**

❶ **V71.3 Observation following accident at work**

❶ **V71.4 Observation following other accident**
Examination of individual involved in motor vehicle traffic accident
Coding Clinic: 2006, Q1, P9; 2004, Q1, P6-7

❶ **V71.5 Observation following alleged rape or seduction**
Examination of victim or culprit

❶ **V71.6 Observation following other inflicted injury**
Examination of victim or culprit

❶ **V71.7 Observation for suspected cardiovascular disease**
Coding Clinic: 2004, Q1, P6-7; 1993, 5th Issue, P17-24; 1990, Q1, P19; 1987, Sept-Oct, P10

V01-V89

● **V71.8 Observation and evaluation for other specified suspected conditions**

    Excludes *contact with and (suspected) exposure to (potentially) hazardous substances (V15.84–V15.86, V87.0–V87.31)*

    Coding Clinic: 1990, Q1, P19

❶ **V71.81 Abuse and neglect**

    Excludes *adult abuse and neglect (995.80–995.85)*
    child abuse and neglect (995.50–995.59)

    Coding Clinic: 2000, Q4, P54-55

❶ **V71.82 Observation and evaluation for suspected exposure to anthrax**

❶ **V71.83 Observation and evaluation for suspected exposure to other biological agent**

    Coding Clinic: 2003, Q4, P46-48

❶ **V71.89 Other specified suspected conditions**

    Coding Clinic: 2008, Q3, P6-7; 2003, Q2, P15-16

❶ **V71.9 Observation for unspecified suspected condition**

    Coding Clinic: 2002, Q1, P6-7

● **V72 Special investigations and examinations**

    Includes routine examination of specific system

    Excludes *general medical examination (V70.0–70.4)*
    general screening examination of defined population groups (V70.5, V70.6, V70.7)
    health supervision of newborn 8 to 28 days old (V20.32) ◀
    health supervision of newborn under 8 days old (V20.31) ◀
    routine examination of infant or child over 28 days old (V20.2) ◀▥

Use additional code(s) to identify any special screening examination(s) performed (V73.0–V82.9)

    Coding Clinic: 2004, Q1, P15-16; 1985, Nov-Dec, P13

🅥🅐 **V72.0 Examination of eyes and vision**

● **V72.1 Examination of ears and hearing**

    Coding Clinic: 2004, Q1, P15-16

🅥🅐 **V72.11 Encounter for hearing examination following failed hearing screening**

    Coding Clinic: 2006, Q4, P118

🅥🅐 **V72.12 Encounter for hearing conservation and treatment**

    Coding Clinic: 2007, Q4, P99-101

🅥🅐 **V72.19 Other examination of ears and hearing**

🅥🅐 **V72.2 Dental examination**

● **V72.3 Gynecological examination**

    Excludes *cervical Papanicolaou smear without general gynecological examination (V76.2)*
    routine examination in contraceptive management (V25.40–V25.49)

    Coding Clinic: 2004, Q4, P104-105

🅥🅐 **V72.31 Routine gynecological examination ♀**
    General gynecological examination with or without Papanicolaou cervical smear
    Pelvic examination (annual) (periodic)

    Use additional code to identify:
    human papillomavirus (HPV) screening (V73.81)
    routine vaginal Papanicolaou smear (V76.47)

    Coding Clinic: 2006, Q2, P3,4

🅥🅐 **V72.32 Encounter for Papanicolaou cervical smear to confirm findings of recent normal smear following initial abnormal smear ♀**

    Coding Clinic: 2006, Q2, P3-4

● **V72.4 Pregnancy examination or test**

    Coding Clinic: 2005, Q4, P94-100; 2004, Q4, P105

🅥🅐 **V72.40 Pregnancy examination or test, pregnancy unconfirmed ♀**
    Possible pregnancy, not (yet) confirmed

🅥🅐 **V72.41 Pregnancy examination or test, negative result ♀**

🅥🅐 **V72.42 Pregnancy examination or test, positive result ♀**   **M**

🅥🅐 **V72.5 Radiological examination, not elsewhere classified**
    Routine chest x-ray

    Excludes *examination for suspected tuberculosis (V71.2)*
    radiologic examinations as part of pre-procedural testing (V72.81–V72.84) ◀

    Coding Clinic: 1990, Q1, P8, 10, 19-21; 1985, Nov-Dec, P13

    OGCR Section I.C.18.d.15 *(outpatient)*
    V72.5 is not to be used if any sign or symptoms, or reason for a test is documented.

● **V72.6 Laboratory examination** ◀▥
    Encounters for blood and urine testing ◀

    Excludes *that for suspected disorder (V71.0–V71.9)*

🅥🅐 **V72.60 Laboratory examination, unspecified** ◀

🅥🅐 **V72.61 Antibody response examination** ◀
    Immunity status testing ◀

    Excludes *encounter for allergy testing (V72.7)* ◀

🅥🅐 **V72.62 Laboratory examination ordered as part of a routine general medical examination** ◀
    Blood tests for routine general physical examination ◀

🅥🅐 **V72.63 Pre-procedural laboratory examination** ◀
    Blood tests prior to treatment or procedure ◀
    Pre-operative laboratory examination ◀

🅥🅐 **V72.69 Other laboratory examination** ◀

    Coding Clinic: 2006, Q2, P4; 1994, Q4, P35; 1990, Q1, P22; 1985, Nov-Dec, P13

    OGCR Section I.C.18.d.15 *(outpatient)*
    V72.6 is not to be used if any sign or symptoms, or reason for a test is documented.

🅥🅐 **V72.7 Diagnostic skin and sensitization tests**
    Allergy tests
    Skin tests for hypersensitivity

    Excludes *diagnostic skin tests for bacterial diseases (V74.0–V74.9)*

    Coding Clinic: 1985, Nov-Dec, P13

● **V72.8   Other specified examinations**

> **Excludes**   *pre-procedural laboratory examinations (V72.63)* ◄
>
> Coding Clinic: 1995, Q4, P51-52; 1990, Q1, P10; 1985, Nov-Dec, P13

V72.81   Preoperative cardiovascular examination
> Pre-procedural cardiovascular examination
> Coding Clinic: 1995, Q4, P51-52

V72.82   Preoperative respiratory examination
> Pre-procedural respiratory examination
> Coding Clinic: 1996, Q3, P14

V72.83   Other specified preoperative examination
> Examination prior to chemotherapy ◄
> Other pre-procedural examination
> Pre-procedural general physical examination
>
> **Excludes**   *routine general medical examination (V70.0)*
> Coding Clinic: 1996, Q3, P14; 1995, Q4, P52

V72.84   Preoperative examination, unspecified
> Pre-procedural examination, unspecified
> Coding Clinic: 1995, Q4, P52

V72.85   Other specified examination
> Coding Clinic: 2004, Q1, P12-13

V72.86   Encounter for blood typing

■ **V72.9   Unspecified examination**

● **V73   Special screening examination for viral and chlamydial diseases**

V73.0   Poliomyelitis

V73.1   Smallpox

V73.2   Measles

V73.3   Rubella

V73.4   Yellow fever

V73.5   Other arthropod-borne viral diseases
> Dengue fever
> Hemorrhagic fever
> Viral encephalitis:
>   mosquito-borne
>   tick-borne

V73.6   Trachoma

● **V73.8   Other specified viral and chlamydial diseases**

V73.81   Human papillomavirus (HPV)
> Coding Clinic: 2007, Q4, P99-101

V73.88   Other specified chlamydial diseases
> Coding Clinic: 2007, Q4, P124-125

V73.89   Other specified viral diseases

> **OGCR**   Section I.C.1.h.
>
> If a patient is being seen to determine HIV status, use V73.89, Screening for other specified viral disease. Use V69.8, Other problems related to lifestyle, as a secondary code if an asymptomatic patient is in a known high risk group for HIV. Should a patient with signs or symptoms or illness, or a confirmed HIV related diagnosis be tested for HIV, code the signs and symptoms or the diagnosis. An additional counseling code V65.44 may be used if counseling is provided during the encounter for the test.

● **V73.9   Unspecified viral and chlamydial disease**

V73.98   Unspecified chlamydial disease

V73.99   Unspecified viral disease

● **V74   Special screening examination for bacterial and spirochetal diseases**

> **Includes**   diagnostic skin tests for these diseases

V74.0   Cholera

V74.1   Pulmonary tuberculosis

V74.2   Leprosy [Hansen's disease]

V74.3   Diphtheria

V74.4   Bacterial conjunctivitis

V74.5   Venereal disease
> Screening for bacterial and spirochetal sexually transmitted diseases
> Screening for sexually transmitted diseases NOS
>
> **Excludes**   *special screening for nonbacterial sexually transmitted diseases (V73.81–V73.89, V75.4, V75.8)*
> Coding Clinic: 2007, Q4, P124-125

V74.6   Yaws

V74.8   Other specified bacterial and spirochetal diseases
> Brucellosis
> Leptospirosis
> Plague
> Tetanus
> Whooping cough

V74.9   Unspecified bacterial and spirochetal disease

● **V75   Special screening examination for other infectious diseases**

V75.0   Rickettsial diseases

V75.1   Malaria

V75.2   Leishmaniasis

V75.3   Trypanosomiasis
> Chagas' disease
> Sleeping sickness

V75.4   Mycotic infections

V75.5   Schistosomiasis

V75.6   Filariasis

V75.7   Intestinal helminthiasis

V75.8   Other specified parasitic infections

V75.9   Unspecified infectious disease

● **V76   Special screening for malignant neoplasms**

V76.0   Respiratory organs

● **V76.1   Breast**

V76.10   Breast screening, unspecified

V76.11   Screening mammogram for high-risk patient ♀
> Coding Clinic: 2003, Q2, P3-5

V76.12   Other screening mammogram
> Coding Clinic: 2006, Q2, P10; Q2, P3-5

V76.19   Other screening breast examination

V76.2   Cervix ♀
> Routine cervical Papanicolaou smear
>
> **Excludes**   *special screening for human papillomavirus (V73.81) that as part of a general gynecological examination (V72.31)*

V76.3   Bladder

V01-V89

● **V76.4   Other sites**
- ⚕ V76.41   Rectum
- ⚕ V76.42   Oral cavity
- ⚕ V76.43   Skin
- ⚕ V76.44   Prostate ♂
- ⚕ V76.45   Testis ♂
- ⚕ V76.46   Ovary ♀
- ⚕ V76.47   Vagina ♀

     Vaginal pap smear status-post hysterectomy for non-malignant condition

     Use additional code to identify acquired absence of uterus (V88.01–V88.03)

     Excludes   *vaginal pap smear status-post hysterectomy for malignant condition (V67.01)*

- ⚕ V76.49   Other sites
     Coding Clinic: 1999, Q1, P4

● **V76.5   Intestine**
- ⚕ V76.50   Intestine, unspecified
- ⚕ V76.51   Colon
     Excludes   *rectum (V76.41)*
     Coding Clinic: 2004, Q1, P11-12; 2001, Q4, P55-56x2
- ⚕ V76.52   Small intestine

● **V76.8   Other neoplasm**
- ⚕ V76.81   Nervous system
- ⚕ V76.89   Other neoplasm

⚕ **V76.9   Unspecified**

● **V77   Special screening for endocrine, nutritional, metabolic, and immunity disorders**
- ⚕ V77.0   Thyroid disorders
- ⚕ V77.1   Diabetes mellitus
- ⚕ V77.2   Malnutrition
- ⚕ V77.3   Phenylketonuria [PKU]
- ⚕ V77.4   Galactosemia
- ⚕ V77.5   Gout
- ⚕ V77.6   Cystic fibrosis
     Screening for mucoviscidosis
- ⚕ V77.7   Other inborn errors of metabolism
- ⚕ V77.8   Obesity
- ● V77.9   Other and unspecified endocrine, nutritional, metabolic, and immunity disorders
  - ⚕ V77.91   Screening for lipid disorders
     Screening cholesterol level
     Screening for hypercholesterolemia
     Screening for hyperlipidemia
  - ⚕ V77.99   Other and unspecified endocrine, nutritional, metabolic, and immunity disorders

● **V78   Special screening for disorders of blood and blood-forming organs**
- ⚕ V78.0   Iron deficiency anemia
- ⚕ V78.1   Other and unspecified deficiency anemia
- ⚕ V78.2   Sickle-cell disease or trait
- ⚕ V78.3   Other hemoglobinopathies
- ⚕ V78.8   Other disorders of blood and blood-forming organs
- ⚕ V78.9   Unspecified disorder of blood and blood-forming organs

● **V79   Special screening for mental disorders and developmental handicaps**
- ⚕ V79.0   Depression
- ⚕ V79.1   Alcoholism
- ⚕ V79.2   Mental retardation
- ⚕ V79.3   Developmental handicaps in early childhood
- ⚕ V79.8   Other specified mental disorders and developmental handicaps
- ⚕ V79.9   Unspecified mental disorder and developmental handicap

● **V80   Special screening for neurological, eye, and ear diseases**
- ● V80.0   Neurological conditions   ◀▥
  - ⚕ V80.01   Traumatic brain injury   ◀
  - ⚕ V80.09   Other neurological conditions   ◀
- ⚕ V80.1   Glaucoma
- ⚕ V80.2   Other eye conditions
     Screening for:
       cataract
       congenital anomaly of eye
       senile macular lesions
     Excludes   *general vision examination (V72.0)*
- ⚕ V80.3   Ear diseases
     Excludes   *general hearing examination (V72.11–V72.19)*

● **V81   Special screening for cardiovascular, respiratory, and genitourinary diseases**
- ⚕ V81.0   Ischemic heart disease
- ⚕ V81.1   Hypertension
- ⚕ V81.2   Other and unspecified cardiovascular conditions
- ⚕ V81.3   Chronic bronchitis and emphysema
- ⚕ V81.4   Other and unspecified respiratory conditions
     Excludes   *screening for:*
       lung neoplasm (V76.0)
       pulmonary tuberculosis (V74.1)
- ⚕ V81.5   Nephropathy
     Screening for asymptomatic bacteriuria
- ⚕ V81.6   Other and unspecified genitourinary conditions

● **V82   Special screening for other conditions**
- ⚕ V82.0   Skin conditions
- ⚕ V82.1   Rheumatoid arthritis
- ⚕ V82.2   Other rheumatic disorders
- ⚕ V82.3   Congenital dislocation of hip
- ⚕ V82.4   Maternal postnatal screening for chromosomal anomalies ♀
     Excludes   *antenatal screening by amniocentesis (V28.0)*
- ⚕ V82.5   Chemical poisoning and other contamination
     Screening for:
       heavy metal poisoning
       ingestion of radioactive substance
       poisoning from contaminated water supply
       radiation exposure
- ⚕ V82.6   Multiphasic screening
- ● V82.7   Genetic screening
     Excludes   *genetic testing for procreative management (V26.31–V26.39)*
     Coding Clinic: 2006, Q4, P118
  - ⚕ V82.71   Screening for genetic disease carrier status
  - ⚕ V82.79   Other genetic screening

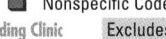

◀ New   ◀▥ Revised   ~~deleted~~ Deleted   ● Use Additional Digit(s)   ■ Nonspecific Code   ❶ First Listed   ⚕ First Listed or Additional
❷ Additional Only   ● Not first-listed DX   OGCR Official Guidelines   Coding Clinic   Excludes   Includes   Use additional   Code first

● **V82.8 Other specified conditions**

    ◐ **V82.81 Osteoporosis**

         Use additional code to identify:
         hormone replacement therapy
         (postmenopausal) status
         (V07.4)
         postmenopausal (natural) status
         (V49.81)

         Coding Clinic: 2000, Q4, P53-54

    ◐ **V82.89 Other specified conditions**

● **V82.9 Unspecified condition**

GENETICS (V83–V84)

OGCR Section I.C.18.d.3

Genetic carrier status indicates that a person carries a gene, associated with a particular disease, which may be passed to offspring who may develop that disease. The person does not have the disease and is not at risk of developing the disease.

● **V83 Genetic carrier status**

  ● **V83.0 Hemophilia A carrier**

    ◐ **V83.01 Asymptomatic hemophilia A carrier**

    ◐ **V83.02 Symptomatic hemophilia A carrier**

  ● **V83.8 Other genetic carrier status**

    ◐ **V83.81 Cystic fibrosis gene carrier**

    ◐ **V83.89 Other genetic carrier status**

OGCR Section I.C.18.d.3

Genetic susceptibility indicates that a person has a gene that increases the risk of that person developing the disease. Codes from category V84, Genetic susceptibility to disease, should not be used as principal or first-listed codes.

● **V84 Genetic susceptibility to disease**

     Includes   Confirmed abnormal gene

     Use additional code, if applicable, for any associated family history of the disease (V16–V19)

  ● **V84.0 Genetic susceptibility to malignant neoplasm**

     Code first, if applicable, any current malignant neoplasms (140.0–195.8, 200.0–208.9, 230.0–234.9)

     Use additional code, if applicable, for any personal history of malignant neoplasm (V10.0–V10.9)

    ❷ **V84.01 Genetic susceptibility to malignant neoplasm of breast**
         Coding Clinic: 2004, Q4, P106-107

    ❷ **V84.02 Genetic susceptibility to malignant neoplasm of ovary ♀**

    ❷ **V84.03 Genetic susceptibility to malignant neoplasm of prostate ♂**

    ❷ **V84.04 Genetic susceptibility to malignant neoplasm of endometrium ♀**

    ❷ **V84.09 Genetic susceptibility to other malignant neoplasm**

  ● **V84.8 Genetic susceptibility to other disease**

    ❷ **V84.81 Genetic susceptibility to multiple endocrine neoplasia [MEN]**
         Coding Clinic: 2007, Q4, P99-101

    ❷ **V84.89 Genetic susceptibility to other disease**

BODY MASS INDEX (V85)

● **V85 Body mass index (BMI)**
     Kilograms per meters squared

     Note: BMI adult codes are for use for persons over 20 years old
     Coding Clinic: 2008, Q4, P191; 2005, Q4, P94-100

  ❷ **V85.0 Body Mass Index less than 19, adult**   A

  ❷ **V85.1 Body Mass Index between 19–24, adult**   A

  ● **V85.2 Body Mass Index between 25–29, adult**

    ❷ **V85.21 Body Mass Index 25.0–25.9, adult**   A

    ❷ **V85.22 Body Mass Index 26.0–26.9, adult**   A

    ❷ **V85.23 Body Mass Index 27.0–27.9, adult**   A

    ❷ **V85.24 Body Mass Index 28.0–28.9, adult**   A

    ❷ **V85.25 Body Mass Index 29.0–29.9, adult**   A

  ● **V85.3 Body Mass Index between 30–39, adult**

    ❷ **V85.30 Body Mass Index 30.0–30.9, adult**   A

    ❷ **V85.31 Body Mass Index 31.0–31.9, adult**   A

    ❷ **V85.32 Body Mass Index 32.0–32.9, adult**   A

    ❷ **V85.33 Body Mass Index 33.0–33.9, adult**   A

    ❷ **V85.34 Body Mass Index 34.0–34.9, adult**   A

    ❷ **V85.35 Body Mass Index 35.0–35.9, adult**   A

    ❷ **V85.36 Body Mass Index 36.0–36.9, adult**   A

    ❷ **V85.37 Body Mass Index 37.0–37.9, adult**   A

    ❷ **V85.38 Body Mass Index 38.0–38.9, adult**   A

    ❷ **V85.39 Body Mass Index 39.0–39.9, adult**   A

  ❷ **V85.4 Body Mass Index 40 and over, adult**   A

  ● **V85.5 Body Mass Index, pediatric**

     Note: BMI pediatric codes are for use for persons age 2–20 years old. These percentiles are based on the growth charts published by the Centers for Disease Control and Prevention (CDC)

    ❷ **V85.51 Body Mass Index, pediatric, less than 5th percentile for age**   P

    ❷ **V85.52 Body Mass Index, pediatric, 5th percentile to less than 85th percentile for age**   P

    ❷ **V85.53 Body Mass Index, pediatric, 85th percentile to less than 95th percentile for age**   P

    ❷ **V85.54 Body Mass Index, pediatric, greater than or equal to 95th percentile for age**   P

ESTROGEN RECEPTOR STATUS (V86)

● **V86 Estrogen receptor status**

     Code first malignant neoplasm of breast (174.0–174.9, 175.0–175.9)

  ❷ **V86.0 Estrogen receptor positive status [ER+]**

  ❷ **V86.1 Estrogen receptor negative status [ER-]**

V01-V89

● V87 Other specified personal exposures and history
        presenting hazards to health

  ● V87.0 Contact with and (suspected) exposure to
            hazardous metals

            Excludes *exposure to lead (V15.86)*
                          toxic effect of metals (984.0-985.9)

    🐾 V87.01 Arsenic
    🐾 V87.09 Other hazardous metals
                Chromium compounds
                Nickel dust

  ● V87.1 Contact with and (suspected) exposure to
            hazardous aromatic compounds

            Excludes *toxic effects of aromatic compounds*
                          (982.0, 983.0)

    🐾 V87.11 Aromatic amines
    🐾 V87.12 Benzene
    🐾 V87.19 Other hazardous aromatic compounds
                Aromatic dyes NOS
                Polycyclic aromatic hydrocarbons

  🐾 V87.2 Contact with and (suspected) exposure to other
            potentially hazardous chemicals
            Dyes NOS

            Excludes *exposure to asbestos (V15.84)*
                          toxic effect of chemicals (980–989)

  ● V87.3 Contact with and (suspected) exposure to other
            potentially hazardous substances

            Excludes *contact with and (suspected) exposure*
                          to potentially hazardous body
                          fluids (V15.85)
                          toxic effect of substances (980–989)

    🐾 V87.31 Exposure to mold
    🐾 V87.32 Contact with and (suspected)
                exposure to algae bloom   ◄
    🐾 V87.39 Contact with and (suspected) exposure to
                other potentially hazardous substances

  ● V87.4 Personal history of drug therapy

            Excludes *long-term (current) drug use*
                          (V58.61-V58.69)

    🐾 V87.41 Personal history of antineoplastic
                chemotherapy
    🐾 V87.42 Personal history of monoclonal drug
                therapy
    ❷ V87.43 Personal history of estrogen therapy   ◄
    ❷ V87.44 Personal history of inhaled steroid
                therapy   ◄
    ❷ V87.45 Personal history of systemic steroid
                therapy   ◄
                Personal history of steroid therapy
                NOS   ◄
    ❷ V87.46 Personal history of
                immunosuppression therapy   ◄

                Excludes *personal history of steroid*
                              therapy (V87.44,
                              V87.45)   ◄

    🐾 V87.49 Personal history of other drug therapy

● V88 Acquired absence of other organs and tissue

  ● V88.0 Acquired absence of cervix and uterus

    ❷ V88.01 Acquired absence of both cervix and
                uterus ♀
                Acquired absence of uterus NOS
                Status post total hysterectomy

    ❷ V88.02 Acquired absence of uterus with
                remaining cervical stump ♀
                Status post partial hysterectomy with
                remaining cervical stump

    ❷ V88.03 Acquired absence of cervix with
                remaining uterus ♀

● V89 Other suspected conditions not found

  ● V89.0 Suspected maternal and fetal conditions not
            found

            Excludes *known or suspected fetal anomalies*
                          affecting management of mother,
                          not ruled out (655.00 655.93,
                          656.00–656.93, 657.00–657.03,
                          658.00–658.93)
                          newborn and perinatal conditions –
                          code to condition

    🐾 V89.01 Suspected problem with amniotic cavity
                and membrane not found ♀   M
                Suspected oligohydramnios not
                found
                Suspected polyhydramnios not
                found
    🐾 V89.02 Suspected placental problem not
                found ♀   M
    🐾 V89.03 Suspected fetal anomaly not
                found ♀   M
    🐾 V89.04 Suspected problem with fetal growth
                not found ♀   M
    🐾 V89.05 Suspected cervical shortening not
                found ♀   M
    🐾 V89.09 Other suspected maternal and fetal
                condition not found ♀   M

V01-V89

1136   ◄ New   ◀▦ Revised   deleted Deleted   ● Use Additional Digit(s)   ■ Nonspecific Code   ❶ First Listed   🐾 First Listed or Additional
        ❷ Additional Only   ● Not first-listed DX   OGCR Official Guidelines   Coding Clinic   Excludes   Includes   Use additional   Code first

SUPPLEMENTARY CLASSIFICATION OF EXTERNAL CAUSES OF INJURY AND POISONING (E000-E999)

This section is provided to permit the classification of environmental events, circumstances, and conditions as the cause of injury, poisoning, and other adverse effects. Where a code from this section is applicable, it is intended that it shall be used in addition to a code from one of the main chapters of ICD-9-CM, indicating the nature of the condition. Certain other conditions which may be stated to be due to external causes are classified in Chapters 1 to 16 of ICD-9-CM. For these, the "E" code classification should be used as an additional code for more detailed analysis.

Machinery accidents [other than those connected with transport] are classifiable to category E919, in which the fourth digit allows a broad classification of the type of machinery involved. ~~If a more detailed classification of type of machinery is required, it is suggested that the "Classification of Industrial Accidents according to Agency," prepared by the International Labor Office, be used in addition; it is included in this publication.~~

Categories for "late effects" of accidents and other external causes are to be found at E929, E959, E969, E977, E989, and E999.

~~Definitions and examples related to transport accidents~~

(a) A transport accident (E800–E848) is any accident involving a device designed primarily for, or being used at the time primarily for, conveying persons or goods from one place to another.

> **Includes** accidents involving:
> aircraft and spacecraft (E840–E845)
> watercraft (E830–E838)
> motor vehicle (E810–E825)
> railway (E800–E807)
> other road vehicles (E826–E829)

In classifying accidents which involve more than one kind of transport, the above order of precedence of transport accidents should be used.

Accidents involving agricultural and construction machines, such as tractors, cranes, and bulldozers, are regarded as transport accidents only when these vehicles are under their own power on a highway [otherwise the vehicles are regarded as machinery]. Vehicles which can travel on land or water, such as hovercraft and other amphibious vehicles, are regarded as watercraft when on the water, as motor vehicles when on the highway, and as off-road motor vehicles when on land, but off the highway.

> **Excludes** *accidents:*
> *in sports which involve the use of transport but where the transport vehicle itself was not involved in the accident*
> *involving vehicles which are part of industrial equipment used entirely on industrial premises*
> *occurring during transportation but unrelated to the hazards associated with the means of transportation [e.g., injuries received in a fight on board ship; transport vehicle involved in a cataclysm such as an earthquake]*
> *to persons engaged in the maintenance or repair of transport equipment or vehicle not in motion, unless injured by another vehicle in motion*

(b) A railway accident is a transport accident involving a railway train or other railway vehicle operated on rails, whether in motion or not.

> **Excludes** *accidents:*
> *in repair shops*
> *in roundhouse or on turntable*
> *on railway premises but not involving a train or other railway vehicle*

(c) A railway train or railway vehicle is any device with or without cars coupled to it, designed for traffic on a railway.

> **Includes** interurban:
> electric car (operated chiefly on its own right-of-way, not open to other traffic)
> streetcar (operated chiefly on its own right-of-way, not open to other traffic)
> railway train, any power [diesel] [electric] [steam]
> funicular
> monorail or two-rail
> subterranean or elevated
> other vehicle designed to run on a railway track

> **Excludes** *interurban electric cars [streetcars] specified to be operating on a right-of-way that forms part of the public street or highway [definition (n)]*

(d) A railway or railroad is a right-of-way designed for traffic on rails, which is used by carriages or wagons transporting passengers or freight, and by other rolling stock, and which is not open to other public vehicular traffic

(e) A motor vehicle accident is a transport accident involving a motor vehicle. It is defined as a motor vehicle traffic accident or as a motor vehicle nontraffic accident according to whether the accident occurs on a public highway or elsewhere.

> **Excludes** *injury or damage due to cataclysm*
> *injury or damage while a motor vehicle, not under its own power, is being loaded on, or unloaded from, another conveyance*

(f) A motor vehicle traffic accident is any motor vehicle accident occurring on a public highway [i.e., originating, terminating, or involving a vehicle partially on the highway]. A motor vehicle accident is assumed to have occurred on the highway unless another place is specified, except in the case of accidents involving only off-road motor vehicles which are classified as nontraffic accidents unless the contrary is stated.

(g) A motor vehicle nontraffic accident is any motor vehicle accident which occurs entirely in any place other than a public highway.

(h) A public highway [trafficway] or street is the entire width between property lines [or other boundary lines] of every way or place, of which any part is open to the use of the public for purposes of vehicular traffic as a matter of right or custom. A roadway is that part of the public highway designed, improved, and ordinarily used, for vehicular travel.

> **Includes** approaches (public) to:
> docks
> public building
> station

> **Excludes** *driveway (private)*
> *parking lot*
> *ramp*
> *roads in:*
> *airfield*
> *farm*
> *industrial premises*
> *mine*
> *private grounds*
> *quarry*

N Newborn Age: 0   **P** Pediatric Age: 0–17   **M** Maternity Age: 12–55   **A** Adult Age: 15–124   ♀ Females Only   ♂ Males Only   1137

E000–E999

(i) A motor vehicle is any mechanically or electrically powered device, not operated on rails, upon which any person or property may be transported or drawn upon a highway. Any object such as a trailer, coaster, sled, or wagon being towed by a motor vehicle is considered a part of the motor vehicle.

Includes automobile [any type]
bus
construction machinery, farm and industrial machinery, steam roller, tractor, army tank, highway grader, or similar vehicle on wheels or treads, while in transport under own power
fire engine (motorized)
motorcycle
motorized bicycle [moped] or scooter
trolley bus not operating on rails
truck
van

Excludes *devices used solely to move persons or materials within the confines of a building and its premises, such as:*
building elevator
coal car in mine
electric baggage or mail truck used solely within a railroad station
electric truck used solely within an industrial plant
moving overhead crane

(j) A motorcycle is a two-wheeled motor vehicle having one or two riding saddles and sometimes having a third wheel for the support of a sidecar. The sidecar is considered part of the motorcycle.

Includes motorized:
bicycle [moped]
scooter
tricycle

(k) An off-road motor vehicle is a motor vehicle of special design, to enable it to negotiate rough or soft terrain or snow. Examples of special design are high construction, special wheels and tires, driven by treads, or support on a cushion of air.

Includes all terrain vehicle [ATV]
army tank
hovercraft, on land or swamp
snowmobile

(l) A driver of a motor vehicle is the occupant of the motor vehicle operating it or intending to operate it. A motorcyclist is the driver of a motorcycle. Other authorized occupants of a motor vehicle are passengers.

(m) An other road vehicle is any device, except a motor vehicle, in, on, or by which any person or property may be transported on a highway.

Includes animal carrying a person or goods
animal-drawn vehicle
animal harnessed to conveyance
bicycle [pedal cycle]
streetcar
tricycle (pedal)

Excludes *pedestrian conveyance [definition (q)]*

(n) A streetcar is a device designed and used primarily for transporting persons within a municipality, running on rails, usually subject to normal traffic control signals, and operated principally on a right-of-way that forms part of the traffic way. A trailer being towed by a streetcar is considered a part of the streetcar.

Includes interurban or intraurban electric or streetcar, when specified to be operating on a street or public highway
tram (car)
trolley (car)

(o) A pedal cycle is any road transport vehicle operated solely by pedals.

Includes bicycle
pedal cycle
tricycle

Excludes *motorized bicycle [definition (i)]*

(p) A pedal cyclist is any person riding on a pedal cycle or in a sidecar attached to such a vehicle.

(q) A pedestrian conveyance is any human powered device by which a pedestrian may move other than by walking or by which a walking person may move another pedestrian.

Includes baby carriage
coaster wagon
heelies
ice skates
perambulator
pushcart
pushchair
roller skates
scooter
skateboard
skis
sled
wheelchair
wheelies

(r) A pedestrian is any person involved in an accident who was not at the time of the accident riding in or on a motor vehicle, railroad train, streetcar, animal-drawn or other vehicle, or on a bicycle or animal.

Includes person:
changing tire of vehicle
in or operating a pedestrian conveyance
making adjustment to motor of vehicle
on foot

(s) A watercraft is any device for transporting passengers or goods on the water.

(t) A small boat is any watercraft propelled by paddle, oars, or small motor, with a passenger capacity of less than ten.

Includes boat NOS
canoe
coble
dinghy
punt
raft
rowboat
rowing shell
scull
skiff
small motorboat

Excludes *barge*
lifeboat (used after abandoning ship)
raft (anchored) being used as a diving platform
yacht

◀ New ◀◀◀ Revised ~~deleted~~ Deleted ● Use Additional Digit(s) ■ Nonspecific Code

OGCR Official Guidelines *Coding Clinic* Excludes Includes Use additional Code first Omit code

(u) An aircraft is any device for transporting passengers or goods in the air.

> **Includes** airplane [any type]
> balloon
> bomber
> dirigible
> glider (hang)
> military aircraft
> parachute

(v) A commercial transport aircraft is any device for collective passenger or freight transportation by air, whether run on commercial lines for profit or by government authorities, with the exception of military craft.

EXTERNAL CAUSE STATUS (E000) ◄

Note: A code from category E000 should be used in conjunction with the external cause code(s) assigned to a record to indicate the status of the person at the time the event occurred. A single code from category E000 should be assigned for an encounter. ◄

● **E000 External cause status** ◄

E000.0 Civilian activity done for income or pay ◄
Civilian activity done for financial or other compensation
> **Excludes** *military activity (E000.1)* ◄

E000.1 Military activity ◄
> **Excludes** *activity of off duty military personnel (E000.8)* ◄

E000.8 Other external cause status ◄
Activity NEC ◄
Hobby not done for income ◄
Leisure activity ◄
Off-duty activity of military personnel ◄
Recreation or sport not for income or while a student ◄
Student activity ◄
Volunteer activity ◄
> **Excludes** *civilian activity done for income or compensation (E000.0)* ◄
> *military activity (E000.1)*

E000.9 Unspecified external cause status ◄

ACTIVITY (E001-E030) ◄

Note: Categories E001 to E030 are provided for use to indicate the activity of the person seeking healthcare for an injury or health condition, such as a heart attack while shoveling snow, which resulted from, or was contributed to, by the activity. These codes are appropriate for use for both acute injuries, such as those from chapter 17, and conditions that are due to the long-term, cumulative effects of an activity, such as those from chapter 13. They are also appropriate for use with external cause codes for cause and intent if identifying the activity provides additional information on the event. ◄

These codes should be used in conjunction with other external cause codes for external cause status (E000) and place of occurrence (E849). ◄

This section contains the following broad activity categories: ◄

E001 Activities involving walking and running ◄
E002 Activities involving water and water craft ◄
E003 Activities involving ice and snow ◄

E004 Activities involving climbing, rappelling, and jumping off ◄
E005 Activities involving dancing and other rhythmic movement ◄
E006 Activities involving other sports and athletics played individually ◄
E007 Activities involving other sports and athletics played as a team or group ◄
E008 Activities involving other specified sports and athletics ◄
E009 Activity involving other cardiorespiratory exercise ◄
E010 Activity involving other muscle strengthening exercises ◄
E011 Activities involving computer technology and electronic devices ◄
E012 Activities involving arts and handcrafts ◄
E013 Activities involving personal hygiene and household maintenance ◄
E014 Activities involving person providing caregiving ◄
E015 Activities involving food preparation, cooking and grilling ◄
E016 Activities involving property and land maintenance, building and construction ◄
E017 Activities involving roller coasters and other types of external motion ◄
E018 Activities involving playing musical instrument ◄
E019 Activities involving animal care ◄
E029 Other activity ◄
E030 Unspecified activity ◄

● **E001 Activities involving walking and running** ◄
> **Excludes** *walking an animal (E019.0)* ◄
> *walking or running on a treadmill (E009.0)* ◄

E001.0 Walking, marching and hiking ◄
Walking, marching and hiking on level or elevated terrain
> **Excludes** *mountain climbing (E004.0)* ◄

E001.1 Running ◄

● **E002 Activities involving water and water craft** ◄
> **Excludes** *activities involving ice (E003.0-E003.9)* ◄
> *boating and other watercraft transport accidents (E830-E838)* ◄

E002.0 Swimming ◄
E002.1 Springboard and platform diving ◄
E002.2 Water polo ◄
E002.3 Water aerobics and water exercise ◄
E002.4 Underwater diving and snorkeling ◄
SCUBA diving
E002.5 Rowing, canoeing, kayaking, rafting and tubing ◄
Canoeing, kayaking, rafting and tubing in calm and turbulent water
E002.6 Water skiing and wake boarding ◄
E002.7 Surfing, windsurfing and boogie boarding ◄
E002.8 Water sliding ◄
E002.9 Other activity involving water and watercraft ◄
Activity involving water NOS ◄
Parasailing ◄
Water survival training and testing ◄

● **E003   Activities involving ice and snow** ◀
    Excludes *shoveling ice and snow (E016.0)* ◀
  E003.0   Ice skating ◀
     Figure skating (singles) (pairs) ◀
     Ice dancing ◀
      Excludes *ice hockey (E003.1)* ◀
  E003.1   Ice hockey ◀
  E003.2   Snow (alpine) (downhill) skiing, snow boarding, sledding, tobogganing and snow tubing ◀
      Excludes *cross country skiing (E003.3)* ◀
  E003.3   Cross country skiing ◀
     Nordic skiing ◀
  E003.9   Other activity involving ice and snow ◀
     Activity involving ice and snow NOS ◀

● **E004   Activities involving climbing, rappelling and jumping off** ◀
    Excludes *hiking on level or elevated terrain (E001.0)* ◀
        jumping rope (E006.5) ◀
        sky diving (E840-E844) ◀
        trampoline jumping (E005.3) ◀
  E004.0   Mountain climbing, rock climbing and wall climbing ◀
  E004.1   Rappelling ◀
  E004.2   BASE jumping ◀
     Building, Antenna, Span, Earth jumping ◀
  E004.3   Bungee jumping ◀
  E004.4   Hang gliding ◀
  E004.9   Other activity involving climbing, rappelling and jumping off ◀

● **E005   Activities involving dancing and other rhythmic movement** ◀
    Excludes *martial arts (E008.4)* ◀
  E005.0   Dancing ◀
  E005.1   Yoga ◀
  E005.2   Gymnastics ◀
     Rhythmic gymnastics ◀
      Excludes *trampoline (E005.3)* ◀
  E005.3   Trampoline ◀
  E005.4   Cheerleading ◀
  E005.9   Other activity involving dancing and other rhythmic movements ◀

● **E006   Activities involving other sports and athletics played individually** ◀
    Excludes *dancing (E005.0)* ◀
        gymnastic (E005.2) ◀
        trampoline (E005.3) ◀
        yoga (E005.1) ◀
  E006.0   Roller skating (inline) and skateboarding ◀
  E006.1   Horseback riding ◀
  E006.2   Golf ◀
  E006.3   Bowling ◀
  E006.4   Bike riding ◀
      Excludes *transport accident involving bike riding (E800-E829)* ◀
  E006.5   Jumping rope ◀
  E006.6   Non-running track and field events ◀
      Excludes *running (any form) (E001.1)* ◀

  E006.9   Other activity involving other sports and athletics played individually ◀
      Excludes *activities involving climbing, rappelling, and jumping (E004.0-E004.9)* ◀
        activities involving ice and snow (E003.0-E003.9) ◀
        activities involving walking and running (E001.0-E001.9) ◀
        activities involving water and watercraft (E002.0-E002.9) ◀

● **E007   Activities involving other sports and athletics played as a team or group** ◀
    Excludes *ice hockey (E003.1)* ◀
        water polo (E002.2) ◀
  E007.0   American tackle football ◀
     Football NOS ◀
  E007.1   American flag or touch football ◀
  E007.2   Rugby ◀
  E007.3   Baseball ◀
     Softball ◀
  E007.4   Lacrosse and field hockey ◀
  E007.5   Soccer ◀
  E007.6   Basketball ◀
  E007.7   Volleyball (beach) (court) ◀
  E007.8   Physical games generally associated with school recess, summer camp and children ◀
     Capture the flag ◀
     Dodge ball ◀
     Four square ◀
     Kickball ◀
  E007.9   Other activity involving other sports and athletics played as a team or group ◀
     Cricket ◀

● **E008   Activities involving other specified sports and athletics** ◀
  E008.0   Boxing ◀
  E008.1   Wrestling ◀
  E008.2   Racquet and hand sports ◀
     Handball ◀
     Racquetball ◀
     Squash ◀
     Tennis ◀
  E008.3   Frisbee ◀
     Ultimate frisbee ◀
  E008.4   Martial arts ◀
     Combatives ◀
  E008.9   Other specified sports and athletics activity ◀
      Excludes *sports and athletics activities specified in categories E001-E007* ◀

● **E009   Activity involving other cardiorespiratory exercise** ◀
    Activity involving physical training ◀
  E009.0   Exercise machines primarily for cardiorespiratory conditioning ◀
     Elliptical and stepper machines ◀
     Stationary bike ◀
     Treadmill ◀
  E009.1   Calisthenics ◀
     Jumping jacks ◀
     Warm up and cool down ◀
  E009.2   Aerobic and step exercise ◀

E000-E999

◀ New   ◀━ Revised   ~~deleted~~ Deleted   ● Use Additional Digit(s)   ■ Nonspecific Code
OGCR Official Guidelines   Coding Clinic   Excludes   Includes   Use additional   Code first   Omit code

E009.3 Circuit training ◀

E009.4 Obstacle course ◀
    Challenge course ◀
    Confidence course ◀

E009.5 Grass drills ◀
    Guerilla drills ◀

E009.9 Other activity involving other cardiorespiratory exercise ◀
> **Excludes** *activities involving cardiorespiratory exercise specified in categories E001-E008* ◀

● E010 Activity involving other muscle strengthening exercises ◀

E010.0 Exercise machines primarily for muscle strengthening ◀

E010.1 Push-ups, pull-ups, sit-ups ◀

E010.2 Free weights ◀
    Barbells ◀
    Dumbbells ◀

E010.3 Pilates ◀

E010.9 Other activity involving other muscle strengthening exercises ◀
> **Excludes** *activities involving muscle strengthening specified in categories E001-E009* ◀

● E011 Activities involving computer technology and electronic devices ◀
> **Excludes** *electronic musical keyboard or instruments (E018.0)* ◀

E011.0 Computer keyboarding ◀
    Electronic game playing using keyboard or other stationary device ◀

E011.1 Hand held interactive electronic device ◀
    Cellular telephone and communication device ◀
    Electronic game playing using interactive device ◀
> **Excludes** *electronic game playing using keyboard or other stationary device (E011.0)* ◀

E011.9 Other activity involving computer technology and electronic devices ◀

● E012 Activities involving arts and handcrafts ◀
> **Excludes** *activities involving playing musical instrument (E018.0-E018.3)* ◀

E012.0 Knitting and crocheting ◀

E012.1 Sewing ◀

E012.2 Furniture building and finishing ◀
    Furniture repair ◀

E012.9 Activity involving other arts and handcrafts ◀

● E013 Activities involving personal hygiene and household maintenance ◀
> **Excludes** *activities involving cooking and grilling (E015.0-E015.9)*
> *activities involving property and land maintenance, building and construction (E016.0-E016.9)*
> *activity involving persons providing caregiving (E014.0-E014.9)*
> *dishwashing (E015.0)*
> *food preparation (E015.0)*
> *gardening (E016.1)* ◀

E013.0 Personal bathing and showering ◀

E013.1 Laundry ◀

E013.2 Vacuuming ◀

E013.3 Ironing ◀

E013.4 Floor mopping and cleaning ◀

E013.5 Residential relocation ◀
    Packing up and unpacking involved in moving to a new residence ◀

E013.8 Other personal hygiene activity ◀

E013.9 Other household maintenance ◀

● E014 Activities involving person providing caregiving ◀

E014.0 Caregiving involving bathing ◀

E014.1 Caregiving involving lifting ◀

E014.9 Other activity involving person providing caregiving ◀

● E015 Activities involving food preparation, cooking and grilling ◀

E015.0 Food preparation and clean up ◀
    Dishwashing ◀

E015.1 Grilling and smoking food ◀

E015.2 Cooking and baking ◀
    Use of stove, oven and microwave oven ◀

E015.9 Other activity involving cooking and grilling ◀

● E016 Activities involving property and land maintenance, building and construction ◀

E016.0 Digging, shoveling and raking ◀
    Dirt digging ◀
    Raking leaves ◀
    Snow shoveling ◀

E016.1 Gardening and landscaping ◀
    Pruning, trimming shrubs, weeding ◀

E016.2 Building and construction ◀

E016.9 Other activity involving property and land maintenance, building and construction ◀

● E017 Activities involving roller coasters and other types of external motion ◀

E017.0 Rollercoaster riding ◀

E017.9 Other activity involving external motion ◀

● E018 Activities involving playing musical instrument ◀
    Activity involving playing electric musical instrument ◀

E018.0 Piano playing ◀
    Musical keyboard (electronic) playing ◀

E018.1 Drum and other percussion instrument playing ◀

E018.2 String instrument playing ◀

E018.3 Wind and brass instrument playing ◀

● E019 Activities involving animal care ◀
> **Excludes** *horseback riding (E006.1)* ◀

E019.0 Walking an animal ◀

E019.1 Milking an animal ◀

E019.2 Grooming and shearing an animal ◀

E019.9 Other activity involving animal care ◀

● E029 Other activity ◀

E029.0 Refereeing a sports activity ◀

E029.1 Spectator at an event ◀

E029.2 Rough housing and horseplay ◀

E029.9 Other activity ◀

E030 Unspecified activity ◀

E000-E999

TRANSPORT ACCIDENTS (E800-E848)

Definitions and examples related to transport accidents

(a) A transport accident (E800-E848) is any accident involving a device designed primarily for, or being used at the time primarily for, conveying persons or goods from one place to another.

RAILWAY ACCIDENTS (E800-E807)

Note: For definitions of railway accident and related terms see definitions (a) to (d).

Excludes *accidents involving railway train and:*
aircraft (E840.0-E845.9)
motor vehicle (E810.0-E825.9)
watercraft (E830.0-E838.9)

The following fourth-digit subdivisions are for use with categories E800-E807 to identify the injured person:

> **0 Railway employee**
> Any person who by virtue of his employment in connection with a railway, whether by the railway company or not, is at increased risk of involvement in a railway accident, such as:
> catering staff of train
> driver
> guard
> porter
> postal staff on train
> railway fireman
> shunter
> sleeping car attendant
> **1 Passenger on railway**
> Any authorized person traveling on a train, except a railway employee.
>
> > **Excludes** *intending passenger waiting at station (8)*
> > *unauthorized rider on railway vehicle (8)*
>
> **2 Pedestrian**
> See definition (r)
> **3 Pedal cyclist**
> See definition (p)
> **8 Other specified person**
> Intending passenger or bystander waiting at station
> Unauthorized rider on railway vehicle
> **9 Unspecified person**

● **E800 Railway accident involving collision with rolling stock**

Requires fourth digit. See beginning of section E800-E845 for codes and definitions.

Includes collision between railway trains or railway vehicles, any kind
collision NOS on railway
derailment with antecedent collision with rolling stock or NOS

● ■ **E801 Railway accident involving collision with other object**

Requires fourth digit. See beginning of section E800-E845 for codes and definitions.

Includes collision of railway train with:
buffers
fallen tree on railway
gates
platform
rock on railway
streetcar
other nonmotor vehicle
other object

Excludes *collision with:*
aircraft (E840.0-E842.9)
motor vehicle (E810.0-E810.9, E820.0-E822.9)

● **E802 Railway accident involving derailment without antecedent collision**

Requires fourth digit. See beginning of section E800-E845 for codes and definitions.

● **E803 Railway accident involving explosion, fire, or burning**

Requires fourth digit. See beginning of section E800-E845 for codes and definitions.

Excludes *explosion or fire, with antecedent derailment (E802.0-E802.9)*
explosion or fire, with mention of antecedent collision (E800.0-E801.9)

● **E804 Fall in, on, or from railway train**

Requires fourth digit. See beginning of section E800-E845 for codes and definitions.

Includes fall while alighting from or boarding railway train

Excludes *fall related to collision, derailment, or explosion of railway train (E800.0-E803.9)*

● **E805 Hit by rolling stock**

Requires fourth digit. See beginning of section E800-E845 for codes and definitions.

Includes crushed by railway train or part
injured by railway train or part
killed by railway train or part
knocked down by railway train or part
run over by railway train or part

Excludes *pedestrian hit by object set in motion by railway train (E806.0-E806.9)*

● ■ **E806 Other specified railway accident**

Requires fourth digit. See beginning of section E800-E845 for codes and definitions.

Includes hit by object falling in railway train
injured by door or window on railway train
nonmotor road vehicle or pedestrian hit by object set in motion by railway train
railway train hit by falling:
earth NOS
rock
tree
other object

Excludes *railway accident due to cataclysm (E908-E909)*

● ■ **E807 Railway accident of unspecified nature**

Requires fourth digit. See beginning of section E800-E845 for codes and definitions.

Includes   found dead on railway right-of-way NOS
injured on railway right-of-way NOS
railway accident NOS

MOTOR VEHICLE TRAFFIC ACCIDENTS (E810-E819)

Note: For definitions of motor vehicle traffic accident, and related terms, see definitions (e) to (k).

Excludes   *accidents involving motor vehicle and aircraft (E840.0-E845.9)*

The following fourth-digit subdivisions are for use with categories E810-E819 to identify the injured person:

> 0   **Driver of motor vehicle other than motorcycle**
> See definition (l)
> 1   **Passenger in motor vehicle other than motorcycle**
> See definition (l)
> 2   **Motorcyclist**
> See definition (l)
> 3   **Passenger on motorcycle**
> See definition (l)
> 4   **Occupant of streetcar**
> 5   **Rider of animal; occupant of animal-drawn vehicle**
> 6   **Pedal cyclist**
> See definition (p)
> 7   **Pedestrian**
> See definition (r)
> ■8   **Other specified person**
> Occupant of vehicle other than above
> Person in railway train involved in accident
> Unauthorized rider of motor vehicle
> ■9   **Unspecified person**

● **E810 Motor vehicle traffic accident involving collision with train**

Requires fourth digit. See beginning of section E800-E845 for codes and definitions.

Excludes   *motor vehicle collision with object set in motion by railway train (E815.0-E815.9)*
railway train hit by object set in motion by motor vehicle (E818.0-E818.9)

● **E811 Motor vehicle traffic accident involving re-entrant collision with another motor vehicle**

Requires fourth digit. See beginning of section E800-E845 for codes and definitions.

Includes   collision between motor vehicle which accidentally leaves the roadway then re-enters the same roadway, or the opposite roadway on a divided highway, and another motor vehicle

Excludes   *collision on the same roadway when none of the motor vehicles involved have left and re-entered the roadway (E812.0-E812.9)*

● ■ **E812 Other motor vehicle traffic accident involving collision with motor vehicle**

Requires fourth digit. See beginning of section E800-E845 for codes and definitions.

Includes   collision with another motor vehicle parked, stopped, stalled, disabled, or abandoned on the highway
motor vehicle collision NOS

Excludes   *collision with object set in motion by another motor vehicle (E815.0-E815.9)*
re-entrant collision with another motor vehicle (E811.0-E811.9)
Coding Clinic: 2007, Q4, P105-107; 1996, Q4, P36.37

● ■ **E813 Motor vehicle traffic accident involving collision with other vehicle**

Requires fourth digit. See beginning of section E800-E845 for codes and definitions.

Includes   collision between motor vehicle, any kind, and:
other road (nonmotor transport) vehicle, such as:
animal carrying a person
animal-drawn vehicle
pedal cycle
streetcar

Excludes   *collision with:*
object set in motion by nonmotor road vehicle (E815.0-E815.9)
pedestrian (E814.0-E814.9)
nonmotor road vehicle hit by object set in motion by motor vehicle (E818.0-E818.9)

● **E814 Motor vehicle traffic accident involving collision with pedestrian**

Requires fourth digit. See beginning of section E800-E845 for codes and definitions.

Includes   collision between motor vehicle, any kind, and pedestrian
pedestrian dragged, hit, or run over by motor vehicle, any kind

Excludes   *pedestrian hit by object set in motion by motor vehicle (E818.0-E818.9)*
Coding Clinic: 1996, Q4, P36.37

● ■E815 **Other motor vehicle traffic accident involving collision on the highway**

> Requires fourth digit. See beginning of section E800-E845 for codes and definitions.

Includes collision (due to loss of control) (on highway) between motor vehicle, any kind, and:
> abutment (bridge) (overpass)
> animal (herded) (unattended)
> fallen stone, traffic sign, tree, utility pole
> guard rail or boundary fence
> interhighway divider
> landslide (not moving)
> object set in motion by railway train or road vehicle (motor) (nonmotor)
> object thrown in front of motor vehicle
> safety island
> temporary traffic sign or marker
> wall of cut made for road
> other object, fixed, movable, or moving

Excludes *collision with:*
> *any object off the highway (resulting from loss of control) (E816.0-E816.9)*
> *any object which normally would have been off the highway and is not stated to have been on it (E816.0-E816.9)*
> *motor vehicle parked, stopped, stalled, disabled, or abandoned on highway (E812.0-E812.9)*
> *moving landslide (E909.2)*
>
> *motor vehicle hit by object:*
> *set in motion by railway train or road vehicle (motor) (nonmotor) (E818.0-E818.9)*
> *thrown into or on vehicle (E818.0-E818.9)*

● E816 **Motor vehicle traffic accident due to loss of control, without collision on the highway**

> Requires fourth digit. See beginning of section E800-E845 for codes and definitions.

Includes motor vehicle:
> failing to make curve and:
>> colliding with object off the highway
>> overturning
>> stopping abruptly off the highway
> going out of control (due to)
>> blowout and:
>>> colliding with object off the highway
>>> overturning
>>> stopping abruptly off the highway
>> burst tire and:
>>> colliding with object off the highway
>>> overturning
>>> stopping abruptly off the highway
>> driver falling asleep and:
>>> colliding with object off the highway
>>> overturning
>>> stopping abruptly off the highway
>> driver inattention and:
>>> colliding with object off the highway
>>> overturning
>>> stopping abruptly off the highway
>> excessive speed and:
>>> colliding with object off the highway
>>> overturning
>>> stopping abruptly off the highway
>> failure of mechanical part and:
>>> colliding with object off the highway
>>> overturning
>>> stopping abruptly off the highway

Excludes *collision on highway following loss of control (E810.0-E815.9)*
>
> *loss of control of motor vehicle following collision on the highway (E810.0-E815.9)*

● E817 **Noncollision motor vehicle traffic accident while boarding or alighting**

> Requires fourth digit. See beginning of section E800-E845 for codes and definitions.

Includes fall down stairs of motor bus while boarding or alighting
> fall from car in street while boarding or alighting
> injured by moving part of the vehicle while boarding or alighting
> trapped by door of motor bus boarding or alighting while boarding or alighting

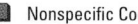

◀ New   ◀▥ Revised   ~~deleted~~ Deleted   ● Use Additional Digit(s)   ■ Nonspecific Code
OGCR Official Guidelines   *Coding Clinic*   Excludes   Includes   Use additional   Code first   Omit code

● ■ **E818**   **Other noncollision motor vehicle traffic accident**

> Requires fourth digit. See beginning of section
> E800-E845 for codes and definitions.

> **Includes**   accidental poisoning from exhaust gas
> generated by motor vehicle while in
> motion
> breakage of any part of motor vehicle
> while in motion
> explosion of any part of motor vehicle
> while in motion
> fall, jump, or being accidentally pushed
> from motor vehicle while in motion
> fire starting in motor vehicle while in
> motion
> hit by object thrown into or on motor
> vehicle while in motion
> injured by being thrown against some part
> of, or object in motor vehicle while
> in motion
> injury from moving part of motor vehicle
> while in motion
> object falling in or on motor vehicle while
> in motion
> object thrown on motor vehicle while in
> motion
> collision of railway train or road vehicle
> except motor vehicle, with object set
> in motion by motor vehicle
> motor vehicle hit by object set in motion by
> railway train or road vehicle (motor)
> (nonmotor)
> pedestrian, railway train, or road vehicle
> (motor) (nonmotor) hit by object set
> in motion by motor vehicle

> **Excludes**   *collision between motor vehicle and:*
> *object set in motion by railway train or*
> *road vehicle (motor) (nonmotor)*
> *(E815.0-E815.9)*
> *object thrown towards the motor vehicle*
> *(E815.0-E815.9)*
> *person overcome by carbon monoxide generated*
> *by stationary motor vehicle off the*
> *roadway with motor running (E868.2)*

● ■ **E819**   **Motor vehicle traffic accident of unspecified nature**

> Requires fourth digit. See beginning of section
> E800-E845 for codes and definitions.

> **Includes**   motor vehicle traffic accident NOS
> traffic accident NOS

> Coding Clinic: 2008, Q4, P96-97; 2006, Q4, P100-102; 2003, Q1, P7;
> 1999, Q4, P11-12; Q1, P10; 1993, Q2, P4-5

MOTOR VEHICLE NONTRAFFIC ACCIDENTS (E820-E825)

> **Note:** For definitions of motor vehicle nontraffic
> accident and related terms see definition (a)
> to (k).

> **Includes**   accidents involving motor vehicles being
> used in recreational or sporting
> activities off the highway
> collision and noncollision motor vehicle
> accidents occurring entirely off the
> highway

> **Excludes**   *accidents involving motor vehicle and:*
> *aircraft (E840.0-E845.9)*
> *watercraft (E830.0-E838.9)*
> *accidents, not on the public highway, involving*
> *agricultural and construction machinery*
> *but not involving another motor vehicle*
> *(E919.0, E919.2, E919.7)*

The following fourth-digit subdivisions are for use
with categories E820-E825 to identify the injured
person:

> 0   **Driver of motor vehicle other than motorcycle**
> See definition (l)
> 1   **Passenger in motor vehicle other than motorcycle**
> See definition (l)
> 2   **Motorcyclist**
> See definition (l)
> 3   **Passenger on motorcycle**
> See definition (l)
> 4   **Occupant of streetcar**
> 5   **Rider of animal; occupant of animal-drawn vehicle**
> 6   **Pedal cyclist**
> See definition (p)
> 7   **Pedestrian**
> See definition (r)
> ■ 8   **Other specified person**
> Occupant of vehicle other than above
> Person on railway train involved in accident
> Unauthorized rider of motor vehicle
> ■ 9   **Unspecified person**

● **E820**   **Nontraffic accident involving motor-driven snow vehicle**

> Requires fourth digit. See beginning of section
> E800-E845 for codes and definitions.

> **Includes**   breakage of part of motor-driven snow
> vehicle (not on public highway)
> fall from motor-driven snow vehicle (not
> on public highway)
> hit by motor-driven snow vehicle (not on
> public highway)
> overturning of motor-driven snow vehicle
> (not on public highway)
> run over or dragged by motor-driven snow
> vehicle (not on public highway)
> collision of motor-driven snow vehicle
> with:
> animal (being ridden) (-drawn vehicle)
> another off-road motor vehicle
> other motor vehicle, not on public
> highway
> railway train
> other object, fixed or movable
> injury caused by rough landing of
> motor-driven snow vehicle (after
> leaving ground on rough terrain)

> **Excludes**   *accident on the public highway involving*
> *motor driven snow vehicle*
> *(E810.0-E819.9)*

N Newborn Age: 0   **P** Pediatric Age: 0–17   **M** Maternity Age: 12–55   **A** Adult Age: 15–124   ♀ Females Only   ♂ Males Only   **1145**

E000-E999

● ■ E821   Nontraffic accident involving other off-road motor vehicle

> Requires fourth digit. See beginning of section E800-E845 for codes and definitions.

> **Includes**   breakage of part of off-road motor vehicle, except snow vehicle (not on public highway)
> fall from off-road motor vehicle, except snow vehicle (not on public highway)
> hit by off-road motor vehicle, except snow vehicle (not on public highway)
> overturning of off-road motor vehicle, except snow vehicle (not on public highway)
> run over or dragged by off-road motor vehicle, except snow vehicle (not on public highway)
> thrown against some part of or object in off-road motor vehicle, except snow vehicle (not on public highway)
> collision with:
>   animal (being ridden) (-drawn vehicle)
>   another off-road motor vehicle, except snow vehicle
>   other motor vehicle, not on public highway
>   other object, fixed or movable

> **Excludes**   *accident on public highway involving off-road motor vehicle (E810.0-E819.9)*
> *collision between motor driven snow vehicle and other off-road motor vehicle (E820.0-E820.9)*
> *hovercraft accident on water (E830.0-E838.9)*

● ■ E822   Other motor vehicle nontraffic accident involving collision with moving object

> Requires fourth digit. See beginning of section E800-E845 for codes and definitions.

> **Includes**   collision, not on public highway, between motor vehicle, except off-road motor vehicle and:
>   animal
>   nonmotor vehicle
>   other motor vehicle, except off-road motor vehicle
>   pedestrian
>   railway train
>   other moving object

> **Excludes**   *collision with:*
> *   motor-driven snow vehicle (E820.0-E820.9)*
> *   other off-road motor vehicle (E821.0-E821.9)*

● ■ E823   Other motor vehicle nontraffic accident involving collision with stationary object

> Requires fourth digit. See beginning of section E800-E845 for codes and definitions.

> **Includes**   collision, not on public highway, between motor vehicle, except off-road motor vehicle, and any object, fixed or movable, but not in motion

● ■ E824   Other motor vehicle nontraffic accident while boarding and alighting

> Requires fourth digit. See beginning of section E800-E845 for codes and definitions.

> **Includes**   fall while boarding or alighting from motor vehicle except off-road motor vehicle, not on public highway
> injury from moving part of motor vehicle while boarding or alighting from motor vehicle except off-road motor vehicle, not on public highway
> trapped by door of motor vehicle while boarding or alighting from motor vehicle except off-road motor vehicle, not on public highway

● ■ E825   Other motor vehicle nontraffic accident of other and unspecified nature

> Requires fourth digit. See beginning of section E800-E845 for codes and definitions.

> **Includes**   accidental poisoning from carbon monoxide generated by motor vehicle while in motion, not on public highway
> breakage of any part of motor vehicle while in motion, not on public highway
> explosion of any part of motor vehicle while in motion, not on public highway
> fall, jump, or being accidentally pushed from motor vehicle while in motion, not on public highway
> fire starting in motor vehicle while in motion, not on public highway
> hit by object thrown into, towards, or on motor vehicle while in motion, not on public highway
> injured by being thrown against some part of, or object in motor vehicle while in motion, not on public highway
> injury from moving part of motor vehicle while in motion, not on public highway
> object falling in or on motor vehicle while in motion, not on public highway
> motor vehicle nontraffic accident NOS

> **Excludes**   *fall from or in stationary motor vehicle (E884.9, E885.9)*
> *overcome by carbon monoxide or exhaust gas generated by stationary motor vehicle off the roadway with motor running (E868.2)*
> *struck by falling object from or in stationary motor vehicle (E916)*

OTHER ROAD VEHICLE ACCIDENTS (E826-E829)

Note: Other road vehicle accidents are transport accidents involving road vehicles other than motor vehicles. For definitions of other road vehicle and related terms see definitions (m) to (o).

Includes　accidents involving other road vehicles being used in recreational or sporting activities

Excludes　*collision of other road vehicle [any] with:*
aircraft (E840.0-E845.9)
motor vehicle (E813.0-E813.9,
E820.0-E822.9)
railway train (E801.0-E801.9)

The following fourth-digit subdivisions are for use with categories E826-E829 to identify the injured person:

> 0　Pedestrian
> 　　See definition (r)
> 1　Pedal cyclist
> 　　See definition (p)
> 2　Rider of animal
> 3　Occupant of animal-drawn vehicle
> 4　Occupant of streetcar
> ■8　Other specified person
> ■9　Unspecified person

● **E826　Pedal cycle accident**
[0-9]　　Requires fourth digit. See beginning of section E800-E845 for codes and definitions.

Includes　breakage of any part of pedal cycle
collision between pedal cycle and:
　animal (being ridden) (herded)
　　(unattended)
　another pedal cycle
　nonmotor road vehicle, any
　pedestrian
　other object, fixed, movable, or moving,
　　not set in motion by motor
　　vehicle, railway train, or aircraft
entanglement in wheel of pedal cycle
fall from pedal cycle
hit by object falling or thrown on the pedal
　cycle
pedal cycle accident NOS
pedal cycle overturned

● **E827　Animal-drawn vehicle accident**
[0,2-4,8,9]　　Requires fourth digit. See beginning of section E800-E845 for codes and definitions.

Includes　breakage of any part of vehicle
collision between animal-drawn vehicle
　and:
　animal (being ridden) (herded)
　　(unattended)
　nonmotor road vehicle, except pedal
　　cycle
　pedestrian, pedestrian conveyance, or
　　pedestrian vehicle
　other object, fixed, movable, or moving,
　　not set in motion by motor
　　vehicle, railway train, or aircraft
fall from animal-drawn vehicle
knocked down by animal-drawn vehicle
overturning of animal-drawn vehicle
run over by animal-drawn vehicle
thrown from animal-drawn vehicle

Excludes　*collision of animal-drawn vehicle with pedal*
cycle (E826.0-E826.9)

● **E828　Accident involving animal being ridden**
[0,2,4,8,9]　　Requires fourth digit. See beginning of section E800-E845 for codes and definitions.

Includes　collision between animal being ridden and:
　another animal
　nonmotor road vehicle, except pedal
　　cycle, and animal-drawn vehicle
　pedestrian, pedestrian conveyance, or
　　pedestrian vehicle
　other object, fixed, movable, or moving,
　　not set in motion by motor
　　vehicle, railway train, or aircraft
fall from animal being ridden
knocked down by animal being ridden
thrown from animal being ridden
trampled by animal being ridden
ridden animal stumbled and fell

Excludes　*collision of animal being ridden with:*
animal-drawn vehicle (E827.0-E827.9)
pedal cycle (E826.0-E826.9)

● ■**E829　Other road vehicle accidents**
[0,4,8,9]　　Requires fourth digit. See beginning of section E800-E845 for codes and definitions.

Includes　accident while boarding or alighting from
　　streetcar
　nonmotor road vehicle not classifiable
　　to E826-E828
blow from object in
　streetcar
　nonmotor road vehicle not classifiable
　　to E826-E828
breakage of any part of
　streetcar
　nonmotor road vehicle not classifiable
　　to E826-E828
caught in door of
　streetcar
　nonmotor road vehicle not classifiable
　　to E826-E828
derailment of
　streetcar
　nonmotor road vehicle not classifiable
　　to E826-E828
fall in, on, or from
　streetcar
　nonmotor road vehicle not classifiable
　　to E826-E828
fire in
　streetcar
　nonmotor road vehicle not classifiable
　　to E826-E828
collision between streetcar or nonmotor
　　road vehicle, except as in E826-E828,
　　and:
　animal (not being ridden)
　another nonmotor road vehicle not
　　classifiable to E826-E828
　pedestrian
　other object, fixed, movable, or moving,
　　not set in motion by motor
　　vehicle, railway train, or aircraft
nonmotor road vehicle accident NOS
streetcar accident NOS

Excludes　*collision with:*
animal being ridden (E828.0-E828.9)
animal-drawn vehicle (E827.0-E827.9)
pedal cycle (E826.0-E826.9)

N Newborn Age: 0　　**P** Pediatric Age: 0–17　　**M** Maternity Age: 12–55　　**A** Adult Age: 15–124　　♀ Females Only　　♂ Males Only

E000-E999

1147

WATER TRANSPORT ACCIDENTS (E830-E838)

Note: For definitions of water transport accident and related terms see definitions (a), (s), and (t).

Includes   watercraft accidents in the course of recreational activities

Excludes   *accidents involving both aircraft, including objects set in motion by aircraft, and watercraft (E840.0-E845.9)*

The following fourth-digit subdivisions are for use with categories E830-E838 to identify the injured person:

> 0 **Occupant of small boat, unpowered**
> 1 **Occupant of small boat, powered**
>   See definition (t)
>   **Excludes** *water skier (4)*
> 2 **Occupant of other watercraft-crew**
>   Persons:
>   engaged in operation of watercraft
>   providing passenger services [cabin attendants, ship's physician, catering personnel]
>   working on ship during voyage in other capacity [musician in band, operators of shops and beauty parlors]
> 3 **Occupant of other watercraft -- other than crew**
>   Passenger
>   Occupant of lifeboat, other than crew, after abandoning ship
> 4 **Water skier**
> 5 **Swimmer**
> 6 **Dockers, stevedores**
>   Longshoreman employed on the dock in loading and unloading ships
> 7 **Occupant of military watercraft, any type** ◄
> 8 **Other specified person**
>   Immigration and custom officials on board ship
>   Person:
>   accompanying passenger or member of crew visiting boat
>   Pilot (guiding ship into port)
> 9 **Unspecified person**

● **E830 Accident to watercraft causing submersion**

Requires fourth digit. See beginning of section E800-E845 for codes and definitions.

Includes   submersion and drowning due to:
        boat overturning
        boat submerging
        falling or jumping from burning ship
        falling or jumping from crushed watercraft
        ship sinking
        other accident to watercraft

● ■ **E831 Accident to watercraft causing other injury**

Requires fourth digit. See beginning of section E800-E845 for codes and definitions.

Includes   any injury, except submersion and drowning, as a result of an accident to watercraft
        burned while ship on fire
        crushed between ships in collision
        crushed by lifeboat after abandoning ship
        fall due to collision or other accident to watercraft
        hit by falling object due to accident to watercraft
        injured in watercraft accident involving collision
        struck by boat or part thereof after fall or jump from damaged boat

Excludes   *burns from localized fire or explosion on board ship (E837.0-E837.9)*

● ■ **E832 Other accidental submersion or drowning in water transport accident**

Requires fourth digit. See beginning of section E800-E845 for codes and definitions.

Includes   submersion or drowning as a result of an accident other than accident to the watercraft, such as:
        fall:
            from gangplank
            from ship
            overboard
        thrown overboard by motion of ship
        washed overboard

Excludes   *submersion or drowning of swimmer or diver who voluntarily jumps from boat not involved in an accident (E910.0-E910.9)*

● **E833 Fall on stairs or ladders in water transport**

Requires fourth digit. See beginning of section E800-E845 for codes and definitions.

Excludes   *fall due to accident to watercraft (E831.0-E831.9)*

● ■ **E834 Other fall from one level to another in water transport**

Requires fourth digit. See beginning of section E800-E845 for codes and definitions.

Excludes   *fall due to accident to watercraft (E831.0-E831.9)*

● ■ **E835 Other and unspecified fall in water transport**

Requires fourth digit. See beginning of section E800-E845 for codes and definitions.

Excludes   *fall due to accident to watercraft (E831.0-E831.9)*

● **E836 Machinery accident in water transport**

Requires fourth digit. See beginning of section E800-E845 for codes and definitions.

Includes   injuries in water transport caused by:
        deck machinery
        engine room machinery
        galley machinery
        laundry machinery
        loading machinery

◄ New   ◄▥ Revised   ~~deleted~~ Deleted   ● Use Additional Digit(s)   ■ Nonspecific Code
OGCR Official Guidelines   Coding Clinic   Excludes   Includes   Use additional   Code first   Omit code

E000-E999

● **E837 Explosion, fire, or burning in watercraft**

     Requires fourth digit. See beginning of section E800-E845 for codes and definitions.

     Includes   explosion of boiler on steamship
                     localized fire on ship

     Excludes   *burning ship (due to collision or explosion) resulting in:*
                 submersion or drowning (E830.0-E830.9)
                 other injury (E831.0-E831.9)

● ■ **E838 Other and unspecified water transport accident**

     Requires fourth digit. See beginning of section E800-E845 for codes and definitions.

     Includes   accidental poisoning by gases or fumes on ship
                 atomic power plant malfunction in watercraft
                 crushed between ship and stationary object [wharf]
                 crushed between ships without accident to watercraft
                 crushed by falling object on ship or while loading or unloading
                 hit by boat while water skiing
                 struck by boat or part thereof (after fall from boat)
                 watercraft accident NOS

AIR AND SPACE TRANSPORT ACCIDENTS (E840-E845)

Note: For definition of aircraft and related terms see definitions (u) and (v).

The following fourth-digit subdivisions are for use with categories E840-E845 to identify the injured person:

   0 Occupant of spacecraft
   1 Occupant of military aircraft, any
       Crew in military aircraft [air force] [army] [national guard] [navy]
       Passenger (civilian) (military) in military aircraft [air force] [army] [national guard] [navy]
       Troops in military aircraft [air force] [army] [national guard] [navy]

       Excludes   *occupants of aircraft operated under jurisdiction of police departments (5)*
                 parachutist (7)

   2 Crew of commercial aircraft (powered) in surface-to-surface transport
■ **3 Other occupant of commercial aircraft (powered) in surface-to-surface transport**
       Flight personnel:
         not part of crew
         on familiarization flight
       Passenger on aircraft (powered) NOS
   4 Occupant of commercial aircraft (powered) in surface-to-air transport
       Occupant [crew] [passenger] of aircraft (powered) engaged in activities, such as:
       aerial spraying (crops) (fire retardants)
       air drops of emergency supplies
       air drops of parachutists, except from military craft
       crop dusting
       lowering of construction material [bridge or telephone pole]
       sky writing

■ **5 Occupant of other powered aircraft**
       Occupant [crew] [passenger] of aircraft [powered] engaged in activities, such as:
       aerobatic flying
       aircraft racing
       rescue operation
       storm surveillance
       traffic surveillance
       Occupant of private plane NOS
   6 Occupant of unpowered aircraft, except parachutist
       Occupant of aircraft classifiable to E842
   7 Parachutist (military) (other)
       Person making voluntary descent

       Excludes   *person making descent after accident to aircraft (.1–.6)*

   8 Ground crew, airline employee
       Persons employed at airfields (civil) (military) or launching pads, not occupants of aircraft
■ **9 Other person**

● **E840 Accident to powered aircraft at takeoff or landing**

     Requires fourth digit. See beginning of section E800-E845 for codes and definitions.

     Includes   collision of aircraft with any object, fixed, movable, or moving while taking off or landing
                 crash while taking off or landing
                 explosion on aircraft while taking off or landing
                 fire on aircraft while taking off or landing
                 forced landing

● ■ **E841 Accident to powered aircraft, other and unspecified**

     Requires fourth digit. See beginning of section E800-E845 for codes and definitions.

     Includes   aircraft accident NOS
                 aircraft crash or wreck NOS
                 any accident to powered aircraft while in transit or when not specified whether in transit, taking off, or landing
                 collision of aircraft with another aircraft, bird, or any object, while in transit
                 explosion on aircraft while in transit
                 fire on aircraft while in transit

● **E842 Accident to unpowered aircraft**
   [6-9]

     Requires fourth digit. See beginning of section E800-E845 for codes and definitions.

     Includes   any accident, except collision with powered aircraft, to:
                 balloon
                 glider
                 hang glider
                 kite carrying a person
                 hit by object falling from unpowered aircraft

● **E843 Fall in, on, or from aircraft**
   [0-9]

     Requires fourth digit. See beginning of section E800-E845 for codes and definitions.

     Includes   accident in boarding or alighting from aircraft, any kind
                 fall in, on, or from aircraft [any kind], while in transit, taking off, or landing, except when as a result of an accident to aircraft

E000-E999

● ■ **E844   Other specified air transport accidents**
   [0-9]
      Requires fourth digit. See beginning of section
      E800-E845 for codes and definitions.

   Includes   hit by aircraft without accident to aircraft
               hit by object falling from aircraft without
                  accident to aircraft
               injury by or from machinery on aircraft
                  without accident to aircraft
               injury by or from rotating propeller
                  without accident to aircraft
               injury by or from voluntary parachute
                  descent without accident to aircraft
               poisoning by carbon monoxide from
                  aircraft while in transit without
                  accident to aircraft
               sucked into jet without accident to aircraft
               any accident involving other transport
                  vehicle (motor) (nonmotor) due to
                  being hit by object set in motion by
                  aircraft (powered)

   Excludes   *air sickness (E903)*
               effects of:
                  high altitude (E902.0-E902.1)
                  pressure change (E902.0-E902.1)
               injury in parachute descent due to accident to
                  aircraft (E840.0-E842.9)

● **E845   Accident involving spacecraft**
   [0,8,9]
      Requires fourth digit. See beginning of section
      E800-E845 for codes and definitions.

   Includes   launching pad accident

   Excludes   *effects of weightlessness in spacecraft (E928.0)*

VEHICLE ACCIDENTS NOT ELSEWHERE CLASSIFIABLE (E846-E848)

**E846   Accidents involving powered vehicles used solely
         within the buildings and premises of industrial or
         commercial establishment**
      Accident to, on, or involving:
         battery-powered airport passenger vehicle
         battery-powered trucks (baggage) (mail)
         coal car in mine
         logging car
         self-propelled truck, industrial
         station baggage truck (powered)
         tram, truck, or tub (powered) in mine or quarry
      Breakage of any part of vehicle
      Collision with:
         pedestrian
         other vehicle or object within premises
      Explosion of powered vehicle, industrial or
         commercial
      Fall from powered vehicle, industrial or commercial
      Overturning of powered vehicle, industrial or
         commercial
      Struck by powered vehicle, industrial or commercial

   Excludes   *accidental poisoning by exhaust gas from*
               vehicle not elsewhere classifiable
               (E868.2)
               injury by crane, lift (fork), or elevator (E919.2)

E847   Accidents involving cable cars not running on rails
      Accident to, on, or involving:
         cable car, not on rails
         ski chair-lift
         ski-lift with gondola
         teleferique
      Breakage of cable
         caught or dragged by cable car, not on rails
         fall or jump from cable car, not on rails
         object thrown from or in cable car not on rails

■ **E848   Accidents involving other vehicles, not elsewhere
         classifiable**
      Accident to, on, or involving:
         ice yacht
         land yacht
         nonmotor, nonroad vehicle NOS

   OGCR   Section I.C.19.b
      Use an additional code from category E849 to
      indicate the Place of Occurrence for injuries and
      poisonings. The Place of Occurrence describes the
      place where the event occurred and not the patient's
      activity at the time of the event. Do not use E849.9 if
      the place of occurrence is not stated.

PLACE OF OCCURRENCE (E849)

● **E849   Place of Occurrence**
      Note: The following category is for use to denote the
               place where the injury or poisoning occurred.

   E849.0   Home
         Apartment
         Boarding house
         Farm house
         Home premises
         House (residential)
         Noninstitutional place of residence
         Private:
            driveway
            garage
            garden
            home
            walk
         Swimming pool in private house or garden
         Yard of home

      Excludes   *home under construction but not yet*
                  occupied (E849.3)
                  institutional place of residence
                  (E849.7)

   E849.1   Farm
         Buildings
         Land under cultivation

      Excludes   *farm house and home premises of farm*
                  (E849.0)

   E849.2   Mine and quarry
         Gravel pit
         Sand pit
         Tunnel under construction

E849.3   Industrial place and premises
Building under construction
Dockyard
Dry dock
Factory
   building
   premises
Garage (place of work)
Industrial yard
Loading platform (factory) (store)
Plant, industrial
Railway yard
Shop (place of work)
Warehouse
Workhouse
Coding Clinic: 2003, Q4, P76-78

E849.4   Place for recreation and sport

Amusement park	Playground, including
Baseball field	school playground
Basketball court	Public park
Beach resort	Racecourse
Cricket ground	Resort NOS
Fives court	Riding school
Football field	Rifle range
Golf course	Seashore resort
Gymnasium	Skating rink
Hockey field	Sports palace
Holiday camp	Stadium
Ice palace	Swimming pool, public
Lake resort	Tennis court
Mountain resort	Vacation resort

> **Excludes**   *that in private house or garden*
> *(E849.0)*

E849.5   Street and highway
Coding Clinic: 1995, Q1, P10

E849.6   Public building
Building (including adjacent grounds) used
   by the general public or by a particular
   group of the public, such as:
   airport
   bank
   cafe
   casino
   church
   cinema
   clubhouse
   courthouse
   dance hall
   garage building (for car storage)
   hotel
   market (grocery or other commodity)
   movie house
   music hall
   nightclub
   office
   office building
   opera house
   post office
   public hall
   radio broadcasting station
   restaurant
   school (state) (public) (private)
   shop, commercial
   station (bus) (railway)
   store
   theater

> **Excludes**   *home garage (E849.0)*
> *industrial building or workplace*
> *(E849.3)*

E849.7   Residential institution
Children's home
Dormitory
Hospital
Jail
Old people's home
Orphanage
Prison
Reform School

■ **E849.8   Other specified places**
Beach NOS
Canal
Caravan site NOS
Derelict house
Desert
Dock
Forest
Harbor
Hill
Lake NOS
Mountain
Parking lot
Parking place
Pond or pool (natural)
Prairie
Public place NOS
Railway line
Reservoir
River
Sea
Seashore NOS
Stream
Swamp
Trailer court
Woods

■ **E849.9   Unspecified place**

ACCIDENTAL POISONING BY DRUGS, MEDICINAL SUBSTANCES, AND BIOLOGICALS (E850–E858)

> **Includes**   accidental overdose of drug, wrong drug
> given or taken in error, and drug
> taken inadvertently
> accidents in the use of drugs and
> biologicals in medical and surgical
> procedures

> **Excludes**   *administration with suicidal or homicidal*
> *intent or intent to harm, or in*
> *circumstances classifiable to E980–E989*
> *(E950.0–E950.5, E962.0, E980.0–E980.5)*
> *correct drug properly administered in*
> *therapeutic or prophylactic dosage, as the*
> *cause of adverse effect (E930.0–E949.9)*

Note: See Alphabetic Index for more complete
list of specific drugs to be classified under
the fourth-digit subdivisions. The American
Hospital Formulary numbers can be used to
classify new drugs listed by the American
Hospital Formulary Service (AHFS). See
Appendix C.

● **E850   Accidental poisoning by analgesics, antipyretics, and antirheumatics**
Coding Clinic: 2008, Q3, P21

E850.0   Heroin
Diacetylmorphine

E850.1   Methadone

E850.2 Other opiates and related narcotics
Codeine [methylmorphine]
Meperidine [pethidine]
Morphine
Opium (alkaloids)

E850.3 Salicylates
Acetylsalicylic acid [aspirin]
Amino derivatives of salicylic acid
Salicylic acid salts

E850.4 Aromatic analgesics, not elsewhere classified
Acetanilid
Paracetamol [acetaminophen]
Phenacetin [acetophenetidin]

E850.5 Pyrazole derivatives
Aminophenazone [amidopyrine]
Phenylbutazone

E850.6 Antirheumatics [antiphlogistics]
Gold salts
Indomethacin

> **Excludes** *salicylates (E850.3)*
> *steroids (E858.0)*

E850.7 Other non-narcotic analgesics
Pyrabital

E850.8 Other specified analgesics and antipyretics
Pentazocine

E850.9 Unspecified analgesic or antipyretic

E851 Accidental poisoning by barbiturates
Amobarbital [amylobarbitone]
Barbital [barbitone]
Butabarbital [butabarbitone]
Pentobarbital [pentobarbitone]
Phenobarbital [phenobarbitone]
Secobarbital [quinalbarbitone]

> **Excludes** *thiobarbiturates (E855.1)*

● E852 Accidental poisoning by other sedatives and hypnotics

E852.0 Chloral hydrate group

E852.1 Paraldehyde

E852.2 Bromine compounds
Bromides
Carbromal (derivatives)

E852.3 Methaqualone compounds

E852.4 Glutethimide group

E852.5 Mixed sedatives, not elsewhere classified

E852.8 Other specified sedatives and hypnotics

E852.9 Unspecified sedative or hypnotic
Sleeping:
drug NOS
pill NOS
tablet NOS

● E853 Accidental poisoning by tranquilizers

E853.0 Phenothiazine-based tranquilizers
Chlorpromazine
Fluphenazine
Prochlorperazine
Promazine

E853.1 Butyrophenone-based tranquilizers
Haloperidol
Spiperone
Trifluperidol

E853.2 Benzodiazepine-based tranquilizers
Chlordiazepoxide   Lorazepam
Diazepam   Medazepam
Flurazepam   Nitrazepam
Coding Clinic: 1991, Q3, P14

E853.8 Other specified tranquilizers
Hydroxyzine
Meprobamate

E853.9 Unspecified tranquilizer

● E854 Accidental poisoning by other psychotropic agents

E854.0 Antidepressants
Amitriptyline
Imipramine
Monoamine oxidase [MAO] inhibitors
Coding Clinic: 1991, Q3, P14

E854.1 Psychodysleptics [hallucinogens]
Cannabis derivatives
Lysergide [LSD]
Marihuana (derivatives)
Mescaline
Psilocin
Psilocybin

E854.2 Psychostimulants
Amphetamine
Caffeine

> **Excludes** *central appetite depressants (E858.8)*

Coding Clinic: 2003, Q2, P11

E854.3 Central nervous system stimulants
Analeptics
Opiate antagonists

E854.8 Other psychotropic agents

● E855 Accidental poisoning by other drugs acting on central and autonomic nervous system

E855.0 Anticonvulsant and anti-Parkinsonism drugs
Amantadine
Hydantoin derivatives
Levodopa [L-dopa]
Oxazolidine derivatives [paramethadione]
[trimethadione]
Succinimides

E855.1 Other central nervous system depressants
Ether
Gaseous anesthetics
Halogenated hydrocarbon derivatives
Intravenous anesthetics
Thiobarbiturates, such as thiopental sodium

E855.2 Local anesthetics
Cocaine
Lidocaine [lignocaine]
Procaine
Tetracaine

E855.3 Parasympathomimetics [cholinergics]
Acetylcholine
Anticholinesterase:
organophosphorus
reversible
Pilocarpine

E855.4 Parasympatholytics [anticholinergics and antimuscarinics] and spasmolytics
Atropine
Homatropine
Hyoscine [scopolamine]
Quaternary ammonium derivatives

E855.5 Sympathomimetics [adrenergics]
    Epinephrine [adrenalin]
    Levarterenol [noradrenalin]

E855.6 Sympatholytics [antiadrenergics]
    Phenoxybenzamine
    Tolazoline hydrochloride

■ E855.8 Other specified drugs acting on central and
    autonomic nervous systems

■ E855.9 Unspecified drug acting on central and
    autonomic nervous systems

E856 Accidental poisoning by antibiotics

■ E857 Accidental poisoning by other anti-infectives

● E858 Accidental poisoning by other drugs
    Coding Clinic: 2008, Q3, P21

E858.0 Hormones and synthetic substitutes

E858.1 Primarily systemic agents

E858.2 Agents primarily affecting blood constituents

E858.3 Agents primarily affecting cardiovascular
    system

E858.4 Agents primarily affecting gastrointestinal
    system

E858.5 Water, mineral, and uric acid metabolism drugs

E858.6 Agents primarily acting on the smooth and
    skeletal muscles and respiratory system

E858.7 Agents primarily affecting skin and
    mucous membrane, ophthalmological,
    otorhinolaryngological, and dental drugs

■ E858.8 Other specified drugs
    Central appetite depressants

■ E858.9 Unspecified drug

ACCIDENTAL POISONING BY OTHER SOLID AND LIQUID SUBSTANCES, GASES, AND VAPORS (E860-E869)

Note: Categories in this section are intended primarily
    to indicate the external cause of poisoning states
    classifiable to 980–989. They may also be used
    to indicate external causes of localized effects
    classifiable to 001–799.

● E860 Accidental poisoning by alcohol, not elsewhere
    classified

E860.0 Alcoholic beverages
    Alcohol in preparations intended for
        consumption
    Coding Clinic: 1996, Q3, P161; 1991, Q3, P14

■ E860.1 Other and unspecified ethyl alcohol and its
    products
    Denatured alcohol
    Ethanol NOS
    Grain alcohol NOS
    Methylated spirit

E860.2 Methyl alcohol
    Methanol
    Wood alcohol

E860.3 Isopropyl alcohol
    Dimethyl carbinol
    Isopropanol
    Rubbing alcohol substitute
    Secondary propyl alcohol

E860.4 Fusel oil
    Alcohol:
        amyl
        butyl
        propyl

■ E860.8 Other specified alcohols

■ E860.9 Unspecified alcohol

● E861 Accidental poisoning by cleansing and polishing
    agents, disinfectants, paints, and varnishes

E861.0 Synthetic detergents and shampoos

E861.1 Soap products

E861.2 Polishes

■ E861.3 Other cleansing and polishing agents
    Scouring powders

E861.4 Disinfectants
    Household and other disinfectants not
        ordinarily used on the person
    Excludes *carbolic acid or phenol (E864.0)*

E861.5 Lead paints

■ E861.6 Other paints and varnishes
    Lacquers
    Oil colors
    Paints, other than lead
    Whitewashes

■ E861.9 Unspecified

● E862 Accidental poisoning by petroleum products, other
    solvents and their vapors, not elsewhere classified

E862.0 Petroleum solvents
    Petroleum:
        ether
        benzine
        naphtha

E862.1 Petroleum fuels and cleaners
    Antiknock additives to petroleum fuels
    Gas oils
    Gasoline or petrol
    Kerosene
    Excludes *kerosene insecticides (E863.4)*

E862.2 Lubricating oils

E862.3 Petroleum solids
    Paraffin wax

■ E862.4 Other specified solvents
    Benzene
    Coding Clinic: 2008, Q3, P6-7

■ E862.9 Unspecified solvent

● E863 Accidental poisoning by agricultural and horticultural
    chemical and pharmaceutical preparations other than
    plant foods and fertilizers
    Excludes *plant foods and fertilizers (E866.5)*

E863.0 Insecticides of organochlorine compounds
    Benzene hexachloride   Dieldrin
    Chlordane   Endrine
    DDT Toxaphene

E863.1 Insecticides of organophosphorus compounds
    Demeton   Parathion
    Diazinon   Phenylsulphthion
    Dichlorvos   Phorate
    Malathion   Phosdrin
    Methyl parathion

E863.2 **Carbamates**
Aldicarb
Carbaryl
Propoxur

E863.3 **Mixtures of insecticides**

⬛ E863.4 **Other and unspecified insecticides**
Kerosene insecticides

E863.5 **Herbicides**
2,4-Dichlorophenoxyacetic acid [2, 4-D]
2,4,5-Trichlorophenoxyacetic acid [2, 4, 5-T]
Chlorates
Diquat
Mixtures of plant foods and fertilizers with
herbicides
Paraquat

E863.6 **Fungicides**
Organic mercurials (used in seed dressing)
Pentachlorophenols

E863.7 **Rodenticides**
Fluoroacetates   Warfarin
Squill and derivatives   Zinc phosphide
Thallium

E863.8 **Fumigants**
Cyanides   Phosphine
Methyl bromide

⬛ E863.9 **Other and unspecified**

⬤ E864 **Accidental poisoning by corrosives and caustics, not elsewhere classified**

> **Excludes** *those as components of disinfectants (E861.4)*

E864.0 **Corrosive aromatics**
Carbolic acid or phenol

E864.1 **Acids**
Acid:
hydrochloric
nitric
sulfuric

E864.2 **Caustic alkalis**
Lye

⬛ E864.3 **Other specified corrosives and caustics**

⬛ E864.4 **Unspecified corrosives and caustics**

⬤ E865 **Accidental poisoning from poisonous foodstuffs and poisonous plants**

> **Includes**   any meat, fish, or shellfish
> plants, berries, and fungi eaten as, or in
> mistake for food, or by a child

> **Excludes** *anaphlyactic shock due to adverse food reaction (995.60–995.69)*
> *food poisoning (bacterial) (005.0–005.9)*
> *poisoning and toxic reactions to venomous plants (E905.6–E905.7)*

E865.0 **Meat**

E865.1 **Shellfish**

⬛ E865.2 **Other fish**

E865.3 **Berries and seeds**

⬛ E865.4 **Other specified plants**

E865.5 **Mushrooms and other fungi**

⬛ E865.8 **Other specified foods**

⬛ E865.9 **Unspecified foodstuff or poisonous plant**

⬤ E866 **Accidental poisoning by other and unspecified solid and liquid substances**

> **Excludes** *these substances as a component of:*
> *medicines (E850.0-E858.9)*
> *paints (E861.5-E861.6)*
> *pesticides (E863.0-E863.9)*
> *petroleum fuels (E862.1)*

E866.0 **Lead and its compounds and fumes**

E866.1 **Mercury and its compounds and fumes**

E866.2 **Antimony and its compounds and fumes**

E866.3 **Arsenic and its compounds and fumes**

⬛ E866.4 **Other metals and their compounds and fumes**
Beryllium (compounds)
Brass fumes
Cadmium (compounds)
Copper salts
Iron (compounds)
Manganese (compounds)
Nickel (compounds)
Thallium (compounds)

E866.5 **Plant foods and fertilizers**

> **Excludes** *mixtures with herbicides (E863.5)*

E866.6 **Glues and adhesives**

E866.7 **Cosmetics**

⬛ E866.8 **Other specified solid or liquid substances**
Coding Clinic: 1990, Q4, P25

⬛ E866.9 **Unspecified solid or liquid substance**

E867 **Accidental poisoning by gas distributed by pipeline**
Carbon monoxide from incomplete combustion of
piped gas
Coal gas NOS
Liquefied petroleum gas distributed through pipes
(pure or mixed with air)
Piped gas (natural) (manufactured)

⬤ E868 **Accidental poisoning by other utility gas and other carbon monoxide**

E868.0 **Liquefied petroleum gas distributed in mobile containers**
Butane or carbon monoxide from incomplete
combustion of these gases
Liquefied hydrocarbon gas NOS or carbon
monoxide from incomplete combustion
of these gases
Propane or carbon monoxide from incomplete
combustion of these gases

⬛ E868.1 **Other and unspecified utility gas**
Acetylene or carbon monoxide from
incomplete combustion of these gases
Gas NOS used for lighting, heating, or
cooking or carbon monoxide from
incomplete combustion of these gases
Water gas or carbon monoxide from
incomplete combustion of these gases

E868.2 Motor vehicle exhaust gas

Exhaust gas from:
- farm tractor, not in transit
- gas engine
- motor pump
- motor vehicle, not in transit
- any type of combustion engine not in watercraft

> **Excludes** *poisoning by carbon monoxide from:*
> *aircraft while in transit (E844.0-E844.9)*
> *motor vehicle while in transit (E818.0-E818.9)*
> *watercraft whether or not in transit (E838.0-E838.9)*

E868.3 Carbon monoxide from incomplete combustion of other domestic fuels

Carbon monoxide from incomplete combustion of:
- coal in domestic stove or fireplace
- coke in domestic stove or fireplace
- kerosene in domestic stove or fireplace
- wood in domestic stove or fireplace

> **Excludes** *carbon monoxide from smoke and fumes due to conflagration (E890.0-E893.9)*

E868.8 Carbon monoxide from other sources

Carbon monoxide from:
- blast furnace gas
- incomplete combustion of fuels in industrial use
- kiln vapor

E868.9 Unspecified carbon monoxide

● **E869 Accidental poisoning by other gases and vapors**

> **Excludes** *effects of gases used as anesthetics (E855.1, E938.2)*
> *fumes from heavy metals (E866.0-E866.4)*
> *smoke and fumes due to conflagration or explosion (E890.0-E899)*

E869.0 Nitrogen oxides

E869.1 Sulfur dioxide

E869.2 Freon

E869.3 Lacrimogenic gas [tear gas]
- Bromobenzyl cyanide
- Chloroacetophenone
- Ethyliodoacetate

E869.4 Second-hand tobacco smoke
Coding Clinic: 1996, Q2, P10

E869.8 Other specified gases and vapors
- Chlorine
- Hydrocyanic acid gas

E869.9 Unspecified gases and vapors

MISADVENTURES TO PATIENTS DURING SURGICAL AND MEDICAL CARE (E870-E876)

> **Excludes** *accidental overdose of drug and wrong drug given in error (E850.0-E858.9)*
> *surgical and medical procedures as the cause of abnormal reaction by the patient, without mention of misadventure at the time of procedure (E878.0-E879.9)*

OGCR Section I.C.19.i.1
Assign a code in the range of E870-E876 if misadventures are stated by the provider.

● **E870 Accidental cut, puncture, perforation, or hemorrhage during medical care**

E870.0 Surgical operation

E870.1 Infusion or transfusion

E870.2 Kidney dialysis or other perfusion

E870.3 Injection or vaccination

E870.4 Endoscopic examination

E870.5 Aspiration of fluid or tissue, puncture, and catheterization
- Abdominal paracentesis
- Aspirating needle biopsy
- Blood sampling
- Lumbar puncture
- Thoracentesis

> **Excludes** *heart catheterization (E870.6)*

E870.6 Heart catheterization

E870.7 Administration of enema

E870.8 Other specified medical care

E870.9 Unspecified medical care

● **E871 Foreign object left in body during procedure**

E871.0 Surgical operation

E871.1 Infusion or transfusion

E871.2 Kidney dialysis or other perfusion

E871.3 Injection or vaccination

E871.4 Endoscopic examination

E871.5 Aspiration of fluid or tissue, puncture, and catheterization
- Abdominal paracentesis
- Aspiration needle biopsy
- Blood sampling
- Lumbar puncture
- Thoracentesis

> **Excludes** *heart catheterization (E871.6)*

E871.6 Heart catheterization

E871.7 Removal of catheter or packing

E871.8 Other specified procedures

E871.9 Unspecified procedure

● **E872 Failure of sterile precautions during procedure**

E872.0   Surgical operation

E872.1   Infusion or transfusion

E872.2   Kidney dialysis and other perfusion

E872.3   Injection or vaccination

E872.4   Endoscopic examination

E872.5   Aspiration of fluid or tissue, puncture, and catheterization
- Abdominal paracentesis
- Aspirating needle biopsy
- Blood sampling
- Lumbar puncture
- Thoracentesis

    Excludes *heart catheterization (E872.6)*

E872.6   Heart catheterization

■ E872.8   Other specified procedures

■ E872.9   Unspecified procedure

● **E873 Failure in dosage**

    Excludes *accidental overdose of drug, medicinal or biological substance (E850.0-E858.9)*

■ E873.0   Excessive amount of blood or other fluid during transfusion or infusion

E873.1   Incorrect dilution of fluid during infusion

E873.2   Overdose of radiation in therapy

E873.3   Inadvertent exposure of patient to radiation during medical care

E873.4   Failure in dosage in electroshock or insulin-shock therapy

E873.5   Inappropriate [too hot or too cold] temperature in local application and packing

E873.6   Nonadministration of necessary drug or medicinal substance

■ E873.8   Other specified failure in dosage

■ E873.9   Unspecified failure in dosage

● **E874 Mechanical failure of instrument or apparatus during procedure**

E874.0   Surgical operation

E874.1   Infusion and transfusion
- Air in system

E874.2   Kidney dialysis and other perfusion

E874.3   Endoscopic examination

E874.4   Aspiration of fluid or tissue, puncture, and catheterization
- Abdominal paracentesis
- Aspirating needle biopsy
- Blood sampling
- Lumbar puncture
- Thoracentesis

    Excludes *heart catheterization (E874.5)*

E874.5   Heart catheterization

■ E874.8   Other specified procedures

■ E874.9   Unspecified procedure

● **E875 Contaminated or infected blood, other fluid, drug, or biological substance**

    Includes presence of:
- bacterial pyrogens
- endotoxin-producing bacteria
- serum hepatitis-producing agent

E875.0   Contaminated substance transfused or infused

E875.1   Contaminated substance injected or used for vaccination

■ E875.2   Contaminated drug or biological substance administered by other means

■ E875.8   Other

■ E875.9   Unspecified

● **E876 Other and unspecified misadventures during medical care**

E876.0   Mismatched blood in transfusion

E876.1   Wrong fluid in infusion

E876.2   Failure in suture and ligature during surgical operation

E876.3   Endotracheal tube wrongly placed during anesthetic procedure

■ E876.4   Failure to introduce or to remove other tube or instrument

    Excludes *foreign object left in body during procedure (E871.0-E871.9)*

E876.5   Performance of ~~inappropriate~~ wrong operation (procedure) on correct patient
- Wrong device implanted into correct surgical site

    Excludes *correct operation (procedure) performed on wrong body part (E876.7)*

    Coding Clinic: 2006, Q3, P9-10

E876.6   Performance of operation (procedure) on patient not scheduled for surgery
- Performance of operation (procedure) intended for another patient
- Performance of operation (procedure) on wrong patient

E876.7   Performance of correct operation (procedure) on wrong side/body part
- Performance of correct operation (procedure) on wrong side
- Performance of correct operation (procedure) on wrong site

■ E876.8   Other specified misadventures during medical care
- Performance of inappropriate treatment, NEC

    Coding Clinic: 2009, Q2, P13x2, 15; 2008, Q4, P152-155

■ E876.9   Unspecified misadventure during medical care

◄ New   ◄ Revised   ~~deleted~~ Deleted   ● Use Additional Digit(s)   ■ Nonspecific Code
OGCR Official Guidelines   Coding Clinic   Excludes   Includes   Use additional   Code first   Omit code

E000-E999

SURGICAL AND MEDICAL PROCEDURES AS THE CAUSE OF ABNORMAL REACTION OF PATIENT OR LATER COMPLICATION, WITHOUT MENTION OF MISADVENTURE AT THE TIME OF PROCEDURE (E878-E879)

Includes procedures as the cause of abnormal reaction, such as:
> displacement or malfunction of prosthetic device
> hepatorenal failure, postoperative
> malfunction of external stoma
> postoperative intestinal obstruction
> rejection of transplanted organ

Excludes *anesthetic management properly carried out as the cause of adverse effect (E937.0-E938.9)*
infusion and transfusion, without mention of misadventure in the technique of procedure (E930.0-E949.9)

OGCR Section I.C.19.i.2
Assign a code in the range of E878-E879 if the provider attributes an abnormal reaction or later complication to a surgical or medical procedure, but does not mention misadventure at the time of the procedure as the cause of the reaction.

● **E878** **Surgical operation and other surgical procedures as the cause of abnormal reaction of patient, or of later complication, without mention of misadventure at the time of operation**

  E878.0 **Surgical operation with transplant of whole organ**
> Transplantation of:
> heart
> kidney
> liver

  E878.1 **Surgical operation with implant of artificial internal device**
> Cardiac pacemaker
> Electrodes implanted in brain
> Heart valve prosthesis
> Internal orthopedic device

  E878.2 **Surgical operation with anastomosis, bypass, or graft, with natural or artificial tissues used as implant**
> Anastomosis:
> arteriovenous
> gastrojejunal
> Graft of blood vessel, tendon, or skin

>   **Excludes** *external stoma (E878.3)*

  E878.3 **Surgical operation with formation of external stoma**
> Colostomy
> Cystostomy
> Duodenostomy
> Gastrostomy
> Ureterostomy

  ■ **E878.4** **Other restorative surgery**

  E878.5 **Amputation of limb(s)**

  ■ **E878.6** **Removal of other organ (partial) (total)**

  ■ **E878.8** **Other specified surgical operations and procedures**

  ■ **E878.9** **Unspecified surgical operations and procedures**

OGCR Section I.C.19.i.2
Assign a code in the range of E878-E879 if the provider attributes an abnormal reaction or later complication to a surgical or medical procedure, but does not mention misadventure at the time of the procedure as the cause of the reaction.

● **E879** **Other procedures, without mention of misadventure at the time of procedure, as the cause of abnormal reaction of patient, or of later complication**

  E879.0 **Cardiac catheterization**

  E879.1 **Kidney dialysis**
> Coding Clinic: 2003, Q4, P60-61; 1994, Q3, P9

  E879.2 **Radiological procedure and radiotherapy**

>   **Excludes** *radio-opaque dyes for diagnostic x-ray procedures (E947.8)*
> Coding Clinic: 2006, Q4, P88-91

  E879.3 **Shock therapy**
> Electroshock therapy
> Insulin-shock therapy

  E879.4 **Aspiration of fluid**
> Lumbar puncture
> Thoracentesis

  E879.5 **Insertion of gastric or duodenal sound**

  E879.6 **Urinary catheterization**

  E879.7 **Blood sampling**

  ■ **E879.8** **Other specified procedures**
> Blood transfusion
> Coding Clinic: 1993, Q2, P3-4

  ■ **E879.9** **Unspecified procedure**

ACCIDENTAL FALLS (E880-E888)

Excludes *falls (in or from):*
> *burning building (E890.8, E891.8)*
> *into fire (E890.0-E899)*
> *into water (with submersion or drowning) (E910.0-E910.9)*
> *machinery (in operation) (E919.0-E919.9)*
> *on edged, pointed, or sharp object (E920.0-E920.9)*
> *transport vehicle (E800.0-E845.9)*
> *vehicle not elsewhere classifiable (E846-E848)*

● **E880** **Fall on or from stairs or steps**

  E880.0 **Escalator**

  E880.1 **Fall on or from sidewalk curb**

>   **Excludes** *fall from moving sidewalk (E885.9)*

  ■ **E880.9** **Other stairs or steps**

● **E881** **Fall on or from ladders or scaffolding**

  E881.0 **Fall from ladder**
> Coding Clinic: 2007, Q1, P3-8

  E881.1 **Fall from scaffolding**
> Coding Clinic: 1999, Q4, P13

N Newborn Age: 0   **P** Pediatric Age: 0–17   **M** Maternity Age: 12–55   **A** Adult Age: 15–124   ♀ Females Only   ♂ Males Only   1157

E000-E999

E882 Fall from or out of building or other structure
Fall from:
    balcony
    bridge
    building
    flagpole
    tower
    turret
    viaduct
    wall
    window
Fall through roof

> **Excludes** *collapse of a building or structure (E916)*
> *fall or jump from burning building (E890.8, E891.8)*

● E883 Fall into hole or other opening in surface

> **Includes** fall into:
>   cavity
>   dock
>   hole
>   pit
>   quarry
>   shaft
>   swimming pool
>   tank
>   well

> **Excludes** *fall into water NOS (E910.9)*
> *that resulting in drowning or submersion without mention of injury (E910.0-E910.9)*

E883.0 Accident from diving or jumping into water [swimming pool]
Strike or hit:
    against bottom when jumping or diving into water
    wall or board of swimming pool
    water surface

> **Excludes** *diving with insufficient air supply (E913.2)*
> *effects of air pressure from diving (E902.2)*

E883.1 Accidental fall into well

E883.2 Accidental fall into storm drain or manhole

■ E883.9 Fall into other hole or other opening in surface

● E884 Other fall from one level to another

E884.0 Fall from playground equipment

> **Excludes** *recreational machinery (E919.8)*
> Coding Clinic: 2007, Q1, P3-8

E884.1 Fall from cliff

E884.2 Fall from chair

E884.3 Fall from wheelchair

E884.4 Fall from bed

E884.5 Fall from other furniture

E884.6 Fall from commode
Toilet

■ E884.9 Other fall from one level to another
Fall from:
    embankment
    haystack
    stationary vehicle
    tree

● E885 Fall on same level from slipping, tripping, or stumbling

E885.0 Fall from (nonmotorized) scooter
Coding Clinic: 2002, Q4, P73

E885.1 Fall from roller skates
Heelies
In-line skates
Wheelies

E885.2 Fall from skateboard
Coding Clinic: 2000, Q4, P61

E885.3 Fall from skis
Coding Clinic: 2007, Q2, P3-4

E885.4 Fall from snowboard

E885.9 Fall from other slipping, tripping, or stumbling
Fall on moving sidewalk

● E886 Fall on same level from collision, pushing, or shoving, by or with other person

> **Excludes** *crushed or pushed by a crowd or human stampede (E917.1, E917.6)*

E886.0 In sports
Tackles in sports

> **Excludes** *kicked, stepped on, struck by object, in sports (E917.0, E917.5)*
> Coding Clinic: 2007, Q2, P3-4

■ E886.9 Other and unspecified
Fall from collision of pedestrian (conveyance) with another pedestrian (conveyance)

■ E887 Fracture, cause unspecified

● E888 Other and unspecified fall
Accidental fall NOS
Fall on same level NOS
Coding Clinic: 1993, Q4, P25-26

E888.0 Fall resulting in striking against sharp object

> Use additional external cause code to identify object (E920)

E888.1 Fall resulting in striking against other object

E888.8 Other fall

E888.9 Unspecified fall
Fall NOS

ACCIDENTS CAUSED BY FIRE AND FLAMES (E890-E899)

> **Includes** asphyxia or poisoning due to conflagration or ignition
> burning by fire
> secondary fires resulting from explosion

> **Excludes** *arson (E968.0)*
> *fire in or on:*
>   *machinery (in operation) (E919.0-E919.9)*
>   *transport vehicle other than stationary vehicle (E800.0-E845.9)*
>   *vehicle not elsewhere classifiable (E846-E848)*

● E890 Conflagration in private dwelling

> **Includes** conflagration in:
>
> | | |
> |---|---|
> | apartment | lodging house |
> | boarding house | mobile home |
> | camping place | private garage |
> | caravan | rooming house |
> | farmhouse | tenement |
> | house | |
>
> conflagration originating from sources classifiable to E893-E898 in the above buildings

E890.0 Explosion caused by conflagration

E890.1 Fumes from combustion of polyvinylchloride [PVC] and similar material in conflagration

■ **E890.2   Other smoke and fumes from conflagration**
> Carbon monoxide from conflagration in private building
> Fumes NOS from conflagration in private building
> Smoke NOS from conflagration in private building
> Coding Clinic: 2005, Q3, P10-11

E890.3   Burning caused by conflagration

■ **E890.8   Other accident resulting from conflagration**
> Collapse of burning private building
> Fall from burning private building
> Hit by object falling from burning private building
> Jump from burning private building

■ **E890.9   Unspecified accident resulting from conflagration in private dwelling**

● **E891   Conflagration in other and unspecified building or structure**
> Conflagration in:
>> barn
>> church
>> convalescent and other residential home
>> dormitory of educational institution
>> factory
>> farm outbuildings
>> hospital
>> hotel
>> school
>> store
>> theater
> Conflagration originating from sources classifiable to E893-E898, in the above buildings

E891.0   Explosion caused by conflagration

E891.1   Fumes from combustion of polyvinylchloride [PVC] and similar material in conflagration

■ **E891.2   Other smoke and fumes from conflagration**
> Carbon monoxide from conflagration in building or structure
> Fumes NOS from conflagration in building or structure
> Smoke NOS from conflagration in building or structure

E891.3   Burning caused by conflagration

■ **E891.8   Other accident resulting from conflagration**
> Collapse of burning building or structure
> Fall from burning building or structure
> Hit by object falling from burning building or structure
> Jump from burning building or structure

■ **E891.9   Unspecified accident resulting from conflagration of other and unspecified building or structure**

E892   Conflagration not in building or structure
> Fire (uncontrolled) (in) (of):
>> forest
>> grass
>> hay
>> lumber
>> mine
>> prairie
>> transport vehicle [any], except while in transit
>> tunnel

● **E893   Accident caused by ignition of clothing**
> **Excludes**   *ignition of clothing:*
>> *from highly inflammable material (E894)*
>> *with conflagration (E890.0-E892)*

E893.0   From controlled fire in private dwelling
> Ignition of clothing from:
>> normal fire (charcoal) (coal) (electric) (gas) (wood) in:
>>> brazier in private dwelling (as listed in E890)
>>> fireplace in private dwelling (as listed in E890)
>>> furnace in private dwelling (as listed in E890)
>>> stove in private dwelling (as listed in E890)

■ **E893.1   From controlled fire in other building or structure**
> Ignition of clothing from:
>> normal fire (charcoal) (coal) (electric) (gas) (wood) in:
>>> brazier in other building or structure (as listed in E891)
>>> fireplace in other building or structure (as listed in E891)
>>> furnace in other building or structure (as listed in E891)
>>> stove in other building or structure (as listed in E891)

E893.2   From controlled fire not in building or structure
> Ignition of clothing from:
>> bonfire (controlled)
>> brazier fire (controlled), not in building or structure
>> trash fire (controlled)
> **Excludes**   *conflagration not in building (E892)*
>> *trash fire out of control (E892)*

■ **E893.8   From other specified sources**
> Ignition of clothing from:
>> blowlamp
>> blowtorch
>> burning bedspread
>> candle
>> cigar
>> cigarette
>> lighter
>> matches
>> pipe
>> welding torch

■ **E893.9   Unspecified source**
> Ignition of clothing (from controlled fire NOS) (in building NOS) NOS

E894   Ignition of highly inflammable material
> Ignition of:
>> benzine (with ignition of clothing)
>> gasoline (with ignition of clothing)
>> fat (with ignition of clothing)
>> kerosene (with ignition of clothing)
>> paraffin (with ignition of clothing)
>> petrol (with ignition of clothing)
> **Excludes**   *ignition of highly inflammable material with:*
>> *conflagration (E890.0-E892)*
>> *explosion (E923.0-E923.9)*

E000-E999

E895　Accident caused by controlled fire in private dwelling

Burning by (flame of) normal fire (charcoal) (coal) (electric) (gas) (wood) in:
    brazier in private dwelling (as listed in E890)
    fireplace in private dwelling (as listed in E890)
    furnace in private dwelling (as listed in E890)
    stove in private dwelling (as listed in E890)

Excludes *burning by hot objects not producing fire or flames (E924.0-E924.9)*
ignition of clothing from these sources (E893.0)
poisoning by carbon monoxide from incomplete combustion of fuel (E867-E868.9)
that with conflagration (E890.0-E890.9)

E896　Accident caused by controlled fire in other and unspecified building or structure

Burning by (flame of) normal fire (charcoal) (coal) (electric) (gas) (wood) in:
    brazier in other building or structure (as listed in E891)
    fireplace in other building or structure (as listed in E891)
    furnace in other building or structure (as listed in E891)
    stove in other building or structure (as listed in E891)

Excludes *burning by hot objects not producing fire or flames (E924.0-E924.9)*
ignition of clothing from these sources (E893.1)
poisoning by carbon monoxide from incomplete combustion of fuel (E867-E868.9)
that with conflagration (E891.0-E891.9)

E897　Accident caused by controlled fire not in building or structure

Burns from flame of:
    bonfire (controlled)
    brazier fire (controlled), not in building or structure
    trash fire (controlled)

Excludes *ignition of clothing from these sources (E893.2)*
trash fire out of control (E892)
that with conflagration (E892)

E898　Accident caused by other specified fire and flames

Excludes *conflagration (E890.0-E892)*
that with ignition of:
    clothing (E893.0-E893.9)
    highly inflammable material (E894)

E898.0　Burning bedclothes
Bed set on fire NOS

E898.1　Other

Burning by:	Burning by:
blowlamp	lamp
blowtorch	lighter
candle	matches
cigar	pipe
cigarette	welding torch
fire in room NOS	

E899　Accident caused by unspecified fire
Burning NOS

ACCIDENTS DUE TO NATURAL AND ENVIRONMENTAL FACTORS (E900-E909)

● E900　Excessive heat

E900.0　Due to weather conditions
Excessive heat as the external cause of:
    ictus solaris
    siriasis
    sunstroke

E900.1　Of man-made origin
Heat (in):
    boiler room
    drying room
    factory
    furnace room
    generated in transport vehicle
    kitchen

E900.9　Of unspecified origin

● E901　Excessive cold

E901.0　Due to weather conditions
Excessive cold as the cause of:
    chilblains NOS
    immersion foot

E901.1　Of man-made origin
Contact with or inhalation of:
    dry ice
    liquid air
    liquid hydrogen
    liquid nitrogen
Prolonged exposure in:
    deep freeze unit
    refrigerator

E901.8　Other specified origin

E901.9　Of unspecified origin

● E902　High and low air pressure and changes in air pressure

E902.0　Residence or prolonged visit at high altitude
Residence or prolonged visit at high altitude as the cause of:
    Acosta syndrome
    Alpine sickness
    altitude sickness
    Andes disease
    anoxia, hypoxia
    barotitis, barodontalgia, barosinusitis, otitic barotrauma
    hypobarism, hypobaropathy
    mountain sickness
    range disease

E902.1　In aircraft
Sudden change in air pressure in aircraft during ascent or descent as the cause of:
    aeroneurosis
    aviators' disease

E902.2　Due to diving
High air pressure from rapid descent in water as the cause of:
    caisson disease
    divers' disease
    divers' palsy or paralysis
Reduction in atmospheric pressure while surfacing from deep water diving as the cause of:
    caisson disease
    divers' disease
    divers' palsy or paralysis

E902.8　Due to other specified causes
Reduction in atmospheric pressure while surfacing from under ground

E902.9　Unspecified cause

E903   Travel and motion

● **E904   Hunger, thirst, exposure, and neglect**

> **Excludes**   *any condition resulting from homicidal intent (E968.0-E968.9)*
>
> *hunger, thirst, and exposure resulting from accidents connected with transport (E800.0-E848)*

E904.0   Abandonment or neglect of infants and helpless persons

Desertion of newborn

Exposure to weather conditions resulting from abandonment or neglect

Hunger or thirst resulting from abandonment or neglect

Inattention at or after birth

Lack of care (helpless person) (infant)

> **Excludes**   *criminal [purposeful] neglect (E968.4)*

> **OGCR** Section I.C.19.e.2
>
> In cases of neglect when the intent is determined to be accidental E code E904.0 should be the first listed E code.

E904.1   Lack of food

Lack of food as the cause of:

    inanition

    insufficient nourishment

    starvation

> **Excludes**   *hunger resulting from abandonment or neglect (E904.0)*

E904.2   Lack of water

Lack of water as the cause of:

    dehydration

    inanition

> **Excludes**   *dehydration due to acute fluid loss (276.51)*

E904.3   Exposure (to weather conditions), not elsewhere classifiable

Exposure NOS

Humidity

Struck by hailstones

> **Excludes**   *struck by lightning (E907)*

E904.9   Privation, unqualified

Destitution

● **E905   Venomous animals and plants as the cause of poisoning and toxic reactions**

> **Includes**   chemical released by animal
>
>   insects
>
>   release of venom through fangs, hairs, spines, tentacles, and other venom apparatus

> **Excludes**   *eating of poisonous animals or plants (E865.0-E865.9)*

E905.0   Venomous snakes and lizards

Cobra

Copperhead snake

Coral snake

Fer de lance

Gila monster

Krait

Mamba

Rattlesnake

Sea snake

Snake (venomous)

Viper

Water moccasin

> **Excludes**   *bites of snakes and lizards known to be nonvenomous (E906.2)*

E905.1   Venomous spiders

Black widow spider

Brown spider

Tarantula (venomous)

E905.2   Scorpion

E905.3   Hornets, wasps, and bees

Yellow jacket

E905.4   Centipede and venomous millipede (tropical)

■ **E905.5   Other venomous arthropods**

Sting of:

    ant

    caterpillar

E905.6   Venomous marine animals and plants

Puncture by sea urchin spine

Sting of:

    coral

    jelly fish

    nematocysts

    sea anemone

    sea cucumber

    other marine animal or plant

> **Excludes**   *bites and other injuries caused by nonvenomous marine animal (E906.2-E906.8)*
>
> *bite of sea snake (venomous) (E905.0)*

■ **E905.7   Poisoning and toxic reactions caused by other plants**

Injection of poisons or toxins into or through skin by plant thorns, spines, or other mechanisms

> **Excludes**   *puncture wound NOS by plant thorns or spines (E920.8)*

■ **E905.8   Other specified**

■ **E905.9   Unspecified**

Sting NOS

Venomous bite NOS

● **E906   Other injury caused by animals**

> **Excludes**   *poisoning and toxic reactions caused by venomous animals and insects (E905.0-E905.9)*
>
> *road vehicle accident involving animals (E827.0-E828.9)*
>
> *tripping or falling over an animal (E885.9)*

E906.0   Dog bite

E906.1   Rat bite

E906.2   Bite of nonvenomous snakes and lizards

■ **E906.3   Bite of other animal except arthropod**

Cats

Moray eel

Rodents, except rats

Shark

E906.4   Bite of nonvenomous arthropod

Insect bite NOS

E906.5   Bite by unspecified animal

Animal bite NOS

■ **E906.8   Other specified injury caused by animal**

Butted by animal

Fallen on by horse or other animal, not being ridden

Gored by animal

Implantation of quills of porcupine

Pecked by bird

Run over by animal, not being ridden

Stepped on by animal, not being ridden

> **Excludes**   *injury by animal being ridden (E828.0-E828.9)*

■ **E906.9   Unspecified injury caused by animal**

E907   Lightning

> **Excludes**   *injury from:*
> *fall of tree or other object caused by*
> *lightning (E916)*
> *fire caused by lightning (E890.0-E892)*

● E908   Cataclysmic storms, and floods resulting from storms

> **Excludes**   *collapse of dam or man-made structure causing*
> *flood (E909.3)*

E908.0   Hurricane
Storm surge
"Tidal wave" caused by storm action
Typhoon

E908.1   Tornado
Cyclone   Twisters

E908.2   Floods
Torrential rainfall   Flash flood

> **Excludes**   *collapse of dam or man-made structure*
> *causing flood (E909.3)*

E908.3   Blizzard (snow) (ice)

E908.4   Dust storm

E908.8   Other cataclysmic storms

E908.9   Unspecified cataclysmic storms, and floods resulting from storms
Storm NOS

● E909   Cataclysmic earth surface movements and eruptions

E909.0   Earthquakes

E909.1   Volcanic eruptions
Burns from lava   Ash inhalation

E909.2   Avalanche, landslide, or mudslide

E909.3   Collapse of dam or man-made structure

E909.4   Tidal wave caused by earthquake
Tidal wave NOS   Tsunami

> **Excludes**   *tidal wave caused by tropical storm*
> *(E908.0)*

E909.8   Other cataclysmic earth surface movements and eruptions

E909.9   Unspecified cataclysmic earth surface movements and eruptions

---

ACCIDENTS CAUSED BY SUBMERSION, SUFFOCATION, AND FOREIGN BODIES (E910-E915)

● E910   Accidental drowning and submersion

> **Includes**   immersion
> swimmers' cramp

> **Excludes**   *diving accident (NOS) (resulting in injury*
> *except drowning) (E883.0)*
> *diving with insufficient air supply (E913.2)*
> *drowning and submersion due to:*
> *cataclysm (E908-E909)*
> *machinery accident (E919.0-E919.9)*
> *transport accident (E800.0-E845.9)*
> *effect of high and low air pressure (E902.2)*
> *injury from striking against objects while in*
> *running water (E917.2)*

E910.0   While water-skiing
Fall from water skis with submersion or drowning

> **Excludes**   *accident to water-skier involving a*
> *watercraft and resulting in*
> *submersion or other injury*
> *(E830.4, E831.4)*

■ **E910.1   While engaged in other sport or recreational activity with diving equipment**
Scuba diving NOS
Skin diving NOS
Underwater spear fishing NOS

■ **E910.2   While engaged in other sport or recreational activity without diving equipment**
Fishing or hunting, except from boat or with diving equipment
Ice skating
Playing in water
Surfboarding
Swimming NOS
Voluntarily jumping from boat, not involved in accident, for swim NOS
Wading in water

> **Excludes**   *jumping into water to rescue another*
> *person (E910.3)*

E910.3   While swimming or diving for purposes other than recreation or sport
Marine salvage (with diving equipment)
Pearl diving (with diving equipment)
Placement of fishing nets (with diving equipment)
Rescue (attempt) of another person (with diving equipment)
Underwater construction or repairs (with diving equipment)

E910.4   In bathtub

■ **E910.8   Other accidental drowning or submersion**
Drowning in:
quenching tank
swimming pool

■ **E910.9   Unspecified accidental drowning or submersion**
Accidental fall into water NOS
Drowning NOS

E911   Inhalation and ingestion of food causing obstruction of respiratory tract or suffocation

Aspiration and inhalation of food [any] (into respiratory tract) NOS
Asphyxia by food [including bone, seed in food, regurgitated food]
Choked on food [including bone, seed in food, regurgitated food]
Suffocation by food [including bone, seed in food, regurgitated food]
Compression of trachea by food lodged in esophagus
Interruption of respiration by food lodged in esophagus
Obstruction of respiration by food lodged in esophagus
Obstruction of pharynx by food (bolus)

> **Excludes**   *injury, except asphyxia and obstruction of*
> *respiratory passage, caused by food*
> *(E915)*
> *obstruction of esophagus by food without*
> *mention of asphyxia or obstruction of*
> *respiratory passage (E915)*

◄ New   ◄▦ Revised   ~~deleted~~ Deleted   ● Use Additional Digit(s)   ■ Nonspecific Code

OGCR Official Guidelines   *Coding Clinic*   Excludes   Includes   Use additional   Code first   Omit code

■ **E912 Inhalation and ingestion of other object causing obstruction of respiratory tract or suffocation**
Aspiration and inhalation of foreign body except food (into respiratory tract) NOS
Compression by foreign body in esophagus
Foreign object [bean] [marble] in nose
Interruption of respiration by foreign body in esophagus
Obstruction of pharynx by foreign body
Obstruction of respiration by foreign body in esophagus

> **Excludes** *injury, except asphyxia and obstruction of respiratory passage, caused by foreign body (E915)*
> *obstruction of esophagus by foreign body without mention of asphyxia or obstruction in respiratory passage (E915)*

● **E913 Accidental mechanical suffocation**

> **Excludes** *mechanical suffocation from or by:*
> *accidental inhalation or ingestion of:*
> *food (E911)*
> *foreign object (E912)*
> *cataclysm (E908-E909)*
> *explosion (E921.0-E921.9, E923.0-E923.9)*
> *machinery accident (E919.0-E919.9)*

E913.0 In bed or cradle

> **Excludes** *suffocation by plastic bag (E913.1)*

E913.1 By plastic bag

E913.2 Due to lack of air (in closed place)
Accidentally closed up in refrigerator or other airtight enclosed space
Diving with insufficient air supply

> **Excludes** *suffocation by plastic bag (E913.1)*

E913.3 By falling earth or other substance
Cave-in NOS

> **Excludes** *cave-in caused by cataclysmic earth surface movements and eruptions (E909.8)*
> *struck by cave-in without asphyxiation or suffocation (E916)*

■ **E913.8 Other specified means**
Accidental hanging, except in bed or cradle

■ **E913.9 Unspecified means**
Asphyxia, mechanical NOS
Strangulation NOS
Suffocation NOS

E914 Foreign body accidentally entering eye and adnexa

> **Excludes** *corrosive liquid (E924.1)*

■ **E915 Foreign body accidentally entering other orifice**

> **Excludes** *aspiration and inhalation of foreign body, any, (into respiratory tract) NOS (E911-E912)*

OTHER ACCIDENTS (E916-E928)

E916 Struck accidentally by falling object
Collapse of building, except on fire
Falling:
rock
snowslide NOS
stone
tree
Object falling from:
machine, not in operation
stationary vehicle

> *Code first* collapse of building on fire (E890.0-E891.9)
> falling object in:
> cataclysm (E908-E909)
> machinery accidents (E919.0-E919.9)
> transport accidents (E800.0-E845.9)
> vehicle accidents not elsewhere classifiable (E846-E848)
> object set in motion by:
> explosion (E921.0-E921.9, E923.0-E923.9)
> firearm (E922.0-E922.9)
> projected object (E917.0-E917.9)

● **E917 Striking against or struck accidentally by objects or persons**

> **Includes** bumping into or against
> object (moving) (projected) (stationary)
> pedestrian conveyance
> person
> colliding with
> object (moving) (projected) (stationary)
> pedestrian conveyance
> person
> kicking against
> object (moving) (projected) (stationary)
> pedestrian conveyance
> person
> stepping on
> object (moving) (projected) (stationary)
> pedestrian conveyance
> person
> struck by
> object (moving) (projected) (stationary)
> pedestrian conveyance
> person

> **Excludes** *fall from:*
> *collision with another person, except when caused by a crowd (E886.0-E886.9)*
> *stumbling over object (E885.9)*
> *fall resulting in striking against object (E888.0-E888.1)*
> *injury caused by:*
> *assault (E960.0-E960.1, E967.0-E967.9)*
> *cutting or piercing instrument (E920.0-E920.9)*
> *explosion (E921.0-E921.9, E923.0-E923.9)*
> *firearm (E922.0-E922.9)*
> *machinery (E919.0-E919.9)*
> *transport vehicle (E800.0-E845.9)*
> *vehicle not elsewhere classifiable (E846-E848)*

E917.0 In sports without subsequent fall
Kicked or stepped on during game (football) (rugby)
Struck by hit or thrown ball
Struck by hockey stick or puck
Coding Clinic: 2007, Q2, P3-4; 2006, Q1, P8; 2004, Q1, P9

E917.1 Caused by a crowd, by collective fear or panic without subsequent fall
Crushed by crowd or human stampede
Pushed by crowd or human stampede
Stepped on by crowd or human stampede

E917.2 In running water without subsequent fall
Excludes *drowning or submersion (E910.0-E910.9) that in sports (E917.0, E917.5)*

E917.3 Furniture without subsequent fall
Excludes *fall from furniture (E884.2, E884.4–E884.5)*

E917.4 Other stationary object without subsequent fall
Bath tub
Fence
Lamp-post

E917.5 Object in sports with subsequent fall
Knocked down while boxing
Coding Clinic: 2007, Q2, P3-4

E917.6 Caused by a crowd, by collective fear or panic with subsequent fall

E917.7 Furniture with subsequent fall
Excludes *fall from furniture (E884.2, E884.4–E884.5)*

■ E917.8 Other stationary object with subsequent fall
Bath tub
Fence
Lamp-post

■ E917.9 Other striking against with or without subsequent fall

E918 Caught accidentally in or between objects
Caught, crushed, jammed, or pinched in or between moving or stationary objects, such as:
escalator
folding object
hand tools, appliances, or implements
sliding door and door frame
under packing crate
washing machine wringer

Excludes *injury caused by:*
cutting or piercing instrument (E920.0-E920.9)
machinery (E919.0-E919.9)
mechanism or component of firearm and air gun (E928.7) ◄
transport vehicle (E800.0-E845.9)
vehicle not elsewhere classifiable (E846-E848)
struck accidentally by:
falling object (E916)
object (moving) (projected) (E917.0-E917.9)

● E919 Accidents caused by machinery
Includes burned by machinery (accident)
caught between machinery and other object
caught in (moving parts of) machinery (accident)
collapse of machinery (accident)
crushed by machinery (accident)
cut or pierced by machinery (accident)
drowning or submersion caused by machinery (accident)
explosion of, on, in machinery (accident)
fall from or into moving part of machinery (accident)
fire starting in or on machinery (accident)
mechanical suffocation caused by machinery (accident)
object falling from, on, in motion by machinery (accident)
overturning of machinery (accident)
pinned under machinery (accident)
run over by machinery (accident)
struck by machinery (accident)
thrown from machinery (accident)
machinery accident NOS

Excludes *accidents involving machinery, not in operation (E884.9, E916-E918)*
injury caused by:
electric current in connection with machinery (E925.0-E925.9)
escalator (E880.0, E918)
explosion of pressure vessel in connection with machinery (E921.0-E921.9)
mechanism or component of firearm and air gun (E928.7) ◄
moving sidewalk (E885.9)
powered hand tools, appliances, and implements (E916-E918, E920.0-E921.9, E923.0-E926.9)
transport vehicle accidents involving machinery (E800.0-E848.9)
poisoning by carbon monoxide generated by machine (E868.8)

E919.0 Agricultural machines
Animal-powered agricultural machine
Combine
Derrick, hay
Farm machinery NOS
Farm tractor
Harvester
Hay mower or rake
Reaper
Thresher

Excludes *that being towed by another vehicle on the highway (E810.0-E819.9, E827.0-E827.9, E829.0-E829.9)*
that in transport under own power on the highway (E810.0-E819.9)
that involved in accident classifiable to E820-E829 (E820.0-E829.9)

E000-E999

E919.1   Mining and earth-drilling machinery
     Bore or drill (land) (seabed)
     Shaft hoist
     Shaft lift
     Under-cutter
     Excludes   *coal car, tram, truck, and tub in mine*
              (E846)

E919.2   Lifting machines and appliances
     Chain hoist except in agricultural or mining
         operations
     Crane except in agricultural or mining
         operations
     Derrick except in agricultural or mining
         operations
     Elevator (building) (grain) except in
         agricultural or mining operations
     Forklift truck except in agricultural or mining
         operations
     Lift except in agricultural or mining
         operations
     Pulley block except in agricultural or mining
         operations
     Winch except in agricultural or mining
         operations
     Excludes   *that being towed by another vehicle on*
              the highway (E810.0-E819.9,
              E827.0-E827.9, E829.0-E829.9)
            that in transport under own power on
              the highway (E810.0-E819.9)
            that involved in accident classifiable to
              E820-E829 (E820.0-E829.9)

E919.3   Metalworking machines
     Abrasive wheel   Metal:
     Forging machine   milling machine
     Lathe   power press
     Mechanical shears   rolling-mill
     Metal: sawing machine
        drilling machine
     Coding Clinic: 2003, Q4, P76-78

E919.4   Woodworking and forming machines
     Band saw   Overhead plane
     Bench saw   Powered saw
     Circular saw   Radial saw
     Molding machine   Sander
     Excludes   *hand saw (E920.1)*

E919.5   Prime movers, except electrical motors
     Gas turbine
     Internal combustion engine
     Steam engine
     Water driven turbine
     Excludes   *that being towed by other vehicle on*
              the highway (E810.0-E819.9,
              E827.0-E827.9, E829.0-E829.9)
            that in transport under own power on
              the highway (E810.0-E819.9)

E919.6   Transmission machinery
     Transmission: Transmission:
       belt   pinion
       cable   pulley
       chain   shaft
       gear

E919.7   Earth moving, scraping, and other excavating
     machines
     Bulldozer   Steam shovel
     Road scraper
     Excludes   *that being towed by other vehicle on*
              the highway (E810.0-E819.9)
            that in transport under own power on
              the highway (E810.0-E819.9)

■ **E919.8   Other specified machinery**
     Machines for manufacture of:
       clothing
       foodstuffs and beverages
       paper
     Printing machine
     Recreational machinery
     Spinning, weaving, and textile machines

■ **E919.9   Unspecified machinery**

● **E920   Accidents caused by cutting and piercing instruments**
     or objects
     Includes   accidental injury (by) object:
                 edged
                 pointed
                 sharp
     Excludes   *injury caused by mechanism or component of*
              firearm and air gun (E928.7) ◄

E920.0   Powered lawn mower

■ **E920.1   Other powered hand tools**
     Any powered hand tool [compressed air]
       [electric] [explosive cartridge] [hydraulic
       power], such as:
       drill
       hand saw
       hedge clipper
       rivet gun
       snow blower
       staple gun
     Excludes   *band saw (E919.4)*
              bench saw (E919.4)

E920.2   Powered household appliances and implements
     Blender
     Electric:
       beater or mixer
       can opener
       fan
       knife
       sewing machine
     Garbage disposal appliance

E920.3   Knives, swords, and daggers

■ **E920.4   Other hand tools and implements**
     Axe
     Can opener NOS
     Chisel
     Fork
     Hand saw
     Hoe
     Ice pick
     Needle (sewing)
     Paper cutter
     Pitchfork
     Rake
     Scissors
     Screwdriver
     Sewing machine, not powered
     Shovel

E920.5 **Hypodermic needle**
Contaminated needle
Needle stick

E920.8 **Other specified cutting and piercing instruments or objects**

Arrow Nail
Broken glass Plant thorn
Dart Splinter
Edge of stiff paper Tin can lid
Lathe turnings

Excludes *animal spines or quills (E906.8)*
flying glass due to explosion (E921.0-E923.9)

Coding Clinic: 2001, Q3, P10

E920.9 **Unspecified cutting and piercing instrument or object**

● E921 **Accident caused by explosion of pressure vessel**

Includes accidental explosion of pressure vessels, whether or not part of machinery

Excludes *explosion of pressure vessel on transport vehicle (E800.0-E845.9)*

E921.0 **Boilers**
Coding Clinic: 2005, Q3, P10-11

E921.1 **Gas cylinders**
Air tank
Pressure gas tank

E921.8 **Other specified pressure vessels**
Aerosol can
Automobile tire
Pressure cooker

E921.9 **Unspecified pressure vessel**

● E922 **Accident caused by firearm and air gun missile**

Excludes *injury caused by mechanism or component of firearm and air gun (E928.7)* ◀

E922.0 **Handgun**
Pistol
Revolver

Excludes *Verey pistol (E922.8)*

E922.1 **Shotgun (automatic)**

E922.2 **Hunting rifle**

E922.3 **Military firearms**
Army rifle
Machine gun

E922.4 **Air gun**
BB gun
Pellet gun

E922.5 **Paintball gun**
Coding Clinic: 2002, Q4, P74

E922.8 **Other specified firearm missile**
Verey pistol [flare]

E922.9 **Unspecified firearm missile**
Gunshot wound NOS
Shot NOS

● E923 **Accident caused by explosive material**

Includes flash burns and other injuries resulting from explosion of explosive material
ignition of highly explosive material with explosion

Excludes *explosion:*
in or on machinery (E919.0-E919.9)
on any transport vehicle, except stationary motor vehicle (E800.0-E848)
with conflagration (E890.0, E891.0, E892)
injury caused by mechanism or component of firearm and air gun (E928.7) ◀
secondary fires resulting from explosion (E890.0-E899)

E923.0 **Fireworks**

E923.1 **Blasting materials**
Blasting cap Explosive [any]
Detonator used in blasting
Dynamite operations

E923.2 **Explosive gases**
Acetylene
Butane
Coal gas
Explosion in mine NOS
Fire damp
Gasoline fumes
Methane
Propane

E923.8 **Other explosive materials**
Bomb Torpedo
Explosive missile Explosion in munitions:
Grenade dump
Mine factory
Shell

E923.9 **Unspecified explosive material**
Explosion NOS

● E924 **Accident caused by hot substance or object, caustic or corrosive material, and steam**

Excludes *burning NOS (E899)*
chemical burn resulting from swallowing a corrosive substance (E860.0-E864.4)
fire caused by these substances and objects (E890.0-E894)
radiation burns (E926.0-E926.9)
therapeutic misadventures (E870.0-E876.9)

E924.0 **Hot liquids and vapors, including steam**
Burning or scalding by:
boiling water
hot or boiling liquids not primarily caustic or corrosive
liquid metal
other hot vapor
steam

Excludes *hot (boiling) tap water (E924.2)*

E924.1 **Caustic and corrosive substances**
Burning by:
acid [any kind]
ammonia
caustic oven cleaner or other substance
corrosive substance
lye
vitriol

E924.2 **Hot (boiling) tap water**

E924.8 **Other**
Burning by:
heat from electric heating appliance
hot object NOS
light bulb
steam pipe

E924.9 **Unspecified**

E000-E999

● **E925   Accident caused by electric current**

     Includes   electric current from exposed wire, faulty appliance, high voltage cable, live rail, or open electric socket as the cause of:

         burn
         cardiac fibrillation
         convulsion
         electric shock
         electrocution
         puncture wound
         respiratory paralysis

     Excludes   *burn by heat from electrical appliance (E924.8)*
               lightning (E907)

E925.0   Domestic wiring and appliances

E925.1   Electric power generating plants, distribution stations, transmission lines
        Broken power line

E925.2   Industrial wiring, appliances, and electrical machinery
        Conductors
        Control apparatus
        Electrical equipment and machinery
        Transformers

■ **E925.8   Other electric current**
        Wiring and appliances in or on:
           farm [not farmhouse]
           outdoors
           public building
           residential institutions
           schools

■ **E925.9   Unspecified electric current**
        Burns or other injury from electric current NOS
        Electric shock NOS
        Electrocution NOS

● **E926   Exposure to radiation**

     Excludes   *abnormal reaction to or complication of treatment without mention of misadventure (E879.2)*
               atomic power plant malfunction in water transport (E838.0-E838.9)
               misadventure to patient in surgical and medical procedures (E873.2-E873.3)
               use of radiation in war operations (E996-E997.9)

E926.0   Radiofrequency radiation
        Overexposure to:
           microwave radiation from:
               high-powered radio and television transmitters
               industrial radiofrequency induction heaters
               radar installations
           radar radiation from:
               high-powered radio and television transmitters
               industrial radiofrequency induction heaters
               radar installations
           radiofrequency from:
               high-powered radio and television transmitters
               industrial radiofrequency induction heaters
               radar installations
           radiofrequency radiation [any] from:
               high-powered radio and television transmitters
               industrial radiofrequency induction heaters
               radar installations

E926.1   Infra-red heaters and lamps
        Exposure to infra-red radiation from heaters and lamps as the cause of:
           blistering   charring
           burning   inflammatory change

     Excludes   *physical contact with heater or lamp (E924.8)*

E926.2   Visible and ultraviolet light sources
        Arc lamps
        Black light sources
        Electrical welding arc
        Oxygas welding torch
        Sun rays
        Tanning bed

     Excludes   *excessive heat from these sources (E900.1-E900.9)*

     Coding Clinic: 1996, Q3, P6

E926.3   X-rays and other electromagnetic ionizing radiation
        Gamma rays
        X-rays (hard) (soft)

E926.4   Lasers

E926.5   Radioactive isotopes
        Radiobiologicals
        Radiopharmaceuticals

■ **E926.8   Other specified radiation**
        Artificially accelerated beams of ionized particles generated by:
           betatrons
           synchrotrons

■ **E926.9   Unspecified radiation**
        Radiation NOS

● **E927   Overexertion and strenuous and repetitive movements or loads**

     Use additional code to identify activity (E001-E030) ◀
     Coding Clinic: 2008, Q3, P21

E927.0   Overexertion from sudden strenuous movement
        Sudden trauma from strenuous movement

E927.1   Overexertion from prolonged static position
        Overexertion from maintaining prolonged positions, such as:
           holding
           sitting
           standing

E927.2   Excessive physical exertion from prolonged activity

E927.3   Cumulative trauma from repetitive motion
        Cumulative trauma from repetitive movements

E927.4   Cumulative trauma from repetitive impact

■ **E927.8   Other overexertion and strenuous and repetitive movements or loads**

■ **E927.9   Unspecified overexertion and strenuous and repetitive movements or loads**

● **E928   Other and unspecified environmental and accidental causes**

E928.0   Prolonged stay in weightless environment
        Weightlessness in spacecraft (simulator)

E928.1   Exposure to noise
        Noise (pollution)
        Sound waves
        Supersonic waves

E928.2   Vibration

E928.3   Human bite

E928.4   External constriction caused by hair

N Newborn Age: 0   **P** Pediatric Age: 0–17   **M** Maternity Age: 12–55   **A** Adult Age: 15–124   ♀ Females Only   ♂ Males Only   **1167**

E000-E999

E928.5 External constriction caused by other object

E928.6 Environmental exposure to harmful algae and toxins
    Algae bloom NOS
    Blue-green algae bloom
    Brown tide
    Cyanobacteria bloom
    Florida red tide
    Harmful algae bloom
    Pfiesteria piscicida
    Red tide
    Coding Clinic: 2007, Q4, P101-102

E928.7 Mechanism or component of firearm and air gun ◄
    Injury due to: ◄
        explosion of gun parts ◄
        recoil ◄
    Pierced, cut, crushed, or pinched by slide trigger mechanism, scope or other gun part ◄
    Powder burn from firearm or air gun ◄

    Excludes *accident caused by firearm and air gun missile (E922.0-E922.9)* ◄

E928.8 Other

E928.9 Unspecified accident
    Accident NOS stated as accidentally inflicted
    Blow NOS stated as accidentally inflicted
    Casualty (not due to war) stated as accidentally inflicted
    Decapitation stated as accidentally inflicted
    Injury [any part of body, or unspecified] stated as accidentally inflicted, but not otherwise specified
    Killed stated as accidentally inflicted, but not otherwise specified
    Knocked down stated as accidentally inflicted, but not otherwise specified
    Mangled stated as accidentally inflicted, but not otherwise specified
    Wound stated as accidentally inflicted, but not otherwise specified

    Excludes *fracture, cause unspecified (E887)*
        injuries undetermined whether accidentally or purposely inflicted (E980.0-E989)
    Coding Clinic: 1996, Q3, P7; 1985, Nov-Dec, P15; 1984, Nov-Dec, P15

LATE EFFECTS OF ACCIDENTAL INJURY (E929)

Note: This category is to be used to indicate accidental injury as the cause of death or disability from late effects, which are themselves classifiable elsewhere. The "late effects" include conditions reported as such or as sequelae, which may occur at any time after the acute accidental injury.

● E929 Late effects of accidental injury
    Excludes *late effects of:*
        surgical and medical procedures (E870.0-E879.9)
        therapeutic use of drugs and medicines (E930.0-E949.9)

E929.0 Late effects of motor vehicle accident
    Late effects of accidents classifiable to E810-E825
    Coding Clinic: 2008, Q4, P102-109; 1997, Q3, P12-13; 1995, Q1, P10; 1994, Q3, P4

E929.1 Late effects of other transport accident
    Late effects of accidents classifiable to E800-E807, E826-E838, E840-E848

E929.2 Late effects of accidental poisoning
    Late effects of accidents classifiable to E850-E858, E860-E869

E929.3 Late effects of accidental fall
    Late effects of accidents classifiable to E880-E888

E929.4 Late effects of accident caused by fire
    Late effects of accidents classifiable to E890-E899

E929.5 Late effects of accident due to natural and environmental factors
    Late effects of accidents classifiable to E900-E909

E929.8 Late effects of other accidents
    Late effects of accidents classifiable to E910-E928.8

E929.9 Late effects of unspecified accident
    Late effects of accidents classifiable to E928.9

OGCR Section I.C.17.e.1
Adverse Effect: When the drug was correctly prescribed and properly administered, code the reaction plus the appropriate code from the E930-E949 series. Codes from the E930-E949 series must be used to identify the causative substance for an adverse effect of drug, medicinal and biological substances, correctly prescribed and properly administered. The effect, such as tachycardia, delirium, gastrointestinal hemorrhaging, vomiting, hypokalemia, hepatitis, renal failure, or respiratory failure, is coded and followed by the appropriate code from the E930-E949 series.

DRUGS, MEDICINAL AND BIOLOGICAL SUBSTANCES CAUSING ADVERSE EFFECTS IN THERAPEUTIC USE (E930-E949)

Includes correct drug properly administered in therapeutic or prophylactic dosage, as the cause of any adverse effect including allergic or hypersensitivity reactions

Excludes *accidental overdose of drug and wrong drug given or taken in error (E850.0-E858.9)*
    accidents in the technique of administration of drug or biological substance such as accidental puncture during injection, or contamination of drug (E870.0-E876.9)
    administration with suicidal or homicidal intent or intent to harm, or in circumstances classifiable to ~~E980-E989~~ *(E950.0-E950.5, E962.0, E980.0-E980.5)* ◄
    See Alphabetic Index for more complete list of specific drugs to be classified under the fourth-digit subdivisions. The American Hospital Formulary numbers can be used to classify new drugs listed by the American Hospital Formulary Service (AHFS). See appendix C.

● E930 Antibiotics
    Excludes *that used as eye, ear, nose, and throat [ENT], and local anti-infectives (E946.0-E946.9)*
    Coding Clinic: 2008, Q3, P21

E930.0 Penicillins
    Natural
    Synthetic
    Semisynthetic, such as:
        ampicillin
        cloxacillin
        nafcillin
        oxacillin
    Coding Clinic: 2008, Q4, P128-131

◄ New   ◄▥ Revised   ~~deleted~~ Deleted   ● Use Additional Digit(s)   ▣ Nonspecific Code
OGCR Official Guidelines   Coding Clinic   Excludes   Includes   Use additional   Code first   Omit code

E930.1 Antifungal antibiotics
    Amphotericin B
    Griseofulvin
    Hachimycin [trichomycin]
    Nystatin

E930.2 Chloramphenicol group
    Chloramphenicol
    Thiamphenicol

E930.3 Erythromycin and other macrolides
    Oleandomycin
    Spiramycin

E930.4 Tetracycline group
    Doxycycline
    Minocycline
    Oxytetracycline
    Coding Clinic: 1988, Q2, P9-10

E930.5 Cephalosporin group
    Cephalexin
    Cephaloglycin
    Cephaloridine
    Cephalothin

E930.6 Antimycobacterial antibiotics
    Cycloserine
    Kanamycin
    Rifampin
    Streptomycin

E930.7 Antineoplastic antibiotics
    Actinomycins, such as:
      bleomycin
      cactinomycin
      dactinomycin
      daunorubicin
      mitomycin

    Excludes *other antineoplastic drugs (E933.1)*
    Coding Clinic: 2007, Q2, P9-10

■ E930.8 Other specified antibiotics
    Coding Clinic: 1993, Q1, P29

■ E930.9 Unspecified antibiotic

● E931 Other anti-infectives
    Excludes *ENT, and local anti-infectives (E946.0-E946.9)*

E931.0 Sulfonamides
    Sulfadiazine
    Sulfafurazole
    Sulfamethoxazole

E931.1 Arsenical anti-infectives

E931.2 Heavy metal anti-infectives
    Compounds of:
      antimony
      bismuth
      lead
      mercury

    Excludes *mercurial diuretics (E944.0)*

E931.3 Quinoline and hydroxyquinoline derivatives
    Chiniofon
    Diiodohydroxyquin

    Excludes *antimalarial drugs (E931.4)*

E931.4 Antimalarials and drugs acting on other blood protozoa
    Chloroquine phosphate
    Cycloguanil
    Primaquine
    Proguanil [chloroguanide]
    Pyrimethamine
    Quinine (sulphate)

■ E931.5 Other antiprotozoal drugs
    Emetine

E931.6 Anthelmintics
    Hexylresorcinol
    Male fern oleoresin
    Piperazine
    Thiabendazole

E931.7 Antiviral drugs
    Methisazone

    Excludes *amantadine (E936.4)*
      cytarabine (E933.1)
      idoxuridine (E946.5)

■ E931.8 Other antimycobacterial drugs
    Ethambutol
    Ethionamide
    Isoniazid
    Para-aminosalicylic acid derivatives
    Sulfones

■ E931.9 Other and unspecified anti-infectives
    Flucytosine
    Nitrofuran derivatives

● E932 Hormones and synthetic substitutes

E932.0 Adrenal cortical steroids
    Cortisone derivatives
    Desoxycorticosterone derivatives
    Fluorinated corticosteroids
    Coding Clinic: 2008, Q4, P91-95; 2003, Q4, P108-109; 2000, Q3, P4-5

E932.1 Androgens and anabolic congeners
    Nandrolone phenpropionate
    Oxymetholone
    Testosterone and preparations
    Coding Clinic: 1985, July-Aug, P8

E932.2 Ovarian hormones and synthetic substitutes
    Contraceptives, oral
    Estrogens
    Estrogens and progestogens combined
    Progestogens

E932.3 Insulins and antidiabetic agents
    Acetohexamide
    Biguanide derivatives, oral
    Chlorpropamide
    Glucagon
    Insulin
    Phenformin
    Sulfonylurea derivatives, oral
    Tolbutamide

    Excludes *adverse effect of insulin administered for shock therapy (E879.3)*

E932.4 Anterior pituitary hormones
    Corticotropin
    Gonadotropin
    Somatotropin [growth hormone]
    Coding Clinic: 1995, Q3, P15

E932.5 Posterior pituitary hormones
    Vasopressin

    Excludes *oxytocic agents (E945.0)*

E932.6 Parathyroid and parathyroid derivatives

E932.7 Thyroid and thyroid derivatives
    Dextrothyroxine
    Levothyroxine sodium
    Liothyronine
    Thyroglobulin

E932.8 Antithyroid agents
    Iodides
    Thiouracil
    Thiourea

■ E932.9 Other and unspecified hormones and synthetic substitutes

E000-E999

● **E933 Primarily systemic agents**

E933.0 Antiallergic and antiemetic drugs
Antihistamines
Chlorpheniramine
Diphenhydramine
Diphenylpyraline
Thonzylamine
Tripelennamine

Excludes *phenothiazine-based tranquilizers (E939.1)*

Coding Clinic: 1997, Q2, P9-10

E933.1 Antineoplastic and immunosuppressive drugs
Azathioprine
Busulfan
Chlorambucil
Cyclophosphamide
Cytarabine
Fluorouracil
Mechlorethamine hydrochloride
Mercaptopurine
Triethylenethiophosphoramide [thio-TEPA]

Excludes *antineoplastic antibiotics (E930.7)*

Coding Clinic: 2008, Q2, P6, 10-11; 2006, Q4, P69-73; Q2, P20; 2005, Q3, P11-12; 1999, Q3, P6-7; Q2, P9; 1996, Q2, P12; 1985, Mar-April, P14

E933.2 Acidifying agents

E933.3 Alkalizing agents

E933.4 Enzymes, not elsewhere classified
Penicillinase

E933.5 Vitamins, not elsewhere classified
Vitamin A
Vitamin D

Excludes *nicotinic acid (E942.2)*
vitamin K (E934.3)

E933.6 Oral bisphosphonates
Coding Clinic: 2007, Q4, P91-92, 102

E933.7 Intravenous bisphosphonates
Coding Clinic: 2007, Q4, P102

■ **E933.8 Other systemic agents, not elsewhere classified**
Heavy metal antagonists

■ **E933.9 Unspecified systemic agent**

● **E934 Agents primarily affecting blood constituents**
Coding Clinic: 1993, 5th Issue, P16

E934.0 Iron and its compounds
Ferric salts
Ferrous sulphate and other ferrous salts

■ **E934.1 Liver preparations and other antianemic agents**
Folic acid

E934.2 Anticoagulants
Coumarin
Heparin
Phenindione
Prothrombin synthesis inhibitor
Warfarin sodium
Coding Clinic: 2008, Q4, P134-136; 2006, Q3, P12-P13; Q2, P17; 2004, Q3, P7; 1994, Q1, P22; 1990, Q3, P14

E934.3 Vitamin K [phytonadione]

E934.4 Fibrinolysis-affecting drugs
Aminocaproic acid
Streptodornase
Streptokinase
Urokinase

■ **E934.5 Anticoagulant antagonists and other coagulants**
Hexadimethrine bromide
Protamine sulfate

E934.6 Gamma globulin

E934.7 Natural blood and blood products
Blood plasma
Human fibrinogen
Packed red cells
Whole blood
Coding Clinic: 2006, Q4, P91-92; 2000, Q3, P9; 1997, Q2, P11

■ **E934.8 Other agents affecting blood constituents**
Macromolecular blood substitutes

■ **E934.9 Unspecified agent affecting blood constituents**

● **E935 Analgesics, antipyretics, and antirheumatics**

E935.0 Heroin
Diacetylmorphine

E935.1 Methadone

■ **E935.2 Other opiates and related narcotics**
Codeine [methylmorphine]
Morphine
Opium (alkaloids)
Meperidine [pethidine]

E935.3 Salicylates
Acetylsalicylic acid [aspirin]
Amino derivatives of salicylic acid
Salicylic acid salts
Coding Clinic: 1984, Nov-Dec, P15

E935.4 Aromatic analgesics, not elsewhere classified
Acetanilid
Paracetamol [acetaminophen]
Phenacetin [acetophenetidin]

E935.5 Pyrazole derivatives
Aminophenazone [aminopyrine]
Phenylbutazone
Coding Clinic: 1990, Q4, P26

E935.6 Antirheumatics [antiphlogistics]
Gold salts
Indomethacin

Excludes *salicylates (E935.3)*
steroids (E932.0)

■ **E935.7 Other non-narcotic analgesics**
Pyrabital

■ **E935.8 Other specified analgesics and antipyretics**
Pentazocine
Coding Clinic: 1992, Q3, P16-17

■ **E935.9 Unspecified analgesic and antipyretic**

● **E936 Anticonvulsants and anti-Parkinsonism drugs**

E936.0 Oxazolidine derivatives
Paramethadione
Trimethadione

E936.1 Hydantoin derivatives
Phenytoin

E936.2 Succinimides
Ethosuximide
Phensuximide

■ **E936.3 Other and unspecified anticonvulsants**
Beclamide
Primidone

E936.4 Anti-Parkinsonism drugs
Amantadine
Ethopropazine [profenamine]
Levodopa [L-dopa]

◄ New   ◄▦ Revised   ~~deleted~~ Deleted   ● Use Additional Digit(s)   ■ Nonspecific Code

OGCR Official Guidelines   Coding Clinic   Excludes   Includes   Use additional   Code first   Omit code

● **E937**   **Sedatives and hypnotics**

     E937.0   **Barbiturates**
          Amobarbital [amylobarbitone]
          Barbital [barbitone]
          Butabarbital [butabarbitone]
          Pentobarbital [pentobarbitone]
          Phenobarbital [phenobarbitone]
          Secobarbital [quinalbarbitone]
          Excludes   *thiobarbiturates (E938.3)*

     E937.1   **Chloral hydrate group**

     E937.2   **Paraldehyde**

     E937.3   **Bromine compounds**
          Bromide
          Carbromal (derivatives)

     E937.4   **Methaqualone compounds**

     E937.5   **Glutethimide group**

     E937.6   **Mixed sedatives, not elsewhere classified**

     ■ **E937.8**   **Other sedatives and hypnotics**

     ■ **E937.9**   **Unspecified**
          Sleeping:
            drug NOS
            pill NOS
            tablet NOS

● **E938**   **Other central nervous system depressants and anesthetics**

     E938.0   **Central nervous system muscle-tone depressants**
          Chlorphenesin (carbamate)
          Mephenesin
          Methocarbamol

     E938.1   **Halothane**

     ■ **E938.2**   **Other gaseous anesthetics**
          Ether
          Halogenated hydrocarbon derivatives, except
            halothane
          Nitrous oxide

     E938.3   **Intravenous anesthetics**
          Ketamine
          Methohexital [methohexitone]
          Thiobarbiturates, such as thiopental sodium

     ■ **E938.4**   **Other and unspecified general anesthetics**

     E938.5   **Surface and infiltration anesthetics**
          Cocaine
          Lidocaine [lignocaine]
          Procaine
          Tetracaine

     E938.6   **Peripheral nerve- and plexus-blocking anesthetics**

     E938.7   **Spinal anesthetics**
          Coding Clinic: 2004, Q2, P18; 2003, Q3, P12; 1987, Jan-Feb,
            P13-14

     ■ **E938.9**   **Other and unspecified local anesthetics**

● **E939**   **Psychotropic agents**

     E939.0   **Antidepressants**
          Amitriptyline
          Imipramine
          Monoamine oxidase [MAO] inhibitors
          Coding Clinic: 2003, Q4, P75-76; 1992, Q3, P16

     E939.1   **Phenothiazine-based tranquilizers**
          Chlorpromazine   Prochlorperazine
          Fluphenazine   Promazine
          Phenothiazine

     E939.2   **Butyrophenone-based tranquilizers**
          Haloperidol
          Spiperone
          Trifluperidol

     ■ **E939.3**   **Other antipsychotics, neuroleptics, and major tranquilizers**
          Coding Clinic: 2006, Q4, P76-78

     E939.4   **Benzodiazepine-based tranquilizers**
          Chlordiazepoxide   Lorazepam
          Diazepam   Medazepam
          Flurazepam   Nitrazepam

     ■ **E939.5**   **Other tranquilizers**
          Hydroxyzine
          Meprobamate

     E939.6   **Psychodysleptics [hallucinogens]**
          Cannabis (derivatives)
          Lysergide [LSD]
          Marihuana (derivatives)
          Mescaline
          Psilocin
          Psilocybin

     E939.7   **Psychostimulants**
          Amphetamine
          Caffeine
          Excludes   *central appetite depressants (E947.0)*

     ■ **E939.8**   **Other psychotropic agents**

     ■ **E939.9**   **Unspecified psychotropic agent**

● **E940**   **Central nervous system stimulants**

     E940.0   **Analeptics**
          Lobeline
          Nikethamide

     E940.1   **Opiate antagonists**
          Levallorphan
          Nalorphine
          Naloxone

     ■ **E940.8**   **Other specified central nervous system stimulants**

     ■ **E940.9**   **Unspecified central nervous system stimulant**

● **E941**   **Drugs primarily affecting the autonomic nervous system**

     E941.0   **Parasympathomimetics [cholinergics]**
          Acetylcholine
          Anticholinesterase:
            organophosphorus
            reversible
          Pilocarpine

     E941.1   **Parasympatholytics [anticholinergics and antimuscarinics] and spasmolytics**
          Atropine
          Homatropine
          Hyoscine [scopolamine]
          Quaternary ammonium derivatives
          Excludes   *papaverine (E942.5)*

     E941.2   **Sympathomimetics [adrenergics]**
          Epinephrine [adrenalin]
          Levarterenol [noradrenalin]
          Coding Clinic: 2002, Q3, P12

     E941.3   **Sympatholytics [antiadrenergics]**
          Phenoxybenzamine
          Tolazoline hydrochloride
          Coding Clinic: 2007, Q4, P77-79

     ■ **E941.9**   **Unspecified drug primarily affecting the autonomic nervous system**

E000-E999

● **E942 Agents primarily affecting the cardiovascular system**

E942.0 Cardiac rhythm regulators
Practolol
Procainamide
Propranolol
Quinidine
Coding Clinic: 1986, Mar-April, P11-12

E942.1 Cardiotonic glycosides and drugs of similar action
Digitalis glycosides
Digoxin
Strophanthins

E942.2 Antilipemic and antiarteriosclerotic drugs
Cholestyramine
Clofibrate
Nicotinic acid derivatives
Sitosterols

Excludes   *dextrothyroxine (E932.7)*

E942.3 Ganglion-blocking agents
Pentamethonium bromide

E942.4 Coronary vasodilators
Dipyridamole
Nitrates [nitroglycerin]
Nitrites
Prenylamine

■ **E942.5 Other vasodilators**
Cyclandelate
Diazoxide
Hydralazine
Papaverine

■ **E942.6 Other antihypertensive agents**
Clonidine
Guanethidine
Rauwolfia alkaloids
Reserpine

E942.7 Antivaricose drugs, including sclerosing agents
Monoethanolamine
Zinc salts

E942.8 Capillary-active drugs
Adrenochrome derivatives
Bioflavonoids
Metaraminol

■ **E942.9 Other and unspecified agents primarily affecting the cardiovascular system**

● **E943 Agents primarily affecting gastrointestinal system**

E943.0 Antacids and antigastric secretion drugs
Aluminum hydroxide
Magnesium trisilicate

E943.1 Irritant cathartics
Bisacodyl
Castor oil
Phenolphthalein

E943.2 Emollient cathartics
Sodium dioctyl sulfosuccinate

■ **E943.3 Other cathartics, including intestinal atonia drugs**
Magnesium sulfate

E943.4 Digestants
Pancreatin
Papain
Pepsin

E943.5 Antidiarrheal drugs
Bismuth subcarbonate
Kaolin
Pectin

Excludes   *anti-infectives (E930.0-E931.9)*

E943.6 Emetics

■ **E943.8 Other specified agents primarily affecting the gastrointestinal system**

■ **E943.9 Unspecified agent primarily affecting the gastrointestinal system**

● **E944 Water, mineral, and uric acid metabolism drugs**

E944.0 Mercurial diuretics
Chlormerodrin
Mercaptomerin
Mercurophylline
Mersalyl

E944.1 Purine derivative diuretics
Theobromine
Theophylline

Excludes   *aminophylline [theophylline ethylenediamine] (E945.7)*

E944.2 Carbonic acid anhydrase inhibitors
Acetazolamide

E944.3 Saluretics
Benzothiadiazides
Chlorothiazide group

■ **E944.4 Other diuretics**
Ethacrynic acid
Furosemide

E944.5 Electrolytic, caloric, and water-balance agents

■ **E944.6 Other mineral salts, not elsewhere classified**

E944.7 Uric acid metabolism drugs
Cinchophen and congeners
Colchicine
Phenoquin
Probenecid

● **E945 Agents primarily acting on the smooth and skeletal muscles and respiratory system**

E945.0 Oxytocic agents
Ergot alkaloids
Prostaglandins

E945.1 Smooth muscle relaxants
Adiphenine
Metaproterenol [orciprenaline]

Excludes   *papaverine (E942.5)*

E945.2 Skeletal muscle relaxants
Alcuronium chloride
Suxamethonium chloride

■ **E945.3 Other and unspecified drugs acting on muscles**

E945.4 Antitussives
Dextromethorphan
Pipazethate hydrochloride

E945.5 Expectorants
Acetylcysteine
Cocillana
Guaifenesin [glyceryl guaiacolate]
Ipecacuanha
Terpin hydrate

E945.6   Anti-common cold drugs

E945.7   Antiasthmatics
     Aminophylline [theophylline ethylenediamine]

■ E945.8   Other and unspecified respiratory drugs

● E946   Agents primarily affecting skin and mucous membrane, ophthalmological, otorhinolaryngological, and dental drugs

E946.0   Local anti-infectives and anti-inflammatory drugs

E946.1   Antipruritics

E946.2   Local astringents and local detergents

E946.3   Emollients, demulcents, and protectants

E946.4   Keratolytics, keratoplastics, other hair treatment drugs and preparations

E946.5   Eye anti-infectives and other eye drugs
     Idoxuridine

E946.6   Anti-infectives and other drugs and preparations for ear, nose, and throat

E946.7   Dental drugs topically applied

■ E946.8   Other agents primarily affecting skin and mucous membrane
     Spermicides

■ E946.9   Unspecified agent primarily affecting skin and mucous membrane

● E947   Other and unspecified drugs and medicinal substances

E947.0   Dietetics

E947.1   Lipotropic drugs

E947.2   Antidotes and chelating agents, not elsewhere classified

E947.3   Alcohol deterrents

E947.4   Pharmaceutical excipients

■ E947.8   Other drugs and medicinal substances
     Contrast media used for diagnostic x-ray procedures
     Diagnostic agents and kits

■ E947.9   Unspecified drug or medicinal substance

● E948   Bacterial vaccines

E948.0   BCG vaccine

E948.1   Typhoid and paratyphoid

E948.2   Cholera

E948.3   Plague

E948.4   Tetanus

E948.5   Diphtheria

E948.6   Pertussis vaccine, including combinations with a pertussis component

■ E948.8   Other and unspecified bacterial vaccines

E948.9   Mixed bacterial vaccines, except combinations with a pertussis component

● E949   Other vaccines and biological substances

     Excludes   *gamma globulin (E934.6)*

     Coding Clinic: 2008, Q3, P21

E949.0   Smallpox vaccine

E949.1   Rabies vaccine

E949.2   Typhus vaccine

E949.3   Yellow fever vaccine

E949.4   Measles vaccine

E949.5   Poliomyelitis vaccine

■ E949.6   Other and unspecified viral and rickettsial vaccines
     Mumps vaccine

E949.7   Mixed viral-rickettsial and bacterial vaccines, except combinations with a pertussis component

     Excludes   *combinations with a pertussis component (E948.6)*

■ E949.9   Other and unspecified vaccines and biological substances

SUICIDE AND SELF-INFLICTED INJURY (E950-E959)

     Includes   injuries in suicide and attempted suicide self-inflicted injuries specified as intentional

● E950   Suicide and self-inflicted poisoning by solid or liquid substances

E950.0   Analgesics, antipyretics, and antirheumatics
     Coding Clinic: 1998, Q4, P50-51

E950.1   Barbiturates

■ E950.2   Other sedatives and hypnotics

E950.3   Tranquilizers and other psychotropic agents

■ E950.4   Other specified drugs and medicinal substances

■ E950.5   Unspecified drug or medicinal substance

E950.6   Agricultural and horticultural chemical and pharmaceutical preparations other than plant foods and fertilizers

E950.7   Corrosive and caustic substances
     Suicide and self-inflicted poisoning by substances classifiable to E864

E950.8   Arsenic and its compounds

■ E950.9   Other and unspecified solid and liquid substances

● E951   Suicide and self-inflicted poisoning by gases in domestic use

E951.0   Gas distributed by pipeline

E951.1   Liquefied petroleum gas distributed in mobile containers

■ E951.8   Other utility gas

● E952   Suicide and self-inflicted poisoning by other gases and vapors

E952.0   Motor vehicle exhaust gas

■ E952.1   Other carbon monoxide

■ E952.8   Other specified gases and vapors

■ E952.9   Unspecified gases and vapors

● **E953 Suicide and self-inflicted injury by hanging, strangulation, and suffocation**

   E953.0 **Hanging**

   E953.1 **Suffocation by plastic bag**

■ E953.8 **Other specified means**

■ E953.9 **Unspecified means**

E954 Suicide and self-inflicted injury by submersion [drowning]

● **E955 Suicide and self-inflicted injury by firearms, air guns and explosives**

   E955.0 **Handgun**

   E955.1 **Shotgun**

   E955.2 **Hunting rifle**

   E955.3 **Military firearms**

■ E955.4 **Other and unspecified firearm**
         Gunshot NOS
         Shot NOS

   E955.5 **Explosives**

   E955.6 **Air gun**
         BB gun
         Pellet gun

   E955.7 **Paintball gun**

■ E955.9 **Unspecified**

E956 Suicide and self-inflicted injury by cutting and piercing instrument

● **E957 Suicide and self-inflicted injuries by jumping from high place**

   E957.0 **Residential premises**

■ E957.1 **Other man-made structures**

   E957.2 **Natural sites**

■ E957.9 **Unspecified**

● **E958 Suicide and self-inflicted injury by other and unspecified means**

   E958.0 **Jumping or lying before moving object**

   E958.1 **Burns, fire**

   E958.2 **Scald**

   E958.3 **Extremes of cold**

   E958.4 **Electrocution**

   E958.5 **Crashing of motor vehicle**

   E958.6 **Crashing of aircraft**

   E958.7 **Caustic substances, except poisoning**

         Excludes *poisoning by caustic substance (E950.7)*

■ E958.8 **Other specified means**

■ E958.9 **Unspecified means**

E959 Late effects of self-inflicted injury

   Note: This category is to be used to indicate circumstances classifiable to E950-E958 as the cause of death or disability from late effects, which are themselves classifiable elsewhere. The "late effects" include conditions reported as such or as sequelae which may occur at any time after the attempted suicide or self-inflicted injury.

OGCR Section I.C.19.e

When the cause of an injury or neglect is intentional child or adult abuse, the first listed E code should be assigned from categories E960-E968, Homicide and injury purposely inflicted by other persons, (except category E967). An E code from category E967, Child and adult battering and other maltreatment, should be added as an additional code to identify the perpetrator, if known.

HOMICIDE AND INJURY PURPOSELY INFLICTED BY OTHER PERSONS (E960-E969)

   Includes   injuries inflicted by another person with intent to injure or kill, by any means

   Excludes   *injuries due to:*
            legal intervention (E970-E978)
            operations of war (E990-E999)
            terrorism (E979)

● **E960 Fight, brawl, rape**

   E960.0 **Unarmed fight or brawl**
         Beatings NOS
         Brawl or fight with hands, fists, feet
         Injured or killed in fight NOS

         Excludes *homicidal:*
               injury by weapons (E965.0-E966, E969)
               strangulation (E963)
               submersion (E964)

   E960.1 **Rape**
         Coding Clinic: 1999, Q3, P15

E961 Assault by corrosive or caustic substance, except poisoning
   Injury or death purposely caused by corrosive or caustic substance, such as:
   acid [any]
   corrosive substance
   vitriol

         Excludes *burns from hot liquid (E968.3)*
               chemical burns from swallowing a corrosive substance (E962.0-E962.9)

● **E962 Assault by poisoning**

   E962.0 **Drugs and medicinal substances**
         Homicidal poisoning by any drug or medicinal substance

■ E962.1 **Other solid and liquid substances**

■ E962.2 **Other gases and vapors**

■ E962.9 **Unspecified poisoning**

E963 Assault by hanging and strangulation
   Homicidal (attempt):
         garrotting or ligature
         hanging
         strangulation
         suffocation

E964 Assault by submersion [drowning]

◀ New   ◀▥ Revised   ~~deleted~~ Deleted   ● Use Additional Digit(s)   ■ Nonspecific Code

OGCR Official Guidelines   Coding Clinic   Excludes   Includes   Use additional   Code first   Omit code

● **E965 Assault by firearms and explosives**

     E965.0 Handgun
             Pistol
             Revolver

     E965.1 Shotgun

     E965.2 Hunting rifle

     E965.3 Military firearms

     ■ **E965.4 Other and unspecified firearm**

     E965.5 Antipersonnel bomb

     E965.6 Gasoline bomb

     E965.7 Letter bomb

     ■ **E965.8 Other specified explosive**
             Bomb NOS (placed in):
                car
                house
             Dynamite

     ■ **E965.9 Unspecified explosive**

E966 Assault by cutting and piercing instrument
     Assassination (attempt), homicide (attempt) by any
         instrument classifiable under E920
     Homicidal:
         cut any part of body
         puncture any part of body
         stab any part of body
     Stabbed any part of body
     Coding Clinic: 1993, Q2, P4-5

● **E967 Perpetrator of child and adult abuse**

     Note: selection of the correct perpetrator code
         is based on the relationship between the
         perpetrator and the victim.

     E967.0 By father, stepfather, or boyfriend
             Male partner of child's parent or guardian

     ■ **E967.1 By other specified person**
             Coding Clinic: 1999, Q3, P14-15

     E967.2 By mother, stepmother, or girlfriend
             Female partner of child's parent or guardian
             Coding Clinic: 1996, Q4, P43-44

     E967.3 By spouse or partner
             Abuse of spouse or partner by ex-spouse or
                ex-partner
             Coding Clinic: 1996, Q4, P43-44

     E967.4 By child

     E967.5 By sibling

     E967.6 By grandparent

     ■ **E967.7 By other relative**

     ■ **E967.8 By non-related caregiver**

     ■ **E967.9 By unspecified person**

● **E968 Assault by other and unspecified means**

     E968.0 Fire
             Arson
             Homicidal burns NOS

         Excludes *burns from hot liquid (E968.3)*

     E968.1 Pushing from a high place

     E968.2 Striking by blunt or thrown object
             Coding Clinic: 1996, Q4, P43-44

     E968.3 Hot liquid
             Homicidal burns by scalding

     E968.4 Criminal neglect
             Abandonment of child, infant, or other
                helpless person with intent to injure or
                kill

     E968.5 Transport vehicle
             Being struck by other vehicle or run down
                with intent to injure
             Pushed in front of, thrown from, or dragged
                by moving vehicle with intent to injure

     E968.6 Air gun
             BB gun
             Pellet gun

     E968.7 Human bite

     ■ **E968.8 Other specified means**
             Coding Clinic: 1999, Q3, P14-15x2

     ■ **E968.9 Unspecified means**
             Assassination (attempt) NOS
             Homicidal (attempt):
                injury NOS
                wound NOS
             Manslaughter (nonaccidental)
             Murder (attempt) NOS
             Violence, non-accidental

E969 Late effects of injury purposely inflicted by other person

     Note: This category is to be used to indicate
         circumstances classifiable to E960-E968 as the
         cause of death or disability from late effects,
         which are themselves classifiable elsewhere.
         The "late effects" include conditions reported
         as such, or as sequelae which may occur at
         any time after the injury purposely inflicted by
         another person.

N Newborn Age: 0   **P** Pediatric Age: 0–17   **M** Maternity Age: 12–55   **A** Adult Age: 15–124   ♀ Females Only   ♂ Males Only   **1175**

E000-E999

LEGAL INTERVENTION (E970-E978)

Includes　injuries inflicted by the police or other
law-enforcing agents, including
military on duty, in the course
of arresting or attempting to
arrest lawbreakers, suppressing
disturbances, maintaining order, and
other legal action
legal execution

Excludes　*injuries caused by civil insurrections
(E990.0-E999)*

E970　Injury due to legal intervention by firearms
Gunshot wound
Injury by:
　machine gun
　revolver
　rifle pellet or rubber bullet
　shot NOS

E971　Injury due to legal intervention by explosives
Injury by:
　dynamite
　explosive shell
　grenade
　motor bomb

E972　Injury due to legal intervention by gas
Asphyxiation by gas
Injury by tear gas
Poisoning by gas

E973　Injury due to legal intervention by blunt object
Hit, struck by:
　baton (nightstick)
　blunt object
　stave

E974　Injury due to legal intervention by cutting and piercing instrument
Cut
Incised wound
Injured by bayonet
Stab wound

■**E975　Injury due to legal intervention by other specified means**
Blow
Manhandling

■**E976　Injury due to legal intervention by unspecified means**

E977　Late effects of injuries due to legal intervention

Note: This category is to be used to indicate
circumstances classifiable to E970-E976 as the
cause of death or disability from late effects,
which are themselves classifiable elsewhere.
The "late effects" include conditions reported
as such, or as sequelae which may occur at any
time after the injury due to legal intervention.

E978　Legal execution
All executions performed at the behest of the judiciary
or ruling authority [whether permanent or
temporary] as:
asphyxiation by gas
beheading, decapitation (by guillotine)
capital punishment
electrocution
hanging
poisoning
shooting
other specified means

TERRORISM (E979)

●**E979　Terrorism**
Injuries resulting from the unlawful use of force or
violence against persons or property to intimidate
or coerce a Government, the civilian population,
or any segment thereof, in furtherance of political
or social objective
Coding Clinic: 2002, Q4, P74-77

E979.0　Terrorism involving explosion of marine weapons
Depth-charge
Marine mine
　Mine NOS, at sea or in harbour
Sea-based artillery shell
Torpedo
Underwater blast

E979.1　Terrorism involving destruction of aircraft
Aircraft:
　burned
　exploded
　shot down
Aircraft used as a weapon
Crushed by falling aircraft

■**E979.2　Terrorism involving other explosions and fragments**
Antipersonnel bomb (fragments)
Blast NOS
Explosion (of):
　artillery shell
　breech-block
　cannon block
　mortar bomb
　munitions being used in terrorism
　NOS
Fragments from:
　artillery shell
　bomb
　grenade
　guided missile
　land-mine
　rocket
　shell
　shrapnel
Mine NOS

E979.3 **Terrorism involving fires, conflagration and hot substances**
    Burning building or structure:
        collapse of
        fall from
        hit by falling object in
        jump from
    Conflagration NOS
    Fire (causing):
        asphyxia
        burns
        NOS
        other injury
    Melting of fittings and furniture in burning
    Petrol bomb
    Smouldering building or structure

E979.4 **Terrorism involving firearms**
    Bullet:
        carbine
        machine gun
        pistol
        rifle
        rubber (rifle)
    Pellets (shotgun)

E979.5 **Terrorism involving nuclear weapons**
    Blast effects
    Exposure to ionizing radiation from nuclear
        weapon
    Fireball effects
    Heat from nuclear weapon
    Other direct and secondary effects of nuclear
        weapons

E979.6 **Terrorism involving biological weapons**
    Anthrax
    Cholera
    Smallpox

E979.7 **Terrorism involving chemical weapons**
    Gases, fumes, chemicals
    Hydrogen cyanide
    Phosgene
    Sarin

■ E979.8 **Terrorism involving other means**
    Drowning and submersion
    Lasers
    Piercing or stabbing instruments
    Terrorism NOS

■ E979.9 **Terrorism secondary effects**

    Note: This code is for use to identify conditions occurring subsequent to a terrorist attack not those that are due to the initial terrorist attack

    Excludes *late effect of terrorist attack (E999.1)*

INJURY UNDETERMINED WHETHER ACCIDENTALLY OR PURPOSELY INFLICTED (E980-E989)

Note: Categories E980-E989 are for use when it is unspecified or it cannot be determined whether the injuries are accidental (unintentional), suicide (attempted), or assault.

● E980 **Poisoning by solid or liquid substances, undetermined whether accidentally or purposely inflicted**

    E980.0 **Analgesics, antipyretics, and antirheumatics**

    E980.1 **Barbiturates**

 ■ E980.2 **Other sedatives and hypnotics**

    E980.3 **Tranquilizers and other psychotropic agents**

 ■ E980.4 **Other specified drugs and medicinal substances**

 ■ E980.5 **Unspecified drug or medicinal substance**

    E980.6 **Corrosive and caustic substances**
        Poisoning, undetermined whether accidental or purposeful, by substances classifiable to E864

    E980.7 **Agricultural and horticultural chemical and pharmaceutical preparations other than plant foods and fertilizers**

    E980.8 **Arsenic and its compounds**

 ■ E980.9 **Other and unspecified solid and liquid substances**

● E981 **Poisoning by gases in domestic use, undetermined whether accidentally or purposely inflicted**

    E981.0 **Gas distributed by pipeline**

    E981.1 **Liquefied petroleum gas distributed in mobile containers**

 ■ E981.8 **Other utility gas**

● E982 **Poisoning by other gases, undetermined whether accidentally or purposely inflicted**

    E982.0 **Motor vehicle exhaust gas**

 ■ E982.1 **Other carbon monoxide**

 ■ E982.8 **Other specified gases and vapors**

 ■ E982.9 **Unspecified gases and vapors**

● E983 **Hanging, strangulation, or suffocation, undetermined whether accidentally or purposely inflicted**

    E983.0 **Hanging**

    E983.1 **Suffocation by plastic bag**

 ■ E983.8 **Other specified means**

 ■ E983.9 **Unspecified means**

    E984 **Submersion [drowning], undetermined whether accidentally or purposely inflicted**

N Newborn Age: 0   **P** Pediatric Age: 0–17   **M** Maternity Age: 12–55   **A** Adult Age: 15–124   ♀ Females Only   ♂ Males Only   **1177**

E000-E999

● **E985 Injury by firearms, air guns and explosives, undetermined whether accidentally or purposely inflicted**

    E985.0   **Handgun**

    E985.1   **Shotgun**

    E985.2   **Hunting rifle**

    E985.3   **Military firearms**

    ■ E985.4   **Other and unspecified firearm**

    E985.5   **Explosives**

    E985.6   **Air gun**
             BB gun
             Pellet gun

    E985.7   **Paintball gun**

E986 Injury by cutting and piercing instruments, undetermined whether accidentally or purposely inflicted

● **E987 Falling from high place, undetermined whether accidentally or purposely inflicted**

    E987.0   **Residential premises**

    ■ E987.1   **Other man-made structures**

    E987.2   **Natural sites**

    ■ E987.9   **Unspecified site**

● **E988 Injury by other and unspecified means, undetermined whether accidentally or purposely inflicted**

    E988.0   **Jumping or lying before moving object**

    E988.1   **Burns, fire**

    E988.2   **Scald**

    E988.3   **Extremes of cold**

    E988.4   **Electrocution**

    E988.5   **Crashing of motor vehicle**

    E988.6   **Crashing of aircraft**

    E988.7   **Caustic substances, except poisoning**

    ■ E988.8   **Other specified means**

    ■ E988.9   **Unspecified means**

E989 Late effects of injury, undetermined whether accidentally or purposely inflicted

    Note: This category is to be used to indicate circumstances classifiable to E980-E988 as the cause of death or disability from late effects, which are themselves classifiable elsewhere. The "late effects" include conditions reported as such or as sequelae which may occur at any time after injury, undetermined whether accidentally or purposely inflicted.

INJURY RESULTING FROM OPERATIONS OF WAR (E990-E999)

    Includes   injuries to military personnel and civilians caused by war and civil insurrections and occurring during the time of war and insurrection, and peacekeeping missions ◄▥

    Excludes   *accidents during training of military personnel, manufacture of war material and transport, unless attributable to enemy action*

● **E990 Injury due to war operations by fires and conflagrations**

    Includes   asphyxia, burns, or other injury originating from fire caused by a fire-producing device or indirectly by any conventional weapon

    E990.0   **From gasoline bomb**
             Incendiary bomb ◄

    E990.1   **From flamethrower** ◄

    E990.2   **From incendiary bullet** ◄

    E990.3   **From fire caused indirectly from conventional weapon** ◄

        Excludes   *fire aboard military aircraft (E994.3)* ◄

    ■ E990.9   **From other and unspecified source**

● **E991 Injury due to war operations by bullets and fragments**

    Excludes   *injury due to bullets and fragments due to war operations, but occurring after cessation of hostilities (E998.0)* ◄
             injury due to explosion of artillery shells and mortars (E993.2) ◄
             injury due to explosion of improvised explosive device [IED] (E993.3-E993.5) ◄
             injury due to sea-based artillery shell (E992.3) ◄

    E991.0   **Rubber bullets (rifle)**

    E991.1   **Pellets (rifle)**

    ■ E991.2   **Other bullets**
             Bullet [any, except rubber bullets and pellets]
             carbine
             machine gun
             pistol
             rifle
             shotgun

    E991.3   **Antipersonnel bomb (fragments)**

    E991.4   **Fragments from munitions** ◄
             Fragments from: ◄
             artillery shell ◄
             bombs, except antipersonnel ◄
             detonation of unexploded ordnance [UXO] ◄
             grenade ◄
             guided missile ◄
             land mine ◄
             rockets ◄
             shell ◄

◄ New   ◄▥ Revised   ~~deleted~~ Deleted   ● Use Additional Digit(s)   ■ Nonspecific Code

OGCR Official Guidelines   Coding Clinic   Excludes   Includes   Use additional   Code first   Omit code

E991.5 Fragments from person-borne improvised explosive device [IED] ◄

E991.6 Fragments from vehicle-borne improvised explosive device [IED] ◄
       IED borne by land, air, or water transport vehicle ◄

E991.7 Fragments from other improvised explosive device [IED] ◄
       Roadside IED ◄

E991.8 Fragments from weapons ◄
       Fragments from: ◄
         artillery ◄
         autocannons ◄
         automatic grenade launchers ◄
         missile launchers ◄
         mortars ◄
         small arms ◄

■ **E991.9 Other and unspecified fragments**
       ~~Fragments from:~~
         ~~artillery shell~~
         ~~bombs, except antipersonnel~~
         ~~grenade~~
         ~~guided missile~~
         ~~land mine~~
         ~~rockets~~
         ~~shell~~
       Shrapnel NOS ◄◁

● **E992 Injury due to war operations by explosion of marine weapons** ◁
       ~~Depth charge~~
       ~~Marine mines~~
       ~~Mine NOS, at sea or in harbor~~
       ~~Sea-based artillery shell~~
       ~~Torpedo~~
       ~~Underwater blast~~

E992.0 Torpedo ◄

E992.1 Depth charge ◄

E992.2 Marine mines ◄
       Marine mines at sea or in harbor ◄

E992.3 Sea-based artillery shell ◄

E992.8 Other by other marine weapons ◄

E992.9 Unspecified marine weapon ◄
       Underwater blast NOS

● **E993 Injury due to war operations by other explosion** ◁
       ~~Accidental explosion of munitions being used in war~~
       ~~Accidental explosion of own weapons~~
       ~~Air blast NOS~~
       ~~Blast NOS~~
       ~~Explosion NOS~~
       ~~Explosion of:~~
         ~~artillery shell~~
         ~~breech block~~
         ~~cannon block~~
         ~~mortar bomb~~
       ~~Injury by weapon burst~~
       Injuries due to direct or indirect pressure or air blast of an explosion occurring during war operations ◄

> **Excludes** *injury due to fragments resulting from an explosion (E991.0-E991.9)* ◄
> *injury due to detonation of unexploded ordnance but occurring after cessation of hostilities (E998.0-E998.9)* ◄
> *injury due to nuclear weapons (E996.0-E996.9)* ◄

E993.0 Aerial bomb ◄

E993.1 Guided missile ◄

E993.2 Mortar ◄
       Artillery shell ◄

E993.3 Person-borne improvised explosive device [IED] ◄

E993.4 Vehicle-borne improvised explosive device [IED] ◄
       IED borne by land, air, or water transport vehicle ◄

E993.5 Other improvised explosive device [IED] ◄
       Roadside IED ◄

E993.6 Unintentional detonation of own munitions ◄
       Unintentional detonation of own ammunition (artillery) (mortars) ◄

E993.7 Unintentional discharge of own munitions launch device ◄
       Unintentional explosion of own:
         Autocannons ◄
         Automatic grenade launchers ◄
         Missile launchers ◄
         Small arms ◄

E993.8 Other specified explosion ◄
       Bomb ◄
       Grenade ◄
       Land mine ◄

E993.9 Unspecified explosion ◄
       Air blast NOS ◄
       Blast NOS ◄
       Blast wave NOS ◄
       Blast wind NOS ◄
       Explosion NOS ◄

● **E994 Injury due to war operations by destruction of aircraft** ◁
       ~~Airplane:~~
         ~~burned~~
         ~~exploded~~
         ~~shot down~~
       ~~Crushed by falling airplane~~

E994.0 Destruction of aircraft due to enemy fire or explosives ◄
       Air to air missile ◄
       Explosive device placed on aircraft ◄
       Rocket propelled grenade [RPG] ◄
       Small arms fire ◄
       Surface to air missile ◄

E994.1 Unintentional destruction of aircraft due to own onboard explosives ◄

E994.2 Destruction of aircraft due to collision with other aircraft ◄

E994.3 Destruction of aircraft due to onboard fire ◄

E994.8 Other destruction of aircraft ◄

E994.9 Unspecified destruction of aircraft ◄

● **E995 Injury due to war operations by other and unspecified forms of conventional warfare** ◁
       ~~Battle wounds~~
       ~~Bayonet injury~~
       ~~Drowned in war operations~~

E995.0 Unarmed hand-to-hand combat ◄

> **Excludes** *intentional restriction of airway (E995.3)* ◄

E995.1 Struck by blunt object ◄
       Baton (nightstick) ◄
       Stave ◄

E995.2 Piercing object ◄
       Bayonet ◄
       Knife
       Sword

N Newborn Age: 0   **P** Pediatric Age: 0–17   **M** Maternity Age: 12–55   **A** Adult Age: 15–124   ♀ Females Only   ♂ Males Only   1179

E000-E999

E995.3 **Intentional restriction of air and airway** ◄
   Intentional submersion ◄
   Strangulation ◄
   Suffocation ◄

E995.4 **Unintentional drowning due to inability to surface or obtain air** ◄
   Submersion ◄

E995.8 **Other forms of conventional warfare** ◄

E995.9 **Unspecified form of conventional warfare** ◄

● E996 **Injury due to war operations by nuclear weapons** ◀▥
   ~~Blast effects~~
   ~~Exposure to ionizing radiation from nuclear weapons~~
   ~~Fireball effects~~
   ~~Heat~~
   ~~Other direct and secondary effects of nuclear weapons~~
   Dirty bomb NOS ◄

   Excludes *late effects of injury due to nuclear weapons (E999.1, E999.0)* ◄

E996.0 **Direct blast effect of nuclear weapon** ◄
   Injury to bodily organs due to blast pressure ◄

E996.1 **Indirect blast effect of nuclear weapon** ◄
   Injury due to being thrown by blast ◄
   Injury due to being struck or crushed by blast debris ◄

E996.2 **Thermal radiation effect of nuclear weapon** ◄
   Burns due to thermal radiation ◄
   Fireball effects ◄
   Flash burns ◄
   Heat effects ◄

E996.3 **Nuclear radiation effects** ◄
   Acute radiation exposure ◄
   Beta burns ◄
   Fallout exposure ◄
   Radiation sickness ◄
   Secondary effects of nuclear weapons ◄

E996.8 **Other effects of nuclear weapons** ◄

E996.9 **Unspecified effect of nuclear weapon** ◄

● E997 **Injury due to war operations by other forms of unconventional warfare**

E997.0 **Lasers**

E997.1 **Biological warfare**

E997.2 **Gases, fumes, and chemicals**

E997.3 **Weapon of mass destruction [WMD], unspecified** ◄

▥ E997.8 **Other specified forms of unconventional warfare**

▥ E997.9 **Unspecified form of unconventional warfare**

● E998 **Injury due to war operations but occurring after cessation of hostilities** ◀▥
   Injuries due to operations of war but occurring after cessation of hostilities by any means classifiable under E990-E997
   Injuries by explosion of bombs or mines placed in the course of operations of war, if the explosion occurred after cessation of hostilities

E998.0 **Explosion of mines** ◄

E998.1 **Explosion of bombs** ◄

E998.8 **Injury due to other war operations but occurring after cessation of hostilities** ◄

E998.9 **Injury due to unspecified war operations but occurring after cessation of hostilities** ◄

● E999 **Late effect of injury due to war operations and terrorism**

   Note: This category is to be used to indicate circumstances classifiable to E979, E990-E998 as the cause of death or disability from late effects, which are themselves classifiable elsewhere. The "late effects" include conditions reported as such or as sequelae which may occur at any time after injury resulting from operations of war or terrorism.

E999.0 **Late effect of injury due to war operations**
   Coding Clinic: 1998, Q1, P4; 1996, Q2, P12

E999.1 **Late effect of injury due to terrorism**

MORPHOLOGY OF NEOPLASMS

The World Health Organization has published an adaptation of the International Classification of Diseases for Oncology (ICD-O). It contains a coded nomenclature for the morphology of neoplasms, which is reproduced here for those who wish to use it in conjunction with Chapter 2 of the International Classification of Diseases, 9th Revision, Clinical Modification.

The morphology code numbers consist of five digits; the first four identify the histological type of the neoplasm and the fifth indicates its behavior. The one-digit behavior code is as follows:

/0   Benign
/1   Uncertain whether benign or malignant
       Borderline malignancy
/2   Carcinoma in situ
       Intraepithelial
       Noninfiltrating
       Noninvasive
/3   Malignant, primary site
/6   Malignant, metastatic site
       Secondary site
/9   Malignant, uncertain whether primary or metastatic site

In the nomenclature below, the morphology code numbers include the behavior code appropriate to the histological type of neoplasm, but this behavior code should be changed if other reported information makes this necessary. For example, "chordoma (M9370/3)" is assumed to be malignant; the term "benign chordoma" should be coded M9370/0. Similarly, "superficial spreading adenocarcinoma (M8143/3)" described as "noninvasive" should be coded M8143/2 and "melanoma (M8720/3)" described as "secondary" should be coded M8720/6.

The following table shows the correspondence between the morphology code and the different sections of Chapter 2:

Morphology Code Histology/Behavior			ICD-9-CM Chapter 2
Any	0	210-229	Benign neoplasms
M8000-M8004	1	239	Neoplasms of unspecified nature
M8010+	1	235-238	Neoplasms of uncertain behavior
Any	2	230-234	Carcinoma in situ
Any	3	140-195 200-208	Malignant neoplasms, stated or presumed to be primary
Any	6	196-198	Malignant neoplasms, stated or presumed to be secondary

The ICD-O behavior digit /9 is inapplicable in an ICD context, since all malignant neoplasms are presumed to be primary (/3) or secondary (/6) according to other information on the medical record.

Only the first-listed term of the full ICD-O morphology nomenclature appears against each code number in the list below. The ICD-9-CM Alphabetical Index (Volume 2), however, includes all the ICD-O synonyms as well as a number of other morphological names still likely to be encountered on medical records but omitted from ICD-O as outdated or otherwise undesirable.

A coding difficulty sometimes arises where a morphological diagnosis contains two qualifying adjectives that have different code numbers. An example is "transitional cell epidermoid carcinomas." "Transitional cell carcinoma NOS" is M8120/3 and "epidermoid carcinoma NOS" is M8070/3. In such circumstances, the higher number (M8120/3 in this example) should be used, as it is usually more specific.

CODED NOMENCLATURE FOR MORPHOLOGY OF NEOPLASMS

M800	**Neoplasms NOS**
M8000/0	*Neoplasm, benign*
M8000/1	*Neoplasm, uncertain whether benign or malignant*
M8000/3	*Neoplasm, malignant*
M8000/6	*Neoplasm, metastatic*
M8000/9	*Neoplasm, malignant, uncertain whether primary or metastatic*
M8001/0	*Tumor cells, benign*
M8001/1	*Tumor cells, uncertain whether benign or malignant*
M8001/3	*Tumor cells, malignant*
M8002/3	*Malignant tumor, small cell type*
M8003/3	*Malignant tumor, giant cell type*
M8004/3	*Malignant tumor, fusiform cell type*
M801-M804	**Epithelial neoplasms NOS**
M8010/0	*Epithelial tumor, benign*
M8010/2	*Carcinoma in situ NOS*
M8010/3	*Carcinoma NOS*
M8010/6	*Carcinoma, metastatic NOS*
M8010/9	*Carcinomatosis*
M8011/0	*Epithelioma, benign*
M8011/3	*Epithelioma, malignant*
M8012/3	*Large cell carcinoma NOS*
M8020/3	*Carcinoma, undifferentiated type NOS*
M8021/3	*Carcinoma, anaplastic type NOS*
M8022/3	*Pleomorphic carcinoma*
M8030/3	*Giant cell and spindle cell carcinoma*
M8031/3	*Giant cell carcinoma*
M8032/3	*Spindle cell carcinoma*
M8033/3	*Pseudosarcomatous carcinoma*
M8034/3	*Polygonal cell carcinoma*
M8035/3	*Spheroidal cell carcinoma*
M8040/1	*Tumorlet*
M8041/3	*Small cell carcinoma NOS*
M8042/3	*Oat cell carcinoma*
M8043/3	*Small cell carcinoma, fusiform cell type*
M805-M808	**Papillary and squamous cell neoplasms**
M8050/0	*Papilloma NOS (except Papilloma of urinary bladder M8120/1)*
M8050/2	*Papillary carcinoma in situ*
M8050/3	*Papillary carcinoma NOS*
M8051/0	*Verrucous papilloma*
M8051/3	*Verrucous carcinoma NOS*
M8052/0	*Squamous cell papilloma*
M8052/3	*Papillary squamous cell carcinoma*
M8053/0	*Inverted papilloma*
M8060/0	*Papillomatosis NOS*
M8070/2	*Squamous cell carcinoma in situ NOS*
M8070/3	*Squamous cell carcinoma NOS*
M8070/6	*Squamous cell carcinoma, metastatic NOS*
M8071/3	*Squamous cell carcinoma, keratinizing type NOS*
M8072/3	*Squamous cell carcinoma, large cell, nonkeratinizing type*
M8073/3	*Squamous cell carcinoma, small cell, nonkeratinizing type*
M8074/3	*Squamous cell carcinoma, spindle cell type*
M8075/3	*Adenoid squamous cell carcinoma*
M8076/2	*Squamous cell carcinoma in situ with questionable stromal invasion*
M8076/3	*Squamous cell carcinoma, microinvasive*
M8080/2	*Queyrat's erythroplasia*
M8081/2	*Bowen's disease*
M8082/3	*Lymphoepithelial carcinoma*
M809-M811	**Basal cell neoplasms**
M8090/1	*Basal cell tumor*
M8090/3	*Basal cell carcinoma NOS*
M8091/3	*Multicentric basal cell carcinoma*
M8092/3	*Basal cell carcinoma, morphea type*
M8093/3	*Basal cell carcinoma, fibroepithelial type*
M8094/3	*Basosquamous carcinoma*
M8095/3	*Metatypical carcinoma*
M8096/0	*Intraepidermal epithelioma of Jadassohn*
M8100/0	*Trichoepithelioma*
M8101/0	*Trichofolliculoma*
M8102/0	*Tricholemmoma*
M8110/0	*Pilomatrixoma*

M812-M813	**Transitional cell papillomas and carcinomas**
M8120/0	Transitional cell papilloma NOS
M8120/1	Urothelial papilloma
M8120/2	Transitional cell carcinoma in situ
M8120/3	Transitional cell carcinoma NOS
M8121/0	Schneiderian papilloma
M8121/1	Transitional cell papilloma, inverted type
M8121/3	Schneiderian carcinoma
M8122/3	Transitional cell carcinoma, spindle cell type
M8123/3	Basaloid carcinoma
M8124/3	Cloacogenic carcinoma
M8130/3	Papillary transitional cell carcinoma
M814-M838	**Adenomas and adenocarcinomas**
M8140/0	Adenoma NOS
M8140/1	Bronchial adenoma NOS
M8140/2	Adenocarcinoma in situ
M8140/3	Adenocarcinoma NOS
M8140/6	Adenocarcinoma, metastatic NOS
M8141/3	Scirrhous adenocarcinoma
M8142/3	Linitis plastica
M8143/3	Superficial spreading adenocarcinoma
M8144/3	Adenocarcinoma, intestinal type
M8145/3	Carcinoma, diffuse type
M8146/0	Monomorphic adenoma
M8147/0	Basal cell adenoma
M8150/0	Islet cell adenoma
M8150/3	Islet cell carcinoma
M8151/0	Insulinoma NOS
M8151/3	Insulinoma, malignant
M8152/0	Glucagonoma NOS
M8152/3	Glucagonoma, malignant
M8153/1	Gastrinoma NOS
M8153/3	Gastrinoma, malignant
M8154/3	Mixed islet cell and exocrine adenocarcinoma
M8160/0	Bile duct adenoma
M8160/3	Cholangiocarcinoma
M8161/0	Bile duct cystadenoma
M8161/3	Bile duct cystadenocarcinoma
M8170/0	Liver cell adenoma
M8170/3	Hepatocellular carcinoma NOS
M8180/0	Hepatocholangioma, benign
M8180/3	Combined hepatocellular carcinoma and cholangio-carcinoma
M8190/0	Trabecular adenoma
M8190/3	Trabecular adenocarcinoma
M8191/0	Embryonal adenoma
M8200/0	Eccrine dermal cylindroma
M8200/3	Adenoid cystic carcinoma
M8201/3	Cribriform carcinoma
M8210/0	Adenomatous polyp NOS
M8210/3	Adenocarcinoma in adenomatous polyp
M8211/0	Tubular adenoma NOS
M8211/3	Tubular adenocarcinoma
M8220/0	Adenomatous polyposis coli
M8220/3	Adenocarcinoma in adenomatous polyposis coli
M8221/0	Multiple adenomatous polyps
M8230/3	Solid carcinoma NOS
M8231/3	Carcinoma simplex
M8240/1	Carcinoid tumor NOS
M8240/3	Carcinoid tumor, malignant
M8241/1	Carcinoid tumor, argentaffin NOS
M8241/3	Carcinoid tumor, argentaffin, malignant
M8242/1	Carcinoid tumor, nonargentaffin NOS
M8242/3	Carcinoid tumor, nonargentaffin, malignant
M8243/3	Mucocarcinoid tumor, malignant
M8244/3	Composite carcinoid
M8250/1	Pulmonary adenomatosis
M8250/3	Bronchiolo-alveolar adenocarcinoma
M8251/0	Alveolar adenoma
M8251/3	Alveolar adenocarcinoma
M8260/0	Papillary adenoma NOS
M8260/3	Papillary adenocarcinoma NOS
M8261/1	Villous adenoma NOS
M8261/3	Adenocarcinoma in villous adenoma

M8262/3	Villous adenocarcinoma
M8263/0	Tubulovillous adenoma
M8270/0	Chromophobe adenoma
M8270/3	Chromophobe carcinoma
M8280/0	Acidophil adenoma
M8280/3	Acidophil carcinoma
M8281/0	Mixed acidophil-basophil adenoma
M8281/3	Mixed acidophil-basophil carcinoma
M8290/0	Oxyphilic adenoma
M8290/3	Oxyphilic adenocarcinoma
M8300/0	Basophil adenoma
M8300/3	Basophil carcinoma
M8310/0	Clear cell adenoma
M8310/3	Clear cell adenocarcinoma NOS
M8311/1	Hypernephroid tumor
M8312/3	Renal cell carcinoma
M8313/0	Clear cell adenofibroma
M8320/3	Granular cell carcinoma
M8321/0	Chief cell adenoma
M8322/0	Water-clear cell adenoma
M8322/3	Water-clear cell adenocarcinoma
M8323/0	Mixed cell adenoma
M8323/3	Mixed cell adenocarcinoma
M8324/0	Lipoadenoma
M8330/0	Follicular adenoma
M8330/3	Follicular adenocarcinoma NOS
M8331/3	Follicular adenocarcinoma, well differentiated type
M8332/3	Follicular adenocarcinoma, trabecular type
M8333/0	Microfollicular adenoma
M8334/0	Macrofollicular adenoma
M8340/3	Papillary and follicular adenocarcinoma
M8350/3	Nonencapsulated sclerosing carcinoma
M8360/1	Multiple endocrine adenomas
M8361/1	Juxtaglomerular tumor
M8370/0	Adrenal cortical adenoma NOS
M8370/3	Adrenal cortical carcinoma
M8371/0	Adrenal cortical adenoma, compact cell type
M8372/0	Adrenal cortical adenoma, heavily pigmented variant
M8373/0	Adrenal cortical adenoma, clear cell type
M8374/0	Adrenal cortical adenoma, glomerulosa cell type
M8375/0	Adrenal cortical adenoma, mixed cell type
M8380/0	Endometrioid adenoma NOS
M8380/1	Endometrioid adenoma, borderline malignancy
M8380/3	Endometrioid carcinoma
M8381/0	Endometrioid adenofibroma NOS
M8381/1	Endometrioid adenofibroma, borderline malignancy
M8381/3	Endometrioid adenofibroma, malignant
M839-M842	**Adnexal and skin appendage neoplasms**
M8390/0	Skin appendage adenoma
M8390/3	Skin appendage carcinoma
M8400/0	Sweat gland adenoma
M8400/1	Sweat gland tumor NOS
M8400/3	Sweat gland adenocarcinoma
M8401/0	Apocrine adenoma
M8401/3	Apocrine adenocarcinoma
M8402/0	Eccrine acrospiroma
M8403/0	Eccrine spiradenoma
M8404/0	Hidrocystoma
M8405/0	Papillary hydradenoma
M8406/0	Papillary syringadenoma
M8407/0	Syringoma NOS
M8410/0	Sebaceous adenoma
M8410/3	Sebaceous adenocarcinoma
M8420/0	Ceruminous adenoma
M8420/3	Ceruminous adenocarcinoma
M843	**Mucoepidermoid neoplasms**
M8430/1	Mucoepidermoid tumor
M8430/3	Mucoepidermoid carcinoma
M844-M849	**Cystic, mucinous, and serous neoplasms**
M8440/0	Cystadenoma NOS
M8440/3	Cystadenocarcinoma NOS
M8441/0	Serous cystadenoma NOS
M8441/1	Serous cystadenoma, borderline malignancy
M8441/3	Serous cystadenocarcinoma NOS

M8450/0	*Papillary cystadenoma NOS*
M8450/1	*Papillary cystadenoma, borderline malignancy*
M8450/3	*Papillary cystadenocarcinoma NOS*
M8460/0	*Papillary serous cystadenoma NOS*
M8460/1	*Papillary serous cystadenoma, borderline malignancy*
M8460/3	*Papillary serous cystadenocarcinoma*
M8461/0	*Serous surface papilloma NOS*
M8461/1	*Serous surface papilloma, borderline malignancy*
M8461/3	*Serous surface papillary carcinoma*
M8470/0	*Mucinous cystadenoma NOS*
M8470/1	*Mucinous cystadenoma, borderline malignancy*
M8470/3	*Mucinous cystadenocarcinoma NOS*
M8471/0	*Papillary mucinous cystadenoma NOS*
M8471/1	*Papillary mucinous cystadenoma, borderline malignancy*
M8471/3	*Papillary mucinous cystadenocarcinoma*
M8480/0	*Mucinous adenoma*
M8480/3	*Mucinous adenocarcinoma*
M8480/6	*Pseudomyxoma peritonei*
M8481/3	*Mucin-producing adenocarcinoma*
M8490/3	*Signet ring cell carcinoma*
M8490/6	*Metastatic signet ring cell carcinoma*

M850-M854 **Ductal, lobular, and medullary neoplasms**

M8500/2	*Intraductal carcinoma, noninfiltrating NOS*
M8500/3	*Infiltrating duct carcinoma*
M8501/2	*Comedocarcinoma, noninfiltrating*
M8501/3	*Comedocarcinoma NOS*
M8502/3	*Juvenile carcinoma of the breast*
M8503/0	*Intraductal papilloma*
M8503/2	*Noninfiltrating intraductal papillary adenocarcinoma*
M8504/0	*Intracystic papillary adenoma*
M8504/2	*Noninfiltrating intracystic carcinoma*
M8505/0	*Intraductal papillomatosis NOS*
M8506/0	*Subareolar duct papillomatosis*
M8510/3	*Medullary carcinoma NOS*
M8511/3	*Medullary carcinoma with amyloid stroma*
M8512/3	*Medullary carcinoma with lymphoid stroma*
M8520/2	*Lobular carcinoma in situ*
M8520/3	*Lobular carcinoma NOS*
M8521/3	*Infiltrating ductular carcinoma*
M8530/3	*Inflammatory carcinoma*
M8540/3	*Paget's disease, mammary*
M8541/3	*Paget's disease and infiltrating duct carcinoma of breast*
M8542/3	*Paget's disease, extramammary (except Paget's disease of bone)*

M855 **Acinar cell neoplasms**

M8550/0	*Acinar cell adenoma*
M8550/1	*Acinar cell tumor*
M8550/3	*Acinar cell carcinoma*

M856-M858 **Complex epithelial neoplasms**

M8560/3	*Adenosquamous carcinoma*
M8561/0	*Adenolymphoma*
M8570/3	*Adenocarcinoma with squamous metaplasia*
M8571/3	*Adenocarcinoma with cartilaginous and osseous metaplasia*
M8572/3	*Adenocarcinoma with spindle cell metaplasia*
M8573/3	*Adenocarcinoma with apocrine metaplasia*
M8580/0	*Thymoma, benign*
M8580/3	*Thymoma, malignant*

M859-M867 **Specialized gonadal neoplasms**

M8590/1	*Sex cord-stromal tumor*
M8600/0	*Thecoma NOS*
M8600/3	*Theca cell carcinoma*
M8610/0	*Luteoma NOS*
M8620/1	*Granulosa cell tumor NOS*
M8620/3	*Granulosa cell tumor, malignant*
M8621/1	*Granulosa cell-theca cell tumor*
M8630/0	*Androblastoma, benign*
M8630/1	*Androblastoma NOS*
M8630/3	*Androblastoma, malignant*
M8631/0	*Sertoli-Leydig cell tumor*
M8632/1	*Gynandroblastoma*
M8640/0	*Tubular androblastoma NOS*
M8640/3	*Sertoli cell carcinoma*

M8641/0	*Tubular androblastoma with lipid storage*
M8650/0	*Leydig cell tumor, benign*
M8650/1	*Leydig cell tumor NOS*
M8650/3	*Leydig cell tumor, malignant*
M8660/0	*Hilar cell tumor*
M8670/0	*Lipid cell tumor of ovary*
M8671/0	*Adrenal rest tumor*

M868-M871 **Paragangliomas and glomus tumors**

M8680/1	*Paraganglioma NOS*
M8680/3	*Paraganglioma, malignant*
M8681/1	*Sympathetic paraganglioma*
M8682/1	*Parasympathetic paraganglioma*
M8690/1	*Glomus jugulare tumor*
M8691/1	*Aortic body tumor*
M8692/1	*Carotid body tumor*
M8693/1	*Extra-adrenal paraganglioma NOS*
M8693/3	*Extra-adrenal paraganglioma, malignant*
M8700/0	*Pheochromocytoma NOS*
M8700/3	*Pheochromocytoma, malignant*
M8710/3	*Glomangiosarcoma*
M8711/0	*Glomus tumor*
M8712/0	*Glomangioma*

M872-M879 **Nevi and melanomas**

M8720/0	*Pigmented nevus NOS*
M8720/3	*Malignant melanoma NOS*
M8721/3	*Nodular melanoma*
M8722/0	*Balloon cell nevus*
M8722/3	*Balloon cell melanoma*
M8723/0	*Halo nevus*
M8724/0	*Fibrous papule of the nose*
M8725/0	*Neuronevus*
M8726/0	*Magnocellular nevus*
M8730/0	*Nonpigmented nevus*
M8730/3	*Amelanotic melanoma*
M8740/0	*Junctional nevus*
M8740/3	*Malignant melanoma in junctional nevus*
M8741/2	*Precancerous melanosis NOS*
M8741/3	*Malignant melanoma in precancerous melanosis*
M8742/2	*Hutchinson's melanotic freckle*
M8742/3	*Malignant melanoma in Hutchinson's melanotic freckle*
M8743/3	*Superficial spreading melanoma*
M8750/0	*Intradermal nevus*
M8760/0	*Compound nevus*
M8761/1	*Giant pigmented nevus*
M8761/3	*Malignant melanoma in giant pigmented nevus*
M8770/0	*Epithelioid and spindle cell nevus*
M8771/3	*Epithelioid cell melanoma*
M8772/3	*Spindle cell melanoma NOS*
M8773/3	*Spindle cell melanoma, type A*
M8774/3	*Spindle cell melanoma, type B*
M8775/3	*Mixed epithelioid and spindle cell melanoma*
M8780/0	*Blue nevus NOS*
M8780/3	*Blue nevus, malignant*
M8790/0	*Cellular blue nevus*

M880 **Soft tissue tumors and sarcomas NOS**

M8800/0	*Soft tissue tumor, benign*
M8800/3	*Sarcoma NOS*
M8800/9	*Sarcomatosis NOS*
M8801/3	*Spindle cell sarcoma*
M8802/3	*Giant cell sarcoma (except of bone M9250/3)*
M8803/3	*Small cell sarcoma*
M8804/3	*Epithelioid cell sarcoma*

M881-M883 **Fibromatous neoplasms**

M8810/0	*Fibroma NOS*
M8810/3	*Fibrosarcoma NOS*
M8811/0	*Fibromyxoma*
M8811/3	*Fibromyxosarcoma*
M8812/0	*Periosteal fibroma*
M8812/3	*Periosteal fibrosarcoma*
M8813/0	*Fascial fibroma*
M8813/3	*Fascial fibrosarcoma*
M8814/3	*Infantile fibrosarcoma*
M8820/0	*Elastofibroma*

M8821/1	*Aggressive fibromatosis*
M8822/1	*Abdominal fibromatosis*
M8823/1	*Desmoplastic fibroma*
M8830/0	*Fibrous histiocytoma NOS*
M8830/1	*Atypical fibrous histiocytoma*
M8830/3	*Fibrous histiocytoma, malignant*
M8831/0	*Fibroxanthoma NOS*
M8831/1	*Atypical fibroxanthoma*
M8831/3	*Fibroxanthoma, malignant*
M8832/0	*Dermatofibroma NOS*
M8832/1	*Dermatofibroma protuberans*
M8832/3	*Dermatofibrosarcoma NOS*

M884   **Myxomatous neoplasms**

M8840/0	*Myxoma NOS*
M8840/3	*Myxosarcoma*

M885-M888   **Lipomatous neoplasms**

M8850/0	*Lipoma NOS*
M8850/3	*Liposarcoma NOS*
M8851/0	*Fibrolipoma*
M8851/3	*Liposarcoma, well differentiated type*
M8852/0	*Fibromyxolipoma*
M8852/3	*Myxoid liposarcoma*
M8853/3	*Round cell liposarcoma*
M8854/3	*Pleomorphic liposarcoma*
M8855/3	*Mixed type liposarcoma*
M8856/0	*Intramuscular lipoma*
M8857/0	*Spindle cell lipoma*
M8860/0	*Angiomyolipoma*
M8860/3	*Angiomyoliposarcoma*
M8861/0	*Angiolipoma NOS*
M8861/1	*Angiolipoma, infiltrating*
M8870/0	*Myelolipoma*
M8880/0	*Hibernoma*
M8881/0	*Lipoblastomatosis*

M889-M892   **Myomatous neoplasms**

M8890/0	*Leiomyoma NOS*
M8890/1	*Intravascular leiomyomatosis*
M8890/3	*Leiomyosarcoma NOS*
M8891/1	*Epithelioid leiomyoma*
M8891/3	*Epithelioid leiomyosarcoma*
M8892/1	*Cellular leiomyoma*
M8893/0	*Bizarre leiomyoma*
M8894/0	*Angiomyoma*
M8894/3	*Angiomyosarcoma*
M8895/0	*Myoma*
M8895/3	*Myosarcoma*
M8900/0	*Rhabdomyoma NOS*
M8900/3	*Rhabdomyosarcoma NOS*
M8901/3	*Pleomorphic rhabdomyosarcoma*
M8902/3	*Mixed type rhabdomyosarcoma*
M8903/0	*Fetal rhabdomyoma*
M8904/0	*Adult rhabdomyoma*
M8910/3	*Embryonal rhabdomyosarcoma*
M8920/3	*Alveolar rhabdomyosarcoma*

M893-M899   **Complex mixed and stromal neoplasms**

M8930/3	*Endometrial stromal sarcoma*
M8931/1	*Endolymphatic stromal myosis*
M8932/0	*Adenomyoma*
M8940/0	*Pleomorphic adenoma*
M8940/3	*Mixed tumor, malignant NOS*
M8950/3	*Mullerian mixed tumor*
M8951/3	*Mesodermal mixed tumor*
M8960/1	*Mesoblastic nephroma*
M8960/3	*Nephroblastoma NOS*
M8961/3	*Epithelial nephroblastoma*
M8962/3	*Mesenchymal nephroblastoma*
M8970/3	*Hepatoblastoma*
M8980/3	*Carcinosarcoma NOS*
M8981/3	*Carcinosarcoma, embryonal type*
M8982/0	*Myoepithelioma*
M8990/0	*Mesenchymoma, benign*
M8990/1	*Mesenchymoma NOS*

M8990/3	*Mesenchymoma, malignant*
M8991/3	*Embryonal sarcoma*

M900-M903   **Fibroepithelial neoplasms**

M9000/0	*Brenner tumor NOS*
M9000/1	*Brenner tumor, borderline malignancy*
M9000/3	*Brenner tumor, malignant*
M9010/0	*Fibroadenoma NOS*
M9011/0	*Intracanalicular fibroadenoma NOS*
M9012/0	*Pericanalicular fibroadenoma*
M9013/0	*Adenofibroma NOS*
M9014/0	*Serous adenofibroma*
M9015/0	*Mucinous adenofibroma*
M9020/0	*Cellular intracanalicular fibroadenoma*
M9020/1	*Cystosarcoma phyllodes NOS*
M9020/3	*Cystosarcoma phyllodes, malignant*
M9030/0	*Juvenile fibroadenoma*

M904   **Synovial neoplasms**

M9040/0	*Synovioma, benign*
M9040/3	*Synovial sarcoma NOS*
M9041/3	*Synovial sarcoma, spindle cell type*
M9042/3	*Synovial sarcoma, epithelioid cell type*
M9043/3	*Synovial sarcoma, biphasic type*
M9044/3	*Clear cell sarcoma of tendons and aponeuroses*

M905   **Mesothelial neoplasms**

M9050/0	*Mesothelioma, benign*
M9050/3	*Mesothelioma, malignant*
M9051/0	*Fibrous mesothelioma, benign*
M9051/3	*Fibrous mesothelioma, malignant*
M9052/0	*Epithelioid mesothelioma, benign*
M9052/3	*Epithelioid mesothelioma, malignant*
M9053/0	*Mesothelioma, biphasic type, benign*
M9053/3	*Mesothelioma, biphasic type, malignant*
M9054/0	*Adenomatoid tumor NOS*

M906-M909   **Germ cell neoplasms**

M9060/3	*Dysgerminoma*
M9061/3	*Seminoma NOS*
M9062/3	*Seminoma, anaplastic type*
M9063/3	*Spermatocytic seminoma*
M9064/3	*Germinoma*
M9070/3	*Embryonal carcinoma NOS*
M9071/3	*Endodermal sinus tumor*
M9072/3	*Polyembryoma*
M9073/1	*Gonadoblastoma*
M9080/0	*Teratoma, benign*
M9080/1	*Teratoma NOS*
M9080/3	*Teratoma, malignant NOS*
M9081/3	*Teratocarcinoma*
M9082/3	*Malignant teratoma, undifferentiated type*
M9083/3	*Malignant teratoma, intermediate type*
M9084/0	*Dermoid cyst*
M9084/3	*Dermoid cyst with malignant transformation*
M9090/0	*Struma ovarii NOS*
M9090/3	*Struma ovarii, malignant*
M9091/1	*Strumal carcinoid*

M910   **Trophoblastic neoplasms**

M9100/0	*Hydatidiform mole NOS*
M9100/1	*Invasive hydatidiform mole*
M9100/3	*Choriocarcinoma*
M9101/3	*Choriocarcinoma combined with teratoma*
M9102/3	*Malignant teratoma, trophoblastic*

M911   **Mesonephromas**

M9110/0	*Mesonephroma, benign*
M9110/1	*Mesonephric tumor*
M9110/3	*Mesonephroma, malignant*
M9111/1	*Endosalpingioma*

M912-M916   **Blood vessel tumors**

M9120/0	*Hemangioma NOS*
M9120/3	*Hemangiosarcoma*
M9121/0	*Cavernous hemangioma*
M9122/0	*Venous hemangioma*
M9123/0	*Racemose hemangioma*
M9124/3	*Kupffer cell sarcoma*

M9130/0	Hemangioendothelioma, benign
M9130/1	Hemangioendothelioma NOS
M9130/3	Hemangioendothelioma, malignant
M9131/0	Capillary hemangioma
M9132/0	Intramuscular hemangioma
M9140/3	Kaposi's sarcoma
M9141/0	Angiokeratoma
M9142/0	Verrucous keratotic hemangioma
M9150/0	Hemangiopericytoma, benign
M9150/1	Hemangiopericytoma NOS
M9150/3	Hemangiopericytoma, malignant
M9160/0	Angiofibroma NOS
M9161/1	Hemangioblastoma

M917 Lymphatic vessel tumors

M9170/0	Lymphangioma NOS
M9170/3	Lymphangiosarcoma
M9171/0	Capillary lymphangioma
M9172/0	Cavernous lymphangioma
M9173/0	Cystic lymphangioma
M9174/0	Lymphangiomyoma
M9174/1	Lymphangiomyomatosis
M9175/0	Hemolymphangioma

M918-M920 Osteomas and osteosarcomas

M9180/0	Osteoma NOS
M9180/3	Osteosarcoma NOS
M9181/3	Chondroblastic osteosarcoma
M9182/3	Fibroblastic osteosarcoma
M9183/3	Telangiectatic osteosarcoma
M9184/3	Osteosarcoma in Paget's disease of bone
M9190/3	Juxtacortical osteosarcoma
M9191/0	Osteoid osteoma NOS
M9200/0	Osteoblastoma

M921-M924 Chondromatous neoplasms

M9210/0	Osteochondroma
M9210/1	Osteochondromatosis NOS
M9220/0	Chondroma NOS
M9220/1	Chondromatosis NOS
M9220/3	Chondrosarcoma NOS
M9221/0	Juxtacortical chondroma
M9221/3	Juxtacortical chondrosarcoma
M9230/0	Chondroblastoma NOS
M9230/3	Chondroblastoma, malignant
M9240/3	Mesenchymal chondrosarcoma
M9241/0	Chondromyxoid fibroma

M925 Giant cell tumors

M9250/1	Giant cell tumor of bone NOS
M9250/3	Giant cell tumor of bone, malignant
M9251/1	Giant cell tumor of soft parts NOS
M9251/3	Malignant giant cell tumor of soft parts

M926 Miscellaneous bone tumors

M9260/3	Ewing's sarcoma
M9261/3	Adamantinoma of long bones
M9262/0	Ossifying fibroma

M927-M934 Odontogenic tumors

M9270/0	Odontogenic tumor, benign
M9270/1	Odontogenic tumor NOS
M9270/3	Odontogenic tumor, malignant
M9271/0	Dentinoma
M9272/0	Cementoma NOS
M9273/0	Cementoblastoma, benign
M9274/0	Cementifying fibroma
M9275/0	Gigantiform cementoma
M9280/0	Odontoma NOS
M9281/0	Compound odontoma
M9282/0	Complex odontoma
M9290/0	Ameloblastic fibro-odontoma
M9290/3	Ameloblastic odontosarcoma
M9300/0	Adenomatoid odontogenic tumor
M9301/0	Calcifying odontogenic cyst
M9310/0	Ameloblastoma NOS
M9310/3	Ameloblastoma, malignant
M9311/0	Odontoameloblastoma
M9312/0	Squamous odontogenic tumor

M9320/0	Odontogenic myxoma
M9321/0	Odontogenic fibroma NOS
M9330/0	Ameloblastic fibroma
M9330/3	Ameloblastic fibrosarcoma
M9340/0	Calcifying epithelial odontogenic tumor

M935-M937 Miscellaneous tumors

M9350/1	Craniopharyngioma
M9360/1	Pinealoma
M9361/1	Pineocytoma
M9362/3	Pineoblastoma
M9363/0	Melanotic neuroectodermal tumor
M9370/3	Chordoma

M938-M948 Gliomas

M9380/3	Glioma, malignant
M9381/3	Gliomatosis cerebri
M9382/3	Mixed glioma
M9383/1	Subependymal glioma
M9384/1	Subependymal giant cell astrocytoma
M9390/0	Choroid plexus papilloma NOS
M9390/3	Choroid plexus papilloma, malignant
M9391/3	Ependymoma NOS
M9392/3	Ependymoma, anaplastic type
M9393/1	Papillary ependymoma
M9394/1	Myxopapillary ependymoma
M9400/3	Astrocytoma NOS
M9401/3	Astrocytoma, anaplastic type
M9410/3	Protoplasmic astrocytoma
M9411/3	Gemistocytic astrocytoma
M9420/3	Fibrillary astrocytoma
M9421/3	Pilocytic astrocytoma
M9422/3	Spongioblastoma NOS
M9423/3	Spongioblastoma polare
M9430/3	Astroblastoma
M9440/3	Glioblastoma NOS
M9441/3	Giant cell glioblastoma
M9442/3	Glioblastoma with sarcomatous component
M9443/3	Primitive polar spongioblastoma
M9450/3	Oligodendroglioma NOS
M9451/3	Oligodendroglioma, anaplastic type
M9460/3	Oligodendroblastoma
M9470/3	Medulloblastoma NOS
M9471/3	Desmoplastic medulloblastoma
M9472/3	Medullomyoblastoma
M9480/3	Cerebellar sarcoma NOS
M9481/3	Monstrocellular sarcoma

M949-M952 Neuroepitheliomatous neoplasms

M9490/0	Ganglioneuroma
M9490/3	Ganglioneuroblastoma
M9491/0	Ganglioneuromatosis
M9500/3	Neuroblastoma NOS
M9501/3	Medulloepithelioma NOS
M9502/3	Teratoid medulloepithelioma
M9503/3	Neuroepithelioma NOS
M9504/3	Spongioneuroblastoma
M9505/1	Ganglioglioma
M9506/0	Neurocytoma
M9507/0	Pacinian tumor
M9510/3	Retinoblastoma NOS
M9511/3	Retinoblastoma, differentiated type
M9512/3	Retinoblastoma, undifferentiated type
M9520/3	Olfactory neurogenic tumor
M9521/3	Esthesioneurocytoma
M9522/3	Esthesioneuroblastoma
M9523/3	Esthesioneuroepithelioma

M953 Meningiomas

M9530/0	Meningioma NOS
M9530/1	Meningiomatosis NOS
M9530/3	Meningioma, malignant
M9531/0	Meningotheliomatous meningioma
M9532/0	Fibrous meningioma
M9533/0	Psammomatous meningioma
M9534/0	Angiomatous meningioma

M9535/0	Hemangioblastic meningioma
M9536/0	Hemangiopericytic meningioma
M9537/0	Transitional meningioma
M9538/1	Papillary meningioma
M9539/3	Meningeal sarcomatosis

M954-M957   **Nerve sheath tumor**

M9540/0	Neurofibroma NOS
M9540/1	Neurofibromatosis NOS
M9540/3	Neurofibrosarcoma
M9541/0	Melanotic neurofibroma
M9550/0	Plexiform neurofibroma
M9560/0	Neurilemmoma NOS
M9560/1	Neurinomatosis
M9560/3	Neurilemmoma, malignant
M9570/0	Neuroma NOS

M958   **Granular cell tumors and alveolar soft part sarcoma**

M9580/0	Granular cell tumor NOS
M9580/3	Granular cell tumor, malignant
M9581/3	Alveolar soft part sarcoma

M959-M963   **Lymphomas, NOS or diffuse**

M9590/0	Lymphomatous tumor, benign
M9590/3	Malignant lymphoma NOS
M9591/3	Malignant lymphoma, non Hodgkin's type
M9600/3	Malignant lymphoma, undifferentiated cell type NOS
M9601/3	Malignant lymphoma, stem cell type
M9602/3	Malignant lymphoma, convoluted cell type NOS
M9610/3	Lymphosarcoma NOS
M9611/3	Malignant lymphoma, lymphoplasmacytoid type
M9612/3	Malignant lymphoma, immunoblastic type
M9613/3	Malignant lymphoma, mixed lymphocytic-histiocytic NOS
M9614/3	Malignant lymphoma, centroblastic-centrocytic, diffuse
M9615/3	Malignant lymphoma, follicular center cell NOS
M9620/3	Malignant lymphoma, lymphocytic, well differentiated NOS
M9621/3	Malignant lymphoma, lymphocytic, intermediate differentiation NOS
M9622/3	Malignant lymphoma, centrocytic
M9623/3	Malignant lymphoma, follicular center cell, cleaved NOS
M9630/3	Malignant lymphoma, lymphocytic, poorly differentiated NOS
M9631/3	Prolymphocytic lymphosarcoma
M9632/3	Malignant lymphoma, centroblastic type NOS
M9633/3	Malignant lymphoma, follicular center cell, noncleaved NOS

M964   **Reticulosarcomas**

M9640/3	Reticulosarcoma NOS
M9641/3	Reticulosarcoma, pleomorphic cell type
M9642/3	Reticulosarcoma, nodular

M965-M966   **Hodgkin's disease**

M9650/3	Hodgkin's disease NOS
M9651/3	Hodgkin's disease, lymphocytic predominance
M9652/3	Hodgkin's disease, mixed cellularity
M9653/3	Hodgkin's disease, lymphocytic depletion NOS
M9654/3	Hodgkin's disease, lymphocytic depletion, diffuse fibrosis
M9655/3	Hodgkin's disease, lymphocytic depletion, reticular type
M9656/3	Hodgkin's disease, nodular sclerosis NOS
M9657/3	Hodgkin's disease, nodular sclerosis, cellular phase
M9660/3	Hodgkin's paragranuloma
M9661/3	Hodgkin's granuloma
M9662/3	Hodgkin's sarcoma

M969   **Lymphomas, nodular or follicular**

M9690/3	Malignant lymphoma, nodular NOS
M9691/3	Malignant lymphoma, mixed lymphocytic-histiocytic, nodular
M9692/3	Malignant lymphoma, centroblastic-centrocytic, follicular
M9693/3	Malignant lymphoma, lymphocytic, well differentiated, nodular
M9694/3	Malignant lymphoma, lymphocytic, intermediate differentiation, nodular
M9695/3	Malignant lymphoma, follicular center cell, cleaved, follicular
M9696/3	Malignant lymphoma, lymphocytic, poorly differentiated, nodular
M9697/3	Malignant lymphoma, centroblastic type, follicular
M9698/3	Malignant lymphoma, follicular center cell, noncleaved, follicular

M970   **Mycosis fungoides**

M9700/3	Mycosis fungoides
M9701/3	Sezary's disease

M971-M972   **Miscellaneous reticuloendothelial neoplasms**

M9710/3	Microglioma
M9720/3	Malignant histiocytosis
M9721/3	Histiocytic medullary reticulosis
M9722/3	Letterer-Siwe's disease

M973   **Plasma cell tumors**

M9730/3	Plasma cell myeloma
M9731/0	Plasma cell tumor, benign
M9731/1	Plasmacytoma NOS
M9731/3	Plasma cell tumor, malignant

M974   **Mast cell tumors**

M9740/1	Mastocytoma NOS
M9740/3	Mast cell sarcoma
M9741/3	Malignant mastocytosis

M975   **Burkitt's tumor**

M9750/3	Burkitt's tumor

M980-M994   **Leukemias**

M980   **Leukemias NOS**

M9800/3	Leukemia NOS
M9801/3	Acute leukemia NOS
M9802/3	Subacute leukemia NOS
M9803/3	Chronic leukemia NOS
M9804/3	Aleukemic leukemia NOS

M981   **Compound leukemias**

M9810/3	Compound leukemia

M982   **Lymphoid leukemias**

M9820/3	Lymphoid leukemia NOS
M9821/3	Acute lymphoid leukemia
M9822/3	Subacute lymphoid leukemia
M9823/3	Chronic lymphoid leukemia
M9824/3	Aleukemic lymphoid leukemia
M9825/3	Prolymphocytic leukemia

M983   **Plasma cell leukemias**

M9830/3	Plasma cell leukemia

M984   **Erythroleukemias**

M9840/3	Erythroleukemia
M9841/3	Acute erythremia
M9842/3	Chronic erythremia

M985   **Lymphosarcoma cell leukemias**

M9850/3	Lymphosarcoma cell leukemia

M986   **Myeloid leukemias**

M9860/3	Myeloid leukemia NOS
M9861/3	Acute myeloid leukemia
M9862/3	Subacute myeloid leukemia
M9863/3	Chronic myeloid leukemia
M9864/3	Aleukemic myeloid leukemia
M9865/3	Neutrophilic leukemia
M9866/3	Acute promyelocytic leukemia

M987   **Basophilic leukemias**

M9870/3	Basophilic leukemia

M988   **Eosinophilic leukemias**

M9880/3	Eosinophilic leukemia

M989   **Monocytic leukemias**

M9890/3	Monocytic leukemia NOS
M9891/3	Acute monocytic leukemia
M9892/3	Subacute monocytic leukemia

M9893/3	Chronic monocytic leukemia
M9894/3	Aleukemic monocytic leukemia
M990-M994	**Miscellaneous leukemias**
M9900/3	Mast cell leukemia
M9910/3	Megakaryocytic leukemia
M9920/3	Megakaryocytic myelosis
M9930/3	Myeloid sarcoma
M9940/3	Hairy cell leukemia

M995-M997	**Miscellaneous myeloproliferative and lymphoproliferative disorders**
M9950/1	Polycythemia vera
M9951/1	Acute panmyelosis
M9960/1	Chronic myeloproliferative disease
M9961/1	Myelosclerosis with myeloid metaplasia
M9962/1	Idiopathic thrombocythemia
M9970/1	Chronic lymphoproliferative disease

GLOSSARY OF MENTAL DISORDERS

Deleted as of October 1, 2004

APPENDIX C

CLASSIFICATION OF DRUGS BY AMERICAN HOSPITAL FORMULARY SERVICES LIST NUMBER AND THEIR ICD-9-CM EQUIVALENTS

The coding of adverse effects of drugs is keyed to the continually revised Hospital Formulary of the American Hospital Formulary Service (AHFS) published under the direction of the American Society of Hospital Pharmacists.

The following section gives the ICD-9-CM diagnosis code for each AHFS list.

AHFS List		ICD-9-CM Diagnosis Code
4:00	**ANTIHISTAMINE DRUGS**	**963.0**
8:00	**ANTI-INFECTIVE AGENTS**	
8:04	Amebicides	961.5
	hydroxyquinoline derivatives	961.3
	arsenical anti-infectives	961.1
8:08	Anthelmintics	961.6
	quinoline derivatives	961.3
8:12.04	Antifungal Antibiotics	960.1
	nonantibiotics	961.9
8:12.06	Cephalosporins	960.5
8:12.08	Chloramphenicol	960.2
8:12.12	The Erythromycins	960.3
8:12.16	The Penicillins	960.0
8:12.20	The Streptomycins	960.6
8:12.24	The Tetracyclines	960.4
8:12.28	Other Antibiotics	960.8
	antimycobacterial antibiotics	960.6
	macrolides	960.3
8:16	Antituberculars	961.8
	antibiotics	960.6
8:18	Antivirals	961.7
8:20	Plasmodicides (antimalarials)	961.4
8:24	Sulfonamides	961.0
8:26	The Sulfones	961.8
8:28	Treponemicides	961.2
8:32	Trichomonacides	961.5
	hydroxyquinoline derivatives	961.3
	nitrofuran derivatives	961.9
8:36	Urinary Germicides	961.9
	quinoline derivatives	961.3
8:40	Other Anti-Infectives	961.9
10:00	**ANTINEOPLASTIC AGENTS**	**963.1**
	antibiotics	960.7
	progestogens	962.2
12:00	**AUTONOMIC DRUGS**	
12:04	Parasympathomimetic (Cholinergic) Agents	971.0
12:08	Parasympatholytic (Cholinergic Blocking) Agents	971.1
12:12	Sympathomimetic (Adrenergic) Agents	971.2
12:16	Sympatholytic (Adrenergic Blocking) Agents	971.3
12:20	Skeletal Muscle Relaxants	975.2
	central nervous system muscle-tone depressants	968.0
16:00	**BLOOD DERIVATIVES**	**964.7**
20:00	**BLOOD FORMATION AND COAGULATION**	
20:04	Antianemia Drugs	964.1
20:04.04	Iron Preparations	964.0
20:04.08	Liver and Stomach Preparations	964.1
20:12.04	Anticoagulants	964.2
20:12.08	Antiheparin agents	964.5
20:12.12	Coagulants	964.5
20.12.16	Hemostatics	964.5
	capillary-active drugs	972.8
	fibrinolysis-affecting agents	964.4
	natural products	964.7

24:00	**CARDIOVASCULAR DRUGS**	
24:04	Cardiac Drugs	972.9
	cardiotonic agents	972.1
	rhythm regulators	972.0
24:06	Antilipemic Agents	972.2
	thyroid derivatives	962.7
24:08	Hypotensive Agents	972.6
	adrenergic blocking agents	971.3
	ganglion-blocking agents	972.3
	vasodilators	972.5
24:12	Vasodilating Agents	972.5
	coronary	972.4
	nicotinic acid derivatives	972.2
24:16	Sclerosing Agents	972.7
28:00	**CENTRAL NERVOUS SYSTEM DRUGS**	
28:04	General Anesthetics	968.4
	gaseous anesthetics	968.2
	halothane	968.1
	intravenous anesthetics	968.3
28:08	Analgesics and Antipyretics	965.9
	antirheumatics	965.6
	aromatic analgesics	965.4
	non-narcotics NEC	965.7
	opium alkaloids	965.00
	heroin	965.01
	methadone	965.02
	specified type NEC	965.09
	pyrazole derivatives	965.5
	salicylates	965.1
	specified type NEC	965.8
28:10	Narcotic Antagonists	970.1
28:12	Anticonvulsants	966.3
	barbiturates	967.0
	benzodiazepine-based tranquilizers	969.4
	bromides	967.3
	hydantoin derivatives	966.1
	oxazolidine derivative	966.0
	succinimides	966.2
28:16.04	Antidepressants	969.0
28:16.08	Tranquilizers	969.5
	benzodiazepine-based	969.4
	butyrophenone-based	969.2
	major NEC	969.3
	phenothiazine-based	969.1
28:16.12	Other Psychotherapeutic Agents	969.8
28:20	Respiratory and Cerebral Stimulants	970.9
	analeptics	970.0
	anorexigenic agents	977.0
	psychostimulants	969.7
	specified type NEC	970.8
28:24	Sedatives and Hypnotics	967.9
	barbiturates	967.0
	benzodiazepine-based tranquilizers	969.4
	chloral hydrate group	967.1
	glutethimide group	967.5
	intravenous anesthetics	968.3
	methaqualone	967.4
	paraldehyde	967.2
	phenothiazine-based tranquilizers	969.1
	specified type NEC	967.8
	thiobarbiturates	968.3
	tranquilizer NEC	969.5
36:00	**DIAGNOSTIC AGENTS**	**977.8**
40:00	**ELECTROLYTE, CALORIC, AND WATER BALANCE AGENTS NEC**	**974.5**
40:04	Acidifying Agents	963.2

APPENDIX D

CLASSIFICATION OF INDUSTRIAL ACCIDENTS ACCORDING TO AGENCY

Annex B to the Resolution concerning Statistics of Employment Injuries adopted by the Tenth International Conference of Labor Statisticians on 12 October 1962

1 MACHINES

11 Prime-Movers, except Electrical Motors
111 *Steam engines*
112 *Internal combustion engines*
119 *Others*

12 Transmission Machinery
121 *Transmission shafts*
122 *Transmission belts, cables, pulleys, pinions, chains, gears*
129 *Others*

13 Metalworking Machines
131 *Power presses*
132 *Lathes*
133 *Milling machines*
134 *Abrasive wheels*
135 *Mechanical shears*
136 *Forging machines*
137 *Rolling-mills*
139 *Others*

14 Wood and Assimilated Machines
141 *Circular saws*
142 *Other saws*
143 *Molding machines*
144 *Overhand planes*
149 *Others*

15 Agricultural Machines
151 *Reapers (including combine reapers)*
152 *Threshers*
159 *Others*

16 Mining Machinery
161 *Under-cutters*
169 *Others*

19 Other Machines Not Elsewhere Classified
191 *Earth-moving machines, excavating and scraping machines, except means of transport*
192 *Spinning, weaving and other textile machines*
193 *Machines for the manufacture of foodstuffs and beverages*
194 *Machines for the manufacture of paper*
195 *Printing machines*
199 *Others*

2 MEANS OF TRANSPORT AND LIFTING EQUIPMENT

21 Lifting Machines and Appliances
211 *Cranes*
212 *Lifts and elevators*
213 *Winches*
214 *Pulley blocks*
219 *Others*

22 Means of Rail Transport
221 *Inter-urban railways*
222 *Rail transport in mines, tunnels, quarries, industrial establishments, docks, etc.*
229 *Others*

23 Other Wheeled Means of Transport, Excluding Rail Transport
231 *Tractors*
232 *Lorries*
233 *Trucks*
234 *Motor vehicles, not elsewhere classified*
235 *Animal-drawn vehicles*
236 *Hand-drawn vehicles*
239 *Others*

24 Means of Air Transport

25 Means of Water Transport
251 *Motorized means of water transport*
252 *Non-motorized means of water transport*

26 Other Means of Transport
261 *Cable-cars*
262 *Mechanical conveyors, except cable-cars*
269 *Others*

3 OTHER EQUIPMENT

31 Pressure Vessels
311 *Boilers*
312 *Pressurized containers*
313 *Pressurized piping and accessories*
314 *Gas cylinders*
315 *Caissons, diving equipment*
319 *Others*

32 Furnaces, Ovens, Kilns
321 *Blast furnaces*
322 *Refining furnaces*
323 *Other furnaces*
324 *Kilns*
325 *Ovens*

33 Refrigerating Plants

34 Electrical Installations, Including Electric Motors, but Excluding Electric Hand Tools
341 *Rotating machines*
342 *Conductors*
343 *Transformers*
344 *Control apparatus*
349 *Others*

35 Electric Hand Tools

36 Tools, Implements, and Appliances, Except Electric Hand Tools
361 *Power-driven hand tools, except electric hand tools*
362 *Hand tools, not power-driven*
369 *Others*

37 Ladders, Mobile Ramps

38 Scaffolding

39 Other Equipment, Not Elsewhere Classified

4 MATERIALS, SUBSTANCES, AND RADIATIONS

41 Explosives

42 Dusts, Gases, Liquids and Chemicals, Excluding Explosives
421 *Dusts*
422 *Gases, vapors, fumes*
423 *Liquids, not elsewhere classified*
424 *Chemicals, not elsewhere classified*

43 Flying Fragments

44 Radiations
441 *Ionizing radiations*
449 *Others*

49   **Other Materials and Substances Not Elsewhere Classified**

---

5 WORKING ENVIRONMENT

51   **Outdoor**
      511 *Weather*
      512 *Traffic and working surfaces*
      513 *Water*
      519 *Others*

52   **Indoor**
      521 *Floors*
      522 *Confined quarters*
      523 *Stairs*
      524 *Other traffic and working surfaces*
      525 *Floor openings and wall openings*
      526 *Environmental factors (lighting, ventilation, temperature, noise, etc.)*
      529 *Others*

53   **Underground**
      531 *Roofs and faces of mine roads and tunnels, etc.*
      532 *Floors of mine roads and tunnels, etc.*
      533 *Working-faces of mines, tunnels, etc.*
      534 *Mine shafts*
      535 *Fire*
      536 *Water*
      539 *Others*

---

6 OTHER AGENCIES, NOT ELSEWHERE CLASSIFIED

61   **Animals**
      611 *Live animals*
      612 *Animals products*

69   **Other Agencies, Not Elsewhere Classified**

---

7 AGENCIES NOT CLASSIFIED FOR LACK OF SUFFICIENT DATA

APPENDIX E

LIST OF THREE-DIGIT CATEGORIES

1. INFECTIOUS AND PARASITIC DISEASES

Intestinal infectious diseases (001–009)
001 Cholera
002 Typhoid and paratyphoid fevers
003 Other salmonella infections
004 Shigellosis
005 Other food poisoning (bacterial)
006 Amebiasis
007 Other protozoal intestinal diseases
008 Intestinal infections due to other organisms
009 Ill-defined intestinal infections

Tuberculosis (010–018)
010 Primary tuberculous infection
011 Pulmonary tuberculosis
012 Other respiratory tuberculosis
013 Tuberculosis of meninges and central nervous system
014 Tuberculosis of intestines, peritoneum, and mesenteric glands
015 Tuberculosis of bones and joints
016 Tuberculosis of genitourinary system
017 Tuberculosis of other organs
018 Miliary tuberculosis

Zoonotic bacterial diseases (020–027)
020 Plague
021 Tularemia
022 Anthrax
023 Brucellosis
024 Glanders
025 Melioidosis
026 Rat-bite fever
027 Other zoonotic bacterial diseases

Other bacterial diseases (030–041)
030 Leprosy
031 Diseases due to other mycobacteria
032 Diphtheria
033 Whooping cough
034 Streptococcal sore throat and scarlet fever
035 Erysipelas
036 Meningococcal infection
037 Tetanus
038 Septicemia
039 Actinomycotic infections
040 Other bacterial diseases
041 Bacterial infection in conditions classified elsewhere and of unspecified site

Human immunodeficiency virus (042)
042 Human immunodeficiency virus [HIV] disease

Poliomyelitis and other non-arthropod-borne viral diseases of central nervous system (045–049)
045 Acute poliomyelitis
046 Slow virus infection of central nervous system
047 Meningitis due to enterovirus
048 Other enterovirus diseases of central nervous system
049 Other non-arthropod-borne viral diseases of central nervous system

Viral diseases accompanied by exanthem (050–059)
050 Smallpox
051 Cowpox and paravaccinia
052 Chickenpox
053 Herpes zoster
054 Herpes simplex
055 Measles
056 Rubella
057 Other viral exanthemata
058 Other human herpesvirus
059 Other poxvirus infections

Arthropod-borne viral diseases (060–066)
060 Yellow fever
061 Dengue
062 Mosquito-borne viral encephalitis
063 Tick-borne viral encephalitis
064 Viral encephalitis transmitted by other and unspecified arthropods
065 Arthropod-borne hemorrhagic fever
066 Other arthropod-borne viral diseases

Other diseases due to viruses and Chlamydiae (070–079)
070 Viral hepatitis
071 Rabies
072 Mumps
073 Ornithosis
074 Specific diseases due to Coxsackie virus
075 Infectious mononucleosis
076 Trachoma
077 Other diseases of conjunctiva due to viruses and Chlamydiae
078 Other diseases due to viruses and Chlamydiae
079 Viral infection in conditions classified elsewhere and of unspecified site

Rickettsioses and other arthropod-borne diseases (080–088)
080 Louse-borne [epidemic] typhus
081 Other typhus
082 Tick-borne rickettsioses
083 Other rickettsioses
084 Malaria
085 Leishmaniasis
086 Trypanosomiasis
087 Relapsing fever
088 Other arthropod-borne diseases

Syphilis and other venereal diseases (090–099)
090 Congenital syphilis
091 Early syphilis, symptomatic
092 Early syphilis, latent
093 Cardiovascular syphilis
094 Neurosyphilis
095 Other forms of late syphilis, with symptoms
096 Late syphilis, latent
097 Other and unspecified syphilis
098 Gonococcal infections
099 Other venereal diseases

Other spirochetal diseases (100–104)
100 Leptospirosis
101 Vincent's angina
102 Yaws
103 Pinta
104 Other spirochetal infection

Mycoses (110–118)
110 Dermatophytosis
111 Dermatomycosis, other and unspecified
112 Candidiasis
114 Coccidioidomycosis
115 Histoplasmosis
116 Blastomycotic infection
117 Other mycoses
118 Opportunistic mycoses

Helminthiases (120–129)
120 Schistosomiasis [bilharziasis]
121 Other trematode infections
122 Echinococcosis
123 Other cestode infection
124 Trichinosis
125 Filarial infection and dracontiasis
126 Ancylostomiasis and necatoriasis
127 Other intestinal helminthiases

128 Other and unspecified helminthiases
129 Intestinal parasitism, unspecified

Other infectious and parasitic diseases (130–136)
130 Toxoplasmosis
131 Trichomoniasis
132 Pediculosis and phthirus infestation
133 Acariasis
134 Other infestation
135 Sarcoidosis
136 Other and unspecified infectious and parasitic diseases

Late effects of infectious and parasitic diseases (137–139)
137 Late effects of tuberculosis
138 Late effects of acute poliomyelitis
139 Late effects of other infectious and parasitic diseases

2. NEOPLASMS

Malignant neoplasm of lip, oral cavity, and pharynx (140–149)
140 Malignant neoplasm of lip
141 Malignant neoplasm of tongue
142 Malignant neoplasm of major salivary glands
143 Malignant neoplasm of gum
144 Malignant neoplasm of floor of mouth
145 Malignant neoplasm of other and unspecified parts of mouth
146 Malignant neoplasm of oropharynx
147 Malignant neoplasm of nasopharynx
148 Malignant neoplasm of hypopharynx
149 Malignant neoplasm of other and ill-defined sites within the lip, oral cavity, and pharynx

Malignant neoplasm of digestive organs and peritoneum (150–159)
150 Malignant neoplasm of esophagus
151 Malignant neoplasm of stomach
152 Malignant neoplasm of small intestine, including duodenum
153 Malignant neoplasm of colon
154 Malignant neoplasm of rectum, rectosigmoid junction, and anus
155 Malignant neoplasm of liver and intrahepatic bile ducts
156 Malignant neoplasm of gallbladder and extrahepatic bile ducts
157 Malignant neoplasm of pancreas
158 Malignant neoplasm of retroperitoneum and peritoneum
159 Malignant neoplasm of other and ill-defined sites within the digestive organs and peritoneum

Malignant neoplasm of respiratory and intrathoracic organs (160–165)
160 Malignant neoplasm of nasal cavities, middle ear, and accessory sinuses
161 Malignant neoplasm of larynx
162 Malignant neoplasm of trachea, bronchus, and lung
163 Malignant neoplasm of pleura
164 Malignant neoplasm of thymus, heart, and mediastinum
165 Malignant neoplasm of other and ill-defined sites within the respiratory system and intrathoracic organs

Malignant neoplasm of bone, connective tissue, skin, and breast (170–176)
170 Malignant neoplasm of bone and articular cartilage
171 Malignant neoplasm of connective and other soft tissue
172 Malignant melanoma of skin
173 Other malignant neoplasm of skin
174 Malignant neoplasm of female breast
175 Malignant neoplasm of male breast

Kaposi's sarcoma (176)
176 Kaposi's sarcoma

Malignant neoplasm of genitourinary organs (179–189)
179 Malignant neoplasm of uterus, part unspecified
180 Malignant neoplasm of cervix uteri
181 Malignant neoplasm of placenta

182 Malignant neoplasm of body of uterus
183 Malignant neoplasm of ovary and other uterine adnexa
184 Malignant neoplasm of other and unspecified female genital organs
185 Malignant neoplasm of prostate
186 Malignant neoplasm of testis
187 Malignant neoplasm of penis and other male genital organs
188 Malignant neoplasm of bladder
189 Malignant neoplasm of kidney and other and unspecified urinary organs

Malignant neoplasm of other and unspecified sites (190–199)
190 Malignant neoplasm of eye
191 Malignant neoplasm of brain
192 Malignant neoplasm of other and unspecified parts of nervous system
193 Malignant neoplasm of thyroid gland
194 Malignant neoplasm of other endocrine glands and related structures
195 Malignant neoplasm of other and ill-defined sites
196 Secondary and unspecified malignant neoplasm of lymph nodes
197 Secondary malignant neoplasm of respiratory and digestive systems
198 Secondary malignant neoplasm of other specified sites
199 Malignant neoplasm without specification of site

Malignant neoplasm of lymphatic and hematopoietic tissue (200–208)
200 Lymphosarcoma and reticulosarcoma
201 Hodgkin's disease
202 Other malignant neoplasm of lymphoid and histiocytic tissue
203 Multiple myeloma and immunoproliferative neoplasms
204 Lymphoid leukemia
205 Myeloid leukemia
206 Monocytic leukemia
207 Other specified leukemia
208 Leukemia of unspecified cell type

Neuroendocrine tumors (209)
209 Neuroendocrine tumors

Benign neoplasms (210–229)
210 Benign neoplasm of lip, oral cavity, and pharynx
211 Benign neoplasm of other parts of digestive system
212 Benign neoplasm of respiratory and intrathoracic organs
213 Benign neoplasm of bone and articular cartilage
214 Lipoma
215 Other benign neoplasm of connective and other soft tissue
216 Benign neoplasm of skin
217 Benign neoplasm of breast
218 Uterine leiomyoma
219 Other benign neoplasm of uterus
220 Benign neoplasm of ovary
221 Benign neoplasm of other female genital organs
222 Benign neoplasm of male genital organs
223 Benign neoplasm of kidney and other urinary organs
224 Benign neoplasm of eye
225 Benign neoplasm of brain and other parts of nervous system
226 Benign neoplasm of thyroid gland
227 Benign neoplasm of other endocrine glands and related structures
228 Hemangioma and lymphangioma, any site
229 Benign neoplasm of other and unspecified sites

Carcinoma in situ (230–234)
230 Carcinoma in situ of digestive organs
231 Carcinoma in situ of respiratory system
232 Carcinoma in situ of skin
233 Carcinoma in situ of breast and genitourinary system
234 Carcinoma in situ of other and unspecified sites

Other disorders of the central nervous system (340–349)
340 Multiple sclerosis
341 Other demyelinating diseases of central nervous system
342 Hemiplegia and hemiparesis
343 Infantile cerebral palsy
344 Other paralytic syndromes
345 Epilepsy
346 Migraine
347 Cataplexy and narcolepsy
348 Other conditions of brain
349 Other and unspecified disorders of the nervous system

Disorders of the peripheral nervous system (350–359)
350 Trigeminal nerve disorders
351 Facial nerve disorders
352 Disorders of other cranial nerves
353 Nerve root and plexus disorders
354 Mononeuritis of upper limb and mononeuritis multiplex
355 Mononeuritis of lower limb
356 Hereditary and idiopathic peripheral neuropathy
357 Inflammatory and toxic neuropathy
358 Myoneural disorders
359 Muscular dystrophies and other myopathies

Disorders of the eye and adnexa (360–379)
360 Disorders of the globe
361 Retinal detachments and defects
362 Other retinal disorders
363 Chorioretinal inflammations and scars and other disorders of choroid
364 Disorders of iris and ciliary body
365 Glaucoma
366 Cataract
367 Disorders of refraction and accommodation
368 Visual disturbances
369 Blindness and low vision
370 Keratitis
371 Corneal opacity and other disorders of cornea
372 Disorders of conjunctiva
373 Inflammation of eyelids
374 Other disorders of eyelids
375 Disorders of lacrimal system
376 Disorders of the orbit
377 Disorders of optic nerve and visual pathways
378 Strabismus and other disorders of binocular eye movements
379 Other disorders of eye

Diseases of the ear and mastoid process (380–389)
380 Disorders of external ear
381 Nonsuppurative otitis media and Eustachian tube disorders
382 Suppurative and unspecified otitis media
383 Mastoiditis and related conditions
384 Other disorders of tympanic membrane
385 Other disorders of middle ear and mastoid
386 Vertiginous syndromes and other disorders of vestibular system
387 Otosclerosis
388 Other disorders of ear
389 Hearing loss

7. DISEASES OF THE CIRCULATORY SYSTEM

Acute rheumatic fever (390–392)
390 Rheumatic fever without mention of heart involvement
391 Rheumatic fever with heart involvement
392 Rheumatic chorea

Chronic rheumatic heart disease (393–398)
393 Chronic rheumatic pericarditis
394 Diseases of mitral valve
395 Diseases of aortic valve
396 Diseases of mitral and aortic valves
397 Diseases of other endocardial structures
398 Other rheumatic heart disease

Hypertensive disease (401–405)
401 Essential hypertension
402 Hypertensive heart disease
403 Hypertensive renal disease
404 Hypertensive heart and renal disease
405 Secondary hypertension

Ischemic heart disease (410–414)
410 Acute myocardial infarction
411 Other acute and subacute form of ischemic heart disease
412 Old myocardial infarction
413 Angina pectoris
414 Other forms of chronic ischemic heart disease

Diseases of pulmonary circulation (415–417)
415 Acute pulmonary heart disease
416 Chronic pulmonary heart disease
417 Other diseases of pulmonary circulation

Other forms of heart disease (420–429)
420 Acute pericarditis
421 Acute and subacute endocarditis
422 Acute myocarditis
423 Other diseases of pericardium
424 Other diseases of endocardium
425 Cardiomyopathy
426 Conduction disorders
427 Cardiac dysrhythmias
428 Heart failure
429 Ill-defined descriptions and complications of heart disease

Cerebrovascular disease (430–438)
430 Subarachnoid hemorrhage
431 Intracerebral hemorrhage
432 Other and unspecified intracranial hemorrhage
433 Occlusion and stenosis of precerebral arteries
434 Occlusion of cerebral arteries
435 Transcient cerebral ischemia
436 Acute but ill-defined cerebrovascular disease
437 Other and ill-defined cerebrovascular disease
438 Late effects of cerebrovascular disease

Diseases of arteries, arterioles, and capillaries (440–448)
440 Atherosclerosis
441 Aortic aneurysm and dissection
442 Other aneurysm
443 Other peripheral vascular disease
444 Arterial embolism and thrombosis
445 Atheroembolism
446 Polyarteritis nodosa and allied conditions
447 Other disorders of arteries and arterioles
448 Diseases of capillaries

Diseases of veins and lymphatics, and other diseases of circulatory system (451–459)
451 Phlebitis and thrombophlebitis
452 Portal vein thrombosis
453 Other venous embolism and thrombosis
454 Varicose veins of lower extremities
455 Hemorrhoids
456 Varicose veins of other sites
457 Noninfective disorders of lymphatic channels
458 Hypotension
459 Other disorders of circulatory system

8. DISEASES OF THE RESPIRATORY SYSTEM

Acute respiratory infections (460–466)
460 Acute nasopharyngitis [common cold]
461 Acute sinusitis
462 Acute pharyngitis
463 Acute tonsillitis
464 Acute laryngitis and tracheitis
465 Acute upper respiratory infections of multiple or unspecified sites
466 Acute bronchitis and bronchiolitis

Other diseases of upper respiratory tract (470–478)

470 Deviated nasal septum
471 Nasal polyps
472 Chronic pharyngitis and nasopharyngitis
473 Chronic sinusitis
474 Chronic disease of tonsils and adenoids
475 Peritonsillar abscess
476 Chronic laryngitis and laryngotracheitis
477 Allergic rhinitis
478 Other diseases of upper respiratory tract

Pneumonia and influenza (480–488)

480 Viral pneumonia
481 Pneumococcal pneumonia [*Streptococcus pneumoniae* pneumonia]
482 Other bacterial pneumonia
483 Pneumonia due to other specified organism
484 Pneumonia in infectious diseases classified elsewhere
485 Bronchopneumonia, organism unspecified
486 Pneumonia, organism unspecified
487 Influenza
488 Influenza due to identified avian influenza virus

Chronic obstructive pulmonary disease and allied conditions (490–496)

490 Bronchitis, not specified as acute or chronic
491 Chronic bronchitis
492 Emphysema
493 Asthma
494 Bronchiectasis
495 Extrinsic allergic alveolitis
496 Chronic airways obstruction, not elsewhere classified

Pneumoconioses and other lung diseases due to external agents (500–508)

500 Coalworkers' pneumoconiosis
501 Asbestosis
502 Pneumoconiosis due to other silica or silicates
503 Pneumoconiosis due to other inorganic dust
504 Pneumopathy due to inhalation of other dust
505 Pneumoconiosis, unspecified
506 Respiratory conditions due to chemical fumes and vapors
507 Pneumonitis due to solids and liquids
508 Respiratory conditions due to other and unspecified external agents

Other diseases of respiratory system (510–519)

510 Empyema
511 Pleurisy
512 Pneumothorax
513 Abscess of lung and mediastinum
514 Pulmonary congestion and hypostasis
515 Postinflammatory pulmonary fibrosis
516 Other alveolar and parietoalveolar pneumopathy
517 Lung involvement in conditions classified elsewhere
518 Other diseases of lung
519 Other diseases of respiratory system

9. DISEASES OF THE DIGESTIVE SYSTEM

Diseases of oral cavity, salivary glands, and jaws (520–529)

520 Disorders of tooth development and eruption
521 Diseases of hard tissues of teeth
522 Diseases of pulp and periapical tissues
523 Gingival and periodontal diseases
524 Dentofacial anomalies, including malocclusion
525 Other diseases and conditions of the teeth and supporting structures
526 Diseases of the jaws
527 Diseases of the salivary glands
528 Diseases of the oral soft tissues, excluding lesions specific for gingiva and tongue
529 Diseases and other conditions of the tongue

Diseases of esophagus, stomach, and duodenum (530–538)

530 Diseases of esophagus
531 Gastric ulcer
532 Duodenal ulcer
533 Peptic ulcer, site unspecified
534 Gastrojejunal ulcer
535 Gastritis and duodenitis
536 Disorders of function of stomach
537 Other disorders of stomach and duodenum
538 Gastrointestinal mucositis (ulcerative)

Appendicitis (540–543)

540 Acute appendicitis
541 Appendicitis, unqualified
542 Other appendicitis
543 Other diseases of appendix

Hernia of abdominal cavity (550–553)

550 Inguinal hernia
551 Other hernia of abdominal cavity, with gangrene
552 Other hernia of abdominal cavity, with obstruction, but without mention of gangrene
553 Other hernia of abdominal cavity without mention of obstruction or gangrene

Noninfective enteritis and colitis (555–558)

555 Regional enteritis
556 Ulcerative colitis
557 Vascular insufficiency of intestine
558 Other noninfective gastroenteritis and colitis

Other diseases of intestines and peritoneum (560–569)

560 Intestinal obstruction without mention of hernia
562 Diverticula of intestine
564 Functional digestive disorders, not elsewhere classified
565 Anal fissure and fistula
566 Abscess of anal and rectal regions
567 Peritonitis
568 Other disorders of peritoneum
569 Other disorders of intestine

Other diseases of digestive system (570–579)

570 Acute and subacute necrosis of liver
571 Chronic liver disease and cirrhosis
572 Liver abscess and sequelae of chronic liver disease
573 Other disorders of liver
574 Cholelithiasis
575 Other disorders of gallbladder
576 Other disorders of biliary tract
577 Diseases of pancreas
578 Gastrointestinal hemorrhage
579 Intestinal malabsorption

10. DISEASES OF THE GENITOURINARY SYSTEM

Nephritis, nephrotic syndrome, and nephrosis (580–589)

580 Acute glomerulonephritis
581 Nephrotic syndrome
582 Chronic glomerulonephritis
583 Nephritis and nephropathy, not specified as acute or chronic
584 Acute renal failure
585 Chronic renal failure
586 Renal failure, unspecified
587 Renal sclerosis, unspecified
588 Disorders resulting from impaired renal function
589 Small kidney of unknown cause

Other diseases of urinary system (590–599)

590 Infections of kidney
591 Hydronephrosis
592 Calculus of kidney and ureter
593 Other disorders of kidney and ureter
594 Calculus of lower urinary tract
595 Cystitis

596 Other disorders of bladder
597 Urethritis, not sexually transmitted, and urethral syndrome
598 Urethral stricture
599 Other disorders of urethra and urinary tract

Diseases of male genital organs (600–608)
600 Hyperplasia of prostate
601 Inflammatory diseases of prostate
602 Other disorders of prostate
603 Hydrocele
604 Orchitis and epididymitis
605 Redundant prepuce and phimosis
606 Infertility, male
607 Disorders of penis
608 Other disorders of male genital organs

Disorders of breast (610–611)
610 Benign mammary dysplasias
611 Other disorders of breast
612 Deformity and disproportion of reconstructed breast

Inflammatory disease of female pelvic organs (614–616)
614 Inflammatory disease of ovary, fallopian tube, pelvic cellular tissue, and peritoneum
615 Inflammatory diseases of uterus, except cervix
616 Inflammatory disease of cervix, vagina, and vulva

Other disorders of female genital tract (617–629)
617 Endometriosis
618 Genital prolapse
619 Fistula involving female genital tract
620 Noninflammatory disorders of ovary, fallopian tube, and broad ligament
621 Disorders of uterus, not elsewhere classified
622 Noninflammatory disorders of cervix
623 Noninflammatory disorders of vagina
624 Noninflammatory disorders of vulva and perineum
625 Pain and other symptoms associated with female genital organs
626 Disorders of menstruation and other abnormal bleeding from female genital tract
627 Menopausal and postmenopausal disorders
628 Infertility, female
629 Other disorders of female genital organs

11. COMPLICATIONS OF PREGNANCY, CHILDBIRTH, AND THE PUERPERIUM

Ectopic and molar pregnancy and other pregnancy with abortive outcome (630–639)
630 Hydatidiform mole
631 Other abnormal product of conception
632 Missed abortion
633 Ectopic pregnancy
634 Spontaneous abortion
635 Legally induced abortion
636 Illegally induced abortion
637 Unspecified abortion
638 Failed attempted abortion
639 Complications following abortion and ectopic and molar pregnancies

Complications mainly related to pregnancy (640–649)
640 Hemorrhage in early pregnancy
641 Antepartum hemorrhage, abruptio placentae, and placenta previa
642 Hypertension complicating pregnancy, childbirth, and the puerperium
643 Excessive vomiting in pregnancy
644 Early or threatened labor
645 Prolonged pregnancy
646 Other complications of pregnancy, not elsewhere classified
647 Infective and parasitic conditions in the mother classifiable elsewhere but complicating pregnancy, childbirth, and the puerperium

648 Other current conditions in the mother classifiable elsewhere but complicating pregnancy, childbirth, and the puerperium
649 Other conditions or status of the mother complicating pregnancy, childbirth, or the puerperium

Normal delivery, and other indications for care in pregnancy, labor, and delivery (650–659)
650 Normal delivery
651 Multiple gestation
652 Malposition and malpresentation of fetus
653 Disproportion
654 Abnormality of organs and soft tissues of pelvis
655 Known or suspected fetal abnormality affecting management of mother
656 Other fetal and placental problems affecting management of mother
657 Polyhydramnios
658 Other problems associated with amniotic cavity and membranes
659 Other indications for care or intervention related to labor and delivery and not elsewhere classified

Complications occurring mainly in the course of labor and delivery (660–669)
660 Obstructed labor
661 Abnormality of forces of labor
662 Long labor
663 Umbilical cord complications
664 Trauma to perineum and vulva during delivery
665 Other obstetrical trauma
666 Postpartum hemorrhage
667 Retained placenta or membranes, without hemorrhage
668 Complications of the administration of anesthetic or other sedation in labor and delivery
669 Other complications of labor and delivery, not elsewhere classified

Complications of the puerperium (670–677)
670 Major puerperal infection
671 Venous complications in pregnancy and the puerperium
672 Pyrexia of unknown origin during the puerperium
673 Obstetrical pulmonary embolism
674 Other and unspecified complications of the puerperium, not elsewhere classified
675 Infections of the breast and nipple associated with childbirth
676 Other disorders of the breast associated with childbirth, and disorders of lactation
677 Late effect of complication of pregnancy, childbirth, and the puerperium

Other Maternal and Fetal Complications (678-679)
678 Other fetal conditions
679 Complications of in utero procedures

12. DISEASES OF THE SKIN AND SUBCUTANEOUS TISSUE

Infections of skin and subcutaneous tissue (680–686)
680 Carbuncle and furuncle
681 Cellulitis and abscess of finger and toe
682 Other cellulitis and abscess
683 Acute lymphadenitis
684 Impetigo
685 Pilonidal cyst
686 Other local infections of skin and subcutaneous tissue

Other inflammatory conditions of skin and subcutaneous tissue (690–698)
690 Erythematosquamous dermatosis
691 Atopic dermatitis and related conditions
692 Contact dermatitis and other eczema
693 Dermatitis due to substances taken internally
694 Bullous dermatoses

695   Erythematous conditions
696   Psoriasis and similar disorders
697   Lichen
698   Pruritus and related conditions

Other diseases of skin and subcutaneous tissue (700–709)
700   Corns and callosities
701   Other hypertrophic and atrophic conditions of skin
702   Other dermatoses
703   Diseases of nail
704   Diseases of hair and hair follicles
705   Disorders of sweat glands
706   Diseases of sebaceous glands
707   Chronic ulcer of skin
708   Urticaria
709   Other disorders of skin and subcutaneous tissue

13. DISEASES OF THE MUSCULOSKELETAL SYSTEM AND CONNECTIVE TISSUE

Arthropathies and related disorders (710–719)
710   Diffuse diseases of connective tissue
711   Arthropathy associated with infections
712   Crystal arthropathies
713   Arthropathy associated with other disorders classified elsewhere
714   Rheumatoid arthritis and other inflammatory polyarthropathies
715   Osteoarthrosis and allied disorders
716   Other and unspecified arthropathies
717   Internal derangement of knee
718   Other derangement of joint
719   Other and unspecified disorder of joint

Dorsopathies (720–724)
720   Ankylosing spondylitis and other inflammatory spondylopathies
721   Spondylosis and allied disorders
722   Intervertebral disc disorders
723   Other disorders of cervical region
724   Other and unspecified disorders of back

Rheumatism, excluding the back (725–729)
725   Polymyalgia rheumatica
726   Peripheral enthesopathies and allied syndromes
727   Other disorders of synovium, tendon, and bursa
728   Disorders of muscle, ligament, and fascia
729   Other disorders of soft tissues

Osteopathies, chondropathies, and acquired musculoskeletal deformities (730–739)
730   Osteomyelitis, periostitis, and other infections involving bone
731   Osteitis deformans and osteopathies associated with other disorders classified elsewhere
732   Osteochondropathies
733   Other disorders of bone and cartilage
734   Flat foot
735   Acquired deformities of toe
736   Other acquired deformities of limbs
737   Curvature of spine
738   Other acquired deformity
739   Nonallopathic lesions, not elsewhere classified

14. CONGENITAL ANOMALIES

Congential anomalies (740–759)
740   Anencephalus and similar anomalies
741   Spina bifida
742   Other congenital anomalies of nervous system
743   Congenital anomalies of eye
744   Congenital anomalies of ear, face, and neck
745   Bulbus cordis anomalies and anomalies of cardiac septal closure

746   Other congenital anomalies of heart
747   Other congenital anomalies of circulatory system
748   Congenital anomalies of respiratory system
749   Cleft palate and cleft lip
750   Other congenital anomalies of upper alimentary tract
751   Other congenital anomalies of digestive system
752   Congenital anomalies of genital organs
753   Congenital anomalies of urinary system
754   Certain congenital musculoskeletal deformities
755   Other congenital anomalies of limbs
756   Other congenital musculoskeletal anomalies
757   Congenital anomalies of the integument
758   Chromosomal anomalies
759   Other and unspecified congenital anomalies

15. CERTAIN CONDITIONS ORIGINATING IN THE PERINATAL PERIOD

Maternal causes of perinatal morbidity and mortality (760–763)
760   Fetus or newborn affected by maternal conditions which may be unrelated to present pregnancy
761   Fetus or newborn affected by maternal complications of pregnancy
762   Fetus or newborn affected by complications of placenta, cord, and membranes
763   Fetus or newborn affected by other complications of labor and delivery

Other conditions originating in the perinatal period (764–779)
764   Slow fetal growth and fetal malnutrition
765   Disorders relating to short gestation and unspecified low birthweight
766   Disorders relating to long gestation and high birthweight
767   Birth trauma
768   Intrauterine hypoxia and birth asphyxia
769   Respiratory distress syndrome
770   Other respiratory conditions of fetus and newborn
771   Infections specific to the perinatal period
772   Fetal and neonatal hemorrhage
773   Hemolytic disease of fetus or newborn, due to isoimmunization
774   Other perinatal jaundice
775   Endocrine and metabolic disturbances specific to the fetus and newborn
776   Hematological disorders of fetus and newborn
777   Perinatal disorders of digestive system
778   Conditions involving the integument and temperature regulation of fetus and newborn
779   Other and ill-defined conditions originating in the perinatal period

16. SYMPTOMS, SIGNS, AND ILL-DEFINED CONDITIONS

Symptoms (780–789)
780   General symptoms
781   Symptoms involving nervous and musculoskeletal systems
782   Symptoms involving skin and other integumentary tissue
783   Symptoms concerning nutrition, metabolism, and development
784   Symptoms involving head and neck
785   Symptoms involving cardiovascular system
786   Symptoms involving respiratory system and other chest symptoms
787   Symptoms involving digestive system
788   Symptoms involving urinary system
789   Other symptoms involving abdomen and pelvis

Nonspecific abnormal findings (790–796)
790   Nonspecific findings on examination of blood
791   Nonspecific findings on examination of urine
792   Nonspecific abnormal findings in other body substances
793   Nonspecific abnormal findings on radiological and other examination of body structure
794   Nonspecific abnormal results of function studies

795 Nonspecific abnormal histological and immunological findings
796 Other nonspecific abnormal findings

Ill-defined and unknown causes of morbidity and mortality (797–799)
797 Senility without mention of psychosis
798 Sudden death, cause unknown
799 Other ill-defined and unknown causes of morbidity and mortality

17. INJURY AND POISONING

Fracture of skull (800–804)
800 Fracture of vault of skull
801 Fracture of base of skull
802 Fracture of face bones
803 Other and unqualified skull fractures
804 Multiple fractures involving skull or face with other bones

Fracture of spine and trunk (805–809)
805 Fracture of vertebral column without mention of spinal cord lesion
806 Fracture of vertebral column with spinal cord lesion
807 Fracture of rib(s), sternum, larynx, and trachea
808 Fracture of pelvis
809 Ill-defined fractures of bones of trunk

Fracture of upper limb (810–819)
810 Fracture of clavicle
811 Fracture of scapula
812 Fracture of humerus
813 Fracture of radius and ulna
814 Fracture of carpal bone(s)
815 Fracture of metacarpal bone(s)
816 Fracture of one or more phalanges of hand
817 Multiple fractures of hand bones
818 Ill-defined fractures of upper limb
819 Multiple fractures involving both upper limbs, and upper limb with rib(s) and sternum

Fracture of lower limb (820–829)
820 Fracture of neck of femur
821 Fracture of other and unspecified parts of femur
822 Fracture of patella
823 Fracture of tibia and fibula
824 Fracture of ankle
825 Fracture of one or more tarsal and metatarsal bones
826 Fracture of one or more phalanges of foot
827 Other, multiple, and ill-defined fractures of lower limb
828 Multiple fractures involving both lower limbs, lower with upper limb, and lower limb(s) with rib(s) and sternum
829 Fracture of unspecified bones

Dislocation (830–839)
830 Dislocation of jaw
831 Dislocation of shoulder
832 Dislocation of elbow
833 Dislocation of wrist
834 Dislocation of finger
835 Dislocation of hip
836 Dislocation of knee
837 Dislocation of ankle
838 Dislocation of foot
839 Other, multiple, and ill-defined dislocations

Sprains and strains of joints and adjacent muscles (840–848)
840 Sprains and strains of shoulder and upper arm
841 Sprains and strains of elbow and forearm
842 Sprains and strains of wrist and hand
843 Sprains and strains of hip and thigh
844 Sprains and strains of knee and leg
845 Sprains and strains of ankle and foot
846 Sprains and strains of sacroiliac region
847 Sprains and strains of other and unspecified parts of back
848 Other and ill-defined sprains and strains

Intracranial injury, excluding those with skull fracture (850–854)
850 Concussion
851 Cerebral laceration and contusion
852 Subarachnoid, subdural, and extradural hemorrhage, following injury
853 Other and unspecified intracranial hemorrhage following injury
854 Intracranial injury of other and unspecified nature

Internal injury of chest, abdomen, and pelvis (860–869)
860 Traumatic pneumothorax and hemothorax
861 Injury to heart and lung
862 Injury to other and unspecified intrathoracic organs
863 Injury to gastrointestinal tract
864 Injury to liver
865 Injury to spleen
866 Injury to kidney
867 Injury to pelvic organs
868 Injury to other intra-abdominal organs
869 Internal injury to unspecified or ill-defined organs

Open wound of head, neck, and trunk (870–879)
870 Open wound of ocular adnexa
871 Open wound of eyeball
872 Open wound of ear
873 Other open wound of head
874 Open wound of neck
875 Open wound of chest (wall)
876 Open wound of back
877 Open wound of buttock
878 Open wound of genital organs (external), including traumatic amputation
879 Open wound of other and unspecified sites, except limbs

Open wound of upper limb (880–887)
880 Open wound of shoulder and upper arm
881 Open wound of elbow, forearm, and wrist
882 Open wound of hand except finger(s) alone
883 Open wound of finger(s)
884 Multiple and unspecified open wound of upper limb
885 Traumatic amputation of thumb (complete) (partial)
886 Traumatic amputation of other finger(s) (complete) (partial)
887 Traumatic amputation of arm and hand (complete) (partial)

Open wound of lower limb (890–897)
890 Open wound of hip and thigh
891 Open wound of knee, leg [except thigh], and ankle
892 Open wound of foot except toe(s) alone
893 Open wound of toe(s)
894 Multiple and unspecified open wound of lower limb
895 Traumatic amputation of toe(s) (complete) (partial)
896 Traumatic amputation of foot (complete) (partial)
897 Traumatic amputation of leg(s) (complete) (partial)

Injury to blood vessels (900–904)
900 Injury to blood vessels of head and neck
901 Injury to blood vessels of thorax
902 Injury to blood vessels of abdomen and pelvis
903 Injury to blood vessels of upper extremity
904 Injury to blood vessels of lower extremity and unspecified sites

Late effects of injuries, poisonings, toxic effects, and other external causes (905–909)
905 Late effects of musculoskeletal and connective tissue injuries
906 Late effects of injuries to skin and subcutaneous tissues
907 Late effects of injuries to the nervous system
908 Late effects of other and unspecified injuries
909 Late effects of other and unspecified external causes

Superficial injury (910–919)
910 Superficial injury of face, neck, and scalp except eye
911 Superficial injury of trunk
912 Superficial injury of shoulder and upper arm

913 Superficial injury of elbow, forearm, and wrist
914 Superficial injury of hand(s) except finger(s) alone
915 Superficial injury of finger(s)
916 Superficial injury of hip, thigh, leg, and ankle
917 Superficial injury of foot and toe(s)
918 Superficial injury of eye and adnexa
919 Superficial injury of other, multiple, and unspecified sites

Contusion with intact skin surface (920–924)
920 Contusion of face, scalp, and neck except eye(s)
921 Contusion of eye and adnexa
922 Contusion of trunk
923 Contusion of upper limb
924 Contusion of lower limb and of other and unspecified sites

Crushing injury (925–929)
925 Crushing injury of face, scalp, and neck
926 Crushing injury of trunk
927 Crushing injury of upper limb
928 Crushing injury of lower limb
929 Crushing injury of multiple and unspecified sites

Effects of foreign body entering through orifice (930–939)
930 Foreign body on external eye
931 Foreign body in ear
932 Foreign body in nose
933 Foreign body in pharynx and larynx
934 Foreign body in trachea, bronchus, and lung
935 Foreign body in mouth, esophagus, and stomach
936 Foreign body in intestine and colon
937 Foreign body in anus and rectum
938 Foreign body in digestive system, unspecified
939 Foreign body in genitourinary tract

Burns (940–949)
940 Burn confined to eye and adnexa
941 Burn of face, head, and neck
942 Burn of trunk
943 Burn of upper limb, except wrist and hand
944 Burn of wrist(s) and hand(s)
945 Burn of lower limb(s)
946 Burns of multiple specified sites
947 Burn of internal organs
948 Burns classified according to extent of body surface involved
949 Burn, unspecified

Injury to nerves and spinal cord (950–957)
950 Injury to optic nerve and pathways
951 Injury to other cranial nerve(s)
952 Spinal cord injury without evidence of spinal bone injury
953 Injury to nerve roots and spinal plexus
954 Injury to other nerve(s) of trunk excluding shoulder and pelvic girdles
955 Injury to peripheral nerve(s) of shoulder girdle and upper limb
956 Injury to peripheral nerve(s) of pelvic girdle and lower limb
957 Injury to other and unspecified nerves

Certain traumatic complications and unspecified injuries (958–959)
958 Certain early complications of trauma
959 Injury, other and unspecified

Poisoning by drugs, medicinals and biological substances (960–979)
960 Poisoning by antibiotics
961 Poisoning by other anti-infectives
962 Poisoning by hormones and synthetic substitutes
963 Poisoning by primarily systemic agents
964 Poisoning by agents primarily affecting blood constituents
965 Poisoning by analgesics, antipyretics, and antirheumatics
966 Poisoning by anticonvulsants and anti-Parkinsonism drugs
967 Poisoning by sedatives and hypnotics
968 Poisoning by other central nervous system depressants and anesthetics

969 Poisoning by psychotropic agents
970 Poisoning by central nervous system stimulants
971 Poisoning by drugs primarily affecting the autonomic nervous system
972 Poisoning by agents primarily affecting the cardiovascular system
973 Poisoning by agents primarily affecting the gastrointestinal system
974 Poisoning by water, mineral, and uric acid metabolism drugs
975 Poisoning by agents primarily acting on the smooth and skeletal muscles and respiratory system
976 Poisoning by agents primarily affecting skin and mucous membrane, ophthalmological, otorhinolaryngological, and dental drugs
977 Poisoning by other and unspecified drugs and medicinals
978 Poisoning by bacterial vaccines
979 Poisoning by other vaccines and biological substances

Toxic effects of substances chiefly nonmedicinal as to source (980–989)
980 Toxic effect of alcohol
981 Toxic effect of petroleum products
982 Toxic effect of solvents other than petroleum-based
983 Toxic effect of corrosive aromatics, acids, and caustic alkalis
984 Toxic effect of lead and its compounds (including fumes)
985 Toxic effect of other metals
986 Toxic effect of carbon monoxide
987 Toxic effect of other gases, fumes, or vapors
988 Toxic effect of noxious substances eaten as food
989 Toxic effect of other substances, chiefly nonmedicinal as to source

Other and unspecified effects of external causes (990–995)
990 Effects of radiation, unspecified
991 Effects of reduced temperature
992 Effects of heat and light
993 Effects of air pressure
994 Effects of other external causes
995 Certain adverse effects, not elsewhere classified

Complications of surgical and medical care, not elsewhere classified (996–999)
996 Complications peculiar to certain specified procedures
997 Complications affecting specified body systems, not elsewhere classified
998 Other complications of procedures, not elsewhere classified
999 Complications of medical care, not elsewhere classified

SUPPLEMENTARY CLASSIFICATION OF FACTORS INFLUENCING HEALTH STATUS AND CONTACT WITH HEALTH SERVICES (V01–V86)

Persons with potential health hazards related to communicable diseases (V01–V09)
V01 Contact with or exposure to communicable diseases
V02 Carrier or suspected carrier of infectious diseases
V03 Need for prophylactic vaccination and inoculation against bacterial diseases
V04 Need for prophylactic vaccination and inoculation against certain viral diseases
V05 Need for other prophylactic vaccination and inoculation against single diseases
V06 Need for prophylactic vaccination and inoculation against combinations of diseases
V07 Need for isolation and other prophylactic measures
V08 Asymptomatic human immunodeficiency virus [HIV] infection status
V09 Infection with drug-resistant microorganisms

Persons with potential health hazards related to personal and family history (V10–V19)
V10 Personal history of malignant neoplasm
V11 Personal history of mental disorder
V12 Personal history of certain other diseases
V13 Personal history of other diseases

V14 Personal history of allergy to medicinal agents
V15 Other personal history presenting hazards to health
V16 Family history of malignant neoplasm
V17 Family history of certain chronic disabling diseases
V18 Family history of certain other specific conditions
V19 Family history of other conditions

Persons encountering health services in circumstances related to reproduction and development (V20–V29)
V20 Health supervision of infant or child
V21 Constitutional states in development
V22 Normal pregnancy
V23 Supervision of high-risk pregnancy
V24 Postpartum care and examination
V25 Encounter for contraceptive management
V26 Procreative management
V27 Outcome of delivery
V28 Antenatal screening
V29 Observation and evaluation of newborns and infants for suspected condition not found

Liveborn infants according to type of birth (V30–V39)
V30 Single liveborn
V31 Twin, mate liveborn
V32 Twin, mate stillborn
V33 Twin, unspecified
V34 Other multiple, mates all liveborn
V35 Other multiple, mates all stillborn
V36 Other multiple, mates live- and stillborn
V37 Other multiple, unspecified
V39 Unspecified

Persons with a condition influencing their health status (V40–V49)
V40 Mental and behavioral problems
V41 Problems with special senses and other special functions
V42 Organ or tissue replaced by transplant
V43 Organ or tissue replaced by other means
V44 Artificial opening status
V45 Other postsurgical states
V46 Other dependence on machines
V47 Other problems with internal organs
V48 Problems with head, neck, and trunk
V49 Problems with limbs and other problems

Persons encountering health services for specific procedures and aftercare (V50–V59)
V50 Elective surgery for purposes other than remedying health states
V51 Aftercare involving the use of plastic surgery
V52 Fitting and adjustment of prosthetic device
V53 Fitting and adjustment of other device
V54 Other orthopedic aftercare
V55 Attention to artificial openings
V56 Encounter for dialysis and dialysis catheter care
V57 Care involving use of rehabilitation procedures
V58 Other and unspecified aftercare
V59 Donors

Persons encountering health services in other circumstances (V60–V69)
V60 Housing, household, and economic circumstances
V61 Other family circumstances
V62 Other psychosocial circumstances
V63 Unavailability of other medical facilities for care
V64 Persons encountering health services for specific procedures, not carried out
V65 Other persons seeking consultation without complaint or sickness
V66 Convalescence and palliative care
V67 Follow-up examination
V68 Encounters for administrative purposes
V69 Problems related to lifestyle

Persons without reported diagnosis encountered during examination and investigation of individuals and populations (V70–V82)
V70 General medical examination
V71 Observation and evaluation for suspected conditions
V72 Special investigations and examinations
V73 Special screening examination for viral and chlamydial diseases
V74 Special screening examination for bacterial and spirochetal diseases
V75 Special screening examination for other infectious diseases
V76 Special screening for malignant neoplasms
V77 Special screening for endocrine, nutritional, metabolic, and immunity disorders
V78 Special screening for disorders of blood and blood-forming organs
V79 Special screening for mental disorders and developmental handicaps
V80 Special screening for neurological, eye, and ear diseases
V81 Special screening for cardiovascular, respiratory, and genitourinary diseases
V82 Special screening for other conditions

Genetics (V83–V84)
V83 Genetic carrier status
V84 Genetic susceptibility to malignant neoplasm

Body Mass Index (V85)
V85 Body mass index

Estrogen Receptor Status (V86)
V86 Estrogen receptor status

Other specified personal exposures and history presenting hazards to health (V87)
V87 Other specified personal exposures and history presenting hazards to health

Acquired absence of other organs and tissue (V88)
V88 Acquired absence of other organs and tissue

Other suspected conditions not found (V89)
V89 Other suspected conditions not found

SUPPLEMENTARY CLASSIFICATION OF EXTERNAL CAUSES OF INJURY AND POISONING (E800–E899)

Railway accidents (E800–E807)
E800 Railway accident involving collision with rolling stock
E801 Railway accident involving collision with other object
E802 Railway accident involving derailment without antecedent collision
E803 Railway accident involving explosion, fire, or burning
E804 Fall in, on, or from railway train
E805 Hit by rolling stock
E806 Other specified railway accident
E807 Railway accident of unspecified nature

Motor vehicle traffic accidents (E810–E819)
E810 Motor vehicle traffic accident involving collision with train
E811 Motor vehicle traffic accident involving re-entrant collision with another motor vehicle
E812 Other motor vehicle traffic accident involving collision with another motor vehicle
E813 Motor vehicle traffic accident involving collision with other vehicle
E814 Motor vehicle traffic accident involving collision with pedestrian
E815 Other motor vehicle traffic accident involving collision on the highway
E816 Motor vehicle traffic accident due to loss of control, without collision on the highway
E817 Noncollision motor vehicle traffic accident while boarding or alighting
E818 Other noncollision motor vehicle traffic accident
E819 Motor vehicle traffic accident of unspecified nature

Motor vehicle nontraffic accidents (E820–E825)

E820 Nontraffic accident involving motor-driven snow vehicle
E821 Nontraffic accident involving other off-road motor vehicle
E822 Other motor vehicle nontraffic accident involving collision with moving object
E823 Other motor vehicle nontraffic accident involving collision with stationary object
E824 Other motor vehicle nontraffic accident while boarding and alighting
E825 Other motor vehicle nontraffic accident of other and unspecified nature

Other road vehicle accidents (E826–E829)

E826 Pedal cycle accident
E827 Animal-drawn vehicle accident
E828 Accident involving animal being ridden
E829 Other road vehicle accidents

Water transport accidents (E830–E838)

E830 Accident to watercraft causing submersion
E831 Accident to watercraft causing other injury
E832 Other accidental submersion or drowning in water transport accident
E833 Fall on stairs or ladders in water transport
E834 Other fall from one level to another in water transport
E835 Other and unspecified fall in water transport
E836 Machinery accident in water transport
E837 Explosion, fire, or burning in watercraft
E838 Other and unspecified water transport accident

Air and space transport accidents (E840–E845)

E840 Accident to powered aircraft at takeoff or landing
E841 Accident to powered aircraft, other and unspecified
E842 Accident to unpowered aircraft
E843 Fall in, on, or from aircraft
E844 Other specified air transport accidents
E845 Accident involving spacecraft

Vehicle accidents, not elsewhere classifiable (E846–E849)

E846 Accidents involving powered vehicles used solely within the buildings and premises of an industrial or commercial establishment
E847 Accidents involving cable cars not running on rails
E848 Accidents involving other vehicles, not elsewhere classifiable
E849 Place of occurrence

Accidental poisoning by drugs, medicinal substances, and biologicals (E850–E858)

E850 Accidental poisoning by analgesics, antipyretics, and antirheumatics
E851 Accidental poisoning by barbiturates
E852 Accidental poisoning by other sedatives and hypnotics
E853 Accidental poisoning by tranquilizers
E854 Accidental poisoning by other psychotropic agents
E855 Accidental poisoning by other drugs acting on central and autonomic nervous systems
E856 Accidental poisoning by antibiotics
E857 Accidental poisoning by anti-infectives
E858 Accidental poisoning by other drugs

Accidental poisoning by other solid and liquid substances, gases, and vapors (E860–E869)

E860 Accidental poisoning by alcohol, not elsewhere classified
E861 Accidental poisoning by cleansing and polishing agents, disinfectants, paints, and varnishes
E862 Accidental poisoning by petroleum products, other solvents and their vapors, not elsewhere classified
E863 Accidental poisoning by agricultural and horticultural chemical and pharmaceutical preparations other than plant foods and fertilizers
E864 Accidental poisoning by corrosives and caustics, not elsewhere classified
E865 Accidental poisoning from poisonous foodstuffs and poisonous plants

E866 Accidental poisoning by other and unspecified solid and liquid substances
E867 Accidental poisoning by gas distributed by pipeline
E868 Accidental poisoning by other utility gas and other carbon monoxide
E869 Accidental poisoning by other gases and vapors

Misadventures to patients during surgical and medical care (E870–E876)

E870 Accidental cut, puncture, perforation, or hemorrhage during medical care
E871 Foreign object left in body during procedure
E872 Failure of sterile precautions during procedure
E873 Failure in dosage
E874 Mechanical failure of instrument or apparatus during procedure
E875 Contaminated or infected blood, other fluid, drug, or biological substance
E876 Other and unspecified misadventures during medical care

Surgical and medical procedures as the cause of abnormal reaction of patient or later complication, without mention of misadventure at the time of procedure (E878–E879)

E878 Surgical operation and other surgical procedures as the cause of abnormal reaction of patient, or of later complication, without mention of misadventure at the time of operation
E879 Other procedures, without mention of misadventure at the time of procedure, as the cause of abnormal reaction of patient, or of later complication

Accidental falls (E880–E888)

E880 Fall on or from stairs or steps
E881 Fall on or from ladders or scaffolding
E882 Fall from or out of building or other structure
E883 Fall into hole or other opening in surface
E884 Other fall from one level to another
E885 Fall on same level from slipping, tripping, or stumbling
E886 Fall on same level from collision, pushing, or shoving, by or with other person
E887 Fracture, cause unspecified
E888 Other and unspecified fall

Accidents caused by fire and flames (E890–E899)

E890 Conflagration in private dwelling
E891 Conflagration in other and unspecified building or structure
E892 Conflagration not in building or structure
E893 Accident caused by ignition of clothing
E894 Ignition of highly inflammable material
E895 Accident caused by controlled fire in private dwelling
E896 Accident caused by controlled fire in other and unspecified building or structure
E897 Accident caused by controlled fire not in building or structure
E898 Accident caused by other specified fire and flames
E899 Accident caused by unspecified fire

Accidents due to natural and environmental factors (E900–E909)

E900 Excessive heat
E901 Excessive cold
E902 High and low air pressure and changes in air pressure
E903 Travel and motion
E904 Hunger, thirst, exposure, and neglect
E905 Venomous animals and plants as the cause of poisoning and toxic reactions
E906 Other injury caused by animals
E907 Lightning
E908 Cataclysmic storms, and floods resulting from storms
E909 Cataclysmic earth surface movements and eruptions

Accidents caused by submersion, suffocation, and foreign bodies (E910–E915)
E910   Accidental drowning and submersion
E911   Inhalation and ingestion of food causing obstruction of respiratory tract or suffocation
E912   Inhalation and ingestion of other object causing obstruction of respiratory tract or suffocation
E913   Accidental mechanical suffocation
E914   Foreign body accidentally entering eye and adnexa
E915   Foreign body accidentally entering other orifice

Other accidents (E916–E928)
E916   Struck accidentally by falling object
E917   Striking against or struck accidentally by objects or persons
E918   Caught accidentally in or between objects
E919   Accidents caused by machinery
E920   Accidents caused by cutting and piercing instruments or objects
E921   Accident caused by explosion of pressure vessel
E922   Accident caused by firearm missile
E923   Accident caused by explosive material
E924   Accident caused by hot substance or object, caustic or corrosive material, and steam
E925   Accident caused by electric current
E926   Exposure to radiation
E927   Overexertion and strenuous movements
E928   Other and unspecified environmental and accidental causes

Late effects of accidental injury (E929)
E929   Late effects of accidental injury

Drugs, medicinal and biological substances causing adverse effects in therapeutic use (E930–E949)
E930   Antibiotics
E931   Other anti-infectives
E932   Hormones and synthetic substitutes
E933   Primarily systemic agents
E934   Agents primarily affecting blood constituents
E935   Analgesics, antipyretics, and antirheumatics
E936   Anticonvulsants and anti-Parkinsonism drugs
E937   Sedatives and hypnotics
E938   Other central nervous system depressants and anesthetics
E939   Psychotropic agents
E940   Central nervous system stimulants
E941   Drugs primarily affecting the autonomic nervous system
E942   Agents primarily affecting the cardiovascular system
E943   Agents primarily affecting gastrointestinal system
E944   Water, mineral, and uric acid metabolism drugs
E945   Agents primarily acting on the smooth and skeletal muscles and respiratory system
E946   Agents primarily affecting skin and mucous membrane, ophthalmological, otorhinolaryngological, and dental drugs
E947   Other and unspecified drugs and medicinal substances
E948   Bacterial vaccines
E949   Other vaccines and biological substances

Suicide and self-inflicted injury (E950–E959)
E950   Suicide and self-inflicted poisoning by solid or liquid substances
E951   Suicide and self-inflicted poisoning by gases in domestic use
E952   Suicide and self-inflicted poisoning by other gases and vapors
E953   Suicide and self-inflicted injury by hanging, strangulation, and suffocation
E954   Suicide and self-inflicted injury by submersion [drowning]
E955   Suicide and self-inflicted injury by firearms and explosives
E956   Suicide and self-inflicted injury by cutting and piercing instruments
E957   Suicide and self-inflicted injuries by jumping from high place

E958   Suicide and self-inflicted injury by other and unspecified means
E959   Late effects of self-inflicted injury

Homicide and injury purposely inflicted by other persons (E960–E969)
E960   Fight, brawl, and rape
E961   Assault by corrosive or caustic substance, except poisoning
E962   Assault by poisoning
E963   Assault by hanging and strangulation
E964   Assault by submersion [drowning]
E965   Assault by firearms and explosives
E966   Assault by cutting and piercing instrument
E967   Child and adult battering and other maltreatment
E968   Assault by other and unspecified means
E969   Late effects of injury purposely inflicted by other person

Legal intervention (E970–E978)
E970   Injury due to legal intervention by firearms
E971   Injury due to legal intervention by explosives
E972   Injury due to legal intervention by gas
E973   Injury due to legal intervention by blunt object
E974   Injury due to legal intervention by cutting and piercing instruments
E975   Injury due to legal intervention by other specified means
E976   Injury due to legal intervention by unspecified means
E977   Late effects of injuries due to legal intervention
E978   Legal execution
E979   Terrorism

Injury undetermined whether accidentally or purposely inflicted (E980–E989)
E980   Poisoning by solid or liquid substances, undetermined whether accidentally or purposely inflicted
E981   Poisoning by gases in domestic use, undetermined whether accidentally or purposely inflicted
E982   Poisoning by other gases, undetermined whether accidentally or purposely inflicted
E983   Hanging, strangulation, or suffocation, undetermined whether accidentally or purposely inflicted
E984   Submersion [drowning], undetermined whether accidentally or purposely inflicted
E985   Injury by firearms and explosives, undetermined whether accidentally or purposely inflicted
E986   Injury by cutting and piercing instruments, undetermined whether accidentally or purposely inflicted
E987   Falling from high place, undetermined whether accidentally or purposely inflicted
E988   Injury by other and unspecified means, undetermined whether accidentally or purposely inflicted
E989   Late effects of injury, undetermined whether accidentally or purposely inflicted

Injury resulting from operations of war (E990–E999)
E990   Injury due to war operations by fires and conflagrations
E991   Injury due to war operations by bullets and fragments
E992   Injury due to war operations by explosion of marine weapons
E993   Injury due to war operations by other explosion
E994   Injury due to war operations by destruction of aircraft
E995   Injury due to war operations by other and unspecified forms of conventional warfare
E996   Injury due to war operations by nuclear weapons
E997   Injury due to war operations by other forms of unconventional warfare
E998   Injury due to war operations but occurring after cessation of hostilities
E999   Late effects of injury due to war operations

TABLE A

TABLE OF BACTERIAL FOOD POISONING

Bacteria Responsible	Description	Habitat	Types of Foods	Symptoms	Cause	Temperature Sensitivity
Staphylococcus aureus	Produces a heat-stable toxin.	Nose and throat of 30 to 50 percent of healthy population; also skin and superficial wounds.	Meat and seafood salads, sandwich spreads, and high salt foods.	Nausea, vomiting, and diarrhea within 4 to 6 hours. No fever.	Poor personal hygiene and subsequent temperature abuse.	No growth below 40° F. Bacteria are destroyed by normal cooking, but toxin is heat-stable.
Clostridium perfringens	Produces a spore and prefers low oxygen atmosphere. Live cells must be ingested.	Dust, soil, and gastrointestinal tracts of animals and man.	Meat and poultry dishes, sauces and gravies.	Cramps and diarrhea within 12 to 24 hours. No vomiting or fever.	Improper temperature control of hot foods and recontamination.	No growth below 40° F. Bacteria are killed by normal cooking, but a heat-stable spore can survive.
Clostridium botulinum	Produces a spore and requires a low oxygen atmosphere. Produces a heat-sensitive toxin.	Soils, plants, marine sediments, and fish.	Home-canned foods.	Blurred vision, respiratory distress, and possible DEATH.	Improper methods of home-processing foods.	Type E and Type B can grow at 38° F. Bacteria destroyed by cooking and the toxin is destroyed by boiling for 5 to 10 minutes. Heat-resistant spore can survive.
Vibrio parahaemolyticus	Requires salt for growth.	Fish and shellfish.	Raw and cooked seafood.	Diarrhea, cramps, vomiting, headache, and fever within 12 to 24 hours.	Recontamination of cooked foods or eating raw seafood.	No growth below 40° F. Bacteria killed by normal cooking.

PART V

2009 Inpatient Procedures

2009 FINAL INPATIENT PROCEDURES

The following list is part of the changes to the Hospital Outpatient Prospective Payment System for Calendar Year 2009. Specifically, the file is Addendum E that lists the codes that are only payable as inpatient procedures as displayed at http://www.cms.hhs.gov/HospitalOutpatientPPS/HORD/list.asp#TopOfPage

For the 2010 updates, see the companion website in December 2009 at: http://codingupdates.com

00176	01632	21147	22207	22857	27138	27470	31380	32653
00192	01634	21151	22208	22861	27140	27472	31382	32654
00211	01636	21154	22210	22862	27146	27477	31390	32655
00214	01638	21155	22212	22864	27147	27485	31395	32656
00215	01652	21159	22214	22865	27151	27486	31584	32657
00452	01654	21160	22216	23200	27156	27487	31587	32658
00474	01656	21179	22220	23210	27158	27488	31725	32659
00524	01756	21180	22224	23220	27161	27495	31760	32660
00540	01990	21182	22226	23221	27165	27506	31766	32661
00542	11004	21183	22318	23222	27170	27507	31770	32662
00546	11005	21184	22319	23332	27175	27511	31775	32663
00560	11006	21188	22325	23472	27176	27513	31780	32664
00561	11008	21193	22326	23900	27177	27514	31781	32665
00562	15756	21194	22327	23920	27178	27519	31786	32800
00567	15757	21196	22328	24900	27179	27535	31800	32810
00580	15758	21247	22532	24920	27181	27536	31805	32815
00604	16036	21255	22533	24930	27185	27540	32035	32820
00622	19271	21256	22534	24931	27187	27556	32036	32850
00632	19272	21268	22548	24940	27222	27557	32095	32851
00670	19305	21343	22554	25900	27226	27558	32100	32852
00792	19306	21344	22556	25905	27227	27580	32110	32853
00794	19361	21346	22558	25909	27228	27590	32120	32854
00796	19364	21347	22585	25915	27232	27591	32124	32855
00802	19367	21348	22590	25920	27236	27592	32140	32856
00844	19368	21366	22595	25924	27240	27596	32141	32900
00846	19369	21395	22600	25927	27244	27598	32150	32905
00848	20661	21422	22610	26551	27245	27645	32151	32906
00864	20664	21423	22630	26553	27248	27646	32160	32940
00865	20802	21431	22632	26554	27253	27702	32200	32997
00866	20805	21432	22800	26556	27254	27703	32215	33015
00868	20808	21433	22802	26992	27258	27712	32220	33020
00882	20816	21435	22804	27005	27259	27715	32225	33025
00904	20824	21436	22808	27025	27268	27724	32310	33030
00908	20827	21510	22810	27030	27269	27725	32320	33031
00932	20838	21615	22812	27036	27280	27727	32402	33050
00934	20930	21616	22818	27054	27282	27880	32440	33120
00936	20931	21620	22819	27070	27284	27881	32442	33130
00944	20936	21627	22830	27071	27286	27882	32445	33140
01140	20937	21630	22840	27075	27290	27886	32480	33141
01150	20938	21632	22841	27076	27295	27888	32482	33202
01212	20955	21705	22842	27077	27303	28800	32484	33203
01214	20956	21740	22843	27078	27365	28805	32486	33236
01232	20957	21750	22844	27079	27445	31225	32488	33237
01234	20962	21810	22845	27090	27447	31230	32491	33238
01272	20969	21825	22846	27091	27448	31290	32500	33243
01274	20970	22010	22847	27120	27450	31291	32501	33250
01402	21045	22015	22848	27122	27454	31360	32503	33251
01404	21141	22110	22849	27125	27455	31365	32504	33254
01442	21142	22112	22850	27130	27457	31367	32540	33255
01444	21143	22114	22852	27132	27465	31368	32650	33256
01486	21145	22116	22855	27134	27466	31370	32651	33257
01502	21146	22206	22856	27137	27468	31375	32652	33258

33259	33517	33774	33976	35276	35583	37617	43123	43843
33261	33518	33775	33977	35281	35585	37618	43124	43845
33265	33519	33776	33978	35301	35587	37660	43135	43846
33266	33521	33777	33979	35302	35600	37788	43279	43847
33300	33522	33778	33980	35303	35601	38100	43300	43848
33305	33523	33779	34001	35304	35606	38101	43305	43850
33310	33530	33780	34051	35305	35612	38102	43310	43855
33315	33533	33781	34151	35306	35616	38115	43312	43860
33320	33534	33786	34401	35311	35621	38380	43313	43865
33321	33535	33788	34451	35331	35623	38381	43314	43880
33322	33536	33800	34502	35341	35626	38382	43320	43881
33330	33542	33802	34800	35351	35631	38562	43324	43882
33332	33545	33803	34802	35355	35632	38564	43325	44005
33335	33548	33813	34803	35361	35633	38724	43326	44010
33400	33572	33814	34804	35363	35634	38746	43330	44015
33401	33600	33820	34805	35371	35636	38747	43331	44020
33403	33602	33822	34806	35372	35637	38765	43340	44021
33404	33606	33824	34808	35390	35638	38770	43341	44025
33405	33608	33840	34812	35400	35642	38780	43350	44050
33406	33610	33845	34813	35450	35645	39000	43351	44055
33410	33611	33851	34820	35452	35646	39010	43352	44110
33411	33612	33852	34825	35454	35647	39200	43360	44111
33412	33615	33853	34826	35456	35650	39220	43361	44120
33413	33617	33860	34830	35480	35651	39499	43400	44121
33414	33619	33861	34831	35481	35654	39501	43401	44125
33415	33641	33863	34832	35482	35656	39502	43405	44126
33416	33645	33864	34833	35483	35661	39503	43410	44127
33417	33647	33870	34834	35501	35663	39520	43415	44128
33420	33660	33875	34900	35506	35665	39530	43425	44130
33422	33665	33877	35001	35508	35666	39531	43460	44132
33425	33670	33880	35002	35509	35671	39540	43496	44133
33426	33675	33881	35005	35510	35681	39541	43500	44135
33427	33676	33883	35013	35511	35682	39545	43501	44136
33430	33677	33884	35021	35512	35683	39560	43502	44137
33460	33681	33886	35022	35515	35691	39561	43520	44139
33463	33684	33889	35045	35516	35693	39599	43605	44140
33464	33688	33891	35081	35518	35694	41130	43610	44141
33465	33690	33910	35082	35521	35695	41135	43611	44143
33468	33692	33915	35091	35522	35697	41140	43620	44144
33470	33694	33916	35092	35523	35700	41145	43621	44145
33471	33697	33917	35102	35525	35701	41150	43622	44146
33472	33702	33920	35103	35526	35721	41153	43631	44147
33474	33710	33922	35111	35531	35741	41155	43632	44150
33475	33720	33924	35112	35533	35800	42426	43633	44151
33476	33722	33925	35121	35535	35820	42845	43634	44155
33478	33724	33926	35122	35536	35840	42894	43635	44156
33496	33726	33930	35131	35537	35870	42953	43640	44157
33500	33730	33933	35132	35538	35901	42961	43641	44158
33501	33732	33935	35141	35539	35905	42971	43644	44160
33502	33735	33940	35142	35540	35907	43045	43645	44187
33503	33736	33944	35151	35548	36660	43100	43770	44188
33504	33737	33945	35152	35549	36822	43101	43771	44202
33505	33750	33960	35182	35551	36823	43107	43772	44203
33506	33755	33961	35189	35556	37140	43108	43773	44204
33507	33762	33967	35211	35558	37145	43112	43774	44205
33510	33764	33968	35216	35560	37160	43113	43800	44210
33511	33766	33970	35221	35563	37180	43116	43810	44211
33512	33767	33971	35241	35565	37181	43117	43820	44212
33513	33768	33973	35246	35566	37182	43118	43825	44227
33514	33770	33974	35251	35570	37215	43121	43832	44300
33516	33771	33975	35271	35571	37616	43122	43840	44310

44314	46716	47802	50125	50830	56634	59325	61514	61609
44316	46730	47900	50130	50840	56637	59350	61516	61610
44320	46735	48000	50135	50845	56640	59514	61517	61611
44322	46740	48001	50205	50860	57110	59525	61518	61612
44345	46742	48020	50220	50900	57111	59620	61519	61613
44346	46744	48100	50225	50920	57112	59830	61520	61615
44602	46746	48105	50230	50930	57270	59850	61521	61616
44603	46748	48120	50234	50940	57280	59851	61522	61618
44604	46751	48140	50236	51060	57296	59852	61524	61619
44605	47010	48145	50240	51525	57305	59855	61526	61624
44615	47015	48146	50250	51530	57307	59856	61530	61630
44620	47100	48148	50280	51550	57308	59857	61531	61635
44625	47120	48150	50290	51555	57311	60254	61533	61680
44626	47122	48152	50300	51565	57531	60270	61534	61682
44640	47125	48153	50320	51570	57540	60505	61535	61684
44650	47130	48154	50323	51575	57545	60521	61536	61686
44660	47133	48155	50325	51580	58140	60522	61537	61690
44661	47135	48400	50327	51585	58146	60540	61538	61692
44680	47136	48500	50328	51590	58150	60545	61539	61697
44700	47140	48510	50329	51595	58152	60600	61540	61698
44715	47141	48520	50340	51596	58180	60605	61541	61700
44720	47142	48540	50360	51597	58200	60650	61542	61702
44721	47143	48545	50365	51800	58210	61105	61543	61703
44800	47144	48547	50370	51820	58240	61107	61544	61705
44820	47145	48548	50380	51840	58267	61108	61545	61708
44850	47146	48551	50400	51841	58275	61120	61546	61710
44899	47147	48552	50405	51865	58280	61140	61548	61711
44900	47300	48554	50500	51900	58285	61150	61550	61735
44950	47350	48556	50520	51920	58293	61151	61552	61750
44955	47360	49000	50525	51925	58400	61154	61556	61751
44960	47361	49002	50526	51940	58410	61156	61557	61760
45110	47362	49010	50540	51960	58520	61210	61558	61850
45111	47380	49020	50545	51980	58540	61250	61559	61860
45112	47381	49040	50546	53415	58548	61253	61563	61863
45113	47400	49060	50547	53448	58605	61304	61564	61864
45114	47420	49062	50548	54125	58611	61305	61566	61867
45116	47425	49203	50600	54130	58700	61312	61567	61868
45119	47460	49204	50605	54135	58720	61313	61570	61870
45120	47480	49205	50610	54390	58740	61314	61571	61875
45121	47550	49215	50620	54411	58750	61315	61575	62005
45123	47570	49220	50630	54417	58752	61316	61576	62010
45126	47600	49255	50650	54430	58760	61320	61580	62100
45130	47605	49425	50660	54650	58822	61321	61581	62115
45135	47610	49428	50700	55605	58825	61322	61582	62116
45136	47612	49605	50715	55650	58940	61323	61583	62117
45395	47620	49606	50722	55801	58943	61332	61584	62120
45397	47700	49610	50725	55810	58950	61333	61585	62121
45400	47701	49611	50728	55812	58951	61340	61586	62140
45402	47711	49900	50740	55815	58952	61343	61590	62141
45540	47712	49904	50750	55821	58953	61345	61591	62142
45550	47715	49905	50760	55831	58954	61440	61592	62143
45562	47720	49906	50770	55840	58956	61450	61595	62145
45563	47721	50010	50780	55842	58957	61458	61596	62146
45800	47740	50040	50782	55845	58958	61460	61597	62147
45805	47741	50045	50783	55862	58960	61470	61598	62148
45820	47760	50060	50785	55865	59120	61480	61600	62161
45825	47765	50065	50800	55866	59121	61490	61601	62162
46705	47780	50070	50810	56630	59130	61500	61605	62163
46710	47785	50075	50815	56631	59135	61501	61606	62164
46712	47800	50100	50820	56632	59136	61510	61607	62165
46715	47801	50120	50825	56633	59140	61512	61608	62180

62190	63087	63198	63281	63704	75952	99255	0075T	0195T
62192	63088	63199	63282	63706	75953	99356	0076T	0196T
62200	63090	63200	63283	63707	75954	99357	0077T	G0341
62201	63091	63250	63285	63709	75956	99462	0078T	G0342
62220	63101	63251	63286	63710	75957	99468	0079T	G0343
62223	63102	63252	63287	63740	75958	99469	0080T	G0406
62256	63103	63265	63290	64752	75959	99471	0081T	G0407
62258	63170	63266	63295	64755	92970	99472	0092T	G0408
63043	63172	63267	63300	64760	92971	99475	0095T	G0412
63044	63173	63268	63301	64809	92975	99476	0098T	G0414
63050	63180	63270	63302	64818	92992	99477	0157T	G0415
63051	63182	63271	63303	64866	92993	99478	0158T	
63076	63185	63272	63304	64868	99190	99479	0163T	
63077	63190	63273	63305	65273	99191	99480	0164T	
63078	63191	63275	63306	69155	99192	0048T	0165T	
63081	63194	63276	63307	69535	99251	0050T	0166T	
63082	63195	63277	63308	69554	99252	0051T	0167T	
63085	63196	63278	63700	69950	99253	0052T	0169T	
63086	63197	63280	63702	75900	99254	0053T	0184T